AF700445

Brief Contents

Pharmacology

Connections to Nursing Practice

FIFTH EDITION

Michael Patrick Adams
Adjunct Professor of Anatomy and Physiology
Hillsborough Community College
Formerly Dean of Health Professions
Pasco-Hernando State College

Carol Quam Urban
Associate Professor
George Mason University

Rebecca E. Sutter
Associate Professor
George Mason University

Pearson

Content Management: Kevin Wilson
Content Production: Michael Giacobbe
Product Management: Patrick Barbera
Project Management: Straive
Rights and Permissions: Ben Ferrini

Please contact https://support.pearson.com/getsupport/s/ with any queries on this content

Cover Image by SciePro/Shutterstock

Library of Congress Cataloging-in-Publication Data

Cataloging-in-Publication Data is available on file at the Library of Congress.

8 2025

Pearson

ISBN-10: 0-13-531100-4
ISBN-13: 978-0-13-531100-4

About the Authors

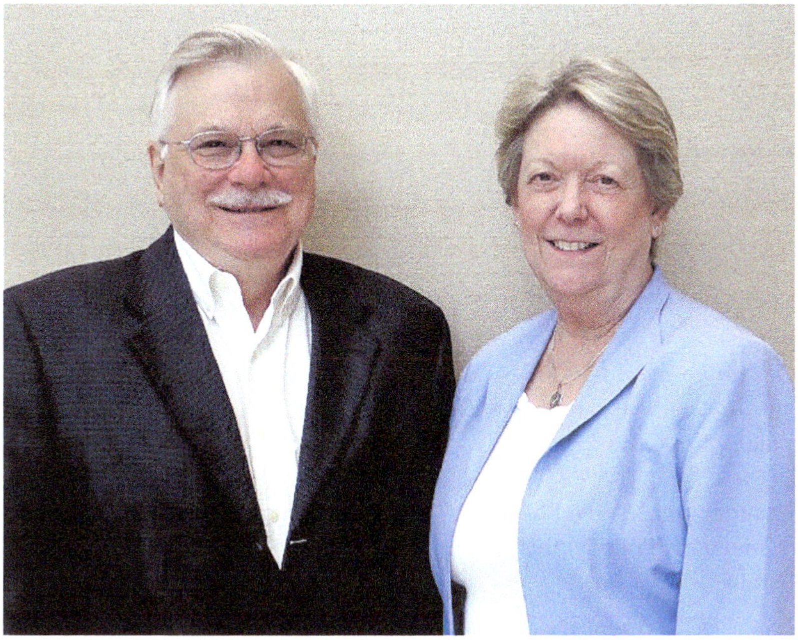

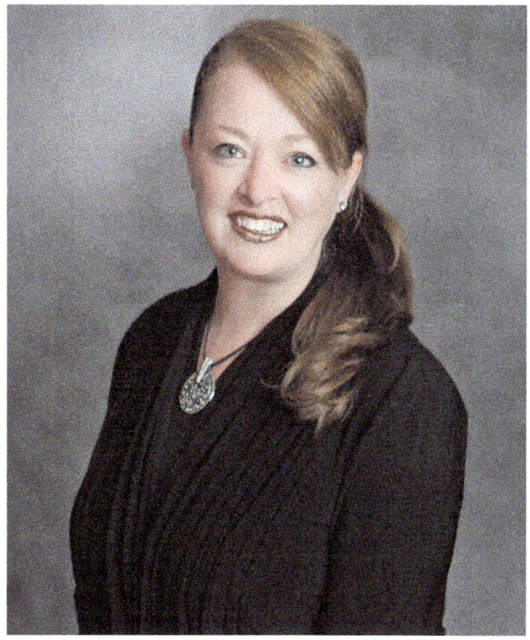

Michael Patrick Adams, PhD, is an accomplished educator, author, and national speaker. The National Institute for Staff and Organizational Development in Austin, Texas, named Dr. Adams a Master Teacher. He has published two other textbooks with Pearson Education: *Core Concepts in Pharmacology* and *Pharmacology for Nurses: A Pathophysiologic Approach*.

Dr. Adams obtained his master's degree in pharmacology from Michigan State University and his doctorate in education from the University of South Florida. Dr. Adams was on the faculty of Lansing Community College and St. Petersburg College, and was Dean of Health Professions at Pasco-Hernando State College for over 19 years. He is currently Adjunct Professor of Anatomy and Physiology at Hillsborough Community College.

I dedicate this book to nursing educators, who contribute every day to making the world a better and more caring place.

—MPA

Carol Quam Urban, PhD, RN, Associate Professor, is the Director of COVID Screening and Testing in the office of Safety, Emergency, and Enterprise Risk Management at George Mason University in Fairfax, Virginia. She has published the Pearson textbook *Pharmacology for Nurses: A Pathophysiologic Approach* with Dr. Adams and Dr. Holland.

To my daughter, Joy, an extraordinary nurse who continues to change the world for the better, and in memory of my son, Keith, and my husband, Mike.

—CQU

Rebecca E Sutter, DNP, BC-FNP, is Associate Professor in the School of Nursing and one of the directors of an academic nurse-managed clinic within the College of Health and Human Services at George Mason University in Fairfax, Virginia. She has been on the nursing faculty for over 15 years at community colleges and universities, and has practiced for over 20 years as a pediatric ICU nurse and a board-certified family nurse practitioner.

To my husband, Lee, and my parents, Jane and Ellis, who have given me the foundation to reach for my dreams, and to my amazing children Andrew, Sarah, and Emily, who have made me stronger, better, and more fulfilled than I could have ever imagined. I love you to the moon and back.

—RES

Thank You

First Edition Contributors

We extend a heartfelt thanks to our contributors, who gave their time, effort, and expertise so tirelessly to the development and writing of chapters and resources that helped foster our goal of preparing student nurses for evidence based practice.

Diane Benson, RN, EdD
Humboldt State University, Arcata, California
Chapter 29

Rebecca Boehne, RN, PhD
Linfield College, Portland, Oregon
Chapter 74

Jacqueline Rosenjack Burchum, APRN, BC
The University of Tennessee Health Science Center, Memphis, Tennessee
Chapter 73

Pamela Evans-Smith, RN, MSN
University of Missouri-Columbia, Columbia, Missouri
Chapter 57

Geralyn Frandsen, RN, MSN, EdD
Maryville University, St. Louis, Missouri
Chapters 26, 27, 28, 30, and 44

Denise Marie McEnroe-Ayers, RN, MSN
Kent State University at Tuscarawas, New Philadelphia, Ohio
Chapters 67, 72, 75, 76, and 77

Mariann Montgomery, RN, MSN
Kent State University at Tuscarawas, New Philadelphia, Ohio
Chapters 66, 67, 68, 75, 76, and 77

Kim Alexander Noble, RN, PhD
Temple University, Philadelphia, Pennsylvania
Chapter 46

G. Elaine Patterson, RNC, MA, FNP-C EdD
Ramapo College of New Jersey, Mahwah, New Jersey
Chapters 10, 11, 12, 70, and 71

Janice Lynn Reilley, RN, C, MSN, EdD
Widener University, Chester, Pennsylvania
Chapter 63

Luann G. Richardson, RN, PhD
Duquesne University, Pittsburgh, Pennsylvania
Chapter 60

Roberta Shea, RN, CCNS, MSN
Indiana University School of Nursing Bloomington, Indiana
Chapters 9, 66, 67, and 68

Pat Teasley, RN, MSN, APRN, BC
Central Texas College, Killeen, Texas
Chapters 22, 23, 24, 25, 57, and 58

Third Edition Reviewers

Our heartfelt thanks go out to our colleagues from schools of nursing across the country who have given their time generously to help create this exciting new edition of our pharmacology textbook. These individuals helped us plan and shape our book and resources by reviewing chapters, art, design, and more. *Pharmacology: Connections to Nursing Practice* has reaped the benefit of your collective knowledge and experience as nurses and teachers, and we have improved the materials due to your efforts, suggestions, objections, endorsements, and inspiration. Among those who gave their time generously to help us are the following:

Wanda Barlow, MSN, RN, FNP-BC
Instructor
Winston-Salem State University
Winston-Salem, North Carolina

Carole Berube, MA, MSN, BSN, RN
Professor Emerita
Bristol Community College
Fall River, Massachusetts

Sophia Beydoun, MSN, RN
Instructor
Henry Ford College
Dearborn, Michigan

Staci M. Boruff, PhD, RN
Professor
Walters State Community College
Morristown, Tennessee

Sharon Burke, EdD, MSN, RNC
Assistant Professor
The Pennsylvania State University
Abington, Pennsylvania

Judy Callicoatt, RN, MS, CNS
ADN Instructor
Trinity Valley Community College
Kaufman, Texas

Katrina Coggins, MSN, RN, CEN
Assistant Professor
Western Carolina University
Cullowhee, North Carolina

Tamara Condrey, DNP, RN, ACNS-BC, CCRN, CNE
Assistant Professor
Columbus State University
Columbus, Georgia

Rebecca A. Crane, MSN, RN, CHPN, CLNC
Assistant Professor
Ivy Tech Community College
Bloomington, Indiana

Lynette DeBellis, RN, MA
Assistant Professor
Westchester Community College
Valhalla, New York

Debra Dickman, MS, RN, CNE
Assistant Professor
Blessing-Rieman College of Nursing
Quincy, Illinois

Teresa Dobrzykowski, PhD, APRN, BC
Assistant Professor
Indiana University
South Bend, Indiana

Deborah Dye, RN, MSN
Department Chair and Assistant Professor
Ivy Tech Community College
Lafayette, Indiana

Nancy W. Ebersole, PhD, RN
Direct-Entry MSN Program Coordinator
Salem State University
Salem, Massachusetts

Anita Fitzgerald, RN, A/GNP
Lecturer, Director, Learning Center
California State University
Long Beach, California

Suzanne Franzoni-Kleeman, MSN, RN, CEN
Assistant Professor
American International College
Springfield, Massachusetts

Lola Goodson, RN, MSN, CRNI
Instructor
Ivy Tech Community College
Sellersburg, Indiana

Amy C. Graham, RN, MSN, FNP-BC
Assistant Professor
James Madison University
Harrisonburg, Virginia

Crystal Graham, RN, CHSE, MSN-Ed
Simulation Lab Director/Instructor of Nursing
Francis Marion University
Florence, South Carolina

Yolanda J. Green, RN, MSN
Associate Professor
Chattanooga State Community College
Chattanooga, Tennessee

Susan Growe, DNP, RN
Lecturer
Nevada State College
Henderson, Nevada

Jeanne Hately, PhD, MSN, RN
Owner
Professional Nurse Consultants, LLC
Aurora, Colorado

Antonie Hiemer, MS, RN
Assistant Professor
Morrisville State College
Morrisville, New York

Susan Holland, MSN, APRN, GNP-BC
Clinical Assistant Professor
Sam Houston State University
Huntsville, Texas

Molly Jackson, RN, MSN APRN, NP-C
Instructor
Case Western Reserve University
Cleveland, Ohio

Sara K. Kaylor, EdD, RN
Assistant Professor
The University of Alabama
Tuscaloosa, Alabama

Amy Mitchell Kennedy, MSN, RN
Adjunct Faculty, RN and PN Program
ECPI University
Newport News, Virginia

Alice Kindschuh, DNP, RN, APRN-CNS, CNE
Adjunct Instructor
Nebraska Methodist College
Omaha, Nebraska

Vicky J. King, RN, MS, CNE
Nursing Faculty
Cochise College
Sierra Vista, Arizona

Julie Ann Koch, DNP, RN, FNP-BC
Assistant Professor and DNP Program Coordinator
Valparaiso University
Valparaiso, Indiana

Angela M. Koller, DNP, MSN, RN
Dean
Ivy Tech Community College
Indianapolis, Indiana

Stephen D. Krau, PhD, RN, CNE
Associate Professor
Vanderbilt University Medical Center, School of Nursing
Nashville, Tennessee

Elizabeth L. Law, MSN, NP-C, RN
Assistant Professor
Ivy Tech Community College
Indianapolis, Indiana

Connie Lawrence, MS, FNP-BC, DNP
Director of RN-BSN Program
The College at Brockport
Brockport, New York

Dr. Euphemia Marlene C. Lazarus
Professor
Camden County College
Blackwood, New Jersey

Carol Isaac MacKusick, PhDc, RN, CNN, CNE
Assistant Professor
Western Carolina University
Cullowhee, North Carolina

Shayne A. Mason, RN, BSN, PMHNP(BC)
Instructor
University of San Francisco
San Francisco, California

Vicki McCalmont RN, MS, ANP-BC, CNS, CCTC
Professor
San Diego State University
San Diego, California

Bethany Mello, DNP, MS, NP-C
Assistant Professor
University of Jamestown
Jamestown, North Dakota

James Mendez, MSN, CRNP
Adjunct Instructor
Villanova University
Villanova, Pennsylvania

Toby Nishikawa, MSN, RN
Assistant Professor
Weber State University
Ogden, Utah

Nola Ormrod, RN, MSN
Department Chair
Centralia College
Centralia, Washington

Mechelle Perea-Ryan, MS, FNP-BC, PHN
Associate Professor
California State University, Stanislaus
Turlock, California

Beth Rowlands, DNP, GNP-BC
Clinical Professor
University of Massachusetts
Boston, Massachusetts

Janet Czermak Russell, APN-BC
Professor
Essex County College
Newark, New Jersey

Jennifer Brindisi Sipe, MSN, RN
Assistant Professor
LaSalle University
Philadelphia, Pennsylvania

Michelle Taylor Skipper, DNP, FNP-BC
Clinical Associate Professor
Director, A/GNP and FNP Concentrations
East Carolina University
Greenville, North Carolina

Sabra H. Smith, DNP, MS, FNP-BC
Clinical Assistant Professor
University of South Carolina
Columbia, South Carolina

Rebecca E. Sutter, DNP, APRN, BC-FNP
Assistant Dean and Assistant Professor
George Mason University
Fairfax, Virginia

Nanci Swan, RN, MSN, CCRN
Instructor
The University of Alabama
Birmingham, Alabama

Valerie Taylor, RN, C, MEd, MSN
Assistant Professor
Lorain County Community College
Elyria, Ohio

Angela Trawick, MSN, RN
Clinical Coordinator
Florida SouthWestern State College
Fort Myers, Florida

Diana White, RN, MS
Professor
Tuskegee University
Tuskegee, Alabama

Carol S. Whiteman, MSN, RN, CCRN
Assistant Professor
Ivy Tech Community College
South Bend, Indiana

Toni C. Wortham, RN, BSN, MSN
Part-time Instructor
Madisonville Community College
Madisonville, Kentucky

Benson Kar Leung Yeung, MSN, RN
Full-time Instructor
California State University
Los Angeles, California

Preface

Pharmacology is one of the most challenging and dynamic subjects for professional nurses. Each month new drugs are being introduced, and new indications are continually being developed for existing medications. Some medications that were considered preferred drugs only a decade ago are now rarely prescribed. Current knowledge of drug actions, mechanisms, interactions, and legislation is mandatory for nurses to provide safe and effective patient care in all healthcare settings. Pharmacotherapeutics remains a critical and ever-changing component of patient care.

The subtitle of this text, *Connections to Nursing Practice*, has guided its continued development. At a fundamental level, pharmacology is a series of interrelated essential concepts. Some key concepts are shared with the natural and applied sciences. Prediction of drug action requires a thorough knowledge of anatomy, physiology, chemistry, and pathology as well as the social sciences of psychology and sociology. This interdisciplinary nature of pharmacology makes the subject difficult to learn but fascinating to study.

However, the discipline of pharmacology is far more than a collection of isolated facts. To effectively learn this discipline, the student must make connections to nursing practice and, ultimately, connections to patient care. Patients expect to receive effective and safe medication administration from a nurse who is competent in the study of pharmacology. *Pharmacology: Connections to Nursing Practice* identifies key pharmacologic concepts and mechanisms and clearly connects them to current nursing theory and practice for providing optimal patient care.

Pharmacology: Connections to Nursing Practice recognizes that pharmacology is not an academic discipline to be learned for its own sake but is a critical tool to prevent disease and promote healing. This connection to patients, their assessment, diagnoses, and interventions supports basic nursing practice. Like other core nursing subjects, the focus of pharmacology must be to teach and promote wellness for patients.

Structure of the Text

This text is organized according to body systems (units) and diseases (chapters). Unit 1, the first seven chapters, identifies fundamental pharmacologic principles that are applied throughout the text. Although new drugs are constantly being developed, these chapters build the structural framework for understanding the applications of all drugs. The role of complementary and alternative therapies, which are used by many patients, is included in the context of holistic care.

Unit 2 connects pharmacology, the nurse, and the patient, with an emphasis on positive patient outcomes. The four chapters in this unit recognize the essential role of nurse-patient interactions in providing optimal patient care throughout the lifespan. The fact that individuals vary in their responses to drug action is an important theme introduced in this unit.

Units 3 through 11 provide the concepts and connections that are necessary to understand the actions and adverse effects of individual drugs on different body systems. Many of the units begin with a chapter that briefly reviews relevant anatomy and physiology, which is a useful feature for the student when studying drug actions. Each chapter clearly identifies the concepts and connections necessary for safe and effective pharmacotherapy. Pharmacology is intimately related to the study of disease processes. The connections between pharmacology and pathophysiology are clearly established for each drug class in every chapter.

Resources for Faculty

Pearson is pleased to offer a suite of resources to support teaching and learning, including:

- **TestGen Test Bank**
- **Lecture Note PowerPoints**
- **Instructor's Resource Manual**

A Practical Approach to Learning Pharmacology

◀ **Disease and Body System Approach.** The organization by body systems (units) and diseases (chapters) places the drugs in context with how they are used therapeutically. This organization connects pharmacology and pathophysiology to nursing care.

PROTOTYPE DRUG **Amiodarone (Nexterone, Pacerone)**

Classification **Therapeutic:** Antidysrhythmic, Class III
Pharmacologic: Potassium channel blocker

Therapeutic Effects and Uses: Approved in 1985, amiodarone is the most frequently prescribed Class III antidysrhythmic. It is considered a broad-spectrum antidysrhythmic because it is effective in terminating both atrial and ventricular dysrhythmias. It is approved for the treatment of resistant ventricular tachycardia and recurrent fibrillation that may prove life-threatening, and it has become a preferred medication for the treatment of atrial dysrhythmias in patients with HF.

▶ **Prototype Approach.** The vast number of drugs that the practicing nurse must learn is staggering. To facilitate learning, this text uses a prototype approach in which the most representative medications in each classification are introduced in detail. This edition features 194 prototype drugs that include detailed information on therapeutic effects, mechanism of action, pharmacokinetics, adverse effects, contraindications, drug interactions, pregnancy data, and treatment of overdose.

Adverse Effects: Potentially serious adverse effects limit the use of amiodarone. This drug may cause nausea and vomiting, anorexia, fatigue, dizziness, and hypotension. Visual disturbances are common in patients taking amiodarone for extended periods and include blurred vision due to cornea deposits, photophobia, xerostomia, cataracts, and macular degeneration. Rashes, photosensitivity, and other skin reactions occur in 10 to 15% of patients taking the drug. Certain tissues concentrate this medication; thus, adverse effects may be slow to resolve, persisting long after the drug has been discontinued. **Black Box Warnings:** Amiodarone has been associated with severe and sometimes fatal pulmonary toxicity. It has prodysrhythmic action and may cause bradycardia, cardiogenic shock, or AV block. Liver injury is frequent with amiodarone.

◀ **Updated! Black Box Warnings.** The latest black box warnings issued by the U.S. Food and Drug Administration are clearly identified for all prototype medications. In this edition, black box warnings have been added for non-prototype drugs.

▶ **Updated! Drug Tables.** Every drug table has been revised to add newly-approved drugs and drug classes and remove withdrawn medications. Unique to this text is a listing of the most common and the most serious adverse effects for each drug or drug class. This allows the student to immediately recognize important safety information regarding the drug(s) he or she is administering.

Table 38.5 Antiplatelet Drugs

Drug	Route and Adult Dose (Maximum Dose Where Indicated)	Adverse Effects
anagrelide (Agrylin)	PO: 0.5 mg qid or 1 mg bid (max: 10 mg/day)	*Nausea and vomiting, diarrhea, abdominal pain, dizziness, headache* Increased bleeding, CNS effects (dipyridamole), anaphylaxis (aspirin), interstitial lung disease (anagrelide)
aspirin (ASA, acetylsalicylic acid)	PO: 80 mg daily to 650 mg bid	
dipyridamole (Persantine)	PO: 75–100 mg qid as adjunct to warfarin therapy	
vorapaxar (Zontivity)	PO: 2.08 mg/day	
ADP Receptor Blockers		
cangrelor (Kengreal)	IV: 30 mcg/kg single dose followed immediately by 4 mcg/kg/minute continuous infusion	*Minor bleeding* Serious bleeding, hypersensitivity, dyspnea
clopidogrel (Plavix)	PO: 75 mg/day (max: 300 mg/day for life-threatening cases)	*Minor bleeding, dyspepsia, abdominal pain, headache, rash, diarrhea* Increased clotting time, GI bleeding, blood dyscrasias, angina
prasugrel (Effient)	PO: 60-mg loading dose followed by 10 mg/day	
ticagrelor (Brilinta)	PO: 180-mg loading dose followed by 90 mg bid	
Glycoprotein IIb/IIIa Receptor Antagonists		
eptifibatide (Integrilin)	IV: 180 mcg/kg initial bolus over 1–2 min, then 2 mcg/kg/min for 24–72 h (max: 180 mcg/kg bolus, 2 mcg/kg/min infusion)	*Dyspepsia, dizziness, pain at injection site, hypotension, bradycardia, minor bleeding* Major hemorrhage, thrombocytopenia
tirofiban (Aggrastat)	IV: 0.4 mcg/kg/min for 30 min, then 0.1 mcg/kg/min for 12–24 h	
Drugs for Intermittent Claudication		
cilostazol	PO: 100 mg bid	*Dyspepsia, nausea and vomiting, dizziness, myalgia, headache* Tachycardia and palpitations (cilostazol), CNS effects (pentoxifylline), HF, MI
pentoxifylline (Trental)	PO: 400 mg tid (max: 1200 mg/day)	

Note: *Italics* indicate common adverse effects. Underline indicates serious adverse effects.

Pregnancy: Animal studies show that lorazepam may cause fetal harm. Neonates born to mothers taking benzodiazepines during pregnancy may experience withdrawal symptoms. Because this drug is secreted in human milk, breastfeeding is not recommended.

◀ **NEW to This Edition:** Pregnancy data for each drug in this text now clearly states known or suspected harm to the embryo or fetus based on laboratory animal and/or human research. Also included is information stating potential harm for the neonate from lactation while the mother is taking the drug. When applicable, this section includes data on recommendations for pregnancy testing prior to and during drug therapy and for the use of contraception while taking the medication.

Connections to Nursing Practice

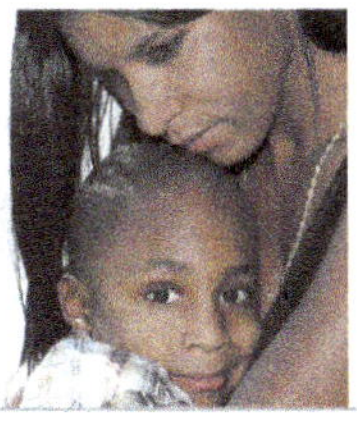

"The school nurse recommended we consider Adderall for Jonathon. He's just doing poorly in school and hates to do his homework. Why would he need a drug for that?"
—*Patient "Jonathon Hogan's" mother*

Chapter 24
Central Nervous System Stimulants and Drugs for Attention-Deficit/Hyperactivity Disorder

Chapter Outline

- Characteristics of Central Nervous System Stimulants
- Etiology and Pathophysiology of Attention-Deficit/Hyperactivity Disorder
- Pharmacotherapy of Attention-Deficit/Hyperactivity Disorder
  - Psychostimulants
  - **PROTOTYPE** *Amphetamine and Dextroamphetamine (Adderall, Adderall XR), p. 377*
  - Nonstimulants
  - **PROTOTYPE** *Atomoxetine (Strattera), p. 379*
- Pharmacotherapy of Narcolepsy
  - **PROTOTYPE** *Modafinil (Provigil), p. 381*
- Methylxanthines
  - **PROTOTYPE** *Caffeine (Cafcit), p. 382*

Learning Outcomes

After reading the chapter, the student should be able to:

1. Describe the general actions and pharmacotherapeutic applications of central nervous system stimulants.
2. Identify the signs and symptoms of attention-deficit/hyperactivity disorder and narcolepsy.
3. Compare and contrast the central nervous system stimulants and nonstimulants in treating attention-deficit/hyperactivity disorder.
4. Describe the role of stimulant medication in the treatment of narcolepsy.
5. Describe the nurse's role in the pharmacologic management of attention-deficit/hyperactivity disorder and narcolepsy.
6. For each class shown in the chapter outline, identify the prototype and representative drugs and explain the mechanism(s) of drug action, primary indications, contraindications, significant drug interactions, pregnancy data and important adverse effects.
7. Apply clinical judgement to care for patients receiving pharmacotherapy with central nervous system stimulants.

372

◀ **Making the Patient Connection** is a feature that opens each chapter with a quote and a photo of a patient. It reinforces to the student that the focus of pharmacology must always be on the patient. To drive this important message home, the patient who is introduced at the start of the chapter is revisited at the end with critical thinking exercises. These questions assist the student to apply the content learned in the chapter to a realistic patient scenario. An additional case study is also included for further application of knowledge learned.

CASE STUDY: Making the Patient Connection

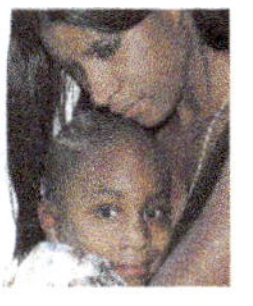

Remember the patient "Jonathon Hogan" at the beginning of the chapter? Now read the remainder of the case study. Based on the information presented within this chapter, respond to the critical thinking questions that follow.

Jonathon Hogan has had trouble at school beginning in kindergarten and for the past year. His teachers have consistently reported that he is easily distracted and wanders around the classroom, even during a lesson. Getting him to do his homework after school has been a struggle. Jonathon loves art and does well at video games. Because he is a happy-go-lucky child, his parents have assumed that Jonathon's right-brain dominance has created trouble with left-brain logical work. With more homework now in second grade, Jonathon is struggling to keep up in school. The school nurse suspects he may have ADHD. She has recommended an appointment with Jonathon's healthcare provider and told his parents that Adderall may help him focus on his schoolwork.

Critical Thinking Questions

1. What is ADHD and why would Jonathon be experiencing more difficulty as he becomes older?
2. How might amphetamine sulfate and dextroamphetamine (Adderall) help Jonathon with his ADHD?
3. What caregiver education would be appropriate regarding dextroamphetamine and amphetamine sulfate (Adderall)?
4. What are other nonpharmacologic treatments for ADHD?

▶ **Expanded! Connections: Advanced Practice Applications.** Dramatic changes in the delivery of healthcare have placed an increased emphasis on developing the critical thinking skills and clinical decision-making abilities of nurses at both the undergraduate and graduate levels. Through case studies, the authors use strategies that promote the clinical decision-making skills of advanced practice nurses. Particular attention is paid to advanced practice nurses who are preparing to work within specialty practice settings and with vulnerable populations.

CONNECTIONS: Advanced Practice Application

Chronic Kidney Disease and Prescribing Considerations

Case

Nolan is a 71-year-old Black male who was admitted to the hospital for altered mental status. His daughter Renee reported that her father had become progressively confused and had been having visual and auditory hallucinations. In the past 24 hours, Nolan's symptoms had become more persistent and she became more concerned. Nolan has a 9-year history of heart failure and type 2 diabetes and was diagnosed 10 months ago with stage V CKD.

On admission, the nurse practitioner hospitalist, his bedside nurse, and the unit's pharmacist. reviewed his medications with Renee. Nolan was taking aspirin, atenolol, metformin, atorvastatin, and gabapentin for the diabetes neuropathy. On physical examination, he was sleepy but arousable. His blood pressure was 136/86 mmHg; pulse was 72 beats/min (regular); respiratory rate was 14 breaths/min; and oxygen saturation 96%. What pharmacologic factors should the team be considering for Nolan?

Discussion

Kidney disease, both AKI and CKD, affects every organ system in the body. The number of patients with AKI and CKD has increased due to the aging population and medical advancements. With the significant increase in polypharmacy over the last decade, it is increasingly important to understand potentially inappropriate medication use by patients with CKD. For prescribing purposes, CKD is divided into three grades:

- Mild: GFR 20–50 mL/min; serum creatinine 150–300 µmol/L
- Moderate: GFR 10–20 mL/min; serum creatinine 300–700 µmol/L
- Severe: GFR less than 10 mL/min; serum creatinine more than 700 µmol/L (GFR above 50 mL/min does not usually require any dosage adjustment.)

Drugs to which particular attention should be given include histamine H_2-receptor antagonists, specific antibiotics, anticonvulsants, digoxin, and NSAIDs. Prescribing any medication that increases potassium levels, such as potassium supplements and potassium-sparing diuretics, is potentially very dangerous. Additionally, methotrexate, enoxaparin, and metformin should no longer be prescribed even with a mild grade of CKD. With cardiovascular (e.g., atenolol) antidiabetic (e.g., metformin) or anticonvulsive (e.g., gabapentin) drugs, the recommendation is to use alternative medications, such as lisinopril, glyburide, or carbamazepine. Drug dose adjustments should be considered with antimicrobial (e.g., ampicillin), antiviral (e.g., acyclovir), and some chemotherapeutic and cytotoxic drugs (e.g., cisplatin). Products with a high sodium content (e.g., antacids) should be avoided because they may cause sodium and water retention in patients with CKD (Kurani et al., 2019).

CONNECTIONS: Treating the Diverse Patient

Ethnic Differences in Thyroid Hormone Replacement

As more is learned in the quest for personalized medicine, the influence of ethnic differences on replacement therapies is also being discovered. In a study of Jewish and non-Jewish children, Oron et al. (2020) discovered that the level of TSH was influenced by both body mass index (BMI) and ethnicity. While thyroid dosing is usually based on weight or BMI, TSH was found to be lower in the Jewish population that was studied than in the non-Jewish population. While BMI remains an appropriate consideration for thyroid replacement dosing, ethnic differences in TSH should also be considered to fine-tune the dose.

◀ **Connections: Treating the Diverse Patient** features identify gender, cultural, and ethical influences that are important modifiers of drug action.

▶ **Connections: Complementary and Alternative Therapies** features present herbal therapies and dietary supplements that may be considered as alternatives to conventional drugs. These features include a description of the herb or supplement, history of use, standardization of dose, and brief description of the scientific evidence supporting (or not supporting) the use of the product.

CONNECTIONS: Complementary and Alternative Therapies

Probiotics for Diarrhea

Description

Probiotics are live microorganisms that are taken in specified amounts to confer a health benefit on the host. Most commercial probiotics are bacteria from the genera *Lactobacillus* and *Bifidobacterium*; however, yeast such as *Saccharomyces* are also sometimes used.

History and Claims

Although probiotics have been used for thousands of years, only in the past 20 years has research begun to confirm their health benefits. Probiotics are claimed to improve immune function, decrease cancer risk, lower blood cholesterol, reduce blood pressure, and prevent vaginal infections. Probiotics are available in yogurts, fermented foods, added to some drinks, and as tablets. Although probiotics are safe, care must be taken not to exceed recommended doses.

Standardization

Supplements include capsules, tablets, and granules, as well as cultured dairy products that contain the probiotic bacteria. Doses are not standardized. Tablet doses range from 50 to 500 mg, and not all dairy products contain active cultures.

Evidence

Most of the evidence supporting the efficacy of probiotics is related to their effects on the intestinal tract microbiome. Both *Lactobacillus* and *Bifidobacterium* are normal nonpathogenic inhabitants of a healthy digestive tract. These are considered to be protective flora, inhibiting the growth of potentially pathogenic species such as *E. coli*, *Candida albicans*, *Helicobacter pylori*, and *Gardnerella vaginalis*. Probiotics are useful in restoring the normal flora of the intestine following diarrhea, particularly diarrhea resulting from antibiotic therapy, and have shown positive effects for a wide variety of other conditions such as allergies, dental problems, and some infections (National Center for Complementary and Integrative Health, 2019).

Although probiotics have been used for many years, they are not without risk. Infections (including sepsis), lactic acidosis, and other serious adverse effects have been noted and probiotic supplements should be used with caution in critically ill patients.

Updated! Connections: Applied Clinical Judgment. Formerly called Nursing Practice Applications, These sections have been totally revised to better reflect the role of the nurse in applying clinical judgment. Based on student feedback, the Applied Clinical Judgment Connections are more concise and in a single column to allow student to rapidly find the essential information they need. Collaboration with other disciplines, such as social support services or dietary services, is also included in the interventions. Important lifespan and diverse patient considerations are noted throughout. The Applied Clinical Judgment features are organized to help students learn to think like a nurse as they take students through the processes of drug administration, nursing care, and teaching that are necessary in pharmacotherapy.

CONNECTIONS: APPLIED CLINICAL JUDGMENT

Patients Receiving Pharmacotherapy for Hyperlipidemia

Key Assessment Data

- History of current condition, baseline vital signs, physical exam findings; history of cardiovascular, musculoskeletal (preexisting conditions that might result in muscle or joint pain), GI (peptic ulcer disease, hemorrhoids, inflammatory bowel disease, chronic constipation, gallbladder disease, dysphagia, or esophageal strictures); drug history including allergies, current prescription and OTC drugs, herbal preparations, and alcohol use; pregnancy status.
- Ongoing assessment during drug therapy includes laboratory findings, especially liver function studies, lipid profiles, and CK.

Desired Therapeutic Outcomes

Improvement is observed and measurable in improved lipid profile levels (lowered total cholesterol and LDL-C levels, increased HDL-C levels).

Minimizing Adverse Effects

- Abnormal liver function tests or increased CK levels may indicate drug-induced adverse hepatic effects or myopathy and should be reported.
- Lipid-lowering drugs often adversely affect the liver but may also cause drug-specific adverse effects, especially musculoskeletal, hepatic, and GI. Lipid-lowering drugs given in combination increase this risk.
- If statins are used, report unusual or unexplained muscle tenderness, increasing muscle pain, numbness or tingling of extremities, or effects that hinder normal ADLs.
- If bile acid resins are used, report severe nausea, heartburn, constipation, or straining with passing stools. Any tarry stools or yellowing of the sclera or skin should also be reported.
- If fibric acid drugs are used, report unusual bleeding or bruising, right upper quadrant pain, muscle cramping, or changes in the color of the stool. Patients with diabetes on PO medications may need a change in their dosage and should monitor their glucose more frequently in early therapy.

Lifespan Considerations

- Monitor liver function and CK tests more frequently in the older adult because age-related physiologic changes may affect the drug's metabolism or excretion.
- Statins should not be used during pregnancy, if pregnancy is suspected, or while breastfeeding.
- If fibric acid drugs are used, the older adult is at increased risk for dizziness and may require assistance with ambulation to prevent falls.

Diversity Considerations

- Because statins metabolize through the CYP450 system, they may interact with other drugs. Observe for less-than-optimal therapeutic effects, especially in ethnically diverse patients.

Patient and Caregiver Education

- Adopt appropriate lifestyle changes: lowered fat intake, increased exercise, limited alcohol intake, and smoking cessation. Increase intake of foods rich in omega-3 and Coenzyme Q10: fish such as salmon and sardines, nuts, extra-virgin olive and canola oils, beef, chicken, and pork. Supplementation may be needed but seek the advice of a healthcare provider before taking supplements. A dietitian consultation may be helpful.
- Take the drug following appropriate guidelines:
  - **Statins:** Most are taken with the evening meal; avoid grapefruit and grapefruit juice, which could inhibit the drug's metabolism, leading to toxic levels.
  - **Bile acid resins:** Take before meals with plenty of fluids, mixing powders or granules thoroughly with liquid. Take other medications 1 h before or 4 h after the bile acid resin is taken.
  - **Niacin:** Take with cold water to decrease the sensation of flushing associated with the drug. Take one adult-strength (325-mg) aspirin 30 min before the niacin dose.
  - **Fibric acid drugs:** Take with a meal.

Prescribing Considerations

- Obtain baseline laboratory tests of renal and liver function before prescribing.
- Combining lipid-lowering agents requires close monitoring of liver function tests and CK levels; discontinue if serum transaminase (ALT) is more than three times the normal level, in the presence of elevated CPK levels, if myopathy occurs, or if there is a predisposition to renal failure.
- Niacin should be started at a low dose, and any increases in dosage should be made very slowly in order to minimize adverse effects.
- When combining niacin with a statin, a smaller dose of niacin should be used in order to lower patients' risk of developing hepatotoxicity, myopathy, and rhabdomyolysis.

CONNECTIONS: Patient Safety

Incorrect Insulin Dose

A patient with diabetes has 30 units of Humulin R (regular) insulin ordered for the morning dose. There are several patients with diabetes on the unit and the nurse has given many doses of insulin that morning. The nurse prepares the insulin but draws up Humalog 30 units instead. The patient begins experiencing symptoms of hypoglycemia within 15 minutes and is treated successfully.

What errors occurred and how could they be prevented in the future?

Connections: Patient Safety, a QSEN competency, is a feature that presents a brief patient–nurse scenario that illustrates potential pitfalls encountered by nurses that can lead to medication errors. Most scenarios end with a question asking the student to identify what went wrong, what the nurse should do in the situation, what the nurse should question about the order, or what the nurse should do differently in order to prevent medication administration errors.

Updated! Connections: Using Research in Practice features illustrate connections to nursing or pharmacology research and discuss the directions of pharmacotherapeutics.

CONNECTIONS: Using Research in Practice

Fecal Microbiota Transplant

The role that normal intestinal flora, or *intestinal microbiota*, plays in maintaining body health and immunity is becoming more apparent—and appreciated. Multiple organisms populate the intestinal tract. Their functions include boosting immune protection against toxins produced by some pathogenic bacteria and guarding against septic shock. In addition, they may play a role in preventing obesity.

When normal intestinal flora is disrupted, such as by antibiotic therapy, the pathogenic bacteria may overgrow and cause serious infection. *Clostridioides difficile*–associated diarrhea (CDAD) is a serious bowel infection that most often results from antibiotic therapy. It results in watery diarrhea that contains blood and pus, and rapid dehydration may occur because of fluid loss. The standard treatment for CDAD includes fluid replacement; for severe and recurrent cases, PO vancomycin may be prescribed. Recent research, however, has supported the process called fecal microbiota transplant (FMT), which involves transplanting small amounts of healthy intestinal flora from a donor into a recipient who has CDAD. The outcomes have been positive.

(*continued*)

CONNECTIONS: Lifespan Considerations

Miscarriage Prevention with Anticoagulants

Miscarriage in pregnancy is devastating, and recurrent miscarriage even more so. Autoimmune diseases are related to poorer obstetric outcomes than that of the general population, especially in mothers with undiagnosed thrombophilia (genetic hypercoagulability disorders) such as antiphospholipid syndrome. In a study of women who had experienced recurrent miscarriages, after controlling for other potential causes of miscarriage (e.g., metabolic, anatomical, or chromosomal), the prevalence of thrombophilia was found to be higher in women with recurrent miscarriages, compared to the general population (Nahas et al., 2018).

Research on treatment recommendations for the use of heparin, LMWH, or aspirin for recurrent miscarriage before 10 weeks of pregnancy is ongoing and the use of anticoagulant therapy has shown mixed results for prevention of such miscarriages (Lin et al., 2019). It is recommended that a woman experiencing such loss discuss the situation with her provider and whether genetic testing should be conducted. If genetic coagulation abnormalities are found, heparin, LMWH, or aspirin may be considered an option.

◀ **Connections: Lifespan Considerations** features clearly identify important considerations to ensure safe and effective pharmacotherapy in the older adult and pediatric populations.

CONNECTION Checkpoint 21.3

The cholinesterase inhibitors for Alzheimer's disease are used for their central actions. From what you learned in Chapter 13, what are the indications for cholinesterase inhibitors that act peripherally? What drug is the prototype peripheral cholinesterase inhibitor?

▲ **Connection Checkpoints** ask the student to recall past concepts from previous chapters that are related to current study. Unique to this text, these reinforce material learned in previous chapters that has direct application to the current chapter.

▶ **PharmFacts** connect relevant statistics to the presented material. They add interest to the subject and place it in perspective with other nursing concepts.

PharmFACT

In 2015 to 2017, 53% of sexually active female teens (age 15 to 19) used oral contraceptives to prevent pregnancy. Emergency contraception in this group was used by 19% (Martinez & Abma, 2020).

▼ **Connections: Community-Oriented Practice** features provide important information that nurses need to convey to their patients to ensure that they receive effective pharmacotherapy after leaving the hospital or clinical setting.

CONNECTIONS: Community-Oriented Practice

Lessons Learned from COVID-19 May Aid in TB Control

The response to the pandemic caused by SARS-CoV-2 (COVID-19) overwhelmed the public health communities and shifted attention and resources away from other diseases still very much present and spreading, such as TB. As a leading cause of death, TB remains in the top 10 causes worldwide (WHO, 2020a). Tuberculosis has not disappeared as the COVID-19 pandemic continues and South-East Asia and Africa account for almost 70% of cases worldwide (WHO, 2020b). As testing, tracing, and drug therapies are diverted to COVID-19 and away from TB control, the potential for the spread of the disease, as well as drug-resistant organisms, rises.

But even as the focus of attention moves away from TB and other global diseases to mitigation and management of COVID-19, lessons learned from the response to the pandemic may help to change the way TB is managed and controlled. Social distancing to prevent the spread of TB, contact-tracing measures to determine others in the community who may also need treatment, and the use of modeling to predict disease severity or successful treatment options may be more fully implemented as strategies for TB control. The hope is that communities, public health professionals, and governments can work together and learn from the efforts used for COVID-19 to improve control of other worldwide diseases (Togun et al., 2020).

Learning Through Visuals

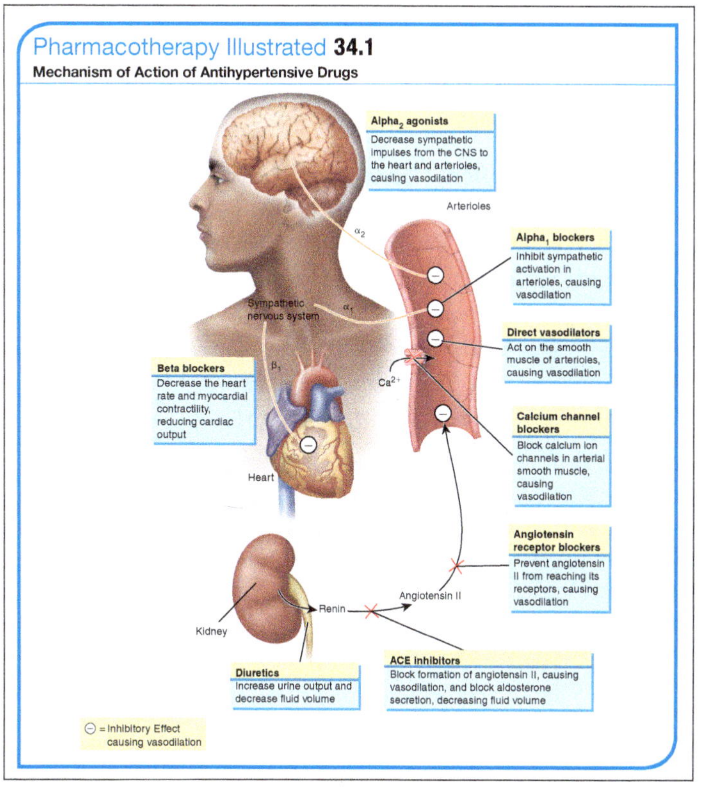

▶ **Pharmacotherapy Illustrated** features visually present the mechanism of action for many of the prototype drugs, showing students specifically how drugs counteract the effects of disease.

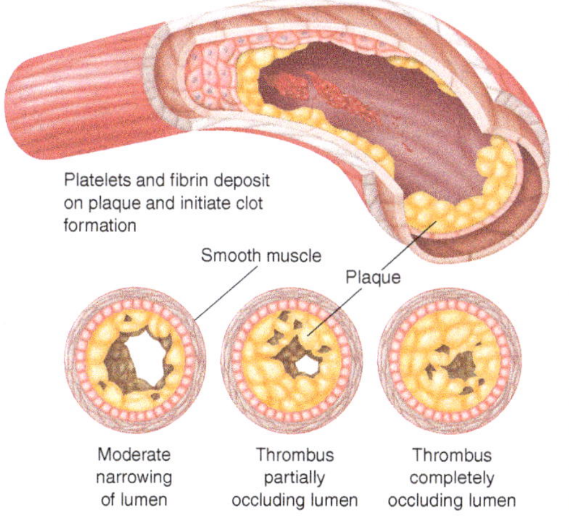

Figure 35.1 Atherosclerosis in the coronary arteries.

◀ **Vivid, Colorful, and Effective Illustrations** help students review the anatomy, physiology, and pathophysiology of a body system to better understand the impact of disease on that system.

Understanding the Chapter

The most comprehensive chapter review in its class! **Understanding the Chapter** begins with a **Key Concepts Summary**, which quickly identifies the numbered key concepts from the chapter. Based on student feedback, answers to all the case study and review questions are now included in the text in Appendix A!

▶ **Making the Patient Connection** reconnects the student to the patient presented in the scenario at the chapter opening. The student learns additional details about the patient's health history and participates in critical thinking questions about the scenario. This allows application of knowledge obtained in the chapter.

CASE STUDY: Making the Patient Connection

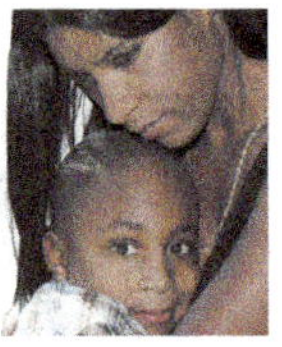

Remember the patient "Jonathon Hogan" at the beginning of the chapter? Now read the remainder of the case study. Based on the information presented within this chapter, respond to the critical thinking questions that follow.

Jonathon Hogan has had trouble at school beginning in kindergarten and for the past year. His teachers have consistently reported that he is easily distracted and wanders around the classroom, even during a lesson. Getting him to do his homework after school has been a struggle. Jonathon loves art and does well at video games. Because he is a happy-go-lucky child, his parents have assumed that Jonathon's right-brain dominance has created trouble with left-brain logical work. With more homework now in second grade, Jonathon is struggling to keep up in school. The school nurse suspects he may have ADHD. She has recommended an appointment with Jonathon's healthcare provider and told his parents that Adderall may help him focus on his schoolwork.

Critical Thinking Questions

1. What is ADHD and why would Jonathon be experiencing more difficulty as he becomes older?
2. How might amphetamine sulfate and dextroamphetamine (Adderall) help Jonathon with his ADHD?
3. What caregiver education would be appropriate regarding dextroamphetamine and amphetamine sulfate (Adderall)?
4. What are other nonpharmacologic treatments for ADHD?

Additional Case Study

Anna Steinmetz has graduated from nursing school and is working nights. She is having difficulty adjusting to her night schedule. Her healthcare provider suggested she utilize a medication to assist with her adjustment to shift work. She has been prescribed modafinil (Provigil).

1. What effect does modafinil (Provigil) have on the patient's ability to maintain alertness during shift work?
2. What teaching will you provide to the patient regarding this medication?
3. The patient reports feelings of lightheadedness with position changes. What interventions will assist in maintaining patient safety?

◀ An **Additional Case Study** gives students another opportunity to apply their knowledge to patient care.

▶ **Chapter Review** prepares students for course exams on chapter content.

Chapter Review

1. An elementary school nurse is providing education to the faculty on the use of central nervous system stimulants to treat attention-deficit/hyperactivity disorder. Of the following, which is most important for the nurse to convey to the faculty?
   1. Have the child bring the drug dose in a lunch bag and come to the office to take it to avoid being teased.
   2. Request that the parents leave an extra copy of the prescription at the school in case the dose runs out.

better off without me." Which action would the nurse take for this patient?

1. Tell the patient to stop taking atomoxetine immediately and not to take it until checking with the provider.
2. Assure the patient that these are normal symptoms because the drug may take 3 or 4 weeks to work.
3. Alert the family or caregiver that immediate attention and treatment are needed for these symptoms.

References

Arthritis Foundation (n.d.). *Glucosamine and chondroitin for osteoarthritis pain*. https://www.arthritis.org/health-wellness/treatment/complementary-therapies/supplements-and-vitamins/glucosamine-chondroitin-osteoarthritis-pain

Bethel, M. (2020). *Osteoporosis*. Medscape. http://emedicine.medscape.com/article/330598- overview#a0156

Kremer, P. A., Laughlin, G. A., Shadyab, A. H., Crandall, C. J., Masaki, K., Orchard, T., et al. (2019). Association between soft drink consumption and osteoporotic fractures among postmenopausal women: The Women's Health Initiative. *Menopause, 26*, 1234–1241. https://doi.org/10.1097/GME.0000000000001389

Zhu, X., Wu, D., Sang, L., Wang, Y., Shen, Y., Zhuang, X., et al. (2018). Comparative effectiveness of glucosamine, chondroitin, acetaminophen or celecoxib for the treatment of knee and/or hip osteoarthritis: a network meta-analysis. *Clinical and Experimental Rheumatology, 36*(4), 595–602.

Selected Bibliography

Arthritis Foundation. (2019). *Arthritis by the numbers*. https://www.arthritis.org/getmedia/e1256607-fa87-4593-aa8a-8db4f291072a/2019-abtn-final-march-2019.pdf

Centers for Disease Control and Prevention (CDC). (2020a). *Gout*. https://www.cdc.gov/arthritis/basics/gout.html

Centers for Disease Control and Prevention (CDC). (2020b). *Rheumatoid arthritis*. https://www.cdc.gov/arthritis/basics/rheumatoid-arthritis.html

Cotts, K. G., & Cifu, A. S. (2018). Treatment of osteoporosis. *Journal of the American Medical Association, 319*(10), 1040–1041. https://doi.org/10.1001/jama.2017.21995

Eastell, R., Rosen, C. J., Black, D. M., Cheung, A. M., Murad, M. H., & Shoback, D. (2019). Pharmacological management of osteoporosis in postmenopausal women: An Endocrine Society clinical practice guideline. *Journal of Clinical Endocrinology and Metabolism, 104*(5), 1595–1622. https://doi.org/10.1210/jc.2019-00221

FitzGerald, J. D., Dalbeth, N., Mikuls, T., Brignardello-Petersen, R., Guyatt, G., Abeles, A. M., et al. (2020). 2020 American College of Rheumatology guideline for the management of gout. *Arthritis Care & Research, 72*(6), 744–760. https://doi.org/10.1002/acr.24180

Köhler, B. M., Günther, J., Kaudewitz, D., & Lorenz, H. M. (2019). Current therapeutic options in the treatment of rheumatoid arthritis. *Journal of Clinical Medicine, 8*(7), 938. https://doi.org/10.3390/jcm8070938

National Institutes of Health (NIH). (2020a). *Calcium: Fact sheet for health professionals*. https://ods.od.nih.gov/factsheets/Calcium-HealthProfessional

National Institutes of Health (NIH). (2020b). *Vitamin D Fact sheet for health professionals*. https://ods.od.nih.gov/factsheets/VitaminD-HealthProfessional/

Rothschild, B. M. (2020). *Gout and pseudogout*. Medscape. http://emedicine.medscape.com/article/329958-overview

Saadeh, C. K. (2020). *Calcium pyrophosphate deposition disease*. Medscape. http://emedicine.medscape.com/article/330936-overview#a5

Smith, H. R. (2020). *Rheumatoid arthritis*. Medscape. http://emedicine.medscape.com/article/331715-overview

Tangpricha, V. (2020). *Vitamin D deficiency and related disorders*. Medscape. http://emedicine.medscape.com/article/128762-overview

◀ Updated **References** and **Bibliography** provide the foundation for evidence-based nursing practice and support the currency and accuracy of the textbook content.

New to the Fifth Edition

- **New Connection features:** Twenty new Connection features have been added to this edition to reflect changes in nursing practice and pharmacotherapeutics.
- **Updated Connections:** Advanced Practice Application features have been completely revised to help students develop critical thinking and clinical decision-making skills.
- **New Connections:** Applied Clinical Judgment features are now included in most chapters to give students concise instructions on caring for patients taking medications.
- **New:** All answers to case study questions and end of chapter review questions are now included in the textbook so that students can get immediate feedback on key concepts contained within each chapter.
- **Completely Revised:** More than 120 new drugs have been added to update medications approved by the FDA since the previous edition.
- **Current references:** All references have been updated to reflect current nursing practice and pharmacotherapeutics.
- **New:** Pregnancy data for each drug in this text reflects current FDA guidelines. This information includes known or suspected harm to the embryo or fetus based on laboratory animal and/or human research. Also included is information stating potential harm for the neonate from lactation while the mother is taking the drug. When applicable, recommendations are included regarding pregnancy testing prior to and during drug therapy and for the use of contraception while taking the medication.

MyLab Nursing

MyLab Nursing is an online learning and practice environment that works with the text to help students master key concepts, prepare for the NCLEX-RN exam, and develop clinical reasoning skills. Through a new mobile experience, students can study Pharmacology: Connections to Nursing Practice anytime, anywhere. New adaptive technology with remediation personalizes learning, moving students beyond memorization to true understanding and application of the content. MyLab Nursing contains the following features:

Dynamic Study Modules

New adaptive learning modules with remediation that personalize the learning experience by allowing students to increase both their confidence and their performance while being assessed in real time.

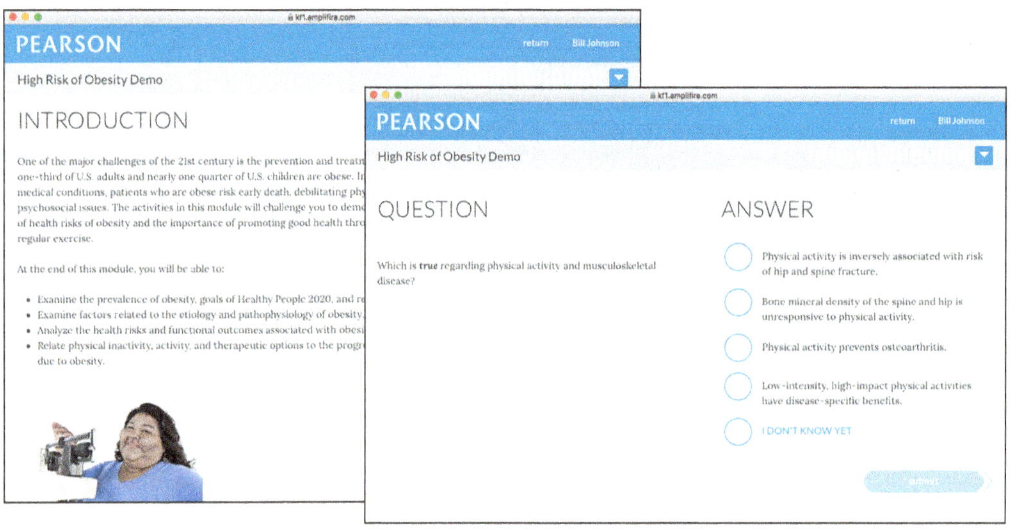

NCLEX-Style Questions

Practice tests with more than 1000 NCLEX-style questions of various types build student confidence and prepare them for success on the NCLEX-RN exam. Questions are organized by Chapter.

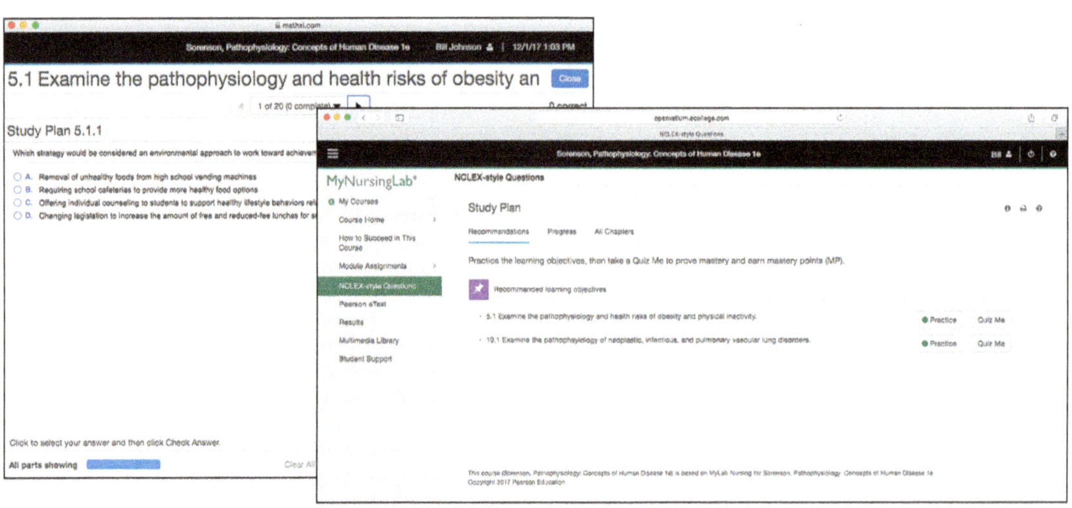

Decision Making Cases

Clinical case studies that provide opportunities for students to practice analyzing information and making important decisions at key moments in patient care scenarios. These 10 unfolding case studies are designed to help prepare students for clinical practice.

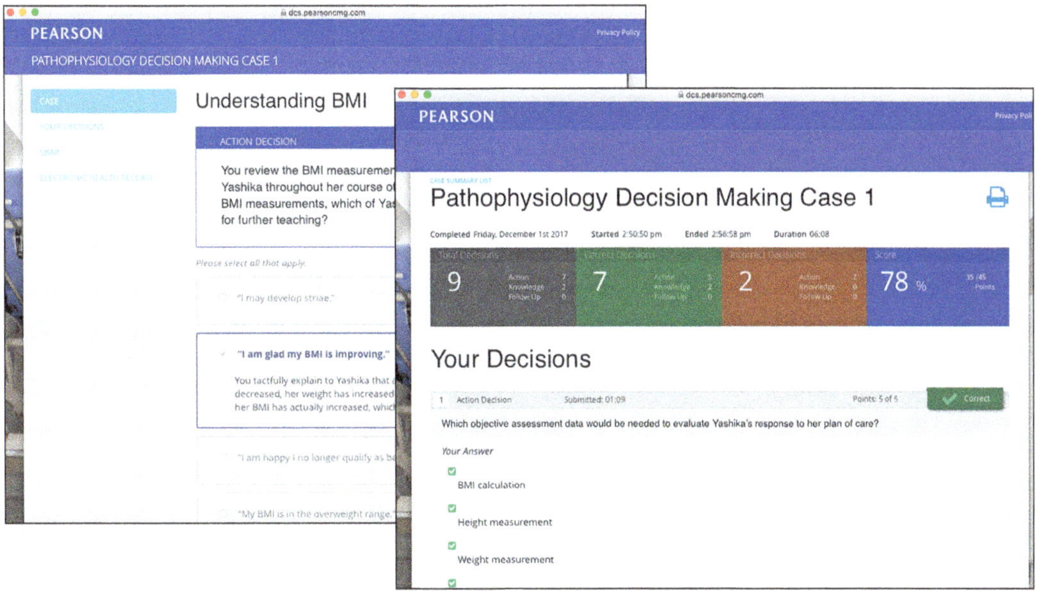

Pearson eText

Enhances student learning both in and outside the classroom. Students can take notes, highlight, and bookmark important content, or engage with interactive and rich media to achieve greater conceptual understanding of the text content. Interactive features include audio clips, pop-up definitions, figures, questions and answers, the nursing process, hotspots, and video animations.

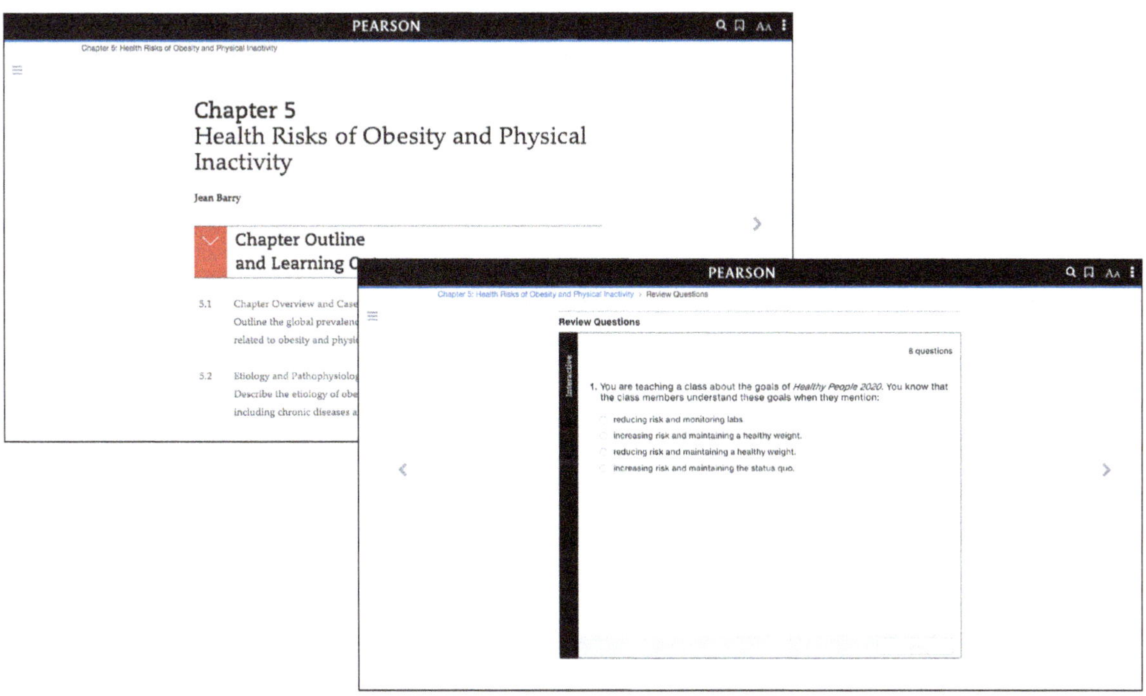

Contents

Unit 1

Fundamental Principles of Pharmacology

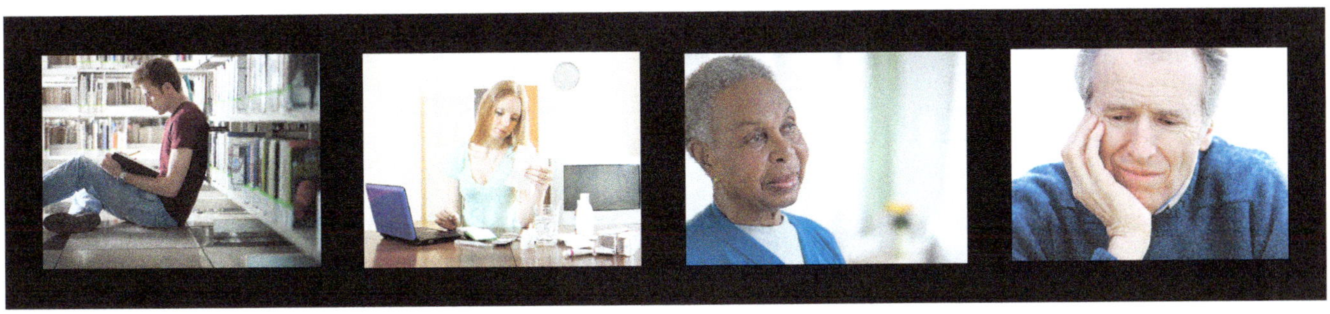

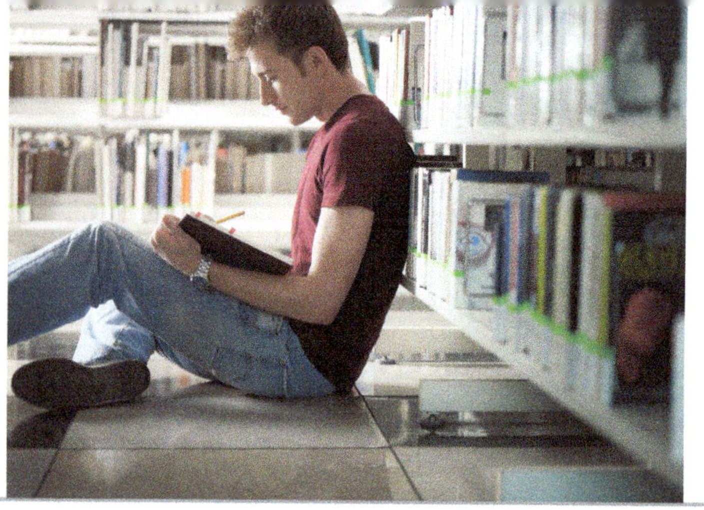

"Wow, I just left my first pharmacology class and my head is swirling. How will I ever remember all this?"
—*Student "Josh Remming"*

Chapter 1
Introduction to Pharmacology: Concepts and Connections

Chapter Outline

- Brief History of Pharmacology
- Pharmacology: The Study of Medicines
- Characteristics of an Ideal Drug
- Classification of Drugs
- Prototype Drugs
- Naming Drugs
- Connecting Pharmacology to Clinical Nursing Practice

Learning Outcomes

After reading this chapter, the student should be able to:

1. Identify key events in the history of pharmacology.
2. Compare and contrast the terms *drug*, *pharmacology*, and *pharmacotherapy*.
3. Explain the importance of pharmacotherapy to clinical nursing practice.
4. Using specific examples, explain the difference between the pharmacologic and therapeutic methods of classifying drugs.
5. Identify the advantages of using prototype drugs to study pharmacology.
6. Classify drugs by their chemical, generic, and trade names.
7. Discuss the rationale for a pharmaceutical company receiving exclusivity for the marketing of a new drug.
8. Analyze possible differences between generic drugs and their trade-name equivalents.
9. Identify differences between biosimilar drug, interchangeable drugs and reference product.
10. Identify the responsibilities of the nurse in drug administration as part of an interprofessional team.

Key Terms

Definitions of the terms in bold may be found in the Glossary.

More drugs are being administered to consumers than ever before. Over 5.8 billion prescriptions were dispensed in the United States in 2018, at a rate of more than 17 prescriptions per person (IQVIA Institute, 2019). Sales of prescription medications at retail pharmacies in the United States exceeded $344 billion in 2018. The number and complexity of medications being approved each year bring exciting challenges for nurses and their patients. The purpose of this chapter is to introduce fundamental concepts of pharmacology and to emphasize the connections between drug therapy and clinical nursing practice.

Brief History of Pharmacology

1.1 The practice of applying products to relieve suffering has been recorded throughout history by virtually every culture.

The story of pharmacology is rich and exciting, filled with accidental discoveries and landmark events. Its history likely began when a human first used a plant to relieve symptoms of disease. One of the oldest forms of healthcare, herbal medicine has been practiced in virtually every culture dating to antiquity. The Babylonians recorded the earliest surviving "prescriptions" on clay tablets in 3000 BC, although magic and the art of reading omens were probably considered just as legitimate to healing as the use of herbal remedies. At about the same time, the Chinese recorded the *Pen Tsao* (Great Herbal), a 40-volume compendium of plant remedies dating to 2700 BC. The Egyptians followed in 1500 BC by archiving their remedies on a document known as the Eber's papyrus, which contains over 700 magical formulas and remedies. Galen, the famous Greek physician, described over 1000 healing preparations using plant products before his death in AD 201.

Little is known about pharmacology during the Dark Ages. Although it is likely that herbal medicine continued to be practiced, especially in monasteries and in centers of Arabic culture, few historical events related to drug therapy were recorded. Pharmacology, and indeed medicine, could not advance until the discipline of science was eventually viewed differently than magic and superstition.

The first recorded reference to the word *pharmacology* was found in a text titled "Pharmacologia sen Manuductio and Materiam Medicum" by Samuel Dale in 1693. Before this date, the study of herbal remedies was called "Materia Medica." The term *Materia Medica* likely originated from a Latin term meaning "medical matters," and use of this term continued into the early 20th century.

Although the exact starting date is obscure, modern pharmacology is thought to have begun in the early 1800s. At that time, chemists were making remarkable progress in separating specific substances from complex mixtures. This enabled chemists to isolate the active agents morphine, colchicine, curare, cocaine, and other early drugs from their natural plant products. Pharmacologists could then study their effects in animals more precisely, using standardized amounts. Some of the early researchers even used themselves as test subjects. Friedrich Sertürner, who first isolated morphine from opium in 1805, injected himself and three of his friends with a huge dose of 100 mg of his new product. He and his cohorts experienced acute morphine intoxication for several days afterward.

Pharmacology as a distinct discipline was officially recognized when the first Department of Pharmacology was established in Estonia in 1847. John Jacob Abel, who is considered the father of American pharmacology due to his many contributions to the field, founded the first pharmacology department in the United States at the University of Michigan in 1890.

In the 20th century, the pace of change in all areas of medicine became exponential. Pharmacologists no longer needed to rely on the slow, laborious process of isolating active agents from scarce natural products. They could synthesize drugs "from scratch" in a laboratory. Hundreds of new drugs could be synthesized and tested in a relatively short time span. More importantly, it became possible to understand how drugs produced their effects, right down to their molecular mechanism of action.

The current practice of pharmacology is extremely complex and has progressed far beyond its early, primitive history. The nurses and other health professionals who administer medications, however, must never forget the early roots of pharmacology: the application of products to relieve or prevent human suffering. Whether a substance is extracted from the Pacific yew tree, isolated from a fungus, or created in a laboratory, the central purpose of pharmacology is focused on the patient and improving the quality of life.

CONNECTION Checkpoint 1.1

Some modern drugs used in the treatment of diabetes, cardiovascular disorders, and other conditions have unique sources. Using an online dictionary or search engine, what are the natural sources for exenatide (Byetta), captopril (Capoten), and hyaluronic acid? What conditions are they used to treat?

Pharmacology: The Study of Medicines

1.2 Pharmacology is the study of medicines.

The word *drug* has already been used numerous times in this text. What exactly is a drug? Is everything a drug, including water, vitamin C, or perhaps a can of cola? What about substances naturally found in the body, such as estrogen or testosterone? Is it even possible to define a drug?

The definition of a drug is indeed difficult but is nevertheless important to the healthcare profession. There are many definitions, but perhaps the clearest is that a **drug** is any substance that is taken to prevent, cure, or reduce symptoms of a medical condition. Considering the substances listed earlier, which, then, are drugs? Although it may seem vague, the correct answer is "it depends."

- The caffeine consumed in a cup of coffee is not considered a drug. Yet caffeine is included in several therapies for headache pain, including Excedrin and Fioricet. For the patient trying to get pain relief, caffeine is a drug.
- Vitamin C, if ingested as part of an orange or tomato, is food. Food is not a drug. However, someone with a vitamin C deficiency may be administered vitamin C to cure scurvy. For this patient, vitamin C is then considered a drug.
- A can of cola is certainly not listed in any drug guide. However, if a patient with diabetes is experiencing a hypoglycemic reaction, the glucose in a can of soda may raise the patient's blood sugar and prevent a coma; thus, the glucose in the cola may be considered a drug in this example.
- Substances normally found in the body are not considered drugs unless they are administered to treat a condition. For example, the hormone estrogen circulating in the blood is not a drug. However, when it is taken as an oral contraceptive to prevent pregnancy, estrogen is considered a drug.

Once the meaning of the term *drug* is understood, the next essential term is *pharmacology*. The word *pharmacology* is derived from two Greek words, *pharmakon*, which means "medicine" or "drug," and *logos*, which means "study." Thus, **pharmacology** is most simply defined as the study of medicines. Pharmacology is an expansive subject, ranging from understanding how drugs are administered, to where they travel in the body, to the actual responses they produce. **Pharmacotherapy**, or pharmacotherapeutics, is the application of drugs for the purpose of disease prevention and treatment of suffering.

Drugs are a form of medical intervention given to improve a patient's condition or to prevent harm. Pharmacotherapy often begins when the patient experiences signs or symptoms that cause dissatisfaction with current or future health status. A major role of the nurse is to design interventions that meet the desired health goals of the patient. Pharmacotherapy is a critical intervention for many conditions. The rationale for pharmacotherapy is illustrated in Figure 1.1.

Over 20,000 prescription drugs and combination products are available for pharmacotherapy (U.S. Food and Drug Administration [FDA], 2019) and 40–50 new drugs are approved each year. Each has its own characteristic set of therapeutic applications, interactions, and adverse effects. Many drugs are prescribed for more than one disease and most produce multiple effects on the body. Further complicating the study of pharmacology is the fact that drugs may elicit different responses depending on individual patient factors such as age, gender, race, body mass, health status, and genetics. Indeed, learning the applications of existing medications and staying current with newly approved drugs can be an enormous challenge for the nurse. The task, however, is a critical one for both the patient and the healthcare provider. When applied properly, medications can dramatically improve patients' quality of life. If applied improperly, the consequences of drug action can cause permanent disability and even death.

There are important exceptions to the drug definition mentioned earlier. What about crack cocaine, ecstasy, LSD, or the fumes in glues and paint thinners? These are certainly drugs, but they are not taken "to prevent, cure, or reduce

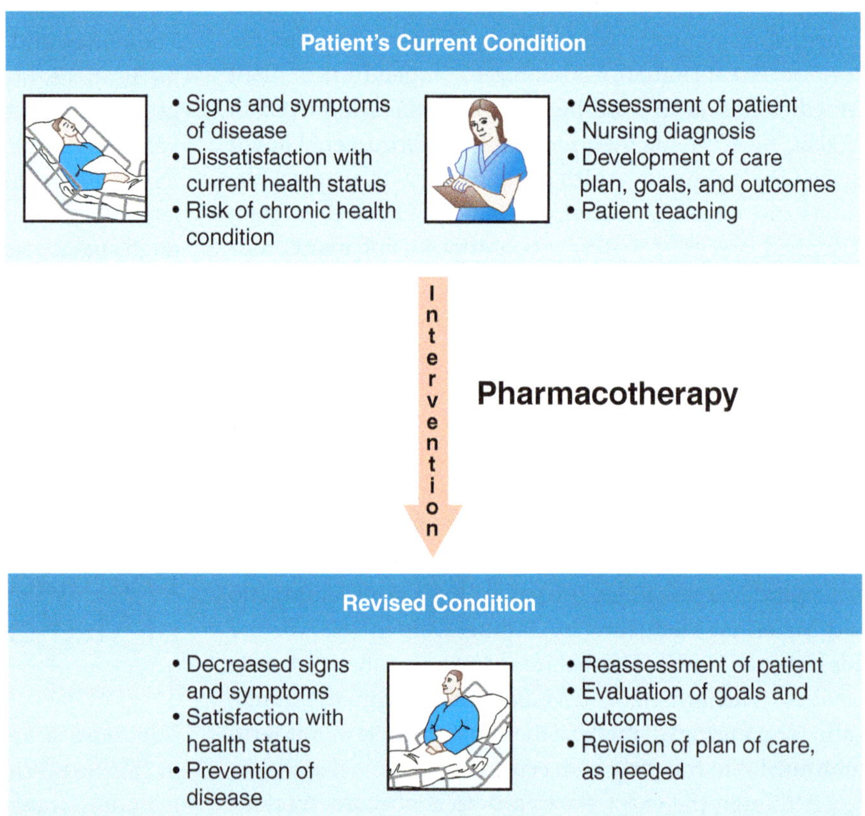

Figure 1.1 Rationale for pharmacotherapy: A partnership between the patient and the healthcare provider.

Based Centers for Disease Control and Prevention. (2016). Prescription opioid overdose data. Retrieved from http://www.cdc.gov/drugoverdose/data/overdose.html.

symptoms of a medical condition." In fact, they are taken to produce a biologic effect viewed as desirable or pleasurable by the user (see Chapter 27). Other exceptions to this definition of the term *drug* will become apparent as the student studies pharmacology.

Characteristics of an Ideal Drug

1.3 The perfect drug is safe and effective.

As they begin their journey in mastering pharmacology, nursing students should start with a notion of the ideal or "perfect drug." Learning the characteristics of an ideal drug gives a basis for comparison to "real drugs." It is always the goal of pharmacotherapy to select the perfect or ideal drug for the patient. Just what is a perfect drug? It is one that:

- Effectively treats, prevents, or cures the patient's condition.
- Produces a rapid, predictable response at relatively low doses.
- Produces no adverse effects.
- Can be taken conveniently, usually by mouth.
- Can be taken infrequently, usually once a day, and for a short length of time.
- Is inexpensive and easily accessible.
- Is quickly eliminated by the body after it produces its beneficial effect.
- Does not interact with other medications or food.

After reading this description, it should appear clear to the student that there is really no such thing as a perfect drug. Some drugs meet most of the criteria, whereas others meet very few. At the very least, all prescription medications are expected to have some degree of effectiveness at treating or preventing a health condition. The conditions for which a drug is approved are its **indications**. Every medication has at least one indication, and most have multiple indications. Some drugs are used for conditions for which they have not been approved; these are called *unlabeled* or *off-label indications*.

As a general rule, the more a medicine strays from the perfect drug profile, the less commonly it is used. This is because whenever possible, healthcare providers strive to prescribe the most effective, safest, and most convenient medication for the patient. In the home care setting, drugs that cause annoying adverse effects, have inconvenient dosing schedules, or are expensive are often not taken by patients, potentially worsening their condition and causing failure of treatment outcomes. Of course, some essential drugs do produce serious adverse effects or must be given by invasive routes, such as intravenously. In these cases, the drug is either administered in a clinical setting by a nurse or the patient receives careful instructions and regular monitoring on an outpatient basis.

CONNECTIONS: Patient Safety

Preventing Interactions

A patient has tried to manage symptoms of depression naturally with St. John's wort, an herbal over-the-counter product, without any improvement in symptoms. After over 6 months on St. John's wort he decided to talk to his primary care family nurse practitioner (FNP) about his options. After a thorough assessment, the FNP gives him a prescription for the antidepressant paroxetine (Paxil). It is important for the patient to be educated on any possible interactions. What will this patient need to know about St. John's wort and paroxetine to ensure safe and effective medication therapy? (Refer to this textbook or a drug reference guide for information about paroxetine and potential interactions.)

Classification of Drugs

1.4 Drugs may be organized by their therapeutic classification or pharmacologic classification.

The U.S. Food and Drug Administration (2020a) document *Approved Drug Products with Therapeutic Equivalence Evaluations*, informally called the "Orange Book," lists over 11,000 drugs. With the vast number of drugs available, it is essential that methods be used to group similar agents to aid in their study and understanding. The two basic classifications of drugs are therapeutic and pharmacologic. Both categories are widely used in classifying prescription and nonprescription drugs. The key difference is that the **therapeutic classification** describes what is being treated by the drug, whereas the **pharmacologic classification** describes how the drug acts.

Drugs are placed into therapeutic classes based on their usefulness in treating a specific disease. Table 1.1 shows the method of therapeutic classification, using cardiovascular drugs as an example. Many different types of drugs affect cardiovascular function. Some drugs influence blood coagulation, whereas others lower cholesterol levels or prevent the onset of stroke. Drugs may be used to treat hypertension, heart failure, abnormal cardiac rhythm, chest pain, myocardial infarction (MI), or circulatory shock. Thus,

Table 1.1 Organizing Drug Information by Therapeutic Classification

THERAPEUTIC FOCUS: DRUGS AFFECTING CARDIOVASCULAR DISEASE

Therapeutic Usefulness	Therapeutic Classification
Influence blood clotting	Anticoagulants
Lower blood cholesterol	Antihyperlipidemics
Lower blood pressure	Antihypertensives
Restore normal cardiac rhythm	Antidysrhythmics
Treat angina	Antianginals

drugs that treat cardiovascular disorders may be placed in several therapeutic classes, for example, anticoagulants, antihyperlipidemics, and antihypertensives. The key to therapeutic classification is to simply state what condition is being treated by the particular drug. Other examples of therapeutic classifications include antidepressants, antipsychotics, drugs for erectile dysfunction, and antineoplastics. Notice how the prefix *anti-* often refers to a therapeutic classification.

The pharmacologic classification addresses a drug's mechanism of action or how a drug produces its effect in the body. Table 1.2 illustrates the use of pharmacologic classification, using hypertension as an example. A diuretic treats hypertension by lowering plasma volume. Calcium channel blockers treat this disorder by decreasing the force of cardiac contractions. Other drugs block components of the renin-angiotensin system. Notice that each example describes how hypertension might be controlled. A drug's pharmacologic classification is more specific than its therapeutic classification and requires an understanding of biochemistry and physiology. Pharmacologic classifications may use a drug's chemical name.

Although classifications help to organize drugs, the process is by no means easy or standardized. Most drugs have multiple classifications. For example, the drug epinephrine is classified as a vasoconstrictor, an autonomic nervous system agent, an adrenergic agonist, a sympathomimetic, a bronchodilator, an agent for anaphylaxis, an ocular mydriatic, an antiglaucoma agent, a catecholamine, and a topical hemostatic. This is clearly a mix of therapeutic (e.g., antiglaucoma) and pharmacologic (e.g., catecholamine) classifications. Which one(s) should the student remember? Unfortunately for nursing students, the answer is all of them. The classification chosen primarily depends on the specific clinical use of the drug (What condition is being treated?). Sometimes the classification of choice is simply a preference of the healthcare provider. Although challenging, remembering the different classifications will pay dividends as the student's pharmacology course progresses.

Table 1.2 Organizing Drug Information by Pharmacologic Classification

FOCUS ON HOW A DRUG WORKS: PHARMACOTHERAPY OF HYPERTENSION

Mechanism of Action	Pharmacologic Classification
Lowers plasma volume	Diuretic
Blocks heart calcium channels	Calcium channel blocker
Blocks hormonal activity	Angiotensin-converting enzyme inhibitor
Blocks physiologic reactions to stress	Adrenergic antagonist (or blocker)
Dilates peripheral blood vessels	Vasodilator

CONNECTION Checkpoint 1.2

State whether each of the following classifications for aspirin is therapeutic or pharmacologic: anticoagulant, salicylate, central nervous system agent, analgesic, antipyretic. Use a drug guide, if needed.

Prototype Drugs

1.5 A prototype drug is the agent to which all other medications in a class are compared.

As discussed in the previous section, learning thousands of drugs is simplified, at least somewhat, by grouping similar drugs together into broad classifications. Just knowing its therapeutic or pharmacologic classification can reveal important information about a drug. For example, simply knowing whether a drug is used to treat cancer or epilepsy tells you something important about the medication.

An additional strategy is helpful when learning pharmacology. One common and useful practice is to select a single drug from a class and compare all other medications in the class to this representative medication. This is called a **prototype drug**. By learning about the prototype drug in depth, the actions and adverse effects of other drugs in the same class can be predicted. For example, by learning the actions and effects of penicillin V, students can extend this knowledge to all other drugs in the penicillin class of antibiotics. In this textbook, the drug prototypes are clearly identified, and detailed information regarding their therapeutic effects, mechanism of action, adverse effects, contraindications, precautions, and nursing responsibilities, including patient and family education, is presented.

Selecting a drug to serve as the prototype for a class is not always a simple matter; healthcare providers and textbooks sometimes disagree. The traditional prototype approach uses the oldest and best understood drug in the class. For example, atropine has been used for thousands of years and still remains a prototype drug for certain indications (see Figure 1.2). Sometimes, however, newer drugs are

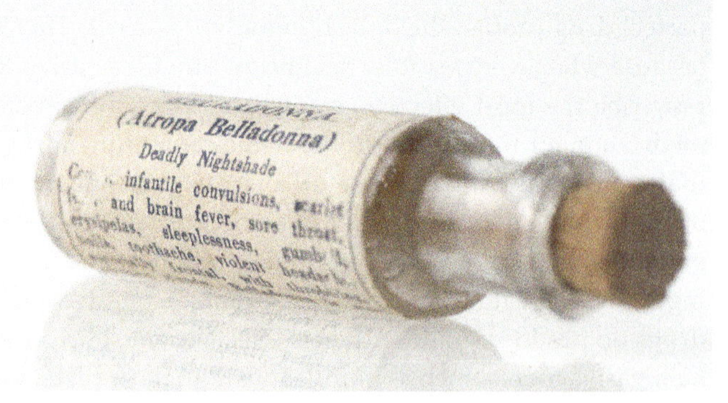

Figure 1.2 Obtained from the deadly nightshade plant *Atropa belladonna*, atropine remains a traditional prototype drug.
Heike Falkenberg/Fotolia.

developed in the same class that are more effective or have a more favorable safety profile. Over time, an older prototype drug may be infrequently prescribed and a different, more clinically useful prototype may be chosen for the class. This textbook uses a practical approach to prototype drugs, selecting a combination of traditional drugs and those most widely used. Regardless of the approach, the student must remember that the prototype is the drug to which all others in a class are compared.

Naming Drugs

1.6 Drugs have chemical, generic, and trade names.

Despite the utility of using drug classes and prototypes when studying pharmacology, learning thousands of drug names remains a challenge. Adding to this difficulty is that most drugs have multiple names. The three basic types of drug names are chemical, generic, and trade names.

Chemical names are assigned using standard nomenclature established by the International Union of Pure and Applied Chemistry (IUPAC). A drug has only one chemical name. This chemical name is sometimes helpful in predicting a drug's physical and chemical properties. Although chemical names convey a clear and concise meaning about the nature of a drug to the chemist, these names are often complicated and difficult to remember or pronounce. For example, it is unlikely that the nurse would remember that the chemical name for alprazolam (Xanax) is 8-chloro-1-methyl-6-phenyl-4H-s-triazolo[4,3-α][1,4]-benzodiazepine. In only a few cases, usually when the name is brief and easily remembered, will nurses use chemical names. Examples of easy-to-remember chemical names of common drugs include lithium carbonate, calcium gluconate, and sodium chloride.

Drugs are sometimes named and classified by a *portion* of their chemical structure, known as the chemical group name. In the Xanax example, a portion of the chemical name, benzodiazepine, is used as a drug class. Other examples include the fluoroquinolones, aminoglycosides, phenothiazines, and thiazides. Although these names may seem complicated when first encountered, knowledge of chemical group names will become invaluable as the nursing student begins to learn and understand the actions of the drugs in the major drug classes.

The **generic name** of a drug is assigned by the United States Adopted Names Council. With few exceptions, generic names are less complicated and easier to remember than chemical names. Many organizations, including the FDA, the United States Pharmacopeial Convention, and the World Health Organization, routinely describe a medication by its generic name. Because each drug has only one generic name, healthcare providers often use this name, and students must memorize it. Fortunately, sometimes components of a generic name can help a student recognize other drugs in that same class. For example, the ending *-lol* is used in the generic name of beta-adrenergic blockers, and the ending *-statin* denotes a lipid-lowering drug.

A drug's **trade name**, sometimes called the *proprietary*, *product*, or *brand name*, is assigned by the pharmaceutical company marketing the drug. The trade name is intentionally selected to be short and easy to remember so that patients will remember it and ask for it by name. The term *proprietary* suggests ownership. Indeed, many times a manufacturer holds a legal patent on the drug.

Trade names are a challenge for students to learn because there may be dozens of products that contain the same drug. For example, if the nurse is looking for aspirin, it may be listed under many trade names, including Acuprin, Aggrenox, Anacin, Aspergum, Bayer, Bufferin, Durlaza, Ecotrin, Excedrin Migraine, Fiorinal, Lanorinal, Percodan, Salocol, Vanquish, Vazalore, and Zorprin, formulated alone or in combination with other active ingredients. Acetaminophen is an additional example of a drug that appears in multiple combination products with dozens of different trade names. Further complicating the naming of proprietary drugs is that trade names change very frequently. To avoid this confusion, generic names should be used when naming the active ingredients in a combination product. When referring to a drug, it is conventional to write the generic name in lowercase first, followed by the trade name in parentheses with the first letter capitalized. Examples include alprazolam (Xanax) and acetaminophen (Tylenol).

Drugs with two or more active generic ingredients are called **combination products**. These products are usually formulated into a single tablet, capsule, solution, prefilled syringe, or inhaler. It is more convenient for the patient to take a single combination product rather than two or more different medications separately. Combination products are especially common in over-the-counter cold remedies, antihypertensives, vaccines, and therapies for HIV infection.

1.7 Generic drugs are less expensive than trade-name drugs, but they may differ in bioavailability.

In the United States, the pharmaceutical company marketing the medication determines the price of a medication. When a drug is newly marketed, there is no competition and the price can be very high. Once competing companies begin to market the generic equivalent drug, consumer savings may be substantial. In many states, pharmacists may routinely substitute a generic drug when the prescription calls for a trade name, a practice called **pharmacy-level substitution**. In other states, the pharmacist must dispense drugs directly as written by a healthcare provider or obtain approval before providing a generic substitute.

Are there significant differences in quality between a trade-name drug and its generic equivalent? The key to comparing trade-name drugs and their generic equivalents lies in measuring the **bioavailability** of the two agents. Bioavailability is defined by the Food, Drug, and Cosmetic Act (see Chapter 2) as the rate and extent to which the active ingredient is absorbed from a drug product and becomes available at the site of drug action to produce its effect. Bioavailability is affected by many factors, including inert ingredients and tablet compression. Anything that affects the absorption of a drug or its travel to its target cells can certainly affect drug action. Measuring how long a drug takes to exert its effect (onset time) gives pharmacologists a crude measure of bioavailability. If the trade and generic products have the same rate of absorption and have the same onset of therapeutic action, they are said to be *bioequivalent*.

The importance of bioavailability differences between a trade-name drug and its generic equivalent depends on the specific circumstances of pharmacotherapy. For example, if a patient is in circulatory shock and the generic equivalent drug takes 5 minutes longer to produce its effect, that may indeed be significant. However, if a generic medication for arthritis pain relief takes 45 minutes to act, compared to 40 minutes for the trade-name drug, it probably does not matter which drug is used, and the inexpensive product should be prescribed to provide cost savings to the consumer. As a general rule, bioavailability is of most concern when using critical-care drugs and those with a narrow safety margin. In these cases, the patient should continue taking the trade-name drug and *not* switch to a generic equivalent, unless approved by the healthcare provider. For most other drugs, the generic equivalent may be safely substituted for the trade-name drug.

In the age of internet pharmacies, the issue of marketing rights has drastically changed. Other countries are not bound by U.S. drug laws, and patients sometimes obtain medications through the mail at a fraction of the cost in the United States. For example, a pharmaceutical company may have the exclusive rights to sell Cialis in the United States, but companies in India and China are able sell the identical drug through internet pharmacies and ship it to customers in the United States. In some cases, they may sell the drug to consumers without a prescription. Some countries do not have the same high-quality manufacturing standards as the United States, and the patient may be purchasing a useless or even harmful product. Furthermore, although some internet sites may appear to be based in the United States, they may instead be obtaining their medications from sources outside the United States. Nurses must urge their patients not to purchase drugs from overseas pharmacies because there is no assurance that the drugs are safe or effective.

PharmFACT

Nine out of every 10 prescriptions dispensed in the United States are for generic drugs, and 95% of these costs $20 or less (Association for Accessible Medicines, 2020).

1.8 Biologic products are drugs produced from living cells.

Biologic products (BPs) are substances made by living cells obtained from humans, animals, plants, or microorganisms. These include a diverse range of products produced through biotechnology, gene therapy and tissue research. Because of their natural origin, BPs are often complex mixtures in which individual chemical structures cannot be easily identified or characterized. In recent years, some BPs have become cutting-edge treatments for rheumatoid arthritis, multiple sclerosis, and cancer. Although effective medications, they are usually very expensive. For example, some of the newer BPs for cancer cost thousands of dollars per dose.

Several laws have been passed in an attempt to increase the availability of biologics and lower their costs. These laws created two new categories: biosimilar BPs and interchangeable BPs.

As defined by the FDA (2020b), "A **biosimilar drug** is a biological product that is highly similar to and has no clinically meaningful differences from an existing FDA-approved reference product." The **reference product** is the original BP that underwent rigorous testing and was approved by the FDA based on a thorough evaluation of its safety and effectiveness.

Is a biosimilar drug the same thing as a generic drug? Recall that a generic drug is an identical chemical copy of the brand-name drug. Because a biosimilar is *not* an exact, duplicate copy of the original medication (reference product), it is not called a generic medication. Biosimilars are not required to undergo the same rigorous preclinical and clinical testing as their reference products; therefore, they are less expensive to bring to market. To be approved as a biosimilar, however, the manufacturer must demonstrate to the FDA that the drug differs very little from the approved reference product. The biosimilar must have the same route of administration, dosage forms, mechanism of action, and clinical indications as the reference product. The first biosimilar, Zarxio, was approved by the FDA with the same indications as filgrastim (Neupogen), the reference product. More than 26 biosimilars have since been approved, and dozens are in the approval process. The FDA gathers information on BPs in the "Purple Book." This is actually not a book at all but an online list of licensed biological products with reference products and biosimilars (FDA, 2020c).

The FDA created an additional category for BPs called **interchangeable products**. An interchangeable product is a biosimilar that has undergone a higher standard of *additional* testing. This testing must show that the interchangeable product produces the same clinical result as the reference product in any given patient. If the product is to be administered more than once, the manufacturer must show that the safety and effectiveness is not changed if the interchangeable product is switched back and forth with the reference product.

Why would a manufacturer provide additional time-consuming (and expensive) testing to the FDA so its product can be classified as an interchangeable product instead of a biosimilar? The answer lies at the pharmacy counter. Recall that in most states, when a practitioner writes a prescription for a trade-name drug, the pharmacist has the authority to substitute a generic medication. However, if a practitioner writes a prescription for a BP that is a reference product, the pharmacist *cannot* substitute a biosimilar. The pharmacist, however, *can* substitute an interchangeable product for the reference product. Of course, laws on pharmacy-level substitution differ among states and the topic of pharmacy-level substitution of biosimilars is rapidly evolving.

The naming of biological products and biosimilars is different than other drugs. When a new biosimilar is approved by the FDA, it receives a product name followed by a hyphen and a four-letter suffix. For example, adalimumab (Humira) was approved in 2002 and is a reference drug. The following are approved biosimilars:

adalimumab-atto (Amjevita) approved in 2016
adalimumab-adbm (Cyltezo) approved in 2017
adalimumab-adaz (Hyrimoz) approved in 2018
adalimumab-afzb (Abrilada) and adalimumab-bwwb (Hadlima) approved in 2019

The four-letter suffix does not denote any property of the BP; in fact, it is purposely meant to be devoid of meaning. It is assigned to track each specific biosimilar, in the event unusual adverse events occur or other differences between products appear during clinical use.

In 2019, adalimumab was the best-selling drug in the world and the retail cost for 26 injector pens (1 year's medication) was over $120,000 in the United States. Will the existence of biosimilars affect the cost of therapy with adalimumab? The answer is unknown in the United States because patent lawsuits have kept all five adalimumab biosimilars from reaching the market. The United Kingdom and Scandinavian countries, however, have experienced a 70–80% drop in cost due to biosimilar use.

Connecting Pharmacology to Clinical Nursing Practice

1.9 Effective pharmacotherapy depends on a thorough understanding of pharmacology.

Pharmacotherapy has become a mainstay of modern medical treatment, and a thorough understanding of expected drug effects, the associated monitoring required, and the care and teaching associated with drugs that are prescribed in patient care is crucial to effective practice. As a member of an interprofessional team, nurses, physicians, advanced practice nurses, pharmacists, and, most importantly, the patient work together to achieve optimal therapeutic outcomes from drug therapy. The importance of pharmacology to clinical practice cannot be overstated and will be emphasized throughout this textbook.

One major goal of this text is to provide a solid foundation in the knowledge of pharmacology and pharmacotherapeutics. Chapters 2 through 4 provide the legal and scientific bases for pharmacotherapeutics. As a member of an interprofessional healthcare team, it is most often the nurse who serves as the connection between a prescription and the patient's safe use of the prescribed drug. Monitoring the patient's condition before and during drug use, evaluating drug effects, teaching the patient about self-administration, and conducting a medication reconciliation are key nursing responsibilities. For the advanced practice nurse, an understanding of the pathophysiology underlying the patient's current condition, excellent assessment skills, and clinical decision-making skills aimed at choosing the best treatment options are required.

A major goal in studying pharmacology is to eliminate medication errors and to limit the number and severity of adverse drug events. Many adverse effects are preventable. We, as healthcare providers, can routinely avoid many serious adverse drug effects in patients by applying experience and knowledge of pharmacotherapeutics to clinical practice. Unfortunately, though, some adverse effects are simply not preventable. It is critical that the entire interprofessional team be prepared to recognize and respond to potential adverse effects of medications. The management of adverse effects and medication errors are discussed in Chapters 5 and 6, respectively.

Before any drug is administered, it is important to ask about pertinent information regarding the patient's medical history, complete a thorough physical assessment, and assess learning needs and capabilities. Growth and developmental factors must always be considered. It is important to remember that a large number of variables influence a patient's response to drugs throughout the lifespan. Having a firm understanding of these variables can increase treatment success. Chapters 8 through 11 of this textbook address these aspects of pharmacotherapy.

Knowledge of pharmacology is an ongoing, lifelong process that builds with clinical practice and chooses of specific clinical areas. Early in practice, learning prototype drugs that represent a specific classification of drugs, recognizing key similarities in generic names, and always looking up unknown or new drugs will help build this knowledge base. As experience grows, anticipating drug effects and care and teaching needs becomes integrated into practice. For an advanced practice nurse working as a nurse practitioner, this clinical experience helps to enhance the new information acquired to prepare for prescriptive authority. Chapters 12 through 75 present the foundational knowledge needed for effective pharmacotherapy. Each unit begins with a review of the anatomy and physiology underlying the mechanism of action of drugs discussed in the unit, followed by detailed information about specific classifications of drugs and nursing responsibilities for those classifications.

Despite its essential nature, the study of pharmacology should be viewed in the proper perspective. Although pharmacology is a key intervention in many cases, all healthcare providers must use all the healing sciences in treating their patients. The effectiveness of a drug in treating disease can never substitute for skilled, compassionate care. Too much reliance on drug therapy can diminish the importance of the nurse–patient relationship.

Understanding Chapter 1

Key Concepts Summary

1.1 The practice of applying products to relieve suffering has been recorded throughout history by virtually every culture.

1.2 Pharmacology is the study of medicines.

1.3 The perfect drug is safe and effective.

1.4 Drugs may be organized by their therapeutic classification or pharmacologic classification.

1.5 A prototype drug is the agent to which all other medications in a class are compared.

1.6 Drugs have chemical, generic, and trade names.

1.7 Generic drugs are less expensive than trade-name drugs, but they may differ in bioavailability.

1.8 Biologic products are drugs produced from living cells.

1.9 Effective pharmacotherapy depends on a thorough understanding of pharmacology.

CASE STUDY: Making the Patient Connection

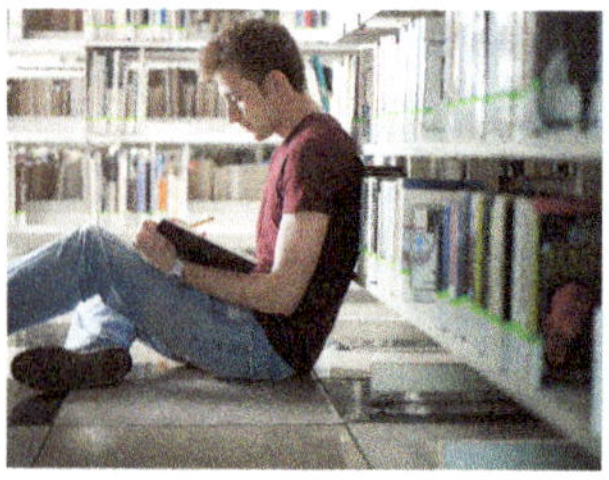

Remember the student "Josh Remming" at the beginning of the chapter? Now read the remainder of the case study. Based on the information presented within this chapter, respond to the critical thinking questions that follow.

Josh Remming, a 23-year-old student, is in his first semester of nursing school. He thought that nursing would provide him with a great career and lots of opportunity. He enjoys helping people and has always been fascinated with healthcare. However, after the first pharmacology class, Josh is worried because there seems to be an overwhelming amount of content to learn in just one semester.

At the end of the class, Josh talks with other students who are concerned and a bit anxious. Much of the conversation centers around lecture content provided by the professor. Following are some of the questions from Josh's classmates. How would you respond?

Critical Thinking Questions

1. What is the difference between therapeutic classification and pharmacologic classification?
2. What classification is a barbiturate? Macrolide? Birth control pills? Laxatives? Folic acid antagonist? Antianginal agent?
3. What is a prototype drug, and what advantages does a prototype approach to studying pharmacology offer?
4. Why do nurses need to know all this pharmacology?

Additional Case Study

Sarah Hawkins, an older woman who lives on a fixed income, is on multiple medications. She says that all her friends are taking the generic form of their medications. During her appointment, she asks, "What do you think of generic medicines? Are they safe? Are they as good? Are they worth it?"

1. How do generic equivalent drugs differ from a proprietary (trade-name) drug?
2. What would you recommend that Sarah do about accepting generic drugs?

Chapter Review

1. While using a drug handbook to determine the indications for the drug furosemide (Lasix). The term *indications* is defined as the:
    1. Way a drug works on the target organs.
    2. Amount of the drug to be administered.
    3. Conditions for which a drug is approved.
    4. Reason that the drug should not be given.

2. In reviewing the patient's medication record, the nurse does not recognize the medication, filgrastim-sndz (Zarxio). Consulting a drug guide, it is listed as a "biosimilar" to filgrastim (Neupogen). Which of the following best describes the definition of a biosimilar drug?
    1. It is another term for a "generic" drug when the two drugs exert similar biologic effects.
    2. It is a drug that has similar effects on the body but belongs in a different chemical and therapeutic classification.
    3. It is a drug that is derived from living cells, such as yeast, and has comparable effectiveness and safety to the reference product drug.
    4. It is a drug that is identical to the reference product drug and thus does not require FDA approval.

3. As a member of an interprofessional team, what key responsibilities does the nurse have to ensure effective pharmacotherapy? (Select all that apply.)
    1. Monitoring the patient's condition before and during pharmacotherapy
    2. Teaching the patient about self-administration and any required monitoring of drug effects
    3. Ensuring that all drug and treatment options have been considered before beginning pharmacotherapy
    4. Frequently conducting a medication reconciliation to verify current medications in use
    5. Determining the ideal drug to be prescribed to the patient to treat the current condition

4. Which patient characteristics, if noted in the patient's medical record, should you consider important information that may affect the physiologic response to various types of drug therapy? (Select all that apply.)
    1. 82-year-old and female
    2. Asian and obese
    3. Past medical history of kidney disease
    4. Mother and sister with diabetes
    5. Has no medical insurance

5. Which of the following would indicate a therapeutic classification?
    1. Beta-adrenergic antagonist
    2. Antihypertensive
    3. Diuretic
    4. Calcium channel blocker

6. Why would a manufacturer provide additional time-consuming (and expensive) testing to the FDA so its product could be classified as an interchangeable product instead of a biosimilar?
    1. So the pharmacist could substitute a generic medication.
    2. So that the pharmacist could substitute a biosimilar product for the reference product.
    3. Because federal laws dictate a pharmacy-level substitution for a biosimilar.
    4. Biosimilars are exact, duplicate copies of the original medication and therefore are interchangeable, so additional testing wouldn't be needed.

See Appendix A for answers to critical thinking questions, case study questions and review questions.

References

Association of Accessible Medicines. (2020). *Generic drug savings in the U.S.* https://accessiblemeds.org/resources/fact-sheets/generic-drug-savings-us

IQVIA Institute. (2019). *Medicine use and spending in the US.* https://www.iqvia.com/insights/the-iqvia-institute/reports/medicine-use-and-spending-in-the-us-a-review-of-2018-and-outlook-to-2023

U.S. Food and Drug Administration. (2019). *Fact sheet: FDA at a glance.* https://www.fda.gov/about-fda/fda-basics/fact-sheet-fda-glance

U.S. Food and Drug Administration. (2020a). *Approved drug products with therapeutic equivalence evaluations (Orange book).* http://www.fda.gov/Drugs/InformationOnDrugs/ucm129662.htm

U.S. Food and Drug Administration. (2020b). *Biological product definitions.* https://www.fda.gov/media/108557/download

U.S. Food and Drug Administration. (2020c). *Purple Book: Lists of licensed biological products with reference product exclusivity and biosimilarity or interchangeability evaluations.* https://www.fda.gov/drugs/therapeutic-biologics-applications-bla/purple-book-lists-licensed-biological-products-reference-product-exclusivity-and-biosimilarity-or

Selected Bibliography

Barbier, L., Ebbers, H., Declerck, P., Simoens, S., Vulto, A. G., & Huys, I. (2020). The efficacy, safety and immunogenicity of switching between reference biopharmaceuticals and biosimilars: a systematic review. *Clinical Pharmacology & Therapeutics.* https://doi.org/10.1002/cpt.1836

Batta, A., Kalra, B. S., & Khirasaria, R. (2020). Trends in FDA drug approvals over last 2 decades: An observational study. *Journal of Family Medicine and Primary Care, 9*(1), 105–114. https://doi.org/10.4103/jfmpc.jfmpc_578_19

Chazin, H., Woo, J., Han, J., Grosser, S., & Luan, J. (2019). FDA's generic drug program: Decreasing time to approval and number of review cycles. *Therapeutic Innovation & Regulatory Science, 54*, 758–763.

Gámez-Belmonte, R., Hernández-Chirlaque, C., Arredondo-Amador, M., Aranda, C. J., González, R., Martínez-Augustin, O., & de Medina, F. S. (2018). Biosimilars: Concepts and controversies. *Pharmacological Research, 133*, 251–264. https://doi.org/10.1016/j.phrs.2018.01.024

Gupta, R., Shah, N. D., & Ross, J. S. (2019). Generic drugs in the United States: Policies to address pricing and competition. *Clinical Pharmacology & Therapeutics, 105*(2), 329–337. https://doi.org/10.1002/cpt.1314

Lau, D. T. (2019). Is prescribing by PAs and NPs comparable to physician prescribing? *Journal of the American Academy of Physician Assistants, 32*(2), 52.

U.S. Food and Drug Administration. (2018). *Facts about generic drugs.* https://www.fda.gov/drugs/generic-drugs/generic-drug-facts

U.S. Food and Drug Administration. (2020). *Frequently asked questions on patents and exclusivity.* https://www.fda.gov/drugs/development-approval-process-drugs/frequently-asked-questions-patents-and-exclusivity

VandeWaa, E. A., & Dolan, C. (2020). Mindful prescribing: Drug development, drug selection, and advanced nursing practice. *Journal for Nurse Practitioners, 16*(3), 186–190. https://doi.org/10.1016/j.nurpra.2019.12.014

"This headache medicine I bought at the grocery store must be safe because I didn't need a prescription."
—*Patient "Gertrude Stone"*

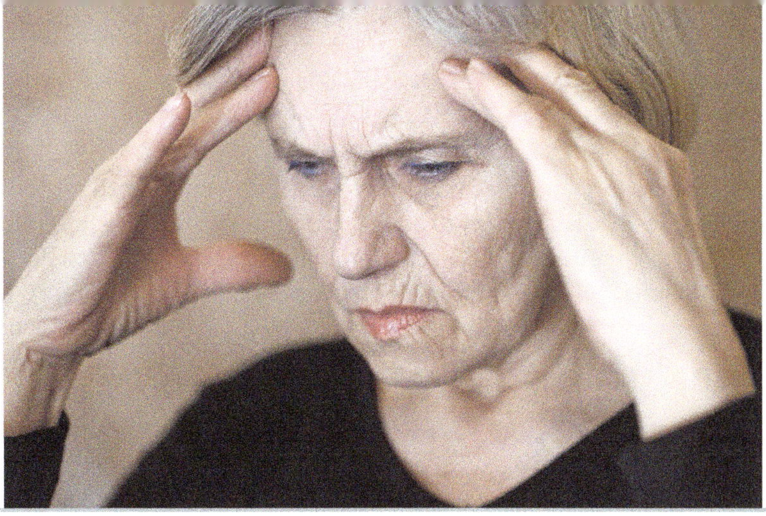

Chapter 2
Drug Regulations

Chapter Outline

- Patent Medicines
- Brief History of Drug Legislation
- Drug Standards
- The U.S. Food and Drug Administration
- Drug Approval
- Changes to the Drug Approval Process
- Prescription and Over-the-Counter Drugs
- Drug Schedules
- Prescriptive Authority for Nurses

Learning Outcomes

After reading this chapter, the student should be able to:

1. Explain the role of patent medicines in the history of pharmacology and the legislation of drugs.
2. Outline the key U.S. drug regulations and explain how each has contributed to the safety and effectiveness of medications.
3. Describe how the *United States Pharmacopeia-National Formulary* (USP-NF) controls drug purity and standards.
4. Evaluate the role of the U.S. Food and Drug Administration in the drug approval process.
5. Categorize the four stages of new drug approval.
6. Explain the role of a placebo in new drug testing.
7. Discuss how changes to the approval process have increased the speed at which new drugs reach consumers.
8. Compare and contrast prescription and over-the-counter drugs.
9. Explain how scheduled drugs are classified and regulated.
10. Explain how advanced practice nurses are helping to fill the primary care workforce gap.

Key Terms

Definitions of the terms in bold may be found in the Glossary.

Laws govern all aspects of the drug approval, labeling, marketing, manufacturing, and distribution process. The primary purpose of this legislation is to protect the public from unsafe and ineffective products. This chapter examines standards and legislation regulating drugs in the United States.

Patent Medicines

2.1 Early American history saw the rise of patent medicines and the lack of adequate drug regulations.

People have an expectation that the medication they are taking is effective at treating their condition, whether it is asthma, diabetes, or a headache. They expect the label to contain clear and accurate instructions on how the product should be taken. They expect that the drug will be safe when the instructions are correctly followed. Are these reasonable assumptions? In the United States and Canada, the answer is yes. But Americans have not always had this reassurance. Although drugs have been used for thousands of years, it was not until the 20th century that extensive standards and regulations were developed to protect the public from unsafe and ineffective products.

In early America, there were few attempts to regulate drugs. This period saw the rise of **patent medicines**. Although the term *patent* implies a legal right to manufacture or sell a drug, this was not the case. Patent medicines contained a trade name that clearly identified the product, such as William Radam's Microbe Killer, Stanley's Snake Oil, Dr. Kilmer's Swamp Root, or Dr. Moore's Indian Root Pills. Because there were no laws to the contrary, these products went untested and could claim to cure nearly any symptom or disease. Dr. William's Pink Pills for Pale People, which contained iron oxide and magnesium sulfate, claimed to cure rheumatism, nervous headache, palpitations, grippe, neuralgia, locomotor ataxia, partial paralysis, sallow complexion, and all forms of weakness in men or women. A typical advertisement from this era is shown in Figure 2.1.

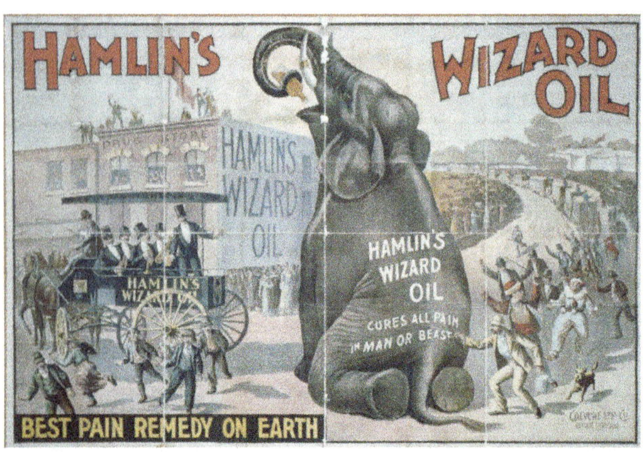

Figure 2.1 Patent medicines contained a trade name that clearly identified the product and claimed to cure just about any symptom or disease.

Library of Congress Prints and Photographs Division Washington [LC-USZC4-1032].

Patent medicines were often harmless (and ineffective), containing coloring, flavoring, and an aromatic substance that "smelled like medicine." At their worst, some contained hazardous levels of dangerous or addictive substances. In fact, cocaine, heroin, and morphine were freely distributed in patent medicines; some elixirs contained up to 50% morphine, which indeed caused many painful disorders to "disappear." Addictive ingredients were purposely added to guarantee repeat customers for their products. (Note the similarity with nicotine added to tobacco and caffeine added to soft drinks.) In the late 1800s, the familiar Coca-Cola soft drink was a patented beverage that contained an estimated 9 mg of cocaine per serving and was claimed to cure headache, dyspepsia, hysteria, morphine addiction, and impotence. The need for stricter regulation became more apparent in the 1860s as cocaine was synthesized, and the use of opiates as painkillers during the Civil War caused thousands of soldiers to become addicted.

Although the marketing and use of patent medicines may seem humorous and even unbelievable to modern consumers, a few of these products are still available over the counter (OTC). Examples of patent medicines that survived the drug regulations of the 1900s include Smith Brothers Throat Drops, Fletcher's Castoria, Doan's Pills, Vick's VapoRub, and Phillip's Milk of Magnesia. Of course, the ingredients of these products have changed over time so that they conform to modern regulations regarding labeling, safety, and effectiveness.

Brief History of Drug Legislation

2.2 In the 1900s, drug legislation was enacted to make drugs safer and more effective.

Although individual states attempted to regulate drugs, the first national law was the Drug Importation Act, passed in 1848, which attempted to stop the entry of unsafe drugs into the United States. In the early 1900s, the United States began to develop and enforce tougher drug legislation to protect the public. This was spurred, in part, by the tragic deaths of 13 children in St. Louis in 1901 who were given diphtheria antitoxin that was contaminated with tetanus. In 1902, the Biologics Control Act was passed to standardize the quality of sera, antitoxins, and other blood-related products. Passed shortly thereafter, the Pure Food and Drug Act (PFDA) of 1906 was a significant and powerful piece of drug legislation that gave the government authority to regulate the labeling of medicines. Essentially, this law required that drug labels accurately reflect the contents. Prior to this date, many labels did not contain any indication of the active ingredient within the bottle or its amount. Although the ingredients had to be accurately labeled, a drug could still be marketed for any disease.

In 1912, the Sherley Amendment to the PFDA prohibited the sale of drugs labeled with false therapeutic claims that were intended to defraud the consumer. A major weakness, as borne out in subsequent legal battles, was the difficulty of proving that the false claim made by the seller was intentional.

It is surprising that up to this point in American history no attempt had been made to legislate the use of addictive drugs. The Harrison Narcotic Act of 1914 was passed to require prescriptions for high doses of narcotic drugs and to mandate that pharmacists and healthcare providers keep narcotic records. Since 1914, hundreds of additional state and federal laws have been passed to regulate drugs with abuse potential, including the landmark Comprehensive Drug Abuse Prevention and Control Act (see Section 2.8). Additional details on the history of the regulation of controlled substances are included in Chapter 27.

Unfortunately, two essential components were still missing from the regulation of drugs in the early 20th century. Although the PFDA and other legislation required that ingredients be listed on the label and prohibited intentional false claims, manufacturers did not have to prove that the drug was effective. Furthermore, product safety did not have to be tested before the drug was marketed. Bringing the issue to the forefront was an incident in 1937 in which an elixir of sulfanilamide containing a poisonous chemical (diethylene glycol) killed 107 people, mostly children.

In 1938, Congress passed the landmark Food, Drug, and Cosmetic Act (FDCA), which corrected certain loopholes in previous laws. This was the first law preventing the sale of newly developed drugs that had not been thoroughly tested for safety. Drug labels were required to contain instructions for safe use. The FDCA was also the first attempt at regulating cosmetics and medical devices. Unfortunately, the FDCA did not clearly define "prescription" or specify which drugs required a prescription. Most drugs, including many addictive and harmful substances, were sold by the corner druggist, sometimes legally, other times illegally. In 1951, the Durham-Humphrey Amendment to the FDCA delineated the difference between safer drugs, which were allowed to be sold OTC, and more dangerous drugs, which required prescriptions.

In the late 1950s, the drug thalidomide was found to produce severe birth defects in the children of women taking the drug as a sleeping pill and to treat morning sickness during pregnancy. Although the drug was not approved in the United States, it is estimated that over 20,000 Americans received the drug because it was widely distributed to healthcare providers without U.S. Food and Drug Administration (FDA) approval. As with other drug legislation, it took a tragedy to convince Congress to pass tougher regulations. Passage of the Kefauver-Harris Amendment to the FDCA in 1962 mandated that manufacturers prove their drugs were effective for specific purposes, as well as safe, through the conduct of "adequate and well-controlled" studies. This law was applied retroactively to all drugs introduced since the passage of the FDCA. This amendment also required that all significant adverse reactions be reported to the FDA and that complete information about adverse effects be included in literature distributed to healthcare providers. For the first time, informed consent was required from patients participating in experimental drug research.

The emphasis on effectiveness continued as the FDA contracted with the National Academy of Sciences and the National Research Council in 1966 to evaluate the effectiveness of 4000 drugs that were approved between 1938 and 1962 based only on their safety. Approximately 40% of all drugs introduced between 1938 and 1962 were found to be ineffective and were subsequently removed from the market. In 1972, a review of OTC drugs began to examine the safety and effectiveness of these products.

In the 1980s, the public placed considerable political pressure on the FDA to find drugs to treat rare or unusual disorders. Pharmaceutical companies were reluctant to develop drugs for these disorders because there would not be enough sales to recoup their research and development costs. To encourage development of such drugs, the Orphan Drug Act became law in 1983. An **orphan product** is a drug or biologic for treating rare diseases that affect fewer than 200,000 people in the United States. Drug manufacturers are now offered development grants, tax credits for clinical investigation expenses, and 7 years of exclusive marketing for an orphan drug. Over 600 medications have been approved as orphan drugs since the passage of this act (Pharmaceutical Processing World, 2019).

A major focus in the 1990s was to speed the drug approval process, which was often prolonged for many years. The Prescription Drug User Fee Act (PDUFA) of 1992 assessed fees from drug manufacturers to be used specifically for reducing the review time for new drug applications. The PDUFA was reauthorized in 1997 with the passage of the Food and Drug Administration Modernization Act, which also included provisions to accelerate the review of medical devices, regulate the advertising of unapproved uses of drugs, and regulate health claims for foods. The PDUFA has been reauthorized every 5 years. It is estimated that PDUFA fees collected in 2020 will amount to over $2.6 billion, accounting for approximately 40% of the total FDA budget (Congressional Research Service, 2020).

In reaction to the rising popularity of dietary supplements, Congress passed the Dietary Supplement Health and Education Act of 1994 to control misleading industry claims. Due in part to intense lobbying from the dietary supplement industry, the regulation of these products remains less stringent than that for prescription or OTC drugs. The regulation of herbal products and dietary supplements is discussed in detail in Chapter 7.

In early 2000, the focus of drug regulation turned to access. Advocacy groups claimed that the high cost of drugs caused unequal access to adequate healthcare for the poor, the uninsured, the underinsured, and older adults. In 2003, the Medicare Prescription Drug, Improvement, and Modernization Act (also called the Medicare Modernization

Table 2.1 Historical Timeline of Regulatory Acts, Standards, and Organizations

Year	Regulatory Acts, Standards, and Organizations
1820	Physicians establish the first comprehensive publication of drug standards, the *United States Pharmacopeia (USP)*.
1848	The Drug Importation Act requires that all drugs (as defined by the newly established pharmacopeia) entering the United States be inspected and analyzed for "quality, purity, and fitness for medical purposes."
1852	Pharmacists found the American Pharmaceutical Association (APhA). The APhA establishes the *National Formulary (NF)*, a standardized publication focusing on pharmaceutical ingredients. The USP continues to catalog all drug-related substances and products.
1862	The Federal Bureau of Chemistry, established under the administration of President Lincoln, eventually becomes the U.S. Food and Drug Administration (FDA).
1902	The Biologics Control Act controls the quality of sera and other blood-related products.
1906	The Pure Food and Drug Act prohibits the manufacture and sale of adulterated or misbranded foods, drugs, and medications.
1912	The Sherley Amendment makes medicines safer by prohibiting the sale of drugs labeled with false therapeutic claims.
1914	The Harrison Narcotics Act requires those who dispense opium, cocaine, and related substances to keep records of the drugs they dispense and makes it illegal to possess narcotics without a prescription. This act allows physicians to prescribe narcotics only for treatment, not to addicts.
1938	The Food, Drug, and Cosmetic Act is the first law preventing the marketing of drugs not thoroughly tested.
1970	The Comprehensive Drug Abuse Prevention and Control Act (also known as the Controlled Substances Act) organizes regulated drugs (including opiates, cocaine, cannabis, stimulants, depressants, and hallucinogens) into five schedules and imposes restrictions and penalties.
1975	The *United States Pharmacopeia* and *National Formulary* become a single standardized publication, the USP-NF.
1986	The Anti-Drug Abuse Act increases sentences and imposes mandatory minimum sentences for those convicted of illegal drug activity based on the type and quantity of drug involved.
1986	The Childhood Vaccine Act authorizes the FDA to acquire information about patients taking vaccines, to recall biologics, and to recommend civil penalties if guidelines regarding biologic use were not followed.
1988	The FDA is officially established as an agency of the U.S. Department of Health and Human Services.
1992	The Prescription Drug User Fee Act requires that nongeneric drug and biologic manufacturers pay fees to be used for improvements in the drug review process.
1994	The Dietary Supplement Health and Education Act requires clear labeling of dietary supplements and gives the FDA the power to remove supplements that cause a significant public risk.
1997	The FDA Modernization Act reauthorizes the Prescription Drug User Fee Act, representing the largest reform effort of the drug review process since 1938.
2002	The Best Pharmaceuticals for Children Act improves the safety and efficacy of medicines for children and continues the exclusivity provisions for pediatric drugs as mandated under the Food and Drug Administration Modernization Act of 1997.
2003	The Medicare Prescription Drug, Improvement, and Modernization Act provides older adults and those with disabilities a prescription drug benefit and better benefits under Medicare.
2007	The FDA Amendments Act (FDAAA) of 2007 reauthorizes and expands the Prescription Drug User Fee Act, the Modernization Act, the Best Pharmaceuticals for Children Act, and the Pediatric Research Equity Act.
2009	The Biologics Competition and Innovation Act of 2009 creates an abbreviated approval pathway for biosimilars and interchangeables
2012	The FDA Safety and Innovation Act (FDASIA) of 2012 reauthorizes the Prescription Drug User Fee Act. This requires the FDA to implement a structured benefit–risk framework in the new drug approval process.
2020	Over-the Counter Monograph Safety, Innovation and Reform Act of 2020 streamlines the process for approval of OTC medications

Act) was passed. This Act created a new prescription drug benefit (called Medicare Part D) for seniors and younger people with disabilities. A brief timeline of major events in U.S. drug regulation is shown in Table 2.1.

Drug Standards

2.3 The standardization of drug purity and strength is specified by the *United States Pharmacopeia-National Formulary.*

Until the 1800s, drugs were prepared from plants that were available in the natural environment. The strength and purity of the products varied considerably because they were entirely dependent on the experience (and integrity) of the druggist preparing the product and the quality of the local ingredients. Potency and safety varied from region to region and, indeed, from batch to batch. Consider the simple analogy of baking. If 100 people across the world were asked to bake a loaf of bread, the final products would vary considerably in size, taste, and nutritional value. It is likely that no two loaves would be the same. It is obvious that a standard recipe must be followed. Similarly, to obtain consistency in the preparation and potency of drugs, standards (recipes) are needed.

Among the first standards used by pharmacists was the **formulary**, or list of pharmaceutical products and drug recipes. In the United States, the first comprehensive publication of drug standards, the *United States Pharmacopeia (USP)*, was established in 1820. A **pharmacopeia** is a medical reference summarizing standards of drug purity, strength, and directions for synthesis. From 1852 until 1975, two major

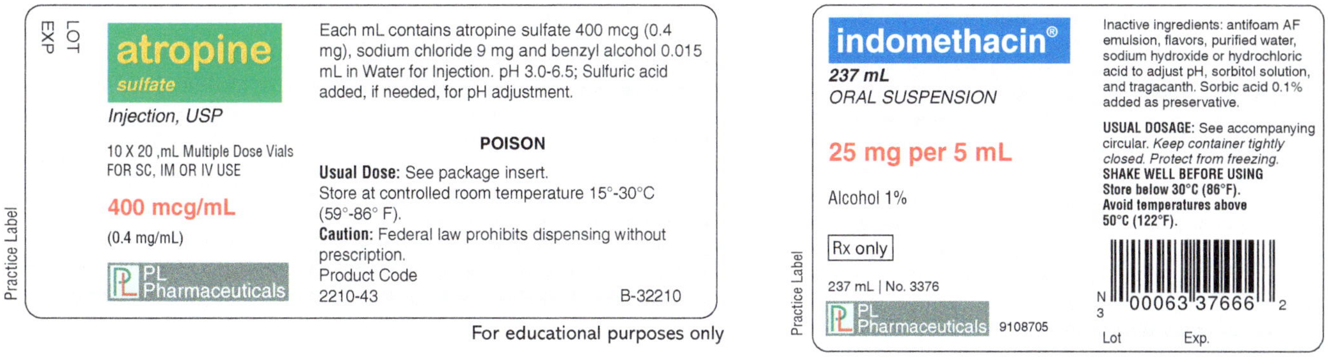

Figure 2.2 Medication with the USP label (left) and without the USP label (right). Practice labels "for educational purposes only."

compendia maintained drug standards in the United States, the USP and the *National Formulary (NF)*. All drug products were covered in the USP, whereas the NF focused on non-drug ingredients. In 1975, the two were merged into a single publication named the *United States Pharmacopeia–National Formulary (USP-NF)*. Recent versions have contained more than 300 chapters and 4900 drug monographs. The USP-NF is published annually. Today, the USP label can be found on many medications verifying the purity and exact amounts of ingredients found within the container. Drugs marketed in the United States must conform to USP-NF standards to avoid possible charges of adulteration and misbranding. Sample labels are illustrated in Figure 2.2. The USP also provides a voluntary program for verifying the label accuracy of dietary supplements (see Chapter 7).

The U.S. Food and Drug Administration

2.4 The regulatory agency responsible for ensuring that drugs and medical devices are safe and effective is the U.S. Food and Drug Administration.

The establishment of a regulatory agency for food and drugs in the United States began with a single chemist appointed by President Abraham Lincoln in 1862. The **U.S. Food and Drug Administration (FDA)** was established by the PFDA of 1906 and later expanded to carry out the provisions of the FDCA of 1938. It is one of the oldest drug regulatory agencies in the world. The FDA mission is:

- Protecting the public health by ensuring the safety, efficacy, and security of human and veterinary drugs, biologic products, medical devices, the nation's food supply, cosmetics, and products that emit radiation.
- Regulating the manufacturing, marketing, and distribution of tobacco products.
- Advancing the public health by helping to speed innovations that make medical products more effective, safer, and more affordable.
- Helping the public get the accurate, science-based information they need to use medical products and foods to maintain and improve their health.
- Ensuring the security of the food supply and fostering development of medical products to respond to deliberate and naturally emerging public threats.

With such an important and diverse mission, the FDA is organized around seven branches, as shown in Figure 2.3. The three that have the most importance to pharmacology are the Center for Drug Evaluation and Research (CDER), Center for Biologics Evaluation and Research (CBER), and the Center for Food Safety and Applied Nutrition (CFSAN).

The mission of the CDER is to ensure the availability of safe, effective drugs; promote the safe use of marketed drugs; and ensure the quality and integrity of marketed drug products. All new drugs must be approved by the CDER before they can be marketed. This includes prescription drugs,

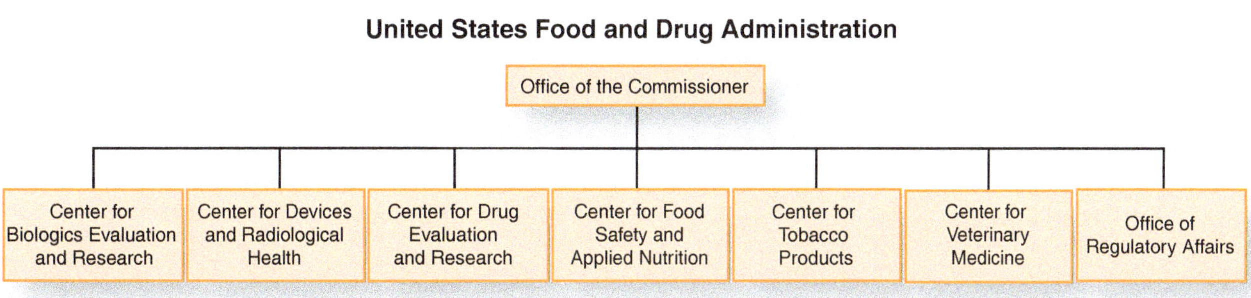

Figure 2.3 Organization of the Food and Drug Administration showing the seven centers that regulate human and veterinary drugs, biologic products, medical devices, the nation's food supply, cosmetics, tobacco, and products that emit radiation.

OTC drugs, and all generic equivalents. After marketing, the CDER is responsible for continued monitoring of safety and may issue additional warnings to healthcare providers or consumers as additional information becomes available.

The CBER regulates the use of *biological products*, including vaccines, allergenics, tissues, cellular and gene therapies, vaccines, and blood. All new biological products are reviewed by the CBER and must be approved by this agency before marketing.

The CFSAN oversees the administration of herbal products, dietary supplements, and cosmetics. Although the CFSAN does not require testing of herbal products, dietary supplements, or cosmetics prior to marketing, the CFSAN is responsible for taking action against any of these products that are deemed unsafe or mislabeled.

Cosmetics are legally defined by the FDCA of 1938 as "articles intended to be rubbed, poured, sprinkled, or sprayed on, introduced into, or otherwise applied to the human body . . . for cleansing, beautifying, promoting attractiveness, or altering the appearance." Examples of products considered cosmetics are skin moisturizers, perfumes, lipsticks, fingernail polishes, eye and facial makeup preparations, shampoos, toothpastes, and deodorants. Can a product be both a cosmetic and a drug? In most cases, cosmetics are not drugs; however, it depends on a product's intended use. For example, if a shampoo is marketed to treat a condition such as dandruff, the active ingredient is considered a drug. If a skin cream claims to provide sunscreen protection, it may be considered a drug. Manufacturers of cosmetics are generally careful not to promote unwarranted therapeutic claims, such as that a product prevents or treats a condition or disease. This would cause the product to be considered a drug by the FDA and it would be subject to tighter regulations.

Drug Approval

2.5 The drug approval process established by the U.S. Food and Drug Administration ensures that drugs sold in the United States are safe and effective.

Drugs are discovered in any number of ways. Penicillin was discovered purely by accident while the scientist was studying an unrelated topic. Many drugs have been isolated from natural substances, including plants and bacteria. Some medications are "me too" drugs, whereby the pharmacologist took a well-known drug and slightly modified the chemical structure to produce a very similar agent. As molecular biology and genetics have progressed into the modern era, drugs have been purposefully designed to fit into specific receptor sites on enzymes or cells.

Regardless of the path to discovery, all medications must be approved by the FDA before they can be sold in the United States. (Medical marijuana, discussed in Chapter 27, has become an exception to this approval process.) The FDA drug review and approval process follows a well-developed and organized plan, as summarized in Figure 2.4.

The first stage of drug development is **preclinical research**, which involves extensive laboratory testing by the pharmaceutical company. Scientists perform testing on human and microbial cells cultured in a laboratory. Studies include several species of animals to examine the drug's effectiveness at different doses and to look for adverse effects. The goals of this extensive testing on cells and in animals are to determine drug action and to predict whether the drug will cause harm to humans. Because laboratory tests do not accurately reflect the precise way the human body will respond to the drug, preclinical research results are always inconclusive. Most potential drugs do not proceed past the preclinical research stage because they are either too toxic or simply not effective. The FDA does not regulate preclinical testing.

If a drug appears promising, the pharmaceutical company submits an **Investigational New Drug (IND)** application to the FDA that contains all the animal and cell testing data. Scientists at the FDA examine the IND and must be convinced that the drug is safe enough to allow human testing. Approval from the FDA is necessary before human testing can begin.

Clinical investigation, the second stage of drug testing, takes place in three different stages termed **clinical phase trials**. These clinical trials are the longest part of the drug approval process and occur in sequential stages.

- **Phase 1.** Testing is conducted on 20 to 80 healthy volunteers for several months to determine proper dosage and to assess for adverse effects. The focus of the phase 1 trial is on *safety*. If unacceptable levels of toxicity are noted, the clinical trials are stopped.

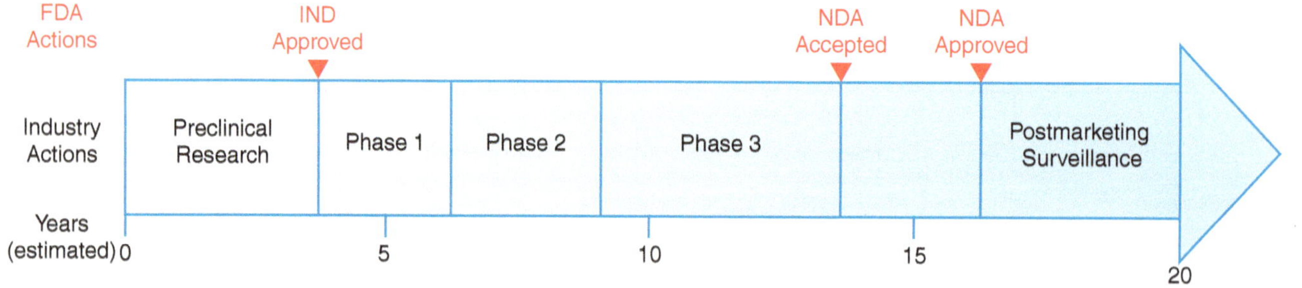

Figure 2.4 Drug development timeline.

- **Phase 2.** In phase 2, an average 12 to 350 participants with the disease are treated with the experimental drug. The primary focus of the phase 2 trial is on *effectiveness*, although safety data continue to be recorded. In most cases, the effectiveness of the new drug is compared to an inert substance, or **placebo**, which serves as a control "nontreatment" group. In other cases, the new drug is compared to a standard drug used for the same condition. For example, a new drug for reducing fever may be compared to acetaminophen (Tylenol). If the new drug is found to have the same (or less) effectiveness and safety profile compared to the standard drug, the pharmaceutical company may stop the clinical trials. This phase may take several years.
- **Phase 3.** In phase 3, large numbers of patients with the disease are given the drug to determine variability of response in different populations. Potential drug–drug interactions are examined. Patients with chronic conditions such as cardiac, renal, or hepatic impairment are given the drug to determine safety in these important populations. Assessment of effectiveness and safety continues for several years, and the average number of patients varies from several hundred to about 3000.

If the drug continues to show promise through the clinical phase trials, a **New Drug Application (NDA)** is submitted to the FDA. The NDA signals that the pharmaceutical company is ready to market the new drug. During the NDA review, the FDA examines all preclinical and clinical data to assess whether the proposed drug is safe and effective. By law, the CDER is obligated to act on at least 90% of the NDAs for standard drugs within 10 months of submission. If the NDA is approved, the manufacturer may begin marketing the new drug. If the NDA is rejected, the FDA indicates whether the drug is "approvable" or "not approvable." "Approvable" means that the drug will likely be approved if the pharmaceutical company conducts additional testing or addresses specific issues identified by the FDA. A designation of "not approvable" indicates that the drug has significant barriers to approval.

Each year, the FDA approves a diverse range of new drugs and biological products. Some of the approved products, however, closely resemble existing medications and do not represent major advances in pharmacotherapy. A better way to track advances in drug therapy is to monitor how many of the approved drugs are **new molecular entities (NMEs)**, medications that are truly unique and structurally different from existing drugs (FDA, 2020c). From 2015 until 2019, the number of new molecular entities varied from 25 to 59 per year.

In the United States, the FDA grants the pharmaceutical company exclusive rights to name and market a drug for a certain number of years after it approves the NDA. During this period of **exclusivity**, competing companies are not allowed to market generic versions of the product (FDA, 2020b). The rationale for exclusivity is that the developing pharmaceutical company needs sufficient time to recoup the millions of dollars in research and development costs involved in designing and testing the new drug. Without the guarantee of exclusivity, pharmaceutical companies have little incentive to develop new and unique drugs. When exclusivity expires, competing companies may sell a generic equivalent drug, sometimes using a different name, which the FDA must approve. The typical length of exclusivity for a new drug is 5 years; however, this may be extended if the drug is determined to have a new indication, can be delivered by a different route, or is made available in a different dosage form. If, for example, a pharmaceutical company completes pediatric studies and determines the dosage and safety of a drug in this population, the FDA adds 6 months of exclusivity. Orphan drugs have 7 years of exclusivity. Expiration dates for the exclusivity of specific drugs are listed by the FDA in its *Approved Drug Products with Therapeutic Equivalence Evaluations* publication.

Postmarketing surveillance, stage 4 of the drug approval process, begins after the NDA review has been completed. The purpose of stage 4 testing is to assess for harmful drug effects in a larger population. Some adverse effects are very subtle, take longer to appear, and are not identified until a drug is prescribed for large numbers of people. Adverse drug reactions are reported by the manufacturers, healthcare providers, and patients to the FDA Adverse Event Reporting System (FAERS), a computerized database designed to support the FDA's postmarketing surveillance program.

The FDA holds public meetings annually to receive comments from patients, professional organizations, and pharmaceutical companies regarding the effectiveness and safety of new drug therapies. If the FDA discovers a serious problem, it will mandate that a drug be withdrawn from the market. Examples of successful postmarketing surveillance include the removal of two cholesterol-lowering drugs in 2016 because long-term clinical trials revealed that the medications were ineffective at reducing adverse cardiovascular events. In these cases, the withdrawals were not prompted by serious safety concerns. The benefits of the drugs were found to no longer outweigh their risks.

The drug approval process has several important limitations. Historically, drug trials have used White men as their test population. Because gender and racial differences may affect how drugs are handled by the body, pharmaceutical companies are now including a more diverse population in their clinical trials. Most drugs have not been tested in children: Pediatric doses and responses are often based on experience rather than research data. Although clinical trials test drugs in pregnant laboratory animals and examine for possible birth defects, these data may not be representative of how drugs affect pregnant women or their fetuses. Finally, adverse effects may occur at such a low level that they are statistically insignificant in clinical trials using a few thousand patients. Several million patients may need to take the drug before these effects can be identified.

Another limitation of the drug approval process relates to off-label uses. A new drug is always approved for a *specific indication* at doses that are demonstrated to be safe and effective. After several years of clinical experience, however, healthcare providers may find that the drug is also useful for indications not approved by the FDA. Or, the prescriber may find that the drug works better at a different dosage level or by a different route of administration. Once initially approved by the FDA, *healthcare providers may legally prescribe the drug for any indications* they feel are appropriate, despite the fact that the drug was never tested or approved for these additional conditions. How widespread is off-label prescribing? It is estimated that over 20% of prescriptions are for indications not approved by the FDA (Agency for Healthcare Research and Quality, 2020). The use of off-label drugs is particularly prevalent in cancer treatment and in pediatric patients (Yackey et al., 2019). The FDA prohibits pharmaceutical companies from advertising or promoting their drugs for off-label uses.

PharmFACT

The median cost for research and development to bring a new drug to market is $985 million. (Wouters et al., 2020).

CONNECTION Checkpoint 2.1

In 2016, granisetron (Sustol), an antiemetic drug, and daclizumab (Zinbryta), an interleukin-2 blocking monoclonal antibody for treating relapsing multiple sclerosis, were approved. Are these considered therapeutic or pharmacologic classifications?

Changes to the Drug Approval Process

2.6 The U.S. Food and Drug Administration has sped up the process of drug review.

The process of synthesizing a new drug and testing it in cells, experimental animals, and humans takes many years. The NDA can include dozens of volumes of experimental and clinical data that must be examined during the FDA review process. Some NDAs contain thousands of pages of data. Even after all experiments have been concluded and clinical data have been gathered, final approval can take several years, or even be denied.

With the high expenses associated with development of a new drug, pharmaceutical companies are justifiably anxious to get the drug marketed. The public is also anxious to receive new medications, particularly for diseases that have a high mortality rate. Although the criticisms of government regulatory agencies are certainly understandable, the fundamental priority of the FDA is to ensure the safety of medications. Without an exhaustive review of scientific data, the public could be exposed to dangerous or ineffective drugs.

In 1992 and in 2012, legislation was passed to allow the FDA to speed up the review and approval of drugs intended to treat serious conditions. The following are four strategies used by the FDA to accelerate the review process (FDA, 2010a).

- **Fast track.** A fast track designation means that the new drug has the *potential* to meet an unmet need for a condition in which there is no current therapy, or the drug may offer significant improvement over existing therapies. The request for a fast track is made by the pharmaceutical company and the designation is reviewed by the FDA within 60 days.
- **Breakthrough therapy.** A breakthrough therapy means that trials suggest there is *clinical evidence* that the drug may demonstrate substantial improvement over existing therapies for a serious or life-threatening condition. Like the fast track, a request for a breakthrough therapy designation is made by the pharmaceutical company and reviewed by the FDA within 60 days.
- **Priority review.** When an NDA is received, the FDA makes a decision to perform a standard review (average 10 months) or a priority review (average 6 months). The decision is based on whether the new drug would offer a significant improvement over existing therapies for a serious condition.
- **Accelerated approval.** It may take many years to demonstrate that a drug provides real clinical benefit: improved patient survival or how a patient feels or functions. In these cases, the FDA may approve the drug based on "intermediate clinical endpoints." The best example is a new anticancer drug. The new drug may show positive evidence of tumor shrinkage in clinical trials and receive accelerated approval based on this evidence. The new drug can be marketed at this point. However, it may take several years before it is known whether the drug actually improves patient survival. The drug company can continue to market the new drug, but must perform follow-up studies, known as *confirmatory trials*. If the confirmatory trials show the drug did not improve survival, the FDA may withdraw the accelerated approval.

Prescription and Over-the-Counter Drugs

2.7 Over-the-counter drugs are usually safe and effective when used according to label instructions.

The 1951 Durham-Humphrey Amendment to the FDCA clearly established the difference between prescription and OTC drugs. To obtain a prescription drug, an order must be given authorizing the patient to receive the medication. Prescription medications are judged by the FDA to be potentially addictive or too harmful for self-administration. In some cases, they are used to treat conditions too complex for self-diagnosis by the consumer or the drug may require a skilled nurse or healthcare provider to administer it.

The advantages of requiring a prescription are numerous. The healthcare provider has an opportunity to examine the patient and determine a specific diagnosis. The prescriber can maximize therapy by ordering the proper drug for the patient's condition and by controlling the amount and frequency of the drug to be dispensed. In addition, the healthcare provider has an opportunity to teach the patient proper use of the drug and its expected adverse effects.

In contrast to prescription drugs, OTC drugs do not require an order from a healthcare provider. In most cases, patients may treat themselves safely if they carefully follow instructions included with the medication. A key point to remember is that no drug is without risk; if patients do not follow the guidelines on the label, serious adverse effects may result.

Patients prefer to take OTC medications for many reasons. OTC drugs are obtained more easily than prescription drugs. No appointment with a healthcare provider is required, thus saving time and money. Without the assistance of a healthcare provider, however, choosing the proper medication for a specific problem can be challenging. OTC drugs may interact with foods, herbal products, prescription drugs, or other OTC drugs. Patients may not be aware that some OTC medications can impair their ability to function safely. Self-treatment is sometimes ineffective, and the potential for harm may increase if the disease is allowed to progress.

The approval process for an OTC product differs from prescription products and may proceed by several paths. The manufacturer may choose to submit an NDA, as described in Section 2.5. However, the company may instead choose to switch a prescription product to an OTC product. In these cases, the FDA reviews existing consumer data to assess drug safety. Products that have changed from prescription to OTC include nicotine patches and gum, famotidine (Pepcid AC), cimetidine (Tagamet HB), omeprazole (Prilosec), cetirizine (Zyrtec), budesonide (Rhinocort), fluticasone (Flonase), and loratadine (Claritin).

An additional path for OTC product approval involves **drug monographs** prepared by the FDA. For OTC products previously approved by the FDA, the detailed monographs describe the active ingredient, its acceptable forms (e.g., capsule, liquid, topical cream), dosages or concentrations, and required labeling. Manufacturers may market an OTC drug *without preapproval of the FDA* if the product falls within the parameters described in the monograph (FDA, 2020d). In 2020 Congress passed the Over-the Counter Monograph Safety, Innovation and Reform Act, which makes it easier to revise monographs so they include up-to-date safety data, dosage changes, and other innovative changes to these medications (Pew Charitable Trust, 2020).

Herbal products and dietary supplements are also widely available OTC. Herbal products and dietary supplements are not considered drugs; they are not marketed to treat any disease, and they are not subject to the same regulatory process as medications. Yet some of these products can cause adverse effects and interact with medications.

CONNECTIONS: Lifespan Considerations

The Association of Cost-Related Medication Nonadherence and Food Insecurity in Older Adults

It is known that the cost of prescription drugs may be a major cause for medication nonadherence in the older adult, but are there other factors that impact nonadherence? Studies suggest that *food insecurity*—the lack of access to sufficient, nutritious, and affordable food—may also predict nonadherence (Afulani et al., 2015; Herman et al., 2015). Afulani et al. (2015) found that as the severity of food insecurity increased, nonadherence also increased. Older adult women and older adults with chronic conditions were more likely to report nonadherence. However, having insurance coverage, particularly Medicare and Medicaid, decreased nonadherence. Food security-related nonadherence is not just a problem for the older adult. Herman et al. (2015) found a similar relationship in the nonelderly adult population. In that study, female adults and adults with chronic conditions, low income, no or insufficient health insurance, severe mental illness, or functional limitations had an increased risk of cost-related medication nonadherence.

Nurses should assess factors other than cost that may increase the risk of nonadherence, particularly food insecurity. Recognizing that patients who are unable to afford or access adequate and nutritious food places them at risk for medication nonadherence may help the healthcare team improve health.

Nurses should always inquire about their patients' use of herbal products and dietary supplements and caution them that the FDA has not tested these products for effectiveness or safety (see Chapter 7).

Drug Schedules

2.8 Drugs with a potential for abuse are categorized into schedules.

Dependence is a powerful physiologic or psychologic need for a substance. Some drugs are frequently abused or have a high potential for dependence; thus, the selling and distribution of these drugs are highly restricted. Drugs that have a significant potential for abuse are placed into five categories called *schedules*. These **scheduled drugs** are classified and regulated according to their potential for abuse, as shown in Table 2.2. Concepts of dependence and drug schedules are discussed in detail in Chapter 27.

In the United States, **controlled substances** are drugs whose use is restricted by the Comprehensive Drug Abuse Prevention and Control Act of 1970 and its later revisions. Every healthcare provider or entity that produces, distributes, dispenses, or prescribes such substances must register with the Drug Enforcement Administration (DEA). Registrants must maintain complete records of all quantities purchased and sold and report suspicious orders of unusual size or frequency. Drugs with the highest abuse potential have additional restrictions. For example, providers must use a special order form to obtain Schedule II drugs, and orders must be written and signed by the provider. Telephone orders to a pharmacy are not permitted. Refills for Schedule II drugs are not permitted; patients must visit their healthcare provider to receive a new prescription. Healthcare providers convicted of unlawful manufacturing, distributing, and dispensing of controlled substances face severe penalties.

CONNECTION Checkpoint 2.2

Once a new drug is approved, it is assigned names. What are the two basic types of drug names and who assigns them?

Prescriptive Authority for Nurses

2.9 Advanced practice nurses are helping to fill the primary care workforce gap.

The Future of Nursing: Leading Change, Advancing Health identified that the changing healthcare landscape, the changing profile of the U.S. population, and notable shortage of primary care health professionals in the United States would require fundamental shifts in the care delivery system (Institute of Medicine, 2011). In particular, the report suggested that advanced practice registered nurses (APRNs), if permitted to practice to the full extent of their education and training, could help build the workforce necessary to meet the country's primary care needs and contribute their unique skills to the delivery of patient-centered, community-based healthcare. At least twenty-two states plus Washington, D.C., the Veterans Administration, and Indian Health Services grant nurse practitioners (NPs) the right to practice to the top of their education without physician oversight. Today the APRN is viewed as an essential member of the healthcare system's ability to deliver affordable care.

NPs hold prescriptive privileges, including controlled substances, in all 50 states and D.C. According to the 2019 AANP National Nurse Practitioner Sample Survey, nurse practitioners in full-time practice write an average of 20 prescriptions per day (American Association of Nurse Practitioners, 2020). The ability to prescribe drugs, a key component of most treatment plans, ensure that patients are provided the best and most cost-effective care possible. This text includes a focus on preparing for prescriptive authority, and Connections features detail specific information the APRN needs to know to prepare for this authority.

Table 2.2 U.S. Drug Schedules and Examples

Drug Schedule	Abuse Potential	Examples	Therapeutic Use
I	Highest	Heroin, GHB, LSD, marijuana, MDMA, mescaline, methaqualone, methcathinone, peyote, and psilocybin	No currently acceptable medical use; high potential for abuse
II	High	Potent opioids (such as codeine in high doses, fentanyl, methadone, morphine, oxycodone, meperidine), amphetamine, cocaine, methamphetamine, methylphenidate, PCP, and short-acting barbiturates	Have currently accepted medical use but use may be severely restricted; normally no refills are permitted (but there are exceptions)
III	Moderate	Anabolic steroids, buprenorphine ketamine, codeine (less than 90 mg per dosage unit), hydrocodone (lower doses compounded with aspirin or acetaminophen), and intermediate-acting barbiturates	Have currently accepted medical use; less stringent controls than Schedule II drugs; five refills allowed in a 6-month period
IV	Low	Benzodiazepines (such as alprazolam, diazepam, midazolam, temazepam), long-acting barbiturates, meprobamate, pentazocine, tramadol, and zolpidem	Have currently accepted medical use; similar controls to Schedule III drugs; five refills allowed in a 6-month period
V	Lowest	Cough medicines with codeine, antidiarrheal medicines with small amounts of opioids	Have currently accepted medical use; similar controls to Schedule III and IV drugs

Controlled Substance Schedules, U.S. Department of Justice, n.d. Retrieved from http://www.deadiversion.usdoj.gov/schedules.

Understanding Chapter 2

Key Concepts Summary

2.1 Early American history saw the rise of patent medicines and the lack of adequate drug regulations.

2.2 In the 1900s, drug legislation was enacted to make drugs safer and more effective.

2.3 The standardization of drug purity and strength is specified by the *United States Pharmacopeia-National Formulary*.

2.4 The regulatory agency responsible for ensuring that drugs and medical devices are safe and effective is the U.S. Food and Drug Administration.

2.5 The drug approval process established by the U.S. Food and Drug Administration ensures that drugs sold in the United States are safe and effective.

2.6 The U.S. Food and Drug Administration has sped up the process of drug review.

2.7 Over-the-counter drugs are usually safe and effective when used according to label instructions.

2.8 Drugs with a potential for abuse are categorized into schedules.

2.9 Advanced practice nurses are helping to fill the primary care workforce gap.

CASE STUDY: Making the Patient Connection

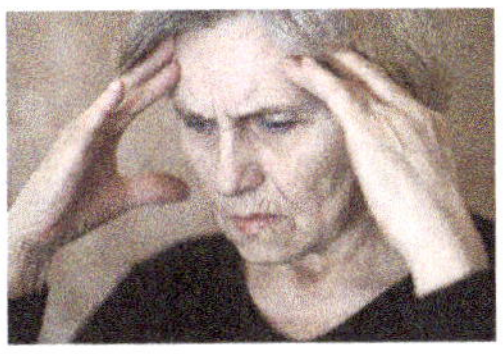

Remember the patient "Gertrude Stone" at the beginning of the chapter? Now read the remainder of the case study. Based on the information presented within this chapter, respond to the critical thinking questions that follow.

Gertrude Stone lives alone in the house she has owned for 46 years. Although she is seldom sick, when she needs to see a healthcare provider, she must ride the public bus system. The trip requires two bus transfers and can be tiring.

Because Gertrude lives only one block from a grocery store, she often self-medicates using OTC drugs. She strongly believes in the use of herbs, vitamins, and home remedies.

As a parish nurse, you are organizing a community health fair at the church where Gertrude is an active member.

Critical Thinking Questions

1. How would you counsel Gertrude about the safety of OTC drugs?
2. What are the advantages and disadvantages of OTC medications?
3. How can Gertrude be certain that OTC medications are safe for her?

Additional Case Study

Your 12-year-old nephew is preparing a report for school about the FDA and the drug approval process. You, as a healthcare provider, are often called on by family members to answer questions about anything health related. Following are his questions. How would you respond?

1. What is the role of the FDA?
2. What role does the FDA play in regulating herbal and dietary supplements?
3. How quickly can a new drug be approved by the FDA?

Answers to Additional Case Study questions are available on the faculty resources site. Please consult with your instructor.

Chapter Review

1. The governmental drug legislation requires the drug manufacturer to prove that a drug is both safe and:
   1. Free of adverse effects and potential reactions.
   2. Effective for a specified purpose.
   3. Reasonable in cost and easily accessible.
   4. Beneficial to various population groups.
2. The drug research participant with a particular disease is taking part in an investigative study to examine the effects of a new drug. Previously, this drug was tested using healthy volunteers. The next phase of the clinical trial investigation in which the patient will be participating is:
   1. Phase 1
   2. Phase 2
   3. Phase 3
   4. Phase 4
3. A drug that is being prescribed "off-label" means that the drug:
   1. Is available in Europe or Canada but not in the United States.
   2. Has FDA approval for one use but is being prescribed for another purpose.
   3. Is under an accelerated approval process and full indications have not yet been discovered.
   4. Is a generic drug being used instead of a trade-name drug.
4. The patient requests that a refill prescription of a Schedule II controlled substance be telephoned to the drug store. When responding to the patient, you would consider which factor? Refills of Schedule II drugs:
   1. Are less costly than the original prescription.
   2. Must be listened to by at least two people.
   3. Are verified through the local DEA office.
   4. Are not permitted under federal law.
5. In 1992 and in 2012, legislation was passed to allow the FDA to speed up the review and approval of drugs intended to treat serious conditions. When would the following accelerated review processes be applicable?
   1. Fast track
   2. Breakthrough therapy
   3. Priority review
   4. Accelerated approval
6. While in the clinic, you note that multiple patients had a reaction to the same medication, a drug that has been available for several years. Which action should you take? (Select all that apply.)
   1. File an Adverse Event Report with the FDA.
   2. Note the reaction in the patient's chart.
   3. Notify the healthcare provider who ordered the drug.
   4. Wait until the FDA sends a notification of the drug's recall before informing the patient.
   5. Compare each patient's reaction to determine if it is the same.

See Appendix A for answers to critical thinking questions, case study questions and review questions.

References

Afulani, P., Herman, D., Coleman-Jensen, A., & Harrison, G. G. (2015). Food insecurity and health outcomes among older adults: The role of cost-related medication underuse. *Journal of Nutrition in Gerontology and Geriatrics*, *34*, 319–342. https://doi.org//10.1080/21551197.2015.1054575

Agency for Healthcare Research and Quality (2020). *Off-label drugs: What you need to know.* https://www.ahrq.gov/patients-consumers/patient-involvement/off-label-drug-usage.html

American Association of Nurse Practitioners (AANP) News Center. (2020). *More than 290,000 Nurse Practitioners Licensed in the United States.* https://www.aanp.org/news-feed/290-000-nps-licensed-in-us

Congressional Research Service. (2020). *The Food and Drug Administration (FDA) budget: Fact sheet.* https://crsreports.congress.gov/product/pdf/R/R44576

Herman, D., Afulani, P., Coleman-Jensen, A., & Harrison, G. G. (2015). Food insecurity and cost-related medication underuse among nonelderly adults in a nationally representative sample. *American Journal of Public Health*, *105*(10), e48–e59. https://doi.org/10.2105/AJPH.2015.302712

Institute of Medicine (IOM). (2011). *The future of nursing: Leading change, advancing health.* National Academies Press.

National Council of State Boards of Nursing. (2016). *Implementation status map: NCSBN's APRN Campaign for Consensus: State progress toward uniformity.* https://www.ncsbn.org/5397.htm

Pew Charitable Trust. (2020). *Congress passes legislation to reform over-the-counter drug regulation.* https://www.pewtrusts.org/en/research-and-analysis/articles/2020/03/27/congress-passes-legislation-to-reform-over-the-counter-drug-regulation

Pharmaceutical Processing World. (2019). *Orphan drug sales to reach $262 billion by 2024.* https://www.pharmaceuticalprocessingworld.com/orphan-drug-sales-to-reach-262-billion-by-2024/

U.S. Food and Drug Administration. (2020a). *Fast track, breakthrough therapy, accelerated approval and priority review.* https://www.fda.gov/patients/learn-about-drug-and-device-approvals/fast-track-breakthrough-therapy-accelerated-approval-priority-review

U.S. Food and Drug Administration. (2020b). *Frequently asked questions on patents and exclusivity.* https://www.fda.gov/drugs/development-approval-process-drugs/frequently-asked-questions-patents-and-exclusivity#whenshould

U.S. Food and Drug Administration. (2020c). *New drugs at FDA: CDER's new molecular entities and new therapeutic biological products.* https://www.fda.gov/drugs/development-approval-process-drugs/new-drugs-fda-cders-new-molecular-entities-and-new-therapeutic-biological-products

U.S. Food and Drug Administration. (2020d). *OTC nonprescription drugs.* https://www.fda.gov/drugs/how-drugs-are-developed-and-approved/otc-nonprescription-drugs

Wouters, O., McKee, M., & Luyten, J. (2020). Estimated research and development investment needed to bring a new medicine to market, 2009–2018. *Journal of the American Medical Association, 323*(9), 844–853. https://doi.org/10.1001/jama.2020.1166

Yackey, K., Stukus, K., Cohen, D., Kline, D., Zhao, S., & Stanley, R. (2019). Off-label medication prescribing patterns in pediatrics: An update. *Hospital Pediatrics, 9*(3), 186–193. https://doi.org/10.1542/hpeds.2018-0168

Selected Bibliography

Congressional Research Service. (2019). *The Controlled Substances Act (CSA): A legal overview for the 116th Congress.* Federation of American Scientists. https://fas.org/sgp/crs/misc/R45948.pdf

Eguale, T., Buckeridge, D. L., Verma, A., Winslade, N. E., Benedetti, A., Hanley, J. A., & Tamblyn, R. (2016). Association of off-label drug use and adverse drug events in an adult population. *JAMA Internal Medicine, 176*, 55–63. https://doi.org/10.1001/jamainternmed.2015.6058

Hamner, C. E. (Ed.). (2019). *Drug development.* CRC Press.

Kesselheim, A. S., Woloshin, S., Lu, Z., Tessema, F. A., Ross, K. M., & Schwartz, L. M. (2019). Physicians' perspectives on FDA approval standards and off-label drug marketing. *JAMA Internal Medicine, 179*(5), 707–709. https://doi.org/10.1001/jamainternmed.2018.8121

U.S. Food and Drug Administration. (2018). *Understanding unapproved use of approved drugs "off label."* https://www.fda.gov/patients/learn-about-expanded-access-and-other-treatment-options/understanding-unapproved-use-approved-drugs-label

U.S. Food and Drug Administration. (2020). *Prescription drug user fee amendments.* https://www.fda.gov/industry/fda-user-fee-programs/prescription-drug-user-fee-amendments

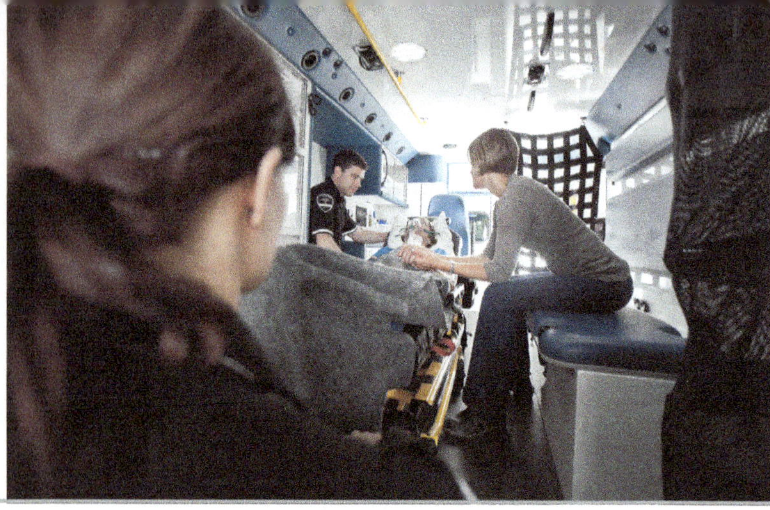

"I'm terribly worried about my father, John Kessler. He's been so ill for so long. I don't know if his body can take much more."

—Patient's daughter, "Emily Kessler Myers"

Chapter 3
Pharmacokinetics

Chapter Outline

- Introduction to Pharmacokinetics
- Primary Processes of Pharmacokinetics
  - Absorption
  - Distribution
  - Metabolism
  - Excretion
- Time–Response Relationships
  - Drug Plasma Levels
  - Drug Half-Life
  - Loading and Maintenance Doses

Learning Outcomes

After reading this chapter, the student should be able to:

1. Identify the four primary processes of pharmacokinetics.
2. Explain mechanisms by which drugs cross plasma membranes.
3. Discuss factors affecting drug absorption.
4. Discuss how drugs are distributed throughout the body.
5. Describe how plasma proteins affect drug distribution.
6. Explain the metabolism of drugs and its applications to pharmacotherapy.
7. Identify major processes by which drugs are excreted.
8. Explain how enterohepatic recirculation affects drug activity.
9. Explain how a drug reaches and maintains its therapeutic range in the plasma.
10. Explain the applications of a drug's plasma half-life ($t_{1/2}$) to pharmacotherapy.
11. Differentiate between loading and maintenance doses.

Key Terms

Definitions of the terms in bold may be found in the Glossary.

Most drugs produce their effects by causing a physiologic or chemical change in specific target cells in the body. To produce a therapeutic effect, a drug must reach its target cells in sufficient quantities. For topical agents used to treat superficial skin conditions, this is an easy task. For most medications, however, the process of reaching target cells to cause a physiologic change is complex. Drugs are exposed to a myriad of barriers and destructive processes after they enter the body. The purpose of this chapter is to examine factors that act on the drug as it attempts to reach its target cells and to provide examples of how the nurse can use this information to optimize pharmacotherapeutic outcomes.

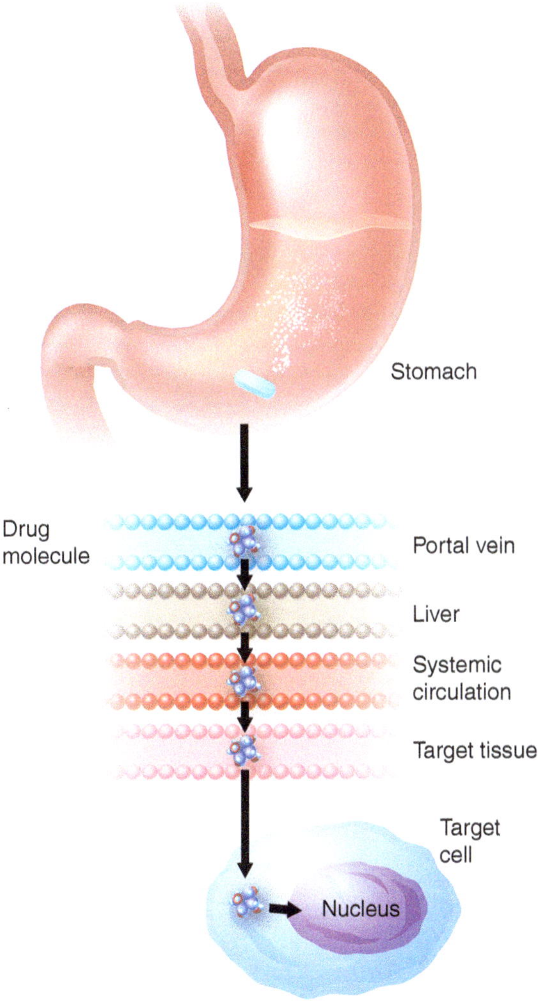

Figure 3.1 Barriers that a drug administered by the oral route must cross before interacting with a target cell.

Introduction to Pharmacokinetics

3.1 Pharmacokinetics focuses on what the body does to drugs after they are administered.

The term **pharmacokinetics** is derived from the root words *pharmaco*, which refers to medicines, and *kinetics*, which means "movement" or "motion." Pharmacokinetics is thus the study of drug movement throughout the body. In practical terms, it describes *what the body does to the medication after it is administered*. Pharmacokinetics is a core subject in pharmacology, and a firm grasp of this topic allows nurses to better understand and predict the actions and adverse effects of medications in their patients.

Drugs face numerous obstacles in reaching their target cells. For most medications, the greatest barrier is crossing the many membranes that separate the drug from its target cells. When taken by mouth, for example, the drug must cross the plasma membranes of the mucosal cells of the gastrointestinal (GI) tract and the endothelial cells of the capillaries to enter the bloodstream. To leave the bloodstream, it must again cross capillary cells, travel through interstitial fluid, and perhaps enter target cells by passing through their plasma membranes. Depending on the mechanism of action, the drug may also need to enter cellular organelles such as nuclei, which are surrounded by additional membranes. Some of the membranes and barriers that many drugs must successfully penetrate before they can elicit a response are illustrated in Figure 3.1.

While seeking their target cells drugs are subjected to numerous physiologic processes. When given by the oral route, stomach acid and digestive enzymes may destroy the drug molecules. Phagocytes may attempt to remove the drug, or an immune response may be triggered. The kidneys, large intestine, and other organs attempt to rapidly excrete the drug from the body.

The preceding examples all illustrate pharmacokinetic processes: how the body handles drugs. The many processes of pharmacokinetics are grouped into four categories: absorption, distribution, metabolism, and excretion, which are illustrated in Figure 3.2. All four of these processes have drug *movement* in common.

3.2 Drugs use diffusion and active transport to cross plasma membranes to reach their target cells.

With few exceptions, drugs must cross plasma membranes and interact with cells to produce their effects. Plasma membranes are composed of a lipid bilayer, with proteins and other molecules interspersed in the membrane. Like other chemicals, drugs use two primary processes to cross membranes: diffusion and active transport.

Simple **diffusion**, or passive transport, is the movement of a chemical from an area of higher concentration to an area of lower concentration. For example, when first administered, a drug given by the intravenous (IV) route is in high concentration in the blood. The drug will move quickly by passive diffusion from its region of high concentration (blood)

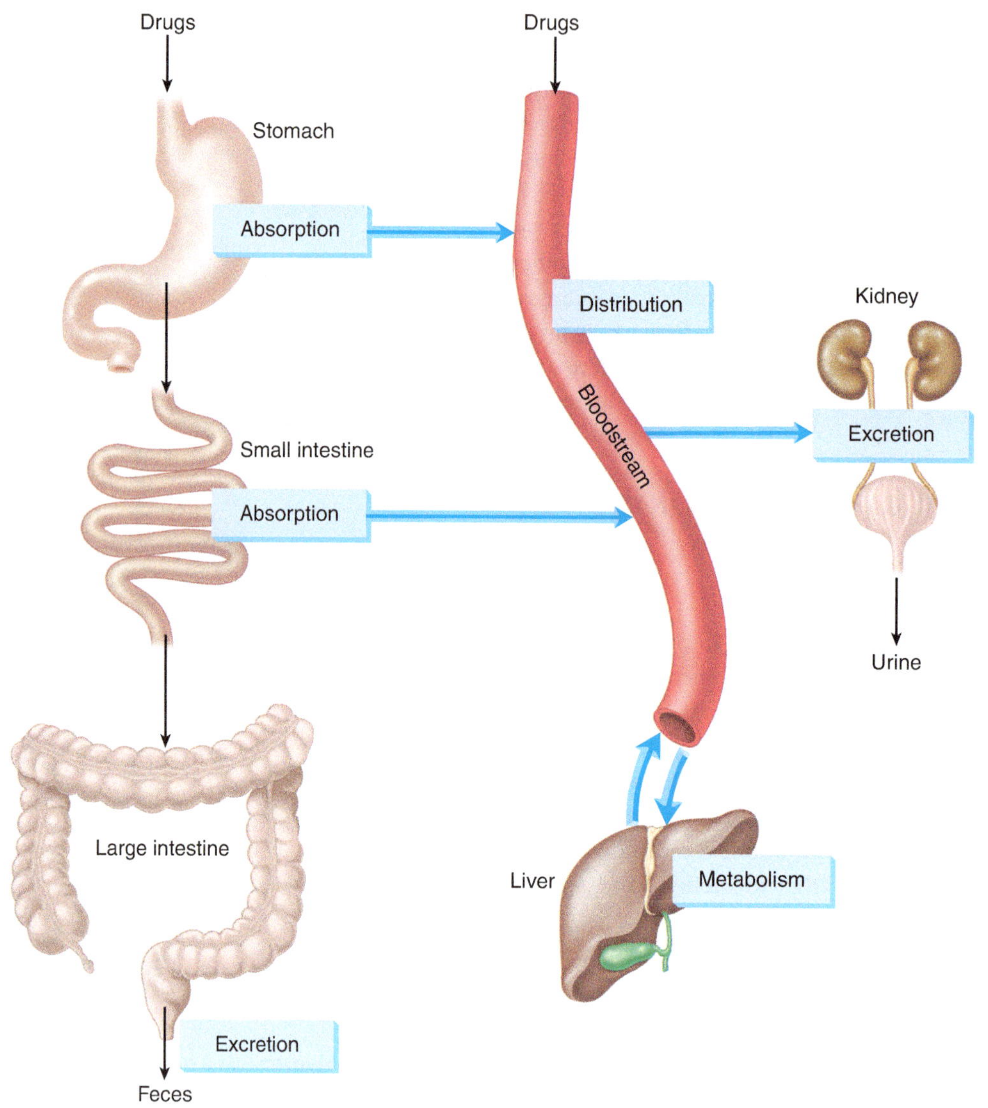

Figure 3.2 The four processes of pharmacokinetics: absorption, distribution, metabolism, and excretion.

to a region of low concentration (target tissue) to produce its action. With time the concentration of drug will diminish at the target tissue. Giving additional doses will create a continual concentration gradient from blood to target tissue.

Diffusion assumes that the chemical is able to freely cross plasma membranes. This, however, is not always the case. Drug molecules that are small, nonionized, and lipid soluble will usually pass through plasma membranes by simple diffusion and easily reach their target cells. This process is illustrated in Figure 3.3. Very small molecules, such as urea, alcohol, and water, may also enter through open channels or pores in the plasma membrane.

Large molecules, ionized drugs, and water-soluble agents have difficulty crossing plasma membranes by simple diffusion and may require carrier, or transport, proteins. A drug that moves into a cell along its concentration gradient utilizing a membrane carrier protein is using the process of facilitated diffusion. This process does not require energy expenditure from the cell, but it does require that a specific carrier protein be present on the plasma membrane. Transport proteins are selective and only carry molecules that have specific structures.

Some drugs cross membranes against their gradient, from low concentration to high concentration, through the process of active transport. This requires expenditure of energy on the part of the cell and a carrier protein. Carrier proteins that assist in active transport are sometimes called *pumps*.

Primary Processes of Pharmacokinetics

3.3 Absorption is the process of moving a drug from the site of administration to the bloodstream.

For most medications the first step toward reaching target cells is **absorption**, the process by which drug molecules move from their site of administration to the blood. With the

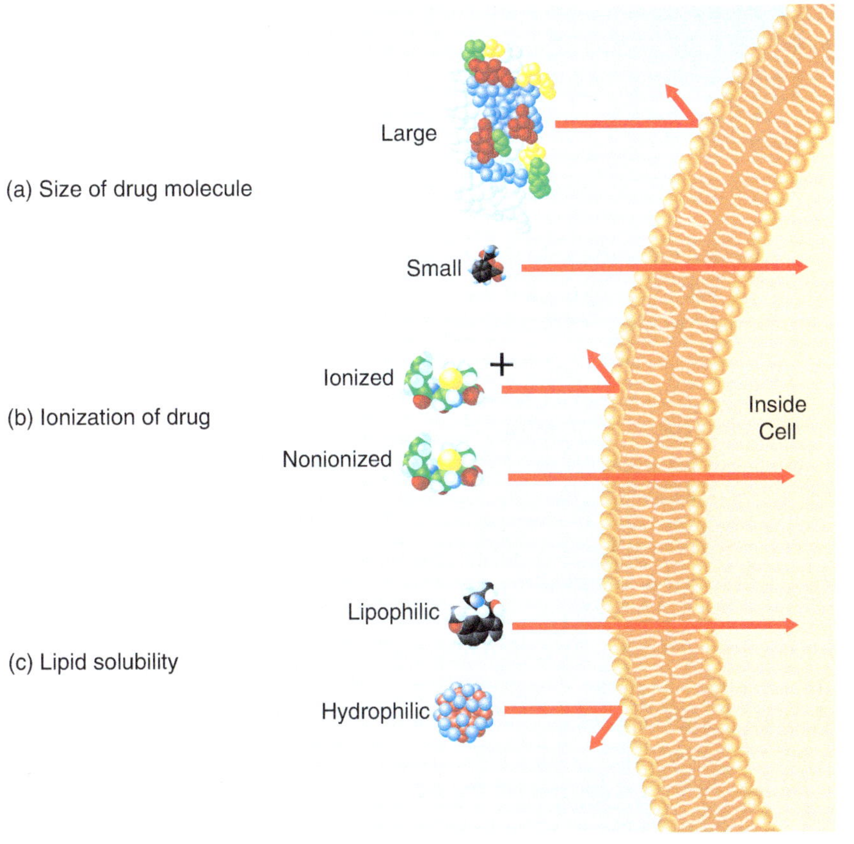

Figure 3.3 Passage of drugs across plasma membranes. (a) Small drugs, (b) nonionized drugs, and (c) lipophilic drugs are more likely to cross membranes.

exception of a few topical medications, local anesthetics, anti-infectives for intestinal parasites, and some radiologic contrast agents, the majority of drugs must be absorbed in order to produce an effect. Of course, drugs administered directly into blood vessels by IV or intra-arterial routes are not absorbed because they are placed directly in the bloodstream.

Absorption is the primary pharmacokinetic factor determining the *onset* of drug action—the length of time it takes a drug to produce its effect. In general, the more rapid the absorption, the faster the onset of drug action. Drugs used in critical care are designed to be absorbed within seconds or minutes, or they are given intravenously. At the other extreme is Mirena, which is absorbed slowly from a polyethylene tube placed in the uterus to provide contraceptive protection for up to 5 years.

Route of Administration

The route of administration is a key factor affecting drug absorption. The three broad categories of routes of drug administration are enteral, topical, and parenteral. Each route has advantages as well as disadvantages. Whereas some drugs are formulated to be given by several routes, others are specific to only one route.

Enteral Route: The **enteral route** includes drugs delivered to the GI tract, either orally (PO) or through nasogastric or gastrostomy tubes. Most enteral medications are intended for absorption to the general circulation, taking advantage of the combined absorptive surfaces of the oral mucosa, stomach, and small intestine. A few enteral medications are administered for local effects, such as infections of the GI tract.

Tablets and Capsules: Tablets and capsules are the most common form of enteral medications. Patients prefer them because of their ease of use. Tablets may be scored, allowing for one-half or one-quarter dosing. The oral route is considered one of the safest because the skin barrier is not compromised. In cases of overdose, drugs remaining in the stomach can be retrieved by inducing vomiting or by suctioning out the stomach contents.

Tablets and capsules must dissolve before the drug is available for absorption; thus, their onset time is relatively slow. The dissolution rate of a tablet or capsule is often the slowest part of the absorption process of an oral medication. Liquid formulations are absorbed faster than tablets or capsules.

The strongly acidic contents of the stomach can destroy some enteral medications. To overcome this obstacle, tablets may have a hard, waxy coating that enables them to resist acidity. These **enteric-coated** tablets are designed to dissolve in the alkaline environment of the small intestine. Some drugs are enteric coated because the medications will irritate the stomach mucosa should they dissolve in the stomach.

As the number of doses per day increases, patients sometimes forget to take their medication. **Extended-release** (XR, XL) tablets or capsules are designed to dissolve slowly, resulting in a longer duration of action for the medication. Also called *long-acting (LA)* or *sustained-release (SR)* medications, these forms allow for the convenience of once- or twice-a-day dosing.

Some patients, particularly children, have difficulty swallowing tablets and capsules. Crushing tablets or opening capsules and sprinkling the medication over food or mixing it with juice may make the drug easier to swallow. The nurse should not crush tablets or open capsules, however, unless the manufacturer specifically states that this is permissible. In general, the following types of drugs should not be chewed, crushed, or opened:

- **Extended-release formulations.** These drugs contain a high dose of medication that is intended to be released over an extended period. Opening the capsule or crushing the tablet will release the entire drug immediately, possibly resulting in adverse effects.
- **Enteric-coated drugs.** When crushed or opened, these drugs are exposed to stomach acid, which may inactivate them. In addition, the drugs may irritate the stomach mucosa and cause nausea and/or vomiting.
- **Oral cavity effects.** Drugs that have a bitter taste are often coated with a thin layer of glucose or inert material to mask their taste. If crushed or opened, the bitter taste is experienced. Other drugs stain the teeth, irritate the oral mucosa, or cause an anesthetic-like effect on the tongue if crushed and exposed to the oral cavity.

As an alternative to crushing, some drugs are available in liquid form for patients who have difficulty swallowing tablets or capsules. Liquid forms include elixirs, syrups, and suspensions. Liquid drugs are usually heavily flavored and sweetened to mask their bitter taste.

Tablets, liquids, and capsules have certain disadvantages. The patient must be conscious and able to swallow properly. Certain types of drugs, including proteins such as insulin, are inactivated by the digestive enzymes in the stomach and small intestine. Furthermore, drugs absorbed from the stomach and small intestine first travel to the liver, where they may be inactivated before they ever reach their target organs—a process called *first-pass effect*, which is described in Section 3.5. There is also significant variation among patients in the motility of the GI tract and in its ability to absorb medications.

Oral Transmucosal Routes: The mucosa of the oral cavity contains extensive capillaries that provide an excellent absorptive surface. Medications given by this route are not subjected to destructive stomach acid, and they bypass the hepatic first-pass effect. The transmucosal drugs include sublingual and buccal tablets, orally disintegrating tablets, and soluble films.

For the *sublingual* method, the medication is placed under the tongue and allowed to slowly dissolve. Because of the rich blood supply to the region, the sublingual route results in a rapid onset of drug action. After moistening the oral cavity, the patient should be instructed not to move the drug with the tongue or to eat or drink anything until the medication has completely dissolved. The sublingual mucosa is not suitable for extended-release formulations because it is a relatively small area that is constantly bathed by saliva that will remove these drugs from the region.

A *buccal* drug is placed in the oral cavity between the gum and cheek. The patient is instructed not to manipulate the drug with the tongue; otherwise it could get displaced to the sublingual area, where it will be more rapidly absorbed, or to the back of the throat, where it could be swallowed. The buccal mucosa is thicker and less permeable to medications than the sublingual area, providing for slower absorption. The buccal route is preferred over the sublingual route for sustained-release delivery because of its greater mucosal surface area. Drugs formulated for buccal administration generally do not cause irritation and are small enough to not cause discomfort to the patient. Like the sublingual route, drugs administered by the buccal route avoid the first-pass effect by the liver as well as the destructive enzymes of the stomach and small intestine.

In recent years, two alternatives to tablets, capsules, and liquids have been developed. *Orally disintegrating tablets (ODTs)* and *soluble films* are designed to dissolve in the oral cavity in less than 30 seconds, without the need to drink water. These dosage forms are convenient and especially appropriate for patients who have difficulty chewing or swallowing and patients who are nauseated, uncooperative, or have a mental impairment. ODTs and soluble films are now available for dozens of medications.

PharmFACT

Medicated lollipops are an emerging technology. The patient sucks or rotates a stick coated with the flavored medication, which dissolves slowly in the mouth (Vangara & Samala, 2015).

Nasogastric and Gastrostomy Tubes: Patients with a nasogastric (NG) tube or a gastrostomy (G) tube may have their medications administered through these devices. Drugs administered through these tubes are usually in liquid form. Although solid drugs can be crushed or dissolved, they tend to clog the tubes. Sustained-release medications should not be crushed and administered through NG or G tubes. Drugs administered by these routes are exposed to the same physiologic processes as those given PO.

Topical Route: The **topical route** of drug administration includes medications applied to the skin or mucous membranes. Topical medications applied to the skin are absorbed very slowly because the drug must penetrate the thick, keratin layer of the epidermis.

Topical drugs are also applied to mucous membranes of the eye, ear, nose, respiratory tract, urinary tract, vagina, or rectum. Some of these medications are absorbed very rapidly because these membranes are thin and have a rich blood supply.

Many drugs are applied topically to produce a *local* effect. For example, antibiotics are applied topically to treat skin infections. Antineoplastic agents may be instilled into the urinary bladder via catheter to treat tumors of the bladder mucosa. Corticosteroids are sprayed into the nostrils to reduce inflammation of the nasal mucosa due to allergic rhinitis. Topical delivery produces few serious adverse effects because drugs are absorbed slowly and only small amounts reach the systemic circulation. The most common adverse events resulting from topical administration are transient burning, stinging, or redness of the area where the medication is applied.

Some drugs are given topically to provide for slow release and absorption of the drug to the general circulation. These medications are given for their *systemic*, rather than local, effects. For example, a nitroglycerin patch is applied to treat coronary artery disease. Likewise, prochlorperazine (Compazine) suppositories are inserted rectally not to treat a disease of the rectum but to alleviate nausea.

The distinction between topical drugs given for local effects and those administered for systemic effects is an important one for the nurse. In the case of local drugs, absorption is undesirable and may result in adverse effects if the drug reaches the systemic circulation in significant amounts. For systemic drugs, absorption across the skin or mucous membrane is essential for the therapeutic action of the drug. Neither type of topical agent should be applied to abraded or denuded skin because it could affect drug absorption.

The use of **transdermal patches** provides an effective means of delivering certain medications. Examples include norelgestromin/ethinyl estradiol (Xulane) to prevent pregnancy, testosterone for hypogonadism, and scopolamine (Transderm Scop) for motion sickness. Transdermal patches contain a specified amount of medication, although the rate of delivery and the actual dose received can vary. Patches are changed on a regular dosing schedule, often daily or weekly, depending on the medication. Medications administered by this route bypass digestive enzymes and the first-pass effect in the liver.

The *ophthalmic route* is used to treat local conditions of the eye and surrounding structures. Common indications include excessive dryness, eye infections, glaucoma, and dilation of the pupil during eye examinations. Ophthalmic drugs are absorbed into the systemic circulation via drainage of the drug into the nasolacrimal ducts and subsequently to the nasopharynx and the GI tract. This is generally a slow process and only small amounts reach the systemic circulation; thus, ophthalmic drugs cause few systemic adverse effects. Infants are an exception. The concentration of drugs reaching the systemic circulation is higher than in an adult, giving a greater chance for adverse drug events.

The *otic route* is used to treat local conditions of the ear, including infections and accumulations of earwax in the auditory canal. Otic medications should always be brought to room temperature before administration because cold medications may cause dizziness or nausea. Systemic adverse effects from otic preparations are not observed unless the drug is applied to areas of open abrasions or injury, such as a ruptured tympanic membrane.

Drugs are applied by the intranasal route for their local effects on the nasal mucosa or for systemic absorption. Advantages of this route include convenience and rapid onset of action. Local indications include drops or sprays to shrink swollen nasal mucous membranes, loosen secretions, and facilitate drainage. For example, decongestant nasal sprays bring immediate relief from the nasal congestion caused by the common cold (see Chapter 45). Intranasal formulations of corticosteroids are first-line drugs for the treatment of allergic rhinitis due to their effectiveness and high safety margin.

The nasal mucosa also provides an excellent absorptive surface for certain medications to produce systemic actions. Advantages of this route include bypassing digestive enzymes and the first-pass effect in the liver. For example, an intranasal form of vitamin B_{12} (Nascobal) is available that is used for patients lacking intrinsic factor, a substance required for the absorption of this vitamin in the GI tract. Intranasal calcitonin is available to treat osteoporosis. Being a protein, calcitonin would be destroyed by stomach enzymes if given PO (see Chapter 72).

Although the nasal mucosa provides an excellent surface for drug delivery, there is a potential for damage to the ciliated cells within the nasal cavity and mucosal irritation may occur. In addition, large amounts of mucus may block a drug from reaching the nasal mucosa.

The *vaginal route* is used to treat local conditions such as vaginal infections, pain, and itching. The vagina has a rich blood supply, and drugs may be absorbed across the mucosa and produce systemic effects. For example, vaginal creams containing estrogen not only produce local effects on the vagina but also result in significant levels of this hormone in the circulation. The contraceptive NuvaRing, inserted into the vagina, contains estrogen and progestin, which are absorbed and provide contraception protection for a month.

The *rectal route* may be used for either local or systemic drug delivery. It is a safe and effective means of delivering medications to comatose patients or to those who are experiencing nausea and vomiting. Rectal medications are normally in suppository form, although a few laxatives and diagnostic agents are given via enema. Although absorption is slower than by other routes, the rectal route is reliable provided the medication can be retained by the patient. Venous blood from the lower rectum is not transported to the circulation by way of the liver; thus, the first-pass effect is avoided as are the digestive enzymes of the upper GI tract.

Parenteral Route: The **parenteral route** uses needles to deliver drugs into the skin layers, subcutaneous tissue, muscles, or veins. Less common parenteral delivery methods include administration into arteries (intra-arterial), bone (intraosseous), body cavities (intrathecal), or organs (intracardiac). Parenteral drug administration is more invasive than topical or enteral because of the potential for introducing pathogenic microbes directly into the blood or body tissues.

Intradermal and Subcutaneous Administration: Injection into the skin delivers drugs to the blood vessels that supply the various layers of the skin. Medications may be injected either intradermally or subcutaneously. The major difference between these methods is the depth of injection. An advantage of both methods is that they offer a means of administering drugs to patients who are unable to take medications PO. Drugs administered by these routes avoid digestive enzymes and the hepatic first-pass effect. However, only small volumes can be administered by these routes, and injections can result in pain and swelling at the injection site.

The *intradermal (ID) route* administers drugs into the dermis layer of the skin. Because the dermis contains more blood vessels than the deeper subcutaneous layer, drugs are more readily absorbed. This route is usually employed for allergy and disease screening or for local anesthetic delivery prior to venous cannulation. ID injections are limited to very small volumes of medication, usually only 0.1 to 0.2 mL.

The *subcutaneous route* delivers drugs to the deepest layers of the skin. Insulin, heparin, vitamins, some vaccines, and other medications are given in this area because the sites are easily accessible and provide for rapid absorption. Subcutaneous doses are small in volume, usually ranging from 0.5 to 1 mL.

Intramuscular Administration: The *intramuscular (IM) route* delivers drugs directly into large muscles. Because muscle tissue has a rich blood supply, drugs are quickly absorbed and produce a more rapid onset of action than with oral, ID, or subcutaneous administration. In a few cases, the drug is formulated in an oily, viscous base that promotes slow and continuous absorption from the muscle.

The anatomic structure of muscle permits this tissue to receive a larger volume of drug than the subcutaneous region. Adults with well-developed muscles can tolerate up to 3 mL in the gluteus maximus and gluteus medius muscles. In the deltoid muscle, volumes of 0.5 to 1 mL are recommended.

Intravenous Administration: The *intravenous (IV) route* delivers drugs and fluids directly into the bloodstream for immediate distribution throughout the body. The IV route is used when a very rapid onset of action is desired. Unlike other routes in which absorption may be unpredictable, an exact level of drug in the bloodstream can be attained by fine adjustments to the IV flow rate. Like other parenteral routes, IV drugs bypass the enzymatic processes of the alimentary canal and avoid the first-pass effect of the liver. The IV route is useful for patients who are comatose or otherwise unable to take oral medications.

Although the IV route offers the fastest onset of drug action, it is also the most dangerous. Once injected, the medication cannot be retrieved. If the drug solution or the needle is contaminated, pathogens have a direct route to the bloodstream and body tissues. Patients receiving IV injections must be closely monitored for adverse reactions. Although some adverse reactions occur immediately after injection, others may take hours or days to appear. Antidotes for drugs that can cause potentially dangerous or fatal reactions must always be readily available.

CONNECTION Checkpoint 3.1

Pharmaceutical companies are always exploring novel methods of drug delivery, such as the new soluble films, so that the period of exclusivity of a medication can be extended. From what you learned in Chapter 1, why is exclusivity important to a pharmaceutical company?

Drug Concentration and Dose

For almost all drugs, higher doses produce a faster and greater response. This is because a higher dose produces a greater concentration gradient for diffusion. As an example, consider the antihypertensive drug diltiazem (Cardizem) given as a 100-mg tablet, which is about 50% absorbed. Half of the drug (50 mg) will reach the bloodstream for distribution to target cells. If the dose of diltiazem is doubled to 200 mg, greater amounts of the drug (100 mg) will be absorbed in the bloodstream. Although the percentage absorbed remains the same (50%), the higher dose results in a greater quantity of drug in the blood and, subsequently, more drug is available to produce an action at its target cells. This concept is further explained in Chapter 4.

GI Tract Environment

For medications given by the enteral route, physical and chemical conditions within the GI tract can affect drug absorption. Most absorption occurs in the small intestine because this portion of the GI tract is longer, and the absorptive surfaces of the microvilli are much more extensive as compared to the stomach. Furthermore, the time spent by food and drugs in the stomach is brief, and the thick mucus layer in that organ discourages absorption.

Digestive motility is variable among patients; very rapid motility may speed the drug through the GI tract before complete absorption occurs. Abnormally slow motility may cause the drug to be retained in the stomach, where it is exposed for a longer time to destructive enzymes and high acidity. Fatty foods in the stomach nearly always slow drug absorption. With few exceptions, absorption is most complete when the drug is taken between meals; the presence of food in the stomach may lessen the incidence of nausea and vomiting, but it also slows absorption. All these factors contribute to wide patient variability with regard to absorption and onset of drug action when drugs are administered PO.

Blood Flow to the Absorption Site

Drugs are absorbed faster from areas of the body where blood flow is high. IM injections are placed into large muscles because they have a high blood flow that maximizes absorption. During heart failure or shock, the amount of blood flow to certain tissues is reduced and absorption from the GI tract or IM sites may be diminished. Topical drugs placed on the skin have slow absorption due to the poor blood supply to the upper layers of the skin.

In some circumstances blood flow can be manipulated to purposely slow absorption. For example, local anesthetics can be toxic if absorbed too quickly. To purposely slow absorption, a vasoconstrictor (epinephrine) is sometimes added to local anesthetics to reduce blood flow to the treated region. As another example, applying ice packs to the site can slow the absorption of a drug to the region; adding heat can cause the opposite effect.

Drug Ionization

Ionized molecules are those that carry a positive or a negative charge. Most drugs can exist in either a charged or an uncharged state, depending on the pH of the surrounding fluid. The ionization of a drug affects its ability to cross plasma membranes and to be excreted by the body (see Section 3.6). Aspirin, or acetylsalicylic acid, provides an example of the effects of ionization on absorption, as depicted in Figure 3.4. In the highly acidic environment of the stomach, aspirin is in its nonionized form and is thus readily absorbed and distributed in the bloodstream. As aspirin enters the alkaline environment of the small intestine, however, it becomes ionized. In its ionized form, the aspirin molecule is less likely to be absorbed. Unlike acidic drugs such as aspirin, medications that are weakly basic are in their nonionized form in an alkaline environment; therefore, basic drugs are much more likely to be absorbed in alkaline environments such as the small intestine. In simplest terms, it may help the student to remember the following:

- Acids are absorbed in acids because they are nonionized.
- Bases are absorbed in bases because they are nonionized.

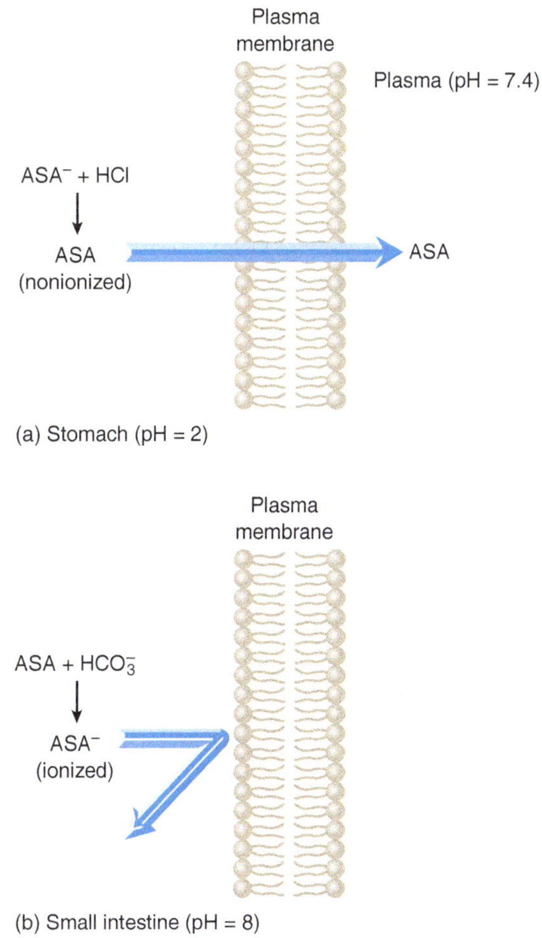

Figure 3.4 Effect of pH on drug absorption. (a) A weak acid such as aspirin (ASA) is in a nonionized form in an acidic environment and absorption occurs. (b) In a basic environment, aspirin is mostly in an ionized form and absorption is prevented.

Drug Interactions

Drug–drug and drug–food interactions have the potential to affect absorption. For example, administering oral tetracyclines with food or drugs containing calcium, iron, or magnesium can significantly delay absorption of the antibiotic. High-fat meals can slow stomach motility significantly and delay the absorption of oral medications taken with the meal. The mechanisms and types of drug interactions are presented in detail in Chapter 5.

Distribution

3.4 Distribution describes how drugs are transported throughout the body.

Distribution is the phase of pharmacokinetics describing the *movement* of medications throughout the body after they are absorbed or injected. Drugs are not simply passive agents, being swept along an inert path to their target tissues. Rather, drugs may interact with blood components and may be chemically and physically changed before reaching their targets. Several key factors influence drug distribution: blood flow to the tissues, drug solubility, tissue storage, and drug–protein binding.

Blood flow to the tissues: The simplest factor determining drug distribution is the amount of blood flow to body tissues. Because the heart, liver, and kidneys receive a great percentage of the blood supply, these organs receive the highest exposure to absorbed or injected drugs. Skin, bone, and adipose tissue receive a meager blood flow; therefore, it is more difficult to deliver high concentrations of drugs to these areas.

Blood flow should also be considered at the local level. For example, after traumatic injury, the blood supply to a fractured bone may be reduced due to damaged blood vessels or blocked by cellular debris from the inflammatory process. Antibiotics may have difficulty reaching the injured area until blood flow can be restored. The delivery of high concentrations of drugs to injured, necrotic, or abscessed areas that have inadequate perfusion is always challenging.

Drug solubility: The physical properties of a drug greatly influence how it moves throughout the body after administration. Lipid solubility is an important characteristic because it determines how quickly a drug is absorbed, mixes within the bloodstream, crosses membranes, and becomes localized in body tissues. Lipid-soluble agents are not limited by the barriers that normally stop water-soluble drugs; thus, they are more completely distributed to body tissues.

Tissue storage: Some tissues have the ability to accumulate and store drugs in high concentrations relative to other tissues. The bone marrow, teeth, eyes, and adipose tissue have an especially high **affinity**, or attraction, for certain medications. Examples of agents that are stored in adipose tissue are diazepam (Valium), lipid-soluble vitamins, and tetracycline, which binds to calcium salts and accumulates in bones and teeth. Once stored in tissues, drugs may remain in the body for many months and be released very slowly back to the circulation. For example, the therapeutic effects of alendronate (Fosamax), a drug for osteoporosis, will continue for 4 to 7 months after the drug is discontinued.

Drug–protein binding: Many drugs bind reversibly to plasma proteins, particularly albumin, to form **drug–protein complexes**. These complexes are too large to cross capillary membranes; the drugs continue circulating in the bloodstream and are unavailable for distribution to their site of action. Medications will remain trapped in the bloodstream bound to plasma proteins until they are released or displaced from the drug–protein complex. Only unbound, or free, drugs can reach their target cells or be excreted by the kidneys. This concept is illustrated in Figure 3.5. Some drugs, such as the anticoagulant warfarin (Coumadin), are highly bound; 99% of the drug in the plasma exists in drug–protein complexes, and only 1% exists as a free drug available to reach target cells.

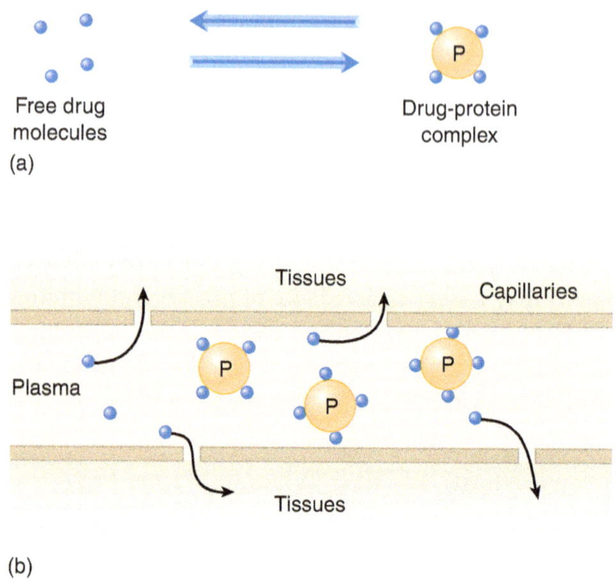

Figure 3.5 Plasma protein binding and drug availability.
(a) The drug exists in a free state or is bound to plasma protein.
(b) Drug–protein complexes are too large to cross membranes.

The number of binding sites on a plasma protein such as albumin is limited. What happens when two or more drugs compete for the same binding sites? The drug that has the greater affinity for these binding sites binds first. This competition for binding sites may result in drug–drug and drug–food interactions when one medication displaces another from plasma proteins. The displaced medication may quickly reach high levels in the blood and produce adverse effects. This is especially important for drugs such as warfarin that have a narrow margin of safety. Most drug guides give the percentage of the drug bound to plasma proteins; when giving multiple medications that are highly bound, the nurse should monitor for potential adverse effects. This topic is discussed further in Chapter 5.

Special barriers to drug distribution: Most capillaries in the body are relatively porous due to spaces between the endothelial cells. Many drugs can exit the bloodstream by traveling through those spaces and enter the interstitial fluid with relative ease. The brain and placenta, however, possess special anatomic barriers that inhibit many chemicals and drugs from exiting the blood. These barriers are referred to as the **blood–brain barrier** and **fetal–placental barrier**.

Unlike other capillaries, those in the brain have endothelial cells that are sealed by tight junctions and a thick basement membrane. The purpose of the blood–brain barrier is obvious: to protect the brain from pathogens and toxic substances. Some highly lipid-soluble agents such as general anesthetics, sedatives, antianxiety agents, and anticonvulsant drugs readily cross the blood–brain barrier to produce their actions on the central nervous system.

In contrast, many antitumor medications and antibiotics do not easily cross this barrier, making brain cancers and infections difficult to treat. The blood–brain barrier becomes more permeable when it is inflamed due to infections such as meningitis.

The fetal–placental barrier prevents certain potentially harmful substances from passing from the mother's bloodstream to the fetus. In reality, the placenta is an inefficient barrier because substances such as alcohol, cocaine, caffeine, and certain prescription medications can easily cross the placental barrier. Consequently, no prescription medication, over-the-counter drug, or herbal therapy should be taken by a pregnant woman without first consulting a healthcare provider. Substances that cause birth defects, or teratogens, are presented in Chapter 5. Chapter 8 discusses special concerns related to pharmacotherapy of pregnant and lactating patients.

Metabolism

3.5 Metabolism is a process that changes the activity of a drug and makes it more likely to be excreted.

Drug **metabolism**, also called *biotransformation*, involves hundreds of complex biochemical pathways and reactions that alter the structure and function of drugs, nutrients, vitamins, and minerals. Although every tissue has the ability to metabolize drugs, the liver is the primary organ of drug metabolism. The kidneys and gastrointestinal tract also have high metabolic rates. The types and rates of metabolic reactions are specific to each type of tissue: Reactions occurring in liver cells are very different from those in skin cells or brain cells.

In most cases, metabolic reactions change the structure of a molecule so that it can be more easily excreted by the body. This often changes the drug from lipid soluble (easily absorbed and distributed) to water soluble (easily excreted by the kidneys). In addition, once the molecule has been changed to water soluble, it is less able to enter tissues. The products of drug metabolism, called *metabolites*, usually have less pharmacologic activity than the original molecule. In this way, metabolism provides an essential *detoxifying effect* for drugs and other substances entering the body.

For a few medications, a metabolite may exhibit a *greater* therapeutic action than the original drug. This is the case for codeine. Although 90% of codeine is changed to inactive metabolites by the liver, 10% is converted to morphine, which has significantly greater ability to relieve severe pain. The metabolite may also have greater toxicity than the original drug. Probably the most common example of this is acetaminophen (Tylenol), which is converted to a metabolite that is highly toxic to the liver.

CONNECTION Checkpoint 3.2

Both codeine and morphine are scheduled drugs. From Chapter 2, which law was enacted to control the manufacturing, importation, possession, and distribution of these drugs?

In a few cases, the drug administered to the patient has no pharmacologic activity at all until it undergoes metabolism. Medications that must undergo metabolism to produce their therapeutic actions are called **prodrugs**. For example, the antihypertensive enalapril (Vasotec) is converted in the liver to a metabolite called enaliprat, which has considerably more ability to lower blood pressure than the original drug. Examples of other prodrugs include benazepril (Lotensin) and losartan (Cozaar).

As shown in Pharmacotherapy Illustrated 3.1, drugs absorbed from the stomach or small intestine cross directly into the hepatic-portal circulation, which carries blood to the liver before it is distributed to other body tissues. Some drugs can be completely metabolized to an inactive form on their first pass through the liver *before they even reach the general circulation*. This **first-pass effect** is important to pharmacology because a large number of oral drugs can be rendered inactive by metabolic reactions in the liver. Alternate routes of delivery, such as the sublingual, rectal, or parenteral routes that bypass the first-pass effect, may be necessary for these drugs.

Hepatic microsomal enzymes: Most metabolism in the liver is accomplished by the **hepatic microsomal enzyme system**. This complex is known as the CYP450 enzyme system, named after cytochrome P450 (CYP450), which is a key component of the system. Although very complex, a key point to remember is that CYP450 is simply an enzyme that metabolizes drugs, as well as toxins, nutrients, and other endogenous substances.

At one time researchers thought that a single CYP450 enzyme was responsible for all drug metabolism, but scientists have since identified more than 50 of them. These different forms are called **isozymes** of CYP450. Although quite similar, each isozyme performs slightly different metabolic functions. CYP450 enzymes are named by assigning numbers to indicate their subfamily, such as CYP1, CYP2, CYP3, and so on. Additional letters and numbers are added to further identify the specific gene, such as CYP1A1, CYP3A4, and CYP26C1. Fortunately for nursing students, only about five of the 50-plus isozymes are responsible for the majority of drug metabolism, as shown in Table 3.1. Indeed, a single isozyme, CYP3A4, is responsible for 30–50% of all drug metabolism in the liver.

Why are the CYP450 enzymes important to pharmacotherapy? They determine the rate at which most drugs are metabolized. In addition, they contribute significantly to drug–drug interactions, possessing the potential to increase or decrease drug action, depending on the specific

Pharmacotherapy Illustrated 3.1

FIRST-PASS EFFECT: Oral Drug Is Metabolized to an Inactive Form Before It Has an Opportunity to Reach Target Cells

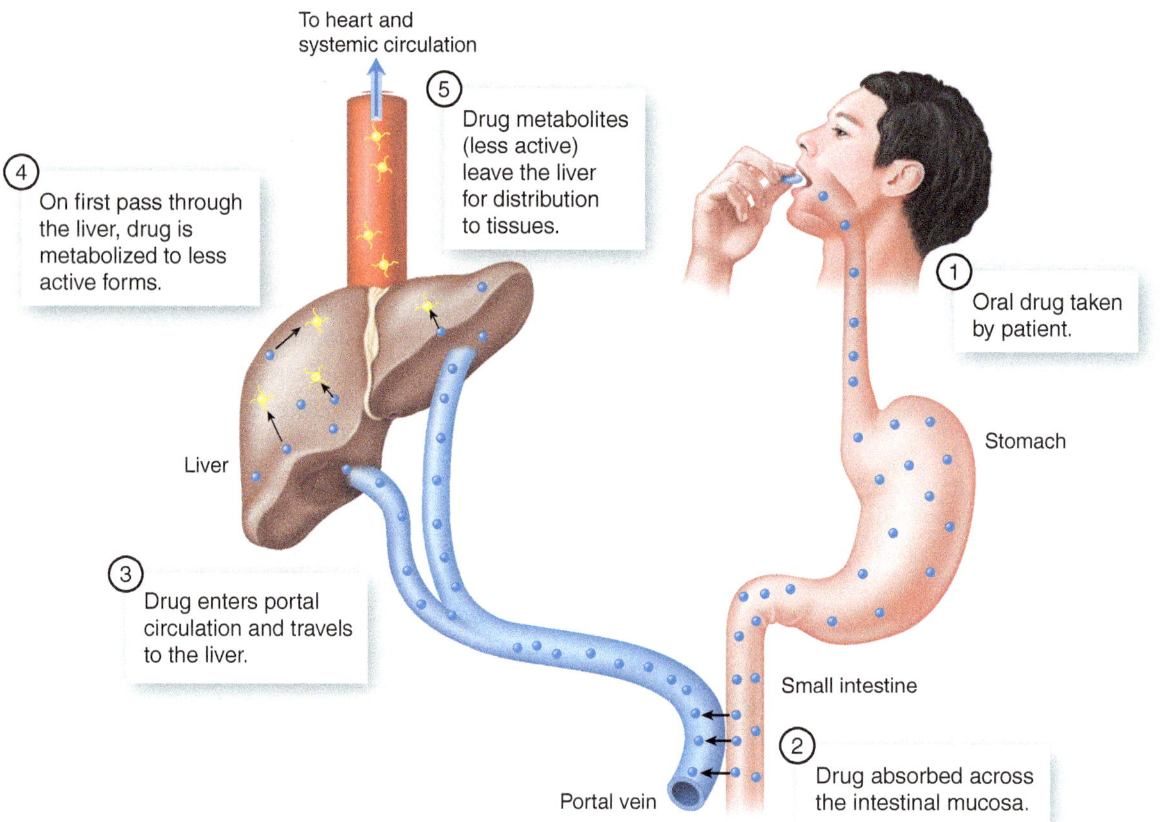

Table 3.1 Selected Isozymes of Cytochrome P450: Substrates, Inducers, and Inhibitors

Isozyme	Substrates	Inducers	Inhibitors
CYP1A2	Caffeine, clozapine, duloxetine, estradiol, naproxen, ondansetron, propranolol tacrine, tamoxifen, tricyclic antidepressants, verapamil, warfarin, zileuton, zolmitriptan	Broccoli, brussels sprouts, carbamazepine, insulin, omeprazole, tobacco	Amiodarone, cimetidine, ciprofloxacin, fluoroquinolones, fluvoxamine, St. John's wort
CYP2C9	Celecoxib, fluoxetine, losartan, nonsteroidal anti-inflammatory drugs (NSAIDs), phenytoin, rosiglitazone, sulfonylureas, tamoxifen, tricyclic antidepressants, valproic acid, warfarin	Carbamazepine, rifampin, secobarbital, St. John's wort	Amiodarone, azole antifungals, fluvoxamine, isoniazid, ritonavir, sertraline, statins, sulfamethoxazole, valproic acid
CYP2C19	Antiepileptics, citalopram, clopidogrel, diazepam, indomethacin, progesterone, propranolol, proton pump inhibitors, sertraline, tricyclic antidepressants, warfarin	Aspirin, carbamazepine, norethindrone, prednisone, ritonavir	Cimetidine, fluvoxamine, isoniazid, ketoconazole, oral contraceptives, proton pump inhibitors
CYP2D6	Amphetamine, antipsychotics, aripiprazole, beta blockers, duloxetine, fluoxetine, lidocaine, metoprolol, ondansetron, opioids, paroxetine, ritonavir, tamoxifen, tramadol, tricyclic antidepressants, venlafaxine	Dexamethasone, rifampin	Bupropion, celecoxib, cimetidine, citalopram, cocaine, diphenhydramine, duloxetine, escitalopram, fluoxetine, paroxetine, ritonavir, sertraline
CYP3A4	Alprazolam, amiodarone, antidepressants, azole antifungals, calcium channel blockers, carbamazepine, chlorpromazine, cocaine, cyclosporine, erythromycin, estradiol, hydrocortisone, lidocaine, methadone, prednisone, propranolol, ritonavir, sildenafil, statins, tamoxifen, testosterone,	Carbamazepine, corticosteroids, efavirenz, nevirapine, oxcarbazepine, phenobarbital, phenytoin, rifampin, St. John's wort	Amiodarone, aprepitant, azole antifungals, cimetidine, ciprofloxacin, diltiazem, erythromycin, fluoxetine, fluvoxamine, grapefruit juice, norfloxacin, protease inhibitors, verapamil

interaction. There are three major possible consequences of CYP 450 drug interactions.

- **Drugs as substrates.** When a drug is metabolized by a CYP450 enzyme, it is said to be a **substrate** for the enzyme. For example, warfarin and NSAIDs such as naproxen are substrates for CYP2C9. Codeine and amphetamine are substrates for a different isozyme, CYP2D6. Each isozyme of CYP450 can metabolize many different drugs, and a drug may be metabolized by multiple CYP450 enzymes. Because of this overlap, two drugs that are administered concurrently may compete for binding sites on the same CYP450 isozyme, resulting in a drug–drug interaction.
- **Drugs as enzyme inhibitors.** Some drugs are able to *inhibit* the action of CYP450 isozymes. The inhibition may affect all hepatic microsomal enzymes or it may be specific to a single isozyme. Inhibiting a CYP450 enzyme could affect the amount of active drug available. For example, ciprofloxacin (Cipro) inhibits CYP1A2. Administering ciprofloxacin concurrently with naproxen (a substrate for CYP1A2) could result in less metabolism of naproxen, higher amounts of naproxen in the blood, and a prolonged drug effect. Giving ciprofloxacin with a more toxic drug such as warfarin (also a substrate for CYP1A2) has the potential to increase levels of warfarin and cause a serious drug interaction. The dose of warfarin would need to be adjusted downward to avoid toxicity. It is important to note that CYP450 enzyme inhibition can occur after a *single dose* of an inhibitor.
- **Drugs as enzyme inducers.** A few drugs have the ability to *increase* metabolic activity in the liver, a process called **enzyme induction**. For example, carbamazepine (Tegretol) causes the liver to synthesize greater amounts of CYP1A2, CYP3A4, and CYP2C9. By doing so, carbamazepine accelerates the metabolism (inactivation) of most drugs metabolized in the liver. Indeed, carbamazepine is contraindicated with most antiviral drugs used to treat human immunodeficiency virus because the interaction may cause loss of therapeutic response to the antiviral drug. Unlike CYP450 inhibition, which can occur after a single dose, enzyme induction generally takes from days to weeks of pharmacotherapy.

Patient variation in metabolism: The baseline level of hepatic microsomal enzyme function is genetically determined. Some patients metabolize at a faster rate, others at a slower rate. Certain genetic disorders have been recognized in which patients lack specific metabolic enzymes. In these "slow metabolizers" average drug doses may cause toxicity. Genetic differences are not always predictable, although some occur at a higher rate in certain ethnic populations (see Chapter 4).

Certain age groups and patients with certain pathologic conditions exhibit diminished hepatic metabolic activity, which may result in altered drug action. Infants do not develop a mature microsomal enzyme system until at least 1 year of age. Hepatic enzyme activity is generally reduced in older adults; thus, these patients may require lower doses. Patients with liver impairment will require reductions in drug dosage because of the decreased metabolic activity.

Chronic alcohol consumption and tobacco use induce certain CYP450 enzymes. St. John's wort, a popular herbal remedy for depression, is an enzyme inducer and can affect the therapeutic response to certain medications. On the other hand, grapefruit juice is an inhibitor of CYP3A4 activity. These examples underscore the importance of obtaining a thorough patient history prior to initiating drug therapy.

Excretion

3.6 Excretion processes remove drugs from the body.

Drugs will continue to act on the body until they are either metabolized to an inactive form or removed from the body by **excretion**. The rate at which a drug is excreted determines its concentration in the blood and, ultimately, its duration of action. Pathologic states, especially liver or kidney disease, often increase the duration and intensity of drug action in the body because they interfere with normal excretion mechanisms.

Renal excretion: The primary site of drug excretion is the kidney. Unbound (free) drugs, water-soluble agents, electrolytes, and small molecules easily pass through the pores of the glomerulus and enter the filtrate in the renal tubule. Proteins, blood cells, and drug–protein complexes are not filtered because of their large size.

After filtration at the renal corpuscle, drugs may undergo reabsorption in the renal tubule. Mechanisms of reabsorption are the same as absorption elsewhere in the body. Nonionized and lipid-soluble drugs cross renal tubular membranes more easily and return to the circulation; ionized and water-soluble drugs generally remain in the filtrate.

Drug–protein complexes and other substances too large to be filtered at the glomerulus are sometimes secreted into the distal tubule of the nephron. For example, only 10% of a dose of penicillin G is filtered; 90% is secreted into the renal tubule. As with metabolic enzyme activity, secretion mechanisms are less active in infants and in older adults.

The renal excretion of drugs is greatly influenced by the pH of the filtrate in the renal tubule. Weak acids like aspirin are excreted more efficiently when the filtrate is slightly alkaline. This is because aspirin is ionized in an alkaline environment, and the ionized drug will remain in the filtrate to be excreted in the urine. Weakly basic drugs such as diazepam (Valium) are excreted more quickly if the filtrate is slightly acidic because they are ionized in that environment. The pH of the filtrate may be intentionally manipulated to speed up renal excretion. For example, following an overdose of an acidic drug such as aspirin, sodium bicarbonate may be administered to make the urine more basic. This basic filtrate ionizes the aspirin molecule, facilitating its urinary excretion. The excretion of diazepam, on the other hand, can be enhanced by giving a drug such as ammonium chloride, which acidifies the filtrate and ionizes the diazepam molecule.

Impairment of kidney function can dramatically affect pharmacokinetics. Patients with renal impairment may retain drugs for extended periods, thus doses for these patients must be reduced to prevent drug toxicity. Because small to moderate changes in renal function can cause rapid increases in serum drug levels, kidney function must be constantly monitored in patients receiving nephrotoxic drugs or medications that have a narrow margin of safety.

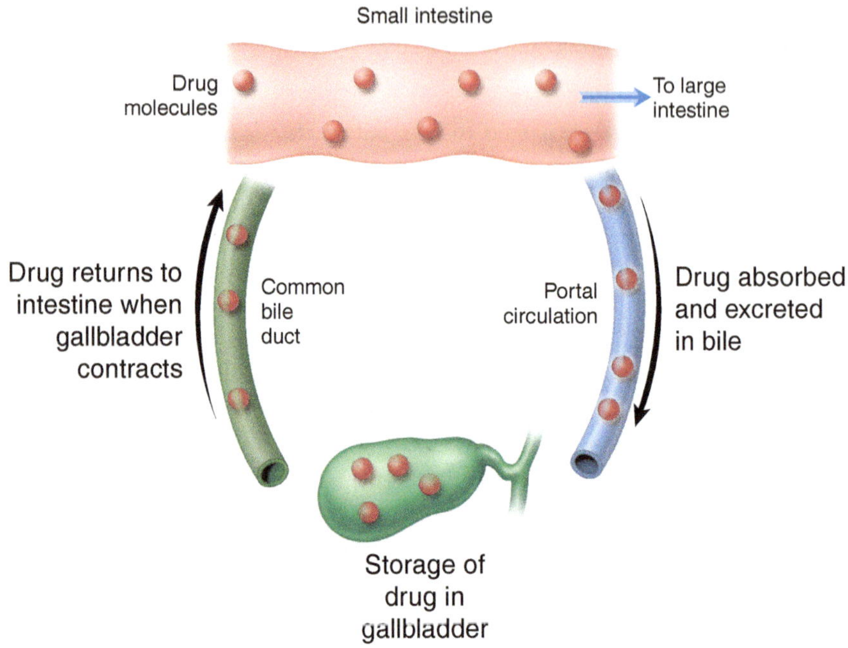

Figure 3.6 Enterohepatic recirculation of a drug can increase its half-life in the body and prolong its duration of action.

Pulmonary excretion: Anesthetics delivered by gas or volatile liquid (liquids that vaporize at room temperature) are especially suited for excretion by the respiratory system. The rate of respiratory excretion is dependent on diffusion, gas solubility, and blood flow to the lungs. The elimination of gaseous and volatile anesthetics following surgery is primarily dependent on respiratory activity: The faster the breathing rate, the more rapid the excretion. On the other hand, the respiratory removal of water-soluble agents such as alcohol is more dependent on blood flow to the lungs: The greater the blood flow through lung capillaries, the greater the pulmonary excretion. In contrast with other methods of excretion, the lungs excrete most drugs in their original unmetabolized form.

Glandular secretion: Some water-soluble drugs are secreted into the saliva, sweat, or breast milk. The "funny taste" that patients experience when given certain drugs is an example of the secretion of medications into saliva. Another example is the garlic smell that can be detected when standing next to a perspiring person who has recently eaten garlic. Excretion into breast milk is of considerable importance for basic drugs such as morphine or codeine because these can achieve high concentrations and potentially affect the nursing infant. Drugs of special concern to the pregnant or breastfeeding patient are discussed in Chapter 8.

Fecal and biliary excretion: After being metabolized, many drugs end up excreted in the feces. Certain oral drugs travel through the GI tract without being absorbed or metabolized. Examples include mebendazole (Vermox), a drug used to kill intestinal worms, and barium sulfate, a radiologic contrast agent.

Some drugs are secreted in bile, a process known as *biliary excretion*. Upon contraction of the gallbladder, drugs in the bile will enter the duodenum and eventually leave the body in the feces. However, some substances in bile are reabsorbed and circulated back to the liver by **enterohepatic recirculation**, as illustrated in Figure 3.6. This is a normal physiologic mechanism for salvaging and reusing useful substances.

Drugs or their metabolites may recirculate numerous times within the bile. This has the result of extending their half-life and possibly prolonging drug action. This is an important route of excretion for tamoxifen, barbiturates, carbamazepine, rifampicin, and oral contraceptives. Recirculated drugs are eventually metabolized by the liver and may be excreted by the kidneys. Recirculation and elimination of drugs through biliary excretion may continue for several weeks after therapy has been discontinued.

Time–Response Relationships

Drug Plasma Levels

3.7 The therapeutic response of most drugs depends on their concentration in the plasma.

The therapeutic response from most drugs is directly related to their concentration in the plasma. Although the concentration of the drug at its target tissue is more predictive of drug action, this quantity is impossible to measure. For example,

CONNECTIONS: Treating the Diverse Patient

Pharmacogenomics: Precisely Prescribing

Pharmacogenomics (PGx) is the use of patient-specific genetic variations to guide medication use and can be a powerful tool for prescribers in the selection of the most effective drugs for patients and to predict increased risks of adverse or subtherapeutic responses to medications. PGx guidance is used in many areas of medicine, including psychiatry, cardiology, and pain management. Today there are hundreds of medications that have been investigated for links to genetic variants. The Food and Drug Administration (FDA; 2018) currently provides information for 284 biomarkers in 214 medications, including multiple boxed warnings that recommend PGx testing before initiating therapy. The PGx tests analyze a subset of variants (also called *single-nucleotide variants*, or *SNPs*) known to be relevant for determining PGx haplotypes of clinical significance. Testing can be performed as either a single-gene assay or as a panel of genes. The price of testing ranges from $250 to $500 and in many cases is covered by insurance plans. Using pharmacogenomics can help healthcare providers look deeper into the genetic codes that promote diseases and potentially make a drug more effective. This has implications for future research into the etiology of diseases and the ability to develop strategies to *prevent* the disease or to halt its progression, not just to provide treatment with the best drug that works with an individual patient's genetic makeup.

although it is possible to conduct a laboratory test that measures the serum level of lithium carbonate (Eskalith) by taking a blood sample, it is a far different matter to measure the quantity of this drug in neurons within the brain.

It is common practice to monitor the plasma levels of drugs that have a low safety margin and to use these data to predict drug action or toxicity. Results of **therapeutic drug monitoring** are used by the healthcare provider to keep the drug dose within a predetermined therapeutic range. For example, the therapeutic range for the antibiotic vancomycin (Vancocin) is 20 to 40 mcg/mL and the toxic level is considered to be greater than 80 mcg/mL. For patients with severe infections, the nurse should carefully monitor these laboratory results to be certain that serum levels of vancomycin fall within the therapeutic range. Dosages would be adjusted upward or downward based on laboratory results and the patient's clinical response. The nurse should always remember, however, that individual responses to drugs are highly variable and patients may experience toxic effects (or no effects) even if the serum concentration of the drug lies in the normal range.

A number of important pharmacokinetic principles can be illustrated by measuring the drug plasma level following a single oral dose. These pharmacokinetic values for a hypothetical drug are shown graphically in Figure 3.7. In this example, the plasma drug level slowly increased and took about 2 hours before the **minimum effective concentration** was reached. The minimum effective drug plasma concentration, the amount of drug required to produce a therapeutic effect, is 6 mcg/mL. The level of drug then entered the **therapeutic range**, which for this drug lies between 6 and 12 mcg/mL. In this range, the drug produced its desired therapeutic action. After peaking, the drug plasma level slowly began to fall out of the therapeutic range due to excretion processes. A higher dose might have caused the drug plasma level to reach a **toxic concentration**, the level of drug that results in serious adverse effects. The goal of pharmacotherapy is to reach and maintain a plasma drug level in the therapeutic range while avoiding the toxic concentration.

These values have great clinical significance. For example, if the patient has a severe headache and is given half of an aspirin tablet, the plasma drug level will likely remain *below* the minimum effective concentration, and the patient will not experience pain relief. Two or three tablets will increase the plasma level of aspirin into the therapeutic range, and the pain will subside. Taking six or more tablets may result in the drug reaching a toxic concentration as evidenced by adverse effects, such as GI bleeding or tinnitus. The goal is to keep each drug's plasma concentration in the therapeutic range. For some drugs, this therapeutic range is quite wide; for others, the difference between a minimum effective dose and a toxic dose can be extremely narrow.

Drug Half-Life

3.8 The drug half-life estimates the duration of action for most medications.

In the example illustrated in Figure 3.7, the serum concentration of the drug reached a peak and then fell back below the therapeutic range. The length of time a drug concentration remains in the therapeutic range is its *duration of action*. In this example, the duration of action was 6 hours. The duration of action is an important pharmacokinetic variable that is determined by how rapidly the drug is metabolized and excreted.

The most common description of a drug's duration of action is its **plasma half-life ($t_{1/2}$)**, the length of time required for the plasma concentration of a drug to decrease by one half after administration. Some drugs have a half-life of only a few minutes, whereas others have a half-life of several hours or days. A few drugs have exceptionally long half-lives; for example, amiodarone (Cordarone) has a $t_{1/2}$ of 40 to 55 days.

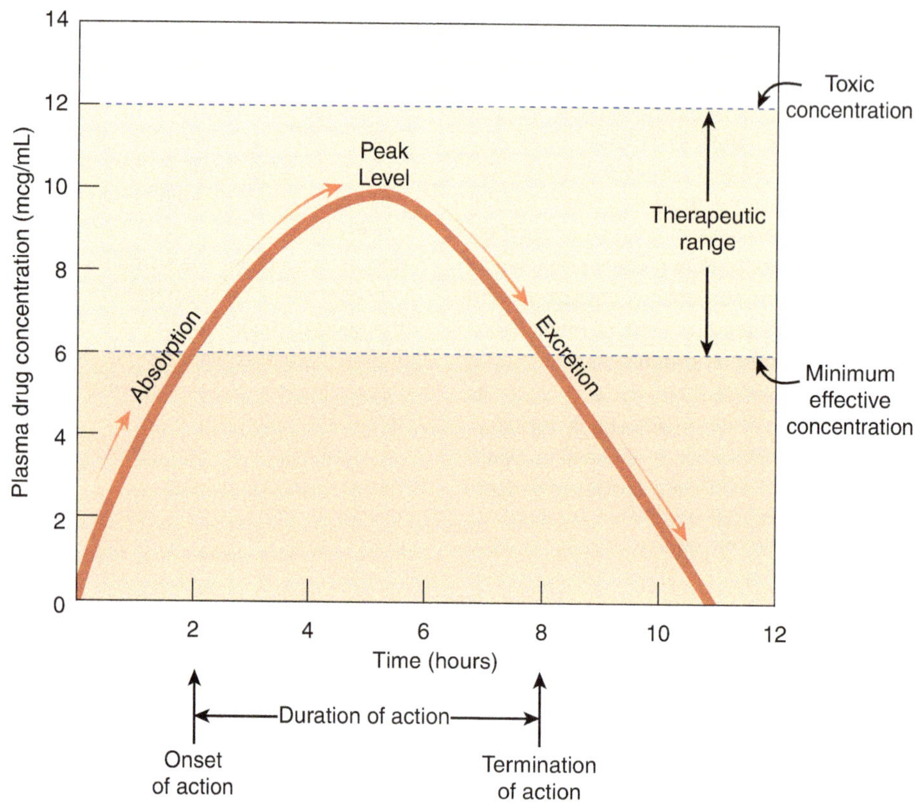

Figure 3.7 Single-dose drug administration. Pharmacokinetic values for this drug are as follows: onset of action = 2 hours; duration of action = 6 hours; termination of action = 8 hours after administration; peak plasma concentration = 10 mcg/mL; time to peak drug effect = 5 hours; $t_{1/2}$ = 4 hours.

Is it better to administer a drug with a short or long half-life? The answer depends on the patient's condition and the treatment goal. Drugs with short half-lives are ideal for conditions and procedures having a brief duration. For example, during a dental procedure, local anesthesia may only be needed for 15 to 20 minutes; thus, procaine, with a half-life of 8 minutes, may be sufficient. Giving a drug with a long duration of action could cause adverse effects after the patient leaves the office. As another example, a simple headache can be relieved with a short-acting drug such as aspirin ($t_{1/2}$ = 15 to 20 minutes), rather than a drug with a 10- or 12-hour duration. Because short-acting drugs are rapidly excreted, the risk of long-term adverse effects is reduced.

Long-duration drugs do have certain advantages. In the preceding example, procaine would not be suitable for a dental procedure that lasts 2 hours because multiple injections would be necessary. Long-duration drugs are beneficial in treating chronic conditions such as heart failure or hypertension and for the prevention of conditions such as migraine headaches, seizures, or pregnancy. Short-acting drugs such as aspirin must be given every 3 to 4 hours, whereas medications with longer half-lives, such as felodipine ($t_{1/2}$ = 10 hours), need to be given only once a day. As drugs stay in the body for prolonged periods, however, the risk for long-term adverse effects increases. This can become particularly serious for patients with significant renal or hepatic impairment; diminished metabolism and excretion will cause the plasma half-life of a drug to increase, and the concentration may reach toxic levels. In these patients, medications must be given less frequently or the dosages must be reduced.

As a rule of thumb, when a drug is discontinued it takes approximately four half-lives before the agent is considered "functionally" eliminated. After four half-lives, 94% of the drug has been eliminated. In the case of procaine with a half-life of only 8 minutes, the drug is considered eliminated in 32 minutes. Although some drug remains, the amount is too small to produce any beneficial or toxic effect. In the example of felodipine ($t_{1/2}$ = 10 hours), the drug would take 40 hours to be eliminated. Note, however, that this "rule of thumb" does not apply to all drugs; it certainly does not apply to medications administered to patients with renal or hepatic impairment.

Loading and Maintenance Doses

3.9 Repeated dosing allows a plateau drug plasma level to be reached.

Few drugs are administered as a single dose. When multiple doses are administered over an extended period, the goal is to keep the drug plasma level *continuously* within the therapeutic range. In other words, the next dose should be administered *before* the drug plasma level falls below the minimum effective concentration.

Multiple doses result in steady concentration of the drug in the bloodstream, as shown in Figure 3.8. When doses are correctly timed, a plateau drug plasma level will be reached and maintained within the therapeutic range. From a pharmacokinetic perspective, at the plateau level the amount of drug absorbed equals the amount of drug being excreted, resulting in a steady therapeutic level of drug being distributed to body tissues. Theoretically, it takes approximately four half-lives to reach this equilibrium. If the medication is given as a continuous infusion, the plateau can be reached very quickly and maintained with little or no fluctuation in drug plasma levels.

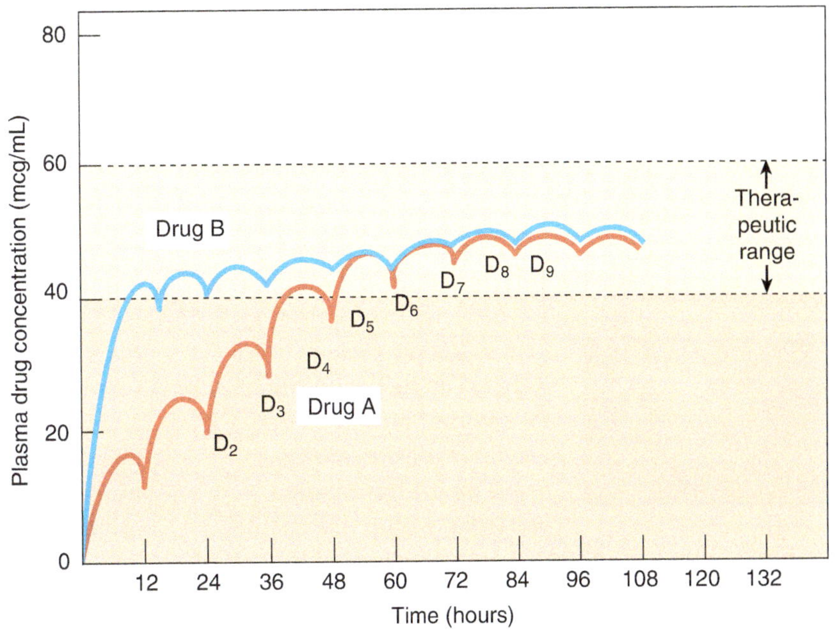

Figure 3.8 Multiple-dose drug administration. Drug A and drug B are administered every 12 hours. Drug B reaches the therapeutic range faster because the first dose is a loading dose.

Note that in Figure 3.8, plasma drug levels are not necessarily smooth and continuous: There are peaks as well as troughs. When giving enteral drugs, there is always some degree of fluctuation in peak concentration and trough concentration levels. A key point is that the peak should not rise into the toxic range, nor should the trough fall below the therapeutic range. Sustained- or extended-release formulations are designed to slowly release the drug so peak and trough fluctuations are minimized. Changing the dosing schedule can also reduce fluctuations. For example, rather than giving 60 mg of codeine once daily, 30 mg bid or 20 mg tid may be given to reduce the possibility of breakthrough pain caused by a wide variation in the peak and trough levels.

The plateau may be reached faster by administration of loading doses followed by regular maintenance doses. A **loading dose** is a higher amount of drug, often given only once or twice, that is administered to "prime" the bloodstream with a level sufficient to quickly induce a therapeutic response. Before plasma levels drop back toward zero, intermittent **maintenance doses** are given to keep the plasma drug concentration in the therapeutic range. Although blood levels of the drug fluctuate with this approach, the equilibrium state can be reached almost as rapidly as with a continuous infusion. Loading doses are particularly important for drugs with prolonged half-lives and for situations in which it is critical to raise drug plasma levels quickly, as might be the case when administering an antibiotic for a severe infection. In Figure 3.8, it took almost five doses (48 hours) before a therapeutic level was reached using a routine dosing schedule. With a loading dose, a therapeutic level was reached within 12 hours.

Understanding Chapter 3

Key Concepts Summary

3.1 Pharmacokinetics focuses on what the body does to drugs after they are administered.

3.2 Drugs use diffusion and active transport to cross plasma membranes to reach their target cells.

3.3 Absorption is the process of moving a drug from the site of administration to the bloodstream.

3.4 Distribution describes how drugs are transported throughout the body.

3.5 Metabolism is a process that changes the activity of a drug and makes it more likely to be excreted.

3.6 Excretion processes remove drugs from the body.

3.7 The therapeutic response of most drugs depends on their concentration in the plasma.

3.8 The drug half-life estimates the duration of action for most medications.

3.9 Repeated dosing allows a plateau drug plasma level to be reached.

CASE STUDY: Making the Patient Connection

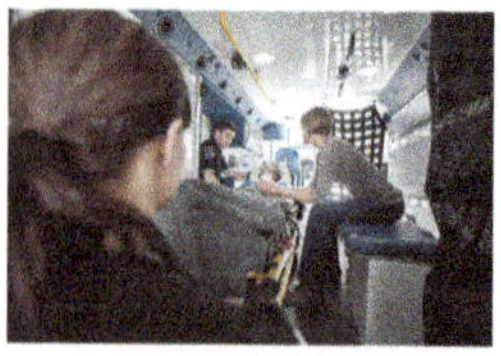

Remember the patient "John Kessler" at the beginning of the chapter? Now read the remainder of the case study. Based on the information presented within this chapter, respond to the critical thinking questions that follow.

John Kessler has been ill for a long time and his prognosis is poor. He is 84 years old with multiple debilitating and chronic conditions. He has had uncontrolled diabetes for more than 20 years and has experienced many complications due to this condition. Three years ago, he developed chronic kidney disease and requires dialysis three times a week. To further complicate his condition, John has continued to consume alcohol every day and smokes one pack of cigarettes per day. He has a long history of both alcohol and tobacco use.

Five days ago, John's daughter noticed that he was becoming increasingly weak and lethargic. Last night when his temperature reached 38.8°C (102°F) and he became confused, his daughter took him to the emergency department, and he was admitted to the medical unit. A chest x-ray this morning revealed bilateral pneumonia. John is receiving multiple medications through both the IV and inhalation routes.

Critical Thinking Questions

1. What factors may influence drug metabolism or excretion in this patient?
2. Discuss why drug elimination for this patient may complicate the pharmacotherapy.
3. How will the IV or inhalation drug therapy affect the absorption of his medications?
4. John will receive a loading dose of IV antibiotic and then be placed on maintenance doses every 6 hours. What is the purpose of this regimen? Why would this patient be a candidate for a loading dose?

Additional Case Study

Janice Albertson is a student nurse caring for a patient on the unit in which you are the RN. She has researched every drug her patient will be receiving and is familiar with the dose, mechanism of action, and possible adverse effects. Now she comes to you and asks, "Why is the drug's plasma half-life listed in the drug reference book? What is the value of this information?"

1. How would you respond to Janice's questions?
2. When is the use of drugs with short half-lives indicated?
3. List the indications for the use of a drug with a long half-life.

Chapter Review

1. The nurse is teaching the patient about a newly prescribed medication. Which statement made by the patient would indicate the need for further medication education?
   1. "The liquid form of the drug will be absorbed faster than the tablets."
   2. "If I take more, I'll have a better response."
   3. "Taking this drug with food will decrease how much drug gets into my system."
   4. "I can consult my healthcare provider if I experience unexpected adverse effects."

2. The nurse is caring for several patients. Which patient will the nurse anticipate is most likely to experience an alteration in drug metabolism?
   1. A 3-day-old premature infant
   2. A 22-year-old pregnant woman
   3. A 32-year-old man with kidney stones
   4. A 50-year-old executive with hypertension

3. The patient is receiving multiple medications, including one drug specifically used to stimulate gastric peristalsis. The nurse knows that this drug could have what influence on additional oral medications?
   1. Increased absorption
   2. Reduced excretion
   3. Decreased absorption
   4. Enhanced distribution

4. A patient is being discharged from the hospital with a nebulizer for self-administration of inhalation medication. Which statement made by the patient indicates to the nurse that patient education has been successful?
   1. "Inhaled medications should only be taken in the morning."
   2. "Doses for inhaled medication are larger than those taken orally."
   3. "Medicines taken by inhalation produce a very rapid response."
   4. "Inhaled drugs are often rendered inactive by hepatic metabolic reactions."

5. The nurse is caring for a patient with hepatitis and resulting hepatic impairment. The nurse would expect the duration of action for most medications to:
   1. Decrease.
   2. Improve.
   3. Be unaffected.
   4. Increase.

6. The nurse is monitoring the therapeutic drug level for a patient on vancomycin (Vancocin) and notes that the level is within the accepted range. What does this indicate to the nurse? (Select all that apply.)
   1. The drug should cause no toxicities or adverse effects.
   2. The drug level is appropriate to exert therapeutic effects.
   3. The dose will not need to be changed for the duration of treatment.
   4. The nurse will need to continue monitoring because each patient response to a drug is unique.
   5. This drug will effectively treat the patient's condition.

See Appendix A for answers to critical thinking questions, case study questions and review questions.

References

Insel, T. (2014). *Blog post by former NIMH Director Thomas Insel: Are children overmedicated?* National Institute of Mental Health, National Institutes of Health. https://www.nimh.nih.gov/about/director/2014/are-children-overmedicated.shtml

U.S. Food and Drug Administration, (2018). *FDA authorizes first direct-to-consumer test for detecting genetic variants that may be associated with medication metabolism.* https://www.fda.gov/NewsEvents/Newsroom/PressAnnouncements/ucm624753.htm

Vangara, K. K., & Samala, S. (2015). Oral transmucosal delivery for improved drug bioavailability and patient compliance. *Journal of Bioequivalence & Bioavailability, 7,* e58. https://doi.org/10.4172/jbb.10000e58

Selected Bibliography

Allen, L. V. (2018). *Ansel's pharmaceutical dosage forms and drug delivery systems* (11th ed.). Wolters Kluwer

Brunton, L. L., Hilal-Dandan, R., & Knollmann, B. C. (Eds.). (2018). *Goodman & Gilman's the pharmacological basis of therapeutics* (13th ed.). McGraw-Hill.

Durendorf, H., & Schmidt, S. (2019). *Rowland & Tozer's clinical pharmacokinetics and pharmacodynamics: Concepts and applications* (5th ed.). Wolters Kluwer.

Faheem, A. M., & Abdelkader, D. H. (2020). Novel drug delivery systems. In A. Seyfoddin, S. M. Dezfooli, & C. A. Greene (Eds.), *Engineering drug delivery systems* (pp. 1–16). Woodhead Publishing.

Rosenbaum, S. E. (2016). *Basic pharmacokinetics and pharmacodynamics: An integrated textbook and computer simulations* (2nd ed.). Wiley.

Shargell, L., & Yu, A. (2016). *Applied biopharmaceutics and pharmacokinetics* (7th ed.). McGraw-Hill.

Southwood, R., Fleming, V. & Huckaby, G. (2018). *Concepts in clinical pharmacokinetics* (7th ed.). American Society of Health-Systems Pharmacists.

Tornio, A., & Backman, J. T. (2018). Cytochrome P450 in pharmacogenetics: An update. In K. Brosen & P. Damkier (Eds.), *Advances in pharmacology: Vol. 83. Pharmacogenetics* (pp. 3–32). Academic Press.

van den Anker, J., Reed, M. D., Allegaert, K., & Kearns, G. L. (2018). Developmental changes in pharmacokinetics and pharmacodynamics. *Journal of Clinical Pharmacology, 58,* S10–S25. https://doi.org/10.1002/jcph.1284

"I am totally confused by all the antacid commercials on television. Some say their medication is the most efficient and others claim their brand is the most potent. What does it all mean?"
—*Patient "Katherine Hunter"*

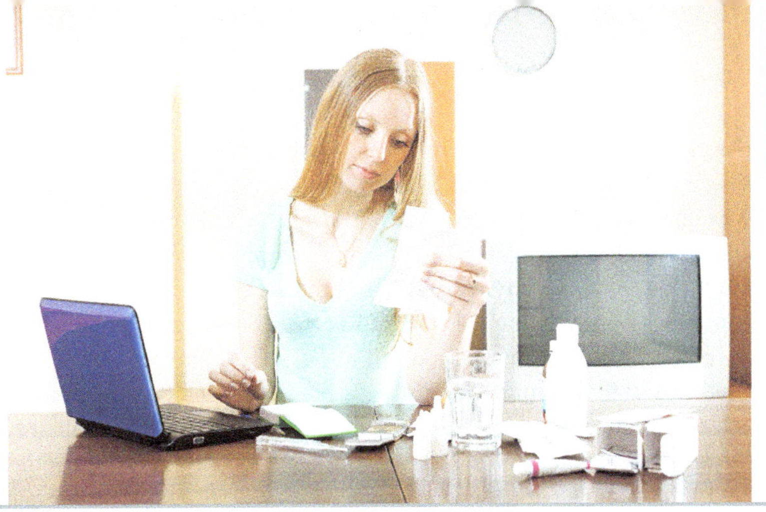

Chapter 4
Pharmacodynamics

Chapter Outline

- Interpatient Variability
- Therapeutic Index
- Dose–Response Relationship
- Potency and Efficacy
- Receptor Theory
- Agonists and Antagonists
- Pharmacogenetics

Learning Outcomes

After reading this chapter, the student should be able to:

1. Apply frequency distribution curves to explain interpatient variability in medication response.
2. Explain the importance of the median effective dose (ED_{50}) to clinical practice.
3. Compare and contrast median lethal dose (LD_{50}) and median toxicity dose (TD_{50}).
4. Relate a drug's therapeutic index to its margin of safety.
5. Identify the significance of the dose–response relationship to clinical practice.
6. Compare and contrast the terms *potency* and *efficacy*.
7. Describe the relationship between receptors and drug action.
8. Distinguish between an agonist, partial agonist, and antagonist.
9. Explain possible future developments in the field of pharmacogenetics.

Key Terms

Definitions of the terms in bold may be found in the Glossary.

The term *pharmacodynamics* comprises the root words *pharmaco*, which refers to medicines, and *dynamics*, which means "change." In simplest terms, pharmacodynamics refers to *how a drug changes the body*. A more complete definition defines **pharmacodynamics** as the branch of pharmacology concerned with the mechanisms of drug action and the relationships between drug concentration and responses in the body. This chapter examines the mechanisms by which drugs affect patients and how the nurse can apply these principles to clinical practice.

Interpatient Variability

4.1 Patients have widely different responses to drugs, which can be depicted on a frequency distribution curve.

The principles of pharmacodynamics have important clinical applications. Healthcare providers must be able to predict whether a given dose of medication will produce a therapeutic change in their patients. Why does the "average" dose obtained from a drug guide sometimes produce a hyperresponse and at other times no response at all? Knowledge of dose–response relationships, therapeutic indexes, and drug–receptor interactions—all topics of pharmacodynamics—can help nurses provide safer and more effective treatment.

The interpatient variability observed during drug therapy can be illustrated by examining a frequency distribution curve. Shown in Figure 4.1, a **frequency distribution curve** is a graphic representation of the number of patients responding with a particular drug action at different doses. On the horizontal axis, notice the wide range in doses that produced the patient responses shown on the curve. A few patients responded to the drug at very low doses (10 to 20 mg). As the dose was increased, more and more patients responded. The peak of the curve (50 mg) indicates the largest number of patients responding to the drug. Some patients required very high doses (80 to 90 mg) to elicit the desired response. The curve does not show the magnitude of the response, only whether or not a measurable response occurred among the patients. As an example, think of possible patient responses to an antihypertensive drug as defined by a reduction of 20-mm in systolic blood pressure. Every patient on the graph experienced this 20-mm reduction. A few patients experienced the desired 20-mm reduction at a dose of only 10 mg; a 50-mg dose gave the largest number of patients the 20-mm blood pressure reduction. However, a few patients needed as much as 90 mg of the drug to produce the same 20-mm reduction.

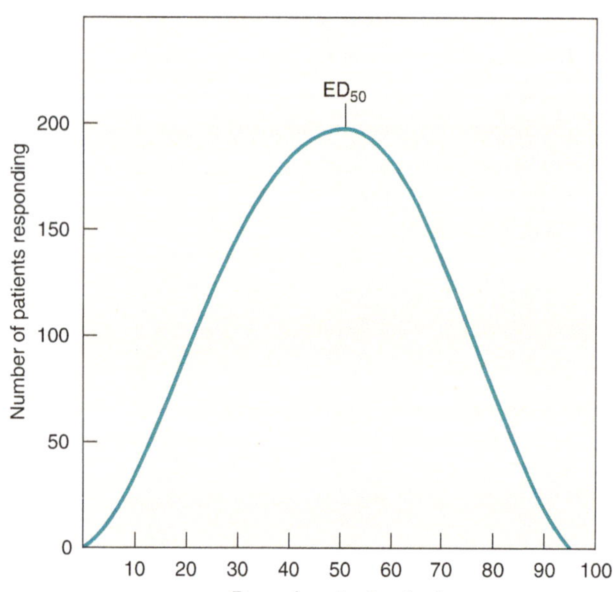

Figure 4.1 Frequency distribution curve: Interpatient variability in drug response.

The dose in the middle of the frequency distribution curve represents the drug's **median effective dose (ED_{50})**. The ED_{50} is the dose required to produce a specific therapeutic response in 50% of a group of patients. Drug guides usually use the ED_{50} as the "average" or standard dose for a drug.

The interpatient variability illustrated in Figure 4.1 has important clinical implications. First, the nurse should realize that the standard or average dose may predict a satisfactory therapeutic response for only about half the population. Many patients will require more or less than the average dose for optimal pharmacotherapy. Using the systolic blood pressure example, assume that a large group of patients is given the average dose of 50 mg. Some of these patients will experience toxicity at this level because they need only 10 mg to achieve blood pressure reduction. A few patients in this group will probably have no reduction in blood pressure at all. By monitoring the patient, taking vital signs, and interpreting any associated laboratory data, the nurse is key in determining whether the average dose is effective for the patient. *It is not enough to simply memorize an average dose for a drug; the nurse must have the skills to know when and how this dose should be adjusted to obtain the optimal therapeutic response.*

Therapeutic Index

4.2 The therapeutic index describes a drug's margin of safety.

Selecting a dose that produces an optimal therapeutic response for each individual is certainly important, but the nurse must also be able to predict whether that dose is safe for that patient. Frequency distribution curves can also be used to illustrate the safety of a drug.

The **median lethal dose (LD_{50})** is a value determined in laboratory animals in preclinical experiments during the drug development process. The LD_{50} is the dose of drug that will kill 50% of a group of animals. Just as with ED_{50}, a population of animals will exhibit considerable variability in lethal dosage; what may be a nontoxic dose for one animal may kill another.

To examine the safety of a particular drug, the LD_{50} is compared to ED_{50}, as shown in Figure 4.2a. In this example, 10 mg of drug is the average effective dose, and 40 mg is the average lethal dose. The ED_{50} and LD_{50} are used to calculate an important value in pharmacology, a drug's therapeutic index. The **therapeutic index (TI)** is defined as the ratio of a drug's LD_{50} to its ED_{50}.

The larger the difference between the two doses, the greater the TI. In Figure 4.2a, the TI is 4 (40 mg ÷ 10 mg). Essentially, this means that it would take an error in magnitude of approximately four times the average dose to be lethal to an average patient. In terms of dosage, this would be considered a relatively safe drug because small to moderate medication errors or changes in the drug's bioavailability would likely not be fatal. Thus, the TI is a measure of a drug's **margin of safety**: the higher the value, the safer the medication. Drugs exhibit a wide range of TIs, from 1 to 2 to greater than 100.

As another example, the TI of a second drug is shown in Figure 4.2b. Drug Z has the same ED_{50} as drug X but shows a different LD_{50}. The TI for drug Z is only 2 (20 mg ÷ 10 mg). The difference between an effective dose and a lethal dose is very small for drug Z; thus, the drug has a narrow safety margin. Small medication errors or changes in the drug's metabolism or excretion could have lethal consequences. The TI offers the nurse practical information on the safety of a drug and a means to compare one drug to another.

In Figure 4.2b, notice that the two curves overlap. Some patients required a dose of 15 to 20 mg to produce the desired effect, yet this same dose was lethal in other patients. This type of drug would require careful assessment of hepatic and renal function prior to the initiation of therapy. With drugs exhibiting a low TI, it is prudent to begin with the lowest dose possible and then increase the amount of drug with careful monitoring.

Because the LD_{50} cannot be experimentally determined in humans, other estimates of drug safety are available. The **median toxicity dose (TD_{50})** is the dose that will produce a given toxicity in 50% of a group of patients. The TD_{50} value may be extrapolated from animal data or based on adverse effects recorded in patient clinical trials.

CONNECTION Checkpoint 4.1

From what you learned in Chapter 2, before a pharmaceutical company tests a drug in patients after preclinical trials have been completed, what document must be submitted to the U.S. Food and Drug Administration (FDA)?

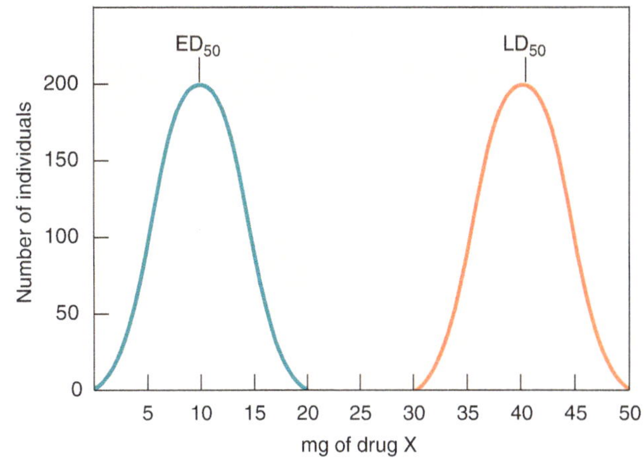

(a) Drug X : $TI = \frac{LD_{50}}{ED_{50}} = \frac{40}{10} = 4$

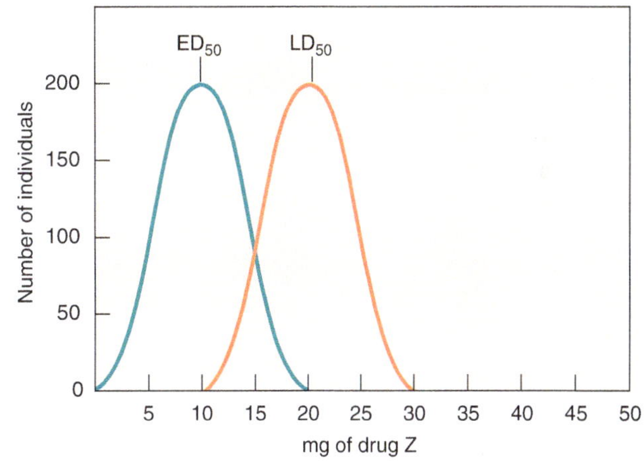

(b) Drug Z : $TI = \frac{LD_{50}}{ED_{50}} = \frac{20}{10} = 2$

Figure 4.2 Therapeutic index. (a) Drug X has a therapeutic index of 4. (b) Drug Z has a therapeutic index of 2.

Dose–Response Relationship

4.3 The dose–response relationship describes how the actions of a drug change with increasing dose.

In the preceding section, frequency distribution curves were used to graphically visualize interpatient differences in responses to medications in a *population*. Pharmacodynamics is also used to study the variability in responses in a *single patient*.

How does a patient respond to varying doses of a drug? Common sense would suggest that a larger dose would produce more drug effect. For example, an antibiotic would kill more bacteria if the dose was increased from 10 to 20 mg. An antihypertensive drug would cause a greater reduction in blood pressure if the dose was increased from 50 to 100 mg. These simple examples describe the **dose–response relationship**, one of the most fundamental concepts in pharmacology. A graphic representation of this relationship, the *dose–response curve*, is illustrated in Figure 4.3. Examining

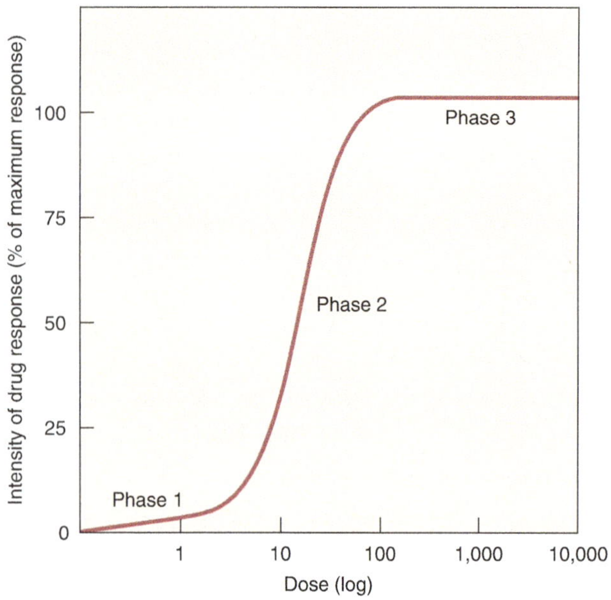

Figure 4.3 Dose–response relationship.

and comparing dose–response curves can yield a large amount of information about a drug.

A dose–response curve illustrates the dose administered versus the degree of response obtained. A dose–response curve has three distinct phases that indicate essential pharmacodynamic principles. Phase 1 occurs at the lowest doses. The flatness of this portion of the curve indicates that few target cells have been affected by the drug; doses that are too small will not produce a therapeutic effect. Phase 2 is the rising, straight-line portion of the curve. In this portion, there is a linear relationship between the amount of drug administered and the degree of response obtained from the patient. For example, if the dose is doubled, twice as much response may be obtained. This is the most desirable range of doses for pharmacotherapeutics because giving more drug results in proportionately more effect; a lower drug dose gives less effect. In phase 3 increasing the drug dose produces no additional therapeutic response—a plateau has been reached. This may occur for a number of reasons. One possible explanation is that all the target receptors for the drug are occupied. It could also mean that the drug has brought 100% relief, such as when a migraine has been terminated; giving higher doses produces no *additional* relief. Although increasing the dose during phase 3 does not result in additional therapeutic effects, the nurse should be mindful that increasing the dose may produce more adverse effects.

The dose–response curve in Figure 4.3 is smooth and continuous; thus, it is sometimes called a *graded* dose–response curve. This is important to pharmacotherapeutics because, by adjusting the dose in small increments, the prescriber is able to attain virtually any degree of therapeutic response (0–100%) within the linear range of drug doses. This is especially true when using the intravenous (IV) route, during which the nurse can adjust the infusion rate in very small increments.

Many types of adverse effects *also* follow a graded dose–response relationship: the higher the dose, the more intense the adverse effect. By adjusting the dose lower, while still keeping it within the therapeutic range, adverse effects may be lessened. Some adverse effects, such as anaphylaxis, are independent of dose in that even the smallest amount of drug may trigger a serious adverse response (see Chapter 5).

Potency and Efficacy

4.4 Potency and efficacy are fundamental concepts of pharmacodynamics that describe a drug's activity.

Within a pharmacologic class, not all drugs are equally effective at treating a disorder. For example, some antineoplastic drugs kill more cancer cells than others; some antihypertensive medications lower blood pressure to a greater extent than others; and some analgesics are more effective at relieving severe pain than others in the same class. Furthermore, drugs in the same class are effective at different doses: One antibiotic may be effective at a dose of 1 mg/kg, whereas another is most effective at 100 mg/kg. Nurses need a method to compare one drug to another so that they can administer treatment effectively.

There are two fundamental ways to compare medications within therapeutic and pharmacologic classes. First is the concept of **potency**, which is the *amount of drug needed to produce a specified effect*. When compared to another drug in the same class, a drug that is more potent will produce its therapeutic effect at lower doses. As an example, consider two calcium channel blockers used for hypertension: amlodipine (Norvasc) and nifedipine (Procardia). Amlodipine produces its decrease in blood pressure at a dose of 10 mg/day and nifedipine at 60 mg/day. Amlodipine is clearly more potent than nifedipine because it takes a lower dose (six times less) to produce its antihypertensive effect.

Thus, potency is a way to compare the doses of two independently administered drugs in terms of how much is needed to produce a particular response. A useful way to visualize the concept of potency is by examining dose–response curves. When comparing the two drugs shown in Figure 4.4a, drug A is more potent because it requires a lower dose to produce the same response.

A second method used to compare drugs is by **efficacy**, which is defined as the *maximum response that can be produced* from a particular drug. In the example in Figure 4.4b, drug A has greater efficacy because it produces a higher maximal response.

Which is more important to the outcomes of pharmacotherapy: potency or efficacy? Perhaps the best way to understand these important concepts is to use the specific example of headache pain. Two common over-the-counter (OTC)

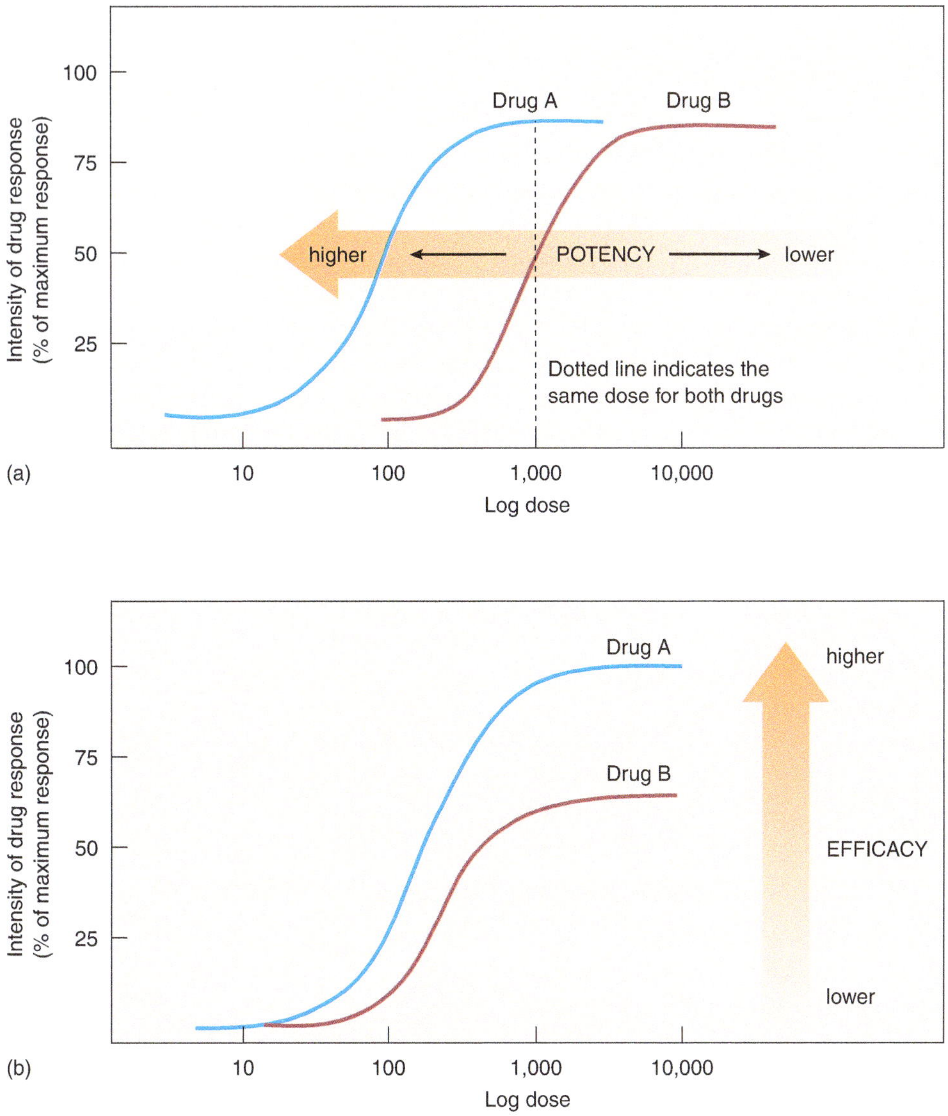

Figure 4.4 Potency and efficacy. (a) Drug A has a higher potency than drug B. (b) Drug A has a higher efficacy than drug B.

analgesic therapies are ibuprofen (200 mg) and aspirin (650 mg). The fact that ibuprofen relieves pain at a lower dose indicates that it is more potent than aspirin. At their average doses, however, both are equally effective at relieving headaches; thus, they have the same efficacy. If the patient is experiencing severe pain, however, neither aspirin nor ibuprofen has sufficient efficacy to bring relief. Narcotic analgesics, such as morphine, have a greater efficacy than aspirin or ibuprofen and could effectively treat this type of pain. From a pharmacotherapeutic perspective, efficacy is almost always more important than potency. In the preceding example, the average dose is unimportant to the patient, but headache relief is essential. As another comparison, the patient with cancer is much more concerned with how many cancer cells have been killed (efficacy) than with the dose the nurse administered (potency). In the comparison of Norvasc to Procardia, although Norvasc is clearly more potent, both drugs reduce blood pressure to the same degree; thus, they have the same efficacy. Although the nurse will often hear claims that one drug is more potent than another, a more compelling concern is which drug has greater efficacy.

A word of caution is necessary at this point. In Section 4.3, it is stated that many adverse effects are related to dose—that higher doses produce more intense adverse effects. This is true only when comparing doses of the *same* drug. For example, a therapeutic dose for amlodipine is 10 mg/day. Giving 20 or 30 mg of amlodipine will most certainly increase the risk of experiencing an adverse effect. Can the dose of amlodipine be compared to a dose of nifedipine, which is 60 mg/day? The answer is *absolutely not*. In fact, 10 mg of amlodipine gives the same risk of adverse effects as 60 mg of nifedipine. *The point is that when two different drugs are compared, one cannot assume that the drug with the lower dose gives fewer adverse effects.*

An additional word of caution is necessary. In clinical practice the term *potency* is often misused to indicate a more effective drug. The nurse should remember the correct definitions of the words *potency* and *efficacy* and try to incorporate them into clinical practice.

Receptor Theory

4.5 Most drugs produce their actions by activating or inhibiting specific cellular receptors.

Drugs rarely create new actions in the body; instead, they enhance or inhibit *existing* physiologic and biochemical processes. To cause these changes, the drug must interact with specific chemicals that are normally found in the body. A cellular molecule to which a medication binds to produce its effects is called a **receptor**. A receptor may be thought of as the drug's specific target. The concept of a drug binding to a receptor and causing a change in physiology is a fundamental concept in pharmacology. Receptor theory predicts that the response of a drug is proportional to the concentration of receptors that are bound or occupied by the drug. Receptor theory explains the mechanisms by which most drugs produce their effects.

It is important to understand, however, that receptors do not exist in the body solely to bind drugs; their normal function is to bind endogenous molecules such as hormones, neurotransmitters, and growth factors. The drug simply uses *existing* targets to cause its effects. When drugs bind to the receptor they either enhance or inhibit a normal cellular function. The binding is usually reversible and the action of the drug is terminated once the drug leaves its receptor. In a few cases, binding of the drug is irreversible. Drugs that have the ability to bind to a receptor and produce a strong action are said to have high **intrinsic activity**. Intrinsic activity and efficacy are related. Drugs that have high intrinsic activity have high efficacy.

Although a drug receptor can be any type of molecule, the vast majority are proteins. As shown in Figure 4.5, a receptor may be depicted as a three-dimensional protein spanning across the plasma membrane. The extracellular component of a receptor often consists of subunits arranged in a specific shape that will bind the specific drug or endogenous chemical (sometimes called a *ligand*). The receptor may form a membrane channel that regulates substances entering and leaving the cell.

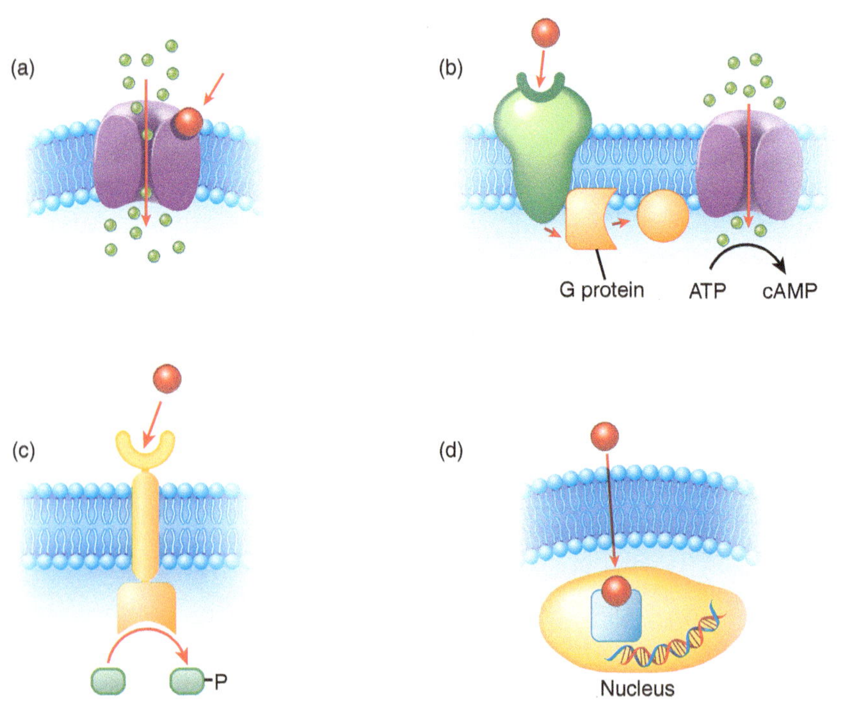

Figure 4.5 Types of cellular receptors. (a) Drug binds to the receptor opening channel. (b) Drug binds to the receptor, causing a G protein–mediated reaction in the cell. (c) Drug binds to the transmembrane receptor to signal a change inside the cell. (d) Drug enters the cell nucleus to increase synthesis of specific proteins.

A drug binds to its receptor in a very selective manner, much like a lock and key. Once the receptor is occupied, a series of **second-messenger** events is triggered within the cell, such as the conversion of adenosine triphosphate (ATP) to cyclic adenosine monophosphate (cyclic AMP), the release of intracellular calcium, or the activation of specific G proteins and associated enzymes. These cascades of biochemical events initiate the drug's action by either stimulating or inhibiting the normal activity of the cell. Small changes to the structure of a drug, or its receptor, may weaken or even eliminate binding between the two molecules, rendering the drug ineffective.

Not all receptors are proteins bound to the plasma membrane. Some are intracellular molecules such as DNA, RNA, or enzymes in the cytoplasm. By interacting with these types of receptors, medications are able to inhibit protein synthesis or regulate events such as cell division and metabolism. Examples of agents that bind intracellular components include steroid hormones and certain vitamins.

Receptor *subtypes* have been discovered that permit the "fine-tuning" of pharmacotherapy. For example, the first drugs affecting the autonomic nervous system affected *all* types of autonomic receptors. These agents were not very useful because they produced such a broad range of therapeutic and adverse effects. Later, it was discovered that two basic receptor types existed in the body, alpha and beta, and drugs were then developed that were selective for only one type. This permitted more specific drug therapy (and fewer adverse effects). Still later, several subtypes of alpha and beta receptors, including alpha-1, alpha-2, beta-1, and beta-2, were discovered that allowed even more specificity in pharmacotherapy. In recent years, researchers have further divided and refined various drug receptor subtypes.

Some drugs act independently of cellular receptors. These medications are associated with other mechanisms, such as changing the permeability of cellular membranes, depressing membrane excitability, or altering the activity of cellular pumps. Actions such as these are often described as *nonspecific* cellular responses. Ethyl alcohol, general anesthetics, and osmotic diuretics are examples of agents that act by nonspecific mechanisms.

Agonists and Antagonists

4.6 Agonists, partial agonists, and antagonists compete for cellular receptors and can modify drug action.

When a drug binds to a receptor, several possible consequences can result. In simplest terms, some specific action in the cell is either enhanced or inhibited. The actual biochemical mechanism underlying the therapeutic effect may be extremely complex and, in some cases, the mechanism of drug action is not known.

When a drug binds to its receptor, it may produce a response that mimics the effect of the endogenous regulatory molecule. For example, when the drug bethanechol is administered, it binds to acetylcholine receptors in the autonomic nervous system and produces the same actions as acetylcholine. A drug that activates a receptor and produces the *same* type of response as the endogenous substance is called an **agonist**. Agonists sometimes produce a greater maximal response than the endogenous chemical. The term **partial agonist** is used to describe a medication that produces a weaker response than a full agonist.

A second possibility is that a drug will occupy a receptor and *prevent* the endogenous chemical from binding to produce its action. This type of drug, an **antagonist**, often competes with agonists for receptor binding sites. For example, the drug atropine competes with acetylcholine for certain receptors in the autonomic nervous system. If the dose is high enough, atropine may completely block the effects of acetylcholine because acetylcholine can no longer reach its receptors. Antagonists may be used as medications when the body is producing too much of a response from an endogenous chemical or from a drug overdose, such as high blood pressure, fast heart rate, secretion of excess stomach acid, or sedation. Giving an antagonist in these situations may reverse the adverse effects. An antagonist has no intrinsic activity; the actions observed after administering an antagonist are caused by lack of agonist action.

Not all antagonism is associated with receptors. *Functional* antagonists inhibit the effects of an agonist, not by competing for a receptor but by changing pharmacokinetic factors. For example, antagonists may slow the absorption of an agonist, resulting in less pharmacologic effect. An antagonist may change the pH of the surrounding fluid and neutralize the agonist before it is even absorbed. By speeding up metabolism or excretion, an antagonist can enhance the removal of an agonist from the body. The relationships that occur between agonists and antagonists explain many of the drug–drug and drug–food interactions that occur in the body (described in Chapter 5). Figure 4.6 illustrates the concept of agonist and antagonist drug action.

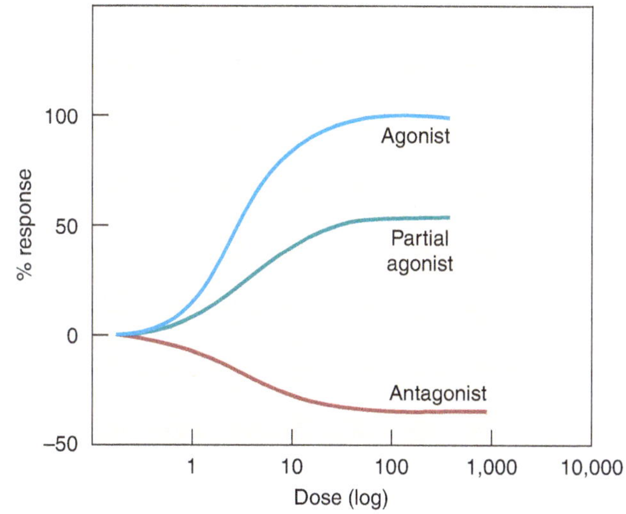

Figure 4.6 Effects of agonists, partial agonists, and antagonists on drug response. (a) An agonist results in maximum response. (b) A partial agonist results in less than maximum response. (c) An antagonist results in diminished response.

CONNECTION Checkpoint 4.2

From what you learned in Chapter 3, phenytoin is an inducer of CYP1A2, the enzyme that metabolizes acetaminophen. Would phenytoin be considered a functional agonist or an antagonist to acetaminophen?

Pharmacogenetics

4.7 In the future, pharmacogenetics may allow customization of drug therapy.

As discussed earlier in this chapter, patients can have widely differing responses to medications. A significant portion of the population either develops unacceptable adverse effects to certain drugs or is unresponsive to them. Is it possible to predict, in advance, which patients will experience these types of responses? For example, is it possible to predict which of 100 antineoplastic drugs will be most effective at killing a tumor without major adverse effects, or which of 50 antidiabetic drugs will be most effective at maintaining a particular patient's blood glucose levels?

Pharmacogenetics is the branch of pharmacology that studies how people respond differently to drug therapy based on their genetic makeup. The most important advances in pharmacogenetics so far have been the identification of genetic differences in drug-metabolizing enzymes and target receptors. The FDA has identified over 400 pharmacogenetic biomarkers that have the potential to influence drug therapy. These biomarkers are included in drug labeling information (FDA, 2020). In some cases, the biomarker information in the drug label includes specific action that the prescriber should take if their patient has a specific biomarker. For example, the recommendation may include changing the dose or selecting an alternative drug for patients exhibiting the biomarker.

CONNECTIONS: Treating the Diverse Patient

Enzyme Deficiencies in Ethnic Populations

The 2019 coronavirus disease (COVID-19) pandemic presented serious adverse implications for populations and the health-care and public health systems. Early indications suggest that there is an association between ethnic ancestry, and outcomes of COVID-19. While there is limited research available, a possible association between glucose-6-phosphate dehydrogenase (G6PD) deficiency and COVID-19 has been suggested (Al-Abdi & Al-Aamri, 2020). G6PD deficiency is a common, recessive genetic condition, with about 400 million people affected worldwide.

A study published in 2008 looked at another human coronavirus, HCoV229E, and its effect on patients with G6PD. The investigators found that patients with G6PD-deficient cells were indeed more susceptible to HCoV229E infection (Wu et al., 2008). COVID-19 is even more concerning for G6PD-deficient patients since hydroxychloroquine has been proposed as a treatment. Hydroxychloroquine has oxidative properties and for G6BD-deficient patients certain oxidative drugs cause an acute hemolysis of red blood cells (RBCs) due to the breaking of chemical bonds in the hemoglobin molecule, leading to large numbers of circulating RBCs being destroyed (La Vieille et al., 2019). If hydroxychloroquine is found to be a standard treatment for COVID-19, this could be a challenge for G6PD-deficient patients.

Understanding Chapter 4

Key Concepts Summary

4.1 Patients have widely different responses to drugs, which can be depicted on a frequency distribution curve.

4.2 The therapeutic index describes a drug's margin of safety.

4.3 The dose–response relationship describes how the actions of a drug change with increasing dose.

4.4 Potency and efficacy are fundamental concepts of pharmacodynamics that describe a drug's activity.

4.5 Most drugs produce their actions by activating or inhibiting specific cellular receptors.

4.6 Agonists, partial agonists, and antagonists compete for cellular receptors and can modify drug action.

4.7 In the future, pharmacogenetics may allow customization of drug therapy.

CASE STUDY: Making the Patient Connection

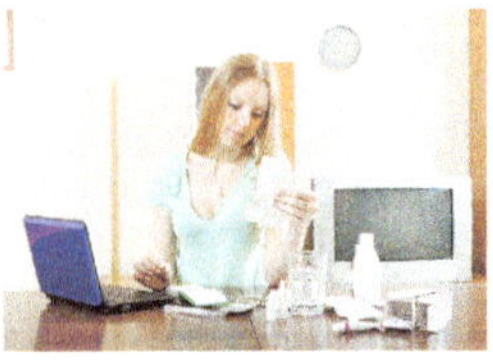

Remember the patient "Katherine Hunter" at the beginning of the chapter? Now read the remainder of the case study. Based on the information presented within this chapter, respond to the critical thinking questions that follow.

Katherine Hunter prides herself on being a wise consumer and cautiously examines the claims by manufacturers for all her purchases. She researches everything she buys, such as automobiles, household appliances, and medications. Recently, Katherine has begun to seriously consider assertions made by the advertisements for various types of antacids. Most brands claim to be the most effective in relieving the symptoms of indigestion. Others say that their brand is the most potent antacid available without a prescription. Some products claim that they not only relieve heartburn but also supply the body with needed vitamins and minerals. When purchasing an OTC medication, all Katherine wants is something that will work quickly with few adverse effects.

Critical Thinking Questions

1. How would you teach Katherine the difference between potency and efficacy?
2. Which of the two concepts (potency and efficacy) would be most important for selecting a drug? Why?
3. What are the drawbacks of comparing two different medications?

Additional Case Study

As the nurse practicing in a middle school, you have been asked to speak to the eighth-grade pre-health professionals' class. The topic for today's discussion is "how drugs work in the body." The teacher has provided you with an outline of concepts that you will need to address.

1. Describe the link between a drug's action and drug receptors.
2. Why do people respond differently to medication?
3. What are drug agonists and drug antagonists?

Chapter Review

1. What parameters would the nurse use to determine whether the average dose of a medication is effective for a patient? (Select all that apply.)
   1. Physical examination
   2. Vital signs
   3. Laboratory values
   4. Dosage time
   5. Efficacy
2. The nurse knows that a drug with a high therapeutic index is:
   1. Probably safe.
   2. Often dangerous.
   3. Frequently risky.
   4. Most likely effective.
3. While reviewing a drug manufacturer's package insert, the nurse reads about the dose–response curve. The purpose of the dose–response curve is to illustrate the relationship between:
   1. The amount of a drug administered and the degree of response it produces.
   2. The prevalence of toxic effects in a given population.
   3. The degree of response and the total duration of action of the drug.
   4. The peak serum drug level when half the dose is administered.
4. A research nurse is discussing the TD_{50} of a drug with the other members of the investigation team. On which of the following would the discussion focus?
   1. Effectiveness
   2. Dose response
   3. Receptor subtypes
   4. Toxicity
5. A patient with myasthenia gravis has been receiving neostigmine, a cholinergic agonist, for the past 2 years. The nurse is ready to administer benztropine, a cholinergic antagonist. Which result will likely occur when these drugs are combined?
   1. Neostigmine will exhibit a greater effect.
   2. Neostigmine will exhibit a lesser effect.
   3. Neostigmine will not be affected by the administration of benztropine.
   4. Neostigmine will first exhibit a greater effect, followed by a lesser effect.
6. When considering pharmacodynamic principles for a patient's drug therapy, the nurse is aware that affinity for a receptor is most closely associated with a drug's:
   1. Potency.
   2. Efficacy.
   3. Metabolism.
   4. First-pass effect.

See Appendix A for answers to critical thinking questions, case study questions and review questions.

References

Al-Abdi, S., & Al-Aamri, M. (2020). G6PD deficiency in the COVID-19 pandemic: Ghost within ghost. *Hematology Oncology and Stem Cell Therapy*. [EPub ahead of print] https://doi.org/10.1016/j.hemonc.2020.04.002

La Vieille, S., Lefebvre, D. E., Khalid, A. F., Decan, M. R., & Godefroy, S. (2019). Dietary restrictions for people with glucose-6-phosphate dehydrogenase deficiency. *Nutrition Reviews*, *77*, 96–106. https://doi.org/10.1093/nutrit/nuy053

Malaria Genomic Epidemiology Network. (2014). Reappraisal of known malaria resistance loci in a large multicenter study. *Nature Genetics*, *46*, 1197–1204. https://doi.org/10.1038/ng.3107

U.S. Food and Drug Administration. (2020). *Table of pharmacogenomic biomarkers in drug labeling*. https://www.fda.gov/drugs/science-and-research-drugs/table-pharmacogenomic-biomarkers-drug-labeling

Wu, Y., Tseng, C., Cheng, M., Ho, H., Shih, S., & Chiu, D. T. (2008). Glucose-6-phosphate dehydrogenase deficiency enhances human coronavirus 229E infection. *Journal of Infectious Diseases*, 197(6), 812–816. https://doi.org/10.1086/528377

Selected Bibliography

Bell, W. R. (2019). Therapeutic agents—pharmacokinetics and pharmacodynamics. *Reviews in Cardiovascular Medicine*, *3* (Suppl. 2), 34–44.

Brunton, L. L., Hilal-Dandan, R., & Knollmann, B. C. (Eds.). (2018). *Goodman & Gilman's the pharmacological basis of therapeutics* (13th ed.). McGraw-Hill.

Durendorf, H., & Schmidt, S. (2019). *Rowland & Tozer's clinical pharmacokinetics and pharmacodynamics: Concepts and applications* (5th ed.). Wolters Kluwer.

Hughes, G. (2016). Friendly pharmacodynamics: A simple introduction. *Nurse Prescribing*, *14*, 34–43. https://doi.org/10.12968/npre.2016.14.1.34

Osanlou, O., Pirmohamed, M., & Daly, A. K. (2018). Pharmacogenetics of adverse drug reactions. In K. Brosen & P. Damkier (Eds.), *Advances in pharmacology: Vol. 83. Pharmacogenetics* (pp. 155–190). Academic Press.

Tornio, A., & Backman, J. T. (2018). Cytochrome P450 in pharmacogenetics: An update. In K. Brosen & P. Damkier (Eds.), *Advances in pharmacology: Vol. 83. Pharmacogenetics* (pp. 3–32). Academic Press.

van den Anker, J., Reed, M. D., Allegaert, K., & Kearns, G. L. (2018). Developmental changes in pharmacokinetics and pharmacodynamics. *Journal of Clinical Pharmacology*, *58*, S10–S25. https://doi.org/10.1002/jcph.1284

"I was told to watch for drug reactions. But with all the drugs I take, how would I ever know if I'm having a reaction or not?"
—*Patient "Elizabeth Washington"*

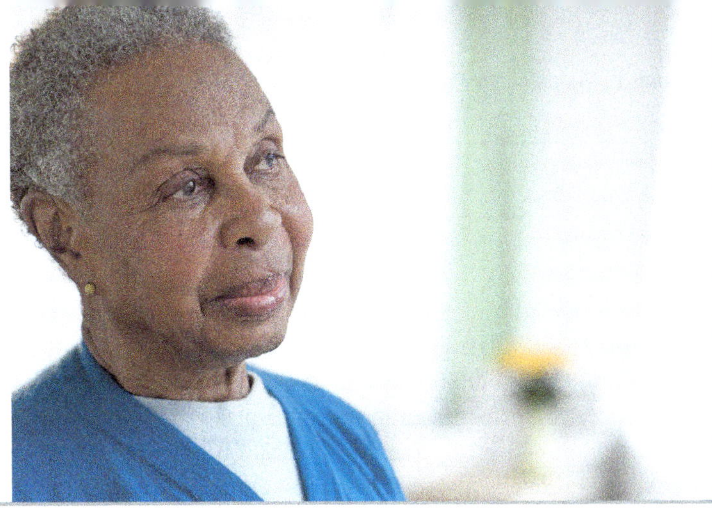

Chapter 5
Adverse Drug Effects and Drug Interactions

Chapter Outline

- Adverse Drug Effects
  - The Nurse's Role in Managing Adverse Drug Effects
  - The FDA's Role in Monitoring Adverse Drug Effects
  - Allergic Reactions
  - Idiosyncratic Responses
  - Carcinogenicity and Teratogenicity
  - Organ-Specific Drug Toxicity
- Drug Interactions
  - Pharmacotherapeutic Outcomes
  - Pharmacokinetic Drug Interactions
  - Pharmacodynamic Drug Interactions
  - Drug Interactions with Food and Dietary Supplements

Learning Outcomes

After reading this chapter, the student should be able to:

1. Differentiate between adverse effects and side effects.
2. Create a plan to minimize or prevent adverse drug events in patients.
3. Explain the advantages and disadvantages of the FDA Adverse Event Reporting System.
4. Describe the incidence and characteristics of drug allergies.
5. Explain how idiosyncratic reactions differ from other types of adverse effects.
6. Explain why certain drugs with carcinogenic or teratogenic potential are used in pharmacotherapy.
7. Report the characteristic signs, symptoms, and treatment for each of the following organ-specific adverse events: nephrotoxicity, neurotoxicity, hepatotoxicity, dermatologic toxicity, bone marrow toxicity, cardiotoxicity, and skeletal muscle and tendon toxicity.
8. Use examples to explain the importance of drug interactions to pharmacotherapy.
9. Describe the mechanisms of drug interactions that alter absorption, distribution, metabolism, or excretion.
10. Differentiate between additive, synergistic, and antagonistic drug interactions.
11. Identify examples of drug–food interactions that may impact pharmacotherapeutic outcomes.

Key Terms

Definitions of the terms in bold may be found in the Glossary.

Medications are administered with the goal of producing a therapeutic effect. All drugs, however, have the potential to produce unintended effects as well as therapeutic effects. An **adverse drug effect** is an undesirable and potentially harmful action caused by the administration of medication. Adverse effects, also called *adverse events*, are a significant component of pharmacotherapy and, when severe, may cause treatment to be discontinued or result in permanent harm to the patient. The purpose of this chapter is to examine the different types of adverse effects and drug interactions, so that the nurse can minimize their impact on treatment outcomes.

Adverse Drug Effects

5.1 The nurse plays a key role in preventing and managing adverse drug effects.

Although every medication has the *potential* to produce adverse events, most pharmacotherapy can be conducted without significant undesirable effects. Indeed, drugs that produce serious adverse effects are screened and removed from consideration during the drug development and approval process or are restricted for treating serious health conditions such as cancer. Patients expect that their drugs—including over-the-counter (OTC) medications, herbal products, and dietary supplements—will be free from serious adverse effects when taken as directed. Although the majority of drugs are very safe, adverse effects cannot be entirely avoided.

Side effects are types of drug effects that are predictable and that may occur even at therapeutic doses. Side effects are less serious than adverse effects. Patients are often willing to tolerate annoying side effects if they believe the drug will improve their condition or prevent a disease. The distinction between an adverse effect and a side effect, however, is often unclear. For example, is headache a side effect or an adverse effect? What about nausea? The answer lies in the severity of the symptoms. Headache or nausea may be minor (side effects), or they may become intense and disabling (adverse effects).

Adverse drug events may be specific to a single type of tissue or affect multiple organ systems. The most common adverse events are serious nausea and vomiting, which may occur when drugs are administered by any route. Severe headache and significant changes in blood pressure are also very common adverse drug events. Some adverse effects, though rare, are serious enough to warrant regular or continuous monitoring. Examples of serious events include impairment or failure of entire organs, such as cardiac, hepatic, or renal failure or loss of vision or hearing. Anaphylaxis, Stevens–Johnson syndrome (SJS), cancer, and birth defects are additional rare, adverse drug events that occur with certain medications. The U.S. Food and Drug Administration (FDA; 2019) defines serious adverse drug events as those that:

- Result in a patient's death.
- Cause a congenital abnormality.
- Cause a life-threatening event.
- Result in hospitalization.
- Result in significant incapacity or substantial disruption of the ability to conduct normal life functions.
- Require medical or surgical intervention to prevent permanent damage.

Many adverse effects are extensions of a drug's pharmacologic actions. These types of events are considered *dose dependent*: As the drug dose increases, the risk for adverse effects also increases. For example, antihypertensive drugs are given to lower blood pressure, but high doses cause hypotension, which may manifest as dizziness or fainting. Drugs for treating insomnia or anxiety may depress brain activity too much at higher doses, resulting in drowsiness or daytime sedation. Knowing the therapeutic actions of the drug enables the nurse to predict the signs and symptoms of many of the adverse effects that occur during treatment. It is important for nurses and their patients to understand that the difference between a drug being a beneficial medication or a toxic substance is often simply a matter of dose.

Can adverse effects be prevented? Although nurses play a key role in minimizing the number and severity of adverse events in their patients, some adverse effects simply cannot be predicted or prevented. Skilled healthcare providers, however, have multiple ways to minimize or prevent adverse effects, from having expert knowledge of how a drug acts to obtaining a comprehensive medical history from their patients. The following are means that nurses use to minimize or prevent adverse drug events in their patients:

- **Obtain a thorough medical history.** The medical history of the patient may reveal drug allergies or conditions that contraindicate the use of certain drugs. The history may also identify prescription drugs, OTC drugs, dietary supplements, and herbal products taken by the patient that could negatively interact with the prescribed medication. At each healthcare visit, a medication reconciliation should be conducted, comparing medications that the patient is taking currently to those that were recorded at the last visit.

- **Conduct a thorough assessment of the patient and all diagnostic data.** Assessment may reveal underlying hepatic or renal impairment that will affect the way a drug is handled by the body. Very young children and older adults are most susceptible to adverse drug reactions because metabolism and excretion of drugs in these populations are less predictable. To prevent adverse effects, average drug doses should be adjusted based on careful patient assessment.
- **Prevent medication errors.** Administering the incorrect dose or giving the drug to the wrong patient may cause unnecessary adverse effects. Methods of preventing medication errors are described in detail in Chapter 6.
- **Monitor pharmacotherapy carefully.** Monitor patient signs and symptoms regularly, especially at the beginning of pharmacotherapy or when doses are increased. This is especially critical when caring for patients who are very ill or when giving parenteral medications. Patients receiving drugs that have frequent or potentially severe adverse effects should be monitored continuously until the baseline effects of the drug have been established.
- **Know the drugs.** It is essential for nurses to know the most frequent and most serious adverse effects for every drug administered. A comprehensive knowledge of the drugs, herbal products, and supplements taken by their patients helps nurses to monitor for and identify adverse effects and provide the necessary interventions before they become serious.
- **Be prepared for the unusual.** Anaphylaxis may occur immediately and unpredictably (see Section 5.3). Other adverse effects may be delayed, occurring days, weeks, or months after therapy is initiated. Some medications produce actions opposite to those expected (see Section 5.4). Patients may be reluctant to report certain adverse effects (such as impotence) without prompting by the nurse.
- **Question unusual orders.** If the nurse suspects that the wrong dose has been ordered or the pharmacy has filled the order incorrectly, the drug should not be administered until the prescriber or the pharmacy has been contacted.
- **Teach patients about adverse effects.** The patient is the nurse's ally in identifying and preventing adverse effects. Teaching patients what therapeutic and adverse effects to expect from the drug and which types of symptoms to report to their healthcare provider are important in self-management and preventing serious adverse events. Furthermore, inadequate teaching may result in poor patient adherence to the drug regimen and suboptimal treatment outcomes.

5.2 The FDA continues to monitor for new adverse events after a drug is approved and marketed.

Before approving a new medication, the FDA carefully examines all clinical information supplied by the manufacturer regarding drug effectiveness and safety. Although extensive testing may have been conducted, clinical research has certain limitations and the FDA's decision is based on a relatively small number of clinical trials. Once marketed, the drug is disseminated to a larger and more diverse patient population, at which point adverse effects that were not discovered during clinical trials may begin to surface. For this reason, the FDA continues to monitor the safety of drugs after they are approved.

Established in 1993, the FDA's MedWatch Safety Information and **Adverse Event Reporting System (FAERS)** is a voluntary program that encourages healthcare providers and consumers to report suspected adverse effects directly to the FDA or the product manufacturer. By law, reports received by the manufacturers are forwarded to the FDA to be added to the computerized information database.

Data from the FAERS are analyzed by clinical reviewers, usually a physician, pharmacist, or nurse, at the Center for Drug Evaluation and Research of the FDA. If a potential safety concern is identified, the FDA may take one of the following actions:

- Conduct additional epidemiologic studies to determine the validity or extent of the safety concern.
- Require changes to a product's labeling information.
- Require a **black box warning** in the drug insert that warns prescribers that the drug carries a risk for a serious adverse effect or death.
- Restrict the use of the drug in specific populations (such as certain age groups or those with comorbid conditions).
- Communicate safety information to healthcare providers and consumers.
- Recall a product that may have quality or performance concerns.
- Remove the product from the market.

The FDA disseminates changes in safety information through its MedWatch website. Interested parties may subscribe to podcasts, electronic newsletters, and even cell phone text message alerts giving them the latest drug safety information.

The FAERS provides a national database for making safety decisions about drugs, but it does have limitations. Because the system relies on voluntary reports, not all adverse events are reported. Furthermore, the filing of a report does not establish causation. The suspected adverse effect may have been caused by some other factor involved in the treatment of an underlying disease. Reports sometimes contain insufficient or vague details regarding the incident.

A word of caution is necessary regarding the reporting of adverse drug events. The placebo effect predicts that a certain percentage of patients will respond with positive therapeutic outcomes to a treatment, even if the substance is inert and has no pharmacologic properties (essentially a "sugar pill"). The same holds true for side and adverse effects. A certain percentage of patients will experience headache, nausea and vomiting, rash, changes in blood pressure, or pain following the administration of a placebo. Thus, when examining drug information, the nurse should always examine the incidence of adverse effects that occur over and above that caused by a placebo. It is important to understand that patients are not faking symptoms caused by a placebo; they truly believe they are experiencing the side effects and may even be visibly exhibiting them. However, the drug itself may not be responsible for the self-reported effects.

5.3 Allergic reactions are caused by a hyper-response of the immune system.

Drug allergies are common, comprising 6–10% of all adverse drug effects. Although drug allergies may elicit a diverse range of patient symptoms, all are caused by a hyper-response of body defenses. Depending on the type of allergic response, basophils, mast cells, eosinophils, or lymphocytes secrete chemical mediators that trigger the allergic response. Specific chemical mediators of allergy include histamine, serotonin, leukotrienes, prostaglandins, and complement.

Several characteristics define a drug allergy. Allergies typically occur with very small amounts of drug; the severity of allergy symptoms is usually not proportional to the dose. The symptoms of allergy are unrelated to the pharmacologic actions of the drug; anaphylaxis has the same symptoms regardless of the drug that induces it. Patients often exhibit cross-allergy, an allergic reaction to drugs with a similar structure, such as those from the same pharmacologic class. Drug allergies require a previous exposure to the drug (or a very similar drug). This sensitizes the patient to subsequent exposures, during which a hyper-response of body defenses is rapidly mounted upon re-exposure to the drug.

The signs and symptoms of drug allergy are variable and range from minor to life-threatening. Symptoms may appear within minutes after the drug is administered or they may develop after prolonged pharmacotherapy. Because the signs and symptoms of drug allergy are nonspecific, it is sometimes difficult to attribute an allergy symptom to a specific drug in patients receiving multiple medications. Complicating an accurate diagnosis is that symptoms of drug allergy are the same as those of allergy to environmental triggers, such as peanuts, seafood, insect stings, animal dander, or dust mites. It is important to determine the source of allergy, especially in patients with severe reactions, so that the offending drug or environmental substance can be avoided in the future. The pharmacologic treatment of allergy is presented in Chapter 45.

Although allergic reactions are possible with most drugs, some exhibit a higher incidence. The medications most likely to cause allergic reactions include penicillins and related antibiotics (monobactams and cephalosporins); radiologic contrast media containing iodine; insulin; nonsteroidal anti-inflammatory drugs (NSAIDs), including aspirin; sulfonamides; cancer chemotherapy agents; preservatives (sulfites and paraben); and certain antiseizure drugs. The use of biological products such as monoclonal antibodies has greatly increased in recent years, and these agents have been shown to produce a high incidence of allergic reactions.

Patients are usually unaware of the true definition of allergy and often report any adverse effect as a drug allergy. For example, many patients experience acute nausea and vomiting with narcotic analgesics such as codeine and will report that they have an allergy to codeine during a drug history. In fact, these symptoms are not caused by an overactive immune response and are thus not a true allergy. Inaccurate reporting of allergies may lead to the healthcare provider avoiding the use of entire drug classes and prescribing more expensive second-line medications that could be less effective or produce more adverse effects.

5.4 Idiosyncratic reactions are unusual drug responses often caused by genetic differences among patients.

An **idiosyncratic response** is an adverse drug effect that produces unusual and unexpected symptoms that are not related to the pharmacologic action of the drug. Idiosyncratic reactions are not classified as allergies because they are not immune related. They are rare, unpredictable, and vary from patient to patient.

Many, though not all, idiosyncratic reactions are due to unique, individual genetic differences among patients. For example, mutations involving specific metabolic enzymes may cause certain patients to be extremely sensitive to the effects of a drug. The drug may be handled by a different metabolic pathway, resulting in the accumulation of a metabolite that gives a different and unexpected response from the original drug.

Historically, the term *idiosyncratic* has been used to denote any drug effect that could not be explained. With advances in the understanding of drug mechanisms and pharmacogenetics, more and more drug responses are now understood. With improved reporting of adverse drug events, rare "unexpected" events are now documented and may be "expected." Thus, use of the term *idiosyncratic*, although still common in clinical practice, will likely continue to diminish with time.

5.5 Some drugs have the ability to induce cancer or cause birth defects.

Most adverse effects occur within minutes or hours after a drug is administered; some develop after several days or weeks of pharmacotherapy. In a few instances, the adverse effect may occur years or even decades after the medication was administered. Such is the case with drug-induced cancer.

Why would the FDA approve a medication if it is known to cause cancer in humans? In most cases, drugs that produce cancer or birth defects in laboratory animals during preclinical trials are not submitted for approval to the FDA. However, there are a few conditions that may warrant the approval of a drug with carcinogenic potential. The answer lies in the **risk–benefit ratio**. If a patient has a condition that is likely to cause premature death or disability if left untreated, the benefits of taking a medication with carcinogenic potential may outweigh the long-term risks. This assumes, of course, that effective, safer alternatives are not available.

Of the thousands of drugs and combination products approved for pharmacotherapy, only a few increase the risk of acquiring cancer. Most of these drugs, shown in Table 5.1, fall into three primary classes: antineoplastics, immunosuppressants, and hormonal agents.

Table 5.1 Selected Drugs Suspected of Causing Cancer in Humans

Class	Drug	Type of Cancer
Antineoplastic	chlorambucil cisplatin cyclophosphamide dacarbazine doxorubicin etoposide metronidazole nitrosoureas phenytoin propylthiouracil teniposide	Leukemia, urinary bladder
Hormones and hormone antagonists	anabolic steroids estrogen replacement therapy and oral contraceptives progesterone tamoxifen	Uterus, breast, hepatic
Immunosuppressants	azathioprine cyclosporine	Lymphoma, skin

Some of the antineoplastics are known chemical carcinogens. With the goal of eliminating cancer cells, some of these drugs cause molecular damage or mutations in deoxyribonucleic acid (DNA). Although much of the DNA damage in normal cells is repaired by enzymes, some mutations persist and accumulate in cells as an individual ages, increasing cancer risk. The initial damage done by the medication may take decades to manifest as cancer. Leukemia is the type of cancer with the greatest cancer risk from antineoplastic therapy. However, the patient may never develop cancer as a result of these medications; indeed, the majority of patients receiving antineoplastic drugs do not develop the disease. Furthermore, if the cancer treatment is successful, the patient may benefit from additional years of life due to pharmacotherapy. Because pharmacotherapy combined with surgery and radiation therapy can result in a total cure for some patients, the benefit of antineoplastic therapy may outweigh the small risk of developing cancer later in life.

The second class of drugs that can induce cancer is the immunosuppressants. These medications are administered to dampen the immune system of patients receiving transplanted tissues or who have serious inflammatory disorders. Because a natural function of the immune system is to remove cancer cells that form in the body, any drug that inhibits this system would be expected to have some degree of cancer risk. Lymphoma is the most frequent type of cancer resulting from immunosuppressant use. Again, the risk of cancer is compared to the potential benefits provided by these immunosuppressants.

The third group that may cause cancer consists of hormones or hormone antagonists. The mechanisms by which hormone imbalances lead to cancer is a topic of ongoing research. In some cases, hormones protect the patient from cancer, or they may reduce the incidence of one type of cancer but increase the risk of another type. Probably the best studied of the hormone mechanisms is how estrogen binds to its intracellular receptors. About 70% of patients with breast cancer are estrogen receptor (ER) positive: The hormone promotes tumor formation in the mammary gland. Cancers caused by hormones or hormone antagonists tend to affect reproductive organs, such as the vagina, uterus, or breast.

A similar question might be asked regarding drugs that cause birth defects, or **teratogens**. Why would a drug be approved by the FDA if it was shown to produce birth defects in laboratory animals during the preclinical stage of drug testing? The answer to this question, however, is very different from that for cancer-inducing drugs.

Teratogens affect a small percentage of the overall population: those who are pregnant or who become pregnant during pharmacotherapy. In most cases these drugs are safe for use by men and postmenopausal women. Thus, known teratogens may be FDA-approved for indications in patients who do not have the potential to become pregnant. For example, finasteride (Proscar) is a known teratogen and it is only approved to treat men with benign prostatic hyperplasia.

When approved for women with childbearing *potential*, however, drugs with teratogenic effects have increased risks. In some cases, a negative pregnancy test may be required prior to pharmacotherapy and the patient should be advised to discontinue the medication if pregnancy is suspected. In women with childbearing potential, teratogenic drugs are not prescribed unless they have clear benefits that outweigh the possible risk of birth defects. All healthcare providers must carefully assess patient compliance with instructions against this potential risk. In extreme cases, such as with the drug isotretinoin (Amnesteem, others), women of childbearing potential must provide two negative pregnancy tests prior to receiving the drug and another one each month the prescription is refilled.

Although new drugs are tested for teratogenicity in laboratory animals, the results cannot predict with great accuracy the effects on the human fetus. In some cases, the risks to a human embryo or fetus have been determined *after* a drug has been approved. The FDA requires manufacturers to provide written information on drug labels estimating the risks to the pregnant mother and her fetus during pregnancy and lactation. (see Chapter 8). Because information on teratogenicity is very limited, all drug use should be assumed to be potentially hazardous during pregnancy, unless data have otherwise demonstrated the drug to be safe. No woman should take a drug, herbal product, or dietary supplement during pregnancy or lactation unless approved by her healthcare provider.

5.6 Drug toxicity may be specific to particular organs.

Very few drugs produce adverse effects in every organ system; these agents would be too toxic for safe pharmacotherapy. Instead, adverse effects are often organ specific, targeting one or a few organs. It is important to learn these specific toxicities so that appropriate signs, symptoms, and diagnostic tests can be carefully monitored. Selected organ-specific toxicities are summarized in Table 5.2.

Table 5.2 Organ-Specific Toxicity

Toxicity	Example Drugs and Classes
Bone marrow	ACE inhibitors, antimalarials, antineoplastics, antiseizure drugs (carbamazepine, phenytoin), antithyroid drugs, cephalosporins, chloramphenicol, chlorpromazine, cimetidine, furosemide, immunosuppressants, methotrexate, NSAIDs, ribavirin, sulfonamides, zidovudine
Cardiotoxicity	5-flourouracil, anthracycline antineoplastics (daunorubicin, doxorubicin, epirubicin, idarubicin, mitoxantrone), paclitaxel
Dermatologic	allopurinol, antiseizure drugs (carbamazepine, phenobarbital, phenytoin), cephalosporins, erythromycin, NSAIDs, penicillin, radiologic contrast media, sulfonamides, tetracyclines
Hepatotoxicity	allopurinol, amoxicillin-clavulanate, anabolic steroids, carbamazepine, chlorpromazine, statins (HMG CoA reductase inhibitors)
Nephrotoxicity	ACE inhibitors, acyclovir, aminoglycosides, amphotericin B, cisplatin and other platinum-based antineoplastics, cocaine, cyclosporine, NSAIDs, protease inhibitors, radiologic contrast media, sulfonamides, tacrolimus, tenofovir
Neurotoxicity	aminoglycosides, cisplatin, ethanol, loop diuretics, MDMA (Ecstasy), salicylates, vincristine
Skeletal muscle and tendon toxicity	ethanol, heroin, fluoroquinolone antibiotics, statins

Bone marrow toxicity: Drugs affecting the bone marrow are of great concern due to the possibility of serious and perhaps fatal outcomes. The bone marrow serves as a nursery for the production of red blood cells, white blood cells, and platelets. Drugs may affect only one of these types of cells or all three. When all three groups are affected, drug-induced pancytopenia or aplastic anemia occurs, and the patient is at great risk for serious illness. Loss of white blood cells may cause agranulocytosis or neutropenia, which places the patient at risk for serious infections. The drug class most likely to cause bone marrow toxicity is the antineoplastics. Bone marrow toxicity, also called *myelosuppression*, is a dose-limiting factor with many of these drugs (see Chapter 57).

To prevent bone marrow toxicity, laboratory data must be carefully monitored and impending toxicity recognized by reporting decreases in red blood cells, white blood cells, or platelets. In many cases, bone marrow toxicity can be quickly reversed if the condition is recognized early and the drug is discontinued. Furthermore, the nurse should carefully monitor the therapeutic regimen of patients who have preexisting blood cell disorders because adding a drug with bone marrow toxicity may worsen these conditions.

Cardiotoxicity: A few medications damage cardiac muscle cells, affecting the ability of the heart to effectively pump blood to the tissues. The most common cardiotoxic drugs belong to a chemical class called the anthracyclines, which include daunorubicin (Cerubidine), doxorubicin (Adriamycin), epirubicin (Ellence), idarubicin (Idamycin), and mitoxantrone (Novantrone). These are all antineoplastic medications. The cardiotoxicity of these drugs can be severe and lead to bradycardia, tachycardia, heart failure, and acute left-ventricular failure. The nurse administering cardiotoxic drugs must be vigilant in observing for signs of cardiotoxicity such as excessive fatigue, cough, shortness of breath (especially when recumbent), weight gain, or peripheral edema.

A second type of cardiotoxicity is manifested as prolongation of the QT interval on an electrocardiogram (ECG). The QT interval represents the time needed to depolarize and repolarize the ventricles. Lengthening of the QT interval is associated with a rare type of ventricular tachycardia called *torsade de pointes*, which can cause sudden cardiac death. More than 100 drugs have been shown to cause QT prolongation and several have been removed from the market because of this adverse effect. Because the QT interval represents the dysrhythmia potential of a drug, the FDA now requires new medications to be tested for QT prolongation prior to approval. When administering drugs that prolong the QT interval, nurses should carefully monitor cardiac function, especially in patients with preexisting heart disease.

Dermatologic toxicity: Drug reactions affecting the skin are some of the most common types of adverse effects. These reactions may be caused by an allergic (hypersensitivity) reaction or by nonimmune-type responses. Rash, the most common cutaneous medication reaction, usually occurs within 1 to 2 weeks of initiation of drug therapy and resolves without serious complications. Drug-induced rash is sometimes accompanied by itching (pruritus). Although almost any drug can cause rash, antibiotics are the most frequent drug class causing this condition. Urticaria (hives) are raised welts that are often accompanied by intense pruritus and, although less common than rash, are a symptom of a potential allergic reaction that could lead to anaphylaxis.

Serious and even fatal dermatologic toxicity can occur. In angioedema, swelling occurs in the dermis, periorbital region, and around the mouth and throat. Angioedema is a severe drug reaction because the swelling may impair breathing and may be fatal. SJS and toxic epidermal necrosis are drug-induced conditions that can be fatal. These syndromes cause severe blistering of the skin and sloughing of the epidermis, usually accompanied by mucous membrane erosion and fever.

Phototoxicity is a type of drug-induced dermatologic toxicity in which certain drugs cause the skin to absorb excess ultraviolet radiation from the sun or heat lamps. Symptoms resemble sunburn and are best prevented by advising patients to avoid direct sunlight. Phototoxicity resolves when the drug is discontinued.

Many types of drug-induced dermatologic toxicity do not require pharmacologic treatment. If pruritus is prominent, an antihistamine or a corticosteroid may be administered. In all cases of serious drug-induced hypersensitivity, the nurse should discontinue the drug until the cause of the skin condition can be diagnosed.

Hepatotoxicity: The liver receives all drugs absorbed across the stomach and intestinal mucosa via the hepatic-portal vein. A major function of the liver is to metabolize and detoxify drugs and other chemicals that enter the body; thus, it should not be surprising that hepatotoxicity is one of the most common adverse drug effects. Effects of hepatotoxic drugs range from minor, transient increases in liver enzyme values to fatal hepatitis.

Liver enzyme tests should be monitored regularly when administering hepatotoxic drugs because changes in these laboratory values are early signs of liver toxicity. Symptoms of liver impairment are often vague and nonspecific and include right upper quadrant pain, anorexia, bloating, fatigue, and nausea and/or vomiting. During chronic hepatotoxicity, jaundice, itching, and easy bruising are evident. In serious cases, the liver will be unable to metabolize other drugs, resulting in high serum drug levels. Extreme care must be taken when administering potentially hepatotoxic drugs to patients with preexisting liver disease.

PharmFACT

It is estimated that 20% of drug-induced injuries in the United States are due to dietary supplements. About half of these are caused by bodybuilding and weight loss products (Ronis et al., 2018)

Nephrotoxicity: The kidneys are one of the most common organs affected by drugs. This is because these organs filter large volumes of blood, and most drugs are excreted by the renal route. Some drugs are reabsorbed or secreted by the kidney, exposing renal tubule cells to high concentrations of these medications and their metabolites. A few obstruct the urinary system by causing crystalluria in the urinary tract. Drug-induced nephrotoxicity may cause both acute kidney injury or chronic kidney disease.

It is critical for the healthcare provider to identify at-risk patients and attempt to prevent drug-induced nephrotoxicity. Means for prevention include providing proper hydration, monitoring urinary lab values, and adjusting doses appropriately for patients with renal impairment. Patients with serious renal impairment should not receive nephrotoxic drugs unless other therapeutic options have been exhausted.

Neurotoxicity: Although the blood–brain barrier prevents many drugs from reaching the brain, neurotoxicity is a relatively common adverse effect of certain drug classes. This is because the brain receives a large percentage of the blood supply and is especially sensitive to small amounts of toxic substances. For sedatives, antidepressants, antianxiety drugs, antiseizure drugs, and antipsychotics, the difference between a therapeutic dose and one that produces adverse effects may be very small. Indeed, drowsiness is seen in a majority of patients receiving these medications. Signs and symptoms of toxicity in the central nervous system (CNS) include depression, mania, sedation, behavioral changes, suicidal feelings, hallucinations, and seizures. The special senses may be affected, including visual changes, loss of balance, and hearing impairment. Hearing impairment, or **ototoxicity**, can result from drug-induced damage to the eighth cranial nerve.

Effective teaching is essential when patients are starting therapy with potentially neurotoxic drugs. Patients should be warned to not drive vehicles or perform other hazardous tasks until they are familiar with the effects of these drugs. Caregivers should be taught to report changes in patient behavior because the individual receiving the medication may have difficulty recognizing these signs. The nurse should be aware that neurotoxic drugs can significantly worsen preexisting mental health disorders. Serious symptoms such as seizures, delirium, suicidal ideation, or significant visual or hearing impairment should be immediately reported to the prescriber.

Skeletal muscle and tendon toxicity: Skeletal muscle is relatively resistant to the effects of drugs, despite its extensive blood supply. Although the incidence of drug-induced myopathy is low, it may be serious when it does occur. The most severe myopathy is rhabdomyolysis, a syndrome characterized by extensive muscle necrosis with the release of muscle enzymes and other constituents into the circulation. Rhabdomyolysis is a rare, though serious adverse effect of statins, common medications used to treat excessive lipid levels in the blood.

Some of the fluoroquinolone antibiotics exhibit toxicity to cartilage and tendons. This is most often manifested as rupture of the Achilles tendon and is most apparent in adults over age 65. Patients under age 18 should not take these medications because they may interfere with cartilage growth.

To prevent skeletal muscle or tendon toxicity, the nurse should assess for unexplained muscle or joint soreness or pain during therapy. Laboratory tests such as creatine kinase should be evaluated regularly during therapy with drugs that have muscle toxicity.

Drug Interactions

5.7 Drug interactions may significantly affect pharmacotherapeutic outcomes.

A **drug interaction** occurs when a substance significantly alters a drug's actions. The substance causing the interaction may be another drug, a dietary supplement, an herbal product, or food. The substance participating in the drug interaction must be external to the body and is usually taken concurrently with the medication. Although substances that are naturally found in the body (endogenous substances) routinely interact with drugs, these are *not* considered drug interactions because they are part of the body's normal response to the drug.

Because most patients take multiple drugs or dietary supplements concurrently, drug interactions occur continually. Even if only one drug is taken, the potential for a drug–food interaction still exists. Drug interactions are impossible to totally eliminate; most go unnoticed and treatment outcomes are rarely affected. Indeed, it is likely that most drug interactions have yet to be documented or researched because they do not cause clinically noticeable effects or harm to the patient.

Some drug interactions are important to pharmacology because they are known to cause adverse effects or otherwise affect treatment outcomes. By understanding the mechanisms of potential drug interactions, the nurse can prevent certain adverse effects and optimize treatment outcomes. For example, if the patient is receiving gentamicin, the nurse should use caution when administering acyclovir because the drug combination can cause higher-than-normal levels of acyclovir in the blood. The prescriber should reduce the dose of acyclovir or substitute a different drug. Understanding drug interactions can directly affect the success of pharmacotherapy.

Drug interactions occur by dozens of different mechanisms. To simplify their study, it may be helpful to remember that drug interactions can have three basic effects on the action of a medication:

- The actions of the medication can be *inhibited*, resulting in less therapeutic action. For example, milk interferes with the absorption of tetracycline, causing a lower serum level of antibiotic, thus diminishing its therapeutic effects.
- The actions of the medication may be *enhanced*, causing a greater therapeutic response. For example, coadministration of the two antiviral drugs lopinavir and ritonavir causes a greater reduction in levels of human immunodeficiency virus (HIV) than occurs when either drug is used alone.
- The interaction may produce a totally *new and different response*. For example, when used alone disulfiram (Antabuse) has no pharmacologic effects. When taken with alcohol, however, the combination produces dramatic, new actions such as severe headache, flushing, dyspnea, palpitations, and blurred vision (see Chapter 27).

5.8 Pharmacokinetic drug interactions include changes in the absorption, distribution, metabolism, or excretion of medications.

Recall from Chapter 3 that *pharmacokinetics* is the branch of pharmacology dealing with how the body acts on a drug after it is administered. Many drug interactions involve some aspect of pharmacokinetics. When studying drug interactions, it is convenient to use the same categories for pharmacokinetics that are presented in Chapter 3. The general types of pharmacokinetic interactions are illustrated in Figure 5.1.

Absorption: Most drugs need to be absorbed to produce their actions; thus, any substance that affects absorption has the potential to influence drug response. In fact, this is

Pharmacokinetic Variable	Type of Interaction	Potential Drug Effect
Absorption	Presence of food	Decreased
	Alteration of pH	Variable
	Drug–drug binding	Decreased
	Increased peristalsis	Variable
	Slowed gastric emptying	Variable
Distribution	Displacement of drug from plasma protein binding site	Increased
Metabolism	Stimulation of CYP: enzyme induction	Decreased
	Inhibition of CYP: enzyme inhibition	Increased
Excretion	Increased excretion	Decreased
	Decreased excretion	Increased

Figure 5.1 Types of pharmacokinetic drug–drug interactions.

one of the most common mechanisms of drug interactions. By interfering with normal absorption, drug action may be inhibited or enhanced. Increasing absorption will raise drug serum levels and produce an enhanced effect; substances inhibiting absorption have the opposite effect.

The simplest way to affect absorption is to change the speed of substances moving through the gastrointestinal (GI) tract. Opioids such as morphine or heroin will slow peristalsis, giving drugs additional time for absorption. Laxatives and drugs that stimulate the parasympathetic nervous system will speed substances through the GI tract, diminishing the absorption time of other drugs. The bile acid resins such as cholestyramine (Prevalite) bind other drugs and prevent their absorption.

Many drug–drug interactions caused by changes in absorption may be prevented by taking the two medications at least 2 to 3 hours apart. In the case of drug–food interactions, the interacting food should be avoided or the drug may be taken on an empty stomach. Taking drugs on an empty stomach, however, may increase the incidence of nausea and/or vomiting, which could result in loss of the drug before complete absorption occurs. The nurse must teach patients with drug-induced nausea not to take drugs with antacids or milk unless approved by the prescriber. Antacids are alkaline (basic) substances that raise the pH of the GI contents and have the potential to change the percentage of ionized drug. Ionized forms of drugs are less able to cross the intestinal mucosa than nonionized forms.

Distribution: Distribution is the movement of a drug from its site of absorption to its site of action. Many drugs travel through the blood bound to plasma proteins and, when bound, the drug is unable to leave the blood to reach its target. Drugs may compete for available binding sites on plasma proteins; one drug may prevent another from binding to plasma proteins or may displace a drug from its binding sites. If this occurs, the amount of unbound or free drug increases, potentially raising the drug serum concentration to toxic levels. For example, diazepam displaces phenytoin from plasma proteins, causing a rapid increase in the plasma concentration of free phenytoin and an increased risk of adverse effects. Medications that have a high potential for displacing other drugs from protein binding sites include aspirin and other NSAIDs, phenylbutazone, and sulfonamides.

A second potential drug–drug interaction involving distribution can occur if the pH of the plasma is altered by a drug. For example, when an alkaline substance such as sodium bicarbonate is infused, the pH of plasma increases, causing acidic drugs to become ionized. The ionized acidic drugs are less able to cross membranes and they accumulate in the extracellular spaces, creating an ionization (pH) gradient. The pH gradient moves acidic drugs from inside cells to the extracellular spaces, thus altering distribution.

Metabolism: A large number of drugs are metabolized by hepatic microsomal (CYP) enzymes. Drug metabolites generally have less activity than the original drug and are more readily excreted by the kidneys. Any drug-induced change in the activity of hepatic enzymes has the potential to cause drug–drug interactions.

As discussed in Chapter 4, certain drugs have the ability to increase (induce) or decrease (inhibit) CYP enzyme activity. Inducers such as phenobarbital will increase drug metabolism, thus promoting the inactivation and excretion of many drugs. Clinically, this will be observed as diminished drug effectiveness. For example, if phenobarbital is administered concurrently with the antihypertensive drug nifedipine, less blood pressure reduction will result. The dose of nifedipine will need to be increased to produce an optimal therapeutic effect. However, care must be taken if the inducer is discontinued because hepatic enzyme activity will return to baseline levels in a few days or weeks. Once CYP enzyme levels return to normal, the dose of nifedipine will have to be adjusted downward to avoid toxicity. Also, remember that a few drugs (prodrugs) are *activated* by metabolism. Increasing the metabolism of prodrugs will cause an increase, rather than a decrease, in therapeutic response.

Inhibitors of hepatic metabolism will cause drug interactions that are *opposite* to those of inducers. For example, ritonavir inhibits CYP3A4 and will decrease the metabolism of other drugs that are substrates for this enzyme. Giving ritonavir concurrently with nifedipine causes an increased blood pressure reduction due to the diminished metabolism of the antihypertensive. The nifedipine dose must be lowered to avoid toxicity. After ritonavir is discontinued, CYP3A4 enzyme levels return to baseline and the nifedipine dose must be adjusted once again to maintain blood pressure control.

Drug interactions involving hepatic metabolism are some of the most complex in pharmacology. Although many of these interactions are not clinically significant, others clearly have the potential to cause adverse effects and affect therapeutic outcomes. The nurse will need to remember which drugs are inducers, inhibitors, and substrates of CYP enzymes to optimize pharmacotherapeutic outcomes and minimize adverse effects (see Chapter 3).

CONNECTION Checkpoint 5.1

From what you learned in Chapter 3, explain the significance of the first-pass effect on pharmacotherapy.

Excretion: The majority of medications are eliminated from the body through renal excretion. A drug interaction may occur if a substance changes the glomerular filtration rate (GFR), the amount of blood filtered (in milliliters) by the kidney per minute. The higher the GFR, the more rapid the excretion of other drugs.

A second type of excretion-related interaction may occur if one drug changes the secretion or reabsorption of another drug in the renal tubule. For example, methotrexate competes with NSAIDs for the same secretion mechanism. If taken concurrently, NSAIDs will block the renal secretion of methotrexate, thus raising drug serum levels and increasing the potential for methotrexate toxicity.

Renal elimination may also be affected by drugs that change the pH of the filtrate in the renal tubules. Changing the pH causes drugs to become more (or less) ionized. The excretion of weak acids can be significantly increased by alkalinizing the urine through the administration of sodium bicarbonate. This drug interaction may be used therapeutically to promote more rapid excretion of acidic drugs such as aspirin during overdose situations. Similarly, excretion of weak bases can be increased by acidifying the urine through the administration of ammonium chloride.

Not all excretion-related drug interactions involve the kidneys. Some drugs are extensively excreted by the biliary system and two drugs excreted in this way may interact through this mechanism. For example, pravastatin and cyclosporine use the same carrier protein to move drug molecules from the liver to bile. Giving the two drugs concurrently will slow the biliary excretion of pravastatin and raise its serum concentration to potentially toxic levels. Because biliary excretion is not the dominant form of elimination for most drugs, this type of drug–drug excretion interaction is far less common than those involving the kidneys.

5.9 Pharmacodynamic drug interactions include additive, synergistic, or antagonistic effects.

Recall from Chapter 4 that *pharmacodynamics* is the branch of pharmacology examining the mechanisms of drug action, meaning how a drug changes the body. Many drugs produce their actions by binding to specific receptors. When two drugs compete for the same receptor, or activate receptors that produce opposite effects, drug interactions are possible. Many common interactions encountered in clinical practice are pharmacodynamic in nature.

During a pharmacodynamic drug interaction, drug action may be either enhanced or inhibited. The result

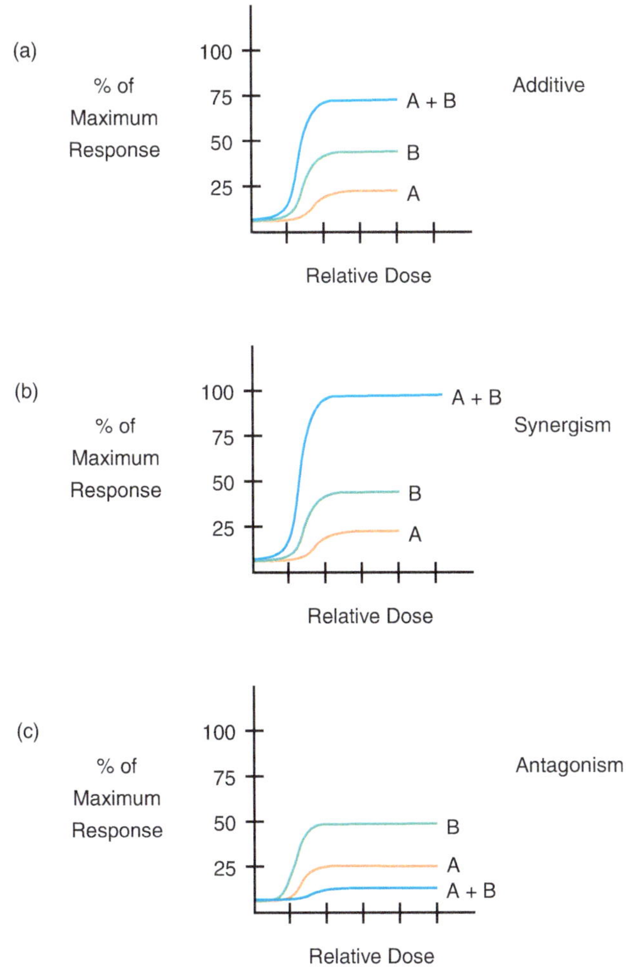

Figure 5.2 Additive, synergistic, and antagonistic drug interactions: (a) additive response, (b) synergistic response, (c) antagonistic response.

of the interaction may be desirable (increased therapeutic response or decreased adverse effect) or undesirable (decreased therapeutic response or increased adverse effect). The basic pharmacodynamic drug–drug interactions are illustrated in Figure 5.2.

The pharmacodynamic drug interaction that is easiest to visualize is the **additive effect**. In this interaction, two drugs from a similar therapeutic class produce a combined summation response. This is used extensively in treating hypertension. For example, a diuretic may be used to lower systolic blood pressure by 10 mmHg, and a beta blocker may be added to the regimen to produce another 15-mmHg reduction. Combined, the two drugs produce a 25-mmHg reduction. Why would two drugs be prescribed, rather than a single drug? There are two rationales. First, to produce a 25-mmHg reduction using only the diuretic, the dose would have to be increased. Keeping the doses of both the diuretic and beta blocker low and taking advantage of their additive effect reduces the potential for adverse drug events caused by higher medication doses. Second, some medications have low efficacy and it may not be possible to achieve a 25-mmHg reduction with a single drug. The maximum effect from the diuretic may have been a 10-mmHg reduction, and another drug would need to be added to the regimen to achieve a greater response. In this example, the two drugs act at very different types of receptors to produce the additive therapeutic response: beta blockers in cardiac muscle and diuretics in the renal tubules.

Remember that additive effects also apply to adverse effects. This is seen frequently in drugs that affect the CNS. For example, narcotic analgesics, antidepressants, antiseizure drugs, and antianxiety drugs all may cause sedation as a side effect. When taken concurrently, drugs from these classes can cause additive sedation that could profoundly affect the ability to safely operate a vehicle. Caution must always be used when administering multiple medications that have similar adverse effects such as nephrotoxicity, hepatotoxicity, or bone marrow toxicity.

Another pharmacodynamic drug interaction that produces an enhanced response is a **synergistic effect**. In this interaction, the effect of the two drugs is greater than would be expected from simply adding the two individual drugs' responses. This type of interaction is used extensively in treating infections. For example, Synercid is a combination drug that contains quinupristin and dalfopristin, two antibiotics that are effective against resistant *Staphylococcus* infections. Both drugs bind to the bacterial ribosome and produce greater killing than would be predicted from adding the two individual drugs' effects. Another example is the combination antibiotic Bactrim, which combines trimethoprim and sulfamethoxazole to produce a synergistic effect on bacterial cell killing.

A third type of pharmacodynamic interaction occurs when adding a second drug results in a *diminished* pharmacologic response. This **antagonistic effect** can result in drug actions being "cancelled." For example, drugs activating the sympathetic nervous system, such as epinephrine, will increase the heart rate and dilate the bronchi. A drug such as carvedilol (Coreg) will have the opposite effects: slowed heart rate and bronchoconstriction. Thus, carvedilol is considered an antagonist to epinephrine and may cancel its actions, depending on the doses of the two drugs. Why would a nurse administer drugs with opposite actions? This is generally done to reduce the adverse effects of a drug. For example, if a medication given to treat hypertension has a potential adverse effect of increasing heart rate, an antagonist may be given to slow the heart rate, keeping it within normal limits. When given intentionally, an antagonist does not necessarily reverse *all* actions of the first drug; it may selectively inhibit an undesirable action.

In some cases, antagonists are used to treat symptoms of drug overdose. For example, patients taking an overdose of narcotics, such as morphine or heroin, experience coma and life-threatening CNS depression. The administration of naloxone, a specific narcotic antagonist, can quickly reverse some of the serious adverse effects of morphine.

Pharmacodynamic interactions can be indirect and complex. The well-documented drug interaction between digoxin (Lanoxin) and diuretics, such as furosemide (Lasix), is an excellent example of an indirect effect. Furosemide enhances the excretion of potassium ion (hypokalemia), which increases the cardiotoxicity of digoxin. This can be a life-threatening interaction. Another example is the inhibition of vitamin K production in the intestine caused by antibiotics. If the patient is also taking warfarin (Coumadin), bleeding may occur because the liver is prevented from producing certain clotting factors. Again, the antibiotic did not directly interact with warfarin, yet the combination produced a serious adverse effect.

CONNECTION Checkpoint 5.2

The types of curves shown in Figure 5.2 are called dose–response curves. From what you learned in Chapter 4, explain the three phases of these curves.

5.10 Food, nutrients, and dietary supplements may interact with medications and affect their actions.

Historically, interactions between drugs and food, dietary supplements, and herbal products have been largely dismissed as clinically unimportant. Although a few interactions, such as tetracyclines with calcium products, have been documented for decades, only recently have drug–food interactions been recognized as important to maximizing pharmacotherapeutic outcomes. The interaction that prompted the increased interest in this topic was that of a benign and healthy substance: grapefruit juice. The interaction was discovered by chance in a research study designed to examine the effects of alcohol on felodipine, a calcium channel blocker. The researchers used grapefruit juice incidentally to disguise the taste of the alcohol.

Patients often take medications with juice because it covers up the bitter taste of a drug and provides a plentiful source of vitamins and minerals. Unfortunately, grapefruit juice also contains substances that increase the metabolism of certain oral drugs. This occurs because grapefruit juice inhibits the enzyme CYP3A4 in the wall of the intestinal tract. As drugs are absorbed, they are not inactivated by CYP3A4, and higher amounts reach the circulation. Surprisingly, the inhibition from grapefruit juice may last up to 3 days after drinking the juice. The substances in the juice inhibiting CYP3A4 enzymes are called *furanocoumarins*. Fortunately, only a few drug classes interact with grapefruit juice. Examples include benzodiazepines, certain calcium channel blockers, and statins (HMG CoA reductase inhibitors).

Most of the drug–food interactions act by either increasing or decreasing the absorption or bioavailability of the drug. Some of these interactions are shown in Table 5.3. Drug–food interactions are easily avoided by timing the drug dose appropriately with the food or supplement. In most cases, there should be a minimum 2-hour time gap between ingestion of the food and drug. In a few cases, the drug should be administered with food to increase its absorption.

Table 5.3 Selected Drug–Food and Drug–Herbal Interactions

Drug	Potential Interaction
antiplatelet and anticoagulant drugs	Garlic can increase the risk of bleeding.
atovaquone (Malarone)	Fatty food enhances absorption.
azithromycin (Zithromax)	Food reduces absorption.
calcium channel blockers and cyclosporine	Grapefruit juice enhances absorption.
cholestyramine (Prevalite)	Drug binds iron, folic acid, and vitamin A to decrease their absorption.
CNS depressants	Valerian can increase drowsiness and sedation.
fluoroquinolones	Calcium, iron, and other metal ions bind the drug and decrease absorption.
lovastatin (Altoprev)	Food increases absorption.
MAO inhibitors	Foods containing tyramine can cause hypertensive crisis.
NSAIDs	Food reduces the incidence of side effects.
penicillin G	Food (milk) and metal ions reduce absorption.
selective serotonin reuptake inhibitors (SSRIs)	St. John's wort and grapefruit juice increase risk of adverse effects (serotonin syndrome).
sucralfate (Carafate)	Food protein binds the drug to decrease absorption.
tetracyclines	Dairy products and iron reduce absorption.
warfarin (Coumadin)	Vitamin K antagonizes the action of warfarin; ginkgo, garlic, and St. John's wort may increase risk of bleeding.
zidovudine (AZT)	Food reduces bioavailability.

Very few clinically significant interactions of drugs with herbal products have been documented. As more patients take these products, however, research is demonstrating that certain drug–herb combinations may impact pharmacotherapy. Because patients view herbal products as natural, they do not usually mention them when recording their medication history; thus, the healthcare provider must ask specific questions about their use.

One of the most widely studied herbs is St. John's wort, which is taken by patients as a complementary or alternative therapy for depression. The herb induces hepatic metabolic enzymes, which can reduce the effectiveness of certain prescription medications, including antidepressants, warfarin, and benzodiazepines. A second herb that has been extensively studied is ginkgo biloba, which is taken to improve circulation and memory. Ginkgo may produce additive anticoagulant effects when taken with warfarin or antiplatelet drugs. It can also antagonize the effects of antiseizure drugs, thus increasing the risk for seizures. Because both St. John's wort and ginkgo can significantly affect drug action, the nurse should assess for the use of these substances when obtaining the patient's health history. Other effects of herbal products are presented in Chapter 7.

CONNECTIONS: Community-Oriented Practice

Food–Drug Interactions

Patient education related to food–drug interactions is one of the most common educational needs a patient will have. Most medications can be administered with food, but there are some foods that contain naturally occurring substances or are fortified with vitamins that do not mix well with certain medications. Sometimes the drug ingredients do not work as well as they should when certain foods are taken concurrently. We also know that some food nutrients affect absorption, metabolism, or elimination of a drug by binding with ingredients in the medication.

As mentioned in this chapter, a common food–drug interaction may occur when a patient eats grapefruit or drinks grapefruit juice with select medications. However, other compounds in food or beverages may also alter pharmacokinetic processes and, thus, drug effects. Other juices such as apple, orange, pomegranate, and tomato and other foods including tea, licorice, chocolate, and cruciferous vegetables have compounds that may also impact pharmacokinetic processes or the way in which the drugs work in the body, and not as much is known yet about these interactions or how to predict them. A detailed dietary recall is needed in addition to a medication history, especially when reactions to medications seem to relate to certain foods (Nicoteri, 2016). Because research into the influence of foods and juices other than grapefruit is limited, unless ordered otherwise, the safest way to take a medication is with a glass of water.

Understanding Chapter 5

Key Concepts Summary

5.1 The nurse plays a key role in preventing and managing adverse drug effects.

5.2 The FDA continues to monitor for new adverse events after a drug is approved and marketed.

5.3 Allergic reactions are caused by a hyper-response of the immune system.

5.4 Idiosyncratic reactions are unusual drug responses often caused by genetic differences among patients.

5.5 Some drugs have the ability to induce cancer or cause birth defects.

5.6 Drug toxicity may be specific to particular organs.

5.7 Drug interactions may significantly affect pharmacotherapeutic outcomes.

5.8 Pharmacokinetic drug interactions include changes in the absorption, distribution, metabolism, or excretion of medications.

5.9 Pharmacodynamic drug interactions include additive, synergistic, or antagonistic effects.

5.10 Food, nutrients, and dietary supplements may interact with medications and affect their actions.

CASE STUDY: Making the Patient Connection

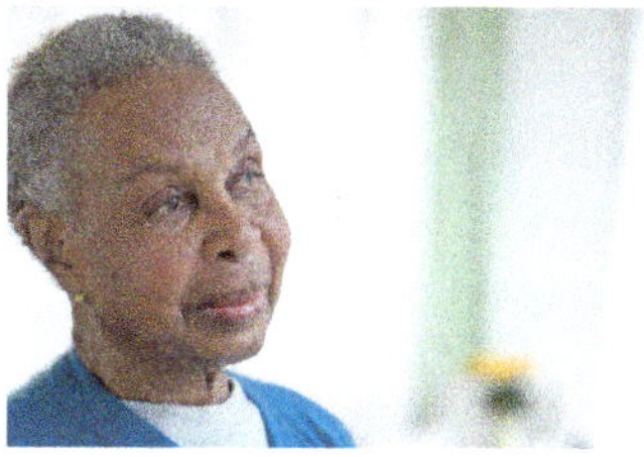

Remember the patient "Elizabeth Washington" at the beginning of the chapter? Now read the remainder of the case study. Based on the information presented within this chapter, respond to the critical thinking questions that follow.

The more medication an individual takes, the more likely it is that an adverse reaction may occur. For Elizabeth Washington this is a real possibility because she takes multiple medications for various physical problems. Elizabeth is a 77-year-old woman with several chronic conditions that require pharmacotherapy, including diabetes, heart failure, arthritis, and depression. She has been wheelchair bound since her stroke 2 years ago and has lost functional ability of her left side.

Unfortunately, she does not have a regular healthcare provider. Elizabeth obtains all her healthcare from a clinic operated for lower-income individuals. The primary healthcare providers in the clinic are medical residents and interns who rotate every month as part of their medical training. Therefore, it is unlikely that she will see the same prescriber more than a couple of times. Her medical record is quite extensive and spans her health history for the past 15 years. Because her medical history record is so lengthy, Elizabeth fears that the new doctors will not take the time to read the entire chart before prescribing the newest treatment or therapy.

Critical Thinking Questions

1. Identify ways that you can minimize or prevent adverse drug events in this patient.
2. What existing conditions make Elizabeth more susceptible to a drug reaction?
3. Discuss how drug reactions can affect pharmacokinetics.
4. Differentiate among additive, synergistic, and antagonist drug effects.

Additional Case Study

As the triage nurse in the emergency department, you determine the patient's chief complaint, obtain vital signs, collect past medical history information, and ask about drug and food allergies. While assessing a patient with a suspected ankle fracture, she tells you that she is allergic to codeine because it makes her nauseated and sleepy.

1. What further questions would you ask the patient about drug allergies?
2. Differentiate between an adverse effect, a side effect, and drug allergy.
3. Is this patient experiencing an idiosyncratic reaction? Explain.

Chapter Review

1. Prior to the administration of an antibiotic, the patient informs you that 4 years ago he experienced an allergic reaction. Based on this information, what should you do first?

1. Ask the patient to describe the reaction further.
2. Notify the healthcare provider on call about the patient's statements.
3. Administer the dose and observe the patient for a reaction.
4. Check the medical administration record for documented allergies.

2. While researching a new drug prior to administration, you see that the drug handbook states that the adverse effects are "dose related," which means that:

1. As the dose increases, the risk of adverse effects also increases.
2. The adverse effects should be expected after the first dose.
3. Oral preparations will produce the most adverse effects.
4. The timing of each dose should be correlated with the presence of adverse effects.

3. The patient is receiving a medication that may cause nephrotoxicity. To decrease the risk of this adverse reaction, the nurse should encourage the patient to:

1. Avoid sunbathing and exposure to direct sunlight.
2. Increase the intake of potassium-enriched foods.
3. Abstain from alcoholic beverages.
4. Increase fluid intake to promote adequate hydration.

4. On physical examination, you observe raised hivelike welts covering the patient's trunk and arms. The patient also reports intense itching after receiving a new medication. You will document which dermatologic adverse effect?

1. Angioedema
2. Stevens–Johnson syndrome
3. Urticaria
4. Photosensitivity

5. When observing a patient for bone marrow toxicity, you should monitor for:

1. Increased reports of muscle and bone pain in the lower extremities.
2. Decrease in red blood cells, white blood cells, and platelets.
3. Decrease in the range of motion of the upper and lower extremities.
4. Increase in hepatic enzymes.

6. The patient is receiving a medication that causes hepatotoxicity. What symptoms would alert you that this drug-related toxicity has occurred?

1. Black furry tongue and vaginal yeast infection
2. A sudden reduction in blood pressure on rising
3. Right upper quadrant pain and anorexia
4. Uncontrollable movements in the face, arms, and legs

See Appendix A for answers to critical thinking questions, case study questions and review questions.

References

Nicoteri, J. A. (2016). Food–drug interactions: Putting the evidence into practice. *The Nurse Practitioner*, *41*(2), 1–7. https://doi.org/10.1097/01.NPR.0000476374.12244.0a

Ronis, M. J., Pedersen, K. B., & Watt, J. (2018). Adverse effects of nutraceuticals and dietary supplements. *Annual Review of Pharmacology and Toxicology*, *58*, 583–601. https://doi.org/10.1146/annurev-pharmtox-010617-052844

U.S. Food and Drug Administration. (2019). *Code of federal regulations, Title 21, Volume 5*. https://www.accessdata.fda.gov/scripts/cdrh/cfdocs/cfcfr/cfrsearch.cfm?fr=312.32

Selected Bibliography

Abbott, K. L., Flannery, P. C., Gill, K. S., Boothe, D. M., Dhanasekaran, M., Mani, S., & Pondugula, S. R. (2020). Adverse pharmacokinetic interactions between illicit substances and clinical drugs. *Drug Metabolism Reviews*, *52*(1), 44–65. https://doi.org/10.1080/03602532.2019.1697283

Amadi, C. N., & Mgbahurike, A. A. (2018). Selected food/herb–drug interactions: Mechanisms and clinical relevance. *American Journal of Therapeutics*, *25*(4), e423–e433. https://doi.org/10.1097/MJT.0000000000000705

Awortwe, C., Bruckmueller, H., & Cascorbi, I. (2019). Interaction of herbal products with prescribed medications: A systematic review and meta-analysis. *Pharmacological Research*, *141*, 397–408. https://doi.org/10.1016/j.phrs.2019.01.028

Choi, J. G., Eom, S. M., Kim, J., Kim, S. H., Huh, E., Kim, H., et al. (2016). A comprehensive review of recent studies on herb–drug interaction: A focus on pharmacodynamic interaction. *Journal of Alternative and Complementary Medicine*, *22*(4), 262–279. https://doi.org/10.1089/acm.2015.0235

Dmitriev, A. V., Lagunin, A. A., Karasev, D. A., Rudik, A. V., Pogodin, P. V., Filimonov, D. A., & Poroikov, V. V. (2019). Prediction of drug–drug interactions related to inhibition or induction of drug-metabolizing enzymes. *Current Topics in Medicinal Chemistry*, *19*(5), 319–336. https://doi.org/10.2174/1568026619666190123160406

Eguale, T., Buckeridge, D. L., Verma, A., Winslade, N. E., Benedetti, A., Hanley, J. A., & Tamblyn, R. (2016). Association of off-label drug use and adverse drug events in an adult population. *JAMA Internal Medicine*, *176*(1), 55–63. https://doi.org/10.1001/jamainternmed.2015.6058

Naples, J. G., Hanlon, J. T., Schmader, K. E., & Semla, T. P. (2016). Recent literature on medication errors and adverse drug events in older adults. *Journal of the American Geriatrics Society*, *64*, 401–408. https://doi.org/10.1111/jgs.13922

Niu, J., Straubinger, R. M., & Mager, D. E. (2019). Pharmacodynamic drug–drug interactions. *Clinical Pharmacology & Therapeutics*, *105*(6), 1395–1406. https://doi.org/10.1002/cpt.1434

Oga, E. F., Sekine, S., Shitara, Y., & Horie, T. (2016). Pharmacokinetic herb–drug interactions: Insight into mechanisms and consequences. *European Journal of Drug Metabolism and Pharmacokinetics*, *41*, 93–108. https://doi.org/10.1007/s13318-015-0296-z

Roberts, A. G., & Gibbs, M. E. (2018). Mechanisms and the clinical relevance of complex drug–drug interactions. *Clinical Pharmacology: Advances and Applications*, *10*, 123–134. https://doi.org/10.2147/CPAA.S146115

U.S. Department of Health and Human Services, National Toxicology Program. (2016). *14th Report on carcinogens*. http://ntp.niehs.nih.gov/pubhealth/roc/index-1.html

Zheng, W. Y., Richardson, L. C., Li, L., Day, R. O., Westbrook, J. I., & Baysari, M. T. (2018). Drug-drug interactions and their harmful effects in hospitalised patients: A systematic review and meta-analysis. *European Journal of Clinical Pharmacology*, *74*(1), 15–27. https://doi.org/10.1007/s00228-017-2357-5

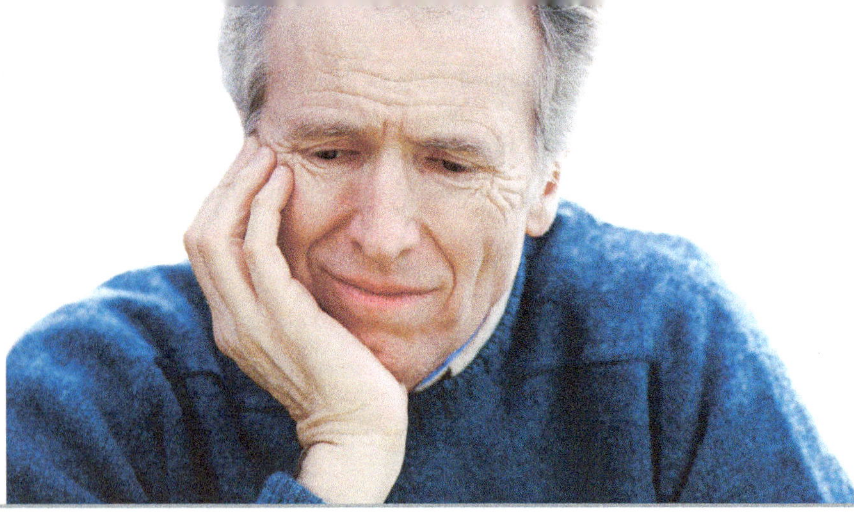

"He was always so cautious about everything. Isn't it amazing . . . he survived a war, worked in a hazardous occupation, and never even got a traffic ticket. Yet all it took was one trip to the hospital for a simple procedure. Now, it's all over."
—*Friend of "Ross Holland"*

Chapter 6
Medication Errors and Risk Reduction

Chapter Outline

- Medication Errors and Their Impact on Healthcare
- Factors Contributing to Medication Errors
- Drug Names and Medication Errors
- Reporting Medication Errors
- Strategies for Reducing Medication Errors

Learning Outcomes

After reading this chapter, the student should be able to:

1. Critique the following statement: "All medication errors can be prevented."
2. Describe the potential impact of a medication error on all aspects of healthcare delivery, including patients, nurses, and healthcare agencies.
3. Using specific examples, analyze major types of medication errors and how they can be prevented.
4. Describe procedures for reporting and documenting medication errors and incidents.
5. Explain how rules, policies, and procedures can help prevent medication errors.
6. Develop a list of strategies that the nurse can implement in practice to reduce medication errors.
7. Explain how medication reconciliation can lead to a reduction in medication errors.
8. Design patient teaching information that can be used to reduce medication errors.
9. Identify strategies that healthcare agencies use to prevent medication errors.

Key Terms

Definitions of the terms in bold may be found in the Glossary.

Medication errors occur throughout the medication-use system including while prescribing, upon entering information into a computer system, when the drug is being prepared or dispensed, or during drug administration. Each of these requires multiple complex steps to be accomplished by prescribers, pharmacists, nurses, and patients and can never be 100% error free. Occasionally, medication errors are made that can significantly impact treatment outcomes. The purpose of this chapter is to examine the reasons for medication errors and explore strategies that nurses may use to prevent them.

PharmFACT

The U.S. Food and Drug Administration (FDA) receives more than 100,000 U.S. reports each year associated with a suspected medication error. The reports come from drug manufacturers, healthcare professionals, and consumers through MedWatch, the FDA's safety information and adverse event reporting program. The FDA (2020) reviews the reports and classifies them to determine the cause and type of error.

Medication Errors and Their Impact on Healthcare

6.1 Medication errors are preventable events that may significantly impact treatment outcomes.

According to the National Coordinating Council for Medication Error Reporting and Prevention (NCC MERP, 2020), a **medication error** is:

> any preventable event that may cause or lead to inappropriate medication use or patient harm while the medication is in the control of the healthcare professional, patient, or consumer. Such events may be related to professional practice, healthcare products, procedures, and systems, including prescribing, order communication, product labeling, packaging, and nomenclature, compounding, dispensing, distribution, administration, education, monitoring, and use.

Whereas most medication errors do not result in patient harm, when they do, it may be devastating to the patient and to those healthcare providers involved in the error. The NCC MERP has developed a **medication error index** that categorizes medication errors by evaluating the extent of harm an error can cause, as shown in Figures 6.1 and 6.2.

The Joint Commission, an accrediting body for many healthcare agencies, considers certain categories of risk to patients to be sentinel events. A **sentinel event** is defined as a risk to patient safety that is so significant that it may result in death, permanent harm, or severe temporary harm (The Joint Commission, 2020c). These events pose such a risk to patient safety that The Joint Commission requires healthcare agencies to immediately conduct a review of any sentinel event and to take appropriate action to ensure it does not occur again. The definition of sentinel events was recently revised by The Joint Commission to highlight the need for healthcare partners to work with the commission to protect the patient and prevent further harm by improving the systems in place. The term *near miss*, also known as *close call* or *no harm*, is used to represent unexpected occurrences that posed a *risk* of harm, or occurrences that resulted in injury that did not rise to the same level of significance as a sentinel event. Both sentinel events and near misses are categorized as "patient safety events." A **patient safety event** is an event, incident, or condition that could have resulted or did result in harm to a patient (The Joint Commission, 2020b). Healthcare agencies are expected to conduct reviews of patient safety events and are strongly encouraged to report such events to the commission, although reporting is not mandatory.

Medication errors may have significant impact beyond just the patient's involvement. Errors may extend the length of hospitalization, which increases medical costs for the patient and agency. Undue harm to the patient due to medication errors is a potential cause of expensive legal challenges for the healthcare industry, physicians, and nurses. If frequent medication errors occur, the accreditation of the facility may be scrutinized and revoked. The agency also suffers loss of reimbursement as well as being perceived by the public as unsafe or delivering substandard care.

There is no acceptable occurrence rate for medication errors. The goal of every healthcare organization should be to improve medication administration systems to prevent harm to patients due to medication errors. All errors, whether or not they affect the patient, should be investigated with the goal of identifying policies and procedures that can improve the medication administration process to prevent future errors. The investigation of errors should be conducted in a nonpunitive manner that encourages staff to report errors, thereby building a culture of safety within an organization. Medication errors, especially those types that occur repeatedly, can alert nurses and healthcare administrators that a new policy, procedure, or process needs to be implemented to maximize patient safety.

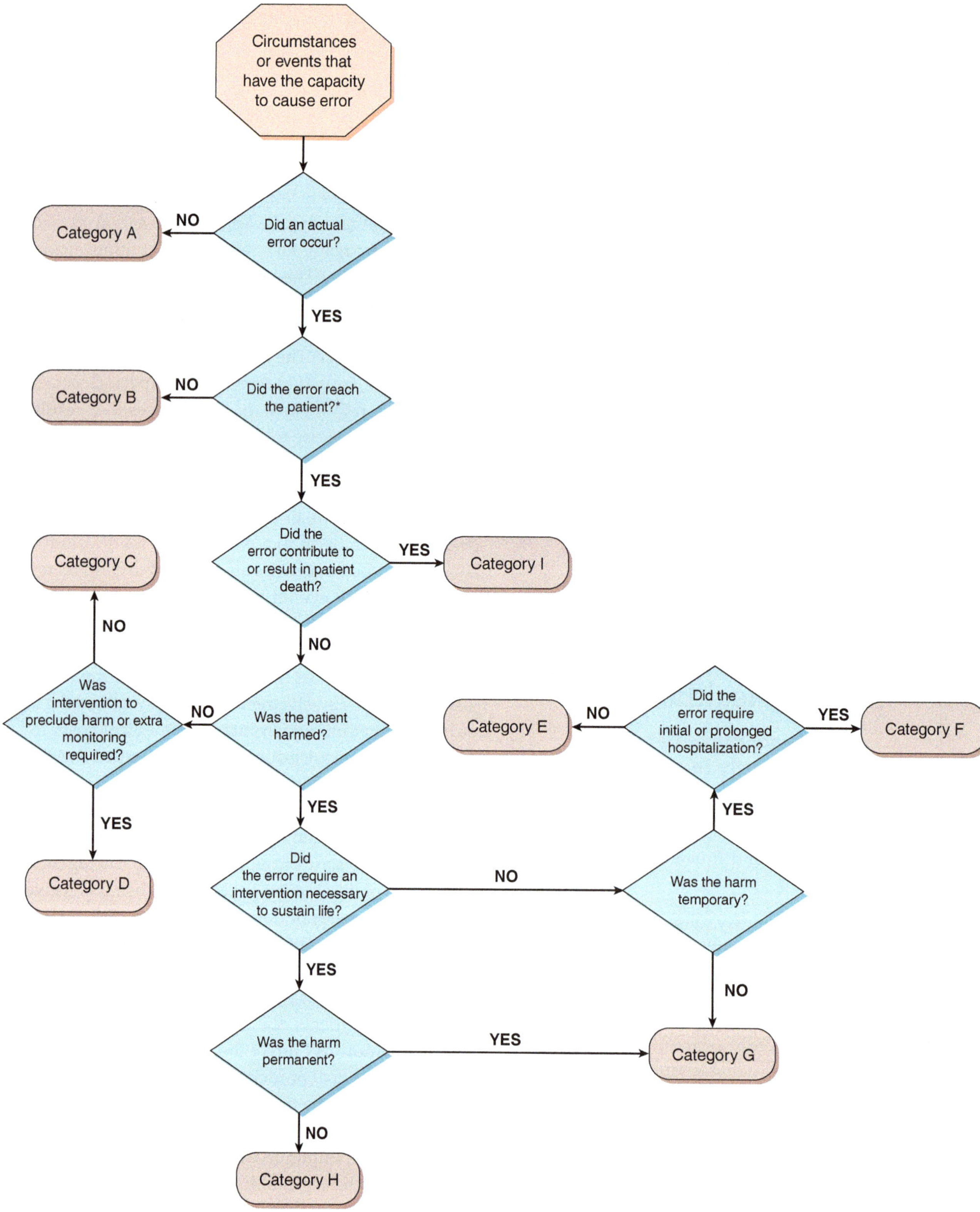

*An error of omission does reach the patient.

Figure 6.1 NCC MERP Index for categorizing medication errors algorithm.

From National Coordinating Council for Medication Error Reporting and Prevention,

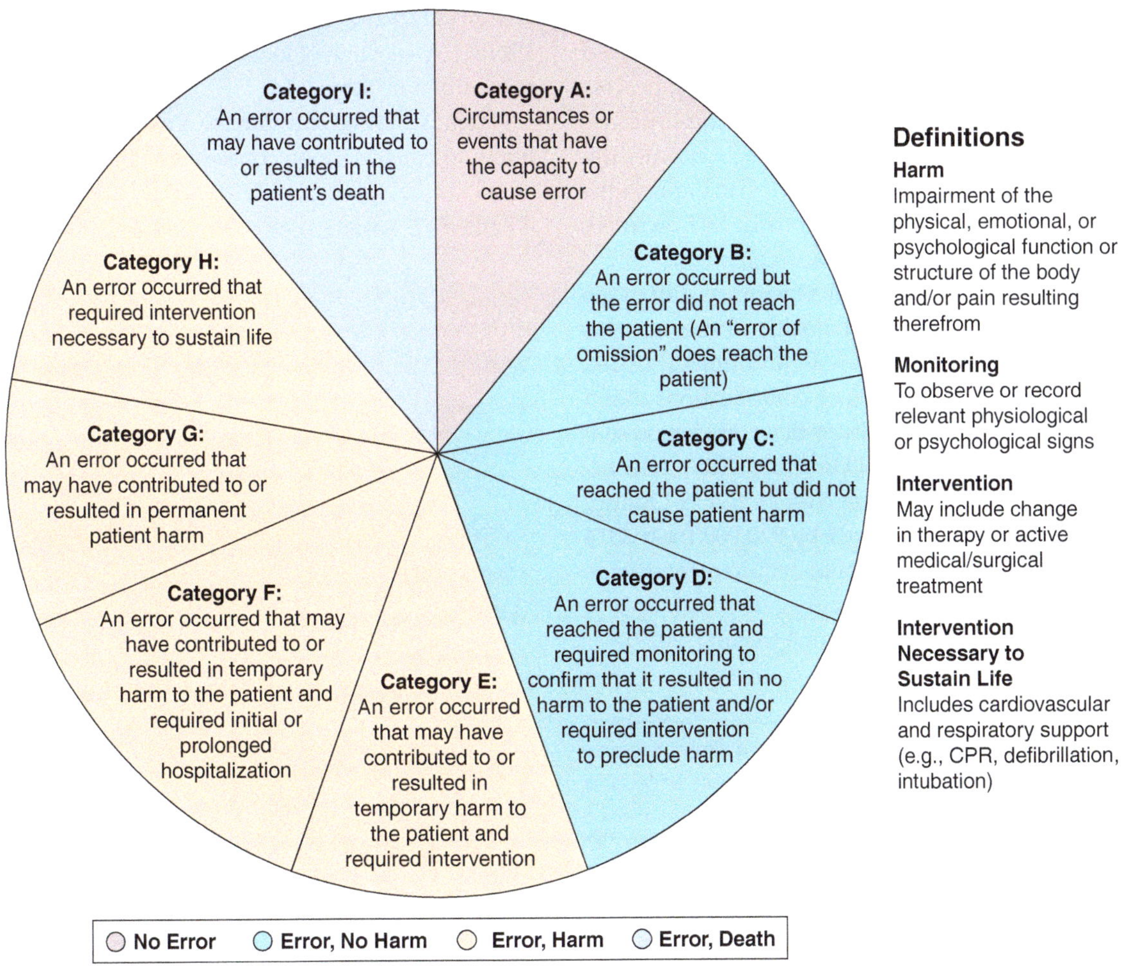

Figure 6.2 NCC MERP Index for categorizing medication errors.
From National Coordinating Council for Medication Error Reporting and Prevention, © 2001a. All rights reserved.

Factors Contributing to Medication Errors

6.2 Medication errors may be caused by human factors, inadequate communication, or confusing labels, packaging, or drug names.

Many different factors contribute to medication errors. When considering the number of healthcare personnel involved, from medication order to administration, patient-related factors, packaging, and other non-human-related elements, there are many opportunities for a medication error to occur. It is not surprising that research into the causes of medication errors has found that the majority stem from human factors—such as deficient knowledge, prescribing or administration errors, and errors of omission—across all healthcare settings (Chu, 2016; Farzi et al., 2017). The most frequent categories of errors include the following.

- Errors in patient assessment (e.g., inadequate medication history, incomplete physical assessment)
- Inaccurate prescribing (e.g., wrong drug, incorrect dose)
- Errors in administration (e.g., route or time of administration, omissions).

Most medication errors involve a breach of one of the cardinal "five rights" of medication administration: the right patient, drug, dosage, route, and time. Labeling designs, changes in packaging, and problems with dispensing devices are other factors contributing to errors. In many settings, the nurse remains the last line of defense to prevent an error from occurring.

Studying the types and causes of medication errors allows agencies and facilities to design ways to prevent them. Once a common source of error is identified, the U.S. Food and Drug Administration (FDA) works with healthcare agencies to determine changes that may be made to prevent that error in the future. For example, if two drug names sound too similar and are causing medication errors, the FDA may mandate a change in name. The FDA may also request pharmaceutical companies to more clearly label or package a drug to avoid confusion. Other forms of intervention include educating healthcare professionals and consumers about common errors and how to prevent them.

Health information technology (HIT) has become an increasingly powerful tool over the past few decades for improving medication safety. Different tools have been developed to support the prescribing process (e.g., computerized prescribing with decision support), the dispensing process (e.g., barcoding or automated dispensing and unit-dose systems), and the administering process (e.g., electronic medication administration records and smart pumps) to improve the medication process at all stages. Additionally, HIT increases the quality and transparency of the documentation.

The Affordable Care Act created a historical shift in the U.S. healthcare system. One early positive outcome was a declining rate of hospital-acquired conditions (HACs). HACs include medical conditions or complications that a patient develops during a hospital stay that were not present on admission (American Hospital Directory, 2017). According to the Agency for Healthcare Research and Quality (AHRQ, 2019), HACs were reduced by 910,000 from 2014 to 2017. The estimated rate of hospital-acquired conditions dropped 13%, from 99 per 1,000 acute care discharges to 86 per 1,000 during the same time frame (AHRQ, 2019).

CONNECTION Checkpoint 6.1

From what you learned in Chapter 5, describe the similarities and differences between a synergistic effect and an additive effect and how they might contribute to a medication error.

Drug Names and Medication Errors

6.3 Certain drugs have higher rates of medication errors.

Some types of medication errors are independent of the drug being administered. For example, failure to perform adequate medication order checks, forgetting to give a dose, or administering the medication to the wrong patient can occur with any medication. Some drugs, however, have higher error rates than others. Furthermore, when an error does occur, certain medications have greater potential to cause harm. Learning which drugs have the highest error rates and produce the most serious consequences can help the nurse to be more vigilant when administering these agents.

With thousands of generic and trade names for drugs, it is inevitable that some will look or sound similar; for example, *hydroxyzine* and *hydralazine* or *Novalin* and *NovoLog*. It is easy to understand how a verbal order given in a hurry over a cell phone could result in the wrong drug. It is likely that hundreds of medication errors occur each year because of look-alike or sound-alike drugs. This is a primary reason why verbal drug orders should always be confirmed in writing before being administered. The Institute for Safe Medication Practices (ISMP, 2019) publishes a list of confused drug names and recommends the use of "Tall Man Letters" as a method to reduce the chance that one drug will be mistaken for another. For example, hydroxyzine would be written as "hydrOXYzine" to avoid confusion with hydralazine (which is recommended as "hydrALAZINE"). A selection of look-alike or sound-alike drug names is included in Table 6.1.

Drugs that have a narrow therapeutic index are more likely to cause serious consequences should a medication

Table 6.1 Selected Look-Alike and Sound-Alike Drug Names

acetazolamide	acetaminophen
AcipHex	Aricept
Adderall	Inderal
alprazolam	clonazepam
bupropion	Buspirone
carboplatin	cisplatin
Celebrex	Cerebyx
chlorpromazine	chlorpropamide
cycloserine	cyclosporine
daunorubicin	doxorubicin
dimenhydramine	diphenhydramine
Diprivan	Ditropan
dobutamine	dopamine
Humalog	Humulin
hydromorphone	morphine
infliximab	rituximab
isotretinoin	tretinoin
Kaletra	Keppra
Lamisil	Lamictal
lamivudine	lamotrigine
leucovorin	Leukeran
Lexapro	Loxitane
MS Contin	OxyContin
Neulasta	Neumega
oxycodone	oxymorphone
paroxetine	fluoxetine
Retrovir	ritonavir
Seroquel	Sinequan
sumatriptan	zolmitriptan
tiagabine	tizanidine
TobraDex	Tobrex
tramadol	trazodone
Trental	tegretol
valacyclovir	valganciclovir
vinblastine	vincristine
Viracept	Viramune
Zantac	Zyrtec
Zestril	Zetia
Zyprexa	Celexa

error occur. These drugs are not necessarily more error prone than others, but the nurse should give extra care when administering them due to their toxicity. The ISMP maintains lists of **high-alert medications** and defines these as "drugs that bear a heightened risk of causing significant patient harm when used in error" (ISMP, 2018). Lists are available for both institutional and inpatient settings as well as community and ambulatory agencies. Healthcare agencies may build in additional safeguards with these medications such as independent double-checks or automated alerts. Each patient care unit may include its own, additional list of high-alert medications. For example, high-alert drugs on a cancer unit or a pediatric unit may differ from those on a medical–surgical unit. A selected list of high-alert medications is included in Appendix B of this text.

PharmFACT

Although medication errors occur at a similar rate in adults and children, pediatric errors are three times more likely to cause harm. Studies have shown that hospitals using computerized provider order entry (CPOE) with clinical decision support (CDS) tended to have lower rates of medication errors (Gates et al., 2019).

Reporting Medication Errors

6.4 Medication errors must be properly documented and reported.

Although some medication errors go unreported, it is always the nurse's legal and ethical responsibility to document all occurrences. In severe cases, adverse reactions caused by medication errors may require the initiation of lifesaving interventions for the patient, including available antidotes. After such an incident, the patient may require close supervision, and additional medical treatments may be warranted.

The FDA has coordinated the reporting of medication errors at the federal level. The FDA Safety Information and Adverse Event Reporting Program, known as MedWatch, provides important and timely clinical information about safety issues involving medical products, including prescription and over-the-counter (OTC) drugs, biologics, medical- and radiation-emitting devices, and special nutritional products. The FDA encourages nurses and other healthcare providers to report medication errors to its database, which is used to assist other professionals in avoiding similar mistakes. Medication errors, or situations that can lead to errors, may be reported anonymously directly to the FDA by telephone or online.

In conjunction with the U.S. Pharmacopeial Convention (USPC), the ISMP operates the voluntary NCC MERP, which accepts reports from consumers and healthcare professionals related to medication safety. Medication errors from the NCC MERP voluntary reporting system are shared with the FDA. Establishment of the NCC MERP has resulted in dozens of medication-related patient safety changes, including nationwide hazard alerts; packaging, labeling, and nomenclature changes; and healthcare system changes.

The USPC also offers MEDMARX, a national, internet-accessible database that hospitals and healthcare systems use to track adverse drug events and medication errors. Agencies participate in MEDMARX voluntarily subscribe to it on an annual basis. MEDMARX is operated as a quality improvement tool, which facilitates productive and efficient documentation, reporting, analysis, tracking, trending, and prevention of adverse drug events.

All medical facilities have policies and procedures that provide guidance to the nurse on reporting medication errors. Documentation of the error should occur in a factual manner and must include specific nursing interventions that were implemented following the error to protect patient safety, such as monitoring vital signs and assessing the

CONNECTIONS: Advanced Practice Application

Medication Errors

Case

A 4-year-old male with no significant medical history presented with his parents to your pediatric office with flulike symptoms. He has a chief complaint of generalized body ache and a fever of 38.7°C (101.6°F) oral. For the past week, his parents had been giving over-the-counter (OTC) diphenhydramine (Benadryl) liquid (12.5 mg/5 mL). The product label indicated the recommended dose for a child younger than 6 years old was 1 to 2 teaspoons (12.5 to 25 mg). However, the dosage cup that came with the medication was marked in teaspoons and milliliters (mL), not in milligrams (mg). On review of the dose given with the father, you realize he had mistakenly been giving the wrong dose and had missed the mL versus mg distinction. Although the child had no adverse events, the father was very concerned he had caused harm to his young son. As the provider you spent time reviewing the correct dose and provided a marked syringe for the parents to use.

Discussion

Errors measuring medicine using dosing cups are not uncommon and have led to serious consequences. Recently, a death occurred when a nurse confused two dosing scales that appeared on a plastic oral liquid dosing cup. To prevent confusion between variable measurement systems, devices should be marked with calibrated units of liquid measurement (tablespoon, teaspoon, milliliter) that are the same as the units of liquid measure specified on the product label and there should not be any unnecessary markings on the dosing device (ISMP, 2020; Pan et al., 2019).

patient for possible complications. Documentation does not simply record that a medical error occurred. Failure to document nursing actions taken related to the error could be interpreted as either negligence or failure to acknowledge that the incident occurred. The nurse should record the names of all individuals who were notified of the error and any follow-up monitoring or treatment prescribed or needed. The patient's **medication administration record (MAR)** should also contain information about what medication was given or omitted. If a medication error should occur, it is important to complete a written occurrence report. The occurrence report allows the opportunity to identify factors that contributed to the medication error. The occurrence report is not usually included in the patient's health record but providers should learn the specific policies applicable to the agency of employment about the methods used to report errors.

CONNECTION Checkpoint 6.2

Additional important functions of the U.S. Pharmacopeial Convention are presented in Chapter 2. What is the role of the USPC in drug regulation?

Strategies for Reducing Medication Errors

6.5 Multiple strategies can be used for reducing medication errors.

What can be done in the clinical setting to avoid medication errors and promote safe drug administration?

1. **Assessment.** Obtain a thorough medication history every time the patient enters the healthcare setting or transfers to another unit or agency. Ask the patient about food or medication allergies, current health concerns, and use of OTC medications and herbal supplements. Assess renal and hepatic functions and determine if other body systems are impaired and could affect pharmacotherapy. Identify areas of needed patient education with regard to medications.
2. **Planning.** Minimize factors that contribute to medication errors: Avoid using abbreviations that could be misunderstood, question unclear orders, do not accept verbal orders, and follow specific facility policies and procedures related to medication administration. Be aware of situations or settings that may increase the risk of errors, such as a busy environment.
3. **Implementation.** When engaged in a medication-related task, focus entirely on the task. Noise, other events, and talking coworkers can distract the nurse's attention and result in a medication error. Keep the following points in mind as well:
   - Positively verify the identity of each patient before administering the medication, according to facility policy and procedures. Never bypass safeguards when checking for identification such as barcoded patient ID bands, which require scanning at the bedside.
   - Use the correct procedures and techniques for all routes of administration. Use sterile materials and techniques when administering parenteral medications.
   - Calculate medication doses correctly and measure liquid drugs carefully. Some medications, such as heparin, have a narrow safety margin for producing serious adverse effects. When giving these medications, ask a colleague or a pharmacist to check the calculations to make certain the dosage is correct and follow any agency-required nomograms as appropriate. Always double-check pediatric calculations prior to administration.
   - Open medication packages or bottles immediately prior to administering the drug and in the presence of the patient.
   - Record the medication and all dosing information on the MAR immediately after administration.
   - Always confirm that the patient has swallowed an oral medication. Do not leave the medication at the bedside unless there is a specific order that it may be left there.
   - Be alert for long-acting oral dosage forms with indicators such as SR, LA, XL, and XR. These tablets or capsules usually must remain intact for the extended-release feature to remain effective. Instruct the patient not to crush, chew, or break the medication in half because doing so could cause an overdose.
4. **Evaluation.** Assess the patient for expected therapeutic outcomes and determine if any adverse effects have occurred. The nurse should be especially vigilant in observing for adverse effects if this is the first time the patient has ever taken the drug or if the dosage is being increased. Because antibiotics have the highest rate of drug allergy, the nurse must be especially observant for signs and symptoms of allergy following administration of these agents. All adverse effects noted should be reported to the healthcare provider, documented in the healthcare record, and reported to the next shift's nurse along with any additional orders from the provider. Have the patient restate information about the drug and dosing directions, including the correct dose of medication and the right time to take it. Asking the patient to demonstrate an understanding of the goals of pharmacotherapy assists the nurse in determining whether additional patient education is necessary.

Nurses and nurse practitioners must stay current on pharmacotherapeutics and should never prescribe or administer a medication unless they are familiar with its uses and adverse effects. There are many sources to obtain updated medication knowledge. Having current electronic or printed drug references available is essential for every level of practice. A word of caution is necessary, however: Drug references may sometimes give incorrect information. Teams must rely on common sense and good judgment. If a dose appears to be inaccurate in a reference source, nurses should always check with the prescriber or pharmacist before administering. In addition, some EHRs may have an automated drug reference available that may be accessed directly from the administration record. Whenever errors in drug references are encountered, nurses have a duty to contact the publisher of the inaccurate data, so that future medication errors may be prevented.

Utilizing inpatient and outpatient pharmacists on teams is an important tool and has become a trend around the country in an effort to decrease medication errors and improve patient outcomes. Pharmacists on interprofessional teams are able to conduct full medication reconciliation from hospital admission through discharge and offer prescribing recommendations, such as eliminating unnecessary or harmful medications and optimizing dosing, and may suggest alternative therapies. They also assist with care coordination and patient navigation near the time of discharge, provide patient education, and schedule follow-up visits for medication management services. These high-touch interventions around transitions between care teams have been shown to improve outcomes and decrease readmission rates (Edlin, 2019; Nuffer et al., 2019).

6.6 Thorough medication reconciliation is an important means of reducing medication errors.

One of The Joint Commission's (2020a) high-priority patient safety goals is to provide medication reconciliation for all patients. **Medication reconciliation** is the "process of comparing the medications a patient is taking (and should be taking) with newly ordered medications. The comparison addresses duplications, omissions, and interactions and the need to continue current medications. The types of information that clinicians use to reconcile medications include (among others) medication name, dose, frequency, route, and purpose. Organizations should identify the information that needs to be collected to reconcile current and newly ordered medications and to safely prescribe medications in the future" (The Joint Commission, 2020a). Medication reconciliation should occur anytime there is a change in the site of the patient's care: admission to, transfer, or discharge from a healthcare facility and, with more care being given in community settings, anytime the patient seeks care from a provider.

The Joint Commission is responsible for monitoring healthcare safety for the public and evaluating healthcare organizations for safety standards. They are responsible for reviewing every patient safety event report to determine whether it relates to one or more Joint Commission standards. Medication reconciliation has been incorporated into The Joint Commission's National Patient Safety Goal 3, "Improve the safety of using medications." This national patient safety goal (NPSG) focuses on the risk points of medication reconciliation and is designed to help organizations reduce negative patient outcomes associated with medication discrepancies.

The Joint Commission 2020 recommendations on medication reconciliation under NPSG.03.06.01 include the following:

- Obtain information on the medications the patient is currently taking when he or she is admitted to the hospital or in an outpatient setting with each interaction and appointment. Include a list of current medications taken at scheduled times and those taken on an as-needed basis. Examples of medication information that may be collected include name, dose, route, frequency, and purpose.
- Compare the medication information the patient brought to the hospital or clinic with the medications ordered for the patient by the hospital or clinic and resolve any discrepancies. Discrepancies include omissions, duplications, contraindications, unclear information, and changes.
- Provide written information about all medications the patient should be taking when he or she is discharged from the hospital or at the end of an outpatient clinic encounter.
- Take the time to explain the importance of managing medication information when the patient is discharged from the hospital or at the end of an outpatient encounter. Examples include instructing the patient to give a list to their primary care physician; to update the information when medications are discontinued, doses are changed, or new medications are added; and to carry medication information at all times in the event of emergency situations.

Many older adults have several chronic medical disorders concurrently, each of which may be treated by individual specialists. It is common for patients to receive multiple prescriptions, sometimes for the same condition, that have conflicting pharmacologic actions, a condition termed **polypharmacy**. Although not unique to older patients, polypharmacy is most often seen in the older age group. Keeping track of multiple medications and their doses, indications, routes, and frequency of administration is a major challenge for both patients and healthcare providers. Failure to properly record medication information and to communicate that information to healthcare providers is a potential cause of medication errors.

6.7 Adequate patient education and adherence are essential strategies for safe medication usage.

In the hospital setting, the physician, advanced practice nurse, nurse, and pharmacist are largely responsible for preventing medication errors, and they collaborate to ensure that the patient is receiving the correct drug in the manner designated by the prescriber. In the home setting, this responsibility relies on proper patient adherence to drug therapy. For prescription drugs, healthcare providers provide patients with verbal and written instructions on how and when to take the medication. Labels for OTC medications, herbal products, and dietary supplements indicate the correct method of taking the agent; however, patients do not always read or understand the information given.

Adherence is a major factor affecting pharmacotherapeutic outcomes and for increasing the risk of medication errors. As it relates to pharmacotherapy, **adherence** is defined as taking medications in the manner prescribed by the healthcare provider. In the case of OTC products, adherence means correctly following the instructions on the label. Patient nonadherence ranges from not taking the medication at all to taking it at the wrong time or at the wrong dose.

Many factors can influence patient adherence with pharmacotherapy. One of the most common sources of nonadherence is simply forgetting a dose of medication. This occurs frequently when the drug must be taken more than twice daily. Another source of nonadherence is that the drug may be too expensive or not approved by the patient's health insurance plan. Patients often discontinue the use of drugs that have annoying adverse effects or those that impair major lifestyle choices. Adverse effects that often prompt nonadherence are headache, dizziness, nausea, diarrhea, and impotence.

Patients often take medications in an unexpected manner, sometimes self-adjusting their doses. Some feel that if one tablet is good, two must be better. Others believe that they will become dependent on the medication if it is taken as prescribed, so they only take half the necessary dose. Still others simply stop taking the medication when they start feeling better. Patients are usually reluctant to admit or report nonadherence for fear of being reprimanded or feeling embarrassed.

The concept of adherence, or compliance, should be expanded to include patient–provider *concordance*. Compliance has been defined as "the extent to which the patient follows the health professionals' advice and takes the treatment"; adherence is "the extent to which a person's behavior—taking medication, following a diet, and executing lifestyle changes—corresponds with agreed recommendations from a healthcare provider"; and concordance as "agreement between the patient and healthcare professional, reached after negotiation that respects the beliefs and wishes of the patient in determining whether, when and how their medicine is taken, and (in which) the privacy of the person is recognized" (Poupoulas, n.d.). Concordance is integrated into a shared decision-making model of care but may take time to develop between patient and provider. Early interactions may retain a paternalistic approach as the patient seeks information about treatment, with the healthcare professional providing treatment and the patient complying and adhering. As the patient learns more about his or her condition, disease, and treatment, a transition to more shared decision making occurs (Mathews et al., 2016).

Because reasons for nonadherence are many and varied, healthcare providers must be vigilant in questioning patients about taking their medications. When pharmacotherapy fails to produce the expected treatment outcomes, nonadherence should always be considered as a possible explanation. There are steps that providers can take to increase the potential for patient adherence to the therapeutic regimen. All of these steps focus on effective teaching. Knowing that patients often feel overwhelmed with the amount of information provided, it is important to discuss the prescription routine with the patient and ask questions: Will the patient be able to fill the prescription? How will it fit into the patient's usual routine or with other medications? Listening for clues that suggest the patient is overwhelmed by the routines, the nurse can ask further questions about what suggestions the patient might have to make the routine workable. Patients may be reluctant to discuss these suggestions with their provider but may feel comfortable doing so with the nurse because of the nurse–patient relationship.

In the plan of care, it is important to address essential information that the patient must know regarding the prescribed medications. This includes factors such as the name of the medication, why it has been ordered, expected drug actions, associated adverse effects, and information regarding interactions with other medications, foods, herbal supplements, or alcohol. Patients should be encouraged to take an active role in ensuring the effectiveness of their medication and their own safety. It is important to remember that, unless diagnosed as mentally incompetent, a well-informed adult always has the legal option of refusal to take any medication. It is the nurse's responsibility, however, to ensure that the patient has all the necessary information to make an informed decision.

For patients receiving outpatient therapy or those being released from a hospital, it is important to carefully assess their ability to take their medications in a safe and effective manner. If it is decided that the patient may have difficulty in properly administering the medications, caregivers should be consulted and other arrangements made to ensure that the patient receives the correct drugs using the proper dosing schedule. With each successive healthcare visit, it is important to review the medication history, asking questions about the prescribed medications. Being alert to reports that the patient is not taking, or is not taking correctly, the prescribed drugs may suggest an overwhelming, complex medication routine that needs to be reassessed if it is to be successful. Economic conditions sometimes result in difficult choices for patients between obtaining medications and other required necessities. Nurses provide medication education and follow-up that will result in positive health outcomes and the prevention of negative health effects and even larger expenditures as a result of poor medication adherence. Special considerations related to drug administration to pediatric and geriatric patients are presented in greater detail in Chapters 9 and 10, respectively.

PharmFACT

In the United States, 133 million Americans, representing more than 40% of the total population of this country, have a diagnosis of at least one chronic condition and almost one-third have a diagnosis of two or more chronic conditions. Of these, as many as 50% do not take their medications as prescribed and this nonadherence is thought to cause at least 100,000 preventable deaths and $100 billion in preventable medical costs per year (Kleinsinger, 2018).

6.8 Healthcare agencies are actively involved in reducing medication errors.

Most healthcare agencies use automated, computerized, locked cabinets for medication storage on patient care units. Each nurse on the unit has a code for accessing the cabinet and removing a medication dose. These automated systems also maintain an inventory of drug supplies. These systems are not foolproof, however, and the nurse must always perform system checks to ensure that the proper medication is in the correct patient drawer.

Large healthcare agencies often have **risk management** departments to examine risks and minimize the number of medication errors. Risk management personnel investigate incidents, track data, identify problems, and provide recommendations for improvement. Nurses collaborate with risk management committees to seek means of reducing medication errors by modifying policies and procedures within the institution. Examples of institutional policies and procedures include the following:

- Store medications under proper conditions (light and temperature control) and separate medications that have look-alike names or packaging.
- Read the drug label to avoid the administration of time-expired medications.
- Avoid the transfer of doses from one container to another.
- Avoid overstocking of medications.
- Monitor adherence to avoiding the use of prohibited prescription abbreviations.
- Remove outdated reference books.

6.9 Analytical tools may be used to identify risk and analyze errors.

Healthcare agencies use analytical tools to assess for the likelihood of errors and to analyze errors once they have occurred. Two such tools are the healthcare failure mode and effect analysis and root-cause analysis. These tools help agencies identify how errors occur and how to take steps to prevent them from occurring again.

In the case of medication administration, **healthcare failure mode and effect analysis (HFMEA)** identifies processes where errors may occur related to prescription, dispensing, and administration. Each process at risk for failure is analyzed and the severity and probability of each is determined. For example, when prescribing, an inaccurate assessment of the patient may occur. The level of the patient's pain may not be adequately assessed or the wrong analgesic may be chosen because of an inadequate consideration of all factors that may affect the use of that medication. The effects of these failures, if they occurred, might include poor pain control or the wrong drug or dose being prescribed. The severity of the failure may be estimated—catastrophic, major, moderate, or minor—and a severity score established. Catastrophic failures would rank as 4, whereas minor failures would rank as 1. The probability of a failure may also be ranked with possibilities ranging from frequent to remote. A "hazard score" is assigned, which is the severity score multiplied by the probability score (Institute for Healthcare Improvement, 2017). In the above example of patient pain and the process of choosing (prescribing) an analgesic, the severity score for selecting an inappropriate analgesic for a patient with undiagnosed hepatic insufficiency may be catastrophic (ranked 4) and the probability of that occurring may be occasional (ranked 3). This would result in a hazard score of 12. The higher the hazard score, the more critical it is to identify strategies to prevent such a failure from occurring. Healthcare organizations use HFMEA as a risk management strategy to prevent health system errors of any kind from occurring.

Once an error has occurred, it is essential to analyze why it happened so that steps can be taken to prevent its recurrence. **Root-cause analysis (RCA)** is a tool to help healthcare organizations retrospectively study events where patient harm or undesired outcomes occurred in order to identify and address the root causes. The Joint Commission has mandated use of RCA to analyze sentinel events since 1997. Through the application of human factors engineering approaches, an analysis of what happened, why it occurred, and how to prevent it from happening again is conducted. RCA of medication errors is often interdisciplinary because of the many opportunities for errors to occur in various departments. An analysis of people, equipment or supplies, policies and procedures, and environmental factors involved in the error is included.

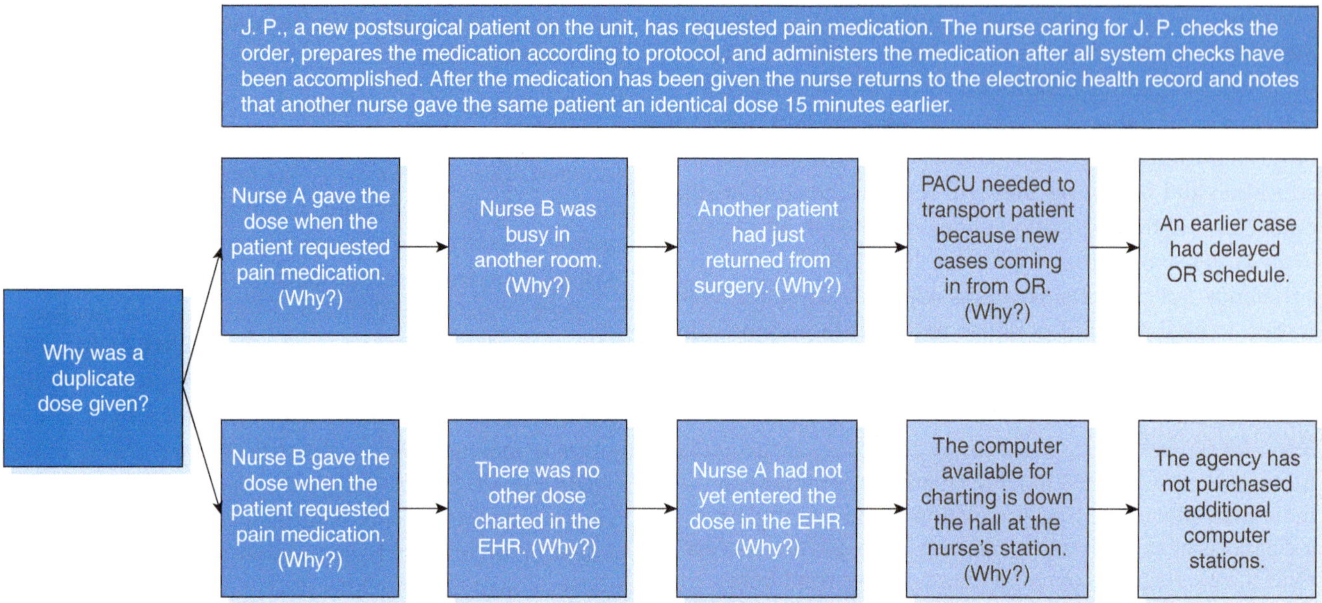

Figure 6.3 Sample root-cause analysis: duplicate dose of a narcotic analgesic.

For each category, "Why did the error occur?" is asked, with each question's answer prompting a further "Why?" question. This technique is sometimes called the "Five Whys" for this reason (iSixSigma, n.d.). There are many ways to diagram the analysis, and the nurse should utilize the tool(s) used in the specific healthcare agency. Figure 6.3 illustrates the beginning of a diagram for an error in which a duplicate dose of a narcotic analgesic was given after the patient returned from the recovery unit from surgery. Note that after asking "why" questions, causes are identified that involve equipment, procedures, and other departments. Each of those causes would also be examined to determine all possible remedies to prevent a recurrence.

The aim is always to maximize patient safety by striving to be 100% accurate when prescribing and administering medications. Drug administration, however, requires multiple complex steps accomplished by the entire healthcare team and can never be 100% error free. Being aware of potential areas that may increase medication errors and employing strategies to mitigate risk are integral components of the nursing role to ensure that pharmacotherapy provides maximum therapeutic effects with minimal harm.

Understanding Chapter 6

Key Concepts Summary

6.1 Medication errors are preventable events that may significantly impact treatment outcomes.

6.2 Medication errors may be caused by human factors, inadequate communication, or confusing labels, packaging, or drug names.

6.3 Certain drugs have higher rates of medication errors.

6.4 Medication errors must be properly documented and reported.

6.5 Multiple strategies can be used for reducing medication errors.

6.6 Thorough medication reconciliation is an important means of reducing medication errors.

6.7 Adequate patient education and adherence are essential strategies for safe medication usage.

6.8 Healthcare agencies are actively involved in reducing medication errors.

6.9 Analytical tools may be used to identify risk and analyze errors.

CASE STUDY: Making the Patient Connection

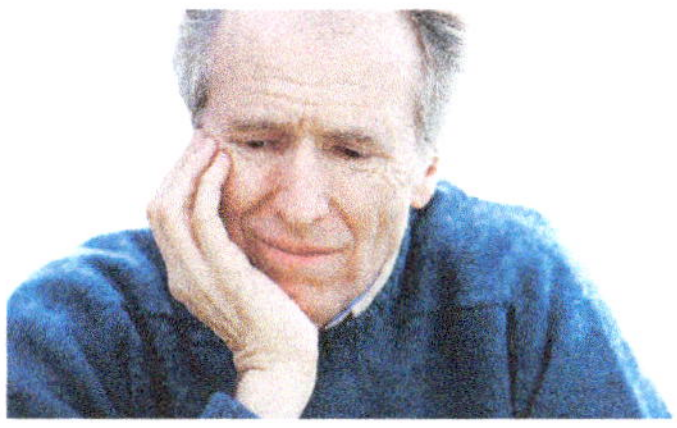

Remember the patient "Ross Holland" at the beginning of the chapter? Now read the remainder of the case study. Based on the information presented within this chapter, respond to the critical thinking questions that follow.

What happened to Ross Holland was truly a tragedy. He entered the hospital for simple sinus surgery and never recovered. Ironically, Ross was a super-vigilant man. As a Vietnam veteran, he had seen the worst of combat for 4 years. During the last 6 months of the conflict, he survived in a prisoner-of-war camp. When Ross returned home, he took a job as a safety inspector in the automobile industry.

From a previous physical examination, Ross knew that he had a slightly irregular heartbeat, but he never really took it seriously. In fact, he never mentioned it to the nurse when she took his preoperative history. This condition became apparent soon after surgery though. The nurse caring for Ross noticed a series of cardiac dysrhythmias on the monitor and contacted the healthcare provider. The healthcare provider ordered Ross to receive a cardiac antidysrhythmic medication stat to correct the problem. In haste, the nurse never clarified the route that the medication was to be given. Additionally, the nurse was not familiar with the medication's usual dose or any precautions that needed to be taken. As a result, the medication was given by direct intravenous administration without being diluted as directed on the medication bottle. Ross was given 100 times the normal dose. Consequently, he experienced seizure activity that lasted 5 minutes followed by respiratory arrest. All efforts to resuscitate him were unsuccessful.

Critical Thinking Questions

1. Ultimately, who was responsible for this medication error? Ross? The healthcare provider? The nurse? Explain.
2. Identify the contributing factors that resulted in the error.
3. What strategies should the nurse have used to prevent the medication error?
4. What common policies should healthcare facilities implement to avoid medication errors?
5. What are the required reporting requirements for a medication error?

Additional Case Study

A young mother brings her 6-month-old infant to the emergency department with a 3-day history of fevers, congestion, and increased irritability at night. The nurse practitioner diagnoses acute otitis media (ear infection) and prescribes an oral antibiotic and acetaminophen (Tylenol) every 4 hours for pain and fever. The young mother appears weepy and concerned. When asked why, she says, "Medications frighten me. When I give any of my children medications, I worry that I will make an error. There is so much that can go wrong."

1. How would you respond to this mother's concern?
2. Create a list of strategies that parents can use to prevent medication errors.
3. What referral resources could help reduce her anxiety?

Chapter Review

1. It is 2:45 a.m. and the nurse has telephoned the prescriber to report that the patient is experiencing an acute episode of postoperative pain. How can the nurse avoid medication errors when receiving a telephone order from a prescriber?
   1. Decline to accept the telephone order.
   2. Refuse to call the prescriber but attempt to comfort the patient.
   3. Instruct the patient's family to call the prescriber.
   4. Repeat the order verbally to ensure accuracy.
2. The nurse cannot read the number of milligrams (mg) to be administered in a drug order written by the healthcare provider. The nurse cannot determine whether 125 mg, 1.25 mg, or 12.5 mg should be administered. What action would be most appropriate to prevent a medication error?
   1. Telephone the healthcare provider about the illegible medication order.
   2. Ask another nurse to read the questionable medication order.
   3. Contact the pharmacist about the medication order.
   4. Consult a drug handbook and administer the normal dose.

3. While counseling a patient on a medication taken daily which strategy should be included that might prevent a medication error?
    1. Insist on trade-name drugs rather than generic drugs.
    2. Have all prescriptions filled at one pharmacy.
    3. Request all prescriptions be placed in easily opened containers.
    4. Consult the internet about possible adverse effects.

4. When given a medication, the patient states, "I've never seen this pill before. It's not like the others I take." Which would be the most appropriate action to take?
    1. Instruct the patient that different brands are frequently used.
    2. Administer the medication in the existing form.
    3. Verify the order and double-check the drug label.
    4. Advise the patient to talk with the healthcare provider and give the drug.

5. While administering medication to several patients, you suddenly realize that the wrong medication has been given to a patient. Which would be the *first* priority action taken?
    1. Assess the patient in order to monitor for adverse effects.
    2. Call the healthcare provider and report the error.
    3. Complete the hospital's drug error form.
    4. Report the medication error to the FDA.

6. As you enter the room to administer medication, the patient states, "I'm in the bathroom. Please leave the medication on my bedside table, and I will take it when I come out." Which would be the appropriate response?
    1. "I will leave the medication and follow up with you in 30 minutes."
    2. "You must take the medication now or refuse the dose."
    3. "Let me know when you are ready, and I will then return with your medicine."
    4. "I've given the drug to your visitors. Take it when you come out of the bathroom."

See Appendix A for answers to critical thinking questions, case study questions and review questions.

References

Agency for Healthcare Research and Quality. (2019). *Analysis finds hospital-acquired conditions declined by nearly 1 million from 2014–2017.* https://www.ahrq.gov/news/newsroom/press-releases/hac-rates-declined.html

American Hospital Directory. (2017). *Quality definitions and methodology: Hospital acquired conditions.* https://www.ahd.com/definitions/hqi_acq_cond_measures.html

Chu, R. (2016). Simple steps to reduce medication errors. *Nursing, 46*(8), 63–65.

Edlin, M. (2019). How health systems use pharmacists to reduce readmissions. *Managed Healthcare Executive, 29*(5), 6–8.

Farzi, S., Irajpour, A., Saghaei, M., & Ravaghi, H. (2017). Causes of medication errors in intensive care units from the perspective of healthcare professionals. *Journal of Research in Pharmacy Practice, 6*(3), 158–165. https://doi.org/10.4103/jrpp.JRPP_17_47

Gates, P. J., Baysari, M. T., Gazarian, M., Raban, M. Z., Meyerson, S., & Westbrook, J. I. (2019). Prevalence of medication errors among paediatric inpatients: Systematic review and meta-analysis. *Drug Safety, 42*(11), 1329–1342. https://doi.org/10.1007/s40264-019-00850-1

Institute for Healthcare Improvement. (2017). *QI Essentials Toolkit: Failure Modes and Effects Analysis (FMEA) tool.* http://www.ihi.org/resources/Pages/Tools/FailureModesandEffectsAnalysisTool.aspx

Institute for Safe Medication Practices. (2018). *ISMP high-alert medications in acute care settings.* https://www.ismp.org/recommendations/high-alert-medications-acute-list

Institute for Safe Medication Practices. (2019). *ISMP's list of confused drug names.* https://www.ismp.org/recommendations/confused-drug-names-list

Institute for Safe Medication Practices. (2020). *Targeted medication safety best practices for hospitals.* https://www.ismp.org/guidelines/best-practices-hospitals

iSixSigma. (n.d.). *Determine the root cause: 5 whys.* http://www.isixsigma.com/tools-templates/cause-effect/determine-root-cause-5-whys

Kleinsinger, F. (2018). The unmet challenge of medication nonadherence. *Permanente Journal, 22*, 18–33. https://doi.org/10.7812/TPP/18-033

Mathews, A. L., Coleska, A., Burns, P. B., & Chung, K. C. (2016). Evolution of patient decision-making regarding medical treatment of rheumatoid arthritis. *Arthritis*

Care & Research, 68, 318–324. https://doi.org/10.1002/acr.22688

National Coordinating Council for Medication Error Reporting and Prevention. (2020). *About medication errors: What is a medication error?* https://www.nccmerp.org/about-medication-errors

Nuffer, W., Dye, L., & Decker, S. (2019). Integrating pharmacist MTM services into medical clinics as part of a health department partnership project. *Innovations in Pharmacy, 10*(4). https://doi.org/10.24926/iip.v10i4.2129

Pan, J., Curran, J., Fitzpatrick, E., Breneol, S., Bennett, C., & Hurley, K. (2019). Interventions to assist parents and caregivers in accurately dosing liquid medications for their children: A scoping review. *Drugs & Therapy Perspectives, 35*(5), 230–240. https://doi.org/10.1007/s40267-019-00615-x

Poupoulas, V. (n.d.). *From compliance to adherence to concordance: The evolution from paternalistic medicine to patient empowerment.* HPS. http://www.hps.com.au/knowledge-centre/clinical-articles/clinical-article-from-compliance-to-adherence-to-concordance

The Joint Commission. (2020a). *National patient safety goals.* https://www.jointcommission.org/-/media/tjc/documents/standards/national-patient-safety-goals/npsg_chapter_ahc_jan2020.pdf

The Joint Commission. (2020b). *Patient safety systems chapter for the hospital program.* https://www.jointcommission.org/patient_safety_systems_chapter_for_the_hospital_program

The Joint Commission. (2020c). *Sentinel event policy and procedures.* https://www.jointcommission.org/en/resources/patient-safety-topics/sentinel-event/sentinel-event-policy-and-procedures

U.S. Food and Drug Administration. (2020). *Medwatch: The FDA safety information and adverse event reporting program.* https://www.fda.gov/safety/medwatch-fda-safety-information-and-adverse-event-reporting-program

Vecchione, A. (2016). Pharmacists take aim at med errors during care transitions. *Drug Topics, 160*(7), 23–25. http://drugtopics.modernmedicine.com/drug-topics/news/pharmacists-take-aim-med-errors-during-care-transitions?page=0,0

Selected Bibliography

Institute for Safe Medication Practices. (2017). *ISMP Building a Smart Infusion System Drug Library.* https://www.ismp.org/sites/default/files/attachments/2017-11/Building-Smart-Infusion-System-Drug-Library.pdf

National Coordinating Council for Medication Error Reporting and Prevention. (2001a). *NCC MERP index for categorizing medication errors.* http://www.nccmerp.org/sites/default/files/indexBW2001-06-12.pdf

National Coordinating Council for Medication Error Reporting and Prevention. (2001b). *NCC MERP index for categorizing medication errors algorithm.* http://www.nccmerp.org/sites/default/files/algorColor2001-06-12.pdf

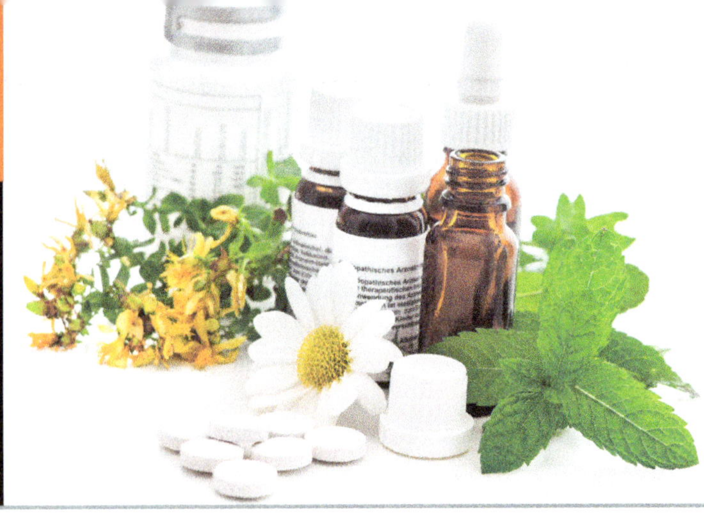

"My daughter is getting so frustrated with me. It seems that I can't remember anything. Just last week I forgot to take my medications twice and failed to pick up my grandson at his weekly tae kwon do lesson."
—*Patient "Larry Bunch"*

Chapter 7
The Role of Complementary and Alternative Therapies in Pharmacotherapy

Chapter Outline

- Types of Complementary and Alternative Therapies
- History of Herbal Therapies
- Standardization of Herbal Products
- Dietary Supplement Regulation
- Herb–Drug Interactions
- Specialty Supplements

Learning Outcomes

After reading this chapter, the student should be able to:

1. Identify specific types of complementary and alternative therapies that are used by patients to promote wellness.
2. Analyze why dietary supplements have steadily increased in popularity.
3. Explain why it is important to standardize herbal products based on specific active ingredients.
4. Describe legislation that governs the use of dietary supplements.
5. Describe drug interactions and adverse effects that are associated with dietary supplements.
6. Distinguish between an herbal product and a specialty supplement.
7. Discuss the role of the nurse in teaching patients about complementary and alternative therapies.

Key Terms

Definitions of the terms in bold may be found in the Glossary.

Complementary and alternative medicine represents a multibillion-dollar industry. About 77% of all adults in the United States take a dietary supplement (Council for Responsible Nutrition, 2019). One out of every three Americans uses complementary therapies (Clarke et al., 2015). Despite the fact that these therapies have not been subjected to the same robust scientific scrutiny as prescription medications, consumers have turned to them for a variety of reasons. The availability of herbal and dietary supplements at a reasonable cost has convinced many consumers to try them, sometimes in lieu of prescription medications. This chapter focuses on the role of complementary and alternative therapies in the prevention and treatment of disease.

Types of Complementary and Alternative Therapies

7.1 Complementary and alternative therapies are used by a large number of people to prevent and treat disease.

Complementary and alternative medicine (CAM) comprises an extremely diverse set of therapies and healing systems that are considered to be outside of mainstream healthcare. Although diverse, the major CAM systems have certain common characteristics:

- Focus on treating the health of the whole individual
- Emphasis on the integration of mind and body
- Emphasis on disease prevention, self-care, and self-healing
- Recognition of the role of spirituality in health and healing

Because of the widespread use of CAM by the public, the scientific community has focused on determining the effectiveness, or lack of effectiveness, of these therapies. Compared to prescription medications, few CAM therapies have been subjected to rigorous, controlled clinical studies. It is likely that some of these therapies will be found ineffective, whereas others will become mainstream treatments. If a nonmainstream practice is used *along with* conventional medical therapies, it is called *complementary*. If the nonmainstream practice is used *instead of* conventional medical therapies, it is called *alternative*. Table 7.1 lists the common CAM therapies.

Healthcare providers have long respected the role of CAM in preventing and treating certain conditions. Prayer, meditation, massage, and yoga have been used to treat both body and spirit for centuries. From a pharmacologic perspective the value of CAM therapies lies in their ability to reduce the need for medications. For example, if a patient can find anxiety relief through massage, deep breathing, or biofeedback therapy, the use of antianxiety drugs may be reduced or even eliminated. Reduction of drug dose leads to fewer adverse effects and better adherence to drug therapy.

Table 7.1 Complementary and Alternative Therapies

Healing Method	Examples
Biologic-based therapies	Herbal therapies
	Dietary supplements
	Special diets
Alternative healthcare systems	Naturopathy
	Homeopathy
	Chiropractic
	Native American medicine (e.g., sweat lodges, medicine wheel)
	Chinese traditional medicine (e.g., acupuncture, Chinese herbs)
Manual healing	Massage
	Pressure-point therapies
	Hand-mediated biofield therapies
Mind–body interventions	Yoga, Pilates, or tai chi
	Meditation
	Hypnotherapy
	Guided imagery
	Biofeedback
	Movement-oriented therapies (e.g., music, dance)
	Deep breathing
Spiritual	Shamans
	Faith and prayer
Others	Bioelectromagnetics
	Detoxifying therapies
	Animal-assisted therapy

This chapter focuses on products used as dietary supplements. **Dietary supplements** are products available over the counter (OTC) that are intended to add to or supplement the nutritional value of the diet. The two subcategories of dietary supplements presented in this chapter include herbal products and specialty supplements. Vitamins and minerals, also considered dietary supplements, are presented in Chapter 61.

History of Herbal Therapies

7.2 Herbal products have been used as medicines for thousands of years.

An **herb** is technically a **botanical** (plant-based substance) that does not contain woody tissue such as stems or bark. In common usage, however, consumers tend to use "herb" to refer to a wide variety of products including substances such as ginkgo biloba (which is a tree) and rosemary (which has woody stems). Over time, the term *herb* has come to refer to any plant product with some useful application either as a food enhancer, such as flavoring or spice, or as a medicine.

The use of herbs has been recorded for thousands of years. One of the earliest recorded uses was a prescription for garlic written in 3000 BC. Eastern and Western medicine have recorded thousands of herbs and herb combinations reputed to have therapeutic value. Over time, the popularity of specific herbs and remedies has varied, depending on the availability of the botanical (i.e., geographical region) and its perceived effectiveness. Popular herbals and their primary uses are shown in Table 7.2.

With the birth of the pharmaceutical industry in the late 1800s, the interest in herbal medicine began to wane. Synthetic drugs could be standardized and produced more cheaply than natural herbal products. Regulatory agencies required that products be safe and effective. The focus of healthcare was on diagnosing and treating specific diseases, rather than promoting wellness and holistic care. Most alternative therapies were no longer taught in medical or nursing schools. Botanical therapies were criticized as being unscientific relics of the past, with evidence of their effectiveness based on folklore instead of science.

Botanicals have reemerged as a CAM, such that a majority of adult Americans are either currently taking herbal therapies on a regular basis or have taken them in the past. Why would people turn to folk remedies and products with uncertain effectiveness when effective prescription medications are available? This increased popularity is due to a number of factors:

- Dietary supplements were once available only in specialty health food stores but can now be purchased in virtually all supermarkets and pharmacies.

Table 7.2 Popular Herbal Supplements

Herb	Medicinal Part	Possible Use(s)	Herb Feature (Chapter)
Acai	Berries	Vitamin and mineral supplement, antioxidant, possible weight loss	—
Aloe vera	Leaves	Topical application for minor skin irritations and burns	73
Bilberry	Berries and leaves	Terminate diarrhea, improve and protect vision, antioxidant	—
Black cohosh	Roots	Relieve symptoms of premenstrual syndrome and menopause	—
Chlorophyll/chlorella	Leaves	Improve digestion, vitamin and mineral supplement	—
Cranberry	Berries/juice	Prevent urinary tract infection	50
Echinacea	Entire plant	Enhance immune system, treat the common cold	42
Elderberry	Berries and flowers	Relieve congestion in respiratory system due to colds and flu	—
Evening primrose	Oil extracted from seeds	Relieve symptoms of premenstrual syndrome and menopause; relieve symptoms of rheumatoid arthritis and other inflammatory symptoms; source of essential fatty acids	—
Flaxseed (ground or oil)	Seeds and oil	Reduce blood cholesterol, laxative	—
Garlic	Bulbs	Reduce blood cholesterol, reduce blood pressure, anticoagulation	38
Ginger	Root	Antiemetic, antithrombotic, diuretic, promote gastric secretions, anti-inflammatory, increase blood glucose, stimulate peripheral circulation	—
Ginkgo	Leaves and seeds	Improve memory, reduce dizziness	—
Ginseng	Root	Relieve stress, enhance immune system, decrease fatigue	—
Grape seed	Seeds/oil	Source of essential fatty acids, antioxidant, restore microcirculation to tissues	—
Green tea	Leaves	Antioxidant; lower LDL cholesterol; prevent cancer; relieve stomach problems, nausea and/or vomiting	63
Horny goat weed	Leaves and roots	Enhance sexual function	—
Milk thistle	Seeds	Antitoxin, protection against liver disease	—
Red rice yeast extract	Dried in capsules	Reduce blood cholesterol	—
Saw palmetto	Berries	Reduce symptoms of benign prostatic hyperplasia	71
Soy	Beans	Source of protein, vitamins, and minerals; relieve symptoms of menopause, prevent cardiovascular disease, anticancer	69
St. John's wort	Flowers, leaves, stems	Reduce symptoms of depression and anxiety, anti-inflammatory	19
Stevia	Leaves	Natural sweetener	—
Valerian	Roots	Relieve stress, promote sleep	—
Wheat or barley grass	Leaves	Improve digestion, vitamin and mineral supplement	—

- Complementary therapies are aggressively marketed by the supplement industry as viable and natural alternatives to conventional medicine. The increased availability of the internet as a marketing tool has led to some sites advertising misleading claims about the effectiveness of herbal and dietary supplements.
- The Baby Boom generation has demonstrated a renewed interest in natural alternatives and preventive medicine.
- The gradual aging of the population has led people to seek therapeutic alternatives for chronic conditions such as pain, arthritis, anxiety, depression, hormone replacement therapy, and prostate difficulties.
- People have the impression that natural substances are safer than synthetic pharmaceuticals.
- The high cost of prescription medicines has driven people to seek less expensive alternatives.
- Nurses and other healthcare providers have been more proactive in promoting self-care and recommending CAM for their patients.

This text emphasizes CAM by the use of Connection features that appear throughout the chapters. The inclusion of these therapies is not an endorsement, nor does it imply their effectiveness. They are included because the nurse will frequently need to teach specific natural therapies, and because some of them have the potential to impact pharmacotherapy (see Section 7.5). The student should refer to the current medical literature for complete dosing and safety information. Several excellent sources of reliable information are available. The National Center for Complementary and Integrative Health (NCCIH) is a branch of the National Institutes of Health (NIH) that offers current information on research involving these products (NCCIH, 2020).

Standardization of Herbal Products

7.3 Herbal products are available in a variety of formulations, some containing standardized extracts and others containing whole herbs.

The pharmacologically active chemicals in an herbal product may be present in only one specific part or in all parts of the plant. For example, the active chemicals in chamomile are in the leaves, stems, or flowers. For other herbs, such as ginger, the roots are used for their healing properties. It is, therefore, essential to know which portion of the plant contains the active chemicals if growing or collecting herbs for home use.

Most prescription drugs contain only one active chemical. This chemical can be standardized and measured, so that the amount of drug received by the patient is precisely known. Herbs, however, may contain dozens of active chemicals, many of which have not yet been isolated, studied, or even identified. It is possible that some of these substances work together synergistically and may not have the same activity if isolated. Furthermore, the strength of an herbal preparation can vary from batch to batch, depending on where it was grown and how it was collected, prepared, and stored. How is it possible, then, for consumers to know the strength of an herbal product, given so much potential variability in ingredients?

To achieve consistency in the strength or dose of an herbal product, scientists have attempted to standardize herbal products. This standardization is based on one of the following methods:

- **Active ingredient extracts.** These standardize the amount of *biologically active substances* in the herb. For example, the active ingredient in saw palmetto has been determined to be fatty acids; therefore, these are used to standardize extracts of this herb.
- **Marker extracts.** These standardize the potency of the herb *based on a common substance* in the whole herb that may not be the active ingredient. For example, ginseng is standardized on the percent of ginsenosides in the extract.

Regardless of which method is used, standardization allows the consumer to compare products and have an indication of the strength of the herb. Some of these standardizations are shown in Table 7.3. Note that the active ingredient in an herb is not always known and there may be more than one. Furthermore, the active ingredient may be different, depending on the indication for which the herb is being used. Until science can better characterize these substances, it is best to conceptualize the active ingredient of an herb as being the *entire herb*. An example of the ingredients and standardization of ginkgo biloba using a marker substance is shown in Figure 7.1. As explained in Section 7.4, it should not be assumed that an herb is safe or effective simply because it contains the standard amount of extract.

Table 7.3 Standardization of Selected Herbal Products

Herb	Standardization	Percent
Black cohosh rhizome	Triterpene glycosides	2.5
Cascara sagrada bark	Anthocyanosides	25
Echinacea purpurea, whole herb	Echinacosides	4
Ginger rhizome	Pungent compounds (gingerols)	>10
Ginkgo leaf	Flavone glycosides	24–25
	Lactones	6
Ginseng root	Ginsenosides	5–15
Milk thistle root	Silymarin	80
Saw palmetto berries	Fatty acids and sterols	80–90
St. John's wort, whole herb	Hypericins	0.3–0.5
	Hyperforin	3–5

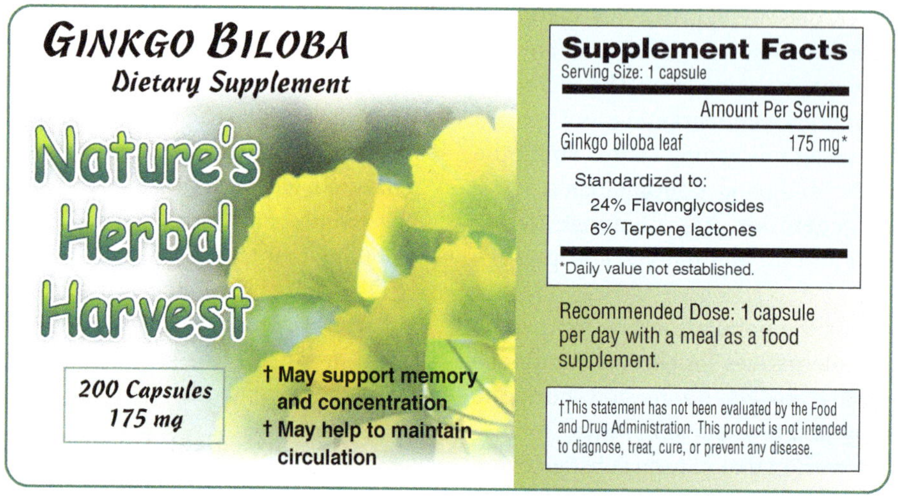
GINKGO BILOBA
Dietary Supplement
Nature's
Herbal
Harvest
200 Capsules
175 mg
† May support memory and concentration
† May help to maintain circulation
Supplement Facts
Serving Size: 1 capsule
Amount Per Serving
Ginkgo biloba leaf 175 mg*
Standardized to:
24% Flavonglycosides
6% Terpene lactones
*Daily value not established.
Recommended Dose: 1 capsule per day with a meal as a food supplement.
†This statement has not been evaluated by the Food and Drug Administration. This product is not intended to diagnose, treat, cure, or prevent any disease.

Figure 7.1 Ginkgo biloba label. This label indicates the product is standardized to percentages of the two active ingredients, flavonglycosides and terpenes, that are found in the ginkgo leaf. Also note the health claims on the label, which have not been evaluated by the FDA.

PharmFACT

A global DNA analysis of herbal products revealed that 27% were adulterated and did not contain what was claimed on the label. The adulterated products contained contaminants, substitutes, filler species, or none of the labeled species. In Australia 79% of the tested products were adulterated compared to 33% in North America (Ichim, 2019).

The two basic formulations of herbal products are solid and liquid. Solid products include pills, tablets, and capsules made from the dried herbs. Other solid products are salves and ointments that are administered topically. Liquid formulations are made by extracting the active chemicals from the plant using solvents such as water, alcohol, or glycerol. The liquids are then concentrated in various strengths and ingested. The types of liquid herbal formulations are described in Table 7.4. Figure 7.2 illustrates some of the formulations of ginkgo biloba, one of the most popular herbals.

Table 7.4 Liquid Formulations of Herbal Products

Product	Description
Decoction	Fresh or dried herbs are boiled in water for 30–60 min until much of the liquid has boiled off; very concentrated
Extract	Active ingredients are extracted using organic solvents to form a highly concentrated liquid or solid form; solvent may be removed or be part of the final product
Infusion	Fresh or dried herbs are soaked in hot water for long periods, at least 15 min; stronger than teas
Tea	Fresh or dried herbs are soaked in hot water for 5–10 min before ingestion; convenient
Tincture	Active ingredients are extracted using alcohol by soaking the herb; alcohol remains as part of the liquid

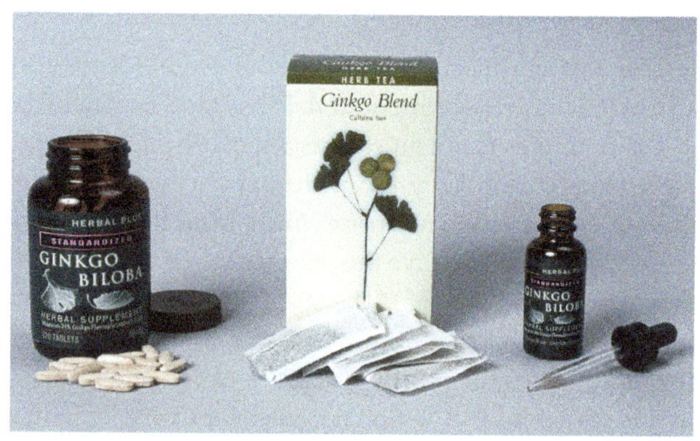

Figure 7.2 Three different ginkgo formulations: tablets, tea bags, and liquid extract.
Adams, Michael P.

Dietary Supplement Regulation

7.4 Dietary supplements are not regulated in the same manner as prescription medications.

Since the passage of the Food, Drug, and Cosmetic Act in 1936, Americans have come to expect that all approved prescription and OTC drugs have passed rigid standards of safety prior to being marketed. Furthermore, it is expected that these drugs have been tested for effectiveness and that they truly provide the medical benefits claimed by the manufacturer. Indeed, most people would be outraged if they found out that the drug they purchased for pain relief or to cure an infectious disease was totally ineffective. For dietary supplements, however, Americans cannot and should not expect the same quality standards. These products are regulated by a far less rigorous law, the **Dietary Supplement Health and Education Act (DSHEA)**.

The DSHEA specifically exempts dietary supplements from regulations under the Food, Drug, and Cosmetic Act.

Because dietary supplements are not classified as drugs or approved by the U.S. Food and Drug Administration (FDA), they are not subjected to the same degree of scrutiny as drugs.

A strength of the DSHEA is that it gives the FDA the authority to remove from the market any dietary supplement that poses a "significant or unreasonable" risk to the public. The FDA used this legislative authority when the dietary supplement ephedra was removed from the market because of reported serious side effects in some people. However, it took 7 years from the time the FDA first warned consumers of the dangers of ephedra until it was removed. Unfortunately, the FDA must wait until possible harm has been caused before it can take legal action.

The DSHEA requires these products to be clearly labeled as "dietary supplements." The product label must state that the dietary supplement is not intended to diagnose, treat, cure, or prevent any disease. However, the label is allowed to make claims about the product's effect on body structure and function, such as the following:

- Helps promote healthy immune systems.
- Reduces anxiety and stress.
- Helps to maintain cardiovascular function.
- May reduce pain and inflammation.

An example of a dietary supplement label for L-carnitine is shown in Figure 7.3.

The health claim on all dietary supplement labels must also state: "This statement has not been evaluated by the U.S. Food and Drug Administration."

Unfortunately, the DSHEA has significant flaws that lead to a lack of standardization in the dietary supplement industry and less protection for the consumer. These flaws include the following:

- The manufacturer does not have to test the safety of a dietary supplement prior to marketing. If it is to be removed from the market, the FDA has the burden of proving that the dietary supplement is harmful.
- Effectiveness does not have to be demonstrated by the manufacturer.

Additional legislation has been passed to address weaknesses in the DSHEA. In 2007, Congress passed the **Dietary Supplement and Nonprescription Drug Consumer Protection Act** of 2010. This requires companies that market dietary supplements to include their contact information (address and phone number) on the product labels so consumers can report adverse events. Companies must notify the FDA of any serious adverse event reports within 15 days of receiving such reports. Under this act, a "serious adverse event" is defined as any adverse reaction resulting in death, a life-threatening experience, inpatient hospitalization, a persistent or significant disability or incapacity, or a congenital anomaly or birth defect, as well as any event requiring medical or

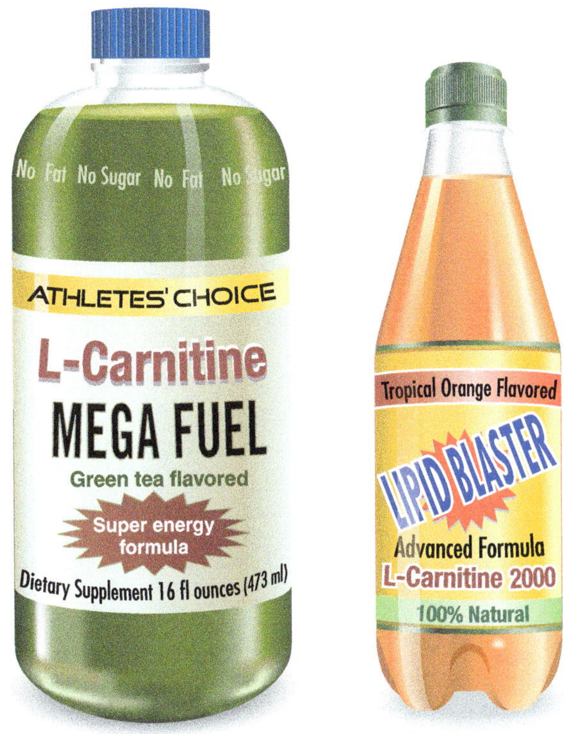

Figure 7.3 L-carnitine is a popular dietary supplement. Notice the labels imply that their use may improve athletic performance and cause weight loss, neither of which has been supported by the scientific literature.

surgical intervention to prevent one of these conditions based on reasonable medical judgment. Companies must keep records of such events for at least 6 years, and the records are subject to inspection by the FDA.

In addition, the manufacturers of dietary supplements are now required to evaluate the identity, purity, potency, and composition of their products. The labels must accurately reflect the content of the products, which must be free of contaminants such as pesticides, toxins, glass, or heavy metals. Still absent from legislation: the company does not have to prove the effectiveness or safety of its products.

The U.S. Pharmacopeial Convention (USPC) is a nonprofit public health organization that has attempted to raise the standards and quality of pharmaceuticals and dietary supplements (see Chapter 1). The organization publishes a large compendium of drug information annually, called the *United States Pharmacopoeia (USP)*. The USPC has developed a voluntary process by which a manufacturer may submit a product for the **USP Verification Program**. Using a multistep approach, the USPC examines the manufacturing processes used to create a supplement and tests the product to see if it contains the ingredients specified on the label and whether the product will break down and release its ingredients in the body (bioavailability). If the product meets the stringent standards of the USP, it may then carry the USP-verified dietary supplement mark on the label. The verification mark indicates to consumers that the product has been manufactured under acceptable standards of purity, has been tested for active ingredients stated on the label, and is free of harmful contaminants. However, it does not indicate that the product is safe or effective.

PharmFACT

A examination of the use of dietary supplements included the following statistics (Interlandi, 2016):

- Supplement sales have increased by 81% in the past 10 years.
- In a physician survey, 45% responded that they recommend herbal supplements.
- Each year 23,000 people end up at emergency departments after taking a supplement.
- There are 15,000 manufacturers of dietary supplements, but fewer than 400 have been inspected since 2010.

CONNECTION Checkpoint 7.1

From what you learned in Chapter 2, what is a pharmacopeia? What function does it serve in the United States?

Herb–Drug Interactions

7.5 Herbal products may have pharmacologic actions and can interact with conventional drugs.

A key concept to remember when learning about alternative therapies is that "natural" is not synonymous with "better" or "safe." It is likely that some botanicals do indeed contain active chemicals that are as powerful as, and perhaps more effective than, some currently approved medications. Thousands of years of experience, combined with current scientific research, have shown that some of these herbal remedies have therapeutic actions. Just because a substance comes from a natural product, however, does not make it safe or effective. For example, poison ivy is natural, but it certainly is not safe or therapeutic. The dried seed pods of the poppy plant yield opium, which has therapeutic effects but can also kill if taken inappropriately. Some natural products may not offer an improvement over conventional therapy in treating certain disorders and, indeed, may be of no value whatsoever. Furthermore, a patient who substitutes an unproven alternative therapy for an established, effective medical treatment may delay healing and cause irreparable harmful effects.

Some herbal products contain ingredients that may cause additive, synergistic, or antagonistic interactions with prescription or OTC drugs. For example, ginkgo biloba and ginger have the ability to increase bleeding time. If used concurrently with anticoagulants, these herbs may increase the potential for adverse bleeding events. St. John's wort, kava, and valerian cause relaxation and may result in excessive sedation if taken concurrently with central nervous system (CNS) depressants. A few herbals have organ-specific toxicity. The herb comfrey given concurrently with large doses of acetaminophen may increase the patient's risk of hepatotoxicity. Herbals such as psyllium, aloe, and flaxseed may bind to drugs in the gastrointestinal (GI) tract, thus slowing their absorption.

The true extent of herb–drug interactions is unknown. Most reports in the medical literature are anecdotal, often given as a case report on a single individual. It is often impossible to know the exact amount of herb taken because there is such a wide variation in the quality of products on the market or even to know what chemical within the herb (either active ingredients or contaminants) may have caused the reported interaction. Relatively few controlled scientific studies of herb–drug or dietary supplement–drug interactions have been conducted. The majority of the information regarding these interactions is theoretical rather than clinically based.

Questions on the use of herbal supplements are important because these products are contraindicated for certain patients. Patients taking medications with potentially serious adverse effects such as insulin, warfarin (Coumadin), antiepileptic drugs, antineoplastic agents, or digoxin (Lanoxin) should be warned to never take any dietary supplement without first discussing their needs with a healthcare provider. Pregnant or lactating women should not take these products without approval of their healthcare provider. The nurse should also remember that the potential for any drug interaction increases in older adults, especially those with hepatic or renal impairment. Potential drug interactions with selected herbs are shown in Table 7.5.

Another warning that must be heeded with natural products is to beware of allergic reactions. It is not unusual to find dozens of different chemicals in teas and infusions made from the flowers, leaves, or roots of a plant. Patients who have known allergies to food products or medicines should seek medical advice before taking a new herbal product. It is always wise to take the smallest amount possible when starting herbal therapy, even less than the recommended dose, to see if adverse effects occur.

Nurses have an obligation to seek the latest medical information on herbal products because there is a good possibility that their patients are using them to supplement traditional medicines. Each patient who takes an herbal product does so for a reason. The nurse needs to listen, assess, and understand the patient's goals for taking the supplement. Does the patient have an accurate understanding of the actions of the herb? Are there more effective therapies, either pharmacologic or nonpharmacologic, for the patient's condition? Is there a potential for harmful effects from the product due to high doses or herb–drug interactions? Establishing a supportive attitude toward the use of CAM is important. Nurses often need to educate their patients on the role of alternative therapies in the treatment

Table 7.5 Documented Herb–Drug Interactions

Common Name (Scientific Name)	Interacts with	Effects of Interaction
Echinacea (*Echinacea purpurea*)	amiodarone, anabolic steroids, ketoconazole, methotrexate	May increase hepatotoxicity when taken with known hepatotoxic drugs
Feverfew (*Tanacetum parthenium*)	aspirin and other nonsteroidal anti-inflammatory drugs (NSAIDs), heparin, warfarin	May increase bleeding risk when taken with drugs that slow blood clotting
Flaxseed (*Linum usitatissimum*)	most drugs	Decreases absorption of oral drugs
Flaxseed oil (*Linum usitatissimum*)	aspirin and other NSAIDs, heparin, warfarin	May increase bleeding risk when taken with drugs that slow blood clotting
	antidiabetic drugs	Increases hypoglycemic effects
	antihypertensives	May lower blood pressure
Garlic (*Allium sativum*)	aspirin and other NSAIDs, heparin, warfarin	May increase bleeding risk when taken with drugs that slow blood clotting
	estrogen contraceptives	May lower drug effectiveness
	isoniazid	Reduces absorption of oral drugs
Ginger (*Zingiber officinale*)	aspirin and other NSAIDs, heparin, warfarin	May increase bleeding risk when taken with drugs that slow blood clotting
Ginkgo (*Ginkgo biloba*)	antiseizure drugs such as valproic acid, gabapentin, and carbamazepine	May increase seizures by decreasing drug effectiveness
	alprazolam, antidepressants	May decrease drug effectiveness
	aspirin and other NSAIDs, heparin, warfarin	May increase bleeding risk when taken with drugs that slow blood clotting
	trazodone	Increases drug effects
Ginseng (*Panax quinquefolius/ Eleutherococcus senticosus*)	antihypertensives	May lower blood pressure
	caffeine	Increases side effects such as nervousness and insomnia
	insulin, oral antidiabetic drugs	May increase hypoglycemic effects
	monoamine oxidase (MAO) inhibitors	May cause hypertensive crisis
	aspirin and other NSAIDs, heparin, warfarin	May increase bleeding risk when taken with drugs that slow blood clotting
Goldenseal (*Hydrastis canadensis/ Eleutherococcus senticosus*)	many drugs metabolized by the liver such as opioids, azole antifungals, tricyclic antidepressants, fluoxetine, and ondansetron	Increases drug effects
Green tea	amiodarone, anabolic steroids, ketoconazole, methotrexate	May increase hepatotoxicity when taken with known hepatotoxic drugs
	aspirin and other NSAIDs, heparin, warfarin	May increase bleeding risk when taken with drugs that slow blood clotting
	beta blockers such as propranolol and metoprolol	May increase blood pressure
Kava kava (*Piper methysticum*)	alcohol, benzodiazepines and other CNS depressants	Potentiates sedation
	levodopa/carbidopa	Reduces drug effectiveness
	phenothiazines	Increases risk and severity of dystonic reactions
Soy	Warfarin	Decreases anticoagulant effects
St. John's wort (*Hypericum perforatum*)	opioids, alcohol, and other CNS depressants	Potentiates sedation
	immunosuppressants	May decrease drug effectiveness
	HIV drugs	Decreases antiretroviral activity
	MAO inhibitors	May cause hypertensive crisis
	oral contraceptives	Decreases drug effectiveness
	selective serotonin reuptake inhibitors, tricyclic antidepressants	Increases risk of side effects and serotonin syndrome
	warfarin	Decreases anticoagulant effects
Valerian (*Valeriana officinalis*)	alcohol, benzodiazepines, tricyclic antidepressants, valproic acid and other CNS depressants	Potentiates sedation

CONNECTIONS: Advanced Practice Application

Older Adults at Risk for Polyherbacy

Case

Mrs. Danville is an 84-year-old woman who came to the Geriatric Primary Care Clinic with new complaints of general fatigue and frequent falls. While taking her health history and conducting her medication reconciliation, you discover she has a history of hypertension, hyperlipidemia, glaucoma, and stroke. Her medications include lisinopril (Prinivil) and hydrochlorothiazide (Microzide), glaucoma eyedrops, low-dose aspirin, and OTC dietary supplements. She is cognitively and functionally intact, with vital signs showing a pulse rate of 76 beats/min lying down and 94 beats/min standing up. Blood pressure was 138/72 mmHg lying down and 130/70 mmHg standing up; respiratory rate, 16 breaths/min; and temperature, 37.2°C (99°F). Examination of her neurologic system, lungs, heart, abdomen, and extremities were all within normal limits for her age. Laboratory work showed a normal complete blood count without any signs of infection or anemia. Vitamin B_{12} level, electrolytes, and renal and liver laboratory findings were normal. Her thyroid-stimulating hormone (TSH) was decreased.

On consultation and further review of her OTC dietary supplements with the community pharmacist, you discover her specific dietary supplements include sea algae, alfalfa, bee pollen, barley malt, licorice, ginseng, ginkgo biloba, and many other herbs. You begin researching these herbs and wonder if they may be contributing to her complaints.

Discussion

Although healthcare providers assess for polypharmacy, older patients may not divulge the use of herbs and supplements. **Polyherbacy**, the use of multiple herbs or dietary supplements, may also be present. Healthcare providers should always inquire about herbal use as a routine part of history taking and medication reconciliation and should be aware of the side effects that may result from the use of such products (Gardenier et al., 2016).

In older adults potential risk for adverse herb–disease interactions can be significant. The following potential adverse herb–disease interactions were identified in Mrs. Danville's case:

- Ginseng may exacerbate hypotension (Kutt et al., 2016).
- Ginkgo biloba may increase the risk of bleeding in a patient with falls and those using aspirin (Kutt et al., 2016).
- Licorice and ginseng have been linked to hypertension (Kutt et al., 2016).
- Sea algae may precipitate hyperthyroidism due to its high iodine content (Gherbon et al., 2019).

of their disorder and discuss which treatment or combination of treatments will best meet their patients' health goals. Patients should be advised to be skeptical of marketing claims for herbal products and to seek health information from reputable sources.

CONNECTION Checkpoint 7.2

St. John's wort induces hepatic CYP metabolic enzymes. From what you learned in Chapter 5, how could this herb affect therapy with antidepressants or benzodiazepines that are substrates for CYP enzymes?

Specialty Supplements

7.6 Specialty supplements are nonherbal dietary products that are widely used to promote wellness.

Specialty supplements are dietary products used to enhance or complement a specific function in the body, such as supporting joint health or immune function. These supplements form a diverse group of products obtained from plant and animal sources that include probiotics, fish oils, amino acids, and enzymes. Like herbal therapies, they are available OTC and are widely used by patients to enhance wellness. However, they are more specific in their action than herbal products and are generally targeted for one condition or a smaller group of related conditions. Popular specialty supplements are listed in Table 7.6.

In general, specialty supplements have a legitimate rationale for their use. For example, chondroitin and glucosamine are natural substances in the body necessary for cartilage growth and maintenance. Amino acids are natural building blocks of muscle protein. Fish oils contain omega fatty acids that have been shown to reduce the risk of heart disease in certain patients.

As with botanicals, the link between most specialty supplements and their intended benefits is unclear. In most cases, the body already has sufficient quantities of the substance; thus, taking additional amounts may be of no benefit. In other cases, the supplement may be marketed for conditions for which the supplement has no proven effect. The good news is that these substances are generally not harmful unless taken in large amounts. The bad news, however, is that they can give patients false hopes of an easy cure for chronic conditions such as heart disease or the pain of arthritis. As with herbal products, the healthcare provider should advise patients to be cautious about the health claims regarding the use of specialty supplements.

Table 7.6 Selected Specialty Supplements

Name	Primary Uses	Supplement Feature (Chapter)
Amino acids	Build protein, muscle strength, and endurance	—
Carnitine	Enhance energy and sports performance, heart health, memory, immune function, and male fertility	—
Chromium	Treat diabetes	—
Coenzyme Q10	Prevent heart disease, provide antioxidant therapy	29
DHEA	Boost immune and memory functions	—
Fish oil	Reduce cholesterol levels, enhance brain function, and increase visual acuity	68
Glucosamine and chondroitin	Reduce the pain of arthritis and other joint conditions	72
Lactobacillus acidophilus	Maintain intestinal health	60
Melatonin	Reduce sleeplessness and jet lag during travel	18
Methyl sulfonyl methane (MSM)	Reduce allergic reactions to pollen and foods, relieve pain and inflammation of arthritis	—
Selenium	Reduce the risk of certain types of cancer	—
Vitamin C	Prevent colds	45

Understanding Chapter 7

Key Concepts Summary

7.1 Complementary and alternative therapies are used by a large number of people to prevent and treat disease.

7.2 Herbal products have been used as medicines for thousands of years.

7.3 Herbal products are available in a variety of formulations, some containing standardized extracts and others containing whole herbs.

7.4 Dietary supplements are not regulated in the same manner as prescription medications.

7.5 Herbal products may have pharmacologic actions and can interact with conventional drugs.

7.6 Specialty supplements are nonherbal dietary products that are widely used to promote wellness.

CASE STUDY: Making the Patient Connection

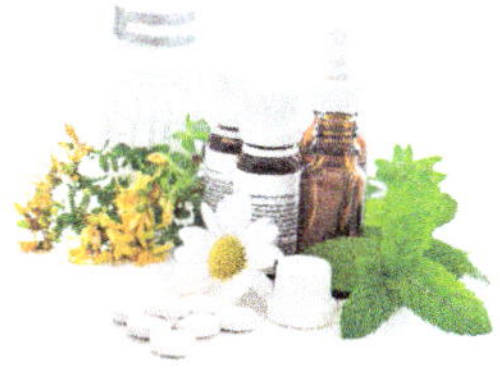

Remember the patient "Larry Bunch" at the beginning of the chapter? Now read the remainder of the case study. Based on the information presented within this chapter, respond to the critical thinking questions that follow.

Sixty-nine-year-old Larry Bunch was not only frustrating his daughter, but his forgetfulness was annoying him as well. Since the death of his wife 2 years ago, his forgetfulness seemed to be worsening. To remedy the situation, he purchased a bottle of ginkgo biloba at the health food store and began taking the supplement about 6 months ago.

Larry was hospitalized 3 years ago for atrial fibrillation. When he was discharged from the hospital, he was placed on an anticoagulant therapy to decrease his risk for a stroke. Today, Larry comes to his healthcare provider's office for a scheduled blood test to determine the effectiveness of his anticoagulant.

When the results from the blood test return, it is noted that Larry's coagulation time is abnormally high and he is at high risk of hemorrhaging. As the nurse, you note that his vital signs are within normal limits, and he states he feels well. However, you also observe some large bruises on Larry's arms, which he cannot explain.

Critical Thinking Questions

1. What is the relationship between this patient's use of ginkgo and the laboratory results?
2. What instructions should this patient receive about taking the supplement?
3. Discuss the hazards that patients face when using complementary and alternative therapies.
4. What should the healthcare provider do concerning Larry's forgetfulness?

Additional Case Study

"It must be safe, after all, it is sold in the grocery store!" exclaimed Linda. As you, the nurse, talk with the patient, Linda Thomas, she explains to you that she takes multiple OTC dietary supplements. Because the bottle states that the ingredients are "all natural," she knows it must be good for her.

1. What are the hazards associated with believing that all medication-type substances sold in the supermarket are safe?
2. Discuss how the words "all-natural ingredients" can be confusing.
3. Identify the nurse's role in working with patients who participate in complementary and alternative therapies.

Chapter Review

1. A patient asks why all healthcare providers do not rely on complementary and alternative medicine. When talking to this patient, the nurse knows that many complementary and alternative therapies:
   1. Have not been subjected to rigorous clinical studies.
   2. Consist only of old wives' tales and fables.
   3. Only provide a placebo effect.
   4. Are costly and not worth the risk.
2. Which health teaching concept should be included in the instructions for a patient taking echinacea?
   1. Dosage can be doubled if symptoms fail to resolve in 48 hours.
   2. Limit fluid intake while taking this supplement.
   3. Take the smallest amount possible when starting herbal therapy.
   4. Allergic reactions are not possible with natural supplements.
3. Which patient is most likely to experience drug toxicity while taking dietary supplements?
   1. An 80-year-old with cirrhosis
   2. A 58-year-old with cardiac irregularities
   3. A 30-year-old with pneumonia
   4. An 18-year-old with chronic acne
4. The patient asks the nurse, "Why are dietary supplements so popular?" The nurse's answer is based on which factors? (Select all that apply.) Herbal supplements:
   1. Can now be purchased in virtually all supermarkets.
   2. Are aggressively marketed by the herbal and supplement industry.
   3. Cost less than prescription medicines.
   4. Are safer than synthetic pharmaceuticals.
   5. Appeal to the aging population.
5. The nurse is teaching at a community wellness seminar when one participant asks, "How can I be sure that my herbal supplement is pure?" Which of the following labeling marks indicates that the product meets acceptable standards of purity?
   1. USP-verified dietary supplement mark
   2. DEA prescriber number
   3. FDA identification and regulation code
   4. U.S. Customs Service integers
6. Polyherbacy may be of concern in the older adult population. A pharmacokinetic factor for this concern is that the older adult:
   1. Is more likely to have difficulty using herbal products correctly.
   2. May spend too much on herbal products rather than prescriptions.
   3. May hold unrealistic expectations for the outcomes of herbal therapy.
   4. May have age-related changes in liver or kidney function.

See Appendix A for answers to critical thinking questions, case study questions and review questions.

References

Clarke, T. C., Black, L. I., Stussman, B. J., Barnes, P. M., & Nahin, R. L. (2015). Trends in the use of complementary health approaches among adults: United States, 2002–2012. *National Health Statistics Reports*, *79*, 1–14. http://www.cdc.gov/nchs/data/nhsr/nhsr079.pdf

Council for Responsible Nutrition (CRN). (2019). *2019 CRN consumer survey of dietary supplements.* https://www.crnusa.org/resources/2019-crn-consumer-survey-dietary-supplements-consumer-intelligence-enhance-business

Gardenier, D., Woods, M. J., & Earp, J. K. (2016). Should nurse practitioners prescribe complementary and alternative medicine? *Journal for Nurse Practitioners*, *12*, 152–153. https://doi.org/10.1016/j.nurpra.2015.12.010

Gherbon, A., Frandes, M., Lungeanu, D., Nicula, M., & Timar, R. (2019). Transient hyperthyroidism following the ingestion of complementary medications containing kelp seaweed: A case-report. *Medicine*, *98*(37), e17058. https://doi.org/10.1097/MD.0000000000017058

Ichim, M. C. (2019). The DNA-based authentication of commercial herbal products reveals their globally widespread adulteration. *Frontiers in Pharmacology*, *10*, 1227. https://doi.org/10.3389/fphar.2019.01227

Interlandi, J. (2016). Supplements: A complete guide to safety. *Consumer Reports*, *81*(9) 20–33.

Kutt, A., Girard, L., Necyk, C., Gardiner, P., Boon, H., Barnes, J., & Vohra, S. (2016). Natural health product–drug interaction tool. *Canadian Pharmacists Journal*, *149*, 75–82. https://doi.org/10.1177/1715163516629156

National Center for Complementary and Integrative Health (NCCIH). (2020). *What does the NCCIH do?* https://www.nccih.nih.gov

Selected Bibliography

Balbontín, Y. M., Stewart, D., Shetty, A., Fitton, C. A., & McLay, J. S. (2019). Herbal medicinal product use during pregnancy and the postnatal period: A systematic review. *Obstetrics and Gynecology*, *133*(5), 920–932. https://doi.org/10.1097/AOG.0000000000003217

Bhusnure, O. G., Suryawanshi, S., Swamy, S. V., Gholve, S. B., Girm, P. S., & Birajdar, M. J. (2019). Standardization and quality evaluation of herbal drugs. *Journal of Drug Delivery and Therapeutics*, *9*(3, Suppl.), 1058–1063. https://doi.org/10.22270/jddt.v9i3-s.2941

Bruno, L. O., Simoes, R. S., de Jesus Simoes, M., Girão, M. J. B. C., & Grundmann, O. (2018). Pregnancy and herbal medicines: An unnecessary risk for women's health—A narrative review. *Phytotherapy Research*, *32*(5), 796–810. https://doi.org/10.1002/ptr.6020

Consumer Healthcare Products Association. (2020). *Regulation of dietary supplements.* https://www.chpa.org/RegulationDS.aspx

Fontaine, K. L. (2020). *Complementary and integrative therapies for nursing practice* (5th ed.). Hoboken, NJ: Pearson.

Illamola, S. M., Amaeze, O. U., Krepkova, L. V., Birnbaum, A. K., Karanam, A., Job, K. M., et al. (2019). Use of herbal medicine by pregnant women: What physicians need to know. *Frontiers in Pharmacology*, *10*, 1483. https://doi.org/10.3389/fphar.2019.01483

Lapenna, S., Gemen, R., Wollgast, J., Worth, A., Maragkoudakis, P., & Caldeira, S. (2015). Assessing herbal products with health claims. *Critical Reviews in Food Science and Nutrition*, *55*, 1918–1928. https://doi.org/10.1080/10408398.2012.726661

National Center for Complementary and Integrative Health. (2020). *Complementary, alternative or integrative health. What's in a name?* https://www.nccih.nih.gov/health/complementary-alternative-or-integrative-health-whats-in-a-name

Onakpoya, I. (2019). Use of herbal products in pregnancy: Harms are reported but the benefit to harm balance is uncertain. *BMJ Evidence-Based Medicine.* http://dx.doi.org/10.1136/bmjebm-2019-111240

Pereira, K. (2016). Herbal supplements: Widely used, poorly understood. *Nursing2016*, *46*(2), 54–59. https://doi.org/10.1097/01.NURSE.0000476233.80384.53

Pizzorno, J. E., & Murray, M. T. (2020). *Textbook of natural medicine.* Churchill Livingstone.

Ruiz, G. G., Nelson, E. O., Kozin, A. F., Turner, T. C., Waters, R. F., & Langland, J. O. (2016). A lack of bioactive predictability for marker compounds commonly used for herbal medicine standardization. *PLoS ONE*, *11*(7), e0159857. https://doi.org/10.1371/journal.pone.0159857

Smeriglio, A., Tomaino, A., & Trombetta, D. (2014). Herbal products in pregnancy: Experimental studies and clinical reports. *Phytotherapy Research*, *28*, 1107–1116. https://doi.org/10.1002/ptr.5106

Unit 2

Pharmacology and the Nurse–Patient Relationship

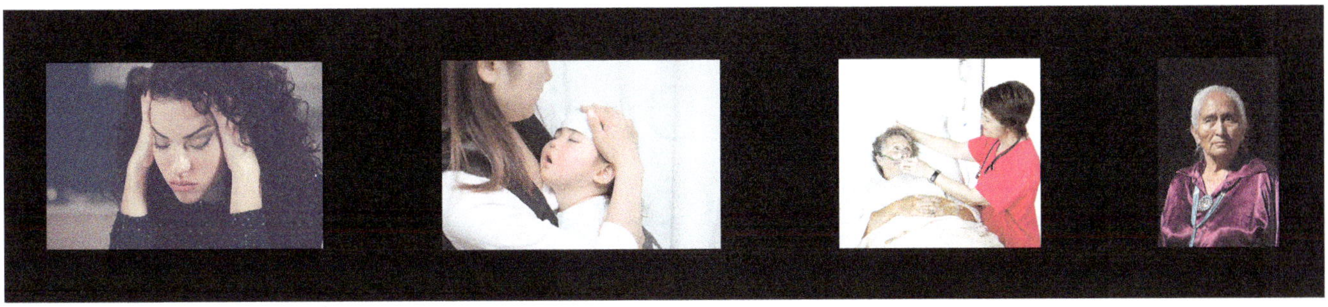

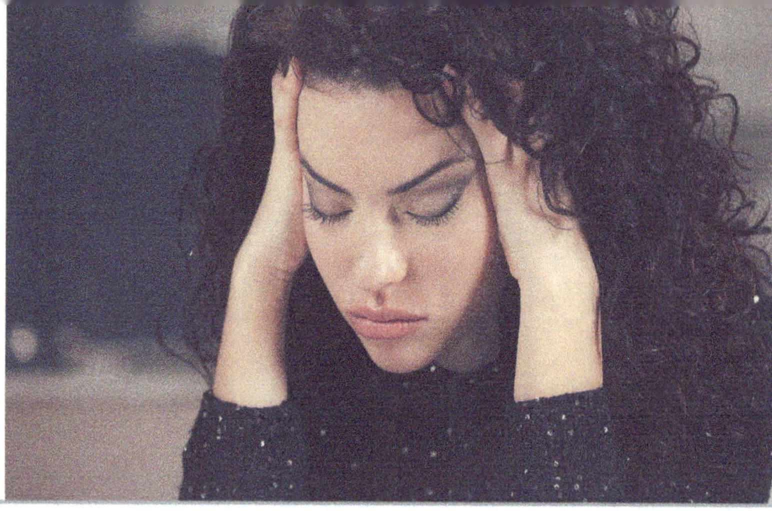

"I've been so nauseated every morning during the past 3 weeks and I'm late with my period. Please tell me I'm not pregnant. I just can't deal with a baby right now."
—*Patient "May David"*

Chapter 8
Pharmacotherapy During Pregnancy and Lactation

Chapter Outline

Learning Outcomes

After reading this chapter, the student should be able to:

1. Discuss the rationale for using drugs during pregnancy and lactation.
2. Describe physiologic changes during pregnancy that may affect the absorption, distribution, metabolism, and excretion of drugs.
3. Describe the placental transfer of drugs from mother to infant.
4. Differentiate among the U.S. Food and Drug Administration pregnancy risk categories.
5. Explain how the Pregnancy and Lactation Labelling Rule (PLLR) has changed the type of pregnancy data required on drug labels.
6. Explain how drugs administered during the different stages of fetal development affect the potential for teratogenic effects.
7. Identify factors that influence the transfer of drugs into breast milk.
8. Describe signs of adverse drug reactions in the breastfeeding infant.
9. Outline important points in patient and family education regarding drug use during pregnancy and lactation.

Key Terms

Definitions of the terms in bold may be found in the Glossary.

The prescribing and administration of medications during pregnancy requires special precautions. Healthcare providers must be aware of the physiologic changes occurring in the woman along with the developmental stage of the fetus. It is important to identify potential adverse drug events occurring in both the mother and the fetus. This chapter describes the pharmacokinetic changes that occur during pregnancy and explains the importance of carefully monitoring the pharmacotherapy during pregnancy and lactation. Emphasis is placed on drugs to avoid or use cautiously, strategies to prevent adverse effects, and the importance of patient and family education.

Rationale for Drug Use During Pregnancy and Lactation

8.1 Women frequently use drugs during pregnancy and lactation.

Healthcare providers caring for the pregnant or lactating woman have the challenge of concurrently being responsible for the health and safety of two people, knowing that most medications cross the placenta and are secreted in breast milk. Almost 1 in 4 pregnant women and nearly half of non-pregnant women between 15 and 44 years of age reported using prescription medications in the last 30 days. About 9 in 10 women take at least one medication during pregnancy, and 7 in 10 take at least one prescription medication (Centers for Disease Control and Prevention, 2020).

Healthcare providers always exercise great caution when initiating pharmacotherapy during pregnancy or lactation. Drug therapy is often postponed until after delivery and lactation; if that is not possible, safer nonpharmacologic alternatives may be implemented. Certain acute and chronic conditions, however, must be managed with medications during pregnancy. These include the following:

- **Treatment of certain preexisting illnesses.** If the patient has preexisting epilepsy, asthma, hypertension, or a psychiatric disorder, it would be unwise to discontinue pharmacotherapy during pregnancy.
- **Treatment of complications related to pregnancy.** Thromboembolic disorders, gestational diabetes, and gestational hypertension may occur during pregnancy and must be treated for the safety of both the mother and growing fetus.
- **Treatment of conditions unrelated to pregnancy.** Antibiotics may be necessary to treat infections acquired during pregnancy. Acute urinary tract infections and sexually transmitted infections have the potential to harm the mother or fetus if undetected or inadequately treated.

The goal of pharmacotherapy during pregnancy is to treat the mother without causing ill effects for the fetus. Often, pharmacotherapy can be safely conducted with the same drugs and dosage levels as in nonpregnant patients. In other cases, a medication may need to be discontinued, changed to a lower dose, or replaced with a safer drug. In all pregnant patients, healthcare providers must carefully consider the therapeutic value of a given medication against its potential adverse effects.

Pharmacotherapy During Pregnancy

8.2 Physiologic changes during pregnancy can alter normal pharmacokinetic responses.

Most body systems undergo predictable changes during pregnancy. Some organs increase in size. Some physiologic activities speed up while others slow down, altering the pharmacokinetic responses to drugs. The healthcare provider must understand these changes in maternal physiology when prescribing drugs for the pregnant woman (Figure 8.1).

Absorption: During pregnancy, increased levels of progesterone cause a decrease in gastric tone and intestinal motility, resulting in delayed gastric emptying. Drugs remain longer in the gastrointestinal (GI) tract, leading to extended time for absorption of oral drugs. High estrogen levels in the pregnant woman cause increased hydrochloric acid production in the stomach, which may affect the absorption of certain acid labile drugs. Furthermore, as the enlarging uterus rises into the abdomen it presses up against the stomach, leading to slower gastric emptying. Medications may take a longer time to be absorbed and distributed, thus prolonging their onset and durations of

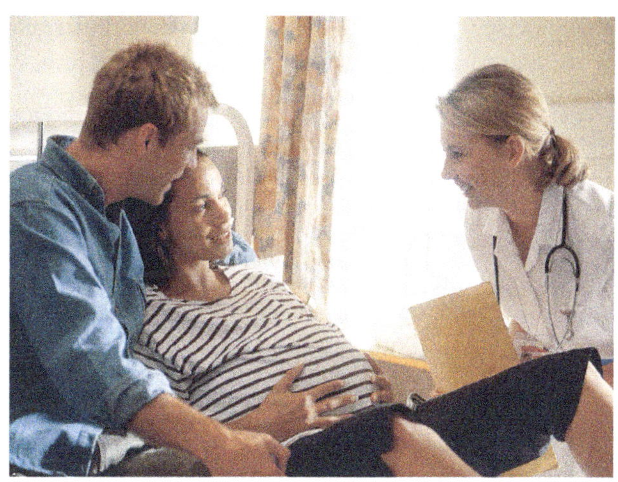

Figure 8.1 Teaching women about the safety of drug use during pregnancy is an essential component of nursing care.
Flying Colors/Photodisc/Getty Images.

action. Some women experience nausea and vomiting and are unable to take oral medications during early pregnancy.

Progesterone also increases pulmonary blood flow, respiratory tidal volume, and minute volume by 40%. As a result, respiratory drugs may be absorbed in larger quantities, leading to higher serum drug levels.

Distribution: Distribution of drugs during pregnancy is affected by changes in total body water, which may increase by over 50%. This increase leads to greater hemodilution of plasma proteins and drugs. Because the plasma proteins are diluted, fewer are available to bind with drugs, thus causing a higher concentration of "free" drug in the plasma. This results in more drug molecules being available for transfer across the placenta or to be secreted in breast milk. Highly lipophilic drugs are distributed into the lipid-rich breast milk and are ultimately passed to the breastfeeding infant. A woman's heart rate may increase up to 15 beats per minute during pregnancy, leading to greater drug distribution.

Metabolism: It was originally thought that metabolism was the pharmacokinetic process least affected by pregnancy. Evidence, however, suggests that metabolism is significantly altered throughout pregnancy.

Some of the cytochrome P450 enzymes increase, noticeably CYP2D6 and CYP3A4, whereas others such as CYP1A2 decrease. Researchers have also found that a single CYP enzyme system may have multiple alleles that express different genetic forms of the same enzyme. Because of these unique differences among individuals, even knowing the pathway through which a drug is metabolized will not always accurately predict how that drug will be metabolized. The fetal liver is still developing throughout this time and lacks the ability to metabolize most drugs received from the mother's system. Lifestyle factors, such as smoking and eating broccoli or other cruciferous vegetables, may also alter how an enzyme system metabolizes a drug. Until more is learned about how drug metabolism is affected during pregnancy, providers should use caution when prescribing any drug during this time and limit prescriptions to those drugs known to have demonstrated a low-risk safety profile.

Excretion: Excretion of drugs during pregnancy is enhanced by renal plasma flow, which can increase 50–70% during the first two trimesters. This increased flow leads to a higher glomerular filtration rate and marked decreases in blood urea nitrogen and creatinine levels. Because these changes result in the increased renal elimination of drugs, doses of many medications must be adjusted.

CONNECTION Checkpoint 8.1

From what you learned in Chapter 3, what effects on drug metabolism may occur if a woman required any of the following drugs during pregnancy: acetaminophen, sertraline, or propranolol? (See Table 3.1 for a list of specific CYP450 enzymes.)

8.3 Many drugs pass from mother to infant via the placenta.

The **placenta** is a temporary organ that allows for nutrition and gas exchange between the mother and fetus. As much as 10% of the mother's cardiac output circulates through the placenta. Although the blood of the mother does not circulate through the fetus, capillary-like structures in the placenta allow an extensive exchange of substances. The placenta offers a degree of protective filtration of the maternal blood, preventing certain harmful substances from reaching the fetus. Nutritional substances such as vitamins, fatty acids, glucose, and electrolytes freely pass from mother to fetus.

Most drugs cross the placenta and pass from mother to fetus by simple diffusion. A few drugs cross by way of active transport. Metabolic enzymes are present in the placenta and likely contribute to drug metabolism. Some drugs may be metabolized extensively and presumably have little or no effect on the developing fetus, whereas other drugs may be changed and become toxic metabolites capable of harm. It should be understood that drugs may cause fetal harm without crossing the placenta or entering the fetal blood. For example, certain drugs may cause constriction of placental blood vessels, impairing nutrient exchange. Other drugs can alter maternal physiology to such an extent that the fetus is affected.

Multiple factors impact the transfer of drugs across the placenta. These variables are the same as those affecting the movement of substances across other biological membranes (see Chapter 3):

- **Plasma drug level in the mother.** In general, the higher the dose taken by the mother, the greater the amount of drug available to cross the placenta and affect the fetus. This is the rationale for prescribing the lowest effective doses of drugs during pregnancy.
- **Solubility of the drug.** Highly lipid-soluble drugs will cross the placental barrier more easily than water-soluble drugs.
- **Molecular size.** Small molecules such as alcohol with molecular weights (MW) less than 300 easily cross the placental barrier; those with MW greater than 500 are slower to cross. Large drugs such as heparin, with MW greater than 1000, do not generally cross the placenta to the fetus.
- **Protein binding.** When a drug is bound to maternal plasma proteins, the drug–protein complex is too large to cross the placental membrane. Thus, drugs that are highly protein bound are more likely to cross the placenta more slowly and in lower doses compared to nonbound drugs.
- **Drug ionization.** Nonionized drugs cross the placenta more easily than ionized drugs. The maternal serum pH

is slightly higher than that of the fetus. Upon reaching the relatively acidic environment of the fetus, drugs that are weak bases become ionized. This effectively traps them on the fetal side of the placenta because ionized drugs cannot recross the placental membrane back to the mother (ion trapping). An example is nicotine (a weak base), which can appear in higher concentrations in the fetus than in the mother due to ion trapping.

- **Blood flow to the placenta.** Decreased uterine blood flow may cause drugs to remain trapped in the fetus for extended periods, resulting in fetal adverse effects. During labor the patient is usually instructed to remain in the lateral position during active uterine contractions to prevent pressure on the aorta and vena cava. Pressure on these vessels will obstruct uterine blood flow and may cause drug accumulation in the fetus.

PharmFACT

The most common antidepressants, the selective serotonin reuptake inhibitors (SSRIs), when taken by pregnant women, have been shown to increase the risk of preterm labor and may cause withdrawal symptoms in newborns that include agitation, irritability, trouble feeding, sleep disturbances, and convulsions (Saccone et al., 2016). Dosages of SSRIs are tapered during the third trimester so that the fetus receives no drug through the placenta for at least 7 to 10 days prior to birth.

8.4 The U.S. Food and Drug Administration drug-labeling information has been revised to provide more detailed information on risks during pregnancy and lactation.

Determining the safety of medications in pregnant and breastfeeding women has always been a challenging endeavor. Testing drugs in humans to estimate their ability to cause birth anomalies is, of course, unethical and prohibited by law. Although most medications are tested in pregnant laboratory animals prior to U.S. Food and Drug Administration (FDA) approval, the structure of the human placenta is unique among mammals. Because most of the FDA pregnancy drug information is extrapolated from these animal data, it is likely only a crude approximation of the actual risk to a human fetus. In only a few cases are human data available to show pregnancy risks. It is important to remind women that no prescription drug, over-the-counter (OTC) medication, or dietary supplement should be taken during pregnancy or breastfeeding unless the healthcare provider verifies that the therapeutic benefits to the mother clearly outweigh the potential risks for the unborn.

Table 8.1 FDA Pregnancy Category Ratings with Examples

Risk Category	Interpretation
A	Adequate, well-controlled studies in pregnant women have not shown an increased risk of fetal abnormalities in any trimester of pregnancy.
B	Animal studies have revealed no evidence of harm to the fetus; however, there are no adequate and well-controlled studies in pregnant women OR animal studies have shown an adverse effect, but adequate and well-controlled studies in pregnant women have failed to demonstrate risk to the fetus in any trimester.
C	Animal studies have shown an adverse effect and there are no adequate and well-controlled studies in pregnant women OR no animal studies have been conducted and there are no adequate and well-controlled studies in pregnant women.
D	Adequate well-controlled or observational studies in pregnant women have demonstrated a risk to the fetus. However, the benefits of therapy may outweigh the potential risk. For example, the drug may be acceptable if needed in a life-threatening situation or serious disease for which safer drugs cannot be used or are ineffective.
X	Adequate well-controlled or observational studies in animals or pregnant women have demonstrated positive evidence of fetal abnormalities or risks. The use of the product is contraindicated in women who are or may become pregnant. There is no indication for use in pregnancy.

Due in part to several high-profile teratogenic events, the FDA introduced **pregnancy categories** in 1979 to inform physicians and the public of risks associated with medications. This labeling used the letters *A*, *B*, *C*, *D*, and *X* to indicate the pregnancy risk category of the medication. This system, shown in Table 8.1, was simple and easily understood by healthcare providers and their patients.

In 1994, in response to criticism that the letter system was too simplistic and did not provide enough safety information to providers or their patients, the FDA began a process of developing a new labeling system. The revision process included input from all interested parties and lasted almost 20 years.

In 2015 the FDA implemented the **Pregnancy and Lactation Labeling Rule (PLLR)**, which replaced the pregnancy risk letter system with narrative sections and subsections (FDA, n.d.). Subsection changes on the drug label include the following:

- The prior Pregnancy subsection is now Pregnancy, Labor, and Delivery. This subsection provides information about dosing adjustments and potential risks to the developing fetus and data on how pregnant women may be affected when they use the medication.
- The prior Nursing Mothers subsection is changed to Lactation and provides data regarding the amount of drug and drug metabolites in breast milk and potential clinical effects on the breastfed infant.

- A new subsection is titled Females and Males of Reproductive Potential. This subsection includes relevant information on pregnancy testing or recommendations to use contraception before, during, or after drug therapy and a medication's effect on fertility or pregnancy loss.

The new labeling began in 2015 for all newly approved drugs and biologics. All medications approved between 2001 and 2015 were required to implement the new format by 2019. Drugs approved before 2001 are not required to use the new format but the manufacturers were directed to remove the letter categories. Examples of selected pregnancy-related statements for drugs approved since 2015 are shown in Table 8.2. This is not a comprehensive list of all statements and only shows representative samples.

Table 8.2 Selected Medications Approved Since 2015 with Pregnancy-Related Statements

Medication	Indication	Label Statement
bremelanotide	Hypoactive sexual desire disorder	Based on findings in animal studies, use in pregnant women may be associated with the potential for fetal harm. Use during pregnancy is not recommended. Advise females of reproductive potential to use effective contraception and to discontinue the medication if pregnancy is suspected.
buprenorphine and naloxone	Opioid dependence	Neonatal opioid withdrawal syndrome may occur in newborn infants of mothers who are receiving treatment.
cannabidiol	Epilepsy	Administration of cannabidiol to pregnant animals produced evidence of developmental toxicity (increased embryo/fetal mortality in rats and decreased fetal body weights in rabbits; decreased growth, delayed sexual maturation, long-term neurobehavioral changes, and adverse effects on the reproductive system in rat offspring).
cenobamate	Epilepsy	Women of reproductive potential using oral contraceptives should use additional or alternative nonhormonal birth control.
glecaprevir and pibrentasvir (Mavyret)	Hepatitis C infection	In animal reproduction studies, no adverse developmental effects were observed when the components of Mavyret were administered separately during organogenesis at exposures up to 53 times the human exposures at the recommended dose of Mavyret.
lasmiditan	Migraine	Excretion of lasmiditan and/or metabolites into milk, at levels approximately three times those in maternal plasma, was observed in lactating rats following oral administration of lasmiditan.
lefamulin	Pneumonia	Based on findings from animal studies, lefamulin may cause fetal harm when administered to pregnant women. Verify pregnancy status in females of reproductive potential.
lemborexant (Dayvigo)	Insomnia	Lemborexant and its metabolites are present in the milk of lactating rats. When a drug is present in animal milk, it is likely that the drug will be present in human milk.
methylphenidate (Adhansia)	Attention-deficit/hyperactivity disorder	Limited published literature, based on breast milk sampling from five mothers, reports that methylphenidate is present in human milk, which resulted in infant doses of 0.16–0.7% of the maternal weight-adjusted dosage. There are no reports of adverse effects on the breastfed infant and no effects on milk production.
ozanimod	Multiple sclerosis	Before initiation of treatment, women of childbearing potential should be counseled on the potential for a serious risk to the fetus and the need for contraception during treatment. Because of the time it takes to eliminate the drug from the body after stopping treatment, the potential risk to the fetus may persist and women of childbearing age should also use effective contraception for 3 months after stopping.
risperidone	Psychosis	Extrapyramidal and/or withdrawal symptoms, including agitation, hypertonia, hypotonia, tremor, somnolence, respiratory distress, and feeding disorder have been reported in neonates who were exposed to antipsychotic drugs, including risperidone, during the third trimester of pregnancy.
tucatinib (Tukysa)	Breast cancer	Based on findings from animal studies, Tukysa may impair male and female fertility. Advise females of reproductive potential to use effective contraception during treatment and for at least 1 week after the last dose. Verify the pregnancy status of females of reproductive potential prior to initiating treatment.
voxelotor	Sickle cell disease	Because of the potential for serious adverse reactions in the breastfed child, including changes in the hematopoietic system, advise patients that breastfeeding is not recommended during treatment and for at least 2 weeks after the last dose.

Of course, drug warnings and labeling are only required for medications approved by the FDA. Many illegal substances likely affect the pregnant mother and her fetus. Selected abused substances and their effects on the fetus are listed in Table 8.3.

8.5 The stage of development has an important influence on adverse drug effects in the embryo and fetus.

The effects of drugs on the fetus depend on the stage of fetal development and the dosage received by the fetus. For the vast majority of medications, very little scientific data are available on the effects of drugs on the human fetus. Lack of knowledge does not mean they are safe; these drugs have the potential to cause adverse drug reactions in the fetus and, in some cases, may cause fetal malformations.

A **teratogen** is any substance, organism, or physical agent that interferes with growth or development of the embryo or fetus and produces a permanent abnormality or death. The word derives from the Greek *gennan* ("to produce") and *terata* ("monster"). The baseline incidence of teratogenic events is approximately 3% of all pregnancies. Potential fetal consequences of drug use include intrauterine fetal death, physical malformations, growth impairment, behavioral abnormalities, and neonatal toxicity.

There are no "absolute" teratogens. Whether or not a drug produces a teratogenic effect depends on multiple, complex factors. Like other effects of drugs, there is a dose–response relationship, with risk increasing with higher doses. The timing of drug therapy and the stage of fetal development critically affect the risk for possible fetal consequences. Because of the constant changes that occur during fetal development, the specific risk is dependent on when during gestation the drug is administered. A well-known example is the drug thalidomide, which causes its fetal effects from day 35 to day 49 after the last menstrual period. The specific malformation is linked to the time of exposure: 35 to 37 days, no ears; 39 to 41 days, no arms; 41 to 43 days, no uterus; 45 to 47 days, no tibia; and 47 to 49 days, triphalangeal thumbs.

Preimplantation Period: Weeks 1 to 2 of the first trimester are known as the preimplantation phase. Before implantation, the developing embryo has not yet established a blood supply with the mother. This is sometimes called the "all-or-none" period because exposure to a teratogen either causes death of the embryo or has no effect. Drugs are less likely to cause congenital malformations during this period because the baby's organ systems have not yet begun to form. Drugs such as nicotine, however, can create a negative environment for the embryo and potentially cause intrauterine growth retardation.

Embryonic Period: During the embryonic period, from 3 to 8 weeks postconception, internal structures develop rapidly. This is the period of maximum sensitivity to

Table 8.3 Street Drugs and Their Potential Effects During Pregnancy

Drug	Potential Effects
Amphetamines/ methamphetamine	Increased risk of pregnancy complications, such as premature birth and placental problems Possible birth defects, including heart defects and cleft lip or palate After delivery, the infant may have withdrawal-like symptoms such as jitteriness, drowsiness, and breathing problems
Cannabis/marijuana	Reduced fertility in both men and women Slowed fetal growth Slightly decreased length of pregnancy After delivery, the infant may have withdrawal-like symptoms such as excessive crying and trembling
Club drugs such as PCP, ketamine, and LSD	After delivery, the infant may have withdrawal symptoms Increased risk of learning and behavioral problems
Cocaine	Increased risk of miscarriage or premature birth Low birth weight with increased risk of health problems such as intellectual disability and cerebral palsy, and even death Increased risk of birth defects involving the urinary tract and possibly other birth defects May cause an unborn baby to have a stroke, which can result in irreversible brain damage or a heart attack, and sometimes death Placental problems, including placental abruption, which can lead to heavy bleeding that can be life-threatening for both mother and baby After delivery, the infant may have mild behavioral disturbances, jitteriness, and irritability; may startle and cry at the gentlest touch or sound Increased risk of sudden infant death syndrome (SIDS)
Heroin	Increased risk of serious pregnancy complications, including poor fetal growth, premature rupture of the membranes, premature birth, and stillbirth Low birth weight often combined with breathing problems and possibility of lifelong disabilities Increased risk of birth defects After delivery, the infant may have withdrawal symptoms such as fever, sneezing, trembling, irritability, diarrhea, vomiting, continual crying, and, occasionally, seizures Increased risk of SIDS
Inhalants, glues, and solvents	Miscarriage, slow fetal growth, preterm birth, and birth defects

Source: Data from "Street Drugs and Pregnancy," March of Dimes, 2020.

teratogens. Teratogenic drugs taken during this phase can lead to structural malformation and spontaneous abortion. The specific abnormality depends on which organ is forming at the time of exposure.

Fetal Period: The fetal phase is from 9 to 40 weeks postconception or until birth. During this time there is continued growth and maturation of the baby's organ systems. Blood flow to the placenta increases and placental vascular membranes become thinner. Such alterations maximize the transfer of substances from the maternal circulation to the fetal blood. As a result, the fetus may receive larger doses of medications and other substances taken by the mother. Because the fetus lacks mature metabolic enzymes and efficient excretion mechanisms, medications will have a prolonged duration of action within the unborn child. Exposure to teratogens during the fetal period is more likely to produce slowed growth or impaired organ function, rather than gross structural malformations.

The nurse caring for the pregnant woman must differentiate adverse drug effects from the normal symptoms of pregnancy. Nausea and vomiting, abdominal cramps, flushed skin, or diaphoresis may indeed be either normal symptoms of pregnancy or adverse drug effects. Fetal tachycardia may be due to drugs being taken by the mother or a fetal cardiac anomaly. During all stages of pregnancy, the nurse should help the mother assess medications and dietary supplements to determine if they are necessary and if adjustments are required. Impairments in the functioning of the mother's liver or kidneys may have a profound impact on maternal and fetal safety. Healthcare providers must consider these factors, so as to minimize the risk of toxicity to the mother and child. Through careful assessments, the nurse contributes greatly to this risk–benefit analysis, which is essential for protecting both the mother and her baby.

PharmFACT

Most medications commonly used in pregnancy have insufficient data available to allow a full understanding of their fetal risk. This limits the ability of providers to make informed clinical decisions on the management of acute and chronic disorders that require medication use during pregnancy. Common preexisting (chronic) disorders that warrant pharmacological intervention during pregnantcy include diabetes, asthma, depression, cardiovascular conditions, and renal disease (Wyszynski & Shields, 2016).

CONNECTION Checkpoint 8.2

From what you learned in Chapter 5, explain why the FDA might approve a drug even though it is a known teratogen and can cause fetal abnormalities.

Pharmacotherapy During Lactation

8.6 Transfer of drugs from mother to infant may occur through breast milk.

According to the *Breastfeeding Report Card 2018* by the Centers for Disease Control and Prevention (2018), 83% of mothers breastfeed their infants and about 57% continue to breastfeed for at least 6 months. Breastfeeding is highly recommended as a means of providing nutrition, emotional bonding, and immune protection to the neonate (Figure 8.2).

The majority of drugs are secreted into breast milk to some extent. Fortunately, there are relatively few instances in which breastfeeding must be discontinued due to medication use. For the few drugs that are absolutely contraindicated during lactation, equally effective, safer alternatives are usually available. Some of these drugs are shown in Table 8.4. Although most medications probably cause no harm to the breastfeeding baby, their effects have not been fully studied.

Drugs enter breast milk primarily by passive diffusion. In the first week of life, the alveolar cells in the breast have large gaps between them, allowing drugs and other substances to penetrate the milk. By the second week of life the alveolar cells swell, closing the intracellular gaps and limiting the drug's access to the milk.

It is important for the nurse to understand factors that influence the amount of drug secreted into breast milk. This allows the nurse to aid the patient in making responsible choices regarding lactation and in reducing exposure of her newborn to potentially harmful substances. The amount of

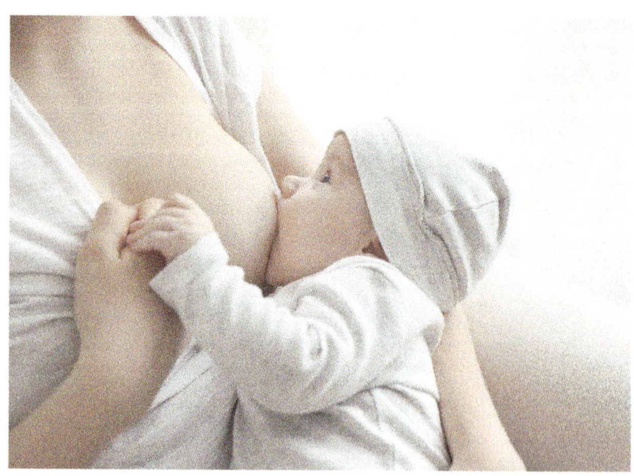

Figure 8.2 Nurses should teach lactating women to avoid all drugs, herbal products, or dietary supplements unless approved by their healthcare provider.
Africa Studio/Shutterstock.

Table 8.4 Selected Drugs Compatible with Breastfeeding

Class	Compatible Drugs	Drugs to Be Avoided
Analgesics (nonopioid)	acetaminophen, aspirin (low dose), ibuprofen	—
Analgesics (opioids)	codeine and morphine (low doses or epidural)	hydrocodone, oxycodone
Anti-infectives	acyclovir, aminoglycosides, cephalosporins, fluconazole, isoniazid, macrolides, penicillins, trimethoprim, sulfisoxazole, tetracyclines (short-term use)	ciprofloxacin, metronidazole
Antimigraine drugs	propranolol	ergotamine
Antiseizure drugs	carbamazepine, diazepam (single dose), phenytoin, valproic acid	buspirone, ethosuximide
Cardiovascular drugs	digoxin, furosemide, heparin, iron salts, lidocaine, nifedipine, prazosin, spironolactone, verapamil, warfarin	ACE inhibitors, atenolol, clonidine, hydrochlorothiazide, statins
Central nervous system drugs	paroxetine, sertraline, tricyclic antidepressants	lithium carbonate
Cytotoxic drugs and immunosuppressants	—	All drugs in this class should be avoided
Gastrointestinal drugs	aluminum hydroxide, magnesium hydroxide, promethazine (single dose)	cimetidine, metoclopramide
Hormones	hydrocortisone (single dose), insulin, oxytocin (short term), prednisone, thyroid hormone	estrogens, oral contraceptives, testosterone

Source: Data from Drugs and Lactation database (LactMed), n.d., National Institutes of Health, U.S. National Library of Medicine. Retrieved from https://www.ncbi.nlm.nih.gov/books/NBK501922/.

drug that passes to the infant during lactation depends on multiple factors:

- **Plasma drug level in the mother.** The higher the dose of drug taken by the mother, the more will be secreted into breast milk. It is therefore standard practice that if a drug must be prescribed during breastfeeding the lowest effective dose should be ordered.
- **Solubility of the drug.** Highly lipid-soluble drugs enter the milk at higher concentrations. Milk at the end of a feed contains considerably more fat and may have a higher concentration of lipid-soluble drugs. Furthermore, the percentage of lipids in milk increases progressively from day 1 to day 84 of lactation. Drugs that act on the central nervous system are usually lipophilic and have a tendency to penetrate milk at higher concentrations.
- **Molecular size and protein binding.** Some drugs, such as heparin and insulin, are simply too large to pass through membranes by passive diffusion. In addition, when drugs are highly protein bound, they are less likely to enter the milk than those that are free. The healthcare provider may choose drugs with greater protein binding capacity for the lactating mother to limit the amount secreted in milk.
- **Drug ionization.** Milk is slightly more acidic than plasma; the pH of milk is 7.2 and plasma 7.4. This pH gradient allows weakly basic drugs to transfer more readily into breast milk and accumulate due to ion trapping (see Chapter 4).
- **Drug half-life.** Drugs with short half-lives will be metabolized and eliminated quickly by the mother. This results in smaller amounts being secreted into milk.

Once ingested by the infant, a drug is subjected to the usual pharmacokinetic influences. The infant's stomach content is quite acidic; therefore, some drugs may be destroyed and have reduced bioavailability. Additionally, some drugs are inactivated when ingested with calcium and protein-rich nutrients in the mother's milk. Some drugs by their nature are likely removed by the infant's liver during first-pass metabolism and never get to the plasma. It is important to remember that the baby's organs responsible for metabolizing and eliminating medications are immature and are not able to perform all the functions of adult organs.

Considering the many variables, it is not surprising that it is difficult to accurately predict the amount of maternal drug that will transfer to the infant plasma during lactation. Estimates of drug transference to breast milk range from less than 1% to 3%. Regardless of the amount, it is imperative for the nurse to teach the mother that many prescription medications, OTC drugs, and herbal products are secreted in breast milk and have the potential to affect her child. The same guidelines for drug use during pregnancy apply during lactation—drugs should be taken only if the benefits to the mother clearly outweigh the potential risks to the infant.

PharmFACT

Because the negative effects of tobacco smoking on the fetus are well documented, the American College of Obstetricians and Gynecologists recommends that healthcare providers counsel their pregnant patients on smoking-cessation techniques and provide resources to support their efforts. Because the safety and efficacy of nicotine replacement therapy (NRT) during pregnancy have not been established, ACOG (2020b) recommends that NRT only be used under the close supervision of a healthcare provider.

8.7 Drugs present in breast milk may cause adverse effects in the breastfeeding infant.

Although the concentration of drugs and their metabolites in breast milk is often very low, their effects on the infant have the potential to be serious. Common drug effects seen in breastfeeding infants are nonspecific and include diarrhea, constipation, sedation, and irritability. The healthcare provider has an important responsibility to monitor for adverse drug effects in breastfeeding infants and to teach new mothers to do the same. Selected drugs that enter the breast milk and are believed to produce adverse effects are shown in Table 8.5.

The nurse must inform the mother that all drugs of abuse are contraindicated during both pregnancy and breastfeeding. If she takes such drugs, her infant may experience withdrawal symptoms and test positive for the drug for several weeks to months following exposure.

In general, topical medications applied to the mother's skin are safe to use during lactation. The nurse must remind the mother, however, that the breastfeeding infant may ingest substances like vitamins E, A, or D in creams that are rubbed on her nipples to soften them.

The National Institutes of Health maintains a searchable Drugs and Lactation Database (LactMed) that is updated monthly and contains clinical data on drug effects on infants during lactation. Healthcare providers should consult this source for current information when counseling their breastfeeding patients.

Table 8.5 Classes of Medications that May Cause Serious Effects in a Baby Following Breastfeeding

Drug Class	Potential Adverse Effect
Antiepileptics (e.g., phenobarbital, ethosuximide)	Sedation
Antineoplastics	Neutropenia
Beta blockers	Lethargy and bradycardia
Benzodiazepines	Sedation and weight loss
Ergot alkaloids	Vomiting and diarrhea
Opioids	Sedation and withdrawal symptoms
Phenothiazines	Sedation
Pseudoephedrine	Inhibition of milk production

CONNECTION Checkpoint 8.3

From what you learned in Chapter 3, how long would it take a 600-mg dose of a drug with a $t_{1/2}$ of 8 hours to reach five half-lives and be safe for a lactating patient concerned about passing the drug through her breast milk? How much drug would be left at that time?

CONNECTIONS: Advanced Practice Application

Zika Virus

Case

Maria is a healthy 22-year-old pregnant woman who came to the free clinic for care. She is new to the country from Brazil. During her first appointment a complete history was taken and blood was drawn to test for human immunodeficiency virus (HIV), cytomegalovirus, rubella, and hepatitis B and C. All laboratory tests came back negative. Maria appears healthy with no cause for concern. After her first appointment at 12 weeks, she was thrilled to hear her baby's heartbeat and left excited to tell her husband. Maria continued to come to the clinic for care and at her 16-week appointment she was given a referral for a routine ultrasound.

At 18 weeks, an ultrasound showed that the fetus's weight was significantly lower than expected. Subsequent ultrasounds performed between 18 and 28 weeks continued to show additional fetal abnormalities. At week 32, labor was induced and resulted in a stillbirth. Laboratory tests later showed that the Zika virus was present in the fetus's tissue. At her postpartum appointment Maria asks if there are any medications she could have taken to prevent the stillbirth. What do we know about medications and the Zika virus?

Discussion

The Zika virus continues to be a problem in many parts of the world. There is no vaccine to prevent infection. It is spread mostly by the bite of an infected *Aedes* species mosquito. The Zika virus can be passed from a pregnant woman to her fetus. Infection during pregnancy poses significant risks to pregnant women because it can cause a birth defect called *microcephaly*, which results in babies born with undersized heads and underdeveloped brains.

No specific antiviral treatment for the Zika virus exists. Treatment is aimed at relieving symptoms with rest, fluids, and medications such as acetaminophen (Tylenol). However, already existing drugs may offer pregnant women and their developing fetuses protection against the damaging effects of the Zika virus (Kincaid, 2016; Li et al., 2017).

Niclosamide is used to treat tapeworm and appears to also have antiviral properties that inhibit the Zika virus from replicating. PHA-690509 is an antiviral drug that potentially may have an effect against the virus by interfering with its gene expression. Emricasan works by inhibiting a natural process that causes viral cell death (Kincaid, 2016; Li et al., 2017). These medications still must undergo extensive testing to determine if they are effective and if they are safe to take during pregnancy.

Understanding Chapter 8

Key Concepts Summary

8.1 Women frequently use drugs during pregnancy and lactation.

8.2 Physiologic changes during pregnancy can alter normal pharmacokinetic responses.

8.3 Many drugs pass from mother to infant via the placenta.

8.4 The U.S. Food and Drug Administration drug-labeling information has been revised to provide more detailed information on risks during pregnancy and lactation.

8.5 The stage of development has an important influence on adverse drug effects in the embryo and fetus.

8.6 Transfer of drugs from mother to infant may occur through breast milk.

8.7 Drugs present in breast milk may cause adverse effects in the breastfeeding infant.

CASE STUDY: Making the Patient Connection

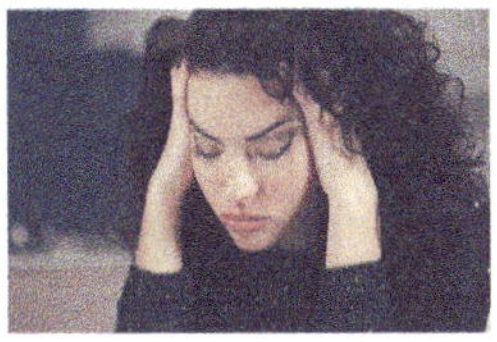

Remember the patient "May David" at the beginning of the chapter? Now read the remainder of the case study. Based on the information presented within this chapter, respond to the critical thinking questions that follow.

May David, a 22-year-old woman, comes to the clinic to obtain a pregnancy test. She has not had her menstrual period for the past 6 weeks but claims that infrequent menses are not unusual for her. She feels nauseous in the mornings, but the feeling is only temporary. You ask May, "Is it possible that you might be pregnant?" May's response is "I doubt it, since we have always used a condom during intercourse." She goes on to explain that she has been taking an antiseizure medication for several years to control her epilepsy and is taking some herbal medicines for a feeling of well-being.

May's vital signs are as follows: temperature, 36.7°C (98°F); pulse, 68 beats/min; respiration, 18 breaths/min; and blood pressure, 110/70 mmHg. She is 1.7 m (5 feet 6 inches) tall and is surprised that she has gained 2.3 kg (5 lb) in the past 4 weeks, bringing her weight to 65.8 kg (145 lb). A urine specimen is sent to the laboratory for human chorionic gonadotropin (HCG). A complete physical examination is performed, followed by a vaginal examination via speculum. All physical findings were within normal limits except for the urine qualitative HCG, which is positive and quantitative HCG = 550, indicating pregnancy. May smokes approximately a half pack of cigarettes per day.

Critical Thinking Questions

1. What are some key points you should discuss with May regarding her condition and the medication she is taking?
2. What education should you provide for May regarding the use of medication during pregnancy?
3. While caring for May, you must consider FDA pregnancy risk categories. In your own words, explain these categories.
4. What effect does May's tobacco use possibly have on her unborn baby? What are the recommendations from ACOG on the use of NRT?

Additional Case Study

You are caring for Irina, an 18-year-old mother of a 6-month-old baby boy. She confides in you that she has experienced postpartum depression since her child was born. She tries to take care of herself but just does not feel very good most of the time. Her husband insists that she continue breastfeeding, but she is now having doubts. After a lengthy discussion, Irina states, "The only time I feel good is when I smoke a joint (marijuana) before feeding my son."

1. How should you respond to Irina?
2. What teaching should you carry out at this time?
3. Should Irina ask her provider for an antidepressant medication?

Chapter Review

1. A patient in her first trimester of pregnancy asks which medications should be avoided during pregnancy. Your response is based on the knowledge that during pregnancy:
    1. Most over-the-counter medications are safe.
    2. When possible, drug therapy is postponed until after pregnancy and lactation.
    3. It is wise to discontinue all drugs used in treating medical conditions.
    4. The decision whether or not to take medication is the responsibility of the woman.
2. When discussing drug use during pregnancy with a group of nursing students, the main topic is the FDA pregnancy drug classifications. The FDA's newly revised Pregnancy and Lactation Labeling Rule (PLLR) will include: (Select all that apply.)
    1. A five-letter system (A, B, C, D, and X)
    2. Helpful information about a medication's risks to the expectant mother, the developing fetus, and the breastfed infant.
    3. Updated information about lactation and the potential for drug effects in the infant.
    4. A subsection that will provide information about pregnancy testing, birth control, and a medication's effect on fertility.
    5. A list of safe drugs that may be used during pregnancy and lactation.
3. A pregnant patient asks what factors determine if a drug will cross the placenta. Your response will be based on which of the following principles?
    1. Highly lipid-soluble drugs cross the placental membrane more easily than low lipids.
    2. The lower the lipid content of a drug, the easier it crosses the placental membrane.
    3. Drugs with large molecular weight pass rapidly through the placental membrane.
    4. Highly protein-bound drugs pass rapidly through the placental membrane.
4. At which stage of fetal development are congenital malformations *least* likely to occur?
    1. 1 to 2 weeks
    2. 3 to 4 weeks
    3. 5 to 6 weeks
    4. 7 to 8 weeks
5. While seeing a postpartum mother who is breastfeeding her 3.2-kg (7-lb) infant daughter, which of the following statements, if made by the mother, indicates that further teaching is necessary? (Select all that apply.)
    1. "When using over-the-counter medication, I should take only the lowest effective dose."
    2. "The higher the dose of medication, the more likely it will be secreted into breast milk."
    3. "I shouldn't take any drug during breastfeeding, even my prescriptions."
    4. "Medication in liquid form should be avoided since it more readily enters the breast milk."
    5. "Now that I'm no longer pregnant, I don't need to worry about the medicines affecting my baby."
6. Before prescribing medications to a patient who is 32 weeks pregnant, you must consider the following normal physiologic principles associated with pregnancy that will affect drug absorption?
    1. Medications are absorbed and distributed more quickly in pregnant women.
    2. There is greater hemoconcentration of drugs in pregnant patients.
    3. Drugs remain longer in the gastrointestinal tract, leading to extended time for absorption.
    4. Drug metabolism is highly affected by pregnancy.

See Appendix A for answers to critical thinking questions, case study questions and review questions.

References

American College of Obstetricians and Gynecologists. (2020b). *Tobacco and nicotine cessation during pregnancy*. https://www.acog.org/clinical/clinical-guidance/committee-opinion/articles/2020/05/tobacco-and-nicotine-cessation-during-pregnancy

Centers for Disease Control and Prevention. (2018). *Breastfeeding report card 2018*. https://www.cdc.gov/media/releases/2018/p0820-breastfeeding-report-card.html

Centers for Disease Control and Prevention. (2020). *Research on medicines and pregnancy*. https://www.cdc.gov/pregnancy/meds/treatingfortwo/research.html

Kincaid, E. (2016). A second look: Efforts to repurpose old drugs against Zika cast a wide net. *Nature Medicine*, *22*, 824–825. https://doi.org/10.1038/nm0816-824

Li, Z., Brecher, M., Deng, Y. Q., Zhang, J., Sakamuru, S., Liu, B., et al. (2017). Existing drugs as broad-spectrum and potent inhibitors for Zika virus by targeting NS2B-NS3 interaction. *Cell Research*, *27*(8), 1046–1064. https://doi.org/10.1038/cr.2017.88

March of Dimes. (2020). *Street drugs and pregnancy*. Retrieved from https://www.marchofdimes.org/pregnancy/street-drugs-and-pregnancy.aspx

Moon, M. A. (2015). Late pregnancy SSRI exposure ups PPHN risk slightly. *OB GYN News*, *50*(7), 21.

National Institutes of Health, U.S. National Library of Medicine. (n.d.). *LactMed: A Toxnet database*. Retrieved from http://toxnet.nlm.nih.gov/newtoxnet/lactmed.htm

National Library of Medicine. (n.d.). *Drugs and Lactation database (LactMed)*. National Institutes of Health. https://www.ncbi.nlm.nih.gov/books/NBK501922/

Saccone, G., Eke, A. C., & Berghella, V. B. (2016). 850: Selective serotonin reuptake inhibitor (SSRI) use during pregnancy and risk of preterm birth: A systematic review and metaanalysis. *American Journal of Obstetrics and Gynecology*, *214*(1, Suppl.), S443. https://doi.org/10.1016/j.ajog.2015.10.900

Singh Joy, S. D. (2014). SSRI use in pregnancy and pulmonary hypertension risk in newborns. *American Journal of Nursing*, *114*(6), 53–53. doi:10.1097/01.NAJ.0000450431.05007.7a

U.S. Food and Drug Administration. (n.d.) *Pregnancy and Lactation Labeling Final Rule*. http://www.fda.gov/Drugs/DevelopmentApprovalProcess/DevelopmentResources/Labeling/ucm093307.htm

Wyszynski, D., & Shields, K. (2016). Frequency and type of medications and vaccines used during pregnancy. *Obstetric Medicine*, *9*(1), 21–27. https://doi.org/10.1177/1753495X15604099

Selected Bibliography

Briggs, G. G., Freeman, R. K., Towers, C.V., & Forinash, A.B. (2017). *Drugs in pregnancy and lactation* (11th ed.). Lippincott Williams & Wilkins.

Centers for Disease Control and Prevention. (2020). *Folic acid* https://www.cdc.gov/ncbddd/folicacid/index.html

Hale, T. W., & Rowe, H. E. (2017). *Medications and mother's milk* (17th ed.). Springer.

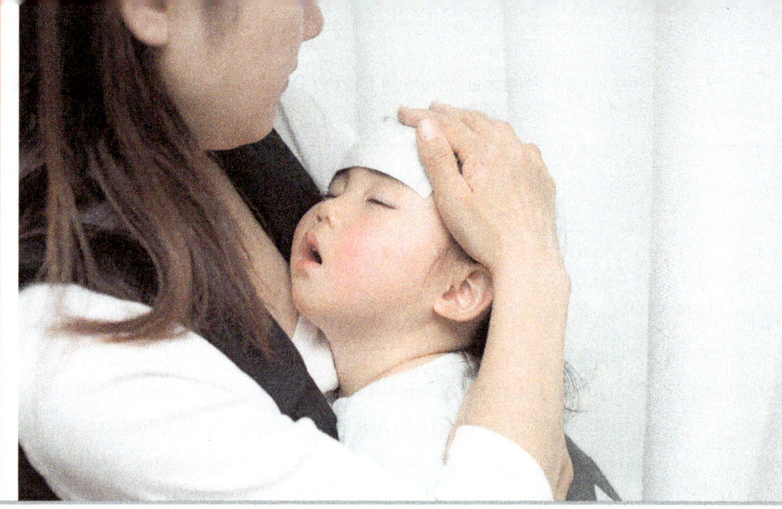

"Last evening my Liam suddenly started vomiting and refused to eat. This morning he had two large, loose, green stools. Please help him."
—*Patient "Liam's" mother, Ms. Nguyen*

Chapter 9
Pharmacotherapy of the Pediatric Patient

Chapter Outline

- Testing and Labeling of Pediatric Drugs
- Pharmacokinetic Variables in Pediatric Patients
- Pharmacologic Implications Associated with Growth and Development
- Medication Safety for Pediatric Patients
- Determining Pediatric Drug Dosages
- Adverse Drug Reactions in Children and Promoting Adherence

Learning Outcomes

After reading this chapter, the student should be able to:

1. Identify the purposes of the U.S. Food and Drug Administration Modernization Act of 1997, the Best Pharmaceuticals for Children Act of 2002, and the Pediatric Research Equity Act of 2003.
2. Explain how differences in pharmacokinetic variables can impact drug response in pediatric patients.
3. Discuss the nursing and pharmacologic implications associated with each of the pediatric developmental age groups.
4. Describe safe methods and techniques appropriate for administering medications to pediatric patients.
5. Explain several methods for accurately calculating drug doses in pediatric patients.
6. Describe nursing interventions for minimizing adverse effects during pediatric pharmacotherapy.
7. Propose appropriate teaching strategies to enhance medication adherence in pediatric patients.

Key Terms

Definitions of the terms in bold may be found in the Glossary.

It is true that children are not just little adults. Beginning with conception, and continuing throughout the lifespan, the organs and systems within the body undergo predictable physiologic changes that influence the absorption, metabolism, distribution, and elimination of medications. A child's body systems are in a constant state of development; therefore, the effects of drugs can often be unpredictable. Healthcare providers must recognize such changes to ensure that drugs are delivered in a safe and effective manner to children and patients of all ages.

The purpose of this chapter is to examine how principles of developmental physiology and lifespan psychology apply to drug administration. Emphasis is placed on determining drug dosages, maximizing therapeutic effects, and minimizing adverse effects. There is strong focus on patient and family education as well as on the importance of promoting adherence with pharmacotherapy.

Testing and Labeling of Pediatric Drugs

9.1 Legislation has attempted to improve the testing and labeling of pediatric drugs.

Pediatric patients receive large numbers of drugs, nearly all of which are the same as those given to adults. The distribution of the drug classes, however, is different in children. Cardiovascular drugs are the most commonly prescribed class in adults, whereas children are more likely to receive respiratory drugs and anti-infectives due to the high incidence of infectious diseases in this population. Table 9.1 provides a summary of the top drug prescriptions by age given to patients by outpatient providers (Qato et al., 2018; Ziesenitz et al., 2016).

Antibiotics are the most commonly prescribed drugs, followed by drugs for asthma. As the child's age increases, prescriptions for drugs used for attention-deficit/hyperactivity disorder (ADHD) increase.

Until the 1990s very little drug information was specifically targeted for the pediatric patient. Drug trials with pediatric patients were virtually unheard of, and data regarding the pharmacokinetics and adverse effects of most drugs were not well documented in this population. Most pediatric drugs were not available in dosage and delivery forms compatible with neonates or infants. Few drugs contained labeling information specifically for pediatric patients. Drugs that were found to be effective in adults were assumed to also be effective in children.

In 1997, the **U.S. Food and Drug Administration (FDA) Modernization Act** was passed, which established the pediatric exclusivity (PE) program that provided financial incentives to drug sponsors in exchange for studying products used in children. This gave pharmaceutical companies

Table 9.1 Common Medications for Children

Drug	Use
albuterol (Proventil)	Asthma
amoxicillin (Amoxil)	Antibiotic
azithromycin (Zithromax)	Antibiotic
beclomethasone	Allergies, inflammation
cetirizine (Zyrtec)	Allergies
clonidine	ADHD
fluticasone (Flonase)	Allergies
ibuprofen	Pain, inflammation, fever
methylphenidate (Ritalin) and amphetamine-dextroamphetamine (Adderal)	ADHD
montelukast (Singulair)	Asthma
omeprazole (Prilosec)	Peptic ulcers, gastroesophageal disease

a financial incentive to conduct the much-needed pediatric research in pharmacology requested by the FDA. In exchange for providing pediatric labeling, the legislation provided drug companies with an additional 6 months of exclusivity, giving them the ability to market the drug with no competition.

Although the exclusivity provision has been highly effective in generating pediatric studies on many drugs and in providing useful information for product labeling, several flaws in the FDA Modernization Act were quickly noted (Olson & Yin, 2018). Many of the medications studied by the drug companies were chosen not for their potential value in children but instead to extend their exclusivity and generate higher profits. The act gave no incentives for studying off-patent (generic) drugs or those that have smaller markets. In 2002, Congress passed the **Best Pharmaceuticals for Children Act (BPCA)**, which authorized the FDA to contract for the testing of already approved pediatric drugs or when the pharmaceutical company declines the option of exclusivity. This act was reauthorized by Congress in 2007 with several new provisions. The **Pediatric Research Equity Act of 2003 (PREA)** authorized the FDA to require research of pediatric uses for new drugs when an approved use includes a condition or conditions applicable to pediatric patients. In addition to studying drugs, this mandate was extended to biologics in 2010, recognizing the increased development and use of these therapeutic drugs in recent years. The U.S. Food and Drug Administration Safety and Innovation Act (FDASIA), enacted in 2012, made BPCA and PREA permanent. This has led to enormous progress in obtaining pediatric studies and has permitted new pediatric labeling of more than 600 products, 149 of which occurred since the passage of FDASIA (Best Pharmaceuticals for Children Act [BPCA] Priority List of Needs in Pediatric Therapeutics, 2019).

Table 9.2 shows some of the changes that resulted from research studies conducted under these acts.

Table 9.2 Examples of Labeling Changes

Potential Risks or Hazards	Drug Name	Disease or Condition Treated	Summary of New Information Contained in Drug Labeling
Unnecessary exposure to ineffective therapies	sumatriptan (Imitrex)	Migraines	Five studies did not establish safety and effectiveness, and postmarketing experience showed that children were having serious adverse effects, such as stroke and vision loss. The product is not recommended for children under age 18 years.
	tolterodine (Detrol)	Overactive bladder and urge incontinence	The drug was not shown to be effective for children and appeared to show a possible increase in aggressive, hyperactive, and abnormal behavior.
	irinotecan (Camptosar)	Tumors	Children had more rapid disease progression and died more quickly. The labeling states that the drug should not be used to treat children with a particular kind of tumor.
	temozolomide (Temodar)	Astrocytoma	Effectiveness in children is not demonstrated.
Ineffective dosing	oxcarbazepine (Trileptal)	Partial seizures	Dose for children age 2 to 4 and weighing less than 44 lb is twice the dose per body weight compared to adults.
	methylphenidate (Ritalin)	ADHD	Children age 13 to 17 eliminated the drug from their bodies faster than the comparison age group. Therefore, the dosing regimen may be increased to prevent ineffective dosing.
Overdosing	leflunomide (Arava)	Juvenile rheumatoid arthritis	Children weighing less than 88 lb require a lower-than-expected dose. Overdosing on leflunomide, which has significant toxicity, could make the drug's risks to children outweigh its benefits.
Previously unlabeled adverse effects, including effects on growth and development	venlafaxine (Effexor)	Depression, generalized anxiety disorder	This drug is associated with an increased risk of suicidal thinking and behavior.
	ciprofloxacin (Cipro)	Complicated urinary tract infection or kidney infection	This drug is associated with increased adverse effects to joints or surrounding tissues for children.
	fentanyl (Duragesic)	Chronic pain	This drug should be used only for children age 2 or older who are opioid tolerant. Use by others can lead to life-threatening respiratory depression and death.
	budesonide (Pulmicort Respules)	Asthma	This drug is now labeled with safety information in patients as young as 6 months. Drug can cause growth suppression and pneumonia.
	fluoxetine (Prozac)	Depression, obsessive–compulsive disorder (OCD)	Effectiveness established in age 7 to 17 with OCD and age 8 to 17 with depression. Drug can cause height and weight suppression. It also has a possible link to suicide ideation.
	fluticasone	Flonase: allergic rhinitis (intranasal)	Effectiveness and safety have been established in age 3 to 9 years with no effect on bone function.
		Cutivate: dermatoses (topical)	Subnormal adrenal function was noted. Drug is not recommended for children.

From Pediatric Drug Research: Studies Conducted Under Best Pharmaceuticals for Children Act, from the U.S. Government Accountability Office, 2007. Retrieved from http://www.gao.gov/new.items/d07557.pdf.

PharmFACT

Off-label prescribing is common practice in pediatrics. One study, looking at the characteristics of off-label prescribing and adverse drug reaction occurrence in a sample of pediatric outpatients treated by general practitioners, found that at least one drug in four was prescribed off label (28.1%) at patient visits during the study period (Yackey et al., 2019). Younger age, longer hospital stays, and mortality were associated with higher rates of off-label medication prescribing. Additionally, the researchers found that rates of off-label medication use were higher in observational (45.5%), inpatient (53.9%), and ambulatory (54.2%) settings (Yackey et al., 2019).

Pharmacokinetic Variables in Pediatric Patients

9.2 Pharmacokinetic responses in children differ from those in adults.

As discussed in Chapters 3 and 4, drugs must reach their target cells in sufficient quantities to produce therapeutic effects. This depends on what the body does to the medication after it is administered (pharmacokinetics) and the mechanisms by which a drug changes the body (pharmacodynamics). The normal physiologic changes of growth and development markedly affect pharmacokinetics and pharmacodynamics. The nurse must understand the unique actions of drugs in their pediatric patients to deliver safe and effective pharmacotherapy.

Absorption: Two primary factors have the potential to influence the oral absorption of drugs in pediatric patients: increased gastric pH and delayed gastric emptying. Low gastric acid production may enhance the absorption of acid-labile drugs such as ampicillin and penicillin and slow the absorption of weak acids like phenobarbital. This is especially true for premature infants and neonates. Gastric acid production may not reach adult levels until age 2 or 3.

Slowed gastric motility in very young children will retain the drug in the stomach longer. This will increase the absorption of drugs that are absorbed across the stomach mucosa but slow the rate of drug absorption for drugs that rely on the intestine for absorption. The rate of bile salt secretion is diminished in premature infants and neonates, which will delay the absorption of lipid-soluble drugs and vitamins.

In infanst, relatively low blood flow to skeletal muscles leads to slow and erratic absorption of drugs administered by the intramuscular (IM) and subcutaneous routes. Weak muscle contractions may also contribute to the delayed absorption and distribution of IM drugs. IM injections are generally avoided due to their unpredictable absorption rates and their associated pain.

The skin of infants is thin and highly permeable, allowing lotions and topical drugs to be absorbed at a more rapid rate than in adults. For example, use of topical corticosteroids in infants may cause systemic effects such as adrenal insufficiency, hyperglycemia, and glaucoma. Care must be taken to prevent accidental overdose.

CONNECTION Checkpoint 9.1

From what you learned in Chapter 3, what effect does food in the stomach have on drug absorption? What effect might this have on neonates who are given frequent feedings?

Distribution: Three main factors affecting drug distribution in children are the proportion of water to fat, immature liver function, and the underdeveloped blood–brain barrier.

Approximately 80% of a newborn's body weight is due to water. This gradually decreases to 60%, that of an adult, during the first year. The higher proportion of water dilutes water-soluble drugs such as furosemide (Lasix). In addition, water-soluble drugs will move out of the serum to other areas of the infant's body where water concentration is high. The overall effect is lower serum drug levels; higher doses may be needed to maintain adequate serum levels of the drug.

What about lipid-soluble drugs? Infants have a low percentage of body fat compared to adults. Lipid-soluble drugs that would normally be distributed to fat tend to stay in the blood, raising serum drug levels.

Prior to age 6 months, the child's immature liver produces very small amounts of plasma proteins. Drugs that normally bind to plasma proteins will now be present as "free" drugs in the serum. Drugs and endogenous substances such as bilirubin compete for the few available protein-binding sites. In some cases, previously bound substances or drugs may be displaced into the serum, leading to potential toxicity. Drugs with high levels of protein binding include ampicillin, morphine, phenytoin (Dilantin), and propranolol (Inderal).

The blood–brain barrier is a network of capillaries in the central nervous system (CNS) that form tight junctions, which prevent the passage of certain medications into the brain. Because the child's blood–brain barrier is not fully developed at birth, drugs and other chemicals can easily penetrate the CNS, resulting in heightened responses. The nurse caring for neonates taking drugs such as barbiturates that affect CNS functions should assess for potential toxicity. It is also possible that some drugs not intended for CNS penetration may access the brain, causing adverse CNS effects such as seizures, drowsiness, or dizziness.

Metabolism: The rate at which drugs are metabolized in children is impacted by the immaturity of the hepatic cytochrome P450 (CYP450) enzyme system. Metabolism is significantly slower in children, leading to reduced clearance rates and extended half-lives for drugs extensively metabolized by the liver. To avoid toxicity, drug doses must be accurately determined and administered at adequately spaced intervals to allow sufficient time for metabolic handling of the drug. The metabolic rate reaches adult levels by ages 3 to 5 years. Until then, the nurse should remain vigilant for signs of toxicity in patients taking drugs such as salicylates that are metabolized primarily in the liver.

The enzyme alcohol dehydrogenase is markedly reduced at birth, gradually increasing until age 5. This enzyme is responsible for detoxifying benzyl alcohol, a preservative found in some parenteral drug formulations. Newborns are especially sensitive to the effects of benzyl alcohol and can develop "gasping syndrome," which can lead to respiratory and cardiovascular failure. The nurse must ensure that neonates do not receive products containing benzyl alcohol.

Excretion: The child's ability to effectively excrete most drugs depends on the maturity and function of the kidneys. For drugs to be excreted efficiently, the kidneys must have an adequate glomerular filtration rate and active tubular secretion and reabsorption functions. Young children have immature renal systems with slower renal clearance, resulting in accumulation of drugs excreted by the kidneys. Signs of nephrotoxicity include oliguria, urinary frequency, hematuria, cloudy urine, rising blood urea nitrogen (BUN) and creatinine, and fever. Although standard pediatric doses can be administered at approximately 3 to 5 months of age when the infant is able to concentrate urine, serum levels of nephrotoxic drugs such as gentamicin must be monitored closely to prevent adverse reactions.

Pharmacologic Implications Associated with Growth and Development

9.3 The role of the nurse in administering medications changes with each developmental age group.

When administering pediatric medications, the age, weight, and developmental level of the child must be considered. For the purposes of medication administration, the pediatric patient is defined as being any age from birth to 16 years and weighing less than 50 kg (110 lb). Additionally, children are classified as neonates, infants, toddlers, preschoolers, school-age children, and adolescents.

Growth is a term that characterizes the progressive increase in physical (body) size. *Development* refers to the functional evolution of the physical, psychomotor, and cognitive capabilities of a living being. Stages of growth and physical development usually go hand in hand in a predictable sequence, whereas psychomotor and cognitive development have a tendency to be more variable in nature.

From birth through adolescence, the growth and development of the pediatric patient mandate adjustments in pharmacotherapeutics above and beyond the calculation of doses. The child's ability to become an active (and willing) partner in his or her own wellness has important implications to nursing care and pharmacotherapeutics.

Pharmacotherapy of the infant: Infancy is the period from birth to 12 months of age. The first 28 days of life are referred to as the neonatal period. During this time, nursing care and pharmacotherapy are directed toward safety of the infant, proper dosing of prescribed drugs, and teaching parents how to administer medications properly. A primary goal is to have the child ingest the entire dose of medication without spitting it out because it is difficult to estimate the amount lost. If the child vomits immediately after taking the drug, the dose may be reordered. The following nursing interventions and parental teaching points are important for this age group:

- The infant should be held and cuddled while administering medications and offered a pacifier if the infant is on fluid restrictions caused by vomiting or diarrhea.
- Medications are often administered to infants via droppers into the eyes, ears, nose, or mouth. Oral medications should be directed to the inner cheek and the child given time to swallow the drug to avoid aspiration. If rectal suppositories are administered, the buttocks should be held together for 5 to 10 minutes to prevent expulsion of the drug before absorption has occurred.
- Special considerations must be observed when administering IM or intravenous (IV) injections to infants. Unlike adults, infants lack well-developed muscle masses, so the smallest needle appropriate for the drug should be used. For volumes less than 1 mL a tuberculin syringe is appropriate. The vastus lateralis is a preferred site for IM injections because it has few nerves and is relatively well developed in infants. The gluteal site is usually contraindicated because of potential damage to the sciatic nerve, injury to which may result in permanent disability.
- Because of the lack of choices for injection sites, the nurse must rotate injection sites from one leg to the next to avoid overuse and to prevent inflammation and excessive pain.
- For IV sites, the feet and scalp veins may provide good venous access.

Pharmacotherapy of the toddler: Toddlerhood ranges from 1 to 3 years of age. By age 1 most of the pharmacokinetic responses are similar to that of the adult. The 2-year-old is able to metabolize drugs at a very rapid rate; therefore, the healthcare provider must adjust drug doses accordingly to maintain therapeutic levels.

During this period, a toddler displays a tremendous sense of curiosity. The child begins to explore, wants to try new things, and tends to place everything in the mouth. This becomes a major concern for medication and household product safety. Toddlers can swallow liquids and may be able to chew solid medications. When prescription drugs are supplied as flavored elixirs, it is important to teach parents that the child not be given access to the medications. Poisoning is extremely common at this age. Some of the most common poisonous substances involved in the exposure of children less than 6 years are analgesics, cough and cold preparations, topical ointments, and vitamins.

Administering medications to toddlers can be challenging. At this stage, the child is rapidly developing increased motor ability and learning to assert independence but has extremely limited ability to reason or understand the relationship of medicines to health. Giving long, detailed explanations to the toddler will prolong the procedure and create additional anxiety. Short, concrete explanations followed by immediate drug administration are best for this age group. Physical comfort in the form of touching, hugging, or verbal praise following drug administration is important.

- Pharmaceutical companies often formulate pediatric medicines in sweet syrups to facilitate drug administration. Extra caution should be observed when medications are flavored. Toddlers may not differentiate between a food product and the medication and may ingest an overdose if the medication is not kept in a child-safe location.

- Unpleasant-tasting oral medications should be mixed with more appetizing food such as jam, syrup, or fruit puree, if possible. The medication may be followed with a carbonated beverage or mint-flavored candy. Parents should be taught to avoid placing medicine in milk, orange juice, or cereals because children may associate these healthy foods with unpleasant-tasting medications in the future.
- IM injections for toddlers may be given into the vastus lateralis muscle. For IV medications, the nurse may choose to access the scalp or feet veins. Additional peripheral site options become available in late toddlerhood.
- Suppositories may be difficult to administer due to the child's resistance. For these invasive administration procedures, having a parent close by will usually reduce the toddler's anxiety and increase cooperation.

Pharmacotherapy of preschoolers: The preschool child ranges in age from 3 to 5 years. In general, principles of medication administration that pertain to the toddler also apply to this age group. Preschoolers tend to cooperate better in taking oral medications if they are crushed or mixed with food or flavored beverages.

- After a child has been walking for about a year, the ventrogluteal site may be used for IM injections because it causes less pain than the vastus lateralis site. Use of the dorsogluteal site has declined due to the risk of affecting the sciatic nerve. The scalp veins can no longer be used for IV access; peripheral veins are used for IV access.
- Like the toddler, the preschooler often physically resists medication administration. A brief explanation followed immediately by medication administration is usually the best method. Uncooperative children may need to be restrained, and patients over 4 years of age may require two adults to administer the medication.
- Before and after medication procedures, the child may benefit from opportunities to play-act troubling experiences with dolls. When the child plays the role of doctor or nurse by giving a "sick" doll a pill or injection, comforting the doll, and explaining that the doll will now feel better, the little actor feels safer and more in control of the situation.

Pharmacotherapy of the school-age child: The school-age child is between 6 and 12 years of age. Some refer to this period as the middle childhood years. Rapid physical, mental, and social development occur and early ethical–moral development begins to take shape. During this time, most children remain relatively healthy, with respiratory infections and gastrointestinal upsets being the most common complaints. When serious illness occurs at this age, the child may become confused and depressed because it is important for the child to be like his peers during this developmental age. When caring for an ill child, the nurse must be aware of possible nonadherence to treatment regimens.

The nurse is usually able to gain considerable cooperation from school-age children. Detailed explanations of the effects and importance of medications in maintaining wellness may be of value because the child has developed some reasoning ability and can understand the relationship between receiving the medicine and feeling better. When children are old enough to welcome choices, they can be offered limited dosing alternatives to provide a sense of control and encourage cooperation. The option of taking one medication before another or the chance to choose which drink will follow a chewable tablet helps to distract children from the issue of whether they will take the medication at all. It also makes an otherwise strange or unpleasant experience a little more tolerable.

- Allowing children to feel that they are willing participants, rather than victims, in medication administration is an important foundation for adherence.
- Praise for cooperation is appropriate for any pediatric patient and will set the stage for successful medication administration in the future.
- School-age children can take chewable tablets and may be able to swallow tablets or capsules. Many still resist injections; however, an experienced pediatric nurse can usually administer parenteral medications quickly and compassionately without the need for restraining the child.
- The ventrogluteal site is preferred for IM injections, although the muscles of older children are developed enough for the nurse to use other sites.

Pharmacotherapy of the adolescent: Adolescence occurs between age 13 and 16 years. Rapid physical growth and psychologic maturation have a great impact on personality development. The adolescent strongly relates to peers, wanting and needing their support, approval, and presence. Physical appearance and conformity with peers in terms of behavior, dress, and social interactions are important. The strong sense of independence leads teens to self-medicate, either with or without their parents' knowledge. Treatment objectives for the nurse should include teaching parents to keep their medications safely stowed out of sight of inquisitive, experiment-minded adolescents. Parents should also be taught the signs and symptoms of drugs commonly abused by teens such as marijuana, inhalants, and methamphetamine.

The most common needs for the pharmacotherapy of teens are for skin problems, headaches, menstrual

CONNECTIONS: Advanced Practice Application

Ingestion of Suspected Poison

Case

Nancy, the mother of a 17-month-old toddler named Sammy, heard a cry and ran into the bathroom to find her son on the floor next to a spilled container of bleach. The toddler was drooling, his lips were blue, and there were blisters on his chin and chest. Desperate, Sammy's mother phoned the poison control center in Washington, DC, where you work as a nurse specialist. You tell Nancy not to induce vomiting because bleach is a caustic substance that could severely damage the esophagus when it comes back up. You then instruct her to call for an ambulance immediately.

Shortly after Sammy arrives at the hospital, an endoscopy was done and showed burns to the esophagus and trachea. He was intubated to protect his airway and transferred to the pediatric intensive care unit. Sammy was hospitalized for several weeks before he was finally well enough to go home. What important actions are needed when ingestion of a poison is suspected?

Discussion

When a child presents with suspected poisoning, start with an assessment of the emergency ABCs (airway, breathing, circulation), and administer oxygen if the child shows signs of respiratory distress. Chart the patient's age, weight, medications, and existing medical conditions. Find out what substance was ingested, the quantity, and when it was taken. Pay close attention to arterial blood gases and blood glucose levels in a child with depressed consciousness and continue to monitor vital signs. When information about what was ingested is incomplete or inaccurate, the physical examination, laboratory tests, and a toxicologic screen should be used to determine treatment.

This case is far from unique and occurs daily in emergency departments (EDs) and poison control centers. The incident could have been avoided by having child-protective locks on the cabinets.

Children younger than 6 years comprise nearly half of the poison exposures each year reported to Poison Control Centers. Pain medications are the single most common cause of pediatric fatalities. (National Capital Poison Center, 2018). Because most of these incidents occur in the home, teaching parents how to minimize the risks of poisoning is essential. It has been shown that poison-prevention counseling, which is recommended by the American Academy of Pediatrics as well as the Academy of Family Physicians, as part of routine pediatric care, results in greater prevention efforts at home. When preventive strategies are overlooked or efforts fail, rapid action is required. Knowing the causes, signs, and symptoms of pediatric poisoning is key for any nurse who cares for young children.

---

symptoms, sex-related concerns, eating disorders, contraception, alcohol and tobacco use, and sports-related injuries.

- Of primary concern to the adolescent are the initiation of sexual intercourse and the avoidance of pregnancy and sexually transmitted infections. The nurse must be prepared to address a variety of topics related to sexuality, including the importance of responsible sexual practices and contraceptive methods.
- Eating disorders commonly occur in this population. The nurse should carefully question adolescents about their eating habits and their use of over-the-counter (OTC) appetite suppressants or laxatives that may be contributing to bulimia or anorexia.
- Alcohol, tobacco use, and other illicit drug experimentation are prevalent in this population. Teenage athletes may use amphetamines to delay the onset of fatigue as well as anabolic steroids to enhance performance. The nurse assumes a key role in educating adolescent patients about the hazards of tobacco use and illicit drugs.
- The adolescent has a need for privacy and control in drug administration. The nurse should communicate with the teen more in the manner of an adult rather than as a child. Teens usually appreciate thorough explanations of their treatment, and ample time should be allowed for them to ask questions.
- Despite their need to have independence and the desire to self-medicate, teens have a very poor understanding of medication information. Adolescents are reluctant to admit their lack of knowledge, so the nurse should carefully explain important information regarding their medications and expected adverse effects, even if these patients claim to understand.

CONNECTION Checkpoint 9.2

The nurse educator is teaching a group of new graduate nurses about the use of the anticoagulant heparin in pediatric patients admitted to the ICU. From what you learned in Chapter 6, what should the nurse include in her instructions about the necessary precautions for this type of drug?

Medication Safety for Pediatric Patients

9.4 The nurse is a key member of the healthcare team in ensuring medication safety in pediatric patients.

The nurse is often responsible for administering medications to children. The importance of accurate drug dosage calculations, proper administration techniques, proper efforts to minimize adverse effects, and the need for overall safety cannot be overemphasized.

Principles of safe medication practice for pediatric patients are identical to those of adult patients. Medication safety is a team approach. Every level of responsibility is involved, including hospital-wide (or corporation-wide) policies, prescriber actions, pharmacy guidelines, nursing interventions, and patient and family adherence. Responsibility for preventing medication errors in pediatric patients is shared by every member of the team.

The safety and effectiveness of a medication regimen depends on proper procurement, storage, and administration of the drug. In the hospital setting, nurses are responsible for adherence to the basic rules of drug administration: right patient, right drug, right route, right dose, at the right time. Younger pediatric patients may not be able to accurately identify themselves; thus, it is imperative that the nurse use precautions to ensure that the right child receives the prescribed medication. The child's identification band must always be checked against the medication record. Most hospitals' policies require that drugs such as digoxin, heparin, insulin, chemotherapeutic drugs, opioid analgesics, and barbiturates be double-checked with another nurse prior to administration. If it is suspected that a dose of medication ordered by the prescriber is outside the normal range, it is the nurse's responsibility to question the order because some drugs can be lethal to pediatric patients. Online drug information sources should be frequently checked for the most recent information on pediatric drugs.

The American Academy of Pediatrics established guidelines in 2007 to prevent pediatric medication errors in the inpatient setting (American Academy of Pediatrics, 2007). Since that time, computerized physician order entry programs, electronic health records, programmable infusion pumps, and other technologies have been implemented. Because no system is fail-safe, the following nursing actions and guidelines should be followed to maximize patient safety:

- Check medication calculations with another professional member of the healthcare team.
- Confirm patient identity before administration of each dose.
- Be familiar with medication ordering and dispensing systems.
- Verify drug orders before medication administration.
- Verify unusually large or small volumes or dosage units for a single patient dose.
- When a patient, a parent, or a caregiver questions whether a drug should be administered, listen attentively, answer questions, and double-check the medication order.
- Remain familiar with the operation of medication administration devices and the potential for errors with such devices, particularly patient-controlled analgesia (PCA) or infusion pumps.

Nursing Education and Communication

- Develop and maintain continuous education programs for nursing competencies in devices used for pediatric medication administration, particularly PCA and infusion pumps.
- Develop and maintain a pediatric medications knowledge base.
- Discuss medication orders with the prescriber whenever possible.
- Integrate and provide education for the patient and caregiver regarding the medication regimen.
- Record and verify patient identity, weight, allergies, and previous medication use.
- Be aware of and be involved in ongoing error-tracking systems and pharmacy programs. Encourage blame-free error reporting. Ensure that all staff members understand the method of reporting and are knowledgeable about the healthcare agency's system for reporting errors.

Determining Pediatric Drug Dosages

9.5 Calculating drug dosages accurately is essential for pediatric patients.

Drug dosage calculation for pediatric patients should be individualized and nurses should take into consideration the child's age, height, weight, maturational state, and body surface area. All drug calculations for pediatric patients in critical care settings should be double-checked by the pharmacist and another nurse prior to administration.

Two common procedures of calculating pediatric dosages are the body weight method and body surface area method. Utilization of the **body weight method** requires a calculation of the number of milligrams of drug, based on the child's weight in kilograms (mg/kg). A unit of time is usually included; for example, gentamicin 5 mg/kg/24 h. The body weight method is simple, and a dose can be calculated quickly. However, the serum concentrations of many drugs are not proportional to body weight, and body weight does not take into consideration pharmacokinetic variables such as changes in metabolism and elimination rates, as discussed in Section 9.2.

The **body surface area (BSA) method** uses an estimate of the child's BSA. This method is believed to be the most valid basis for dosage because it is related to certain physiologic functions that account for the pharmacokinetic differences in pediatric patients. The BSA method better estimates blood volume, metabolism, and the effects of drugs. Measurements of the fluid volume compartment and the serum concentrations of drugs also correlate well with the BSA. Several different formulas have been used to calculate BSA, and each gives slightly different results. There is a lack of consensus as to which calculation method gives the most accurate results.

Calculators are readily available online to calculate BSA. The child's height (in centimeters) and weight (in kilograms) is entered and the body mass is calculated in square meters. The BSA can then be used to calculate a correct dose (Medscape, 2020).

CONNECTIONS: Patient Safety

A Tenfold Error

The nurse is caring for a 6-year-old boy newly diagnosed with seizures, tonic-clonic type. In reviewing the written orders, valproic acid (Depakene) 150 mg/kg/day is ordered. The pharmacist calls the unit to verify the order and the nurse contacts the prescriber. The order is corrected to 15 mg/kg/day. What could be done to prevent this error from recurring?

Adverse Drug Reactions in Children and Promoting Adherence

9.6 Pediatric patients are more susceptible than adults to adverse drug effects.

Because of their smaller size and immature or developing organ systems, pediatric patients are more susceptible to adverse effects. Identifying adverse effects may be challenging because infants and young children do not have the maturity or verbal skills to accurately describe their feelings following the medication administration. Identifying pediatric adverse effects will depend on the ability of the nurse to assess subtle changes in patient response. For example, a child on diuretics should have strict intake and output measurements to help determine if the drug is working properly. Excessive weight gain could be caused by edema resulting from poor kidney excretion or weight loss might be due to excessive diuresis. Signs of ototoxicity may go unnoticed for a long time unless someone checks that the child no longer responds to verbal commands. It may be necessary to consult a psychologist to identify signs of suicidal ideation from antidepressant use in adolescents.

Most types of adverse effects that occur in children age 1 or older are the same as those in adults. Like adults, the majority of adverse effects are dose related. Knowing specific drugs and their adverse effects in the adult population will help the nurse quickly identify signs and symptoms in pediatric patients. For example, antibiotics such as amoxicillin frequently result in diarrhea in both adults and children. Antianxiety drugs, antidepressants, and antipsychotic drugs that cause CNS depression will likely cause drowsiness in patients of all ages.

A few types of adverse effects are specific to children due to their immature or developing organs and tissues. For example, tetracycline must be avoided in the neonate because of the potential for permanent staining of the teeth. Sulfonamides can cause jaundice in neonates, and aspirin is contraindicated in children with fever due to the potential for Reye's syndrome. Glucocorticoids can inhibit growth. Table 9.3 illustrates a list of commonly used drugs and their adverse effects on the pediatric patient.

CONNECTION Checkpoint 9.3

The nurse gives a preschooler a sedative but, rather than sleep, the child becomes excited and experiences insomnia. From what you learned in Chapter 5, this reaction is most likely classified as what type of effect?

Like adults, children may experience drug interactions. Drugs that are most likely to contribute to drug interactions in pediatric patients are those with high potency, narrow therapeutic index, and extensive protein binding and those that affect vital organ functions or hepatic metabolism.

Often parents' first response to their child's illness is to provide home remedies such as OTC and herbal treatments in the household. The nurse should be familiar with commonly used OTC and herbal remedies in order to advise the families about the proper treatment. Parents must understand that OTC and herbal therapies may have adverse effects of their own and may interact with prescription medications. Herbal remedies commonly used in homes include St. John's wort, echinacea, ginseng, licorice, and sassafras.

A drug will fail to achieve optimal therapeutic outcomes if it is not taken properly. *Adherence*, also called *compliance*, is taking the drug according to the instructions on the label or as directed by the prescriber. Maximizing adherence to the medication regimen is a major goal of the pediatric nurse. The nurse must assess the patient and family to determine factors that could affect the family's ability to assist the child with the medication regimen and develop strategies that will enhance medication adherence. The more complex, expensive, and inconvenient the medication regimen, the less likely the child and family will adhere. Children are most likely to adhere to their medication regimen if the following conditions exist:

- High expectations of successful outcomes of the therapy
- Supportive family members who are able to communicate with the prescriber
- Positive interactions with the nurse and caregivers
- Minimal adverse effects from the medications
- Simple, short-term, inexpensive regimen with minimum disruption to daily routine.

The patient and family should be asked directly if they have doubts about their ability to adhere to the regimen. If there is doubt, the nurse should explore the areas of concern with the family and discuss the importance of the drug, route of administration, expected outcomes, and possible adverse effects. Follow-up appointments may be necessary to assess drug responses or to administer the oral drug(s) to the child and observe the drug being swallowed. This technique is known as **directly observed therapy (DOT)**. In extreme cases when the child does not appear to be responding appropriately to the prescribed regimen, periodic measurement of plasma drug levels can help determine the amount of drug ingested and whether it has been taken as prescribed.

Table 9.3 Selected Pediatric Drugs for Which Specific Indications and Dosage Guidelines Exist

Drug	Dosage/Route (Maximum Dose Where Indicated)	Adverse Effects
acetaminophen (Tylenol)	PO: 10–15 mg/kg q4–6h for children under age 12, not to exceed 2.6 g/day	Methemoglobinemia, hepatotoxicity
acyclovir (Zovirax)	PO: 200 mg 5 times daily for genital herpes	*Diarrhea, nausea* Renal failure, seizures
amoxicillin (Amoxil) or amoxicillin/clavulanate (Augmentin)	PO: 20–40 mg/kg/day	*Diarrhea* Anaphylaxis
amphetamine and dextroamphetamine (Adderall)	PO: 2.5–5 mg once or twice daily (regular release) or 10 mg once daily (extended release)	*Insomnia, anorexia, headache* Tachycardia, psychotic episodes, abuse potential
ampicillin	PO: 50–100 mg/kg/day	*Diarrhea* Anaphylaxis
atomoxetine (Strattera)	PO: 40–80 mg once daily	*Dry mouth, anorexia, insomnia, headache* Depression, suicidal ideation
azithromycin (Zithromax)	PO: 5–10 mg/kg/day	*Diarrhea* Hepatotoxicity
budesonide (Rhinocort)	Intranasal: 2 sprays in each nostril bid for allergies	*Headache, fatigue* Paresthesia
ceftriaxone	IV/IM: 50–100 mg/kg/day	*Diarrhea* Colitis
cephalexin (Keflex)	PO: 25–50 mg/kg/day q6h	*Diarrhea* Anaphylaxis, angioedema
clarithromycin	PO: 15 mg/kg/day	*Vomiting, diarrhea* Colitis
diphenoxylate and atropine (Lomotil)	PO: 1/2–1 tsp, up to 4 doses/day	*Dizziness, sedation* Paralytic ileus
erythromycin (EryC, Erythrocin)	PO: 30–50 mg/kg/day	*Nausea and vomiting* Hepatotoxicity
ferrous sulfate (Feosol, Fergon, others)	PO: 0.5–1 mg/kg/day maintenance	*Nausea, black stools* Shock
fluconazole (Diflucan)	PO: 6 mg/kg/day first dose, then 3 mg/kg/day	*Headache, nausea* Hepatotoxicity
fluticasone (Flonase)	Intranasal: 1 spray in each nostril once a day; may increase to 2 sprays daily	*Nasal dryness* Epistaxis
gentamicin	IV/IM: 6–7.5 mg/kg/day (2–2.5 mg/kg administered q8h)	*Pain at injection site* Neurotoxicity, nephrotoxicity
ibuprofen (Advil, Motrin)	PO: 5–10 mg/kg/dose given q6–8h	*Nausea, heartburn* GI bleeding
imipramine (Tofranil)	PO: 25–50 mg/day for nocturnal enuresis	*Urinary retention* Angioedema
methylphenidate (Ritalin)	PO: 5–10 mg/day (dose not to exceed 60 mg/day, depending on trade name)	*Nervousness, insomnia* Palpitations
minocycline (Minocin)	PO: 4 mg/kg/day bid	*Dizziness, nausea*
oxcarbazepine (Trileptal)	PO: 8–10 mg/kg/day not to exceed 600 mg/day	*Fatigue* Somnolence
penicillin G	PO: 25–50 mg/kg/day q3–4h	*Diarrhea* Anaphylaxis
trimethoprim-sulfamethoxazole (Bactrim, Septra)	PO: 8 mg/kg/day trimethoprim, 40 mg/kg/day sulfamethoxazole q12h	*Nausea, rash, anemia* Exfoliative dermatitis
valproic acid (Depakene, Depakote)	PO: 10–15 mg/kg/day initially (dose not to exceed 60 mg/kg/day)	*Drowsiness, nausea* Bone marrow suppression

Note: *Italics* indicate common adverse effects. Underline indicates serious adverse effects.

Understanding Chapter 9

Key Concepts Summary

9.1 Legislation has attempted to improve the testing and labeling of pediatric drugs.

9.2 Pharmacokinetic responses in children differ from those in adults.

9.3 The role of the nurse in administering medications changes with each developmental age group.

9.4 The nurse is a key member of the healthcare team in ensuring medication safety in pediatric patients.

9.5 Calculating drug dosages accurately is essential for pediatric patients.

9.6 Pediatric patients are more susceptible than adults to adverse drug effects.

CASE STUDY: Making the Patient Connection

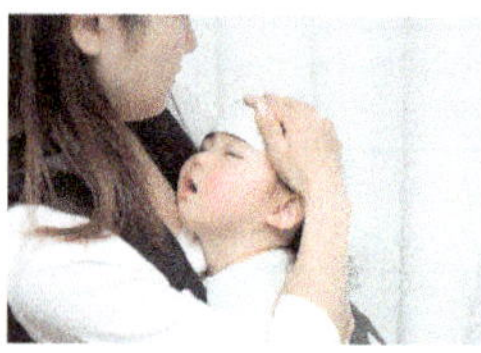

Remember 7-month-old "Liam," the patient introduced at the beginning of the chapter? Now read the remainder of the case study. Based on the information presented within this chapter, respond to the critical thinking questions that follow.

Ms. Nguyen reports that Liam has not been eating well for the past 48 hours. Last night he vomited three times after drinking sips of water and also had several very loose, green, foul-smelling bowel movements. He voided only once in the past 12 hours. For the past 5 days Liam has been taking amoxicillin for an ear infection. Liam lies still on the examination table but responds to his mother's commands. The nurse prepares Liam for examination.

Liam's preliminary diagnosis is gastroenteritis with mild dehydration. His vital signs are as follows: temperature, 39.1°C (102.4°F); heart rate, 160 beats/min; respiration, 38 breaths/min; blood pressure, 100/57 mmHg; and weight, 8.6 kg (19 lb). His skin is dry and warm to touch, and there is slight tenting. The following laboratory studies were performed: serum electrolytes, complete blood count, blood urea nitrogen, creatinine, urinalysis, and stool for culture and sensitivity. Electrolytes were as follows: sodium, 136 mEq/L; potassium, 4.2 mEq/L; chloride, 114 mEq/L; bicarbonate, 9 mEq/L.

An IV line was inserted immediately and a solution of D_5W in 1/3 NSS was started to infuse at 30 mL/h. Liam was placed on NPO.

Critical Thinking Questions

1. What primary factors are contributing to Liam's risk for deficient fluid balance?
2. What are some physical signs to assess when evaluating dehydration in this infant?
3. What would best explain the cause for diarrhea in this patient?
4. What are some key points to focus on when monitoring the infant's IV fluid intake?

Additional Case Study

Sinead, a 3-year-old girl, arrives at the ED in status asthmaticus. Her mother informs you that she was diagnosed with asthma 9 months ago and since then has been back to the ED for treatment twice. Two hours prior to admission, Sinead started coughing and wheezing and then an hour ago started having difficulty breathing. Her mother attempted to relieve the symptoms by giving steam and fluids, but the condition only worsened. Sinead has an audible expiratory wheeze, nasal flaring, and inter- and substernal retractions.

1. What nursing actions would take priority?
2. What nursing assessment should the nurse carry out immediately?
3. What immediate outcomes could be expected from treatment?

Chapter Review

1. Which factor(s) is/are true regarding the pharmacokinetics in the pediatric population? (Select all that apply.)
    1. Slower gastric motility in young children will keep the drug in the stomach longer.
    2. Before 6 months of age, there is greater plasma protein binding of drugs, and drug distribution will be lower in this age group.
    3. Before age 5, the liver may not metabolize drugs as readily as an adult's liver and doses must be adjusted accordingly.
    4. Drug excretion by the kidneys will not equal an adult's until the child is at least 2 years of age.
    5. Drugs with CNS effects have little to no effect in infants and very young children.
2. A mother calls the urgent care center and frantically tells you that her toddler drank a bottle of cleaning fluid. Which of the following is the priority instruction that should be given to the parent?
    1. Contact the poison control center.
    2. Watch the child closely and call back if there are signs of respiratory distress.
    3. Take the child immediately to the emergency department.
    4. Give the child syrup of ipecac.
3. The experienced pediatric nurse is teaching a new nursing student about injections in the pediatric population. Which statement by the student would indicate that teaching was effective?
    1. "Intramuscular (IM) injections in infants are absorbed slowly."
    2. "Children experience rapid absorption of IM medications."
    3. "IM injections are encouraged due to their predictable absorption rate."
    4. "Strong muscle contractions result in delayed absorption of IM medication."
4. It is time to give a 3-year-old oral medication. Which comment is most therapeutic?
    1. "This is the medicine that makes you better."
    2. "If you don't take your medicine you can't go home."
    3. "Would you like to take your medicine with water or juice?"
    4. "See how easily your roommate has taken his medicine?"
5. Drugs that are most likely to create drug interactions in pediatric patients are those with:
    1. Low potency.
    2. Wide therapeutic index.
    3. Extensive protein binding.
    4. Effects on the skin.
6. The healthcare provider knows that the pediatric patient and parents will most likely adhere to the medication regimen if the:
    1. Regimen is simple and inexpensive.
    2. Medications are costly but well known.
    3. Medications are prescribed for a long period.
    4. Medications are taken at different times each day.

See Appendix A for answers to critical thinking questions, case study questions and review questions.

References

American Academy of Pediatrics. (2007). AAP Publications Reaffirmed, January 2007. Policy statement: Prevention of medication errors in the pediatric inpatient setting. *Pediatrics, 119*(5), 1031. https://doi.org/10.1542/peds.2007-0471

Best Pharmaceuticals for Children Act (BPCA) Priority List of Needs in Pediatric Therapeutics. (2019). https://www.nichd.nih.gov/sites/default/files/inline-files/Priority_List_07082014.pdf

Medscape. (2020). *Body surface area based dosing*. http://reference.medscape.com/calculator/bsa-dosing

National Capital Poison Center (2018). Poison statistics, National Data 2018. https://www.poison.org/poison-statistics-national

Olson, M., & Yin, N. (2018). Examining firm responses to R&D policy: An analysis of pediatric exclusivity. *American Journal of Health Economics*, *4*(3), 321–357. https://doi.org/10.1162/ajhe_a_00104

Qato, D., Alexander, G., Guadamuz, J., & Lindau, S. (2018). Prescription medication use among children and adolescents in the United States. *Pediatrics (Evanston)*, *142*(3), e20181042. https://doi.org/10.1542/peds.2018-1042

Yackey, K., & Stanley, R. (2019). Off-label prescribing in children remains high: A call for prioritized research. *Pediatrics (Evanston)*, *144*(4), e20191571. https://doi.org/10.1542/peds.2019-1571

Yackey, K., Stukus, K., Cohen, D., Kline, D., Zhao, S., & Stanley, R. (2019). Off-label medication prescribing patterns in pediatrics: An update. *Hospital Pediatrics*, *9*(3), 186–193. https://doi.org/10.1542/hpeds.2018-0168

Ziesenitz, V. C., van den Anker, J. N., & Amirshahi, M. (2016). Availability of pediatric formulations for the 100 most prescribed drugs in pediatric ambulatory care—2002 vs. 2010. *Archives of Disease in Childhood*, *101*(1), e1. https://doi.org/10.1136/archdischild-2015-310148.12

Selected Bibliography

American Association of Family Physicians. (2019). *Clinical practice guideline: Otitis media* https://www.aafp.org/family-physician/patient-care/clinical-recommendations/all-clinical-recommendations/otitis-media.html

Benjamin, L., Frush, K., Shaw, K., Shook, J. E., Snow, S. K., American Academy of Pediatrics Committee on Pediatric Emergency Medicine, & Emergency Nurses Association Pediatric Emergency Medicine Committee. (2018). Pediatric medication safety in the emergency department. *Pediatrics*, *141*(3), e20174066. https://doi.org/10.1542/peds.2017-4066

Chonmaitree, T., Trujillo, R., Jennings, K., Alvarez-Fernandez, P., Patel, J., Loeffelholz, M., et al. (2016). Acute otitis media and other complications of viral respiratory infection. *Pediatrics*, *137*(4). https://doi.org/10.1542/peds.2015-3555

Committee on Drugs. (2015). Metric units and the preferred dosing of orally administered liquid medications. *Pediatrics*, *135*(4), 784–787. https://doi.org/10.1542/peds.2015-0072

Coppini, R., Simons, S., Mugelli, A., & Allegaert, K. (2016). Clinical research in neonates and infants: Challenges and perspectives. *Pharmacological Research*, *108*, 80–87. https://doi.org/10.1016/j.phrs.2016.04.025

De Bie, S., Ferrajolo, C., Straus, S., Verhamme, K., Bonhoeffer, J., Wong, I., & Sturkenboom, M. (2015). Pediatric drug safety surveillance in FDA-AERS: A description of adverse events from GRiP project. *PLoS ONE*, *10*(6), e0130399. https://doi.org/10.1371/journal.pone.0130399

Hoon, D., Taylor, M. T., Kapadia, P., Gerhard, T., Strom, B. L., & Horton, D. B. (2019). Trends in off-label drug use in ambulatory settings: 2006–2015. *Pediatrics*, *144*(4), e20190896. https://doi.org/10.1542/peds.2019-0896

Kliegman, R. M., Stanton, B., St. Geme, J., Schor, N., & Behrman, R. E. (Eds.). (2016). *Nelson textbook of pediatrics* (19th ed.). W. B. Saunders.

Meyers, R. (2020). A wish list for drug development in pediatrics. *Journal of Pharmaceutical Sciences*, *109*(2), 939–943. https://doi.org/10.1016/j.xphs.2019.10.029

Mueller, B. U., Neuspiel, D. R., & Fisher, E. R. S. (2019). Principles of pediatric patient safety: Reducing harm due to medical care. *Pediatrics*, *143*(2). https://doi.org/10.1542/peds.2018-3649

Mary Smith, 80 years old, is being transported via ambulance to the emergency department. She looks pale and thin with sunken eyes and chapped, dry lips. "I'm so relieved my neighbor came by to check on me. I have not been able to get out of bed for 2 days."

—*Patient "Mary Smith"*

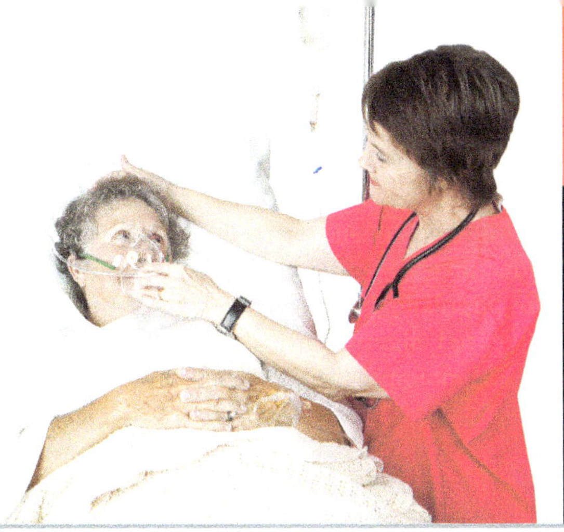

Chapter 10
Pharmacotherapy of the Geriatric Patient

Chapter Outline

- Polypharmacy
- Physiologic Changes Related to Aging
- Pharmacokinetic and Pharmacodynamic Changes in Older Adults
- Adherence and Drug Misuse Among Older Adults
- Adverse Drug Reactions in Older Adults

Learning Outcomes

After reading this chapter, the student should be able to:

1. Describe factors that lead to polypharmacy in older adults.
2. Identify age-related physiologic changes in the older adult.
3. Explain how age-related physiologic changes alter pharmacokinetics and pharmacodynamics and affect drug response in older adults.
4. Explain strategies that the nurse may implement to improve adherence with drug therapy in geriatric patients.
5. Explain why older adults are more likely to experience adverse drug reactions and interactions.
6. Identify specific drugs that are particularly hazardous for use in older patients.
7. Differentiate medication responses that result from age-related alterations in specific body systems from those that occur in younger individuals.
8. Develop nursing interventions that maximize pharmacotherapeutic outcomes in older adults.
9. Generate key points for family and patient education regarding drug pharmacotherapy for older adults.

Key Terms

Definitions of the terms in bold may be found in the Glossary.

There is no universally accepted age that is considered old. The older adult, or an elderly individual, is typically defined as someone over age 65. Of this age group, those older than 84 years are the fastest-growing segment of the population. The average age of the population has increased significantly during the past few decades because of improved access to healthcare, people choosing healthier lifestyles, and more effective treatment of chronic diseases. With the increase in lifespan, however, has come an increased reliance on medications to maintain health. This chapter focuses on aspects of pharmacology unique to geriatric patients and provides steps that the nurse can take to provide safe, effective pharmacotherapy for this population.

PharmFACT

The number of Americans age 65 and older is projected to nearly double, from 52 million in 2018 to 95 million by 2060, and the 65-and-older age group of the total population will rise from 16% to 23% (U.S. Census Bureau, n.d.).

Polypharmacy

10.1 Older adults take more medications than any other segment of the population.

The pharmacotherapy of older adults is more challenging than that of their middle-age or younger counterparts. To deliver safe and effective treatment for patients in this age group, the nurse must consider many age-related variables that affect pharmacotherapy. In addition, older adults generally experience more chronic conditions than their younger counterparts. Most of these conditions require drug therapy to treat and prevent complications. Finally, many older adults self-medicate for minor conditions that do not require prescription drug therapy.

Longevity inevitably leads to increased illnesses, which, in turn, results in the use of increased numbers of medications. Comorbidity, the presence of several chronic medical disorders concurrently, is common among older adults. By about age 65, half the older population has two or more chronic disorders, the most prevalent being a combination of hypertension and arthritis. Other comorbidities that occur in a significant number of older adults are heart disease with arthritis, hypertension with diabetes, and depression with nearly any other chronic disorder.

Comorbidities often result in the need for multiple drugs, a condition termed **polypharmacy**. Although not unique to older patients, polypharmacy is prevalent in this age group because of these comorbidities. The higher the number of drugs taken by a patient, the greater the possibility of experiencing adverse effects and drug interactions. As presented in Chapter 5, drugs that may be safe when used as monotherapy can have additive adverse effects when combined with other drugs. For example, taking multiple drugs that cause central nervous system (CNS) depression can lead to excessive sedation, thus increasing the risk for injuries due to falls. Taking two or more drugs that cause renal or liver impairment can result in additive organ damage in older adults who may already have some degree of function loss due to normal aging processes.

Polypharmacy may also occur when the patient takes over-the-counter (OTC) drugs, herbal products, and dietary supplements in conjunction with prescribed medications. For example, older adults frequently seek OTC medications to treat constipation and minor aches and pains. Many also take vitamins, alternative therapies, and dietary supplements. Most patients are unaware that these agents can interact with prescription medications.

Patients who visit multiple healthcare providers and use different pharmacies may experience polypharmacy because each provider or pharmacist may not be aware of all the drugs ordered by other prescribers. Nurses should urge patients to report all prescription and OTC products at each office visit and teach them to use one pharmacy for their prescription needs.

In addition to polypharmacy, many other factors can alter a geriatric patient's response to medication. These include physiologic changes associated with aging, changes in pharmacokinetics and pharmacodynamics, and patient adherence with the therapeutic regimen.

CONNECTION Checkpoint 10.1

From what you learned in Chapter 5, state the differences between additive, synergistic, and antagonistic effects.

Physiologic Changes Related to Aging

10.2 Anatomic and physiologic changes associated with aging may alter the patient's response to medications.

With advancing age, certain anatomic and physiologic changes occur. These predictable changes should be considered a normal part of the aging process, rather than as diseases or pathologic conditions. Awareness of the physiologic changes that occur during the lifespan is critically important in properly assessing and caring for the older adult (Figure 10.1). Failure to recognize these changes may lead to less than optimal therapeutic outcomes and may endanger patient safety.

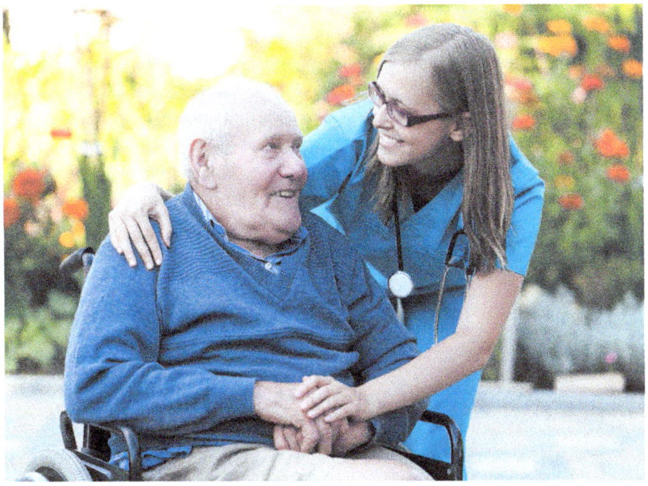

Figure 10.1 Pharmacology of the older adult can be challenging due to physiologic changes that occur with aging.
Barabasa/Shutterstock.

Giving an "average dose" of a drug to an older adult may produce a very different response compared to the same dose given to a younger patient, even if the two patients weigh the same. The pharmacologic action of the drug in older adults may be enhanced or diminished. The adverse effects may be more severe or entirely different from those observed in younger patients. The older patient may experience more drug interactions. What factors are responsible for this wide variation in drug response in the geriatric population?

In general, physiologic processes slow down with advancing age. For example, the rate of absorption of nutrients from the gastrointestinal (GI) system tends to slow due to the decrease in GI motility and reduced GI blood flow. Metabolism also diminishes due to decreased liver size and reduced blood flow to this organ. Additionally, as a person ages, the production of serum albumin by the liver declines. The older adult has a decreased volume of total body water, leading to higher concentrations of substances in the serum.

Cardiovascular system changes in the older adult are related to changes in cardiac muscle and increased peripheral resistance (hypertension). These physiologic changes lead to decreased contractile force, which diminishes cardiac output and slows the circulation of nutrients and drugs.

In the nervous system, conduction velocity slows and sensory functions such as vision, hearing, and smell begin to diminish. Brain mass begins to decline, resulting in a progressive loss of cognitive ability. Additionally, the efficiency of the blood–brain barrier declines, allowing more substances to enter the CNS and affect the brain, as a person ages.

Older adults undergo a progressive decline in renal function as a result of decreased renal blood flow, decreased glomerular filtration rate, and decreased numbers of nephrons. The kidneys begin to lose their ability to effectively excrete creatinine and other wastes from the body. The body retains drugs and other substances for longer periods.

Normal, age-related physiologic changes in organ systems can greatly affect responses to medications. Selected changes, and their effects on drug response, are shown in Table 10.1.

Pharmacokinetic and Pharmacodynamic Changes in Older Adults

10.3 Normal aging processes can alter pharmacokinetic and pharmacodynamic responses to drugs.

To produce therapeutic effects, most drugs must reach their target cells in sufficient quantities. To a large extent, this depends on what the body does to the medications after they are administered, a process known as pharmacokinetics. Drug response is also dependent on pharmacodynamic factors: the mechanisms by which drugs change the body. The normal physiologic changes of aging affect pharmacokinetics and pharmacodynamics. Knowing about these changes when administering medications to the older adult helps the nurse to understand the unique actions of drugs in these patients and to predict and prevent adverse effects.

Absorption: In general, absorption of nutrients and drugs tends to slow with aging. Fortunately, although the rate slows, absorption is usually complete because most drugs are absorbed by passive diffusion.

Because of the increased gastric pH in older adults, oral tablets and capsules that require high levels of acid for absorption may dissolve more slowly and take longer to reach their target tissues. Furthermore, decreased blood flow to and from the GI tract in the older adult delays the absorption and subsequent distribution of medications. Slowed motility allows drugs to remain longer in the GI tract, increasing the length of time for absorption and raising the risk for adverse effects such as nausea and vomiting. Physiologic changes that lead to alterations in the rate and quantity of drug absorption are listed in Table 10.1.

Distribution: As the body ages, the proportion of body fat increases, which can cause lipid-soluble drugs such as diazepam (Valium) to be stored in the body for extended periods. This may lead to lower plasma levels and increased drug concentrations in the tissues. The longer a drug remains in the tissues, the more significant the response to the drug will be and the greater the potential for adverse effects.

Table 10.1 Physiologic Factors Affecting Medication Responses in Older Adults

Body System	Changes in Physiologic Factors	Effect on Medication Response
Cardiovascular system	• Decreased force of contraction and stroke volume • Decreased oxygen uptake by tissues • Decreased serum albumin and serum-binding capacity	• Reduced cardiac output and slowed distribution • Decreased metabolism • Changed drug distribution, producing unpredictable and toxic levels of highly protein-bound drugs such as phenytoin
Central nervous system	• Decreased brain size, number of neurons, and peripheral nerve function • Declining efficiency of blood–brain barrier	• Decreased drug distribution • Increased penetration of drug in the brain
Endocrine system	• Alterations in carbohydrate metabolism • Decreased growth hormone production and altered corticosteroid activity, leading to increased body fat, decreased muscle, and decreased bone mass	• Reduced insulin secretion and increased insulin resistance, manifesting as type 2 diabetes mellitus • Increased absorption of fat-soluble drugs
Gastrointestinal system	• Decreased GI motility • Decreased emptying of gastric contents • Reduced gastric acid production • Increased gastric pH • Decreased blood flow to the GI tract • Decreased thirst perception, leading to risk for dehydration, electrolyte imbalance, and poor nutritional intake	• Slowed rate of absorption • Increased potential for adverse effects
	• Decreased liver size • Decreased blood flow to the liver • Decreased ability of the liver to metabolize drugs	• Slowed metabolism • Prolonged drug half-life, increasing the potential for adverse effects
Musculoskeletal system	• Decreased lean muscle mass and increased and redistributed body fat	• Extended and increased effect of fat-soluble drugs such as diazepam
Respiratory system	• Decreased muscle strength and endurance	• Decreased chest and lung expansion and response to hypoxia, resulting in altered rate of absorption and excretion of some respiratory drugs
Urinary system	• Decreased total fluid volume • Decreased renal blood flow, glomerular filtration, and tubular secretory function • Decreased creatinine clearance	• Higher concentrations of water-soluble drugs • Reduced rate of excretion and decreased drug clearance • Decreased drug excretion

As the body ages, there may be a reduction in total body water resulting in water-soluble drugs such as gentamicin (Garamycin) and hydrochlorothiazide (Microzide) having less body fluid for dilution. Therefore, water-soluble drugs have higher serum concentrations and may produce more intense actions. To prevent toxicity, the peak and trough levels of drugs with a low safety index such as gentamicin are checked periodically, and drug dosages are adjusted accordingly.

Because of declining liver function, plasma protein levels are reduced in the older adult. This decrease results in fewer binding sites for certain drugs and higher concentrations of free drugs, which may lead to toxicity. In older adults taking highly protein-bound drugs such as phenytoin (Dilantin) and warfarin (Coumadin), the nurse must carefully assess for signs of toxicity, even when the patient is receiving therapeutic doses.

Higher levels of drugs are able to enter the brain in older adults due to the inefficient blood–brain barrier. Patients taking drugs such as benzodiazepines, antipsychotic drugs, antiepileptic drugs, or tranquilizers that affect the CNS must be assessed for signs of adverse effects that often manifest as reduced cognitive function, drowsiness, confusion, and even hallucinations and psychoses.

Metabolism: Although most tissues metabolize drugs to some extent, the liver is by far the most important organ performing this function. Age-related changes in the liver include reduced hepatic function, decreased liver mass, diminished blood flow, and alteration in the activity of some hepatic enzymes.

Age-related changes in liver function are often unpredictable, causing the level of some metabolic enzymes to be reduced, whereas others remain unchanged. In general, blood flow to the liver decreases and metabolic activity of the CYP450 enzymes is diminished. Reduced metabolism means that drugs will have extended durations of action. Drugs with a long half-life such as gentamicin, digoxin (Lanoxin), and acetaminophen (Tylenol) remain longer in the body with the potential for accumulation in tissues. Such drugs should be prescribed with longer intervals between doses or in reduced dosages, and the patient should be monitored closely.

CONNECTIONS: Lifespan Considerations

Drug Monitoring in the Older Adult

To avoid toxicity, a number of drug dosage changes should be made for the older adult:

- The older adult should be started on the smallest effective dose of medication and then be titrated upward.
- Observe the older patient for signs of drug accumulation about 3 to 5 days after new drug initiation. Consider any change in physical or emotional behavior as possible drug intoxication.
- Monitor hydration and nutritional status, especially among older patients, because dehydration and low protein in the diet are primary causes of drug toxicity in this age group.

Excretion: The kidneys are the primary site for excretion of most drugs. Renal function declines with aging, resulting in a slower clearance of drugs from the body. The half-life of drugs is increased, and the dosages or frequency of administration should be decreased to avoid toxicity due to drug accumulation. Patients who are taking drugs that are excreted primarily by the kidneys should receive periodic serum creatinine tests to assess renal function. Dosages of drugs must be carefully adjusted in patients with impaired renal function. Unlike hepatic function, which is often unpredictable in older adults, diminished renal function is mostly consistent from patient to patient.

Pharmacodynamic changes: Pharmacodynamic changes are usually associated with drug receptors. Evidence suggests that older adults have decreased numbers of receptors and, possibly, changes in receptor sensitivity. In assessing the older adult, the nurse will find a decreased response to beta-adrenergic agonists and antagonists and, at the same time, an increased response to anticholinergics, CNS depressants, and drugs such as warfarin. There is limited information on how pharmacodynamic alterations actually occur in older adults.

CONNECTION Checkpoint 10.2

From what you learned in Chapter 3, what are CYP450 enzymes? State the differences between a substrate and an inducer of CYP450 enzymes.

Adherence and Drug Misuse Among Older Adults

10.4 Adherence with the therapeutic regimen is a major challenge for many older adults.

Drug adherence is the willingness and ability to take medications as instructed on the label or by the healthcare provider. Medication nonadherence accounts for approximately 450,000 emergency department visits every year and 10% of hospitalizations in older adults. Healthcare providers often assume that patients leaving the clinic or hospital will be adherent by filling their prescriptions and taking their medicines as directed. It may be surprising to learn that over a third of patients report they are often nonadherent with drug therapy. Reasons for nonadherence are many and varied and, although nonadherence is not unique to older adults, this population is especially vulnerable. Older adult patients are more likely to have visual impairment, functional disabilities, and cognitive dysfunction that may be sources of medication errors and nonadherence. Functional hearing loss can prevent older adults from understanding the verbal instructions given by the healthcare provider. The large number of drugs taken by some older adults makes for a complicated dosing schedule that can be confusing for patients of any age.

Successful management of medical problems depends on a patient's adherence with the regimen. One of the main responsibilities of the nurse is to assess barriers to medication adherence in the older adult. Studies suggest that nonadherence is affected by three factors: the individual patient, the healthcare provider, and the patient's social support network.

Adherence at the patient level requires the patient's comprehension and commitment to the treatment. The patient must be able to afford the medication, believe in its efficacy, appropriately self-administer, and adjust to lifestyle changes that may be required. The healthcare provider must be able to effectively instruct the patient regarding a medication's efficacy, prescribe cost-effective medication, decrease the complexity of the regimen, and provide manageable and understandable instructions. Nurses play a key role in assessing the patient's understanding of the medications that have been ordered and for assessing patient concerns with cost or effects.

The nurse should provide the older adult's spouse or caregiver with adequate information regarding the patient's medication regimen, expected lifestyle changes, and the need for emotional support and monitoring. Table 10.2 lists reasons that patients give for nonadherence and provides suggestions for the nurse to promote adherence.

Drug misuse is a specific form of nonadherence that is common among older adults. Misuse includes overuse, underuse, or, in some cases, erratic use. This misuse may be unintentional or deliberate. Self-adjusting the medication dose is a common practice: Patients change their dose level depending on how they feel. Some believe that taking extra doses will speed their recovery. Uninsured or underinsured patients who cannot afford their medications may try to make the medications last longer by splitting doses. Patients rarely report such practices to their healthcare provider.

Table 10.2 Promoting Adherence in the Older Adult

Reasons for nonadherence	• Unpleasant adverse effects • Forgetfulness • Cognitive or physical impairment • Poor or misunderstood instructions • Complicated regimens • Inability or refusal to purchase the medication • Health beliefs about medications
Ways the nurse can promote adherence	• Assist the older adult in comprehending and committing to the drug treatment regimen. • Communicate the instructions in such a manner that the older patient fully understands the purpose of the treatment. • Provide the older patient with social support services to obtain the medications. • Work with a pharmacist to ensure that the medication is dispensed in containers that are easily opened and in formulations that are easily taken. • Make sure all drugs are clearly labeled with instructions. • Simplify the regimen to reduce the number of drugs and doses per day. • Suggest that the older patient use a daily or weekly pill counter. • Provide the patient with a check-off calendar to document each time a medication is taken. • Engage family members or friends in supporting the older patient in efforts to comply. • Encourage the older patient to report signs of adverse effects. • Schedule periodic tests to determine plasma drug levels. • Place follow-up calls to high-risk patients.

Drug misuse may have serious consequences: Many older adult visits to emergency departments are drug related, with nonadherence accounting for a substantial percentage.

CONNECTION Checkpoint 10.3

From what you learned in Chapter 2, describe some of the benefits to older adults created by the Medicare Prescription Drug, Improvement, and Modernization Act of 2003.

Adverse Drug Reactions in Older Adults

10.5 Older adults are at high risk for experiencing adverse drug reactions and interactions.

An adverse drug effect is an undesirable and potentially harmful action caused by the administration of medications (see Chapter 5). Although older adults have many factors that predispose them to an increased risk of adverse effects, the number of drugs prescribed is probably the most important. The risk of an adverse effect greatly increases with the number of drugs taken. A survey in the United States of 2206 adults aged 62 to 85 showed that at least one prescription medication was used by 87% of the older adults, five or more prescription medications were used by 36%, and 38% used OTC medications (Qato et al., 2016).

To minimize adverse effects, prescribers should order drugs only when they are needed and for the shortest length of time necessary to produce a therapeutic effect. Medications and doses should be reviewed on a regular basis to ensure that the intervention is still necessary.

Age-related physiologic changes in renal and hepatic function are often responsible for placing older patients at greater risk for adverse effects. As the ability of the kidney to excrete drugs diminishes, serum drug levels may rise to cause toxicity. Loss of the ability of the liver to metabolize drugs can also raise serum drug levels and cause adverse effects. The nurse must be vigilant in assessing laboratory results of renal and hepatic function in older adult patients. Doses of most drugs must be adjusted with renal or hepatic impairment to prevent adverse effects.

It often becomes difficult for the healthcare provider to differentiate between behaviors that may be a natural part of aging and symptoms caused by adverse effects. For example, a frail older adult who walks with an ataxic gait might be wrongly suspected of having an adverse effect from benzodiazepines or phenytoin, although the condition might be caused by normal aging. Older adults are more likely to experience CNS drug adverse effects such as dizziness and drowsiness, which are also symptoms that are often associated with normal aging processes. Medications should be considered as an underlying cause of the following symptoms in older patients:

- Sudden change in mental status
- Rapid weight loss
- Dehydration
- Restlessness
- Falls
- Anorexia
- Urinary retention or fluid retention
- Change in bowel habits
- Major change in functional status of any organ system.

The American Geriatrics Society (AGS) Beers Criteria is an explicit list of Potentially Inappropriate Medications (PIM) that should be avoided by older adults or should only be prescribed under very specific situations for certain diseases or conditions. Along with a panel of experts in geriatric care, the AGS has been responsible for monitoring the list and criteria and produces updates about every 3 years. For the 2019 update, an interdisciplinary expert panel reviewed evidence published since the last update and each of the five types of criteria in the 2015 update were retained. These include medications that are potentially inappropriate in most older adults, those that should typically be avoided in older adults with certain conditions, drugs to use with caution, drug–drug interactions, and drug dose adjustment

Table 10.3 Selected High-Risk Drugs for Older Adults

Drug	Adverse Response or Rationale
Anticholinergics (e.g., chlorpheniramine, diphenhydramine, hydroxyzine, promethazine)	Sedation, confusion, other anticholinergic effects
Antipsychotic drugs (e.g., chlorpromazine, clozapine, risperidone)	Increased mortality (in patients with dementia, stroke)
Antispasmodics (e.g., atropine, hyoscyamine, scopolamine)	Highly anticholinergic, uncertain effectiveness
Anxiolytics: benzodiazepines (e.g., alprazolam, lorazepam, oxazepam) and nonbenzodiazepines (e.g., eszopiclone, zaleplon, zolpidem)	Cognitive impairment, depression, falls and other accidents
Cardiovascular: alpha-1 blockers (e.g., doxazosin, prazosin, terazosin)	Orthostatic hypotension, alternative drugs have higher safety profile
Cardiovascular: CNS alpha-2 agonists (clonidine, methyldopa)	CNS adverse effects, orthostatic hypotension, bradycardia
Cardiovascular: heart failure (e.g., diltiazem, verapamil, cilostazol)	Fluid retention, risk for worsening heart failure
Digoxin (Lanoxin) as first-line treatment for atrial fibrillation or heart failure	Reduced renal clearance, alternative drugs are safer and more effective
GI drugs: proton pump inhibitors (e.g., esomeprazole, lansoprazole, omeprazole)	Risk of *C. difficile* infection, bone loss, fractures
Nonsteroidal anti-inflammatory drugs (NSAIDs) (e.g., aspirin over 325 mg/day), ibuprofen, naproxen)	Nephrotoxicity, upper GI bleeding
Skeletal muscle relaxants (e.g., carisoprodol, cyclobenzaprine, methocarbamol)	Sedation, fractures, anticholinergic effects
Tricyclic antidepressants (e.g., amitriptyline, doxepin, imipramine)	Sedation, confusion, highly anticholinergic

based on kidney function. Providers should use this list to help guide prescribing for older patients (Fick et al., 2019).

Table 10.3 provides a select list of PIMs that should be avoided in older adults along with their specific adverse effects of concern.

A drug interaction occurs when a medication interacts with another substance and the drug's actions are affected. The other substance causing the drug interaction may be another drug, a dietary supplement, an herbal product, or a food (see Chapter 5). The large number of prescription drugs and OTC products taken by older adults predisposes this population to a high risk for drug interactions.

Another factor contributing to the increased risk for drug interactions is the presence of comorbidities (see Section 10.2). For example, the patient with both arthritis and heart disease may be using nonsteroidal anti-inflammatory

CONNECTIONS: Advanced Practice Application

Complicated Medication Routines and Older Adults

Case

Mr. Barkins is an 88-year-old who is a frequent patient in our community geriatric clinic. He has lived alone since his wife died and visits the clinic often because he is lonely and looking for conversation and company. He is a favorite patient to most of the staff. In addition to the social isolation, Mr. Barkins has many medical issues including type 2 diabetes mellitus, hypertension, chronic kidney disease, peptic ulcer disease, and anemia. In fact, while doing his medication reconciliation you realize he is on 18 different medications! He tells you that he is having difficulty managing "all these pills" at home and is not taking all his prescribed medications. You inquire further and find out he is missing doses because it is "too hard to take all of them" and that by skipping some of the medications every day, he keeps the costs down. What are some of the things you can do to optimize adherence? What community resources are available for Mr. Barkins?

Discussion

Oftentimes, older patients may decide to skip doses or stop taking their medication without telling their provider until they are asked. Medication adherence should be one of the routine health history questions for older patients. Medication reconciliation is the first step in assisting older adults to manage their medications. A "medication check-in" should be conducted annually or more often to review all the patient's medications and to determine which medications and dosage adjustments are needed.

Older patients are more likely to adhere to a prescribed medication that has a simpler dosing schedule, such as once daily, compared to another medication that has a more complex dosing schedule, such as twice daily.

Many pharmaceutical companies offer medication assistance programs to low-income older patients. These programs typically require a provider form and proof of financial status from the patient.

BenefitsCheckUp is a free service of the National Council on Aging (n.d.), a nonprofit service and advocacy organization in Washington, DC. The online service asks a series of questions and then identifies programs that could help patients pay for prescriptions, healthcare, food, and other expenses.

Table 10.4 Nursing Responsibilities Related to Adverse Drug Reactions and Drug Interactions in Older Adults

Nursing Responsibilities	Rationales
• Review the patient's medications to determine the potential for adverse effects and drug interactions. Consider cultural and dietary issues.	• Adverse effects are common in older patients because of physiologic changes in body composition, multiple illnesses, polypharmacy, and nonadherence. • Some dietary practices may lead to adverse effects and interactions (e.g., low salt intake may lead to lithium toxicity).
• Instruct the patient about potential adverse effects.	• A well-informed patient is better able to notify the healthcare provider as early as possible to minimize adverse effects.
• Assess the patient's fluid volume.	• Alteration in fluid volume could lead to increased sensitivity to alpha antagonists and other drugs with effects on blood pressure.
• Instruct the patient about the proper time to administer medications.	• Taking medications at the proper time will ensure optimal effectiveness and lower the chance for adverse effects.
• Ensure that the fewest number and lowest doses of medications with the simplest regimens have been prescribed for the patient.	• Polypharmacy may lead to drug toxicity.
• Monitor the patient for expected responses and any changes from normal.	• Adverse effects may not always be predictable because they may arise from sudden changes in the patient's condition.
• Discard all unused and expired medications and instruct the patient to do the same.	• Drug effects diminish after the expiration date and some drugs can become toxic over time.
• Assess and monitor the patient's mental status for any alterations that may be caused by adverse effects.	• Delirium or confusion may be caused by adverse effects of psychoactive drugs.
• Periodically review the patient's OTC medications, nutritional supplements, and prescribed medications.	• Review of all drugs and alternative therapies can reduce the chances of adverse effects.

drugs (NSAIDs) for pain and warfarin (Coumadin) to prevent blood clots. The NSAID may increase the effect of the warfarin, thus raising the potential for bleeding. The patient with both diabetes and hypertension may be taking thiazides and insulin. The thiazides reduce the effectiveness of insulin, thus affecting glycemic control.

The nurse plays a key role in optimizing pharmacotherapy outcomes in older adult patients, including addressing adverse effects, drug interactions, and issues of polypharmacy. One of the primary nursing responsibilities is to make a connection between the patient and family and the medication regimens. This entails assessing the level of comprehension, cultural beliefs, dietary practices, and physiologic conditions of the patient and family. Advanced age does not negate the patient's right to know the names of the prescribed medications, the reasons they are being prescribed, and the potential adverse effects. Table 10.4 highlights nursing responsibilities and rationales regarding adverse effects and drug–drug interactions in older patients.

PharmFACT

Annual flu vaccinations are important for the older adult. There are two types recommended for older adults: a high-dose flu vaccine (Fluzone) and an adjuvanted flu vaccine (Fluad). The adjuvanted flu vaccine includes a substance that creates a stronger immune response. Both vaccines are designed to be more effective in older adults (Centers for Disease Control and Prevention, 2019).

Understanding Chapter 10

Key Concepts Summary

10.1 Older adults take more medications than any other segment of the population.

10.2 Anatomic and physiologic changes associated with aging may alter the patient's response to medications.

10.3 Normal aging processes can alter pharmacokinetic and pharmacodynamic responses to drugs.

10.4 Adherence with the therapeutic regimen is a major challenge for many older adults.

10.5 Older adults are at high risk for experiencing adverse drug reactions and interactions.

CASE STUDY: Making the Patient Connection

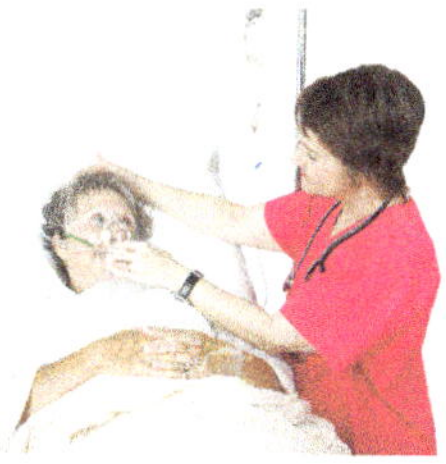

Remember the patient "Mary Smith" at the beginning of the chapter? Now read the remainder of the case study. Based on the information presented within this chapter, respond to the critical thinking questions that follow.

Mary has an IV solution of normal saline infusing in her left arm and oxygen by mask at 2 L/min. Last week she heard that her older cousin had passed away, and since then she has become extremely depressed. Mary refuses to eat or drink but continues to take her medications on a regular basis. This 80-year-old woman is dehydrated and somewhat confused. Her neighbor provides the history. The nurse finds that Mary has been taking a diuretic (hydrochlorothiazide), an antihypertensive (atenolol), and multivitamins daily.

Vital signs are as follows: temperature, 38.6°C (101.4°F); apical pulse, 100 beats/min; respiratory rate, 32 breaths/min; and blood pressure, 92/62 mmHg. Mary's skin is dry and warm to the touch, and her lips are pale, dry, and chapped. She weighs 51.3 kg (113 lb) and her height is 1.7 m (5′7″). Her speech is quiet and slurred. Mary has not eaten anything during the past 24 hours and has only taken sips of water during the past 12 hours. She has voided once in 12 hours.

The following laboratory tests are completed: urinalysis, blood urea nitrogen and creatinine, complete blood count, and basal metabolic panel. Mary is prescribed IV rehydration fluid and is stabilized in the emergency department before being admitted to the hospital unit.

Critical Thinking Questions

1. What are some potential predisposing factors that could lead to this patient's condition? (The student may need to consult later chapters or a drug reference book for the drugs included.)
2. What are the most immediate patient care priorities for the nurse to address at this time?
3. What priority areas will the nurse assess?
4. What are some of the expected patient outcomes, including changes in vital signs, following management of dehydration?

Additional Case Study

Ms. Haynes, 88 years of age, is fiercely independent and lives in her own apartment in an assisted living facility, with meals taken in a group dining room, which she clearly enjoys. She has a history of diabetes controlled with an oral antidiabetic drug, hypertension controlled with an antihypertensive drug and a mild diuretic, and occasional stomach upset for which she takes antacids. Her daughter suspects that her mother has not been taking any of her medications regularly because her blood sugar and blood pressure have been extremely variable lately and she asks the nurse for assistance.

1. What should the nurse do to assess whether Ms. Haynes is taking her medications regularly? What laboratory test will help determine diabetic control over a period of time?
2. If Ms. Haynes is not taking her medications, what would the nurse's next action be?
3. What recommendation should be given to Ms. Haynes's daughter?

Chapter Review

1. In general, drug absorption in the older adult is somewhat slowed. What physiologic changes may account for this? (Select all that apply.)
   1. Increased gastric pH
   2. Decreased rate of blood flow to the GI tract
   3. Increased gastrointestinal motility
   4. Increased body surface area
   5. Decreased cardiac output
2. While completing an initial home assessment of an independent 82-year-old woman recently diagnosed with type 2 diabetes mellitus managed with insulin injections, what action is most appropriate for insulin administration for this patient?
   1. Teach the daughter how to administer the insulin to her mother.
   2. Instruct the patient how to administer the insulin.

3. Recommend daily visits by a home health aide to give the insulin.
4. The order should be changed to an oral antidiabetic medication.

3. Which age-related change in the older patient makes it necessary to reduce drug dosages?
   1. Decrease in total body fat
   2. Decrease in renal blood flow
   3. Increase in plasma protein levels
   4. Increase in total body water

4. Older adults experience adverse effects more frequently than young adults due to which of the following? (Select all that apply.)
   1. Excessive prescribing
   2. Multiple-drug therapy
   3. Increased drug sensitivity
   4. Increased body mass
   5. Lack of consistent exercise

5. One-third of older adult patients report that they are often nonadherent with drug therapy. Which response is given most frequently for nonadherence?
   1. "The drugs prevented me from doing other things I wanted to do."
   2. "I didn't have my medicine with me."
   3. "I wanted to save money."
   4. "I didn't believe the drugs were effective."

6. Which statement by the patient would require more teaching prior to discharge?
   1. "It doesn't matter if the medication works as long as the doctor prescribed it."
   2. "This medication is fully covered by my health insurance."
   3. "I have been taking my medications by myself all my life."
   4. "I don't mind making changes to my lifestyle while I am on this drug."

See Appendix A for answers to critical thinking questions, case study questions and review questions.

References

Centers for Disease Control and Prevention. (2019). *People 65 years and older & influenza.* https://www.cdc.gov/flu/highrisk/65over.htm.

Fick, D., Semla, T., Steinman, M., Beizer, J., Brandt, N., Dombrowski, R., et al. (2019). American Geriatrics Society 2019 Updated AGS Beers Criteria® for potentially inappropriate medication use in older adults. *Journal of the American Geriatrics Society, 67*(4), 674–694. https://doi.org/10.1111/jgs.15767

National Council on Aging. (n.d.). *Find my benefits.* https://www.benefitscheckup.org

Qato, D. M., Wilder, J., Schumm, P., Gillet, V., & Alexander, G. C. (2016). Changes in prescription and over-the-counter medication and dietary supplement use among older adults in the United States, 2005 vs 2011. *JAMA Internal Medicine, 176*, 473–482. https://doi.org/10.1001/jamainternmed.2015.8581

U.S. Census Bureau. (n.d.). *Population projections.* https://www.census.gov/programs-surveys/popproj/data.html

Selected Bibliography

Chou, J., Tong, M., & Brandt, N. J. (2019). Combating polypharmacy through deprescribing potentially inappropriate medications. *Journal of Gerontological Nursing, 45*(1), 9–15. https://doi.org/10.3928/00989134-20190102-01

Forman, D. E., & Zieman, S. J. (2019). "Doc, I think my meds are killing me! Please help . . . ": Transdisciplinary forces unite to refocus pharmacotherapy for older adults. *Journal of the American Geriatrics Society, 67*(2), 205–207. https://doi.org/10.1111/jgs.15706

Jacobs, L. G. (2019). For older adults, medications are common: An Updated AGS Beers Criteria® aims to ensure they are appropriate, too. *Journal of Gerontological Nursing, 45*(5), 47–48. https://doi.org/10.3928/00989134-20190319-01

Schwartz, J. B., Schmader, K. E., Hanlon, J. T., Abernethy, D. R., Gray, S., Dunbar-Jacob, J., et al. (2019). Pharmacotherapy in older adults with cardiovascular disease: Report from an American College of Cardiology, American Geriatrics Society, and National Institute on Aging Workshop. *Journal of the American Geriatrics Society, 67*(2), 371–380. https://doi.org/10.1111/jgs.15634

"It was so humiliating. When I was in the hospital, no one ever called me by name. I overheard someone refer to me as 'the Indian woman in room 425.' No one really tried to communicate with me."
—*Patient "Aponi Nampeyo"*

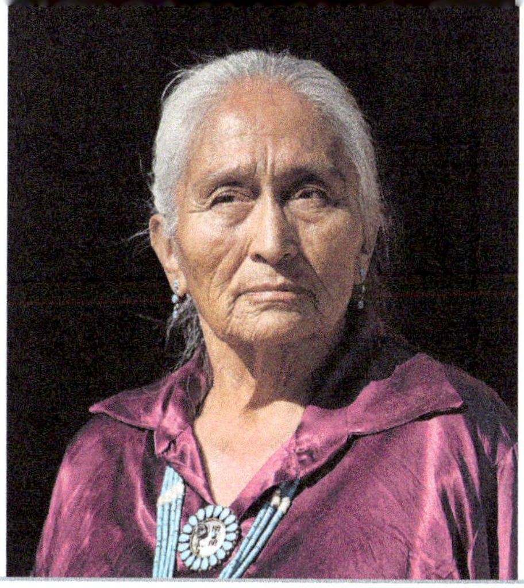

Chapter 11
Individual Variations in Drug Responses

Chapter Outline

- Psychosocial Influences
- Cultural and Ethnic Variables
- Pharmacogenetic Factors
- Gender Influences

Learning Outcomes

After reading this chapter, the student should be able to:

1. Describe the fundamental concepts underlying a holistic approach to patient care and their importance to pharmacotherapy.
2. Identify psychosocial and spiritual factors that can affect pharmacotherapeutics.
3. Explain how ethnicity can affect pharmacotherapeutic outcomes.
4. Identify examples of how cultural values and beliefs can influence pharmacotherapeutic outcomes.
5. Convey how genetic mutations can influence pharmacotherapy.
6. Explain how pharmacogenomics may be used to customize drug therapy.
7. Explain how gender can influence the actions of certain drugs.

Key Terms

Definitions of the terms in bold may be found in the Glossary.

Pharmacotherapy would indeed be simplified if the "average" dose given in a drug guide produced the same response in every patient. However, as presented in Chapter 4, patients can respond very differently to drug administration. For example, the same dose of an antihypertensive drug can result in a desired therapeutic effect in one patient and produce no effect or profound hypotension in other patients. The purpose of this chapter is to examine some of the factors that may cause this variability, including psychosocial influences, culture and ethnicity, genetics, and gender. Knowledge of these factors can contribute to safer and more effective pharmacotherapy.

Psychosocial Influences

11.1 Many psychosocial influences impact pharmacotherapy.

The term **psychosocial** is used in healthcare to describe the interaction between one's psychologic development and one's social environment. Psychosocial nursing is part of a holistic model that includes the examination of patients' social roles, environmental stressors, culture, values, and family, all of which contribute to health and wellness.

Psychosocial also includes the spiritual nature of an individual. *Psycho-social-spiritual* is a term that appears in the healthcare literature. Studies have established that these factors have a tremendous impact on health and well-being. Healthcare providers recognize that the close relationship among the psychologic, social, and spiritual nature of individuals strongly influences their illness and wellness.

The psychosocial history of the patient, which is often collected during the initial assessment, can influence the success of pharmacotherapy. Important assessment data include developmental needs, environmental stressors, and life transitions that could require major adaptations by the patient. The nurse also considers the patient's level of motivation to correct the health issue because nonadherence to medication regimens and recommended lifestyle adjustments could impede the success of pharmacotherapy. For example, a highly stressed, middle-aged patient who is struggling with a new business might find it difficult to focus on wellness goals associated with maintaining normal blood pressure and cholesterol levels.

A thorough psychosocial assessment should provide the healthcare provider with a clear picture of the patient's living arrangements, family involvement and interaction, financial resources, emotional condition, physical condition, and cognitive functioning. For example, does the patient have a trusting and empathetic family relationship? Would the family be able and willing to help the patient through some difficult challenges with adverse effects or long-term therapy? Is the patient emotionally stable enough to receive prescription drugs that have a possible suicidal risk? All of this information is important to developing effective health goals and pharmacotherapeutic outcomes.

In some cases, the patient assessment may indicate a need to address psychosocial interventions before pharmacotherapy is begun. Behavioral or cognitive therapies may be employed to reduce negative thoughts and behaviors that could impact therapy. In children or adolescents, attempts at psychosocial therapies may be a prerequisite to initiating pharmacotherapy for conditions such as attention-deficit/hyperactivity disorder, major depressive disorder, or bipolar disorder. The integrated use of pharmacologic and psychosocial therapies is believed to increase therapeutic success in addiction treatment.

CONNECTION Checkpoint 11.1

Patients may have widely different responses to drugs and the average recommended dosage does not produce the same results in all people. From what you learned in Chapter 4, what does a frequency distribution (dose–response) curve represent? What is the median effective dose (ED_{50})?

Cultural and Ethnic Variables

11.2 Cultural and ethnic variables can influence pharmacotherapy.

Although they are sometimes used interchangeably, culture and ethnicity differ in their exact definitions. **Ethnicity** refers to the social and historical experiences that apply to a community of people of common heritage and ancestry. **Culture** is a set of beliefs, values, and norms that provide meaning for an individual or group. People within a culture have common rituals, religious beliefs, language, and certain expectations of behavior. Cultural and ethnic variables are important aspects of patient care that directly relate to pharmacotherapy. Both can influence the occurrence of specific drug effects and patient treatment outcomes.

For most of the history of pharmacology, the impact of cultural and ethnic variables was unknown or regarded as unimportant. This was primarily caused by a lack of diversity in the conduct of clinical trials and follow-up reporting. For example, older clinical trials enrolled mostly White males. Little attention was focused on identifying differences in pharmacologic effects in diverse ethnic or cultural groups.

The protocol for clinical trials now includes participants of different ages, genders, and ethnic groups whenever possible. Indeed, much research specifically examines differences among these populations, and findings are included in drug labels, as appropriate.

CONNECTIONS: Treating the Diverse Patient

Medication Refusal for Religious, Moral, or Dietary Reasons

One of the "rights" of medication administration is refusal. Patients have the right to refuse their medications due to religious or other reasons. Perhaps most familiar is the refusal to accept blood or blood products by a Jehovah's Witness member because of religious beliefs. Less familiar is refusal due to the fact that the medication or treatment contains animal-derived products. For example, acceptance or refusal of porcine (pork) and bovine (beef) drugs or surgical products by members of the Jewish, Muslim, and Hindu faiths is common (Ogden, 2016); however, this may vary among individual members of the faith. People who follow vegetarian or vegan diets may also shun the use of animal-based products.

Many medications contain animal-based products, including inactive ingredients such as gelatin or lactose. Depending on the religious tradition, beef, pork, chicken, fish, shellfish, or all meat may be refused on religious or moral grounds or for dietary reasons. It may be difficult to determine the source of the animal product unless the manufacturer identifies the source on the container. When a substitution can be made, the alternate product should be used. Sensitivity to a patient's religious beliefs, traditions, moral reasoning, or dietary needs should be maintained. When a patient questions whether to use an essential drug or treatment and an alternate is not available, encourage the patient to discuss the information with healthcare providers and informed religious leaders before making the decision to refuse the treatment.

Certainly, there are many more cultures and subcultures than ethnic groups. To have complete knowledge about the many variations in culture among a population of patients is impossible. However, nurses can strive to understand the significance of the cultural traditions and their potential impact on patients' pharmacologic regimens. Patients bring cultural (religious or ideological) beliefs that may challenge or conflict with what the healthcare provider believes to be in their best interests. How illness is defined is sometimes based on the cultural beliefs of an individual. One example that illustrates this point is the difference in belief systems between age groups—each with its own unique culture.

PharmFACT

The infant mortality rate of American Indians and Alaska Natives is twice that of non-Hispanic Whites. Twelve percent of American Indians and Alaska Natives received late or no prenatal care, compared to 4.5% of non-Hispanic Whites (U.S. Department of Health and Human Services, 2019).

The nurse must keep in mind the following variables when treating patients from different cultural and ethnic groups.

- **Dietary considerations.** Cultures vary in their dietary preferences and practices, with diets that include some foods and exclude others. Patients need to understand that foods can increase or decrease the effectiveness of certain medications. Spices and herbs can be important to a patient's culture but may affect pharmacologic therapies. For example, some cultures include a diet high in foods such as cheese, pickled fish, or wine that can interact with medications to cause adverse events. Certain herbs can affect anticoagulants, beta blockers, and antidepressants. Assessing the primary foods of a patient's culture is an important component of the patient's psychosocial history.
- **Complementary and alternative medicine (CAM).** Various cultural groups use CAM therapies, such as vitamins, herbs, or acupuncture, either along with or in place of modern medicines. Some folk remedies and traditional treatments have existed for thousands of years and helped form the foundation for modern medical practice. Other healing practices such as rhythmic drumming, the use of gemstones and crystals, cleansing purification ceremonies, or surrounding one with herbal smoke (smudging) may seen quite foreign to healthcare providers. The nurse can assess the treatments used and interpret the effect of these CAM therapies on the prescribed medications to maximize positive outcomes. The nurse can explain that certain herbs or supplements may cause potential health risks when combined with prescribed drugs.
- **Beliefs about health and disease.** Cultures view health and illness in different ways. Individuals may seek assistance from people in their own community whom they believe have healing powers. Consultation with traditional healers, prayer or laying-on of hands, or other culturally based strategies may be utilized as a primary source or as a supplement to more traditional Western-based medicine practices such as drug therapy. The nurse's understanding of the patient's trust in alternative healers is important. The more nurses know about the various cultural beliefs, the better support and guidance they can provide to patients.

Pharmacogenetic Factors

11.3 Pharmacogenetics can reveal important information about a drug's safety and effectiveness.

The field of **pharmacogenomics**, the study of how genes influence a person's response to drugs, has made incredible progress over the past decade. The goal of pharmacogenomics is to identify genetic variants that may require prescribing action to impact the success of drug therapy. It is expected that this type of data will someday allow drug therapy that is customized for each individual patient based on his or her genetic profile, as illustrated in Figure 11.1. The following are examples of actions that may be taken, based on the results of pharmacogenetic testing:

- The dose of a drug may need to be increased to achieve the desired therapeutic outcome.
- The dose of a drug may need to be decreased to avoid a serious adverse effect.
- An alternative drug should be substituted to prevent a toxic reaction or a fatal response.

Pharmacogenetic testing is now widely available for some (but not all) medications. Because of the high cost, testing is usually reserved for medications with a high potential risk, when determining the proper dose (or an alternative drug) is essential to patient safety or therapeutic success. In known cases of significant gene–drug interactions, the U.S. Food and Drug Administration (FDA) has included this information in the drug label.

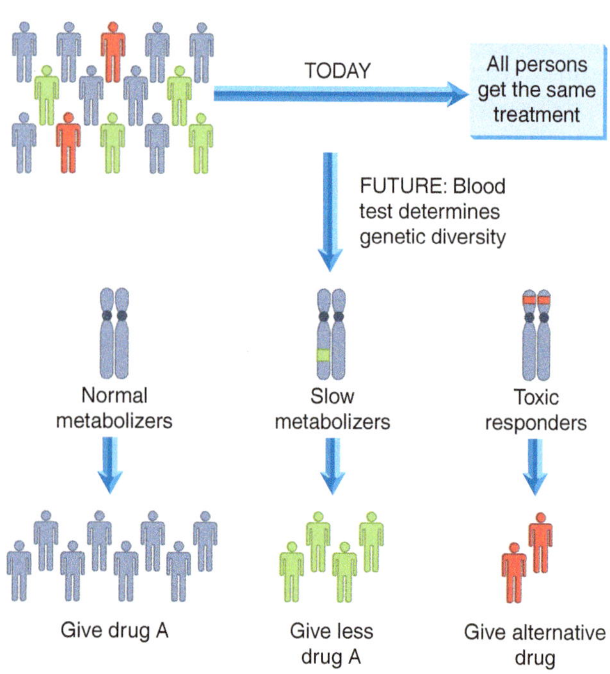

Figure 11.1 Pharmacogenomics and the future of pharmacotherapy.

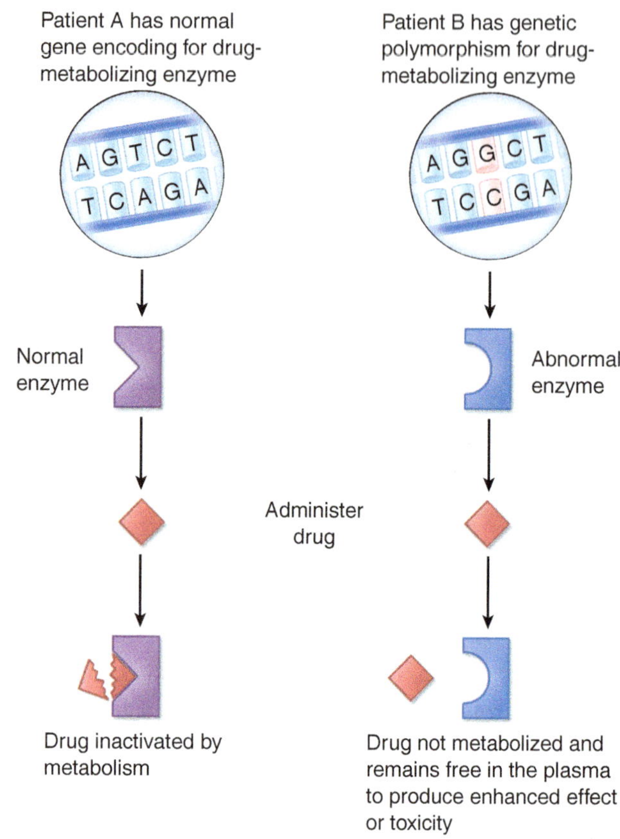

Figure 11.2 Consequences of genetic polymorphisms.

Pharmacogenetic testing has required intervention from the FDA to ensure test results and claims are based on sound science (FDA, 2020a). The FDA now maintains a website where current information is available on specific pharmacogenetic testing and the guidelines for interpretation of the results.

What are the mechanisms by which genetic variations, called **polymorphisms**, result in changes in an individual's drug responses? Some of these possible mechanisms were presented in Chapter 3, Section 3.5. A genetic variant occurs when a mutation occurs in the portion of the DNA that encodes for a certain protein. This produces two or more versions of the same protein (essentially a "normal" protein and an "abnormal protein"), as shown in Figure 11.2. The abnormal protein can alter:

- Enzymes that metabolize drugs (deactivation of the drug)
- Enzymes that convert a drug to a more active form (activation of a prodrug)
- Target molecules (e.g., inability or enhanced ability for a drug to bind to its receptor)
- Immune responses to drugs (e.g., hypersensitivity)

As a well-known example, over 100 different genetic variants have been discovered in the enzyme acetyltransferase, which metabolizes (deactivates) isoniazid (INH), a drug prescribed for tuberculosis. The altered form of the enzyme performs its metabolic process, known as acetylation, more slowly in people who have this mutation. The reduced acetylation can cause INH to accumulate in the blood to toxic levels. These patients, who are frequently Whites or African Americans, are known as slow acetylators. In contrast, mutations in many people of Japanese descent have a genetic variant of this enzyme that results in *rapid* acetylation. These patients will inactivate the drug so quickly that it will not produce a therapeutic effect (Ma, Woo, & Mcleod, 2002).

Another well-researched example involves the narcotic analgesic codeine. Codeine is a prodrug that is metabolized by hepatic microsomal enzyme CYP2D6 to morphine, a much more potent and potentially dangerous analgesic. More than other groups, people of Asian and African descent may carry genetic mutations that impair the action of CYPD26. These variants, called poor metabolizers, will experience less (or no) analgesic effect because codeine is not metabolized to morphine. On the other hand, a percentage of North Africans and Arabs have a variant that makes them ultra-rapid metabolizers. These patients may experience severe or life-threatening toxicity after normal codeine doses due to the formation of large amounts of morphine (Dean, 2017).

The hundreds of different pharmacogenetic variants vary in their importance to patient safety and in the amount of research evidence supporting their effect on drug therapy (Clinical Pharmacogenetics Implementation Consortium, 2019). Selected examples are shown in Table 11.1. Four levels of importance appear on FDA-approved drug labels. These actions are:

- **Testing required:** The drug label states that genetic testing *should be conducted* before using the drug. This may apply to all patients or only a specific subset of patients.
- **Testing recommended:** The drug label states that genetic testing *should be considered* before using the drug. This implies that either the genetic variant has a more limited effect on patient safety or drug action or that sufficient research has not yet accumulated to require testing.
- **Actionable pharmacogenetics:** This label states that changes in effectiveness, dosage, or metabolism may occur due to a genetic variant. The label may mention a contraindication of the drug for a specific subset of patients, but it does not recommend or require testing.
- **Informative pharmacogenetics:** The label states that some pharmacogenetic data may be available, but that data is not clinically significant enough to change the effectiveness, dosage, or metabolism of the drug.

Table 11.1 Selected Drugs with Safety Recommendations Based on Pharmacogenetic Data

Drug	Testing	Gene	Description
abacavir	Required	*HLA-B*	Higher risk for hypersensitivity reaction
amphetamine	No recommendation	*CYP2D6*	May increase adverse effects in poor metabolizers; consider lower starting dose
aripiprazole	No recommendation	*CYP2D6*	May increase adverse effects in poor metabolizers; consider dosage adjustment
azathioprine	Required	*TPMT*, *NUDT15*	Higher risk for myelosuppression in poor metabolizers
carbamazepine	Required	*HLA-B*	Higher risk for severe skin reactions
clopidogrel	No recommendation	*CYP2C19*	Lower antiplatelet response may increase adverse effects in poor metabolizers; consider alternative drug
codeine	No recommendation	*CYP2D6*	Higher risk for serious adverse effects in ultra-rapid responders
eliglustat	Recommended	*CYP2D6*	Higher systemic drug concentrations cause increased risk for QT prolongation
isoniazid	No recommendation	*NAT*	Higher risk for adverse reactions in poor metabolizers
mercaptopurine	Required	*TPMT*, *NUDT15*	Higher risk for myelosuppression in poor metabolizers
oxcarbazepine	Required	*HLA-B*	Higher risk for severe skin reactions
pimozide	Recommended	*CYP2D6*	Higher systemic drug concentrations in poor metabolizers
siponimod	Required	*CYP2C9*	Higher systemic drug concentrations
tetrabenazine	Recommended	*CYP2D6*	Higher systemic drug concentrations in poor metabolizers
thioguanine	Required	*TPMT*, *NUDT15*	Higher risk for myelosuppression in poor metabolizers
tramadol	No recommendation	*CYP2D6*	Higher systemic drug levels and breast milk metabolites in ultra-rapid metabolizers; breastfeeding not recommended
warfarin	No recommendation	*CYP2C9*, *CYP4F2*, *VKORC1*	Alters systemic dosage requirements; monitor and adjust dosages using INR

Source: Food and Drug Administration. (2020B). Table of Pharmacogenetic Associations. Retrieved from https://www.fda.gov/medical-devices/precision-medicine/table-pharmacogenetic-associations.

CONNECTION Checkpoint 11.2

The best-known genetic variants are those involving hepatic CYP450 enzymes. From what you learned in Chapter 3, explain the type of drug–drug interaction that might occur if drug A induced CYP450 enzymes and drug B was inactivated by the same enzymes.

Gender Influences

11.4 Men and women may respond differently to drugs.

There are well-established differences in the patterns of disease between men and women. Women tend to pay more attention to changes in health patterns and seek healthcare earlier than their male counterparts. However, many women do not seek medical attention for potential cardiac problems because heart disease has traditionally been considered to be a "man's disease." Alzheimer's disease affects both men and women, but studies in various populations have shown that 1.5 to 3 times as many women have the disease. Alzheimer's disease is now recognized as a primary "woman's health issue," along with osteoporosis, breast cancer, and fertility disorders (Escoffery, 2018).

Adherence to the medication regimen of a particular drug class may be influenced by gender because the adverse effects affect only one gender. A common example is certain antihypertensive drugs that produce male impotence. Men may experience strokes if they abruptly stop taking their medication to avoid impotence. Some drugs can cause gynecomastia, an increase in breast size, which can be embarrassing for men. Similarly, certain drugs can cause masculine adverse effects such as hirsutism (abnormal increase in hair growth), which can be a cause of nonadherence in women taking these medications. Also, in women, the estrogen contained in oral contraceptives causes an elevated risk of thromboembolic disorders.

Research has found many examples of differences in drug response between men and women. If males and females contain nearly all the same genes, how can these differences be explained? Although they may have identical genes, the "expression" of the genes differs greatly. For example, both males and females possess the same genes for hepatic metabolic enzymes, but one gender may produce more of a certain enzyme, thus producing a different degree of drug action. An example of a gender difference in a pharmacologic outcome is aspirin, which is more effective at preventing heart attack in men than in women.

PharmFACT

A study of 1750 patients with psoriatic arthritis taking tumor necrosis factor inhibitors showed that males were strongly associated with better treatment outcomes than females. Females also had a much higher withdrawal rate during therapy due to both lack of drug effectiveness and more frequent adverse events (Højgaard et al., 2018).

Some of the gender differences in drug response may be explained by differences in body composition, such as the fat-to-muscle ratio. Cerebral blood flow variances in genders can alter patient response to specific analgesics. An example is the benzodiazepines given for anxiety. Women experience slower elimination rates and this difference becomes more significant if a woman is concurrently taking oral contraceptives.

In the past, the majority of drug research studies were conducted using only male participants. These studies assumed that there were no differences between genders and conclusions would apply to both women and men. Current research, however, recognizes that gender differences in drug response may exist, and new drug development research now includes both males and females, as appropriate. Gender consideration is necessary in the analyses of clinical data and assessment of potential pharmacokinetic and pharmacodynamic differences.

Understanding Chapter 11

Key Concepts Summary

11.1 Many psychosocial influences impact pharmacotherapy.

11.2 Cultural and ethnic variables can influence pharmacotherapy.

11.3 Pharmacogenetics can reveal important information about drug safety and effectiveness.

11.4 Men and women may respond differently to drugs.

CASE STUDY: Making the Patient Connection

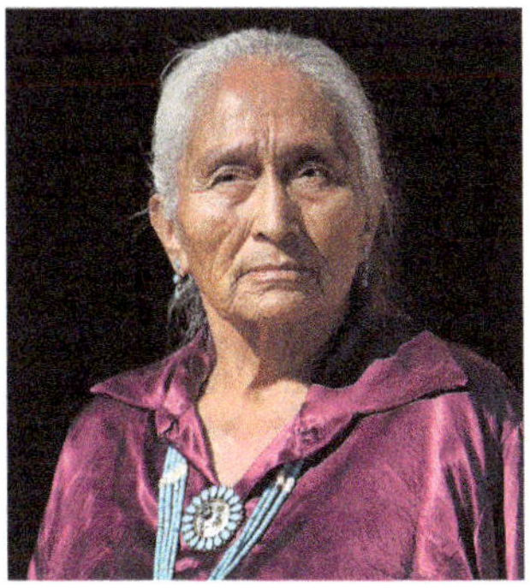

Remember the patient "Aponi Nampeyo" at the beginning of the chapter? Now read the remainder of the case study. Based on the information presented within this chapter, respond to the critical thinking questions that follow.

While traveling out of state with her husband to visit her children and grandchildren, Aponi Nampeyo became ill and was hospitalized. After being examined in the emergency department, she was diagnosed with appendicitis and underwent an emergency appendectomy. Aponi is a native of the United States and has lived most of her life in Arizona. She is well educated but she is not overly talkative and is comfortable with silence.

Aponi willingly accepts Western medical treatments. However, she also relies on traditional herbs and remedies from her youth. As the nurse caring for this patient, you are curious about her culture and health practices. However, you do not want to appear nosy or intrusive.

Critical Thinking Questions

1. Should nurses discuss cultural beliefs with patients? Explain your answer.
2. Describe how the nurse could learn about Mrs. Nampeyo's culture.
3. Are most healthcare workers culturally competent? Why? Why not?

Additional Case Study

Marjorie, a 30-year-old woman, is a single parent with three small children. She works as a self-employed housekeeper and earns minimum wage. Her annual income is $25,600, which pays for her family's housing, groceries, bus transportation, and clothing. Marjorie needs a job that pays benefits such as medical insurance. However, she fears that she will not be able to secure one because she never finished high school. She is constantly trying to save money. She has just been diagnosed with diabetes and requires insulin therapy.

1. Is it likely that Marjorie will be able to adequately care for her diabetes?
2. List the psychosocial factors that will influence this patient's ability to adhere to the therapy for her diabetes.
3. What can the nurse do to help this patient?

Chapter Review

1. In initiating holistic care with a patient who has chronic headaches, which action would the nurse take?
   1. Tell the patient to take Tylenol as directed on the label.
   2. Ask the patient what he or she believes may be contributing to the problem.
   3. Monitor the patient's pupil response to light.
   4. Refer the patient to an ophthalmologist for an eye exam.
2. Various psychosocial variables may influence nonadherence to pharmacotherapy. An example of this would occur when the patient reports that the prescribed drug:
   1. Produces an unpleasant aftertaste.
   2. Is a very large tablet and difficult to swallow.
   3. Is too expensive for the patient to afford.
   4. Potentially causes hepatotoxicity.
3. A patient of Native American descent states, "I will only take medications that are approved by the Shaman." The nurse understands that this statement reflects the patient's:
   1. Ethnicity.
   2. Cultural belief.
   3. Genetic polymorphisms.
   4. Health-related bias.

4. A patient is known to have a genetic variant that causes slow acetylation. If this patient must start on isoniazid (INH), a drug that is metabolized by acetyltransferase, what is a likely outcome?
    1. The patient will be more prone to drug toxicity.
    2. The patient will require more time to absorb enteral medications.
    3. The patient must be given liquid medication forms only.
    4. The patient should be advised to decrease protein intake.
5. Which of the following is considered a gender factor that may influence effective pharmacotherapy? (Select all that apply.)
    1. Fat-to-muscle ratio
    2. Cerebral blood flow
    3. Limited drug research on females
    4. Health beliefs
    5. Dietary considerations
6. Which is the most effective method for a nurse to recognize patient-specific genetic influences?
    1. Ask the patient if there have been drug–dose-related problems in the past.
    2. Consult reference books and the internet for information.
    3. Observe the effects with other patients of similar racial-ethnic background.
    4. Be cautious with all drugs and observe for individual patient responses.

See Appendix A for answers to critical thinking questions, case study questions and review questions.

References

Clinical Pharmacogenetics Implementation Consortium. (2019). *Genes-Drugs.* https://cpicpgx.org/genes-drugs/

Dean, L. (2017) Codeine therapy and CYP2D6 genotype. In *Medical Genetics Summaries.* National Institutes of Health. https://www.ncbi.nlm.nih.gov/books/NBK100662/

Escoffery, C. (2018). Gender similarities and differences for e-health behaviors among U.S. adults. *Telemedicine Journal and e-Health, 24,* 335–343. doi:10.1089/tmj.2017.0136

Højgaard, P., Ballegaard, C., Cordtz, R., Zobbe, K., Clausen, M., Glintborg, B., et al. (2018). Gender differences in biologic treatment outcomes—a study of 1750 patients with psoriatic arthritis using Danish Health Care Registers. *Rheumatology, 57*(9), 1651–1660. https://doi.org/10.1093/rheumatology/key140

Ma, M. K., Woo, M. H., & Mcleod, H. L. (2002). Genetic basis of drug metabolism. *American journal of health-system pharmacy, 59*(21), 2061–2069.

Ogden, J. (2016). Religious constraints on prescribing medications. *Prescriber, 27*(12), 47–51.

U.S. Department of Health and Human Services, Office of Minority Health. (2019). *Profile: American Indian/Alaska Native.* https://minorityhealth.hhs.gov/omh/browse.aspx?lvl=4&lvlid=38

U.S. Food and Drug Administration. (2020a). *FDA announces collaborative review of scientific evidence to support associations between genetic information and specific medications.* https://www.fda.gov/news-events/press-announcements/fda-announces-collaborative-review-scientific-evidence-support-associations-between-genetic

U.S. Food and Drug Administration. (2020b). *Table of pharmacogenetic associations.* https://www.fda.gov/medical-devices/precision-medicine/table-pharmacogenetic-associations

Selected Bibliography

Collins, S. L., Carr, D. F., & Pirmohamed, M. (2016). Advances in the pharmacogenomics of adverse drug reactions. *Drug Safety, 39,* 15–27. https://doi.org/10.1007/s40264-015-0367-8

Fulton, C. R., Swart, M., De Luca, T., Liu, S. N., Collins, K. S., Desta, Z., et al. (2018). Pharmacogenetics and practice: Tailoring prescribing for safety and effectiveness. *Journal for Nurse Practitioners, 14*(10), 697–704. https://doi.org/10.1016/j.nurpra.2018.09.021

Johannessen Landmark, C., & Johannessen, S. I. (2016). Pharmacotherapy in epilepsy—does gender affect safety? *Expert Opinion on Drug Safety, 15,* 1–4. https://doi.org/10.1517/14740338.2016.1117606

Kautzky-Willer, A., & Harreiter, J. (2017). Sex and gender differences in therapy of type 2 diabetes. *Diabetes Research and Clinical Practice, 131,* 230–241. https://doi.org/10.1016/j.diabres.2017.07.012

Kazdin, A. E. (2017). Addressing the treatment gap: A key challenge for extending evidence-based psychosocial interventions. *Behaviour Research and Therapy*, *88*, 7–18. https://doi.org/10.1016/j.brat.2016.06.004

Krau, S. D. (2016). The role of pharmacogenomics: The same medications do not work the same on everyone. *Nursing Clinics*, *51*, ix–x. https://doi.org/10.1016/j.cnur.2015.12.002

Orlando, V., Mucherino, S., Guarino, I., Guerriero, F., Trama, U., & Menditto, E. (2020). Gender differences in medication use: A drug utilization study based on real world data. *International Journal of Environmental Research and Public Health*, *17*(11), 3926. https://doi.org/10.3390/ijerph17113926

Parve, J., Carlile, J., & Parve, J. (2019). Pharmacogenetic testing in primary care. *The Nurse Practitioner*, *44*(10), 44–49. https://doi.org/10.1097/01.NPR.0000580780.66980.85

Sesel, A. L., Sharpe, L., & Naismith, S. L. (2018). Efficacy of psychosocial interventions for people with multiple sclerosis: A meta-analysis of specific treatment effects. *Psychotherapy and Psychosomatics*, *87*(2), 105–111. https://doi.org/10.1159/000486806

Weitzel, K. W., Duong, B. Q., Arwood, M. J., Owusu-Obeng, A., Abul-Husn, N. S., Bernhardt, B. A., et al. (2019). A stepwise approach to implementing pharmacogenetic testing in the primary care setting. *Pharmacogenomics*, *20*(15), 1103–1112. https://doi.org/10.2217/pgs-2019-0053

Youssef, E., Buck, J., & Wright, D. (2020). Understanding pharmacogenomic testing and its role in medicine prescribing. *Nursing Standard*. https://doi.org/10.7748/ns.2020.e11543

Unit 3

Pharmacology of the Autonomic Nervous System

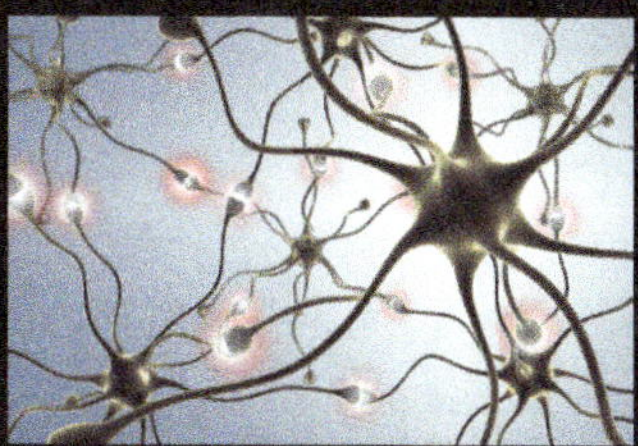
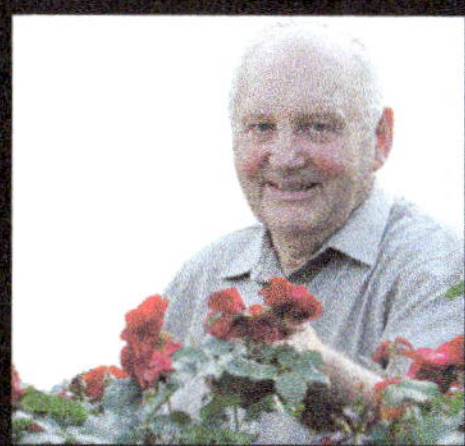
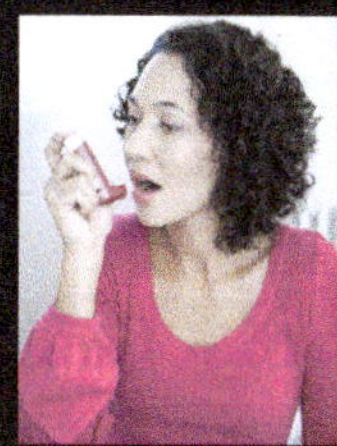
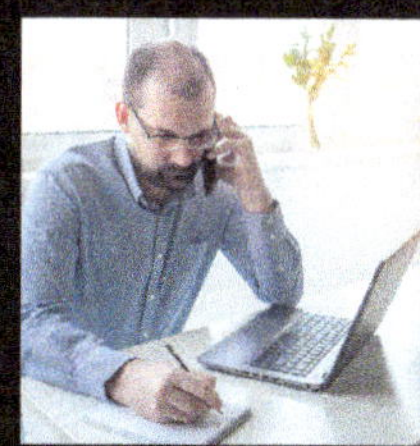

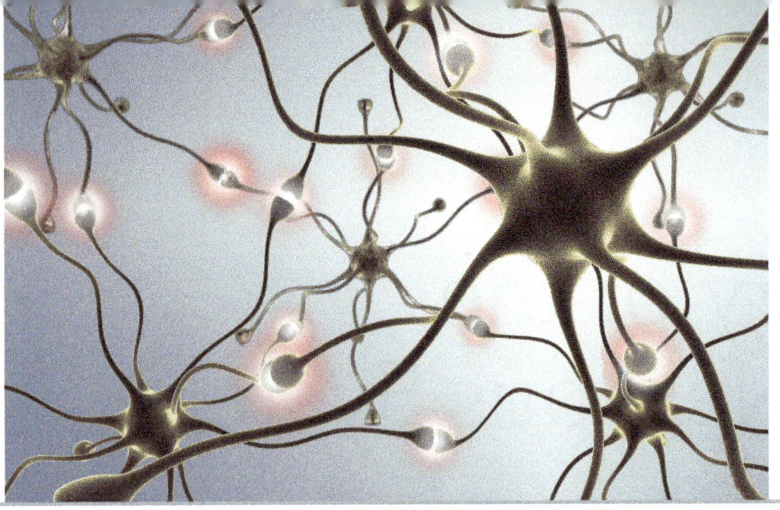

Chapter 12
Review of Neurotransmitters and the Autonomic Nervous System

Chapter Outline

Learning Outcomes

After reading this chapter, the student should be able to:

1. Distinguish between the functions of the central and peripheral nervous systems.
2. Compare and contrast the two divisions of the peripheral nervous system.
3. Compare and contrast the actions of the sympathetic and parasympathetic divisions of the autonomic nervous system.
4. Explain the process of synaptic transmission.
5. Explain mechanisms by which drugs affect synaptic transmission.
6. Describe the actions of acetylcholine at cholinergic synapses.
7. Describe the actions of norepinephrine at adrenergic synapses.
8. Compare the actions of the adrenal medulla with those of other sympathetic effector organs.
9. Explain how higher centers in the brain can influence autonomic function.
10. Design a method for classifying autonomic drugs based on which receptors are affected.

Key Terms

Definitions of the terms in bold may be found in the Glossary.

Neuropharmacology represents one of the largest, most complicated, and least understood branches of pharmacology. Nervous system drugs are used to treat a large and diverse set of conditions, including pain, anxiety, depression, schizophrenia, insomnia, and seizures. Through their action on nerves, these medications are used to treat disorders affecting other body systems such as abnormalities in heart rate and rhythm, hypertension, glaucoma, asthma, and even a runny nose.

Traditionally, the study of neuropharmacology begins with the autonomic nervous system. This is because autonomic physiology lays the foundation for understanding nervous, cardiovascular, and respiratory pharmacology. This chapter serves two purposes. First, it provides a concise review of autonomic nervous system physiology. Second, it introduces the four fundamental classes of autonomic medications, which are presented in depth in Chapters 13 through 16.

Overview of the Nervous System

12.1 The two major subdivisions of the nervous system are the central nervous system and the peripheral nervous system.

The nervous system is the master controller of most activities occurring within the body. Compared to the other major regulator, the endocrine system, the nervous system has the ability to act instantaneously to maintain homeostasis. The brain, spinal cord, and peripheral nerves act as a smoothly integrated whole to accomplish rapid, continuous changes in essential functions such as heart rate, blood pressure, pupil size, and intestinal movement. The fundamental functions of the nervous system are to:

- *Monitor* the internal and external environment of the body and alert the brain of important changes.
- *Process* and integrate the environmental changes that are perceived and determine an appropriate response.
- *Respond* to the environmental changes by producing an action or a response.

The nervous system has two major divisions: the central nervous system (CNS) and the peripheral nervous system. The CNS is made up of the brain and spinal cord, whereas the peripheral division consists of spinal nerves that carry messages to and from the CNS. Drugs used to treat disorders and conditions of the CNS are discussed in Chapters 17 through 26. The functional divisions of the nervous system are illustrated in Figure 12.1.

12.2 The peripheral nervous system is divided into somatic and autonomic components.

With its immense potential and complexity, the human brain requires a continuous flow of information to accomplish its functions. In addition, the brain would be useless without a means to carry out its commands. The peripheral nervous system provides the brain the means to communicate with and receive sensory messages from the outside world.

Neurons in the peripheral nervous system *recognize* changes to the environment (sensory division) and *respond* to those changes by moving muscles or secreting chemicals (motor division). The sensory division consists of specialized nerves that recognize touch, pain, heat, body position, light, or specific chemicals in body fluids. These sensory neurons send their messages to the spinal cord. Based on this information, the brain prioritizes the messages, determines whether an action is needed, and plans an appropriate response.

The motor division is divided into two components. The **somatic nervous system** consists of nerves that provide for the *voluntary* control of skeletal muscle. The nerves of the **autonomic nervous system (ANS)** provide for the *involuntary* control of vital functions of the cardiovascular, digestive, respiratory, and genitourinary systems. The ANS controls vital life activities without people being aware of its functions. The three main activities of the ANS are:

- Contraction of smooth muscle of the bronchi, blood vessels, gastrointestinal (GI) tract, eye, and genitourinary tract
- Contraction of cardiac muscle
- Secretion of salivary, sweat, gastric, and bronchial glands.

The ANS is particularly important to pharmacology because a large number of medications affect autonomic nerves. Some of these drug actions produce desirable, therapeutic effects, whereas others produce adverse effects. The remainder of this chapter reviews the structure and function of this complex system.

Structure and Function of the Autonomic Nervous System

12.3 The autonomic nervous system is divided into two mostly opposing components: the sympathetic and parasympathetic branches.

The ANS has two distinct divisions: the *sympathetic* nervous system and the *parasympathetic* nervous system. Most organs and glands receive nerves from both branches, and the two divisions have opposing actions. For example, one branch causes cardiac muscle to contract faster and with greater force; the other causes it to relax. The ultimate action of the cardiac muscle, smooth muscle, or gland depends on which branch is sending the most signals at any given time. The major actions of the two divisions are shown

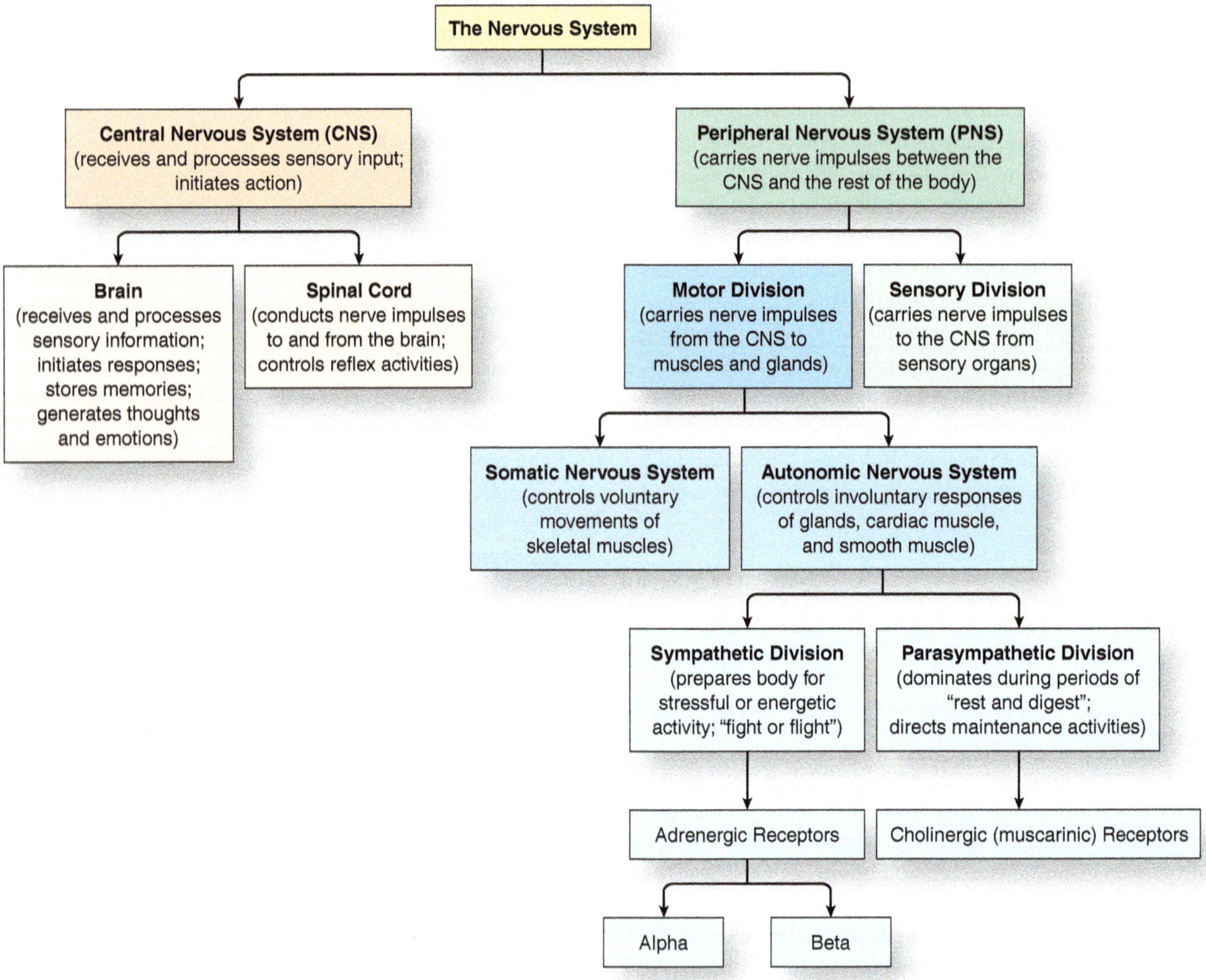

Figure 12.1 Functional divisions of the nervous system.

in Figure 12.2. It is essential for the student to learn these actions early in the study of pharmacology because knowledge of autonomic effects is used to predict the actions and adverse effects of many drugs.

The **sympathetic nervous system** is activated under emergency conditions or stress and produces a set of actions called the **fight-or-flight response**. Activation of this branch prepares the body for heightened activity and for an immediate response to a threat. The brain experiences an increase in alertness and readiness. Heart rate and blood pressure increase and blood is shunted to skeletal muscles, thus preparing the body for sudden, intense physical activity. The liver immediately produces more glucose for energy. The bronchi dilate to allow maximum airflow into the lungs, and breathing becomes faster and deeper. The pupils dilate to provide better vision for dealing with the emergency. The body warms and perspiration increases. At the same time the body is preparing for the threat, nonemergency maintenance functions such as peristalsis and urine formation are temporarily reduced.

The **parasympathetic nervous system** is activated under less stressful conditions and produces a set of actions known as **rest-and-digest responses**, which promote relaxation and body maintenance activities. Digestive secretions increase, peristalsis propels substances along the alimentary canal, and defecation is promoted. Heart rate and blood pressure decline. Because less air is needed, the bronchi constrict and respiration slows. The student should notice that the actions of the parasympathetic division are opposite to those of the sympathetic division.

Under most conditions, the two branches of the ANS cooperate to achieve a balance of readiness and relaxation. Because they have opposite effects, homeostasis may be achieved by changing one or both branches. For example, heart rate can be increased by either increasing the firing of sympathetic nerves or by decreasing the firing of

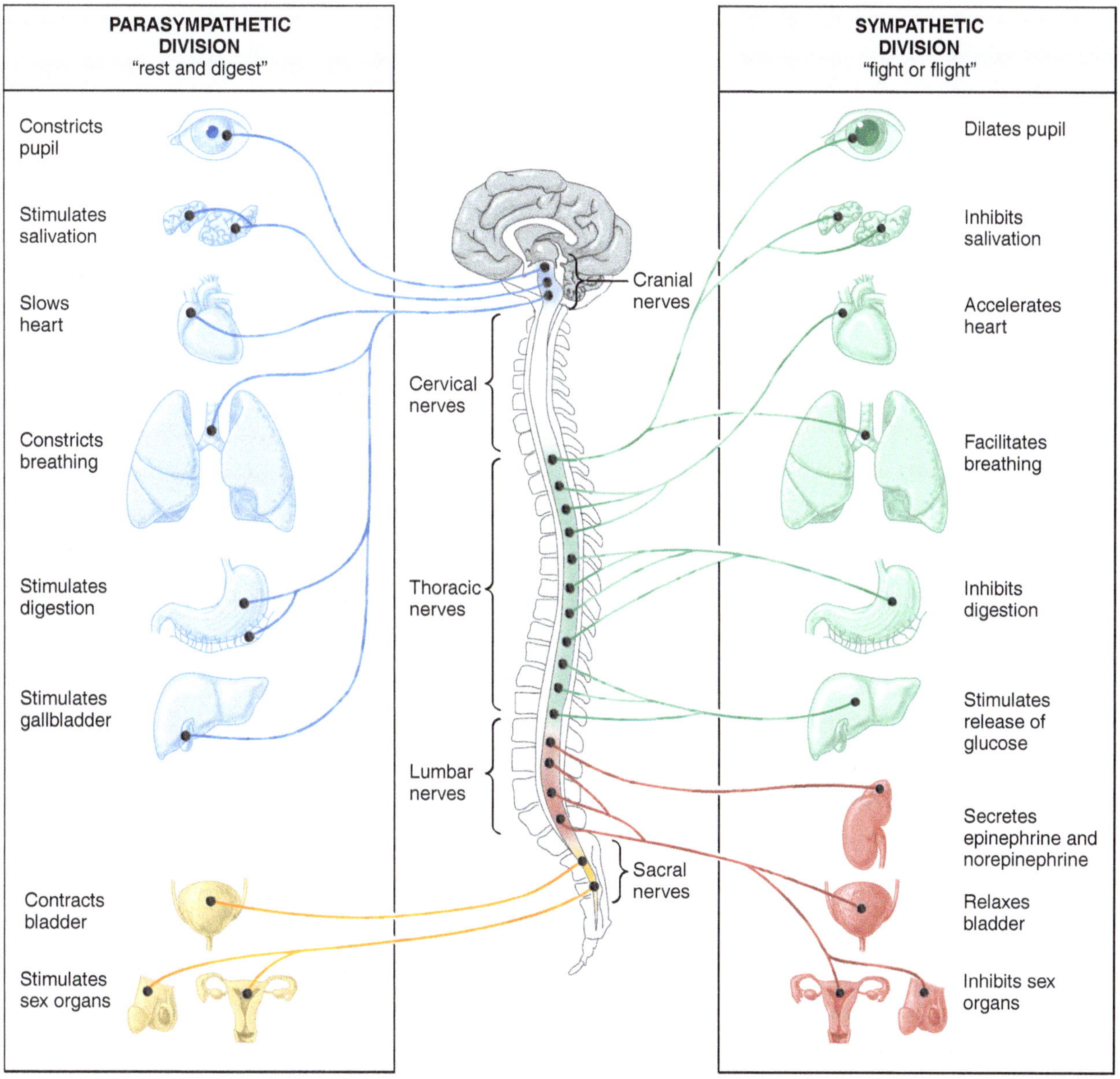

Figure 12.2 Effects of the sympathetic and parasympathetic nervous systems.

parasympathetic nerves. This allows the body to fine-tune its essential organ systems.

Some degree of autonomic activity is always occurring even in the absence of stimuli. This background level of activity is known as **autonomic tone**. For example, sympathetic nerves are constantly firing, keeping arterioles in a constant state of constriction. This sympathetic tone allows for faster changes in blood pressure because the vessels are in a constant state of readiness. On the other hand, parasympathetic tone on the smooth muscle of the alimentary and urinary tracts maintains continuous contractions and keeps intestinal peristalsis and urine flow steady. With the important exception of the vascular system, the predominant tone of autonomic tissues is from the parasympathetic nervous system.

The sympathetic and parasympathetic divisions do not always have opposite effects. For example, the constriction of arterioles is controlled entirely by the sympathetic branch. Sympathetic stimulation causes constriction of arterioles, whereas lack of stimulation causes vasodilation. Only sympathetic nerves control the adrenal medulla and the sweat glands. The sympathetic division is also solely responsible for the release of renin by the kidneys, an action that increases blood pressure. Metabolic effects such as increases in blood glucose and mobilization of lipids for energy are uniquely sympathetic functions. In the male reproductive system, the roles are complementary. Erection of the penis is a function of the parasympathetic division, and the sympathetic branch controls ejaculation.

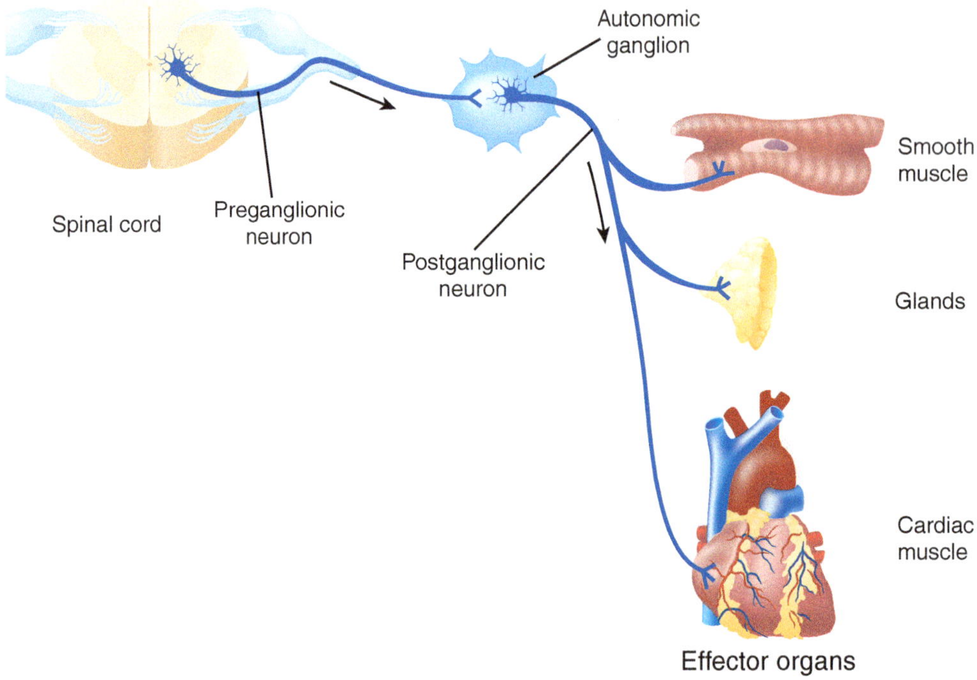

Figure 12.3 Basic structure of an autonomic pathway.

Synaptic Transmission

12.4 Synaptic transmission allows information to be communicated between two nerves or from nerves to muscles or glands.

For information to be transmitted throughout the nervous system, neurons must communicate with each other and with muscles and glands. The basic unit of the ANS is a two-neuron chain. The first neuron, called the preganglionic neuron, originates in the CNS. The preganglionic neuron connects with the second nerve outside the CNS in structures called **ganglia**. A ganglion (singular of *ganglia*) contains the cell body of the postganglionic neuron, which is waiting to receive the action potential. The basic structure of an autonomic pathway is shown in Figure 12.3.

Before the message can be communicated from one nerve to another, however, it must cross the **synapse**, a physical space between the two neurons. The transfer of the message from one cell to another, or synaptic transmission, utilizes chemical messengers called **neurotransmitters**. It is important to study the details of synaptic transmission because a large number of drugs affect this process. The process of synaptic transmission is illustrated in Pharmacotherapy Illustrated 12.1.

The second (postganglionic) neuron terminates on smooth muscle, cardiac muscle, or a gland at a specialized synapse called the **neuroeffector junction**. Synaptic transmission across the neuroeffector junction occurs in several steps.

1. Synthesis of the neurotransmitter. The neurotransmitter is synthesized in the cell body of the neuron or in the axon terminal where the synapse is located. Over 50 different neurotransmitters have been identified, the most common of which are shown in Table 12.1. Each neurotransmitter is associated with a unique set of functions and responses. The two primary neurotransmitters of the ANS are **norepinephrine (NE)** and **acetylcholine (ACh)**.
2. Storage of the neurotransmitter. Because nerve impulses travel rapidly from neuron to neuron, there must be an ample and continuous supply of the neurotransmitter. At the terminal ends of each axon lie millions of granules or vesicles loaded with neurotransmitters, waiting for an action potential to release them.
3. Release of the neurotransmitter. When the nerve impulse reaches the end of the axon, it stimulates vesicles to release their stored neurotransmitter into the synapse. The neurotransmitter enters the **synaptic cleft**, which must be bridged for the impulse to reach the postganglionic neuron or organ.
4. Binding to the receptor. The neurotransmitter diffuses across the synaptic cleft to reach receptors waiting on the surface of the postsynaptic cell. There is a brief delay in impulse conduction of about 0.2 to 0.5 msec for the neurotransmitter to cross the synapse. Once the neurotransmitter binds to its receptor, the message is conveyed to the postsynaptic cell. The neurotransmitter induces the target muscle cell, glandular cell, or another neuron tissue to elicit its characteristic response.

Pharmacotherapy Illustrated **12.1**

Synaptic Transmission

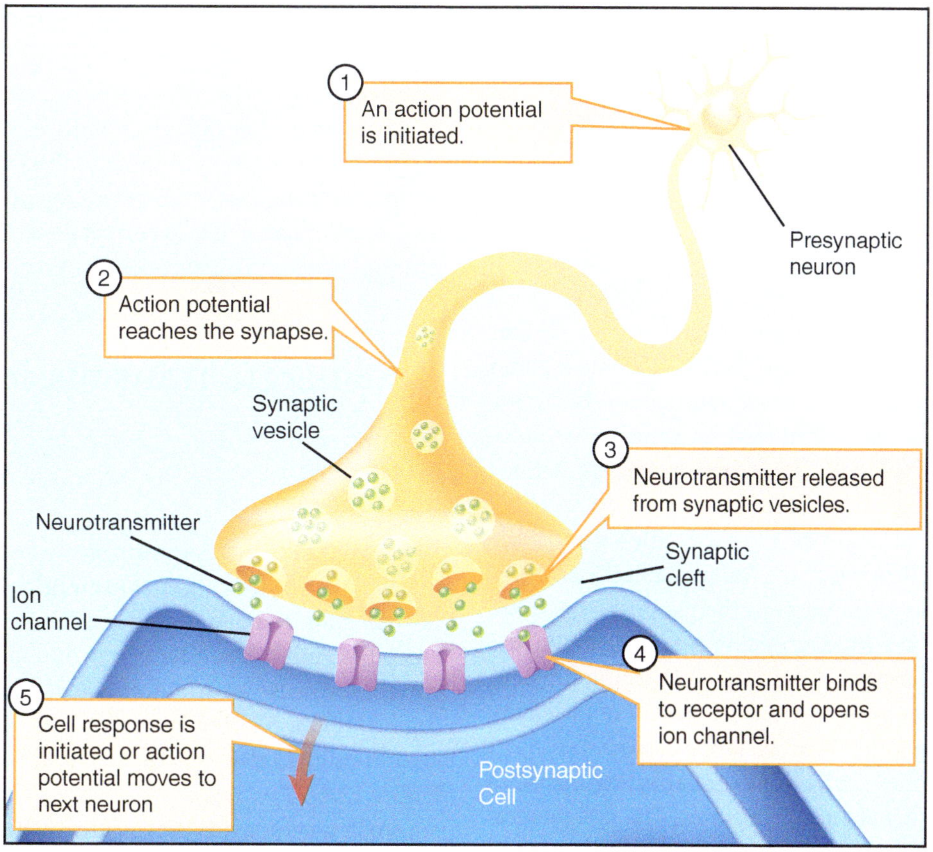

Generally, the more neurotransmitter released into the synapse, the more intense and longer lasting the response.

5. Termination of neurotransmitter action. Once the message is transmitted, the neuron and the effector cell must quickly return to baseline conditions and ready themselves for future messages. This is accomplished by removal of the neurotransmitter. The neurotransmitter is either degraded in the synaptic cleft by enzymes, or it diffuses back into the preganglionic neuron, thus stopping the action of the muscle or gland.

Table 12.1 Selected Neurotransmitters and Their Receptors: Effects and Clinical Applications

Neurotransmitter	Primary Locations of Receptors	Clinical Application (Chapter Number)
Acetylcholine	Synapses throughout the CNS; preganglionic neurons ending in the ganglia in both the sympathetic and parasympathetic nervous systems (nicotinic); postganglionic neurons ending in neuroeffector target tissues in the parasympathetic nervous system (muscarinic)	Alzheimer's disease (21); myasthenia gravis (13)
Dopamine	Limbic system and hypothalamus; some sympathetic ganglia	Attention-deficit/hyperactivity disorder (24); Parkinson's disease (21); psychoses (20)
Gamma aminobutyric acid (GABA)	Throughout the CNS	Anesthesia (26); anxiety (18); seizures (22)
Glutamate	Throughout the CNS	Seizures (22)
Nitric oxide	CNS, adrenal gland, and nerves to the penis	Impotence (71)
Norepinephrine	Throughout the CNS; most neuroeffector target junctions in the sympathetic nervous system	Attention-deficit/hyperactivity disorder (24); cocaine and amphetamine abuse (27); depression (19)
Serotonin (5-HT)	Limbic system and hypothalamus; primary neurotransmitter in the extrapyramidal system; GI tract	Anxiety (18); depression (19); nausea and vomiting (60); psychoses (20)
Substance P	Pain pathways in the spinal cord; brain and sensory neurons	Analgesia (25)

Conduction of action potentials in the ANS is much slower than in the somatic nervous system. Because somatic nerves are myelinated and have no ganglia, impulses more quickly reach their target tissues. Autonomic messages must cross the synaptic cleft, and postganglionic nerves are unmyelinated, which slows the action potential.

12.5 Autonomic drugs exert their effects by acting at synapses.

The student may be wondering why it is necessary to learn ANS anatomy and physiology in such depth. The reason is that a large number of drugs act by altering neurotransmitter activity in the ANS. Some medications are identical to endogenous neurotransmitters or have a very similar chemical structure and are able to directly activate a gland or muscle. Other drugs are used to stimulate or block the actions of natural neurotransmitters. A firm grasp of autonomic physiology is essential to understanding the actions and adverse effects of hundreds of drugs.

The two-neuron chain of the ANS allows multiple locations at which drugs can act. Some medications affect the outflow of nervous impulses at their source—the CNS. A second potential site for drug action is at the ganglia, the synapse where the preganglionic and postganglionic neurons meet. Yet a third possible site is at the end of the chain, at the neuroeffector junction of the target organs.

Although complex, actions of drugs affecting this ANS can be grouped into just a few categories. The five general mechanisms by which drugs affect synaptic transmission in the ANS are as follows:

- Medications may affect the *synthesis* of the neurotransmitter in the preganglionic nerve. Drugs that decrease neurotransmitter synthesis inhibit autonomic responses. Those that increase neurotransmitter synthesis have the opposite effect.
- Medications can prevent the *storage* of the neurotransmitter in vesicles within the preganglionic nerve. Prevention of neurotransmitter storage inhibits autonomic actions.
- Medications can influence the *release* of the neurotransmitter from the preganglionic nerve. Promoting neurotransmitter release stimulates autonomic responses, whereas preventing neurotransmitter release has the opposite effect.
- Medications can bind to the *neurotransmitter receptors* on the postganglionic cell. Drugs that bind to receptors and stimulate the cell will increase autonomic responses. Those that attach to the postganglionic cell and prevent the natural neurotransmitter from reaching its receptors will inhibit autonomic actions.
- Medications can *prevent the destruction or reuptake* of the neurotransmitter. These drugs cause the neurotransmitter to remain in the synapse for a longer time and will stimulate autonomic actions.

It is important to understand that autonomic drugs are rarely given to correct physiologic defects in the ANS itself. Compared to other body systems, the ANS has remarkably little disease. Rather, medications are used to stimulate or inhibit target organs or glands of the ANS, such as the heart, lungs, or digestive tract. With few exceptions, the disorder lies in the target organ, not the ANS. Thus, when an autonomic drug is administered, the goal is not to treat an autonomic disease; it is to correct disorders of target organs through its effects on autonomic nerves.

Cholinergic Transmission

12.6 Acetylcholine is the neurotransmitter released at cholinergic receptors, which may be nicotinic or muscarinic.

ACh was the first neurotransmitter to be identified. Neurons releasing ACh are called **cholinergic** nerves. Located on postganglionic or neuroeffector cell membranes, cholinergic receptors bind ACh and either continue the impulse (at the ganglia) or cause an autonomic action (at the neuroeffector organ). When reading the following sections, the student should refer to the sites of ACh and NE action shown in Figure 12.4.

ACh is synthesized in the preganglionic nerve terminal and stored in synaptic vesicles. A preganglionic neuron may contain 300,000 vesicles, each housing as many as 50,000 ACh molecules. When an action potential reaches the nerve terminal, a brief burst of ACh is released into the synaptic cleft, where it diffuses across to attach to its receptors on the postganglionic cell.

Cholinergic Receptors and Neurotransmitters

Two types of cholinergic receptors bind ACh. These are named after certain chemicals that bind to them:

- **Nicotinic receptors.** Located at preganglionic neurons ending in the ganglia in both the sympathetic and parasympathetic nervous systems
- **Muscarinic receptors.** Located at postganglionic neurons ending in neuroeffector target tissues in the parasympathetic nervous system.

Early research on laboratory animals found that the actions of ACh at the ganglia resembled those of nicotine, the active chemical in tobacco products. Because of this similarity, receptors for ACh in the ganglia are called **nicotinic** receptors. Nicotinic receptors are also found in skeletal

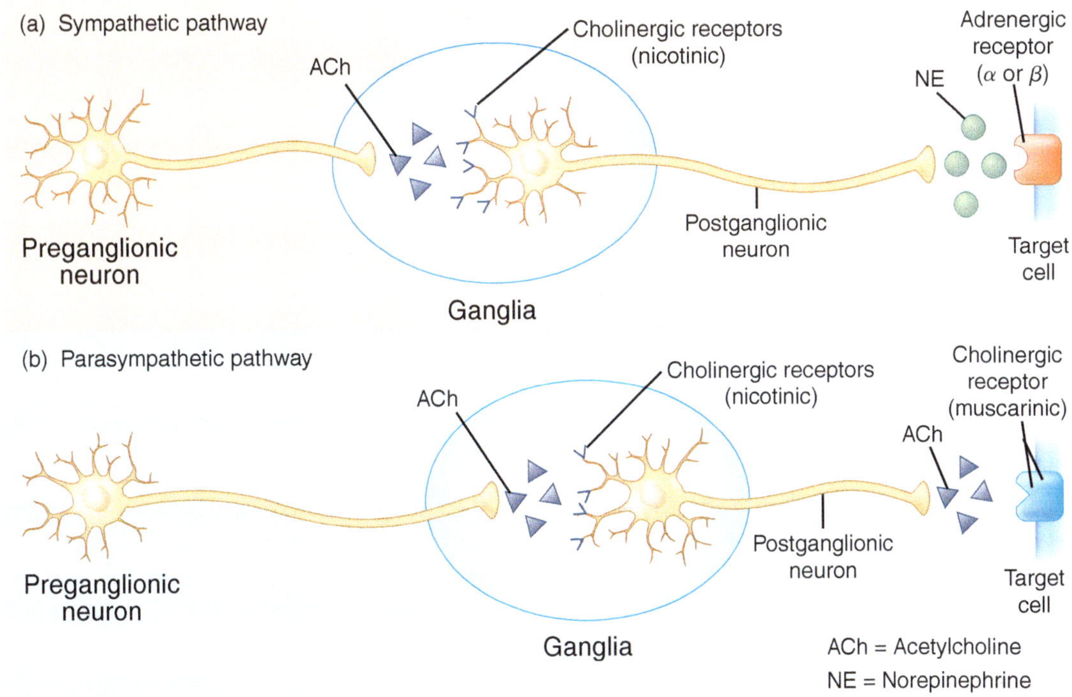

Figure 12.4 Receptors in the autonomic nervous system. (a) Sympathetic pathway: ACh is released at the ganglia (nicotinic receptor) and NE at the effector organ (adrenergic receptor). (b) Parasympathetic pathway: ACh is released at both the ganglia (nicotinic receptor) and effector organ (cholinergic receptor).

muscle, which is controlled by the somatic nervous system, and in the adrenal medulla. Because nicotinic receptors are present in so many locations, drugs affecting these receptors produce profound effects on both the ANS and somatic nervous system. Activation of ACh nicotinic receptors always produces stimulatory actions. Nicotinic actions include increased sweat production, increased release of adrenal medullary hormones, and enhanced nerve conduction in the ganglia and tachycardia, hypertension, and increased tone and motility in the digestive tract. Although nicotinic receptor blockers were some of the first drugs used to treat hypertension, they are rarely used for this purpose today due to the discovery of safer drugs. The primary current therapeutic application of these drugs is to produce skeletal muscle relaxation (a somatic effect) during surgical procedures. A complete discussion of nicotinic blockers can be found in Chapter 14.

CONNECTION Checkpoint 12.1

Nicotine induces hepatic microsomal (CYP450) enzymes. From what you learned in Chapter 5, how can this induction affect the actions of medications?

Activation of ACh receptors at postganglionic nerve endings in the parasympathetic nervous system results in the classic symptoms of parasympathetic stimulation shown in Figure 12.2. Early research determined that these actions closely resembled those produced after eating the poisonous mushroom *Amanita muscaria*. The active substance in this mushroom is the chemical muscarine; thus, these ACh receptors were named **muscarinic** receptors. Muscarinic receptors are also found in most sweat glands and in blood vessels serving skeletal muscles. The locations of nicotinic and muscarinic receptors are illustrated in Figure 12.4.

Unlike the actions of ACh at nicotinic receptors, which are always stimulatory, ACh action at muscarinic receptors may be stimulatory or inhibitory, depending on the target organ. For example, activation of muscarinic receptors in the heart will *decrease* the heart rate, but activation of muscarinic receptors in the intestine will *increase* peristalsis. Drugs that affect muscarinic receptors have more pharmacologic applications than those affecting nicotinic receptors. Medications that block muscarinic receptors are used during ophthalmic procedures, as preanesthetic drugs, and in the pharmacotherapy of asthma and bradycardia (see Chapter 16).

Although ACh itself can stimulate both muscarinic and nicotinic receptors, some drugs are selective to only one type. Table 12.2 summarizes the types of responses produced by activation of the two types of ACh receptors.

Termination of Acetylcholine Action

The goal of nerve transmission is to produce an immediate, though transient, response. To accomplish this, ACh must be rapidly removed from the synaptic cleft after producing its effect. The enzyme that resides in the synaptic cleft and catalyzes the destruction of ACh is called **acetylcholinesterase**

Table 12.2 Types of Autonomic Receptors

Neuro-transmitter	Receptor	Primary Locations	Selected Responses
Acetylcholine (cholinergic)	Muscarinic	Parasympathetic target organs (other than the heart) Heart	Stimulation of smooth muscle and exocrine gland secretions Decreased heart rate and force of contraction
	Nicotinic	Postganglionic neurons and neuromuscular junctions of skeletal muscle	Stimulation of smooth muscle and gland secretions
Norepinephrine (adrenergic)	Alpha$_1$	All sympathetic target organs except the heart	Constriction of blood vessels; dilation of pupils
	Alpha$_2$	Presynaptic adrenergic nerve terminals	Inhibition of norepinephrine release
	Beta$_1$	Heart and kidneys	Increased heart rate and force of contraction; release of renin
	Beta$_2$	All sympathetic target organs except the heart	Inhibition of smooth muscle contraction

(AChE), or cholinesterase (*Note:* The suffix *-erase* can be thought of as "wiping out" the ACh.) AChE is quite efficient at performing its task. It is estimated that over half the ACh molecules released from the vesicles are destroyed before they have a chance to reach their receptors. Following the breakdown of ACh, choline is re-formed and is taken up by the preganglionic neuron, where it is used to synthesize more ACh. The recycling of ACh in the neuron is shown in Figure 12.5.

Medications can interfere with the lifecycle of ACh. Some drugs (and poisons) can prevent the inactivation of ACh by blocking the acetylcholinesterase enzyme. These drugs will cause a prolonged action of ACh at the synapse. Other medications will prevent ACh from reaching its receptors, thus blocking its actions. Medications that interfere with the lifecycle of ACh are presented in Chapters 13 and 14.

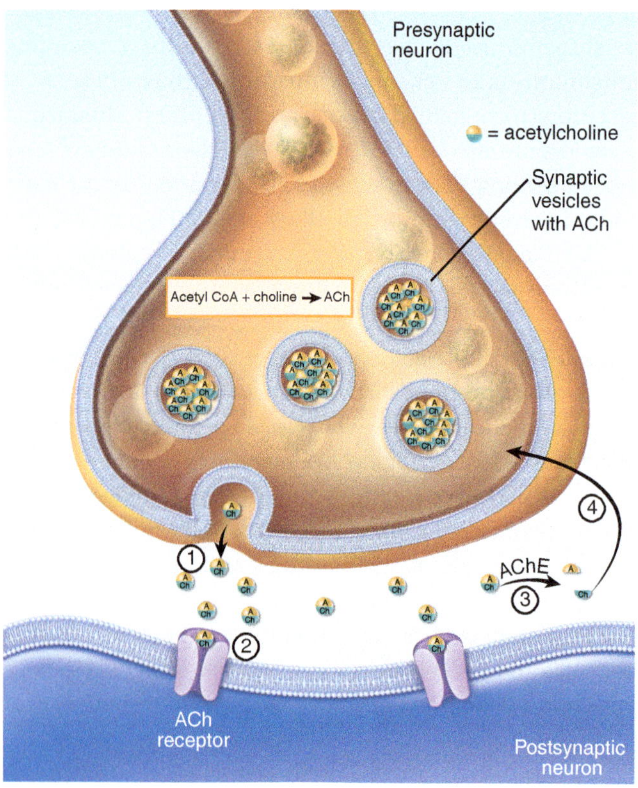

Figure 12.5 Lifecycle of acetylcholine (ACh). (1) ACh is released into the synaptic cleft. (2) ACh binds to receptors on the postsynaptic membrane. (3) ACh is broken down into acetate and choline. (4) Choline is returned to the presynaptic neuron and recycled to make additional ACh.

Pseudocholinesterase, also known as plasma cholinesterase, is another enzyme that destroys ACh. Found primarily in the liver, pseudocholinesterase rapidly inactivates ACh and drugs with a chemical structure similar to ACh as they circulate in the plasma. Some people are born with a genetic deficiency of this enzyme and are unable to inactivate succinylcholine, a surgical drug structurally similar to ACh. These patients are particularly sensitive to the effects of succinylcholine (see Chapter 26).

Adrenergic Transmission

12.7 Norepinephrine is the primary neurotransmitter released at adrenergic receptors, which may be alpha or beta.

In the sympathetic nervous system, NE is the neurotransmitter released at almost all postganglionic nerves. NE belongs to a class of hormones called **catecholamines**, all of which are involved in neurotransmission. Other endogenous catecholamines include epinephrine (adrenalin) and dopamine. The receptors at the ends of postganglionic sympathetic neurons are called **adrenergic**, which is derived from the word *adrenaline*.

NE is synthesized in the nerve terminal and stored in vesicles until an action potential triggers its release into the synaptic cleft. NE then diffuses across the cleft to bind to its receptors on the effector cell.

Adrenergic receptors are of two basic types: alpha (α) and beta (β). These receptors are further divided into the subtypes beta$_1$, beta$_2$, alpha$_1$, and alpha$_2$. Activation of each type of subreceptor results in a characteristic set of physiologic responses, which are summarized in Table 12.2.

PharmFACT

According to Aronson (2000), adrenaline was isolated and identified by John Jacob Abel in 1897, who founded the very first Department of Pharmacology at the University of Michigan. The name was changed to "epinephrine" in the United States because Parke, Davis, and Co. owned the trademark rights to the word *adrenalin* (without the final *e*). It is still known as adrenaline in the rest of the world.

Alpha-Adrenergic Receptors

When alpha receptors are stimulated, enzymes on the inside of the plasma membrane are activated and a cascade of changes occurs within the cell. These changes occur due to the production of a second messenger, the G-protein, which initiates the cascade. In $alpha_1$ receptors intracellular calcium stores are released, causing excitatory effects such as smooth muscle contraction or sphincter closure. Drugs affecting $alpha_1$ receptors are primarily used for their effects on vascular smooth muscle in the treatment of hypertension (see Chapters 16 and 34). Drugs that block the $alpha_1$ receptor are used to treat benign prostatic hyperplasia (see Chapters 14 and 71).

Stimulation of $alpha_2$ receptors causes different effects due to the activation of a separate cascade of events in the target cells. By increasing cyclic adenosine monophosphate (cAMP) within the cell, activation of $alpha_2$ receptors inhibits NE release from sympathetic nerve endings, causing mostly *inhibitory* actions. In addition, activation of $alpha_2$ receptors in the CNS can suppress the outflow of sympathetic activity from the brain. Indeed, as is discussed in Chapter 15, drugs that affect $alpha_2$ receptors are usually used for their ability to decrease blood pressure due to their effects on the CNS, not the ANS.

Beta-Adrenergic Receptors

Three subtypes of beta-adrenergic receptors have been identified, although only $beta_1$ and $beta_2$ have pharmacologic importance. Beta receptors act by increasing the second-messenger cAMP in target cells. The specific response caused by activation of the beta receptor depends on its location.

The primary tissues served by $beta_1$ receptors are the heart, coronary vessels, and kidneys. Activation of these receptors increases the heart rate and strength of contraction and dilates the coronary arteries, thus preparing the heart for fight or flight. $Beta_1$ receptors in the kidney respond by releasing renin, which helps to maintain (increase) blood pressure.

$Beta_2$ receptors are more widely distributed than $beta_1$ receptors, with locations in the smooth muscle in arterioles, the GI tract, and the lungs. Activation of these receptors will dilate arteries to skeletal muscles, dilate bronchioles, slow peristalsis, and decrease urine production.

The significance of adrenergic receptor subtypes to pharmacology cannot be overstated. Some drugs are selective and activate only one type of adrenergic receptor, whereas others affect all of them. Furthermore, a drug may activate one type of receptor at low doses and begin to affect other receptor subtypes as the dose is increased. Committing the receptor types and their responses to memory is an essential step in learning autonomic pharmacology.

Other types of adrenergic receptors exist. Although the functional role of dopamine was once thought to be only a chemical precursor to NE, research has determined that this agent serves a larger role as a neurotransmitter. Five dopaminergic receptors (D1 through D5) have been identified in the CNS. Dysfunction of dopamine transmission is associated with several disorders, including Parkinson's disease, Alzheimer's dementia, schizophrenia, attention-deficit/hyperactivity disorder, and Tourette's syndrome. Medications affecting the dopamine receptor have been developed to treat certain antipsychotic medicines (see Chapter 20) and Parkinson's disease (see Chapter 21). Dopamine receptors in the peripheral nervous system are located in the arterioles of the kidney and other viscera. Although these receptors likely have a role in autonomic function, their therapeutic importance has yet to be discovered.

Termination of Norepinephrine Action

The termination of NE action occurs through mechanisms different from those of ACh. The majority of the NE (50–80%) is taken back into the nerve terminal, a process known as *reuptake*. Following its reuptake, NE is repackaged in vesicles for future use or destroyed enzymatically by **monoamine oxidase (MAO)**. NE entering the circulation, such as that secreted by the adrenal glands or given as medication, is destroyed by the enzyme **catechol-O-methyltransferase (COMT)** in kidney and liver cells. Many drugs affect autonomic function by influencing the synthesis, storage, release, reuptake, or destruction of NE. The lifecycle of NE is shown in Figure 12.6.

Activation of the sympathetic division produces longer lasting effects than those of parasympathetic activation. This is because NE acts *indirectly* through a second-messenger mechanism. Its effects are produced more slowly than ACh, which acts directly at cholinergic sites. Furthermore, the primary means of inactivation of NE is through reuptake, which is a slower process than the direct enzymatic destruction of ACh.

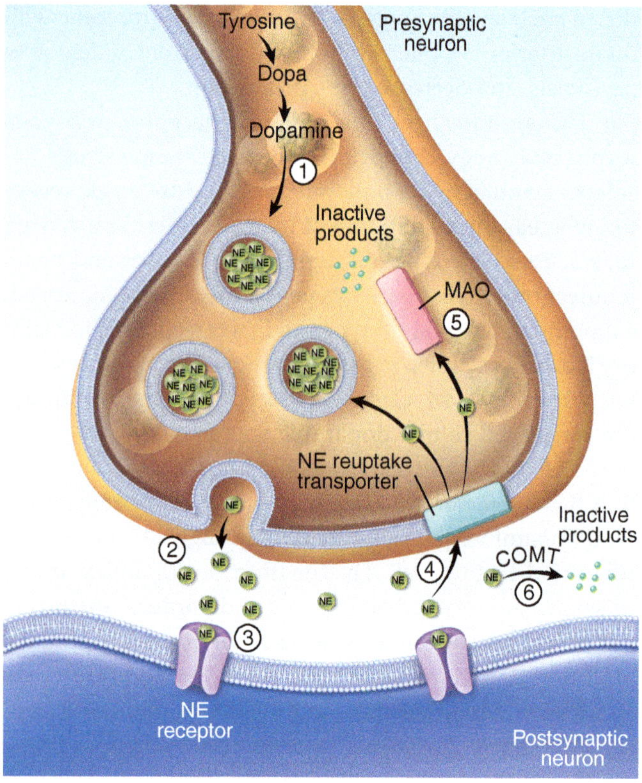

Figure 12.6 Lifecycle of norepinephrine (NE). (1) NE is synthesized from the amino acid tyrosine. (2) NE is released into the synaptic cleft. (3) NE binds to receptors on the postsynaptic membrane. (4) NE is taken back into the presynaptic neuron. (5) NE is degraded by MAO. (6) Small amounts of NE are degraded by COMT.

CONNECTION Checkpoint 12.2

The herb St. John's wort is believed to inhibit the reuptake of serotonin into presynaptic nerve terminals in the CNS. From what you learned in Chapter 7, what is the most common indication for using this herb?

12.8 The adrenal medulla is a specialized type of sympathetic nervous system tissue that secretes epinephrine and norepinephrine.

Lying in the inner portion of each adrenal gland, the adrenal medulla is closely associated with the sympathetic nervous system but has a different anatomic and physiologic arrangement than the rest of the sympathetic branch. Early in embryonic life, the adrenal medulla is part of the neural tissue that is destined to become the sympathetic nervous system. This primitive tissue splits, however, and the adrenal medulla becomes its own functional division. Preganglionic neurons from the spinal cord terminate in the adrenal medulla and release the neurotransmitters epinephrine and NE *directly* into the blood. Approximately 80% of the secretion is epinephrine, with the other 20% being NE. Once released, these agents are widely distributed to target organs, where they elicit the classic fight-or-flight symptoms.

Once released into the systemic circulation by the adrenal gland, epinephrine and NE produce more diffuse and longer-lasting effects than those produced by activation of sympathetic neurons in the ANS. In addition, the bloodstream distributes these agents to all body cells, not just those innervated by the ANS. Significant concentrations of epinephrine and NE may persist for as long as 30 seconds, and their effects on tissues may continue for several minutes until the liver eventually deactivates the hormones. It is estimated that 25–50% of all sympathetic nervous system responses at any given time are due to circulating hormones from the adrenal medulla.

Regulation of Autonomic Functions

12.9 The autonomic nervous system is influenced by higher levels of control in the cerebral cortex and hypothalamus.

Although it is often stated that control of the ANS is involuntary, this is an oversimplification. For example, strong emotions such as rage are seated in the brain, but they trigger the heart to race, the blood pressure to rise, and the respiration rate to increase. Mental depression can have the opposite effects. The smell of steak or chicken cooking on the grill can increase peristalsis, resulting in "grumbling" of the stomach and increased salivation. Clearly, autonomic actions can be modified by higher brain centers.

The roles of higher centers in regulating the ANS are shown in Figure 12.7. The hypothalamus is thought to be the main integration center of the ANS. This tissue receives signals from the cerebrum and sensory input, such as emotions, from the limbic system of the brain. The hypothalamus interprets the information and responds by sending messages to the various portions of the ANS, such as increasing peristalsis and salivation when the sights, sounds, and smells of the grilled steak are experienced. Messages from the hypothalamus travel along the medulla oblongata, the brainstem, and the spinal cord.

Drugs can affect the ANS by influencing these higher centers. For example, drugs that decrease anxiety or diminish the incidence of panic attacks can slow the heart rate and lower blood pressure through their ability to affect conscious thought. It is important to understand that these drugs do not necessarily act on autonomic receptors, nor do patients consciously lower their blood pressure or heart rate. The autonomic effect is indirect, caused by a reduction of stress, and it is at a subconscious level. Controlling autonomic activity through conscious thought is the principle underlying biofeedback therapy.

Classification of Autonomic Drugs

12.10 Autonomic drugs are classified by which receptors they stimulate or block.

At this point of the chapter, it is normal for students to feel overwhelmed by the complexity of the various autonomic receptors and their actions. It is the existence of

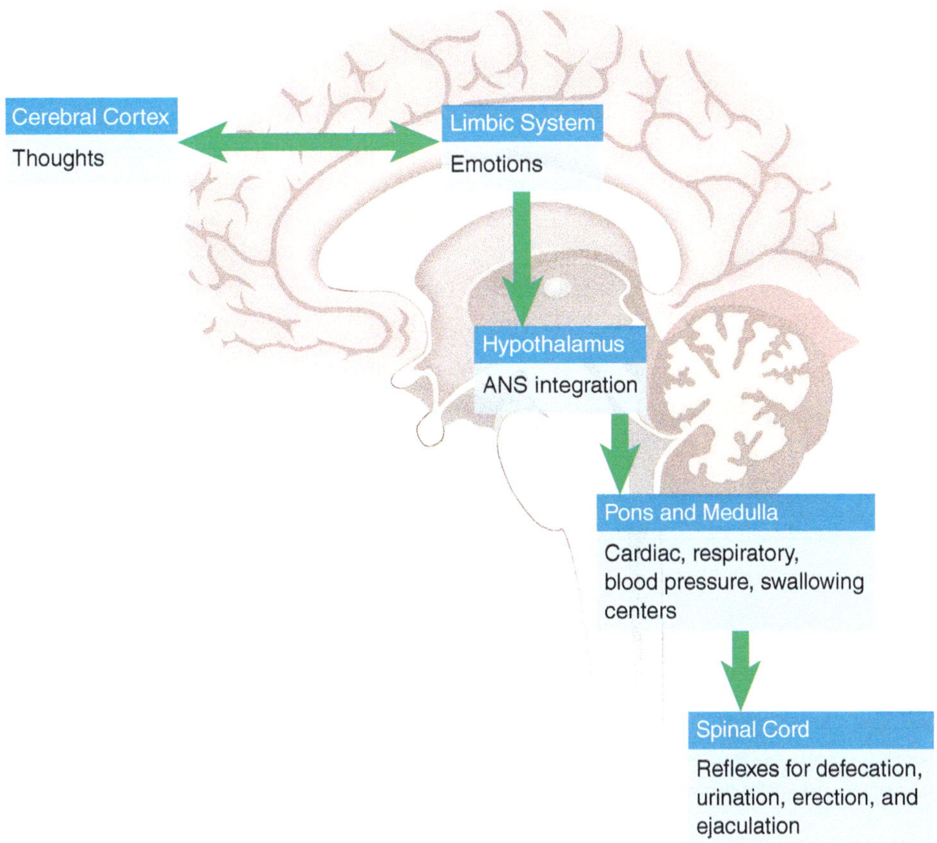

Figure 12.7 Higher centers influencing autonomic function.

these different receptors, however, that allows drugs to cause very specific therapeutic actions. For example, it is desirable to have drugs that affect blood pressure without increasing heart rate or drugs that dilate bronchi without causing hypertension. At this stage in the study of pharmacology, the student can just memorize the receptor types and actions because applications in the coming chapters provide clarity to this subject.

Given the opposite actions of the sympathetic and parasympathetic nervous systems, autonomic drugs are classified based on one of four possible actions:

1. Stimulation of the sympathetic nervous system. These drugs are called *sympathomimetics* or *adrenergic agonists* and they produce the classic symptoms of the fight-or-flight response.
2. Stimulation of the parasympathetic nervous system. These drugs are called *parasympathomimetics* or *muscarinic agonists* and they produce the characteristic symptoms of the rest-and-digest response.
3. Inhibition of the sympathetic nervous system. These drugs are called *adrenergic antagonists* or *adrenergic blockers* and they produce actions opposite to those of the sympathomimetics.
4. Inhibition of the parasympathetic nervous system. These drugs are called *anticholinergics*, *parasympatholytics*, or *muscarinic blockers* and they produce actions opposite to those of the parasympathomimetics.

Table 12.3 Indications for Autonomic Drugs

Indication	Autonomic Class	Chapter
Allergic rhinitis and the common cold	$Alpha_1$-adrenergic agonists	45
Alzheimer's disease	Cholinergic agonists	21
Angina pectoris	Beta-adrenergic blockers	35
Asthma and COPD	Beta-adrenergic agonists Anticholinergics	44
Benign prostatic hyperplasia	$Alpha_1$-adrenergic blockers	71
Cardiac arrest	Adrenergic agonists	35
Dysrhythmias	Beta-adrenergic blockers	37
Eye examinations	Anticholinergics	74
Glaucoma	Alpha-adrenergic blockers Beta-adrenergic blockers Cholinergic agonists	74
Heart failure	Beta-adrenergic blockers Beta-adrenergic agonists	36
Hypertension	$Alpha_1$-adrenergic blockers $Alpha_2$-adrenergic agonists Beta-adrenergic blockers	34
Hypotension and shock	Beta-adrenergic agonists	15
Myasthenia gravis	Cholinergic agonists	13
Myocardial infarction	Beta-adrenergic blockers	35
Overactive bladder	Anticholinergics	14
Parkinson's disease	Anticholinergics	21
Peptic ulcer disease	Anticholinergics	59
Thyroid crisis (storm)	Beta-adrenergic blockers	67

There is a method for simplifying the learning of autonomic pharmacology. On examining the preceding four drug classes, it is evident that only one group need be learned because the others are logical extensions of the first. If the fight-or-flight symptoms of the sympathomimetics are learned, the other three groups are either the same or opposite. For example, both the sympathomimetics and the anticholinergics increase heart rate and dilate the pupils. The other two groups, the parasympathomimetics and the adrenergic antagonists, have the opposite effects of slowing heart rate and constricting the pupils. Although this is an oversimplification and exceptions exist, it is a time-saving means of learning the basic actions and adverse effects of dozens of drugs affecting the ANS. It should be emphasized again that mastering the actions and terminology of autonomic drugs early in the study of pharmacology will reap rewards later in the course when these drugs are applied to various systems. Table 12.3 shows the many applications of autonomic drugs in medicine and the chapter in this text in which each is covered.

Understanding Chapter 12

Key Concepts Summary

12.1 The two major subdivisions of the nervous system are the central nervous system and the peripheral nervous system.

12.2 The peripheral nervous system is divided into somatic and autonomic components.

12.3 The autonomic nervous system is divided into two mostly opposing components: the sympathetic and parasympathetic branches.

12.4 Synaptic transmission allows information to be communicated between two nerves or from nerves to muscles or glands.

12.5 Autonomic drugs exert their effects by acting at synapses.

12.6 Acetylcholine is the neurotransmitter released at cholinergic receptors, which may be nicotinic or muscarinic.

12.7 Norepinephrine is the primary neurotransmitter released at adrenergic receptors, which may be alpha or beta.

12.8 The adrenal medulla is a specialized type of sympathetic nervous system tissue that secretes epinephrine and norepinephrine.

12.9 The autonomic nervous system is influenced by higher levels of control in the cerebral cortex and hypothalamus.

12.10 Autonomic drugs are classified by which receptors they stimulate or block.

References

Aronson, J. K. (2000). Where name and image meet—the argument for "adrenaline." *British Medical Journal, 320*, 506–509. https://doi.org/10.1136/bmj.320.7233.506

Krogh, D. (2011). *Biology: A guide to the natural world* (5th ed.). Pearson.

Selected Bibliography

Bear, M. F., Connors, B. W., & Paradiso, M. A. (2020). *Neuroscience: Exploring the brain* (Enhanced 4th ed.). Jones & Bartlett.

Brunton, L. L., Hilal-Dandan, R., & Knollman, B. C. (2017). *Goodman and Gilman's The pharmacological basis of therapeutics* (13th ed.). McGraw-Hill.

Hall, J. E. (2020). *Guyton & Hall textbook of medical physiology* (14th ed.). Elsevier.

Martini, F. H., Nath, J. L., & Bartholomew, E. F. (2018). *Fundamentals of human anatomy and physiology* (11th ed.). Pearson.

Silverthorn, D. U. (2019). *Human physiology: An integrated approach* (8th ed.). Pearson.

Thorp, A. A., & Schlaich, M. P. (2015). Relevance of sympathetic nervous system activation in obesity and metabolic syndrome. *Journal of Diabetes Research*, 2015, 341583. https://doi.org/10.1155/2015/341583

Zalewski, P., Słomko, J., & Zawadka-Kunikowska, M. (2018). Autonomic dysfunction and chronic disease. *British Medical Bulletin, 128*(1), 61–74. https://doi.org/10.1093/bmb/ldy036

"It's rather embarrassing, but I'm having some "accidents" these past two days since my surgery and they say I'm not passing my urine as I should. When I was released from the hospital, they sent me home on this new prescription. What do I need to know about this bladder medicine I'm supposed to take?"

—*Patient "Patricia Sparks"*

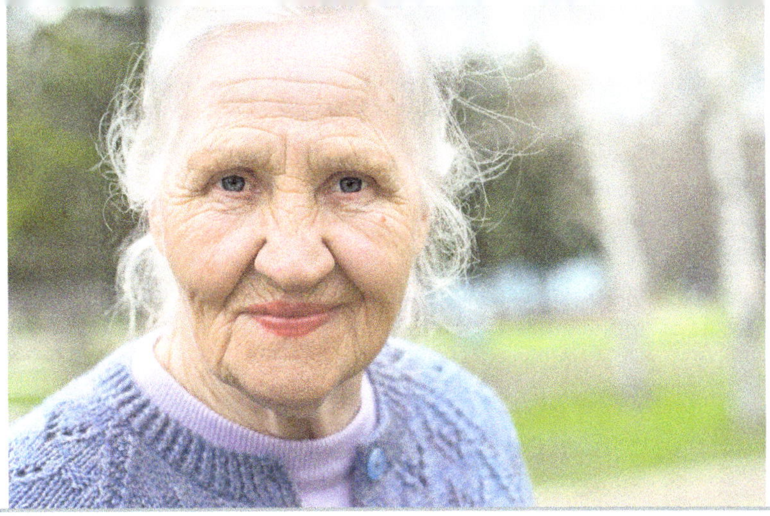

Chapter 13
Cholinergic Agonists

Chapter Outline

Learning Outcomes

After reading this chapter, the student should be able to:

1. Compare and contrast the mechanisms of action for direct- and indirect-acting cholinergic agonists.
2. Identify the actions of muscarinic agonists and their pharmacologic uses.
3. Describe the pharmacotherapy of myasthenia gravis.
4. Differentiate between the treatment of cholinergic crisis and myasthenic crisis.
5. Explain the actions and pharmacologic applications of nicotine.
6. For each of the classes shown in the chapter outline, identify the prototype and representative drugs and explain the mechanism(s) of drug action, primary indications, contraindications, significant drug interactions, pregnancy category, and important adverse effects.
7. Apply the clinical judgment to care for patients receiving pharmacotherapy with cholinergic agonists.

Key Terms

Definitions of the terms in bold may be found in the Glossary.

Of the four classes of autonomic drugs, the cholinergic agonists comprise the smallest and least prescribed group. Because cholinergic synapses are so widely dispersed throughout the central and peripheral nervous systems, drugs affecting these receptors will have diverse effects. A few have applications in the treatment of glaucoma, myasthenia gravis, and early Alzheimer' disease.

Cholinergic Receptors

13.1 Drugs can activate cholinergic receptors either directly or indirectly.

Recall from Chapter 12 that cholinergic receptors are located throughout the peripheral nervous system. To understand the effects of cholinergic drugs, it is important to review these locations. In the autonomic nervous system:

- At the *neuroeffector junctions* in the parasympathetic division
- At the *ganglia* in both the parasympathetic and sympathetic divisions.

In the somatic nervous system:

- At the *neuromuscular junctions*, which result in skeletal muscle contraction.

In addition, cholinergic synapses are present throughout the central nervous system (CNS). These locations are summarized in Figure 13.1.

All of these locations use acetylcholine as the neurotransmitter. The degree of activation at a cholinergic synapse is dependent on the *amount* of ACh interacting with its receptors. Drugs and other chemicals that increase the action of ACh at cholinergic receptors will initiate rest-and-digest types of responses. These substances are called **cholinergic agonists**, or parasympathomimetics.

Also recall from Chapter 12 that there are two primary types of cholinergic receptors: muscarinic and nicotinic. Although ACh itself stimulates both types of receptors, drugs may be selective for only one type. For example, bethanechol is selective for muscarinic receptors and thus it is called a **muscarinic agonist**. On the other hand, nicotine is selective for nicotinic receptors and therefore is classified as a **nicotinic agonist**. Note that both bethanechol and nicotine are considered cholinergic agonists: The terms *muscarinic* and *nicotinic* are used to specify which cholinergic synapses are activated. If the student has not yet learned the differences between muscarinic and nicotinic receptors, then Section 12.6 should be reviewed before continuing. A summary of the differences is provided in Table 13.1.

Cholinergic agonists can activate cholinergic receptors directly or indirectly. *Direct-acting* drugs, such as bethanechol, enter the synaptic cleft and bind to ACh receptors to produce typical rest-and-digest responses. Some of these direct-acting drugs cause the release of additional ACh into the synaptic cleft, thus enhancing the normal

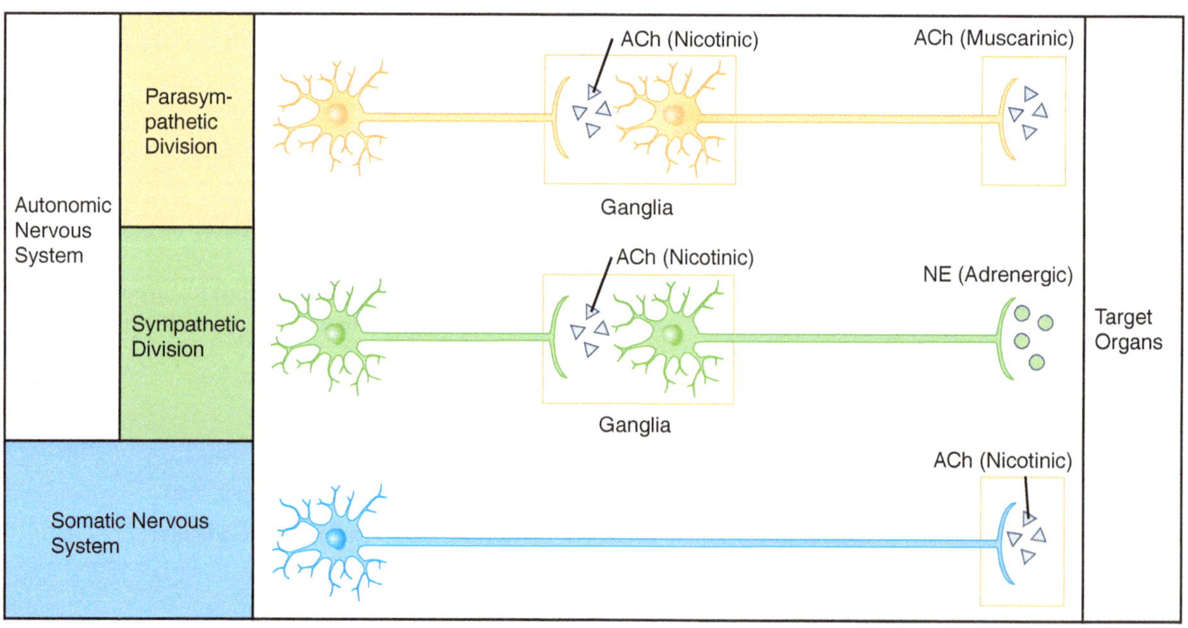

Figure 13.1 Locations of cholinergic synapses. Acetylcholine is released at the ganglia in both the parasympathetic and sympathetic divisions, at the neuroeffector junctions in the parasympathetic division, and in the somatic nervous system at neuromuscular synapses.

Table 13.1 Types of Cholinergic Receptors and Their Actions

	Muscarinic	Nicotinic
Receptor location	Glands, smooth muscle, cardiac muscle	Skeletal muscle, autonomic ganglia, brain, adrenal gland
General actions	Pupil constriction Decreased accommodation of the eye Increased GI motility Decreased heart rate Decreased blood pressure Increased glandular secretions (salivary, lacrimal, and sweat) Constriction of bronchial smooth muscle Release of urine	Skeletal muscle contraction Initial stimulation of glandular secretion, followed by inhibition Increased heart rate Increased blood pressure

physiologic responses caused by ACh. The direct-acting cholinergic agonists essentially act by the same mechanism as ACh itself. The direct mechanism of cholinergic activation is shown in Figure 13.2a.

Indirect-acting drugs inhibit acetylcholinesterase (AChE; also called cholinesterase), the enzyme in cholinergic synapses that destroys ACh. By blocking the destruction of ACh, the neurotransmitter accumulates and remains in the

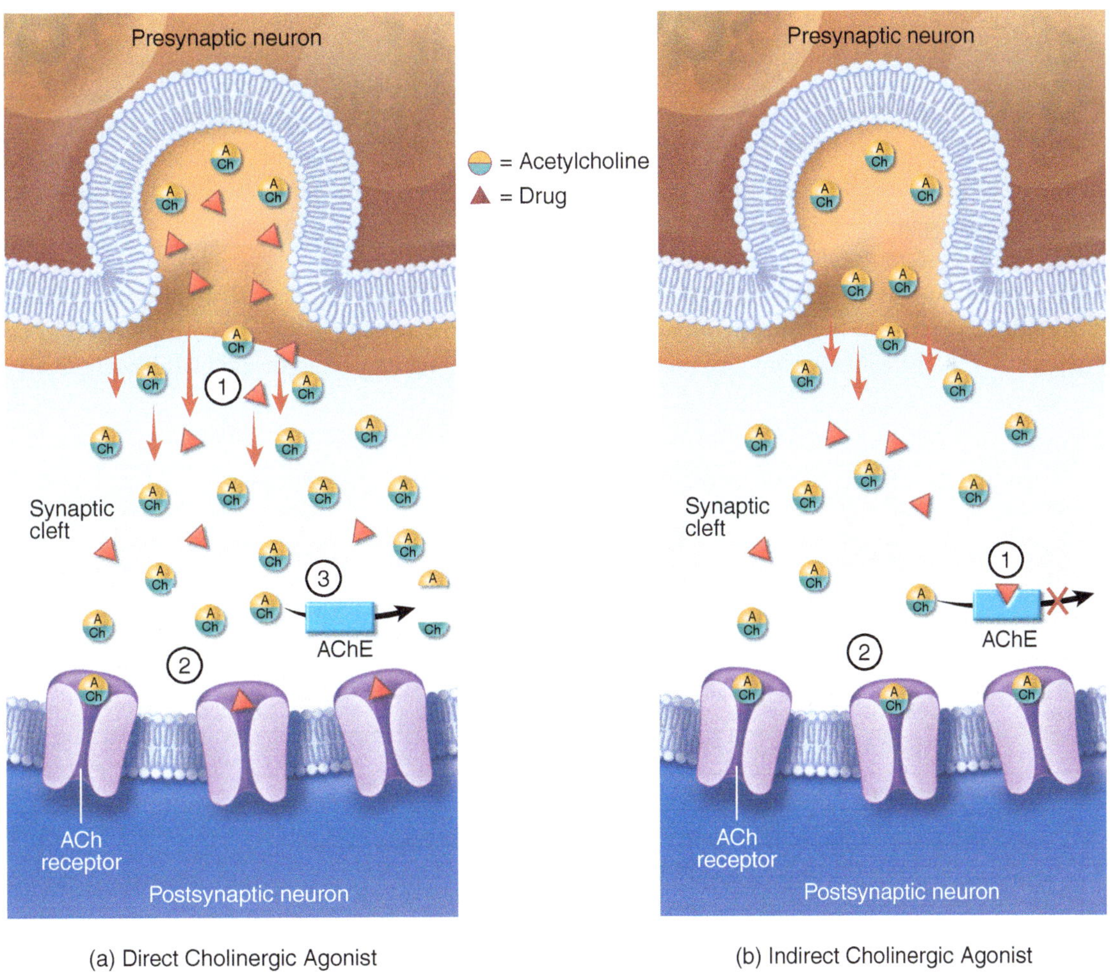

Figure 13.2 (a) Mechanisms of action for direct cholinergic agonists. Direct cholinergic agonists can activate the cholinergic receptor by two mechanisms: (1) The drug can cause more acetylcholine (ACh) to be released into the synaptic cleft, resulting in additional ACh occupying ACh receptors. (2) The drug can bind to ACh receptors, enhancing the action potential on the postsynaptic neuron. Inactivation of drug action is achieved by acetylcholinesterase (AChE). (b) Mechanism of action for indirect cholinergic agonists: (1) The drug binds the enzyme (AChE), which prevents the ACh from being destroyed. This increases the amount of ACh remaining in the synaptic cleft, (2) thus enhancing the action potential on the postsynaptic neuron.

synaptic cleft for a longer time to produce enhanced rest-and-digest responses. Some indirect drugs such as neostigmine bind only briefly to AChE and exhibit short durations of action. These drugs are called *reversible* acetylcholinesterase inhibitors.

Certain chemicals bind *irreversibly* to AChE. For example, certain insecticides and nerve gas agents bind to AChE for excessively prolonged periods and can cause death if ingested or absorbed. Because of the hazardous nature of these chemicals, irreversible acetylcholinesterase inhibitors are not widely used in medicine.

Note that physiologically it does not matter whether the cholinergic synapse was activated directly or indirectly: The parasympathetic responses are the same. There are some important differences, however, as is discussed in Section 13.3. The indirect mechanism of cholinergic activation is shown in Figure 13.2b.

Muscarinic Agonists

13.2 Muscarinic agonists produce their effects by directly stimulating cholinergic receptors.

Muscarinic agonists are drugs that activate cholinergic receptors located at the *neuroeffector junctions* in the parasympathetic nervous system. By definition, ACh itself is a muscarinic agonist; however, it has no clinical value because it is rapidly destroyed both in the bloodstream and in synapses (by AChE). Muscarinic agonists used as medications are relatively resistant to destruction by AChE and exhibit a longer duration of action than ACh. Muscarinic agonists are poorly absorbed across the gastrointestinal (GI) tract and generally do not cross the blood–brain barrier. They have minimal effects on ACh nicotinic receptors in the ganglia. Because of the potential for serious adverse effects, few muscarinic agonists are widely used in pharmacotherapy. Available drugs are listed in Table 13.2.

Muscarinic agonists have widespread effects on the body, nearly all of which are due to parasympathetic activation. All of these drugs can increase the degree of smooth muscle tone and contractions of the GI tract. When administered before meals, stomach emptying is promoted due to increased peristalsis of the alimentary canal. Muscarinic agonists should never be administered to patients with suspected obstructive disease of the GI tract because the increased peristaltic contractions could lead to injury or rupture to the mucosa.

CONNECTION Checkpoint 13.1

From what you learned in Chapter 12, would you expect the cholinergic agonists to have similar or opposite effects to the following: adrenergic agonists, adrenergic antagonists, cholinergic antagonists?

Muscarinic agonists also stimulate the smooth muscle of the urinary tract, increasing ureteral peristalsis and promoting emptying of the bladder. These are considered

Table 13.2 Cholinergic Agonists

Drug	Route and Adult Dose (Maximum Dose Where Indicated)	Adverse Effects
Direct Acting (Muscarinic Agonists)		
bethanechol (Duvoid, Urecholine)	PO: 10–50 mg tid or qid (max: 200 mg/day)	*Increased salivation, abdominal cramping, sweating, flushing of the skin, miosis, blurred vision, nausea and vomiting* Orthostatic hypotension with possible syncope, bradycardia, reflex tachycardia, complete heart block, acute bronchospasm
cevimeline (Evoxac)	PO: 30 mg tid (max: 90 mg/day)	
pilocarpine (Isopto-Carpine, Salagen)	Topical: 1–2 drops in affected eye tid or qid for chronic glaucoma	
	PO: 5–10 mg tid for xerostomia (max: 10 mg/dose, 30 mg/day)	
Indirect Acting (Acetylcholinesterase Inhibitors)		
donepezil (Aricept)	PO or orally disintegrating tablet (ODT): 5–10 mg (max: 10 mg/day)	*Involuntary contraction or twitching of muscles, nausea and vomiting, miosis, increased salivation* Bradycardia, hypotension, dyspnea, seizures, bronchospasm, cholinergic crisis, death due to paralysis of respiratory muscles
galantamine (Razadyne)	PO: 4 mg bid for 4 wk; may increase by 4 mg bid q4wk to target dose of 12 mg bid (max: 24 mg/day)	
neostigmine (Bloxiverz)	IV: 0.5–2.5 mg (max: 5 mg/day)	
physostigmine (Antilirium)	IM/IV: 0.5–2 mg (IV not faster than 1 mg/min); repeat as needed	
pyridostigmine (Mestinon, Regonol)	PO: 60 mg–1.5 g/day; sustained release: 180–540 mg 1–2 times/day at intervals of at least 6 h IV: 0.1–0.25 mg/kg	
rivastigmine (Exelon)	PO: Start with 1.5 mg bid; may increase to target dose of 3–6 mg bid (max: 12 mg/day) Transdermal: Start with one 4.6-mg patch daily (max: one 9.5-mg patch daily)	

Note: *Italics* indicate common adverse effects. Underline indicates serious adverse effects.

therapeutic actions in patients with urinary retention. Care must be taken not to administer muscarinic agonists when obstructive uropathy is present, however, because the increased smooth muscle contractions of the ureters and bladder could aggravate pain and bleeding.

Muscarinic agonists stimulate most exocrine glands, increasing lacrimal, sweat, digestive, and salivary secretions. This action has been used to advantage in treating patients with **xerostomia** (dry mouth) or those with **Sjögren syndrome**, a chronic autoimmune disorder characterized by excessive dryness of mucous membranes, which is associated with rheumatoid arthritis in menopausal women. In addition to creating discomfort for the patient, xerostomia can promote dental caries, periodontal disease, oral ulcers, and candidiasis.

In the eye, muscarinic agonists cause the muscles of the iris to contract, resulting in pupillary constriction, or miosis. Miosis has no therapeutic application and is considered an adverse effect of muscarinic agonists. A second effect on the eye is contraction of the ciliary muscle, which causes loss of ability to focus for near vision. Although this action may cause blurred vision, ciliary muscle contraction has an indirect, beneficial effect: It allows fluid to drain from the anterior chamber of the eye, reducing intraocular pressure. When applied topically to the eye, cholinergic agonists, such as pilocarpine, can be of value in treating glaucoma. Cholinergic agonists are considered second-line drugs for glaucoma therapy, however, having been replaced by safer, more effective alternatives (see Chapter 74).

Muscarinic agonists contract bronchial smooth muscle, causing the airways to narrow. In patients with respiratory disease, bronchoconstriction may trigger episodes of breathlessness or an asthma attack. This is why muscarinic agonists are contraindicated in patients with a history of asthma.

When activated, muscarinic receptors in the cardiovascular system slow the heart rate and lower blood pressure. Baroreceptors in the carotid arteries and aortic arch, however, recognize the falling blood pressure and signal the vasomotor center in the medulla to increase the heart rate. This phenomenon, known as **reflex tachycardia**, is not unique to the cholinergic agonists; it can occur with any drug that causes blood pressure to fall. When administering cholinergic agonists by the oral (PO) or parenteral routes, the patients' heart rate must be closely monitored to avoid bradycardia. Blood pressure must also be monitored to prevent serious hypotension, particularly in those with preexisting cardiovascular disease. Patients with hyperthyroidism may experience atrial fibrillation. Serious heart disease is a contraindication to therapy with cholinergic agonists.

Occasionally, patients experience acute poisoning from eating certain species of mushrooms containing high amounts of muscarine, the original cholinergic agonist isolated from the mushroom *Amanita muscaria*. *A. muscaria* itself has only small amounts of muscarine, but several other species of fungi possess significant amounts of this toxin that can cause severe illness if ingested. Symptoms of acute poisoning appear 30 to 90 minutes after ingestion and resemble an overdose of cholinergic agonists: an exaggerated parasympathetic response. Symptoms may persist for 24 hours. *Amanita* species are sometimes intentionally ingested to obtain psychotic effects, reportedly to expand or alter spatiotemporal awareness.

PharmFACT

Muscarinic receptors are named after muscarine, which is obtained from the mushroom *Amanita muscaria*. The actual chemical that causes poisoning in patients eating this mushroom, however, is primarily ibotenic acid, which causes excitement, hallucinations, and confusion. Death from *Amanita* mushroom poisoning is rare (Rolston-Cregler, 2017).

Symptoms of parasympathetic stimulation, whether caused by medications or poisoning, may be reversed by administering an anticholinergic drug. Atropine is considered the specific antidote for these conditions. Acute symptoms of parasympathetic stimulation will begin to resolve within minutes after a subcutaneous injection of atropine. Atropine is a prototype cholinergic antagonist presented in Chapter 14.

PROTOTYPE DRUG Bethanechol (Duvoid, Urecholine)

Classification **Therapeutic:** Drug to treat urinary retention
Pharmacologic: Cholinergic agonist, muscarinic agonist (direct acting)

Therapeutic Effects and Uses: Approved in 1948 by the U.S. Food and Drug Administration (FDA), bethanechol is available in tablet form. Effects of bethanechol are most noted in the digestive and urinary tracts, where it stimulates smooth muscle contraction. In the urinary tract, bethanechol relaxes the sphincters and causes the detrusor muscle of the bladder to contract. These combined actions result in voiding; thus, it is used to treat nonobstructive urinary retention in patients with atony of the bladder. Off-label uses include the treatment of adynamic ileus and gastric atony.

Mechanism of Action: Structurally similar to ACh, bethanechol interacts directly with muscarinic receptors to cause body responses typical of parasympathetic stimulation. This drug is selective for muscarinic receptors. Bethanechol is not destroyed by AChE; therefore, its actions are more prolonged than those of ACh.

Pharmacokinetics:

Route(s)	PO
Absorption	Poorly absorbed
Distribution	Widely distributed; does not cross the blood–brain barrier
Primary metabolism	Unknown
Primary excretion	Renal
Onset of action	30–60 min
Duration of action	1–6 h

Adverse Effects: The adverse effects of bethanechol are predictable knowing its parasympathetic actions. Common adverse effects include increased salivation, abdominal cramping, sweating, flushing of the skin, miosis, blurred vision, and nausea and vomiting. Serious effects include orthostatic hypotension with possible syncope, bradycardia, reflex tachycardia, complete heart block, and acute bronchospasm.

Contraindications/Precautions: Bethanechol should be used with extreme caution in patients with disorders that could be aggravated by increased contractions of the GI tract, such as suspected bowel obstruction, recent GI surgery, an active ulcer, or an inflammatory disease. Patients with suspected urinary obstruction or those who have had recent bladder surgery should not receive this drug because the increased smooth muscle contractions could worsen these conditions. Patients with cystitis should not be given bethanechol because contractions of the bladder may force urine up the ureters to the kidneys if the sphincter fails to open. Because of the possibility of bronchoconstriction, administration of bethanechol to patients with asthma or chronic obstructive pulmonary disease (COPD) is contraindicated. Muscarinic agonists such as bethanechol can slow the heart rate; thus, they are contraindicated in patients with recent myocardial infarction (MI), severe bradycardia, hypotension, or hypertension. Patients with hyperthyroidism can experience dysrhythmias with bethanechol use. Other contraindications include peritonitis, epilepsy, and Parkinson's disease.

Drug Interactions: Concurrent therapy with AChE inhibitors should be avoided because this class also stimulates muscarinic receptors, and excessive parasympathetic activity will result. Procainamide, quinidine, atropine, and epinephrine antagonize the effects of bethanechol. Concurrent administration with ganglionic blockers may result in a rapid fall in blood pressure. **Herbal/Food:** Unknown.

Pregnancy: Category C.

Treatment of Overdose: Overdose will result in serious cholinergic symptoms such as nausea and vomiting, abdominal cramping, diarrhea, salivation, and hypotension. Administration of subcutaneous atropine quickly reverses most symptoms.

Clinician Responsibilities: Key clinical implications for patients receiving bethanechol are included in Applied Clinical Judgment: Patients Receiving Pharmacotherapy with Cholinergic Agonists.

Drugs Similar to Bethanechol (Duvoid, Urecholine)

Other direct-acting cholinergic agonists include cevimeline and pilocarpine.

Cevimeline (Evoxac): Cevimeline is a direct-acting cholinergic drug whose only indication is the treatment of xerostomia in patients with Sjögren syndrome. Given orally, cevimeline increases saliva flow, relieving dry mouth. The most common adverse effect is excessive sweating, although this occurs less frequently than with pilocarpine. Other signs of parasympathetic stimulation are possible, such as diarrhea, runny nose, miosis, and bradycardia. This drug is pregnancy category C.

Pilocarpine (Isopto-Carpine, Salagen): Pilocarpine is a direct cholinergic agonist that is administered orally or as an ophthalmic solution. Salagen is an oral preparation of pilocarpine given for xerostomia due to its ability to stimulate salivary flow. When given orally, the adverse effects of pilocarpine are those expected of parasympathetic stimulation, which include diarrhea, runny nose, miosis, and bradycardia. Excessive sweating occurs in 30–60% of patients taking oral pilocarpine.

Pilocarpine is also approved as eyedrops to treat certain types of glaucoma and to counteract the effects of mydriatics and cycloplegics following eye examinations. This drug is pregnancy category C.

13.3 Acetylcholinesterase inhibitors are used to treat Alzheimer' disease and myasthenia gravis.

The indirect-acting cholinergic agonists inhibit the enzymatic destruction of ACh, allowing the neurotransmitter to remain on cholinergic receptors for a longer time. Like the direct-acting (muscarinic) agonists, these drugs essentially prolong the actions of ACh. Unlike the direct-acting agonists, however, the **acetylcholinesterase (AChE) inhibitors** are *nonselective* and affect ACh synapses located at the autonomic ganglia, muscarinic receptors, neuromuscular junctions, and synapses in the CNS.

The muscarinic actions of the AChE inhibitors are identical to those described for the direct-acting drugs. As such, these drugs would be expected to increase peristalsis in the GI and urinary tracts, and some can decrease intraocular pressure.

The AChE inhibitors have some additional *nonautonomic* indications due to their actions in the CNS and on motor nerve endings in skeletal muscle. AChE inhibitors used to treat mild to moderate Alzheimer' disease include galantamine (Razadyne), donepezil (Aricept), and rivastigmine (Exelon). These drugs increase the amount of

ACh in cholinergic synapses in the brain, which improves memory and cognitive function. The AChE inhibitors do not cure Alzheimer' disease; improvement is limited and short lived. Donepezil is presented as a prototype drug for Alzheimer' disease in Chapter 21.

Some cholinergic agonists are used in the pharmacotherapy of myasthenia gravis. This indication is presented in Section 13.5.

Cholinergic Crisis

13.4 A cholinergic crisis may develop with overdoses of AChE inhibitors or with certain toxins.

When cholinergic receptors are overstimulated, a medical emergency known as a **cholinergic crisis** may result. Overdoses of acetylcholinesterase inhibitors, or exposure to toxic nerve gases (such as Sarin) or organophosphate insecticides (such as Malathion), may cause an acute accumulation of ACh at cholinergic synapses. The use of nerve gases as a bioterrorist threat is discussed in Chapter 75.

A cholinergic crisis is recognized by signs of intense parasympathetic stimulation such as miosis, nausea and vomiting, urinary incontinence, increased exocrine secretions, abdominal cramping, and diarrhea. As the crisis progresses, signs of sympathetic and nicotinic stimulation appear, including tachycardia, hyperglycemia, and muscle twitching, with progressive muscle weakness and possibly flaccid paralysis. In massive overdoses, mechanical ventilation is necessary and paralysis of respiratory muscles may cause death. CNS effects are prominent with the organophosphates and include headache, blurred vision, anxiety, delirium, convulsions, and coma. In general, overdose with AChE drugs produces less severe and shorter-duration effects than does poisoning with organophosphates.

The treatment of cholinergic crisis includes administration of atropine, the specific antidote that reverses muscarinic effects. Subcutaneous atropine can act within minutes. Because some insecticides have long-lasting effects, atropine therapy may continue for several weeks.

Pralidoxime (Protopam) is a cholinergic agonist that has primarily antinicotinic action, which can reverse muscle twitching and increase muscle strength. It is a specific antidote for poisoning by organophosphate insecticides and is used to control overdoses of the AChE inhibitors used to treat myasthenia gravis. In acute poisoning, pralidoxime is administered by IV infusion over 15 to 30 minutes. To be most effective, pralidoxime must be given as soon as possible after the suspected poisoning or overdose. Furthermore, it should always be administered concurrently with atropine (which blocks muscarinic sites). DuoDote is a drug that contains both pralidoxime and atropine combined in a single intramuscular (IM) injection.

Pharmacotherapy of Myasthenia Gravis

13.5 Acetylcholinesterase inhibitors are used in the pharmacotherapy of myasthenia gravis to increase the strength of muscular contraction.

Myasthenia gravis (MG), which literally means "grave muscular weakness," first appeared in medical reports in 1672 and afflicts about 125 of 1 million people in the United States. It is one of the best understood autoimmune diseases of the nervous system. The disease occurs when antibodies *attack nicotinic synapses* on skeletal muscles, resulting in symptoms of extreme fatigue, double vision, speech impairment, and difficulty chewing or swallowing. The most visible symptom is an obvious drooping of the eyelids (ptosis) due to muscular weakness. The ocular muscles may become so fatigued that the patient is unable to open the eyelids. Muscle fatigue worsens after exercise, or late in the day. MG is considered a progressive disease, although the severity of symptoms fluctuates over time.

PharmFACT

The mean age of onset of MG is 28 years in women and 42 years in men. Most mortality from the disease occurs within 3 years following diagnosis. Worsening of the disease is uncommon after 3 years (Jowkar, 2018).

MG is diagnosed by the anti–acetylcholine receptor (AChR) antibody test. An individual without MG should have virtually no antibodies to the acetylcholine receptor. In a patient with MG, the body forms antibodies to the ACh receptor, and these can be measured in the blood with an accuracy of almost 100%. For confirmation, an electromyelography test may be conducted to test for muscle activity and fatigue.

For patients with suspected MG, it is important to perform an accurate baseline physical assessment of neuromuscular and respiratory function. The patient's swallowing ability should be assessed prior to medication administration due to decreased muscle strength caused by the disease process. Subsequent assessments are important for monitoring the progress of pharmacotherapy.

Management of MG is divided into symptomatic control and immunosuppression, as shown in Pharmacotherapy Illustrated 13.1. In the early stages of the disease, symptoms can be controlled successfully with AChE inhibitors, usually pyridostigmine. These drugs are effective for mild symptoms, act rapidly, and produce few serious adverse effects at low to moderate doses. Muscarinic side effects such as diarrhea and abdominal cramps are common, and muscle twitching can occur. High doses should not be used because AChE inhibitors can begin to affect ACh nicotinic receptors, worsening the degree of muscle weakness.

Pharmacotherapy Illustrated 13.1

Myasthenia Gravis

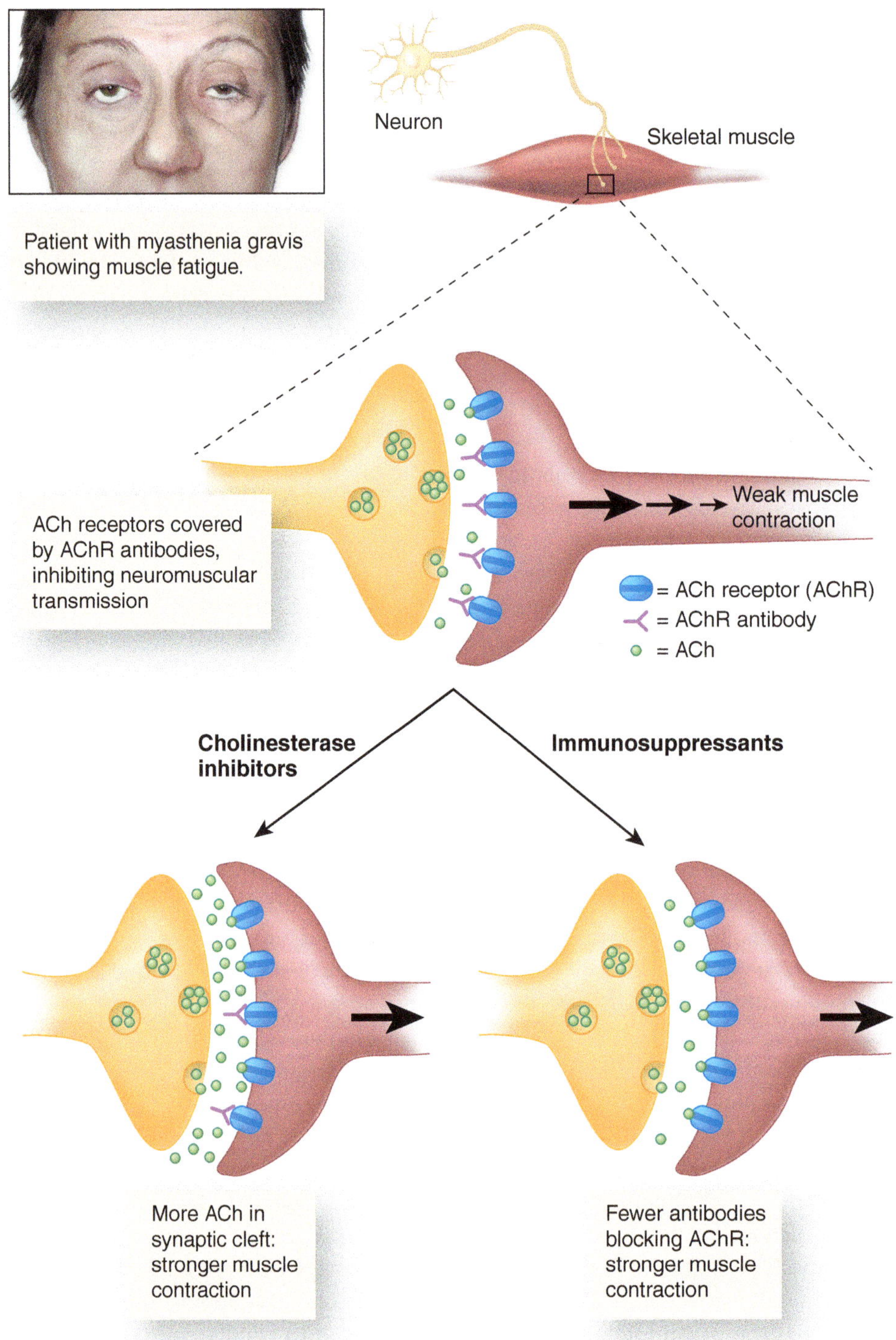

As MG progresses, immunosuppressant drugs such as corticosteroids are added to the regimen. Corticosteroids such as prednisone reduce AChE receptor antibody levels and result in symptomatic improvement. Care must be taken when initiating corticosteroid therapy because patient symptoms may dramatically worsen during the first few days of therapy. Doses of prednisone are gradually increased until the desired therapeutic effect is obtained. Unfortunately, improvement may take weeks or even months, and corticosteroids can exhibit considerable toxicity when given on a long-term basis (see Chapter 68). Therapy with corticosteroids is limited to the shortest time necessary, although some patients may require these drugs for the rest of their life.

Other immunosuppressants such as azathioprine (Imuran), cyclosporine (Sandimmune), methotrexate or mycophenolate mofetil (CellCept) may be administered as alternatives to corticosteroids. Occasionally, these alternatives are administered concurrently with prednisone to allow for lower doses of the corticosteroid. Immunosuppressants are discussed in Chapter 42. Eculizumab (Soliris) is a monoclonal antibody given by IV infusion once a week for 1 month, followed by a fifth dose 1 week later, then ongoing infusions biweekly. The high cost of this drug (about $500,000 per year) limits its use.

A **myasthenic crisis** may occur if a patient with MG abruptly discontinues their medication. This leads to extreme muscular weakness and symptoms similar to those of a cholinergic crisis. Rapid, correct diagnosis is essential, however, because antidotes for the myasthenic crisis and the cholinergic crisis are very different. Weakness that appears approximately 1 hour after drug administration that is accompanied by signs of muscarinic overstimulation suggests cholinergic crisis (overdose) and is treated by prompt withdrawal of neostigmine and immediate administration of atropine. Weakness that occurs 3 hours or more after drug administration without muscarinic overstimulation is more likely due to myasthenic crisis (underdose, abrupt discontinuation, or drug resistance) and is treated by more intensive AChE therapy.

It should be clearly understood that MG is a disease affecting skeletal muscle; it is not a disorder of the autonomic nervous system. It is presented in this chapter dealing with the autonomic nervous system because the primary pharmacotherapy for the disease is AChE inhibitors. Although these drugs provide symptomatic relief, they do not cure or slow the progression of MG. With treatment, however, patients may experience a near-normal life expectancy.

PROTOTYPE DRUG Pyridostigmine (Mestinon, Regonol)

Classification **Therapeutic:** Drug for myasthenia gravis
Pharmacologic: Indirect-acting cholinergic agonist, AChE inhibitor

Therapeutic Effects and Uses: Approved in 1955, pyridostigmine is available by both oral and parenteral routes for the symptomatic treatment of MG. Affecting the neuromuscular synapses, pyridostigmine increases the strength of skeletal muscle contraction and delays fatigue. An average dose is ten 60-mg tablets per day, spaced apart to provide for maximum muscle strength. The extended-release form consists of 180-mg tablets that are taken once or twice daily.

Pyridostigmine is also approved for military personnel with potential exposure to certain nerve gases. Pyridostigmine is only effective if administered several hours prior to nerve gas exposure. If exposure occurs, pyridostigmine is discontinued and the antidotes (atropine and pralidoxime) are administered.

The intravenous (IV) form of pyridostigmine (Regonol) is administered to reverse the neuromuscular blocking action of nondepolarizing muscle relaxants. When given by the IV route, extreme caution should be used to avoid overdosage, which can worsen neuromuscular blockade.

Mechanism of Action: Pyridostigmine reversibly inhibits the action of AChE at cholinergic synapses, which allows ACh to accumulate and cause a greater effect. Its use in treating MG is due to its effects on nicotinic ACh receptors in skeletal muscle.

Pharmacokinetics:

Route(s)	PO and IV
Absorption	PO: only 1–2% is absorbed; the oral dose is much higher than the parenteral dose
Distribution	Distributed to most tissues; crosses the placenta; does not cross the blood–brain barrier
Primary metabolism	Hepatic and plasma, by cholinesterases
Primary excretion	Kidneys
Onset of action	PO: 30–45 min; IV: 2–5 min
Duration of action	3–6 h (regular), 6–12 h (extended release)

Adverse Effects: In addition to its effects on nicotinic receptors, pyridostigmine also affects muscarinic receptors. At muscarinic synapses, pyridostigmine will enhance the parasympathetic response, resulting in increased peristalsis, bronchoconstriction, bradycardia, and hypotension. Common adverse effects include involuntary contraction or twitching of muscles, nausea and vomiting, miosis, and increased salivation. Potentially serious adverse effects include those of cholinergic crisis.

Patients with obstructive disorders of the GI or urinary tracts should not receive this drug because the increased smooth muscle contractions could worsen these conditions. This drug should be used with caution in patients with asthma, bradycardia, recent MI, or heart failure. This drug is pregnancy category C.

Contraindications/Precautions: Pyridostigmine should be used with caution in patients with disorders that could be aggravated by increased contractions of the GI tract, such as suspected bowel obstruction or active ulcers. Patients with suspected urinary obstruction should not receive this drug because the increased smooth muscle contractions could worsen this condition. Because of the potential for bronchoconstriction, patients with asthma or COPD should be treated cautiously with cholinergic agonists. Cholinergic agonists such as pyridostigmine can cause bradycardia; thus, they are used cautiously in patients with recent MI or heart failure.

Drug Interactions: Because of the potential for additive effects, other cholinergic agonists should not be administered concurrently with pyridostigmine. Drugs that interfere with neuromuscular transmission such as local anesthetics, some general anesthetics, and antidysrhythmic drugs should be used cautiously in patients with MG because severe muscular weakness may result. If administered to patients with MG, the dose of pyridostigmine should be increased. Cholinergic drugs increase gastric acid secretion and should be used with caution with other ulcer-promoting drugs such as corticosteroids or nonsteroidal anti-inflammatory drugs (NSAIDs).

Pregnancy: Category C.

Treatment of Overdose: Overdose with pyridostigmine may be life-threatening because the drug can cause a cholinergic crisis leading to respiratory failure. The administration of atropine reverses most overdose symptoms.

Clinician Responsibilities: Key clinical implications for patients receiving pyridostigmine are included in Applied Clinical Judgment: Patients Receiving Pharmacotherapy with Cholinergic Agonists.

Drugs Similar to Pyridostigmine (Mestinon, Regonol)

The other AChE inhibitor for MG is neostigmine.

Neostigmine (Bloxiverz): Neostigmine has a shorter duration of action than pyridostigmine and causes a higher frequency of adverse effects. The adverse effects result from its ability to stimulate the parasympathetic nervous system. Common adverse effects include involuntary contraction or twitching of muscles, nausea and vomiting, miosis, and increased salivation. Potentially serious adverse effects include those of cholinergic crisis. If using large doses of neostigmine to treat MG, atropine (an anticholinergic) is sometimes administered concurrently to reverse the muscarinic adverse effects of neostigmine.

CONNECTIONS: APPLIED CLINICAL JUDGMENT

Patients Receiving Pharmacotherapy with Cholinergic Agonists

Key Assessment Data

- History of current condition, baseline vital signs, physical exam findings; history of CV, GI, GU disease or diabetes; pregnancy status.
- Bowel sounds, urinary output, muscle strength, mental status, and the patient's ability to swallow should be assessed depending on the condition being treated.
- Monitor hepatic function laboratory values for up to 6 weeks after starting the drug and periodically thereafter.

Desired Therapeutic Outcomes

Improvement is observed and measurable in patient's ability to carry out activities of daily living (ADLs); urinary elimination and output; musculoskeletal weakness, ptosis, diplopia, chewing, and swallowing.

Minimizing Adverse Effects

- Monitor for signs of excessive ANS stimulation: Tremors, palpitations, changes in blood pressure, dizziness, urinary retention, abdominal pain, or changes in behavior (e.g., confusion, depression, or drowsiness).
- For patients treated for MG: Note periods of muscle weakness and their association to dosage time to determine whether overdosage (cholinergic crisis), or underdosage or drug resistance (myasthenic crisis) may be occurring.

Lifespan Considerations

- Subtle changes during the day in the older adult's muscle strength, voice quality, or slurred speech, especially if timed around drug peaks or troughs, may indicate underdosage rather than age-related changes.
- The male older adult is at higher risk for mechanical obstruction due to an enlarged prostate and the drug should be given cautiously, or not prescribed if obstruction is severe.
- Dizziness related to drug therapy may increase the risk of falls in the older adult.

Patient Education

- Have bathroom facilities nearby after the drug is administered. Assistance to the toilet or commode may be needed if dizziness occurs.
- Maintain a diary of variations in muscle strength, particularly periods of weakness, and plan activities according to muscle strength and fatigue and to allow for frequent and adequate rest periods. Immediately report extreme fatigue or any severe muscle weakness that occurs 1 hour after taking the drug or 3 or more hours after drug administration.
- Follow appropriate administration techniques, and a teach-back session should occur before patient self-administration. Any difficulty in swallowing of sustained-release tablets should be reported. To avoid under- or overdosage, self-regulation of dosage should not occur.
- Rise from lying or sitting to standing slowly and avoid prolonged standing in one place so as not to cause dizziness or falls.
- Exercise caution during driving in low-light conditions, at night, or if vision is blurred. Nightlight use at home and safety measures may be needed to prevent falls.
- Obtain and wear a medical alert bracelet or other device describing the disease and the medications used.

Prescribing Considerations

- A pharmacist consult is beneficial; the pharmacist can verify dosing, look for drug–drug interactions, perform medication reconciliation, and report back to the prescriber if there are issues.

CONNECTIONS: Advanced Practice Application

Myasthenia Gravis: Future Treatments

Case

Jane Richard is an active, busy 26-year-old mother of two young children, Amy, age 1, and Grant, age 4. One day she began to have facial weakness and reports that her "lower jaw gets tired and begins to twitch" when she chews. She has even had episodes of choking. Jane also mentions having double vision when she reads, especially late at night. Of most concern, however, is that she is experiencing muscle weakness and has a hard time caring for Amy, her 1-year-old. Jane is afraid she will drop her when she picks her up.

Jane's neurologic examination showed ptosis, drooping of both eyelids. Electromyographic testing further revealed that she had progressive weakness and decreased contraction of the distal arm muscles on repeated mild shocks (5 shocks per second) of the ulnar and median nerves. Blood testing revealed high levels of an anti–acetylcholine receptor antibody in her plasma, and a diagnosis of myasthenia gravis was made.

Jane began treatment with pyridostigmine, a long-acting acetylcholinesterase inhibitor and was given a prescription for prednisone to suppress the immune system and promote the formation of new acetylcholine receptors in muscle cell membranes. She also underwent occasional plasmapheresis when her symptoms became especially severe. Jane was given a prescription of atropine as needed to reduce the nausea, abdominal cramps, diarrhea, and excessive salivation she experienced as side effects of the pyridostigmine.

Discussion

MG is no longer considered a fatal disease, and most patients lead near normal lives with the help of either drugs or surgery. Corticosteroids suppress the immune system and may promote the formation of new acetylcholine receptors in muscle cell membranes. Patients taking corticosteroids such as prednisone for an extended time may be susceptible to bone thinning. Taking adequate amounts of calcium and vitamin D is important. Foods to include are milk products, cooked dark green vegetables, salmon, dried beans, and calcium-fortified juices and cereals. Because corticosteroids can cause fluid retention, salt substitutes or spices may be healthy alternatives to table salt. Cured or smoked meats, canned vegetables and soups, salty snacks, and pickled foods should be avoided.

Plasmapheresis, or taking the fluid part of the blood (plasma) containing the abnormal antibodies out and replacing it with other fluids, can be life-changing for MG patients. Because the effects of plasmapheresis often last only 2 weeks, a series of treatments is usually necessary.

The current standard of care in MG mainly consists of generalized immunosuppression. However, the future of MG treatment will be based on increased understanding of the immune function and use of immunosuppressive drugs. Immunosuppressive drugs that were originally developed to prevent immune rejection of transplanted organs have been useful in treating MG. Additionally, the long-awaited study results from a randomized trial of thymectomy in myasthenia gravis compared patients who received a thymectomy plus prednisone to a group that received only prednisone (Wolfe et al., 2016). Those who received surgery plus prednisone had an overall reduction in muscle weakness and required lower daily doses of prednisone (Kaufman et al., 2016). Based on this, treatment of MG with combined surgery and medication for those who meet surgical criteria should be considered.

Nicotinic Agonists

13.6 Nicotine acts by activating ACh receptors at the ganglia.

Very few drugs are used for their effects on ACh nicotinic receptors located in the autonomic ganglia. These ganglia synapse with neurons leading to skeletal muscles (nicotinic receptors) as well as those leading to effector organs (muscarinic receptors). Drugs affecting the ganglia have the potential to produce widespread, nonselective effects on the entire autonomic nervous system.

The only common drug that activates ganglionic receptors is nicotine. The most active component of tobacco products, nicotine is well absorbed from the GI and respiratory mucosa as well as from the skin. Because nicotine acts at the ganglia, both parasympathetic and sympathetic responses are stimulated. Stimulation of organ activity generally occurs with low doses, such as those acquired from cigarette smoking. Within seconds after smoking, activation of the CNS increases alertness. The heart rate and blood pressure increase, although these parameters may subsequently decrease due to the baroreceptor reflex. The emetic center in the CNS is triggered, causing a feeling of nausea. As the level of nicotine in the blood falls, these same organ systems become depressed. Nicotine is pregnancy category D.

Nicotine is an extremely dangerous substance. Acute toxicity, which can occur due to the unintentional ingestion of insecticides containing nicotine, may cause death due to paralysis of the respiratory muscles. The chronic effects of nicotine in tobacco smokers such as lung cancer and emphysema are well documented and presented in Chapter 27.

As a drug, nicotine is used as nicotine replacement therapy (NRT) in tobacco cessation programs. Delivery systems include chewing gum (Nicorette), transdermal patches (Habitrol, NicoDerm), and nasal spray (Nicotrol). Use of these products reduces the uncomfortable symptoms of nicotine withdrawal, such as difficulty sleeping, lack of concentration, depression, headaches, and food cravings. As tobacco use diminishes over an 8- to 12-week period, these products are gradually withdrawn.

The goal of NRT is to gradually reduce the patient's physical dependence on nicotine. The nurse should remember, however, that psychologic dependence also occurs with nicotine and that most successful smoking cessation programs include behavioral modification therapy such as self-help groups. The consistent use of NRT roughly doubles a patient's chances of quitting smoking, but a great deal of persistence and motivation is required.

CONNECTION Checkpoint 13.2

Some cholinergic agonists activate both muscarinic and nicotinic receptors. From what you learned in Chapter 12, give the locations where each of these receptors may be found.

Understanding Chapter 13

Key Concepts Summary

13.1 Drugs can activate cholinergic receptors either directly or indirectly.

13.2 Muscarinic agonists produce their effects by directly stimulating cholinergic receptors.

13.3 Acetylcholinesterase inhibitors are used to treat Alzheimer' disease and myasthenia gravis.

13.4 A cholinergic crisis may develop with overdoses of AChE inhibitors or with certain toxins.

13.5 Acetylcholinesterase inhibitors are used in the pharmacotherapy of myasthenia gravis to increase the strength of muscular contraction.

13.6 Nicotine acts by activating ACh receptors at the ganglia.

CASE STUDY: Connection to Practice

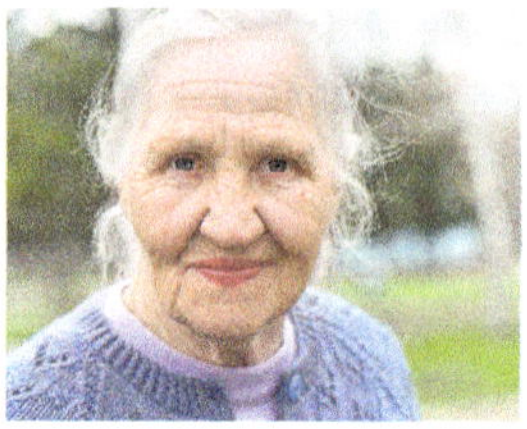

Remember the patient "Patricia Sparks" at the beginning of the chapter? Now read the remainder of the case study. Based on the information presented within this chapter, respond to the critical thinking questions that follow.

Patricia Sparks is an 82-year-old patient who lives alone in a two-story house. She has been in excellent health and has required no medications other than an occasional aspirin for osteoarthritis pain. Due to the osteoarthritis, she has had a left knee replacement. Patricia bounced back relatively quickly after surgery but required two straight-catheterizations due to urinary retention in the postoperative period.

During the past 2 days, Patricia noticed leakage of urine and felt as if she was not emptying her bladder. When she returned to her provider on her third postoperative day, she reported these symptoms. A bladder scan confirmed that Patricia was retaining a significant amount of urine, estimated at 900 mL on this visit, and a diagnosis of "overflow incontinence" is made. Her provider gives her a short-term prescription for bethanechol, and she is to return to the office in 3 days.

Critical Thinking Questions

1. As Patricia's nurse, you will be reviewing her medications before she leaves the office. What pertinent information should she receive about bethanechol?
2. Patricia states, "Sometimes, my memory is not so good and I forget to take my medication." What should she do if she forgets a dose? List suggestions that you could provide this patient to help remember her medication times and to ensure safe and effective administration.
3. What parameters would you use to determine the effectiveness of this drug therapy?

Additional Case Study

The patient has smoked cigarettes for the past 25 years. She tells the nurse that she has been using nicotine replacement therapy (Nicorette) as prescribed for the past week. However, she continues to think about and crave cigarettes, especially when she is with a group of her coworkers who smoke.

1. What should the nurse tell this patient about her continued thoughts and cravings for cigarettes?
2. Identify two websites with helpful tips that might aid this patient with smoking cessation.

Chapter Review

1. The nurse is reviewing the adverse effects associated with a muscarinic agonist. The nurse recognizes that reflex tachycardia may occur with this drug because:

1. Baroreceptors acknowledge transient hypotension and signal the medulla to increase the heart rate.
2. This drug stimulates the sinoatrial node in the right atrium.
3. Aortic receptors identify episodes of systolic hypertension and stimulate heart rhythms.
4. This drug stimulates bronchial smooth muscle contraction and a narrowing of the airway.

2. The nurse is preparing a plan of care for a patient with myasthenia gravis. Which of the following outcome statements would be appropriate for a patient receiving a cholinergic agonist such as pyridostigmine (Mestinon) for this condition? The patient will exhibit:

1. An increase in pulse rate, blood pressure, and respiratory rate.
2. Enhanced urinary elimination.
3. A decrease in muscle weakness, ptosis, and diplopia.
4. Prolonged muscle contractions and proprioception.

3. The nurse is discussing the therapeutic effects of bethanechol (Duvoid, Urecholine) with a patient who is receiving this drug for urinary retention. The nurse understands that bethanechol:

1. Changes the diameter of the urethral opening.
2. Increases the amount of urine made in the kidneys.
3. Improves blood flow to the kidney.
4. Increases the contractions of the bladder and structures that promote urination.

4. The nurse is monitoring the patient for which of the common adverse effects associated with bethanechol (Duvoid, Urecholine)? (Select all that apply.)

1. Abdominal discomfort
2. Sweating
3. Flushed skin
4. Constipation
5. Blurred vision

5. Neostigmine has been ordered for each of these patients. The order would be questioned for which patient?

1. A patient with postoperative abdominal distention
2. A patient who is experiencing urinary retention
3. A patient who has chronic obstructive pulmonary disease
4. A patient who has received nondepolarizing muscle relaxants

6. A patient has been treated with pyridostigmine (Mestinon) for myasthenia gravis and has been well managed until today. He is taken to the emergency department with symptoms of a cholinergic crisis. As the nurse caring for this patient, what symptom would be indicative of this complication?

1. Nausea and vomiting
2. Miosis
3. Drooling
4. Progressively severe muscle weakness

See Appendix A for answers to critical thinking questions, case study questions and review questions.

References

Jowkar, A. (2018). *Myasthenia gravis*. Medscape. https://emedicine.medscape.com/article/1171206-overview

Kaufman, A. J., Palatt, S., Sivak, M., Raimondi, P., Lee, D.-S., Wolf, A., . . . Flores, R. M. (2016). Thymectomy for myasthenia gravis: Complete stable remission and associated prognostic factors in over 1000 cases. *Seminars in Thoracic and Cardiovascular Surgery*, *28*, 561–568. https://doi.org/10.1053/j.semtcvs.2016.04.002

Rolston-Cregler, L. (2017). *Hallucinogenic mushroom toxicity*. Medscape. http://emedicine.medscape.com/article/817848-overview

Wolfe, G. I., Kaminski, H. J., Aban, I. B., Minisman, G., Kuo, H. C., Marx, A., . . . Cutter, G. R. (2016). Randomized trial of thymectomy in myasthenia gravis. *New England Journal of Medicine*, *375*, 511–522. https://doi.org/10.1056/NEJMoa1602489

Selected Bibliography

Asalu, A. F., Oloche, J., Itodo, S. O., & Arubi, P. O. (2019). Update on clinical evaluation and management of organophosphate poisoning. *Journal of Research in Basic and Clinical Sciences*, *1*(2), 116–121.

Goldenberg, W. D. (2018). *Emergent management of myasthenia gravis*. Medscape. https://emedicine.medscape.com/article/793136-overview

Guptill, J. T., Soni, M., & Meriggioli, M. N. (2016). Current treatment, emerging translational therapies, and new therapeutic targets for autoimmune myasthenia gravis. *Neurotherapeutics*, *13*, 118–131. https://doi.org/10.1007/s13311-015-0398-y

Katzung, B. G. (2018). Introduction to autonomic pharmacology. In B. G. Katzung (Ed), *Basic and clinical pharmacology* (13th ed., pp. 89–106). McGraw-Hill.

"I felt fine 2 days ago while working in the garden. How did I end up in this emergency room?"

—Patient "Pete Elbertson"

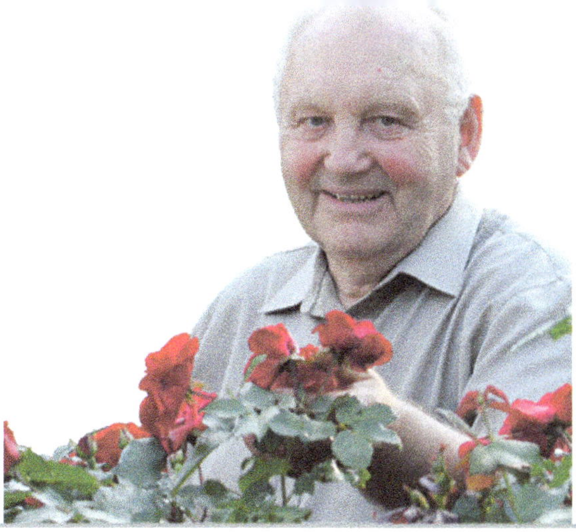

Chapter 14
Cholinergic Antagonists

Chapter Outline

- Classification of Cholinergic Antagonists
- Muscarinic Antagonists

  PROTOTYPE *Atropine (Atropen), p. 175*
- Nicotinic Antagonists: Ganglionic Blockers
- Nicotinic Antagonists: Neuromuscular Blockers

  Neuromuscular Blockers: Depolarizing Type

  PROTOTYPE *Succinylcholine (Anectine, Quelicin), p. 179*

  Neuromuscular Blockers: Nondepolarizing Type

Learning Outcomes

After reading this chapter, the student should be able to:

1. Describe how the therapeutic actions and adverse effects of the cholinergic antagonists can be explained by their blockade of muscarinic or nicotinic receptors.
2. Identify indications for muscarinic antagonists.
3. Identify symptoms of anticholinergic syndrome.
4. Identify indications for ganglionic blockers.
5. Compare and contrast the actions of the depolarizing and nondepolarizing neuromuscular blockers.
6. Compare and contrast the indications for drugs that block nicotinic receptors at the ganglia versus those that block nicotinic receptors at the neuromuscular junction.
7. For each of the classes shown in the chapter outline, identify the prototype and representative drugs and explain the mechanism(s) of drug action, primary indications, contraindications, significant drug interactions, pregnancy category, and important adverse effects.
8. Apply the nursing process to care for patients receiving pharmacotherapy with cholinergic antagonists.

Key Terms

Definitions of the terms in bold may be found in the Glossary.

Cholinergic antagonists, or anticholinergics, are drugs that inhibit the action of the neurotransmitter acetylcholine (ACh) at cholinergic synapses. Because there are two different types of cholinergic synapses, muscarinic and nicotinic, the actions and therapeutic uses of these drugs are dependent on their specific site of action. Though not as widely used as the adrenergic antagonists, several anticholinergics are important to pharmacotherapy.

Classification of Cholinergic Antagonists

14.1 Cholinergic antagonists act by blocking the effects of acetylcholine at muscarinic or nicotinic receptors.

As discussed in Chapter 13, cholinergic receptors in the autonomic nervous system are found in three anatomic locations, illustrated in Figure 14.1. This results in two primary classes of cholinergic antagonists:

- **Muscarinic antagonists** are drugs that block receptors at cholinergic synapses in the parasympathetic nervous system and at a few target organs in the sympathetic nervous system.
- **Nicotinic antagonists** are drugs that block receptors at cholinergic synapses in the ganglia or in the somatic nervous system at the neuromuscular junction.

Drugs that block the action of ACh at muscarinic receptors have more therapeutic applications than those that block nicotinic receptors. These drugs are known by a number of names, including anticholinergics, cholinergic blockers, muscarinic antagonists, and parasympatholytics. Although the term *anticholinergic* is commonly used in clinical practice, the most accurate term for this group of drugs is *muscarinic antagonists*. This is because these drugs are selective for ACh muscarinic receptors at therapeutic doses and have little effect on nicotinic receptors. The muscarinic antagonists are shown in Table 14.1.

The muscarinic antagonists compete with ACh for binding to muscarinic receptors. When ACh is prevented

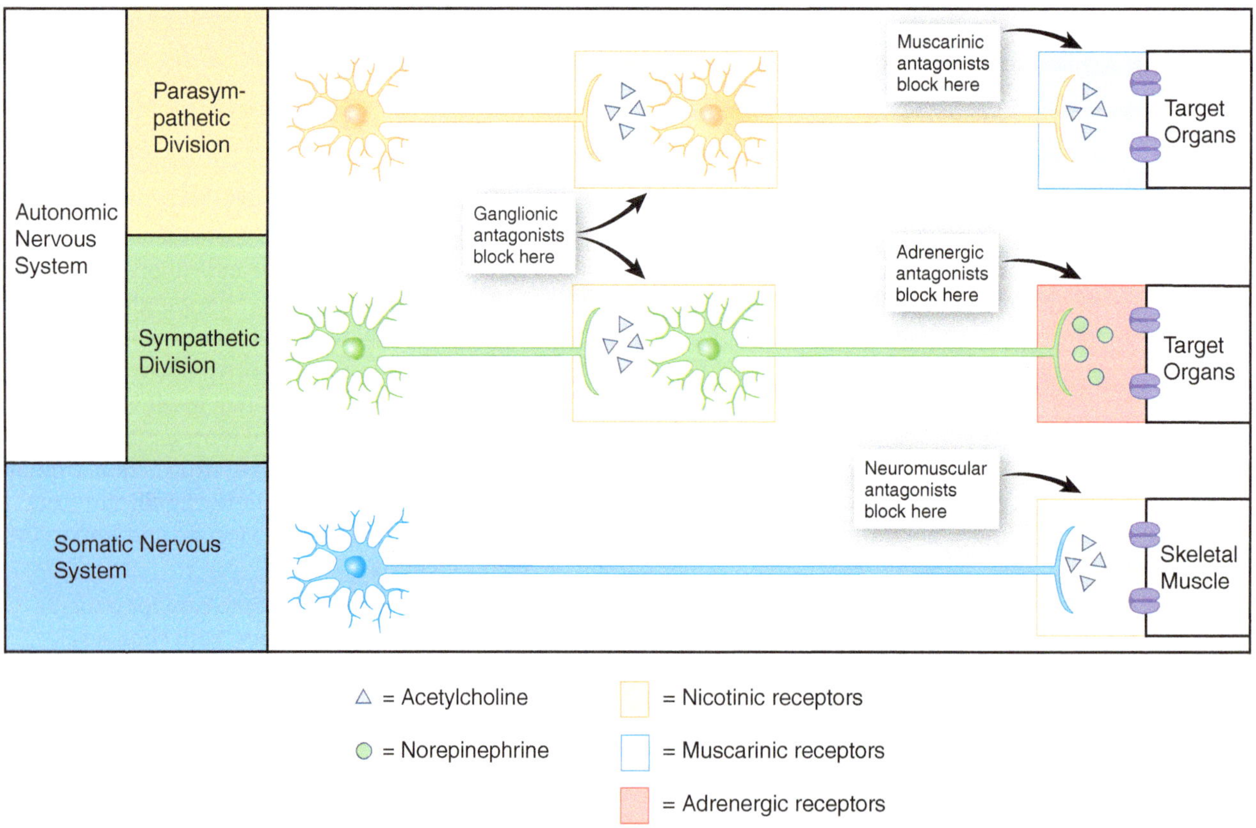

Figure 14.1 Sites of cholinergic antagonist actions. Muscarinic antagonists block cholinergic receptors in the parasympathetic nervous system. Nicotinic antagonists block cholinergic receptors at ganglia, or in the somatic nervous system at the neuromuscular junction.

from binding, parasympathetic responses are diminished at the neuroeffector organs. Suppressing the effects of ACh at muscarinic receptors will allow symptoms of sympathetic nervous system activation to predominate (fight-or-flight response). Most therapeutic uses of the muscarinic antagonists are predictable extensions of their parasympathetic-blocking actions: dilation of the pupils, increase in heart rate, drying of secretions, and bronchodilation. Note that these are the same symptoms as fight-or-flight sympathetic activation; thus, blocking the parasympathetic division causes actions similar to those that result when activating the sympathetic division. Their actions are also *opposite* those of the cholinergic agonists discussed in Chapter 13.

Nicotinic antagonists can act at two locations. **Ganglionic blockers** inhibit transmission at the ganglia in the sympathetic and parasympathetic nervous systems, thus affecting both autonomic divisions. **Neuromuscular blockers** do not act on the autonomic nervous system at all but instead inhibit transmission at the neuromuscular junctions on skeletal muscles in the somatic nervous system. The therapeutic uses of nicotinic antagonists are more limited than those of muscarinic antagonists due to their widespread and diverse actions on body function. The specific sites of action of the ganglionic and nicotinic blockers are illustrated in Figure 14.1.

Muscarinic Antagonists

14.2 Muscarinic antagonists have been used for a diverse number of conditions, but they are rarely first-line drugs due to their adverse effects.

Anticholinergics are very old drugs that have been used for a large number of disorders over many centuries. The deadly nightshade plant, *Atropa belladonna*, grows

Table 14.1 Muscarinic Antagonists (Anticholinergics)

Drug	Route and Adult Dose (Maximum Dose Where Indicated)	Adverse Effects
aclidinium (Tudorza Pressair)	Inhalation: 1 inhalation (400 mcg) bid	*Headache, cough, dry mouth, blurred vision, mydriasis, constipation, insomnia, urinary retention, burning, nasopharyngitis (inhalation forms), or stinging (eyedrop forms)* Worsening of glaucoma, tachycardia, paradoxical bradycardia, dysrhythmias, paralytic ileus, urinary retention; inhalation forms may cause sinusitis, paradoxical bronchospasm, and oropharyngeal candidiasis
atropine (Atropen)	Preanesthesia: IV/IM/subcutaneous: 0.4–0.6 mg 30–60 min before surgery Dysrhythmias: IV/IM: 0.5–1 mg q1–2h prn (max: 3 mg) Cholinergic crisis: IV: 1–2 mg, repeated every 20–30 min	
benztropine (Cogentin)	PO: 0.5–1 mg/day (max: 6 mg/day) IM/IV: 1–4 mg once or twice daily	
cyclopentolate (Cyclogyl)	Topical: 1 drop of 0.5–2% solution in the eye 40–50 min before the procedure, followed by 1 drop in 5 min	
darifenacin (Enablex)	PO: 7.5–15 mg once daily	
dicyclomine (Bentyl)	PO: 20–40 mg qid IM: 10–20 mg qid	
fesoterodine (Toviaz)	PO: 4–8 mg once daily	
glycopyrrolate (Cuvposa, Lonhala Magair, Qbrexa)	PO (for peptic ulcer): 1–2 mg tid–bid (max: 8 mg/day) PO (for excessive drooling): 0.02 mg/kg tid (max: 0.1 mg/kg tid) IM/IV: 0.1–0.2 mg tid–qid Topical (Qbrexa): one cloth applied to axilla daily Inhalation (Lonhala Magair): 25 mcg bid	
ipratropium (Atrovent)	Metered-dose inhaler (MDI): 2 inhalations qid (max: 12 inhalations/day) Nebulizer: 500 mcg q6–8h	
methscopolamine	PO: 2.5 mg tid	
oxybutynin (Ditropan XL, Oxytrol)	PO (Ditropan XL): 5–10 mg once daily (max: 30 mg/day) Transdermal (Oxytrol): 1 patch twice weekly	
propantheline	PO: 7.5–15 mg tid–qid	
revefenacin (Yupelri)	Inhalation: one vial (175 mcg) once daily	
scopolamine (Transderm-Scop)	Transdermal: 1 patch q72h starting 12 h before travel	
solifenacin (VESIcare)	PO: 5–10 mg once daily	
tiotropium (Spiriva)	Inhalation/HandiHaler: 1 capsule inhaled/day	
tolterodine (Detrol)	PO (extended release): 2–4 mg once daily	
trihexyphenidyl	PO: 1 mg/day gradually increased to 6–10 mg/day (max: 15 mg/day)	
tropicamide (Mydriacyl)	Topical: 1–2 drops of 0.5–1% solution in each eye	
trospium	PO: 20 mg bid (regular release) or 60 mg once daily (extended release)	
umeclidinium (Incruse Ellipta)	Dry-powder inhaler (DPI): one inhalation (62.5 mcg) once daily	

Note: *Italics* indicate common adverse effects. Underline indicates serious adverse effects.

throughout the world and has been a natural source of alkaloids with anticholinergic activity. References to the use of **belladonna** date back to the ancient Hindus, the Roman Empire, and the Middle Ages. The name *belladonna* is Latin for "pretty woman." Roman women applied extracts of belladonna to the face and to the eyes to create the preferred female attributes of that era—pink cheeks and dilated doe-like eyes. Because of its extreme toxicity, extracts of belladonna were sometimes used for intentional poisoning, including suicide.

Although once widely prescribed, the development of safer and more effective medications has greatly decreased the current usage of muscarinic antagonists. Most muscarinic antagonists are now prescribed as alternative medications when the preferred drug is contraindicated or not well tolerated. Potential therapeutic applications of these drugs include the following:

- **Gastrointestinal (GI) disorders.** Muscarinic antagonists suppress the secretion of gastric acid and can be used to treat peptic ulcer disease (see Chapter 59). These drugs also slow intestinal motility and can reduce cramping and diarrhea associated with irritable bowel syndrome (IBS) (see Chapter 60).
- **Ophthalmic procedures.** Topical application of muscarinic antagonists to the eye causes pupil dilation (mydriasis) and paralysis of accommodation (cycloplegia), actions that are beneficial during ophthalmic examinations (see Chapter 74).
- **Cardiac rhythm abnormalities.** Muscarinic antagonists accelerate the heart rate, which is beneficial for patients experiencing bradycardia.
- **Adjuncts to anesthesia.** Combined with drugs from other classes, muscarinic antagonists can decrease excessive salivary and respiratory secretions and reverse the bradycardia caused by general anesthetics (see Chapter 26).
- **Asthma and chronic obstructive pulmonary disease (COPD).** Muscarinic antagonists are useful in treating asthma and COPD due to their ability to dilate the bronchi (see Chapter 44).
- **Antidotes for poisoning or overdose.** These drugs are specific antidotes for overdoses with muscarinic agonists or for poisoning with muscarinic mushrooms or organophosphate insecticides (see Chapter 13).
- **Urge incontinence (overactive bladder).** A newer indication for muscarinic antagonists such as oxybutynin (Ditropan XL, Oxytrol), darifenacin (Enablex), and solifenacin (VESIcare) is to prevent involuntary voiding due to their antispasmodic effects on the smooth muscle of the bladder and detrusor muscle.
- **Parkinson's disease.** Although muscarinic antagonists are generally considered for their effects on the peripheral nervous system, several of these drugs cross the blood–brain barrier and are used for their actions on the central nervous system (CNS). They are usually prescribed to treat mild symptoms of Parkinson's disease (see Chapter 21).

CONNECTION Checkpoint 14.1

From what you learned in Chapter 13, describe the symptoms of a cholinergic crisis and explain why muscarinic antagonists are first-line drugs in reversing this condition.

Muscarinic antagonists exhibit a relatively high incidence of adverse effects, most of which are predictable because they are associated with inhibition of the parasympathetic nervous system. Adverse effects that limit their usefulness include tachycardia and CNS stimulation. Men with prostate disorders should avoid muscarinic antagonists due to the increased risk of urinary retention. Adverse effects such as xerostomia (dry mouth) and dry eyes occur in many patients due to the blockade of muscarinic receptors on the salivary glands and lacrimal glands, respectively. Blockade of muscarinic receptors can inhibit sweating, which may lead to hyperthermia. In the eye, muscarinic antagonists can paralyze the ciliary muscle and the sphincter of the iris. These ocular effects can cause photophobia (sensitivity to bright light) and increased intraocular pressure; therefore, these drugs are usually avoided in patients with glaucoma.

Overdose with anticholinergic substances produces a set of symptoms known as **anticholinergic syndrome**. Symptoms of anticholinergic syndrome include dry mouth, blurred vision, photophobia, visual changes, difficulty swallowing, agitation, and altered mental status. Although uncommon, death may result with high doses. Drugs from several other classes have cholinergic-blocking effects, including antihistamines, antipsychotics, and tricyclic antidepressants, and can trigger these same symptoms. Certain plants (including belladonna) also trigger anticholinergic syndrome. Children sometimes eat the colorful, purple berries of the deadly nightshade plant, mistaking them for cherries. Plants such as henbane and angel's trumpet are sometimes intentionally ingested for their hallucinogenic effects.

The specific antidote for anticholinergic toxicity is physostigmine, a reversible cholinesterase inhibitor. Most patients, however, recover from anticholinergic syndrome without drug treatment. Physostigmine is generally only administered to patients showing severe symptoms of anticholinergic syndrome such as seizures or psychoses.

PROTOTYPE DRUG **Atropine (Atropen)**

Classification **Therapeutic:** Drug for treatment of bradycardia, antidote for cholinergic agonist overdose
Pharmacologic: Anticholinergic, muscarinic antagonist

Therapeutic Effects and Uses: Atropine has been used for centuries for a wide variety of disorders; however, it remains a preferred drug for very few conditions because adverse effects are so common. The actions of atropine are predictable based on its ability to block muscarinic receptors.

One of the most important actions of atropine is to increase the heart rate, which can be used to therapeutic advantage when administered to patients with bradycardia. However, this increase in heart rate is considered an adverse effect when atropine is administered for other indications. The drug should be used with caution in patients with dysrhythmias because it can cause tachycardia.

Like other muscarinic antagonists, atropine can relax smooth muscle in the GI, genitourinary (GU), and respiratory tracts. This action has led to its use in treating hypermotility or spastic disorders of the GI tract including dysentery, abdominal cramping, and IBS. Slowing peristalsis too much, however, can lead to constipation. In the urinary tract, decreased smooth muscle tone can lead to urinary retention.

Because atropine decreases the quantity of exocrine secretions, the drug has been used to suppress secretions of the salivary glands and respiratory tract during surgical procedures. Excessive drying and thickening of bronchial secretions, however, can worsen asthma. Once widely used to produce bronchodilation in patients with asthma, atropine is now rarely prescribed for this disorder due to the development of safer drugs.

Topical administration of atropine to the eye will cause mydriasis and paralyze the ciliary muscle, causing cycloplegia. This may be used to advantage in ophthalmic examinations. When used for other indications, however, these actions on the eye are considered adverse effects and can result in blurred vision and photophobia.

Atropine is an antidote used to reverse symptoms of toxicity due to overdose of cholinergic agonists, including organophosphate insecticides and ingestion of mushrooms containing muscarine. AtroPen is an intramuscular (IM) autoinjection delivery system for poisonings due to toxic nerve agents or insecticides. Improvement in symptoms is usually noted within minutes.

Mechanism of Action: By occupying muscarinic receptors, atropine blocks the parasympathetic activation by ACh and induces symptoms of the fight-or-flight response. At therapeutic doses, atropine is specific for muscarinic receptors. At high doses, the drug may block nicotinic receptors in the ganglia and on skeletal muscle.

Pharmacokinetics:

Route(s)	PO, IV, IM, subcutaneous, inhalation, or ophthalmic
Absorption	Well absorbed by all routes
Distribution	Completely distributed; crosses the blood–brain barrier and placenta; small amounts are secreted in breast milk
Primary metabolism	Hepatic
Primary excretion	Renal
Onset of action	Subcutaneous/IM: 15 min; PO: 30 min; IV: 2–4 min
Duration of action	Half-life: 4 h

Adverse Effects: Common adverse effects include drying of the oral and nasal mucosa, constipation, urinary retention, increased heart rate, blurred vision, and photophobia. Serious adverse effects include ventricular fibrillation, delirium, and coma.

Contraindications/Precautions: Atropine is contraindicated in patients with acute closed-angle glaucoma because the drug may cause paralysis of the iris muscle, which can increase intraocular pressure. Safety has not been established for pregnancy and lactating mothers. Anticholinergics may cause fetal tachycardia.

Atropine should be used with caution in patients with COPD because drying of the bronchial mucosa can cause viscous mucous plugs. Blockade of cardiac muscarinic receptors can accelerate heart rate and exacerbate preexisting cardiovascular disease. Patients with hyperthyroidism should not be given atropine because the heart rate in these patients is generally high and administration of anticholinergics can induce dysrhythmias. Atropine is contraindicated for patients with serious GI conditions such as ulcerative colitis and ileus because blockade of muscarinic receptors can decrease the tone and motility of intestinal smooth muscle, which can exacerbate intestinal conditions. Patients with gastroesophageal reflux disease (GERD) and hiatal hernia experience decreased muscle tone in the lower esophageal sphincter and delayed stomach emptying. Atropine exacerbates these symptoms, increasing the risk of esophageal injury and aspiration. Patients with Down syndrome are more sensitive to the effects of atropine due to structural differences in the CNS caused by the trisomy chromosomal abnormality. Patients with Down syndrome also tend to have disorders such as GERD and heart disease, which may be adversely affected by anticholinergics.

Drug Interactions: Care must be taken when administering atropine concurrently with other drugs with anticholinergic actions, such as antihistamines, tricyclic antidepressants, quinidine, and phenothiazines, because their anticholinergic effects will be additive. Because atropine slows GI motility, the absorption of orally (PO) administered drugs may be altered. **Herbal/Food:** Some herbal supplements have atropine-like effects that potentiate the medication and can be harmful to the patient. For example, aloe, senna, buckthorn, and cascara sagrada may increase the effect of atropine, particularly if the herbs are used chronically.

Pregnancy: Category C.

Treatment of Overdose: Overdose with atropine is serious, with signs of parasympathetic blockade that include respiratory depression and circulatory collapse. Central signs such as hallucinations, seizures, and mania may be evident. Treatment is mostly supportive and may include drugs to control seizures and to increase respirations and heart rate.

Clinician Responsibilities: Key clinical implications for patients receiving atropine are included in the Applied Clinical Judgment: Patients Receiving Pharmacotherapy with Cholinergic (Muscarinic) Antagonists.

Drugs Similar to Atropine (Atropen)

The muscarinic antagonists are listed in Table 14.1.

Antisecretory drugs: Glycopyrrolate (Cuvposa), methscopolamine, and propantheline reduce gastric acid secretions in patients with peptic ulcer disease. Drugs with greater effectiveness and fewer adverse effects have replaced the anticholinergics for the first-line therapy of peptic ulcer disease.

Although an older drug, glycopyrrolate has been reformulated for several diverse indications. An IV form is available to reverse neuromuscular blockade following surgery. An oral form (Cuvposa) is available to reduce excessive drooling in children ages 3 to 16 years with certain neurologic conditions. As monotherapy and also combined with the beta-adrenergic agonist formoterol, glycopyrrolate is indicated to treat symptomatic COPD (Chapter 44). In 2018 a closely related form of this drug (glycopyrronium) was approved as a topical treatment for axillary hyperhidrosis (excessive underarm sweating).

Antispasmodic drugs: All anticholinergics slow motility in the GI tract. Dicyclomine is approved by the U.S. Food and Drug Administration (FDA) to slow GI motility and for the adjunctive treatment of peptic ulcer disease and IBS. Dicyclomine (Bentyl) is given for its ability to relax bowel spasms in patients with IBS. Antispasmodic drugs should not be administered to patients with suspected obstructive disease of the GI or GU tract because they can worsen these conditions by decreasing motility and tone.

Bronchodilation drugs: Aclidinium (Tudorza Pressair), ipratropium (Atrovent), revefenacin (Yupelri), tiotropium (Spiriva), and umeclidinium (Incruse Ellipta), are used for patients with asthma or COPD. Their primary action is relaxation of bronchial smooth muscle, which dilates the airways. Delivered via inhalation, these drugs produce more localized action with fewer systemic adverse effects than atropine.

Centrally acting drugs: Benztropine (Cogentin) and trihexyphenidyl are prescribed to reduce the muscular tremor and rigidity associated with Parkinson's disease. They may be used alone for mild forms of the disease or in combination with other medications to reduce symptoms of advanced Parkinson's. Benztropine tends to produce less CNS stimulation than does trihexyphenidyl. A parenteral form of benztropine is available for treating symptoms of acute parkinsonism associated with the use of certain antipsychotic medications. Their use is limited by adverse effects such as sedation and confusion.

Ophthalmic drugs: Anticholinergics may be applied topically to the eye to produce cycloplegia and mydriasis during ophthalmic procedures. Drugs used for this purpose include tropicamide (Mydriacyl) and cyclopentolate (Cyclogyl).

Scopolamine (Transderm-Scop): Scopolamine is very similar to atropine, although scopolamine crosses the blood–brain barrier and is more likely to cause sedation at therapeutic doses. Scopolamine is very effective for preventing motion sickness. For this indication, a transdermal patch containing scopolamine is applied to the skin, usually behind the ear, for slow release of the drug. The most common adverse effect from the transdermal product is dry mouth, although sedation may be a problem in some patients. This drug is pregnancy category C.

Urge incontinence (overactive bladder) drugs: Darifenacin (Enablex), fesoterodine (Toviaz), oxybutynin (Ditropan XL, Oxytrol), solifenacin (VESIcare), tolterodine (Detrol), and trospium are anticholinergics used for their ability to relax smooth muscle in the urinary bladder. In patients with urge incontinence, this action limits smooth muscle spasms in the bladder, thus diminishing incidences of involuntary voiding. Oxybutynin is a first-line drug for this condition and is available as immediate-release and extended-release (XL) tablets and transdermal formulations (Gelnique, Oxytrol).

Tolterodine is an alternative to oxybutynin and is also available in an extended-release (LA) formulation. More recently approved medications include darifenacin (Enablex), solifenacin (VESIcare), and trospium. These newer drugs are more selective for muscarinic receptors in the urinary bladder and thus have a more favorable side effect profile than the older drugs.

CONNECTION Checkpoint 14.2

From what you learned in Chapter 12, which of the following classes would give physiologic responses similar to the muscarinic antagonists: adrenergic agonists, adrenergic antagonists, or cholinergic agonists?

Nicotinic Antagonists: Ganglionic Blockers

14.3 Ganglionic blockers act at the autonomic ganglia to lower blood pressure in emergency situations.

Ganglionic blockers are drugs that interrupt the transmission of nerve impulses at nicotinic receptors at the autonomic ganglia. As discussed in Chapter 12, both the sympathetic and parasympathetic nervous systems have ganglia. This means that, unlike the muscarinic antagonists that selectively block parasympathetic actions, nicotinic antagonists nonselectively *inhibit the entire autonomic nervous system*. If parasympathetic and sympathetic actions are both inhibited, what types of effects will be observed?

In most cases, inhibiting the ganglia in both systems will affect the parasympathetic system more than the sympathetic. This is because the predominant, baseline autonomic tone to most organs is from the parasympathetic nervous system. When ganglionic blockers slow parasympathetic nerve impulses, symptoms characteristic of anticholinergic drugs—such as urinary retention, constipation, blurred vision, increased heart rate, and dry mouth—occur.

Although they affect all autonomic organs, the ganglionic blockers' only action that has therapeutic usefulness is vasodilation. By reducing sympathetic vasomotor tone at the arterioles, ganglionic blockers are capable of causing profound hypotension. Emergency kits must be readily available so that a vasoconstrictor such as epinephrine may be administered if blood pressure falls to a dangerous level.

Because of their potential toxicity, only one ganglionic blocker, mecamylamine, is approved for use. Mecamylamine is a long-acting nicotinic receptor antagonist that was one of the first oral antihypertensives approved by the FDA in the 1950s. Because mecamylamine produces significant adverse effects at therapeutic doses and has been replaced by safer antihypertensives. Newer potential uses (off label) include the treatment of nicotine dependence and Tourette syndrome that is unresponsive to other medications. Dosage information for mecamylamine is given in Table 14.2.

Table 14.2 Nicotinic Antagonists

Drug	Route and Adult Dose (Maximum Dose Where Indicated)	Adverse Effects
Ganglionic Blocker		
mecamylamine	PO: 2.5 mg, with increments of 2.5 mg until desired blood pressure reduction is achieved	*Orthostatic hypotension, anorexia, nausea and vomiting, constipation, dry mouth* Adynamic ileus, seizures, choreiform movement
Neuromuscular Blockers		
atracurium	IV: 0.4–0.5 mg/kg initial dose, then 0.08–0.1 mg/kg 20–45 min after the first dose, if necessary; reduce doses if used with general anesthetics	*Transient flushing of the face, neck, or chest; rash, weakness, increased salivation* Respiratory depression, anaphylaxis, prolonged apnea, cardiac arrest, bradycardia, dysrhythmias, hypotension, increases and decreases in heart rate, malignant hyperthermia, muscle paralysis
cisatracurium (Nimbex)	IV: 0.15 or 0.20 mg/kg for intubation; 0.03 mg/kg every 20 min prn or 1–2 mcg/kg/min for maintenance	
pancuronium	IV: 0.04–0.1 mg/kg initial dose; may give additional doses of 0.01 mg/kg at 30- to 60-min intervals	
rocuronium	IV: 0.6 mg/kg initially followed by continuous infusion of 0.01–0.012 mg/kg/min	
succinylcholine (Anectine, Quelicin)	IV: 0.3–1.1 mg/kg over 10–30 sec	
vecuronium	IV: 0.04–0.1 mg/kg initially, then after 25–40 min, 0.01–0.15 mg/kg every 12–15 min or 0.001 mg/kg/min by continuous infusion	

Note: *Italics* indicate common adverse effects. Underline indicates serious adverse effects.

Nicotinic Antagonists: Neuromuscular Blockers

14.4 Muscle contraction occurs when the motor end plate is depolarized.

The neuromuscular junction is a specialized cholinergic synapse that allows for communication between the nervous system and skeletal muscle. This synapse on the muscle, known as a **motor end plate**, receives an action potential from the axon of a motor neuron. Like other cholinergic synapses, the action potential causes the release of ACh, which travels across the synaptic cleft to its receptors on skeletal muscle. Anatomically, the neuromuscular junction is part of the somatic nervous system (not the autonomic).

Binding of ACh to its receptors changes the permeability of the muscle cell membrane and opens sodium channels, allowing sodium ions to rush in. Being a positive ion, sodium causes the inside of the muscle cell to depolarize and acquire a positive charge. This depolarization at the motor end plate triggers the release of calcium ions from internal storage areas within the muscle cell. The intense, though brief, release of calcium is quickly followed by skeletal muscle contraction.

As presented in Chapter 12, destruction of ACh by the enzyme acetylcholinesterase (AChE) removes the neurotransmitter from the motor end plate, allowing the muscle cell membrane to repolarize. Calcium returns to its internal storage depots, and muscle relaxation occurs. This process by which the action potential causes muscular contraction is known as *excitation-contraction coupling*.

When multiple action potentials arrive at a specific motor end plate, the muscle cell undergoes a series of repeated depolarizations and repolarizations. This causes a continuous depolarized state in which calcium does not return to its storage depots, and a *sustained* muscle contraction is achieved. This contraction, however, can only be sustained by a continuous cycle of depolarizations and repolarizations. If the cell is simply depolarized (without undergoing repolarization), calcium will return to its storage areas and contraction will totally cease, resulting in a flaccid muscle. This paralyzed condition is necessary when performing certain surgical procedures. The depolarization of the motor end plate is illustrated in Figure 14.2.

Neuromuscular Blockers: Depolarizing Type

14.5 Depolarizing neuromuscular blockers are given to produce muscle paralysis during short medical–surgical procedures.

The nicotinic synapse at the neuromuscular junction can be affected by drugs that can act by either a depolarizing

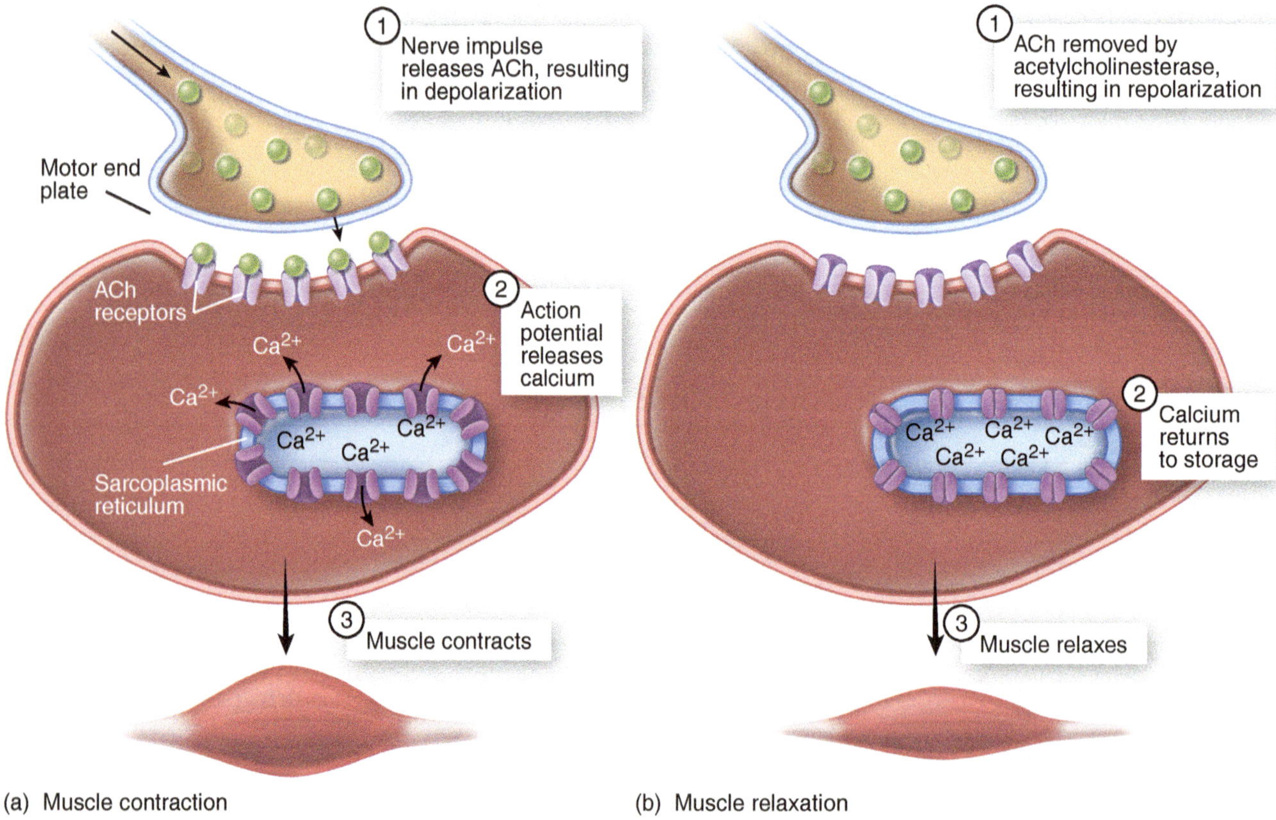

Figure 14.2 Normal depolarization of the motor end plate: (a) Depolarization: ACh causes calcium to be released from storage, resulting in muscle contraction. (b) Repolarization: ACh is destroyed by acetylcholinesterase, calcium returns to storage, and muscle relaxation results.

or nondepolarizing mechanism. These depolarizing and nondepolarizing neuromuscular blockers produce the same result: total skeletal muscle relaxation or muscle paralysis.

Succinylcholine is the sole member of the depolarizing neuromuscular blocker class of drugs. This drug competes with ACh for nicotinic receptors on the motor end plates of skeletal muscle. Once bound to ACh receptors, succinylcholine produces muscle contraction by the same mechanism as ACh. However, succinylcholine is not destroyed by AChE, and the drug causes a prolonged and continuous depolarization of the muscle cell. Without repolarization, calcium returns to its internal storage depots and the muscle relaxes. The mechanism of action of succinylcholine is illustrated in Figure 14.3a.

It is important to note that succinylcholine does not enter the CNS. Although the drug causes muscle paralysis, it does not produce anesthesia or loss of consciousness. The patient is still able to feel pain and is aware of his or her surroundings. Thus, succinylcholine is only one component of balanced anesthesia, as discussed in Chapter 26.

CONNECTION Checkpoint 14.3

Pyridostigmine also affects nicotinic receptors in skeletal muscle. From what you learned in Chapter 13, would you expect this drug to interact with neuromuscular blockers? What is the primary indication for pyridostigmine?

PROTOTYPE DRUG Succinylcholine (Anectine, Quelicin)

Classification **Therapeutic:** Skeletal muscle relaxant
Pharmacologic: Neuromuscular blocker (depolarizing type)

Therapeutic Effects and Uses: Effects of succinylcholine are first noted as muscle weakness and muscle spasms. Eventually muscle paralysis occurs. The drug is primarily used as an adjunct to surgical anesthesia to cause complete skeletal muscle relaxation of the abdominal muscles. It may also be used to relax muscles during the insertion of an endotracheal tube and to assist in the management of mechanical ventilation. Administration of succinylcholine reduces the amount of general anesthetic needed for surgical procedures.

When given IV, succinylcholine induces muscle relaxation in less than a minute. When the infusion is discontinued, muscle control returns in a few minutes because the drug is rapidly destroyed in the plasma by the enzyme **pseudocholinesterase** (also called plasma cholinesterase). This makes the drug ideal for very short procedures, such as intubation or electroconvulsive shock therapy.

Some patients have a genetic deficiency in plasma cholinesterase. In these patients, succinylcholine will

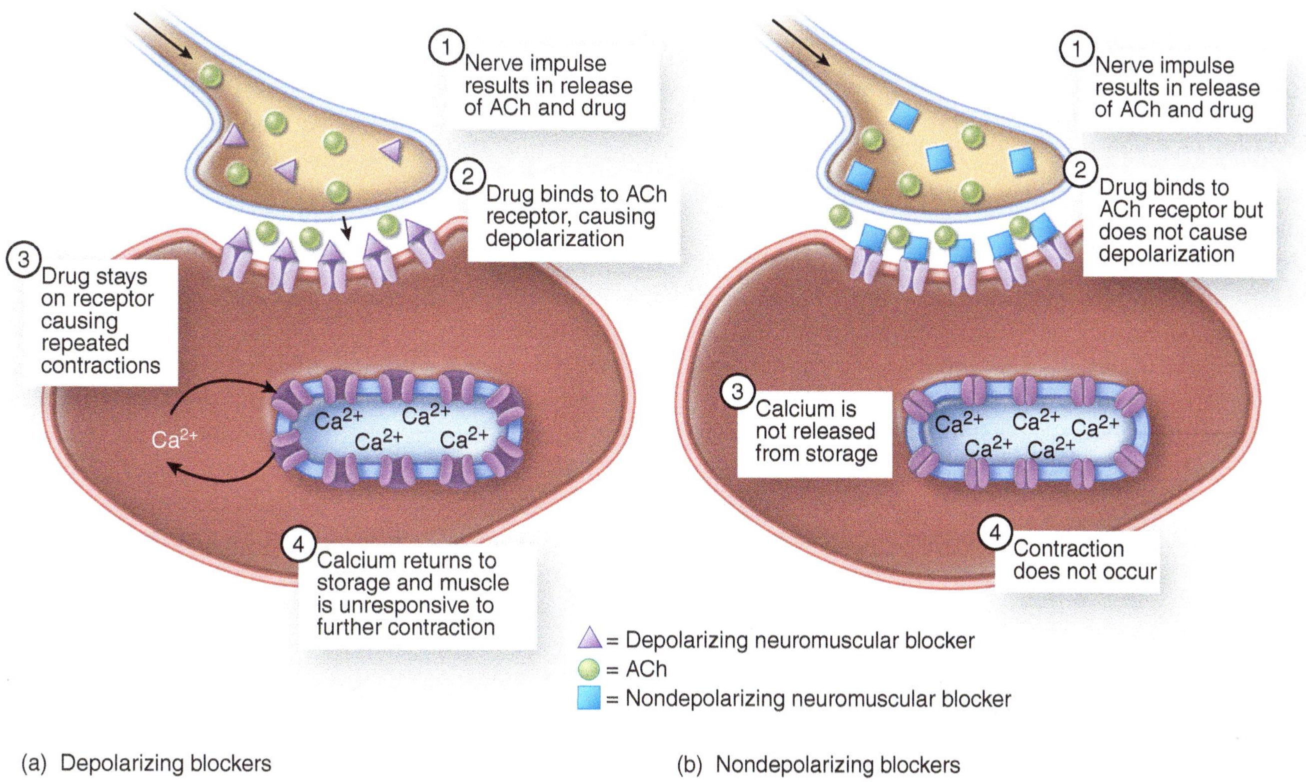

Figure 14.3 Mechanism of action of neuromuscular blockers: (a) Depolarizing neuromuscular blocker occupies ACh receptors and causes depolarization and muscle paralysis. (b) Nondepolarizing neuromuscular blocker occupies ACh receptors and causes muscle paralysis without depolarization.

have an unusually prolonged duration of action, and paralysis may persist for hours. Because there is no specific antidote for succinylcholine overdose, the patient must receive supportive treatment until the drug is metabolized and removed by the body. This adverse effect may be avoided by assessing plasma cholinesterase levels prior to surgery. If low, succinylcholine may be contraindicated, or the dose lowered to prevent prolonged muscle paralysis.

In addition to genetic deficiency, pseudocholinesterase levels may be decreased during therapy with acetylcholinesterase inhibitors such as pyridostigmine, which is a preferred drug for treating patients with myasthenia gravis (see Chapter 13). Patients having this genetic deficiency will exhibit a prolonged duration of muscle paralysis if given succinylcholine.

Mechanism of Action: Like endogenous ACh, succinylcholine binds to cholinergic receptor sites at neuromuscular junctions (nicotinic). After repeated contractions the skeletal muscle membranes are unable to repolarize as long as the drug stays on the receptor. The result is total muscle relaxation or paralysis.

Pharmacokinetics:

Route(s)	IM, IV
Absorption	Well-absorbed IM
Distribution	Completely, including crossing the placenta
Primary metabolism	Plasma by pseudocholinesterase
Primary excretion	Renal
Onset of action	IV: less than 1 min; IM: 2–3 min
Duration of action	IV: 2–3 min; IM: 10–30 min

Adverse Effects: Succinylcholine can cause complete paralysis of the diaphragm and intercostal muscles; thus, mechanical ventilation is necessary during surgery. If doses are high, succinylcholine will also inhibit nerve transmission at the ganglia, causing tachycardia, hypotension, and urinary retention. In certain susceptible patients, a rapid onset of extremely high fever with muscle rigidity may occur, a serious condition known as **malignant hyperthermia**. The high temperature is caused by excessive metabolic activity in muscles, triggered by the drug. Although rare, malignant hyperthermia may be fatal. Other serious adverse effects include respiratory depression, apnea, and dysrhythmias. **Black Box Warning:** Children with certain congenital musculoskeletal diseases (e.g., Duchenne muscular dystrophy) are at greater risk for cardiac arrest when this drug is used and should be monitored especially closely. Because there is no way to predict which patients are at risk, the use of succinylcholine in children should be reserved for emergency intubation or instances where immediate securing of the airway is necessary.

Contraindications/Precautions: Because succinylcholine is an essential component of balanced surgical anesthesia, there are few absolute contraindications. Patients with a personal or family history of malignant hyperthermia should not receive this drug. Succinylcholine should be used cautiously in patients with preexisting electrolyte imbalances or heart failure because this drug can cause a sudden release of intracellular potassium, resulting in hyperkalemia. Patients with pulmonary or metabolic disorders should be monitored carefully because succinylcholine can cause respiratory depression and acidosis. Due to its renal excretion, succinylcholine should be used cautiously in patients with kidney disease. Because the drug can increase intraocular pressure, it is contraindicated in patients with glaucoma.

Drug Interactions: Additive skeletal muscle inhibition will occur if succinylcholine is given concurrently with clindamycin, phenothiazine, aminoglycosides, furosemide, lithium, quinidine, or lidocaine. If succinylcholine is given concurrently with the anesthetics halothane or nitrous oxide, the risk of dysrhythmias, sinus arrest, apnea, and malignant hyperthermia is increased. Use with digoxin can increase the risk of dysrhythmias due to the hyperkalemia caused by the neuromuscular blocker. If opioid analgesics are given concurrently with succinylcholine, there is an increased risk of bradycardia and sinus arrest. **Herbal/Food:** Melatonin may increase the neuromuscular blocking action of succinylcholine.

Pregnancy: Category C.

Treatment of Overdose: Overdose can lead to serious or fatal respiratory depression. The drug is discontinued and assisted ventilation is provided until the drug's effects wear off.

Nursing Responsibilities:

- Monitor vital signs frequently and keep the airway free of secretions.
- Obtain baseline laboratory tests such as serum electrolytes. Imbalances in potassium, calcium, and magnesium can potentiate the actions of neuromuscular blockers.
- Monitor for transient apnea, which usually occurs at the point of maximal drug effect (1 to 2 minutes); spontaneous respiration should return in a few seconds or, at most, 3 or 4 minutes.
- Prepare for emergency endotracheal intubation, artificial respiration, and assisted or controlled respiration with oxygen.
- Monitor temperature frequently in the postoperative patient when succinylcholine has been used.
- Provide emotional support and pain relief, if needed. The drug will cause paralysis without analgesia or sedation.

Lifespan and Diversity Considerations:

- Because of postprocedural stiffness or muscle weakness, extra caution should be exercised when assisting the older patient with ambulation or activities of daily living (ADLs) to prevent falls or injury.
- When used in children, monitor vital signs, especially heart rate and rhythm, frequently due to increased risk of cardiac arrest related to certain congenital musculoskeletal diseases. The existence of these diseases may not always be known and the drug is usually avoided in children when possible.

Patient and Family Education:

- Muscle stiffness and pain that may last for as long as 24 to 30 hours may occur after the procedure.
- Understand that sore throat and hoarseness are common even when the pharyngeal airway has not been used.
- Report persistent muscle weakness.

Drugs Similar to Succinylcholine (Anectine, Quelicin)

Succinylcholine is the only depolarizing neuromuscular blocker.

Neuromuscular Blockers: Nondepolarizing Type

14.6 Nondepolarizing neuromuscular blockers are given to produce muscle paralysis during longer surgical procedures.

The first neuromuscular blocker was **curare**, which was initially extracted from different plant species native to the rain forests of South America. Indians of the region cooked the roots and stems to produce a thick, tarry substance that could be rubbed on the tips of arrows. Once shot into the muscle of an animal, curare would rapidly cause muscle weakness, allowing the Indians to overcome and kill the game. It is these same properties that allowed medical science to use curare to reduce muscle spasms and to cause skeletal muscle paralysis during operative procedures. The active chemical extracted from curare is called tubocurarine. Tubocurarine is no longer used for medical procedures, but there are six **nondepolarizing neuromuscular blockers (NDNBs)** that have similar uses, actions, and adverse effects (see Table 14.2).

Like succinylcholine, the NDNBs are nicotinic antagonists that bind to ACh receptors at motor end plates in skeletal muscle. However, the NDNBs do not cause depolarization of the muscle cell; they act by preventing ACh from reaching its receptors. The mechanism of action of the NDNBs is illustrated in Figure 14.3b.

All NDNBs have identical actions, with their primary application being to relax skeletal muscles during operative procedures. These drugs may also be used to facilitate management of mechanical ventilation by suppressing contractions of respiratory muscles, thus eliminating resistance to mechanical ventilation. Suppressing muscular reflexes allows smoother insertion of an endotracheal tube, which is an additional indication for the use of these drugs. For patients undergoing electroconvulsive shock therapy or those who have tetanus, neuromuscular blockers can reduce the intensity and pain of severe muscle contractions.

The NDNBs are charged molecules that do not readily cross membranes. Thus, they are almost always administered IV. Because they do not cross the blood–brain barrier, they do not induce sedation, analgesia, or loss of consciousness. This allows for complete skeletal muscle paralysis without loss of consciousness. Administration of an anesthetic is necessary when diminished consciousness or analgesia is desired, such as during surgical anesthesia.

The NDNBs differ in their durations of action. This is a critical difference because the muscular relaxation induced by the drug must last long enough to complete the specific surgical procedure. All NDNBs have a very rapid onset of action, inducing paralysis within 1 to 2 minutes.

The most common adverse effects of the NDMBs are tachycardia, urticaria, and hypotension, which occur when these drugs trigger the release of histamine. Some neuromuscular blockers such as pancuronium and vecuronium cause less histamine release. Pretreatment with an antihistamine can lessen the risk for these adverse effects

The most serious concern when using NDNBs is paralysis of respiratory muscles, leading to laryngeal collapse and possible respiratory arrest. For atracurium, cisatracurium, and pancuronium, these adverse effects can be prevented or reversed by administering a combination of neostigmine and glycopyrralate. For rocuronium and vecuronium, sugammadex (Bridion) is administered. Sugammadex was approved in 2015 and produces fewer side effects than neostigmine.

Short-acting drugs: Rocuronium has the shortest duration of action, about 15 to 20 minutes. A continuous infusion may be used to maintain the neuromuscular block for a longer time.

Intermediate-acting drugs: Atracurium, cisatracurium (Nimbex), and vecuronium have durations of action of 30 to 45 minutes. Atracurium and cisatracurium are not eliminated by the liver or kidneys and may be better choices for patients with hepatic or renal disease. Vecuronium has the advantage of causing no histamine release.

Long-acting drugs: The only long-acting drug in this class, pancuronium, has a duration of 60 to 90 minutes.

CONNECTIONS: Patient Safety

Medication Errors During Transitions of Care

The risk for a medication error increases during transitions of care, also known as "handoffs." These errors may occur with transfers between patient care units in a healthcare agency or at time of discharge (Dusek et al., 2015; Robins & Dai, 2015; Ruggiero et al., 2015). As a nurse working in the postanesthesia care unit (PACU), how could the chance for a medication error be decreased when transferring a patient from the PACU to a surgical unit?

CONNECTION Checkpoint 14.4

From what you learned in Chapter 13, explain why a patient with myasthenia gravis might be particularly susceptible to the actions of neuromuscular blockers.

CONNECTIONS: APPLIED CLINICAL JUDGMENT

Patients Receiving Pharmacotherapy with Cholinergic (Muscarinic) Antagonists

Key Assessment Data

- History of current condition, baseline vital signs, physical exam findings; history of CV, GI, GU disease, acute (closed-angle) glaucoma; medication history; pregnancy status. Bowel sounds, urinary output, and cardiac rhythm should be assessed depending on the condition being treated.
- Ongoing assessment during drug therapy should include monitoring for excessive ANS stimulation (tremors, palpitations, changes in blood pressure, dizziness, urinary retention, abdominal pain) or changes in behavior (e.g., confusion, depression, or drowsiness). Monitor for abdominal distention and auscultate for bowel sounds. Palpate for bladder distention and monitor output.

Desired Therapeutic Outcomes

Improvement is observed and measurable by patient's pulse, BP, respiratory rate and ease of breathing within acceptable parameters; gastric motility and cramping have slowed; involuntary voiding has diminished or eased.

Minimizing Adverse Effects:

- Notify the healthcare provider if BP or pulse exceeds established parameters. Continue frequent cardiac monitoring as appropriate (e.g., electrocardiogram) and urine output.
- Because anticholinergics may decrease tone and motility of intestinal and bladder smooth muscle, monitor the patient for abdominal distention and auscultate for bowel sounds. Palpate for bladder distention and monitor output.
- Minimize exposure to heat and strenuous exercise to avoid heatstroke because anticholinergics can inhibit sweat gland secretions.
- Provide for eye comfort such as a darkened room, soft cloth over eyes, sunglasses, or lubricating eyedrops if mydriasis occurs.

Lifespan Considerations

- Children and older adults may be more sensitive to the effects of anticholinergic drugs and require frequent monitoring.
- "Atropine fever"—hyperpyrexia due to suppression of perspiration and heat loss—increases the risk of heatstroke in young children and older adults. Children and older adults should be monitored frequently.
- The older adult is at increased risk of constipation due to slowed peristalsis, and the male older adult is at higher risk for mechanical obstruction due to an enlarged prostate.
- Older and debilitated patients should report excessive drowsiness or CNS stimulation, even at usual doses of anticholinergics.

Patient Education

- Provide for eye comfort such as a darkened room, soft cloth over eyes, sunglasses, or lubricating eyedrops.
- Encourage the use of sips of water, ice chips, oral rinses free of alcohol, or hard candies, which may ease mouth dryness.
- Minimize exposure to heat and strenuous exercise. Dizziness, change in mental status, pale skin, muscle cramping, and nausea are signs of impending heat exhaustion or heatstroke and should be reported immediately.
- Photosensitivity may occur and sunglasses may be needed in bright light or for outside activities. Lubricating eyedrops may soothe dryness. Caution should be taken with driving until drug effects are known.
- Increase fluids and fiber to ease constipation. Report difficulty with urination.
- Teach appropriate administration techniques; a teach-back session should occur before patient self-administration.

Prescribing Considerations

- Patients who are on a cholinesterase inhibitor should be seen for follow-up at 3 and 6 months to assess drug response and tolerance and to prevent any symptoms of cholinergic excess.
- Patients should receive education, in detail, regarding the common potential adverse effects of all new medications.
- A pharmacist consult is beneficial; the pharmacist can verify dosing, look for drug–drug interactions, and perform medication reconciliation and report back to the prescriber if there are issues.
- An interprofessional team approach is essential in cholinergic therapy to achieve optimal patient results.

Understanding Chapter 14

Key Concepts Summary

14.1 Cholinergic antagonists act by blocking the effects of acetylcholine at muscarinic or nicotinic receptors.

14.2 Muscarinic antagonists have been used for a diverse number of conditions, but they are rarely drugs of choice due to their adverse effects.

14.3 Ganglionic blockers act at the autonomic ganglia to lower blood pressure in emergency situations.

14.4 Muscle contraction occurs when the motor end plate is depolarized.

14.5 Depolarizing neuromuscular blockers are given to produce muscle paralysis during short medical–surgical procedures.

14.6 Nondepolarizing neuromuscular blockers are given to produce muscle paralysis during longer surgical procedures.

CASE STUDY: Making the Patient Connection

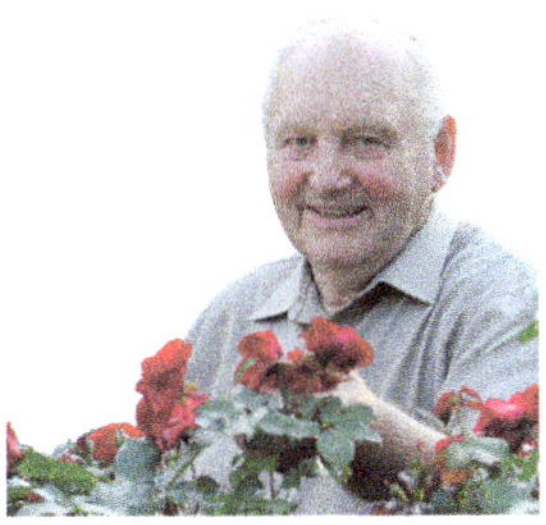

Remember the patient "Pete Elbertson" at the beginning of the chapter? Now read the remainder of the case study. Based on the information presented within this chapter, respond to the critical thinking questions that follow.

Pete Elbertson is a 60-year-old man who enjoys working in his large vegetable garden. Two days ago, while watering his tomatoes, he noticed that insects had infested the plants. To avoid further damage, Pete powdered the plants with an insecticide. In his rush to finish, he unintentionally contaminated himself with the insecticide and kept working for several hours before showering.

Now, Pete presents to the local emergency department (ED) with nausea, dizziness, sweating, excessive salivation, weepy eyes, and a runny nose. He reports intermittent twitching of his upper extremities and uncoordinated movement.

His initial assessment reveals an 84-kg (185-lb) White male with a past medication history of hypertension diagnosed 5 years ago. He is married and has two adult children. He smokes one pack of cigarettes per day and does not use alcohol. Pete's vital signs are blood pressure, 158/94 mmHg; heart rate, 58 beats/min; respiratory rate, 30 breaths/min; and temperature, 37.3°C (99.2°F). His skin is pale and moist. He exhibits copious lacrimation and rhinorrhea. Both pupils are constricted. Crackles are heard bilaterally in all lung fields on inspiration. Since admission to the ED he has vomited twice and had one large diarrhea stool.

Pete is diagnosed with acute organophosphate poisoning. The patient is started on oxygen therapy, and the nurse will observe him closely for further respiratory distress. Atropine 2 mg is administered IV every 15 minutes over the next hour.

Critical Thinking Questions

1. Discuss the mechanism of action associated with atropine.
2. Why is this drug being given to Pete?
3. What adverse effects should you expect for the patient from the administration of atropine?

Additional Case Study

You are caring for Nick, a 56-year-old man, in the intensive care unit. During the past 2 hours, you have been closely monitoring him due to increased respiratory distress. When the healthcare provider arrives, he informs you that Nick will need to be placed on a mechanical ventilator. The patient will be given a neuromuscular blocking drug to assist with the insertion of an endotracheal tube.

1. Describe the mechanism of action associated with this drug classification.
2. What is the rationale for the administration of neuromuscular blocking drugs for this patient?
3. Identify the problems associated with the administration of neuromuscular blocking drugs.

Chapter Review

1. Which health teaching concept should the nurse review with a patient receiving tolterodine (Detrol) for urge incontinence?
   1. Exercise daily to avoid muscle atrophy.
   2. Increase dietary fiber and water intake to avoid constipation.
   3. Consume foods high in iron to increase red blood cell production.
   4. Monitor the heart rate for bradycardia.

2. The nurse is aware that the therapeutic uses for cholinergic antagonists include (select all that apply):
   1. Ophthalmic procedures.
   2. Cardiac rhythm abnormalities.
   3. Asthma.
   4. Poisonings.
   5. Urinary retention.

3. Which factor in the patient's history would cause the nurse to question a medication order for atropine?
   1. A 42-year-old woman with a history of drug abuse
   2. An 85-year-old man with benign prostatic hyperplasia
   3. An 18-year-old man with irritable bowel syndrome
   4. A 22-year-old woman on the second day of her menstrual cycle

4. Muscarinic antagonists, such as benztropine (Cogentin), are most often contraindicated in glaucoma because these drugs can:
   1. Increase intraocular pressure.
   2. Promote ocular infections.
   3. Cause miosis, which leads to blindness.
   4. Detach the retina.

5. The patient will be taking cholinergic antagonists following discharge from the healthcare agency. Which statement, made by the patient, would indicate that additional teaching is needed?
   1. "To relieve dry mouth, I should drink plenty of water."
   2. "I will avoid activities requiring mental alertness until I know the effects of this drug."
   3. "The use of lubricating eyedrops should be avoided. I should see an eye doctor for dry eyes."
   4. "I will not breastfeed while taking this drug without consulting my healthcare provider."

6. The nurse administering succinylcholine knows that this drug causes:
   1. Muscle paralysis; it does not produce anesthesia or loss of consciousness.
   2. Loss of consciousness, along with muscle paralysis and anesthesia.
   3. Deep muscle relaxation and relief from pain.
   4. Increased mental alertness with muscle paralysis.

See Appendix A for answers to critical thinking questions, case study questions and review questions.

References

Dusek, B., Pearce, N., Harripaul, A., & Lloyd, M. (2015). Care transitions: A systematic review of best practices. *Journal of Nursing Care Quality*, *30*, 233–239. https://doi.org/10.1097/NCQ.0000000000000097

Robins, H. M., & Dai, F. (2015). Handoffs in the postoperative anesthesia care unit: Use of a checklist for transfer of care. *AANA Journal*, *83*, 264–268.

Ruggiero, J., Smith, J., Copeland, J., & Boxer, B. (2015). Discharge time out: An innovative nurse-driven protocol for medication reconciliation. *Medsurg Nursing*, *24*(3), 165–172.

Selected Bibliography

Buhl, R., & Hamelmann, E. (2019). Future perspectives of anticholinergics for the treatment of asthma in adults and children. *Therapeutics and Clinical Risk Management, 15*, 473–485. https://doi.org/10.2147/TCRM.S180890

Clar, D. T., & Liu, M. (2020). *Non-depolarizing neuromuscular blockers*. StatPearls Publishing.

Kachru, N., Carnahan, R. M., Johnson, M. L., & Aparasu, R. R. (2015). Potentially inappropriate anticholinergic medication use in older adults with dementia. *Journal of the American Pharmacists Association, 55*, 603–612. https://doi.org/10.1331/JAPhA.2015.14288

Katz, K. D. (2018). *Organophosphate toxicity*. Medscape. http://emedicine.medscape.com/article/167726-overview

Leron, E., Weintraub, A. Y., Mastrolia, S. A., & Schwarzman, P. (2017). Overactive bladder syndrome: Evaluation and management. *Current Urology, 11*(3), 117–125. https://doi.org/10.1159/000447205

Nishtala, P. S., Salahudeen, M. S., & Hilmer, S. N. (2016). Anticholinergics: Theoretical and clinical overview. *Expert Opinion on Drug Safety, 15*(6), 753–768. https://doi.org/10.1517/14740338.2016.1165664

Ramnarine, M. (2019). *Anticholinergic toxicity*. Medscape. https://emedicine.medscape.com/article/812644-overview

Stawicki, N., & Gessner, P. (2018). Residual neuromuscular blockade in the critical care setting. *AACN Advanced Critical Care, 29*(1), 15–24. https://doi.org/10.4037/aacnacc2018384

Thiagamoorthy, G., Cardozo, L., & Robinson, D. (2016). Current and future pharmacotherapy for treating overactive bladder. *Expert Opinion on Pharmacotherapy, 17*, 1317–1325. https://doi.org/10.1080/14656566.2016.1186645

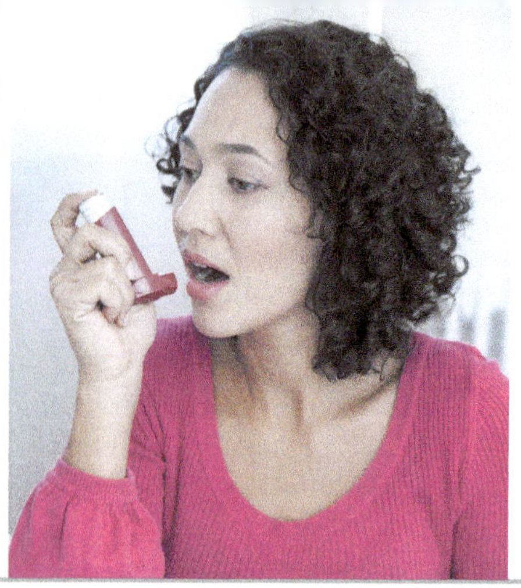

"I woke up this morning having difficulty breathing. I think my asthma is acting up again."
—*Patient "Alexia Howard"*

Chapter 15
Adrenergic Agonists

Chapter Outline

Learning Outcomes

After reading this chapter, the student should be able to:

1. Identify the physiologic responses produced when a drug activates adrenergic receptors.
2. Explain the direct and indirect mechanisms by which adrenergic agonists act.
3. Compare and contrast the characteristics of catecholamines and noncatecholamines.
4. Identify indications for pharmacotherapy with adrenergic agonists.
5. Compare and contrast the types of responses that occur when a drug activates $alpha_1$-, $alpha_2$-, $beta_1$-, or $beta_2$-adrenergic receptors.
6. For each of the classes shown in the chapter outline, identify the prototype and representative drugs and explain the mechanism(s) of drug action, primary indications, contraindications, significant drug interactions, pregnancy data and important adverse effects.
7. Apply clinical judgement to care for patients receiving pharmacotherapy with adrenergic agonists.

Key Terms

Definitions of the terms in bold may be found in the Glossary.

Adrenergic agonists are drugs that activate the sympathetic nervous system and induce symptoms of the fight-or-flight response. The pharmacology of adrenergic drugs is more complex than their cholinergic counterparts due to the existence of the receptor subtypes alpha and beta. Drugs that activate these subtypes have widespread applications to the pharmacotherapy of shock, hypotension, asthma, and symptoms of the common cold.

Actions of Adrenergic Agonists

15.1 Adrenergic agonists activate the sympathetic nervous system to produce fight-or-flight symptoms.

Adrenergic agonists, also called **sympathomimetics**, are agents that activate adrenergic receptors in the sympathetic nervous system. Drugs in this class include naturally occurring (endogenous) substances such as norepinephrine (NE), epinephrine, and dopamine. NE is the major neurotransmitter in the sympathetic nervous system, whereas epinephrine is the primary hormone released by the adrenal medulla. Dopamine is the immediate biochemical precursor to NE and is a key neurotransmitter in certain regions of the central nervous system (CNS). In addition to their natural physiologic roles in the body, NE, epinephrine, and dopamine are available as prescription drugs. A number of synthetic adrenergic agonists that mimic the effects of these natural neurotransmitters are also available.

When administered as drugs, the adrenergic agonists induce symptoms of the fight-or-flight response. Clinically, their most important actions are on the cardiovascular and respiratory systems. Activation of adrenergic receptors in the myocardium increases the heart rate (positive chronotropic effect) and the force of contraction (positive inotropic effect). Cardiac output increases. Constriction of vascular smooth muscle causes a rapid increase in blood pressure. Administration by the parenteral or inhalation routes immediately relaxes bronchial smooth muscle, resulting in bronchodilation. Activation of adrenergic receptors in the smooth muscle of the gastrointestinal (GI) and urinary tracts slows peristalsis. Metabolic effects include increased oxygen consumption and increased blood glucose and lactate levels. Other adrenergic actions include reduction of glandular secretory activity and mydriasis.

It is important to remember that the symptoms of the fight-or-flight response elicited by the adrenergic agonists may be considered as therapeutic or adverse, depending on the condition of the patient and the goals of pharmacotherapy. For example, if the patient is in shock, increased blood pressure is a key therapeutic effect. However, if the patient is taking an adrenergic agonist to treat nasal congestion, an increase in blood pressure is an adverse effect. Furthermore, a therapeutic effect may become an adverse effect if taken to extreme, such as raising blood pressure too much or causing excessive drying of the nasal or oral mucosa.

The actions produced by adrenergic agonists are similar to those of cholinergic (muscarinic) antagonists (see Chapter 14). This is because blocking muscarinic receptors in the parasympathetic nervous system allows sympathetic nerve impulses to predominate. However, because the sympathetic nervous system has alpha- and beta-receptor subtypes, the actions of many adrenergic agonists are more specific than the cholinergic blockers, allowing for wider therapeutic applications with a lower incidence of adverse effects.

CONNECTION Checkpoint 15.1

From what you learned in Chapter 12, where are most dopaminergic receptors located? Dopaminergic drugs would most likely be prescribed for what disorders?

PharmFACT

Pheochromocytomas are tumors of the adrenal medulla that secrete large amounts of adrenergic agonists including dopamine, epinephrine, and norepinephrine. As expected, signs and symptoms are those of sympathetic nervous system hyperactivity: increased heart rate and blood pressure and anxiety resembling that of a panic attack. Treatment includes pharmacotherapy with antihypertensives until surgery can be performed to remove the tumor (Blake, 2018).

Mechanisms of Action of Adrenergic Agonists

15.2 Adrenergic agonists may act directly by binding to adrenergic receptors or indirectly by increasing the amount of norepinephrine at synapses.

Sympathomimetics exert their effects by two distinct mechanisms. Most act *directly* by binding to and activating adrenergic receptors. Examples include the three endogenous hormones epinephrine, NE, and dopamine.

Some adrenergic agonists act *indirectly* by increasing the amount of NE neurotransmitter in adrenergic synapses. Any substance that increases the amount of NE in the synaptic cleft will produce an intense and prolonged fight-or-flight response. A few drugs, such as ephedrine, act by both direct and indirect mechanisms. The mechanisms of indirect-acting agents are shown in Figure 15.1. NE can be increased at the synapse by the following three means:

- **Stimulating the release of NE from its storage vesicles on the presynaptic neuron.** Drugs that act by this mechanism include ephedrine and amphetamine.
- **Inhibiting the reuptake of NE from the synaptic cleft back to the presynaptic neuron.** Examples of drugs

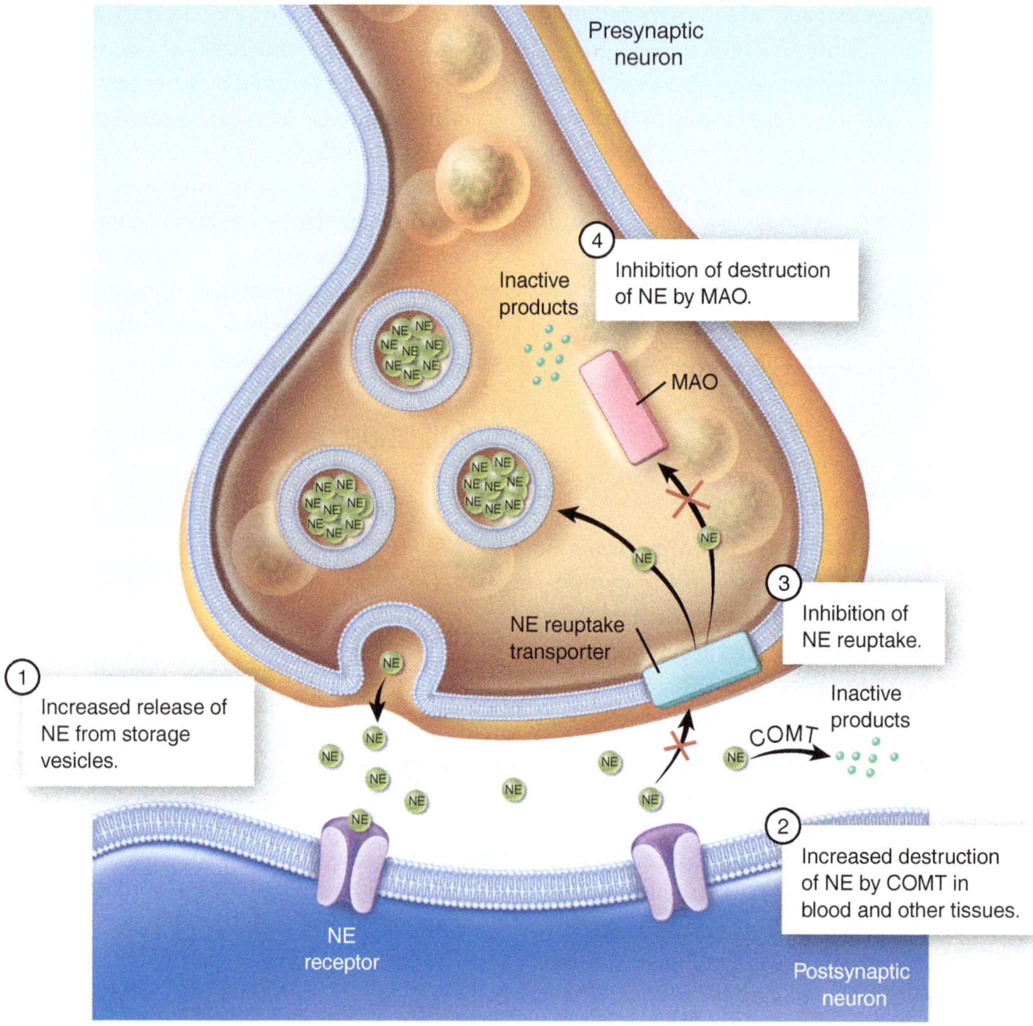

Figure 15.1 Mechanisms of action of adrenergic agonists: (1) stimulation of the release of norepinephrine (NE); (2) increased destruction of NE by catechol-O-methyltransferase (COMT); (3) inhibition of the reuptake of NE; (4) inhibition of the destruction of NE by MAO.

that inhibit reuptake of NE include the antidepressant imipramine (Tofranil) and cocaine.

- **Inhibiting the destruction of NE by the enzyme monoamine oxidase (MAO).** Phenelzine (Nardil) is an example of a MAO inhibitor (MAOI).

Indirect adrenergic agonists are less commonly prescribed than the direct agents due to a higher incidence of serious adverse effects. Some indirect-acting agents such as amphetamine and cocaine are controlled substances that are abused for their central effects on the brain rather than their autonomic effects.

Classification of Adrenergic Agonists

15.3 Adrenergic agonists may be classified as catecholamines or noncatecholamines.

The first adrenergic agonist to be identified, epinephrine, was isolated from extracts of the adrenal gland in the late 1890s. The chemical structure of epinephrine was found to have an aromatic (6-carbon) ring with two OH groups, similar to a common organic chemical known as catechol. Because the molecule also has an NH or amino group, the term *catecholamine* was assigned to epinephrine by physiologists. Several other adrenergic agonists share this core chemical structure, including NE, dopamine, isoproterenol, and dobutamine. This has led to a simple chemical classification of adrenergic agonists as catecholamines or noncatecholamines. Examples of noncatecholamines include phenylephrine, terbutaline, and ephedrine. The fundamental chemical structure of a catecholamine is shown in Figure 15.2.

Catecholamines and noncatecholamines have important pharmacokinetic differences. Catecholamines have a short duration of action because they are destroyed rapidly by the enzymes **monoamine oxidase (MAO)** and catechol-O-methyltransferase (COMT) (see Figure 15.1). Because these destructive enzymes are active in the mucosa of the intestinal tract, catecholamines cannot be given orally (PO) and must be administered parenterally or by inhalation.

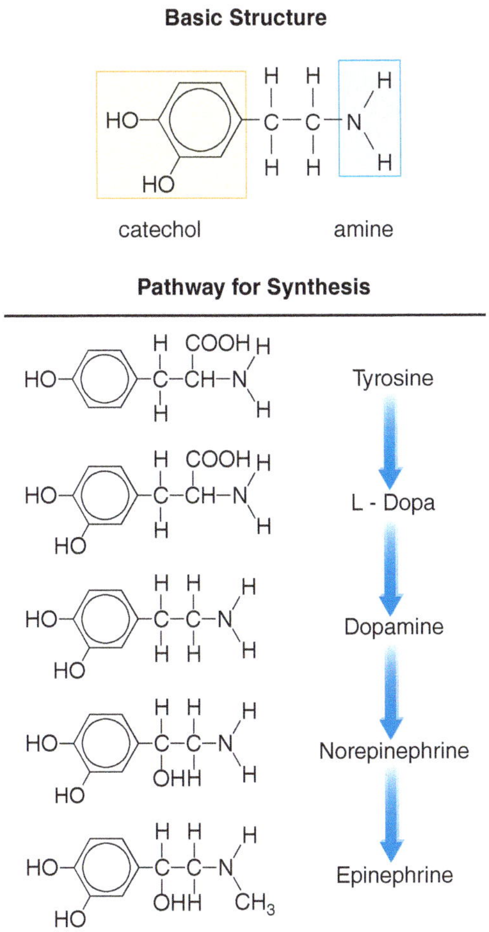

Figure 15.2 Basic chemical structure and synthesis of catecholamines. The synthesis of norepinephrine occurs in the neuron near the neuroeffector junction.

Furthermore, the OH groups on the catechol portion of the molecule make these drugs polar and prevent them from crossing the blood–brain barrier.

On the other hand, the noncatecholamines may be taken PO because they are not destroyed as readily by MAO or COMT. This also extends their duration of action. These drugs are less polar than the catecholamines; thus, they more easily enter the brain and affect the CNS.

CONNECTION Checkpoint 15.2

From what you learned in Chapter 3, how does the ionization of a drug molecule affect its absorption? How does it affect its distribution to tissues?

Nonselective Adrenergic Agonists

15.4 The nonselective adrenergic agonists activate both alpha and beta receptors and are used to treat bronchospasm, cardiac arrest, and hypotension.

Although the general actions of adrenergic agonists are predictable, based on their activation of the sympathetic nervous system, the specific effects of each drug are dependent on which receptor subtypes are stimulated. As discussed in Chapter 12, adrenergic receptors include alpha$_1$, alpha$_2$, beta$_1$, and beta$_2$ subtypes. Because the receptor responses are very different and critical to understanding drug action, the student will need to remember the specific subclass(es) of receptors activated by each adrenergic agonist drug. Therapeutic applications and adverse effects for the different receptor activations are summarized in Table 15.1.

Some sympathomimetics are *nonselective*, stimulating two or more adrenergic-receptor subtypes. For example, epinephrine and ephedrine stimulate all four types of adrenergic receptors. In doing so, these drugs cause widespread activation of the sympathetic nervous system and an intense fight-or-flight response (resulting in many adverse effects).

One of the most important applications of the nonselective adrenergic agonists is for the pharmacotherapy of shock and other life-threatening cardiac disorders. In certain types of shock, the most serious medical challenge facing the patient is hypotension, which may become so severe as to collapse the circulatory system. In the early stages of shock, the body compensates by activating the sympathetic nervous system; blood pressure is raised, and the rate and force of myocardial contraction are increased. These compensatory measures maintain blood flow to vital organs such as the heart and brain and decrease flow to "less vital" organs, including the kidneys and liver.

The body's ability to compensate for severe shock is limited, however, and profound hypotension may develop as the condition progresses. In minor to moderate shock, fluid replacement agents are the preferred drugs for raising

Table 15.1 Summary of Adrenergic Agonist Subtypes

Receptor Subtype	Indications	Adverse Effects
Alpha$_1$-receptor	Hypotension Mydriasis Nasal congestion	Headache Hypertension Nervousness Reflex bradycardia Urinary retention
Alpha$_2$-receptor	Hypertension	Hypotension Sedation Xerostomia
Beta$_1$-receptor	Cardiac arrest Cardiogenic shock Heart failure	Dysrhythmias Hypertension Nervousness Palpitations Tachycardia
Beta$_2$-receptor	Asthma Chronic obstructive pulmonary disease (COPD)	Nervousness Palpitations Tachycardia Tremor
Beta$_3$-receptor	Overactive bladder	Hypertension Urinary retention

blood pressure (see Chapter 33). Should fluid replacement agents prove ineffective, however, adrenergic agonists are administered to maintain blood pressure. When given intravenously (IV), these drugs immediately increase blood pressure. Because rapid, intense vasoconstriction can cause serious hypoperfusion of tissues with potential organ damage, these drugs are generally used when safer alternatives have failed to produce the desired therapeutic outcome. Epinephrine, NE, and dopamine are nonselective drugs for shock or anaphylaxis when blood pressure and heart rate need to be restored quickly to normal levels. The nonselective adrenergic agonists are shown in Table 15.2.

The nonselective adrenergic agonists cause more autonomic-related adverse effects than the selective drugs. Most of these adverse effects are extensions of their autonomic actions. Cardiovascular effects such as tachycardia, hypertension (HTN), and dysrhythmias are particularly troublesome and may limit therapy. Blood pressure and heart rate must be monitored continuously during parenteral administration of these drugs. Large doses can induce CNS excitement and seizures. Patients with diabetes may experience a significant increase in blood glucose levels due to an increased breakdown of glycogen in the liver and skeletal muscle. Care must be taken to avoid extravasation because this can cause severe tissue injury. Should extravasation occur, the antidote is phentolamine, an alpha-adrenergic blocker, which will help to counteract the vasoconstriction caused by the catecholamine at the site. Other adverse effects associated with sympathetic activation include dry mouth and nausea and vomiting.

Amphetamine is a nonselective adrenergic agonist with a marked CNS stimulant effect. Amphetamine also causes anorexia, which has led to its historical use as an appetite suppressant. Because of prominent cardiovascular adverse effects, nervous system effects such as paranoia and psychosis, and the risk of physical dependence, the drug is no longer routinely prescribed for weight loss. In 2015, amphetamine (Evekeo) was approved as an adjunct for the short-term (a few weeks) treatment of obesity when combined with a strict dietary regimen. Amphetamine and amphetamine-like drugs are widely prescribed to treat attention-deficit/hyperactivity disorder. In children with this disorder, amphetamine has less stimulatory effect; instead, it increases children's attention span, allowing them to focus more on tasks. Additional details on amphetamine may be found in Chapters 24 and 27.

PROTOTYPE DRUG Epinephrine (Adrenalin)

Classification **Therapeutic:** Antishock and antianaphylaxis drug, bronchodilator
Pharmacologic: Nonselective adrenergic agonist, catecholamine

Therapeutic Effects and Uses: Epinephrine has several therapeutic applications, all of which are the result of

Table 15.2 Selected Adrenergic Agonists

Drug	Adrenergic receptor(s)	Route and Adult Dose (Maximum Dose Where Indicated)
albuterol (Proventil HFA, Ventolin HFA, VoSpire ER)	β_2	Metered-dose inhaler (MDI): 2 inhalations q4–6h prn PO (Vospire ER): 8 mg bid (max: 32 mg/day)
arformoterol (Brovana)	β_2	Nebulizer: 15 mcg bid (max: 30 mcg/day)
dobutamine	β_1	IV: Infused at a rate of 2.5–40 mcg/kg/min for a max of 72 h
dopamine	α_1	IV: 2–5 mcg/kg/min initial dose; may be increased to 20–50 mcg/kg/min (max: 50 mcg/kg/min)
droxidopa (Northera)	α_1, α_2, β_1, β_2	PO: 100 mg tid (max: 600 mg tid)
ephedrine (Corphedra)	α_1, α_2, β_1, β_2	IV: 5–10 mg bolus, followed by additional boluses as needed
epinephrine (Adrenalin)	α_1, α_2, β_1, β_2	Subcutaneous: 0.1–0.5 mL of 1:1000 every 10–15 min prn IV: 0.1–0.25 mL of 1:1000 every 10–15 min
isoproterenol (Isuprel)	β_1, β_2	IV: 0.01–0.02 mg
levalbuterol (Xopenex)	β_2	Nebulizer: 0.63 mg tid–qid MDI: 90 mcg (2 inhalations) q4–6h
midodrine (Orvaten)	α_1	PO: 10 mg tid (max: 20 mg/dose)
mirabegron (Myrbetriq)	β_3	PO: 25–50 mg q8h
norepinephrine (Levophed)	α_1, α_2, β_1	IV: Initially 0.5–1 mcg/min, titrate slowly to therapeutic response; usual range 8–30 mcg/min
olodaterol (Striverdi Respimat)	β_2	Inhalation: 2 inhalations daily
phenylephrine (Neo-Synephrine, Vazculep)	α_1	IV (Vazculep): 0.1–0.18 mg/min until blood pressure stabilizes, then 0.04–0.06 mg/min for maintenance Intranasal: 1–2 sprays per nostril once daily

adrenergic-receptor activation. It can be administered parenterally, topically, by inhalation, or by instillation.

Epinephrine is a first-line drug for cardiac arrest after cardiopulmonary resuscitation (CPR) has failed. Given as an IV infusion or by intracardiac injection, the drug has the potential to immediately restore cardiac rhythm. Epinephrine also constricts arterioles, raising cerebral and cardiac perfusion pressure, which discourages cardiovascular collapse. The intracardiac route is used only under extreme conditions, usually during open cardiac massage, or when no other route is possible.

Epinephrine can quickly reverse many of the distressing symptoms of anaphylaxis. Almost immediately after injection, blood pressure increases due to stimulation of $alpha_1$ receptors. Activation of $beta_2$ receptors in the bronchi dilates the airways to relieve shortness of breath. Epinephrine can also be administered by inhalation, which has the potential to immediately terminate acute bronchospasm.

Epinephrine is sometimes added to cartridges of local anesthetics to cause vasoconstriction of local vessels. This forces the anesthetic to remain localized in the tissues for a longer period, prolonging analgesia and slowing the absorption of anesthetic. Epinephrine can also be applied topically to control superficial bleeding along a surgical incision. Repeated injection or application to the same site can result in tissue necrosis due to the diminished blood supply to the area.

Ophthalmic administration of epinephrine causes mydriasis and the outflow of fluid from the anterior chamber of the eye, making the drug an adjunct to the pharmacotherapy of open-angle glaucoma. Intranasal administration can be used to reduce nasal congestion.

Mechanism of Action: Epinephrine is a nonselective adrenergic agonist, stimulating both alpha- and beta-adrenergic receptors throughout the body. Actions typical of the fight-or-flight response are induced.

Pharmacokinetics:

Route(s)	Subcutaneous, IV, intramuscular (IM), inhalation, topical, ophthalmic
Absorption	Not absorbed PO; minimal absorption by inhalation; rapidly absorbed by IM and subcutaneous routes
Distribution	Widely distributed; does not cross the blood–brain barrier; crosses the placenta; secreted in breast milk
Primary metabolism	Rapidly metabolized by MAO and COMT in the liver and most tissues
Primary excretion	Small amount excreted unchanged in the kidneys
Onset of action	Subcutaneous: 3–5 min; IM: 5–10 min; inhalation: 1 min (for local respiratory effects); IV: immediate onset
Duration of action	1–4 h

Adverse Effects: The most common adverse effects of epinephrine are nervousness, tremors, palpitations, tachycardia, dizziness, headache, and stinging at the site of application. Serious adverse effects include HTN, dysrhythmias, pulmonary edema, and cardiac arrest. Intense CNS stimulation including hallucinations, panic attacks, and aggression may occur, especially in patients with preexisting psychiatric disorders. Extravasation of epinephrine can produce an injection site reaction, causing severe tissue damage and necrosis.

Contraindications/Precautions: Contraindications for epinephrine include hypersensitivity to other adrenergic agonists, closed-angle glaucoma, severe shock (other than anaphylaxis), and dysrhythmias. The drug should be used with caution in patients with coronary artery disease because intense angina symptoms may result. Due to its ability to relax uterine smooth muscle, epinephrine will delay labor. Patients with hyperthyroidism or HTN are very sensitive to the effects of administered epinephrine and other catecholamines. In life-threatening conditions such as anaphylaxis or cardiac arrest, there are no absolute contraindications for the use of epinephrine.

Drug Interactions: Additive cardiovascular effects will occur if epinephrine is used concurrently with other sympathomimetics or antihypotensive drugs. MAOIs block the destruction of catecholamines and will intensify the effects of epinephrine. Tricyclic antidepressants block the reuptake of catecholamines, which is the primary way by which epinephrine is inactivated; thus, doses of epinephrine should be lowered in patients using these depressants. Alpha- and beta-adrenergic antagonists inhibit the actions of epinephrine. Epinephrine will decrease the effects of beta blockers. Digoxin and some general anesthetics may sensitize the heart to the effects of epinephrine. Two drugs used for Parkinson's disease, entacapone and tolcapone, are inhibitors of COMT, the enzyme that degrades epinephrine; concurrent use may cause increased effects of epinephrine on the heart and blood pressure.

Herbal/Food: Caffeine should be avoided because it may increase blood pressure and heart rate.

Pregnancy: Animal reproduction studies show evidence of teratogenicity and fetal cardiac effects. Large numbers of pregnant women have received this drug without evidence of adverse fetal effects. High doses can reduce milk production and milk letdown but the effects on breastfed infants are unknown.

Treatment of Overdose: Overdose of epinephrine is life-threatening and the immediate administration of an alpha- or beta-adrenergic blocker is indicated. If blood pressure remains high, a direct vasodilator may be administered.

Clinician Responsibilities: Key clinical implications for patients receiving epinephrine are included in the Applied Clinical Judgment: Patients Receiving Pharmacotherapy with Adrenergic Agonists.

Drugs Similar to Epinephrine (Adrenalin)

Other nonselective adrenergic agonists include dopamine, droxidopa, ephedrine, and NE.

Dopamine: Approved as a drug by the U.S. Food and Drug Administration (FDA) in 1974, dopamine is an endogenous catecholamine that has both alpha- and beta-agonist activity. It is administered by the IV route and has a brief 10-minute duration of action. Doses are slowly increased until the desired therapeutic effects have been achieved. Vital signs should be monitored continuously during the infusion.

Dopamine is primarily used to treat hypovolemic and cardiogenic shock. Whenever possible, hypovolemia is corrected with fluid-expanding agents before starting a dopamine infusion. At low doses (1–5 mcg/kg/min), the drug selectively stimulates dopaminergic receptors, especially in the kidneys, leading to vasodilation and thus increasing renal blood flow and enhancing urine output. This helps to prevent renal failure, which can occur during shock conditions. At higher doses (more than 10 mcg/kg/min), dopamine stimulates $beta_1$-adrenergic receptors, causing the heart to beat more forcefully, increasing cardiac output. Also, at higher doses, dopamine stimulates $alpha_1$-adrenergic receptors, causing vasoconstriction and increased blood pressure.

Headache and nausea and vomiting are common adverse effects. High doses can produce ventricular tachycardia. Severe necrosis or gangrene can result if extravasation occurs; thus, phentolamine should be readily available. Animal studies show that dopamine may cause fetal harm. This drug can reduce milk production and milk letdown but the effects on breastfed infants are unknown.

Droxidopa (Northera): Approved in 2014, droxidopa is a prodrug that is metabolically converted to NE after oral administration. As such, it shares the same vasoconstrictor action as NE. The drug is approved to treat neurogenic orthostatic hypotension that is associated with disorders such as Parkinson's disease and autonomic neuropathy. The most common adverse events of droxidopa include headache, dizziness, nausea, HTN, and fatigue. The drug carries a black box warning that the patient should be monitored carefully for potentially fatal supine HTN during therapy. Animal studies show that droxidopa may cause fetal harm. Due to the potential for adverse reactions, breastfeeding is not recommended.

Ephedrine (Corphedra): Ephedrine is a noncatecholamine, originally obtained from the Ephedra plant species, that activates both alpha and beta receptors. Although ephedrine was approved by the FDA in 1939, extracts from the ephedra plant have been used to treat various ailments for thousands of years. In Chinese medicine, the herb ma huang contains ephedrine as one of its active ingredients. In the past, ephedrine has been used to relieve respiratory congestion, prevent bronchospasm, suppress appetite, improve athletic performance, and reverse the CNS depression caused by opioid or barbiturate overdose. The FDA has banned all over-the-counter (OTC) products containing ephedrine, and the major Athletic Associations prohibit its use. Serious side effects now limit the use of this drug to the treatment of serious hypotension, usually in the setting of surgical anesthesia.

Ephedrine acts by two mechanisms: directly, by binding to adrenergic receptors, and indirectly, by causing the release of NE from storage vesicles in the nerve terminals. This strong stimulatory effect is the cause of major adverse effects of the drug such as nervousness, insomnia, palpitations, and tachycardia. Like the closely related drug pseudoephedrine, ephedrine is highly regulated because it can be used to make methamphetamine. Animal reproduction studies have not been conducted with ephedrine. Neonates should be monitored for lactic acidosis. This drug is secreted in human milk but effects on the breastfed infant are unknown.

Norepinephrine (Levophed): Approved in 1938, NE is a nonselective catecholamine that has actions similar to epinephrine, except that is does not activate $beta_2$ receptors. Approved to treat shock and hypotension, NE acts directly on alpha-adrenergic receptors in vascular smooth muscle to immediately raise blood pressure. It also stimulates $beta_1$ receptors in the heart to increase cardiac output. It is given by the IV route and has a duration of only 1 to 2 minutes after the infusion is terminated. Because NE is a powerful vasoconstrictor, continuous monitoring of blood pressure is required to avoid HTN. When first administered, reflex bradycardia is sometimes experienced, and the drug has the ability to produce various dysrhythmias. Blurred vision and photophobia are signs of overdose. Like other drugs in this class, NE produces symptoms of CNS stimulation such as nervousness, insomnia, and confusion. Severe tissue necrosis can result if extravasation occurs; thus, phentolamine should be readily available. The primary indications for NE are acute shock and cardiac arrest. Animal reproduction studies have not been conducted with ephedrine. Neonates should be monitored for lactic acidosis. Effects on the breastfed infant are unknown.

CONNECTIONS: Patient Safety

Appropriate Use of the Epinephrine Autoinjector

Epinephrine autoinjectors are used to prevent and treat anaphylaxis and severe allergic reactions to insect stings, foods, or drugs. The devices are designed to be easy to operate, although the word *auto* sometimes gives people a false sense of security that the injector is foolproof. It is crucial that a potential anaphylactic reaction be treated as quickly as possible, and often an adult may administer the injection to a child, particularly in a school setting.

Written or voice instructions were given to adults participating in a research study on the use of two types of epinephrine autoinjectors, the Auvi-Q or EpiPen Jr. While all adults successfully completed an injection on a child-size manikin after training, significantly more digital/hand errors were noted with the EpiPen Jr. than the Auvi-Q injector (Kessler et al., 2019). Overall, participants also preferred the Auvi-Q to the EpiPen Jr. This study highlights the importance of education on both the use of the epinephrine autoinjector, as well as on appropriate administration techniques. Because there are choices as to type of injector, patients or caregivers should use the type they find the easiest to use to ensure proper injection technique.

Alpha-Adrenergic Agonists

15.5 Alpha-adrenergic agonists are used to relieve nasal decongestion and elevate blood pressure.

Activation of alpha-adrenergic receptors causes a number of important physiologic responses, most of which relate to contraction of vascular smooth muscle. Like the nonselective adrenergic agonists, several of the selective alpha agonists are used to treat hypotension associated with shock and other critical care conditions. Alpha agonists may also be administered to treat patients who are susceptible to orthostatic hypotension.

A second application of alpha-adrenergic agonists is for the treatment of nasal congestion. During upper respiratory infections or allergic rhinitis, arterioles in the nose dilate and produce excess mucus. Alpha$_1$ agonists relieve nasal congestion by constricting vessels of the nasal mucosa. Intranasal drugs such as phenylephrine work within minutes and are highly effective at clearing the nasal passages. The intranasal route causes few systemic side effects because absorption is limited. Oral decongestants take longer to act and the risk for systemic side effects is higher; however, they are less damaging to the nasal mucosa than the intranasal drugs. The pharmacotherapy of upper respiratory congestion is presented in Chapter 45.

Topical instillation of alpha$_1$ agonists to the eye has two applications. Alpha$_1$-adrenergic receptors are present on the radial muscle of the iris. When these receptors are activated, the radial muscle contracts and the pupil dilates, allowing for a better examination of the interior structures of the eye. Another ophthalmic application of alpha$_1$ agonists is to relieve conjunctival congestion and redness. The mechanism behind this effect is through alpha$_1$-receptor activation of arterioles in the eye, causing vasoconstriction. Tetrahydrozoline (Tyzine) is widely used for minor eye irritation and redness and is available OTC. The pharmacotherapy of ophthalmic conditions is discussed in detail in Chapter 74.

Most adverse effects of the alpha$_1$-adrenergic agonists are logical extensions of their autonomic actions. Their intense vasoconstrictive effect can lead to HTN. This increase in blood pressure can activate the baroreceptor reflex, causing reflex bradycardia. Because of the potential for cardiovascular adverse effects, patients should be continuously monitored when receiving high doses or infusions of these drugs. Should extravasation occur, the intense local vasoconstriction caused by these drugs can lead to tissue necrosis. Major adverse effects or overdose may be treated by administering a specific alpha-adrenergic antagonist such as phentolamine. Bradycardia can be prevented or reversed by administration of an anticholinergic drug such as atropine. In low doses, many of the alpha agonists can be safely used as OTC drugs for symptoms of the common cold, minor allergies, or minor ophthalmic conditions.

Activation of alpha$_2$-adrenergic receptors produces very different responses than alpha$_1$ activation. The most important responses to alpha$_2$-receptor agonists occur in the brain rather than the peripheral nervous system. Unlike alpha$_1$ agonists, which increase sympathetic nervous system activity, alpha$_2$ agonists act in the CNS to *decrease* sympathetic activity. Methyldopa (Aldomet) and clonidine (Catapres, Duraclon) are two drugs in this class. Because they decrease blood pressure, their primary therapeutic application is for the treatment of HTN (see Chapter 34).

PROTOTYPE DRUG **Phenylephrine (Neo-Synephrine, Vazculep, Others)**

Classification **Therapeutic:** Nasal decongestant, vasoconstrictor
Pharmacologic: Alpha-adrenergic agonist

Therapeutic Effects and Uses: Approved in 1938, the actions and indications of phenylephrine are predictable extensions of its sympathetic activation. Its most frequent application is for the relief of congestion associated with the common cold and allergies. Historically, pseudoephedrine was the preferred drug for these indications. Phenylephrine has now largely replaced pseudoephedrine in OTC multisystem cold, allergy, and sinus remedies because it cannot be used by illicit drug dealers to synthesize methamphetamine. For congestion, phenylephrine is available via oral and intranasal routes. When applied intranasally by spray or drops, it reduces nasal congestion by constricting small blood vessels in the nasal mucosa.

Parenteral administration of phenylephrine causes systemic vasoconstriction that can prevent or reverse acute hypotension caused by spinal anesthesia or vascular shock. Its long duration of activity and lack of significant cardiac adverse effects gives phenylephrine advantages over epinephrine or NE in treating acute hypotension. Unlike epinephrine, which markedly increases the heart rate, phenylephrine tends to slow the heart rate, probably due to reflex bradycardia. In situations in which reflex bradycardia is undesirable, this action may be blocked by the administration of atropine. In 2019, the FDA approved Biorphen, the first ready-to-use injectable form of phenylephrine.

Phenylephrine is also available for topical use. Applied topically to the eye during ophthalmic examinations, phenylephrine can dilate the pupil without causing significant cycloplegia. Applied to swollen hemorrhoidal tissue, the drug can relieve itching and burning associated with hemorrhoids.

Mechanism of Action: Phenylephrine directly activates $alpha_1$-adrenergic receptors in the peripheral nervous system. It has weak beta-adrenergic activity at high doses, but this is usually not of clinical significance.

Pharmacokinetics:

Route(s)	PO, IM, subcutaneous, IV, intranasal, and ophthalmic solutions
Absorption	Readily absorbed in the GI tract; well absorbed when given IM or subcutaneously
Distribution	Widely distributed; does not cross blood–brain barrier or enter breast milk in significant amounts
Primary metabolism	Intestinal and hepatic by MAO
Primary excretion	Unknown
Onset of action	Oral: peaks in 1–2 h; subcutaneous/IM: 10–15 min; IV: immediate
Duration of action	Oral: 3 h; subcutaneous/IM: 30–120 min; IV: 15–20 min

Adverse Effects: Phenylephrine causes few serious adverse effects when taken by the PO, intranasal, or ophthalmic routes. Common adverse effects with intranasal phenylephrine use include stinging of the nasal mucosa, sneezing, and rebound congestion. Ophthalmic use can cause closed-angle glaucoma or photophobia. Parenteral use can lead to symptoms of CNS stimulation such as anxiety, restlessness, and tremor. Serious adverse effects include reflex bradycardia and reduced blood flow to peripheral tissues due to severe vasoconstriction. OTC cough and cold products containing phenylephrine or pseudoephedrine should not be given to children under age 2 years because overdose may cause serious illness or death.

Contraindications/Precautions: Phenylephrine is contraindicated in patients with severe HTN because the drug will raise blood pressure to dangerous levels. Because it causes reflex bradycardia, patients with preexisting bradycardia should not receive phenylephrine. Phenylephrine causes vasoconstriction, which can reduce coronary blood flow in patients with advanced coronary artery disease, inducing angina attacks. Phenylephrine also reduces the effectiveness of nitrates such as nitroglycerin that are taken to prevent anginal episodes. Because of its effects on the eye, it should not be administered to patients with closed-angle glaucoma. Phenylephrine should be used with caution in patients with hyperthyroidism or diabetes because these patients are more sensitive to the potential cardiac adverse effects.

Drug Interactions: Phenylephrine will reduce the effectiveness of antihypertensive medications. A hypertensive crisis may occur in patients receiving MAOIs; phenylephrine should not be administered within 21 days of a MAOI. Increased effects of phenylephrine may occur in patients taking ergot alkaloids and tricyclic antidepressants. Additive effects may occur if phenylephrine is given concurrently with other adrenergic agonists, including amphetamines or cocaine. Concurrent administration with oxytocin during the postpartum period may cause persistent HTN. Concurrent use with halothane or digoxin may increase the risk of dysrhythmias.

Herbal/Food: Phenylephrine should be used with caution with St. John's wort because this combination may result in HTN. Ingestion of substances with high amounts of caffeine will worsen the CNS stimulation caused by phenylephrine.

Pregnancy: Based on animal data phenylephrine may cause fetal harm. Adverse effects during human pregnancy or breastfeeding are not clearly established.

Treatment of Overdose: When given by the parenteral route, overdose will result in HTN and possible dysrhythmias. Phentolamine is a specific alpha antagonist that can be used to lower blood pressure, and antidysrhythmic drugs may be indicated.

Clinician Responsibilities: Key clinical implications for patients receiving phenylephrine are included in the Applied Clinical Judgment: Patients Receiving Pharmacotherapy with Adrenergic Agonists.

Drugs Similar to Phenylephrine (Neo-Synephrine, Vasculep)

Most drugs with predominant alpha-adrenergic agonist activity can be grouped into subclasses based on their indications: intranasal or ocular decongestants.

Intranasal Decongestants: Oxymetazoline (Afrin), pseudoephedrine (Sudafed), xylometazoline (Neo-Synephrine II, Long-Acting), and tetrahydrozoline (Tyzine) are given by the intranasal route to diminish nasal congestion caused by allergies or the common cold. Use of these medications is generally limited to 3 to 5 days. If intranasal decongestants are abruptly discontinued, congestion may worsen, a phenomenon known as rebound congestion. Although these drugs may also have some beta-adrenergic activity, they are only used for their effects on alpha-adrenergic receptors in the nasal mucosa. The pharmacotherapy of nasal decongestants is presented in Chapter 45.

Pseudoephedrine is an intranasal decongestant that deserves special attention because of its potential for misuse. Pseudoephedrine is the starting chemical for the synthesis of illegal methamphetamine by drug traffickers. Most states have enacted laws to regulate the sale of solid tablet formulations containing pseudoephedrine, requiring that pseudoephedrine be placed behind the pharmacy counter so that only pharmacists can provide the product. Most states also require the pharmacist to record the name and address of the buyer. Note that these precautions are not being taken because pseudoephedrine itself is a dangerous drug, but to limit the availability of the drug to illicit makers of methamphetamine. A prototype feature for pseudoephedrine can be found in Chapter 45.

Ocular Decongestants: Naphazoline (Naphcon, Clear Eyes), oxymetazoline (Afrin 12 Hour), and tetrahydrozoline (Visine) are available as ophthalmic solutions to relieve redness due to minor eye irritations, such as those caused by the common cold, swimming, allergies, or contact lenses. These drugs act by constricting arteries in the conjunctiva. Other than local stinging, they rarely cause adverse effects. The pharmacotherapy of ocular medications is presented in Chapter 74.

Midodrine (Orvaten): Approved in 1996, midodrine is converted into an active metabolite that has alpha$_1$-agonist actions. It is given PO for the symptomatic treatment of orthostatic hypotension. The drug increases standing, sitting, and supine systolic and diastolic blood pressure. Because marked elevation of supine blood pressure can occur, midodrine carries a black box warning that supine and sitting blood pressures should be monitored during therapy and that it should not be used in patients with an initial supine systolic pressure greater than 180 mmHg. Signs of supine HTN include pounding sensations in the ears or chest, blurred vision, and headache. The most common adverse effects are paresthesia, goose bumps, dysuria, and pruritus of the scalp. Midodrine is contraindicated in patients with heart failure, severe cardiac or renal disease, or excessive supine HTN. Based on animal data midodrine may cause fetal harm. Adverse effects during human pregnancy or breastfeeding are unknown.

CONNECTION Checkpoint 15.3

Parenteral phenylephrine can cause reflex bradycardia. From what you learned in Chapter 14, would the administration of an anticholinergic such as atropine improve or worsen this condition?

Beta-Adrenergic Agonists

15.6 Beta-adrenergic agonists are used to treat asthma, shock, and heart failure.

Activation of beta-adrenergic receptors can produce a wide variety of physiologic responses, depending on the location of the receptor and which subtype is stimulated. Some beta-adrenergic agonists are selective for beta$_1$ receptors, whereas others affect primarily beta$_2$. The indications for the beta$_1$ activators are very different from those of the beta$_2$ activators:

- **Beta$_1$ applications:** cardiac arrest, heart failure, atrioventricular (AV) heart block, and shock
- **Beta$_2$ applications:** asthma, chronic obstructive pulmonary disease (COPD), and delay of preterm labor.

Beta$_1$-Adrenergic Agonists: Pharmacologically, the most significant site having beta$_1$ receptors is cardiac muscle. Activation of beta$_1$ receptors results in cardiac actions typical of the fight-or-flight response: increased heart rate (positive chronotropic effect), force of contraction (positive inotropic effect), and velocity of impulse conduction across the myocardium (positive dromotropic effect). These cardiac effects may be considered beneficial or adverse, depending on the condition of the patient and the therapeutic goals.

Drugs used for their beta$_1$-agonist actions are sometimes called **cardiotonic drugs** because they increase the force of contraction of the heart. In the treatment of heart failure or shock, they are administered to increase cardiac output. Another name applied to these drugs is **inotropic drugs** because they reverse the cardiac symptoms of shock by increasing the strength of myocardial contraction. The use of beta$_1$ agonists in treating heart failure is presented in Chapter 36.

Most drugs used for their strong beta$_1$-agonist activity are nonselective and activate other receptor subtypes. For example, although epinephrine is often used for its beta$_1$ activation of the heart following cardiac arrest, the drug has effects on all receptor subtypes. Similarly, although NE is used for its beta$_1$-agonist actions during cardiac arrest, the drug also activates alpha receptors. Dopamine is somewhat unique in that at low doses the drug activates dopamine receptors, and at moderate doses it stimulates both beta$_1$ and dopamine receptors. At high doses dopamine activates all three receptor types: dopamine, alpha, and beta$_1$.

Dobutamine is selective for $beta_1$ receptors and isoproterenol activates both $beta_1$ and $beta_2$ receptors.

Beta₂-Adrenergic Agonists: $Beta_2$-adrenergic receptors are more widely distributed than $beta_1$ receptors. Pharmacologically, the most important site is in the lung, where activation of $beta_2$ receptors leads to relaxation of bronchial smooth muscle. $Beta_2$-adrenergic agonists, commonly referred to as bronchodilators, are used extensively in the treatment of asthma, COPD, and other pulmonary disorders. The following discussion is limited to autonomic bronchodilators; information on other classes of drugs used in the pharmacotherapy of asthma is presented in Chapter 44.

Autonomic drugs used as bronchodilators include both nonselective and selective $beta_2$ adrenergic agonists. Epinephrine is the best example of a nonselective drug that is an effective bronchodilator. Unfortunately, epinephrine exhibits a high incidence of adverse effects, such as HTN and dysrhythmias, due to its stimulation of multiple receptor subtypes throughout the body. Likewise, isoproterenol is an effective bronchodilator; however, it also affects both $beta_1$ and $beta_2$ receptors, which increases the incidence of cardiovascular adverse effects. Selective $beta_2$ agonists such as albuterol were developed to minimize these adverse effects and they have become first-line drugs in the pharmacotherapy of conditions characterized by bronchospasm. A drug prototype feature for albuterol can be found in Chapter 44.

When given for asthma, $beta_2$ agonists are usually administered by the inhalation or PO routes. Inhalation administration with metered-dose inhalers, nebulizers, or dry powder inhalers can relieve acute bronchospasm within minutes. The PO route exhibits a longer onset of action and causes more systemic side effects than the inhaled drugs.

Adverse effects of the $beta_2$ agonists are predictable extensions of their autonomic activation. Tachycardia, palpitations, flushing, insomnia, and tremor are possible adverse effects with all $beta_2$ agonists. The oral forms have some $beta_1$ activity; thus, systemic adverse effects are more common than the inhaled drugs, which act locally and produce few systemic adverse effects. Beta agonists should be used cautiously in patients with dysrhythmias or heart failure. These drugs antagonize the actions of beta-adrenergic blockers.

PROTOTYPE DRUG | Isoproterenol (Isuprel)

Classification **Therapeutic:** Bronchodilator, drug for shock

Pharmacologic: Nonselective beta-adrenergic agonist

Therapeutic Effects and Uses: Isoproterenol is a catecholamine that has been available as a drug for over 50 years. The drug activates both $beta_1$- and $beta_2$-adrenergic receptors but has minimal effect on alpha receptors. Given by the IV route, isoproterenol immediately activates $beta_1$ receptors to increase the strength of myocardial contraction and improve cardiac output. The cardiac actions of isoproterenol are used to advantage in the pharmacotherapy of cardiogenic or bacteremic shock, cardiac arrest, Adams–Stokes syndrome, and certain types of ventricular dysrhythmias. Dobutamine has largely replaced isoproterenol as a cardiac drug because it is more specific to $beta_1$ receptors in the heart.

Isoproterenol was once available by inhaler for asthma pharmacotherapy and was a preferred drug due to its bronchodilation effects caused by activation of $beta_2$ receptors in the airways. The development of selective $beta_2$ agonists with fewer cardiac adverse effects, however, led to a significant decline in the use of isoproterenol for treating asthma. This drug is no longer available via inhalation devices. Other types of acute bronchospasm, such as that caused by anesthesia, may be reversed by IV isoproterenol.

Mechanism of Action: Isoproterenol is a potent activator of both $beta_1$- and $beta_2$-adrenergic receptors throughout the body.

Pharmacokinetics:

Route(s)	IV
Absorption	N/A
Distribution	Distributed to most tissues; it is unknown if it crosses the placenta or is secreted in breast milk
Primary metabolism	Hepatic by COMT
Primary excretion	Renal: 40–50% unchanged
Onset of action	Immediate
Duration of action	Less than 1 h

Adverse Effects: Adverse effects of isoproterenol are predictable based on its activation of beta-adrenergic receptors. Common adverse effects include headache, nausea and vomiting, and symptoms of CNS stimulation such as tremors, anxiety, and insomnia. Adverse effects affecting the heart include serious dysrhythmias.

Contraindications/Precautions: Because isoproterenol increases the myocardial workload, it should be used with extreme caution in patients with severe cardiac disease, dysrhythmias, or HTN. The drug should be used with caution in patients with hyperthyroidism or diabetes because these patients are more sensitive to the potential cardiac adverse effects.

Drug Interactions: Concurrent administration with a beta-adrenergic blocker diminishes the bronchodilation effect of isoproterenol and may induce bronchospasm in patients with asthma. Use with other bronchodilators or adrenergic agonists such as epinephrine or dopamine may result in additive effects. MAOIs and tricyclic antidepressants should be discontinued at least 2 weeks prior to isoproterenol therapy to avoid possible hypertensive crisis. Isoproterenol should not be concurrently administered with potassium-wasting diuretics because hypokalemia may result. Isoproterenol may lower serum levels of digoxin and induce dysrhythmias.

Pregnancy: Animal reproduction studies have shown adverse fetal effects. Adverse effects during human pregnancy or breastfeeding are unknown.

Treatment of Overdose: Overdose with isoproterenol will cause tachycardia and other dysrhythmias. Blood pressure usually falls. Due to the relatively short half-life of the drug, discontinuing the infusion is often enough to reverse symptoms, although supportive cardiac drugs may be necessary.

Clinician Responsibilities: Key clinical implications for patients receiving isoproterenol are included in the Applied Clinical Judgment: Patients Receiving Pharmacotherapy with Adrenergic Agonists.

Drugs Similar to Isoproterenol (Isuprel)

Beta-adrenergic agonists may be grouped into two primary subclasses: bronchodilators and tocolytics.

Bronchodilators: The majority of the beta$_2$ agonists are used to treat asthma and/or COPD. The classification of these drugs is based on onset of action.

- Short-acting beta agonists (SABAs): These are first-line drugs to relieve acute bronchospasm. Patients can be dosed every 20 to 30 minutes until control is achieved. Onset of action is under 3 to 5 minutes and the bronchodilation effect lasts 3 to 6 hours. Examples include albuterol (Proventil HFA, Ventolin HFA), levalbuterol (Xopenex), pirbuterol (Maxair), and terbutaline.
- Long-acting beta$_2$ agonists (LABAs): The LABAs are often combined with inhaled corticosteroids to boost their effectiveness. The long onset of action of these drugs makes them unsuitable for relieving acute bronchospasm. Onset of action is greater than 5 minutes; however, the bronchodilation effect lasts 12 hours or more. Examples include formoterol (Perforomist) and salmeterol (Serevent).
- Ultra-long-acting beta$_2$ agonists (ULABs): The major benefit of the ULABs is their 24-hour duration of action that allows once daily dosing. Examples include vilanterol and olodaterol (Striverdi Respimat).

Dobutamine: Dobutamine is a beta$_1$-adrenergic agonist that also has some weak beta$_2$ and alpha a$_1$ activity. Its only indication is for the short-term treatment of certain types of shock due to its ability to cause the heart to beat more forcefully. Dobutamine is especially beneficial in cases where the primary cause of shock is related to heart failure, not hypovolemia. In fact, hypovolemia should be corrected before administering adrenergic agonists such as dobutamine. The resulting increase in cardiac output assists in maintaining blood flow to vital organs; renal blood flow is enhanced and urine output is increased. Dobutamine has a brief half-life of 2 minutes and is only given as an IV infusion. The patient should be monitored continuously during the infusion for abnormal changes in heart rate or rhythm. Animal studies have not shown evidence of fetal toxicity. Adverse effects during human pregnancy or breastfeeding are unknown.

Tocolytics: Terbutaline not only activates beta$_2$ receptors in the lung, but also in the uterus. In the lungs, terbutaline relaxes bronchial smooth muscle and is approved for asthma. In the uterus, it relaxes uterine smooth muscle and has been used to delay preterm contractions. Drugs used to delay preterm labor are called **tocolytics**. Although not approved by the FDA as a tocolytic, terbutaline is sometimes used off-label for this purpose. It is administered as an IV infusion, subcutaneous injection, or by a portable infusion pump programmed to deliver small amounts of the drug at prescribed intervals. Tocolytics may cause the fetus to experience transient tachycardia. Tocolytics are presented in greater detail in Chapter 69.

Beta$_3$-Adrenergic Agonists: The beta$_3$-adrenergic receptor has been known for over a decade but has largely been ignored as a pharmacologic target. This receptor is primarily located in adipose tissue and skeletal muscle, though it has subsequently been found in the gallbladder and the urinary bladder. The first drug acting on the beta$_3$ receptor, mirabegron (Myrbetriq), is an oral drug approved in 2012 for the treatment of overactive bladder. The most commonly observed side effects are HTN, nasopharyngitis, urinary tract infection, and headache. This drug causes fetal harm in laboratory animals. Because it is secreted in animal milk, caution should be used if breastfeeding.

CONNECTION Checkpoint 15.4

A patient has severe bronchoconstriction due to an acute allergic attack. From what you learned in Chapter 3, which route of administration—oral, subcutaneous, or inhalation—would likely give the fastest onset of drug action for this patient?

CONNECTIONS: APPLIED CLINICAL JUDGEMENT

Patients Receiving Pharmacotherapy with Adrenergic Agonists

Key Assessment Data

- History of current condition, baseline vital signs, physical exam findings; history of cardiovascular disease, cerebrovascular disease, respiratory disease, diabetes; medication history; pregnancy status. Baseline ECG, urinary output, and cardiac output should be assessed, depending on the condition being treated.
- Ongoing assessment during drug therapy should include monitoring for excessive autonomic nervous system stimulation (tachycardia, hypertension, tremors, headache).
- If given IV, the insertion site should be monitored frequently during infusion. Blanching of the area may indicate vasoconstriction from extravasation of the drug, requiring prompt discontinuation of the infusion and additional intervention.
- When given as a nasal decongestant, inspect nasal mucosa for irritation, rhinorrhea, or bleeding.

Desired Therapeutic Outcomes

Improvement is observed and measurable by patient's pulse, BP, respiratory rate, and ease of breathing within acceptable parameters; nasal congestion has diminished or eased.

Minimizing Adverse Effects

- Closely monitor the IV infusion site when using IV adrenergic agonists. Stop the infusion if extravasation occurs and notify the provider for further treatment orders to prevent tissue damage.
- Continue to monitor blood glucose level as patients with diabetes may need a change in diabetic medication or dosing if glucose remains elevated.

Lifespan Considerations

- Older adults may be more sensitive to the effects of adrenergic drugs due to existing cardiovascular disease and require more frequent monitoring.
- Nasal sprays and other decongestants are not recommended for children and should be used only on recommendation by the provider.

Patient Education

Short-Term Drug Use (Inhalants and Topicals)

- Limit use of nasal spray to no longer than five days to avoid rebound congestion.

Long-Term Drug Use

- All education as above.
- Ensure appropriate use of the inhaler and provide instructions on the differences in the duration of action (e.g., SABA, LABA) if different inhalers are ordered.
- Photosensitivity may occur and sunglasses may be needed in bright light or for outside activities. Lubricating eyedrops may soothe irritation. Caution should be taken with driving until drug effects are known.
- Teach appropriate administration techniques; a teach-back session should occur before patient self-administration. If an epinephrine autoinjector is needed and used, 911/EMS and the healthcare provider should be called immediately after use.

Prescribing Considerations

- There is a broad variation in the therapeutic index of adrenergic drugs given the large number of medications.
- A pharmacist consult is essential if there is any question about the use of an adrenergic agent; the pharmacist can look for drug–drug interactions, recommend appropriate dosing based on the condition treated, and perform medication reconciliation.

Understanding Chapter 15

Key Concepts Summary

15.1 Adrenergic agonists activate the sympathetic nervous system to produce fight-or-flight symptoms.

15.2 Adrenergic agonists may act directly by binding to adrenergic receptors or indirectly by increasing the amount of norepinephrine at synapses.

15.3 Adrenergic agonists may be classified as catecholamines or noncatecholamines.

15.4 The nonselective adrenergic agonists activate both alpha and beta receptors and are used to treat bronchospasm, cardiac arrest, and hypotension.

15.5 Alpha-adrenergic agonists are used to relieve nasal decongestion and elevate blood pressure.

15.6 Beta-adrenergic agonists are used to treat asthma, shock, and heart failure.

CASE STUDY: Making the Patient Connection

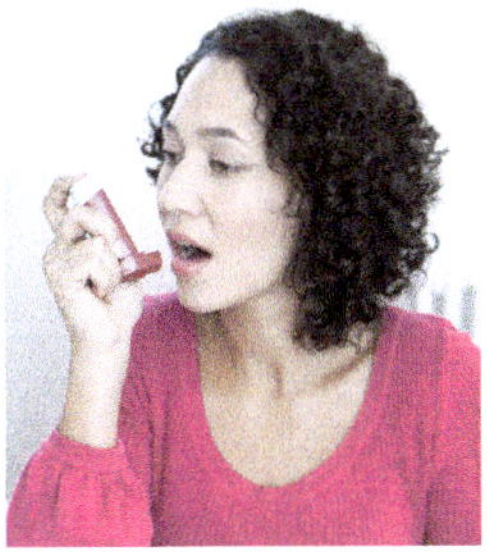

Remember the patient "Alexia Howard" at the beginning of the chapter? Now read the remainder of the case study. Based on the information presented within this chapter, respond to the critical thinking questions that follow.

Alexia Howard is a 22-year-old woman with a history of asthma since childhood. She is presently a student at the local university where she lives in a dormitory. Since the beginning of the semester, Alexia has experienced tremendous stress trying to manage school and part-time employment. Her roommate, an animal lover, has kept stray dogs and cats in their room several times during the past few months until she could find them good homes.

Today Alexia arrives at the University Health Center with tachypnea and acute shortness of breath with audible wheezing. She has not consistently taken her prescribed medications to avoid asthma attacks. A physical examination revealed a heart rate of 110 beats/min and a respiratory rate of 40 breaths/min with signs of accessory muscle use. Auscultation revealed decreased breath sounds with inspiratory and expiratory wheezing. The patient was coughing up small amounts of white sputum. Her saturated oxygen is 93% on room air.

An aerosol treatment with albuterol (Proventil) was ordered, using a small-volume nebulizer for 15 minutes. Peak flow measures after the treatment showed marked improvement of airflow. On auscultation there was clearing of bilateral breath sounds. Alexia's respiratory rate at the time of discharge was 20 breaths/min and her heart rate was 108 beats/min. The patient verbalized that she felt much better but a little nervous.

Alexia was discharged from the University Health Center. She was given a prescription for inhaled steroids and instructed to resume her home medications and use them consistently.

Critical Thinking Questions

1. Discuss the mechanism of action associated with albuterol (Proventil).
2. Why is albuterol being given to Alexia, and why is this route of administration being used?
3. What adverse effects is Alexia demonstrating as a result of the administration of albuterol (Proventil)?

Additional Case Study

Bill Jennings, a 55-year-old man, has been using an epinephrine inhaler for asthma for several months. He is attending a community health fair at a local church, and you are the nurse screening his blood pressure.

When you take Bill's blood pressure, you discover it is 172/94 mmHg. As you talk with him, the patient reveals that he is also self-medicating with OTC pseudoephedrine 60 mg three times per day for seasonal allergies. Bill says his blood pressure is usually 120/80 mmHg.

1. Explain why the increased blood pressure might be related to the drug combination.
2. What patient teaching should occur in this situation?

Chapter Review

1. Why would epinephrine (Adrenalin) be the preferred drug in cardiac arrest situations when CPR has failed?
    1. It may restore heart rhythm and, because of peripheral vasoconstriction, prevent cardiovascular collapse.
    2. It causes bronchodilation, allowing for better oxygenation during ventilation.
    3. It increases renal blood flow by increasing cardiac output, thus preserving kidney function.
    4. It has selective cardiac effects, preventing systemic vasoconstriction and tissue damage.
2. The nurse is teaching the patient about the use of phenylephrine (Neo-Synephrine) nasal spray at home. What patient teaching is needed related to this medication? (Select all that apply.)
    1. Do not share the nasal spray with another individual.
    2. Use this drug only for 3 to 5 days unless directed otherwise by a healthcare provider.
    3. Symptoms of excessive use of this drug are lethargy and fatigue.
    4. Infants and children should not use this medication unless directed to do so by a healthcare provider.
    5. This drug can be safely used by individuals with diabetes.

3. The healthcare provider has prescribed epinephrine by autoinjector for a patient who was stung by several wasps several minutes ago. The nurse knows that the primary purpose of this medication for this patient is to:
   1. Stop the systemic release of histamine produced by the mast cells.
   2. Counteract the formation of antibodies in response to an invading antigen.
   3. Increase the number of white blood cells produced to fight the primary invader.
   4. Decrease the potential for hypotension and dilate constricting bronchi associated with anaphylaxis.

4. A patient takes a dose of albuterol (Vospire ER) prior to bedtime. Which effect would the nurse consider normal for this drug?
   1. Insomnia
   2. Sleepiness
   3. Urticaria
   4. Tinnitus

5. To evaluate the effectiveness of high-dose dopamine, the nurse would assess the:
   1. Pupillary response.
   2. Blood pressure.
   3. Level of consciousness.
   4. Gag reflex.

6. A beta-adrenergic agonist is prescribed for each of the following conditions. A nurse would question the order for which condition? (Select all that apply.)
   1. Hyperthyroidism
   2. Asthma
   3. Shock
   4. Dysrhythmias
   5. Heart failure

See Appendix A for answers to critical thinking questions, case study questions and review questions.

References

Blake, M. A. (2018). *Pheochromocytoma*. Medscape. http://emedicine.medscape.com/article/124059-overview

Kessler, C., Edwards, E., Dissinger, E., Sye, S., Visich, T., & Grant, E. (2019). Usability and preference of epinephrine autoinjectors: Auvi-Q and EpiPen Jr. *Annals of Allergy, Asthma, and Immunology, 123*, 256–262. https://doi.org/10.1016/j.anai.2019.06.005

Selected Bibliography

Colbert, B. J., & Gonzales, L. S. (2019). *Integrated cardiopulmonary pharmacology* (5th ed.). BVT Publishing.

D'Aragon, F., Belley-Cote, E. P., Meade, M. O., Lauzier, F., Adhikari, N. K., Briel, M., et al. (2015). Blood pressure targets for vasopressor therapy: A systematic review. *Shock, 43*, 530–539. https://doi.org/10.1097/SHK.0000000000000348

Kalil, A. (2019). *Septic shock*. Medscape. http://emedicine.medscape.com/article/168402-overview

Kawagoe, Y. (2020). Maintenance tocolytic therapy. In H. Sameshima (Ed.), *Preterm labor and delivery* (pp. 125–129). Springer.

Kopsaftis, Z. A., Sulaiman, N. S., Mountain, O. D., Carson-Chahhoud, K. V., Phillips, P. A., & Smith, B. J. (2018). Short-acting bronchodilators for the management of acute exacerbations of chronic obstructive pulmonary disease in the hospital setting: systematic review. *Systematic Reviews, 7*(1), 213. https://doi.org/10.1186/s13643-018-0860-0

Mirza, S., Clay, R. D., Koslow, M. A., & Scanlon, P. D. (2018). COPD guidelines: A review of the 2018 GOLD report. *Mayo Clinic Proceedings, 93*(10), 1488–1502).

Moore, C. (2020). Implementing an asthma and COPD overlap protocol in general practice. *Nursing Times, 116*(4), 31–34.

Peacock, S. (2020). Medications used for the respiratory system. In P. Hood & E. Khan (Eds.), *Understanding pharmacology in nursing practice* (pp. 283–317). Springer.

Pleasants, R. A., Radlowski, P. A., & Davidson, H. E. (2019). Optimizing drug therapies in patients with COPD in the US nursing home setting. *Drugs & Aging, 36*(8), 733–745. https://doi.org/10.1007/s40266-019-00680-x

Tian, D. H., Smyth, C., Keijzers, G., Macdonald, S. P., Peake, S., Udy, A., & Delaney, A. (2019). Safety of peripheral administration of vasopressor medications: A systematic review. *Emergency Medicine Australasia, 32*, 220–227. https://doi.org/10.1111/1742-6723.13406

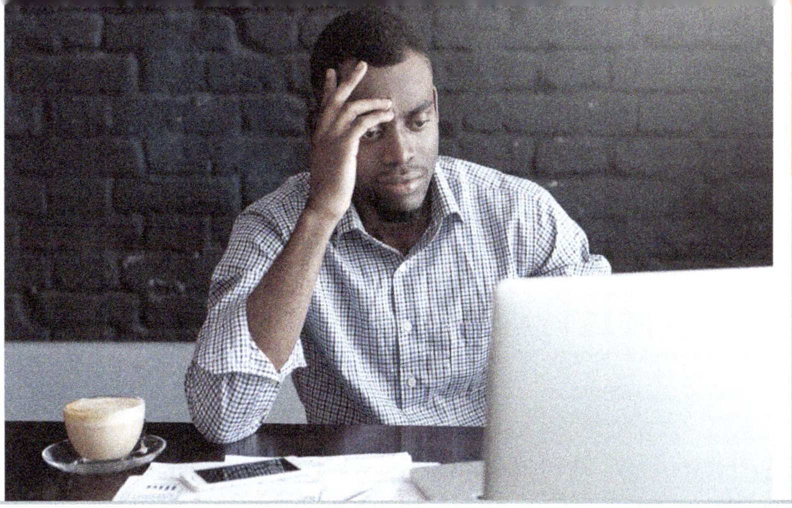

"I have all these reports to finish by Friday. I just don't have time to deal with high blood pressure."
—*Patient "Chris Williams"*

Chapter 16
Adrenergic Antagonists

Chapter Outline

Learning Outcomes

After reading this chapter, the student should be able to:

1. Identify the physiologic responses produced when a drug blocks alpha$_1$-, alpha$_2$-, beta$_1$-, and beta$_2$-adrenergic receptors.
2. Identify indications for pharmacotherapy with alpha$_1$ and alpha$_2$-adrenergic antagonists.
3. Identify indications for pharmacotherapy with nonselective beta-adrenergic antagonists.
4. Identify indications for pharmacotherapy with selective beta$_1$-adrenergic antagonists.
5. Explain the advantages of selective beta antagonists versus nonselective beta antagonists.
6. For each of the classes shown in the chapter outline, identify the prototype and representative drugs and explain the mechanism(s) of drug action, primary indications, contraindications, significant drug interactions, pregnancy data and important adverse effects.
7. Apply clinical judgement to care for patients receiving pharmacotherapy with adrenergic antagonists.

Key Terms

Definitions of the terms in bold may be found in the Glossary.

Adrenergic antagonists inhibit the sympathetic nervous system and produce many of the same rest-and-digest symptoms as the cholinergic agonists. They have wide therapeutic applications in the management of hypertension (HTN), angina pectoris, myocardial infarction, and heart failure (HF). They also serve limited roles in the pharmacotherapy of benign prostatic hyperplasia (BPH), thyroid crisis, and glaucoma.

Actions of Adrenergic Antagonists

16.1 Adrenergic antagonists act by blocking the effects of norepinephrine at adrenergic receptors.

When the adrenergic receptor binds norepinephrine (NE), symptoms typical of the fight-or-flight response are induced. Drugs that activate these receptors are used to treat shock, cardiac arrest, nasal congestion, and asthma. If the student is not yet thoroughly familiar with the actions at the adrenergic receptor, Chapters 12 and 15 should be reviewed before continuing.

Adrenergic antagonists are drugs that compete with NE for adrenergic receptors, as shown in Figure 16.1. By blocking NE from reaching its receptors, symptoms of the fight-or-flight response are *prevented*. With reduced sympathetic activation, nerve impulses from the parasympathetic nervous system will predominate. In fact, most of the symptoms produced by adrenergic antagonists are those of parasympathetic activation. In other words, adrenergic antagonists and cholinergic agonists result in many of the same actions.

CONNECTION Checkpoint 16.1

Although cholinergic agonists and adrenergic antagonists may produce similar physiologic actions, their indications are very different. From what you learned in Chapter 13, what are the primary indications for pharmacotherapy with cholinergic agonists?

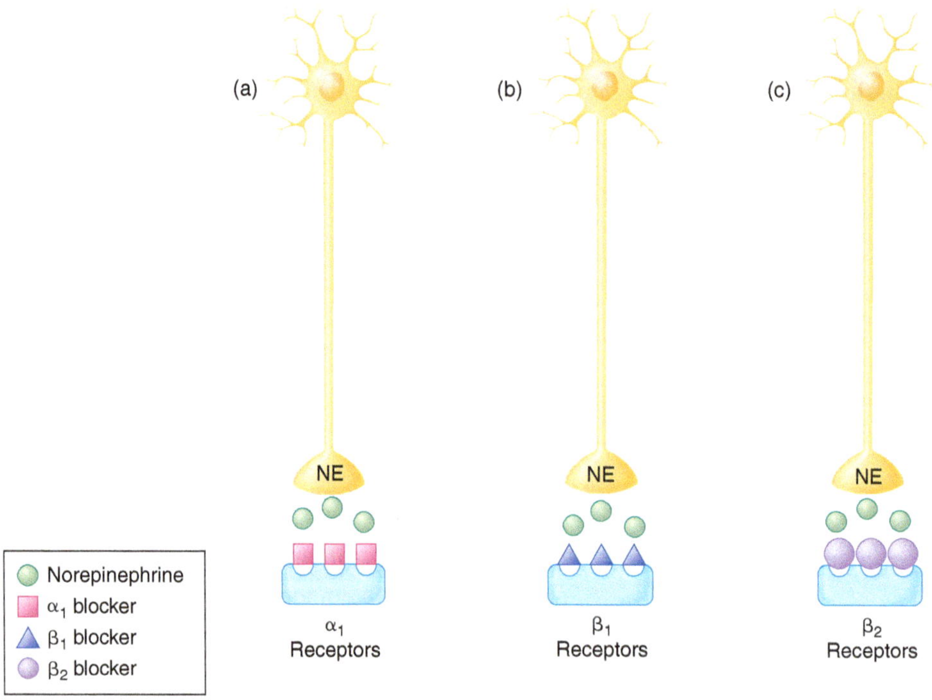

	(a) α_1 Receptors	(b) β_1 Receptors	(c) β_2 Receptors
Pharmacologic Effects	Inhibition of ejaculation Pupil constriction Relaxation of smooth muscles in prostate and bladder neck Vasodilation	Decreased force of cardiac contraction Decreased heart rate Slowed cardiac conduction	Bronchoconstriction Increased intestinal motility Uterine contraction
Indications	Benign prostatic hyperplasia Hypertension Raynaud's disease	Angina pectoris Heart failure Hypertension Myocardial infarction	Dysrhythmias Glaucoma Heart failure Hypertension Migraine Myocardial infarction

Figure 16.1 Pharmacologic effects and indications of adrenergic antagonists: (a) blockade of $alpha_1$ receptors, (b) blockade of $beta_1$ receptors, (c) blockade of $beta_2$ receptors.

Recall that the presence of the alpha- and beta-adrenergic receptor subtypes in the sympathetic nervous system allows for more specific pharmacologic responses. For example, with the adrenergic agonists, epinephrine activates both alpha and beta receptors, whereas albuterol activates only beta$_2$ receptors. The same type of division occurs with adrenergic antagonists. Actions of these drugs are specific to either alpha blockade or beta blockade. Beta blockade is further divided into those drugs that inhibit both beta$_1$ and beta$_2$ receptors and those that selectively inhibit only beta$_1$ receptors. The therapeutic uses and adverse effects of each drug are dependent on which receptor subtype is blocked. Adrenergic antagonists are the most frequently prescribed class of autonomic drugs.

Alpha-Adrenergic Antagonists

16.2 Alpha$_1$-adrenergic antagonists are used to treat hypertension and benign prostatic hyperplasia.

Alpha-adrenergic receptors are primarily located on smooth muscle, and their activation results in contraction (constriction). Most blood vessels, including those serving the myocardium, genitourinary (GU) system, gastrointestinal (GI) system, and brain, have alpha receptors. Because of their key locations on arterial smooth muscle, the **alpha-adrenergic antagonists**, or alpha blockers, have significant effects on the cardiovascular system such as lowering blood pressure.

Alpha-adrenergic antagonists can be classified as drugs that are selective for alpha$_1$, those that are selective for alpha$_2$, and those that affect both alpha$_1$ and alpha$_2$. Drugs affecting alpha$_1$ receptors are listed in Table 16.1.

Phentolamine and phenoxybenzamine (Dibenzyline) are the only alpha blockers that are *nonselective*, activating both alpha$_1$ and alpha$_2$ receptors. These drugs have limited clinical usefulness because they exhibit a high incidence of adverse effects, such as hypotension, tachycardia, nausea and vomiting, and diarrhea.

Selective alpha$_1$ antagonists have two primary indications: HTN and BPH. Their ability to block alpha$_1$ receptors on arterial smooth muscle lowers blood pressure *directly*. Their ability to dilate veins lowers blood pressure *indirectly* by decreasing venous return to the heart. This reduces cardiac output, resulting in a reduction in systemic blood pressure. Alpha blockers for HTN include prazosin, doxazosin, and terazosin. When used to treat HTN, the alpha blockers are often administered concurrently with other classes of antihypertensives, such as diuretics (see Chapter 32).

In addition to dilating vascular smooth muscle, alpha$_1$ blockers relax smooth muscle in the trigone and sphincter muscles at the base of the urinary bladder and in the prostate. Relaxation of these muscles increases urine flow in patients who have difficulty voiding due to strictures in this region. This action has resulted in the use of alpha blockers in the treatment of BPH, a nonmalignant condition in which the prostate gland enlarges to restrict urine flow through the urethra. These medications increase urine flow and decrease residual urine volume in patients with BPH. Selective alpha$_1$ antagonists used for this indication include alfuzosin (Uroxatral), doxazosin (Cardura), silodosin (Rapaflo), tamsulosin (Flomax), and terazosin. Alpha$_1$ blockers do not cure this disorder, and patients with moderate to severe BPH often require surgery to correct the restriction in urinary flow. A complete discussion on the pharmacotherapy of BPH is found in Chapter 71.

Alpha$_1$ antagonists are occasionally used to treat pheochromocytoma and Raynaud's disease. **Pheochromocytoma** is a tumor, usually benign, arising from the adrenal medulla that is characterized by excessive secretion of catecholamines. A patient with a pheochromocytoma will exhibit extreme HTN, palpitations, dyspnea, anxiety, and profuse sweating. All are signs of excessive amounts of catecholamines. Although surgical removal is the usual treatment, alpha$_1$-receptor antagonists may be administered to block

Table 16.1 Alpha-Adrenergic Antagonists

Drug	Route and Adult Dose (Maximum Dose Where Indicated)	Adverse Effects
alfuzosin (Uroxatral)	PO: 10 mg once daily	*Orthostatic hypotension, dizziness, headache, fatigue* First-dose phenomenon, tachycardia, dyspnea
doxazosin (Cardura)	PO (regular release): 1 mg/day (max: 8 mg/day)	
phenoxybenzamine (Dibenzyline)	PO: Initially 10 mg bid, may increase by 10 mg at 4-day intervals to 20–40 mg bid or tid	
phentolamine (OraVerse)	IV/IM: 5 mg 1–2 h prior to surgery Intradermal: 5–10 mg diluted in 10 mL of normal saline injected into the affected area within 12 h of catecholamine extravasation	
prazosin (Minipress)	PO: 1 mg/day; may increase to 1 mg bid–tid (max: 20 mg/day)	
silodosin (Rapaflo)	PO: 8 mg once daily	
tamsulosin (Flomax)	PO: 0.4–0.8 mg/day (max: 0.8 mg/day)	
terazosin	PO: 1–5 mg/day (max: 20 mg/day)	

Note: *Italics* indicate common adverse effects. Underline indicates serious adverse effects.

the peripheral vascular effects of natural (endogenous) catecholamines. This reduces the profound HTN in patients who are high surgical risks.

In **Raynaud's disease**, vasospasms of vessels serving the fingers and toes can lead to intermittent pain and cyanosis of the digits. Emotional stress or cold temperatures usually exacerbate the disorder. The primary treatment is nonpharmacologic: warming techniques and avoidance of cold. For those who require pharmacotherapy, administration of alpha$_1$ antagonists can diminish the vasospasm and bring symptomatic relief. Long-acting calcium channel blockers (see Chapter 30) such as nifedipine (Procardia XL) are also used to relieve Raynaud's vasospasms.

PharmFACT

Raynaud's disease is more common in women than in men and can occur secondary to other diseases, usually autoimmune disorders. For example, 90% of individuals with scleroderma also develop Raynaud's disease. Systemic lupus erythematosus may also occur concurrently with Raynaud's phenomenon (Hansen-Dispenza, 2018).

The adverse effects of alpha$_1$ antagonists are predictable based on their mechanism of action. When the sympathetic nervous system is blocked, parasympathetic tone will predominate; thus, most of the significant adverse effects of alpha blockers are due to increased parasympathetic activity.

The limiting adverse effect of pharmacotherapy with most alpha$_1$ antagonists is hypotension. The vasodilation caused by alpha$_1$ blockers is more intense when the patient is upright, as compared to recumbent. Significant **orthostatic hypotension** can occur when the patient abruptly changes from a recumbent to an upright position, resulting in diminished blood flow to the brain. Much of this effect is caused by blockade of alpha$_1$ receptors in the veins. As the patient moves to an upright position, blood accumulates in the veins, cardiac output decreases, and blood pressure falls. Orthostatic hypotension is especially pronounced at the beginning of pharmacotherapy and when increasing the dose. This adverse effect is called the **first-dose phenomenon**. Because the first-dose phenomenon can cause syncope due to reduced blood flow to the brain, initial therapy is begun with low doses, usually administered at bedtime.

The fall in blood pressure during alpha$_1$-antagonist therapy may be accompanied by reflex tachycardia, which occurs when the baroreceptor reflex is triggered. Reflex tachycardia can be particularly troublesome in patients who are susceptible to dysrhythmias. A beta-adrenergic antagonist is sometimes administered concurrently with alpha blockers to reduce the risk of reflex tachycardia. A less serious, though annoying, adverse effect of alpha antagonists is nasal congestion, which is caused by vasodilation of blood vessels serving the nasal mucosa.

A number of noncardiovascular adverse effects may also occur during alpha$_1$-blocker pharmacotherapy. Because smooth muscle contraction is inhibited in the vas deferens and ejaculatory ducts, these drugs can cause an inability to ejaculate during intercourse. This is a major reason for discontinuation of alpha-antagonist therapy in sexually active men. Increased smooth muscle activity in the GI tract may cause nausea and/or vomiting or abdominal cramping. Incontinence or increased urinary frequency may occur due to more active smooth muscle contractions in the urinary tract. These medications cross the blood–brain barrier and may cause central nervous system (CNS) effects such as depression, lethargy, and vivid dreams. Alpha blockers increase urinary metabolites of vanillylmandelic acid (VMA) and NE, which can result in false-positive test results for pheochromocytoma.

Although a few drugs selectively block alpha$_2$-adrenergic receptors, they currently have no clinical application. Yohimbine, once approved by the U.S. Food and Drug Administration (FDA) for the treatment of erectile dysfunction, selectively blocks alpha$_2$ receptors. Yohimbe (converted to yohimbine in the body) is a natural product obtained from the bark of a West African tree that is available over the counter (OTC) as an herbal supplement. Claims that this herb improves male sexual function have not been supported by controlled research studies. This product is not recommended for this purpose due to the availability of safer and more effective drugs.

PROTOTYPE DRUG **Prazosin (Minipress)**

Classification **Therapeutic:** Antihypertensive
Pharmacologic: Selective alpha$_1$-adrenergic antagonist

Therapeutic Effects and Uses: The primary therapeutic action of prazosin is a rapid decrease in peripheral resistance that reduces blood pressure. The drug has very little effect on cardiac output or heart rate and it causes less reflex tachycardia than some other drugs in this class. Approved in 1976, its most common use is in combination with other drugs, such as beta blockers or diuretics, in the pharmacotherapy of HTN. Optimal therapeutic effects may require 4 to 6 weeks of therapy. Off-label indications include symptomatic BPH, treatment of Raynaud's disease, and nightmares and sleep disruption related to posttraumatic stress disorder. Prazosin has a relatively short half-life that requires it to be administered two to three times per day.

Mechanism of Action: Prazosin competes with NE at alpha-adrenergic receptors on vascular smooth muscle in arterioles and veins. It is selective for alpha$_1$-adrenergic receptors and has no activity at alpha$_2$- or beta-adrenergic receptors.

Pharmacokinetics:

Route(s)	PO
Absorption	Well absorbed
Distribution	Completely distributed; small amounts secreted in breast milk
Primary metabolism	Hepatic
Primary excretion	Primarily bile and feces, with small amounts by the kidneys
Onset of action	2 h
Duration of action	Less than 24 h

Adverse Effects: The most common adverse effects of prazosin include dizziness, drowsiness, fatigue, weakness, palpitations, orthostatic hypotension, and headache. Nausea and vomiting and other GI effects occur in about 5% of patients. Most patients develop tolerance to these adverse effects as therapy progresses. The first-dose phenomenon may cause syncope. Erectile dysfunction, including priapism, is rare but can present a barrier to patient adherence.

Contraindications/Precautions: The only contraindication to the use of prazosin is prior sensitivity to the drug. The drug should be used with caution in older patients and those with renal impairment because these groups tend to exhibit more pronounced orthostatic hypotension and syncope. Patients with coronary artery disease should be treated with caution because prazosin may worsen angina symptoms in these patients.

Drug Interactions: Additive hypotensive effects may occur when prazosin is used concurrently with other antihypertensives and diuretics. This additive effect is used to advantage in the pharmacotherapy of HTN, in which the dose of each individual drug may be lower than if a single drug were used as monotherapy. Ingestion of alcohol or use with erectile dysfunction drugs such as sildenafil (Viagra) may induce hypotension. Use with sympathomimetics having alpha-agonist activity will antagonize the therapeutic effects of prazosin. **Herbal/Food:** Hawthorn may cause an additive drop in blood pressure when used with antihypertensive drugs such as prazosin.

Pregnancy: Animal studies have not shown evidence of fetal abnormalities. The drug is secreted in human milk but effects on the breastfeeding infant are unknown.

Treatment of Overdose: Overdose will lead to hypotension and possibly sudden loss of consciousness; thus, it is important to keep the patient supine. Fluid expanders may be administered to raise blood pressure, and renal function should be monitored. Vasopressors such as levarterenol or dopamine may be necessary to increase blood pressure. Drowsiness may also be prominent.

Clinician Responsibilities: Key clinical implications for patients receiving prazosin are included in the Applied Clinical Judgment: Patients Receiving Pharmacotherapy with Adrenergic Antagonists.

Drugs Similar to Prazosin (Minipress)

Other alpha-adrenergic blockers used for HTN include doxazosin, phenoxybenzamine, phentolamine, silodosin, and terazosin. Two alpha-adrenergic blockers, alfuzosin and tamsulosin, are indicated only for BPH.

Alfuzosin (Uroxatral): Alfuzosin was approved in 2003 to treat BPH as an extended-release tablet that permits once-daily dosing. Both tamsulosin and alfuzosin relax smooth muscle in the bladder and prostate gland, which reduces pressure on the urethra, thus enhancing urine flow. The drug is well tolerated, with the most common adverse effects being dizziness, fatigue, headache, and upper respiratory infection. Hypotension may be a serious problem in patients taking antihypertensive drugs or erectile dysfunction drugs such as sildenafil (Viagra). Caution should be used in patients with moderate or severe hepatic or renal impairment. This drug is not indicated for use in women.

Doxazosin (Cardura): Approved in 1990, doxazosin is an oral drug used to treat both HTN and BPH. The extended-release form of the drug, Cardura XL, is only approved for BPH. It has the longest duration of action of the selective $alpha_1$ blockers, allowing for once-daily dosing. The most frequent adverse effects are dizziness, fatigue, headache, and edema. Orthostatic hypotension occurs in a significant number of patients, especially when therapy is initiated or with changes in dose. Patients who ingest alcohol or use this drug with erectile dysfunction drugs such as sildenafil (Viagra) may experience increased hypotension. The drug should be used cautiously in older adults because they tend to experience more hypotension-related adverse effects. Doxazosin should be taken at bedtime to avoid the first-dose phenomenon. Animal reproduction studies showed no adverse developmental effects. High doses showed reduced fetal survival. The drug is secreted in human milk but effects on the breastfeeding infant are unknown.

Phenoxybenzamine (Dibenzyline): Phenoxybenzamine is an older drug, approved in 1954, that blocks both $alpha_1$- and $alpha_2$-adrenergic receptors. The drug has a very prolonged duration of action, and its effects may last up to a week after the drug is discontinued. Because it has the potential to cause extended alpha blockade and serious cardiovascular adverse effects, its use is limited to managing the HTN caused by pheochromocytoma. Off-label indications include symptomatic BPH, Raynaud's disease, and frostbite. Animal reproduction studies have not been conducted on this drug, and effects on lactation are unknown.

Phentolamine (OraVerse): Like phenoxybenzamine, phentolamine blocks both $alpha_1$ and $alpha_2$ receptors. Approved in 1952, it is the only alpha blocker that is given parenterally. Phentolamine may be administered to treat or prevent hypertensive crises during surgical removal of pheochromocytomas. Phentolamine is an antidote for treating hypertensive emergencies caused by catecholamine overdose. The drug may be injected subcutaneously to prevent or treat dermal necrosis or sloughing caused by extravasation of catecholamines such as NE and dopamine. Although the drug has been used in the past to diagnose pheochromocytoma, safer measures such as urinary or blood assays of catecholamine levels are more accurate indicators of this disease. OraVerse was approved in 2016 for the reversal of dental anesthesia. In animal reproduction studies, high doses of phentolamine resulted in skeletal immaturity and reduced growth of offspring. Effects on breastfeeding are unknown.

Silodosin (Rapaflo): Approved in 2008, silodosin is a selective alpha$_1$-adrenergic antagonist that is indicated for the management of BPH. The most common adverse effects are retrograde ejaculation, dizziness, diarrhea, orthostatic hypotension, headache, nasopharyngitis, and nasal congestion. It should be taken with food to lessen the risk of adverse effects. This drug is not indicated for use in women.

Tamsulosin (Flomax): Like alfuzosin and silodosin, tamsulosin has only one indication: BPH. Approved in 1997, it is administered orally (PO) and should be taken with food to reduce the incidence of orthostatic hypotension. The drug is generally well tolerated and exhibits adverse effects similar to other alpha blockers. Significant numbers of patients may experience headache, rhinitis, and orthostatic hypotension. Tamsulosin is extensively metabolized by hepatic CYP enzymes and may interact with drugs that are inducers or substrates of these enzymes. This drug is not indicated for use in women.

Terazosin: Approved in 1987, terazosin has a long duration of action and is indicated for both HTN and symptomatic BPH. Given PO, its prolonged half-life permits once-daily dosing. Common adverse effects include orthostatic hypotension, dizziness, and fatigue. Tolerance develops to most adverse effects as therapy progresses. Like other drugs in this class, terazosin should be taken at bedtime to avoid the first-dose phenomenon. Older adults are more sensitive to the hypotensive and adverse effects of terazosin, such as dry mouth and drowsiness. In animal reproduction studies terazosin was not teratogenic at relevant doses. Effects on breastfeeding are unknown.

Beta-Adrenergic Antagonists

16.3 Nonselective beta-adrenergic antagonists affect both beta$_1$ and beta$_2$ receptors and are prescribed for HTN, angina, and other cardiovascular disorders.

Beta-adrenergic antagonists, or beta blockers, are classified as nonselective or selective. Nonselective beta-adrenergic antagonists, such as propranolol, block both beta$_1$ and beta$_2$ receptors. Selective drugs that block only beta$_1$ receptors are sometimes called *cardioselective agents* and are discussed in Section 16.4.

Some beta blockers, such as carvedilol (Coreg), also have some alpha-antagonist activity, which adds to their ability to lower blood pressure. A few beta blockers such as pindolol exhibit mixed beta-antagonist and beta-*agonist* activity. This low level of beta-agonist activity is called **intrinsic sympathomimetic activity (ISA)**. Theoretically, the agonist action of these drugs may result in fewer adverse effects in patients who have bradycardia, HF, or compromised pulmonary function. Regardless of their receptor specificity, most therapeutic applications of the beta blockers relate to their effects on the cardiovascular system (Table 16.2).

Because their mechanism of action is to block the effects of endogenous catecholamines, all beta blockers have the potential to reduce the heart rate (negative chronotropic effect), decrease the force of myocardial contraction (negative inotropic effect), and slow conduction velocity through the atrioventricular node (negative dromotropic effect). These effects are modest when the heart is at rest. During periods of stress or exercise, however, beta blockers tend to prevent the normal increase in sympathetic stimulation to the heart, which is intended to bring more blood flow to this organ. In some cases, this results in an undesirable short-term decrease in cardiac output, and the sympathetic nervous system responds by activating alpha receptors and raising blood pressure. In time, peripheral resistance returns to normal or below-normal levels, particularly in patients with HTN, and blood pressure falls.

The primary use of beta-adrenergic antagonists is the treatment of HTN. The following multiple mechanisms are believed to contribute to their antihypertensive effect:

- Diminished myocardial contractility decreases cardiac output.
- The release of renin by the kidney, normally stimulated by catecholamines, is prevented.
- The nonselective adrenergic antagonists block alpha$_1$-adrenergic receptors, relaxing arteriolar smooth muscle.
- Central actions reduce sympathetic output from the vasomotor center in the brain.

The student should refer to Chapter 34 for additional details on the use of beta blockers in HTN management.

Beta-adrenergic antagonists have several other important applications, although they are not always first-line drugs for these conditions. By decreasing cardiac workload and oxygen demand, beta blockers can ease the acute chest pain characteristic of angina pectoris (see the prototype feature for atenolol in Chapter 35). Because they slow cardiac conduction, beta blockers are used in the pharmacotherapy of certain types of dysrhythmias (see Chapter 37). Some nonselective beta blockers have the ability to reduce intraocular pressure when

Table 16.2 Beta-Adrenergic Antagonists

Drug	Route and Adult Dose (Maximum Dose Where Indicated)	Adverse Effects
Selective Beta$_1$-Adrenergic Antagonists		
acebutolol	PO: 200–800 mg/day in divided doses (max: 1200 mg/day)	*Fatigue, insomnia, diarrhea, constipation, drowsiness, impotence or decreased libido, hypotension, bradycardia, confusion* Bronchospasm, Stevens–Johnson syndrome, anaphylaxis, worsening of HF; if the drug is abruptly withdrawn, palpitations, rebound HTN, dysrhythmias, MI
atenolol (Tenormin)	PO: 25–50 mg daily (max: 100 mg/day)	
betaxolol	PO: 10–20 mg daily (max: 40 mg/day)	
bisoprolol	PO: 2.5–5 mg once daily (max: 20 mg/day)	
esmolol (Brevibloc)	IV: 500 mcg/kg loading dose followed by 50 mcg/kg/min; may increase dose every 5–10 min (max: 200 mcg/kg/min)	
metoprolol (Lopressor, Toprol XL)	PO (extended release): 100 mg once daily (max: 200 mg/day for HF; 400 mg/day for HTN or angina)	
nebivolol (Bystolic)	PO: 5 mg once daily (max: 40 mg)	
Alpha$_1$ and Beta Blockers (Centrally Acting)		
nadolol (Corgard)	PO: 40 mg once daily (max: 240–320 mg/day)	*Headache, dizziness, fatigue, drowsiness, anxiety, depression, lethargy, impotence, peripheral vascular insufficiency, hypoglycemia* Bradycardia, bronchospasm, laryngospasm, respiratory disturbances, may worsen HF and mask symptoms of hypoglycemia, Stevens–Johnson syndrome (propranolol), toxic epidermal necrolysis (propranolol), exfoliative dermatitis (propranolol), dysrhythmias (sotalol)
pindolol	PO: 5 mg bid (max: 60 mg/day)	
propranolol (Inderal LA, InnoPran XL)	PO (extended release): 80–120 mg once daily IV: 0.5–3 mg q4h prn for dysrhythmias	
sotalol (Betapace, Sorine, Sotylize)	PO (regular release): Initial dose of 80 mg bid (max: 320–640 mg/day)	
timolol	PO: 10 mg bid (max: 60 mg/day for HTN)	
Mixed Alpha$_1$- and Beta-Adrenergic Antagonists		
carvedilol (Coreg)	PO (regular release): start with 3.125 mg bid (max: 50 mg/day) PO (extended release): start with 10–20 mg once daily (max: 80 mg/day)	Same as the above two classes
labetalol (Trandate)	PO: 100 mg bid (max: 2400 mg/day)	

Note: *Italics* indicate common adverse effects. Underline indicates serious adverse effects.

given as ophthalmic solutions in the pharmacotherapy of glaucoma (see Chapter 74). Other therapeutic uses include the treatment of HF (see Chapter 36), myocardial infarction (MI; see Chapter 35), and migraine prophylaxis (see Chapter 25). Beta blockers such as propranolol have been used off-label to treat the anxiousness, sweating, and tachycardia associated with stage fright and PTSD.

Pharmacotherapy with nonselective beta antagonists usually produces more adverse effects than treatment with selective beta$_1$ antagonists. Because of this, the use of the nonselective drugs has declined. One of the more serious adverse effects with the nonselective beta blockers is that inhibition of beta$_2$ receptors in the lung can cause bronchoconstriction, which can induce acute shortness of breath,

CONNECTIONS: Treating the Diverse Patient

Racial and Ethnic Differences in Antihypertensive Treatment and Control

One of the largest clinical trials of drug therapy for hypertensive disease, the Antihypertensive and Lipid-Lowering Treatment to Prevent Heart Attack Trial (ALLHAT; Gupta et al., 2010), noted differences in response to antihypertensive drugs among Whites, Blacks, and Asian Americans. Although Blacks experienced less of a response to the use of a beta blocker (atenolol) than other patients, adding a diuretic increased the blood pressure–lowering effects. And Asian Americans experienced a greater antihypertensive effect when an ACE inhibitor (perindopril) was added to the medication routine.

Differences also exist in the prevalence and treatment of hypertension across racial/ethnic groups. In a large study investigating racial and ethnic disparities in prevalence, treatment, and hypertensive control, non-Hispanic Blacks were found to have the highest prevalence and highest incidence of unmet treatment goals (e.g., control of BP not achieved to goal level) (Al Kabria, 2019). And Hispanics and other non-White, non-Black racial/ethnic groups had the highest incidence of untreated hypertension.

Understanding the need for differing treatment should be only one part of the overall treatment plan. Recognizing that a significant portion of the population may be untreated or have treatment that does not result in full realization of the treatment goals, especially in different racial/ethnic populations, is equally important to achieve antihypertensive therapy goals.

in patients with chronic obstructive pulmonary disease (COPD) or asthma.

The metabolic effects of beta-adrenergic antagonists can be important for patients with diabetes mellitus. Under normal conditions, catecholamines break down glycogen, which frees glucose to enter the blood to be used as an energy source. Many body tissues, particularly skeletal muscles, must receive a continuous source of glucose, especially during prolonged physical activity or heavy exercise. Beta blockers prevent this hyperglycemic effect of the catecholamines, and patients with diabetes may develop hypoglycemia. In addition, beta blockers will prevent tachycardia, an important warning sign of impending hypoglycemia. Beta-blocker therapy in patients with diabetes must be carefully monitored.

A second metabolic effect of nonselective beta-adrenergic antagonists relates to lipid metabolism. Catecholamines normally stimulate lipolysis, the breakdown of stored lipid in adipose tissue, resulting in the release of free fatty acids into the blood. Like glucose, these fatty acids serve as an essential energy source for skeletal muscle. By blocking the actions of catecholamines, beta antagonists decrease the amount of free fatty acids available during periods of metabolic stress. Nonselective beta blockers may also increase serum triglycerides and decrease high-density lipoproteins. During the course of therapy with beta blockers, patients with preexisting lipid disorders should have their lipid profiles monitored periodically to prevent hyperlipidemia.

Overdoses with nonselective beta blockers are potentially serious and treatment involves maintaining or restoring cardiovascular function. An anticholinergic such as atropine or a beta-adrenergic agonist such as isoproterenol may be administered to reverse severe bradycardia and cause bronchodilation. Cardiac failure caused by beta-antagonist overdose may be treated by administering digoxin (Lanoxin) or diuretics. Severe hypotension may require the administration of a vasopressor such as epinephrine or NE.

Beta blockers should always be withdrawn gradually over several weeks. If discontinued abruptly, the heart displays hypersensitivity to catecholamines, resulting in sweating, palpitations, headache, and tremors. This phenomenon is called *rebound cardiac excitation*. Some of the beta blockers have a black box warning to discontinue the drug gradually because patients with coronary artery disease may experience a worsening of angina symptoms or MIs may occur.

PROTOTYPE DRUG Propranolol (Inderal LA, InnoPran XL)

Classification **Therapeutic:** Antihypertensive, antidysrhythmic
Pharmacologic: Nonselective beta-adrenergic blocker

Therapeutic Effects and Uses: Approved in 1967, propranolol reduces heart rate and slows conduction velocity through the atrioventricular (AV) node by blocking $beta_1$ receptors in cardiac muscle. The decrease in cardiac output, as well as its suppression of renin activity, results in a reduction in blood pressure. Cardiac workload and myocardial oxygen demand decrease due to the slower heart rate and decreased cardiac output. Propranolol is prescribed for a wide variety of indications (some off-label), including the following:

- **Hypertension.** For the treatment of HTN, propranolol has largely been replaced by angiotensin-converting enzyme (ACE) inhibitors and calcium channel blockers, which are more effective at preventing the long-term consequences of HTN such as stroke and MI. Propranolol is still widely used in patients with HTN who have angina, prior MI, or heart failure.
- **Angina pectoris.** Beta blockers are the preferred drugs for treating chronic angina. The nonselective drugs such as propranolol are less frequently used than the cardioselective agents.
- **Dysrhythmias.** Propranolol is one of the few beta-adrenergic antagonists approved to treat dysrhythmias. As an antidysrhythmic, propranolol is most effective at preventing tachycardia caused by excessive sympathetic stimulation.
- **Migraine prophylaxis.** Propranolol has been frequently prescribed for the prevention of migraines.
- **Prophylaxis of MI.** When given following an MI, propranolol reduces cardiovascular mortality and the risk of reinfarction.

Propranolol has a number of other indications. By lowering venous pressure, it may be useful in reducing portal HTN and bleeding due to esophageal varices. Propranolol is sometimes used to reduce the tachycardia, palpitations, tremor, and nervousness associated with thyroid crisis (storm). It has been used to treat panic attacks, PTSD, chronic agitation, and aggressive behavior. Lastly, it has been used to manage involuntary, rhythmic movements of essential tremor.

Both immediate-release and extended-release forms of propranolol are available. InnoPran XL has a timed delivery system that is designed for bedtime dosing, with a peak effect in the morning.

Mechanism of Action: Propranolol is a nonselective beta-adrenergic antagonist, affecting both $beta_1$ receptors in the heart and $beta_2$ receptors in the lung and other locations throughout the body. It has no ISA.

Pharmacokinetics:

Route(s)	Usually PO; IV for severe dysrhythmias
Absorption	Completely absorbed

Distribution	Widely distributed, including the CNS and placenta; secreted in breast milk; 90% bound to plasma protein
Primary metabolism	Hepatic
Primary excretion	90–95% renal
Onset of action	PO: 1–2 h; IV: immediate
Duration of action	Half-life: 3–5 h

Adverse Effects: Propranolol is well tolerated and common adverse effects, such as nausea and vomiting and diarrhea, generally diminish as therapy progresses. Other frequent adverse effects include fatigue, insomnia, drowsiness, bradycardia, and confusion. Impotence or loss of libido occurs in a small percentage of patients. Serious adverse effects include agranulocytosis, bronchospasm, Stevens–Johnson syndrome, and anaphylaxis. If the drug is abruptly withdrawn, palpitations, rebound HTN, life-threatening dysrhythmias, or myocardial ischemia may occur. **Black Box Warning:** Abrupt withdrawal is not advised in patients with angina or heart disease. Dosage should gradually be reduced over 1 to 2 weeks and the drug should be reinstituted if angina symptoms develop during this period.

Contraindications/Precautions: Because of its depressive effects on the heart, propranolol is contraindicated in cardiogenic shock, sinus bradycardia, greater than first-degree heart block, and severe HF. Patients with cardiac impairment must be monitored carefully to prevent worsening of their condition. Due to its constriction of smooth muscle in the airways, the drug is contraindicated in patients with COPD or asthma. Propranolol should be used cautiously in patients with diabetes because it interferes with glucose metabolism and can cause hypoglycemia. The drug can also mask signs of impending hypoglycemia such as tachycardia and tremors. Propranolol should be used with caution in patients with reduced renal output because the drug may accumulate to toxic levels in the blood and cause dysrhythmias.

Drug Interactions: Propranolol interacts with many other drugs. When given with other beta blockers, effects on the cardiovascular system may be additive and bradycardia or hypotension may result. Because both propranolol and calcium channel blockers such as verapamil (Calan) and diltiazem (Cardizem) suppress myocardial contractility, concurrent use may lead to additive bradycardia. Use with antidysrhythmic drugs that slow conduction through the AV node such as amiodarone may lead to AV block. Phenothiazines can add to the hypotensive effects of propranolol. Because monoamine oxidase (MAO) inhibitors deplete endogenous catecholamines, concurrent administration with propranolol could result in severe bradycardia and hypotension.

Use of ethanol or antacids containing aluminum hydroxide gel will slow the absorption of propranolol and reduce its therapeutic effects. Administration of beta-adrenergic agonists such as albuterol (Proventil) will antagonize the antihypertensive action of propranolol. **Herbal/Food:** Hawthorn may cause an additive drop in blood pressure when used with antihypertensive drugs such as propranolol. Large doses of vitamin C may reduce the absorption of propranolol.

Pregnancy: In animal reproduction studies, high doses of propranolol showed embryotoxicity, and increased neonatal deaths. In mothers taking this drug in the third trimester, neonates should be observed for bradycardia and hypoglycemia This drug is secreted in human milk but effects on the breastfed neonate are unknown.

Treatment of Overdose: Overdose will cause bradycardia, hypotension, and bronchospasm. Treatment may require the use of plasma volume expanders or vasopressors to raise blood pressure to normal levels and atropine to counteract the bradycardia. Isoproterenol (a beta agonist) may be administered to reverse bronchospasm.

Clinician Responsibilities: Key clinical implications for patients receiving propranolol are included in the Applied Clinical Judgment: Patients Receiving Pharmacotherapy with Adrenergic Antagonists.

Drugs Similar to Propranolol (Inderal LA, InnoPran XL)

Many beta blockers are available. All nonselective beta-adrenergic blockers have the same actions but differ in their pharmacokinetics and therapeutic applications. Those prescribed for glaucoma, including betaxolol, carteolol, levobunolol, metipranolol, and timolol, are discussed in Chapter 74. Beta-blockers cross the placenta and are also secreted in human breast milk. Caution is advised during pregnancy and lactation.

Carvedilol (Coreg): Approved in 1995, carvedilol is a PO medication approved for the management of HTN and HF and to reduce mortality in patients who have survived the acute phase of an MI. It may be used off-label to treat angina. In addition to being a nonselective beta-receptor blocker, carvedilol blocks $alpha_1$-adrenergic receptors. Because of its alpha-antagonist action, carvedilol shares similar adverse effects, such as orthostatic hypotension, with the $alpha_1$ blockers. Like most beta blockers, fatigue and dizziness are common adverse effects. Patients with asthma or chronic lung disorders may experience dyspnea or wheezing due to the bronchoconstriction effects of the drug.

Labetalol (Trandate): Like carvedilol, labetalol has nonselective beta-blocking action as well as the ability to selectively block alpha$_1$-adrenergic receptors. Approved in 1984, it is available by both the oral and IV routes for the therapy of HTN. When treating HTN, the drug may be given concurrently with a thiazide diuretic. The most common adverse effects are generally mild and include insomnia, drowsiness, fatigue, decreased libido, and tingling of the scalp. Orthostatic hypotension is greatest 2 to 4 hours after the drug is administered. When given by the IV route for hypertensive emergencies, as many as 60% of patients will experience orthostatic hypotension.

Nadolol (Corgard): Approved in 1989, nadolol is a nonselective beta-adrenergic blocker that is used to treat HTN and for the long-term management of angina. Off-label uses of nadolol include suppression of ventricular dysrhythmias, migraine prophylaxis, treatment of essential tremor, and anxiety. Given by the oral route, it has a long half-life of 20 to 24 hours, which offers the benefit of once-daily dosing. Unlike many beta blockers, it is not metabolized by the liver and is excreted mostly unchanged by the kidneys. Adverse effects are generally mild and similar to those of propranolol and include drowsiness, fatigue, and decreased libido. The drug carries a black box warning that abrupt discontinuation can exacerbate ischemic heart disease.

Pindolol: Approved in 1982, pindolol is an oral, nonselective beta blocker that is used in the pharmacotherapy of HTN, usually in combination with a thiazide diuretic. It is used off-label for the management of chronic stable angina. Pindolol has the highest degree of ISA of any beta blocker, which gives it some beta-agonist action in addition to antagonist activity. Adverse effects are generally mild and temporary and include nausea and vomiting, insomnia, fatigue, and dizziness. Maximum antihypertensive action may take up to 2 weeks to achieve.

Sotalol (Betapace, Sorine, Sotylize): Although all nonselective beta blockers affect heart rate and rhythm, sotalol is one of the few drugs in this class used exclusively as an antidysrhythmic. By slowing the action potential crossing the myocardium, the heart is able to regain normal rhythm. Adverse effects are those typical of beta blockers but they occur more frequently: fatigue, dyspnea, and sinus bradycardia are common. Patients with a history of dysrhythmias are more likely to experience serious adverse effects. Initially approved in 1992, the drug carries a black box warning that therapy should be started in a facility with continuous ECG monitoring, that cardiac resuscitation equipment be available, and that the drug can induce life-threatening dysrhythmias. Other adverse effects include insomnia, nausea and vomiting, and drowsiness. The role of sotalol in the pharmacotherapy of dysrhythmias is presented in Chapter 37.

Timolol (Timoptic): When given PO, timolol is indicated for HTN, migraine prophylaxis, and reduction of mortality following an acute MI. Chronic, stable angina is an off-label indication for the drug. Systemic adverse effects are generally mild and transient and include nausea and vomiting, diarrhea, bradycardia, fatigue, and dizziness. The drug carries a black box warning that abrupt discontinuation of PO timolol can exacerbate ischemic heart disease. Approved in 1978, timolol is available as an ophthalmic solution to treat glaucoma and is presented as a prototype for glaucoma in Chapter 74.

16.4 Beta$_1$-adrenergic antagonists are selective for beta$_1$ receptors in the myocardium and are used to treat HTN and other cardiovascular disorders.

Because of their specificity for beta$_1$ receptors in the myocardium, the beta$_1$-adrenergic antagonists exert fewer noncardiac adverse effects than nonselective agents such as propranolol. This selectivity is not absolute, however; some of these drugs affect beta$_2$ receptors at higher doses, and a few have intrinsic sympathomimetic activity.

The primary indication for selective beta$_1$ antagonists is HTN. Some are also used in the pharmacologic management of chronic angina pectoris and HF. Although used for the same indications as the nonselective agents, the beta$_1$ blockers have certain advantages. The major advantage is that they have little effect on beta$_2$ receptors in bronchial smooth muscle. This allows the beta$_1$ blockers to be administered to patients with asthma or COPD with a lower risk of bronchospasm. The beta$_1$ blockers also have less effect on glucose and lipid metabolism than the nonselective drugs.

Beta blockers should be used with great caution in patients with a history of HF because both the nonselective and selective beta$_1$ blockers slow the speed of impulse conduction across the myocardium. In patients with healthy hearts, this effect presents as a clinical problem only at high doses. In patients with diseased hearts, however, this depression can worsen cardiac impairment and lead to HF. This cardiac impairment may develop gradually in patients taking beta blockers for prolonged periods; therefore, the patient should receive regular assessments of cardiac function during therapy. Generally, beta blockers are discontinued or their doses adjusted as soon as HF is suspected.

Overdose with beta$_1$ antagonists is treated in a manner similar to the nonselective beta blockers. An anticholinergic drug such as atropine or a beta agonist such as isoproterenol may be given to promote bronchodilation and increase the heart rate. Digoxin (Lanoxin) or diuretics may be indicated if HF develops. Severe hypotension may require the administration of an emergency vasopressor such as dopamine (a beta agonist).

CONNECTION Checkpoint 16.2

Dopamine is a catecholamine. From what you learned in Chapter 15, identify other catecholamines that are used to quickly raise blood pressure in acute care situations.

PROTOTYPE DRUG **Metoprolol (Lopressor, Toprol XL)**

Classification **Therapeutic:** Antihypertensive
Pharmacologic: Selective $beta_1$-adrenergic antagonist

Therapeutic Effects and Uses: Approved in 1978, the primary indication for metoprolol is HTN, as monotherapy or in combination with other antihypertensives. It is also indicated for angina and for the treatment of stable, symptomatic HF.

The therapeutic actions of metoprolol include decreases in heart rate (both resting and during exercise), cardiac output, and blood pressure (both systolic and diastolic). Fixed-dose combination formulations are available for HTN: Lopressor HCT combines metoprolol with the diuretic hydrochlorothiazide in a single tablet. Because it slows the rate and force of myocardial contraction, metoprolol can reduce oxygen demands on the heart and benefit patients with angina and stable HF. Off-label uses include essential tremor, migraine prophylaxis, and the control of heart rate in patients with atrial dysrhythmias.

Metoprolol reduces the mortality associated with recent MI. Following an acute MI, metoprolol is infused slowly until a target heart rate between 60 and 90 beats/min is reached. This reduces myocardial oxygen demand at a time when the heart is at high risk for a subsequent MI or life-threatening dysrhythmias. On hospital discharge, patients continue metoprolol therapy by switching to the PO form of the drug.

Mechanism of Action: Metoprolol is a selective $beta_1$-adrenergic antagonist that competes with endogenous catecholamines at adrenergic receptors in cardiac muscle. At high doses, it may affect $beta_2$ receptors in bronchial smooth muscle.

Pharmacokinetics:

Route(s)	Usually PO; IV for MI
Absorption	Well absorbed
Distribution	Completely, including CNS and placenta; secreted in breast milk; 12% bound to plasma protein
Primary metabolism	Hepatic
Primary excretion	Renal
Onset of action	PO: 15 min; IV: immediate
Duration of action	13–19 h

Adverse Effects: Metoprolol is well tolerated, and adverse effects generally diminish as therapy progresses. Nausea and vomiting are the most common adverse effects. Other common adverse effects include dizziness, fatigue, insomnia, bradycardia, heartburn, and dyspnea. Serious adverse effects include agranulocytosis, laryngospasm, complete heart block, and thyroid storm in patients with thyrotoxicosis. Bronchospasm and dyspnea are rare because the drug has little effect on $beta_2$ receptors in bronchial smooth muscle. Dysrhythmias, severe HTN, or MI may occur if the drug is abruptly withdrawn. **Black Box Warning:** Abrupt withdrawal is not advised in patients with angina or heart disease. Dosage should gradually be reduced over 1 to 2 weeks and the drug should be reinstituted if angina symptoms develop during this period.

Contraindications/Precautions: Because of its multiple effects on the heart, patients with preexisting cardiac disease such as HF should be carefully monitored. This drug is contraindicated in cardiogenic shock, severe bradycardia, and heart block greater than first degree. Metoprolol should be used with caution in patients with severe hepatic disease because its major route of excretion is the liver. Metoprolol should be used with caution in patients with asthma and those with a history of bronchospasm because the drug may affect $beta_2$ receptors at high doses.

Drug Interactions: $Beta_1$ blockers such as metoprolol have the potential to interact with many drugs. The nurse should always be cautious when administering a beta blocker with any other medication that affects the heart, particularly those that depress AV node conduction. Because certain calcium channel blockers such as verapamil suppress myocardial contractility, concurrent use with metoprolol can lead to additive bradycardia and even heart block. Use with other antihypertensive drugs may cause additive hypotension. Certain drugs, including cimetidine and oral contraceptives, can also add to the hypotensive effect of metoprolol. Metoprolol should not be given with sympathomimetics because the actions of the drugs will cancel each other. Metoprolol can reduce the clearance of lidocaine and cause lidocaine toxicity.

Pregnancy: In animal reproduction studies, high doses of metoprolol showed embryotoxicity, and increased neonatal deaths. No evidence of teratogenicity or carcinogenicity was found. This drug is secreted in human milk but effects on the breastfed neonate are unknown.

Treatment of Overdose: Overdose of metoprolol will induce bradycardia, hypotension, and bronchospasm. Treatment may require the use of plasma volume expanders or vasopressors to raise blood pressure to normal levels and atropine to counteract the bradycardia. Isoproterenol may be administered for bronchospasm.

Clinician Responsibilities: Key clinical implications for patients receiving metoprolol are included in the Applied Clinical Judgment: Patients Receiving Pharmacotherapy with Adrenergic Antagonists.

Drugs Similar to Metoprolol (Lopressor, Toprol XL)

Other $beta_1$-adrenergic antagonists include acebutolol, atenolol, betaxolol, bisoprolol, esmolol, and nebivolol. The $beta_1$-adrenergic antagonists are very similar but differ in their pharmacokinetics and specific indications.

Acebutolol: Approved in 1984, acebutolol is a cardioselective $beta_1$ antagonist similar to metoprolol that is given PO for HTN and recurrent ventricular dysrhythmias. An off-label indication is chronic stable angina. In addition to being a selective $beta_1$ blocker, it exhibits mild ISA. Because of its 3- to 4-hour half-life, it is usually administered twice daily. Common adverse effects include CNS effects such as fatigue, dizziness, and headache. Higher doses can produce hypotension and bradycardia. Like other beta blockers, care must be taken when using acebutolol with other drugs that depress myocardial conduction because bradycardia and hypotension may result. Studies in humans showed that this drug crosses the placenta and may cause reduced birth weight, transient low blood pressure and reduced heart rate. Because this drug is secreted in human milk, breastfeeding is not recommended.

Atenolol (Tenormin): Approved in 1981, atenolol is available PO for HTN and for the long-term management of chronic stable angina. It is also given by the IV route to reduce the risk of sudden death in patients with an acute MI. Off-label indications include migraine prophylaxis and the prevention of symptoms in patients undergoing ethanol withdrawal. Atenolol has a long half-life, which allows for once-daily dosing. Common adverse effects are the same as those of other drugs in this class, such as nausea and vomiting, fatigue, dizziness, and headache. The risk of bradycardia is low at normal doses. Like other beta blockers, care must be taken to avoid abrupt discontinuation of therapy, especially in patients with coronary artery disease. Tenoretic is a combination of atenolol and the diuretic chlorthalidone that is approved for HTN. Atenolol is presented as a prototype drug for angina in Chapter 35. This drug may cause fetal harm and is not recommended during pregnancy or lactation.

Betaxolol: Approved in 1985, betaxolol is available in tablet form for the pharmacotherapy of HTN, sometimes given concurrently with thiazide diuretics. The drug is one of the most potent and selective of the beta blockers; it is nine times more potent than atenolol. It has no ISA, and it inhibits $beta_2$-adrenergic receptors in the lung only at very high doses. When given PO, adverse effects such as nausea and vomiting, dizziness, fatigue, and headache are typical of the beta blockers. The risk of bradycardia increases with higher doses. Like other beta blockers, care must be taken to avoid abrupt discontinuation of therapy, especially in patients with coronary artery disease, because myocardial ischemia, MI, HTN, or dysrhythmias may result. Animal reproduction data showed evidence of embryo loss and increased developmental abnormalities. Bradycardia and hypoglycemia may occur in the fetus and neonate. Betaxolol is secreted in human milk and caution is advised during breastfeeding.

Betaxolol is also available as a 0.25% ophthalmic suspension (Betoptic) for reducing intraocular pressure in patients with chronic open-angle glaucoma. Adverse effects are limited to the eye and include burning and transient blurred vision.

Bisoprolol: Approved in 1992, bisoprolol is approved only for HTN, although HF and chronic stable angina are off-label indications. Given PO, bisoprolol has a longer half-life than metoprolol, which allows for less frequent dosing. The cardioselective nature of bisoprolol action only applies to low doses; at higher doses it also blocks $beta_2$ receptors to cause dyspnea and wheezing. Common adverse effects are the same as those of other drugs in this class, such as fatigue, dizziness, and headache. Like other beta blockers, care must be taken to avoid abrupt discontinuation of therapy, especially in patients with coronary artery disease. Ziac combines bisoprolol with the diuretic hydrochlorothiazide in a single tablet. In animal reproduction studies bisoprolol was embryolethal and fetotoxic at high doses. It is not known if this drug is secreted in human milk.

Esmolol (Brevibloc): Approved in 1986, esmolol is very different from other $beta_1$-adrenergic blockers. It is administered by continuous IV infusion in emergency situations, usually postoperative or perioperative, to rapidly correct supraventricular tachycardia or hypertensive emergency. It has a very short half-life of only 8 minutes, and the patient must be monitored for hypotension and bradycardia during the infusion. Although it has the same actions and adverse effects as other beta blockers, the actions of esmolol begin to diminish within minutes after discontinuation of the infusion. Esmolol should be used with extreme caution in patients with severe bradycardia, AV block, or cardiogenic shock. Hypotension occurs in about 40% of patients receiving the drug but resolves quickly following completion of the infusion. Animal reproduction studies showed no evidence of teratogenicity or embryotoxicity. Esmolol may cause bradycardia in the fetus or newborn. It is not known if this drug is secreted in human milk.

Nebivolol (Bystolic): Approved in 2007, nebivolol is a selective $beta_1$-adrenergic blocker that is indicated for the treatment of HTN, either as monotherapy or in combination with other antihypertensives. Nebivolol is highly cardioselective but may activate $beta_2$ receptors at higher doses. It has no ISA activity. Nebivolol has equal effectiveness to other drugs in its class, but it appears to produce fewer adverse effects. The drug is well tolerated, with the most frequently observed adverse effects being headache, fatigue, paresthesia, dizziness, hypotension, and bradycardia. Like other beta blockers, care must be taken to avoid abrupt discontinuation of therapy, especially in patients with coronary artery disease. Animal reproduction studies showed decreased birth weight and survival. No embryotoxicity or teratogenic effects were observed. Because ebivolol has the potential to cause bradycardia in the breastfed infant, breastfeeding is not recommended.

CONNECTIONS: APPLIED CLINICAL JUDGMENT

Patients Receiving Pharmacotherapy with Adrenergic Antagonists

Key Assessment Data

- History of current condition, baseline vital signs, physical exam findings; history of CV, cerebrovascular, respiratory disease, diabetes; medication history; pregnancy status. Baseline ECG, cardiac output, and urinary output should be assessed, depending on the condition being treated.
- Ongoing assessment during drug therapy should include monitoring for bradycardia, hypotension, reflex tachycardia, dysrhythmias, bronchospasm, decreased urinary output, edema or weight gain over 1 kg (2 lb) per day.

Desired Therapeutic Outcomes

Improvement is observed and measurable in patient's pulse, BP, cardiac rhythm, ease of urination (BPH) within acceptable parameters.

Minimizing Adverse Effects:

- Monitor for orthostatic hypotension. Notify the provider if BP or pulse decreases beyond the established parameters or if hypotension is accompanied by reflex tachycardia.
- Continue cardiac monitoring (e.g., ECG) as ordered for dysrhythmias in the hospitalized patient, promptly reporting dysrhythmias, palpitations, or angina.
- Weigh daily and report weight gain over 1 kg (2 lb) in a 24-hour period or edema. These may signal that the BP has lowered too quickly, stimulating renin release, or is an adverse effect.
- Monitor urine output and symptoms of dysuria such as hesitancy or retention when given for BPH.
- Continue to monitor blood glucose levels and appropriate laboratory work. (Adrenergic antagonists affect a wide range of body systems. They may also interfere with some oral diabetic drugs or change the way a hypoglycemic reaction is perceived.)

Lifespan Considerations

- Older adults may be more sensitive to the effects of adrenergic antagonist drugs and dizziness may increase the risk of falls.

Diversity Considerations

- Differences exist in the response to antihypertensive therapy among various racial/ethnic populations and ongoing assessment is needed to ensure response to drug therapy is adequate.

Patient Education

- Monitor pulse, BP, and daily weight using a diary or log and bring these to each provider visit. Promptly report any weight gain over 1 kg (2 lb) in a 24-hour period, increasing or severe shortness of breath, palpitations, or chest pain to the provider.
- Take the first dose of an antihypertensive at bedtime if possible to avoid excessive dizziness and a first-dose effect with hypotension.
- Rise slowly from lying or sitting to standing, pausing between changes if dizziness occurs. Don't take the medication if dizziness continues, or the BP is below 90/60, or per parameters set by the provider, and contact the provider for further instruction.
- Patients with diabetes should monitor their blood glucose more frequently and be aware of subtle signs of possible hypoglycemia (e.g., nervousness, irritability). Patients on oral antidiabetic drugs should promptly report any consistent changes in their blood sugar levels to the healthcare provider.
- Report any urinary hesitancy, feelings of bladder fullness, or difficulty starting urinary stream to the provider
- Photosensitivity may occur and sunglasses may be needed in bright light or for outside activities. Lubricating eyedrops may soothe dryness. Caution should be taken with driving until drug effects are known.
- The drug should not be stopped abruptly to avoid rebound hypertension. If the patient is unable to take medication for more than one day due to illness, the provider should be contacted.
- Take the drug at the same time(s) every day when possible.
- Teach appropriate administration techniques; a teach-back session should occur before patient self-administration. The drug should be taken at the same time(s) each day when possible.

Prescribing Considerations

- Patients with severe renal impairment or moderate hepatic impairment should begin with a low dose and titrate up slowly.
- Patients should know how they react to this medicine before they operate automobiles, use machinery, or engage in other tasks requiring alertness.
- A pharmacist consult is essential if there is any question about the use of an adrenergic antagonist; the pharmacist can look for drug–drug interactions, recommend appropriate dosing based on the condition treated, and perform medication reconciliation.

Understanding Chapter 16

Key Concepts Summary

16.1 Adrenergic antagonists act by blocking the effects of norepinephrine at adrenergic receptors.

16.2 Alpha$_1$-adrenergic antagonists are used to treat hypertension and benign prostatic hyperplasia.

16.3 Nonselective beta-adrenergic antagonists affect both beta$_1$ and beta$_2$ receptors and are prescribed for HTN, angina, and other cardiovascular disorders.

16.4 Beta$_1$-adrenergic antagonists are selective for beta$_1$ receptors in the myocardium and are used to treat HTN and other cardiovascular disorders.

CASE STUDY: Making the Patient Connection

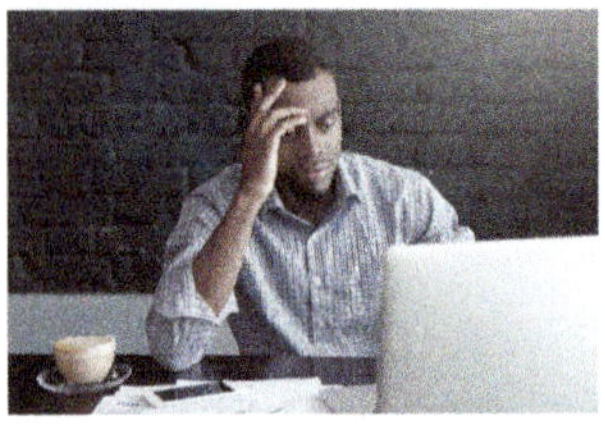

Remember the patient "Chris Williams" from the beginning of the chapter? Now read the remainder of the case study. Based on the information presented within this chapter, respond to the critical thinking questions that follow.

Chris Williams is a 42-year-old executive who lives a very active life. He has a wife and two teenage children. His job requires frequent travel for up to 2 weeks at a time. Every year, Chris's company recommends a complete health physical as part of the executive benefits package. Chris has not taken advantage of this opportunity in the past. However, this year his wife has insisted that he have a checkup.

Chris arrives at the employee health clinic for the physical examination. On arrival he is visibly anxious and has accepted three calls on his cell phone since entering the clinic. During the initial health history session, Chris reveals that he smokes one pack of cigarettes per day and does not drink alcohol. He states that he has no time for exercise and has gained weight during the past year. Most nights Chris sleeps 4 to 6 hours. He states that he frequently wakes up during the night with thoughts of what he needs to do the next day. He finds it difficult to return to sleep after waking.

His medical and family histories indicate that both of his parents died within the past 10 years. His father died of a stroke and his mother died of a heart attack. Chris states that he has been prescribed prazosin (Minipress) in the past but he stopped taking it. When questioned about why he chose not to take the medication, Chris reluctantly confides in you that he suspected that the medication was causing sexual adverse effects.

The physical examination reveals that Chris is 1.9 m (6′2″) tall and weighs 119 kg (262 lb). His body temperature is 37°C (98.6°F), heart rate is 88 beats/min, respiratory rate is 18 breaths/min, and blood pressure is 160/90 mmHg. During the examination an ECG and laboratory test results were all within normal limits.

Critical Thinking Questions

1. Identify the mechanism of action associated with prazosin (Minipress).
2. Discuss the physiology of sexual disorders associated with alpha-adrenergic antagonists.
3. As this patient's nurse, how would you approach the topic of medication-induced sexual dysfunction?

Additional Case Study

Richard Perry is a 64-year-old patient who has been successfully treated for HTN for over 15 years with propranolol (Inderal). He is allergic to cats, and he recently visited his grandson who has a new kitten. Mr. Perry now has weepy eyes and a runny nose. He is considering taking the OTC medication pseudoephedrine (Sudafed) to relieve the allergic symptoms.

1. Is it safe for Mr. Perry to take this OTC medication? Why or why not?
2. Is there another OTC medication that would be safer for this patient?

Chapter Review

1. The patient is started on propranolol (Inderal). Which is the most important action to be included in the plan of care for this patient related to this medication?
   1. Monitor apical pulse and blood pressure.
   2. Elevate the head of the bed during meals.
   3. Take the medication after meals.
   4. Consume foods high in potassium.
2. Which of the following should the nurse instruct a patient with diabetes who is prescribed a beta-adrenergic blocker for the treatment of hypertension to do?
   1. Increase insulin intake by 2 to 3 units daily each morning.
   2. Decrease the intake of carbohydrates while on the antihypertensive medications.
   3. Elevate the lower extremities to promote venous drainage.
   4. Monitor blood glucose levels frequently and report hypoglycemia.

3. To avoid the first-dose phenomenon, the nurse knows that the initial dose of prazosin (Minipress) should be:
   1. Very low and given at bedtime.
   2. Doubled and given before breakfast.
   3. The usual dose and given before breakfast.
   4. Doubled and given immediately after breakfast.

4. A patient who is taking an adrenergic antagonist for hypertension reports being dizzy when first getting out of bed in the morning. The nurse should advise the patient to:
   1. Move slowly from the recumbent to the upright position.
   2. Drink a full glass of water before rising to increase vascular circulatory volume.
   3. Avoid sleeping in a prone position.
   4. Stop taking the medication.

5. A healthcare provider has ordered an alpha$_1$-adrenergic antagonist for each of these patients. A nurse should question the order for the patient with which disorder?
   1. Benign prostatic hyperplasia
   2. Pheochromocytoma
   3. Raynaud's disease
   4. Tachycardia

6. The nurse is caring for a patient with chronic hypertension. The patient is receiving a beta-adrenergic blocker daily. Which patient manifestations would the nurse conclude are adverse effects of this medication? (Select all that apply.)
   1. Anorexia
   2. Increased serum triglycerides
   3. Hypoglycemia
   4. Decreased libido
   5. Thrombocytopenia

See Appendix A for answers to critical thinking questions, case study questions and review questions.

References

Al Kabria, G. M. (2019). Racial/ethnic disparities in prevalence, treatment, and control of hypertension among US adults following application of the 2017 American College of Cardiology/American Heart Association guideline. *Preventative Medicine Reports, 14*, 100850. https://doi.org/10.1016/j.pmedr.2019.100850

Gupta, A. K., Poulter, N. R., Dobson, J., Eldridge, S., Cappuccio, F. P., Caulfield, M., et al. (2010). Ethnic differences in blood pressure response to first- and second-line antihypertensive therapies in patients randomized in the ASCOT Trial. *American Journal of Hypertension, 23*, 1023–1030. https://doi.org/10.1038/ajh.2010.105

Hansen-Dispenza, H. (2018). *Raynaud phenomenon*. Medscape. http://emedicine.medscape.com/article/331197-overview#http://emedicine.medscape.com/article/331197-overview

Selected Bibliography

Cesario, D. A., & Fonarow, G. C. (2019). Beta-blocker therapy for heart failure: The standard of care. *Reviews in Cardiovascular Medicine, 3*(1), 14–21.

Danesh, A., & Gottschalk, P. C. H. (2019). Beta-blockers for migraine prevention: A review article. *Current Treatment Options in Neurology, 21*(4), 20. https://doi.org/10.1007/s11940-019-0556-3

Dézsi, C. A., & Szentes, V. (2017). The real role of β-blockers in daily cardiovascular therapy. *American Journal of Cardiovascular Drugs, 17*(5), 361–373. https://doi.org/10.1007/s40256-017-0221-8

Do Kyung Kim, J. Y. L., Jung, J. H., Kim, J. H., Hah, Y. S., Hong, C. H., & Cho, K. S. (2019). Alpha-1 adrenergic receptor blockers for the treatment of lower urinary tract symptoms in women: A systematic review and meta-analysis. *International Neurourology Journal, 23*(1), 56–68. https://doi.org/10.5213/inj.1836188.094

El Hussein, M. T., Blayney, S., & Clark, N. (2020). ABC's of heart failure management: A guide for nurse practitioners. *Journal for Nurse Practitioners, 16*(4), 243–248. https://doi.org/10.1016/j.nurpra.2019.12.021

Goldberger, J. J., Bonow, R. O., Cuffe, M., Liu, L., Rosenberg, Y., Shah, P. K., et al. (2015). Effect of beta-blocker dose on survival after acute myocardial infarction. *Journal of the American College of Cardiology*, *66*, 1431–1441. https://doi.org/10.1016/j.jacc.2015.07.047

Lauterbach, M. (2019). Clinical toxicology of beta-blocker overdose in adults. *Basic & Clinical Pharmacology & Toxicology*, *125*(2), 178–186. https://doi.org/10.1111/bcpt.13231

Sharma, A. (2018). *Beta-blocker toxicity*. Medscape. http://emedicine.medscape.com/article/813342-overview

Taqueti, V. R., & O'Gara, P. T. (2015). Beta-blocker therapy after myocardial infarction: More questions than answers. *Journal of the American College of Cardiology*, *66*, 1442–1444. https://doi.org/10.1016/j.jacc.2015.08.007

Vu, M., Schleiden, L. J., Harlan, M. L., & Thorpe, C. T. (2020). Hypertension management in nursing homes: Review of evidence and considerations for care. *Current Hypertension Reports*, *22*, 8.

Unit 4
Pharmacology of the Central Nervous System

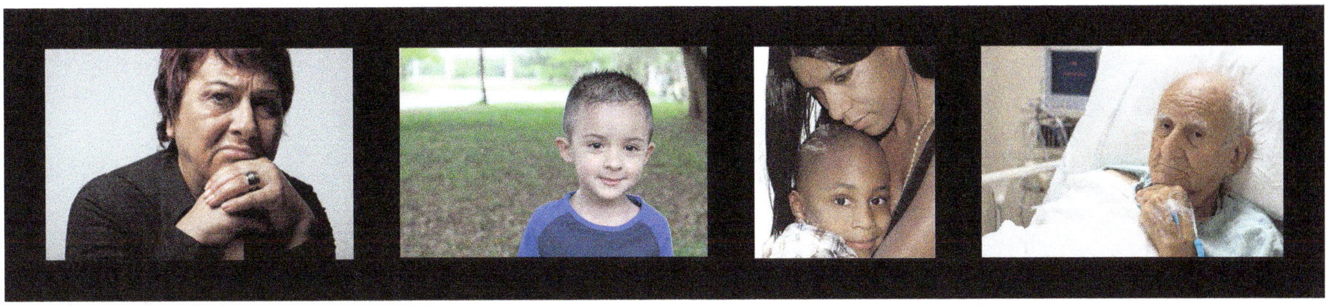

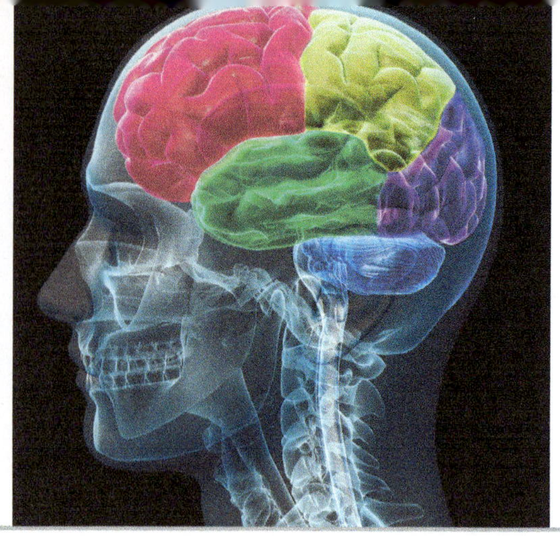

Chapter 17
Review of the Central Nervous System

Chapter Outline

Learning Outcomes

After reading this chapter, the student should be able to:

1. Identify disorders for which central nervous system medications are prescribed.
2. Illustrate the major components of a synapse within the central nervous system.
3. Identify the major neurotransmitters in the central nervous system and their functions.
4. Describe the major structural regions of the brain and their primary functions.
5. Explain the major functional systems of the brain and their primary functions.

Key Terms

Definitions of the terms in bold may be found in the Glossary.

Chapters 12 through 16 introduced the autonomic nervous system (ANS)—the division that provides involuntary control over vital functions of the cardiovascular, digestive, respiratory, and genitourinary systems. This chapter launches Unit 4, which examines the pharmacology of the central nervous system (CNS). The two components of the CNS, the brain and spinal cord, are collectively responsible for receiving all sensory information, interpreting that data, and formulating appropriate responses. Typical responses may include thinking (deciding if the sensory information is harmful or pleasurable), emotions (anger, depression, euphoria), or movement (running away, pounding a fist, or hugging). The purpose of this chapter is to provide a brief review of concepts of CNS anatomy and physiology that are relevant to neuropharmacology.

Scope of Central Nervous System Pharmacology

17.1 Medications affect the central nervous system by stimulating or suppressing the firing of specific neurons.

CNS pharmacology is one of the largest and most important divisions in medicine, encompassing 11 chapters in this text. Medications are administered to treat a large number of neurologic and psychiatric disorders of the CNS. In addition, many drugs cause CNS adverse effects, while others are self-administered to produce pleasurable psychoactive effects. At high doses, a large number of drugs affect the brain, and CNS toxicity is a dose-limiting factor in the pharmacotherapy of many diseases.

Of all divisions of pharmacology, CNS drug mechanisms are the least understood. For some medications, pharmacologists know only that the drug acts on the CNS and produces a therapeutic effect, but its mechanism of action remains largely unknown. There are two primary reasons for this lack of understanding about how CNS drugs produce their effects: the uniqueness of the human brain and the complexity of the disorders affecting it.

The human brain is truly unique, with no other species having the same degree of complexity. It is not known if animals experience the same types of mental disorders as humans, and objective measurement of hallucinations, euphoria, or depression is difficult, if not impossible, in most species. If a drug does induce changes in animal behavior such as depression or anxiety, it is not known whether these data apply to humans because of the enormous differences in brain physiology as well as human social networks that can profoundly influence mental health conditions. Pharmacologists are certainly able to measure changes in brain activity or in the amounts of neurotransmitters in specific regions of the brain, but these do not adequately explain complex changes in thinking, mood, or behavior. Without good animal models, pharmacologists must rely largely on empirical observations—evidence derived from giving the drugs to patients and determining what works rather than how it works.

Also complicating the study of CNS pharmacology is that mental disorders themselves are incompletely understood. The physiologic basis for disorders such as schizophrenia, major depression, bipolar disorder, panic attacks, or post-traumatic stress disorder is not well established. There is great patient variability in symptoms and disease progression with these disorders, and social factors play important roles. Without a complete understanding of the etiology and pathophysiology of mental disorders, pharmacotherapy of these conditions and the development of new drug therapies for CNS disorders will remain challenging.

The next nine chapters present the major classes of drugs whose pharmacotherapeutic goal is to modify the activity of some portion of the CNS. A 10th chapter examines substances that are abused for their effects on the CNS. In a few cases, CNS drugs affect the function of very specific regions of the brain. Most CNS drugs, however, are nonspecific and affect multiple brain regions.

In simplest terms, CNS drugs have two basic actions: They either stimulate (activate) or suppress (inhibit) the firing of neurons. In some cases, CNS drugs may have both actions: activation of some neurons and inhibition of others. The pharmacologic effects of a CNS drug are the result of precisely which neurons are changed and how many are affected. As a result of neuron modification, the following beneficial effects of CNS medications are observed and are studied in this unit:

- Reduction in anxiety
- Improved sleep patterns
- Elevated mood
- Management of psychotic symptoms
- Slowing of the progression of chronic degenerative diseases of the brain
- Termination and prevention of seizures
- Reduction in muscle spasms and spasticity
- Reduction of hyperactivity and mania
- Reduction in pain
- Induction of anesthesia.

CONNECTION Checkpoint 17.1

From what you learned in Chapter 12, what are the two divisions of the peripheral nervous system and what are their primary functions?

Neurons and Neurotransmission

17.2 Neurons in the central nervous system communicate with each other and with body tissues, using neurotransmitters.

The **neuron** is the primary functional cell in all portions of the nervous system. The function of the 100 billion neurons making up the nervous system is to communicate messages through conduction of an action potential. In the CNS, the vast majority of neurons communicate with other neurons. These neuronal pathways or circuits are extremely complex and provide the basis for the higher-level functions of the brain such as thinking, memory, and intelligence. Although a single neuron in the CNS serves no practical function, the interconnections among 100 billion neurons are a major part of what distinguishes the human brain from that of all other species.

Communication between neurons in the brain, as well as that between the brain and other organs, is provided through **synapses**. Synapses are junctions between two neurons, or between a neuron and a muscle or gland. Synapses in the ANS are presented in detail in Chapter 12. The student should review that chapter before proceeding.

Synapses within the CNS operate by the same basic principles as those in the ANS. An action potential from the presynaptic neuron releases a neurotransmitter that moves across the synaptic cleft to activate receptors on the postsynaptic neuron, as illustrated in Figure 17.1a. In some cases, the neuron may be excitatory, enhancing neural transmission (Figure 17.1b). In other cases, the impulse inhibits a neurotransmitter from being released or it causes the release of an inhibitory neurotransmitter that suppresses neuronal conduction (Figure 17.1c). All interconnections in the CNS depend on transmission of the action potential from one neuron to another neuron or to multiple neurons at synapses.

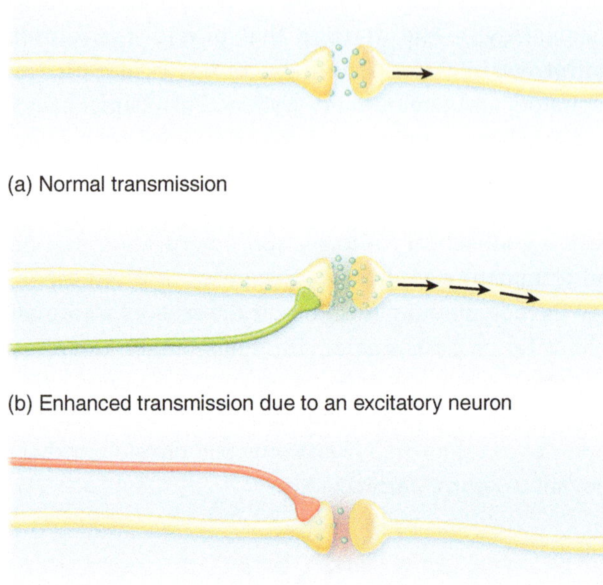

(a) Normal transmission

(b) Enhanced transmission due to an excitatory neuron

(c) Suppressed transmission due to an inhibitory neuron

Figure 17.1 Modification of neural transmission in the central nervous system: (a) normal transmission, (b) enhanced transmission, (c) suppressed transmission.

In the ANS only two neurotransmitters account for nearly all synaptic transmission: acetylcholine (ACh) and norepinephrine (NE). Although these two chemicals are also found in the CNS, more than 30 additional substances have been identified as neurotransmitters in the brain, making the study of neuronal communication in this organ very complex. Some neurotransmitters such as glutamate are primarily stimulatory, whereas others such as gamma aminobutyric acid (GABA) inhibit neuronal activity. NE can activate or inhibit neuronal activity, depending on its location in the brain. A summary of relevant brain neurotransmitters is shown in Table 17.1.

Table 17.1 Selected Central Nervous System Neurotransmitters and Their Functions

Neurotransmitter	Abundance	Effect	Clinical Significance
Acetylcholine (ACh)	Widely distributed in the CNS; a major transmitter in the ANS	CNS: May be excitatory or inhibitory; controls voluntary skeletal muscle movement ANS: Activates the parasympathetic nervous system	Myasthenia gravis, Alzheimer's disease
Dopamine	Basal ganglia and limbic system	Usually excitatory; locomotion, attention, learning, and the reinforcing effects of abused drugs	Parkinson's disease; psychoses; motivation, pleasure
Endorphins and enkephalins	Widely distributed in the CNS and peripheral nervous system (PNS)	Usually inhibitory; reduction of pain	Opioids bind to endorphin receptors
Gamma aminobutyric acid (GABA)	Widely distributed in the CNS	Most common inhibitory CNS neurotransmitter	Seizure and anxiety disorders
Glutamate	Widely distributed in the CNS	Most common excitatory CNS neurotransmitter	Memory
Norepinephrine (NE)	Widely distributed in the CNS; a major transmitter in the ANS	CNS: May be excitatory or inhibitory ANS: Activates the sympathetic nervous system	Depression, memory, panic attacks
Serotonin	Common in the brainstem but also found in the limbic system, gastrointestinal tract, and platelets	Usually inhibitory	Anxiety, bipolar disorder, depression

Adrenergic synapses: Adrenergic synapses utilize NE as the neurotransmitter. Adrenergic synapses in the CNS are abundant in the hypothalamus, the limbic system, and the reticular activating system (RAS). NE activates parts of the brain to heighten alertness and is prominent during waking hours. Adrenergic neurons likely play a role in mood disorders such as depression and anxiety. Drugs used to modify adrenergic synapses in the CNS include caffeine, amphetamines, and tricyclic antidepressants.

Cholinergic synapses: Cholinergic synapses utilize ACh as the neurotransmitter. In the brain, these synapses are most often stimulatory. Cholinergic synapses are abundant in the motor cortex and basal ganglia but are uncommon in other areas. Cholinergic synapses are especially important in the pathophysiology of Parkinson's disease and Alzheimer's disease.

Dopaminergic synapses: These synapses utilize dopamine as the neurotransmitter. **Dopamine** is a chemical precursor in the synthesis of NE and, like epinephrine and NE, is classified chemically as a catecholamine. Dopaminergic synapses are generally excitatory and affect arousal and wakefulness. However, two major receptor subtypes exist: D1 is stimulatory and D2 is inhibitory. Cocaine and amphetamines produce their stimulatory actions by affecting dopamine receptors; marijuana is also thought to exert some of its psychoactive effects by increasing dopaminergic activity. Dopamine receptors are important in the pharmacotherapy of psychosis and Parkinson's disease.

CONNECTION Checkpoint 17.2

The neurotransmitter dopamine is also available as a drug. From what you learned in Chapter 15, what are the indications for dopamine therapy?

Endorphins and enkephalins: Endorphins and enkephalins are small peptides secreted by neurons in the hypothalamus, pituitary, limbic system, and spinal cord. The receptor for these molecules is the opioid receptor, which is involved in pain transmission. Endorphins and enkephalins are sometimes called natural opiates because they produce effects very similar to those of morphine and other opioid drugs. Drugs used to modify the types of synapses in the CNS include opioids such as codeine and morphine.

Gamma aminobutyric acid synapses: These synapses utilize **gamma aminobutyric acid (GABA)** as a neurotransmitter. GABA synapses are the second most common type in the CNS, accounting for 30–40% of all brain synapses. GABA is the primary inhibitory neurotransmitter in the CNS and is found throughout the brain, with greatest abundance in the basal ganglia and hypothalamus. Several GABA receptor subtypes have been identified. GABA receptors are the primary site of action for several classes of drugs, including the benzodiazepines and barbiturates.

Glutamate synapses: Glutamate synapses utilize the amino acid **glutamate** (glutamic acid) as a neurotransmitter. Glutamate is the most common neurotransmitter in the CNS, and its synapses are always excitatory in nature. It is found in nearly all regions of the brain. Several glutamate receptor subtypes have been identified, with the N-methyl-D-aspartate (NMDA) receptor being particularly important to memory and learning. In addition to glutamate, zinc, magnesium, glycine, and even phencyclidine (a hallucinogen) bind to the NMDA receptor, thus modulating neuronal activity. High amounts of glutamate can cause neuron death and may be the mechanism responsible for certain types of neurotoxicity.

Serotonergic synapses: Serotonergic synapses utilize **serotonin**, also known as 5-hydroxytryptamine or 5-HT, as a neurotransmitter. Although some serotonergic synapses are located in the CNS, 98% of the serotonergic receptors are found outside the CNS in platelets, mast cells, and other peripheral cells. Serotonergic receptors are found throughout the limbic (emotional) system of the brain, often in close association with adrenergic synapses. Serotonin is used by the body to synthesize the hormone melatonin in the pineal gland. Low serotonin levels in the CNS are associated with anxiety and impulsive behavior, including suicidal ideation. Serotonergic receptors play an important role in the mechanism of action of antidepressant drugs.

PharmFACT

Conduction of nerve impulses in large-diameter myelinated neurons can reach speeds up to 268 miles/h (120 m/s) (Silverthorn, 2019).

Structural Divisions of the Central Nervous System

17.3 The central nervous system is divided into several major structural components.

The brain consists of dozens of structural divisions that serve common functions. Identification of the many anatomic components in the CNS is complex and beyond the scope of this text. This section focuses on regions of the CNS that have applications to neuropharmacology. For a more complete discussion of CNS anatomy, the student should consult anatomy and physiology textbooks. Basic brain structures are illustrated in Figure 17.2.

Cerebrum: The cerebrum is the "thinking" part of the brain responsible for perception, speech, conscious motor

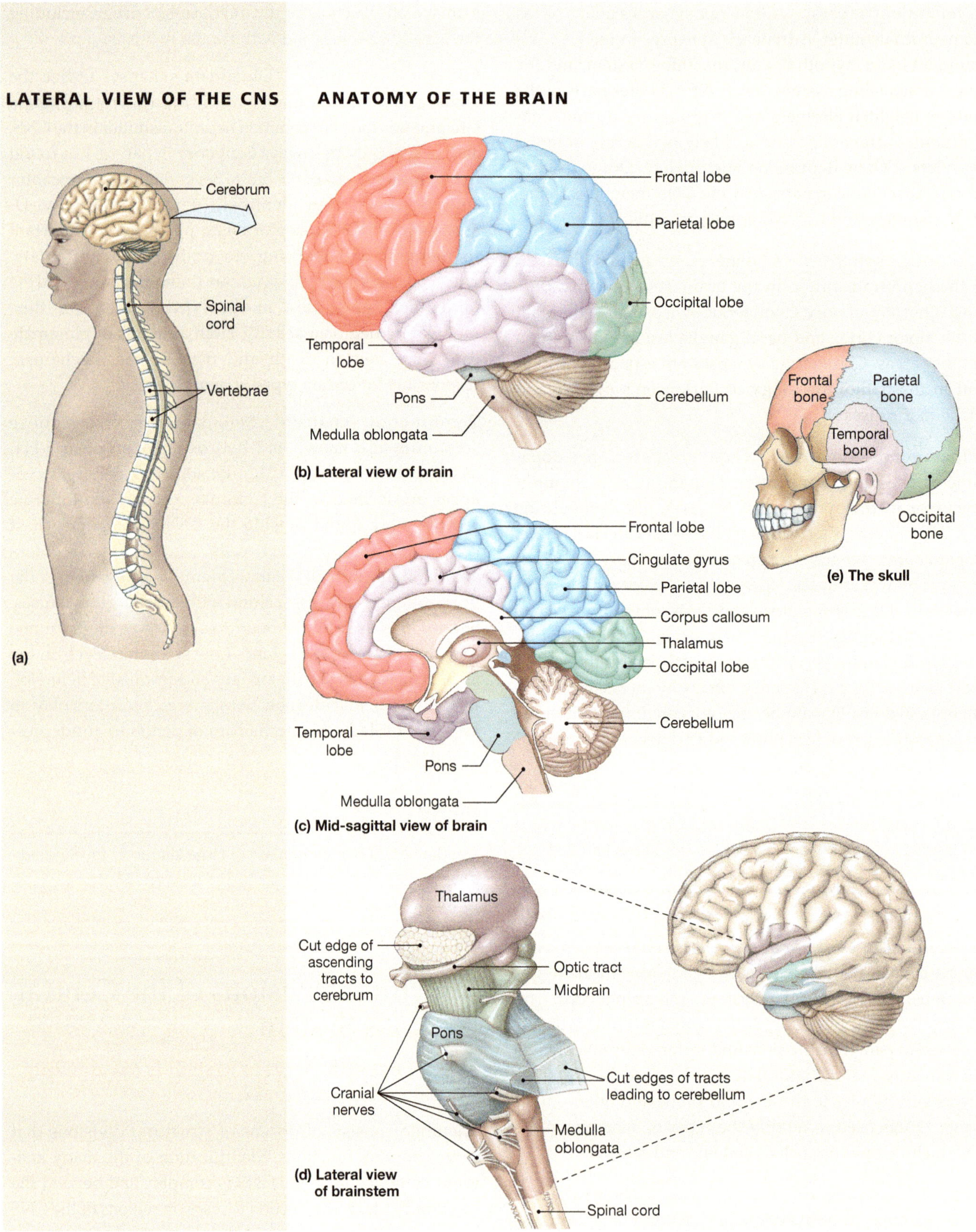

Figure 17.2 Basic anatomy of the brain.

From Human Physiology: An Integrated Approach (2nd ed.) by D. U. Silverthorn, 2001. Reprinted and electronically reproduced by permission of Pearson Education, Inc., Upper Saddle River, NJ.

movement, movement of skeletal muscles, memory, and smell. It is the largest part of the brain, by weight, and the most advanced. Portions of the cerebrum are organized for specialized functions. For example, the occipital lobe is associated with vision and the frontal lobes are concerned with reasoning and planning. Other areas are specific to language, hearing, motor, or sensory functions.

Disorders of the cerebrum may be focal or generalized. Focal abnormalities, often the result of a stroke, occur in specific regions and may affect a single brain function such as vision, hearing, or movement of a particular limb. Generalized disorders of the cerebrum affect widespread areas or multiple regions and can produce drowsiness, coma, hallucinations, depression, or generalized anxiety.

Thalamus: The thalamus is the major relay center in the brain that sends sensory information such as sounds, sights, pain, touch, and temperature to the cerebral cortex for analysis. To reach the cerebrum, all sensory information must travel through the thalamus. Portions of the thalamus comprise the limbic system, an area that controls mood and motivation. Abnormalities of the thalamus have been associated with diverse mood disorders such as obsessive–compulsive disorder, bipolar disorder, anxiety, and panic disorder.

Hypothalamus: The hypothalamus is the major visceral control center in the body. Regulation of hunger, thirst, water balance, and body temperature is a function of this region. The hypothalamus is also part of the limbic system, which is associated with emotional balance. Some neurons in the hypothalamus connect to the brainstem to affect vital centers such as heart rate, respiratory rate, blood pressure, and pupil size. These responses are associated with the fight-or-flight response of the ANS. The There are many endocrine functions of the hypothalamus are discussed in Chapter 65. Disorders of the hypothalamus may affect some or all of these essential functions.

CONNECTION Checkpoint 17.3

From what you learned in Chapter 12, describe the symptoms of the fight-or-flight response.

Cerebellum: The cerebellum controls muscle movement, balance, posture, and tone. It is involved in learning fine motor skills that make muscular movements smooth and continuous. The cerebellum receives sensory information, including vision, position, equilibrium, and touch, and calculates the strength and extent of muscle movement needed to maintain posture and coordinate complex tasks such as walking, driving, or playing a musical instrument. Injury or disease in this region results in uncoordinated, jerky body movements.

Brainstem: The brainstem, consisting of the medulla oblongata, pons, and midbrain, connects the spinal cord to the brain. Because of its critical location, it serves as the major relay center for messages traveling to and from the brain. In addition, it contains major reflex and control centers involving breathing, heart rate, vision, swallowing, coughing, and vomiting. Injury to the brainstem can be fatal if vital centers are disrupted. The brainstem contains clusters of scattered neurons, known as the reticular formation, that help maintain alertness.

Spinal cord: The spinal cord is essentially a conduction pathway to and from the brain. Disruptions of these pathways will prevent transmission of nerve impulses and cause loss of sensory (paresthesia) or motor (paralysis) function.

Blood–brain barrier: The brain must receive a continuous supply of oxygen and glucose; interruptions for even brief periods may cause loss of consciousness. At the same time it needs large quantities of nutrients, the brain must also protect itself from pathogens or toxins that may have entered the blood. Capillaries in most regions of the brain are not as porous as those in other organs; the endothelial cells form tight junctions, creating a seal or barrier to many substances. This is important to pharmacology because CNS drugs must have the ability to penetrate the blood–brain barrier to produce their effects. The blood–brain barrier is illustrated in Figure 17.3.

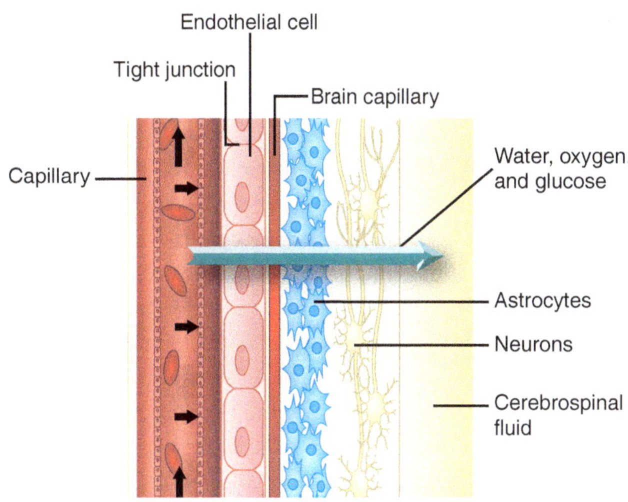

Figure 17.3 Blood–brain barrier.

Functional Systems of the Central Nervous System

17.4 Several functional divisions of the central nervous system are important to pharmacotherapy.

Functional brain systems are clusters of neurons that work together to perform a common function. These clusters may be located far apart from each other in the CNS, but they form a network that acts as a coordinated unit. Some CNS drugs produce their effects by modifying the functions of these systems.

Limbic system: The **limbic system** is a group of structures deep in the brain that are responsible for emotional expression, learning, and memory. Emotional states associated with this system include anxiety, fear, anger, aggression, remorse, depression, sexual drive, and euphoria. Signals routed through the limbic system ultimately connect with the hypothalamus. Through its connection with the hypothalamus, autonomic actions such as rapid heart rate, high blood pressure, or peptic ulcers are associated with intense emotional states. The limbic system also communicates with the cerebrum, which allows people to think and reflect on their emotional states. The connection to the cerebrum allows one to use logic to "override" emotional reactions that might be inappropriate or harmful. Parts of the limbic system also allow people to remember emotional responses. The components of the limbic system are illustrated in Figure 17.4.

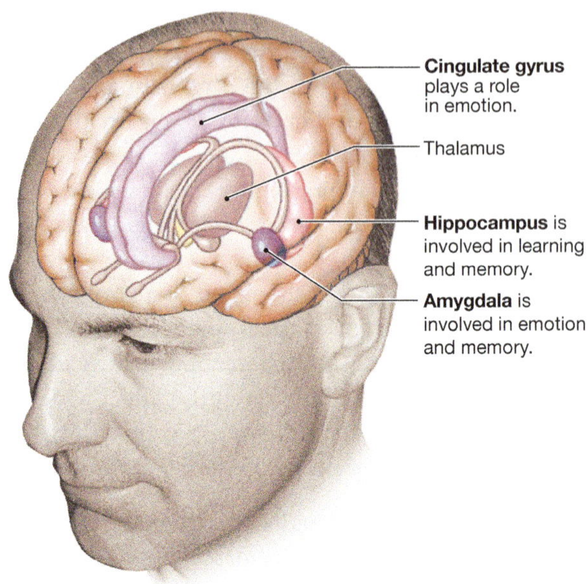

Figure 17.4 Limbic system.
From Human Physiology: An Integrated Approach (4th ed.), by D. U. Silverthorn, 2007. Reprinted and electronically reproduced by permission of Pearson Education, Inc., Upper Saddle River, NJ.

Reticular activating system: The reticular formation, a network of neurons found along the entire length of the brainstem, is shown in Figure 17.5. Stimulation of the reticular formation causes heightened alertness and arousal of the brain as a whole. Inhibition causes general drowsiness and the induction of sleep.

The larger area in which the reticular formation is found is called the **reticular activating system (RAS)**. This structure projects from the brainstem to the thalamus. The RAS is responsible for sleeping and wakefulness and performs an alerting function for the cerebral cortex. It also acts as a filter, allowing people to ignore weak, repetitious, or unimportant sensory stimuli and to focus attention on individual tasks by transmitting information to higher brain centers. This is important in busy, noisy environments when an individual must concentrate on a specific task, such as studying or reading. In any given situation, as much as 99% of all sensory information may be filtered and never reach consciousness.

The RAS has particular importance to pharmacology because many drugs act by decreasing neuronal activity in this system to cause drowsiness or sleep. Examples include alcohol and sedative–hypnotics. Lysergic acid diethylamide (LSD) interferes with portions of the RAS, causing unusual sensory experiences such as seeing odors or hearing colors.

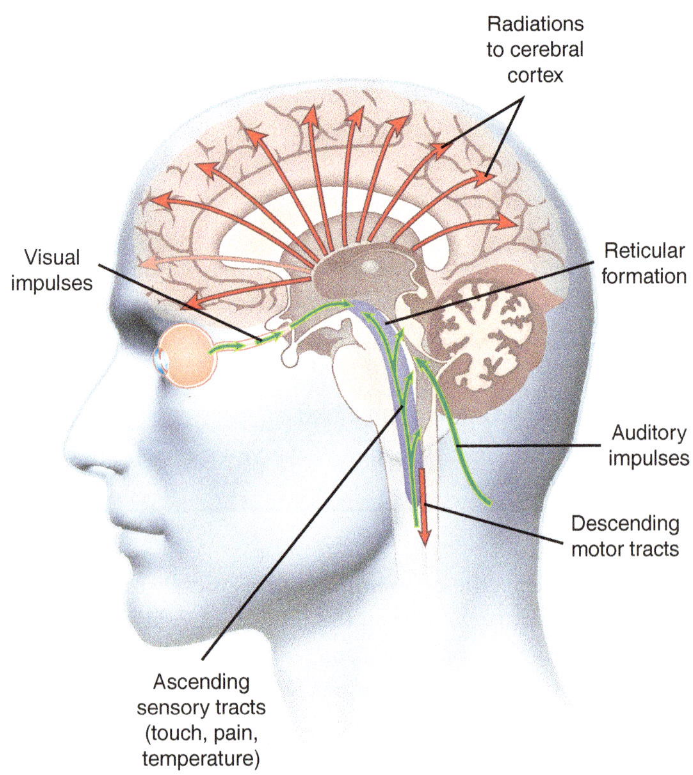

Figure 17.5 With input from sensory neurons, activation of the reticular activating system causes arousal of the cerebral cortex, thus maintaining the awake-and-alert state.

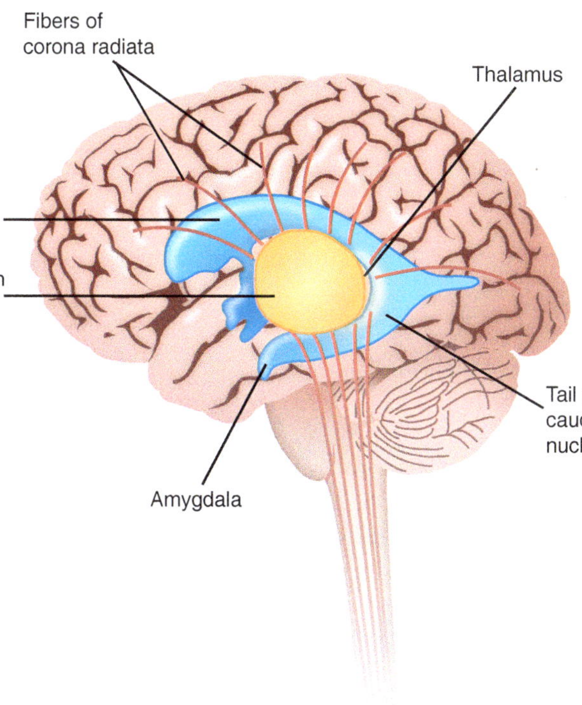

Figure 17.6 The basal ganglia are clusters of gray matter that control learned movement and are involved with the subconscious control of skeletal muscle tone.

Basal nuclei: The **basal nuclei**, also called *basal ganglia*, are a cluster of neurons in the brain that help regulate the initiation and termination of skeletal muscle movement. They also help initiate and terminate certain cognitive functions such as memory, learning, planning, and attention. Connections between the basal ganglia and the limbic system are thought to be associated with psychoses, attention-deficit/hyperactivity disorder, and obsessive–compulsive disorder. Reduced dopaminergic transmission through the basal ganglia is the most common etiology for Parkinson's disease. The basal ganglia are illustrated in Figure 17.6.

Extrapyramidal system: Messages controlling the voluntary movement of skeletal muscle originate in the cerebrum and travel down the CNS in tracts or pathways. The two motor pathways, traveling through the brain, brainstem, and spinal cord, are called pyramidal (direct) and extrapyramidal (indirect). The pyramidal tracts are voluntary tracts involved with the movement of skeletal muscles. The **extrapyramidal system** controls locomotion, complex muscular movements, and posture. The extrapyramidal system has particular importance to pharmacology because it is adversely affected by certain medications, especially the conventional antipsychotic drugs (see Chapter 20). Adverse extrapyramidal symptoms include jerking motions; muscular spasms of the head, face, and neck; and akathisia, an inability to remain at rest. Some extrapyramidal symptoms resemble those of Parkinson's disease (see Chapter 21).

PharmFACT

Some of the postsynaptic neurons connect with and receive information from as many as 150,000 presynaptic neurons (Silverthorn, 2019).

Understanding Chapter 17

Key Concepts Summary

17.1 Medications affect the central nervous system by stimulating or suppressing the firing of specific neurons.

17.2 Neurons in the central nervous system communicate with each other and with body tissues, using neurotransmitters.

17.3 The central nervous system is divided into several major structural components.

17.4 Several functional divisions of the central nervous system are important to pharmacotherapy.

References

Silverthorn, D. U. (2001). *Human physiology: An integrated approach* (2nd ed.). Pearson.

Silverthorn, D. U. (2007). *Human physiology: An integrated approach* (4th ed.). Pearson.

Silverthorn, D. U. (2019). *Human physiology: An integrated approach* (8th ed.). Pearson.

Selected Bibliography

Bear, M. F., Connors, B. W., & Paradiso, M. A. (2020). *Neuroscience: Exploring the brain* (Enhanced 4th ed.). Jones & Bartlett.

Hall, J. E. (2020). *Guyton & Hall textbook of medical physiology* (14th ed.). Elsevier.

Krogh, D. (2014). *Biology: A guide to the natural world* (5th ed.). Benjamin Cummings.

Marieb, E. N., & Hoehn, K. (2019). *Human anatomy and physiology* (11th ed.). Pearson.

Martini, F. H., Nath, J. L., & Bartholomew, E. F. (2018). *Fundamentals of human anatomy and physiology* (11th ed.). Pearson.

"I've always worked hard and enjoyed my work, whether it was helping Joe establish our home, raising our children, or teaching school. Lately, though, it takes all I've got to get out of bed, deal with my family, and get to work. I just don't understand why my life has taken this turn, and I don't think things will ever improve."

—*Patient "Seraphina Alvarez"*

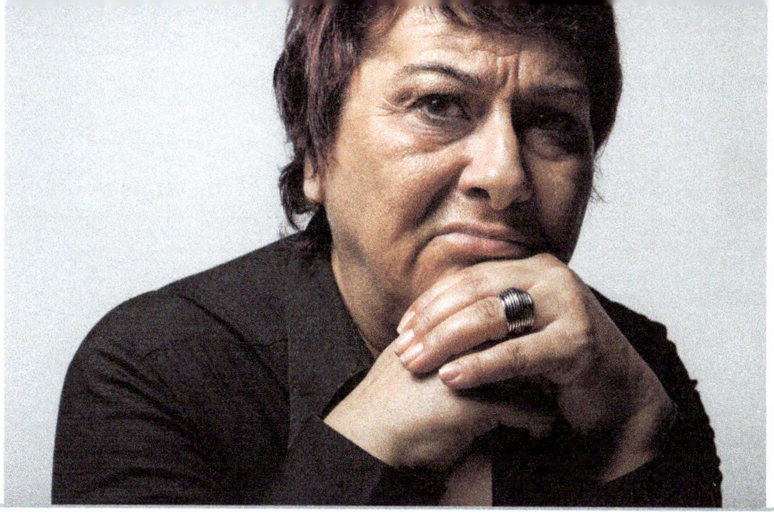

Chapter 18
Pharmacotherapy of Anxiety and Sleep Disorders

Chapter Outline

- Anxiety Disorders
- Sleep Disorders
- Management of Anxiety and Sleep Disorders
- Pharmacotherapy of Anxiety and Insomnia

  Benzodiazepines

  PROTOTYPE *Lorazepam (Ativan), p. 238*

  Nonbenzodiazepine Anxiolytics

  PROTOTYPE *Zolpidem (Ambien, Edluar, Others), p. 241*

  Antidepressants

  Barbiturates

  PROTOTYPE *Phenobarbital (Luminal), p. 245*

Learning Outcomes

After reading this chapter, the student should be able to:

1. Explain why it is important to obtain an accurate diagnosis of anxiety.
2. Compare and contrast the five major categories of anxiety disorders.
3. Identify the regions and systems of the brain associated with anxiety, sleep, and wakefulness.
4. Describe the normal stages of sleep and explain how they are affected by anxiety and stress.
5. Identify sleep disorders that may benefit from pharmacotherapy.
6. Explain the association between insomnia and anxiety.
7. Describe nonpharmacologic methods for managing anxiety and sleep disorders.
8. Identify the major classes of medications used to treat anxiety and sleep disorders.
9. Describe the nurse's role in the pharmacologic and nonpharmacologic management of anxiety and sleep disorders.
10. For each of the classes shown in the chapter outline, identify the prototype and representative drugs and explain the mechanism(s) of drug action, primary indications, contraindications, significant drug interactions, pregnancy data and important adverse effects.
11. Develop a plan of care for patients receiving pharmacotherapy for anxiety and sleep disorders.

Key Terms

Definitions of the terms in bold may be found in the Glossary.

Anxiety is a generalized feeling of worry, fear, or uneasiness over a perceived threat. This threat may be clearly identifiable, such as an upcoming divorce or pharmacology test, or it may be an unfocused, general feeling of worry or dread. Anxiety is a normal, adaptive response to stress that prepares an individual to deal, both physically and emotionally, with a perceived threat. However, when the anxiety is excessive or irrational, the patient's quality of life may become seriously affected and there will be an increased risk of developing chronic gastrointestinal (GI) and cardiovascular disorders. This chapter deals with medications that treat anxiety, cause sedation, or help patients sleep.

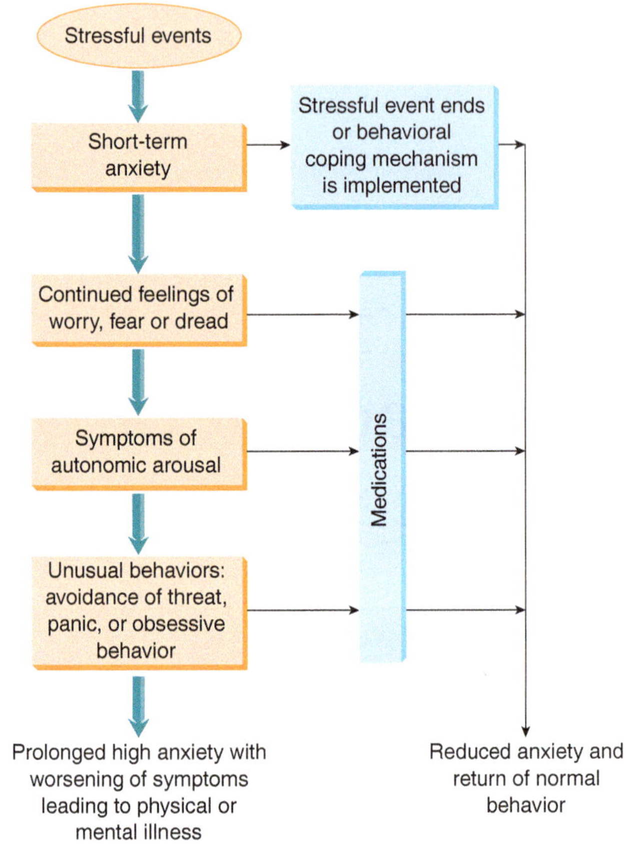

Figure 18.1 Anxiety model. Stressful events lead to physical and mental symptoms, which can be resolved by coping mechanisms or medication.

Anxiety Disorders

18.1 Proper diagnosis of anxiety disorders is important to identifying the most effective treatment option.

Anxiety disorders are the most common mental health illnesses encountered in clinical practice. Patients with anxiety often present with multiple symptoms and describe their condition in diverse ways. They often describe their feelings using terms such as *apprehension*, *dread*, *fear*, or *worry*. Anxiety activates the sympathetic nervous system and triggers symptoms of the flight-or-fright response such as rapid heart rate, shortness of breath, hypertension, excessive sweating, or dry mouth. Many patients recognize that their feelings of anxiety are disproportionate to any real threats or dangers. A diagram of how people typically deal with stressful events is shown in Figure 18.1.

It is often challenging to sort through the many diverse and subjective patient symptoms to determine the etiology of the anxiety. Patients may be unclear as to why they are feeling anxious, or they may be reluctant to discuss the causes because they may be deeply personal. The healthcare provider must accurately diagnose the condition, however, because treatment differs among the various types of anxiety disorders. In some cases, pharmacotherapy may not be the best option. Anxiety is a disorder that may respond to complementary and alternative medicine (CAM) such as stress-reduction techniques. Some patients benefit from individual or group psychotherapy. Some anxiety disorders, however, are debilitating and require effective pharmacotherapy.

When obtaining a comprehensive medication history during the initial patient assessment, the nurse should note any substances that the patient is taking that may worsen or cause anxiety symptoms. Sometimes discontinuing these "anxiety-promoting" medications can reduce patient symptoms. A simple example is substituting decaffeinated beverages for those containing caffeine. In addition, many medical conditions are associated with anxiety symptoms. This is called *substance-induced anxiety disorder*. Drugs and medical conditions associated with anxiety disorders are shown in Table 18.1.

CONNECTION Checkpoint 18.1

From what you learned in Chapter 12, which classes of autonomic drugs would be most likely to cause anxiety as a side effect: sympathomimetics, parasympathomimetics, adrenergic blockers, or cholinergic blockers?

18.2 Anxiety disorders may be divided into five major categories.

The anxiety experienced by people faced with a temporary stressful environment is called **situational anxiety**. Situational anxiety is not considered a major anxiety disorder because it is not disabling or persistent. To a degree,

Table 18.1 Medications and Medical Conditions Associated with Anxiety

Medications
Antibiotics: isoniazid, fluoroquinolones
Antidepressants: bupropion, selective serotonin reuptake inhibitors, tricyclic antidepressants
Antihypertensives: felodipine, methyldopa
Antiseizure drugs: carbamazepine
Bronchodilators: albuterol, theophylline
Hallucinogens: ecstasy, LSD
Hormones: prednisone, thyroid hormone
Nonsteroidal anti-inflammatory drugs: ibuprofen
Stimulants: amphetamines, caffeine, cocaine, methylphenidate
Sympathomimetics: pseudoephedrine
Medical Conditions
Cardiovascular: angina, dysrhythmias, heart failure, myocardial infarction (MI), pulmonary embolus, stroke
Endocrine: Cushing's disease, hyperthyroidism, hypoglycemia
Neurologic: dementia, epilepsy, Parkinson's disease, severe or chronic pain
Others: anemias, cancer, impotence, nausea, vertigo, withdrawal from abused substances
Respiratory: asthma, chronic obstructive pulmonary disease (COPD), pneumonia

situational anxiety is beneficial because it motivates people to accomplish tasks in a prompt manner—if for no other reason than to eliminate the source of nervousness. Situational anxiety generally does not require pharmacotherapy.

Anxiety requires treatment when it becomes chronic, interferes with activities of daily living (ADLs), or begins to result in long-term physical damage such as heart disease. There are multiple methods for classifying anxiety disorders. The American Psychiatric Association (APA; 2017) groups anxiety disorders into six categories: generalized anxiety disorder, panic disorder, social anxiety disorder, specific phobia, agoraphobia, and separation anxiety disorder.

Formerly classified as anxiety disorders, obsessive–compulsive disorder and post-traumatic stress disorder are no longer grouped with anxiety disorders. However, because they are closely related to anxiety disorders and are often treated with the same medications, their pharmacotherapy is included in this chapter.

PharmFACT

About 19% of adult Americans experienced an anxiety disorder in the past year. Of these cases, almost 22% are classified as serious (National Institute of Mental Health [NIMH], 2017)

Generalized anxiety disorder (GAD) is excessive anxiety that persists for 6 months or longer. GAD has a gradual onset and is most prevalent in the 20- to 35-year-old age group. The characteristic feature of GAD is excessive worry or fear regarding life events or activities, frequently focusing on family, money, or health. Symptoms include restlessness, fatigue, muscle tension, nervousness, inability to focus or concentrate, an overwhelming sense of dread, and sleep disturbances. Signs of sympathetic nervous system activation that accompany GAD include blood pressure elevation, heart palpitations, varying degrees of respiratory change, and dry mouth. Parasympathetic responses may consist of abdominal cramping, diarrhea, fatigue, and urinary urgency.

Panic disorder is a type of anxiety characterized by intense feelings of immediate apprehension, fearfulness, terror, or impending doom, accompanied by increased autonomic nervous system activity such as sweating, rapid heart rate, shortness of breath, and trembling. To be diagnosed with panic disorder, the patient must present with at least 1 month of ongoing fear about experiencing subsequent episodes. Panic attacks typically last only 1 to 10 minutes, although one attack may quickly follow another, and patients may perceive the episode as lasting much longer. Up to 5% of the population will experience one or more panic attacks during their lifetime, with women being affected about twice as often as men. Patients with panic disorder usually modify their behavior to try to avoid another attack. Panic attacks are often associated with major depression.

Social anxiety disorder, formerly called *social phobia*, is an unreasonable and persistent fear of being judged, ridiculed, or embarrassed by others. Performing and speaking in public are two common examples of activities that may trigger social anxiety disorder. Patients will either avoid the situation entirely or tolerate it with great discomfort. Symptoms include sweating, blushing, tachycardia, trembling, and bowel cramping or diarrhea. The average age of onset is the midteens, and the disorder may persist for decades before the individual seeks treatment.

Specific (simple) phobia is an irrational and intense fear attached to certain situations or objects. This may include fear of snakes, spiders, high altitudes, exposure to blood, or needles. Panic attacks may occur when individuals encounter their specific phobia.

Agoraphobia is an extreme fear and avoidance of certain places that typically presents between the ages of 20 and 30. These may be closed places such as airplanes, public meetings, or elevators. Some patients express their intense anxiety in open spaces such crowds or public transport. The patient will experience the typical autonomic symptoms of extreme anxiety when encountering their agoraphobia, and panic attacks are common. Agoraphobia can become severe enough that a person will refuse to leave the house.

Separation anxiety disorder nearly always occurs in childhood and is characterized by excessive, inappropriate fear when separated from home or an attachment figure. The child may refuse to sleep away from home or without their attachment figure near. Poor sleep quality with repeated nightmares are common

Obsessive–compulsive disorder (OCD) involves recurrent, intrusive thoughts or repetitive behaviors. To be diagnosed with OCD, the behavior or thought must occupy more than 1 hour each day and negatively impact the patient's normal daily activities. The obsession portion of this behavior involves thoughts, whereas the compulsion portion involves actions. One common example is repetitive thoughts about the fear of exposure to germs. The patient may think about the presence of germs constantly and what can be done to decrease exposure (obsession). The individual may engage in repetitive hand washing (compulsion). OCD activities may occur so frequently that they severely intrude a person's ability to do normal activities, including work or school. Other obsessions or compulsions include viewing sexually explicit pictures, doubting whether the iron or stove was turned off, repeating the same words silently, or repetitive counting. Most commonly, the age of onset is the teen years or early adulthood.

Post-traumatic stress disorder (PTSD) is an intense fear that develops in response to re-experiencing a previous life event. Witnessing or experiencing traumatic events such as combat, physical or sexual abuse, torture, or natural disasters may lead to a sense of helplessness and re-experiencing of the event. The re-experience may take the form of nightmares, hallucinations, or flashbacks, accompanied by uncomfortable physical signs such as tachycardia and extreme nervousness or panic attacks. To be diagnosed with PTSD, the patient must experience distressing symptoms for more than 1 month.

PharmFACT

For three anxiety disorders, women are twice as likely to be affected as men. These disorders include GAD, panic disorder, and specific phobias (Anxiety and Depression Association of America, 2018).

18.3 Specific regions of the brain have been identified that are responsible for anxiety.

The modulation of anxiety is accomplished in specific brain regions and by multiple neurotransmitter systems. Neural pathways associated with GAD, social anxiety disorder, and panic disorder are different.

Neural systems in the brain that are associated with anxiety include the limbic system and the reticular activating system. These are shown in Pharmacotherapy Illustrated 18.1. The student should read Section 17.4 in Chapter 17 for a brief review of these two systems before proceeding.

The limbic system is a cluster of structures in the middle of the brain that is responsible for governing emotions, behavior, and long-term memory. A key part of the limbic system involved in the pathogenesis of anxiety is the **amygdala**, located in the temporal lobe. The amygdala is essential for the ability to feel emotions and to perceive them in other people. The amygdala initiates a fast response to environmental stimuli that could present an immediate danger. Once activated, the amygdala generates feelings of anxiety and fear and stimulates regions of the brain that initiate autonomic stress responses, such as high blood pressure, elevated breathing rate, and dilated pupils. The amygdala can store these fearful memories and, over time, may react to situations that do not represent a real threat.

The amygdala has neural connections to the hippocampus, another memory storage area. It allows us to retrieve specific memories associated with a stressful event. For example, the sight of large crowds may trigger agoraphobia, or a loud firecracker may trigger PTSD. The hippocampus thus can retrieve negative memories that, once sent to the amygdala, can create or worsen anxiety symptoms.

Activation of the amygdala also sends signals to the hypothalamus, an important command center responsible for modulating the fight-or-flight response of the autonomic nervous system. Symptoms of sympathetic activation result, such as increased heart rate and blood pressure. The hypothalamus responds to chronic stress by causing the release of corticosteroids from the adrenal glands. Corticosteroids are major modulators of the long-term stress response (see Chapter 68), keeping the body on continual "high alert" for stressors. High levels of corticosteroids can lead to irritability, anxiety, and depression.

Within the brainstem, the **locus coeruleus** maintains close neural connections to the amygdala and hypothalamus. The locus coeruleus monitors internal and external signals and is the principal site for norepinephrine synthesis in the brain. Release of norepinephrine from this region activates the brain for fight or flight. Dysfunction of the locus coeruleus has been associated with excessive anxiety and PTSD. Certain medications inhibit this area of the brain, preventing anxiety-related behaviors.

The hypothalamus connects with the reticular formation, a collection of neurons found along the core of the brainstem. The reticular formation receives input from nearly all sensory organs as well as from the cerebrum and cerebellum. Ascending fibers project to the cerebrum to form the *reticular activating system (RAS)*. The RAS is responsible for regulating sleep and wakefulness and it performs an alerting function for the entire cerebral cortex.

Signals routed through the RAS proceed to higher brain centers such as the prefrontal cortex. This is the neural mechanism thought to be responsible for feelings of anxiety, fear, restlessness, and an interrupted sleeping pattern. Drugs that stimulate the RAS cause heightened alertness, arousal, and focus. If signals are prevented from passing through the RAS, there is a reduction in general brain activity; thus, inhibitory drugs cause general drowsiness and the induction of sleep.

Pharmacotherapy Illustrated 18.1

Regions of the Brain Affected by Antianxiety Medications

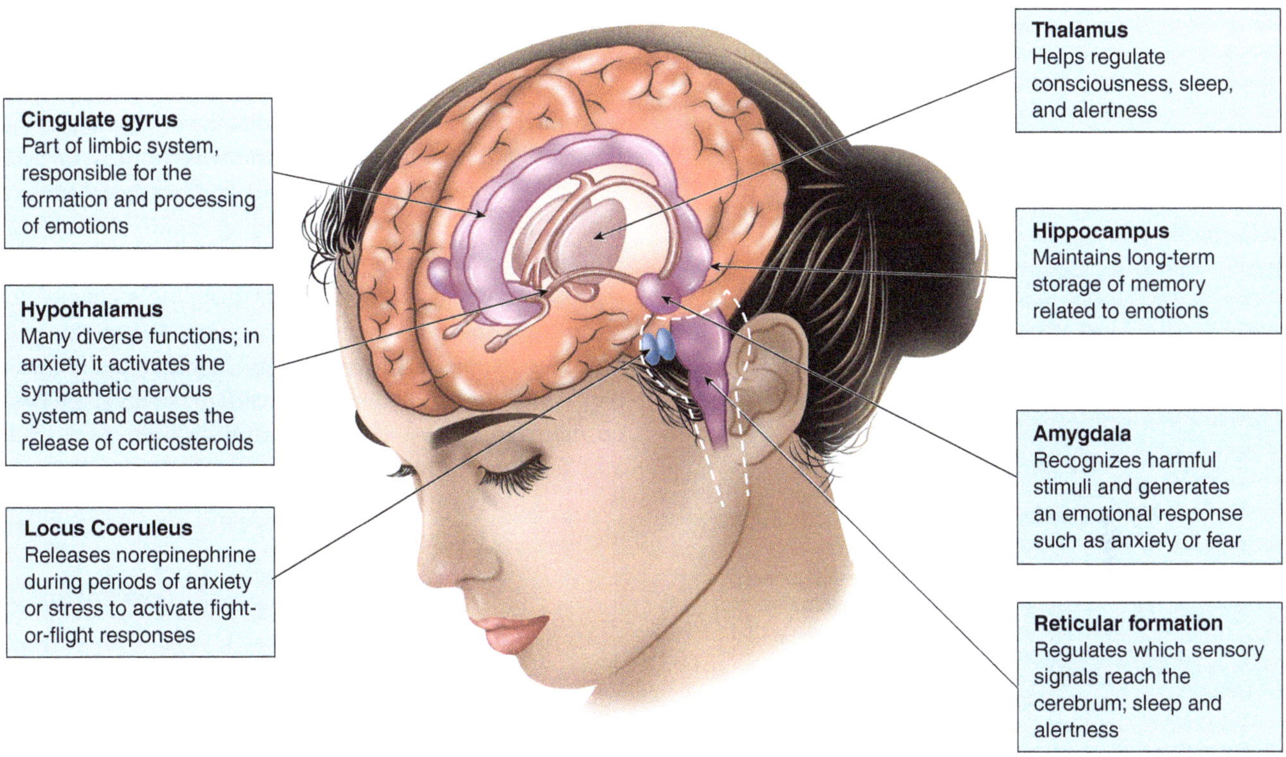

Sleep Disorders

18.4 Sleep occurs in distinct stages.

The process of sleep has been well studied. Although it is known that sleep is essential for wellness, scientists are unsure of its function or how much is needed to maintain optimal health. Following are some theories:

1. Physical inactivity during sleep gives the body time to repair itself.
2. Sleep is a function that evolved as a protective mechanism. Throughout history, nighttime was the safest time of day for resting.
3. Sleep involves electrical charging and discharging of the brain. The brain needs time for processing and filing information collected throughout the day. When this is done without interference from the outside environment, these vast amounts of data can be retrieved later through memory.

Sleep occurs in two basic phases: rapid eye movement (REM) sleep and non–rapid eye movement (NREM) sleep. NREM sleep is further subdivided into four distinct stages based on the depth of sleep. Drugs may affect the length of time spent in the different stages of sleep. Decreases in the neurotransmitters acetylcholine, norepinephrine, and serotonin signal the change from wakefulness to **non–rapid eye movement (NREM) sleep**. During this phase, respirations slow, heart rate and blood pressure decrease, oxygen consumption by muscles decreases, and urine formation decreases. NREM accounts for about 75–85% of total sleep time. The four stages of NREM sleep are described in Table 18.2.

Rapid eye movement (REM) sleep is considered the active dreaming stage of sleep, although dreams may also occur in NREM sleep. The eyes move during this stage, muscle tone diminishes, and heart rate and breathing become irregular. Penile erections and clitoral enlargement may occur. Although adults spend about 25% of their sleep in REM sleep, newborns may spend as much as 80% of their sleep in this phase.

Sleep occurs in cycles, alternating between REM and NREM sleep about four to five times each night, with each sleep cycle lasting approximately 90 minutes. More time is spent in NREM in early cycles, with REM sleep increasing in the later cycles. When the individual moves from NREM to REM sleep, acetylcholine levels increase and serotonin

Table 18.2 Stages of Sleep

Stage of Sleep	Description
NREM stage 1	At the onset of sleep, the patient experiences drowsiness for 1–7 min. During this time, the patient can be easily awakened. This stage of sleep is so light that when awakened from it, individuals often deny that they were asleep. Respirations slow, muscles relax. This stage lasts for about 4–5% of total sleep time.
NREM stage 2	Although deeper than stage 1, the patient can still be easily awakened. This stage constitutes the greatest amount of total sleep time, 45–55%.
NREM stage 3	This is the period in which an individual may experience nightmares, bedwetting, or sleepwalking. Heart rate and blood pressure fall; GI activity rises. This stage lasts for about 4–6% of total sleep time.
NREM stage 4	The deepest stage of sleep, this comprises about 12–15% of total sleep time. Dreams that occur are usually thoughtlike and revolve around current concerns or recent events with little story line. This is the stage during which nightmares occur in children. Sleepwalking is also a common behavior for this stage. Heart rate and blood pressure remain low; GI activity remains high.
REM sleep	This stage, which lasts for about 25% of sleep time, is characterized by eye movement and a loss of muscle tone. Eye movement occurs in bursts of activity. Active dreaming takes place in this stage; dreams are vivid, emotional, story-like, and frequently bizarre. The mind is very active and resembles a normal waking state.

and norepinephrine levels further decrease. As REM sleep continues, the body progressively increases the levels of serotonin and norepinephrine until the amounts are adequate to stop REM sleep. For a brief time, the individual may awaken until the next cycle begins.

Patients who are deprived of stage 4 NREM sleep experience depression and a feeling of apathy and fatigue. Stage 4 NREM sleep appears to be linked to repair and restoration of the physical body, whereas REM sleep is associated with learning, memory, and the capacity to adjust to changes in the environment. The body requires the dream state associated with REM sleep to keep the psyche functioning normally. When deprived of REM sleep, people experience a sleep deficit and become frightened, irritable, paranoid, and even emotionally disturbed. Judgment is impaired, and reaction time is slowed. It is speculated that to make up for their lack of dreaming, these individuals experience far more daydreaming and fantasizing throughout the day. The stages of sleep are shown in Table 18.2.

The sleep patterns of adults vary widely. Some people do very well with less sleep, whereas others require above-average amounts to feel refreshed and mentally alert. Most people awaken at least once during the night; older adults awaken more frequently. The nurse can be a valuable ally to the patient experiencing sleep disturbances by explaining these normal variations and by assisting the patient to reach a desirable sleep pattern.

The acts of sleeping and waking are synchronized with many different bodily functions. Body temperature, blood pressure, hormone levels, and respiration all fluctuate on a cyclic basis throughout the 24-hour day, known as the **circadian rhythm**. Even without realizing it, those who are "day people" or "night people" structure their activities, even their occupations, around what they recognize as their best individual pattern of sleep and wakefulness. *Circadian dysrhythm* refers to the psychologic and biological stress an individual undergoes when traveling rapidly through several time zones, such as during a long airplane journey. "Jet lag" is a very real, and sometimes disabling, phenomenon, although not a permanent dysfunction. When this cycle becomes impaired, pharmacologic or other interventions may be needed to readjust it. Circadian rhythms are based on many complex variables, including light–dark cycles and secretion of hormones such as melatonin. Biological rhythms likely exist in all living things and have even been identified in bacteria.

18.5 Sleep disorders affect a large percentage of the population.

A sleep disorder is a disturbance in the normal pattern, quality, or quantity of sleep. It is estimated that 40 million Americans experience sleep disorders. Although about 70 specific types of sleep-related disorders have been identified, pharmacotherapy is beneficial in treating only a few of them. Examples of common sleep disorders are shown in Table 18.3.

Insomnia is the most common sleep disorder and the one that is the most frequent indication for pharmacotherapy. Insomnia can be simply defined as the lack of adequate sleep; however, the disorder can be better explained by the following terms:

- **Sleep-onset insomnia.** Inability to fall asleep within a reasonable time, usually more than 30 minutes
- **Sleep-maintenance insomnia.** Frequent awakenings during the night or the inability to fall back asleep
- **Sleep-offset insomnia.** Premature, early-morning awakenings
- **Nonrestorative sleep.** Persistent sleepiness during the day, despite adequate sleep duration.

The diagnosis of *chronic* insomnia is determined by its duration (at least 30 days or more) and the degree to which it affects ADLs. The most frequent symptom reported by patients is excessive daytime drowsiness.

Insomnia has multiple causes and often presents secondary to an underlying disorder. Examples of conditions causing *secondary* insomnia are shown in Table 18.4. The best approach to resolving secondary insomnia is to treat the underlying disorder. Insomnia not associated with

Table 18.3 Types of Sleep Disorders

Type	Example(s)
Circadian rhythm sleep disorders	Time zone syndrome (jet lag), shift work sleep disorder
Hypersomnias of central origin	Narcoplexy (with or without cataplexy)
Insomnia	Acute, chronic, transient
Parasomnias	Sleepwalking, sleep terrors, nightmares
Sleep-related breathing disorders	Sleep apnea
Sleep-related movement disorders	Restless leg syndrome

another medical, psychiatric, or medication-related cause is considered to be *primary*.

A thorough medical history can sometimes distinguish between primary and secondary insomnia; however, for objective testing patients are referred to sleep disorder specialists for polysomnography and actigraphy. Polysomnography is a series of tests that record physiologic changes occurring during sleep, including eye movement, muscle tension, respiration, cardiac rhythm, and brain-wave activity. Polysomnography can also determine the amount of REM and NREM sleep. Brain-wave activity is measured using an electroencephalogram (EEG). Actigraphy is another frequently used diagnostic test that measures the motor activity of a patient during waking and sleeping hours. The results of these comprehensive tests can be used to diagnose most sleep disorders.

Narcolepsy is a rare sleep disorder caused by the destruction of **orexin neurons** in portions of the brain. Orexin neurons help regulate the balance between sleep and wakefulness. The disease is believed to have a genetic, autoimmune origin. The symptoms of narcolepsy are believed to result from orexin deficiency.

Narcolepsy is characterized by severe daytime sleepiness such that the patient is unable to stay awake and may fall asleep quickly and at inappropriate times. An episode of narcolepsy, called a "sleep attack," may last from a few seconds to about 30 minutes. In addition to the sleep attack, the following four symptoms are observed in some, but not all, patients with narcolepsy:

- **Cataplexy** is a sudden loss of muscle strength manifested as slurred speech, sagging of the jaw, head nodding, or even complete collapse of the body. The condition is triggered by strong emotions.
- **Hypnagogic hallucinations** are vivid, fearful sensory illusions that may be experienced at the onset of sleep or on awakening.
- **Sleep paralysis** may result in the temporary inability to move or speak on awakening.
- Automatic behavior may include actions such as talking or repetitive movements during the sleep episode. The individual has no memory of the behavior on awakening.

For the patient who experiences narcolepsy *without* cataplexy, pharmacologic options include central nervous system (CNS) stimulants such as methylphenidate, armodafinil (Nuvigil), and modafinil (Provigil). At the doses used to treat narcolepsy, these drugs are generally well tolerated and adverse effects such as headache, nausea, nervousness, and anxiety are often mild. Armodafinil and modafinil are Schedule IV controlled substances: methylphenidate is Schedule II.

In 2019, two new medications were approved to treat the excessive daytime sleepiness associated with narcolepsy. Pitolisant (Wakix) inhibits histamine receptors in the CNS. Its most frequent side effect is headache. Solriamfetol (Sunosi) is a dopamine and norepinephrine reuptake inhibitor that is also approved to improve wakefulness in patients with obstructive sleep apnea. Its most frequent adverse effects are headache and decreased appetite. Neither pitolisant nor solriamfetol are controlled substances.

For patients who experience narcolepsy *with* cataplexy, additional drugs are necessary. Now considered a first-line drug for this disorder, sodium oxybate (gamma hydroxybutyrate [GHB], Xyrem, Xyway) is effective in managing symptoms of both narcolepsy and cataplexy. This substance is very unusual because (as GHB) it has been used illegally to produce euphoria and cause amnesia and has been implicated in sexual assaults as a "date-rape" drug (see Chapter 27). Because of these abuses, GHB is listed as a Schedule I drug. However, the *same* chemical substance, marketed as Xyrem to treat narcolepsy, is a Schedule III drug. It is only available using a limited distribution program, which requires the patient to obtain the drug through a central pharmacy, have regular office visits, and demonstrate understanding about the safety and proper use of the drug. Xyrem is a CNS depressant and is taken immediately

Table 18.4 Causes of Secondary Insomnia

Cause	Description
Drug	Amphetamines, cocaine, caffeinated beverages, corticosteroids, sympathomimetics, antidepressants, alcohol use, nicotine or tobacco use
Medical disorder	Dementia, anxiety disorder, epilepsy, Parkinson's disease, Tourette's syndrome, psychosis, mania, migraines, asthma, sleep apnea, chronic or severe pain, COPD, gastroesophageal reflux, hyperthyroidism
Poor sleep hygiene	Noisy environment; too much light in the bedroom; large meals; working or exercising just prior to sleeping; partner who snores, talks, or moves frequently during sleep
Stressful situation	Major life event such as marriage, divorce, death of a loved one, chronic or terminal disease, stressful job

prior to bedtime because it can cause confusion and loss of motor coordination within the first 6 hours after dosing. When taken with other CNS depressants—such as sedatives, opioids, alcohol, benzodiazepines, antipsychotics, or antiepileptics—severe respiratory depression, syncope, sedation, and death may occur. Common adverse effects include headache, nausea, dizziness, and somnolence. The mechanism by which Xyrem improves wakefulness in patients with narcolepsy is unknown. For resistant cataplexy, older medications such as tricyclic antidepressants (TCAs) or selective serotonin reuptake inhibitors (SSRIs) may be added to the regimen.

Management of Anxiety and Sleep Disorders

18.6 Insomnia and anxiety are closely related.

The student may be wondering why two seemingly different conditions, anxiety and insomnia, are being presented in the same chapter. There are two fundamental reasons. First, there is a pathophysiologic link between sleep and anxiety and, second, many of the drugs used to treat anxiety are also effective for treating insomnia.

Research has shown a high incidence of serious insomnia in patients with comorbid mental health conditions such as depression and anxiety (Khurshid, 2018). Patients with insomnia are likely to report symptoms of nervousness and anxiety. But which comes first, the anxiety or the insomnia? In some patients, insomnia can lead to anxiety and worry about lack of restful sleep. In other patients, anxiety and worry can cause someone to lie awake and experience insomnia. Thus, it is not a matter of which came first or which caused the other. Anxiety and insomnia should be recognized as a continuous, destructive cycle with each "feeding" on the other. Recognizing this link makes insomnia therapy more than just a nighttime problem. It involves treating anxiety during the day while improving sleep at night. The nurse should assess patients for anxiety when they report sleeplessness, and vice versa.

Three primary classes of drugs are used for treating both anxiety and insomnia: benzodiazepines, nonbenzodiazepine antianxiety drugs, and antidepressants. The benzodiazepines are used for the short-term therapy of anxiety and for the treatment of patients who are unable to fall asleep due to excessive worrying at bedtime. Some of the nonbenzodiazepines and antidepressants are effective for the longer-term therapy of insomnia and anxiety. A second approach is to use combined therapy because treating both conditions concurrently may result in better sleep outcomes than treating insomnia only.

Long-term use of sleep medications is likely to worsen insomnia, and many of these medications cause physical or psychologic dependence. Patients may experience a phenomenon referred to as **rebound insomnia**. This condition occurs when a sedative drug is discontinued abruptly after it has been taken for several months or longer. Symptoms of sleeplessness, anxiety, and daytime drowsiness become markedly worse for a few days before the original insomnia symptoms return.

18.7 Management of anxiety and sleep disorders utilizes a combination of pharmacologic and nonpharmacologic therapies.

The choice of therapy for anxiety and insomnia depends primarily on the severity of the symptoms. In some cases, several therapies may be combined to achieve optimal results. The three types of therapies include complementary and alternative therapies, nonprescription drugs, and prescription drugs.

Complementary and alternative therapies: In mild cases of anxiety or insomnia, patients should be encouraged to explore and develop nonpharmacologic coping strategies to deal with the underlying causes. Such strategies may include cognitive-behavioral therapy, counseling, biofeedback techniques, yoga, and meditation. Complementary and alternative treatments that may be useful in reducing anxiety and enhancing sleepiness are listed in Table 18.5.

Many natural products and supplements are claimed to promote relaxation and sleep. The best-studied natural remedy is melatonin, which may improve both sleep onset and sleep duration. Melatonin is a natural hormone; however, taking too much can disrupt homeostasis and cause adverse effects such as headache, mental impairment, and nightmares.

Two herbal products with demonstrated efficacy in promoting relaxation are kava and valerian. Although kava appears to be effective, high doses have been associated with liver damage. This has prompted some countries to withdraw kava from the market. While still available in the United States, the U.S. Food and Drug Administration

Table 18.5 Complementary and Alternative Treatments for Anxiety and Insomnia*

Alternative therapies	Acupuncture, aromatherapy, prayer, massage, meditation, biofeedback therapy, hypnosis, guided imagery, music therapy
Exercise and nutrition	Exercise therapy, nutrition therapy, deep breathing, yoga
Herbal therapies	Kava, valerian, chamomile, ginseng, lemon balm, passionflower, St. John's wort, lavender

*Safety and effectiveness have not been demonstrated for most complementary and alternative therapies.

(FDA) has issued a warning that kava should not be used unless recommended by a healthcare provider.

Valerian is effective at producing drowsiness and promoting sleep and has not been shown to cause serious adverse effects when used at doses on the label. Other herbs are claimed to have relaxation and sleep-promoting properties (often by those marketing the products), but research has not proved their validity or safety in treating anxiety or insomnia.

Nonprescription drugs: Antihistamines are drugs used to treat cold or allergy symptoms. One of the side effects of antihistamines is drowsiness. This is used to advantage in over-the-counter (OTC) sleep aid products such as Sominex and Nytol. In addition, products indicated as "p.m." or "nighttime" contain antihistamines that promote sleep. The two antihistamines most frequently used to produce drowsiness are diphenhydramine and doxylamine.

Because antihistamines have a long duration of action (up to 12 hours), the patient may experience drowsiness the next day. They also cause drying of the nose and mouth, which is the reason they are included in cold and flu remedies. Some patients experience dizziness and blurred vision. Antihistamines should not be taken for prolonged periods for insomnia because patients become tolerant to the drowsiness effect of the drugs. The use of antihistamines in treating allergic rhinitis and the common cold is presented in Chapter 45.

Prescription drugs: The remainder of this chapter examines the classes of prescription drugs used to treat anxiety and insomnia. These medications are used when the anxiety or sleep disorder is severe or when the condition is unresponsive to nonpharmacologic therapies.

The first drugs used to treat anxiety and insomnia were *general* CNS depressants. Ethanol and opium were the two CNS depressants most widely used for treating these disorders until the discovery of the barbiturates in the early 1900s. Other nonselective CNS depressants such as chloral hydrate, methaqualone (Quaalude), and meprobamate (Miltown) were also widely prescribed in the mid-20th century. Because general CNS depressants suppress most neuronal functions, they have serious adverse effects and are very dangerous in overdose situations. Methaqualone was removed from the U.S. market in 1984 because of its addictive potential and widespread illegal use in the 1960s and 1970s. Starting in the 1960s and continuing until present day, more *selective* CNS depressants have been developed that target *specific* areas of the brain controlling anxiety and sleep, without causing the serious adverse effects of the older drugs.

The terminology used to describe these drugs can be confusing. An **anxiolytic** is any drug that has the ability to relieve anxiety. In the broadest definition, anxiolytics include drugs from a large number of different pharmacologic classes. In clinical practice, however, the term *anxiolytic* is often more narrowly defined to include just the benzodiazepine and nonbenzodiazepine antianxiety drugs.

A *sedative* is a CNS depressant that produces relaxation, calmness, and a reduction in anxiety and excitement. *Tranquilizer* is an older term, though still often used, to describe a sedative. A *hypnotic* is a drug that produces sleep. A sedative is most often administered during the day to induce a feeling of calm or relaxation without causing sleep, whereas hypnotics are used during the night to induce sleep. The term **sedative–hypnotic** is used to describe a drug with the ability to produce a calming effect at lower doses and sleep at higher doses. Very high doses

CONNECTIONS: Complementary and Alternative Therapies

Melatonin

Description

Melatonin is a natural hormone produced during the night by the pineal gland. Melatonin production in the brain is related to time of day, falling in the morning with light inhibiting its release and rising in the evening (National Center for Complementary and Integrative Health [NCCIH], 2019).

History and Claims

The secretion of melatonin is stimulated by darkness and inhibited by light. As melatonin production rises, alertness decreases, and body temperature starts to fall, both of which make sleep more inviting. Melatonin production is related to age. Children manufacture more melatonin than older adults; however, melatonin production begins to drop at puberty. Supplemental melatonin, 0.5 to 3 mg at bedtime, is alleged to decrease the time required to fall asleep and to produce a deep and restful sleep.

Standardization

Melatonin is commonly marketed as 1- to 3-mg tablets. Melatonin is one of only two hormones not regulated by the FDA and sold OTC without a prescription (dehydroepiandrosterone [DHEA] is the other).

Evidence

Melatonin appears to somewhat effective for jet lag, delayed sleep-wake phase disorder, anxiety before surgery, and for some children's sleep disorders. The NCCIH (2019) cites evidence that melatonin may be useful in people with insomnia related to disrupted circadian rhythm cycles, such as with shift work, although current evidence is too low to support recommending melatonin. Melatonin appears to be safe for short-term use, although it is not recommended during pregnancy or breastfeeding. Side effects such as dizziness, headache, nausea, and sleepiness may occur (Andersen et al., 2016).

Table 18.6 Benzodiazepines and Nonbenzodiazepine Anxiolytics

Drug	Route and Adult Dose (Maximum Dose Where Indicated)	Adverse Effects
Benzodiazepines for Anxiety		
alprazolam (Xanax)	Anxiety: PO (immediate release): 0.25–0.5 mg tid (max: 4 mg/day) Panic disorder: PO (extended release): 3–6 mg once daily in the morning (max: 10 mg/day)	*Drowsiness, lethargy, ataxia, confusion, dizziness, headache, blurred vision, slurred speech* <u>Physical dependence, seizures (following abrupt withdrawal of high doses), birth defects, suicidal ideation, sleepwalking or sleep-driving (with insomnia therapy). With overdose: coma, respiratory depression, paradoxical anxiety, hypotension, dyspnea, cardiac arrest (IV forms)</u>
chlordiazepoxide (Librium)	PO: 5–25 mg tid or qid	
clonazepam (Klonopin)	PO: 0.25–1 mg/day in divided doses (max: 4 mg/day)	
clorazepate (Tranxene)	PO: 15–30 mg/day (max: 60 mg/day)	
diazepam (Valium)	PO: 2–10 mg bid–qid or 15–30 mg/day sustained release IM/IV: 2–10 mg, repeat if needed in 3–4 h	
lorazepam (Ativan)	PO: 2–4 mg/day at bedtime (max: 10 mg/day)	
oxazepam	PO: 10–30 mg tid or qid	
Benzodiazepines for Insomnia		
estazolam	PO: 0.5–1 mg at bedtime (max: 2 mg/day)	
flurazepam	PO: 15–30 mg at bedtime	
quazepam (Doral)	PO: 7.5–15 mg at bedtime	
temazepam (Restoril)	PO: 7.5–30 mg at bedtime	
triazolam (Halcion)	PO: 0.125–0.25 mg at bedtime (max: 0.5 mg/day)	
Nonbenzodiazepine Anxiolytics		
buspirone	PO: 7.5–15 mg in divided doses; may increase by 5 mg/day every 2–3 days (max: 60 mg/day)	*Dizziness, headache, nausea and vomiting, drowsiness, fatigue, dry mouth, headache, dream disturbances, unpleasant taste (eszopiclone, ramelteon), decreased testosterone and increased prolactin levels (ramelteon)* <u>Paradoxical excitation, mood changes, tachycardia, blurred vision, confusion, myalgia</u>
eszopiclone (Lunesta)	PO: 2–3 mg/day at bedtime	
ramelteon (Rozerem)	PO: 8 mg/day at bedtime (max: 8 mg/day)	
suvorexant (Belsomra)	PO: 5–20 mg once daily 30 min before bedtime	
tasimelteon (Hetlioz)	PO: 20 mg/day at bedtime	
zaleplon (Sonata)	PO: 5–10 mg at bedtime (max: 20 mg/day)	
zolpidem (Ambien, Edluar, others)	PO (immediate release): 5–10 mg at bedtime for 7–10 days (max: 10 mg/day) PO (extended release): 12.5 mg at bedtime SL: 1.75–3.5 mg (Intermezzo) or 5–10 mg (Edluar) once per night	

Note: *Italics* indicate common adverse effects. <u>Underline</u> indicates serious adverse effects.

of sedative–hypnotics may produce coma and death due to respiratory failure. All of these drugs—anxiolytics, tranquilizers, sedatives, and hypnotics—are classified more broadly as CNS depressants.

The overlap in meaning can easily be seen with the preceding definitions. Some medications may be used as an anxiolytic, a sedative, or a hypnotic, depending on the dose administered. This is because CNS depression is a continuum ranging from mild relaxation to sedation to the induction of sleep and anesthesia. To avoid this confusion in terminology, drugs for anxiety and insomnia are usually referred to by their chemical or pharmacologic classifications. The four general classifications of drugs used for patients experiencing anxiety or sleep disorders are as follows:

- Benzodiazepines
- Nonbenzodiazepine anxiolytics
- Antidepressants
- Barbiturates.

Many CNS depressants have the potential to cause physical and psychologic dependence and nearly all of them are controlled substances. The withdrawal syndrome for some CNS depressants such as the barbiturates can cause life-threatening neurologic reactions (see Chapter 27). Drugs for treating anxiety and insomnia are listed in Table 18.6.

CNS depressants are very effective drugs. If a patient does not respond to these medications with improved relaxation or sleep, the presence of a serious underlying psychiatric or medical condition should be considered that requires further assessment by behavioral specialists. This is especially true if the drug worsens insomnia or produces bizarre thinking or unusual behaviors. Examples of such behaviors that should be immediately reported to the healthcare provider include aggressiveness, hallucinations, suicidal thinking, and unusual extroversion or depersonalization.

Table 18.7 Indications for Benzodiazepines

Drug	GAD	Panic Disorder	Insomnia	Seizures	Alcohol Withdrawal	Preanesthetic Medication	Other
alprazolam (Xanax)	A	A	O				Premenstrual dysphoric disorder
chlordiazepoxide (Librium)	A				A	A	
clonazepam (Klonopin)	O	A	O	A			
clorazepate (Tranxene)	A		O	A	A		
diazepam (Valium)	A		O	A	A	A	Muscle spasms
estazolam	O		A				
flurazepam	O		A				
lorazepam (Ativan)	A	O	O	A (IV form)	O	A (IV form)	
midazolam (Versed)				O		A	Conscious sedation
oxazepam	A		O		A		
quazepam (Doral)	O		A				
temazepam (Restoril)			A				
triazolam (Halcion)			A				

Note: A, FDA approved for this indication; O, off-label use. Off-label uses are highly dependent on the prescriber and change frequently. The student should refer to current reference sources for updated information on approved and off-label indications.

Pharmacotherapy of Anxiety and Insomnia

18.8 Benzodiazepines are preferred drugs for generalized anxiety disorder and the short-term therapy of insomnia.

The benzodiazepines are versatile drugs used for a diverse collection of medical conditions, including anxiety, seizure disorders, muscle spasms, premedication for medical procedures and anesthesia, and alcohol withdrawal. Diazepam (Valium) is featured as a prototype drug in Chapter 22 for its use in treating acute seizure disorders.

The benzodiazepines are first-line drugs for GAD and for the short-term management of insomnia. Since the introduction of the first benzodiazepines—chlordiazepoxide (Librium) and diazepam (Valium)—in the 1960s, the class has become one of the most widely prescribed in medicine. Benzodiazepines account for approximately three-fourths of all prescriptions for anxiety because they are effective, have a low incidence of drug interactions, and have less abuse potential compared to the older sedative–hypnotic drugs. There is a relatively wide margin of safety between therapeutic and lethal doses.

Although about 15 benzodiazepines are available, all have very similar actions and adverse effects; the various benzodiazepines differ primarily in their onset and duration of action. Although their actions are similar, drugs in this class have different indications, which are listed in Table 18.7.

Benzodiazepines bind to the gamma-aminobutyric acid (GABA) receptor and intensify the effect of GABA, the natural inhibitory neurotransmitter found throughout the brain. Most are metabolized in the liver to active metabolites and are excreted primarily in urine. One major advantage of the benzodiazepines is that they do not produce respiratory depression when taken in therapeutic doses. Death due to overdose is unlikely unless the benzodiazepines are taken in extreme quantities in combination with other CNS depressants or if the patient has sleep apnea.

The benzodiazepines are categorized as Schedule IV drugs; their use may lead to physical and psychologic dependence. The risk of dependence increases with higher doses and prolonged therapy. Abrupt termination of treatment can result in withdrawal symptoms that include headache, confusion, irritability, insomnia, and restlessness. Preexisting mental health conditions such as depression or suicidal tendencies may emerge or worsen during benzodiazepine therapy.

Most benzodiazepines are given orally (PO). Those that can be given parenterally, such as diazepam (Valium) and lorazepam (Ativan), the prototype drug in this category, should be monitored carefully due to their rapid onset of CNS effects and possible hypotension and respiratory depression. Benzodiazepines are given parenterally for conditions such as status epilepticus or severe symptoms of acute schizophrenia. Midazolam (Versed) is administered parenterally because it can act within minutes to produce conscious sedation in patients undergoing minor medical–surgical procedures.

The benzodiazepines have replaced the barbiturates for the short-term treatment of insomnia caused by anxiety because of their greater margin of safety. Benzodiazepines shorten the length of time it takes to fall asleep and reduce the frequency of interrupted sleep. Initially, patients will report an increase in refreshed, deep sleep. Although most benzodiazepines increase total sleep time, some reduce stage 4 sleep and some affect REM sleep. With chronic use, the patient will experience a gradual increase of REM sleep as tolerance develops to the REM-suppressant effects of the medication.

The benzodiazepines approved to treat short-term insomnia are different from those indicated for GAD (see Table 18.6). The anti-insomnia benzodiazepines are administered as hypnotics to induce sleep. Like other benzodiazepines, tolerance develops to their therapeutic effects, and all have the potential for physical and psychologic dependence. Most produce excessive daytime drowsiness, although this diminishes after a few days of therapy. They are indicated for short-term therapy of insomnia, approximately 4 weeks, although in clinical practice they may be used for longer periods. Rebound insomnia may be significant if these drugs are used for prolonged therapy.

Sedative–hypnotic medications such as the benzodiazepines have the potential to cause sleep-related behaviors that the patient does not remember. These include sleepwalking, sleep-eating, and even making phone calls or driving a car (sleep-driving) while not fully awake. Patients often deny that these events occurred.

Flumazenil (Romazicon) is an antidote for benzodiazepine overdose. Given by rapid IV injection, flumazenil competes with benzodiazepines for the GABA receptor and reverses benzodiazepine-induced sedation within minutes. It has a very short duration of action, and multiple doses, given every 30 to 45 seconds, may be necessary. If there is no response after the maximum dose (3 mg/h) has been administered, the patient's sedation was likely caused by a drug other than a benzodiazepine. Flumazenil must be used cautiously because the patient may awaken abruptly with dysphoria, agitation, and even seizures. Flumazenil does not reverse the depressed respiration characteristic of benzodiazepine overdose and it is not an antidote for the serious CNS depression caused by barbiturates or opioids. It does, however, reverse the CNS effects of some of the nonbenzodiazepine drugs such as zolpidem and eszopiclone.

As a class, all benzodiazepines have the potential to cause fetal harm. Neonates born to mothers taking benzodiazepines during pregnancy or breastfeeding may experience withdrawal symptoms. Benzodiazepines should not be used during pregnancy or breastfeeding unless the potential benefits outweigh the potential risks to the fetus.

PROTOTYPE DRUG Lorazepam (Ativan)

Classification **Therapeutic:** Antianxiety drug, sedative–hypnotic, antiseizure drug
Pharmacologic: Benzodiazepine, GABA receptor agonist

Therapeutic Effects and Uses: Approved in 1977, lorazepam is administered as oral tablets, concentrated oral solution, or by the intramuscular (IM) or intravenous (IV) routes. Lorazepam is approved for the routine management of GAD and to reduce anxiety prior to surgical or medical procedures. As a preanesthetic drug, it is administered by the IV route 15 to 20 minutes prior to surgery or by the IM route 2 hours prior to the procedure. Mechanically ventilated patients may receive lorazepam infusions to manage excessive anxiety and agitation that commonly occur while connected to a ventilation device.

Lorazepam is also used for several off-label indications, including insomnia, seizures, and the prevention or control of acute symptoms associated with ethanol withdrawal. Although used off-label for this indication, it is a preferred drug for treating life-threatening status epilepticus. For this indication it is administered by slow IV injection over a 2- to 4-minute period.

Mechanism of Action: Lorazepam potentiates the actions of GABA, an inhibitory neurotransmitter in the CNS. It is capable of causing all levels of CNS depression, from simple relaxation, to the induction of sleep, to coma.

Pharmacokinetics:

Route(s)	PO, IM, IV
Absorption	Readily absorbed
Distribution	91% bound to plasma proteins; widely distributed, including crossing the placenta; secreted in breast milk
Primary metabolism	Hepatic
Primary excretion	Renal
Onset of action	Peak effect: PO: 1–6 h; IM: 1–1.5 h; IV: 1–5 min
Duration of action	12–24 h

Adverse Effects: The most frequently reported adverse effects include dizziness, ataxia, drowsiness, blurred vision, vertigo, sedation, and confusion. These CNS effects are dose related and tolerance to them may develop as therapy progresses. Less common adverse effects include hepatotoxicity (including jaundice), alopecia, anaphylaxis, orthostatic hypotension, cardiac changes (tachycardia, hypotension, cardiac arrest following rapid IV administration), constipation, dry mouth, nausea and vomiting, and anorexia. Paradoxical CNS stimulation can occur in psychiatric patients, older adults, and hyperactive children. Patients may experience nightmares, talkativeness, mania, sleep disorders, acute rage reactions, anxiety, restlessness, and euphoria.

Contraindications/Precautions: Like other benzodiazepines, use of lorazepam may cause fetal malformations; thus, this drug is contraindicated during pregnancy unless the patient's condition is life-threatening. It is also contraindicated in lactating women because the drug is secreted in breast milk. Those with a hypersensitivity to benzodiazepines or who have closed-angle glaucoma, psychosis, or chronic COPD should not take lorazepam. Precautions must be taken in older adults, those who are debilitated, or those who have hepatic or renal dysfunction. Safe use in children has not been established. Lorazepam is a Schedule IV controlled substance and can cause both physical and psychologic dependence. Those with a history of drug abuse should be monitored carefully.

Drug Interactions: There are many potential drug interactions with lorazepam. Most notably, additive CNS depression will occur if the drug is given concurrently with other CNS depressants, such as alcohol, opiates, or other sedative–hypnotics. Oral contraceptives inhibit the metabolism of benzodiazepines that undergo oxidation (alprazolam, chlordiazepoxide, diazepam, and others); thus, the actions of these antianxiety drugs may be increased. On the other hand, oral contraceptives increase the metabolism of benzodiazepines that undergo conjugation (e.g., lorazepam, oxazepam, and temazepam) such that the antianxiety effects of these drugs may be reduced. Sedation effects may be increased if lorazepam is taken concurrently with disulfiram. Valproic acid may decrease the effects of lorazepam. **Herbal/Food:** Use with kava, melatonin, and valerian may cause excessive drowsiness. Excessive ingestion of caffeinated food and drinks may decrease the effectiveness of lorazepam.

Pregnancy: Animal studies show that lorazepam may cause fetal harm. Neonates born to mothers taking benzodiazepines during pregnancy may experience withdrawal symptoms. Because this drug is secreted in human milk, breastfeeding is not recommended.

Treatment of Overdose: Overdose will cause sedation, lethargy, and coma. Supportive care should be provided while the patient is recovering. Gastric lavage and activated charcoal may be administered. The benzodiazepine antagonist flumazenil may be administered to reverse sedation.

Clinician Responsibilities: Key clinical implications for patients receiving lorazepam are included in Applied Clinical Judgment: Patients Receiving Pharmacotherapy for Anxiety or Sleep Disorders.

Drugs Similar to Lorazepam (Ativan)

Benzodiazepines for anxiety: Benzodiazepines that are primarily used to treat anxiety are discussed next and include alprazolam, chlordiazepoxide, clorazepate, diazepam, and oxazepam. Benzodiazepines that are primarily indicated for seizures (clonazepam, clorazepate, diazepam, and lorazepam) are presented in Chapter 22. Midazolam is used as an adjunct to anesthesia and is presented in Chapter 26.

Alprazolam (Xanax): Approved in 1981, alprazolam is indicated for the management of GAD and panic disorder. It is used off-label for the short-term treatment of insomnia and for premenstrual dysphoric disorder that is unresponsive to nonpharmacologic therapies. An extended-release form (Xanax XR) is administered once daily. An orally disintegrating tablet (ODT) form is also available (Niravam). The drug is well tolerated, with drowsiness being the most common adverse effect. Patients are encouraged to refrain from consuming grapefruit and grapefruit juice while taking alprazolam because the combination may inhibit the metabolism of the drug. Older adults should receive a small dose, which can then be gradually increased as indicated, to prevent ataxia or excessive sedation.

Chlordiazepoxide (Librium): Chlordiazepoxide is a long-acting benzodiazepine that has been available for almost 50 years. It is available as capsules for oral administration; the parenteral formulations are no longer marketed in the United States. It is approved to manage GAD, acute anxiety situations, and symptoms associated with acute alcohol withdrawal. Off-label uses include treatment of panic disorder, tremors, and tension headaches. The use of chlordiazepoxide has markedly declined in favor of the shorter-acting drugs in this class such as lorazepam and alprazolam. Drowsiness is the most common adverse effect. Precautions should be used in those with impaired hepatic or renal function. Children and older adults are more likely to experience adverse effects and should be started with a low dose, which may then be gradually increased as needed.

Clorazepate (Tranxene): Approved in 1972, clorazepate is available by the oral route to treat GAD, partial seizures, and symptoms associated with ethanol withdrawal. It may be used off-label for the short-term management of insomnia. Clorazepate is essentially a prodrug that is converted into the same active metabolites as diazepam; thus, these drugs share the same actions and adverse effects.

Diazepam (Valium): Diazepam is an older benzodiazepine that is available for PO, IM, and IV administration. It is FDA approved to treat GAD, seizures, and muscle spasms and for the relief of symptoms associated with acute alcohol withdrawal. It is also approved to produce relaxation or sedation prior to medical procedures. Off-label uses include reduction of agitation, treatment of acute chloroquine overdose, and treatment of withdrawal symptoms associated with benzodiazepine abuse. Diazepam has the same actions and adverse effects as other drugs in its class.

Oxazepam: Approved in 1965, oxazepam is indicated for managing the symptoms of acute alcohol withdrawal and for treating mild to moderate GAD. It may be used off-label for the short-term management of insomnia associated with situational anxiety. Available only PO, its actions and adverse effects are the same as other benzodiazepines.

Benzodiazepines for insomnia: Benzodiazepines primarily used as hypnotics to treat insomnia include estazolam, flurazepam, quazepam, temazepam, and triazolam. All of the benzodiazepines used for insomnia are contraindicated during pregnancy and breastfeeding.

Estazolam: Approved in 1990, estazolam is an intermediate-duration benzodiazepine approved as a hypnotic in the short-term management of insomnia. This drug should be given at bedtime because it causes significant drowsiness and promotes sleep. The most common adverse effects are somnolence, hypokinesia, abnormal coordination, and dizziness. After several weeks of therapy, patients may exhibit tolerance to the sedative effects of the drug and will experience difficulty sleeping during the early-morning hours.

Flurazepam: Flurazepam, the oldest benzodiazepine hypnotic, was approved in 1970. This drug is only available PO and should be taken immediately before bedtime because it rapidly induces significant drowsiness. Flurazepam has a longer duration of action than some drugs in this class because it is converted to long-acting active metabolites in the liver. Its longer duration has the potential to extend drowsiness into the morning hours. Because of the development of tolerance to the sedative effects of this drug and the potential for physical and psychologic dependence, therapy is usually limited to 4 weeks.

Quazepam (Doral): Approved in 1985, quazepam is a benzodiazepine hypnotic drug available only by the PO route. It is administered just before bedtime because it rapidly produces significant drowsiness. This drug has a long duration of action because it is converted to several active metabolites in the liver that extend the drug's half-life. Patients may experience daytime sedation, although tolerance develops to this adverse effect after a few days. Therapy is usually limited to 4 weeks because of the development of tolerance and the potential for dependence.

Temazepam (Restoril): Approved in 1981, temazepam is indicated for the short-term therapy (7–10 days) of insomnia. It is administered PO and should be taken at bedtime due to its rapid onset of action. Unlike flurazepam and quazepam, the metabolism of temazepam does not result in active metabolites; thus, the drug may be safer for use in patients with hepatic impairment.

Triazolam (Halcion): Approved in 1982, triazolam is similar to other benzodiazepine hypnotics. Because of its rapid onset, it should be taken immediately prior to sleep. It has a relatively short half-life and has no active metabolites. Daytime drowsiness is less of a problem with triazolam because of its relatively short half-life. It is approved for the short-term therapy (7–10 days) of insomnia. Anterograde amnesia may occur more frequently with triazolam than with other benzodiazepine hypnotics.

CONNECTION Checkpoint 18.2

Differences in sleep patterns and ability to sleep may be apparent in different age groups. From what you learned in Chapter 8, should sleeping difficulties in the pregnant or lactating woman be treated with medications?

18.9 Nonbenzodiazepine anxiolytics have become popular choices for treating anxiety and sleep disorders.

Several CNS depressants, chemically unrelated to benzodiazepines, are used for anxiety and sleep disorders. These drugs come from multiple classes and are grouped together as nonbenzodiazepine anxiolytics.

Older CNS depressants, such as paraldehyde (Paracetaldehyde), ethchlorvynol (Placidyl), chloral hydrate, meprobamate (Equanil), and glutethimide (Doriglute), have only historic interest because they are so rarely prescribed due to their potential for serious adverse effects. The student should refer to drug guides or older pharmacology references for information on these medications.

A few nonbenzodiazepine drugs have antianxiety properties but their primary use is for indications other than anxiety. For example, valproic acid (Depakote) is a commonly prescribed antiseizure medication that is used off-label to treat agitation in older adults or anxiety in patients with bipolar disorder. Atenolol (Tenormin), metoprolol (Lopressor, Toprol XL), and propranolol (Inderal) are beta blockers that reduce the autonomic nervous system symptoms of anxiety such as nervousness, tremor, and tachycardia. Similarly, clonidine (Catapres) is an adrenergic antagonist that can block the autonomic symptoms that accompany anxiety. Diphenhydramine (Benadryl) and hydroxyzine are antihistamines that produce drowsiness and may be beneficial in calming patients. They offer the advantage of not causing dependence, although their use is often limited by their anticholinergic adverse effects. Diphenhydramine is a common component of OTC sleep aids and medications used to treat seasonal allergies. Because anxiety is a *secondary* indication for these drugs, they are discussed in other chapters of this text.

The most frequently prescribed nonbenzodiazepine anxiolytics are newer drugs that produce more selective CNS depression. Buspirone is commonly prescribed for its anxiolytic effect. Zolpidem (Ambien, Edluar, others), ramelteon (Rozerem), zaleplon (Sonata), suvorexant (Belsomra), lemborexant (Dayvigo), and eszopiclone (Lunesta) are used for their hypnotic effects. Other than their use in treating anxiety or insomnia, these drugs share little in common with each other and are discussed individually next.

PROTOTYPE DRUG Zolpidem (Ambien, Edluar, Others)

Classification **Therapeutic:** Sedative–hypnotic, drug for insomnia
Pharmacologic: Nonbenzodiazepine anxiolytic

Therapeutic Effects and Uses: Approved in 1992, zolpidem is indicated for the short-term (7–10 days) treatment of insomnia. Zolpidem decreases sleep-onset time and the number of nighttime awakenings and improves the length and quality of sleep. Muscle relaxation and anticonvulsant effects occur at doses much higher than the hypnotic dose. Immediate release (Ambien), extended release (Ambien CR), oral spray (Zolpimist), and sublingual (Edluar, Intermezzo) forms are available. The sublingual and oral spray forms have a more rapid onset than tablets and eliminate the requirement for water or the need to swallow.

Zolpidem should be administered just prior to expected sleep due to its rapid onset of action. Its lack of active metabolites and short half-life reduce the incidences of excessive daytime drowsiness and rebound insomnia.

Mechanism of Action: Zolpidem has a similar mechanism of action as the benzodiazepines: enhancing the action of GABA, the inhibitory neurotransmitter. Whereas the benzodiazepines bind nonselectively to all three known subtypes of the GABA receptors, zolpidem binds to only one specific type (omega-1). This explains why the drug shares some actions of the benzodiazepines, such as anti-anxiety and hypnotic effects, but has no effects on muscle relaxation or reducing seizures.

Pharmacokinetics:

Route(s)	PO
Absorption	70% absorbed
Distribution	Widely distributed; unknown if it crosses the placenta; small amounts are secreted in breast milk; 92% bound to plasma protein
Primary metabolism	Hepatic
Primary excretion	Renal, small amounts in bile and feces
Onset of action	7–27 min; peak effect: 90 min
Duration of action	Duration: 6–8 h; half-life: 1.4–4.5 h

Adverse Effects: Adverse reactions to zolpidem are usually mild and include dizziness, diarrhea, and daytime drowsiness. Other adverse effects include nausea and vomiting, depression, confusion, and amnesia. As with other hypnotic drugs, a small percentage of patients experience abnormal thinking, behavioral changes, sleep-eating, sleep-driving, and hallucinations. Very high doses may cause severe ataxia, bradycardia, altered vision, severe nausea, vomiting, drowsiness, difficulty breathing, and coma. Abrupt withdrawal after long-term use may result in asthenia, diaphoresis, vomiting, tremor, or facial flushing. Zolpidem is a Schedule IV controlled substance that can be abused and lead to dependency. **Black Box Warning:** Zolpidem can cause complex sleep behaviors such as sleepwalking, sleep-driving, and engaging in other activities while not fully awake. Some of these may cause injury or death.

Contraindications/Precautions: Other than hypersensitivity to zolpidem, there are no contraindications to the use of this drug. As with other CNS depressants, it should be used cautiously in patients with respiratory impairment and in older adults, who are generally more sensitive to the depressive effects of the drugs; lower dosages may be necessary. Impaired liver or kidney function can increase serum drug levels and doses should be lowered. Zolpidem should be used with caution in individuals with depression and suicidal ideation because there is a potential for intentional overdose in these patients. The safety and effectiveness in patients under age 18 have not been established.

Drug Interactions: Zolpidem is a substrate for hepatic CYP3A4 enzymes and thus may interact with drugs that induce or inhibit this enzyme system. Concurrent use with other CNS depressants, including alcohol and fentanyl, will cause additive sedation. When given concurrently with certain SSRIs, disorientation or worsening of depression may occur. **Herbal/Food:** The presence of food will reduce absorption of the drug; thus, it should be taken on an empty stomach. St. John's wort may cause confusion and, rarely, hallucinations. Valerian, kava, and melatonin supplements may cause additive sedation.

Pregnancy: Animal reproduction studies suggest that zolpidem may cause fetal harm. Neonates born to mothers taking this drug during pregnancy may experience withdrawal symptoms. Because the drug is secreted in breast milk, caution should be used in breastfeeding.

Treatment of Overdose: Overdose with zolpidem can cause serious impairment of consciousness and may be fatal. The benzodiazepine antagonist flumazenil will reverse the sedative effects of zolpidem but may precipitate seizures. Other treatment involves supportive care, such as gastric lavage.

Clinician Responsibilities: Key clinical implications for patients receiving zolpidem are included in Applied Clinical Judgment: Patients Receiving Pharmacotherapy for Anxiety or Sleep Disorders.

Drugs Similar to Zolpidem (Ambien, Edluar, Others)

Other drugs in this category include buspirone, eszopiclone, lemborexant, ramelteon, suvorexant, tasimelteon, and zaleplon.

Buspirone: Buspirone is a nonbenzodiazepine anxiolytic approved in 1986 for the short-term management (up to 1 month) of GAD. Available PO, taking the drug with food will cause less nausea. Grapefruit juice may increase the effects of the drug and should be avoided. The mechanism of action for buspirone is unclear but appears to involve two pathways: enhancing dopamine (D_2) receptors and suppressing serotonin receptors in the brain. It is less likely to affect cognitive and motor performance than benzodiazepines and rarely interacts with other CNS depressants. The most common adverse effects include dizziness, drowsiness, nausea and vomiting, and headache. When switching from a benzodiazepine to buspirone, the patient may experience withdrawal symptoms or anxiety; therefore, the dose of benzodiazepine should be gradually tapered while buspirone is increased. Unlike other CNS depressants, buspirone does not cause dependence or have withdrawal symptoms. Therapy may take 2–4 weeks to achieve optimal results. Buspirone is sometimes used off-label to treat symptoms of nicotine withdrawal and premenstrual syndrome. Animal reproduction studies did not show teratogenicity. Buspirone is secreted in human milk but the effects on breastfeeding infants are unknown.

Eszopiclone (Lunesta): Although not structurally related to other sedative–hypnotics, eszopiclone shares certain properties with zolpidem and the benzodiazepines. Approved in 2004, eszopiclone has a long elimination half-life, about twice as long as that of zolpidem, which offers an advantage in maintaining sleep and decreasing early-morning awakening. On the other hand, the long half-life is more likely to cause sleepiness to carry over into the morning hours and result in daytime sedation. Adverse effects are mild and include headache, dizziness, dry mouth, and an unpleasant taste that may persist into the following day. It is only available PO and should be taken immediately before bedtime due to its rapid onset of action. Eszopiclone is metabolized by hepatic CYP3A4 enzymes; thus, potential drug–drug and drug–herb interactions exist for substances that induce or inhibit these enzymes. The onset of action may be reduced if taken with or immediately following a high-fat meal. Older adults with impaired hepatic or renal function may need a lower dose. Eszopiclone may be used for the long-term treatment of insomnia. However, tolerance develops to the sedative effects after a few weeks of therapy and rebound insomnia may occur on withdrawal. Eszopiclone is a Schedule IV controlled substance. Like zolpidem, eszopiclone carries a black box warning that the drug can cause complex sleep behaviors such as sleepwalking, sleep-driving, and engaging in other dangerous activities while not fully awake. Animal reproduction studies found no evidence of teratogenicity or structural defects. Neonates born to mothers taking this drug during pregnancy may experience withdrawal symptoms such as hypothermia, feeding difficulties and respiratory depression. No information is available regarding the effects of eszopiclone during lactation.

Lemborexant (Dayvigo): One of the newest drugs for insomnia, lemborexant was approved in 2019 to treat sleep-onset and sleep-maintenance insomnia. This drug is classified as an orexin receptor antagonist. Orexin is a neurotransmitter found in the brain that helps regulate sleep–wake cycles by maintaining wakefulness. By blocking orexin receptors, lemborexant promotes drowsiness and sleep. The most common adverse effects are somnolence, headache, and sleep paralysis, and it is contraindicated in patients with narcolepsy. Complex sleep behaviors such as sleep-walking or sleep-driving have been observed. Lemborexant is a Schedule IV controlled substance. In animal reproduction studies, this drug caused toxicities only at very high doses. This drug is secreted in animal milk but there are no data regarding human lactation.

Ramelteon (Rozerem): Approved in 2005, ramelteon is approved to treat chronic insomnia in people who have problems falling asleep. It appears to be safe for long-term use. Ramelteon has a unique mechanism of action: It activates melatonin receptors, specifically MT1 and MT2, which are mediators of the normal sleep–wake cycle. With an onset of action of 30 minutes and a short duration of action, it is helpful in treating sleep onset but it does not maintain sleep. It is less effective if taken with or immediately after a high-fat meal. There is little next-day residual drowsiness owing to its short half-life. Adverse effects of ramelteon are mild and include dizziness, fatigue, and somnolence. Ramelteon can affect the levels of sex hormones in the body, so the patient may experience amenorrhea, decreased libido, galactorrhea, and problems with fertility. Alcohol should be avoided because it may cause additive CNS depression. Fluvoxamine (Luvox) can greatly increase (more than 50 times) the levels of ramelteon so it should not be used concurrently. Animal reproduction studies showed teratogenicity and decreased viability of offspring at high doses. This drug is secreted in animal milk but there are no data regarding effects on human lactation.

Suvorexant (Belsomra): Like lemborexant, suvorexant is classified as an orexin antagonist used to treat sleep-onset and sleep-maintenance insomnia. Like other drugs for insomnia, the primary side effect is daytime drowsiness. Caution must be used when combining suvorexant with alcohol or other CNS depressants due to additive sedation. Use with inhibitors of hepatic CYP3A4, including grapefruit juice, should be avoided. Complex sleep behaviors such as sleep-walking or sleep-driving have been observed. Suvorexant is a Schedule IV controlled substance. Animal reproduction studies suggest this drug may cause fetal farm at high doses. This drug is secreted in animal milk but there are no data regarding human lactation.

Tasimelteon (Hetlioz): Tasimelteon was approved in 2014 for non-24-hour sleep–wake disorder. This is a condition that occurs in people who are totally blind. Because no light is perceived, these patients are unable to synchronize the timing of sleep to a 24-hour light–dark cycle. This may result in the patient being active when others are sleeping or drowsy when others are awake. Several weeks or months of therapy may be needed to improve the sleep–wake cycle. The most common adverse effects are headache, elevated alanine aminotransferase, and nightmares. Animal reproduction studies suggest this drug may cause fetal farm at high doses. There are no data regarding effects on human lactation.

Zaleplon (Sonata): Approved in 1999, zaleplon is an oral nonbenzodiazepine sedative–hypnotic whose only indication is for the short-term treatment (7–10 days) of insomnia. Zaleplon decreases time to sleep onset. Like zolpidem, it binds specifically to the omega-1 GABA receptor, but it has a faster onset and shorter duration of action than zolpidem. Zaleplon should be taken immediately before bedtime due to its rapid onset of action. Administration immediately following a high-fat meal slows the absorption of zaleplon and reduces its effectiveness. The drug is well tolerated and causes few adverse effects other than headache. High doses produce symptoms characteristic of other sedative–hypnotics such as drowsiness, confusion, dizziness, and lethargy. As with other sedative and hypnotic drugs, worsening of depression or suicidal thinking has been reported. Long-term use does not result in tolerance and, although it is a Schedule IV drug, dependence potential is low. Like zolpidem and eszopiclone, zaleplon carries a black box warning that the drug can cause complex sleep behaviors such as sleepwalking, sleep-driving, and engaging in other dangerous activities while not fully awake. Animal reproduction studies show zaleplon increased stillbirths and postnatal mortality. This drug is secreted in human milk and breastfed infants should be monitored for sedation, increased crying and poor feeding.

Antidepressants

18.10 Antidepressants are widely prescribed for anxiety disorders.

Antidepressants include drugs from five classes that were developed to treat major depressive disorder, a condition characterized by chronic low mood and loss of interest or pleasure in activities that were previously enjoyable (see Chapter 19). In later years, pharmacologists discovered that some antidepressants were effective in treating other conditions, including anxiety and insomnia. Indeed, some have become preferred drugs in treating anxiety-related disorders.

Antidepressants act by altering the levels of two important neurotransmitters in the brain: norepinephrine and serotonin. Restoration of normal neurotransmitter balances reduces symptoms associated with depression, panic attacks, obsessive–compulsive behavior, PTSD, and phobias. A more detailed treatment of these drugs and their use in treating depression is presented in Chapter 19. The following section focuses on their applications to treating anxiety disorders and insomnia.

For most patients, intense anxiety symptoms come in two stages. In the first stage, termed *anticipatory anxiety*, the patient begins to think about an upcoming challenge and starts to experience feelings of dread. The second stage is when physical symptoms such as shortness of breath, accelerated heart rate, and muscle tension start to emerge as a consequence of activation of the autonomic nervous system. If medications are successful at reducing the negative thoughts associated with the anticipatory component of anxiety, then there is less likelihood that the patient will experience excessive stress.

The antidepressants used to reduce symptoms of anxiety-related disorders are the SSRIs, atypical antidepressants and TCAs. Indications for these medications are shown in Table 18.8. Following is a brief summary of additional important considerations for each antidepressant class. Individual drug information, patient teaching, and nursing responsibilities are presented in Chapter 19.

Selective serotonin reuptake inhibitors: This is the most widely prescribed antidepressant class because these drugs are safer than those from other classes and cause fewer sympathomimetic effects (increased heart rate and hypertension) and anticholinergic effects. Some SSRIs can, however, cause weight gain and sexual dysfunction. Overdoses can cause confusion, anxiety, restlessness, hypertension, tremors, sweating, fever, and lack of muscle coordination.

Table 18.8 Indications for Antidepressants Used for Anxiety-Related Disorders or Insomnia

Drug	GAD	Panic Disorder	Social Anxiety Disorder	OCD	PTSD	Insomnia
Atypical Antidepressants, Including the SNRIs						
duloxetine (Cymbalta)	A					
trazodone (Oleptro)	O	O				O
venlafaxine extended release (Effexor XR)	A	A	A	O		
Selective Serotonin Reuptake Inhibitors (SSRIs)						
citalopram (Celexa)		O		O	O	
escitalopram (Lexapro)	A	O	O			
fluoxetine (Prozac)		A	A	A	O	
fluvoxamine (Luvox)		O	O	A	O	
paroxetine (Paxil)	A	A	A	A	A	
sertraline (Zoloft)	O	A	A	A	A	
Tricyclic Antidepressants (TCAs)						
clomipramine (Anafranil)				A		
doxepin (Silenor)	A					A

Note: A, FDA approved for this indication; O, off-label use. Off-label uses are highly dependent on the prescriber and change frequently. The student should refer to current reference sources for updated information on approved and off-label indications.

Five SSRIs are approved for anxiety-related disorders, although other drugs in this class may be used off-label. The indications for each drug are given in Table 18.8.

- **Generalized anxiety disorder.** Paroxetine (Paxil) and escitalopram (Lexapro) are considered first-line drugs for patients with GAD and anxiety that is associated with depressive disorders. Unlike the benzodiazepines that act immediately, onset for the antianxiety effects of the SSRIs may take several weeks.
- **Panic disorder.** The three SSRIs approved for panic disorder—fluoxetine (Prozac), paroxetine (Paxil), and sertraline (Zoloft)—are considered first-line drugs for this disorder. They reduce both the frequency and intensity of panic attacks.
- **Obsessive–compulsive disorder.** Four SSRIs are approved to treat OCD, although others in this class may be used off-label. Paroxetine (Paxil), fluvoxamine (Luvox), fluoxetine (Prozac), and sertraline (Zoloft) are first-line drugs for this disorder. Optimal therapeutic effects may take several months to achieve.
- **Social anxiety disorder.** Paroxetine (Paxil), fluvoxamine (Luvox), and sertraline (Zoloft) are SSRIs approved for the long-term therapy of social anxiety disorder. Because several months may be necessary for optimal therapeutic benefit, the benzodiazepines are better choices for acute symptoms of social anxiety disorder.
- **Post-traumatic stress disorder.** Paroxetine (Paxil) and sertraline (Zoloft) are the two SSRIs approved for the therapy of PTSD. Therapy should be initiated as soon after the traumatic event as possible, and several months may be necessary for optimal results.

Atypical antidepressants: These include serotonin–norepinephrine reuptake inhibitors (SNRIs). Adverse effects are similar to those of the SSRIs and include insomnia, abnormal dreams, sweating, constipation, dry mouth, loss of appetite, weight loss, tremor, abnormal vision, headache, nausea and vomiting, dizziness, and reduced libido. Two atypical antidepressants are used for anxiety disorders:

- **Duloxetine (Cymbalta).** Approved in 2007 for GAD, duloxetine has the potential to become a first-line drug for this disorder due to its safety and effectiveness, especially in patients with accompanying major depression. It is also approved to treat fibromyalgia, chronic musculoskeletal pain, and diabetic peripheral neuropathic pain.
- **Venlafaxine (Effexor XR).** The extended-release form of venlafaxine was the first antidepressant approved for GAD. It is also beneficial in treating panic attacks and social anxiety disorder. It is widely used for anxiety disorders that are accompanied by depression.

Tricyclic antidepressants (TCAs): TCAs are older drugs that, although effective, generally produce more adverse effects than SSRIs. Patients often have annoying anticholinergic effects such as dry mouth, blurred vision, urine retention, and hypertension (see Chapter 14). They are not recommended for patients with a history of heart attack, heart block, or dysrhythmia. Concurrent use with alcohol or other CNS depressants should be avoided, and patients with asthma, GI disorders, alcoholism, schizophrenia, or bipolar disorder should take TCAs with extreme caution. Although several drugs in this class are used off-label, only two TCAs are approved for anxiety disorders:

- **Clomipramine (Anafranil).** The only drug in this class approved for OCD, clomipramine is very effective but tends to cause more adverse effects than SSRIs. It is considered an alternative for patients who are unable to tolerate SSRIs.
- **Doxepin (Silenor).** Originally approved for anxiety associated with depressive disorders, doxepin produces a rapid antianxiety effect. This drug is also approved to treat insomnia characterized by difficulty with sleep maintenance. Because of significant anticholinergic side effects, it is not considered a first-line drug for anxiety.

CONNECTION Checkpoint 18.3

Fluvoxamine, fluoxetine, and duloxetine have similar-sounding names and may look alike when written as prescriptions. From what you learned in Chapter 6, describe means that you should implement to avoid these types of medication errors.

18.11 Barbiturates are effective sedative–hypnotics but have potentially serious adverse effects that limit their use.

Used in pharmacotherapy since the early 1900s, barbiturates are powerful CNS depressants prescribed for their sedative, hypnotic, and antiseizure effects. Until the discovery of the benzodiazepines, barbiturates were the preferred drugs for patients with anxiety and insomnia. They are now rarely prescribed for anxiety or insomnia because of their significant adverse effects and because of the availability of more effective medications. The risk of psychologic and physical dependence is high—several are Schedule II drugs. If a patient does become physically dependent on barbiturates, the withdrawal syndrome is extremely severe and can be fatal. Overdose results in profound respiratory depression, hypotension, and shock. Barbiturates have frequently been used to commit suicide, and death due to overdose was common when these drugs were widely prescribed in the 1960s and 1970s.

Barbiturates are capable of depressing CNS function at all levels. Like benzodiazepines, barbiturates act by binding to GABA receptor–chloride channel molecules, intensifying the effect of GABA throughout the brain. At low doses they reduce anxiety and cause drowsiness. At moderate doses they inhibit seizure activity (see Chapter 22) and promote sleep by inhibiting brain impulses traveling through the limbic system and the RAS. At higher doses, some barbiturates can induce anesthesia (see Chapter 26). Barbiturates are classified by their duration of action: short acting, intermediate acting, or long acting. Selected barbiturates used to treat sleep disorders are shown in Table 18.9.

When taken for prolonged periods, barbiturates induce the synthesis of hepatic CYP450 enzymes and can stimulate their own metabolism as well as that of hundreds of other drugs that use these enzymes for their breakdown. This significantly increases the risk for drug–drug interactions. After 2 weeks, tolerance begins to develop to the sedative effects of barbiturates; this includes cross-tolerance to other CNS depressants such as the opioids. Tolerance does not develop, however, to the respiratory depressant effects. Thus, the patient may take higher and higher doses to produce sleep while approaching dangerous and even lethal dosage levels.

PROTOTYPE DRUG Phenobarbital (Luminal)

Classification **Therapeutic:** Sedative–hypnotic, antiepileptic drug
Pharmacologic: Barbiturate, GABA receptor agonist

Therapeutic Effects and Uses: A Schedule IV drug, phenobarbital is available as tablets or elixir for PO doses and as injection for IM or IV administration. By the IV route, phenobarbital is reserved for emergency conditions such as status epilepticus. It is effective for treating generalized and partial seizures, which may be the most common indications for the use of the drug. The drug is FDA approved for the short-term treatment of insomnia, although there are

Table 18.9 Selected Barbiturates for Insomnia

Drug	Route and Adult Dose (Maximum Dose Where Indicated)	Adverse Effects
butabarbital (Butisol)	Sedative: PO: 15–30 mg tid or qid Hypnotic: PO: 50–100 mg at bedtime	*Somnolence, hangover, confusion, nausea and vomiting, rebound insomnia* CNS depression, coma, death, bradycardia, liver damage, hypocalcemia, Stevens–Johnson syndrome, severe respiratory depression, birth defects
pentobarbital (Nembutal)	Preoperative sedation: IM: 150–200 mg in two divided doses Hypnotic: IM: 150–200 mg IV: 100 mg every 1–3 min up to 500-mg dose	
phenobarbital (Luminal)	Sedative: PO: 30–120 mg/day IV/IM/subcutaneous: 100–320 mg/day	
secobarbital (Seconal)	Sedative: PO: 100–300 mg/day in three divided doses Hypnotic: PO: 100–200 mg	

Note: *Italics* indicate common adverse effects. Underline indicates serious adverse effects.

many safer and equally effective medications available for this indication. Therapeutic serum phenobarbital concentrations range from 15 to 40 mcg/mL. As a sedative–hypnotic, phenobarbital decreases time to sleep onset and lengthens total sleep time. The number of nighttime awakenings diminishes. Significant rebound insomnia occurs when the drug is discontinued.

Mechanism of Action: Phenobarbital binds to GABA receptors, where it enhances the activity of GABA.

Pharmacokinetics:

Route(s)	PO, IM, and IV
Absorption	Well absorbed by all routes
Distribution	Rapidly and widely distributed; may cross the placenta; secreted in breast milk; 20–45% bound to protein
Primary metabolism	Hepatic
Primary excretion	Renal
Onset of action	IV: 5 min; PO: 8–12 h
Duration of action	Half-life: 53–118 h

Adverse Effects: Many adverse effects are possible with phenobarbital. Serious ones include coma, Stevens–Johnson syndrome, angioedema, and thrombophlebitis. Adverse reactions related to CNS depression include oversedation, "hangover" effect, lethargy, and hallucinations. Other adverse effects can include blood dyscrasias, hypocalcemia, hepatic disease, nausea and vomiting, diarrhea, or constipation. Deficiency in folic acid, calcium, and vitamin D may result in osteomalacia. Phenobarbital can cause paradoxical excitation in older adults or children, especially during the first 2 weeks of treatment. If abruptly discontinued after prolonged use, the patient may experience nightmares, insomnia, tremor, hallucinations, and nausea and vomiting.

Contraindications/Precautions: Phenobarbital is contraindicated in patients with hypersensitivity to barbiturates, suicidal ideation or previous suicide attempt, preexisting CNS depression, severe respiratory disease, severe pain, or hyperthyroidism. Patients with impaired hepatic, renal, and cardiovascular function should not receive phenobarbital, or the dose should be lowered to prevent toxicity. Patients with COPD may experience profound respiratory depression, even at therapeutic doses, and should not receive phenobarbital. A patient who has a familial history of porphyria should not be administered phenobarbital. Porphyria is a metabolic disorder in which neurologic disturbances are noted. Phenobarbital should be used cautiously in patients with hyperthyroidism, diabetes mellitus, and severe anemia.

Drug Interactions: Phenobarbital induces CYP450 enzymes and has the potential to interact with drugs that are metabolized by the liver such as corticosteroids, oral contraceptives, and anticonvulsants. Use with other CNS depressants, including alcohol, may cause profound sedation. Valproic acid may increase the risk of phenobarbital toxicity. Phenobarbital may decrease the effectiveness of digoxin, TCAs, metronidazole, quinidine, or oral anticoagulants. **Herbal/Food:** St. John's wort may lead to decreased barbiturate effect. Use of kava, chamomile, eucalyptus, lemon balm, or valerian may increase additive CNS depression.

Pregnancy: Phenobarbital can cause birth defects and physical dependence in the neonate, and thus it is contraindicated during pregnancy. Phenobarbital is secreted in breast milk and can cause profound effects on the neonate; thus, it is contraindicated during lactation.

Treatment of Overdose: Overdosage of phenobarbital is a medical emergency and may be fatal. Activated charcoal is administered followed by gastric lavage. Alkalinization of the urine with sodium bicarbonate increases the renal elimination of phenobarbital.

Clinician Responsibilities: Key clinical implications for patients receiving phenobarbital are included in Applied Clinical Judgment: Patients Receiving Pharmacotherapy for Anxiety or Sleep Disorders.

Drugs Similar to Phenobarbital (Luminal)

The barbiturates are classified by duration of action, and all have the same actions and adverse effects as phenobarbital. None are in common use.

Ultra-short Acting: With a half-life of less than 10 minutes, methohexital (Brevital) is administered by the IV route to induce or maintain anesthesia, as preoperative sedation, or in the emergency management of seizures.

Short Acting: With half-lives of 15 to 40 minutes, secobarbital (Seconal) and pentobarbital are oral drugs that have been used to treat insomnia and as preoperative medications. These are Schedule II drugs and have been the most widely abused barbiturates.

Intermediate Acting: With a slightly longer half-life, butabarbital (Butisol) is an oral drug that has been used as a sedative–hypnotic and for preanesthesia sedation.

Long Acting: Phenobarbital is the only long-acting barbiturate. Mephobarbital (Mebaral) was withdrawn from the U.S. market in 2012.

CONNECTIONS: Advanced Practice Application

Treating Childhood Anxiety Disorders

Case

Frankie, a 16-year-old adolescent, arrives for her follow-up therapy appointment. She had been diagnosed 2 months ago with general anxiety disorder (GAD) after having symptoms of fatigue, irritability, and sleep disturbance. Frankie was having trouble engaging in school, and many days was absent or would leave early. She asked the school counselor for help after she had a panic attack in the school health clinic. Frankie is currently in therapy and continues to have difficulty managing her symptoms. The inability to sleep is interfering with her school success. You and the therapist recognize the importance of a holistic treatment focus and begin working with Frankie on progressive muscle relaxation, breathing techniques, and diet management. What pharmacologic interventions should the provider be considering for Frankie?

Discussion

Children and adolescents may experience intense fear and worry that can lead to the same types of anxiety disorders experienced by adults. Signs may include excessive worrying about ordinary school activities; physical symptoms such as sweating, headache, trembling, and palpitations; social withdrawal; and sleep disturbances. If not recognized and treated, childhood anxiety disorders may lead to low self-esteem, poor interpersonal relationships, drug or alcohol use, or repeated school absences. Worldwide it is estimated that 10–20% of children and adolescents experience mental disorders and 6.5% of 6- to 18-year-olds experience anxiety, girls being affected more than boys (Polanczyk et al., 2015; World Health Organization, 2020).

Cognitive-behavioral therapy and relaxation techniques are usually the first treatments used for childhood anxiety. If medication is indicated in addition to these therapies, the SSRIs are the preferred drugs for children (Cousins & Goodyer, 2015). The use of any antidepressant in children must be carefully considered, with the risks versus benefits weighed before the drugs are prescribed and carefully monitored thereafter. In 2004, the FDA issued a black box warning that applied to most antidepressants, citing the possibility of increased risk of suicide in children and adolescents. In 2007, this warning was extended to include young adults up to age 25. Prescribing of SSRIs has dropped by 20% in the United States since 2004, likely due to increased awareness of this suicide risk (Anxiety and Depression Association of America, 2018; National Institute of Mental Health, n.d.). Caregivers must be diligent in monitoring for signs of potential suicidal thoughts in children taking SSRI antidepressants and report any such changes to the healthcare provider immediately. Signs include unusual changes in behavior, sleeplessness, agitation, and social withdrawal.

Recent studies have shown that the use of vitamin C in the treatment of depression may reduce the severity of symptoms in both children and adult patients (De Oliveira et al., 2015), although further studies are needed to substantiate this finding.

CONNECTIONS: APPLIED CLINICAL JUDGMENT

Patients Receiving Pharmacotherapy for Anxiety or Sleep Disorders

Key Assessment Data

- History of current condition, baseline vital signs, physical exam and mental status findings; history of hepatic, renal, respiratory, cardiovascular, or neurologic disease; sleep history (e.g., quality and quantity of sleep, frequent wakefulness, snoring or apnea); medication and substance use history; pregnancy status.
- Ongoing assessment during drug therapy includes stress and coping patterns; appropriate laboratory findings (e.g., hepatic or renal function studies).

Desired Therapeutic Outcomes

Improvement is observed and measurable by patient statements of improvement in anxiety, coping, appetite, ability to carry out ADLs, and normalized sleep patterns.

Minimizing Adverse Effects

- Excessive drowsiness and dizziness may occur and, for a prolonged period of time, depending on the drug's half-life, increasing the risk of falls and injury. Daytime drowsiness may impair walking or the ability to carry out usual ADLs. Subtle changes in mental alertness and cognitive functioning may occur, even in the absence of sleepiness.
- Neurologic changes such as changes in level of consciousness, agitation, disorientation, or confusion may indicate overmedication or effects of sleep deprivation.
- Drugs used for anxiety and sleep may increase the risk of mental depression, especially in patients with suicidal tendencies. Concurrent use of alcohol and other CNS depressants increases the effects and the risk.
- Avoid abrupt discontinuation of therapy. Withdrawal symptoms, including rebound anxiety and sleeplessness, are possible with abrupt discontinuation after long-term use.

Lifespan Considerations

- Older adults may be at increased risk for falls. Many benzodiazepines and all barbiturates are included on the Beers list of potentially inappropriate drugs for older adults and warrant careful monitoring.

(continued)

CONNECTIONS: APPLIED CLINICAL JUDGMENT *(continued)*

Patients Receiving Pharmacotherapy for Anxiety or Sleep Disorders

Diversity Considerations

- Barbiturates induce CYP450 enzymes and may interact with other drugs. Ethnically diverse populations may also experience less than optimal effects of the drug. Nonbenzodiazepine sedative–hypnotic drugs are also metabolized through the CYP450 pathways.
- Women may metabolize some sublingual drugs (e.g., zolpidem) more slowly, and dosage may need to be halved by the provider.

Patient Education

- Referral for cognitive-behavioral therapy may be useful for developing healthy coping strategies and sleep habits.
- Keep a sleep diary of bedtime, time involved trying to fall asleep, quality and quantity of sleep, daytime sleepiness; bring the diary to each healthcare visit.
- Rise from lying or sitting to standing slowly to avoid dizziness or falls. If dizziness occurs, sit or lie down and do not attempt to stand or walk until the sensation passes.
- Be cautious or avoid driving or other activities requiring mental alertness or physical coordination until the effects of the drug are known.
- Report increasing lethargy, disorientation, confusion, changes in behavior or mood, slurred speech, or ataxia immediately.
- Have caregivers observe for nighttime behavioral activities such as sleepwalking, sleep-eating, or sleep-driving if nonbenzodiazepine sedative–hypnotic drugs are given, and report immediately. The patient may not remember or be aware of these activities.
- Report significant mood changes, especially depression, and avoid alcohol and other CNS depressants while taking the drug. Continued monitoring may be advisable, especially if preexisting depression is present.
- Take the drug exactly as prescribed and to not stop it abruptly. Do not be keep the drug at the bedside to avoid taking additional doses when drowsy.
- Do not open, chew, or crush extended-release tablets (e.g., zolpidem); swallow them whole with plenty of water. Sublingual forms of the drug should be allowed to dissolve under the tongue; water should not be taken.

Prescribing Considerations

- Assess sleep patterns
- Rule out any underlying conditions that may be causing difficulty sleeping
- Prescribe for a limited period of time to determine the benefits and side effects
- May not be safe while pregnant or breast-feeding
- May increase the risk of nighttime falls and injury in older adults, consider a lower dose of medication to reduce risk.
- Patients with kidney disease, hypotension, arrhythmias, or a history of seizures should be monitored closely and may not be appropriate to prescribe for.

Understanding Chapter 18

Key Concepts Summary

18.1 Proper diagnosis of anxiety disorders is important to identifying the most effective treatment option.

18.2 Anxiety disorders may be divided into five major categories.

18.3 Specific regions of the brain have been identified that are responsible for anxiety.

18.4 Sleep occurs in distinct stages.

18.5 Sleep disorders affect a large percentage of the population.

18.6 Insomnia and anxiety are closely related.

18.7 Management of anxiety and sleep disorders utilizes a combination of pharmacologic and nonpharmacologic therapies.

18.8 Benzodiazepines are preferred drugs for generalized anxiety disorder and the short-term therapy of insomnia.

18.9 Nonbenzodiazepine anxiolytics have become popular choices for treating anxiety and sleep disorders.

18.10 Antidepressants are widely prescribed for anxiety disorders.

18.11 Barbiturates are effective sedative–hypnotics but have potentially serious adverse effects that limit their use.

CASE STUDY: Making the Patient Connection

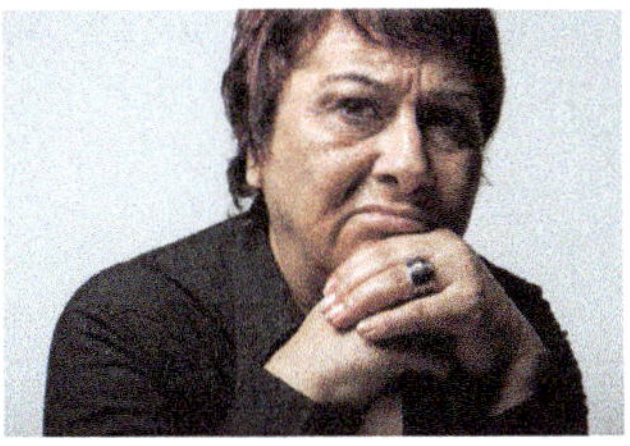

Remember the patient "Seraphina Alvarez" at the beginning of the chapter? Now read the remainder of the case study. Based on the information presented within the chapter, respond to the critical thinking questions that follow.

Seraphina Alvarez, age 59, is an elementary school teacher who has planned on retiring at the end of this academic year. She is the married mother of seven adult children, six of whom live within a 15-mile radius and see her often. Her husband, Joe, has been retired for 3 years. He receives Social Security and a small pension from his former employment as a construction worker. Seraphina and Joe's oldest daughter's two children and two dogs came to live with them approximately 10 months ago because their daughter is unable to provide a home for them. The children, Joseph, age 15, and Mariah, age 12, are good students who are active in school and church activities. They resent having to move from their long-time home and school and are acting out some.

Seraphina resents having to raise her grandchildren. It interferes with plans that she and her husband had made to travel after she retired. In fact, she may not be able to retire as planned because they need the extra income to meet the children's needs. Seraphina loves the children and tries very hard not to let her resentment show. She also has guilt feelings that she did not do all she could or should have done to raise her daughter to be a responsible parent. As a result, she is unable to sleep well and reports having anxiety. Seraphina first turned to herbal remedies common in her Latino culture and to prayer. Neither of these interventions has helped, but she is reluctant to discuss her problems with anyone else. She sees her parish priest on a regular basis. He is very supportive of Seraphina and understanding of her feelings of resentment but does not realize that she is experiencing anxiety and insomnia.

Seraphina, whose health has always been good, has begun having some health issues, including hypertension, diarrhea, and weight loss. She finds herself becoming more anxious, and her family has noticed that she is decreasing time spent with family and friends and does not leave her home other than to go to work and church. Seraphina has lost 16 kg (35 lb) in 2 months and appears to have lost her "zest" for living. Her diet consists of black coffee and fresh fruit. Joe frequently finds her sitting in a rocking chair on their front porch during the night, rather than being in bed. She also has begun missing work, saying, "I just don't feel up to facing the kids today."

Critical Thinking Questions

1. What current factors in Seraphina's life may be interfering with her ability to get a good night's sleep?
2. What medications may Seraphina's healthcare provider order on a short-term or long-term basis?
3. What role may herbal remedies play in anxiety control and sleep induction? What specific herbs might Seraphina be using?

Additional Case Study

Craig Edwards is a 46-year-old sales representative working at a respected car dealership in the community. With the economy, his income has dropped significantly because it is partially based on commission and he is worried that he is not able to provide for his family. Craig begins to experience insomnia, difficulty concentrating, and other symptoms related to his anxiety. His healthcare provider prescribes a short-term course of lorazepam (Ativan) to help him through this difficult period.

1. What adverse effects are associated with this drug therapy?
2. What information should Craig receive about this medication?
3. What nonpharmacologic measures can the nurse recommend to Craig to assist him in feeling better about his current situation?

Chapter Review

1. A nurse should advise a patient who is receiving lorazepam (Ativan) about the adverse effects of this medication, which include:

1. Tachypnea.
2. Astigmatism.
3. Ataxia.
4. Euphoria.

2. The patient with insomnia is being treated with temazepam (Restoril). The nurse monitors for therapeutic effectiveness by noting which of the following?

1. Sleeping in 3-hour intervals, awaking for a short time, and then returning to sleep
2. Feeling less anxiety during activities of daily living
3. Having fewer episodes of panic attacks when stressed
4. Sleeping 7 hours without awakening

3. Which of these statements, if made by a patient, would indicate that further instruction is needed about alprazolam (Xanax)?

1. "I will stop smoking by undergoing hypnosis."
2. "I will not drive immediately after I take this medication."
3. "I will stop the medicine when I feel less anxious."
4. "I will take my medication with food if my stomach feels upset."

4. The nurse should question a healthcare provider's order of phenobarbital for the patient with which condition?

1. Seizure disorder
2. Panic disorder
3. Prior to a bronchoscopy
4. Prior to receiving a general anesthetic

5. The nurse is caring for a patient receiving a sedative–hypnotic. Which adverse effect associated with this drug therapy is the highest priority for the nurse?

1. Urinary incontinence
2. Activity intolerance
3. Fall risk
4. Poor nutritional intake

6. The patient, who is receiving benzodiazepines, is a two-pack-per-day cigarette smoker. The nurse expects to administer a/an _______ dose of this medication.

1. larger
2. smaller
3. extra
4. half

See Appendix A for answers to critical thinking questions, case study questions and review questions.

References

American Psychiatric Association. (2017). *What are anxiety disorders?* https://www.psychiatry.org/patients-families/anxiety-disorders/what-are-anxiety-disorders

Andersen, L. P., Gögenur, I., Rosenberg, J., & Reiter, R. J. (2016). The safety of melatonin in humans. *Clinical Drug Investigation, 36*, 169–175. https://doi.org/10.1007/s40261-015-0368-5

Anxiety and Depression Association of America. (2018). *Facts and statistics.* https://www.adaa.org/about-adaa/press-room/facts-statistics

Cousins, L., & Goodyer, I. M. (2015). Antidepressants and the adolescent brain. *Journal of Psychopharmacology, 29*, 545–555. https://doi.org/10.1177/0269881115573542

De Oliveira, I., De Souza, V., Motta, V., & Da-Silva, S. (2015). Effects of oral vitamin C supplementation on anxiety in students: A double-blind, randomized, placebo-controlled trial. *Pakistan Journal of Biological Sciences, 18*, 11–18. https://doi.org/10.3923/pjbs.2015.11.18

Khurshid, K. A. (2018). Comorbid insomnia and psychiatric disorders: An update. *Innovations in Clinical Neuroscience, 15*(3–4), 28–32.

National Center for Complementary and Integrative Health. (2019). *Melatonin: What you need to know.* https://www.nccih.nih.gov/health/melatonin-what-you-need-to-know

National Institute of Mental Health. (n.d.). *Antidepressant medications for children and adolescents: Information for parents and caregivers.* https://www.nimh.nih.gov/health/topics/child-and-adolescent-mental-health/antidepressant-medications-for-children-and-adolescents-information-for-parents-and-caregivers.shtml

National Institute of Mental Health. (2017). *Any anxiety disorder*. https://www.nimh.nih.gov/health/statistics/any-anxiety-disorder.shtml

Polanczyk, G. V., Salum, G. A., Sugaya, L. S., Caye, A. K., & Rohde, L. A. (2015). Annual research review: A meta-analysis of the worldwide prevalence of mental disorders in children and adolescents. *Journal of Child Psychology and Psychiatry*, *56*, 345–365. https://doi.org/10.1111/jcpp.12381

World Health Organization. (2020). *Child and adolescent mental health*. https://www.who.int/mental_health/maternal-child/child_adolescent/en/

Selected Bibliography

Barateau, L., & Dauvilliers, Y. (2019). Recent advances in treatment for narcolepsy. *Therapeutic Advances in Neurological Disorders*. https://doi.org/10.1177/1756286419875622

Bhatt, N. V. (2019). *Anxiety disorders*. Medscape. http://emedicine.medscape.com/article/286227-overview

Bui, E., King, F., & Melaragno, A. (2019). Pharmacotherapy of anxiety disorders in the 21st century: A call for novel approaches. *General Psychiatry*, *32*(6), e100136. https://doi.org/10.1136/gpsych-2019-100136

Cadet, M., Tucker, L., Allen, D. H., Lawal, E., Dickson, D., & Denis, A. M. (2019). Assessing for and managing chronic insomnia in primary care settings. *The Nurse Practitioner*, *44*(7), 27–35. https://doi.org/10.1097/01.NPR.0000559843.91496.20

Chawla, J. (2020). *Insomnia*. Medscape. https://emedicine.medscape.com/article/1187829-overview

Edmund, S. J., & Sheppard, K. G. (2018). The challenge of generalized anxiety disorder in primary care. *The Nurse Practitioner*, *43*(4), 14–18. https://doi.org/10.1097/01.NPR.0000531075.19182.0b

Gore, T. A. (2018). *Posttraumatic stress disorder*. Medscape. http://emedicine.medscape.com/article/288154-overview

Harris, T., & Nikles, J. (2018). Herbal medicines used in the treatment of chronic insomnia and how they influence sleep patterns: A review. *Journal of Complementary Medicine and Alternative Healthcare*, *6*. https://doi.org/10.19080/JCMAH.2018.06.555680

Hassinger, A. B., Bletnisky, N., Dudekula, R., & El-Solh, A. A. (2020). Selecting a pharmacotherapy regimen for patients with chronic insomnia. *Expert Opinion on Pharmacotherapy*, *21*(9), 1035–1043. https://doi.org/10.1080/14656566.2020.1743265

Janto, K., Prichard, J. R., & Pusalavidyasagar, S. (2018). An update on dual orexin receptor antagonists and their potential role in insomnia therapeutics. *Journal of Clinical Sleep Medicine*, *14*(8), 1399–1408. https://doi.org/10.5664/jcsm.7282

Maruyama, T., Matsumura, M., Sakai, N., & Nishino, S. (2016). The pathogenesis of narcolepsy, current treatments and prospective therapeutic targets. *Expert Opinion on Orphan Drugs*, *4*, 63–82. https://doi.org/10.1517/21678707.2016.1117973

Sateia, M. J., Buysse, D. J., Krystal, A. D., Neubauer, D. N., & Heald, J. L. (2017). Clinical practice guideline for the pharmacologic treatment of chronic insomnia in adults: An American Academy of Sleep Medicine clinical practice guideline. *Journal of Clinical Sleep Medicine*, *13*(2), 307–349. https://doi.org/10.5664/jcsm.6470

Thorpy, M. J., & Bogan, R. K. (2020). Update on the pharmacologic management of narcolepsy: mechanisms of action and clinical implications. *Sleep Medicine*, *68*, 97–109. https://doi.org/10.1016/j.sleep.2019.09.001

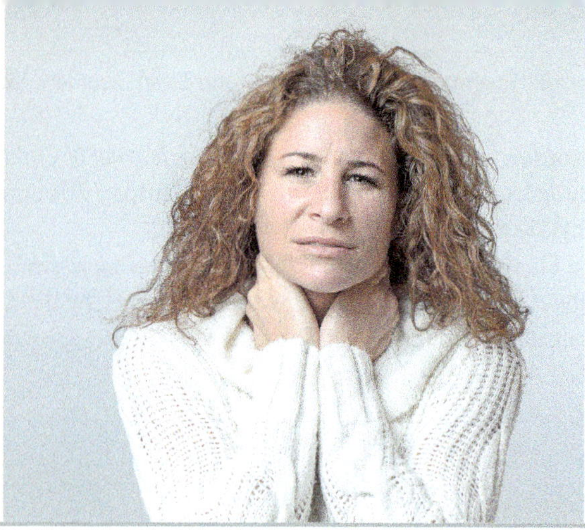

"For the past 4 to 5 weeks my wife, Adelphia, has been having problems. She doesn't get up to see that the children are off to school, dinner is not started when I get home from work at 6:00 p.m., no housework or laundry has been done, she is frequently still in pajamas with her hair uncombed, and obviously has not showered or brushed her teeth. Her friends say that Adelphia has not returned their calls in weeks."

—*"Charlie Williams," Adelphia's husband*

Chapter 19
Pharmacotherapy of Mood Disorders

Chapter Outline

Learning Outcomes

After reading this chapter, the student should be able to:

1. Compare and contrast the major categories of mood disorders and their symptoms.
2. Explain the pathophysiology of major depression and bipolar disorder.
3. Discuss the nurse's role in the assessment of patients with mood disorders.
4. Identify the relationship between suicide and depression.
5. Describe the nurse's role in the pharmacologic and nonpharmacologic management of mood disorders.
6. For each of the classes shown in the chapter outline, identify the prototype and representative drugs and explain the mechanism(s) of drug action, primary indications, contraindications, significant drug interactions, pregnancy data and important adverse effects.
7. Apply clinical judgement to care for patients receiving pharmacotherapy for mood disorders.

Key Terms

Definitions of the terms in bold may be found in the Glossary.

Inappropriate or unusually intense emotions are among the leading mental health disorders. Although mood changes are a normal part of life, a patient may be diagnosed as having a mood disorder when they become prolonged and severe and impair functioning within the family, work environment, or interpersonal relationships,. The purpose of this chapter is to explain the role of pharmacotherapy in treating the two primary categories of mood disorders: major depression and bipolar disorder.

PharmFACT

From 2013 until 2016 over 8% of American adults aged 20 or older experienced depression in the previous 2 weeks. The prevalence of depression decreased as family income increased (Centers for Disease Control and Prevention [CDC], 2018).

Categories of Mood Disorders

19.1 The two primary categories of mood disorders are depression and bipolar disorder.

A **mood disorder** can be broadly defined as a persistent disturbance in mood that impairs an individual's ability to effectively deal with normal activities of daily living (ADLs). Mood disorders affect people of all cultures and ages, from children to older adults. Mood disorders are a major cause of disability and can significantly strain social relationships. They are a leading cause of absenteeism and diminished productivity in the workplace.

The diagnosis of mood disorders is often challenging; the line between normal emotion and a mood disorder is sometimes unclear. Because healthcare providers see patients for such brief periods, they must rely on patient self-reports or caregiver information, both of which are often quite subjective.

Mood disorders can present with a wide range of symptoms, which has resulted in classification of the disorder into the following categories:

- **Major depressive disorder.** When people use the word *depression*, they are most often referring to major depressive disorder. This is sometimes called *clinical depression*.
- **Persistent depressive disorder (dysthymic disorder).** This is mild, chronic depression that persists for at least 2 continuous years.
- **Premenstrual dysphoric disorder.** Depression coinciding 1 week before the onset of menses followed by resolution after onset. Symptoms include irritability, anger, depressed mood, hopelessness, or marked affective lability.
- **Bipolar 1 disorder.** Formerly called *manic depression*, the patient alternates between intense excitement (mania) and a depressive disorder.
- **Bipolar 2 disorder.** Includes less intense mania symptoms (hypomania) that last for at least 1 week and significantly impact social functioning. The patient with bipolar 2 will experience major depression, which may be more prominent than the hypomania.
- **Cyclothymic disorder.** A mild form of bipolar disorder in which the patient alternates between hypomania and mild depression for a period of at least 2 years. Largely undiagnosed, many of these patients will eventually develop bipolar disorder.

Mood disorders often coexist with other conditions. For example, about 50% of patients diagnosed with major depression also meet the criteria for an anxiety disorder (see Chapter 18). Of those patients with mood disorder, 25–40% have a comorbid substance abuse condition. Those with chronic medical conditions such as hypertension (HTN) or arthritis have a higher incidence of depression. The most serious of the comorbid conditions is suicide.

Major Depressive Disorder

19.2 Major depressive disorder is characterized by a depressed mood, with accompanying symptoms, that lasts at least 2 weeks.

Depression is a disorder characterized by a sad or despondent mood that becomes out of proportion to actual life events. Depression can manifest as an extremely diverse set of symptoms, including lack of energy, sleep disturbances, abnormal eating patterns, or feelings of despair, guilt, and hopelessness. Depression is the most common mental health disorder, affecting women between the ages of 25 and 45 more than any other group. Depression may result in suicide, more frequently in men. Many people who are depressed never seek or receive care for their condition.

Major depressive disorder is diagnosed when the patient has a depressed mood that lasts for a minimum of 2 weeks and which is present for most of the day, every day, or almost every day. In addition, at least five of the symptoms shown in Table 19.1 must be present. Depressed moods caused by general medical conditions or by substances such as alcohol or other central nervous system (CNS) depressants do not warrant a diagnosis of major depressive disorder. For the purposes of this text, the terms *depression* and *major depressive disorder* are considered interchangeable unless otherwise specified.

Once a diagnosis of a mood disorder is made, additional details about the condition may be provided by the healthcare provider in the form of "specifiers." The use

Table 19.1 Symptoms of Depression

To be diagnosed with major depressive disorder the patient must have diminished mood and at least five of the following:	
Diminished interest in almost all activities	Fatigue or loss of energy
Significant weight gain or abnormal eating patterns	Feelings of worthlessness
Insomnia or hypersomnia	Reduced ability to concentrate; indecisiveness
Psychomotor agitation or retardation	Obsessed with death; expresses desire to commit suicide
Additional symptoms of depression	
Staying in bed most of the day and night	Lack of interest in personal appearance or sex
Not going to work or unable to function effectively at work	Avoiding psychosocial and interpersonal interactions
Vague physical symptoms (gastrointestinal [GI] pain, joint or muscle pain, or headaches)	Neglecting usual household chores

of specifiers gives mental health professionals more detailed information about the disorder and its treatment. Specifiers are best thought of as subcategories of major depressive disorder and bipolar disorder. Some of the specifiers used with depression include with or without psychotic features, single episode or recurrent, melancholic features, atypical features, and catatonic features. Two additional important specifiers are peripartum onset and seasonal onset.

Up to 80% of new mothers experience brief "baby blues" or **peripartum depression**, which can occur during pregnancy or within 4 weeks after the birth of a baby. About 10–15% of these women will experience major depression within the first 6 months postdelivery, which is likely related to the dramatic hormonal shifts that occur during that period. Along with the hormonal changes, additional situational stresses such as changing responsibilities at work and at home, single parenthood, and caring for children and for aging parents may contribute to the onset of symptoms. Because of the potentially serious consequences of peripartum-onset depression, some states mandate that all new mothers receive information about these mood disorders prior to their discharge after giving birth. All levels of healthcare providers treating new mothers are encouraged to conduct routine screening for symptoms of peripartum mood disorders.

During the dark winter months, some patients experience a type of depression known as **seasonal affective disorder**. Seasonal affective disorder is more common in areas such as Alaska, where the days are very short during the winter months and there is little natural sunlight. This type of depression is associated with a reduced release of the hormone melatonin from the pineal gland. The condition is generally self-limiting and resolves when spring arrives. Exposing patients on a regular basis to specific wavelengths of light may relieve this type of depression and prevent future episodes.

Pathophysiology of Depression

19.3 The pathophysiology of depression has biological, genetic, and environmental components.

Depression is one of the most frequently diagnosed mental health conditions. Although the etiology of depression is incompletely understood, several theories have been proposed to explain the causes of depression and why some people are predisposed to developing the disease. The etiology and pathogenesis are influenced by multiple, complex variables.

Research attempting to identify the biological causes of depression has focused on the levels and function of neurotransmitters in the limbic system of the brain. The limbic system is the region that regulates emotions (see Chapters 17 and 18). Major depression has been associated with abnormally low levels of neurotransmitters such as norepinephrine, serotonin, and dopamine in this region. Although it is well known that some of the antidepressant medications act by increasing the levels of these neurotransmitters, scientists have yet to discover what role each specific neurotransmitter plays in the development of major depressive disorder. Does having depression deplete the brain of these neurotransmitters, or does a loss of neurotransmitters cause depression? The answers remain elusive.

Certain hormonal abnormalities are associated with depression, suggesting that the endocrine system also plays an important role in the pathogenesis of the disease. About half of those who are depressed have abnormally high serum cortisol levels. Cortisol mobilizes the body for stress situations and is thought to reduce serotonin levels in the brain, bringing about symptoms of depression. Recall from Chapter 18, that high cortisol levels are also associated with anxiety. Hypothyroidism is associated with depression. In some patients, therapy with thyroid hormone (T_3) results in a marked improvement in mood.

Depression clearly has a genetic component. Major depression is 1.5 to 3 times more common in individuals who have a first-degree relative (parent or sibling) with depression compared to the general population. In identical twins, when one twin is diagnosed with depression, the other twin has a 50% probability of acquiring the disorder. This relationship holds true whether the twins were raised together or separately. Even fraternal twins have a 19% chance of developing depression when the other twin is diagnosed, which is a percentage higher than that of the general population.

Environmental causes of depression include prolonged stress at work or at home, loss of a loved one, and other traumatic life events. Various childhood events have been associated with an increased risk of adult depression, including sexual or physical abuse and death of, separation from, or mental illness of a parent.

CONNECTION Checkpoint 19.1

From what you learned in Chapter 17, what are the connections between the limbic system, the hypothalamus, and the cerebrum, and how can these connections be used to explain symptoms of depression?

Assessment of Depression

19.4 Assessment and diagnosis of depression are a collaborative effort among healthcare providers.

For proper diagnosis and treatment to occur, the recognition of depression must be a collaborative effort among healthcare providers, patients, and caregivers. The first step in implementing appropriate treatment for depression is a thorough medical examination because the diagnosis of depression begins by ruling out other medical conditions. Certain medications such as corticosteroids, beta blockers, levodopa, antipsychotic drugs, oral contraceptives, and CNS depressants can cause symptoms of depression. Depression may be mimicked by a variety of medical and neurologic disorders, ranging from B-vitamin deficiencies to thyroid gland malfunction to early Alzheimer's disease. If medical causes for the depression are discovered, proper treatment of the underlying disorder may be sufficient to resolve symptoms of depression. If causes for the depression cannot be identified, a mental health professional may be consulted to perform a comprehensive psychologic evaluation.

Because they are comorbid with depression in a significant number of patients, inquiries should be made about alcohol and drug use and any thoughts about suicide. The initial examination should also include questions about any family history of depressive illness. The manifestation of depression that is most obvious to those surrounding someone who is depressed is a change in attitude toward usual daily activities. The patient loses interest in work, school, or other hobbies or activities that he or she previously enjoyed.

Severe depressive illness, particularly that which is recurrent, will require both medication and psychotherapy to achieve optimal outcomes. Daily outpatient visits to a treatment facility may be necessary when beginning treatment, then tapered to a less frequent schedule as improvement is noted. Some patients, especially those at high risk for suicide, will require an initial period of hospitalization where continuous monitoring is provided.

Depression remains greatly underdiagnosed among older adults despite the fact that as many as 6 million Americans over the age of 65 have this disorder. Of this group, only about 10% receive treatment. Older patients may be reluctant to admit to depression, seeing this as a sign of weakness or an inability to continue to care for themselves. Depression in the older adult may be manifested as difficulty making decisions and as a growing reluctance to leave the home. Feelings of despair, lack of self-worth, and guilt are common.

Factors that contribute to depression in the older adult include loss of spouse or children; the need to move from a long-term residence to a smaller home or in with other family or to assisted living; loss of friends and other support systems; being unmarried; living alone; having multiple health challenges; the expense of polypharmacy; decreased finances; and worry about end-of-life issues.

CONNECTIONS: Advanced Practice Application

Perinatal and Postpartum Depression: A Screening Update

According to the Centers for Disease Control and Prevention (CDC) Pregnancy Risk Assessment Monitoring System (PRAMS), a surveillance system designed to identify groups of women and infants at high risk for health problems and to measure progress toward goals in improving the health of mothers and infants, the overall prevalence of depression in women in the United States during pregnancy and within a year after giving birth is around 11.5% (CDC, 2019). The overall incidence is likely to be even higher, given that the PRAMS report reflects only 27 states and 41% of U.S. births (Ko et al., 2017). Characteristics of women with the highest prevalence of developing peripartum and postpartum depression include those under 24 years old; who are unmarried; who smoke; those that are American Indian, Alaskan Native, or Asian/Pacific Islander; who have a history of recent stressful life events; and those who gave birth to newborns with low birth weight or who required care in the neonatal intensive care unit (CDC, 2019; Ko et al., 2017). Evans and colleagues (2015) found that first-time mothers, those with low social support, and those with a history of substance abuse are also at higher risk, with the strongest predictors being a personal history or family history of anxiety and/or depression and low socioeconomic status.

While the American College of Obstetricians and Gynecologists (2017) recommends that clinicians screen women at least once during the perinatal period for mood disorders, the American Academy of Pediatrics, the National Association of Pediatric Nurse Practitioners, and the Centers for Medicare and Medicaid Services all recommend screening women for depression starting at prenatal visits, with screening continuing during well-child visits with pediatricians for at least the first year after delivery.

19.5 The majority of patients who attempt suicide have major depression.

Suicide is defined as the intentional act of ending one's life. Suicide is the 10th leading cause of death in the United States; over 48,000 people take their own lives every year (American Foundation for Suicide Prevention, 2020). No age group, income level, educational level, race, religion, or other demographic group is exempt from it. Comorbid conditions include mood disorders, psychoses, personality disorder, anxiety disorders, severe insomnia, chronic alcohol or substance use, chronic disabling or painful disease, and family history, especially in the same-sex parent.

If major depression or bipolar disorder is left untreated, the risk for suicide is very high. Early studies led the U.S. Food and Drug Administration (FDA) to conclude that the use of antidepressant medications *increased* the suicide rate. This prompted the FDA (2004) to issue a controversial black box warning indicating that antidepressant medications may be associated with an increased risk of suicidal thinking and behavior in children and adolescents. This black box warning was later expanded to include young adults 18 to 25 years of age. When the black box warning was issued, the number of prescriptions for antidepressants declined.

Numerous subsequent studies have been unable to confirm the relationship between antidepressant use and suicide. Indeed, when the use of antidepressants declined, the suicide rate went up. Some have called for a removal of the black box warning because it can lead to healthcare providers undertreating depression in young people (Fornaro et al., 2019).

So what interventions can the healthcare provider implement to reduce the potential for suicidal behavior during antidepressant therapy? Careful monitoring of the patient is the simplest yet most important intervention, especially children and young adults. Weekly patient or caregiver contact may be necessary until the medication begins to effectively elevate mood, which could be as long as 12 weeks. A patient who has had a previous suicide attempt is at higher risk and must be more carefully monitored. Any patient who verbalizes about committing suicide must be taken seriously. The nurse should judiciously monitor all prescribed drugs because suicidal patients often take overdoses of their medications (including those prescribed to treat the depression!). Therapy with multiple CNS depressants such as for pain, anxiety, insomnia, and depression is strongly discouraged because these drugs produce additive sedation. Worsening symptoms of depression must be reported immediately because these may indicate that the drug is not working or that the patient is not compliant with pharmacotherapy. Switching to a different antidepressant or even hospitalization may be necessary for persistent major depression.

Nonpharmacologic Therapies for Depression

19.6 Depression is sometimes treated with nonpharmacologic therapies.

Although pharmacotherapy is the standard treatment for patients with major depression, other therapies may be beneficial for some patients. Indeed, psychotherapy may be the treatment of choice if the patient is willing to participate and the depressive state is mild to moderate in intensity. Other nonpharmacologic therapies for depression are shown in Table 19.2.

Older nonpharmacologic treatments include cognitive–behavioral therapies to help patients change negative styles of thought and behavior that are often associated with their depression. These therapies focus on resolving the patients' internal conflicts by looking at the influence of past experiences on current behavior and how behavior is influenced by emotional factors. These therapies are sometimes postponed until the acute depressive symptoms have improved. **Bright light therapy** (or *phototherapy*), which lasts from 30 to 90 minutes daily and can be conducted in the patient's home, is especially useful for people with seasonal affective disorder.

Table 19.2 Nonpharmacologic Therapies for Major Depression

Type	Definition
Bright light therapy (phototherapy)	Therapy that uses artificial lighting that is 5–20 times brighter than usual indoor lighting; it is used to simulate natural sunlight in areas where there is little natural sunlight for several months of the year.
Cognitive-behavioral therapy	Therapy that helps patients change the negative styles of thought and behavior that are often associated with their depression.
Electroconvulsive therapy	The induction of a brief convulsion by passing an electric current through the brain as therapy, especially in patients who have not responded to pharmacotherapy.
Interpersonal therapy	Therapy focusing on the patient's disturbed personal relationships that both cause and exacerbate the depression.
Psychodynamic therapy	Therapy focusing on resolving a patient's internal conflicts.
Repetitive transcranial magnetic stimulation therapy	Used for treatment-resistant depression; a device administers magnetic pulses through the brain to stimulate neurons regulating emotions.
Vagus nerve stimulation	Places a nerve stimulator into the patient's chest with an electrode with ends wrapped around the left vagus nerve on the patient's neck; the device is programmed for frequency and intensity of stimulus; used for resistant depression that has not responded to at least four other therapies.

In patients with serious and life-threatening mood disorders that are unresponsive to pharmacotherapy and psychotherapy, **electroconvulsive therapy (ECT)** continues to be a useful treatment. ECT induces a brief seizure by passing an electric current into the brain while the patient is anesthetized. A muscle relaxant is given prior to the treatment and the patient is unaware of the treatment or convulsion. Typically, 6 to 12 treatments are needed to relieve depression. In severe, refractory cases ECT may be continued for several years.

Repetitive transcranial magnetic stimulation (rTMS) is an emerging therapy for major depression. rTMS is a noninvasive procedure that passes an electromagnetic pulse through a coil placed on the scalp. Treatments with rTMS devices are generally for 30 to 40 minutes five times a week for 4 to 6 weeks. rTMS has minimal side effects, such as headache, lightheadedness, and scalp discomfort at the sight of administration.

Vagus nerve stimulation (VNS) involves the surgical implantation of a 3- to 4-inch battery-powered device into the patient's chest. An electrode is threaded through the subcutaneous tissue from the device to the vagus nerve on the left side of the neck. The left vagus connects to the brainstem and deep brain structures thought to be involved in epilepsy and some psychiatric disorders such as major depression. Stimulating these fibers affects the concentration of gamma aminobutyric acid (GABA) and other neurotransmitters in that area. VNS is approved in the United States for treating epilepsy and bipolar disorder and for the adjunctive treatment of chronic depression that is unresponsive to antidepressant medications.

Pharmacotherapy of Depression

19.7 The mechanism of action of antidepressants involves modulation of neurotransmitter levels in the brain.

Antidepressants are medications used to enhance, elevate, or stabilize mood. They are used to treat all symptoms of major depressive disorder as well as the depressive phases of bipolar disorder. They are ineffective against the manic phases of bipolar disorder, and other drugs must be used to control those symptoms (see Section 19.12).

The antidepressants act by restoring normal neurotransmitter balances in specific regions of the brain. Depending on the medication, the primary neurotransmitters affected are norepinephrine, serotonin, and, to a lesser degree, dopamine. The two basic mechanisms of action are blocking the enzymatic breakdown of norepinephrine and slowing the reuptake of serotonin into neurons. Although antidepressants may not completely restore chemical balance, they help to manage depressive symptoms while the patient develops effective strategies for coping.

In addition to elevating mood, changing the neurotransmitter balance has a number of other effects on the brain. Some of the antidepressants have become major treatments for anxiety-related disorders such as phobia, obsessive–compulsive behavior, panic disorder, and generalized anxiety disorder, as presented in Chapter 18. Certain antidepressants are also beneficial as adjuvant analgesics in the pharmacotherapy of pain (see Chapter 25). Antidepressants are beneficial in treating depression that is associated with painful, chronic conditions such as fibromyalgia or muscle spasticity (see Chapter 23).

Once patients begin to feel less depressed and more hopeful, many seek to discontinue drug therapy due to the expense of the medication or because they are experiencing uncomfortable adverse effects. Nurses must be aware that many patients taking antidepressants stop taking their medication without notifying their healthcare provider. Unfortunately, about half of these patients will relapse within 6 months of discontinuing antidepressant therapy; the percentage increases to 85% after 3 years. It is important to teach patients that daily antidepressant dosing is required and that adherence to the healthcare provider's instructions is essential for the long-term maintenance of mental health.

When administered at therapeutic doses, all antidepressants have similar effectiveness; therefore, the specific choice of medication is not usually based on this factor. The treatment of depression, however, is highly individualized and patients who are unresponsive to one class of medications may respond favorably to drugs from a different class. In fact, patients may respond differently to drugs within the *same* class. Furthermore, the spectrum of adverse effects differs among the classes, and patients may find that drugs from one class are better tolerated than another. Overall, about 65% of patients will respond favorably to antidepressant pharmacotherapy. Success rates improve to 85% when psychotherapy or alternative or adjunctive medicine is used along with antidepressant medications. The four primary classes of antidepressants, shown in Table 19.3, are as follows:

- Selective serotonin reuptake inhibitors (SSRIs)
- Atypical antidepressants
- Tricyclic antidepressants (TCAs)
- Monoamine oxidase inhibitors (MAOIs)

Therapy with antidepressants is generally begun with low doses of a drug from the SSRI class. If no improvement in mood is noted after about 4 weeks, the dose of the drug is increased. Continued lack of response may indicate that the patient is not taking the medication as prescribed or that a drug from a different class should be used, such as a TCA or an atypical antidepressant. It is important for patients to understand that antidepressant therapy may extend for many years. In general, antidepressant therapy should continue for a minimum of 6 months after the depressive symptoms resolve to prevent uncomfortable withdrawal symptoms and the potential for rebound depression.

Table 19.3 Antidepressant Drugs

<table>
<tr><th>Drug</th><th>Route and Adult Dose (Maximum Dose Where Indicated)</th><th>Adverse Effects</th></tr>
<tr><td colspan="3">Selective Serotonin Reuptake Inhibitors</td></tr>
<tr><td>citalopram (Celexa)</td><td>PO: 20–40 mg once daily (max: 40 mg/day)</td><td rowspan="8">Nausea and vomiting, dry mouth, insomnia, somnolence, headache, nervousness, anxiety, diarrhea, dizziness, anorexia, fatigue, sexual dysfunction, weight changes
<u>Stevens–Johnson syndrome (SJS), serotonin syndrome, suicidal ideation in children and young adults</u></td></tr>
<tr><td>escitalopram (Lexapro)</td><td>PO: 10–20 mg once daily (max: 20 mg/day)</td></tr>
<tr><td>fluoxetine (Prozac)</td><td>PO: 20 mg/day (max: 80 mg/day); when stable may switch to 90-mg sustained-release capsule once weekly (max: 90 mg/wk)</td></tr>
<tr><td>fluvoxamine (Luvox)</td><td>PO (extended release): 100 mg once daily at bedtime (max: 300 mg/day)</td></tr>
<tr><td>paroxetine (Paxil, Pexeva)</td><td>PO (immediate release): 20–50 mg once daily (max: 50 mg/day)</td></tr>
<tr><td></td><td>PO (controlled release): 25–62.5 mg daily (max: 62.5 mg/day)</td></tr>
<tr><td>sertraline (Zoloft)</td><td>PO: Start with 50 mg once daily and increase at weekly intervals as needed (max: 200 mg/day)</td></tr>
<tr><td>vortioxetine (Trintellix)</td><td>PO: 5–20 mg once daily (max: 20 mg/day)</td></tr>
<tr><td colspan="3">Atypical Antidepressants</td></tr>
<tr><td>amoxapine</td><td>PO: Start with 50 mg bid–tid and increase to 100 mg bid–tid by the end of the first wk (max: 400 mg/day)</td><td rowspan="6">Insomnia, nausea and vomiting, dry mouth, constipation, increased blood pressure and heart rate, dizziness, sweating, agitation, blurred vision, headache, tremor, drowsiness, somnolence, increased appetite, orthostatic hypotension
<u>SJS; seizures; vaginal, uterine, or anal hemorrhage; suicidal ideation; priapism; parkinsonism (amoxapine); elevated hepatic enzymes (mirtazapine); bone marrow suppression (mirtazapine); liver failure (nefazodone)</u></td></tr>
<tr><td>bupropion (Forfivo XL, Wellbutrin, others)</td><td>PO: 100 mg tid (immediate release), 150 mg bid (sustained release), or 300 mg once daily (extended release) (max: 450 mg/day)</td></tr>
<tr><td>mirtazapine (Remeron)</td><td>PO: 15 mg/day in a single dose at bedtime (max: 45 mg/day)</td></tr>
<tr><td>nefazodone</td><td>PO: 50–100 mg bid (max: 600 mg/day)</td></tr>
<tr><td>trazodone</td><td>PO: 150 mg/day (max: 600 mg/day)</td></tr>
<tr><td>vilazodone (Viibryd)</td><td>PO: 10–40 mg once daily (max: 40 mg/day)</td></tr>
<tr><td colspan="3">Atypical Antidepressants: Serotonin–Norepinephrine Reuptake Inhibitors</td></tr>
<tr><td>desvenlafaxine (Pristiq)</td><td>PO: 50 mg once daily (max: 100 mg/day)</td><td rowspan="4">Nausea, dry mouth, constipation, sweating, agitation, somnolence, decreased appetite, changes in weight (loss or gain), increased blood glucose level (duloxetine), elevated blood pressure and heart rate (levomilnacipran)
<u>Serotonin syndrome, suicidal ideation, hepatotoxicity, syncope, neuroleptic malignant syndrome, abnormal bleeding, HTN (desvenlafaxine, venlafaxine), seizures</u></td></tr>
<tr><td>duloxetine (Cymbalta)</td><td>PO: 30–60 mg/day in 1–2 divided doses (max: 60–120 mg/day)</td></tr>
<tr><td>levomilnacipran (Fetzima)</td><td>PO: 40–120 mg daily (max: 120 mg/day)</td></tr>
<tr><td>venlafaxine (Effexor)</td><td>PO (immediate release): 75–375 mg/day in divided doses (max: 375 mg/day
PO (extended release): 37.5–225 mg/once daily (max: 225 mg/day)</td></tr>
<tr><td colspan="3">Tricyclic Antidepressants</td></tr>
<tr><td>amitriptyline (Elavil)</td><td>PO: 25–100 mg/day (max: 300 mg/day)</td><td rowspan="11">Drowsiness, sedation, dizziness, orthostatic hypotension, dry mouth, constipation, urinary retention, blurred vision, mydriasis, tachycardia
<u>Bone marrow depression, seizures, dysrhythmias, heart block, myocardial infarction, hepatitis, acute renal failure</u></td></tr>
<tr><td>amoxapine</td><td>PO: 50–100 mg bid–tid (max: 400 mg/day)</td></tr>
<tr><td>clomipramine (Anafranil)</td><td>PO: 25 mg once daily (max: 250 mg/day)</td></tr>
<tr><td>desipramine (Norpramin)</td><td>PO: 75–300 mg/day (max: 300 mg/day)</td></tr>
<tr><td>doxepin (Silenor)</td><td>PO (generic for depression or anxiety): 25–150 mg/day in divided doses (max: 300 mg/day)</td></tr>
<tr><td></td><td>PO (Silenor for insomnia): 3–6 mg at bedtime</td></tr>
<tr><td>imipramine (Tofranil)</td><td>PO: 75–150 mg/day (max: 300 mg/day)</td></tr>
<tr><td>maprotiline</td><td>PO: 75–150 mg/day in divided doses (max: 225 mg/day)</td></tr>
<tr><td>nortriptyline (Pamelor)</td><td>PO: 25 mg tid or qid (max: 150 mg/day)</td></tr>
<tr><td>protriptyline (Vivactil)</td><td>PO: 15–40 mg/day in divided doses (max: 60 mg/day)</td></tr>
<tr><td>trimipramine (Surmontil)</td><td>PO: 50–150 mg/day in divided doses (max: 200 mg/day)</td></tr>
<tr><td colspan="3">Monoamine Oxidase Inhibitors</td></tr>
<tr><td>isocarboxazid (Marplan)</td><td>PO: 10–40 mg/day (max: 60 mg/day)</td><td rowspan="4">Drowsiness, insomnia, orthostatic hypotension, blurred vision, nausea, constipation, anorexia, dry mouth, urinary retention, sexual dysfunction, overactivity
<u>Hypertensive crisis, circulatory collapse, dysrhythmias</u></td></tr>
<tr><td>phenelzine (Nardil)</td><td>PO: 15 mg tid (max: 90 mg/day)</td></tr>
<tr><td>selegiline (Emsam)</td><td>Transdermal: one patch (6 mg/day)</td></tr>
<tr><td>tranylcypromine (Parnate)</td><td>PO: 30 mg/day (max: 60 mg/day)</td></tr>
</table>

Note: *Italics* indicate common adverse effects. <u>Underline</u> indicates serious adverse effects.

Selective Serotonin Reuptake Inhibitors

19.8 Selective serotonin reuptake inhibitors are the preferred drugs for treating depression due to their low incidence of serious adverse effects.

Serotonin is a neurotransmitter in the CNS that is found in high concentrations in certain neurons in the hypothalamus, limbic system, medulla, and spinal cord. It is essential for several body activities, including the cycling between non–rapid eye movement and rapid eye movement sleep, pain perception, and emotions. Lack of adequate serotonin in the limbic regions of the CNS can lead to depression. The actions of serotonin are terminated when it is metabolized to a less active substance by the enzyme monoamine oxidase (MAO). This process is illustrated in Figure 19.1. In the scientific literature, serotonin is commonly referred to by its chemical name, 5-hydroxytryptamine or 5-HT.

In the 1970s, it became increasingly clear that serotonin had a more substantial role in depression than initially thought. Although TCAs and MAOIs had been in use for decades, clinicians did not understand how serotonin levels relieved symptoms of depression. Ongoing efforts to discover antidepressants with fewer adverse effects led to the development of the selective serotonin reuptake inhibitors, which were first introduced in 1987. Whereas the TCAs inhibit the reuptake of *both* norepinephrine and serotonin into presynaptic nerve terminals, the SSRIs *selectively* target serotonin. Increased levels of serotonin in the synaptic spaces induce complex neurotransmitter changes in presynaptic and postsynaptic neurons in the brain. Essentially, presynaptic receptors become less sensitive, and postsynaptic receptors become more sensitive.

SSRIs are as effective in treating depression as the TCAs but exhibit fewer significant adverse effects. Sympathomimetic effects (increased heart rate and HTN) and anticholinergic effects (dry mouth, blurred vision, urinary retention, and constipation) are less common with SSRIs. Sedation occurs less frequently, and cardiotoxicity is not observed. The greater safety profile of the SSRIs has led to their current status as first-line drugs for depression.

One of the most common adverse effects of SSRIs relates to sexual dysfunction. Up to 70% of both men and women can experience decreased libido and inability to reach orgasm. In men, delayed ejaculation and impotence may occur. For patients who are sexually active, these adverse effects may be serious enough to cause nonadherence with pharmacotherapy, and a different antidepressant may be indicated. The SSRIs can cause weight gain, which may also lead to discontinuation. Other common adverse effects include nausea, headache, nervousness, and insomnia.

All drugs in the SSRI class have equal effectiveness and similar adverse effects. In general, SSRIs elevate mood more quickly than TCAs, which is a major advantage when treating acute depressive disorders. The SSRIs are used for a wide variety of other mental health disorders, including obsessive–compulsive disorder (OCD), social anxiety disorder, panic disorder, generalized anxiety disorder (GAD), post-traumatic stress disorder (PTSD), and premenstrual dysphoric disorder. They are one of the most widely prescribed drug classes in the United States.

Serotonin syndrome (SES) is a serious medical condition that can occur when a patient is taking multiple medications that affect the metabolism, synthesis, or reuptake of serotonin, causing this neurotransmitter to accumulate in neurons in the CNS. These drugs include SSRIs, MAOIs, TCAs, lithium, St. John's wort, opioids, and triptans. SES sometimes occurs as a result of illicit drug use because amphetamines, cocaine, MDMA (Ecstasy), and opioids also affect serotonin levels. Symptoms of SES include mental status changes (confusion, anxiety, restlessness, agitation), HTN, tremors or muscle rigidity, sweating, hyperpyrexia, and ataxia. Symptoms may begin as early as 2 hours after taking the first dose or be delayed for several weeks. Conservative treatment is to discontinue all serotonergic drugs and provide supportive care that stabilizes vital signs; the condition usually resolves in 24 hours. In severe cases, mechanical ventilation and administration of muscle relaxants such as benzodiazepines may be necessary. Agitated patients may require sedation and in severe cases serotonin antagonists such as cyproheptadine, risperidone (Risperdal), or olanzapine (Zyprexa) may be administered.

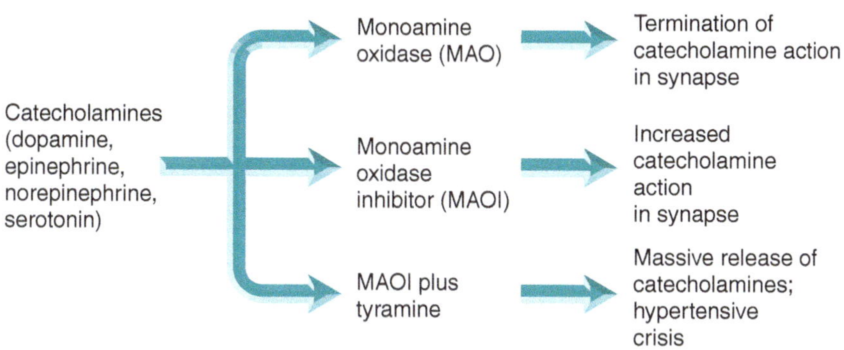

Figure 19.1 Catecholamines and monoamine oxidase.

PROTOTYPE DRUG Fluoxetine (Prozac)

Classification **Therapeutic:** Antidepressant, antianxiety drug
Pharmacologic: Selective serotonin reuptake inhibitor (SSRI)

Therapeutic Effects and Uses: Approved in 1987, fluoxetine was the first SSRI marketed to treat major depressive disorder in the United States. Fluoxetine was subsequently approved as the first medication to treat bulimia nervosa. It was also the first SSRI approved for the treatment of pediatric depression. It is approved for the treatment of OCD in both adults and children, panic disorder, and premenstrual dysphoric disorder.

Fluoxetine is available as tablets, capsules, oral solution, and delayed release capsules. Sarafem is a formulation of fluoxetine specifically marketed for premenstrual dysphoric disorder in a pulvule—a gelatin-based capsule. It is taken daily or for just the 2 weeks prior to an expected menses. Prozac Weekly is a capsule containing enteric-coated granules that allows for only one dose each week. Symbyax is a fixed-dose combination of fluoxetine and olanzapine that is indicated for bipolar disorder. Olanzapine, an antipsychotic drug, is marketed by itself as Zyprexa for schizophrenia and the manic phase of bipolar disorder.

Fluoxetine is used off-label to treat many other disorders involving multiple body systems. Off-label indications include anorexia nervosa, obesity, alcohol dependence in patients with alcoholism, fibromyalgia, autism, refractory orthostatic hypotension, premature ejaculation, and menopausal hot flashes. Although patients gradually begin to feel less depressed after about 2 weeks of therapy, optimal response may take 8 weeks or longer.

Fluoxetine is extensively metabolized in the liver to norfluoxetine, which has about the same pharmacologic activity as the parent drug. Fluoxetine and norfluoxetine have long half-lives; it takes 30 to 60 days after discontinuing the drug for them to be eliminated by the body. This duration is even more prolonged in patients with liver disease.

Mechanism of Action: All SSRIs block the uptake of the neurotransmitter serotonin (but not norepinephrine) at the neuronal presynaptic membrane. This increases the amount of neurotransmitter available at the postsynaptic receptor sites, thus enhancing the actions of serotonin.

Pharmacokinetics:

Route	PO
Absorption	Readily absorbed
Distribution	Widely distributed, including the cerebrospinal fluid; likely crosses the placenta; secreted in breast milk; 94% bound to plasma protein
Primary metabolism	Metabolized in the liver to norfluoxetine, an active metabolite
Primary excretion	Renal, small amounts in feces
Onset of action	Peak plasma level: 6–8 h
Duration of action	Half-life: 2–3 days

Adverse Effects: The most common adverse effects of fluoxetine are headache and nausea and vomiting, which diminish as therapy progresses. Other common GI effects include diarrhea, anorexia, cramping, and flatulence. Fluoxetine does not cause sedation; in fact, insomnia may occur in as many as 25% of patients receiving the drug. Fluoxetine also does not cause the serious cardiotoxicity, orthostatic hypotension, or anticholinergic effects seen with the TCAs. Fluctuations in weight are common. Significant anorexia and weight loss occur in 10–15% of patients, whereas others experience a weight gain of as much as 9 kg (20 lb) or more. Patients may experience various types of sexual dysfunction, including delayed ejaculation, impotence, anorgasmia, decreased libido, and priapism. The drug may induce seizures in patients with preexisting seizure disorders or during overdoses. Other adverse effects include cramping, constipation, poor concentration, diarrhea, hot flashes, palpitations, and nervousness. Serotonin syndrome can occur. Pediatric patients may experience personality disorders or hyperkinesia.

Abrupt withdrawal of fluoxetine or other SSRIs can result in a withdrawal syndrome; the patient may experience dizziness, headache, tremor, anxiety, dysphoria, and sensory disturbances. These symptoms usually begin 1 to 7 days after the last dose and may continue for 1 to 3 weeks. Because fluoxetine has an extended half-life and serum levels diminish gradually, withdrawal symptoms are generally less serious than those of the shorter-acting SSRIs. Tapering the dose over 2 weeks or longer can prevent withdrawal symptoms. **Black Box Warning:** Antidepressants increase the risk of suicidal thinking and behavior in children, adolescents, and young adults. Patients of all ages should be monitored and observed closely during therapy for clinical worsening, suicidal ideation, or unusual changes in behavior.

Contraindications/Precautions: Hypersensitivity to fluoxetine is a contraindication to using the drug. The drug should not be administered to patients with bipolar disorder because it may precipitate a manic episode. It must be used cautiously in patients with cardiac dysfunction (including prolonged QT interval), diabetes, or seizure disorders. Children or young adults with a history of attempted suicide should not receive fluoxetine. There are no known age-related precautions for use in older adults, but children may experience more behavioral adverse effects such as restlessness and insomnia.

Caution must be used when fluoxetine is administered late in pregnancy. The neonate may exhibit symptoms of withdrawal, including irritability, respiratory distress, tremors, abnormal crying, and, possibly, seizures. With supportive care, symptoms of withdrawal in the neonate will disappear in a few days. In most cases, the benefits of treating pregnant women who have major depression with fluoxetine are greater than the potential risks to the neonate.

Drug Interactions: Because fluoxetine inhibits multiple CYP450 isozymes, it has the potential to interact with many other drugs and herbal products. Medications that are metabolized by CYP450 may build to toxic levels due to their impaired metabolism. Some drugs affected by diminished metabolism include TCAs, phenothiazines, most atypical antipsychotics, certain antidysrhythmics, and benzodiazepines. Excessive sedation may occur if fluoxetine is given concurrently with other CNS depressants, including opioids, sedative–hypnotics, or alcohol. Taken concurrently with or within 14 days of MAOIs can result in serotonin syndrome or neuroleptic malignant syndrome. Concurrent use with warfarin, aspirin, or other nonsteroidal anti-inflammatory drugs (NSAIDs) may increase the risk of bleeding. Fluoxetine may cause an increased risk of toxicity to phenytoin, digoxin, or carbamazepine. Concurrent use with certain antipsychotics may lead to increased extrapyramidal symptoms such as akathisia, dystonia, tardive dyskinesia, and pseudoparkinsonism. Fluoxetine can increase the half-life of diazepam. Caution must also be used if the patient is taking lithium because fluoxetine may increase plasma levels of the drug. **Herbal/Food:** Increased CNS effects may occur if fluoxetine is given concurrently with lavender, kava, or hops. There is an increased risk of serotonin syndrome with the concurrent use of St. John's wort. Increased anticholinergic effects may result from the use of jimsonweed or corkwood. Because grapefruit juice may cause elevated serum levels of fluoxetine, it should be avoided during therapy.

Pregnancy: Human data on fluoxetine showed a small risk for cardiovascular malformations in infants whose mothers took the drug during the first trimester. Infants exposed during the third trimester showed a risk for pulmonary hypertension, cyanosis, apnea, feeding difficulty and other signs of distress upon delivery that resemble serotonin syndrome. Fluoxetine should be used during pregnancy and lactation only if the potential benefits justify the potential risks to the fetus and neonate.

Treatment of Overdose: Overdose can result in seizures, tachycardia, somnolence, and, rarely, death. Supportive treatment is indicated, including gastric lavage and activated charcoal. With intentional overdose, the possibility of multiple drug involvement should always be considered.

Clinician Responsibilities: Key clinical implications for patients receiving fluoxetine are included in Applied Clinical Judgment: Patients Receiving Pharmacotherapy with Antidepressants.

Drugs Similar to Fluoxetine (Prozac)

Other SSRIs include citalopram, escitalopram, fluvoxamine, paroxetine, sertraline, and vortioxetine. Unless otherwise noted below, all SSRIs have the same effects on the fetus and neonate and fluoxetine. All the SSRIs should be used during pregnancy and lactation only if the potential benefits justify the potential risks to the fetus and neonate.

Citalopram (Celexa): Citalopram was approved by the FDA in 1998 for the treatment of major depressive disorder in adults. Off-label uses include anxiety-related disorders such as GAD, social anxiety disorder, OCD, panic disorder, and PTSD. Other off-label uses include schizophrenia, binge-eating disorder, premenstrual dysphoric disorder, and menopausal hot flashes. Citalopram is available as regular tablets, as oral disintegrating tablets, or as an oral solution. It is almost identical structurally to escitalopram but is very different from other SSRIs. Older adults are more susceptible to the anticholinergic effects of citalopram than to other SSRIs. It causes fewer drug interactions than does fluoxetine. All other actions and adverse effects are the same as those of fluoxetine and escitalopram (including the black box warning regarding suicidal ideation). Citalopram should not be used with other medications that increase the QTc interval.

Escitalopram (Lexapro): Approved in 2002, escitalopram is one of the most frequently prescribed drugs in the United States. Approved indications include major depressive disorder and GAD in adults and in adolescents age 12 and older. It may be used off-label to treat social anxiety disorder, OCD, insomnia, and menopausal hot flashes. Structurally, it is nearly identical to citalopram, although it is more potent; 20 mg of escitalopram is bioequivalent to 40 mg of citalopram. It is available as a tablet or solution. Escitalopram has the same spectrum of adverse effects as fluoxetine and other SSRIs (including the black box warning regarding suicidal ideation). It elevates mood relatively quickly, in 1 to 2 weeks. Its safety and effectiveness in children younger than age 12 have not been established.

Fluvoxamine (Luvox): Approved in 1994, fluvoxamine is approved to treat OCD. It is the only SSRI not FDA approved to treat major depression, although it may be prescribed off-label for that indication. Other off-label uses include anxiety disorders in children, social anxiety disorder, GAD, PTSD, and panic disorder. It is available as regular-release tablets and extended-release capsules (Luvox CR). Adverse reactions are the same as with fluoxetine except that fluvoxamine causes sedation rather than CNS excitement.

Paroxetine (Paxil, Pexeva): Approved in 1992, paroxetine is available as oral tablets, oral suspension, or controlled-release tablets (Paxil CR). It is approved to treat a large number of mental health conditions, including major depression, OCD, social anxiety disorder, panic disorder, GAD, PTSD, and premenstrual dysphoric disorder. In 2014 paroxetine (Brisdelle) was approved to treat menopausal vasomotor symptoms (hot flashes). Off-label use may include stuttering, fibromyalgia, bipolar disorder (with lithium), and premature ejaculation. Adverse effects are generally mild, dose dependent, and similar to those of other SSRIs. These effects usually diminish or disappear completely in time. A lower starting dosage is recommended for older adults. Precautions are similar to those for other SSRIs (including a black box warning about suicidal ideation). Several human studies suggest that paroxetine is a teratogen and use during pregnancy is not advised.

Sertraline (Zoloft): Approved in 1991, sertraline is one of the most frequently prescribed SSRIs. It is available as tablets or as an oral concentrate that must be diluted before use. Approved indications include major depressive disorder, OCD, panic disorder, PTSD, social anxiety disorder, and premenstrual dysphoric disorder. It may be used off-label to treat GAD and eating disorders. Contraindications and precautions are the same as with escitalopram. The main difference between sertraline and fluoxetine is that sertraline blocks the uptake of dopamine in addition to blocking the uptake of serotonin. Adverse effects, uses, and drug interactions are the same as those of fluoxetine. The oral concentrate contains 12% alcohol, which is contraindicated in patients taking disulfiram (Antabuse).

Vortioxetine (Trintellix): Vortioxetine was approved in 2013 for the treatment of major depression. In 2016, the trade name was changed from Brintellix to Trintellix to avoid confusion with a similar-sounding medication. It has a complex mechanism that enhances serotonin activities in some regions of the brain, while inhibiting the neurotransmitter in other regions. It has the same spectrum of adverse effects as other drugs in this class.

Atypical Antidepressants

19.9 Atypical antidepressants are alternatives to the selective serotonin reuptake inhibitors for depression and anxiety disorders.

Atypical antidepressants are a diverse class of drugs that act by mechanisms other than those of the SSRIs, TCAs, and MAOIs. In effect, this is a "miscellaneous" class of drugs because they have very little in common with each other except their ability to alleviate symptoms of depression. They act by preventing the reuptake of specific neurotransmitters in the CNS or by blocking neurotransmitter receptors. Mechanisms include the following:

- Serotonin–norepinephrine reuptake inhibitors (SNRIs): desvenlafaxine (Pristiq), levomilnacipran (Fetzima), venlafaxine (Effexor), and duloxetine (Cymbalta)
- Norepinephrine and dopamine reuptake inhibitors (NDRIs): bupropion (Wellbutrin)
- Norepinephrine reuptake inhibitors (NRIs): reboxetine (Edronax, Vestra)
- Combined reuptake inhibitor and receptor blocker: trazodone (Desyrel), nefazodone, and mirtazapine (Remeron).

As a group, the atypical antidepressants have similar pharmacologic actions to the SSRIs and exhibit fewer adverse effects than the TCAs and MAOIs. Each drug in the class has certain specific adverse effects, as described next. Some are widely used for indications other than depression, such as neuropathic pain, fibromyalgia, and anxiety disorders. The atypical antidepressants are considered to have equal efficacy to other well-established drugs for the treatment of depression.

Two recently approved "miscellaneous" antidepressants act by very different mechanisms and have specific indications. Esketamine (Spravato) is an intranasal spray approved in 2019 for treatment-resistant depression. Although the mechanism of its antidepressive action remains unknown, it is an antagonist at the N-methyl-D-aspartate receptor, similar to ketamine and the drug memantine. It is given once or twice weekly under the direct supervision of a healthcare provider, who must monitor the patient for 2 hours after dosing for sedation and blood pressure changes. Estimated cost for treatment is $33,000–49,000 annually. Esketamine is a Schedule III controlled substance.

Approved in 2019, brexanolone (Zulresso) is the first medication specifically approved for postpartum depression. The mechanism of its antidepressive action is unclear, but it is known to affect the GABA receptor. Several factors restrict the widespread use of brexanolone. First, it must be given intravenously over a 60-hour period in a healthcare facility. The patient must be continuously monitored for excessive sedation and hypoxia. Second, the expense of treatment is expected to be $34,000 per treatment, plus the cost of hospitalization.

PROTOTYPE DRUG **Venlafaxine (Effexor)**

Classification **Therapeutic:** Atypical antidepressant
Pharmacologic: Serotonin–norepinephrine reuptake inhibitor (SNRI)

Therapeutic Effects and Uses: Venlafaxine is an atypical antidepressant approved by the FDA in 1993 to treat major depression. Later, its approved indications were extended to include panic disorder, GAD, and social anxiety disorder. It has been used off-label to treat a large number of other conditions, including neuropathic pain, premenstrual dysphoric disorder, menopausal hot flashes, migraines, OCD, and fibromyalgia. Venlafaxine XR is an extended-release capsule that permits once-daily dosing. It is metabolized to an active metabolite in the liver. Venlafaxine has pharmacologic effects, drug interactions, and adverse effects very similar to those of the SSRIs.

Like other antidepressants, there is little potential for psychologic dependence with venlafaxine—it is not a drug of abuse. Abrupt discontinuation, however, can cause mild to moderate withdrawal symptoms such as nervousness, headache, agitation, fatigue, drowsiness, tremor, and sweating. Gradual tapering of the dose is a means of preventing withdrawal symptoms.

Mechanism of Action: Venlafaxine inhibits the presynaptic neuronal reuptake of both norepinephrine and serotonin in the CNS.

Pharmacokinetics:

Route(s)	PO
Absorption	92% absorbed from the GI tract
Distribution	Widely distributed; crosses the placenta; secreted in breast milk; 27% bound to plasma protein
Primary metabolism	Metabolized in the liver to desmethylvenlafaxine, an active metabolite; substantial first-pass effect
Primary excretion	Renal
Onset of action	Peak serum level: 5.5 h but the antidepressant action may take 2–3 weeks
Duration of action	Half-life: 5–7 h (9–11 h for the active metabolite)

Adverse Effects: The most common adverse effect of venlafaxine is nausea, which can occur in a large number of patients. Tolerance may develop to the nausea as therapy progresses. The nausea, combined with anorexia, sometimes leads to weight loss. Pediatric patients taking venlafaxine have been shown to have a decrease in overall height as well as weight. Venlafaxine has structural similarities to amphetamines and can cause CNS stimulation, nervousness, and insomnia. Other patients, however, exhibit sedative effects from the drug. Other CNS adverse effects include headache, emotional lability, dizziness, and asthenia. Sustained elevations, 10 to 15 mmHg, of blood pressure may occur. Types of sexual dysfunction seen with venlafaxine include impotence, abnormal ejaculation, and delayed or absent orgasm in women. Rare, life-threatening adverse reactions include rectal, vaginal, or uterine hemorrhage. **Black Box Warning:** Antidepressants increase the risk of suicidal thinking and behavior in children, adolescents, and young adults. Patients of all ages should be monitored and observed closely during therapy for clinical worsening, suicidality, or unusual changes in behavior.

Contraindications/Precautions: Venlafaxine is contraindicated if the patient has hypersensitivity to venlafaxine or an SSRI, if a MAOI is being used concurrently, or during lactation. Caution must be used when administered to patients with cardiac, hepatic, or renal impairment; recent myocardial infarction (MI); seizure disorder; anorexia; or suicidal ideation. Venlafaxine is not administered to patients with bipolar disorder or with a history of mania because it can trigger manic episodes. Safety in children under age 18 has not been established. Patients with hepatic impairment may require as much as a 50% reduction in dose.

Drug Interactions: Venlafaxine is primarily metabolized by the hepatic CYP2D6 isozyme; drugs that inhibit CYP2D6 may cause venlafaxine serum levels to rise. Serotonin syndrome may occur if venlafaxine is given concurrently with SSRIs, MAOIs, lithium, or other drugs that act by increasing serotonin levels. If switching from venlafaxine to a MAOI, venlafaxine must be withdrawn at least 7 days before beginning the MAOI. Alcohol, opioids, sedatives, hypnotics, or antihistamines can cause additive CNS depression. Cimetidine, haloperidol, fluoxetine, sertraline, or phenothiazine can lead to increased toxicity. **Herbal/Food:** No food interactions have been reported, but there are several possible interactions with herbal products. St. John's wort and SAM-e may increase the risk of SES. CNS depression may occur with concurrent use of chamomile, kava, hops, lavender, valerian, or skullcap. Jimsonweed or corkwood may cause increased anticholinergic effects. Yohimbe may increase the risk for HTN.

Pregnancy: Infants exposed during the third trimester showed a risk for pulmonary hypertension, cyanosis, apnea, feeding difficulty and other signs of distress upon delivery that resemble serotonin syndrome. Venlafaxine should be used during pregnancy and lactation only if the potential benefits justify the potential risks to the fetus and neonate.

Treatment of Overdose: Overdoses are generally not fatal but can cause serious symptoms such as CNS depression, seizures, altered level of consciousness, hypotension, and dysrhythmias. General measures include inducing emesis and administering activated charcoal and gastric lavage. The electrocardiogram (ECG) must be monitored and antiseizure drugs administered as necessary.

Clinician Responsibilities: Key clinical implications for patients receiving venlafaxine are included in Applied Clinical Judgment: Patients Receiving Pharmacotherapy with Antidepressants.

Drugs Similar to Venlafaxine (Effexor)

Other atypical antidepressants include bupropion, desvenlafaxine, duloxetine, levomilnacipran, mirtazapine, nefazodone, trazodone, and vilazodone. Unless otherwise noted below, the atypical antidepressants have the same effects on the fetus and neonate as venlafaxine. These medications should be used during pregnancy and lactation only if the potential benefits justify the potential risks to the fetus and neonate.

Bupropion (Aplenzin, Forfivo XL, Wellbutrin, Others): Approved in 1985, bupropion has a chemical structure similar to that of amphetamine. It is approved to treat major depression as well as being the first approved therapy for persistent seasonal affective disorder (Wellbutrin XR). Off-label uses may include neuropathic pain and attention-deficit/hyperactivity disorder (ADHD).

The naming of bupropion has resulted in medication errors. It is available as immediate-release tablets (100 mg, three times daily) and as extended-release formulations, Wellbutrin SR (150 mg, twice daily) and Wellbutrin XL (300 mg, once daily). In pharmacology, the terms *sustained release* (SR) and *extended release* (XL or XR) are usually used interchangeably, but this is not the case for bupropion. Further confusing the naming is that the *U.S. Pharmacopeia* requires that all generic versions of prolonged-release medications be labeled "extended release." In 2008 a new salt form, bupropion hydrobromide (Aplenzin), was approved as a once-daily tablet (348 mg, once daily) for depression. Caution must be used when dispensing bupropion to be certain the correct salt and dosing schedule are used.

Bupropion not only inhibits the reuptake of serotonin, but it may also affect the activity of norepinephrine and dopamine. Like amphetamine, bupropion has stimulant actions and suppresses the appetite. It does not cause weight gain or sexual dysfunction, which makes it appealing to women who are experiencing hypoactive sexual disorder. Indeed, it is sometimes used to counteract the sexual dysfunction that occurs in patients taking SSRIs. Antidepressant action begins in 1 to 3 weeks and is equal to that of the TCAs. Because bupropion has a greater potential for causing seizures than other antidepressants, it should be used with caution in patients with seizure disorders. The risk for seizures is dose dependent and increases for patients drinking alcohol or taking other drugs that lower the seizure threshold. Seizures have been reported in infants receiving breast milk from mothers taking bupropion. Common adverse reactions include CNS stimulation (agitation, insomnia, and restlessness), weight loss, headache, dry mouth, constipation, and GI upset. About 20% of patients taking this drug will develop tremors. Because of its potential adverse effects, bupropion is usually considered an alternative antidepressant for patients who do not respond to SSRIs. Animal reproduction studies showed increased skeletal malformations. Limited human data does not show a clear risk for fetal harm. The drug is secreted in human milk in significant amounts and breastfeeding is not advised.

Desvenlafaxine (Pristiq): An active metabolite of venlafaxine, desvenlafaxine is an SNRI approved in 2008 for the treatment of major depressive disorder. It is available as an extended-release tablet that is taken once daily. Common adverse effects include nausea, dizziness, excessive sweating, constipation, somnolence, anxiety, male function disorders, and decreased appetite. Because this drug can raise blood pressure, preexisting HTN should be corrected before starting therapy. Desvenlafaxine should be discontinued gradually to prevent the appearance of withdrawal symptoms.

Duloxetine (Cymbalta): Like venlafaxine, duloxetine is an atypical antidepressant that is classified as an SNRI. First approved for major depression in 2004, it has since received FDA approval to treat diabetic peripheral neuropathic pain, fibromyalgia, chronic musculoskeletal pain, and GAD. Stress urinary incontinence is an off-label indication. Abnormal vision is the most frequently reported adverse effect, and nausea is a common reason for discontinuation of therapy. Other adverse events include photosensitivity, bruising, anorexia, thrombophlebitis, constipation, diarrhea, dry mouth, insomnia, and anxiety. Postmarketing incidences of liver injury suggest that the drug should be used with great caution in patients with preexisting hepatic impairment or in people with alcoholism. Caution must be exercised when administered to individuals with mania, seizures, HTN, or cardiac, renal, or hepatic disease; older adults; children; or lactating women. When discontinuing therapy, the dose should be tapered slowly to prevent withdrawal symptoms. Patients may begin feeling the antidepressant effects of duloxetine within 2 weeks of beginning treatment. Based on animal data duloxetine may cause fetal harm. The drug is secreted in human milk and breastfeeding is not advised.

Levomilnacipran (Fetzima): Levomilnacipran was approved in 2013 as an extended-release capsule for the treatment of major depression in adults. It has very similar actions and side effects to other SNRIs such as venlafaxine. The most frequently observed side effects include nausea and vomiting, constipation, hyperhidrosis, heart rate increase, erectile dysfunction, and heart palpitations. Levomilnacipran is the isomer of milnacipran (Savella). Despite their close structural similarities, levomilnacipran is approved only for major depression, whereas milnacipran is approved only for fibromyalgia. Based on animal data levomilnacipran may cause fetal harm. Effects on the breastfeeding neonate are unknown.

Mirtazapine (Remeron): Classified as a tetracyclic compound, this drug was approved in 1996 for major depression in adults and may be used off-label to treat PTSD, hot flashes, or insomnia. It blocks presynaptic serotonin and norepinephrine receptors, thereby enhancing release of these neurotransmitters from nerve terminals. Unlike the TCAs, it has few anticholinergic actions. It does carry a higher risk of seizure activity in patients with a previous history of seizures, head injury, or alcoholism. Serious adverse reactions include worsening of psychosis in patients with bipolar disorder, bone fractures, agranulocytosis, serotonin syndrome, and suicidal ideation. Other adverse reactions include dizziness, orthostatic hypotension, QT prolongation, sedation, tachycardia, HTN, or extrapyramidal symptoms in older adults. Mirtazapine should not be used in patients with hypersensitivity to TCAs, seizure disorders, prostatic hypertrophy, serious hepatic impairment, chronic kidney disease, or those who are recovering from MI. Mirtazapine usually elevates mood within 2 to 4 weeks after the initiation of therapy. Animal reproduction studies showed that high doses of mirtazapine can cause adverse fetal effects. Because this drug is secreted in human milk breastfeeding is not recommended.

Nefazodone: Chemically similar to trazodone, nefazodone causes minimal cardiovascular effects, fewer anticholinergic effects, less sedation, and less sexual dysfunction than some of the other antidepressants. The most common adverse effects are xerostomia, drowsiness, nausea and vomiting, dizziness, and constipation. Although FDA approved only for major depression, the medication is used off-label to treat anxiety, panic attacks, premenstrual dysphoric disorder, PTSD, and social anxiety disorder. Nefazodone acts by blocking serotonin receptors and inhibiting serotonin reuptake. It also has some blocking effect on norepinephrine reuptake. Originally approved in 1994, a trade name form of the drug, Serzone, was removed from the market in 2004 due to a possibility of liver damage; generic nefazodone is still available. A black box warning indicates that the drug should not be used in patients with acute liver impairment and that hepatic laboratory values should be regularly monitored during therapy. The drug should be withdrawn if the patient develops signs of hepatic injury such as increased serum aspartate aminotransferase (AST) or serum alanine aminotransferase (ALT) levels greater than three times normal. Animal reproduction studies showed reduced offspring survival. Effects on the breastfeeding neonate are unknown.

Trazodone: Approved in 1981, trazodone works by producing a moderate, selective blockade of serotonin reuptake. It is not very effective when used alone as an antidepressant, but its sedative properties are especially useful in patients who have antidepressant-induced insomnia. In fact, trazodone is most frequently used off-label as a sleep aid, rather than as an antidepressant. Other off-label indications include aggressive behavior, cocaine withdrawal, migraine prevention, and as an adjuvant to reduce cravings for alcohol in patients with alcohol dependency. It causes little cardiac toxicity and few anticholinergic effects so it may be useful for older adults and other individuals for whom either of these may be intolerable. Trazodone should not be used with other medications that increase the QTc interval. Common adverse effects include orthostatic hypotension, nausea, sedation, and dry mouth. Reported sexual effects include priapism, anorgasmia, and ejaculation dysfunctions. Overdose with trazodone is considered to be safer than overdose from MAOIs or TCAs, and there have been no reports of death from trazodone use alone. However, death can occur from overdose when the patient combines trazodone with other CNS depressants. Based on animal data, high doses of trazodone may cause fetal harm. Because this drug is secreted in human milk breastfeeding is not recommended.

Vilazodone (Viibryd): Approved in 2011, vilazodone acts by blocking serotonin reuptake and by demonstrating partial agonist action at serotonin receptors. It appears to have equivalent effectiveness to other drugs in this class. One advantage of vilazodone is that clinical improvement is noted after 7 days of therapy, compared to the 4 to 6 weeks required for some of the other antidepressants. In addition, the drug has only minor adverse effects, with GI-related symptoms being the most common. Like other antidepressants, the drug carries a black box warning about possible increased suicidality in adolescents and young adults. Animal reproduction studies showed reduced offspring survival. Because this drug is secreted in human milk breastfeeding is not recommended..

CONNECTION Checkpoint 19.2

Atypical antidepressants are sometimes used to treat anxiety when drugs from other classes are not effective. From what you learned in Chapter 18, what class of drugs is the traditional choice for the short-term therapy of generalized anxiety disorder?

Tricyclic Antidepressants

19.10 Tricyclic antidepressants were once the mainstay for the treatment of depression, but they have many adverse effects.

The **tricyclic antidepressants (TCAs)** have been available in the United States for more than 60 years. Although no longer preferred drugs, the TCAs are still prescribed for many patients with major depressive disorder. This group of medications is named after its molecular structure, which has a three-ring core. Because this molecular arrangement is very similar to the structure of the phenothiazine antipsychotics, these two classes of drugs share similar adverse effects (see Chapter 20). Several of the TCAs are also prescribed to treat the depressive stage of bipolar disorder, chronic insomnia, OCD, neuropathic pain, and fibromyalgia.

The TCAs act by blocking the reuptake transport of norepinephrine and serotonin at synapses, as shown in Figure 19.2. This blockade results in a greater quantity of neurotransmitters being available in the synaptic space, leading to an intensified action. Some TCAs such as desipramine, maprotiline, and protriptyline are specific to blocking the reuptake of norepinephrine, whereas the other drugs in this class affect both norepinephrine and serotonin. In general, all TCAs have similar effectiveness in treating depression and exhibit the same spectrum of adverse effects.

The advantages of TCAs are that they are inexpensive and their effectiveness in treating depression has been well established for many decades. They are rapidly absorbed when given orally (PO) and widely distributed throughout the body. Relative to the SSRIs and atypical antidepressants, the TCAs have more frequent adverse effects, which has limited their use.

Blockade of muscarinic receptors by TCAs is responsible for causing a high incidence of anticholinergic adverse effects with symptoms such as dry mouth, blurred vision, constipation, urinary retention, and tachycardia. Orthostatic hypotension is common and may be serious enough to cause injury due to falls. Although rare, the most serious adverse effect is the ability of TCAs to cause life-threatening cardiac dysrhythmias, especially if the patient receives an overdose of the medication.

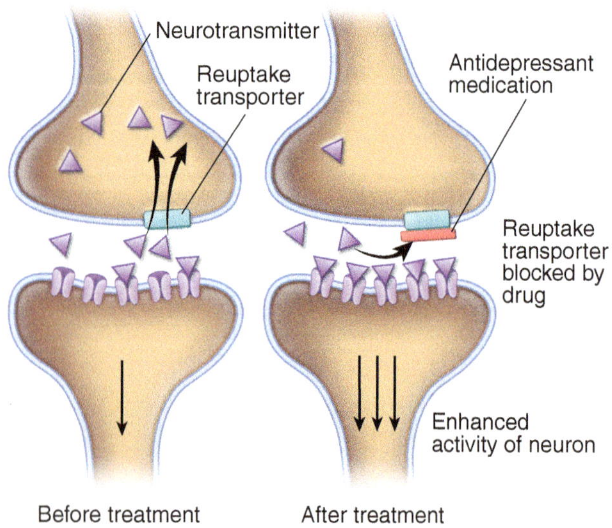

Figure 19.2 Mechanisms of action of antidepressants. (a) In adrenergic and serotonergic neurons the activity of the neurotransmitter is terminated by reuptake. (b) Tricyclic antidepressants and SSRIs produce their effects by inhibiting the reuptake of neurotransmitters. The neurotransmitter accumulates in the synaptic cleft and activates more receptors, thus causing an enhanced effect at the synapse.

A few of the TCAs have central effects that cause sedation, which can be managed by taking the drugs at bedtime. Sedation is worsened by the concurrent use of other CNS depressants such as alcohol. Confusion, dizziness, and fatigue are other possible dose-limiting effects of TCAs. At high doses some cause seizures.

TCAs exhibit a relatively high incidence of sexual dysfunction, including impotence and delayed ejaculation in men, and breast enlargement and impaired orgasm in women. Weight gain is possible. In addition, some patients quickly change mood from depression to hypomania or mania and may begin to display symptoms of bipolar disorder. These patients require a dosage adjustment or a change to a different antidepressant.

Tolerance and psychologic dependence are usually not major problems with TCAs. Once stabilized, therapy may often be conducted for years without requiring a dosage adjustment. Unlike many CNS depressants, the TCAs are not drugs of abuse. Patients on high doses for prolonged periods, however, may exhibit a mild withdrawal syndrome on discontinuation and experience symptoms such as irritability, nausea, sleep impairment, muscle aches, and fatigue. To avoid these symptoms, and to ensure that rebound depression does not occur, it is best that these drugs be withdrawn gradually.

CONNECTION Checkpoint 19.3

Anticholinergic effects are common with TCAs and some other antidepressants. From what you learned in Chapter 14, name the prototype anticholinergic drug. If anticholinergic effects become prominent in a patient, what class of drugs can be used to counteract the cardiovascular adverse effects?

PROTOTYPE DRUG Imipramine (Tofranil)

Classification **Therapeutic:** Tricyclic antidepressant
Pharmacologic: Norepinephrine reuptake inhibitor

Therapeutic Effects and Uses: Approved in 1959 as the first TCA, imipramine is effective in treating major depressive disorder. Like other TCAs, it is given PO and is well absorbed from the GI tract. A drawback to the use of imipramine is that it takes 2 weeks or longer to achieve full therapeutic effect. During the initial weeks of therapy, when blood levels of imipramine have not yet produced their full therapeutic effects, suicide risks may increase, especially in children, adolescents, and young adults. Although it is not a first-line therapy for the disorder, imipramine is one of only two drugs approved for nocturnal enuresis, or bedwetting, in children. The urge to urinate is diminished by the anticholinergic (urinary retention) effects of the drug.

Like other TCAs, imipramine has a number of off-label indications. These include the adjuvant treatment of cancer or neuropathic pain, overactive bladder, ADHD, insomnia, and bulimia nervosa. The use of TCAs in treating social anxiety disorder and panic disorder is presented in Chapter 18. The active metabolite of imipramine is desipramine, which is marketed separately as Norpramin.

Mechanism of Action: Imipramine blocks the reuptake of norepinephrine and serotonin into presynaptic nerve terminals. This results in an increased action of both neurotransmitters in neurons. Imipramine also blocks acetylcholine receptors, which is likely responsible for its effectiveness in treating enuresis.

Pharmacokinetics:

Route(s)	PO, IM (rare)
Absorption	Completely absorbed from the GI tract
Distribution	Widely distributed; crosses the placenta; secreted in breast milk; 85–95% bound to plasma protein
Primary metabolism	Hepatic; metabolized to the active metabolite desipramine
Primary excretion	Renal; small amounts in bile and feces
Onset of action	1–2 h for peak serum level; mood elevation requires 2–3 weeks
Duration of action	Not known

Adverse Effects: Frequent adverse reactions with imipramine include orthostatic hypotension (the most common adverse effect), dizziness, confusion, drowsiness, diarrhea, dry mouth, increased appetite, jaundice, urinary retention, rash, pruritus, and photosensitivity. Serious adverse reactions include seizures, hepatitis, acute renal failure, paralytic ileus, leukopenia, agranulocytosis, thrombocytopenia, or eosinophilia. Serious adverse reactions occur with acute doses when imipramine accumulates in cardiac tissue; dysrhythmias, heart failure, or MI can occur. **Black Box Warning:** Antidepressants increase the risk of suicidal thinking and behavior in children, adolescents, and young adults. Patients of all ages should be monitored and observed closely during therapy for clinical worsening, suicidality, or unusual changes in behavior.

Contraindications/Precautions: Imipramine should not be used by patients with seizure disorders because it lowers the seizure threshold. It must be used with caution in individuals with suicidal tendencies, urinary retention, prostatic hyperplasia, cardiac or hepatic disease, increased intraocular pressure, or hyperthyroidism. Use in patients with Parkinson's disease will induce or worsen parkinsonism symptoms. Patients with cardiac disease such as heart failure, QT prolongation, or history of MI should be carefully monitored during therapy; use in patients recovering from MI has resulted in sudden death. Imipramine should not be used during pregnancy or lactation.

Drug Interactions: Like other TCAs, imipramine is metabolized by hepatic CYP450 enzymes and is highly protein bound; thus, there is a high potential for drug–drug interactions. Increased sedation can occur when imipramine is given concurrently with other CNS depressants, including alcohol. Drug interactions causing decreased effects of imipramine include oral contraceptives, clonidine, carbamazepine, and indirect-acting sympathomimetics. Concurrent use with thyroid hormone may induce dysrhythmias. Imipramine should not be given concurrently with other drugs that prolong the QT interval, such as the Class IA antidysrhythmics, because of the potential for serious cardiac toxicity. Phenothiazines and TCAs are structurally very similar and concurrent use will likely cause additive anticholinergic adverse effects. Concurrent use of MAOIs must be avoided because this combination may cause hypertensive crisis, seizures, or hyperpyretic crisis. SSRIs must not be used concurrently; this can cause increased toxicity of TCAs. **Herbal/Food:** Several commonly used herbal products may lead to increased imipramine effects, including kava, hops, lavender, valerian, skullcap, and chamomile. An increased anticholinergic effect can occur with the use of belladonna, jimsonweed, or henbane. Serotonin syndrome may occur with the use of St. John's wort.

Pregnancy: Animal reproduction studies showed some embryotoxicity but no teratogenicity. Human data do not show malformations. Neonates exposed in utero may experience withdrawal symptoms such as lethargy, cyanosis, tremors and feeding difficulty. Imipramine is secreted in human milk but effects on the breastfeeding neonate are not known.

Treatment of Overdose: Overdoses with TCAs may be life-threatening, with symptoms that include mixed mania and depression followed by coma. Medical management includes treating possible seizures, hypotension, and dysrhythmias.

Clinician Responsibilities: Key clinical implications for patients receiving imipramine are included in Applied Clinical Judgment: Patients Receiving Pharmacotherapy with Antidepressants.

Drugs Similar to Imipramine (Tofranil)

Other TCAs include amitriptyline, amoxapine, clomipramine, doxepin, maprotiline, protriptyline, and trimipramine. Desipramine is an active metabolite of imipramine, and the two drugs have the same actions and adverse effects, as previously described. Unless otherwise noted below, the TCAs have the same effects on the fetus and neonate as imipramine. These medications should be used during pregnancy and lactation only if the potential benefits justify the potential risks to the fetus and neonate.

Amitriptyline and nortriptyline (Pamelor): Amitriptyline has been available by the PO route since 1961 for the therapy of major depression. It has been used for a large number of off-label indications, including neuropathic pain syndromes such as fibromyalgia, and for nocturnal enuresis, social anxiety disorder, ADHD, migraines, persistent hiccups, insomnia, and bulimia nervosa. It produces more sedation than most other TCAs and is thus taken at bedtime. It is metabolized in the liver to nortriptyline, which is marketed as a separate drug. Both amitriptyline and nortriptyline produce significant anticholinergic adverse effects. Like other TCAs, cardiac toxicity is a concern at high doses. Animal studies suggest that amitriptyline is a teratogen and use during pregnancy or breastfeeding is not advised. Studies with nortriptyline are inconclusive.

Amoxapine: Approved in 1980, amoxapine is chemically related to both TCAs and phenothiazines. The drug exhibits potentially serious adverse effects, which limit its use to patients who have major depression accompanied by psychotic symptoms such as agitation. Adverse effects resemble those of TCAs (blood dyscrasias, orthostatic hypotension, sedation, anticholinergic effects, sexual dysfunction, cardiac toxicity) and phenothiazines (neuroleptic malignant syndrome, parkinsonism symptoms). Amoxapine must be used cautiously in those with suicidal ideation. Animal reproduction studies showed amoxapine to be embryotoxic with increased numbers of stillbirths and decreased offspring survival. This drug is secreted in human milk but effects on breastfeeding neonates are unknown.

Clomipramine (Anafranil): Approved in 1991, the only FDA-approved indication for clomipramine is OCD. Depression is an off-label indication. Other off-label uses are premature ejaculation and childhood autism. Because the drug produces significant anticholinergic effects and orthostatic hypotension, it is not a first-line drug for depression. Animal studies did not show teratogenicity. This drug is secreted in human milk but effects on breastfeeding neonates are unknown.

Doxepin (Silenor): Approved in 1969 to treat major depression, doxepin is also approved to treat insomnia and anxiety. Doses used to treat depression (25–150 mg/day) are much higher than those used for insomnia (3–6 mg). When given PO for depression or anxiety, the most common side effect is sedation. Other adverse effects include nausea and upper respiratory tract infection. The drug may cause complex sleep behaviors such as sleep-walking or sleep driving. A topical form of doxepin (Zonalon) is available for pruritus associated with atopic dermatitis. Because doxepin is absorbed through the skin, topical applications can cause systemic adverse effects. Animal data showed doxepin may cause fetal harm. This drug is secreted in human milk but effects on breastfeeding neonates are unknown.

Maprotiline: Maprotiline does not have a tricyclic chemical structure but it is included with the TCAs because it has very similar therapeutic and adverse effects. It was approved to treat major depression in 1980. Off-label indications include bulimia nervosa, neuropathic pain, panic attacks, and enuresis. It has the same adverse effects as other drugs in this class and offers no specific advantages over other TCAs. Animal studies did not show teratogenicity. This drug is secreted in human milk but effects on breastfeeding neonates are unknown.

Protriptyline (Vivactil): Protriptyline is an oral antidepressant that was approved in 1967. It has the same adverse effects as other TCAs except that it tends to produce CNS stimulation rather than sedation. It is the only TCA that has respiratory stimulant activity. These respiratory effects have led to its occasional off-label use for treating chronic obstructive pulmonary disease or sleep apnea. Animal studies did not show teratogenicity. It is not known whether this drug is secreted in human milk and effects on breastfeeding neonates are unknown.

Trimipramine: Trimipramine was approved in 1979 for major depression. Off-label indications include anxiety, schizophrenia, and rheumatoid arthritis. Drowsiness is a serious problem; however, the incidence of anticholinergic effects is one of the lowest of any drug in its class. It offers no major benefits over other TCAs. Animal reproduction studies showed trimipramine to be embryotoxic and fetotoxic at high doses. It is not known whether this drug is secreted in human milk and effects on breastfeeding neonates are unknown.

Monoamine Oxidase Inhibitors

19.11 Monoamine oxidase inhibitors are effective antidepressants but are seldom used due to potentially serious adverse effects.

MAO is a key enzyme located in the liver, intestinal wall, and adrenergic neurons. It is responsible for inactivating monoamines: substances that contain one $-NH_2$ (amine) group. Not only does MAO inactivate natural monoamines such as norepinephrine, dopamine, and serotonin, but it also acts on those present in food and drugs. The **monoamine oxidase inhibitors (MAOIs)** are antidepressants that block the actions of MAO.

In adrenergic neurons, MAOIs slow the destruction of norepinephrine, dopamine, and serotonin. This creates higher levels of these neurotransmitters and enhances their activity in the brain. Through mechanisms incompletely understood, this increase in neurotransmitters creates an antidepressant action.

Although they are as effective in treating depression as the SSRIs or TCAs, serious adverse reactions limit their use. Because of their low safety margin, these drugs are

Table 19.4 Foods High in Tyramine

Category of Food	Specific Foods
Meats	Beef or chicken liver, pate Hot dogs, bologna Pepperoni, salami, sausage
Dairy products	Aged cheese Sour cream Yogurt
Fruits	Avocados Bananas, in large amounts Canned figs Papaya products, including meat tenderizers Raisins
Vegetables	Pods of fava beans Fermented soybeans, soybean paste
Fish	Dried or cured fish Fermented, smoked, aged fish Pickled or kippered herring
Alcohol	Beer Wine, especially red wine
Miscellaneous	Protein dietary supplements Soups (may contain protein extract) Shrimp paste Soy sauce Yeast, brewer's or extracts

reserved for patients with refractory depression that has not responded to TCAs, atypical antidepressants, or SSRIs. They are rarely used for depression in clinical practice.

A serious adverse reaction with MAOIs is their ability to cause a hypertensive crisis if combined with foods that contain **tyramine**. Widely found in nature, tyramine is a type of monoamine that is formed by the metabolism of tyrosine, an amino acid. When a patient is taking an MAOI, the drug blocks the breakdown of dietary tyramine, causing it to accumulate to high levels. In turn, tyramine causes the release of norepinephrine stored in adrenergic neurons. Rapid vasoconstriction occurs with a potential rise of blood pressure of 30 mmHg or more. Table 19.4 contains a list of tyramine-rich foods that must be avoided by patients taking MAOIs. Products containing tyramine are sometimes marketed as dietary supplements to increase fat loss from the body. There is no valid scientific evidence to support this claim, and these supplements must be strictly avoided by patients taking MAOIs.

PROTOTYPE DRUG Phenelzine (Nardil)

Classification **Therapeutic:** Antidepressant
Pharmacologic: Monoamine oxidase inhibitor

Therapeutic Effects and Uses: An older drug approved in 1959, phenelzine was once widely used to treat major depression. It has also been used off-label to treat OCD, panic disorder, social anxiety disorder and migraine prophylaxis. Although very effective in treating these disorders, phenelzine interacts with tyramine in foods and with many other drugs to produce potentially serious interactions.

Like other antidepressants, phenelzine may take up to 4 to 8 weeks to produce a maximum antidepressant response. This drug is changed to active metabolites in the liver.

Mechanism of Action: Phenelzine produces its effects by binding irreversibly to MAO. This intensifies the actions of endogenous epinephrine, norepinephrine, serotonin, and dopamine in the CNS. Increased concentrations of these neurotransmitters result in elevated mood.

Pharmacokinetics:

Route(s)	PO
Absorption	Well absorbed
Distribution	Widely distributed; crosses the placenta
Primary metabolism	Hepatic
Primary excretion	Renal
Onset of action	Peak level: 2–4 h (antidepressant action takes 2–8 weeks)
Duration of action	Half-life: 11 h

Adverse Effects: The most serious adverse effect of phenelzine is hypertensive crisis precipitated by foods containing tyramine, which can induce fatal intracranial bleeding. Dizziness and orthostatic hypotension are common during therapy. Other frequent adverse reactions include drowsiness, sexual dysfunction, and anorexia. Life-threatening adverse reactions include dysrhythmias and a syndrome of inappropriate antidiuretic hormone-like symptoms. **Black Box Warning:** Antidepressants increase the risk of suicidal thinking and behavior in children, adolescents, and young adults. Patients of all ages should be monitored and observed closely during therapy for clinical worsening, suicidal ideation, or unusual changes in behavior.

Contraindications/Precautions: Patients with schizophrenia, cardiovascular or cerebrovascular disease, hepatic impairment or chronic kidney disease, or pheochromocytoma should not take phenelzine. Caution should be used when prescribing phenelzine to a patient with epilepsy, severe or frequent headaches, HTN, dysrhythmias, or suicidal tendencies.

Drug Interactions: Phenelzine interacts with many other drugs. The nurse should consult a current drug guide for a comprehensive list of drug–drug interactions. Other CNS depressants, including alcohol, may lead to additive CNS depression. Concurrent administration with buspirone may increase blood pressure. Use with opioid analgesics may lead to hypotension, hyperpyrexia, vascular collapse, seizures, coma, and death. CNS stimulants and sympathomimetics may increase the cardiac stimulant and vasopressor effects of phenelzine. SES may occur if phenelzine is administered with other drugs such as SSRIs, TCAs, lithium, or dextromethorphan that potentiate the actions of serotonin. **Herbal/Food:** Patients who are taking phenelzine or any MAOI must avoid tyramine-containing foods (see Table 19.4) because these foods may precipitate a hypertensive crisis. Caffeine, including over-the-counter products, should be avoided because they may increase the risk of HTN and dysrhythmias. An increased sympathomimetic effect may occur when phenelzine is combined with capsicum peppers or large amounts of green tea. Ginkgo, nutmeg, and yohimbe use can result in increased effects. Ginseng use can lead to irritability, hallucinations, mania, and increased tension headaches. Decreased effects can occur with the use of valerian. Serotonin syndrome may occur with the use of St. John's wort.

Pregnancy: Animal studies using high doses showed a decrease in the number of viable offspring, but data are limited. It is not known whether this drug is secreted in human milk and effects on breastfeeding neonates are unknown.

Treatment of Overdose: Overdosage with phenelzine is serious and can result in death if untreated. Symptoms may include either CNS stimulation (seizures) or depression (coma). Induction of gastric lavage with activated charcoal may be beneficial. Electrolytes and vital signs must be monitored and the appropriate intervention administered to keep values within normal ranges.

Clinician Responsibilities: Key clinical implications for patients receiving phenelzine are included in Applied Clinical Judgment: Patients Receiving Pharmacotherapy with Antidepressants.

Drugs Similar to Phenelzine (Nardil)

The other MAOIs that are available include isocarboxazid, selegiline, and tranylcypromine.

Isocarboxazid (Marplan): Like phenelzine, isocarboxazid was initially approved by the FDA for depression in the 1950s. Off-label indications may include refractory panic disorder and social anxiety disorder. It is only used when other therapies have failed to produce satisfactory outcomes. The drug has the same precautions and potential interactions as phenelzine, including the possibility of a hypertensive crisis occurring when taken with tyramine-containing products. Animal pregnancy and lactation data are not available for isocarboxazid.

Selegiline (Emsam): Approved in 2006 for major depression, selegiline is a transdermal patch that delivers a controlled amount of the MAOI over 24 hours. Absorption across the skin bypasses MAO located in intestinal cells; thus, there is less risk of a hypertensive crisis when eating foods containing tyramine. The drug is also indicated for the treatment of Parkinson's disease by capsule or orally disintegrating tablets (Zelapar). The various forms of this drug should not be administered concurrently due to the

CONNECTIONS: Complementary and Alternative Therapies

St. John's Wort for Depression

Description

St. John's wort (*Hypericum perforatum*) is an herb found throughout Great Britain, Asia, Europe, and North America.

History and Claims

The herb gets its name from a legend that red spots once appeared on its leaves on the anniversary of St. John's beheading. The word *wort* is a British term for "plant." Use of the herb dates to ancient Greece, and Native Americans used it as an antiseptic or anti-inflammatory agent. Modern uses have focused on the antidepressant properties of the herb.

Standardization

The active substances in St. John's wort are believed to be hyperforin and hypericin. There is no standard dosage; however, some manufacturers are beginning to report dose by the percentage of hypericin in the extract. For example, one commonly used dose is 300 mg of St. John's wort standardized to 0.2–0.3% hypericin. Some studies use 5% hyperforin.

Evidence

Recent studies suggest that St. John's wort produces its effects by increasing the levels of serotonin, norepinephrine, and dopamine in the brain (Busti et al., 2015).

St. John's wort induces hepatic CYP450 enzymes and interacts with many medications, including oral contraceptives, warfarin, digoxin, and cyclosporine. It should not be taken concurrently with antidepressant medications and patients should discuss the use of St. John's wort with their healthcare provider before taking the supplement. St John's wort has not been studied extensively in children or in pregnant women and should be avoided in those populations.

An active ingredient in St. John's wort is a photoactive compound that when exposed to light produces substances that can damage myelin. Patients have reported feeling stinging pain on the hands after sun exposure while taking the herbal remedy. Patients who take this herb should be advised to apply sunscreen or wear protective clothing when outdoors.

risk of hypertensive crisis caused by drug overdose. Common adverse effects include skin irritation at the site of the patch application, headache, sleep disorders, diarrhea, and dry mouth. Animal reproduction studies showed no teratogenic effects but high doses increased stillbirths and reduced offspring survival. It is not known whether this drug is secreted in human milk and effects on breastfeeding neonates are unknown

Tranylcypromine (Parnate): Tranylcypromine was approved in 1961 for the therapy of depression. Off-label indications may include refractory panic disorder and social anxiety disorder. The drug binds reversibly to MAO. This results in a more rapid onset of antidepressant action than phenelzine or isocarboxazid and a more rapid return to normal MAO levels after the drug is discontinued. However, it has the same precautions and potential interactions as phenelzine and is rarely used due to its adverse effects. Animal pregnancy and lactation data are inconclusive. This drug is secreted in human milk but effects on breastfeeding neonates are unknown.

CONNECTIONS: APPLIED CLINICAL JUDGMENT

Patients Receiving Pharmacotherapy with Antidepressants

Key Assessment Data
- History of current condition, including family history of depression or mood disorder, baseline vital signs, weight, physical exam and mental status findings; history of diabetes, hepatic, renal, cardiovascular, or neurologic disease; medication and substance use history; allergies; pregnancy status.
- Ongoing assessment during drug therapy includes CBC, electrolytes, glucose, hepatic, and renal function studies.

Desired Therapeutic Outcomes

Improvement is observed and measurable by increased mood, lessening depression, increased activity level, return to normal ADLs, appetite, and sleep patterns. Drugs used for depression may take 2 to 8 weeks before full effects are realized. Use objective measures (e.g., PHQ-9, Beck Depression Inventory, or Geriatric Depression Scale) when possible to help quantify therapeutic results.

Minimizing Adverse Effects
- Neurologic changes may indicate under- or overmedication, exacerbation of other psychiatric illness, or adverse drug effects. Promptly report increasing lethargy, disorientation, confusion, changes in behavior or mood, agitation or aggression, slurred speech, or ataxia.
- For outpatient therapy, prescriptions may be limited to a 7-day supply of medication. Have patient sign "No Harm/No Suicide" contract as appropriate.
- Some antidepressant drugs may cause hepatotoxicity as an adverse effect. Continue to monitor CBC, electrolytes, and renal and hepatic function.
- Early signs of SES include rapid increases in blood pressure and pulse. Headache, palpitations, fever, and neck stiffness may signal a life-threatening hypertensive crisis in a patient taking MAO inhibitors. Monitor cardiovascular status and immediately report severe headache, dizziness, paresthesia, palpitations, tachycardia, chest pain, nausea and/or vomiting, diaphoresis, or fever.
- TCAs may cause blood dyscrasias and increased chances of bleeding or infection. Promptly report any signs of increased bruising, bleeding, or infections (e.g., sore throat, fever, or skin rash) promptly.
- Anticholinergic-like effects and sexual dysfunction, including loss of libido and impotence, are common antidepressant adverse effects. Symptomatic relief (e.g., ice chips, sips of water, "dry eye" drops) may help to alleviate symptoms.
- Weight gain may be a reason for nonadherence with drug therapy. Continue weekly weights and report gain or loss above 2 kg (5 lb).
- Profound depression, seizures, or withdrawal symptoms may occur with abrupt discontinuation. Avoid abrupt discontinuation of therapy.

Lifespan Considerations
- The older adult may be at increased risk for falls due to drowsiness and dizziness, hypotension, or impaired mental and physical abilities.
- The older adult man with an enlarged prostate is at higher risk for mechanical obstruction and may experience urinary retention due to anticholinergic effects. Tolerance to anticholinergic effects usually develops in 2–4 weeks. Promptly report difficulty with urination, hesitancy, or dysuria.
- Adolescents and older adults may be at risk for anorexia and weight loss. Report gain or loss above 2 kg (5 lb).

Diversity Considerations
- SSRIs are metabolized through the CYP450 system and may result in less than optimal therapeutic results based on differences in enzymes. Monitor ethnically diverse patients more frequently in the early stages of drug therapy.

Patient Education
- Full effects may not occur for a prolonged period, but that some improvement should be noticeable after beginning therapy. Keep all appointments with the therapist and to discuss ongoing symptoms of depression, reporting any suicidal ideations immediately.
- Rise from lying or sitting to standing slowly to avoid dizziness or falls. If dizziness occurs, sit or lie down and do not attempt to stand or walk until the sensation passes.
- Be cautious or avoid driving or other activities requiring mental alertness or physical coordination until the effects of the drug are known.
- Report increasing lethargy, disorientation, confusion, changes in behavior or mood, slurred speech, or ataxia immediately.
- Promptly report any abdominal pain, particularly in the upper quadrants, changes in stool color, yellowing of sclera or skin, or darkened urine.
- Wear or carry medical identification stating the type of drug therapy used, especially if MAOIs are given.
- For patients taking MAO inhibitors, provide explicit instructions, written as well as verbal, on foods and beverages that must be avoided while taking the medication.
- Discuss concerns about sexual functioning and refer to the healthcare provider if concerns affect medication adherence.

Prescribing Considerations
- Antidepressants can react unpredictably with other medicines, including some over-the-counter medicines such as ibuprofen.
- Antidepressants are not usually recommended for most pregnant women, especially during the early stages of a pregnancy.
- The use of antidepressants while breastfeeding is not recommended.
- The use of antidepressants is not usually recommended in children and young people under the age of 18.

Bipolar Disorder

19.12 Bipolar disorder is a serious psychiatric disorder characterized by extreme mood swings from depression to euphoria.

Bipolar disorder, once known as manic depression, is a relatively common and serious psychiatric disorder. Suicide is a major risk; up to 50% of these patients attempt suicide, and 10–20% succeed. Many patients stop taking their medication during the course of pharmacotherapy. The etiology of the disorder is unknown, and symptoms may persist throughout the patient's lifespan.

Mania is characterized by symptoms that are generally the opposite of depressive symptoms. The excessive CNS stimulation that is characteristic of mania can be recognized by the following symptoms:

- Inflated self-esteem or grandiosity, the belief that one's ideas are far superior to anyone else's
- Decreased need for sleep or food
- Distractibility; racing thoughts with attention too easily drawn to irrelevant external stimuli
- Increased psychomotor or goal-directed activity (either socially, at work or at school, or sexually)
- Excessive pursuit of pleasurable activities without consideration of the negative consequences, such as shopping sprees, sexual indiscretions, or unsound business investments
- Increased talkativeness or pressure to keep talking
- With severe disease, delusions, paranoia, hallucinations, and bizarre behavior.

Although the pathophysiology of bipolar disorder is incompletely understood, mania and hypomania likely result from abnormal functioning of neurotransmitters in the brain. Mania may involve an excess of excitatory neurotransmitters (such as glutamate or norepinephrine) or a deficiency of inhibitory neurotransmitters (such as GABA). It is important to distinguish bipolar disorder from drug abuse, severe anxiety disorders, schizophrenia, dementia, or electrolyte disturbances, which can all produce symptoms similar to those of bipolar disorder.

Nonpharmacologic interventions play important roles in the treatment of patients with bipolar disorder. Lack of sleep, excessive stress, and poor nutrition are triggers for manic episodes and should be addressed in the plan of care. Support groups and psychotherapy are helpful for many patients. ECT is effective at treating acute manic and depressive episodes.

Pharmacotherapy of bipolar disorder is highly individualized and dependent on the severity of the condition and whether depression or mania is the predominant symptom. For patients with mild symptoms that cause only slight functional disruption, monotherapy with low doses of a mood stabilizer is indicated. More severely affected patients usually require combination therapy with a mood stabilizer plus an atypical antipsychotic. Antidepressant medications are usually discontinued because they can trigger mania in people with bipolar disorder. Caution must be used in female patients of childbearing potential because some drugs used for bipolar disorder cause fetal malformations.

Like the treatment of major depression, nonadherence with drug therapy is a serious problem in patients with bipolar disorder. As many as 50% of patients discontinue their medication during the first year of therapy. Lack of awareness is the single most common reason for nonadherence; mania is simply not viewed as abnormal by the individual experiencing it. In fact, people with mania are often able to work tirelessly on projects and accomplish many work- and home-related tasks. Surprisingly, the second most common reason for nonadherence is the presence of a comorbid substance abuse disorder, usually alcoholism. Psychotherapy and family support may be necessary to achieve proper adherence.

Drugs for Bipolar Disorder

19.13 Lithium is the conventional therapy for the treatment of bipolar disorder.

Drugs for bipolar disorder are called **mood stabilizers** because they have the ability to moderate extreme shifts in emotion and relieve symptoms of mania and depression during acute episodes. The selection of drug(s) depends on the predominant symptoms in the individual patient. Some of the drugs are better at managing mania, aggression, or agitation, whereas others are more effective at treating the depressive stage. Drugs from the following classes are used to manage bipolar disorder.

- *Lithium carbonate (Eskalith, Lithobid)*, the traditional medication for bipolar disorder, is a mood stabilizer prescribed as monotherapy or in combination with drugs from the classes listed below.
- *Antiseizure mood stabilizers*, such as valproic acid/divalproex (Depakene), have become a first-line therapy for bipolar disorder due to their improved safety profile. Valproic acid and other miscellaneous drugs for bipolar disorder are discussed in Section 19.14.
- *Atypical antipsychotics* are sometimes added to the regimen to control manic episodes, especially when mood stabilizers have proven ineffective.

Drugs used to treat bipolar disorder are shown in Table 19.5.

PROTOTYPE DRUG	Lithium Carbonate (Eskalith, Lithobid)

Classification **Therapeutic:** Antimanic, drug for bipolar disorder
Pharmacologic: Alkali metal ion salt

Table 19.5 Drugs for Bipolar Disorder

Drug	Route and Adult Dose (Maximum Dose Where Indicated)	Adverse Effects
lithium carbonate (Eskalith, Lithobid)	PO: 900–1800 mg/day individualized to patient response (max: 2.4 g/day)	*Headache, lethargy, fatigue, recent memory loss, nausea and vomiting, anorexia, abdominal pain, diarrhea, dry mouth, muscle weakness, nephrogenic diabetes insipidus, fine hand tremors, reversible leukocytosis* Peripheral circulatory collapse, neurotoxicity, seizures, coma
Antiseizure Drugs		
carbamazepine (Tegretol)	PO: 200 mg bid (max: 1600 mg/day)	*Dizziness, ataxia, somnolence, headache, nausea and vomiting, diplopia, blurred vision, sedation, drowsiness, prolonged bleeding time, transient leukopenia* Heart block, aplastic anemia, agranulocytosis, respiratory depression, exfoliative dermatitis, SJS, toxic epidermal necrolysis, deep coma, death (with overdose), liver failure, pancreatitis, bone marrow depression
lamotrigine (Lamictal)	PO: 300–500 mg/day in two divided doses (max: 700 mg/day)	
valproic acid/divalproex (Depakene)	PO: 250–750 mg/day in divided doses (max: 60 mg/kg/day)	
Atypical Antipsychotic Drugs		
aripiprazole (Abilify)	PO: 15–30 mg daily (max: 30 mg daily)	*Tachycardia, sedation, dizziness, headache, lightheadedness, somnolence, anxiety, nervousness, agitation, hostility, insomnia, nausea and vomiting, transient fever, constipation, akathisia, parkinsonism, gynecomastia (risperidone)* Agranulocytosis, neuroleptic malignant syndrome (risperidone, rare), risk of stroke in older adults with dementia-related psychosis (aripiprazole)
asenapine (Saphris)	SL: 5–10 mg bid (max: 20 mg/day)	
cariprazine (Vraylar)	PO: 1–6 mg once daily (max: 6 mg/day)	
lurasidone (Latuda)	PO: 40 mg once daily (max: 160 mg/day)	
olanzapine (Zyprexa)	PO: Start with 10 mg once daily; may increase or decrease in 5 mg/day increments	
quetiapine (Seroquel)	PO: 300–400 mg/day divided bid or tid (max: 800 mg/day)	
risperidone (Risperdal)	PO: 2–3 mg daily (max: 6 mg/day)	
ziprasidone (Geodon)	PO: 40–80 mg bid (max: 80 mg bid	

Note: *Italics* indicate common adverse effects. Underline indicates serious adverse effects.

Therapeutic Effects and Uses: Lithium was approved for use in 1970, although its benefit in treating bipolar disorder had been established since the 1950s. Lithium is a simple inorganic element that is found in the same group as sodium and potassium. It is available for PO administration as tablets, syrup, and controlled-release and slow-release tablets. Onset of action may take 1 to 3 weeks. Dosing is highly individualized and is based on serum drug levels and clinical response. Lithium has a short half-life and must be taken in multiple doses each day.

Lithium is an effective drug for controlling acute manic episodes and for preventing the recurrence of mania or depression. In the patient with mania, lithium decreases euphoria, hyperactivity, and other symptoms without causing sedation. Previously lithium was used for all patients with mania; at the present time it is used primarily for those patients with classic euphoric mania. Lithium, rather than valproic acid, appears to be more effective in reducing suicide risk in people diagnosed with bipolar disorder. Lithium may also be used for off-label indications, including alcoholism, bulimia, neutropenia, schizophrenia, prevention of vascular headaches, and hyperthyroidism.

Mechanism of Action: The precise mechanism of action of lithium is not known. It likely acts by changing neurotransmitter balance in specific brain regions. Lithium increases the synthesis of serotonin.

Pharmacokinetics:

Route(s)	PO
Absorption	Completely absorbed
Distribution	Distributed to all tissues and body fluids; crosses the blood–brain barrier and placenta; secreted in breast milk; not bound to plasma protein
Primary metabolism	Not metabolized
Primary excretion	Renal
Onset of action	Peak levels: 4–12 h (tablets) or 15–60 min (solutions)
Duration of action	Unknown

Adverse Effects: Many potential adverse effects are associated with the use of lithium. These are sometimes divided into those that occur at the initiation of therapy and those that occur with long-term therapy. Initial adverse effects are muscle weakness, lethargy, nausea and vomiting, polyuria, nocturia, headache, dizziness, drowsiness, tremors, and confusion. Many of the initial adverse effects are transient or may be easily managed. Long-term therapy can produce serious toxicity, including kidney impairment (proteinuria, albuminuria, or glycosuria), dysrhythmias, circulatory collapse, and leukocytosis. Lithium interferes with the synthesis of thyroid hormone and can cause hypothyroidism and goiter. **Black Box Warning:** Toxicity from lithium is closely related to serum concentrations and may occur at doses close to therapeutic levels. Facilities should be available to provide prompt and accurate serum concentration data. Serum lithium levels are monitored regularly during therapy and should be maintained within the narrow range of 0.8 to 1.4 mEq/L at the start of therapy and 0.4 to 1 mEq/L during maintenance therapy.

Contraindications/Precautions: Contraindications to the use of lithium include serious cardiovascular impairment, chronic kidney disease, and severe dehydration or sodium depletion. Older adults and debilitated patients must be carefully monitored. Caution must be used when the drug is given to patients with cardiovascular disease, thyroid disease, history of a seizure disorder, diabetes, urinary retention, or a systemic infection. Lithium produces an increased incidence of congenital defects, especially those involving the heart, and is normally not used during pregnancy. Its use should be discouraged during lactation.

Drug Interactions: There are many potential drug interactions, some of which can be serious. Diuretics can increase the risk of lithium toxicity by promoting sodium loss; the body replaces lost sodium with lithium, which is also a salt. NSAIDs and thiazide diuretics can increase lithium levels by increasing the renal reabsorption of lithium. Lithium may cause an increased hypothyroid effect of antithyroid drugs or drugs containing iodine. Concurrent administration with haloperidol may cause increased neurotoxicity. SES may result if lithium is administered with other drugs, such as SSRIs or dextromethorphan, or MAOIs that potentiate the actions of serotonin. **Herbal/Food:** An increased lithium effect may occur with the use of dandelion, goldenrod, juniper, parsley, nettle, or horsetail. Black or green tea, cola nut, or plantain may lead to a decreased lithium effect. Significant changes in sodium intake from foods will alter lithium excretion.

Pregnancy: Human data suggests that lithium carbonate may cause various fetal defects, including cardiac malformations, neural tube defects, increased birth complications, neonatal toxicity and many other adverse effects. All women of childbearing potential should be advised to use effective contraception during therapy. Breastfeeding is not recommended because the infant can develop lithium toxicity.

Treatment of Overdose: Overdose of lithium is treated with supportive measures such as emesis or lavage, maintaining airway and respiratory function, and dialysis, if lithium intoxication is severe.

Clinician Responsibilities:

- Obtain a complete health history and history of depression and mania symptoms. Obtain a medication history, particularly other medications used for depression or bipolar disorder.
- Assess baseline vital signs, weight, and laboratory studies, especially serum sodium, CBC, hepatic, and renal values. Monitor drug levels, weight, CBC, electrolytes, and urinalysis for protein, albumin, and glucose periodically during therapy.
- Report thirst, dizziness, lethargy or confusion, muscle weakness, or polyuria to the provider immediately after the early period of therapy as possible toxic effects.

Lifespan and Diversity Considerations:

- Carefully assess the older adult for signs of sodium imbalance or dehydration and for therapeutic and adverse effects. Monitor the older adult frequently because lithium toxicity may occur at lower therapeutic levels than in a younger patient.
- Monitor ethnically diverse patients closely for signs of lithium toxicity. Evaluate normal diet routines for high-sodium foods or beverages that may affect the therapeutic range of the drug.

Patient and Family Education:

- The full therapeutic effects of lithium may take 2 to 3 weeks or more to appear. Monitor the patient more closely during the early stages of therapy.
- Return regularly for laboratory work. Weigh self weekly and report a gain or loss of 1 kg (2 lb) in a day or 2 kg (5 lb) in a week.
- Maintain a normal-sodium diet and fluid intake without unusual or dramatic increases or decreases, which can affect drug level. Be cautious with exercising or on hot days because excessive sweating will lead to water and sodium loss. Avoid caffeine and alcohol.
- Report excessive thirst, urination, dizziness, muscle weakness, tachycardia, palpitations, or confusion promptly to the healthcare provider.
- Do not abruptly discontinue the drug. If discontinuation of the drug is desired, it should be discussed with the healthcare provider and alternative therapy considered.

Drugs Similar to Lithium Carbonate (Eskalith, Lithobid)

There are no drugs similar to lithium carbonate.

19.14 Antiseizure and atypical antipsychotic drugs are used to control symptoms of bipolar disorder.

Although lithium is well established as an effective treatment for bipolar disorder, many patients are unable to tolerate lithium. Pharmacologists have found several alternatives, some of which are FDA approved for bipolar disorder and others are prescribed off-label. It is relatively common for practitioners to use several drugs concurrently for the management of bipolar disorder. All of these medications have additional primary indications and are presented in other chapters of this textbook. The other classes include antiseizure drugs and atypical antipsychotics.

Antiseizure Drugs. The antiseizure drugs for bipolar disorder are classified as mood stabilizers. These medications have pharmacologic actions similar to lithium: relieving symptoms and preventing the recurrence of mania and depression.

Valproic acid (Depakene) and divalproex sodium (Depakote ER) are FDA approved for mood stabilization and mania suppression. Valproic acid is a preferred drug for many patients because it has fewer adverse effects than lithium, a higher therapeutic index, and a more rapid onset of action. One area in which it does not compare as favorably with lithium is in the ability to prevent suicide. Valproic acid is well tolerated in most patients but can occasionally cause serious toxicity. Rare cases of thrombocytopenia, pancreatitis, and liver failure have occurred and signs of any of these adverse events require immediate withdrawal of the drug. As with lithium, valproic acid is teratogenic and should not be used during pregnancy. It is secreted in breast milk and therefore should not be used during lactation. A prototype feature for this drug is included in Chapter 22.

Carbamazepine (Tegretol) was one of the initial drugs studied as a lithium alternative, but it was not until 2005 that it was approved for that indication. It reduces the symptoms of both manic and depressive phases of bipolar disorder and can reduce recurrence of the condition. It is preferred over lithium for patients who have mixed mania or rapid-cycling bipolar disorder. Neurologic adverse effects such as vertigo, headache, unsteadiness, and ataxia are common during early therapy but usually subside with continued use. Oral contraceptives may be less effective, and pregnant women should not take carbamazepine because this drug may cause birth defects. Increased CNS toxicity can result if carbamazepine is used concurrently with lithium. Carbamazepine is one of the most frequently prescribed antiseizure drugs, and a prototype feature is included in Chapter 22.

The antiseizure drug lamotrigine (Lamictal) is indicated for long-term maintenance therapy of bipolar disorder to prevent or delay relapses. It may be used alone or in combination with other mood stabilizers. The drug is well tolerated, with the most common adverse events being drowsiness, dizziness, ataxia, headache, diplopia, blurred vision, nausea and vomiting, and rash. Because rare cases of SJS have been documented, any appearance of rash calls for discontinuation of the drug. To minimize the risk of serious skin rashes, the dose of lamotrigine is increased gradually. Lamotrigine should be used cautiously in lactating women.

Other antiseizure drugs have been used off-label for bipolar disorder but they do not appear to be more effective than existing medications. These include oxcarbazepine (Trileptal), gabapentin (Neurontin), and topiramate (Topamax). Clonazepam (Klonopin) and lorazepam (Ativan) are benzodiazepines used for seizures that have been used off-label for bipolar disorder in combination with other drugs.

Atypical Antipsychotics. The primary use of antipsychotic drugs is to manage symptoms of severe psychosis, such as those found in patients with schizophrenia (see Chapter 20). However, some of the antipsychotic medications are also effective in controlling acute symptoms of mania and as long-term mood stabilizers in bipolar disorder. These drugs are usually used in combination with lithium or valproic acid, but they are also effective as monotherapy. Atypical antipsychotics approved for use in treating bipolar disorder include aripiprazole (Abilify), asenapine (Saphris), cariprazine (Vraylar), quetiapine (Seroquel), risperidone (Risperdal), and ziprasidone (Geodon). Symbyax a combination medication containing olanzapine and fluoxetine. The only approved indication for lurasidone (Latuda) is bipolar depression. For specific information on atypical antipsychotics, refer to Chapter 20.

Understanding Chapter 19

Key Concepts Summary

19.1 The two primary categories of mood disorders are depression and bipolar disorder.

19.2 Major depressive disorder is characterized by a depressed mood, with accompanying symptoms, that lasts at least 2 weeks.

19.3 The pathophysiology of depression has biological, genetic, and environmental components.

19.4 Assessment and diagnosis of depression are a collaborative effort among healthcare providers.

19.5 The majority of patients who attempt suicide have major depression.

19.6 Depression is sometimes treated with nonpharmacologic therapies.

19.7 The mechanism of action of antidepressants involves modulation of neurotransmitter levels in the brain.

19.8 Selective serotonin reuptake inhibitors are the preferred drugs for treating depression due to their low incidence of serious adverse effects.

19.9 Atypical antidepressants are alternatives to the selective serotonin reuptake inhibitors for depression and anxiety disorders.

19.10 Tricyclic antidepressants were once the mainstay for the treatment of depression, but they have many adverse effects.

19.11 Monoamine oxidase inhibitors are effective antidepressants but are seldom used due to potentially serious adverse effects.

19.12 Bipolar disorder is a serious psychiatric disorder characterized by extreme mood swings from depression to euphoria.

19.13 Lithium is the conventional therapy for the treatment of bipolar disorder.

19.14 Antiseizure and atypical antipsychotic drugs are used to control symptoms of bipolar disorder.

CASE STUDY: Making the Patient Connection

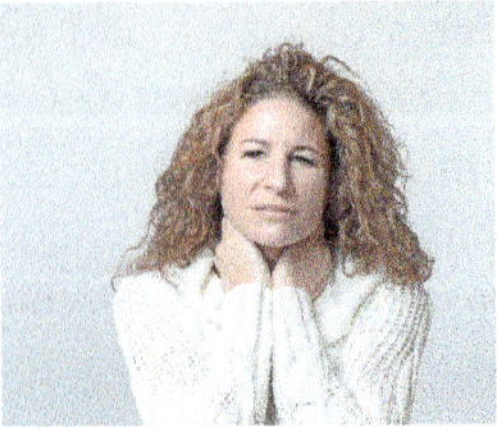

Remember the patient "Adelphia Williams" at the beginning of the chapter? Now read the remainder of the case study. Based on the information presented within this chapter, respond to the critical thinking questions that follow.

Adelphia is a 34-year-old mother of three young children. Before the children were born, she was employed as a corporate attorney, but she and her husband decided prior to the birth of their first child that she would stay at home until the children completed high school. They are financially stable. Adelphia has been a soccer coach, Boy Scout leader, president of the ladies' group at her church, and involved in various other community organizations. Within the past month, she has not participated in any of her previous activities and she has not explained why. Adelphia is in good physical health and had her annual physical examination the previous month. Other than a recent weight gain of 14 kg (31 lb), there has been no change since her last health visit. She takes no routine medications or herbal supplements.

Critical Thinking Questions

1. What first step must Charlie take to aid his wife with her depression?
2. When Adelphia is evaluated by a mental health professional, they begin talking about how antidepressant drug therapy works. Provide a brief explanation of antidepressant therapy.
3. How can a nurse determine if a therapeutic effect from the antidepressant medication is being achieved with Adelphia?

Additional Case Study

Andrew Phillips, age 17, was diagnosed with bipolar illness with acute mania at age 15. He was stabilized with lithium for the manic periods and is also taking valproic acid. This fall, he played football and is looking forward to playing baseball this spring and summer. Although they have a close relationship, his parents have concerns about his dietary habits and post-game festivities, especially now that he is driving and they are not available to monitor the situation.

1. Considering Andrew's activities and eating habits, what risks are possible and what assessments would the nurse make to ensure Andrew's lithium dosage remains effective and within a therapeutic range?
2. What suggestions could the nurse make that would help Andrew participate fully in his sports interests and post-game festivities?
3. What strategies might the nurse suggest for helping Andrew's parents participate in his activities and care?

Chapter Review

1. A healthcare provider has ordered imipramine (Tofranil) for four patients. A nurse would question the order for the patient with:
    1. Seizure disorders.
    2. Depression.
    3. Enuresis.
    4. Neuropathic pain.
2. The nurse determines that the patient understands an important principle in self-administration of fluoxetine (Prozac) when the patient makes which statement?
    1. "I should not decrease my sodium or water intake."
    2. "This drug can be taken concurrently with a monoamine oxidase inhibitor."
    3. "It may take up to 1 month to reach full therapeutic effects."
    4. "There are no problems associated with concurrent use of other central nervous system depressants."
3. The nurse is monitoring the patient for early lithium carbonate (Eskalith) toxicity. Which symptoms, if manifested by the patient, would indicate that toxicity may be developing? (Select all that apply.)
    1. Persistent gastrointestinal upset
    2. Confusion
    3. Polyuria
    4. Convulsions
    5. Ataxia
4. Which statement made by the patient who is taking lithium carbonate (Eskalith) indicates that further teaching is necessary?
    1. "I will be sure to remain on a low-sodium diet."
    2. "I will have blood levels drawn every 2 to 3 months, even when I have no symptoms."
    3. "Lithium has a narrow margin of safety, so toxicity is a very real concern."
    4. "I will not be able to breastfeed my baby."
5. The patient who has been taking venlafaxine (Effexor) for 2 weeks calls the nurse to report that there is no improvement in the depression. The nurse's best response is:
    1. "Call your healthcare provider and see if he or she will change the order to a different medication."
    2. "Are you sure that you are taking it as ordered? Perhaps you should consider increasing the dosage gradually."
    3. "The medication may take up to 3 weeks or longer to be effective. Continue taking the medication as ordered."
    4. "Add an over-the-counter antianxiety agent to your daily medications."
6. A 17-year-old patient is started on fluoxetine (Prozac) for treatment of depression. When teaching the patient and his family, what would the nurse include? (Select all that apply.)
    1. Report any sedation to the provider and exercise caution with activities requiring mental alertness.
    2. Fluctuations in weight may be managed with a healthy diet and adequate amounts of exercise.
    3. Report any thoughts of suicide to the provider immediately, especially during early initiation of the drug.
    4. The drug may be safely stopped if unpleasant side effects occur and reported to the provider at the next scheduled visit.
    5. The drug may cause excessive thirst but dramatic increase in fluid intake should be avoided.

See Appendix A for answers to critical thinking questions, case study questions and review questions.

References

American Foundation for Suicide Prevention. (2020). *Suicide statistics*. Retrieved from https://afsp.org/suicide-statistics/

Busti, A. J., Herrington, J. D., & Nuzum, D. S. (2015). *The mechanism of action of St. John's wort (Hypericum perforatum) in the treatment of depression*. Evidence-Based Medicine Consult. https://www.ebmconsult.com/articles/herbal-supplement-st-john-wort-hypericum-perforatum-mechanism-depression

Centers for Disease Control and Prevention. (2018). *Prevalence of depression among adults aged 20 and older: United States 2013–2016*. https://www.cdc.gov/nchs/products/databriefs/db303.htm

Centers for Disease Control and Prevention. (2019). *About PRAMS*. https://www.cdc.gov/prams/about/prams-faq.htm

Evans, M. G., Phillippi, S., & Gee, R. E. (2015). Examining the screening practices of physicians for postpartum depression: Implications for improving health outcomes. *Women's Health Issues, 25*(6), 703–710. https://doi.org/10.1016/j.whi.2015.07.003

Fornaro, M., Anastasia, A., Valchera, A., Carano, A., Orsolini, L., Vellante, F., et al. (2019). The FDA "black box" warning on antidepressant suicide risk in young adults: More harm than benefits? *Frontiers in Psychiatry, 10*, 294. https://doi.org/10.3389/fpsyt.2019.00294

Kilpatrick, S. J., Papile, L. A., & Macones, G. A. (2017). *Guidelines for perinatal care*. American Academy of Pediatrics.

Ko, J. Y., Rockhill, K. M., Tong, V. T., Morrow, B., & Farr, S. L. (2017). Trends in postpartum depressive symptoms—27 States, 2004, 2008, and 2012. *Morbidity and Mortality Weekly Report, 66*(6), 153–158. https://doi.org/10.15585/mmwr.mm6606a1

U.S. Food and Drug Administration. (2004). *FDA launches a multi-pronged strategy to strengthen safeguards for children treated with antidepressant medications* (FDA Publication No. P04-97). Washington, DC: U.S. Government Printing Office.

Selected Bibliography

Baldessarini, R. J. (2020). Epidemiology of suicide: Recent developments. *Epidemiology and Psychiatric Sciences, 29*, e71. http://doi.org/10.1017/S204579601900067

Byrnes, L. (2018). Perinatal mood and anxiety disorders. *Journal for Nurse Practitioners, 14*(7), 507–513. https://doi.org/10.1016/j.nurpra.2018.03.010

Centers for Disease Control and Prevention. (2017). *Deaths and mortality*. https://www.cdc.gov/nchs/fastats/deaths.htm

Gaynes, B. N., Jackson, W. C., & Rorie, K. D. (2015). Major depressive disorder in the primary care setting: Strategies to achieve remission and recovery. *Journal of Family Practice, 64*(9), S1–S15.

John, R. L., & Antai-Otong, D. (2016). Contemporary treatment approaches to major depression and bipolar disorders. *Nursing Clinics, 51*, 335–351. https://doi.org/10.1016/j.cnur.2016.01.015

Johnson, R. L., & Wilson, C. G. (2018). A review of vagus nerve stimulation as a therapeutic intervention. *Journal of Inflammation Research, 11*, 203–213. https://doi.org/10.2147/JIR.S163248

Karyotaki, E., Smit, Y., Henningsen, K. H., Huibers, M. J. H., Robays, J., de Beurs, D., & Cuijpers, P. (2016). Combining pharmacotherapy and psychotherapy or monotherapy for major depression?: A meta-analysis on the long-term effects. *Journal of Affective Disorders, 194*, 144–152. https://doi.org/10.1016/j.jad.2016.01.036

Morsel, A. M., Morrens, M., & Sabbe, B. (2018). An overview of pharmacotherapy for bipolar I disorder. *Expert Opinion on Pharmacotherapy, 19*(3), 203–222. https://doi.org/10.1080/14656566.2018.1426746

National Institute of Mental Health. (2019). Major depression. https://www.nimh.nih.gov/health/statistics/major-depression.shtml

Parker, G. F. (2014). DSM-5 and psychotic and mood disorders. *Journal of the American Academy of Psychiatry and the Law Online, 42*(2), 182–190.

Potter, D. R. (2019). Major depression disorder in adults: A review of antidepressants. *International Journal of Caring Sciences, 12*(3), 1936–1941.

Richardson, L., & Adams, S. (2018). Cognitive deficits in patients with depression. *Journal for Nurse Practitioners*, 14(6), 437–443. https://doi.org/10.1016/j.nurpra.2018.03.006

Rocha, F. L., Fuzikawa, C., Riera, R., & Hara, C. (2012). Combination of antidepressants in the treatment of major depressive disorder: A systematic review and meta-analysis. *Journal of Clinical Psychopharmacology, 32*, 278–281. https://doi.org/10.1097/JCP.0b013e318248581b

Soreff, S. (2019). *Bipolar disorder*. Medscape. http://emedicine.medscape.com/article/286342-overview

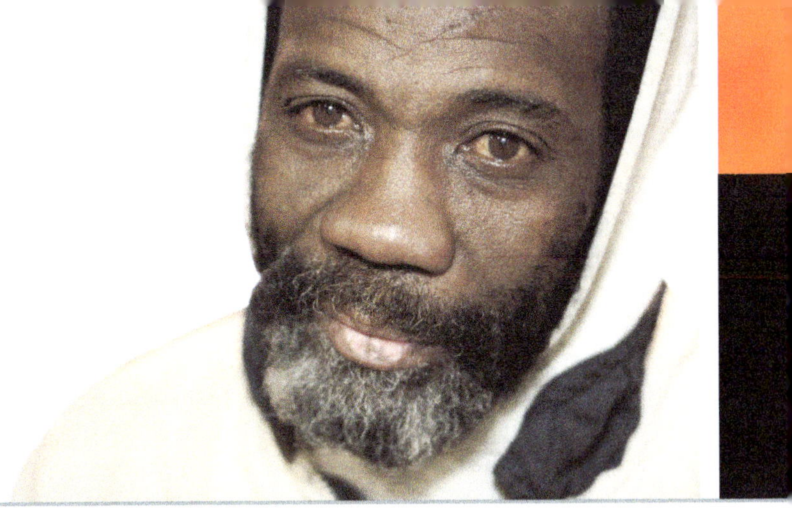

"It started when I was a teenager. I hear voices when there is nobody there. Sometimes, I can ignore them, but other times the voices get louder. You have to watch out because the neighbors may try to steal your soul. You can't let that happen to you. That's not going to happen to me. Don't let it happen to you."
—*Patient "George Watkins"*

Chapter 20
Pharmacotherapy of Psychoses

Chapter Outline

Learning Outcomes

After reading this chapter, the student should be able to:

1. Describe the general symptoms of psychosis.
2. Compare and contrast the positive and negative symptoms of schizophrenia.
3. Explain theories for the etiology of schizophrenia.
4. Describe the initial treatment and maintenance pharmacotherapy of schizophrenia.
5. Explain the importance of patient drug adherence in the pharmacotherapy of psychoses.
6. Explain how antipsychotic drugs are classified.
7. Discuss the rationale for selecting a specific antipsychotic drug for the treatment of schizophrenia.
8. Identify the extrapyramidal adverse effects of antipsychotic drugs.
9. Describe the nurse's role in the pharmacologic management of schizophrenia.
10. For each of the classes shown in the chapter outline, identify the prototype and representative drugs and explain the mechanism(s) of drug action, primary indications, contraindications, significant drug interactions, pregnancy data and important adverse effects.
11. Apply clinical judgement to care for patients receiving pharmacotherapy for psychosis.

Key Terms

Definitions of the terms in bold may be found in the Glossary.

Severe mental illness can be incapacitating for the patient and intensely frustrating for caregivers and healthcare providers. Prior to the 1950s, patients with such illness were institutionalized as soon as symptoms appeared, and often remained that way for their entire lives, with little or no hope of ever improving to the point of being able to function in society. The introduction of chlorpromazine (Thorazine) in the 1950s, and the subsequent development of newer drugs, revolutionized the treatment of mental illness. Many people with schizophrenia and other mental illnesses can now lead productive lives as functioning members of society, as long as their healthcare provider is able to successfully manage their condition. This chapter examines the nature and pharmacotherapy of psychotic illness.

Characteristics of Psychoses

20.1 Psychoses are severe mental disorders characterized by the inability to recognize reality.

Psychosis is a general term used in medicine to describe a loss of contact with reality. A psychosis is a symptom of a mental illness and is not considered a disease in itself. Characteristics of psychosis are relatively easy to recognize and include the following:

- **Delusions. Delusions** are firm ideas and beliefs that are false and not founded in reality. Delusions are sometimes religious in nature, with the individual believing he is a higher power or a messenger of a higher power. They may be grandiose, with the individual believing he is a king or great leader. Some patients with psychosis exhibit paranoid delusions, an extreme suspicion that they are being followed and that others are trying to harm them.
- **Hallucinations. Hallucinations** involve seeing, hearing, or feeling something that is not really there. Hallucinations most often are auditory; patients may hear voices telling them to harm themselves or others, that they are worthless or ugly, or that their behavior is unacceptable. Some patients may have visual hallucinations, seeing people or objects that are not present.
- **Lack of insight and judgment.** Patients are often unaware of their bizarre behavior and truly believe that the voices they hear and the delusions they experience are real.
- **Mood and affect.** During psychotic episodes, the patient's mood and affect may vary widely and be socially inappropriate. The patient may laugh at sad events or show no emotion at all. The patient may rapidly shift between happy and sad moods for no apparent reason.

Psychotic behavior ranges from total inactivity to extreme agitation and combativeness. Because patients are unable to distinguish what is real from what is illusion, they are often labeled as insane.

Psychoses are classified as acute or chronic. Acute psychotic episodes occur over hours or days, whereas chronic psychoses develop over months or years. Sometimes a specific cause may be attributed to the psychosis, such as brain tumors, overdoses of certain medications, extreme depression, electrolyte disorders, chronic alcoholism, or psychoactive drugs. Treating the underlying disorder may cause the psychosis to disappear.

Unfortunately, the vast majority of psychoses have no identifiable cause. These include psychoses associated with schizophrenia, bipolar disorder, and severe clinical depression.

To function in society, people with chronic psychoses require long-term pharmacotherapy. Patients must see their healthcare provider at regular intervals, and medication must be taken for life. Family members and social support groups are important sources of help for patients who cannot function normally in society without continuous drug therapy. One potential difficulty is that family relationships may be fractured secondary to the symptoms of psychosis, the length of time symptoms have been evident, and the tendency for the patients to become nonadherent to drug therapy. If these patients stop taking the antipsychotic medications, then symptoms of psychosis will most assuredly promptly reappear.

PharmFACT

Approximately 3.5 million Americans have schizophrenia, and about 50% of those diagnosed have received no treatment (Schizophrenia and Related Disorders Alliance of America, 2020).

Symptoms of Schizophrenia

20.2 Schizophrenia, the most common psychosis, has both positive and negative symptoms.

Schizophrenia is the most common psychotic disorder. Symptoms generally begin to appear in early adulthood, with a peak incidence in men 15 to 24 years of age and women 25 to 34 years of age. It is present in all cultures and ethnic groups.

Patients with schizophrenia experience a variety of diverse symptoms that may change over time. The disorder is characterized by abnormal thoughts and thought processes, disordered communication, withdrawal from people and the outside environment, an inability to independently perform activities of daily living (ADLs), and a high risk for suicide. Patients have a marked impairment in their ability to work or attend school. Many people with schizophrenia demonstrate all of these symptoms at some time during their illness, whereas others exhibit only one or two. Several subtypes of schizophrenia have been identified based on clinical presentation.

Symptoms of schizophrenia are classified as either positive or negative. **Positive symptoms** are those associated with a distortion in *excess* of normal function. These include hallucinations, delusions, disorganized thought or speech pattern, and movement disorders. **Negative symptoms** are those associated with a *loss* of normal functioning. These symptoms include a lack of interest in social activities, reduced or repetitious speech, loss of desire to perform personal hygiene measures, lack of emotion, unresponsiveness, or lack of pleasure in daily activities. Negative symptoms are characteristic of the indifferent personality exhibited by many patients with schizophrenia. Negative symptoms are harder to associate with schizophrenia and may be mistaken for depression or even laziness. Table 20.1 lists the different categories of schizophrenia symptoms.

Proper diagnosis of positive and negative symptoms is important for selection of the appropriate antipsychotic drug. Positive symptoms are easily recognized and more likely to motivate the patient or caregiver to seek treatment. Indeed, the positive symptoms respond more favorably to pharmacotherapy with antipsychotic drugs. The negative symptoms, however, often prevent a patient with schizophrenia from living independently, holding down a job, and enjoying life. When selecting outcomes for pharmacotherapy, the healthcare provider must address both positive and negative symptoms.

A third category of symptoms exhibited during schizophrenia is called *cognitive symptoms*. These include thinking difficulties, decreased attentiveness or ability to concentrate, and significant learning and memory problems. A retrospective look at the patient diagnosed with schizophrenia will usually reveal that these cognitive symptoms were present for some time but were not recognized as part of schizophrenia until the more obvious positive and negative symptoms appeared.

Schizoaffective disorder is a type of psychosis in which the patient exhibits symptoms of both schizophrenia *and* a mood disorder such as depression or bipolar disorder. An acute schizoaffective reaction may include distorted perceptions, hallucinations, and delusions, followed by extreme depression. Over time both positive and negative psychotic symptoms usually appear.

Many conditions can cause bizarre behavior, and these should be distinguished from schizophrenia. Chronic use of amphetamines or cocaine can create a paranoid syndrome. Certain complex partial seizures can cause unusual symptoms that are sometimes mistaken for psychosis. Brain neoplasms, infections, or hemorrhage can also cause bizarre, psychotic-like symptoms.

Etiology of Schizophrenia

20.3 The precise etiology of schizophrenia remains unknown.

The etiology and pathogenesis of schizophrenia are complex and involve multiple environmental and genetic factors. Early theories of the etiology of schizophrenia focused on specific disturbances in childrearing, such as poor communication between parents and offspring with schizophrenia. This view has been rejected in favor of biological theories. It should be understood, however, that environmental factors such as family dynamics can affect coping skills, which may influence the onset of psychosis, drug response, and adherence to treatment.

There is a definite genetic component to schizophrenia. People have a 5 to 10 times greater risk of getting schizophrenia if they have a first-degree relative with the disorder. In identical twins, if one twin has schizophrenia, the other has nearly a 50% risk of having the disorder. If both parents have schizophrenia, there is a 40% risk that their offspring will have the disorder.

Whether caused by genetics or the environment, schizophrenia is the result of various neurotransmitter

Table 20.1 Categories of Symptoms of Schizophrenia

Positive Symptoms	Negative Symptoms	Cognitive Symptoms
Agitation, anxiety Aggressiveness, combativeness Delusions Disorganized thoughts and speech Hallucinations; may be auditory, visual, tactile, olfactory, or gustatory Illusions Paranoia such as hypervigilance, worry, and vocalizations that everyone is "out to get me"	Lack of follow-through such as staying on schedule to finish a task (avolition) Little or no functional speech such as communicating in rambling statements or made-up words Marked withdrawal from social interactions and interpersonal relationships Lack of awareness or insight Apathy and lack of pleasure (anhedonia) Lack of ability to perform ADLs such as bathing or toileting Diminished or missing affect (affective flattening) Indifference or detachment toward life activities	Difficulty following the thread of a conversation Inability to focus attention Difficulty in identifying the steps needed to complete a task and placing them in the proper sequence Deficits in long-term memory Diminished "working memory": an inability to remember recently learned information and use it right away Difficulty following instructions

imbalances in specific areas of the brain. Abnormal dopaminergic pathways in the mesolimbic region of the brain are thought to be responsible for some of the symptoms of the disorder. Symptoms have been associated with **dopamine type 2 (D_2) receptors**. Most antipsychotic drugs act by entering dopaminergic synapses and competing with dopamine for receptors. By blocking D_2 receptors, antipsychotic drugs reduce the symptoms of schizophrenia. Pharmacotherapy Illustrated 20.1 shows antipsychotic drug action at the dopaminergic receptor.

Other neurotransmitters are also important to the pathogenesis of psychoses. These include serotonin (5-HT) and glutamate receptors.

PharmFACT

Childhood schizophrenia (younger than age 13) is rare but carries a worse prognosis than adult-onset schizophrenia. The majority of these children present with mental health disorders such as anxiety, depression, bipolar disorder, or attention-deficit/hyperactivity disorder 2 years prior to the onset of psychotic symptoms (Ash, 2019).

Management of Psychoses

20.4 Medical management of psychosis is challenging because patients often lack insight into their disease and believe their behavior is normal.

The medical management of severe mental illness is extremely challenging. Many patients do not view their behavior as abnormal and have difficulty understanding the need for drug therapy. When a medication produces undesirable adverse effects, such as severe muscle twitching

Pharmacotherapy Illustrated 20.1

Mechanism of Action of Antipsychotic Drugs

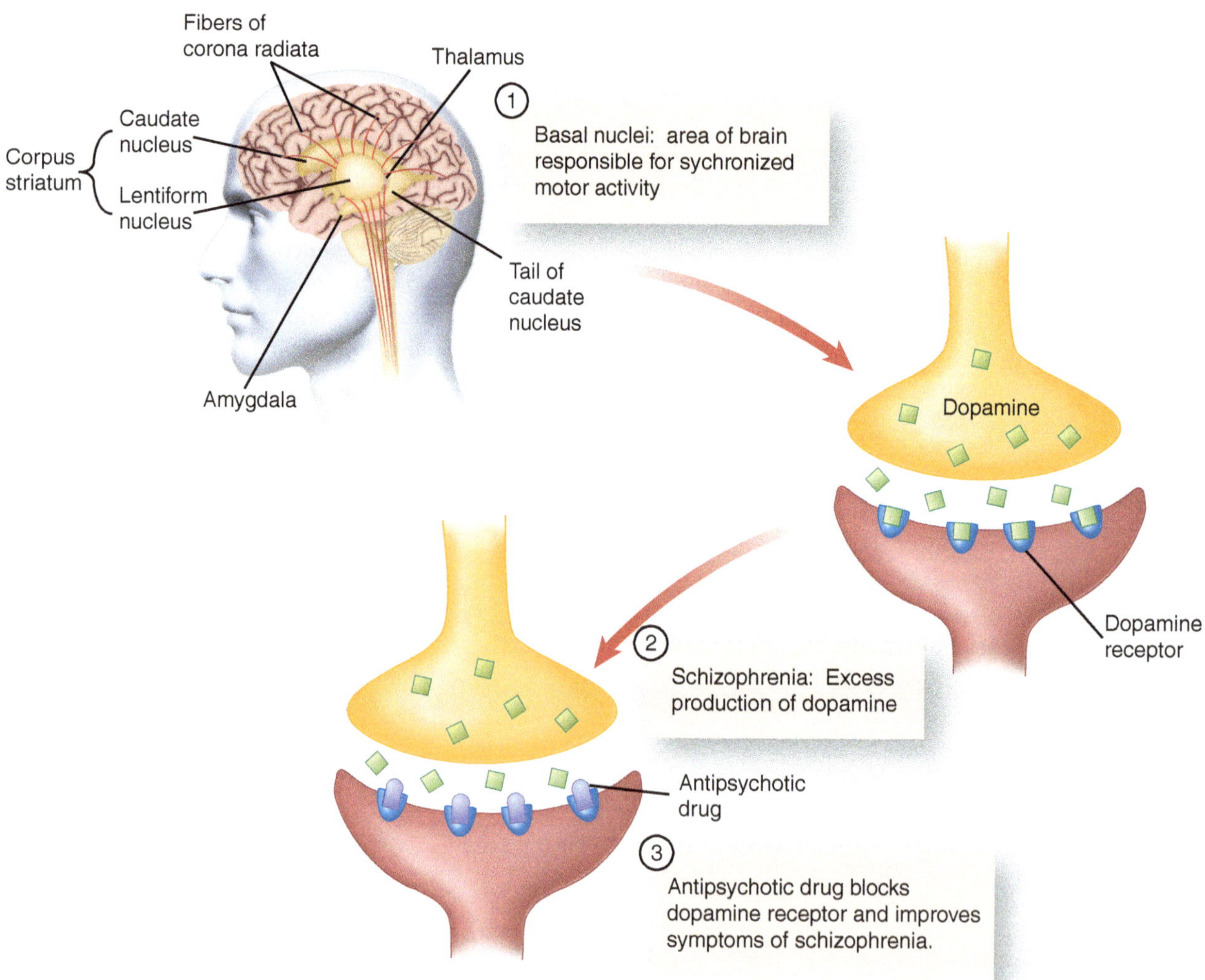

or sexual dysfunction, patients stop taking it and relapse, experiencing their former symptoms. Agitation, distrust, and extreme frustration are common because patients cannot comprehend why others are unable to think as they do or see the same things that they see.

The primary goal in treating psychosis is to manage symptoms such that the patient can function independently and accomplish ADLs with minimum assistance. This includes obtaining and holding employment and maintaining satisfactory interpersonal relationships. This level of success in treatment requires setting many small, realistic benchmarks that the patient, caregiver, and healthcare provider can achieve. These subgoals nearly always involve pharmacotherapy as well as establishing effective psychologic and social support.

Initial Treatment: The first psychotic episode may occur suddenly, or it may be preceded by a long period of subacute symptoms such as depression or withdrawal from normal activities. If the patient is exhibiting agitation or aggressiveness or presenting a physical danger to others, the initial doses of the antipsychotic drug may be higher than normal. High doses produce sedation, which is normally viewed as an adverse effect, but which is therapeutic in combative patients. Although most antipsychotics are given orally (PO), a few are available by the intramuscular (IM) route if the patient is uncooperative or if it is suspected that the patient is "cheeking" the medicine—hiding it in the mouth until the nurse leaves the room. Benzodiazepines such as lorazepam (Ativan) may be administered IM during the initial treatment period to relax or provide sedation for agitated patients. Lorazepam produces fewer serious adverse effects than antipsychotics and allows the dose of the antipsychotic drug to be reduced. Acute symptoms of psychosis usually resolve in 3 to 7 days, at which time the patient is switched to maintenance therapy.

Maintenance Treatment: The pharmacotherapy of chronic psychosis is a long-term process, with symptoms resolving gradually. Some symptoms resolve faster than others, depending on the patient and specific medication used. A patient or caregiver may notice improvement in acute symptoms after less than a week of therapy. After 2 to 4 weeks, mood, socialization, and the ability to provide self-care usually improve. By 6 to 8 weeks, definite improvement should be noted in most symptoms. Patients who have experienced untreated schizophrenia for many years are slower to respond than those experiencing their first episode. As long as symptoms continue to gradually improve, the patient is maintained on a stable dosage.

If substantial improvement is not observed after 8 to 12 weeks of therapy, the healthcare provider must explore reasons for the lack of response. For example, the patient may not be taking the medication or the original diagnosis may have been incorrect. If the patient has been taking the medication at average doses or higher, the healthcare provider will often *not* increase the dose because doing so increases the potential for serious adverse effects. Instead of increasing the dosage, a different antipsychotic drug may be substituted. The nurse, patient, and caregivers must understand that drug therapy is not a cure; in some cases, medications are simply not able to eliminate all psychotic symptoms.

How long does drug maintenance therapy continue? The answer to this is highly individualized, but the most common answer is for the lifetime of the patient. In patients experiencing their first acute episode, healthcare providers may slowly taper the dose after a year of successful therapy. Abrupt cessation of some antipsychotics can cause serious withdrawal symptoms, including nightmares, nausea and vomiting, salivation, sweating, and nervousness. When discontinuation is attempted, the patient should be monitored carefully and the drug restarted at the first sign of relapse. Approximately 15 to 25% of patients with psychoses can successfully stop drug therapy without experiencing their former symptoms. Discontinuation is not usually attempted in patients with long-standing chronic psychosis.

Nonadherence: Patients with serious mental illness have a very high nonadherence rate. Unless they are deemed overtly dangerous to themselves or other people, patients cannot be held for long periods of hospitalization against their wishes. Once the patient returns to the community, he or she may discontinue taking the drug and not return for follow-up appointments.

Reasons for nonadherence are many. Lack of insight into their illness causes patients with psychosis to view their behavior as normal. Patients with paranoia may feel that drug therapy is a plot by others to poison them and keep them from thinking clearly. Adverse effects are common and sometimes serious. Even motivated patients who understand the need for continuous drug therapy may have difficulty tolerating the adverse effects. The nurse must be diligent in teaching caregivers about means of maximizing adherence to the pharmacotherapeutic regimen and how to recognize signs of nonadherence.

Another factor causing nonadherence with medications for schizophrenia is the desire to drink alcohol. Excessive alcohol use is considered a comorbid condition with schizophrenia. Some patients use alcohol in an attempt to elevate their mood or to decrease symptoms of schizophrenia. However, alcohol can interact with some antipsychotic medications and cause a suboptimal response. Because studies have confirmed that alcohol worsens psychotic symptoms, patients should be instructed to avoid alcohol use.

Nonpharmacologic Therapies: Psychotherapy is an essential component of the total care of the patient with psychosis. In addition to individual supportive therapy, occupational therapy is initiated to give patients the requisite technical, social, and behavioral skills to enable them to return to the workforce. Some patients need skills in performing ADLs such as cooking, cleaning, and dressing. Family and caregiver training are included in the plan of care for the treatment of patients with schizophrenia whenever feasible.

Prognosis: Although there is no cure, schizophrenia can be successfully managed in a significant number of patients. Strong family and caregiver support, combined with pharmacotherapy, can decrease hospitalization and relapse rates and increase the potential for recovery. The prognosis for schizophrenia after 10 years of the disease is estimated as follows (Schizophrenia.com, n.d.):

- 25% completely recovered
- 25% much improved, relatively independent
- 25% improved, but require extensive support network
- 15% hospitalized, unimproved
- 10% deceased (mostly suicide).

Antipsychotic Drugs

20.5 Selection of an antipsychotic drug depends on its spectrum of adverse effects and the experience of the healthcare provider.

The pharmacotherapy of psychosis has undergone three major "generations." The first generation appeared in the early 1950s when the original drugs for treating severe mental illnesses were discovered. These drugs include conventional antipsychotics such as chlorpromazine. This essentially ended the era of placing all patients in mental asylums for their lifetimes. Unfortunately, first-generation drugs produced numerous adverse effects that were sometimes as serious as the symptoms of the patient's original disorder.

The second-generation or *atypical* antipsychotic drugs were discovered in the 1970s and 1980s. "Atypical" refers to several characteristics of these drugs compared to the conventional drugs:

- Significantly fewer adverse effects related to the extrapyramidal system
- Better patient adherence due to reduced adverse effects and less cognitive impairment
- More effective at resolving negative psychotic symptoms.

The third generation of antipsychotics began with the approval of the dopamine system stabilizers in 2002 and continues to this day. The drugs in this class have a lower risk of serious adverse effects than the previous two generations.

Two older terms are occasionally used to describe antipsychotic drugs. *Major tranquilizer* was the term used following the introduction of the first-generation drugs because sedation is a prominent action of them. *Neuroleptic* is a term used to denote drugs that have effects on the nervous system, especially those that have Parkinson's-like adverse effects on posture and body movement. Although the student will still encounter reference sources that refer to these drugs as tranquilizers or neuroleptics, *antipsychotic* is more accurate and is the preferred term.

Classification of Antipsychotics: There are two means of classifying antipsychotic medications. The older system uses the conventional versus atypical distinction. The conventional group is further subdivided by chemical classes into phenothiazines and nonphenothiazines. This older classification scheme has flaws because there is not always a clear distinction between a drug that is conventional and one that is atypical. Furthermore, some antipsychotics have an adverse effect profile that appears as if it is atypical at low doses but becomes conventional at high doses.

In recent years, a new system for classification has emerged. This system divides these medications by potency levels: low potency (drugs that require higher doses), moderate potency (drugs that require middle-range dosing), and high potency (drugs able to control symptoms of schizophrenia with low doses). This categorization was made based on the amount of medication necessary to produce an equivalent effect as compared to other drugs in the same category. As an example, 100 mg of chlorpromazine is approximately equivalent to 2 mg of haloperidol (Haldol). According to the categories, haloperidol is a high-potency drug, whereas chlorpromazine is a low-potency drug (although both are conventional antipsychotics). The nurse must not confuse potency with efficacy or effectiveness. *Potency* refers to a quantity, whereas *efficacy* refers to therapeutic response. Unfortunately, the potency classification method does not give any indication of a drug's effectiveness, mechanism of action, or chemical class.

So for the antipsychotic drugs, which classification should the student learn and use? Because the conventional/atypical and potency methods of drug classification are used in clinical practice, the student must be aware of both schemes.

Drug Selection

In terms of *effectiveness*, there is no single preferred drug for the long-term therapy of schizophrenia. Selection is based on clinician experience, the occurrence of adverse effects, and the therapeutic response of each individual patient. For example, patients with both psychosis and Parkinson's disease need an antipsychotic with minimal extrapyramidal symptoms. Those who operate machinery need a drug that does not cause sedation. Men who are sexually active may adhere better to a regimen with a drug that does not cause sexual dysfunction.

Clearly, the second-generation atypical and third-generation antipsychotics result in a lower incidence of serious adverse effects and are preferred drugs for psychosis. The experience and skills of the healthcare provider and mental health nurse are particularly valuable in achieving successful psychiatric pharmacotherapy.

Several long-acting depot preparations are available for patients who exhibit chronic nonadherence to the therapeutic regimen. For example, risperidone (Perseris, Risperdal Consta), paliperidone (Invega Sustenna), and fluphenazine decanoate last 2 to 6 weeks, depending on the dose and patient response.

CONNECTION Checkpoint 20.1

From what you learned in Chapter 4, explain why it is more important to receive an antipsychotic drug that has greater efficacy versus one that has higher potency.

Managing Adverse Effects

Although antipsychotic drug therapy clearly results in significant improvement in clinical symptoms, adverse effects are common and often serious. Managing these adverse effects is an essential component of successful antipsychotic pharmacotherapy.

Extrapyramidal symptoms (EPS) are a particularly serious set of adverse reactions to antipsychotic drugs. The term *extrapyramidal* refers to locations in the central nervous system (CNS) outside the cerebrospinal pyramidal tracts of the brain. Whereas the pyramidal system controls visible, voluntary movements, the extrapyramidal system is associated with postural and automatic movements that are not usually noticeable in a healthy person. EPS include the following:

- **Acute dystonia** occurs early in the course of pharmacotherapy with antipsychotics and involves severe muscle spasms, particularly of the back, neck, tongue, and face. In rare cases, acute dystonia can be so severe as to dislocate joints and impair respiration due to laryngospasm. The risk of acute dystonia is greater with high-potency antipsychotics. Administration of drugs with anticholinergic properties such as diphenhydramine (Benadryl) or benztropine (Cogentin) can reverse acute dystonia symptoms within minutes when administered parenterally. For dystonia refractory to anticholinergic drugs, diazepam (Valium) may be administered.
- **Akathisia**, the most common EPS, is an inability to rest or relax. The patient paces, has trouble sitting or remaining still, and has difficulty sleeping. Repetitive movements such as rocking while standing or sitting and crossing and uncrossing legs may be evident. Akathisia can even be mistaken for anxiety and agitation, possibly resulting in an increase in antipsychotic dose, which will exacerbate these adverse effects. In some cases, akathisia may require symptom management with beta-adrenergic blockers, anticholinergics, or benzodiazepines.
- **Parkinsonism** is induced by antipsychotic drugs and may include tremor, loss of fine motor skills, muscle rigidity, stooped posture, and a shuffling gait. The treatment of antipsychotic drug-induced parkinsonism includes anticholinergic drugs and amantadine (Symmetrel) (see Chapter 21).
- **Tardive dyskinesia (TD)** is characterized by involuntary, unusual tongue and face movements such as lip smacking, rapid eye blinking, and wormlike motions of the tongue. They generally occur during long-term therapy, and symptoms may persist for months or years after the drug is discontinued. Symptoms of TD may worsen or even become permanent when the antipsychotic drug is withdrawn. In 2017 the first drug for treating TD was approved by the U.S. Food and Drug Administration (FDA). Valbenazine (Ingressa) improves the involuntary movements that are characteristic of TD. This drug may cause serious side effects such as drowsiness and QT prolongation.

When EPS are reported early, the drug is usually withdrawn or the dosage reduced so that the symptoms can be eliminated. If allowed to continue for prolonged periods, EPS may become permanent. The nurse must be vigilant in observing and reporting EPS because prevention is the best treatment. Table 20.2 contains further information on the EPS of antipsychotic medications.

A potentially fatal adverse reaction to antipsychotic medications is **neuroleptic malignant syndrome (NMS)**. Symptoms include high fever, diaphoresis, muscle rigidity, tachycardia, and blood pressure fluctuations. Although rare, quick, aggressive treatment is necessary because the condition can rapidly deteriorate to stupor or coma. The most immediate intervention is to discontinue all antipsychotics. Supportive treatment includes antipyretics, electrolytes, and muscle relaxants.

Adverse effects on the reproductive system are a major cause of nonadherence to the drug regimen in some patients. Up to 50 to 60% of men taking antipsychotics may experience ejaculation disorders and erectile dysfunction. In women, decreased libido and inability to achieve orgasm may occur. Many antipsychotics increase serum levels of the hormone prolactin, which can cause secretion of breast

Table 20.2 Extrapyramidal Symptoms of Antipsychotic Medications

Type of Symptom	Time of Onset	Manifestations	Treatment
Acute dystonia	Several hours to 5 days	Severe spasms of the muscles of the tongue, face, neck, or back; involuntary upward deviation of the eyes; arching forward of the trunk while the head and legs are thrust backward	Immediately administer an anticholinergic such as diphenhydramine or benztropine IV or IM. Symptoms usually resolve within 5–20 min.
Akathisia	Within first 2 months of treatment	Pacing, squirming, inability to sit still, uncontrollable need to be moving	Anticholinergics (diphenhydramine, etc.), benzodiazepines (diazepam, alprazolam, etc.), or beta blockers (atenolol, labetalol, etc.).
Antipsychotic-induced parkinsonism	5–30 days	Tremor, rigidity, shuffling gait, masklike facies, drooling, cogwheeling (a jerky or clicking sensation when a limb is moved), stooped posture, bradykinesia. Symptoms cannot be distinguished from true Parkinson's disease.	Anticholinergics (benztropine, diphenhydramine, etc.), amantadine. Treatment should not need to be continued for more than a few months because symptoms should resolve.
Tardive dyskinesia	During long-term therapy	Involuntary, unusual movements of the tongue and face and lip-smacking movements; may include involuntary movements of the arms and legs, fingers, toes, and trunk. Incidence is very high in older patients.	For some patients, decreased doses of antipsychotics, administration of benzodiazepines, or gradual withdrawal of anticholinergics may help. Some patients may benefit from switching to an atypical antipsychotic.

milk (galactorrhea) and breast enlargement (gynecomastia). These events may occur in both men and women. Most women will also experience menstrual dysfunction due to the high prolactin levels.

Unlike many CNS drugs, antipsychotic medications do not cause physical or psychologic dependence. They also have a wide safety margin between a therapeutic and a lethal dose; deaths due to overdoses of antipsychotic drugs are uncommon. They should be gradually discontinued, however, to avoid withdrawal symptoms.

First-Generation Antipsychotics

The first-generation or conventional antipsychotics form two subclasses: the phenothiazines and the nonphenothiazines.

20.6 The phenothiazines are effective at treating schizophrenia symptoms but exhibit a high incidence of adverse effects.

Phenothiazine is a chemical term that refers to compounds with three rings that are joined together by nitrogen and sulfur atoms. Originally developed as a yellow dye in the 1800s, phenothiazine became the starting molecule for a series of drugs, which are recognized by the *-zine* suffix. The student will encounter the term *phenothiazine* in other chapters because several drug classes produce "phenothiazine-like" adverse effects. The phenothiazines are listed in Table 20.3.

At equivalent doses, all phenothiazines have the same effectiveness in treating psychoses, and all produce a similar spectrum of adverse effects. Selection of a specific phenothiazine is determined by the severity and extent of expected adverse effects. For example, if EPS are a major concern, thioridazine may be selected because it gives the lowest incidence of EPS in the class. If the patient is driving or working, fluphenazine may be selected because it produces less sedation and fewer anticholinergic effects than other phenothiazines.

It should be clearly understood at the outset of conventional antipsychotic therapy that it is not always possible to control the disabling symptoms of schizophrenia without producing some degree of EPS or anticholinergic adverse effects. Adjunct drug therapy may be warranted to treat expected adverse effects. For example, concurrent pharmacotherapy with an anticholinergic drug may prevent some of the EPS. For acute dystonias, benztropine (Cogentin) may be given parenterally. Levodopa is usually avoided because its ability to increase dopamine function antagonizes the mechanism of action of the phenothiazines. Beta-adrenergic blockers and benzodiazepines are sometimes given to reduce signs of akathisia.

Some phenothiazines have indications beyond psychiatry. These indications include:

- **Nausea and vomiting.** The phenothiazines reduce nausea and vomiting by blocking dopamine receptors in the chemoreceptor trigger zone in the medulla. Although effective, the use of phenothiazines in treating nausea and vomiting has declined due to the discovery of serotonin antagonists such as ondansetron (Zofran).
- **Cold and allergy symptoms.** Promethazine has antihistamine properties that are of benefit for treating serious cough and symptoms of the common cold. For this indication, promethazine is combined with other medications such as codeine or dextromethorphan.
- **Tourette's syndrome.** This condition is characterized by tics: sudden, loud vocalizations, often cursing, and muscle movements such as twitches, kicking, or hitting. The patient feels a premonitory urge, a type of

Table 20.3 First-Generation Antipsychotic Drugs

Drug	Route(s) and Adult Dose (Maximum Dose Where Indicated)	Adverse Effects
Phenothiazines		
chlorpromazine	PO: 10–25 mg tid initially, with dose gradually increased until response is obtained (max: 1000 mg/day) IM/IV: 25–50 mg (max: 600 mg q4–6h)	*Sedation, drowsiness, dizziness, EPS, constipation, photosensitivity, orthostatic hypotension, anticholinergic effects, seizures* Agranulocytosis, pancytopenia, anaphylaxis, TD, NMS, hypothermia, adynamic ileus, sudden unexplained death
fluphenazine	PO: 1–10 mg/day in 1–4 divided doses (max: 40 mg/day) Subcutaneous/IM: Decanoate 12.5–25 mg every 2–4 wk	
perphenazine	PO: 4–8 mg tid (max: 64 mg/day)	
prochlorperazine	PO: 5–10 mg tid or qid (max: 150 mg/day for psychosis, 40 mg/day for nausea and/or vomiting) IM: 10–20 mg, may repeat q1–4h	
thioridazine	PO: 50–100 mg tid (max: 800 mg/day)	
trifluoperazine	PO: 1–2 mg bid (max: 20 mg/day)	
Nonphenothiazines		
haloperidol (Haldol)	IM (depot): 50–100 mg each month	*Akathisia, sedation, transient drowsiness, EPS, tremor, orthostatic hypotension, weight changes, anticholinergic effects* TD, NMS, acute kidney failure, respiratory depression, laryngospasm, hepatotoxicity, sudden unexplained death, agranulocytosis
loxapine	PO: Start with 20 mg/day and increase to 60–100 mg/day in divided doses (max: 250 mg/day)	
pimozide	PO: 1–2 mg/day (max: 10 mg/day)	
thiothixene	PO: 2 mg tid (max: 60 mg/day)	

Note: *Italics* indicate common adverse effects. Underline indicates serious adverse effects.

warning, that a tic is forthcoming, and the tics may be consciously suppressed for limited periods. Drugs from a large number of classes have been used to suppress tics, including phenothiazines such as fluphenazine. There is no cure for Tourette's syndrome, but the symptoms can be managed in many patients.

- **Organic brain syndrome.** *Organic brain syndrome (OBS)* is a general term that refers to decreased mental function due to physical disorders rather than psychiatric illness. OBS can cause symptoms similar to those of schizophrenia, including delirium, amnesia, and agitation. OBS is a common diagnosis in older adults and is associated with a large number of conditions, including head trauma, brain tumors, stroke, shock, drug interactions, adverse effects, and kidney or hepatic failure. Chronic OBS is known as dementia. Historically, the phenothiazines were the preferred drugs for treating symptoms of OBS; however, atypical antipsychotics such as risperidone (Risperdal) are now more commonly prescribed for this condition.

PROTOTYPE DRUG Chlorpromazine

Classification **Therapeutic:** Antipsychotic (first generation)
Pharmacologic: Phenothiazine, dopamine (D_2) receptor antagonist

Therapeutic Effects and Uses: Approved in 1954, chlorpromazine is a low-potency antipsychotic that blocks several types of receptors within and outside the CNS, including dopamine, histamine, norepinephrine, and acetylcholine receptors. The therapeutic effects in a patient with schizophrenia appear to be due to the blocking of dopamine receptors. Peak antipsychotic effects may take as long as 6 weeks to several months. IM dosing is available for acutely agitated patients. Thorazine was once a popular trade name for this drug, but chlorpromazine is now only available in generic form. The major use of chlorpromazine is to treat the symptoms of schizophrenia and other psychotic disorders. The drug can effectively suppress symptoms of acute psychotic episodes and can greatly decrease the incidence of relapse if it is used consistently. Although once widely prescribed for psychosis, chlorpromazine is rarely used today because of the potential for serious adverse effects. Other approved uses for chlorpromazine include treating schizoaffective disorder and the manic phase of bipolar disorder, as an antiemetic, as an adjunct in the treatment of tetanus, and for intractable hiccups. It is important to understand that chlorpromazine, and the other phenothiazines, do not change the underlying pathology of psychotic disease, but rather deal only with the symptoms.

Mechanism of Action: Chlorpromazine acts by blocking postsynaptic dopamine receptors. Decreases in the function of this neurotransmitter are associated with diminished psychotic symptoms. Decreased dopamine in the chemoreceptor trigger zone in the medulla results in an antiemetic effect.

Pharmacokinetics:

Route(s)	PO, rectal, IM, IV (only for severe conditions)
Absorption	20% absorbed PO; well-absorbed IM
Distribution	Widely distributed; crosses the placenta; secreted in breast milk; 92–97% bound to plasma protein
Primary metabolism	Hepatic; some active metabolites
Primary excretion	Renal
Onset of action	1/2–12 h, depending on route; optimal results will take several months
Duration of action	Half-life: 30 h

Adverse Effects: Common adverse effects of chlorpromazine include headache, anticholinergic symptoms (dry mouth, anorexia, nausea, vomiting, constipation), weight gain, anemia, phototoxicity, blurred vision, dry eyes, and glaucoma. Of all the antipsychotics, phenothiazines are the most likely to produce EPS. Serious or life-threatening adverse effects include tachycardia, cardiac arrest, laryngospasm, respiratory depression, seizures, agranulocytosis, leukopenia, leukocytosis, and NMS. Abrupt withdrawal can induce symptoms such as nausea and vomiting and tremors. **Black Box Warning:** This drug is not indicated for the treatment of dementia-related psychosis. Older adults with dementia-related psychosis treated with antipsychotic drugs are at increased risk of death compared to placebo.

Contraindications/Precautions: There are many contraindications to the use of chlorpromazine; these are coronary artery disease, severe hypertension or hypotension, blood dyscrasias, coma, brain damage, bone marrow depression, alcohol or barbiturate withdrawal, glaucoma, hepatic dysfunction, and children under age 6 months. The drug should be used with caution in patients with cardiovascular disease because it may cause orthostatic hypotension (especially in older adults), increase the heart rate, and prolong the QT interval on the electrocardiogram (ECG). Patients with severe hepatic impairment may experience excessive CNS depression. The drug decreases the seizure threshold; thus, patients with preexisting epilepsy must be carefully monitored. Chlorpromazine may produce drowsiness and lethargy in breastfeeding newborns; thus, use is not recommended during lactation. Older adults are very sensitive to the EPS effects of phenothiazines; thus, the drug must be used with caution in this population. Patients with benign prostatic hyperplasia (BPH) should use this drug with caution because it may cause urinary retention.

Drug Interactions: Many drug interactions are possible with chlorpromazine. Use with other CNS depressants, including alcohol, will cause additive sedation. Use with tricyclic antidepressants or anticholinergic drugs will result in additive anticholinergic adverse effects. Decreased absorption and thus lower serum levels of chlorpromazine will occur if used with antacids, barbiturates, or lithium. Increased serum levels and possible hypotension may occur if administered concurrently with epinephrine. Use with warfarin can lead to decreased anticoagulant effects. Phenothiazines inhibit the therapeutic effects of levodopa and may cause excessive sedation if used concurrently. **Herbal/Food:** Increased action of chlorpromazine may occur with nutmeg, hops, nettle, and cola tree. Increased anticholinergic effects can occur with henbane leaf, kava, and betel palm.

Pregnancy: Animal reproduction studies showed embryotoxicity, fetal toxicity and increased neonatal mortality. Chlorpromazine is secreted in human milk and breastfed neonates should be monitored for drowsiness and lethargy.

Treatment of Overdose: Overdose will cause profound CNS depression, seizures, hypotension, and EPS. Treatment is supportive and may include vasopressors and antiseizure drugs. Airway and gastric lavage are provided if taken PO. Epinephrine should not be administered, and vomiting should not be induced.

Clinician Responsibilities: Key clinical implications for patients receiving chlorpromazine are included in Applied Clinical Judgment: Patients Receiving Pharmacotherapy with Antipsychotics.

Drugs Similar to Chlorpromazine

Similar drugs include fluphenazine, perphenazine, prochlorperazine, thioridazine, and trifluoperazine. Promethazine is chemically classified as a phenothiazine, but the drug has no antipsychotic action and its primary use is as an antihistamine (see Chapter 45). All first-generation phenothiazines carry black box warnings that they are not to be used to treat dementia-related psychosis due to an increased risk of mortality in patients with this disorder. In animal reproduction studies, phenothiazines have been shown to cause fetal harm. Human neonates exposed during the third trimester are at risk to developing severe symptoms such as agitation, tremor, and feeding disorder. These drugs should only be used during pregnancy or lactation when the potential benefits justify the potential risks to the fetus or neonate.

Fluphenazine: Approved in 1959, fluphenazine is a high-potency phenothiazine approved to treat psychotic disorders, including schizophrenia. The drug is most often given as fluphenazine decanoate, a long-acting depot formulation that is given either subcutaneously or IM. Administered at 1- to 4-week intervals, fluphenazine decanoate is advantageous for those patients who are not adherent to taking their PO medications daily. Oral and injectable preparations (fluphenazine hydrochloride) are also available. A stable dose of PO fluphenazine is generally achieved before placing the patient on the depot preparation. The injectable preparations are not recommended for children under age 12. Fluphenazine produces less sedation and fewer anticholinergic effects than chlorpromazine, but EPS are a major concern.

Perphenazine: Approved in 1959, perphenazine is a medium-potency drug used to treat schizophrenia, nausea, and vomiting. EPS are prominent. The drug has the same actions and adverse effects as chlorpromazine. Orthostatic hypotension is common.

Prochlorperazine: Approved in 1956, prochlorperazine is a phenothiazine rarely used as an antipsychotic. Its primary use is for the management of severe nausea and vomiting (see Chapter 60). For this purpose, it may be administered PO, rectally, IM, or IV. When used as an antiemetic, doses are low and phenothiazine-like adverse effects are rare.

Thioridazine: Thioridazine, a low-potency phenothiazine, is approved to treat schizophrenia that has not responded to other antipsychotics. Because of the possibility of fatal dysrhythmias (black box warning), thioridazine should be used only to treat conditions that have not responded to safer drugs. Approved in 1959, thioridazine is available PO and has one of the lowest incidences of EPS of the phenothiazines.

Trifluoperazine: Trifluoperazine is a high-potency phenothiazine approved to treat psychotic disorders. Approved in 1958, it is available in PO form. Trifluoperazine causes less sedation than chlorpromazine but EPS is prominent. All other information is the same as with chlorpromazine, except that it cannot be used in children under age 6. Trifluoperazine was formerly available as Stelazine, but this trade name is no longer marketed.

20.7 The nonphenothiazine first-generation antipsychotics have the same therapeutic applications and similar adverse effects as the phenothiazines.

The nonphenothiazine conventional antipsychotic class consists of drugs whose chemical structures are dissimilar to the phenothiazines. Introduced shortly after the phenothiazines, the nonphenothiazines were initially expected to produce fewer serious adverse events. Unfortunately, this is not the case. The spectrum of adverse effects for the nonphenothiazines is identical to that for the phenothiazines, although the degree to which a particular effect occurs depends on the drug utilized.

In general, the nonphenothiazine drugs cause less sedation and fewer anticholinergic adverse effects than chlorpromazine but exhibit an equal or greater incidence of EPS. Concurrent therapy with other CNS depressants must be carefully monitored because of potential additive sedation.

Drugs in the nonphenothiazine class have the same therapeutic effects and efficacy as the phenothiazines. They are also believed to act by the same mechanism as the phenothiazines; that is, by blocking postsynaptic D_2 dopamine receptors. As a class, they offer no significant advantages over phenothiazines in the treatment of schizophrenia and have largely been replaced by the second-generation, atypical antipsychotics. Doses of the nonphenothiazine antipsychotics are shown in Table 20.3.

PROTOTYPE DRUG Haloperidol (Haldol)

Classification **Therapeutic:** Antipsychotic (first generation)
Pharmacologic: Nonphenothiazine, dopamine (D_2) receptor antagonist

Therapeutic Effects and Uses: Haloperidol, a high-potency antipsychotic approved in 1967, is effective in treating both acute and chronic psychotic disorders as well as Tourette's syndrome. It may be used off-label to treat persistent hiccups, autism, children with severe behavioral problems (short term) and OBS with psychotic features, and for the emergency sedation of patients who are severely agitated or delirious. It may be administered PO or IM but should not be given IV due to the potential for dysrhythmias. Haloperidol decanoate (Haldol LA) is a long-acting IM formulation that is administered once a month. This is an excellent formulation for patients who cannot be independent in their drug regimen, who may become nonadherent to the drug regimen, or who have no family members to assist them in taking their medication on a regular basis. The medication can be administered either in a clinic setting or by a home health nurse.

Mechanism of Action: Haloperidol depresses the cerebral cortex, hypothalamus, and limbic system, which are parts of the brain that control activity and aggression. It blocks neurotransmission at postsynaptic dopamine D_2 receptors and exhibits alpha$_1$-adrenergic blocking and anticholinergic effects.

Pharmacokinetics:

Route(s)	PO, IM
Absorption	Well-absorbed PO and IM
Distribution	Widely distributed; may cross the placenta; secreted in breast milk; 92% bound to plasma protein
Primary metabolism	Hepatic; significant first-pass metabolism
Primary excretion	Renal; small amounts biliary with extensive enterohepatic recycling
Onset of action	Erratic if given PO; 30–45 min IM; decanoate form reaches peak plasma level in 7 days
Duration of action	Half-life: 24 h (PO); 21 h (IM); 3 wk (decanoate)

Adverse Effects: Haloperidol exhibits an adverse effect profile similar to that of other first-generation antipsychotics. Common adverse effects include drowsiness and EPS. Life-threatening adverse effects include TD, NMS, agranulocytosis, respiratory depression, and laryngospasm. Like chlorpromazine, thioridazine, and pimozide, haloperidol increases the QT interval and can pose a risk for dysrhythmias. **Black Box Warning:** This drug is not indicated for the treatment of dementia-related psychosis. Older adults with dementia-related psychosis treated with antipsychotic drugs are at increased risk of death compared to placebo.

Contraindications/Precautions: Contraindications for use of haloperidol include Parkinson's disease, seizure disorders, coma, alcoholism, severe mental depression, CNS depression, or lactation. Patients who are older or debilitated or those with urinary retention, glaucoma, or severe cardiovascular disorders must be given haloperidol cautiously. The drug lowers the seizure threshold; thus, patients with preexisting epilepsy must be carefully monitored.

Drug Interactions: Haloperidol is metabolized by hepatic CYP450 enzymes and can inhibit some isozymes (CYP2D6). Thus, interactions are possible with other drugs affecting these enzymes. For example, carbamazepine, an inducer of CYP450, can reduce the serum level of haloperidol by up to 50%. Increased CNS depression can occur if given concurrently with other CNS depressants, including alcohol, tricyclic antidepressants, or opioids. Anticholinergics that are given concurrently may increase intraocular pressure. Use with methyldopa may precipitate dementia. Haloperidol may increase the QT interval and should be used with caution with other drugs that increase this interval due to the potential for additive cardiotoxicity. A few patients who were taking haloperidol and lithium concurrently experienced irreversible brain damage; thus, the two drugs should not be combined. Haloperidol inhibits the therapeutic effects of levodopa and may cause excessive sedation if used concurrently. **Herbal/Food:** Increased action of haloperidol may occur if chamomile, hops, kava, nutmeg, skullcap, or valerian is used concurrently. An antagonist action may occur with the use jimsonweed. Increased EPS may occur if betel palm or kava is used concurrently.

Pregnancy: Animal reproduction studies showed embryotoxicity, fetal death, and gross malformations. The drug is excreted in human milk and has produced EPS in breastfed infants.

Treatment of Overdose: Overdose will result in sedation, respiratory depression, coma, hypotension, and severe EPS. Treatment is supportive. Antidysrhythmic and vasopressor drugs may be necessary to maintain cardiovascular function.

Clinician Responsibilities: The phenothiazine and nonphenothiazine drug classes are both first-generation antipsychotics with very similar pharmacologic actions and adverse effects. Key clinical implications for patients receiving these drugs are included in Applied Clinical Judgment: Patients Receiving Pharmacotherapy with Antipsychotics.

Drugs Similar to Haloperidol (Haldol)

Similar drugs include loxapine, pimozide, and thiothixene. All first-generation nonphenothiazines carry black box warnings that they are not to be used to treat dementia-related psychosis. In animal reproduction studies, the nonphenothiazines showed embryotoxicity, and human neonates exposed during the third trimester are at risk to developing severe symptoms such as agitation, tremor, and feeding disorder. These drugs should only be used during pregnancy or lactation when the potential benefits justify the potential risks to the fetus or neonate.

Loxapine: Approved in 1975, loxapine is a medium-potency antipsychotic given by the PO route. It is approved to treat schizophrenia, psychotic depression, and other psychotic disorders, and it is used off-label to treat severe behavioral disturbances associated with Parkinson's and Alzheimer's diseases. Use of loxapine is restricted to treating mental illness refractory to treatment from safer drugs. The adverse effect profile of loxapine is the same as that of haloperidol, and EPS frequently occur during therapy. An active metabolite of loxapine is amoxapine, a drug marketed separately as an antidepressant.

Pimozide: Approved in 1984, pimozide is a high-potency PO medication used for treating motor and vocal tics associated with Tourette's syndrome. Although not a true antipsychotic medication, it may be used off-label to treat schizophrenia. The drug has little sedative action and should not be used to control acute psychosis characterized by agitation or hyperexcitability. EPS occur frequently with pimozide. Although effective, the drug exhibits a higher degree of cardiotoxicity than others in its class and is thus only used when other therapies fail to achieve their designated outcomes.

Thiothixene: Thiothixene, a high-potency antipsychotic, is approved to treat psychotic disorders, including schizophrenia, and acute agitation. Approved in 1967, it is available as a PO preparation and has adverse effects that are characteristic of those of other first-generation antipsychotics. It is not a first-line drug for psychosis.

Second-Generation (Atypical) Antipsychotics

20.8 Second-generation antipsychotics have become preferred drugs for the treatment of schizophrenia.

Available since the early 1990s, the second-generation, or atypical, antipsychotics have become preferred drugs for the pharmacotherapy of severe mental illness. The members of this group are diverse and have little in common with each other, except that they all improve negative psychosis symptoms and produce a lower incidence of adverse effects (especially EPS) than the first-generation drugs.

The exact mechanisms of action of the various second-generation antipsychotics are mostly unknown. It is known that atypical antipsychotics bind less tightly to dopamine (D_2) receptors than the first-generation drugs, which may explain the relatively low incidence of EPS with these drugs. Some inhibit different subtypes of dopamine receptors, D_1 and D_4, which are especially prominent in the limbic system of the brain. Some also inhibit serotonin (5-HT) receptors in the CNS. Like the first-generation drugs, some atypical antipsychotics have prominent anticholinergic adverse effects. Doses of the second-generation antipsychotics are listed in Table 20.4.

CONNECTIONS: Lifespan Considerations

Early Diagnosis and Treatment of Psychosis in Children

As in adults, the earlier a serious mental disorder such as schizophrenia is diagnosed in children, the earlier treatment can begin. Symptoms of psychosis may have an acute or insidious onset, and other conditions may also be present, such as bipolar disorder or neurologic conditions, which may cause similar symptoms.

Recent research suggests that prior to the development of psychosis, children may exhibit abnormal, involuntary motor movements (Kindler et al., 2016). Involuntary repetitive movements are most common in the facial area, limbs, and respiratory muscles and appear to be related to changes in the brain's subcortical areas. These movements appear to be related to changes in the brain's subcortical areas (Dean & Mittal, 2015). Increasing declines in verbal functions and impaired executive functioning (e.g., memory, flexible thinking, self-control) have also been noted to be present in children who transitioned to schizophrenia (Mollon et al., 2018; Pontillo et al., 2019).

Although many other conditions, including seizure disorders and neuromuscular diseases, may cause involuntary movements and declines in cognitive functioning, these findings may lead to earlier diagnosis and treatment of children, especially those at high risk for developing psychosis based on a strong family history of the disorder.

Table 20.4 Second-Generation (Atypical) Antipsychotics

Drug	Route and Adult Dose (Maximum Dose Where Indicated)	Adverse Effects
aripiprazole (Abilify)	PO: 10–15 mg/day (max: 30 mg/day) IM (Abilify Maintena): 300–400 mg once monthly	*Sedation, headache, akathisia, confusion, insomnia, depression, tachycardia, dizziness, lightheadedness, anxiety, nervousness, hostility, nausea and vomiting, constipation, somnolence, EPS, asthenia, dry mouth, weight gain, tremor, restlessness, sleep disorders*
asenapine (Saphris, Secuado)	Sublingual (Saphris): 5–10 mg bid Transdermal (Secuado): one patch daily (3.8–7.6 mg/day)	
brexpiprazole (Rexulti)	PO: 0.5–4 mg once daily (max: 4 mg/day)	
cariprazine (Vraylar)	PO: 1.5–6 mg once daily (max: 6 mg/day)	
clozapine (Clozaril)	PO: 300–450 mg/day (max: 900 mg/day)	Agranulocytosis (clozapine), NMS, bone marrow suppression, seizures, suicidal tendencies, TD, diabetes mellitus, ischemia, prolonged QT interval, hypotension, acute dystonia (risperidone)
iloperidone (Fanapt)	PO: 12–24 mg/day (max: 24 mg/day)	
lurasidone (Latuda)	PO: 40 mg once daily (max: 80 mg/day)	
olanzapine (Zyprexa)	PO: 10–20 mg/day (max: 20 mg/day) IM (extended release): 150–405 mg q2–4wk	
paliperidone (Invega, Invega Sustenna, Invega Trinza)	PO (immediate release): 6 mg/day (max: 12 mg/day) IM: 39–234 mg monthly (Invega Sustenna) or 272–819 mg every 3 months (Invega Trinza)	
pimavanserin (Nuplazid)	PO: 34 mg once daily	
quetiapine (Seroquel)	PO (immediate release): 300–400 mg/day in divided doses (max: 800 mg/day) PO (extended release): 300 mg at bedtime (max: 800 mg/day)	
risperidone (Perseris, Risperdal, Risperdal Consta)	PO: 1–8 mg/day (max: 8 mg/day) IM (Risperdal Consta): 12.5–50 mg once q2wk (max 50 mg) SC (Perseris): 90–120 mg once monthly (max: 120 mg/month)	
ziprasidone (Geodon)	PO: 20 mg bid (max: 80 mg bid) IM: 10 mg q2h or 20 mg q4h (max: 40 mg/day)	

Note: *Italics* indicate common adverse effects. Underline indicates serious adverse effects.

PROTOTYPE DRUG Risperidone (Risperdal)

Classification **Therapeutic:** Antipsychotic (second-generation, atypical), antimanic drug
Pharmacologic: Dopamine (D_2) receptor antagonist

Therapeutic Effects and Uses: Risperidone is an atypical antipsychotic available for PO or IM use that has become one of the most frequently prescribed drugs for psychosis. It was initially approved in 1993 to treat negative psychotic symptoms in individuals with schizophrenia and related psychoses. In subsequent years, approved indications were extended to include acute mania associated with bipolar disorder. Risperidone was the first drug approved to treat irritability associated with autism in children ages 5 to 16. Off-label uses include the pharmacotherapy of Tourette's syndrome, attention-deficit/hyperactivity disorder, severely disruptive behavior in children with developmental disabilities, dementia, and psychotic depression. The IM depot form of Risperdal (Risperdal Consta) requires 3 weeks to produce a therapeutic response; the patient is usually placed on PO antipsychotics during this 3-week period. Subsequent IM injections are administered every 2 weeks. In 2018 a subcutaneous depot form (Perseris) was approved as a once-monthly dosage. Risperidone is also available as orally disintegrating tablets (Risperdal M-TAB), which are especially beneficial when treating patients suspected of "cheeking" the drug.

Mechanism of Action: The precise mechanism for risperidone is unknown. It is believed that the drug acts by blocking the binding of dopamine to its receptors in various brain regions. It has highest affinity for type D_2 and has less effect on D_1 receptors. It also blocks 5-HT receptors, alpha$_1$-adrenergic receptors, and histaminergic receptors.

Pharmacokinetics:

Route(s)	PO, IM
Absorption	70% absorbed PO; slowly absorbed IM
Distribution	Widely distributed; crosses both the blood–brain and placental barriers; secreted in breast milk; 90% bound to plasma protein
Primary metabolism	Extensive hepatic metabolism by CYP2D6; changed to the active metabolite 9-hydroxyrisperidone
Primary excretion	Renal, with small amounts in feces
Onset of action	Peak action: 1–3 h (optimal antipsychotic effects may take several months)
Duration of action	Half-life: 20 h

Adverse Effects: The adverse effects of risperidone therapy are similar to those of other atypical antipsychotics. Gastrointestinal (GI) effects such as drowsiness, nausea and vomiting, constipation, and increased salivation are common. Symptoms of parkinsonism may occur in 5 to 10% of patients. The incidence of anticholinergic adverse effects is low, and agranulocytosis is very rare. Risperidone elevates serum prolactin levels, which can result in galactorrhea, impotence, gynecomastia, and menstrual irregularities. Hyperglycemia, including some rare cases of diabetic ketoacidosis, has been reported in patients taking this drug. Orthostatic hypotension is common at the initiation of therapy. Excessive weight gain occurs in children taking risperidone. Adverse effects for the PO and IM depot formulations are the same, except the parenteral form may cause pain and local injection-site reactions. **Black Box Warning:** This drug is not indicated for the treatment of dementia-related psychosis. Older adults with dementia-related psychosis treated with atypical antipsychotics are at increased risk of death compared to placebo.

Contraindications/Precautions: Hypersensitivity to risperidone is a contraindication. The drug should be used with caution in patients with severe CNS depression, seizures, dysrhythmias, hypotension, diabetic ketoacidosis, and suicidal ideation. Patients with chronic kidney disease should be treated with caution. Use during lactation is contraindicated because the drug and its active metabolite are secreted in breast milk.

Drug Interactions: Risperidone is a substrate for hepatic CYP2D6 enzymes; thus, it may interact with drugs that inhibit or induce these enzymes. For example, many of the selective serotonin reuptake inhibitors (SSRIs) inhibit CYP2D6, which reduces the metabolism of risperidone and raises serum drug levels. Concurrent use with alcohol, benzodiazepines, or other CNS depressants can cause severe CNS depression. Antihypertensives and nitrates may potentiate hypotension. Decreased risperidone levels may occur with the use of phenobarbital, rifampin, omeprazole, or carbamazepine. Increased risperidone levels may occur with the use of verapamil, azole antifungals, and lamotrigine. Risperidone antagonizes the actions of levodopa and dopamine agonists. Risperidone should be used with caution with drugs known to prolong the QT interval, such as amiodarone, droperidol, and pimozide. **Herbal/Food:** Increased CNS depression may occur if used with St. John's wort or valerian. Food does not affect the absorption of risperidone.

Pregnancy: In animal reproduction studies, risperidone caused fetal harm. Human neonates exposed during the third trimester are at risk to developing withdrawal symptoms such as agitation, tremor, and feeding disorder. The drug is secreted in human milk and the breastfed neonate may experience sedation, EPS, and failure to thrive.

Risperidone should only be used during pregnancy or lactation when the potential benefits justify the potential risks to the fetus or neonate.

Treatment of Overdose: Symptoms of overdose include confusion, sedation, hypotension, and dysrhythmias. Treatment is supportive and includes gastric lavage and maintenance of cardiovascular function.

Clinician Responsibilities: Key clinical implications for patients receiving risperidone are included in Applied Clinical Judgment: Patients Receiving Pharmacotherapy with Antipsychotics.

Drugs Similar to Risperidone (Risperdal)

Other drugs classified as atypical antipsychotics include asenapine, clozapine, iloperidone, lurasidone, olanzapine, paliperidone, pimavanserin, quetiapine, and ziprasidone. Aripiprazole (Abilify) is an atypical antipsychotic that is a prototype for a different pharmacologic class (see Section 20.9). All the atypical antipsychotics carry a black box warning that they should not be used in older patients with dementia-related psychosis because they may increase mortality in those patients. When taken during the third trimester of pregnancy, many antipsychotics (including the second-generation class) have the potential to produce serious EPS and withdrawal symptoms in the neonate. These drugs should only be taken during pregnancy if the potential benefits justify the potential risks to the fetus or neonate.

Asenapine (Saphris): One of the newer atypical antipsychotics, asenapine is a dopamine antagonist that blocks 5-HT receptors. One unique feature of asenapine is that it is approved to treat both schizophrenia and manic or mixed episodes associated with bipolar disorder, including in pediatric patients ages 10 to 17. A second advantage is that it is administered by the sublingual route, which bypasses hepatic first-pass metabolism. In 2019, the FDA approved Secuado, the first transdermal patch to treat adults with schizophrenia. The types and incidences of adverse effects are similar to those of other drugs in this class. The most common adverse effects include akathisia, oral hypoesthesia, somnolence, dizziness, weight gain, and EPS. Animal reproduction studies showed no developmental defects or teratogenicity. Effects on the nursing infant are unknown.

Clozapine (Clozaril): In 1989, clozapine was the first atypical antipsychotic approved for use in the United States. Clozapine is approved for the management of schizophrenia in patients resistant to standard therapies and to reduce the risk of recurrent suicidal behavior in patients with schizophrenia. Off-label indications include treatment of bipolar disorder, severe obsessive–compulsive disorder, and dementia-related behavioral disorders. Clozapine is available as regular tablets, orally disintegrating tablets, and oral suspension (Versacloz).

Because of potentially severe adverse effects, it is generally reserved for schizophrenia symptoms that have not responded favorably to other drugs. The most serious and limiting adverse effect of clozapine is agranulocytosis, a white blood cell (WBC) count below 500/mm^3. Although it occurs in less than 1% of patients taking the drug, agranulocytosis can be fatal. To avoid toxicity, clozapine therapy requires special monitoring and surveillance requirements. WBC and absolute neutrophil counts (ANCs) are performed weekly for the first 6 months of treatment and reduced in frequency to every 2 weeks for the next 6 months. CNS effects such as sedation, dizziness, confusion, fatigue, and headache are common at the initiation of therapy but may diminish with continued therapy. Clozapine lowers the seizure threshold and can precipitate seizures in 5% of patients taking high doses. Although the incidence of EPS is less than with first-generation drugs, akathisia, tremor, and agitation can still occur. Orthostatic hypotension is common at the initiation of therapy and during dosage changes. Other warnings on the drug label include an increased risk of hyperglycemia leading to diabetic ketoacidosis and increased risk of fatal myocarditis. Animal reproduction studies did not show evidence of impaired fertility or fetal harm. Neonates exposed to this drug during the third trimester should be monitored for EPS and withdrawal symptoms following delivery. Because clozapine is secreted in human milk, caution should be used if breastfeeding.

Iloperidone (Fanapt): Approved to treat acute schizophrenia in 2009, iloperidone is a dopamine antagonist that also blocks 5-HT receptors. Iloperidone is considered a second-line drug because it prolongs the QT interval, which is associated with dysrhythmia and sudden death. The drug should be administered with caution when used in combination with other medications that prolong the QT interval. Another disadvantage is that iloperidone requires 1 to 2 weeks of gradually increasing the dose before a therapeutic drug level is reached. This is because the drug can cause orthostatic hypotension and possible syncope with the first few doses. Other common adverse effects include dry mouth, dizziness, fatigue, nasal congestion, somnolence, tachycardia, and weight gain. Animal reproduction studies showed developmental toxicity and increased stillbirths but no teratogenicity. Because iloperidone is secreted in human milk, caution should be used if breastfeeding.

Lurasidone (Latuda): Approved in 2010, lurasidone is an atypical antipsychotic approved to treat patients with schizophrenia and for treating depressive episodes of bipolar I disorder, often as an adjunct to lithium or valproic acid. Lurasidone blocks dopamine receptors and its effectiveness is similar to that of other atypical antipsychotics. This drug should be taken with food because that will substantially increase drug absorption. Common adverse effects are typical of other drugs in this class: somnolence, akathisia, nausea, agitation, and parkinsonism. Significant orthostatic hypotension may occur early in treatment. Concurrent administration with CYP3A4 inducers (e.g., carbamazepine or St. John's wort) or CYP inhibitors (e.g., azole antifungals or ritonavir) is contraindicated. Patients should be monitored for suicidal thoughts during therapy. Animal reproduction studies did not show adverse developmental effects or teratogenicity. Effects on the breastfeeding infant are unknown.

Olanzapine (Zyprexa): Approved in 1996, olanzapine is a second-generation antipsychotic available as regular tablets, orally disintegrating tablets (Zyprexa, Zydis), and IM in both immediate release and extended release (Zyprexa, Relprevv). It is used to treat both the positive and negative symptoms of schizophrenia, and it is also approved to treat acute agitation and mania associated with bipolar 1 disorder (see Chapter 19). A single IM dose can usually calm patients presenting with acute agitation in about 15 minutes. The combination of olanzapine with fluoxetine (Symbyax) is approved to treat resistant depression and the depressive episodes of bipolar 1 disorder. In 2021 Lybalvi, a combination of olanzapine with samidorphan (an opioid antagonist), was approved to treat schizophrenia and bipolar I disorder. Off-label, olanzapine may be used to treat chemotherapy-induced nausea and vomiting and to reduce severe behavioral symptoms associated with the dementia of Alzheimer's disease.

Like other second-generation antipsychotics, the incidence of EPS with olanzapine is low, with drowsiness being the most frequent adverse effect. Weight gain has been reported in up to 25% of patients and is a frequent cause of discontinuation of the drug. Other common adverse effects include orthostatic hypotension, dizziness, nervousness, insomnia, headache, and hostility. Use with other CNS depressants may cause additive CNS depression. The risk of patients developing type 2 diabetes mellitus is greater with the use of olanzapine than with other atypical antipsychotics. A major advantage of olanzapine is that it rarely causes neutropenia or agranulocytosis, which are major drawbacks to clozapine therapy. Safety and effectiveness in children under age 18 has not been established.

In animal reproduction studies, high doses of olanzapine caused fetal toxicity but no teratogenicity. Because olanzapine is secreted in human milk, caution should be used if breastfeeding.

Paliperidone (Invega): Approved in 2006, paliperidone is indicated for the acute and maintenance therapy of schizophrenia and for schizoaffective disorder. Paliperidone can improve both the positive and negative symptoms of schizophrenia. It is available as an immediate-release tablet, as a monthly IM depot injection (Invega Sustenna), and as a quarterly IM depot injection (Invega Trinza). Invega Trinza is approved only after patients have stabilized on Invega Sustenna for 4 months. Paliperidone is the active metabolite of risperidone, which is the prototype antipsychotic for this class.

The incidence of serious adverse events with paliperidone is low. The drug is not extensively metabolized in the liver; thus, it has less potential for drug–drug interactions than many other antipsychotics. The most common reported adverse effects include EPS, restlessness, akathisia, tachycardia, orthostatic hypotension, syncope, and insomnia. The IM form of the drug can cause injection-site reactions. NMS or TD may occur with the use of paliperidone. Like olanzapine, increased appetite and weight gain are possible. It does not cause neutropenia or agranulocytosis and does not appear to lower the seizure threshold.

In animal reproduction studies, high doses of paliperidone did not cause fetal abnormalities. Because paliperidone is secreted in human milk, caution should be used if breastfeeding.

Pimavanserin (Nuplazid): Approved in 2016, pimavanserin was the first atypical antipsychotic indicated for hallucinations and delusions specifically associated with Parkinson's disease. It is not approved for other types of psychoses. The drug is well tolerated, with nausea, peripheral edema, and confusion being the most common adverse effects. It does not have adverse effects on motor function. Pimavanserin is metabolized by CYP3A4; therefore, caution must be used when this medication is given concurrently with strong inducers or inhibitors of this enzyme. This drug is not pregnancy rated. In animal reproduction studies, no adverse developmental effects or teratogenicity were observed. Effects on the breastfeeding infant are unknown.

Quetiapine (Seroquel): Initially approved in 1997 to treat both positive and negative symptoms of schizophrenia, indications were later extended to include the short-term therapy of acute mania associated with bipolar disorder (in combination with lithium or valproic acid). The drug is also approved to treat major depressive disorder and depression associated with bipolar disorder. It is sometimes used off-label to treat anxiety-related disorders that are unresponsive to other therapies. Quetiapine is available only in tablet form. An extended-release formulation (Seroquel XR) is available.

Like other atypical antipsychotics, the incidence of EPS and other serious adverse effects with quetiapine is low. Unlike clozapine, agranulocytosis has not been reported. Sedation is commonly experienced during the initial stages of therapy. Cautious use is recommended in patients who have a history of cardiovascular disease or seizures, individuals with Alzheimer's disease, those who are taking other CNS depressants, and those who are older or debilitated. Lens changes have occurred during quetiapine use; thus, baseline and 6-month eye examinations are recommended. Other common adverse reactions include weight gain, constipation, postural hypotension, dyspepsia, and xerostomia. Like other antidepressants, quetiapine carries a black box warning that it may increase the risk of suicidal thinking in younger patients. Animal reproduction studies showed embryo-fetal toxicity and maternal toxicity but no teratogenicity. Because quetiapine is secreted in human milk, caution should be used if breastfeeding.

Ziprasidone (Geodon): Approved in 2001, ziprasidone is available in PO or IM formulations to treat schizophrenia and acute mania associated with bipolar 1 disorder. The IM formulation is used to treat acute episodes of agitation with schizophrenia because it can reduce major symptoms in 15 minutes. Ziprasidone may be used off-label to treat Tourette's syndrome. Common adverse effects include somnolence, headache, and nausea. Ziprasidone causes fewer EPS than most other antipsychotics but has the possibility of prolonging the QT interval and thereby increasing the risk for dysrhythmias; it should not be administered concurrently with other medications that increase the QT interval. It must also be used cautiously in patients with seizure history, Alzheimer's disease, or cardiovascular or hepatic disease or who are being treated with antihypertensives. Additive CNS depression may occur if used concurrently with antianxiety drugs, sedative–hypnotics, alcohol, or opiate preparations. Ziprasidone causes less weight gain than other atypical antipsychotics and does not cause agranulocytosis. Animal reproduction studies showed developmental abnormalities, possible teratogenicity, and increase in stillbirths. Effects on the breastfeeding infant are unknown.

CONNECTION Checkpoint 20.2

When atypical antipsychotic drugs are used to treat bipolar disorder, they are usually combined with drugs from other classes. From what you learned in Chapter 19, what two drugs are usually combined with the atypical antipsychotics?

CONNECTIONS: Using Research in Practice

Weight Gain in Children and Adolescents Prescribed Antipsychotic Drugs

Weight gain is a potential adverse effect of both antipsychotic and antidepressant drugs in adult patients. It may be significant enough that some patients stop taking their medication in order to avoid gaining too much weight. Do the drugs used to treat behavioral health and serious mental illness cause weight gain for children and adolescents as well? With the increase in significant behavioral health disorders in children and adolescents, and the rise in type 2 diabetes in these populations, this is an important question.

Reekie et al. (2015) noted that in short-term use, SSRIs, SNRIs, and antipsychotics such as risperidone, used alone or with other antipsychotics, did not cause significant weight gain. However, similar to studies of adults, long-term use of drug therapy, even SSRIs and SNRIs, led to weight gain, with risperidone, olanzapine, and clozapine noted to have the highest risk for significant weight gain.

The weight gain associated with these drugs did not significantly decrease after the drug is stopped. In a study of children with bipolar disorder, Upadhyay et al. (2019) noted a weight loss after drug discontinuation, but little change in body mass index, even a year after the drug regimen was stopped. For patients who were already experiencing weight-management issues, adding drugs such as metformin or topiramate appeared to have some beneficial effects against additional weight gain (Hendrick et al., 2017; Reekie et al., 2015), especially at the initiation of antipsychotic drug therapy.

Dopamine System Stabilizers

20.9 Dopamine system stabilizers are a newer class of atypical antipsychotics.

Dopamine system stabilizers (DSSs) are medications that bind to the D_2 receptor. Unlike the conventional antipsychotics, however, they do not totally block the actions of dopamine. Instead, DSSs act as if a weaker form of dopamine was occupying the receptor, causing a stabilizing, milder effect. In essence, DSSs are *partial* agonists. They reduce the hyperactivity of dopamine in certain regions of the brain (to produce therapeutic effects), while at the same time restoring normal dopamine activity in other regions (to lower the incidence of adverse effects observed with other antipsychotics). The balance between these two activities appears to account for the decrease in observed EPS, relative to other antipsychotics. The DSSs also affect the dopamine D_3 receptor and a variety of different subtypes of the serotonin (5-HT_3) receptor, which explains some of their clinical differences.

The first DSS, aripiprazole, was approved in 2002. Two newer drugs in this class, brexpiprazole (Rexulti) and cariprazine (Vraylar), were approved in 2015. All three DSSs have similar efficacy and spectrum of adverse effects. Aripiprazole is approved for many more indications than the other two.

In 2019 a new antipsychotic, lumateperone (Caplyta), was approved to treat schizophrenia. This drug appears to have some dopamine stabilizing effect, but it has a much greater affinity for serotonin receptors (5-HT_{2A}). In is unclear whether its antipsychotic properties are due to its effects on dopamine receptors or serotonin receptors, or a combination.

PROTOTYPE DRUG **Aripiprazole (Abilify)**

Classification **Therapeutic:** Atypical antipsychotic
Pharmacologic: Dopamine system stabilizer

Therapeutic Effects and Uses: Aripiprazole controls both the positive and negative symptoms of schizophrenia and improves cognition with minimal risk of EPS. In addition to tablet form, the drug is available as an orally disintegrating tablet and a parenteral, extended-release form (Abilify Maintena, Aristada) that permits once-monthly dosing. Aripiprazole exhibits the same level of effectiveness as other atypical antipsychotics but with a lower incidence of adverse effects. An advantage over other atypical drugs is that there is little or no weight gain, hypotension, dysrhythmias, anticholinergic effects, or prolactin release with aripiprazole. It does not appear to lower the seizure threshold.

Since its initial approval, a number of other indications have been added. An IM formulation is approved for the treatment of schizophrenia and for manic or mixed episodes associated with bipolar disorder. Aripiprazole is approved as an add-on for major depressive disorder in patients whose symptoms are not relieved by antidepressants alone. In addition, the drug is approved to treat Tourette's disorder, as well as irritability associated with autistic disorder in children. The drug is approved for pediatric patients age 13 to 17 for schizophrenia, age 10 to 17 for bipolar disorder, and age 6 to 17 for autism.

Mechanism of Action: Aripiprazole is thought to act through a combination of partial agonist activity at dopamine type 2 (D_2 and D_3) and serotonin type 2 ($5\text{-}HT_{1A}$) receptors and antagonist activity at $5\text{-}HT_{2A}$ receptors.

Pharmacokinetics:

Route(s)	PO, IM
Absorption	Well-absorbed PO and IM
Distribution	Widely distributed; unknown if crosses the placenta or is secreted in breast milk
Primary metabolism	Hepatic; metabolized to active metabolite
Primary excretion	Feces, some in urine
Onset of action	Peak effect: 3–5 h (PO); 1–3 h (IM)
Duration of action	Half-life: 75–146 h

Adverse Effects: Frequently reported adverse effects include drowsiness, insomnia, agitation, hyper- or hypotension, lightheadedness, anxiety, headache, restlessness, EPS, akathisia, nausea and vomiting, and constipation. Weight gain may occur in a significant number of patients. Serious adverse effects include seizures, NMS, and blood dyscrasias. About 5% of patients will develop EPS. **Black Box Warning:** This drug is not indicated for the treatment of dementia-related psychosis. Older adults with dementia-related psychosis treated with atypical antipsychotics are at increased risk of death compared to placebo. Antidepressants increase the risk of suicidal thinking and behavior in children, adolescents, and young adults. Patients of all ages should be monitored and observed closely during therapy for clinical worsening, suicidality, or unusual changes in behavior.

Contraindications/Precautions: Lactation, seizure disorders, or hypersensitivity are contraindications to the use of aripiprazole. Precautions must be taken when administering aripiprazole to individuals with cardiovascular or cerebrovascular disease or any condition that predisposes them to hypotension.

Drug Interactions: Aripiprazole is a substrate for several hepatic CYP450 enzymes and induces others; thus, it may interact with drugs that undergo hepatic metabolism. For example, many of the SSRIs inhibit CYP2D6, which can cause reduced metabolism of aripiprazole, raised serum levels, and possible toxicity. Concurrent use of other antipsychotics or lithium may increase the incidence of EPS. Alcohol and other CNS depressants will cause increased CNS depression. Decreased excretion of aripiprazole may occur with the use of drugs such as fluoxetine or paroxetine. **Herbal/Food:** Grapefruit juice may increase the serum levels of aripiprazole and cause toxicity.

Pregnancy: In animal reproduction studies, developmental toxicity, fetal mortality, and teratogenic effects were observed. Because aripiprazole is secreted in human milk, breastfeeding is not recommended.

Treatment of Overdose: Overdose can cause vomiting, tremor, and drowsiness, but fatalities have not been reported. There is no specific treatment for overdose.

Clinician Responsibilities: Key clinical implications for patients receiving aripiprazole are included in Applied Clinical Judgment: Patients Receiving Pharmacotherapy with Antipsychotics.

Drugs Similar to Aripiprazole (Abilify)

Drugs similar to aripiprazole include brexpiprazole, cariprazine, and lumateperone. When taken during the third trimester of pregnancy, most antipsychotics have the potential to produce serious EPS and withdrawal symptoms in the neonate. These drugs should only be taken during pregnancy if the potential benefits justify the potential risks to the fetus or neonate.

Brexpiprazole (Rexulti): Brexpiprazole is believed to have a mechanism similar to that of aripiprazole. In addition to schizophrenia, it is approved as an adjunctive therapy in the treatment of major depressive disorder. It carries the same black box warnings as other antipsychotics (not to be used for dementia-related psychosis) and the antidepressants (possible suicidal risk). It shows similar adverse effects to aripiprazole, including headache, agitation, insomnia, akathisia, sedation, and weight gain. Animal reproduction studies did not find adverse developmental effects or teratogenicity. The effects of brexpiprazole on the breastfed infant are unknown.

Cariprazine (Vraylar): Cariprazine is believed to have a mechanism similar to that of aripiprazole. In addition to schizophrenia, it is approved for the treatment of manic or mixed-episode bipolar I disorder. It carries the same black box warnings as other antipsychotics (not to be used for dementia-related psychosis). Common adverse effects include akathisia, parkinsonism, insomnia, constipation, and somnolence. Animal reproduction studies showed fetal developmental toxicity, skeletal malformations, and decreased postnatal survival. The effects of cariprazine on the breastfed infant are unknown.

Lumateperone (Caplyta): Lumateperone is given PO once daily and exhibits a very low incidence of EPS adverse effects. The most common adverse effects are somnolence, dry mouth, and nausea. It carries the same black box warnings as other antipsychotics (not to be used for dementia-related psychosis). Animal reproduction studies at high doses found developmental abnormalities, early postnatal deaths, and skeletal malformations. Lumateperone may impair male and female fertility. Based on animal studies, this drug is not recommended during breastfeeding.

CONNECTIONS: APPLIED CLINICAL JUDGMENT

Patients Receiving Pharmacotherapy with Antipsychotics

Key Assessment Data

- History of current condition, including family history of depression or mental disorders, baseline vital signs, weight, physical exam and mental status findings; history of diabetes or hepatic, renal, cardiovascular, or neurologic disease (especially Parkinson's disease or seizures), current mental status; medication and substance use history; allergies; pregnancy status.
- Assess for disturbances in thought processes, perception, verbal communication, behavior, affect, interpersonal relationships, and self-care. Use objective measures specific to the healthcare agency when possible to help quantify therapeutic results.
- Ongoing assessment during drug therapy includes mental status assessment, CBC, electrolytes, glucose, hepatic and renal function studies, signs or symptoms of EPS and motor dysfunction.

Desired Therapeutic Outcomes

Improvement is observed and measurable by reduction of positive and negative symptoms of the disorder (e.g., normalizing thought processes, lessening delusions, lessening hallucinations), ability to return to normal ADLs and appetite and sleep patterns; if used for other conditions (e.g., severe hiccups), assess for appropriate therapeutic effects. Drugs used for psychosis and schizophrenia do not cure the underlying disorder.

Minimizing Adverse Effects

- Orthostatic hypotension and reflex tachycardia may occur. Monitor vital signs periodically, especially orthostatic blood pressure. Ensure patient safety; monitor ambulation until the effects of the drug are known.
- Neurologic changes may indicate under- or overmedication, exacerbation of other psychiatric illness, or adverse drug effects. Promptly report increasing lethargy, disorientation, confusion, changes in behavior or mood, agitation or aggression, slurred speech, or ataxia.
- The presence of severe mental disorders may result in nonadherence to prescribed medications. Regular, consistent dosing is essential to correcting the underlying disorder. Because the drugs do not cure the underlying disorder, if regular administration is disrupted, symptoms may return abruptly. Alternative drug forms such as PO disintegrating tablets or IM depot injections may need to be considered if chronic nonadherence continues.
- Motor and EPS effects such as bradykinesia may predispose the patient to falls. Akathisia with pacing may significantly impair the patient's ability to rest and sleep; additional medications may be required to treat it. Anticholinergics or other drugs may be required to stop spasms of acute dystonia. Continue to monitor motor activity, coordination, and balance and for EPS symptoms.
- Severe choreoathetoid tongue movement in tardive dyskinesia (TD) may significantly hinder or prevent adequate nutrition. Ensure adequate nutrition and fluid intake if TDs are present.
- Neuroleptic malignant syndrome (NMS) is a rare but potentially fatal syndrome that must be recognized and treated immediately. Monitor for and immediately report signs and symptoms of NMS: unstable blood pressure, elevated temperature, diaphoresis, muscle rigidity.
- An increased risk of death from cardiovascular events (e.g., heart failure, sudden cardiac death) or from respiratory infection has been noted in some patients, particularly those taking atypical antipsychotic drugs. Monitor cardiovascular and respiratory function more frequently, particularly in the older adult with existing disease or dementia.
- Antipsychotic drugs may cause bone marrow depression, hepatotoxicity, increased glucose levels, or hyperlipidemia as adverse effects. Continue to monitor CBC, electrolytes, glucose, renal and hepatic function, lipid levels, and therapeutic drug levels.
- Anticholinergic symptoms are common adverse effects of antipsychotic drugs. Tolerance to anticholinergic effects usually develops over time. Monitor for anticholinergic effects, including dry mouth, drowsiness, blurred vision, constipation, and urinary retention. Provide symptomatic treatment to ease effects.
- Many antipsychotic drugs cause weight gain and have pituitary effects. Impotence and weight gain may be significant reasons for nonadherence. Monitor for weight gain, gynecomastia (breast enlargement and tenderness in either sex), and changes in secondary sexual characteristics (e.g., amenorrhea, impotence).
- Other substances (alcohol, caffeine, tobacco, or illicit substances), when used concurrently, may have deleterious effects. Alcohol and illicit substances may cause an increased CNS depressant effect or an exacerbation in psychotic symptoms. Use of caffeine-containing substances may negate the effects of antipsychotics. And heavy smoking may decrease metabolism of some antipsychotics such as haloperidol, leading to decreased efficacy. Referral to appropriate support (e.g., Alcoholics Anonymous, smoking-cessation programs, dietitian consult) may be needed.

Lifespan Considerations

- The older adult may be at increased risk for falls due to drowsiness and dizziness, hypotension, or impaired mental and physical abilities.
- The older adult man with an enlarged prostate is at higher risk for mechanical obstruction and may experience urinary retention due to anticholinergic effects. Promptly report difficulty with urination, hesitancy, or dysuria.
- Most antipsychotic drugs are pregnancy category C and the benefits of the use of any particular drug must be weighed against possible fetal effects should a woman be or desire to become pregnant. Monitor for the possibility of pregnancy in women of childbearing age.
- Children and adolescents younger than age 24, and the older adult, particularly with dementia, are at greater risk for suicide than other patients. Monitor adolescents under age 24 and older adults for unusual symptoms or expressed thoughts of suicide.

(continued)

CONNECTIONS: APPLIED CLINICAL JUDGMENT *(continued)*

Patients Receiving Pharmacotherapy with Antipsychotics

Diversity Considerations

- Most antipsychotic drugs are metabolized through the CYP450 system and may result in different effects based on differences in enzymes. Monitor ethnically diverse patients more frequently to ensure optimal therapeutic effects and minimal adverse effects, especially in early stages of drug therapy.

Patient and Caregiver Education

- The drugs do not cure the underlying disorder, but improvement may occur and full effects may not be known for a prolonged period. Some improvement should be noticeable after beginning therapy. Supportive, inpatient care may be required during the acute, early period of therapy.
- Ensure that the patient takes the medication as prescribed. Never leave medications at the bedside for the patient to take. Question the possibility of nonadherence if original symptoms or adverse effects suddenly increase in frequency or severity.
- Rise from lying or sitting to standing slowly to avoid dizziness or falls. If dizziness occurs, sit or lie down and do not attempt to stand or walk until the sensation passes. For patients who are taking the medications at home or at an outpatient clinic, avoid driving or other activities requiring mental alertness or physical coordination until the effects of the drug are known.
- Report new or worsening EPS symptoms for additional treatment. Record weight weekly to ensure that dietary needs are being met if TDs are present.
- Immediately report symptoms of NMS: any changes in level of consciousness, elevated temperature, excessive sweating, severe muscle rigidity, increased respirations, shortness of breath, or incontinence.
- Promptly report any abdominal pain, particularly in the upper quadrants, changes in stool color, yellowing of sclera or skin, or darkened urine.
- Encourage sips of water, ice chips, hard candy, or chewing gum to ease mouth dryness. Avoid alcohol-based mouthwashes, which are drying to the mucosa.
- Weigh the patient daily and report a significant weight gain of 2 kg (5 lb) per week to the healthcare provider. Encourage a healthy diet of increased fruits and vegetables, adequate protein intake, and increased exercise. Promptly report excessive thirst, urination, hunger, unusual weight loss or gain, or other symptoms of diabetes.
- Discuss concerns about sexual functioning and refer to the healthcare provider if concerns affect medication adherence. For women of childbearing age, discuss family planning with the healthcare provider. Teach the patient, family, or caregiver to promptly report a positive pregnancy test or suspicion of pregnancy to the provider.
- Provide referral to outpatient resources (e.g., Alcoholics Anonymous, Narcotics Anonymous, smoking-cessation programs, dietary consult) as needed.
- Switching brands of drugs may result in differing pharmacokinetics and alterations in therapeutic effect. Take the drug exactly as ordered and the same manufacturer's brand each time the prescription is filled. Ensure that all medication is taken as directed. Use of a calendar to track doses may be helpful. If the medication causes drowsiness, take at bedtime. Unless otherwise directed, mix liquid drug solutions with water, milk, or nongrapefruit juices. Do not mix with cola, tea, or caffeine-containing beverages.
- Administer IM injections by deep gluteal injection using enclosed diluent and safety needle if provided by the manufacturer. Check the enclosed directions about refrigerating dosages.
- Do not abruptly discontinue the medication. If unable to take or administer the drug, contact the provider for instructions.

Prescribing Considerations

- Determine the goal of therapy. It may be unrealistic to aim for complete elimination of the responsive behavior. It is important to discuss the intended goal with the family/caretaker and care team. This should be clearly documented in the health record to guide monitoring and assessment.
- Start with the lowest dose. The smallest recommended dose should be the starting point for any antipsychotic medication. Allow 2 weeks between dose increases due to the very slow elimination of metabolites from the brain. This is especially important for older patients where there is a two to three times higher rate of adverse drug effects than patients younger than 30 years of age.
- Monitor and evaluate the response to treatment. Regular monitoring of the responsive behavior is required, and prescribers should evaluate for a change in frequency and intensity of behaviors.
- If symptoms warrant, attempt to slowly lower doses or discontinue medications when possible as risk of adverse events increase over time.

Understanding Chapter 20

Key Concepts Summary

20.1 Psychoses are severe mental disorders characterized by the inability to recognize reality.

20.2 Schizophrenia, the most common psychosis, has both positive and negative symptoms.

20.3 The precise etiology of schizophrenia remains unknown.

20.4 Medical management of psychosis is challenging because patients often lack insight into their disease and believe their behavior is normal.

20.5 Selection of an antipsychotic drug depends on its spectrum of adverse effects and the experience of the healthcare provider.

20.6 The phenothiazines are effective at treating schizophrenia symptoms but exhibit a high incidence of adverse effects.

20.7 The nonphenothiazine first-generation antipsychotics have the same therapeutic applications and similar adverse effects as the phenothiazines.

20.8 Second-generation antipsychotics have become preferred drugs for the treatment of schizophrenia.

20.9 Dopamine system stabilizers are a newer class of atypical antipsychotics.

CASE STUDY: Making the Patient Connection

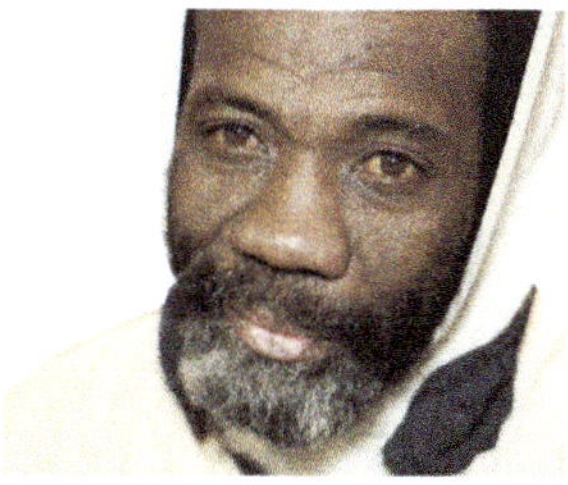

Remember the patient "George Watkins" at the beginning of the chapter? Now read the remainder of the case study. Based on the information presented within this chapter, respond to the critical thinking questions that follow.

George Watkins is a 47-year-old African American man who was admitted to the psychiatric unit this morning. He was diagnosed with schizophrenia at age 20. He looks disheveled, with long, dirty, stringy hair. George's clothes are mismatched and dirty. Although it is summer, he is wearing an overcoat and a winter hat pulled down over his ears. This is George's fourth hospitalization for out-of-control schizophrenia. The last severe episode occurred 4 years ago.

Sheri Watkins, George's wife, states that he quit his job as an assembly-line supervisor about 2 weeks ago. He has also quit coaching softball and soccer games. Sheri and George have been married since they were both 18. Their marriage is basically strong but has had its difficult times, especially when George's schizophrenia is active. About 3 to 4 weeks before each hospitalization for psychosis, he stopped taking his antipsychotic medication. He has taken different antipsychotic medications over the course of his schizophrenia, but none has proved to be successful over a long period.

George and Sheri have two children: Toby, who is 14, and Felecia, who is 10. Both children do well in school, have many friends, and are active in several organizations and sports. As the children get older, they realize that "something is not quite right" with their father. They have never been told of their father's mental illness. The children worry that they will catch whatever it is that causes their father's erratic behavior. George's parents and four siblings live in the same town. George, his father, and his two brothers worked at the same manufacturing plant. His other two siblings are teachers in the local school system, as is Sheri.

Mr. and Mrs. Watkins, George's parents, tell you that their son had a normal childhood. He was active in sports, starred on the high school football team, was an honor student and a Boy Scout, and had many friends. They have always enjoyed many social occasions with their large extended family. George is always welcome at family gatherings, but relatives tend to avoid him when his behavior becomes bizarre. They all know he has schizophrenia but do not fully understand the implications of the diagnosis.

Critical Thinking Questions

1. What are the most likely reasons George gives for discontinuing his medication?
2. What clues do his family and friends have that would indicate that symptoms of his schizophrenia may be returning?
3. What can be done to prevent George's schizophrenia from returning in the future?

Additional Case Study

Suzette Anderson is a 19-year-old patient who has been admitted to the psychiatric unit with newly diagnosed schizophrenia. She is agitated and paces back and forth in the day room until she is called for dinner. She is heard muttering to herself, "I don't know why they put me here. They just don't want me to get my inheritance. Maybe it's because they know I'll leave them all when I get the money. I'll be real rich and can start a new life for myself." Suzette demonstrates no overt threatening behavior toward any of the other patients or toward the staff. Her agitation escalates until she cannot calm herself down and will not listen to staff. She begins hitting her fist into the wall and shouting.

There is an order for haloperidol (Haldol), 4 mg IM every 1 to 4 hours prn for agitation.

1. What is the main use of haloperidol (Haldol) in this situation?
2. As the nurse caring for Suzette, what adverse effects would you monitor for?
3. How long would you expect Suzette to remain hospitalized? Why?

Chapter Review

1. The patient states that he has not taken his antipsychotic drug for the past 2 weeks because it was causing sexual dysfunction. The nurse is aware that the name *antipsychotic* indicates that continuing the medication as prescribed is important because:
    1. Hypertensive crisis may occur with abrupt withdrawal.
    2. Muscle twitching may occur with abrupt withdrawal.
    3. Parkinson-like symptoms will occur with withdrawal.
    4. Symptoms of psychosis are likely to return if the medication is withdrawn.
2. Prior to discharge, the nurse provides teaching related to adverse effects of aripiprazole (Abilify) to the patient and caregivers. Which of the following should be included?
    1. The patient may experience social withdrawal and slowed activity.
    2. Avoid grapefruit and grapefruit juice in the diet because it increases stomach acidity.
    3. Tardive dyskinesia is likely early in therapy.
    4. Additional drugs such as fluoxetine may be needed to prevent adverse effects.
3. The nurse expects that the patient experiencing extrapyramidal symptoms during therapy with phenothiazines will be prescribed:
    1. Benztropine (Cogentin).
    2. Diazepam (Valium).
    3. Haloperidol (Haldol).
    4. Lorazepam (Ativan).
4. Nursing implications of the administration of haloperidol (Haldol) to a patient exhibiting psychotic behavior include which of the following? (Select all that apply.)
    1. Take 1 hour before or 2 hours after antacids.
    2. The incidence of extrapyramidal symptoms is high.
    3. It is therapeutic if ordered on an as-needed basis.
    4. Haldol is contraindicated in Parkinson's disease, seizure disorders, alcoholism, and severe mental depression.
    5. Crush the sustained-release form for easier swallowing.
5. Which statement made by the patient who is taking risperidone (Risperdal) indicates that further teaching is necessary?
    1. "I'll monitor my weight every month."
    2. "I can increase my intake of fluids and fiber if I have any gastrointestinal problems."
    3. "I'll have my blood pressure monitored regularly."
    4. "There is no problem if I want to drink alcohol on the weekends."
6. The development of which symptom(s) in a patient taking an antipsychotic must be reported immediately?
    1. Fever, tachycardia, stupor, and incontinence
    2. Suddenly occurring muscle spasms, especially in the neck and back
    3. Sexual dysfunction
    4. Leg pains, pacing, an inability to sit still

See Appendix A for answers to critical thinking questions, case study questions, and review questions.

References

Ash, M. E. (2019). *Childhood-onset schizophrenia*. Medscape. http://emedicine.medscape.com/article/914840-overview

Dean, D. J., & Mittal, V. A. (2015). Spontaneous parkinsonisms and striatal impairment in neuroleptic free youth at ultrahigh risk for psychosis. *NPJ*

Schizophrenia, *1*, Article No. 14006. https://doi.org/10.1038/npjschz.2014.6

Hendrick, V., Dasher, R., Gitlin, M., & Parsi, M. (2017). Minimizing weight gain for patients taking antipsychotic medications: The potential role for early use of metformin. *Annals of Clinical Psychiatry*, *29*(2), 120–124.

Kindler, J., Schultze-Lutter, F., Michel, C., Martz-Irngartinger, A., Linder, C., Schmidt, S. J., et al. (2016). Abnormal involuntary movements are linked to psychosis-risk in children and adolescents: Results of a population-based study. *Schizophrenia Research*, *174*, 58–64. https://doi.org/10.1016/j.schres.2016.04.032

Mollon, J., David, A.S., Zammit, S., Lewis, G., & Reichenberg, A. (2018). Course of cognitive development from infancy to early adulthood in the psychosis spectrum. *JAMA Psychiatry*, *75*, 270–279. https://doi.org/10.1001/jamapsychiatry2017.4327

Pontillo, M., Menghini, D., & Vicari, S. (2019). Neurocognitive profile and onset of psychosis in children, adolescents, and young adults with 22q11 deletion syndrome: A longitudinal study. *Schizophrenia Research*, *208*, 76–81. https://doi.org/10.1016/j.schres.2019.04.012

Reekie, J., Hosking, S. P. M., Prakash, C., Kao, K.-T., Juonala, M., & Sabin, M. A. (2015). The effect of antidepressants and antipsychotics on weight gain in children and adolescents. *Obesity Reviews*, *16*, 566–580. https://doi.org/10.1111/obr.12284

Schizophrenia.com. (n.d.). *Schizophrenia facts and figures.* http://www.schizophrenia.com/szfacts.htm

Schizophrenia and Related Disorders Alliance of America. (2020). *About schizophrenia: DSM-5 schizophrenia spectrum disorder*. http://www.sardaa.org/resources/about-schizophrenia

Upadhyay, N., Patel, A., Chan, W., Aparasu, R. R., Ochoa-Perez, M., Sherer, J. T., et al. (2019). Reversibility of psychotropic medication induced weight gain among children and adolescents with bipolar disorders. *Psychiatry Research*, *276*, 151–159. https://doi.org/10.1016/j.psychres.2019.05.005

Selected Bibliography

Driver, D. I., Thomas, S., Gogtay, N., & Rapoport, J. L. (2020). Childhood-onset schizophrenia and early-onset schizophrenia spectrum disorders: An update. *Child and Adolescent Psychiatric Clinics*, *29*(1), 71–90. https://doi.org/10.1016/j.chc.2019.08.017

Frankel, J. S., & Schwartz, T. L. (2017). Brexpiprazole and cariprazine: Distinguishing two new atypical antipsychotics from the original dopamine stabilizer aripiprazole. *Therapeutic Advances in Psychopharmacology*, *7*(1), 29–41. https://doi.org/10.1177/2045125316672136

Haygarth, L., & Hemingway, S. (2018). Schizophrenia: Practical prescribing of antipsychotics. *Nurse Prescribing*, *16*(2), 64–70. https://doi.org/10.12968/npre.2018.16.2.64

Jann, M. W., & Penzak, S. R. (2018). Long-acting injectable second-generation antipsychotics: an update and comparison between agents. *CNS Drugs*, *32*(3), 241–257. https://doi.org/10.1007/s40263-018-0508-6

Kowalski, J. M. (2020). *Medication-induced dystonic reactions*. Medscape. https://emedicine.medscape.com/article/814632-overview

Krogmann, A., Peters, L., von Hardenberg, L., Bödeker, K., Nöhles, V. B., & Correll, C. U. (2019). Keeping up with the therapeutic advances in schizophrenia: A review of novel and emerging pharmacological entities. *CNS Spectrums*, *24*(Suppl. 1), 38–69. https://doi.org/10.1017/S109285291900124X

Limandri, B. J. (2019). Clinical use of dopamine modulators as third-generation antipsychotic agents. *Journal of Psychosocial Nursing and Mental Health Services*, *57*(2), 7–11. https://doi.org/10.3928/02793695-20190116-02

Meyer, J. M. (2020). Lumateperone for schizophrenia. *Current Psychiatry*, *19*(2), 33–39.

National Institute of Mental Health. (2020). *Schizophrenia*. https://www.nimh.nih.gov/health/topics/schizophrenia/index.shtml

Olfson, M., King, M., & Schoenbaum, M. (2015). Treatment of young people with antipsychotic medications in the United States. *JAMA Psychiatry*, *72*, 867–874. https://doi.org/10.1001/jamapsychiatry.2015.0500

Stroup, T. S., & Gray, N. (2018). Management of common adverse effects of antipsychotic medications. *World Psychiatry*, *17*(3), 341–356. https://doi.org/10.1002/wps.20567

Widschwendter, C. G., & Hofer, A. (2019). Antipsychotic-induced tardive dyskinesia: Update on epidemiology and management. *Current Opinion in Psychiatry*, *32*(3), 179–184. https://doi.org/10.1097/YCO.0000000000000491

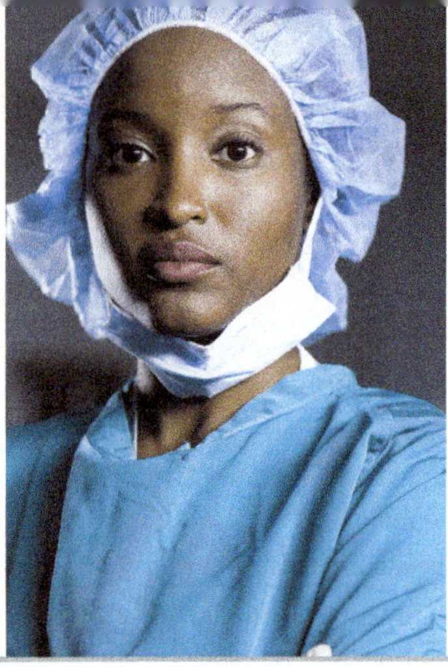

"This just can't happen to me, not now. What is this going to do to my career, my family?"
—*Patient "Althea Taylor"*

Chapter 21
Pharmacotherapy of Degenerative Diseases of the Central Nervous System

Chapter Outline

Learning Outcomes

After reading this chapter, the student should be able to:

1. Identify the most common degenerative diseases of the central nervous system.
2. Distinguish between idiopathic Parkinson's disease and secondary Parkinson's disease.
3. Describe symptoms of Parkinson's disease.
4. Explain the neurochemical basis for Parkinson's disease, focusing on the roles of dopamine and acetylcholine in the brain.
5. Describe symptoms of Alzheimer's disease and explain theories about why these symptoms develop.
6. Describe the nurse's role in the pharmacologic management of Parkinson's disease, Alzheimer's disease, and multiple sclerosis.
7. Discuss the pharmacologic goals for the management of Parkinson's disease, Alzheimer's disease, multiple sclerosis, and other neurodegenerative disorders.
8. For each of the classes shown in the chapter outline, identify the prototype and representative drugs and explain the mechanism(s) of drug action, primary indications, contraindications, significant drug interactions, pregnancy data and important adverse effects.
9. Apply clinical judgement to care for patients receiving pharmacotherapy for degenerative diseases of the central nervous system.

Key Terms

Definitions of the terms in bold may be found in the Glossary.

Degenerative diseases of the central nervous system (CNS) are difficult to treat pharmacologically. In nearly all cases, medications are unable to cure or reverse the progressive nature of these disorders, and the symptomatic relief provided by the drugs is only temporary. The focus of this chapter is on four debilitating and progressive conditions categorized as degenerative diseases of the CNS: Parkinson's disease, Alzheimer's disease, multiple sclerosis, and amyotrophic lateral sclerosis.

Degenerative Diseases of the Central Nervous System

21.1 Degenerative diseases of the central nervous system are characterized by irreversible and progressive loss of neuronal function.

Neurodegenerative diseases include a diverse set of disorders that differ in their causes and outcomes. Each involves a progressive and irreversible loss of neuron function in the brain or spinal cord, or both. Neuron loss is sometimes isolated to specific regions of the CNS, and symptoms will vary by the region(s) most affected by the disorder.

Alzheimer's disease and Parkinson's disease present major challenges for older adults as well as for the health-care industry, which must provide services for the vast numbers of patients with these neurodegenerative disorders. Although less common, Huntington's disease, multiple sclerosis, and amyotrophic lateral sclerosis are equally devastating to patients and their families. These disorders are described in Table 21.1.

The specific etiology of most neurodegenerative diseases is unknown, although the loss of neurons appears to have both genetic and environmental components. Huntington's disease is clearly the result of an autosomal dominant genetic defect. Alzheimer's disease and Parkinson's disease also tend to occur more commonly within families, but this does not account for the majority of cases. It is likely that exposure of neurons to various toxins, genetic predisposition, and normal aging processes all have important roles in the etiology of these disorders.

Most neurodegenerative diseases of the CNS progress from subtle signs and symptoms early in the course of the disease to profound neurologic and cognitive deficits. Because of this, neurodegenerative disorders are quite difficult to diagnose in their early stages. With some of them, diagnosis is made only after other neurologic, infectious, cardiovascular, or traumatic etiologies have been ruled out.

With the exception of Parkinson's disease and multiple sclerosis, pharmacotherapy provides only minimal benefit to patients with neurodegenerative disease, especially in their more advanced stages. Currently, medications are unable to cure or significantly alter the clinical course of any of the degenerative diseases of the CNS.

PharmFACT

About 1 million Americans have Parkinson's disease. Approximately 60,000 new cases are diagnosed each year (Parkinson's Foundation, n.d.).

Parkinson's Disease

21.2 Parkinson's disease is a progressive neurodegenerative disorder characterized by abnormal motor movement.

Named after British physician James Parkinson who identified the condition in 1817, **Parkinson's disease (PD)** is the second most common degenerative disease of the nervous system and

Table 21.1 Major Degenerative Diseases of the Central Nervous System

Disease	Description
Alzheimer's disease	A chronic, progressive disease that profoundly diminishes memory, reasoning ability, and thinking skills and leaves the patient totally dependent on others for all aspects of care; usually affects people over age 60.
Amyotrophic lateral sclerosis (Lou Gehrig's disease)	A degenerative disease of the motor neurons characterized by weakness and atrophy of the muscles of the hands, forearms, and legs, spreading to involve most of the body and face; symptoms usually begin during the middle years, with death occurring within 2–5 years.
Huntington's disease (formerly called Huntington's chorea)	A rare hereditary condition characterized by progressive chorea and mental deterioration resulting in dementia; symptoms usually begin in the 30s–50s with death occurring within 15 years.
Multiple sclerosis	A chronic debilitating autoimmune disease characterized by fatigue, muscle weakness, difficulty with balance and walking, and vision, hearing, and speech abnormalities; symptomatic periods alternate with remissions; symptoms vary depending on which portion of the nervous system is experiencing inflammation.
Parkinson's disease	A debilitating disease characterized by resting tremor, muscle rigidity, hypokinesia, masklike faces, and a slow, shuffling gait. Symptoms usually appear in the 60s.

the third most common neurologic disorder of older adults. The disease peaks between 58 and 62 years of age; however, even teenagers can develop the disorder. Men are affected 1.5 times more often than women. The disease is progressive, with the expression of full symptoms developing over many years.

The two etiologies of PD are idiopathic and secondary. Idiopathic PD, the most common type, has no known cause and is characterized by a progressive destruction of neurons in specific regions of the brain. Some patients with idiopathic parkinsonism have a family history of the disorder, and a genetic link is highly probable.

Secondary parkinsonism is caused by medical conditions such as head trauma, brain infections, brain tumors, and exposure to neurotoxins. The most frequent cause of secondary parkinsonism is treatment with antipsychotic drugs (see Chapter 20). Once a patient on antipsychotic therapy shows signs of parkinsonism, the dosage is adjusted or replaced with a different medication. Symptoms of drug-induced PD are usually reversible but may become permanent if pharmacotherapy is prolonged.

PD begins with subtle symptoms. The patient reports feeling tired and seems to move more slowly, often demonstrating a slight tremor. Diagnosis is based on clinical findings after the presence of other neurologic diseases has been ruled out. Once the disease progresses, the symptoms of PD are quite characteristic and can be easily recognized. The four cardinal signs of PD, or parkinsonism, are summarized as follows:

- **Tremor.** The hands and head develop a palsy-like, continuous motion or shaking when at rest. The tremors may be so pronounced that the individual cannot hold a glass or eating utensils and successfully bring them to his or her mouth. **Pill rolling** is a common behavior in progressive states, in which patients rub the thumb and forefinger together in a circular motion, resembling the motion of rolling a tablet between two fingers.
- **Muscle rigidity.** Resistance to passive movements of the arms and legs develops. The muscle rigidity or stiffness may resemble symptoms of arthritis. Patients often have difficulty bending over and moving limbs. Changes in facial expression, or a lack of facial expression, are due to rigidity of the facial muscles. This rigidity can lead to chewing and swallowing difficulties if the pharyngeal muscles are involved. Uncontrollable drooling may also be evident. A noticeable symptom of PD is a lack of arm swinging while walking; the patient walks with the arms close to the side. Muscle rigidity is present early in the disease process. Although the symptoms may be less noticeable at first, they progress and become obvious in later years.
- **Bradykinesia.** An involuntary slowness of voluntary movement and speech, **bradykinesia** is one of the most noticeable of all symptoms and is marked by difficulty chewing, swallowing, or speaking. Patients with PD have difficulties initiating movement and controlling fine muscle movements. Patients shuffle their feet without taking normal strides, making walking difficult.
- **Postural instability.** Patients may be stooped over and easily lose their balance. Stumbling results in frequent falls with associated injuries.

Although PD is a progressive neurologic disorder primarily affecting muscle movement, other health problems often develop in these patients, including anxiety, major depression, sleep interruptions, and disturbances of the autonomic nervous system such as constipation, difficulty urinating, and sexual dysfunction. Many develop sensory and thought disturbances, and dementia may occur, especially in those over age 70. These associated health problems often require pharmacologic intervention, which increases the potential for drug interactions and adverse effects.

21.3 Parkinson's disease is caused by a lack of sufficient amounts of dopamine produced by the substantia nigra.

Although the precise etiology of PD is incompletely understood, much is known about the effects of the disease on the CNS. Neurotransmitter deficiencies in specific regions of the brain are closely associated with the disease.

Involuntary muscle movements are controlled by the basal nuclei (also called basal ganglia), which are clusters of interconnected neurons in several distinct regions of the brain. The basal nuclei are responsible for regulating the flow of information from the cerebral cortex to the motor neurons in the spinal cord. This region helps to synchronize stopping and starting activity such as that which occurs during walking. Two portions of the basal nuclei that are important to the pathogenesis of PD are the substantia nigra and the striatum. The student should review the functions of the basal nuclei and associated structures in Chapter 17.

The **substantia nigra**, a dark band of gray matter in the midbrain, is a primary producer of the neurotransmitter dopamine. The dopamine travels through axons along the nigrostriatal pathway to the **striatum** (also called corpus striatum), where the neurotransmitter is released. In the striatum, dopamine encounters its receptors and produces multiple actions. One function that is important to the pathogenesis of PD is the planning and modulation of motor pathways responsible for unconscious muscle movement. Dopamine serves an *inhibitory* function, slowing the flow of impulses down spinal neurons.

When dopamine is present, the normal flow of motor impulses from the striatum helps to produce coordinated, unconscious muscle movement. Symptoms of parkinsonism develop when levels of dopamine fall because of the loss of dopamine-producing neurons in the substantia nigra. Remarkably, the body can function normally even when as many as 50% of the neurons stop producing dopamine. When 60 to 80% lose their function, however, symptoms of parkinsonism are observed.

A second neurotransmitter modulates the effects of neuronal outflow from the striatum. Acetylcholine (ACh) serves an *excitatory* function. Under normal conditions, the inhibitory effects of dopamine and the excitatory effects of ACh balance one another to produce smooth, coordinated muscle movement. If dopamine levels decline, ACh has a more dramatic stimulatory effect in this area and the abnormal muscular movements characteristic of PD are observed.

CONNECTION Checkpoint 21.1

Dopamine belongs to a class of natural hormones called catecholamines. From what you learned in Chapter 12, what are the other two major catecholamines found in the nervous system?

Pharmacotherapy of Parkinson's Disease

21.4 The drugs used for Parkinson's disease help to alleviate symptoms but do not cure the disease.

Antiparkinson medications are given to restore the balance between dopamine and ACh in specific regions of the brain. Maintaining a *balance* between the two neurotransmitters offers several means by which drug therapy may be used to manage the symptoms of PD:

- **Dopamine agonists.** These drugs increase the levels of dopamine in the striatum. This may be accomplished by directly replacing dopamine, decreasing the breakdown of dopamine, increasing the release of dopamine from neurons, or activating dopamine receptors.
- **Anticholinergic drugs.** These drugs block the excitatory actions of ACh in the striatum.

The goal of pharmacotherapy for PD is to increase the ability of the patient to perform normal activities of daily living (ADLs) such as eating, walking, dressing, and bathing and decrease the chances of falls that could cause serious injury. Pharmacotherapy is an essential part of the management of PD; drugs decrease symptoms and allow patients to provide for enhanced self-care, have a degree of self-worth, and improve their quality of life. Although pharmacotherapy does not prevent or reverse neuronal degeneration, symptoms can be dramatically reduced in many patients.

Patients receiving prolonged antiparkinson pharmacotherapy may periodically experience a loss of drug effect. This **wearing-off effect** appears gradually near the end of a dosing interval. Symptoms worsen at this time because the concentration of the drug has fallen below the therapeutic level. Adjusting the dosing interval to provide for more frequent dosing can help to reduce this effect.

Another type of loss of drug effect occurs abruptly. The **on–off syndrome** occurs when the patient alternates between symptom-free periods (on) and times when the drugs stop working and symptoms abruptly reappear (off). The on–off time intervals range from just a few minutes to several hours. Off periods may occur even when the serum level of the drug is high. The on–off syndrome is difficult to control. Scheduling doses closer together or using a second, adjunct medication during the off period are strategies used to reduce the on–off syndrome in patients receiving levodopa and carbidopa.

Several classes of antipsychotic drugs can cause symptoms of parkinsonism as major adverse effects. These dyskinesias are referred to as extrapyramidal symptoms (EPS). The term *extrapyramidal* refers to locations in the CNS that contain neurons associated with postural and automatic movements. Recall from Chapter 20 that antipsychotic drugs act through a blockade of dopamine receptors. Thus, EPS develop for the same neurochemical reasons as PD: deficiency of dopamine in the striatum. Antiparkinson drugs may be used to treat these symptoms.

If drug therapy becomes ineffective, alternative treatments can be tried. Again, these treatments may help control symptoms, but they will not cure or prevent the disease from progressing. The four accepted nonpharmacologic treatments for PD are deep brain stimulation (DBS), fetal tissue transplantation, pallidotomy, and thalamotomy. Table 21.2 describes each of these therapies.

Table 21.2 Nondrug Treatments for Parkinson's Disease

Name of Treatment	Type of Treatment	Procedure
Deep brain stimulation (DBS)	Electrical stimulation	An electrode is implanted in the thalamus or subthalamus. It is connected to a device that delivers electric currents to interfere with cells that cause tremors. An implantable generator is inserted under the patient's skin in much the same way as a cardiac pacemaker. The patient can adjust the settings by using a special magnet placed over the implanted generator. DBS is used when medications are no longer controlling symptoms.
Pallidotomy	Surgical and electrical stimulation	The target area is identified with magnetic resonance imaging (MRI). A hollow probe is inserted into the globus pallidum. The probe is used to destroy the targeted brain tissue. Pallidotomy may reduce tremor and alleviate other movement disorders.
Stem cell transplantation	Surgical	Stem cells are transplanted into the caudate nucleus of the brain. The expected outcome is that the patient will show a substantial decrease of motor symptoms. This is considered experimental at this time and although it shows promise, no long-term results are available.
Thalamotomy	Surgical	The target area is identified with magnetic resonance imaging (MRI). Part of the thalamus is destroyed in an attempt to reduce tremor and rigidity. This procedure is rarely done today.

Dopamine Replacement Therapy

21.5 Replacement therapy with levodopa is the most effective therapy for treating Parkinson's disease.

Drug therapy for PD attempts to restore the functional balance of dopamine and ACh in the striatum of the brain. Dopamine replacement drugs are used to directly increase dopamine levels in this region. Dopamine itself cannot be used for this purpose because it is unable to cross the blood–brain barrier after it is administered. Doses for these drugs are listed in Table 21.3.

Levodopa is a dopaminergic drug that has been prescribed more extensively than any other medication for this disorder. As shown in Pharmacotherapy Illustrated 21.1, levodopa is a precursor in the synthesis of dopamine. Unlike dopamine, however, levodopa easily crosses the blood–brain barrier to reach the affected region. Administration of levodopa directly leads to increased biosynthesis of dopamine within the nerve terminals. Carbidopa is nearly

Table 21.3 Drugs for Parkinson's Disease

Drug	Route and Adult Dose (Maximum Dose Where Indicated)	Adverse Effects
Dopamine Replacement Drug		
levodopa-carbidopa (Duopa, Rytary, Sinemet)	PO (Sinemet CR): 50 mg carbidopa/200 mg levodopa or 25 mg carbidopa/100 mg levodopa with dosing based on individual response (max: 1600 mg levodopa/day)	*Involuntary movements (dyskinetic, dystonic, choreiform), orthostatic hypotension, sleep disturbances, anorexia, nausea and vomiting* Neuroleptic malignant syndrome, hallucinations, agranulocytosis, depression with suicidal ideation
Dopamine Agonists		
apomorphine (Apokyn, Kynmobi)	Subcutaneous: 2–4 mg (max: 4 mg)	*Dyskinesias, injection site reactions, somnolence, yawning, orthostatic hypotension* Severe nausea and vomiting, syncope, hallucinations, sleep attacks
bromocriptine (Parlodel)	PO: 1.25–2.5 mg/day (max: 2.5 mg tid)	*Nausea, hypotension, headaches, dizziness, orthostatic hypotension* Shock, acute myocardial infarction (MI), sleep attacks
pramipexole (Mirapex)	PO (immediate release): 0.125 mg tid for 1 wk and gradually increase to 1.5 mg tid PO (extended release): 0.375 mg/day and gradually increase as needed (max: 4.5 mg/day)	*Dizziness, somnolence, insomnia, dyskinesia, orthostatic hypotension, nausea, constipation* EPS, asthenia, sleep attacks, hallucinations
ropinirole (Requip)	PO (immediate release): 0.25 mg tid and gradually increase as needed (max: 24 mg/day) PO (extended release): 2 mg/day and gradually increase as needed (max: dose of 24 mg/day)	*Fatigue, viral infection, dizziness, somnolence, nausea and vomiting, dyspepsia, orthostatic hypotension* Sleep attacks, syncope, hallucinations
rotigotine (Neupro)	Transdermal: 2–8 mg daily (one patch)	*Nausea and vomiting, somnolence, application-site reactions, dizziness, anorexia, hyperhidrosis, insomnia, peripheral edema, and dyskinesia* Hallucinations, hypertension, sleep attacks
COMT Inhibitors		
entacapone (Comtan)	PO: 200 mg administered with each dose of levodopa/carbidopa (max: 1600 mg/day)	*Urine discoloration, hyperkinesia, nausea, diarrhea, dystonia, orthostatic hypotension, sleep disorders* Dyskinesia, liver failure (tolcapone), sleep attacks (opicapone),
opicapone (Ongentys)	PO: 50 mg once daily	
tolcapone (Tasmar)	PO: 100 mg tid (max: 600 mg/day)	
Monoamine Oxidase-B Inhibitors		
rasagiline (Azilect)	PO: 0.5–1 mg once daily	*Nausea, dizziness, confusion, depression, orthostatic hypotension, arthralgia* Dyskinesia, hallucinations, serotonin syndrome
safinamide (Xadago)	PO: 50–100 mg once daily	
selegiline (Zelapar)	PO: 5 mg bid (max: 10 mg/day)	
Miscellaneous Drugs		
amantadine (Gocovri, Osmolex ER)	PO (immediate release): 100 mg 1–2 times/day PO (Osmolex ER): 129–258 once daily (max: 322 mg/day)	*Dizziness, lightheadedness, difficulty concentrating, anxiety, headache, fatigue, nausea and vomiting, orthostatic hypotension* Falling asleep during activities of daily living, suicidal ideation, hallucinations
istradefylline (Nourianz)	PO: 20–40 mg/day (max: 40 mg/day)	*Constipation, nausea, dizziness* Dyskinesia, hallucinations

Note: *Italics* indicate common adverse effects. Underline indicates serious adverse effects.

Pharmacotherapy Illustrated 21.1

Antiparkinson Drugs Focus on Restoring Dopamine Function and Blocking Cholinergic Activity in the Nigrostriatal Pathway

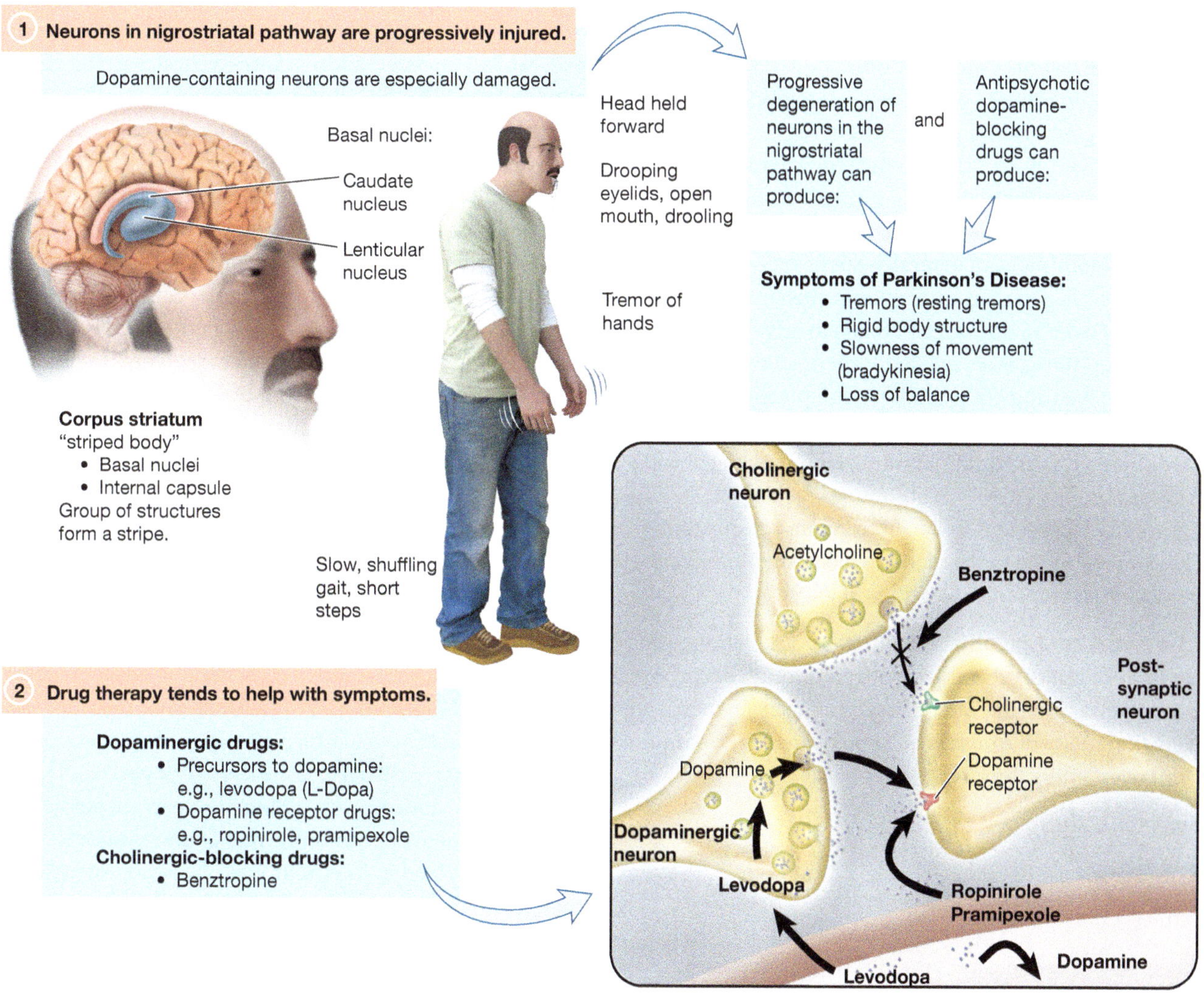

always administered with levodopa. Carbidopa increases the plasma levels and half-life of levodopa.

Two to three weeks of therapy are needed before improvement is observed, and many patients require several months of therapy to achieve optimal therapeutic outcomes. Dramatic improvement in symptoms is often noted early in therapy. As therapy progresses, however, the beneficial effects of the medication tend to diminish. In addition, the on–off syndrome tends to worsen with continued use of the drug.

PROTOTYPE DRUG **Levodopa-Carbidopa (Sinemet)**

Classification **Therapeutic:** Antiparkinson drug
Pharmacologic: Dopamine replacement drug

Therapeutic Effects and Uses: Approved in 1970, levodopa is an oral (PO) drug indicated for the treatment of idiopathic and secondary PD. The drug restores normal dopamine levels in the striatum of the brain. Some symptoms of PD, such as tremor, bradykinesia, gait, and muscle rigidity, respond well to levodopa treatment. Others, such as imbalance, sensory problems, sexual dysfunction, and constipation, do not respond as well. Dosing is highly individualized to deliver the least amount of drug that will resolve the patient's symptoms.

The addition of carbidopa boosts the effectiveness of levodopa. Carbidopa itself has no therapeutic effects of its own because it cannot cross the blood–brain barrier. Instead, carbidopa inhibits the breakdown of levodopa in the intestine and peripheral tissues, which makes more levodopa available to reach the CNS. Without carbidopa, only 1% of the dose of levodopa reaches the CNS. The combination of the two drugs allows for much lower doses of levodopa to be prescribed than when levodopa is used alone; 25 mg of levodopa is used as a combination drug versus 125 mg of levodopa when delivered as monotherapy. Carbidopa also decreases dopamine production in peripheral tissues, leading to reduced nausea and vomiting as well as fewer cardiovascular responses to levodopa.

Various preparations of levodopa-carbidopa are available, including an oral tablet that dissolves on the tongue and is swallowed with saliva, which is a distinct advantage for patients with swallowing difficulties. Sinemet and Rytary are extended-release products containing levodopa-carbidopa. Duodopa is an enteral suspension of levodopa-carbidopa that is pumped directly into the small intestine continuously over 16 hours for patients in advanced stages of the disease. Inbrija is an inhaled form of levodopa that is taken during wearing-off periods. A complete dose is two capsules, each of which is loaded into the Inbrija inhaler and inhaled. Stalevo is a combination of levodopa-carbidopa with entacapone, a COMT inhibitor (see Section 21.7). The addition of entacapone is believed to create a more consistent level of levodopa in the blood, which can minimize the extent and duration of the wearing-off effect.

Mechanism of Action: Levodopa is a metabolic precursor of dopamine. When metabolized through decarboxylation to dopamine, dopamine levels in the brain increase. If given alone, 99% of a dose is decarboxylated to dopamine before it ever enters the CNS.

Pharmacokinetics:

Route(s)	PO
Absorption	Well absorbed from the gastrointestinal (GI) tract; absorption is decreased when given with meals
Distribution	Widely distributed throughout the body
Primary metabolism	Stomach, intestines, and liver (levodopa); carbidopa not extensively metabolized
Primary excretion	Renal
Onset of action	30 min (immediate release); 2 h (extended release)
Duration of action	Half-life: 1 h

Adverse Effects: The adverse effects of this drug combination are due to the levodopa component; carbidopa has no significant adverse effects. Common adverse effects include orthostatic hypotension, nausea and vomiting, anorexia, dysphagia, abdominal distress, fatigue, headache, anxiety, confusion, agitation, nightmares, and insomnia. Life-threatening adverse effects include agranulocytosis, leukopenia, and hemolytic anemia. Other potential adverse effects are related to the anticholinergic properties of levodopa, including urinary retention and dry mouth. Psychosis develops in up to 20% of patients taking levodopa, including hallucinations, paranoia, or nightmares. Drug therapy with an antipsychotic such as clozapine (Clozaril) or quetiapine (Seroquel) may be necessary to control serious psychosis. However, adding antipsychotics to the regimen may worsen EPS side effects of levodopa.

Although the dystonias characteristic of PD are treated with levodopa-carbidopa, this drug also has the potential to *cause* dystonias. Some dystonias such as head bobbing or jaw clenching are considered minor side effects of levodopa therapy, whereas others such as quick jerking movements may be serious. These dystonias may occur just as the optimal dosage level of levodopa is reached, which is extremely discouraging for patients and their caregivers. To reduce the severity of these dystonias, the dose of levodopa and carbidopa must be reduced. This, of course, causes the symptoms of PD to return.

Contraindications/Precautions: Levodopa-carbidopa is contraindicated in patients with hypersensitivity to the drug and those with closed-angle glaucoma, or within 2 weeks of use of a monoamine oxidase inhibitor (MAOI). Caution must be taken if administering levodopa to patients with cardiac, respiratory, endocrine, renal, or hepatic disease; myocardial infarction (MI) with dysrhythmias; seizure disorder; lactation; peptic ulcer; psychiatric disorders; or hypertension. This drug may cause patients to fall asleep during ADLs. The drug should not be abruptly discontinued due to the possibility of the development of neuroleptic malignant syndrome (NMS), such as tachycardia, muscular rigidity, fever, mental status changes, diaphoresis, and tachypnea.

Drug Interactions: Although antipsychotic drugs may be used to control psychosis associated with parkinsonism, conventional antipsychotic drugs block dopamine receptors in the brain and can decrease the therapeutic effects of levodopa. MAOIs can lead to a hypertensive crisis. Increased orthostatic hypotension may occur if used with tricyclic antidepressants. Concurrent use with antihypertensives may cause additive hypotension. Decreased levodopa effects can occur with use of anticholinergics, hydantoins, or pyridoxine. Antacids may increase the effects of levodopa. **Herbal/Food:** Food, especially high-protein foods and vitamin-fortified foods containing vitamin B_6, decreases the rate and extent of levodopa absorption; however, many people must take levodopa with food to decrease the nausea and vomiting that may occur. Kava may worsen symptoms of PD. Indian snakeroot will decrease levodopa action while increasing EPS.

Pregnancy: In animal studies, levodopa-carbidopa was associated with developmental toxicity and visceral and skeletal malformations. Levodopa is secreted in breast milk and breastfed infants should be monitored for adverse effects related to levodopa therapy. Levodopa-carbidopa should only be administered during pregnancy or lactation if the potential benefit to the mother justifies the potential risk to the fetus or neonate.

Treatment of Overdose: No specific treatment.

Clinician Responsibilities: Key clinical implications for patients receiving levodopa and carbidopa are included in Applied Clinical Judgment: Patients Receiving Pharmacotherapy for Neurodegenerative Disorders.

Drugs Similar to Levodopa-Carbidopa

There are no other drugs similar to levodopa and carbidopa.

Dopamine Agonists

21.6 Dopamine agonists may be used as monotherapy for early symptoms of Parkinson's disease or as adjuncts to levodopa in patients with advanced disease.

Dopamine agonists (also called dopaminergic agonists) directly activate dopamine receptors in the CNS. They are used as monotherapy for patients with mild to moderate symptoms of PD and may be used in combination with levodopa in patients with advanced disease. Doses of these drugs are listed in Table 21.3.

Dopamine agonists have certain advantages over levodopa. The drugs do not have to be metabolized to be effective and they are not converted to potentially toxic metabolites. Dietary protein does not interfere with their absorption, so a low-protein diet is not necessary. They exhibit a lower incidence of the wearing-off effect and are less likely to cause dyskinesias in patients younger than age 60.

Certain adverse effects of dopamine agonists may be more serious than those of levodopa. These include orthostatic hypotension, unexpected sleep attacks, and hallucinations. This group of drugs is generally reserved for younger patients, who tend to tolerate adverse effects better than older adult patients.

The dopamine agonists are divided into two subclasses: ergot alkaloids and nonergot drugs. Bromocriptine (Parlodel) is an ergot alkaloid derived from the ergot fungus that grows on rye wheat. Another use of ergot alkaloids is in the treatment of migraines. The nonergot alkaloids include apomorphine (Apokyn), pramipexole (Mirapex), ropinirole (Requip), and rotigotine (Neupro).

PROTOTYPE DRUG **Pramipexole (Mirapex)**

Classification **Therapeutic:** Antiparkinson drug
Pharmacologic: Dopamine receptor agonist, nonergot type

Therapeutic Effects and Uses: Pramipexole is an oral drug indicated for the treatment of idiopathic PD. It is used as monotherapy in early PD and in combination with levodopa in advanced stages of the disease. It can produce significant motor improvement in early PD and decreases fluctuations in motor performance in late disease. Many patients are able to lower their doses of levodopa when they take pramipexole concurrently. It is also approved at low doses for treating symptoms of restless leg syndrome. Several weeks of therapy are necessary for the patient to obtain maximum benefits from pramipexole. An extended duration form of the drug, Mirapex ER, permits a convenient once-daily dosing schedule.

Mechanism of Action: Pramipexole is a selective agonist of the D_2 subfamily of dopamine receptors at both presynaptic and postsynaptic sites in the striatum. The binding helps to restore the balance of dopaminergic effects in the striatum. Binding at D_3 receptors also contributes to the antiparkinson effects.

Pharmacokinetics:

Route(s)	PO
Absorption	90% absorption
Distribution	Widely distributed, especially to red blood cells; 15% bound to plasma proteins
Primary metabolism	Hepatic (minimal)
Primary excretion	Renal, mostly unchanged
Onset of action	2 h
Duration of action	Half-life: 8 h; in the older adult, 12–14 h

Adverse Effects: Pramipexole has many possible adverse effects. The most common are hallucinations, dizziness, drowsiness, and nausea. The incidence of hallucinations increases with age and may cause discontinuation of therapy in older patients. Orthostatic hypotension occurs in over half the patients taking the drug and may contribute to injury due to falls. Life-threatening adverse effects include unexpected sleep attacks, hemolytic anemia, agranulocytosis, and leukopenia. Daytime sleep attacks can occur without warning, regardless of current activity level, and cause unintentional injuries. Agitation, insomnia, hypotension, constipation, anorexia, and dyskinesias are other adverse effects. In 2012 the U.S. Food and Drug Administration (FDA) issued a safety alert that pramipexole may be associated with new-onset heart failure.

Contraindications/Precautions: Pramipexole should not be used in an individual who has hypersensitivity to the drug. The drug should be used cautiously if the patient has renal, hepatic, or cardiac disease; is taking CNS depressants; or has psychosis, dyskinesia, or affective disorders.

Drug Interactions: Concurrent use with antipsychotic drugs will reduce the pharmacologic effects of pramipexole. Caution should be used if the drug is combined with other dopamine agonists such as levodopa or ropinirole. Drugs that may increase pramipexole levels include cimetidine, ranitidine, diltiazem, verapamil, and quinidine. Pramipexole may worsen dyskinesias when used concurrently with levodopa. **Herbal/Food:** Kava may decrease the effects of pramipexole.

Pregnancy: Animal reproduction studies showed embryotoxicity, with no evidence of developmental adverse effects. Pramipexole inhibits prolactin secretion in humans. Adverse effects on nursing infants are unknown.

Treatment of Overdose: No specific treatment is available for overdose. General supportive measures should be implemented.

Clinician Responsibilities: Key clinical implications for patients receiving pramipexole are included in Applied Clinical Judgment: Patients Receiving Pharmacotherapy for Neurodegenerative Disorders.

Drugs Similar to Pramipexole (Mirapex)

Other dopamine agonists used to treat PD include apomorphine, bromocriptine, ropinirole, and rotigotine.

Apomorphine (Apokyn, Kynmobi): Apomorphine, available as a subcutaneous injection, is a nonergot dopamine agonist used as a single dose to treat severe off episodes in patients who have advanced PD. Kynmobi is a sublingual for patients who have difficulty swallowing. It is not intended for use as routine management of PD symptoms. Apomorphine is structurally related to morphine, but it does not bind to opioid receptors or cause morphine-like effects (see Chapter 25). Life-threatening adverse effects include sleep attacks or acute circulatory failure. Sleep attacks are more serious than the general drowsiness or sleepiness that occurs frequently with dopaminergic agonists. They can occur during any activity, including driving and other potentially dangerous activities. The drug causes significant nausea and vomiting, and the manufacturer recommends the administration of trimethobenzamide (Tigan), an antiemetic drug, 3 days prior to the apomorphine injection. The serotonin (5-HT_3) antagonist antiemetics such as ondansetron (Zofran) are contraindicated because they may result in severe hypotension and loss of consciousness. Common adverse effects are orthostatic hypotension, nausea and vomiting, and dyskinesias. Animal reproduction studies showed increased neonatal deaths and malformations. Adverse effects on nursing infants are unknown.

Bromocriptine (Parlodel): Approved in 1978, bromocriptine, available as a tablet, is an ergot alkaloid that has a variety of uses. In addition to being a dopamine agonist used for adjunctive treatment with levodopa for PD, it is approved for pituitary adenoma, acromegaly, type 2 diabetes (Cycloset), and for women with amenorrhea and infertility caused by excessive prolactin secretion. Off-label indications include alcoholism, cocaine withdrawal, mastalgia, NMS, and premenstrual syndrome.

When used concurrently with levodopa-carbidopa, bromocriptine allows a significant dose reduction of levodopa. Life-threatening adverse reactions may include seizures, shock, or MI. The most common dose-limiting adverse effects are psychologic reactions, including confusion, agitation, hallucinations, paranoid delusions, or nightmares. Other adverse effects include orthostatic hypotension, headache, nausea and vomiting, anorexia, and rash on the face and arms. Studies in pregnant women have not shown an increase in abnormalities or direct effects on the fetus. Bromocriptine inhibits lactation and is not recommended during breastfeeding.

Ropinirole (Requip): Approved for PD in 1997, ropinirole is an oral nonergot dopamine receptor agonist used as monotherapy for the treatment of early PD or in combination with levodopa in more advanced disease. The most common adverse effects are syncope, fatigue, drowsiness, nausea and vomiting, and viral infections. A major advantage of ropinirole is that it causes a lower rate of dyskinesias than levodopa. In addition, the patient taking ropinirole rarely experiences sleep attacks. Ropinirole was subsequently approved to treat restless leg syndrome. An extended release form (Requip XL) offers the convenience of once-daily dosing for PD. Common adverse effects include nausea, somnolence, syncope, and asthenia. Animal reproduction studies showed increased fetal death and malformations. Ropinirole inhibits lactation and is secreted in breast milk, therefore it is not recommended during breastfeeding.

Rotigotine (Neupro): Approved in 2007, rotigotine is a transdermal patch available for treating early- and late-stage PD as well as moderate to severe restless leg syndrome. The patch provides for ease of use and is changed daily. Rotigotine can reduce the on–off periods experienced during levodopa therapy. Nausea and vomiting and drowsiness are common during therapy. Care must be taken to prevent injuries due to unexpected sleep attacks. Animal reproduction studies showed increased fetal death and adverse effects on embryo-fetal development. Rotigotine inhibits lactation and may be secreted in breast milk, therefore caution should be used if breastfeeding.

Miscellaneous Dopaminergic Drugs

21.7 Several miscellaneous dopaminergic drugs are used as adjuncts to levodopa therapy.

In addition to levodopa and dopaminergic agonists, several other drugs may be used to increase dopamine levels in the striatum. These drugs act on neurons by either increasing the release of dopamine or by reducing its destruction. Doses of these drugs are listed in Table 21.3.

Amantadine (Gocovri): Amantadine acts by increasing the release of dopamine from storage sites in the presynaptic neurons. It also blocks the reuptake of dopamine into the presynaptic neurons. Both of these mechanisms result in increased dopamine action. Given PO, the drug produces a rapid reduction in parkinsonism symptoms, but its effects begin to diminish after several months of therapy. Adverse effects are primarily CNS related and include confusion, dizziness, irritability, and headache. Care must be taken to prevent injuries due to unexpected sleep attacks. Amantadine should be used with caution in patients with major psychotic disorder because it can exacerbate psychoses and cause hallucinations and suicidal ideation. Gocovri and Osmolex are extended-release forms of amantadine approved for treating dyskinesia in patients with PD receiving levodopa-carbidopa therapy. Amantadine is also an antiviral drug used for the prophylactic and symptomatic treatment of influenza A virus infection. A prototype feature is found in Chapter 54. Animal reproduction studies of rotigotine showed increased embryolethality and teratogenicity. Amantadine inhibits lactation and may be secreted in breast milk; therefore, caution should be used if breastfeeding.

Catechol-O-Methyltransferase Inhibitors: Catechol-O-methyltransferase, or COMT, is the enzyme responsible for metabolizing levodopa to its inactive intermediate, 3-O-methyldopa. The **COMT inhibitors** are drugs that prevent the destruction of levodopa in peripheral tissues, thus increasing the amount of levodopa available to enter the brain. This results in a longer half-life and more consistent serum levels of levodopa. The COMT inhibitors have no therapeutic effects on their own; their beneficial effects are entirely the result of increased levodopa levels.

Three drugs in this category are available. Approved in 1999, entacapone (Comtan) is available as a tablet and is recommended as an adjunct to levodopa and carbidopa. Entacapone can significantly reduce the off time experienced during levodopa therapy. Approved in 1998, tolcapone (Tasmar) is also available as a tablet as an adjunct to levodopa-carbidopa. Tolcapone has a longer duration of action than entacapone and acts on COMT both peripherally and centrally. Opicapone (Ongentys) was approved as a once daily PO therapy to reduce the "off" episodes during levodopa-carbidopa therapy.

Most adverse effects observed during therapy with the COMT inhibitors are those of excessive amounts of levodopa: nausea and vomiting, dyskinesias, orthostatic hypotension, and psychiatric symptoms. Entacapone itself can cause nausea, diarrhea, abdominal pain, and urine discoloration. Tolcapone carries a black box warning regarding the possible development of liver failure, which may be fatal. Regular monitoring of hepatic status must be performed during tolcapone therapy. If improvement is not observed after 3 weeks of tolcapone therapy, the drug should be withdrawn. Entacapone, tolcapone and opicapone are always given with levodopa-carbidopa, which is known to cause visceral and skeletal malformations in pregnant animals. Thus, these drugs should only be administered during pregnancy or lactation if the potential benefit to the mother justifies the potential risk to the fetus or neonate.

Istradefylline (Nourianz): Approved in 2019, istradefylline is indicated to decrease the wearing-off periods in patients taking levodopa-carbidopa. It acts by blocking a specific type of receptor for adenosine called the A_{2A} receptor. Adenosine is best known as one of the four nucleosides composing DNA and as part of the energy carrier adenosine triphosphate (ATP). However, adenosine also plays an important role in neurotransmission throughout the body. When adenosine attaches to its A_{2A} receptor in the basal ganglia in the brain it *inhibits* dopaminergic neurons, resulting in a "shortage" of dopamine. When istradefylline blocks the A_{2A} receptor, adenosine can no longer bind, resulting in more dopamine. This additional dopamine helps to shorten wearing-off periods during levodopa therapy. As an interesting side note, the stimulant effect of caffeine is thought to be caused by a blockade of this same receptor. The most common adverse effect is dyskinesia. Based on animal data, this drug may cause fetal harm when either given alone or with levodopa-carbidopa. Use during pregnancy or lactation is not recommended.

Monoamine Oxidase-B Inhibitors: Monoamine oxidase (MAO) is an enzyme found in synaptic spaces that metabolizes catecholamines to inactive compounds. MAO-A acts on norepinephrine and serotonin, whereas MAO-B inactivates dopamine. Although MAOs are distributed throughout the body, most of the MAO located in the brain is type B. By inhibiting MAO-B these drugs increase the level of dopamine in the striatum, resulting in greater dopaminergic activity in this region.

Approved for PD in 1989, selegiline is available as a tablet, a capsule, and as an orally disintegrating tablet (Zelapar). A selegiline transdermal patch (Emsam) is approved for the treatment of major depression, but not Parkinson's. Selegiline may be used off-label to treat extrapyramidal symptoms or attention-deficit/hyperactivity disorder. A second MAO-B inhibitor, rasagiline (Azilect), was approved in 2006 and offers the convenience of once-daily dosing. The newest drug in this class, safinamide (Xadago), was approved in 2017. Selegiline and rasagiline may be prescribed either as monotherapy for PD or concurrently with levodopa-carbidopa. Safinamide is approved only as an adjunct to levodopa and carbidopa therapy to reduce the frequency of off periods.

The most frequent adverse effects during MAO-B therapy are those that are also associated with levodopa: nausea and vomiting, confusion, orthostatic hypotension, and dyskinesias. Minor adverse effects include insomnia, headache, arthralgia, and dyspepsia. With most MAOIs, the patient must strictly avoid food containing tyramine and certain medications that could result in hypertensive crisis. Because these drugs selectively inhibit MAO-B, this is not a major concern. With high doses, however, they lose their selectivity for MAO-B and begin to affect MAO-A, thus increasing the risk of a hypertensive crisis when high-tyramine foods are eaten. There is a risk of severe CNS toxicity (serotonin syndrome) if MAO-B inhibitors are used concurrently with antidepressants. The MAO-B inhibitors are contraindicated or should be used with extreme caution in patients taking other MAOIs, opioids, selective serotonin reuptake inhibitors, tricyclic antidepressants, methylphenidate, amphetamine, dextromethorphan, or St. John's wort. Based on animal data, MAO-B inhibitors may cause fetal harm and may inhibit milk production. Use during pregnancy or lactation is not recommended.

CONNECTION Checkpoint 21.2

From what you learned in Chapter 19, what is the other major indication for MAO inhibitors? What food nutrient must be strictly avoided in patients taking these drugs?

Anticholinergic Drugs

21.8 Anticholinergic drugs are the oldest of the antiparkinson drugs and are effective at reducing tremor.

Anticholinergic drugs comprise the oldest category of drugs used to treat symptoms of PD, having been used for over 150 years. They help to restore the balance between ACh and dopamine by blocking ACh (muscarinic) receptors in the striatum of the brain. This inhibits the effects of ACh, allowing dopamine to have greater influence.

Anticholinergics are of most benefit to the patients whose primary symptom is tremor; they are less effective at reducing bradykinesia. Overall, they exhibit fewer serious adverse effects than levodopa, but they are less effective. Anticholinergics must be used with caution in older adults because this population often has difficulty with the CNS adverse effects, including confusion, delusion, and hallucinations. The anticholinergic drugs used most often to treat PD are benztropine (Cogentin), diphenhydramine (Benadryl), and trihexyphenidyl. The student should refer to Chapter 14 for a complete discussion on the indications, actions, and adverse effects of this class of medications. Doses of selected anticholinergics used to treat PD are listed in Table 21.4.

PROTOTYPE DRUG Benztropine (Cogentin)

Classification **Therapeutic:** Antiparkinson drug
Pharmacologic: Anticholinergic drug

Therapeutic Effects and Uses: Benztropine is used as combination therapy with trihexyphenidyl or levodopa-carbidopa in the management of PD symptoms. It is also used to treat drug-induced EPS. Although it suppresses tremor and rigidity, it is not effective at alleviating tardive dyskinesia. The patient may notice decreased symptoms after only 2 to 3 days of therapy with benztropine. It is an older medication approved in 1954 that is available by PO and parenteral routes. An off-label indication is to treat hypersalivation in patients who have developmental disabilities.

Mechanism of Action: Benztropine acts by reducing the excess cholinergic effect associated with dopamine deficiency and by restoring neurotransmitter balance in the striatum.

Pharmacokinetics:

Route(s)	PO, intramuscular (IM), intravenous (IV)
Absorption	Rapidly absorbed
Distribution	Wide distribution; 95% bound to plasma proteins
Primary metabolism	Hepatic
Primary excretion	Renal
Onset of action	1–2 h PO; 15 min if given IM or IV
Duration of action	Half-life: 6–10 h

Table 21.4 Anticholinergic Drugs and Drugs with Anticholinergic Activity Used for Parkinsonism

Drug	Route and Adult Dose (Maximum Dose Where Indicated)	Adverse Effects
benztropine (Cogentin)	PO/IM: 0.5–1 mg/day (max: 6 mg/day)	*Nausea, constipation, dry mouth, blurred vision, drowsiness, dizziness, tachycardia, hypotension, nervousness*
diphenhydramine (Benadryl)	PO: 25–50 mg tid–qid (max: 300 mg/day)	
trihexyphenidyl	PO: start with 1 mg and gradually increase to 6–10 mg/day (max: 15 mg/day)	<u>Paralytic ileus, cardiovascular collapse, anaphylactic shock (diphenhydramine)</u>

Note: *Italics* indicate common adverse effects. <u>Underline</u> indicates serious adverse effects.

Adverse Effects: Common adverse reactions to benztropine are related to its anticholinergic effects and include sedation, constipation, blurred vision, dry mouth, decreased sweating, urinary retention, and confusion. Paralytic ileus is the only identified life-threatening adverse reaction.

Contraindications/Precautions: Contraindications to the use of benztropine include closed-angle glaucoma, myasthenia gravis, tardive dyskinesia, GI or urinary obstruction, prostatic hypertrophy, peptic ulcers, tachycardia, and children under age 3. Caution must be taken when benztropine is given to patients with psychiatric diagnoses because it may worsen these conditions.

Drug Interactions: Additive toxicity can occur when benztropine is taken with other drugs that exhibit anticholinergic effects, including antihistamines, tricyclic antidepressants, phenothiazines, MAOIs, or quinidine. Alcohol and other CNS depressants will have an additive sedative effect. Antidiarrheals will slow GI motility and decrease absorption of the medication. **Herbal/Food:** Kava will cause a decreased benztropine effect. Jimsonweed or butterbur may lead to increased benztropine effects.

Pregnancy: Studies on the effects of benztropine during pregnancy and lactation are inadequate. Other anticholinergic drugs have been shown to inhibit lactation.

Treatment of Overdose: Overdose can cause circulatory collapse, respiratory depression, shock, and coma. Physostigmine, 1 to 2 mg subcutaneous or IV, will reverse symptoms of anticholinergic intoxication. If needed, it may be repeated in 2 hours. Other treatment is supportive, according to symptoms being experienced.

Clinician Responsibilities: Key clinical implications for patients receiving benztropine are included in Applied Clinical Judgment: Patients Receiving Pharmacotherapy for Neurodegenerative Disorders in this chapter and in Applied Clinical Judgment: Patients Receiving Pharmacotherapy with Cholinergic (Muscarinic) Antagonists in Chapter 14.

Drugs Similar to Benztropine (Cogentin)

The other anticholinergic widely used for PD is trihexyphenidyl. Diphenhydramine is most often prescribed for allergies and information on this drug can be found in Chapter 45.

Trihexyphenidyl: Approved in 1949, trihexyphenidyl is available in several PO formulations in both regular and extended-release forms. It is indicated for both idiopathic and drug-induced PD and its actions and adverse effects are similar to those of benztropine. It is useful in decreasing involuntary movements and salivation, which are two problems experienced by patients with PD. The most serious adverse effect is paralytic ileus. Other adverse effects include typical anticholinergic reactions such as constipation, dryness of the mouth, nausea, blurred vision, urinary retention, dizziness, and nervousness. In patients over age 60, the dose must be increased gradually to prevent serious side effects. It must not be given to patients with hypersensitivity to the drug, closed-angle glaucoma, severe cardiac impairment, myasthenia gravis, or GI or urinary obstruction. In addition, this drug should be used with caution in older men due to the potential for developing prostatic hyperplasia. Studies on the effects of trihexyphenidyl during pregnancy and lactation are inconclusive. Other anticholinergic drugs have been shown to inhibit lactation.

Alzheimer's Disease

21.9 Alzheimer's disease, the most common dementia, leads to a progressive loss of cognitive function.

Dementia is a chronic, degenerative disorder characterized by progressive memory loss, confusion, and inability to think or communicate effectively. It is usually associated with cerebral atrophy or other degenerative structural changes within the brain. Loss of short-term memory is an early sign. Patients have difficulty finding their way around familiar places and forget where they leave items. Mood swings and changes in behavior or personality eventually develop as patients become angry and frustrated with their condition. They forget how to perform ADLs such as bathing, cooking, or toileting and may not comprehend instructions. They often have an altered sense of time and place. Psychosis occurs in about 10% of patients and 15 to 20% develop major depression as comorbid conditions. Late changes include the inability to walk or feed themselves, incontinence, and inability to swallow.

PharmFACT

Over 5.8 million Americans have Alzheimer's dementia. One in 10 seniors age 65 and older have the disorder (Alzheimer's Association, 2020).

Known causes of dementia include multiple small cerebral infarcts (vascular dementia), toxins (lead), severe infections, metabolic disorders (hypothyroidism and vitamin B_{12} deficiency), and brain tumors. Infection with the human immunodeficiency virus (HIV) causes dementia late in the progress of the disease. Approximately 60 to 80% of the patients with dementia are diagnosed as having Alzheimer's disease.

It should be clearly understood that dementia is not a normal consequence of aging. Although cognitive changes such as memory impairment and a decline in the speed of information recall do occur with aging, these rarely interfere with ADLs and are not considered dementia.

Table 21.5 Symptoms of Alzheimer's Disease

Early (2–4 Years Duration)	Middle (2–12 Years Duration)	Late (2–4 Years Duration and Longer)
Depression Loss of ability to concentrate Increased anxiety and agitation Irritability Weight loss Forgetting the location of common items (car keys, home); blaming others for moving or stealing items Forgetting important dates (family birthdays, healthcare provider appointments) Not paying bills	Lack of ability to recall names of acquaintances Recent memory loss Loss of orientation to time, person, or place Changes in personal habits (may become loud, use profane language, have delusions, or show repetitive behavior) Increasing difficulty with self-care Unable to recall their address, day of the week, or year	Lack of ability to recognize family members Loss of ambulation ability Loss of ability to perform any ADLs Loss of sphincter control Loss of ability to recognize self (e.g., does not recognize self in the mirror) Sundowning syndrome (worsening of symptoms in the evening)

Alzheimer's disease (AD) is a neurodegenerative disease that involves a chronic, progressive loss of cognitive function. The disorder generally begins after age 60 and affects as many as 50% of the population over age 85. AD is a leading cause of death. A summary of the major symptoms of AD is shown in Table 21.5.

AD leads to loss of productivity and wages (both for the patient and the caregivers), and often the patient must be placed in a long-term care facility. In addition to the economics of caring for an individual with AD, there are the psychologic and emotional costs to families and caregivers. Pharmacotherapy has limited success in improving the cognitive function of patients with AD.

Despite many attempts at identifying the etiology of AD, the causes remain largely unknown. Although the cause has been elusive, structural damage in the brains of patients with AD has been well documented. Beta-amyloid protein and **neurofibrillary tangles** are found at autopsy in the brains of nearly all patients with AD. The neurofibrillary tangles are composed of tau and amyloid proteins, and their abundance is proportional to the amount of cognitive impairment observed in the patient. It is suspected that these structural changes are caused by chronic inflammatory or oxidative cellular damage to the surrounding neurons. Environmental, immunologic, and nutritional factors, as well as viruses, are considered possible sources of brain damage. There are losses in both the numbers and functions of neurons.

In addition to structural changes, there are abnormalities in the balance of neurotransmitters in the brains of patients with AD. The best documented change is a deficiency of ACh, which is likely caused by brain atrophy and destruction of neurons. This loss of cholinergic activity is thought to be responsible for decreased cognition, loss of recent memory, and the inability to retain new information. Deficiencies in other brain neurotransmitters are also likely to contribute to the complex symptoms of AD.

Genetic factors likely contribute to the development of AD. Early-onset AD (ages 30–60) has been associated with mutations on chromosomes 1, 14, and 21 that are believed to lead to the development of the neurofibrillary tangles. The contribution of genetics to late-onset AD (after age 65) is less clear but is believed to result from a mutation on chromosome 19, combined with environmental and lifestyle factors.

It is important to assess the degree of cognitive impairment in patients with dementia. Various assessment tools are used to determine a baseline degree of cognition to make decisions on whether pharmacotherapy should be implemented. During pharmacotherapy, these tools are used to determine the progression of dementia and to gauge the effectiveness (or ineffectiveness) of therapy. Tools for assessing the progress of AD include periodic magnetic resonance imaging (MRI) and cognitive tests for memory, problem solving, attention, and language. In 2020 a new radioactive diagnostic agent, flortaucipir F18 (Tauvid) was FDA approved. Given prior to a positron emission tomography (PET) scan, flortaucipir F18 binds to portions of the brain containing tau protein and enables scientists to estimate the amounts of tau neurofibrillary tangles in patients with AD.

Pharmacotherapy of Alzheimer's Disease

21.10 Pharmacotherapy of Alzheimer's disease produces only modest results and is ineffective at stopping the progression of the disorder.

Drugs are used to slow memory loss and other progressive symptoms of dementia. In most cases, the pharmacologic treatment of dementia is the same regardless of its cause. In addition, pharmacotherapy is often required to manage common comorbid conditions such as depression, anxiety, or psychosis.

The FDA has approved only a few drugs for AD. These medications, listed in Table 21.6, do not cure or prevent AD; at best, they may slow progression of memory loss. The pharmacotherapy of AD is shown in Pharmacotherapy Illustrated 21.2.

Table 21.6 Drugs to Treat Alzheimer's Disease

Drug	Route and Adult Dose (Maximum Dose Where Indicated)	Adverse Effects
memantine (Namenda XR)	PO (extended release): 7–28 mg once daily	*Headache, confusion, dizziness, cough, hypertension* No serious adverse effects
Cholinesterase Inhibitors		
donepezil (Aricept)	PO: 5–10 mg at bedtime (max:23 mg/day)	*Nausea and vomiting, anorexia, diarrhea, abdominal pain, dizziness, headache, weight loss, muscle cramps* Hallucinations, depression, confusion, hepatotoxicity, increased mortality in patients with mild cognitive impairment (galantamine)
galantamine (Razadyne ER)	PO (extended release): 8–24 mg once daily	
rivastigmine (Exelon)	PO: 1.5–6 mg bid (max: 6 mg bid) Transdermal: 4.6–13.3 mg (one patch) daily	

Note: *Italics* indicate common adverse effects. Underline indicates serious adverse effects.

Pharmacotherapy Illustrated 21.2

Alzheimer's Drugs Work by Intensifying the Effect of Acetylcholine at the Receptor

1 Alzheimer's disease

Characterized by abnormal structures in the brain:
- Neurons die
- The brain shrinks
- Memory is lost

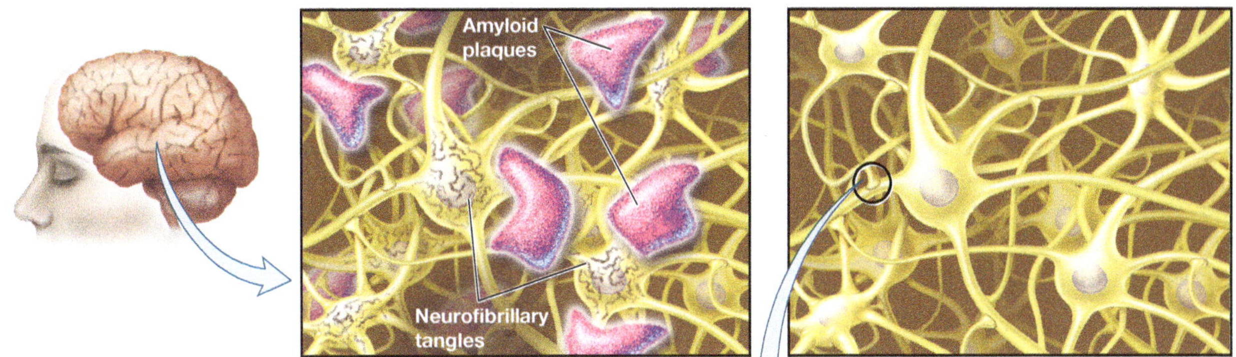

Unhealthy neuronal structure

Healthy neuronal structure

2 Drug therapy focuses on restoring or enhancing acetylcholine's role in the brain

- Cholinesterase inhibitors
  e.g., donepezil

3 Factors responsible for brain cell death include excessive transmission of glutamate

Drug therapy:
- N-methyl-D-aspartate (NMDA) receptor drugs
  e.g., memantine

Combination drug therapy:
- Donepezil and memantine

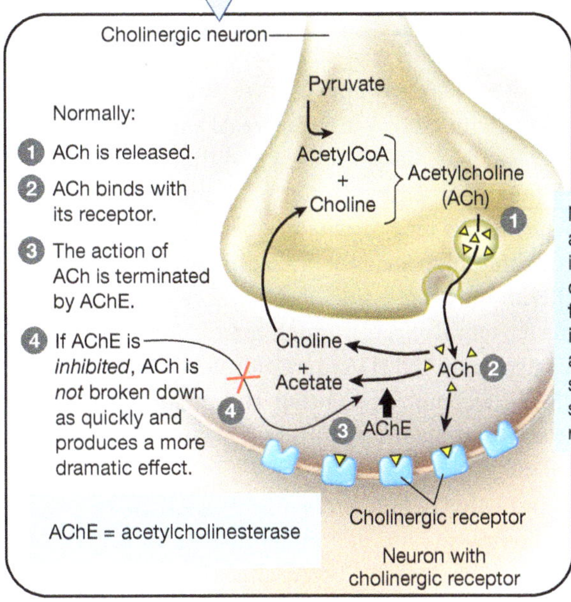

Normal role of acetylcholine in a vast array of brain functions, including the ability to speak, move, see, think, and remember.

The reversible **cholinesterase inhibitors** are the most widely prescribed drug class for treating AD. ACh is naturally degraded in the synaptic cleft by the enzyme cholinesterase. When cholinesterase is inhibited, ACh levels become elevated and produce a more profound effect on ACh receptors. They are similar to the peripheral cholinesterase inhibitors such as neostigmine but demonstrate greater CNS activity.

The goal of pharmacotherapy with reversible cholinesterase inhibitors is to improve function in three domains: ADLs, behavior, and cognition. Although the cholinesterase inhibitors improve all three domains, their effectiveness is modest at best. Therapy is begun as soon as the diagnosis of AD is established. These medications are less effective in treating the severe stages of this disorder, probably because too many neurons have died; increasing the level of ACh is effective only if functioning neurons are present. As the disease progresses and fewer neurons are present, drug effects diminish and the cholinesterase inhibitors may be discontinued; their therapeutic benefit may not justify their expense or the risks of adverse effects.

All cholinesterase inhibitors used to treat AD have similar efficacy. Adverse effects are those expected of drugs that enhance the parasympathetic nervous system (see Chapter 13). The GI system is most often affected, with nausea and vomiting and diarrhea being frequent adverse events. Rivastigmine (Exelon) is associated with weight loss, which is a potentially serious adverse effect in some older adults. When therapy is discontinued, doses of the cholinesterase inhibitors should be tapered gradually.

CONNECTION Checkpoint 21.3

The cholinesterase inhibitors for Alzheimer's disease are used for their central actions. From what you learned in Chapter 13, what are the indications for cholinesterase inhibitors that act peripherally? What drug is the prototype peripheral cholinesterase inhibitor?

Memantine (Namenda) was approved in 2003 for the treatment of patients with moderate to severe AD. It acts by a different mechanism than the centrally acting cholinesterase inhibitors. Memantine reduces abnormally high levels of **glutamate**, which is the major excitatory neurotransmitter of the CNS. Chronic, high levels of brain glutamate have been associated with the progression of AD and cell death. Glutamate exerts its neural effects through interaction with the N-methyl-D-aspartate (NMDA) receptor. Memantine binds to the NMDA receptor, preventing glutamate from causing its destructive excitatory actions and, theoretically, slowing nerve damage.

Caution is indicated when memantine is given to older adults or those with chronic kidney disease or seizure disorder. No life-threatening adverse effects have been identified. Occasional adverse effects have been reported, including dizziness, confusion, vomiting, headache, cough, and hypertension. Because memantine and cholinesterase inhibitors act by different mechanisms, they may be taken in combination. When taken together, these drugs do not interfere with each other's absorption, distribution, metabolism, or elimination. An extended-release form (Namenda XR) offers the convenience of once-daily dosing. Namzaric, a fixed-dose combination of memantine and donepezil, was approved in 2015 to treat moderate to severe AD.

Other medication classes frequently prescribed for symptoms associated with AD include antipsychotics, antidepressants, and antianxiety drugs. Agitation occurs in the majority of patients with AD, which may be accompanied by delusions, paranoia, hallucinations, or other psychotic symptoms. Atypical antipsychotics such as risperidone (Risperdal) and olanzapine (Zyprexa) may be used to control these episodes. The antipsychotic medications are presented in Chapter 20.

Although not as common as agitation, anxiety and depression occur in many patients with AD. Anxiolytics such as buspirone (BuSpar) or benzodiazepines are used to control anxiety. Mood stabilizers such as sertraline (Zoloft), citalopram (Celexa), or fluoxetine (Prozac) are given if major depression interferes with ADLs. The student should refer to Chapters 18 and 19 for information on these drugs.

PROTOTYPE DRUG Donepezil (Aricept)

Classification **Therapeutic:** Anti-Alzheimer's drug
Pharmacologic: Reversible cholinesterase inhibitor

Therapeutic Effects and Uses: Donepezil was approved to treat symptoms of AD in 1996. The drug is available in tablet, PO solution, and PO disintegrating tablet (Aricept ODT) forms. It has an extended duration of action that allows for once-daily dosing. Donepezil is the most frequent drug prescribed for early AD.

There is no evidence that donepezil stops the destruction of neurons or that it alters the course of the underlying dementia. It may, however, prolong the time between diagnosis and the institutionalization of the patient. A caregiver should be present to assist the patient in adhering to the medication regimen.

Mechanism of Action: Donepezil raises ACh concentrations in the brain. Because the drug is moderately selective for cholinesterase in the CNS, it produces fewer peripheral adverse effects than other drugs in this class.

Pharmacokinetics:

Route(s)	PO
Absorption	Completely absorbed
Distribution	Well distributed; crosses the blood–brain barrier; 96% bound to plasma proteins

Primary metabolism	Hepatic; metabolized to active metabolites
Primary excretion	Primarily renal; some feces
Onset of action	3–4 h
Duration of action	Half-life: 10 h, if single dose; 70 h, if multiple dose

Adverse Effects: Common adverse effects of donepezil that cause discontinuation of therapy are diarrhea and nausea and vomiting. Donepezil exhibits typical cholinergic effects such as diaphoresis, bradycardia, salivation, and muscle weakness. Other possible adverse effects are anorexia, muscle cramps, fatigue, arthralgia, abnormal dreams, and headache. Many of these adverse events will diminish with continued therapy or by using a lower dose of the drug. Potential life-threatening adverse effects include atrial fibrillation, sinus bradycardia, and seizures. Abrupt discontinuation of the drug results in a sudden decline of cognitive function and an increase in behavioral disturbances.

Contraindications/Precautions: The only contraindication to the use of donepezil is hypersensitivity to the drug. There is a risk of GI bleeding, especially in patients with a history of peptic ulcers or chronic use of nonsteroidal anti-inflammatory drugs (NSAIDs). It should be used with caution in patients with hyperthyroidism or hepatic dysfunction or those who are lactating. Increased numbers of seizures have been recorded in patients taking donepezil, especially in those patients with a history of seizures.

Drug Interactions: Donepezil is metabolized by CYP2D6 and CYP3A4, and drugs that enhance or inhibit these enzymes have the potential to interact with donepezil. Decreased effects of donepezil will occur with concurrent administration of phenytoin, phenobarbital, rifampin, dexamethasone, and carbamazepine. Concurrent use of NSAIDs may lead to GI ulceration and bleeding. Synergistic effects will occur with cholinergic agonists, cholinesterase inhibitors, and succinylcholine. Because it is a cholinergic agonist, donepezil will decrease the effects of anticholinergic drugs. Metabolism of donepezil may be inhibited by quinidine and ketoconazole. **Herbal/Food:** None known.

Pregnancy: Animal studies suggest that donepezil may cause fetal harm. It is unknown if the drug is secreted in milk or if there are any adverse effects on the breastfed neonate.

Treatment of Overdose: Overdosage will result in signs of cholinergic crisis, such as nausea and vomiting, bradycardia, respiratory depression, hypotension, and seizures. Anticholinergic drugs such as 1 to 2 mg IV atropine may be administered to reverse some of the overdose symptoms.

Clinician Responsibilities: Key clinical implications for patients receiving donepezil are included in Applied Clinical Judgment: Patients Receiving Pharmacotherapy for Neurodegenerative Disorders.

Drugs Similar to Donepezil (Aricept)

Other cholinesterase inhibitors used to treat the symptoms of AD are galantamine and rivastigmine.

Galantamine (Razadyne): Galantamine is an oral cholinesterase inhibitor that has the same uses and actions as donepezil. Approved in 2001, it is indicated for mild to moderate symptoms of dementia. Like other AD medications, it does not alter the progression of the disease. It is available in immediate and extended-release (ER) forms.

The most frequent adverse effects are nausea and vomiting. The drug may be administered with food or with an antiemetic to reduce these effects. Other adverse reactions include diarrhea, bradycardia, chest pain, fatigue, anemia, syncope, vertigo, headache, insomnia, or tremor. Anorexia and weight loss are possible and may be serious effects in patients who are debilitated. In addition, it is not recommended for use in individuals with severe hepatic or renal dysfunction. It must be used cautiously in individuals with respiratory disease, bradycardia, cardiac conduction disorders, seizure history, history of GI bleeding, peptic ulcer disease, or asthma. Animal reproduction studies showed developmental toxicity and reduced offspring growth. It is unknown if the drug is secreted in milk or if there are any adverse effects on the breastfed neonate.

Rivastigmine (Exelon): Like other drugs in this class, rivastigmine inhibits brain cholinesterase more than heart or skeletal muscle cholinesterase. Approved in 2000, it is used to treat mild to moderate symptoms of dementia associated with AD and PD. It has similar effectiveness to donepezil. Rivastigmine is given PO with food to prevent nausea and vomiting, which frequently occur with this medication. Liquid preparations should be mixed only with water, soda, or juice. A once-daily transdermal patch of rivastigmine is available for both PD and AD.

Rivastigmine is contraindicated in patients with hypersensitivity to rivastigmine or carbamate. Nausea and vomiting, anorexia, and diarrhea occur in a significant number of patients. The transdermal patch form of the drug causes a lower incidence of GI adverse effects. Other common adverse effects include headache, vertigo, abdominal pain, and confusion. Cautious use is indicated when given to patients with a hypersensitivity to cholinesterase inhibitors; cardiac, pulmonary, renal, or hepatic disease; diabetes; GI disorders; concurrent use of other cholinergic or anticholinergic drugs; PD; seizure history; or concurrent use of NSAIDs. No potential life-threatening adverse effects have been identified. Animal reproduction studies did not show fetal harm. The drug is secreted in animal milk but effects on human breastfeeding are unknown.

Multiple Sclerosis

21.11 Multiple sclerosis is a chronic, neurodegenerative disease that is treated with immunomodulator drugs.

Multiple sclerosis (MS) is a neurodegenerative disease characterized by demyelination, the destruction or removal of the myelin sheath from a nerve or nerve fiber. The destruction is secondary to an inflammatory response that leads to random areas of demyelination, known as plaques, in the white matter of the CNS. It is believed that a pathogen, such as a latent virus, may trigger an abnormal autoimmune response in patients who are genetically susceptible. The processes of inflammation and neurodegeneration occur simultaneously throughout the disease process. MS is a leading cause of neurologic disability in the 20- to 40-year-old age group, although it may affect individuals of any age (Figure 21.1).

The most common type of MS, relapsing-remitting MS (RRMS) has a typical pattern of progression that is characterized by periods of symptom exacerbation alternating with periods of remission during which symptoms may completely disappear. Remissions may last several months or even years. Less commonly, progression may be continuous without any clear remission periods, a type known as secondary-progressive MS (SPMS). Types that are much less common include primary-progressive MS (PPMS) and progressive-relapsing MS (PRMS) (Multiple Sclerosis Association of America, 2020).

Diagnosis of MS is sometimes difficult because its symptoms mimic those of other neurologic disorders. Early symptoms are frequently vague and nonspecific and include weakness, visual disturbances, paresthesias, and difficulty with bladder control. Symptoms of cognitive impairment such as cognitive deficits, fatigue, mood disturbances, and major depression are common and often appear very early in the course of the disease. Assessment should determine if the symptoms are worsening or are intermittent. Also of note is whether the activity level of the patient has decreased, along with worsening fatigue, activities that aggravate the symptoms (e.g., hot showers or baths, overexertion, stress), and any changes in personality or behavior. A diagnosis is made after other neurologic disorders have been ruled out. Imaging studies such as MRI are useful in identifying the areas of demyelination in the brain.

Like other neurodegenerative disorders, medications are unable to cure MS or reverse the progressive demyelination of nerves. Existing drugs for MS are only partially effective at slowing neurodegeneration and some have serious adverse effects. In general, pharmacotherapy has the following three goals:

- Modify the progression of the disease.
- Treat acute exacerbations.
- Manage symptoms.

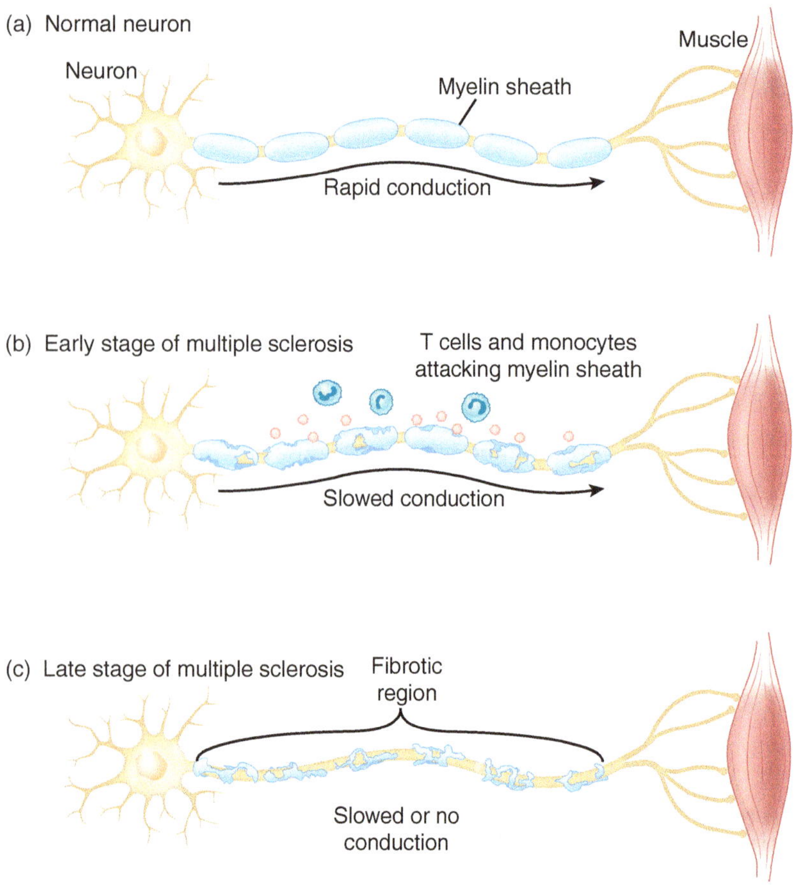

Figure 21.1 Multiple sclerosis.

Disease-Modifying Drugs for MS

Although the exact etiology of MS remains unknown, it is considered an autoimmune disease. The body has mounted an immune attack against its own tissues, in this case, the myelin surrounding nerves. Strategies for slowing the progression of MS have therefore focused on modifying the abnormal immune response of these patients through the application of immunomodulators. **Immunomodulator** is a general term that refers to drugs that affect body defenses. In the context of MS treatment, these medications are called disease-modifying drugs (DMDs). With few exceptions, these medications are only used to treat MS, and all are able to slow the progress of neurodegeneration.

The DMDs are used to prevent irreversible neuronal damage in patients with MS. Therapy with DMDs is initiated soon after the diagnosis of MS is confirmed because early control of disease activity has been demonstrated to delay the progressive phase of MS and prolong the ability of patients to remain active. Treatment normally continues indefinitely and is only changed or discontinued if toxicity develops or there is no apparent clinical benefit. Doses of these drugs are listed in Table 21.7.

There is no "best drug" for treatment of MS. All DMDs have been shown to be effective in treating MS. Over 18 DMDs are available, acting by over 10 different mechanisms. They differ by route of administration, frequency of dosing, and spectrum of adverse effects. Furthermore, the effectiveness of a medication varies greatly from one patient to another and may change for each individual patient as therapy progresses.

PROTOTYPE DRUG Interferon Beta-1b (Betaseron, Extavia)

Classification **Therapeutic:** Drug for relapsing forms of multiple sclerosis
Pharmacologic: Immunomodulator

Therapeutic Effects and Uses: Approved in 1993, interferon (IFN) beta-1b is produced by recombinant DNA

Table 21.7 Drugs for Modifying the Progression of Multiple Sclerosis

Drug	Route and Adult Dose (Maximum Dose Where Indicated)	Adverse Effects
alemtuzumab (Lemtrada)	IV (two infusions, 12 months apart): first course 12 mg/day for 5 days; second course 12 mg/day for 3 days	*Infections, rash, headache, pyrexia, nasopharyngitis, fatigue* Cytopenias, infusion reactions, serious infections, increased risk of malignancies, serious autoimmune conditions
cladribine (Mavenclad)	PO: Two treatment cycles of 20 days, separated by one year. 1.75 mg/kg/course.	*Headache, upper respiratory infection* Lymphopenia, hypersensitivity Contraindicated during pregnancy or lactation
dimethyl fumarate (Tecfidera)	PO: 120 mg bid for 7 days, then 240 mg bid	*Flushing, abdominal pain, diarrhea, and nausea* Lymphopenia
fingolimod (Gilenya)	PO: 0.5 mg once daily	*Headache, back pain, diarrhea, elevated liver transaminase* Macular edema, bradycardia and other dysrhythmias
glatiramer (Copaxone, Glatopa)	Subcutaneous: 20 mg daily or 40 mg 3 times/wk	*Local reactions, arthralgia, back pain, flulike symptoms, infection, anxiety, vasodilation, chest pain, palpitations, rash, pruritus, diarrhea, nausea, dyspnea, rhinitis* Asthenia, lymphadenopathy
interferon beta-1a (Avonex, Rebif) and peginterferon beta-1a (Plegridy)	IM (Avonex): 30 mcg/wk Subcutaneous (Rebif): 4.4–44 mcg 3 times/wk Subcutaneous (Plegridy): 63 mg once on day 1; 94 mcg on day 15; 125 mcg on day 29 and thereafter q2wk	*Myalgia, upper respiratory infection, flulike symptoms, injection-site reactions, headache, fever, nausea, chills* Hepatotoxicity, leukopenia, myelosuppression, severe depression (suicide risk), seizures, anaphylaxis
interferon beta-1b (Betaseron, Extavia)	Subcutaneous: 0.0625–0.25 mg every other day	
mitoxantrone (Novantrone)	IV: 12 mg/m^2 every 3 months (max: lifetime dose 140 mg/m^2)	*Nausea and vomiting, diarrhea, cough, headache, abdominal pain, fever, alopecia* Myelosuppression, renal failure, hepatotoxicity, cardiotoxicity (heart failure, MI, fetal harm)
natalizumab (Tysabri)	IV: 300 mg infused over 1 h every month	*Headache, depression, fatigue, menstrual dysfunction* Anaphylaxis (rare), infections
ocrelizumab (Ocrevus)	IV: 300 mg followed by 300 mg 2 wk later; subsequent dosing is 600 mg every 6 months	*Respiratory and skin infections* Infusion reaction, possible malignancies and teratogenicity
ofatumumab (Kesimpta)	Subcutaneous: 20 mg week 0,1; then 20 mg/month	*Infections, injection site reactions* Fetal harm, hepatitis B reactivation
ozanimod (Zeposia)	PO: 0.23–0.92 mg/day	*Upper respiratory infection, orthostatic hypotension, elevated liver transaminase* Macular edema, bradycardia and other dysrhythmias, serious infections, fetal toxicity
siponimod (Mayzent)	PO: 1–2 mg/day (maintenance dose)	*Headache, hypertension, diarrhea, elevated liver transaminase* Macular edema, bradycardia and other dysrhythmias, fetal toxicity
teriflunomide (Aubagio)	PO: 7–14 mg once daily	*Alopecia, diarrhea, influenza, nausea, paresthesia* Severe hepatotoxicity, teratogenicity, leukopenia, severe skin reactions

Note: *Italics* indicate common adverse effects. Underline indicates serious adverse effects.

technology and is very similar to natural IFN. It was one of the first drugs developed that was found to slow the progression of MS. Patients taking IFN beta-1b experience fewer relapses and a reduction in brain lesions characteristic of MS. This drug is available by subcutaneous injection for the treatment of patients with relapsing MS.

Mechanism of Action: The mechanism of action by which IFN beta-1b produces improvements in the symptoms of MS is unknown. It is believed to act by suppressing the activity of T cells and reducing the inflammatory actions of cytokines, which are substances secreted by activated T cells.

Pharmacokinetics:

Route(s)	Subcutaneous
Absorption	50% absorbed
Distribution	Crosses the blood–brain barrier poorly; crosses placenta and enters breast milk
Primary metabolism	Rapidly metabolized in body tissues
Primary excretion	Unknown
Onset of action	6–12 h
Duration of action	Half-life: 8 min–4 h

Adverse Effects: Adverse effects are very common with IFN beta-1b. Most patients taking interferon beta-1b will experience transient flulike symptoms: Analgesics and antipyretics may be premedicated on injection days to reduce these symptoms. Injection-site reactions also occur in the majority of patients. Patients should be monitored closely for depression and suicidal ideation. Injection-site inflammation occurs in most patients and may progress to necrosis. Severe hepatic injury has occurred with IFN beta-1b and caution should be used when using other hepatotoxic drugs, including alcohol. Common adverse effects include leukopenia, headache, insomnia, asthenia, increased liver enzymes, rash, peripheral edema, and malaise.

Contraindications/Precautions: The only contraindication is history of hypersensitivity to interferon beta, albumin, or mannitol.

Drug Interactions: Zidovudine (AZT) levels may increase to toxic levels during therapy. **Herbal/Food:** None known.

Pregnancy: Animal studies and some human data suggest an increased number of spontaneous abortions. It is unknown if the drug is secreted in milk or it there are any adverse effects on the breastfed neonate. IFN beta-1b should be administered during pregnancy or lactation only if the potential benefit to the mother justifies the potential risk to the fetus or neonate.

Treatment of Overdose: Treatment for overdose of this drug has not been documented.

Clinician Responsibilities: Key clinical implications for patients receiving interferon beta-1b are included in Applied Clinical Judgment: Patients Receiving Pharmacotherapy for Neurodegenerative Disorders.

Drugs Similar to Interferon Beta-1b (Betaseron, Extavia)

Other drugs used to treat the relapsing symptoms of MS are alemtuzumab, cladribine, dimethyl fumarate, diroximel fumarate, fingolimod, glatiramer, IFN beta-1a, mitoxantrone, ozanimod, natalizumab, siponimod, and teriflunomide.

Alemtuzumab (Lemtrada): Alemtuzumab is a monoclonal antibody against CD52 approved in 2014 for relapsing forms of MS. Because of the potential for serious adverse effects, it is used for patients who have had an inadequate response to at least two other MS medications. It is given by two IV infusions, 12 months apart. Because nearly all patients experience infusion reactions, premedicate with a high-dose corticosteroid for the first 3 days of each treatment course. This drug comes with several black box warnings including an increased risk for cytopenias (including fatal pancytopenia), infusion reactions (some of which have been fatal), serious infections (including *Pneumocystis jiroveci*), and malignancies (including thyroid cancer, melanoma, and lymphoproliferative disorders). The patient should be monitored for cytopenias monthly for 48 months after the last infusion. Alemtuzumab is contraindicated in patients infected with human immunodeficiency virus (HIV). This medication can cause serious fetal harm: Women of child-bearing potential should use effective contraception for 4 months after each treatment. Alemtuzumab is secreted in animal milk and due to the potential for serious adverse effects, breastfeeding is not recommended.

Cladribine (Mavenclad): Approved in 2019, cladribine is recommended for patients who have not responded to other MS medications. The drug appears to act by cytotoxicity of B and T lymphocytes. It has an unusual dosing schedule; two annual courses for 20 days over 2 years. Adverse effects include upper respiratory infections, headache, leukopenia, and herpes zoster infection. Cladribine is contraindicated in patients infected with HIV. An IV form of cladribine is approved to treat hairy cell leukemia and may be used off-label to treat other malignancies. This drug carries a black box warning for an increased risk for malignancy and fetal harm. The drug is contraindicated in pregnant women and during lactation. Women of childbearing potential and men should use effective contraception for at least 6 months after the last dose for each treatment course.

Dimethyl Fumarate (Tecfidera), Monomethyl Fumarate (Bafiertam), and Diroximel Fumarate (Vumerity): These three drugs are closely related. All three are given PO, act by the same mechanism, and have similar indications and adverse effects. Approved in 2013, dimethyl fumarate is used for treating relapsing forms of MS. Given PO, its mechanism of action is unknown. Adverse effects include mild to moderate flushing, abdominal pain, diarrhea, and nausea. Lymphocyte counts should be monitored during therapy because dimethyl fumarate can cause significant lymphopenia. In animal reproduction studies, high doses of dimethyl fumarate showed embryotoxicity, delayed sexual maturation, and neurobehavioral impairment. It is unknown if the drug is secreted in milk or if there are any adverse effects on the breastfed neonate. Diroximel fumarate (Vumerity) was approved in 2019 and monomethyl fumarate in 2020. Doses of the three medications are not equivalent.

Fingolimod (Gilenya): Approved in 2010, fingolimod has a unique mechanism of action in that it blocks the capacity of lymphocytes to exit lymph nodes. Because they remain in the nodes, there are fewer lymphocytes in peripheral tissues, including the CNS. The drug can reduce lymphocyte counts to 60% of baseline values within 4 to 6 hours after a single dose. Fingolimod accomplishes its effects by affecting the sphingosine-1-receptor (S1PR) on lymphocytes, therefore it (along with ozanimod and siponimod) is classified as an S1PR modulator.

Fingolimod is approved for the treatment of patients with relapsing forms of MS and was the first drug approved for pediatric MS. A major advantage is that the drug is given PO with once-daily dosing. Unfortunately, fingolimod has the potential to cause serious dysrhythmias: Patients must be carefully monitored for bradycardia and other cardiac rhythm abnormalities during therapy. Due to the diminished lymphocyte count, patients are at risk for infections. Macular edema is an adverse effect that is especially troublesome in patients with a history of uveitis or diabetes. The most common adverse effects are headache, influenza, diarrhea, back pain, cough, and elevated liver transaminase levels. Fingolimod may cause serious fetal harm. The drug is secreted in animal milk but effects on the breastfed neonate are unknown.

Glatiramer (Copaxone, Glatopa): Approved in 1996, glatiramer is one of several first-line drugs in the treatment of relapsing MS, including patients who have experienced their initial clinical episode of the disease. The drug reduces the annual relapse rate for MS and the generation of new lesions in the brain. Administered daily by the subcutaneous route, it is believed to dampen the immune response by activating suppressor T cells. Glatiramer produces an immediate post-injection reaction in many patients that includes chest pain, palpitations, anxiety, dyspnea, and urticaria. The symptoms are usually transient and self-limiting. Other common adverse effects are injection-site reactions, vasodilation, and rash. Animal reproduction studies did not show adverse effects on embryo-fetal development or lactation. Effects on the breastfed neonate are unknown.

IFN beta-1a (Avonex, Rebif) and PEG IFN beta-1a (Plegridy): Approved in 1996, IFN beta-1a is structurally identical to the natural IFN produced by the body. IFN beta-1a decreases the frequency of clinical exacerbations and slows the progression to physical disability. The drug acts by inhibiting the release of proinflammatory cytokines that initiate the autoimmune reaction leading to MS. IFN beta-1a also changes the blood–brain barrier and reduces T-lymphocyte migration into the brain, thereby reducing inflammation. It is available by the subcutaneous (Rebif) and IM (Avonex) routes. Peginterferon beta-1a (Plegridy) has the same actions but has a longer duration of action that allows for dosing once every 2 weeks. Adverse effects are similar to those of other IFNs, with flulike symptoms being observed in the majority of patients. Patients should be monitored for depression and suicidal ideation. Decreased peripheral blood counts, including thrombocytopenia and leukopenia, have been reported. Rare cases of severe hepatotoxicity, including some cases requiring liver transplantation, have been reported in patients taking IFN beta-1a. In animal studies, this drug increased the risk for spontaneous abortions, but did not show teratogenicity or adverse effects of fetal development. Effects on the breastfed neonate are unknown.

Mitoxantrone (Novantrone): Mitoxantrone is an immunomodulator that is approved to treat acute myelogenous leukemia, prostate cancer, and chronic, progressive relapsing forms of MS. In treating MS, mitoxantrone acts by suppressing B and T lymphocytes and macrophages. Fatigue and GI-related adverse effects are common. The drug carries several black box warnings. Mitoxantrone is cardiotoxic and may result in potentially fatal heart failure as long as several years after therapy is discontinued. It may also cause acute myelogenous leukemia. Serious myelosuppression may increase the risk for infections and bleeding. Because of the potential for serious adverse effects, this medication is infrequently used to treat MS. It is only administered by IV infusion. This medication can cause serious fetal harm: Women of childbearing potential should use effective contraception and submit a negative pregnancy test prior to each dose. Mitoxantrone is secreted in milk and breastfeeding is not recommended.

Natalizumab (Tysabri): Administered by IV infusion, natalizumab is a monoclonal antibody that acts by preventing white blood cells from migrating to the CNS. This inhibition reduces the inflammation and demyelination of nerves in the brain. Although effective for treating MS, its use is severely restricted due to a small risk of progressive multifocal leukoencephalopathy (PML), a rare and sometimes fatal demyelinating disease of the CNS (black box warning). Restrictions limit prescribers to those who have special training in PML. In addition, only certain pharmacies can distribute the drug. This drug can cause immunosuppression, resulting in infections. Natalizumab is also indicated for Crohn's disease. Animal reproduction studies have shown reduced offspring survival and hematologic effects on the fetus. The drug is secreted in milk but effects on the breastfed neonate are unknown.

Ocrelizumab (Ocrevus): Approved in 2017, ocrelizumab is a monoclonal antibody that binds to the CD20 receptor on B lymphocytes, resulting in the immune destruction of these cells. It is the only drug approved to treat primary progressive MS, a form of the disease that steadily worsens, without relapses. To reduce the risk for infusion reactions, the patient is premedicated with a corticosteroid and an antihistamine 30 minutes prior to each injection. Other common adverse effects include respiratory infections and skin infections. The first dose of ocrelizumab is followed by a second dose 2 weeks later and subsequent doses at 6-month intervals. Based on animal studies, ocrelizumab may cause fetal harm and neonatal death. Women of childbearing potential should use effective contraception during therapy and for 6 months after the last dose. Ocrelizumab is secreted in animal milk but effects on the breastfed neonate are unknown.

Ozanimod (Zeposia): Approved in 2020, ozanimod is another S1PR modulator that blocks the egress of lymphocytes from lymph nodes. It is approved to treat adults with relapsing forms of MS. It is reported to cause fewer cardiac adverse effects than fingolimod, the original S1PR modulator. Respiratory and urinary infections, elevated liver enzymes, and orthostatic hypotension are common adverse effects. Because the drug lowers lymphocyte counts, the patient is at risk for infections. Ozanimod is contraindicated in patients who have experienced a serious cardiac event in the past 6 months. Based on animal studies, ozanimod may cause fetal harm and teratogenicity. Women of childbearing potential should use effective contraception during therapy and for 3 months after the last dose. Ozanimod is secreted in animal milk but effects on the breastfed neonate are unknown.

Siponimod (Mayzent): Siponimod is a PO medication approved in 2019 to treat relapsing forms of MS. Like fingolimod, it is an S1PR modulator that acts by blocking the ability of lymphocytes to exit lymph nodes. Because the drug lowers lymphocyte counts, the patient is at risk for infections. Siponimod is contraindicated in patients who have experienced a serious cardiac event in the past 6 months. The most frequent adverse effects include headache, hypertension, and changes in liver function tests. Potentially serious adverse effects include macular edema, transient decreases in heart rate, and reduced lung function. Based on animal studies, siponimod may cause fetal harm and teratogenicity. Women of childbearing potential should use effective contraception during therapy and for 10 days after the last dose. Siponimod is secreted in animal milk but effects on the breastfed neonate are unknown.

Teriflunomide (Aubagio): Approved in 2012, teriflunomide is an oral drug for treating relapsing forms of MS. It is an active metabolite of leflunomide (Arava), used for treating rheumatoid arthritis. Teriflunomide acts by suppressing the division of B and T cells. Teriflunomide is generally well tolerated; however, some serious toxicities are associated with the drug. It carries a black box warning that severe and sometimes fatal liver injury may occur. In addition, the drug may cause birth defects. This drug is eliminated very slowly and may take 8 to 24 months to be completely excreted from the body. Because the drug lowers lymphocyte and neutrophil counts, the patient is at risk for infections. Pregnancy is contraindicated. Women of childbearing potential and men should use effective contraception during therapy and for 10 days after the last dose. Teriflunomide is secreted in animal milk but effects on the breastfed neonate are unknown.

In a study of patients with relapsing-remitting MS (RRMS) or secondary-progressive MS (SPMS) receiving treatment with either interferon beta-1a or natalizumab, several quality-of-life concerns were noted by the patients (Buesa-Estelléz et al., 2019). Four main thematic areas emerged: feelings about the injections (e.g., difficulty and discomfort with daily injections, required therapy), coping strategies for the routine of drug therapy (e.g., resignation when results may not be visible, integrating injections into daily routines), other drug forms available such as oral or once-a-month intravenous forms, and dealing with discomfort related to the injectable drug (e.g., pain, bruising). Since many of these concerns may be mitigated by patient education and patient-centered care, clinicians should explore patients' concerns and alternative measures that could be considered, such as switching from an injectable to oral drug form or considering autoinjectors if self-injections are difficult or painful. Working collaboratively with the patient may lead to better adherence overall with what will be a lifelong need for treating the disease.

CONNECTIONS: Using Research in Practice

Drug Therapy for Patients with Multiple Sclerosis and Quality-of-Life Issues

Multiple sclerosis (MS) is a lifelong disease that impacts every aspect of life. In addition, drug therapy needs to be tailored to the type of MS as well as the patient's response to therapy. While newer treatments have made a dramatic difference in delaying the progression of the disease, the pharmacologic treatment also has impact on the patient's quality of life.

Drugs for treating acute exacerbations of MS: Acute exacerbations of the disease are treated with high-dose corticosteroid therapy with prednisone or methylprednisolone. The recommended length of treatment is no longer than 3 weeks and no more than three times a year. Although very high doses are administered, the short-term use of corticosteroids does not usually cause significant adverse effects (see Chapter 68). Another drug that can be used to treat an acute exacerbation is IV gamma globulin. This has proven to be a successful treatment for patients who are unresponsive or unable to tolerate corticosteroids.

Drugs for managing symptoms of MS: Many classes of medications may be ordered to manage symptoms of MS, including antianxiety drugs, antidepressants, antipsychotics, or sedative–hypnotics. These symptomatic medications are used to treat other conditions and are discussed in other chapters of this text. The patient may experience physical symptoms such as muscle spasticity or bladder or bowel dysfunction. Depression is common; it may be the emotional response to a diagnosis of a chronic, progressive, potentially debilitating disease, or it may be secondary to damage to mood-regulating neurons as the disease progresses. Chronic pain may require the use of analgesics and neuropathic pain may respond to treatment with gabapentin or carbamazepine. Approved in 2010, dalfampridine (Ampyra) is specifically indicated to improve walking in patients with MS.

Amyotrophic Lateral Sclerosis

21.12 The pharmacotherapy of amyotrophic lateral sclerosis is limited to a few drugs.

Amyotrophic lateral sclerosis (ALS), commonly known as Lou Gehrig's disease, is the most common degenerative disease of motor neurons. Its symptoms include weakness and atrophy of the muscles of the legs, hands, and forearms that spread to all muscles of the body. Sensory and cognitive functions are not affected. It usually occurs in middle age and progresses rapidly to death in 2 or 3 years due to respiratory failure or pneumonia. There is no known cause or curative treatment for the disease. About 10% of cases have a familial history of the disorder.

Disease-modifying drugs for ALS: Only two drugs have FDA approval specifically for treating patients with ALS, and neither of them is able to cure the disease. Approved in 1995, riluzole (Rilutek) has been shown to extend survival by reducing the degeneration of neurons. It is estimated that survival is prolonged by only 3 months. Riluzole is a tablet that is given every 12 hours on an empty stomach. Seizures are the only serious adverse effect. Common adverse effects include headache, dizziness, poor concentration, confusion, anxiety, hypotension, and edema.

Approved in 2017, edaravone (Radicava) has been shown to slow the progression of ALS and help individuals to preserve function for a longer period of time. Administered by IV infusion, edaravone is administered for 14 consecutive days, followed by a 2-week drug-free period. All cycles thereafter are infused for 10 days, followed by a 2-week drug-free period. The most common adverse effects include bruising, difficulty walking, and headache. This drug is not pregnancy rated but based on animal data it may cause fetal harm.

The patient with ALS experiences painful muscle spasticity. Treatment with muscle relaxants such as baclofen (Lioresal) may bring some relief (see Chapter 23). Anticholinergic drugs such as trihexyphenidyl or benztropine may be administered to decrease saliva production. RimabotulinumtoxinB (Myobloc) may be used off-label to reduce saliva secretion for up to 3 months. Opioids may be necessary to treat severe pain late in the progress of the disease.

CONNECTIONS: APPLIED CLINICAL JUDGMENT

Patients Receiving Pharmacotherapy for Neurodegenerative Disorders

Key Assessment Data

- History of current condition, baseline vital signs, physical exam findings; history of cardiovascular or musculoskeletal disease; medication and allergy history; bowel sounds, urinary output, muscle strength, and mental status as appropriate; pregnancy status.
- Assess for disturbances in thought processes, perception, verbal communication, affect, behavior, interpersonal relationships, and self-care. Use objective screening tools such as the Movement Disorder Society Unified Parkinson's Disease Rating Scale (MDS-UPDRS), the Mini-Mental State Examination (MMSE), or as per healthcare agency. Obtain a history of depression or sleep disorders and current treatments used.
- Ongoing assessment during drug therapy includes laboratory findings such as hepatic or renal function studies, exacerbating conditions, and ability to carry out ADLs, particularly mobility and eating. Consider safety concerns and whether alternative care environments are needed.

Desired Therapeutic Outcomes

Improvement is observed and measurable by decreased musculoskeletal and neurologic symptoms (e.g., tremors, bradykinesia, or rigidity; decreased agitation and fearfulness; and maintenance or improvement of current functioning level).

(continued)

CONNECTIONS: APPLIED CLINICAL JUDGMENT *(continued)*

Patients Receiving Pharmacotherapy for Neurodegenerative Disorders

Minimizing Adverse Effects

- Orthostatic hypotension and reflex tachycardia may occur. Monitor vital signs periodically, especially orthostatic blood pressure. Ensure patient safety; monitor ambulation until the effects of the drug are known.
- Disease-related motor coordination and ambulation, eating, or other essential motor activities may be impaired. Drug therapy improves but does not cure the underlying disorder and drug response may vary as frequently as daily. The ability to carry out ADLs gradually improves with consistent usage of drug therapy. Have the patient request assistance prior to getting out of bed or attempting to walk alone if bradykinesia, rigidity, weakness, or tremors are particularly severe.
- Behavioral or mental changes or a decrease in the ability to perform self-care activities may indicate progression of the disease or ineffectiveness of drug therapy and should be reported to the provider.
- Absorption of levodopa taken for PD decreases with high-protein meals or high consumption of foods or vitamins that contain vitamin B_6 (pyridoxine). Symptoms may dramatically increase if absorption is impaired because the dose does not adequately absorb during the expected time. Take the medication for PD on an empty stomach or avoid taking it with a high-protein meal. Avoid excessive consumption of vitamin B_6-rich foods such as bananas, wheat germ, fortified cereals, green vegetables, meat, and legumes and avoid multivitamins that contain vitamin B_6.

Lifespan Considerations

- The older adult may be at increased risk for falls due to drowsiness and dizziness, hypotension, or impaired mental and physical abilities.
- The older adult man with an enlarged prostate is at higher risk for mechanical obstruction and may experience urinary retention due to anticholinergic effects. Promptly report difficulty with urination, hesitancy, or dysuria.

Patient and Caregiver Education

- The drugs do not cure the underlying disorder, but improvement may occur and full effects may not be known for a prolonged period. Some improvement should be noticeable after beginning therapy. Increasing symptoms or a decrease in the ability to perform self-care activities should be reported.
- Rise from lying or sitting to standing slowly to avoid dizziness or falls. If dizziness occurs, sit or lie down and do not attempt to stand or walk until the sensation passes. Avoid driving or other activities requiring mental alertness or physical coordination until the effects of the drug are known.
- Report new or worsening symptoms (e.g., muscle twitching, including blepharospasm, greatly increasing tremors, rigidity, agitation, or aggression) for additional treatment. Encourage the patient or caregivers to maintain a symptom diary and review the diary with the patient on each healthcare visit.
- Medications for PD should be taken on an empty stomach or avoid taking it with a high-protein meal. Avoid excessive consumption of vitamin B_6-rich foods such as bananas, wheat germ, fortified cereals, green vegetables, meat, and legumes and avoid multivitamins that contain vitamin B_6.
- Patients taking injectable drug forms for the treatment of MS (e.g., interferon beta-1b) should report increasing redness, pain, or blackening of the injection site, which may indicate that tissue necrosis is occurring.
- Encourage the family or caregivers to discuss concerns related to their own health, financial status, or other issues. Provide additional healthcare referrals as required for a support group, counseling, or respite care.

Prescribing Considerations

- In PD, the return or gradual increase of symptoms as the next dose comes due may signal a wearing-off effect and the dose may need to be increased, the interval of dosage adjusted, or an adjunctive drug added. A significant and sudden increase in symptoms may signal an overdose or on–off syndrome where symptoms dramatically increase. If symptoms are significant, hospitalization may be required to assess for the reason behind the exacerbation.
- Continued tremors, rigidity, or other symptoms may require dosage adjustment or a change in drug therapy.
- Ongoing assessment during drug therapy includes laboratory findings such as hepatic or renal function studies.
- PD medications may have interactions with certain foods, other medications, vitamins, herbal supplements, over-the-counter cold pills, and other remedies. It is recommended that all prescriptions be filled at the same pharmacy to avoid interactions between medications.

Understanding Chapter 21

Key Concepts Summary

21.1 Degenerative diseases of the central nervous system are characterized by irreversible and progressive loss of neuronal function.

21.2 Parkinson's disease is a progressive neurodegenerative disorder characterized by abnormal motor movement.

21.3 Parkinson's disease is caused by a lack of sufficient amounts of dopamine produced by the substantia nigra.

21.4 The drugs used for Parkinson's disease help to alleviate symptoms but do not cure the disease.

21.5 Replacement therapy with levodopa is the most effective therapy for treating Parkinson's disease.

21.6 Dopamine agonists may be used as monotherapy for early symptoms of Parkinson's disease or as adjuncts to levodopa in patients with advanced disease.

21.7 Several miscellaneous dopaminergic drugs are used as adjuncts to levodopa therapy.

21.8 Anticholinergic drugs are the oldest of the antiparkinson drugs and are effective at reducing tremor.

21.9 Alzheimer's disease, the most common dementia, leads to a progressive loss of cognitive function.

21.10 Pharmacotherapy of Alzheimer's disease produces only modest results and is ineffective at stopping the progression of the disorder.

21.11 Multiple sclerosis is a chronic, neurodegenerative disease that is treated with immunomodulator drugs.

21.12 The pharmacotherapy of amyotrophic lateral sclerosis is limited to a few drugs.

CASE STUDY: Making the Patient Connection

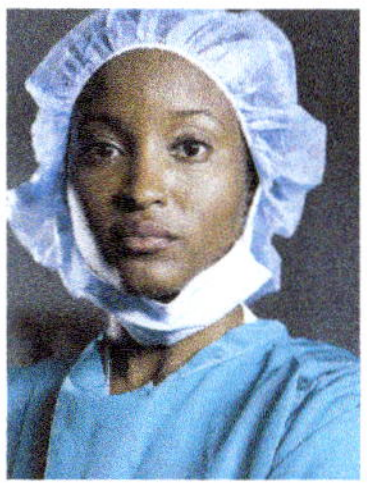

Remember the patient "Althea Taylor" at the beginning of the chapter? Now read the remainder of the case study. Based on the information presented within this chapter, respond to the critical thinking questions that follow.

Althea Taylor is a 45-year-old female nurse who works in the perioperative areas, most often in the operating room. She has always enjoyed the challenges of working in these areas and finds perioperative nursing to draw on the full range of her knowledge, technical skills, and interpersonal abilities. Over the past 8 months, Althea has had symptoms that have progressed from extreme fatigue to numbness and weakness in her hands, an increasingly unsteady gait, and periods of depression that are unusual for her. After several visits to her primary provider, she is referred to a neurologist with a preliminary diagnosis of relapsing-remitting MS (RRMS).

Critical Thinking Questions

1. What are the types of MS and how is a diagnosis determined?
2. What are the goals of drug therapy and why are the disease-modifying drugs (DMDs) so important in the treatment of MS?
3. What should Althea be alert for with regard to her disease and the use of a DMD in its treatment?

Additional Case Study

Michael, at 45 years of age, could not believe his ears when the healthcare provider told him he had PD. "Isn't that an old person's disease?" he asked. However, he knew something had been very wrong for about 3 months. At first, he felt more tired than usual, and he noticed a slight tremor, especially when he became fatigued. Michael's wife pointed out that his "hand shakes" were getting worse. Like many people first diagnosed with a degenerative nervous system disease, Michael has many questions and concerns. Following are just a few of his questions. As his nurse, how would you respond?

1. What physiologic problem causes PD and what is the etiology of this disease? How could a nurse describe this etiology to Michael?
2. Eventually, Michael is prescribed levodopa-carbidopa (Sinemet) for his parkinsonism. How does this medication work? What is the advantage of combining the two medications?
3. After months of drug therapy, Michael reports having periods where "the drug just doesn't seem to be working" and his symptoms worsen during the day. What might be the probable cause? What questions might help rule out other causes? What might be a solution?

Chapter Review

1. The patient is receiving levodopa and carbidopa for parkinsonism. Which drug would the nurse expect to be added to the patient's drug regimen to help control tremors?

1. Amantadine (Gocovri)
2. Benztropine (Cogentin)
3. Haloperidol (Haldol)
4. Donepezil (Aricept)

2. Which statement, if made by the patient, would alert the nurse that the antiparkinson medication is effective?

1. "I'm sleeping a lot more, especially during the day."
2. "My appetite has improved."
3. "I'm able to shower by myself."
4. "My skin doesn't itch anymore."

3. The nurse is counseling the caregivers of a patient with Alzheimer's disease. Which statement, if made by a caregiver, would indicate that the session had been effective?

1. "I should give this medication as symptoms of Alzheimer's disease become noticeable."
2. "If constipation occurs, I will notify the healthcare provider immediately."
3. "The medication may improve symptoms but will not cure the disease."
4. "I will take the patient's vital signs before every dose of the medication."

4. The nurse knows that the use of donepezil (Aricept) to treat the symptoms of early Alzheimer's disease has which of the following advantages? (Select all that apply.)

1. It is not associated with hepatotoxicity.
2. It is taken once per day.
3. It may be used safely in patients with peptic ulcer disease.
4. It may be used safely in patients with cardiac disease.
5. It may increase the time between diagnosis and when memory care is needed.

5. The nurse knows an advantage to rivastigmine (Exelon) over other cholinesterase inhibitors is that it:

1. Has no significant drug interactions.
2. Does not cause cholinergic adverse effects.
3. Is absorbed best on an empty stomach.
4. Does not alter glucose control in patients with diabetes.

6. Interferon beta-1b (Betaseron) has been ordered for the patient with MS. The nurse will instruct the patient on possible adverse effects that may be managed symptomatically by the patient. These include (select all that apply):

1. Flulike symptoms.
2. Insomnia.
3. Depression.
4. Rashes.
5. Pain at the injection site and blackening of the surrounding skin.

See Appendix A for answers to critical thinking questions, case study questions, and review questions.

References

Alzheimer's Association. (2020). *2206 Alzheimer's disease facts and figures*. https://www.alz.org/media/Documents/alzheimers-facts-and-figures.pdf

Buesa-Estelléz, A., Cno-de-la-Cuerda, R., Ortiz-Gutiérrez, R. M., & Palacios-Ceña, D. (2019). The impact of pharmacological treatment on patients with multiple sclerosis. *Disability and Health Journal*, *12*, 615–621. https://doi.org/10.1016/j.dhjo.2019.05.005

Multiple Sclerosis Association of America. (2020). *Types of MS*. https://mymsaa.org/publications/about-ms/types/

Parkinson's Foundation. (n.d.). *Statistics*. https://www.parkinson.org/Understanding-Parkinsons/Statistics

Selected Bibliography

Alzheimer's Association. (2020). *Treatments for sleep changes*. http://www.alz.org/alzheimers_disease_10429.asp#top

Atri, A. (2019, April). Current and future treatments in Alzheimer's disease. *Seminars in Neurology*, *39*(2), 227–240. https://doi.org/10.1055/s-0039-1678581

Baldassari, L. E., & Fox, R. J. (2018). Therapeutic advances and challenges in the treatment of progressive multiple sclerosis. *Drugs*, *78*(15), 1549–1566. https://doi.org/10.1007/s40265-018-0984-5

Carrera, I., & Cacabelos, R. (2019). Current drugs and potential future neuroprotective compounds for Parkinson's disease. *Current Neuropharmacology*, *17*(3), 295–306. https://doi.org/10.2174/1570159X17666181127125704

Costello, K., Halper, J., Kalb, R., Skutnik, L., & Rapp, R. (2019). *The use of disease-modifying therapies in multiple sclerosis: Principles and current evidence*. National Multiple Sclerosis Society. http://www.nationalmssociety.org/NationalMSSociety/media/MSNationalFiles/Brochures/DMT_Consensus_MS_Coalition.pdf

Feinstein, A., Freeman, J., & Lo, A. C. (2015). Treatment of progressive multiple sclerosis: What works, what does not, and what is needed. *The Lancet Neurology*, *14*, 194–207. https://doi.org/10.1016/S1474-4422(14)70231-5

Gholamzad, M., Ebtekar, M., Ardestani, M. S., Azimi, M., Mahmodi, Z., Mousavi, M. J., & Aslani, S. (2019). A comprehensive review on the treatment approaches of multiple sclerosis: currently and in the future. *Inflammation Research*, *68*(1), 25–38. https://doi.org/10.1007/s00011-018-1185-0

Hergesheimer, R., Lanznaster, D., Vourc'h, P., Andres, C., Bakkouche, S., Beltran, S., et al. (2020). Advances in disease-modifying pharmacotherapies for the treatment of amyotrophic lateral sclerosis. *Expert Opinion on Pharmacotherapy*, *21*(9), 1103–1110. https://doi.org/10.1080/14656566.2020.1746270

Khoury, R., Grysman, N., Gold, J., Patel, K., & Grossberg, G. T. (2018). The role of 5 HT6-receptor antagonists in Alzheimer's disease: an update. *Expert Opinion on Investigational Drugs*, *27*(6), 523–533. https://doi.org/10.1080/13543784.2018.1483334

Kumar, K., Kumar, A., Keegan, R. M., & Deshmukh, R. (2018). Recent advances in the neurobiology and neuropharmacology of Alzheimer's disease. *Biomedicine and Pharmacotherapy*, *98*, 297–307. https://doi.org/10.1016/j.biopha.2017.12.053

Leahy, T., & Counihan, T. J. (2018). Physician and advanced nurse practitioner decision-making in the management of multiple sclerosis. *British Journal of Neuroscience Nursing*, *14*(5), 240–248. https://doi.org/10.12968/bjnn.2018.14.5.240

Multiple Sclerosis Association of America. (2020). *Long-term treatments for multiple sclerosis*. https://mymsaa.org/ms-information/treatments/long-term/

Parish, A. L., & Kim, J. (2020). The role of the primary care provider in work-up and management of Parkinson's disease. *Advances in Family Practice Nursing*. https://doi.org/10.1016/j.yfpn.2019.12.004

Rutatangwa, A. K. (2019). *Pediatric multiple sclerosis*. Medscape. https://emedicine.medscape.com/article/2091406-overview#a3

Selway, J. S. (2018). Growing significance of the nurse practitioner in dementia care. *Journal for Nurse Practitioners*, *14*(3), A9.

Skeen, M. B. (2020). *Sphigosine-1-phosphate modulators of multiple sclerosis*. Practical Neurology. https://practicalneurology.com/articles/2020-feb/sphingosine-1-phosphate-modulators-for-multiple-sclerosis

Vucic, S., Rothstein, J. D., & Kiernan, M. C. (2014). Advances in treating amyotrophic lateral sclerosis: Insights from pathophysiological studies. *Trends in Neurosciences*, *37*, 433–442. https://doi.org/10.1016/j.tins.2014.05.006

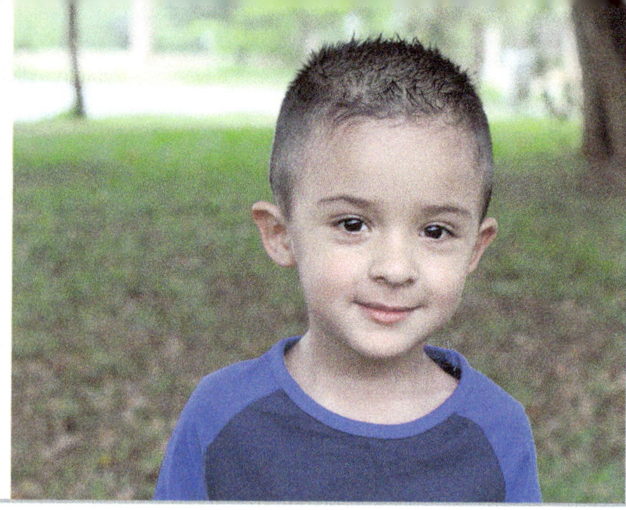

"I'm not sure I can cope with my child having a seizure disorder. The schedule for giving the medicines seems daunting to me. I'm not sure I'll know what to do when he has a seizure or how the medicines work."
—*Patient "Jorge Alvarez's" mother*

Chapter 22
Pharmacotherapy of Seizures

Chapter Outline

Learning Outcomes

After reading this chapter, the student should be able to:

1. Understand the causes of epilepsy.
2. Differentiate among the following terms: epilepsy, seizures, and convulsions.
3. Describe how the presentation and pharmacotherapy of epilepsy change throughout the lifespan.
4. Differentiate the signs, symptoms, and treatment of the different types of seizure disorders.
5. Compare and contrast the pharmacotherapy of generalized and partial seizures.
6. Identify factors that influence the selection of a specific antiepileptic drug by the healthcare provider.
7. Describe the nurse's role in the pharmacologic management of seizures.
8. For each of the classes shown in the chapter outline, identify the prototype and representative drugs and explain the mechanism(s) of drug action, primary indications, contraindications, significant drug interactions, pregnancy data and important adverse effects.
9. Apply clinical judgement to care for patients receiving pharmacotherapy for seizures.

Key Terms

Definitions of the terms in bold may be found in the Glossary.

The word *epilepsy* is derived from the Greek word *epilepsia*, meaning "to take hold" or "seize." Epilepsy is a neurologic condition characterized by recurrent seizures that affects approximately 2 million Americans. Research in the past two decades has resulted in the development of new drugs to treat epilepsy and other seizure disorders. In this chapter the student will study the current medications for seizures and understand the nurse's role in the administration and patient education associated with the medication regimen.

Characteristics of Seizure Disorders

22.1 Epilepsy is characterized by recurrent seizures caused by disturbances in the electrical activity of the brain.

Epilepsy is a disruption of the activity of clusters of neurons in the brain that is characterized by two or more seizures. A **seizure** is a disturbance of the brain's electrical activity that may result in loss of consciousness, sensory malfunction, and an alteration in motor activity. The many diverse symptoms of seizure are caused by abnormal neuronal discharges within the different regions of the brain. Abnormal neuronal discharges can be measured as sharp spikes or waves on an electroencephalogram (EEG), which is a valuable tool in diagnosing seizure disorders.

When a patient presents with symptoms of a seizure, it is important to identify a possible underlying cause of seizure activity so that an appropriate treatment plan can be implemented. Epileptic seizures are sometimes symptoms of an underlying disorder such as a brain tumor, head trauma, brain aneurysm, stroke, alcoholism, or infectious disease of the brain. The diagnosis of epilepsy always begins with a search for an underlying disorder that could explain the seizures. Table 22.1 lists common etiologies for seizure disorders. Successful treatment of the underlying condition often eliminates the seizure activity. If a brain abnormality remains after the acute seizure has resolved, recurrent seizures are likely.

In 50 to 70% of cases, the etiology of a seizure is idiopathic; no specific cause can be identified. These patients may have a lower tolerance to environmental triggers, and seizures may occur when they are sleep deprived, are exposed to strobe or flickering lights, or have a fluid and electrolyte imbalance. Diagnostic tests such as complete blood count (CBC), serum lead levels, and blood glucose are important in excluding the systemic causes of seizures. Virtually anything that changes the homeostatic environment of neurons in the brain has the potential to cause seizures, thus complicating the diagnosis and treatment of epilepsy.

It is important to distinguish between the terms *convulsion* and *seizure*. Most often, patients associate epilepsy with **convulsions**, which are involuntary, violent spasms of the large skeletal muscles of the face, neck, arms, and legs. Convulsions are a characteristic sign of tonic–clonic seizures. Many forms of epilepsy, however, do not involve convulsions. For example, absence seizures

Table 22.1 Etiology of Seizure Disorders

Etiology	Pathophysiology
Fever	Rapid increase in body temperature may result in febrile seizure. This is particularly noted in infants and toddlers.
Infectious disease	Meningitis and encephalitis, which are infections of the brain, result in brain inflammation and seizure development.
Metabolic disorders	Alteration in the fluid and electrolyte levels can result in seizure development. Hypoglycemia, hyponatremia, and water intoxication contribute to the alteration in electrical impulse transmission at the cellular level.
Miscellaneous causative agents	Medication used to treat mood disorders and psychotic episodes and local anesthetics produce increased levels of stimulatory neurotransmitters or toxicity. Drug abuse, such as cocaine addictions alters the neurotransmitters in the brain and produces seizures. Alcohol and sedative–hypnotic drug withdrawal can result in seizure activity.
Neoplastic disorders	Both benign and malignant brain lesions, particularly those that grow rapidly, prevent adequate oxygenated blood supply to the brain tissue and contribute to increased intracranial pressure, which results in seizure development.
Trauma	Head injuries may result in increased intracranial pressure, which results in seizure development. Exposure to toxic fumes or substances, or ingestion of poisons, can result in trauma to brain tissue and resultant seizures.
Vascular disorders	Hypoxia of brain tissue disrupts the electrical transmission of impulses contributing to seizure development. Carbon monoxide poisoning reduces the oxygen-carrying ability of the blood and results in cerebral hypoxia. The related ischemia of brain tissue alters the electrical transmission of impulses and contributes to seizure development. Other vascular causes of seizures include hypotension, stroke, shock, and cardiac dysrhythmias.

do not involve any dramatic movement of the limbs and may be barely noticeable by those observing the affected individual. Thus, it may be stated that all convulsions are seizures, but not all seizures are convulsions. Because of this difference, drugs used to treat epilepsy are best described as antiepileptic drugs (AEDs) or antiseizure medications, rather than anticonvulsants.

PharmFACT

Patients with Alzheimer's disease who develop seizures were more likely to have an earlier age of dementia onset and a shorter time to death (Baumann et al., 2018).

Seizures have the potential to significantly impact one's quality of life. They may cause serious injury if they occur while someone is driving a vehicle or performing a potentially hazardous activity. Without pharmacotherapy, epilepsy can severely limit participation in school, employment, and social activities and affect self-esteem. Chronic depression may accompany poorly controlled seizures. Proper treatment, however, can reduce or completely eliminate seizures in many patients. Important considerations in nursing care include identifying patients at risk for seizures, documenting the pattern and type of seizure activity, and implementing safety precautions. In collaboration with the patient, healthcare provider, and pharmacist, the nurse is instrumental in achieving positive therapeutic outcomes during AED therapy. The nurse must educate patients that effective seizure control is usually achieved through a combination of pharmacotherapy and support from family and caregivers.

22.2 Seizure disorders differ throughout the lifespan.

Seizure disorders occur throughout the lifespan. Of those who experience seizures, about half will experience their first seizure before age 10. Because of this, epilepsy is considered a major disorder of childhood. Fortunately, many patients who have childhood epilepsy experience a reduction in symptoms as they age, and some will no longer require pharmacotherapy as adults. In addition to childhood, epilepsy manifests with higher frequency during pregnancy and in older adults. Treatment of epilepsy differs throughout the lifespan.

Women, pregnancy, and lactation: The pharmacotherapy of epilepsy in women with childbearing potential can be challenging. These patients require special education to prevent conception during AED pharmacotherapy or to safely prevent seizures during pregnancy.

Some AEDs interact with oral contraceptives, diminishing the effectiveness of birth control pills. AEDs that are inducers of hepatic CYP450 enzymes will increase the metabolism of contraceptive hormones, thus decreasing their effectiveness in preventing conception. Antiseizure drugs that induce CYP450 include phenobarbital, carbamazepine, oxcarbazepine, topiramate, and phenytoin. To prevent an unplanned pregnancy, the patient should receive a higher dose of oral contraceptive and be instructed to use a backup method of birth control such as condoms. Therapy with antiseizure drugs that do not induce CYP450 enzymes, such as valproic acid or gabapentin, may be an option for these women.

Pregnancy is a major concern for women with seizure disorders. Women with epilepsy have a higher risk for delivering a child with congenital abnormalities, and some of the AEDs are teratogenic. The risk of birth defects is further increased because some AEDs cause folic acid (folate) deficiency, a condition that has been associated with increased risk of neural tube defects in the embryo. Folic acid supplements (0.4–4 mg/day) should always be recommended for women who are considering pregnancy and those who become pregnant. The use of vitamin supplementation will also reduce the risk of developing cardiac abnormalities and cleft lip or palate. Single-drug therapy should be used whenever possible because therapy with multiple AEDs results in a higher risk of birth defects. Doses are reduced to the lowest possible level that effectively controls the seizures. AEDs such as lamotrigine, gabapentin, and zonisamide should be considered because they appear to have a lower risk of teratogenicity.

Women who have epilepsy have a reduced fertility rate. Epilepsy and AEDs can disrupt the hypothalamus–pituitary axis, causing menstrual irregularities. The length of the menstrual cycle in these patients may vary from 23 to 35 days, and 40% of women with epilepsy have polycystic ovaries. Many women who have epilepsy do not ovulate. Genital blood flow is diminished and libido is reduced, contributing to a reduction in the frequency of intercourse.

During pregnancy, some of the enzyme-inducing AEDs cross the placenta and induce hepatic enzyme metabolism in the fetal liver. This decreases the circulating vitamin K levels, posing an increased risk of hemorrhage in the newborn. It is recommended that prenatal vitamin K be prescribed to women who are taking AEDs during pregnancy to prevent hemorrhagic disease in the newborn; 10 to 20 mg of vitamin K should be administered daily during the last 4 months of pregnancy.

Gestational epilepsy is a rare condition in which the patient experiences her first seizure during pregnancy. Seizures in a pregnant patient who has never been diagnosed with epilepsy may indicate the development of preeclampsia or eclampsia. **Preeclampsia** usually begins after the 20th week of pregnancy and is diagnosed by blood pressure of 140/90 mmHg or higher on two separate occasions, and 300 mg of protein is found in the urine over a 24-hour period. The rate of preeclampsia in the United States is approximately 5 to 7% of all pregnancies, affecting about 1 in every 2000 to 3000 deliveries.

Eclampsia occurs when hypertension (HTN) continues to worsen during pregnancy. Eclampsia is associated with seizures and a high risk of cerebral edema and coma. If the baby is of proper gestational age, delivery is the treatment of choice for eclampsia. When the pregnant woman is diagnosed with preeclampsia or eclampsia and delivery is not imminent, intravenous (IV) magnesium sulfate may be administered to prevent or terminate seizures. Magnesium sulfate acts by decreasing the amount of acetylcholine liberated from the motor nerve terminals and produces a peripheral neuromuscular blockade. It also has the therapeutic effect of increasing uterine blood flow. Because seizures may extend beyond labor and delivery, magnesium sulfate therapy may continue for 24 hours postpartum or until the HTN resolves.

The issue of maternal AEDs during lactation has been addressed by a number of research studies. Many studies have confirmed the safety of AEDs taken during lactation, especially when considering the benefits to the neonate derived from breastfeeding. It is likely that the amounts of AEDs secreted in breast milk are too low to cause ill effects in the baby. Follow-up studies performed 6 years after breastfeeding confirm that breastfeeding does not affect the cognitive development of children exposed to AEDs in breast milk (Haunt, 2016). The exception is valproic acid, which may have a higher risk than other AEDs.

CONNECTION Checkpoint 22.1

From what you learned in Chapter 8, how does each of the following affect the amount of drug that passes to the infant during lactation: lipid solubility of the drug, drug ionization, and drug half-life?

Childhood: Seizures in children are either idiopathic or acquired. Children with idiopathic seizures often have a family history of epilepsy or have an associated serious neurologic abnormality, such as mental retardation or cerebral palsy. Febrile seizures are another form of idiopathic seizure that occurs in children under the age of 2 years. Seizures represent the most common serious neurologic problem affecting children, with an overall incidence of approximately 1% for idiopathic epilepsy.

Acquired seizure disorders may result from injury to the brain during the prenatal, antenatal, or postpartum periods. Infants whose mothers have been exposed to cytomegalovirus during pregnancy are at increased risk of developing an acquired seizure disorder. Other causes of acquired seizures include head trauma, metabolic imbalances, exposure to toxins, and infection.

CONNECTIONS: Complementary and Alternative Therapies

The Ketogenic Diet

Description

Ketogenic diets have become popular for weight loss and control, but the diet has also been used in the treatment of epilepsy, especially when seizures cannot be controlled through pharmacotherapy alone. Before AEDs were developed, this diet was a primary treatment for epilepsy.

History and Claims

The ketogenic diet may be used for babies, children, or adults. With adults, however, it may be harder to develop the ketones that are necessary for the diet.

Standardization

The ketogenic diet is a stringently calculated diet that is high in fat, moderate in protein, and low in carbohydrates. It limits water intake to avoid ketone dilution and carefully controls caloric intake. Each meal has a ketogenic ratio of 3 or 4 g of fat to 1 g of carbohydrate. A modified Atkins diet with a ratio of 1 or 2 g of fat to 1 g of carbohydrate has also been used.

Evidence

Research suggests that these diets produce a success rate, in some cases, that is equivalent to that of modern antiepileptic drugs (Rezaei et al., 2019). The diet appears to be equally effective for every seizure type, and seizure activity has been shown to decrease by 38 to 50% (Dahlin & Prast-Nielsen, 2019). Adverse effects include hyperlipidemia, constipation, vitamin deficiencies, kidney stones, acidosis, and, possibly, slower growth rates.

Not all patients respond to the diet. Several studies suggest that response within the first 3 to 6 months may indicate that the diet has positive results, whereas those patients who fail to respond in that time period are not likely to respond with continued diet therapy for longer periods (Lambrechts et al., 2015; Vehmeijer et al., 2015).

While it has been noted that the ketogenic diet has beneficial effects in controlling seizure activity, the exact mechanism for this benefit is unknown. Recent studies have investigated the effects of the diet on the microbiome of the gut and have noted a change in the microbial environment (microbiota) in the gastrointestinal tract, with an increase in beneficial flora (Dahlin & Prast-Nielsen, 2019; Fan et al., 2019). Additional research is needed to investigate the link between gastrointestinal flora and its association with epilepsy, but at present, the ketogenic diet may be a treatment option for seizure control.

Seizure treatment for infants and children is usually accomplished with pharmacotherapy. The most commonly prescribed pediatric AEDs include valproic acid, phenytoin, carbamazepine, felbamate, lamotrigine, and topiramate. To maintain optimal seizure control, the dosage of AEDs should be increased during periods of rapid growth and development.

Nonpharmacologic treatments for epilepsy are available. One such alternative therapy is the ketogenic diet. The beneficial effects of this diet occur when ketones are eliminated from the body, thus decreasing seizure activity. Other forms of seizure treatment include surgical intervention with an excision of a circumscribed area of the brain affected by the seizure activity. The implantation of a vagal nerve stimulator in the brain is a type of therapy that delivers electrical signals to the vagus nerve to reduce the frequency of seizures.

Older adults: Seizure disorders in the older adult are often associated with an underlying comorbid condition. Stroke accounts for one-third of new-onset cases and is the most common risk factor for the development of epilepsy after age 60. Other conditions associated with epilepsy in the aging patient include progressive Alzheimer's disease, subdural hematoma from a head injury due to falling, central nervous system (CNS) infection, and brain tumors.

The nurse needs to assess the patient's therapeutic response to the AEDs and also monitor the serum drug level. The clinical response should be used to guide the needed dosage changes. When possible, only a single AED is prescribed because the use of multiple AEDs increases the risk of adverse drug events. In most patients, therapy with AEDs begins with low doses followed by careful monitoring for drug effectiveness. Gradual dosage changes are made based on clinical outcomes. It is vital to regularly monitor the liver and kidney functions of the older patient when administering multiple medications because impairment may lead to toxic serum drug levels and possible seizures.

Older patients with memory deficits may have difficulty remembering to take their AEDs. The nurse should teach these patients and their caregivers that these medicines must be taken on a regular basis, at the same time each day, for the most effective seizure prevention. If a dose is forgotten, it is not advisable to take a double dose of an AED because this may cause CNS toxicity. Furthermore, patients need to understand that waiting until the first sign of a seizure before taking their AED is ineffective at stopping the seizure because the drug will not be absorbed quickly enough.

Table 22.2 Changes in Seizure Terminology

Old Term	New Term
Absence seizure or petit mal	Generalized absence
Atonic or drop attack	Focal atonic or generalized atonic
Complex partial	Focal with impaired awareness
Focal motor	Focal motor with awareness or focal motor with impaired awareness
Focal sensory	Focal sensory with awareness or focal sensory with impaired awareness
Grand mal	Generalized tonic–clonic
Infantile spasms	Focal epileptic spasms or generalized epileptic spasms
Limbic	Focal with impaired awareness
Myoclonic	Focal myoclonic or generalized myoclonic
Psychomotor	Focal with impaired awareness
Simple partial	Focal with awareness
Tonic–clonic	Generalized tonic–clonic
Tonic or drop attack	Focal tonic or generalized tonic–clonic
—	Eyelid myoclonia

Classification of Seizure Disorders

Seizures begin with the firing of hyperexcitable neurons in the brain. The area where the abnormal electrical activity starts is known as a focus (plural = foci). As these neurons discharge impulses, the patient begins to exhibit the characteristic signs and symptoms of epilepsy. The specific symptoms depend on the nature of the discharge: the location of the abnormal focus in the brain and the extent of the discharge. It is important to identify and classify the type of seizure because this determines which drugs will be prescribed.

Classifying seizures can be difficult. Sometimes the total seizure is not observed by anyone, or the patient may present with mixed signs and symptoms that are not easy to categorize. Indeed, the patient may not even be aware that a seizure has occurred. In 2017 a new classification method was adopted to better define the types of seizures. Unfortunately, this has led to more confusion, as clinicians continue to use old terminology mixed with the new. Furthermore, most AEDs were FDA-approved using the old terminology, which continues to be used in Drug Guides. This text continues to use the old classification system, while phasing in the new terms as appropriate. Changes in terminology are shown in Table 22.2.

22.3 Most seizures are classified as generalized or partial.

There are two broad categories of seizure activity: generalized and partial (focal). A third category, called unknown, is considered a temporary classification until a seizure can be further observed and studied. Preferred drugs for the management of seizures are shown in Table 22.3.

Generalized Seizures

In **generalized seizures**, multiple foci spread abnormal neuronal discharges across both brain hemispheres simultaneously. The patient often experiences loss of consciousness,

Table 22.3 Drugs Used for the Management of Seizures

Type of Seizure	First-Line Drugs*	Alternative Drugs
Generalized Seizures		
Absence	ethosuximide, lamotrigine, valproic acid	topiramate
Atonic	lamotrigine, valproic acid	clonazepam, levetiracetam, topiramate
Myoclonic	clonazepam, levetiracetam, valproic acid	lamotrigine, phenobarbital, topiramate
Tonic–clonic	lamotrigine, topiramate, valproic acid	clonazepam, diazepam, levetiracetam, oxcarbazepine, perampanel, phenobarbital, phenytoin, zonisamide
Partial Seizures		
Focal-onset	carbamazepine, lamotrigine, phenytoin, valproic acid	brivaracetam, cenobamate, clorazepate, diazepam, eslicarbazepine, ezogabine, felbamate, gabapentin, lacosamide, levetiracetam, oxcarbazepine, perampanel, phenobarbital, pregabalin, tiagabine, topiramate, vigabatrin, zonisamide
Other Seizures		
Alcohol withdrawal	diazepam, lorazepam	carbamazepine
Febrile	acetaminophen (for prophylaxis)	diazepam, phenytoin
Infantile (epileptic) spasms	adrenocorticotropic hormone (ACTH), prednisone	vigabatrin
Lennox–Gastaut	benzodiazepines, valproic acid	cannabidiol, felbamate, lamotrigine, rufinamide, topiramate
Seizure clusters	diazepam (intranasal), midazolam (intranasal)	clonazepam, lorazepam
Status epilepticus	lorazepam, phenobarbital	diazepam, phenytoin, valproic acid

*Selection of first-line drugs varies according to patient age and comorbid conditions, prescriber experiences, institution, and geographic region.

and the seizure may occur with or without convulsions. The four primary types of generalized seizures are tonic–clonic seizures, absence seizures, atonic seizures, and myoclonic seizures.

Generalized tonic–clonic seizures, also referred to as grand mal seizures, are the type of seizure most associated by the public with epilepsy. It is the most common type of seizure in every age group. The seizure may be preceded by an aura, a warning that a seizure is imminent, that some patients describe as a spiritual feeling, flash of light, or special noise. Neurologists consider the aura to be part of the actual seizure. Loss of consciousness and intense muscle contractions indicate the tonic phase. A hoarse cry may occur at the onset of the seizure due to air being forced out of the lungs, and patients may temporarily lose bladder or bowel control. Breathing may become shallow and even stop momentarily. The clonic phase is characterized by alternating contraction and relaxation of muscles that are characteristic of convulsions. The seizure usually lasts 1 to 2 minutes, after which the patient becomes drowsy and disoriented and sleeps deeply. The period following the seizure is known as the **postictal state**.

Generalized absence seizures, formerly called petit mal seizures, most often occur in children and last only a few seconds. It is considered a generalized type of seizure because it begins on *both* hemispheres of the brain simultaneously. Approximately half of the patients with absence seizures may also experience at least one tonic–clonic seizure. Absence seizures involve a reduction of normal brain activity. Staring and transient loss of responsiveness are the most common signs, but there may be slight motor activity with eyelid fluttering or muscular jerking movements. These episodes are subtle and can be mistaken for daydreaming or inattention, such as is seen in attention-deficit/hyperactivity disorder (ADHD). Children with absence seizures may experience poor academic performance because these episodes can occur several times per day. Most children who experience absence seizures will "outgrow" the disorder and become seizure-free in adulthood.

Atonic seizures are sometimes known as drop attacks, due to the fact that the patient will stumble and fall for no apparent reason. The episode is brief, lasting less than 15 seconds. The patient loses control of muscle tone throughout the body. During the episode of weakness, the patient's head will droop forward or the trunk muscles will not support the patient, thus causing the drop attack. Although the seizure itself causes no serious harm, the patient is at risk of injury due to falls. Usually this seizure affects both hemispheres of the brain (generalized-onset atonic seizure) but it may occur in only one hemisphere and affect only part of the body (focal motor atonic seizure).

Myoclonic seizures are generalized seizures characterized by jerking body movements, usually involving the muscles of the neck, shoulders, and upper arms. Major muscle groups contract quickly, usually for only a few seconds, and patients appear unsteady and clumsy. These patients do not lose consciousness but may fall or drop whatever they might be holding. Most patients with myoclonic seizures also exhibit tonic–clonic or absence seizures, or both. Myoclonic seizures usually begin around puberty and comprise 5 to 10% of all epilepsies. Although these seizures continue for the life of the patient, most can be controlled with pharmacotherapy.

Partial (Focal) Seizures

Partial (focal) seizures involve a limited portion of the brain, with the abnormal neuronal discharges starting in one brain hemisphere and traveling only a short distance before they stop. Many partial seizures do not involve loss of consciousness or convulsions. Some symptoms are subtle and reflect the simple nature of neuronal misfiring in limited areas of the brain, whereas other symptoms may be more complex. Sometimes the abnormal focus begins as a partial seizure and subsequently extends to both hemispheres to become a generalized seizure.

Simple partial (focal aware) seizures have an onset that begins at a small, regional focus. The person remains awake and alert during the seizure, which lasts less than 2 minutes. Patients with focal aware seizures experience a wide array of symptoms depending on the specific region of the brain affected. If the motor cortex is affected, jerky, rhythmic contractions of a specific muscle group are noted. Hallucinations affecting hearing, taste, smell, or sensation may not be noticeable to an observer. Patients may feel for a brief moment that their precise location is vague, or that they have been there before (déjà vu). Other patients become emotional and experience a sense of joy, fear, or grief. Consciousness is retained during the seizure, although the patient may express amnesia about the event.

Complex partial (focal impaired awareness) seizures, formerly called psychomotor seizures, originate from a single focus, usually in the temporal lobe of the brain. Patients exhibit some degree of altered or impaired consciousness. Total loss of consciousness may not occur during a complex partial seizure, but a brief period of somnolence or confusion may follow the episode. Focal impaired awareness seizures are usually preceded by an aura that may be described as an unpleasant odor or taste, colored spots, unexplained fear, or tingling. Seizures may start with a blank stare and proceed to repetitive arm movements, leg movements, head rolling, chewing, lip smacking, or swallowing. These repetitive movements are called **automatisms**. Most patients will be unresponsive to verbal commands and act as if they are having hallucinations. Focal impaired awareness seizures occur in about 35% of patients with epilepsy.

22.4 Some types of seizures are called special epileptic seizures.

Not all seizure disorders can be classified neatly into the two broad categories of generalized and partial. These "other" types of seizures are referred to as special epileptic seizures.

Febrile seizures are most likely to occur in the 3-month to 5-year age group. As many as 5% of children experience febrile seizures. These seizures are associated with high fever and are characterized by tonic–clonic motor activity lasting 1 to 2 minutes with rapid return of consciousness. They usually occur only once during any given illness. Febrile seizures may be generalized (occur once and quickly resolve) or complex (occur multiple times in 24 hours and last more than 15 minutes). Pharmacotherapy with AEDs is not necessary with most febrile seizures. Prevention of the onset of fever with acetaminophen is the best method for controlling this disorder.

Acute repetitive seizures include seizure clusters and status epilepticus. **Seizure clusters** may be defined as three or more seizures in a 24-hour period. These types of seizures are common in refractory epilepsy and suggest that seizure management is unsuccessful. Benzodiazepines are the treatment of choice for cluster seizures. Patients are often prescribed rescue medications for home use such as intranasal diazepam (Valtoco) or intranasal midazolam (Nayzilam). Oral benzodiazepines may be prescribed, although these have a slower onset of action than the intranasal forms.

Status epilepticus is a medical emergency that occurs when a seizure continues for more than 30 minutes or when two or more sequential seizures occur without full recovery of consciousness between them. Tonic–clonic symptoms are usually exhibited; however, some forms of this disorder may resemble focal aware or focal awareness impaired seizures. When generalized tonic–clonic seizures are prolonged or continuous, the time in which breathing is affected by muscle contraction is lengthened and hypoxia may develop. The continuous muscle contraction can also lead to hypoglycemia, acidosis, and hypothermia due to increased metabolic needs, lactic acid production, and heat loss during contraction. If untreated, status epilepticus could lead to brain damage and death. Medical treatment involves administration of AEDs by the IV route. In the home setting, valproic acid or diazepam can be administered by the rectal route.

Infantile (epileptic) spasm, also called West syndrome, usually occurs in the first year of life and is characterized by a sudden bending forward, body stiffening, or arching of the torso. Infantile spasms may occur in clusters, often with several dozen separated by 5 to 30 seconds. Prognosis for infants with infantile spasms is poor and most have some degree of mental and developmental delays.

Lennox–Gastaut syndrome is a severe childhood seizure that involves characteristics of tonic–clonic, atonic, and atypical absence seizures. The cause of this syndrome is unknown. This seizure disorder has a mean age of onset of 26 to 28 months and is often associated with intellectual disability and mood instability. In older children, this type of epilepsy is associated with personality disorders and psychotic episodes. Seizures associated with Lennox–Gastaut syndrome are often resistant to pharmacotherapy.

Antiepileptic Drugs

22.5 The selection of antiepileptic drug therapy is dependent on seizure type and characteristics.

There are over 20 FDA-approved AEDs and all are effective at treating seizures. In general, narrow-spectrum AEDs are highly specific for focal-onset seizures, and broad-spectrum AEDs are effective for both generalized and focal-onset seizures. It is common for healthcare providers to prescribe AEDs off-label.

The choice of AED medication is highly individualized for each patient and is dependent on many factors, including the type of seizure; the patient's medical history, including the characteristics and length of the seizure; the results of the EEG and other diagnostic laboratory studies; and the presence of comorbid medical conditions. To prevent adverse drug effects, the prescriber initially chooses the lowest, effective dose of an AED and increases it as necessary. Serum drug levels may be obtained to assist the healthcare provider in determining the most effective drug concentration. To prevent adverse effects and possible worsening of seizures, the discontinuation of an AED or significant dose reductions are extended over 6 to 12 weeks.

In most cases, effective seizure management can be obtained by using a single AED. If seizure activity continues, the initial drug is gradually discontinued and replaced by a medication from a different class. An overlap in dosing the two drugs is necessary. Some patients require multiple AEDs for effective seizure control. However, certain AED drug combinations have the potential to increase the incidence of seizures; thus, it is important for the healthcare provider to consult current literature for drug compatibility and administration guidelines. At the initiation of pharmacotherapy, the patient must be carefully assessed for adverse effects, particularly increased CNS depression, and advised not to drive or engage in hazardous activities until drug levels have stabilized.

Patients who remain symptom free for prolonged periods often believe that they have "outgrown" their seizures and therefore no longer require medication. Although this may indeed be the case, the nurse should teach patients to never stop taking AEDs without the guidance of their healthcare provider. In general, withdrawal of antiepileptic medications is attempted only after the patient has been seizure-free for at least 3 years. The withdrawal of medications requires close monitoring, and doses must be reduced slowly, one medication at a time, over a period of several months. If seizures recur during the withdrawal process, pharmacotherapy is resumed with the same medication previously prescribed. The nurse must educate the patient and family to maintain strict adherence to the pharmacotherapy regimen. Periodic serum drug levels can assist the nurse in assessing adherence: Low serum drug levels in a patient claiming to be taking his or her medication may indicate nonadherence to therapy.

Many patients with epilepsy attempt a nondrug treatment, with stress management techniques and prayer being the most common alternative therapies. Other therapies utilized to manage epilepsy include herbal supplements, chiropractic care, acupuncture, and yoga. The implementation of the ketogenic diet can produce positive effects in some patients by decreasing seizure activity. However, the use of alternative therapies alone for the management of epilepsy is not considered effective and should be discouraged by the nurse.

PharmFACT

Contrary to popular belief, it is impossible to swallow the tongue during a seizure, and one should never force an object into the mouth of someone who is having a seizure (Epilepsy Foundation of America, 2019a).

22.6 Antiepileptic drugs act by suppressing abnormal neuronal discharges.

All antiepileptic medications suppress neuron discharges, thus preventing the abnormal focus from forming or spreading across the cerebrum. AEDs suppress abnormal discharges by at least four mechanisms. The study of AEDs is complicated because some of these drugs act through multiple mechanisms, and a few have unknown mechanisms. These mechanisms are shown in Pharmacotherapy Illustrated 22.1. The basic mechanisms are:

- Electrolyte movement
  Inhibition of the influx of sodium in neurons
  Inhibition of the influx of calcium in neurons
- Neurotransmitter balance
  Enhancement of GABA activity
  Blocking glutamate receptors in the brain.

Control of electrolyte movement. In their resting state, neurons are surrounded by a high extracellular concentration of sodium, calcium, and chloride ions. Potassium levels are higher inside the cell. An influx of sodium or calcium into the neuron enhances neuronal activity, whereas an influx of chloride ions has an inhibitory effect. This affords several mechanisms to dampen abnormal neuronal activity.

The primary target for many AEDs is the *sodium* channel. The sodium channel on the neuronal plasma membrane must open, allowing sodium to rush into the cell, for an action potential to be generated and propagated. Phenytoin, lamotrigine, and carbamazepine bind to the sodium channel, inactivating it and preventing the passage of sodium ion into the neuron. This slows the excitability of neurons, dampening the flow of abnormal, repetitive discharges.

Pharmacotherapy Illustrated 22.1

Mechanisms of Action of Antiepileptic Drugs

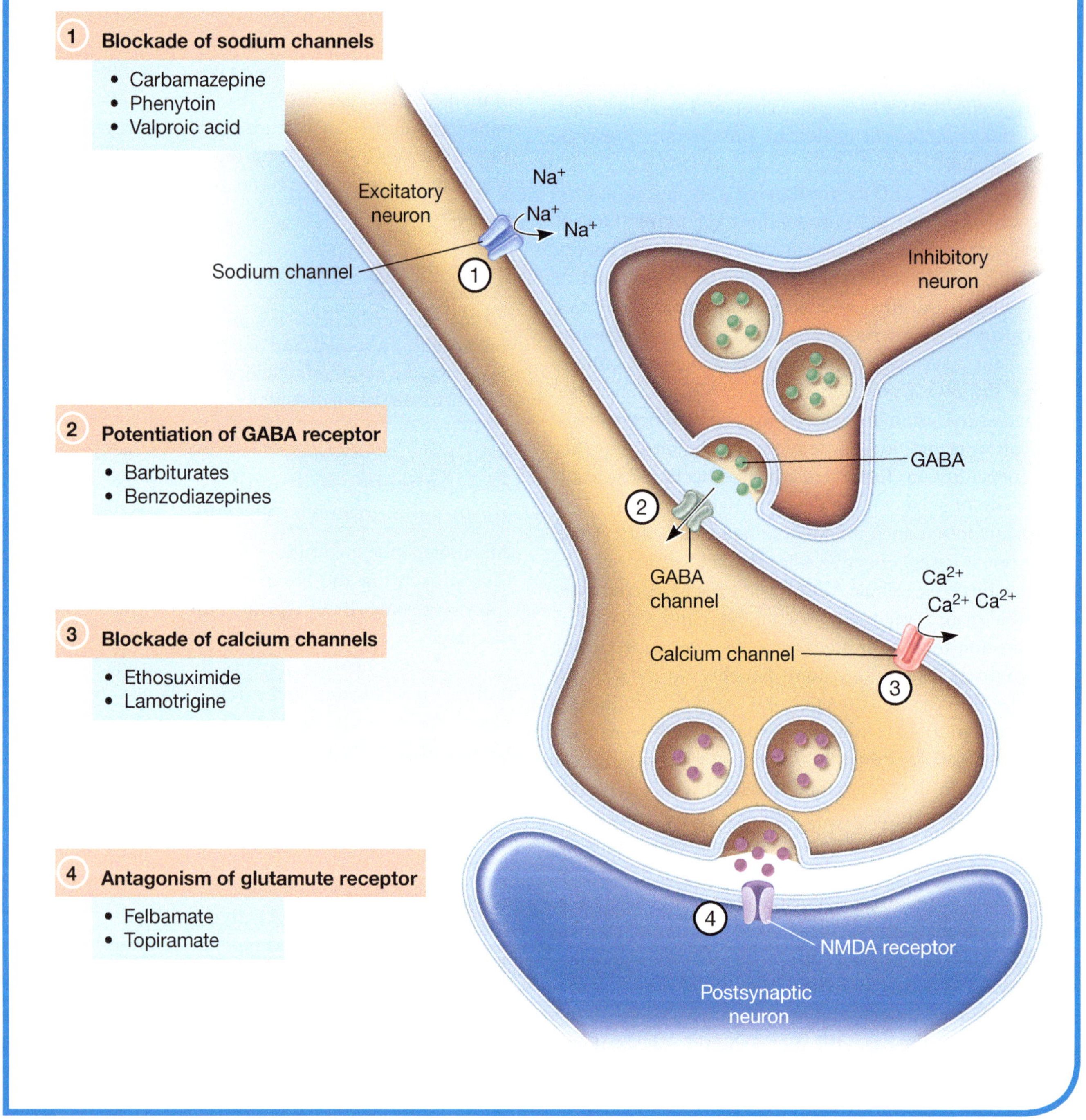

Calcium channels are found at the synaptic terminals. When opened, calcium enters the presynaptic neuron, causing the release of stored neurotransmitter into the synaptic cleft. Blocking calcium channels prevents the release of the neurotransmitter and dampens impulse conduction. The AEDs believed to block calcium channels include ethosuximide, gabapentin, pregabalin, and lamotrigine.

Neurotransmitter balance. Drugs that enhance or inhibit neurotransmitter activity in the CNS will affect neuronal firing. The neurotransmitter most affected by AEDs is gamma aminobutyric acid (GABA), the primary *inhibitory* neurotransmitter in the brain. Increasing the activity of GABA in the CNS will slow neuronal firing, thus suppressing seizure activity. AEDs accomplish this suppression by means of several mechanisms, as illustrated in Figure 22.1:

- **Increased synthesis or amount of GABA in the presynaptic nerve terminal.** Some drugs block the

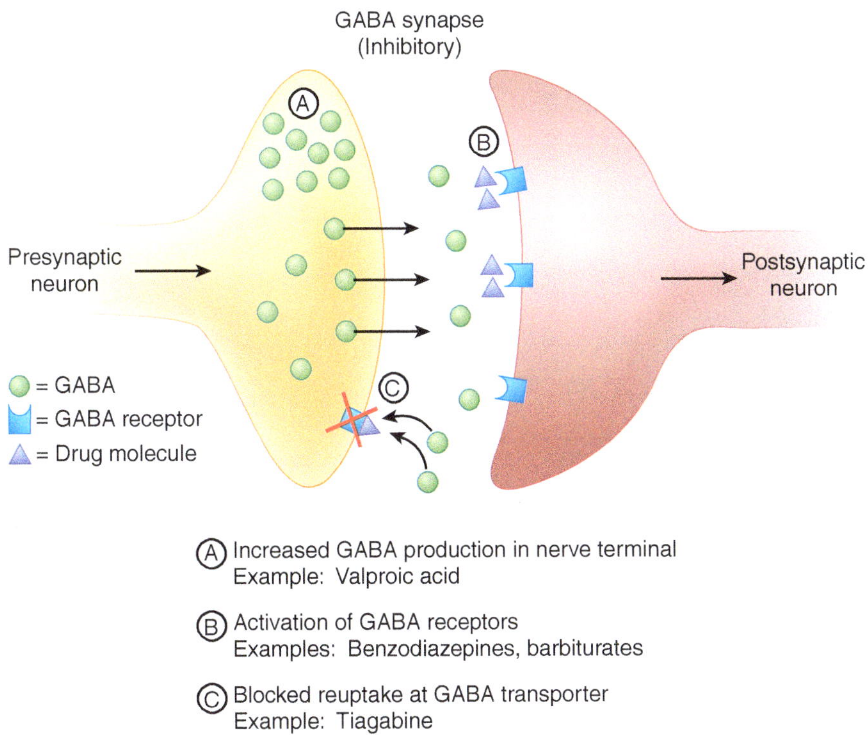

Figure 22.1 Mechanisms of action of antiepileptic drugs that affect GABA.

metabolic breakdown of GABA or enhance its formation. An example is valproic acid.

- **Activation of GABA receptors.** Some drugs mimic GABA and occupy its receptor on the postsynaptic membrane, causing the same inhibitory effect as GABA. This is achieved by stimulating an influx of chloride ion, which causes the neuron to have greater difficulty achieving an action potential. Examples include barbiturates, benzodiazepines, topiramate, and felbamate.
- **Blocked reuptake of GABA.** After GABA produces its action at the synapse, it is normally pumped back into the presynaptic neuron, which terminates its action. Drugs that block this reuptake will keep GABA on its receptors for a longer time, thus causing more neuronal inhibition. An example is tiagabine.

A second neurotransmitter affected by AEDs is glutamate, the primary *excitatory* neurotransmitter in the brain. By blocking glutamate receptors (known as N-methyl-D-aspartate [NMDA] receptors), these drugs serve as antagonists to glutamate and suppress neuronal firing. Examples include topiramate and felbamate.

Antiepileptic medications are difficult to classify. One method is by mechanism of action; however, many AEDs act by multiple means and a few have unknown mechanisms. Another classification scheme groups these drugs into "newer" and "older" generations, but there is no clear distinction between the groups. Grouping by type of seizure is not possible because most of these medications are useful against more than one type. This text uses a combination of chemical classes and mechanisms of action. The student should be aware, however, that other classifications will be encountered in clinical practice. The AEDs are listed in Table 22.4 and, later in the chapter, Table 22.5.

22.7 Barbiturates are traditional drugs for tonic–clonic seizures that have been replaced by newer and safer medications.

The barbiturates have been used to treat seizures for almost 100 years. Barbiturates act biochemically in the brain by enhancing the action of GABA, the inhibitory neurotransmitter responsible for suppressing abnormal neuronal discharges.

Although barbiturates are occasionally prescribed for epilepsy, newer drugs have replaced them as first-line drugs for this indication. As a class, they have a low margin of safety and can cause profound CNS depression, including sedation, coma, and death. Barbiturates will yield significant sedation when combined with alcohol, antidepressants, and other CNS depressants. Children may exhibit hyperkinesis rather than sedation. Cardiovascular and respiratory adverse effects include respiratory depression, bradycardia, syncope, and hypotension. Patients with impaired hepatic, respiratory, renal, and cardiovascular function should not receive barbiturates, or the doses should be lowered to prevent toxicity. Barbiturates also possess a high potential for drug dependence. Barbiturates may cause fetal harm. Women of childbearing potential are advised to use two methods of birth control.

This section highlights only the antiseizure properties of barbiturates. These drugs are also classified as sedative–hypnotics, and a prototype feature for phenobarbital can be found in Chapter 18. Nursing responsibilities, lifespan and diversity considerations, and patient and family education for this drug class may also be found in Chapter 18.

Phenobarbital: Phenobarbital is effective for long-term management of tonic–clonic seizures and partial seizures. It can be administered in patients with status epilepticus or febrile seizures or to treat eclampsia. It is relatively ineffective in treating absence seizures. Although phenobarbital is no longer considered a first-line drug, it may still be prescribed when safer AEDs prove to be ineffective.

Oral (PO) administration of phenobarbital may take several weeks for an optimal level of antiseizure activity to be achieved. The advantages of phenobarbital are that

Table 22.4 Drugs for Seizures: Barbiturates Benzodiazepines, Hydantoins, Dibenzazepines, and Succinimides

Drug	Route and Dose (Maximum Dose Where Indicated)	Adverse Effects
Barbiturates		
phenobarbital	Adult: PO: 50–100 mg bid–tid IV/IM: 200–600 mg (max: 20 mg/kg) Child: PO/IV: 3–8 mg/kg or 125 mg/m²/day	*Drowsiness, dizziness, nausea and vomiting, sedation, confusion, unsteady gait, lethargy, paradoxical excitement, pain at the injection site, hypotension with IV administration* Agranulocytosis, angioedema, Stevens–Johnson syndrome (SJS), respiratory depression, bradycardia, CNS depression, coma
primidone (Mysoline)	Adult: PO: 100–250 mg bid–tid (max: 2 g/day) Child younger than age 8: PO: 50–250 mg tid (max: 2 g/day)	
Benzodiazepines		
clobazam (Onfi, Sympazan)	PO: 5–10 mg/day gradually increased to a target dose of 20–40 mg/day	*Sedation, headache, drowsiness, weakness, vertigo, ataxia, paradoxical excitement, short-term amnesia* Coma, respiratory depression, cardiac arrest, suicidal ideation, blood dyscrasias, physical dependence, cardiovascular collapse (diazepam), status epilepticus with abrupt withdrawal
clonazepam (Klonopin)	Adult: PO: 1.5 mg/day (max: 20 mg/day) Child younger than age 10: PO: 0.01–0.03 mg/kg/day gradually increased until seizures are controlled (max: 0.2 mg/kg/day)	
clorazepate (Tranxene)	Adult: PO: 7.5 mg tid (max: 90 mg/day) Child ages 9–12: PO: 3.75–7.5 mg bid (max: 60 mg/day)	
diazepam (Valium)	Status epilepticus: Adult: IV/IM: 5–10 mg, repeat if needed at 10- to 15-min intervals up to 30 mg Child: IV/IM: 0.2–1 mg slowly q2–5 min up to 5–10 mg	
lorazepam (Ativan)	Adult: IV: 4 mg injected slowly at 2 mg/min; may repeat dose once after 10 min (max: 8 mg during any 12-h period) Status epilepticus: Child: IV: 0.1 mg/kg slowly over 2–5 min; may repeat with 0.05 mg in 10–15 min (max: 4 mg/dose)	
Hydantoins		
fosphenytoin (Cerebyx)	Adult: IV loading dose: 10–20 mg phenytoin equivalents/kg administered at 100–150 mg phenytoin equivalents/min Maintenance IV dose: 4–6 mg PE/kg/day	*Hypotension, nystagmus, ataxia, lethargy, confusion, slurred speech, dizziness, nervousness, headache, nausea and vomiting, gingival hyperplasia, rash, somnolence* Seizures, dysrhythmias, blood dyscrasias, systemic lupus erythematosus, cardiac arrest, cardiovascular collapse, coma, toxic epidermal necrolysis, SJS, osteomalacia
phenytoin (Dilantin, Phenytek)	Adult: PO (extended release): 100 mg tid (max: 600 mg/day) IV: 10–15 mg/kg loading dose, then 100 mg tid Child: PO (extended release): 5 mg/kg/day	
Dibenzazepines		
carbamazepine (Carbatrol, Tegretol, others)	Adult: PO: 200 mg bid gradually increased to 800–1200 mg/day Child younger than age 6: PO: 10-35 mg/kg/day (max: 35 mg/kg/day) Child ages 6–12: PO: 100-800 mg,	*Dizziness, headache, ataxia, fatigue, rash, pruritus, dry mouth, nausea and vomiting, diplopia, abnormal gait* SJS, aggravated absence seizures, hallucinations, aplastic anemia, agranulocytosis, heart block, respiratory depression, exfoliative dermatitis, suicidal ideation, status epilepticus (with abrupt withdrawal)
eslicarbazepine (Aptiom)	PO: 400 mg once daily gradually increased to 1200 mg once daily	
oxcarbazepine (Oxtellar XR, Trileptal)	Adult: PO: 300 mg bid (max: 2400 mg/day as monotherapy) Child ages 4–16: PO: 8–10 mg/kg/day (max: 600 mg/day)	
Succinimides		
ethosuximide (Zarontin)	Adult: PO: 250 mg bid (max: 1.5 g/day) Child ages 3–6: PO: maintenance dose 20 mg/kg/day	*Drowsiness, headache, diarrhea, nausea and vomiting* Anorexia, SJS, psychosis, blood dyscrasias, systemic lupus erythematosus, suicidal ideation
methsuximide (Celontin)	PO: 150–300 mg/day (max: 1.2 g/day)	

Note: *Italics* indicate common adverse effects. Underline indicates serious adverse effects.

it is relatively inexpensive and long acting. The sedation effect of the drug is prominent at the initiation of therapy but often diminishes as treatment progresses.

Phenobarbital is a major inducer of hepatic CYP450 enzymes and will markedly increase the metabolism of other drugs metabolized by these enzymes. This results in a significant potential for drug interactions with other medications metabolized in the liver. Phenobarbital also increases its own metabolism, which leads to significant tolerance as therapy progresses.

Primidone (Mysoline): Primidone is metabolized in the liver to phenobarbital, which is responsible for most of its pharmacologic effects. It is effective for treating all types of seizures except absence seizures. It has no approved indications other than seizure. The actions and adverse effects of primidone are equivalent to those of phenobarbital.

PharmFACT

Twenty to 30% of patients with epilepsy also have psychiatric disturbances, the most common of which is mood or anxiety disorder. The risk of suicide in patients with epilepsy is about 13%, which is almost twice that of the general population (Algreeshah, 2016).

Table 22.5 Miscellaneous Drugs for Seizures

Drug	Route and Dose (Maximum Dose Where Indicated)	Adverse Effects
brivaracetam (Briviact)	PO, oral solution, and IV: 50 mg bid	*Drowsiness, dizziness, nausea and vomiting, fatigue* Suicidal ideation, psychoses
cannabidiol (Epidiolex)	PO: 2.5–20 mg/kg/day	somnolence, infections, decreased appetite, elevated liver transaminases, diarrhea Excessive sedation, suicidal ideation
ezogabine (Potiga)	Adult: PO: 100 mg tid gradually increased to 200–400 mg tid	*Dizziness, fatigue, blurred vision, diplopia, vertigo, tremor* Retinal abnormalities, confusion, memory impairment, urinary retention, psychosis, prolongation of QT interval
felbamate (Felbatol)	Adult: PO: 1200 mg/day gradually increased to 3600 mg/day Child ages 2–14: PO: 15 mg/kg/day (max: 45 mg/kg/day)	*Headache, dizziness, blurred vision, nausea and vomiting, anorexia* Liver failure, aplastic anemia
gabapentin (Neurontin)	Adult: PO: 300 mg tid gradually increased to 1800–2400 mg/day Child ages 3–12: PO: 10–40 mg/kg/day	*Dizziness, drowsiness, fatigue, ataxia, diplopia, nystagmus, tremor, impaired concentration, dry mouth, flulike syndrome* Increased frequency of partial seizures, blurred vision, unintentional injury, suicidal ideation
lacosamide (Vimpat)	Adult: PO: 50 mg bid gradually increased to 200–400 mg/day	*Dizziness, headache, diplopia, nausea* Suicidal ideation, prolongation of QT interval, syncope, hypersensitivity reactions
lamotrigine (Lamictal)	Adult: PO: 25-500 mg/day (max: 700 mg/day without concurrent valproic acid, 200 mg/day with valproic acid) Child ages 2–16: PO: 0.2–5 mg/kg/day (max: 15 mg/kg/day without valproic acid; 5 mg/kg/day or 250 mg/day with concurrent valproic acid)	*Dizziness, headache, ataxia, drowsiness, insomnia, tremor, rash, diplopia, blurred vision, flulike symptoms, infection, nausea and vomiting, back pain* SJS, toxic epidermal necrolysis, emotional lability (children), suicidal ideation
levetiracetam (Keppra)	Adult (regular release): PO: 500 mg bid; gradually increased to 3 g/day Adult (extended release): PO: 1000–3000 mg once daily Child ages 4–16: PO: 20-60 mg/kg/day	*Drowsiness, headache, dizziness, nervousness, flulike symptoms, nausea and vomiting, anorexia, asthenia* Emotional lability and personality disorder (children), unintentional injury, suicidal ideation, blood dyscrasias
perampanel (Fycompa)	PO: 8–12 mg/day	*Dizziness, headache, fatigue, and somnolence* Psychiatric and behavioral changes
pregabalin (Lyrica)	PO: 150-600 mg/day	*Dizziness, confusion, drowsiness, fatigue, weight gain, ataxia, diplopia, nystagmus, tremor, impaired concentration, dry mouth* Increased frequency of partial seizures, blurred vision, unintentional injury, angioedema, suicidal ideation
rufinamide (Banzel)	Adult: PO: 400–800 mg/day gradually increased to 3200 mg/day Child ages 4 and older: PO: 10 mg/kg/day gradually increased to 45 mg/kg/day or 3200 mg/day, whichever is less	*Dizziness, headache, somnolence, nausea, fatigue* Suicidal ideation, shortening of QT interval, hypersensitivity reactions
tiagabine (Gabitril)	Adult: PO: 4-56 mg/day Adolescent ages 12–18: PO: 4-32 mg/day	*Dizziness, asthenia, tremor, somnolence, nervousness, difficulty concentrating* Vasodilation, HTN, palpitations, tachycardia, syncope, peripheral edema
topiramate (Topamax, Trokendi XR, others)	PO: 50 mg/day gradually increased to 400 mg/day	*Paresthesia, anorexia, weight loss, fatigue, dizziness, somnolence, nervousness, psychomotor slowing, difficulty with memory or concentration, confusion* Acute myopia with closed-angle glaucoma, oligohidrosis and hyperthermia, suicidal ideation, hyperammonemia with encephalopathy, teratogenicity
valproic acid (Depakote)	Adult/child: PO/IV: 10–15 mg/kg/day gradually increased to 60 mg/kg/day	*Nausea and vomiting, abdominal cramps, anorexia, dyspepsia, drowsiness, dizziness, asthenia, insomnia, weight gain* Deep coma, hallucinations, hyperammonemia, thrombocytopenia, blurred vision, hepatotoxicity, pancreatitis, bone marrow depression, prolonged bleeding time
vigabatrin (Sabril)	Adult: PO: 500 mg bid gradually increased to 1500 mg/day	*Fatigue, somnolence, nystagmus, tremor, vision changes, memory impairment, weight gain, arthralgia, abnormal coordination* Depression, psychosis, confusion, severe rash, anemia, suicidal ideation
zonisamide (Zonegran)	Adult: PO: 100 mg/day gradually increased to 200–400 mg/day	*Dizziness, ataxia, drowsiness, fatigue, anorexia, speech abnormalities, difficulty in concentrating or remembering, flulike symptoms, headache, abnormal gait, gingivitis, rhinitis* Severe rash including SJS, kidney stones, depression, psychosis

Note: *Italics* indicate common adverse effects. Underline indicates serious adverse effects.

22.8 Benzodiazepines are important drugs in the treatment of status epilepticus.

Benzodiazepines are the first-line drugs for the treatment of certain anxiety disorders and are one of the most widely prescribed drug classes in the United States. Detailed information about the benzodiazepines used for anxiety and a prototype feature for lorazepam (Ativan) are included in Chapter 18. The remainder of this section focuses on the antiseizure properties of drugs in this class.

Benzodiazepines control seizures by acting in the limbic, thalamic, and hypothalamic regions of the CNS. All drugs in this class act by enhancing the inhibitory action of GABA. They accomplish this by increasing the affinity of GABA for its receptors. Sedation can be a limiting adverse effect for the benzodiazepines.

The applications of benzodiazepines in the treatment of seizure disorders are limited. The parenteral benzodiazepines diazepam (Valium) and lorazepam may be utilized in the treatment of status epilepticus. Clonazepam (Klonopin), clobazam (Onfi, Sympazan), and clorazepate (Tranxene) are used for specific types of seizures, usually when other drugs have proven ineffective Benzodiazepines should never be discontinued abruptly because status epilepticus may result.

Two nasal spray formulations offer novel approaches to treating cluster seizures. Diazepam intranasal (Valtoco) was approved in 2020 as a single-dose spray into one nostril. A second dose, which requires an additional spray device, can be given at least 4 hours after the first, if needed. Midazolam intranasal (Nayzilam), approved in 2019, is also available as a single-dose spray, which can be repeated after 10 minutes if the seizure has not been terminated. These formulations offer the convenience of treatment outside of a clinic environment.

PROTOTYPE DRUG Diazepam (Valium)

Classification **Therapeutic:** Antiepileptic drug, antianxiety drug, skeletal muscle relaxant
Pharmacologic: Benzodiazepine, GABA receptor agonist

Therapeutic Effects and Uses: Diazepam was originally approved by the U.S. Food and Drug Administration (FDA) in 1963. In antiseizure therapy, the primary indication for diazepam is status epilepticus. It may also be used to prevent seizures in patients who have received toxic substances or during the acute phase of alcohol or benzodiazepine withdrawal. Oral diazepam may be combined with other AEDs in the treatment of refractory seizures. A newer indication for diazepam is the oral prophylaxis of febrile seizures in children ages 6 months to 5 years.

Diazepam has a large number of other indications. It was once widely prescribed for the management of anxiety disorders, although it has largely been replaced by other drugs such as alprazolam (Xanax). It is administered prior to procedures such as cardioversion or endoscopy to provide relaxation or sedation. Oral or parenteral diazepam may be administered for muscle relaxation in patients with acute inflammation, trauma, tetanus, or spasticity.

Mechanism of Action: Diazepam enhances the action of GABA in the brain, thus inhibiting the abnormal neuronal discharges characteristic of seizures.

Pharmacokinetics:

Route(s)	IV, IM, PO, rectal
Absorption	Rapidly absorbed by the gastrointestinal (GI) tract; erratic absorption with IM administration
Distribution	Widely distributed; crosses the blood–brain barrier and the placenta; 99% bound to protein
Primary metabolism	Hepatic
Primary excretion	Renal
Onset of action	IV: 1–5 min; IM: 15–30 min; PO: 30–60 min
Duration of action	Half-life: 20–50 h

Adverse Effects: The most serious adverse effect of diazepam is cardiovascular collapse. The nurse should assess for hypotension, tachycardia, and edema, which are precursors to cardiovascular collapse. CNS adverse effects include drowsiness, fatigue, ataxia, dizziness, and vertigo. Diazepam can cause urinary retention and menstrual irregularities. The major respiratory adverse effect is laryngeal spasm and cough. Benzodiazepines are Schedule IV drugs and possess a risk for substance abuse in susceptible individuals (see Chapter 27). **Black box warning**: Concurrent use of benzodiazepines with opioids may result in serious sedation, respiratory depression, coma, and death.

Contraindications/Precautions: Diazepam should not be administered to patients with depressed vital signs, those in shock, or those with acute alcohol intoxication. It is also contraindicated in the presence of closed-angle glaucoma because it can increase intraocular pressure. Diazepam should be used cautiously in patients with depression and myasthenia gravis, and a reduced dose should be administered in patients with impaired hepatic or renal function. Patients who have respiratory disorders such as chronic obstructive pulmonary disease (COPD) should be monitored closely due to the risk of respiratory depression. After prolonged therapy, abrupt discontinuation of diazepam may precipitate withdrawal symptoms, including seizures. The drug can cause birth defects and should not be administered to pregnant patients unless benefits clearly outweigh the potential risks. Diazepam is not recommended during lactation because the drug is secreted in breast milk and may cause CNS depression in the neonate.

Drug Interactions: Diazepam is metabolized by hepatic CYP450 enzymes and may interact with drugs that inhibit these enzymes. Other CNS depressants, including alcohol, will intensify the sedative effects of diazepam. Concurrent administration with cimetidine will increase the plasma levels of diazepam. Administration of diazepam with antiparkinsonism medications may worsen the severity of Parkinson's disease symptoms. Diazepam when administered with phenytoin will result in increased phenytoin levels and possible toxicity. Diazepam should never be administered within 14 days of a monoamine oxidase inhibitor (MAOI) due to the risk of hypertensive crisis. **Herbal/Food:** Kava and valerian administered with diazepam will result in additive sedative effects. Echinacea may lower the serum levels of diazepam. Grapefruit juice increases the peak serum concentrations of diazepam by as much as two times.

Pregnancy: Animal studies showed that diazepam may cause fetal harm. Neonates born to mothers taking benzodiazepines during pregnancy may experience withdrawal symptoms. Because diazepam is secreted in human milk, breastfeeding is not recommended.

Treatment of Overdose: Flumazenil (Romazicon) is administered for overdosage of diazepam. This medication is a specific benzodiazepine receptor antagonist that reverses the CNS depression from diazepam.

Clinician Responsibilities: Key clinical implications for patients receiving diazepam are included in Applied Clinical Judgment: Patients Receiving Pharmacotherapy for Seizures and in Applied Clinical Judgment: Patients Receiving Pharmacotherapy for Anxiety or Sleep Disorders in Chapter 18.

Drugs Similar to Diazepam (Valium)

Clobazam, clonazepam, clorazepate, and lorazepam are benzodiazepine antiepileptic medications. All benzodiazepines are controlled substances, and all should be used with extreme caution with opioids. Animal studies show that benzodiazepines may cause fetal harm, and breastfeeding is not recommended because the drugs are secreted in human milk. They should not be used during pregnancy unless the potential benefits to the mother justify the potential risk to the fetus or neonate.

Clobazam (Onfi, Sympazan): Clobazam was approved for the U.S. market in 2013 and is available as tablets, as a suspension, and as an oral film (Sympazan) for one specific indication: seizures associated with Lennox–Gastaut syndrome in patients 2 years of age or older. The drug exhibits the adverse effects typical of benzodiazepines, especially sedation, which can be profound when the drug is used with alcohol or other CNS depressants. Stevens–Johnson syndrome (SJS) is a serious, though rare, adverse effect. Tolerance to the sedation effect, as well as the antiepileptic effect, occurs with continued therapy. The patient should be monitored for suicidal ideation. Clobazam is a Schedule IV controlled substance.

Clonazepam (Klonopin): Approved in 1975, clonazepam is an oral benzodiazepine with strong antiseizure properties. It is approved for the prophylaxis of absence seizures, Lennox–Gastaut syndrome, akinetic and myoclonic seizures, and nocturnal myoclonus. Its primary use as an AED is to treat refractory myoclonic seizures. Clonazepam is also approved for the treatment of panic disorder. It is occasionally prescribed off-label for other anxiety disorders, insomnia, and restless leg syndrome.

Like other benzodiazepines, the most common adverse effect of clonazepam is sedation. Ataxia, abnormal coordination, dizziness, and cardiovascular or respiratory depression are possible. If given for an extended period, the patient may require an increase in dose due to the development of tolerance. Tolerance also develops to the sedative side effects of the drug. Therapeutic serum levels are 20 to 80 mg/mL.

Clorazepate (Tranxene): Approved in 1972, clorazepate is approved for the pharmacotherapy of anxiety, focal seizures, and seizures associated with acute ethanol withdrawal. It may be used off-label to treat insomnia. Clorazepate is administered PO and has a long duration of action. The actions of clorazepate are the same as those of diazepam because the two drugs share the same active metabolite. It is not a first-line drug for epilepsy, but it may be used as an adjunct to control focal seizures. Most adverse effects are CNS related and include mental depression, confusion, fatigue, tremor, and vertigo. The patient should be monitored for suicidal ideation.

Lorazepam (Ativan): Approved in 1977, lorazepam is an important drug for treating status epilepticus because it persists in the cerebrospinal fluid (CSF) longer than diazepam. Whereas diazepam remains active in the brain for 30 to 60 minutes, lorazepam may prevent seizures for up to 12 hours. It is also used to prevent or treat seizures associated with acute ethanol withdrawal. When given orally, lorazepam is indicated for the short-term management of anxiety disorders or anxiety associated with depressive symptoms. It is the most potent of the benzodiazepines and has the ability to produce skeletal muscle relaxation, sedation, and a hypnotic state. Oral, IM, and IV forms are available. A prototype feature for lorazepam is presented in Chapter 18.

CONNECTION Checkpoint 22.2

In addition to epilepsy, what are other indications for benzodiazepines?

22.9 Hydantoins are effective in the management of most types of seizures but have many adverse effects.

First used in 1938, phenytoin (Dilantin) quickly became a preferred drug for many types of epilepsy because it provided effective seizure control without the serious CNS depression and abuse potential associated with barbiturates. With the discovery of newer and safer AEDs, hydantoins are now less commonly prescribed.

Hydantoins act by delaying the influx of sodium ions across neuronal membranes in the brain. Sodium ion movement is the major factor determining the initiation and propagation of a neuron action potential. Hydantoin medications do not block the sodium channels but instead desensitize them. Total blockage of sodium channels would cause neuronal activity to cease as is seen with the administration of local anesthetics. At high doses, the hydantoins begin to exert excitatory CNS effects and can induce seizures.

PROTOTYPE DRUG **Phenytoin (Dilantin, Phenytek)**

Classification **Therapeutic:** Antiepileptic drug
Pharmacologic: Hydantoin, neuronal sodium channel modulator

Therapeutic Effects and Uses: Phenytoin is approved for the prevention of all types of seizures except absence seizures. Phenytoin has been used to prevent seizures that might occur during neurosurgery or eclampsia. The IV form of phenytoin is effective in treating generalized convulsions due to status epilepticus. The action of IV phenytoin is not immediate; therefore, an IV benzodiazepine is often administered prior to, or concurrently with, IV phenytoin to achieve faster seizure control. Phenytoin injections must always be performed slowly (not to exceed 50 mg/min in adults) to prevent cardiovascular collapse. Phenytoin (Phenytek) is an extended-release form of the drug that allows once-daily dosing.

Due to the potential for adverse effects, patients taking phenytoin must be closely monitored and the dosage adjusted based on clinical response and laboratory results. The therapeutic serum range is narrow, 10 to 20 mcg/mL, and small increases in dose can produce large changes in the serum concentration. Thus, the patient should be educated on the importance of maintaining a strict schedule for administration of the medication and for keeping all laboratory appointments. The brand of phenytoin should not be changed without approval of the healthcare provider because differences in bioavailability among brands have been noted.

Phenytoin is also a Class 1B antidysrhythmic and may be used off-label to treat ventricular tachycardia (especially those induced by digoxin) or paroxysmal atrial tachycardia (see Chapter 37). Other off-label indications for phenytoin include the treatment of migraines, diabetic neuropathy, and neuropathic pain.

Mechanism of Action: Phenytoin inhibits seizure activity by delaying the influx of sodium ions in neurons, thus slowing the propagation and spread of abnormal discharges. Unlike some AEDs, phenytoin does not elevate the seizure threshold.

Pharmacokinetics:

Route(s)	PO, IV
Absorption	Slowly but completely absorbed in the GI tract
Distribution	Enters the CSF; crosses the placenta; secreted in breast milk; 95% bound to protein
Primary metabolism	Hepatic
Primary excretion	Renal
Onset of action	PO (with loading dose): 30–120 min
Duration of action	Half-life is highly variable, ranging from 7 to 42 h with an average of 24 h

Adverse Effects: Phenytoin can be a very toxic drug and patients must be monitored carefully. CNS adverse effects are relatively common and include lethargy, headache, drowsiness, and dizziness. High doses can cause nystagmus, confusion, ataxia, coma, and seizures. Cardiovascular adverse effects include bradycardia, ventricular fibrillation, hypotension, and phlebitis. GI adverse effects include gingival hyperplasia (swelling of the gums), weight loss, and liver necrosis. Hematologic adverse effects include agranulocytosis, leukopenia, thrombocytopenia, and aplastic anemia. Rashes and serious dermatologic conditions occur in 5 to 10% of patients taking the drug. Abrupt discontinuation of phenytoin can induce status epilepticus. **Black Box Warning:** When IV infusion rates exceed 50 mg/min in adults, the patient is at risk for hypotension and dysrhythmias. Careful cardiovascular monitoring is needed during and after IV administration.

Contraindications/Precautions: Patients who have developed a rash, sore throat, fever, oral ulcers, or other hypersensitivity reactions to a hydantoin should not receive phenytoin. This medication is contraindicated in patients who have experienced seizures caused by hypoglycemia. Phenytoin should be administered cautiously to patients with impaired liver or kidney function because these may increase the serum concentration of phenytoin to toxic levels. Patients with serious cardiovascular signs and symptoms such as dysrhythmias, bradycardia, and heart failure must be monitored carefully during therapy. Patients with blood dyscrasias should not receive phenytoin because this drug can worsen these conditions.

Drug Interactions: Because phenytoin strongly induces hepatic CYP3A4 enzymes, the metabolism of many other drugs may be affected, and drug–drug interactions are common. Phenytoin increases the metabolism of corticosteroids, warfarin, and oral contraceptives, thus rendering these drugs less effective. Chronic alcohol ingestion, carbamazepine, and barbiturates can increase the metabolism of phenytoin, thus decreasing the antiseizure effects of phenytoin. Amiodarone, chloramphenicol, diazepam, valproic acid, isoniazid, omeprazole, and ticlopidine will increase phenytoin levels when administered concurrently. **Herbal/Food:** The administration or consumption of foods that contain folic acid, calcium, and vitamin D will decrease the absorption of phenytoin. Ginkgo may decrease the antiseizure effectiveness of phenytoin.

Pregnancy: Phenytoin is a known teratogen and is contraindicated during pregnancy. Because the drug is secreted in milk and has the potential to cause adverse effects, breastfeeding is not recommended.

Treatment of Overdose: Overdoses of phenytoin are treated with activated charcoal with gastric lavage.

Clinician Responsibilities: Key clinical implications for patients receiving phenytoin are included in Applied Clinical Judgment: Patients Receiving Pharmacotherapy for Seizures.

Drugs Similar to Phenytoin (Dilantin, Phenytek)

Fosphenytoin is the only other hydantoin.

Fosphenytoin (Cerebyx): Approved in 1996, fosphenytoin is a prodrug that is converted to phenytoin following metabolism. Given only by the parenteral route, it is considered functionally equivalent to phenytoin; their actions and adverse effects are the same. Doses on the label are indicated as phenytoin equivalents (PE). Indications for fosphenytoin include tonic–clonic seizures, status epilepticus, and seizure prophylaxis during neurosurgery. Because the drug is converted to phenytoin, therapeutic serum levels of phenytoin may be monitored during therapy. Potential advantages of fosphenytoin over phenytoin include more rapid IV administration (important during status epilepticus), ability to be administered by the IM route, and less pain and phlebitis at the injection site. The adverse effects are the same as IV phenytoin, except that fosphenytoin may cause intense burning, itching, and paresthesia (not at the site of injection) for several minutes to hours following the IV dose. Fosphenytoin carries the same black box warning as phenytoin. Fosphenytoin is converted to phenytoin, which is a known teratogen that is contraindicated during pregnancy. This drug is secreted in human milk and breastfeeding is not recommended.

> **CONNECTIONS:**
> **Community-Oriented Practice**
> **Epilepsy and Driving Restrictions**
>
> Epilepsy can develop for many reasons but regardless of cause, driving may be restricted, usually for periods of 3 to 6 months, and for up to 1 year in some states, until the person is seizure-free (Epilepsy Foundation of America, 2019b). Some states also require that a medical professional provide periodic medical records to the state as well. In the interest of the public's safety, these restrictions decrease the chance that a driver will experience a seizure while driving, and potentially injure themselves or others. But the impact to the person with the seizure disorder can be significant. Adverse drug effects such as cognitive changes or drowsiness, in addition to state driving restrictions, can have notable effects on employment, limit social interaction, and carry a stigma about the disorder and the need for restrictions. Arcot Jayagopal and colleagues (2018) found that patients were likely to continue driving, ignoring driving restrictions or adverse drug-related effects. Advocating for better public transportation and exploring transportation options for patients with newly diagnosed seizure disorders, or who continue to experience seizures, may help to limit the need to drive or provide alternatives until the patient is seizure-free for the required time.

22.10 Dibenzazepines are the first-line drugs for treating many tonic–clonic and partial seizures.

The dibenzazepines are a small class of drugs that have important applications to seizure management. These drugs have three rings in their structures, which makes them chemically related to the tricyclic antidepressants (see Chapter 19). The drugs in this class, carbamazepine (Carbatrol, Tegretol), eslicarbazepine (Aptiom), and oxcarbazepine (Oxtellar XR, Trileptal), have similar pharmacologic activity.

The mechanisms of action of the dibenzazepines are incompletely understood. Like phenytoin, they affect the sodium channels in cortical neurons, slowing the propagation and spread of repetitive action potentials. These drugs have other actions, however, that are unexplained by the sodium channel mechanism, including analgesic, anticholinergic, antidysrhythmic, antidepressant, and sedative effects. They also have muscle relaxant and neuromuscular-blocking properties. Doses for the dibenzazepines are listed in Table 22.3.

PROTOTYPE DRUG Carbamazepine (Carbatrol, Tegretol, Others)

Classification **Therapeutic:** Antiepileptic drug
Pharmacologic: Dibenzazepine, neuronal sodium channel modulator

Therapeutic Effects and Uses: Approved by the FDA in 1968, carbamazepine is one of the most widely prescribed AEDs in the world because of its effectiveness and relative safety. It is indicated for the management of generalized tonic–clonic seizures, partial seizures with complex symptomatology, and mixed seizure patterns. It is ineffective against absence seizures. Carbamazepine may be administered as monotherapy or in combination with other AEDs. Carbamazepine is also approved for the treatment of acute mania associated with bipolar disorder, either as monotherapy or in combination with lithium (see Chapter 19). Carbamazepine is available as an extended-release form (Tegretol XR and Carbatrol) and as a multiphasic extended-release form (Equetro). PO forms of carbamazepine include Epitol, a chewable tablet, and Teril, an oral suspension.

Prior to its use as an AED, carbamazepine was approved to treat pain associated with trigeminal neuralgia. It remains one of the most effective drugs for this condition. Off-label uses of carbamazepine include the treatment of neuropathic pain associated with diabetic neuropathy and post-herpetic pain. The drug is also used off-label to treat hiccups and for the management of severe symptoms of dementia such as aggression and agitation, which are seen in some patients with Alzheimer's disease.

Although carbamazepine is structurally similar to the tricyclic antidepressants, it does not produce the antidepressant effects of drugs in that class. The medication is metabolized in the liver to an active metabolite and is a potent inducer of CYP450 enzymes that will increase its own metabolism. Long-term administration of carbamazepine will result in the need to increase the dose because its half-life becomes shortened.

For all indications, therapy with carbamazepine must be monitored carefully and the dosage adjusted based on clinical outcomes and drug serum levels. The therapeutic serum concentrations usually range from 4 to 12 mcg/mL. Several weeks of therapy may be required before the optimal dose is determined and the effective plasma drug concentration achieved.

Mechanism of Action: Carbamazepine inhibits sodium channels, blocking the repetitive, sustained firing of neurons that is characteristic of epilepsy. Other mechanisms are likely but are incompletely understood.

Pharmacokinetics:

Route(s)	PO
Absorption	Slowly absorbed across the GI tract
Distribution	Widely distributed; enters the CSF; crosses the placenta; secreted in breast milk; 75–85% bound to proteins
Primary metabolism	Hepatic (induces CYP450 enzymes)
Primary excretion	Primarily renal with some in feces
Onset of action	Slow and variable
Duration of action	Half-life: 14–16 h; 35–40 h for extended release

Adverse Effects: Carbamazepine is well tolerated; adverse effects are usually transient and diminish as therapy progresses. The most frequently observed effects include drowsiness, dizziness, ataxia, and nausea and vomiting. Transient sedation is common at the onset of therapy or following increases in dosage. Other CNS effects include confusion, blurred vision, lethargy, and visual disturbances, although the patient usually develops tolerance to these effects. Other possible adverse effects include myalgia, leg cramps, carbamazepine-induced systemic erythematosus, heart block, aplastic anemia, respiratory depression, phototoxicity, urticaria, and alopecia. Elevated hepatic enzymes occur during therapy, although the patient is usually asymptomatic for hepatic disease. A few rare cases of serious hepatic impairment have been documented. Some patients have reported urinary retention and frequency, and male patients may experience impotence. **Black Box Warning:** Aplastic anemia and agranulocytosis have been reported with this drug. Serious and sometimes fatal dermatologic reactions, including toxic epidermal necrosis and SJS, have also occurred with carbamazepine. Patients testing positive for the *HLA-B 1502* gene (usually found in people of Asian ancestry) are at higher risk for severe dermatologic reactions and should not receive this drug unless the benefit clearly justifies the risk.

Contraindications/Precautions: Patients who are hypersensitive to tricyclic antidepressants should not take carbamazepine. Patients who have been diagnosed with increased intraocular pressure, systemic lupus erythematosus, cardiac disease, hepatic disease, and liver disease should not take carbamazepine. This medication is contraindicated with HTN. Older adults should be monitored closely if they possess a history of cardiac disease because a major adverse effect is heart block.

Drug Interactions: Carbamazepine induces the activity of several hepatic CYP450 enzymes, which can result in decreased serum concentrations of AEDs and other drugs metabolized by the liver. Increased carbamazepine levels have been noted when the drug is administered with verapamil, erythromycin, ketoconazole, or nefazodone. Patients who take carbamazepine with anticoagulants will experience decreased hypoprothrombinemic effects. Carbamazepine may decrease the effectiveness of oral contraceptives. **Herbal/Food:** Ginkgo may decrease the antiepileptic effectiveness of carbamazepine. Grapefruit juice and St. John's wort induce CYP450 enzymes and can decrease serum carbamazepine levels.

Pregnancy: Carbamazepine may cause fetal harm and withdrawal symptoms have been observed in neonates born to mothers taking the drug. This drug causes multiple birth defects in laboratory animals. Because carbamazepine enters milk and has the potential to cause serious adverse effects in the neonate, breastfeeding is not recommended.

Treatment of Overdose: Activated charcoal and gastric lavage are administered with carbamazepine overdose.

Clinician Responsibilities: Key clinical implications for patients receiving carbamazepine are included in Applied Clinical Judgment: Patients Receiving Pharmacotherapy for Seizures.

Drugs Similar to Carbamazepine (Carbatrol, Tegretol, Others)

Other dibenzazepines include eslicarbazepine and oxcarbazepine.

Eslicarbazepine (Aptiom): Eslicarbazepine was approved in 2013 for the treatment of partial-onset seizures. It is usually used as an add-on treatment to therapy with other AEDs. It has a long half-life that allows for once-daily dosing. Eslicarbazepine and oxcarbazepine have very similar actions and adverse effects because both are converted to the same active metabolite. Use of eslicarbazepine with oxcarbazepine is contraindicated due to a synergistic effect. Common adverse effects include dizziness, somnolence, nausea and vomiting, headache, blurred vision, and tremor. Serious adverse effects include suicidal ideation, anaphylaxis, hyponatremia, and severe dermatologic reactions. This drug may decrease the effectiveness of hormonal contraceptives. In animal reproduction studies, eslicarbazepine caused developmental toxicity, embryotoxicity, and teratogenicity. Because the drug enters milk and has the potential to cause serious adverse effects in the neonate, breastfeeding is not recommended.

Oxcarbazepine (Oxtellar XR, Trileptal): Although oxcarbazepine is structurally similar to the tricyclic antidepressants, it does not possess antidepressant activity. Approved in 2000, oxcarbazepine can be administered as monotherapy or in combination with other medications in the treatment of partial seizures, with or without secondary generalization. Off-label uses include the treatment of neuropathic pain and bipolar disorder. A major advantage of oxcarbazepine over carbamazepine is that drug interactions appear less significant and monitoring of drug plasma levels and hematologic values is generally not necessary. Although it induces CYP450 enzymes, it is not as strong an inducer as carbamazepine and it does not induce its own metabolism. An extended-release form of the drug (Oxtellar XR) is available for once-daily dosing.

For checking adherence with the drug regimen or in overdose situations, the therapeutic serum concentration of the drug is 12 to 30 mcg/mL. Adverse effects are similar to those of carbamazepine, with dizziness, drowsiness, headache, and ataxia being the most common effects. Serious adverse effects include suicidal ideation, agranulocytosis, hyponatremia, and severe dermatologic reactions. A serious and sometimes fatal adverse event called drug reaction with eosinophilia and systemic systems (DRESS) has been reported with oxcarbazepine.

In animal reproduction studies, oxcarbazepine caused developmental toxicity, embryotoxicity, and teratogenicity. Because the drug enters milk and has the potential to cause serious adverse effects in the neonate, breastfeeding is not recommended.

22.11 Succinimides are the first-line drugs for the pharmacotherapy of absence seizures.

Succinimides form a small group of AEDs that block T-type calcium channels in neurons in the thalamus. This action decreases the firing of thalamic neurons, which reduces the likelihood of abnormal action potentials. Despite the small size of the class, these drugs have important roles in the pharmacotherapy of absence seizures.

PROTOTYPE DRUG | **Ethosuximide (Zarontin)**

Classification **Therapeutic:** Antiepileptic drug
Pharmacologic: Succinimide, neuronal calcium channel modulator

Therapeutic Effects and Uses: Ethosuximide is the only drug in this class that is commonly prescribed. Approved in 1960, it is a preferred drug for managing absence seizures. Because ethosuximide is ineffective in treating focal seizures and tonic–clonic seizures, combination pharmacotherapy is needed to manage mixed seizures.

Ethosuximide is only administered by the oral route. Therapeutic serum concentrations range from 40 to 100 mcg/mL, although dosing is usually based on clinical response rather than serum levels. It may take 4 to 7 days before optimal therapeutic levels are attained.

Mechanism of Action: Ethosuximide depresses the motor cortex by delaying the calcium influx into the neuron.

Pharmacokinetics:

Route(s)	PO
Absorption	Readily and completely absorbed
Distribution	Widely distributed; very small amounts bound to proteins; crosses the placenta and is secreted in breast milk
Primary metabolism	Hepatic
Primary excretion	Primarily renal, with some in feces and bile
Onset of action	Peak: 4 h
Duration of action	Half-life: 30 h in children; 60 h in adults

Adverse Effects: The most common adverse effects of ethosuximide are GI related, including anorexia, nausea and vomiting, abdominal pain, and diarrhea. Adverse CNS events include drowsiness, dizziness, ataxia, confusion, and night terrors. Hematologic toxicity may include agranulocytosis, pancytopenia, and aplastic anemia. Dermatologic effects include rash, pruritus, and exfoliative dermatitis. Like many AEDs, this drug may increase the risk of suicidal ideation.

Contraindications/Precautions: Ethosuximide is contraindicated in patients who have a known sensitivity to succinimides. It should be administered with caution to patients with liver or kidney impairment. Administration of ethosuximide may increase the frequency of tonic–clonic seizures. Patients with blood dyscrasias or bone marrow suppression should not receive this drug because it can worsen these conditions.

Drug Interactions: Ethosuximide can participate in many drug–drug interactions. When used in combination therapy with other AEDs, serum drug levels should be regularly monitored. CNS depressants and ethanol may cause additive sedation. Ethosuximide administered concurrently with phenobarbital, phenothiazines, or tricyclic antidepressants can increase seizure frequency. Isoniazid administered in combination with ethosuximide can result in increased serum ethosuximide levels. Carbamazepine will cause a decrease in ethosuximide serum levels. Concurrent use of valproic acid will inhibit the metabolism of ethosuximide, leading to possible toxicity. **Herbal/Food:** Unknown.

Pregnancy: There are incomplete data on the safety of this medication during pregnancy. The drug is secreted in milk but the effects on breastfeeding infants are unknown.

Treatment of Overdose: Activated charcoal and gastric lavage are administered with ethosuximide overdose.

Clinician Responsibilities: Key clinical implications for patients receiving ethosuximide are included in Applied Clinical Judgment: Patients Receiving Pharmacotherapy for Seizures.

Drugs Similar to Ethosuximide (Zarontin)

Methsuximide is the only other drug in this class.

Methsuximide (Celontin): Like ethosuximide, methsuximide is indicated for the management of absence seizures. This drug is rarely used in clinical practice because it is less effective and more toxic than ethosuximide. It has the same indications and adverse effects as ethosuximide. There is incomplete data on the safety of this medication during pregnancy. The drug is likely secreted in milk but the effects on breastfeeding infants are unknown.

22.12 Several miscellaneous drugs are important in treating epilepsy.

As explained in Section 22.6, it is difficult to classify AEDs because many act by multiple mechanisms, whereas others are unique and are the only drug in a class. Indeed, the "miscellaneous" class is the largest group of AEDs and several drugs in this group are widely used. Following the discussion of the two prototypes, other miscellaneous drugs and their indications are described. Doses for these drugs are shown in Table 22.5.

PROTOTYPE DRUG Gabapentin (Neurontin)

Classification **Therapeutic:** Antiepileptic drug
Pharmacologic: GABA analog

Therapeutic Effects and Uses: Gabapentin consists of a molecule of the neurotransmitter GABA with an attached side chain. The side chain makes the molecule lipid soluble so that it readily crosses the blood–brain barrier. Approved in 1993, gabapentin is used in combination with other AEDs to control focal seizures with or without secondary generalization. Doses are based on therapeutic response, making it unnecessary to measure serum drug levels during therapy. It is available as capsules, as tablets, and as an oral solution.

Therapy with gabapentin has been found to benefit a number of other conditions. Extended-release forms of gabapentin (Gralise) are approved for the treatment of post-herpetic neuralgia and gabapentin (Horizant) for restless leg syndrome. The extended-release forms are not approved to treat seizures. Gabapentin is used off-label for other conditions with neuropathic pain such as diabetic neuropathy. In fact, the drug may be prescribed more often for the treatment of neuropathic pain than for epilepsy. It has been designated as an orphan drug for the treatment of amyotrophic lateral sclerosis (ALS). Some research has suggested that gabapentin may be useful in treating trigeminal neuralgia, paresthesia, spasticity, and ocular ataxia in patients with multiple sclerosis.

Mechanism of Action: The exact mechanism of anticonvulsant action for gabapentin is unknown. Although closely related structurally to GABA, it does not appear to bind to GABA receptors or to prevent endogenous GABA from binding. It does not appear to affect the binding of other neurotransmitters such as serotonin, dopamine, glutamate, or histamine. It likely affects calcium channels, but its exact mechanism has not been determined.

Pharmacokinetics:

Route(s)	PO
Absorption	50–60% is absorbed from the GI tract
Distribution	Crosses the blood–brain barrier and the placenta; readily passes into the CSF; secreted in breast milk; very small amounts bound to proteins
Primary metabolism	Not metabolized
Primary excretion	Excreted unchanged by the kidneys
Onset of action	1 h
Duration of action	Half-life: 5–6 h

Adverse Effects: Gabapentin is well tolerated, with CNS symptoms such as drowsiness, fatigue, nystagmus, and dizziness being the primary adverse effects. The administration of gabapentin can lead to increased frequency of viral infections, weight gain, and gastric upset. Behavioral problems such as hostility, emotional lability, impaired cognition, aggressiveness, and hyperkinesia have been reported in the pediatric population ages 3 to 12.

Contraindications/Precautions: Gabapentin should not be administered during pregnancy or lactation unless the benefits of pharmacotherapy outweigh the risks. It should not be administered in patients who have experienced a hypersensitivity reaction to GABA-related medications. It should be used cautiously with status epilepticus and with older adults. Gabapentin should be used with caution in patients with chronic kidney disease because the drug could accumulate to toxic levels. The drug should be discontinued gradually to prevent withdrawal-associated seizures.

Drug Interactions: A major advantage of gabapentin is that it does not induce CYP450 enzymes, and thus it exhibits fewer drug interactions than many other AEDs. No interactions with carbamazepine, phenobarbital, phenytoin, or valproic acid have been observed. Morphine and hydrocodone may cause additive CNS depression when administered with gabapentin. **Herbal/Food:** The administration of ginkgo with gabapentin may result in decreased anticonvulsant effects. The use of valerian is contraindicated due to the risk of additive sedation.

Pregnancy: In animal reproduction studies, gabapentin showed embryofetal toxicity and adverse effects on offspring development. The drug is secreted in milk but the effects on breastfeeding infants are unknown.

Treatment of Overdose: Overdose results in dyspnea, sedation, double vision, and slurred speech. Renal dialysis can be utilized to treat gabapentin overdose.

Clinician Responsibilities: Key clinical implications for patients receiving gabapentin are included in Applied Clinical Judgment: Patients Receiving Pharmacotherapy for Seizures.

PROTOTYPE DRUG | **Valproic Acid (Depakote)**

Classification **Therapeutic:** Antiepileptic drug, antimanic drug
Pharmacologic: GABA agonist

Therapeutic Effects and Uses: Approved in 1978, valproic acid has become a first-line drug for treating many types of epilepsy. This medication has several trade names and formulations, which may cause confusion.

- Valproic acid is the delayed-release form of the drug given by the oral route (given twice daily).
- Valproate sodium is the sodium salt of valproic acid given orally or IV.
- Divalproex sodium (Depakote ER) is a sustained-release combination of valproic acid and its sodium salt in a 1:1 mixture. It is given orally once daily and is available in an enteric-coated form.

All three formulations of the drug form valproate after absorption or on entering the brain. The pharmacokinetics of each form varies, and they are not interchangeable. In this text, the name "valproic acid" is used to describe all forms of the drug, unless specifically stated otherwise.

Valproic acid is administered as monotherapy or in combination with other AEDs to treat absence seizures and complex partial (focal, impaired awareness) seizures. Depakote ER is also approved for the prevention of migraines and mania associated with bipolar disorder. Off-label indications include severe behavioral disturbances such as agitation due to dementia, Alzheimer's disease, or explosive temper in patients with ADHD; persistent hiccups; and status epilepticus refractory to IV diazepam. Dosage adjustments for valproic acid are usually based on patient response; normal serum drug levels for epilepsy are 50 to 100 mcg/mL.

Mechanism of Action: Valproic acid increases concentrations of the inhibitory neurotransmitter GABA in the brain. Abnormal neuron discharges are suppressed, leading to decreased seizure activity.

Pharmacokinetics:

Route(s)	IV, PO
Absorption	Rapidly absorbed in the GI tract
Distribution	Crosses the placenta and is secreted in breast milk; 80–90% bound to protein
Primary metabolism	Hepatic
Primary excretion	Renal and GI tract
Onset of action	15–30 min
Duration of action	Half-life: 5–20 h

Adverse Effects: The most common adverse effects are GI related, such as nausea and vomiting, diarrhea, abdominal pain, and diminished appetite. An enteric-coated formulation of valproic acid can be used to reduce these uncomfortable effects. These effects are usually transient and not severe. CNS adverse effects such as headache, tremor, dizziness, and sedation occur in about 25% of patients. High doses of valproic acid cause diminished platelet aggregation, which can result in prolonged bleeding and clotting times. Bone marrow depression, photosensitivity, and pulmonary edema are rare potential adverse effects. Valproic acid may cause hyperammonemic encephalopathy, especially in combination with topiramate, which requires discontinuation of valproic acid therapy. **Black Box Warnings:** Serious hepatotoxicity has been reported in infants younger than age 2 taking valproic acid; Life-threatening pancreatitis has occurred as a result of valproic acid administration; When given during pregnancy, valproic acid can produce neural tube defects and children exposed while in utero demonstrate lower cognitive scores.

Contraindications/Precautions: Patients with hypersensitivity to any formulation of valproic acid should not be administered this drug. Other contraindications include significant hepatic impairment, bleeding disorders, cirrhosis, congenital metabolic disorders, and autoimmune deficiency syndrome. Patients with known or suspected pancreatitis should not receive this drug because life-threatening pancreatitis has been reported. Valproic acid should be administered cautiously in patients with a low serum albumin or chronic kidney disease. Extreme caution should be used in treating patients under age 2 because fatal hepatotoxicity has been reported. The drug should not be administered to patients with known hepatic impairment. Abrupt discontinuation may cause status epilepticus. This drug is a known teratogen and should be used during pregnancy only when benefits of therapy clearly outweigh the risk of birth defects.

Drug Interactions: Valproic acid inhibits CYP450 enzymes, which can result in many drug–drug interactions. Valproic acid administered concurrently with alcohol and other CNS depressants may result in additive sedation. Patients taking enzyme-inducing AEDs such as carbamazepine, phenytoin, and phenobarbital will metabolize valproic acid more rapidly, and dosage adjustment will be necessary. Valproic acid may increase the serum levels of tricyclic antidepressants, requiring a reduction in antidepressant dosage. Aspirin increases the serum drug levels of valproic acid and should not be administered concurrently. Isoniazid will elevate serum valproic acid levels. Cholestyramine will decrease absorption of valproic acid. Cimetidine will increase valproic acid levels and will place the patient at risk for hepatotoxicity. Valproic acid should not be administered with topiramate due to an increased risk of hyperammonemic encephalopathy. **Herbal/Food:** Ginkgo may decrease the antiepileptic effects of valproic acid.

Pregnancy: Animal and human data show that valproic acid can cause birth defects, especially neural tube defects. It is also secreted in milk. Women should use effective contraception during therapy and refrain from breastfeeding.

Treatment of Overdose: The effects from overdose of valproic acid may be serious and include sedation, heart block, deep coma, and death. Naloxone (Narcan) is utilized to reverse the CNS depression, and hemodialysis can lower drug serum levels. Caution must be used when administering naloxone because this drug may also reverse the antiseizure action of valproic acid.

Clinician Responsibilities: Key clinical implications for patients receiving valproic acid are included in Applied Clinical Judgment: Patients Receiving Pharmacotherapy for Seizures.

Other Miscellaneous Drugs

Brivaracetam (Briviact): Approved in 2016, brivaracetam is one of the newer drugs for treating focal seizures in patients 16 years and older. Available by PO or IV administration, this drug acts by a similar mechanism of action to levetiracetam, although its dose is 10 times lower. It is used as an add-on when other AEDs are unable to successfully control seizures. The patient should be carefully monitored for psychiatric adverse reactions, sedation, and suicidal ideation during therapy. Brivaracetam may be administered by either the PO or IV route. Animal studies indicate that brivaracetam may cause fetal harm. The drug is secreted in animal milk but adverse effects on breastfeeding infants are unknown.

Cannabidiol (Epidiolex): Epidiolex is the first FDA-approved drug containing cannabidiol, which is derived from the marijuana plant. It was approved in 2018 for two rare seizure disorders, Lennox-Gastaut syndrome and Dravet syndrome, in patients 2 years and older. Cannabidiol has no psychoactive properties; therefore, it does not cause the same effects as marijuana. The most common side effects include somnolence, infections, decreased appetite, and diarrhea. Use with CNS depressants may cause profound sedation and patients should be monitored for suicidal ideation. Cannabidiol causes significant elevations in hepatic enzymes and liver function should be monitored during therapy. Abrupt discontinuation of cannabidiol will increase seizure frequency and possibly induce status epilepticus. In animal reproduction studies, cannabidiol caused embryofetal mortality and adverse effects on male fertility in offspring. No data are available on the effects of cannabidiol on lactation or the breastfed infant.

Ezogabine (Potiga): Ezogabine was approved in 2011 for the adjunctive treatment of focal-onset seizures in adults. The drug acts by stabilizing potassium channels in the brain, which reduces brain excitability. The drug should be used with caution in patients with benign prostatic hyperplasia because it may cause urinary retention. Dizziness, somnolence, and fatigue are common side effects during therapy. Patients should be observed for the development of neuropsychiatric symptoms such as confusion, psychosis, and hallucinations. Ezogabine is a Schedule V drug. Based on animal studies, this drug may cause embryofetal toxicity. Ezogabine is secreted in animal milk but adverse effects on breastfeeding infants are unknown. Due to potential adverse reactions, breastfeeding is not recommended during therapy.

Felbamate (Felbatol): Approved in 1993, felbamate is an oral drug that is effective against most types of seizures. Serious adverse effects, however, limit its use to severe partial seizures and the treatment of focal and generalized seizures associated with Lennox–Gastaut syndrome in children who have not responded to other therapies. Although the incidence of these adverse effects is rare, they may be serious or fatal. More common adverse effects include nausea and vomiting, anorexia, drowsiness, dizziness, insomnia, and vision changes. This drug carries a black box warning that fatal aplastic anemia and fatal hepatic failure have been associated with felbamate use. Baseline and periodic hematologic and hepatic laboratory tests should be conducted. Effects of felbamate during pregnancy and lactation are unknown. However, due to potential adverse effects relating aplastic anemia and hepatic failure in adults, breastfeeding in not recommended.

Lacosamide (Vimpat): Lacosamide is a miscellaneous AED used in the management of focal-onset seizures in adults whose seizures are not well controlled by other medications. Approved in 2008, its most frequent adverse effects include diplopia, headache, ataxia, dizziness, and nausea. Lacosamide prolongs the PR interval; therefore, it should be used with caution in patients with cardiac conduction abnormalities. In animal reproduction studies, lacosamide increased embryofetal deaths and perinatal mortality. Lacosamide is secreted in animal milk but adverse effects on breastfeeding infants are unknown.

Lamotrigine (Lamictal): Approved in 1994, lamotrigine is a broad-spectrum AED indicated for the adjunctive therapy of focal-onset seizures, Lennox–Gastaut syndrome, absence seizures, and tonic–clonic seizures in adults and pediatric patients 2 years of age or older. It is also used in the maintenance therapy of bipolar disorder. Lamotrigine inhibits the release of glutamate in neurons and inhibits flow through sodium ion channels, which stabilizes neuronal membranes. It is available in regular, extended-release, and oral disintegrating tablets.

Lamotrigine does not induce or inhibit hepatic metabolic enzymes. It is metabolized by CYP450 enzymes, however, and patients who are taking potent inducers of CYP450 enzymes (e.g., carbamazepine, phenytoin, and phenobarbital) will metabolize the drug more rapidly. Doses of lamotrigine will need to be *increased* in these patients to produce an optimal antiseizure response. On the other hand, valproic acid will reduce the elimination of lamotrigine, and the dose of lamotrigine should be *reduced* to prevent toxicity. Oral contraceptives reduce serum levels of lamotrigine, and the dosage of the AED will need to be adjusted when therapy with the hormones is initiated or discontinued and during the "pill-free" week of the month.

Lamotrigine is generally well tolerated with the most common adverse effects being drowsiness, dizziness, ataxia, headache, diplopia, blurred vision, nausea and vomiting, and rash. Patients should be monitored for the development of suicidal ideation. This drug carries a black box warning that serious dermatologic toxicity, including SJS, has been reported, especially in children. Life-threatening rashes normally present during the first 2 to 8 weeks of therapy but may occur during prolonged therapy. Lamotrigine should be discontinued at the first sign of any type of rash. Animal studies suggest that lamotrigine may cause fetal harm. The drug is secreted in milk but adverse effects on breastfeeding infants are unknown. Infants born to breastfeeding mothers should be monitored for lamotrigine toxicity.

Levetiracetam (Keppra): Levetiracetam is a broad-spectrum AED available for both PO and IV routes and is utilized in adjunctive therapy for partial seizures in adults and children age 4 years and older, adjunctive therapy for myoclonic seizures in adults and adolescents age 12 years and older, and adjunctive therapy of primary generalized tonic–clonic seizures in adults and children age 6 years and older. Approved in 1999, the mechanism of its antiseizure activity is unknown. Levetiracetam is excreted unchanged by the kidneys; thus, dosage should be reduced in patients with chronic kidney disease (CKD). Few significant drug interactions have been recorded. An extended-release form of the drug (Keppra XR) is approved to treat partial-onset seizures.

Levetiracetam is generally well tolerated, with the most common adverse effects being drowsiness, dizziness, infections, headache, and asthenia. The nurse must teach the patient to exercise care in performing hazardous tasks because an increase in unintentional injuries is associated with levetiracetam use. Pediatric patients exhibit a relatively high incidence of behavioral effects, including agitation, nervousness, hyperkinesia, hostility, depression, and emotional lability. These effects may be serious enough to necessitate discontinuation of therapy. The patient should be monitored for suicidal ideation, aggressive behavior, and psychiatric symptoms. In animal reproduction studies, levetiracetam produced embryofetal mortality, developmental toxicity, and teratogenicity. This drug is secreted in milk but adverse effects on breastfeeding infants are unknown. Due to the potential for adverse effects, breastfeeding is not recommended.

Perampanel (Fycompa): Approved in 2012, perampanel is indicated as monotherapy or adjunctive use for focal-onset seizures in patients as young as 4 years old and for generalized tonic–clonic seizures in those age 12 and older. It is available as tablets and as an oral suspension. Common side effects include dizziness, headache, fatigue, and somnolence. This drug increases the risk for falls, leading to serious injury and fractures. Perampanel carries a black box warning that serious or life-threatening psychiatric and behavioral changes can occur during therapy such as suicidal ideation, irritability, aggressiveness, and homicidal threats. Perampanel decreases the effectiveness of hormonal contraceptives. Women taking oral contraceptives should be advised to use a nonhormonal form of contraception while on this medication. Animal studies show that this drug may cause embryofetal toxicity. Perampanel is secreted in animal milk but adverse effects on breastfed infants are unknown.

Pregabalin (Lyrica): Approved in 2004, pregabalin is an oral AED that is very similar to gabapentin. Pregabalin is indicated for the adjunctive therapy of adult patients with partial-onset seizures. Like gabapentin, it is used more often for its other approved indications: the management of neuropathic pain associated with diabetic peripheral neuropathy, post-herpetic neuralgia, and fibromyalgia. Off-label uses include the therapy of anxiety and social phobia. The safety of pregabalin in pediatric patients has not been established. Although its mechanism of action has not been clearly demonstrated, it is thought to act by increasing GABA levels by reducing the calcium channel function of neurons in the brain. This drug does not affect CYP450 enzymes; thus, it has fewer drug–drug interactions than many other AEDs. Pregabalin is not bound to plasma proteins and is excreted in an unmetabolized form by the kidneys. Dose reduction in patients with CKD is necessary to avoid toxicity.

Pregabalin is well tolerated by most patients. Dizziness and drowsiness are the most common adverse effects, and these may affect 20 to 40% of patients taking pregabalin, especially at high doses. Other common adverse effects of pregabalin are blurred vision, lethargy, dry mouth, peripheral edema, weight gain, and difficulty with concentration or attention. Patients should be monitored for the development of suicidal ideation. Concurrent administration with other CNS depressants can lead to increased sedation. Because pregabalin is a Schedule V controlled substance that may cause physical and psychologic dependence, it should be used with caution in patients with a known or suspected history of substance abuse. In animal reproduction studies, pregabalin showed developmental toxicity, growth retardation, and skeletal malformations. Pregabalin is secreted in animal milk but adverse effects on breastfed infants are unknown. Due to the potential for adverse reactions, breastfeeding is not recommended during therapy.

Rufinamide (Banzel): Rufinamide is an oral drug approved in 2008 for the adjunctive treatment of seizures associated with Lennox–Gastaut syndrome. It is well tolerated, with dizziness, headache, and fatigue being common adverse effects. The drug acts by regulating the activity of sodium channels in the brain. Rufinamide decreases the effectiveness of hormonal contraceptives. Patients should be monitored for the development of suicidal ideation. Because rufinamide can shorten the QT interval, it is contraindicated in patients with familial short QT syndrome. Animal studies suggest that rufinamide can cause fetal harm, including skeletal malformations and spontaneous abortion. Rufinamide is likely secreted in milk, therefore breastfeeding is not recommended during therapy.

Tiagabine (Gabitril): Tiagabine is given by the oral route for the adjunctive treatment of partial seizures in patients who have not responded to therapy with other AEDs. Safety in patients under age 12 has not been established. Approved in 1997, it acts by inhibiting GABA reuptake into the presynaptic neuron. Tiagabine is extensively metabolized by CYP3A enzymes. Patients who are taking potent inducers of CYP450 enzymes (e.g., carbamazepine, phenytoin, and phenobarbital) will metabolize tiagabine more rapidly. Doses of tiagabine will need to be increased in these patients to produce an optimal antiseizure response. Tiagabine itself does not induce CYP450 enzymes; thus, it has fewer drug–drug interactions than many other AEDs. Tiagabine is 98% bound to plasma proteins and is eliminated in both the urine and feces.

Approximately 10 to 20% of patients taking tiagabine experience adverse effects that require discontinuation of therapy. The most common adverse effects are dizziness, lethargy, confusion, somnolence, nausea, irritability, tremor, asthenia, abdominal pain, and difficulty with concentration or attention. As with other AEDs the nurse should teach patients to avoid injury due to possible sedative effects. Although tiagabine suppresses seizures in patients with epilepsy, it has been found to increase new-onset seizures when given to patients without epilepsy for off-label psychiatric disorders. Because of this, the FDA and the manufacturer have advised prescribers not to administer tiagabine for any indication other than partial seizures in patients 12 years and older. An additional FDA warning advises healthcare providers to monitor carefully for any increase in suicidal behavior or ideation. Animal studies suggest that tiagabine can cause fetal harm, including skeletal malformations and stillbirths. This drug is secreted in animal milk but adverse effects on breastfed infants are unknown.

Topiramate (Topamax, Trokendi XR, Others): Approved in 1996, topiramate is a broad-spectrum AED that has become an important medication in treating a broad range of seizure types in adults and children. It may be used as monotherapy or in combination with other AEDs. It is approved for migraine prophylaxis and may be prescribed off-label for neuropathic pain or bipolar disorder. The drug is usually well tolerated, with the most frequent adverse effects being dizziness, fatigue, paresthesia, anorexia, weight loss, and psychomotor slowing. Extended-release forms (Qudexy XR, Trokendi XR) offer the convenience of once-daily dosing. During therapy, patients should be monitored for visual changes, glaucoma, metabolic acidosis, cognitive dysfunction, and suicidal behavior. Adequate fluid intake should be encouraged to prevent kidney stone formation. Because this drug can decrease sweating, the patient may be susceptible to hyperthermia during hot weather. Topiramate causes fetal harm and may increase the risk of oral clefts in children exposed to the drug while in utero. This drug is secreted in milk but adverse effects on breastfed infants are unknown. Use of topiramate during pregnancy and lactation is not advised unless the potential benefits to the mother justify the potential risks to the fetus and neonate.

Vigabatrin (Sabril): Available PO, vigabatrin was approved in 2009 for adjunctive therapy of refractory complex partial seizures in adults and for infantile spasms in infants 1 month to 2 years of age. Because of potential serious adverse effects, vigabatrin is available in a restricted distribution program and is only prescribed when patients have not responded adequately to other AEDs. This drug contains a black box warning that permanent vision loss can occur during therapy. Other serious adverse effects include anemia, confusion, and memory impairment. Patients should be monitored for the development of suicidal ideation. Based on animal data, vigabatrin can cause fetal harm and is secreted in milk. Use of vigabatrin during pregnancy and lactation is not advised unless the potential benefits to the mother justify the potential risks to the fetus and neonate.

Zonisamide (Zonegran): Approved in 2000, zonisamide is an oral sulfonamide that is effective in combination with other AEDs for partial seizures in adults. Safety in patients under age 16 has not been established, although the drug is sometimes used off-label in children. It produces antiepileptic effects by inhibiting sodium and calcium channels in brain neurons. Zonisamide has a long half-life and 2 weeks may be required before optimal antiseizure activity is achieved.

Zonisamide is well tolerated by most patients. The most common adverse effects are dizziness, ataxia, drowsiness, fatigue, anorexia, speech abnormalities, and difficulty in concentrating or remembering. Because many patients are allergic to sulfonamides, it is important to assess these patients for sulfonamide hypersensitivity prior to the administration of the medication. Sulfonamides can cause fatal skin reactions, including SJS. The medication should be administered cautiously in patients who are receiving drugs that inhibit or reduce CYP3A4 enzymes; phenytoin, carbamazepine, phenobarbital, and valproic acid will decrease the half-life of zonisamide. Doses of zonisamide will need to be increased in these patients to produce an optimal antiseizure response. Zonisamide itself does not induce CYP enzymes; thus, it has fewer drug–drug interactions than many other AEDs. Zonisamide is teratogenic in laboratory animals and is secreted in milk. Use during pregnancy and lactation is not advised unless the potential benefits to the mother justify the potential risks to the fetus and neonate.

CONNECTIONS: APPLIED CLINICAL JUDGMENT

Patients Receiving Pharmacotherapy for Seizures

Key Assessment Data

- History of current condition, baseline vital signs, physical exam findings; history of cardiovascular, hepatic, renal, or neurologic disease; medication and allergy history; mental status as appropriate; pregnancy or breastfeeding status.
- Obtain a seizure history (e.g., frequency, duration, physical symptoms, preseizure symptoms that occur, and length of postictal period).
- Obtain a developmental history in pediatric patients (e.g., DDST-II level of growth and development and school performance). Obtain height and weight.
- Ongoing assessment during drug therapy includes laboratory findings such as CBC, hepatic or renal function studies, height and weight (pediatric patients).

(continued)

CONNECTIONS: APPLIED CLINICAL JUDGMENT (*continued*)

Patients Receiving Pharmacotherapy for Seizures

Desired Therapeutic Outcomes

Improvement is observed and measurable in diminished frequency and severity of seizure activity.

Minimizing Adverse Effects

- Antiseizure drugs may cause drowsiness and dizziness, hypotension, or impaired mental and physical abilities, increasing the risk of falls and injury. Continue to monitor vital signs, mental status, coordination, and balance periodically. Ensure patient safety; monitor ambulation until effects of the drug are known.
- Neurologic changes may indicate overmedication or adverse drug effects. Assess for changes in level of consciousness, disorientation, confusion, or agitation.
- Antiseizure drugs may cause renal and hepatotoxicity, pancreatitis (with valproic acid), blood dyscrasias with increased chances of bleeding or infection, or dermatologic toxicity, including Stevens-Johnson syndrome. Continue to monitor drug levels, CBC, renal and hepatic function, and pancreatic enzymes. Assess for bruising, bleeding, or signs of infection. Monitor for dermatologic effects including red or purplish skin rash, blisters, and sunburn. Immediately report severe rashes, especially associated with blistering.
- Antiseizure drugs may increase the risk of mental depression and suicide. Concurrent use of alcohol or other CNS depressants increases the effects and the risk. Monitor affect and emotional status.
- Caffeine and nicotine may decrease the effectiveness of the benzodiazepines. Barbiturates, drugs with GABA action, and hydantoins and phenytoin-like drugs affect the absorption of vitamins K, D, and B and folic acid. Alcohol and other CNS depressants may increase the adverse effects of antiseizure drugs. Encourage appropriate lifestyle and dietary changes: increased intake of foods that are rich in vitamins K, D, and B and folic acid; lowered caffeine intake including OTC medications that contain caffeine; and limited or no alcohol intake.
- Hydantoins and phenytoin-like drugs may cause gingival hyperplasia, increasing the risk of oral infections. Assess the condition of gums and encourage good oral hygiene measures.
- Treatment with antiseizure drugs may require using combinations of drugs, and seizure activity may diminish but may not be resolved. Social isolation and low self-esteem may occur with continued seizure disorder. Provide for emotional support and appropriate referrals as needed.
- Benzodiazepines, hydantoins, and barbiturates are irritating to the vein when the drug is given IV. Blanching and pain at the IV site are an indicator of extravasation. Closely monitor the IV infusion site when using IV antiseizure drugs and the IV infusion should be immediately stopped. Contact the provider for further treatment orders.
- Status epilepticus may occur with abrupt discontinuation of the drug. Avoid abrupt discontinuation and contact the provider if the drug cannot be taken for longer than a 24-hour period.

Lifespan Considerations

- The older adult may be at increased risk for falls due to drowsiness and dizziness, hypotension, or impaired mental and physical abilities.
- Many antiseizure medications may cause fetal harm and are secreted in milk. Some AEDs decrease the effectiveness of oral contraceptives and additional forms of contraception should be used. Assess women of childbearing potential for the possibility of pregnancy and plans for pregnancy, breastfeeding, and contraceptive use. Alternative contraceptive forms should be considered.
- Adverse effects of antiseizure drugs or unresolved seizures may hinder normal growth and development. Continue to monitor height, weight, and developmental level in pediatric patients. In the school-age child, assess school performance.
- Monitor children for paradoxical response to barbiturates; hyperactivity may occur.

Diversity Considerations

- Some antiseizure drugs induce or inhibit CYP450 enzymes and may interact with other drugs. Observe for less than optimal therapeutic effects, especially in ethnically diverse patients.

Patient and Caregiver Education

- Antiseizure drugs may not completely resolve symptoms but the frequency and severity of seizures should be diminished. Increasing seizures or a decrease in the ability to perform self-care activities should be reported. Keep a seizure diary of frequency, type, length, pre-seizure symptoms, and postictal period and bring it to each healthcare visit.
- Rise from lying or sitting to standing slowly to avoid dizziness or falls. If dizziness occurs, sit or lie down and do not attempt to stand or walk until the sensation passes. Avoid driving or other activities requiring mental alertness or physical coordination until the effects of the drug are known.
- Keep regularly scheduled appointments with the healthcare provider and for pediatric patients, report any developmental lags or concerns.
- Promptly report abdominal pain, particularly in the upper quadrants; changes in stool color, yellowing of sclera or skin, or darkened urine; and increased bruising, bleeding, or infections (e.g., sore throat and fever or skin rash). Report increasing lethargy, disorientation, confusion, changes in behavior or mood, slurred speech, or ataxia immediately.
- Avoid alcohol and other CNS depressants while taking the drug.
- Discuss pregnancy and family planning with women of childbearing age. Explain the effect of medications on pregnancy and breastfeeding and the need to discuss any pregnancy plans with the healthcare provider. Discuss the need for additional forms of contraception, including barrier methods.
- Take the drug:
  - Exactly as ordered and the same manufacturer's brand each time the prescription is filled. Switching brands may result in differing pharmacokinetics and alterations in seizure control.
  - Read label directions for how to take the medication. Some forms may not be opened or chewed; others require chewing thoroughly. When in doubt, consult a pharmacist or other healthcare provider.
  - Take a missed dose as soon as it is noticed but do not take double or extra doses to "catch up." Notify the provider if the drug cannot be taken for over 24 hours.
  - Take with food to decrease GI upset.
  - Do not stop the drug abruptly.
- Carry a wallet identification card or wear medical identification jewelry indicating a seizure disorder and antiseizure medication used.

Prescribing Considerations

- AEDs should be initiated one at a time, with doses increased at intervals of 1 to 2 weeks.
- The optimal dose will vary in every patient and should be based on effective seizure control with minimal side effects.
- If adequate seizure control cannot be attained without unmanageable side effects, then combination therapy should be considered.
- There are no specific protocols for when to discontinue AEDs. Patients that have been seizure-free for at least 3 years may be considered.
- Discontinuation of AEDs should occur gradually over several months by slowly decreasing one medication at a time.

Understanding Chapter 22

Key Concepts Summary

22.1 Epilepsy is characterized by recurrent seizures caused by disturbances in the electrical activity of the brain.

22.2 Seizure disorders differ throughout the lifespan.

22.3 Most seizures are classified as generalized or partial.

22.4 Some types of seizures are called special epileptic seizures.

22.5 The selection of antiepileptic drug therapy is dependent on seizure type and characteristics.

22.6 Antiepileptic drugs act by suppressing abnormal neuronal discharges.

22.7 Barbiturates are traditional drugs for tonic–clonic seizures that have been replaced by newer and safer medications.

22.8 Benzodiazepines are important drugs in the treatment of status epilepticus.

22.9 Hydantoins are effective in the management of most types of seizures but have many adverse effects.

22.10 Dibenzazepines are the first-line drugs for treating many tonic–clonic and partial seizures.

22.11 Succinimides are the first-line drugs for the pharmacotherapy of absence seizures.

22.12 Several miscellaneous drugs are important in treating epilepsy.

CASE STUDY: Making the Patient Connection

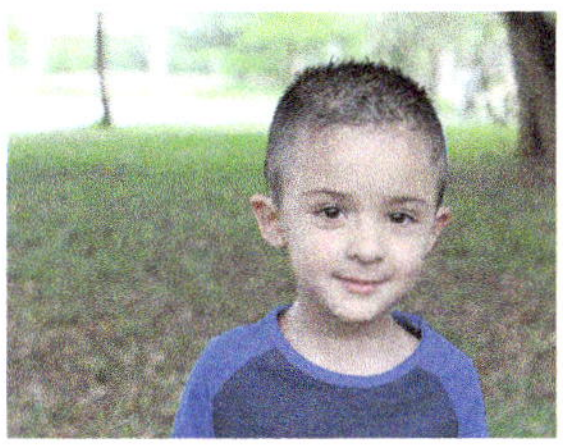

Remember the patient "Jorge Alvarez" at the beginning of the chapter? Now read the remainder of the case study. Based on the information presented within this chapter, respond to the critical thinking questions that follow.

Jorge Alvarez is a 3-year-old boy who has been hospitalized following a seizure. Since being admitted 2 days ago, he has experienced three subsequent generalized tonic–clonic seizures lasting 2 to 2.5 minutes each. Prior to having a seizure, Jorge notices a flash of light. He then loses consciousness, emits a hoarse cry, and has intense muscle contractions. During the clonic phase he is incontinent of bowel and bladder. His postictal phase is characterized by drowsiness, disorientation, and deep sleep.

On admission Jorge was scheduled for a sleep-and-awake EEG. His EEG revealed a high-voltage spike discharge, which is diagnostic of a generalized tonic–clonic seizure. The laboratory studies performed on Jorge included a serum lead level to rule out lead intoxication and a serum glucose level to rule out hypoglycemia. Both the lead level and blood glucose were in the normal range.

Jorge has been started on the following medications to assist in controlling his tonic–clonic seizures: carbamazepine (Tegretol) 300 mg PO tid and phenytoin (Dilantin) 120 mg PO tid.

Critical Thinking Questions

1. Jorge's mother expresses concern about what to do if he has a seizure. Create a list of home safety tips that could be given to her.
2. What will you instruct Jorge's mother about with regard to his medication administration?

Additional Case Study

Matt has had epilepsy since childhood. It seems that his current medications are no longer keeping him seizure-free. Valproic acid (Depakote) is being added to Matt's medication regimen. How would you respond to the following questions from Matt about this new medication?

1. How does valproic acid work to prevent seizures?
2. What adverse effects are associated with this drug?
3. Why should Matt inform his dentist that he is now on valproic acid?

Chapter Review

1. A 10-year-old child has been evaluated for a learning disability and has been diagnosed with generalized absence seizures. Ethosuximide (Zarontin) has been ordered and the nurse is teaching the patient and family about the drug. Because of the patient's age, it is important to include instructions to:
   1. Curtail after-school sports activities because the drug's metabolism may be increased with physical activity.
   2. Increase intake of calcium-rich foods and vitamin D to prevent bone loss.
   3. Monitor height and weight weekly to be sure GI side effects are not hindering nutrition and normal growth.
   4. Increase fluid intake to avoid dehydration caused by the drug.

2. The nurse is caring for a 42-year-old patient who was recently diagnosed with focal seizures with impaired awareness and has been prescribed oxcarbazepine (Trileptal). Which laboratory study would the nurse expect to be ordered?
   1. CBC with differential
   2. Serum albumin and glucose levels
   3. Sedimentation rate and platelet count
   4. Serum sodium and renal function studies

3. An 80-year-old patient is prescribed carbamazepine (Tegretol) for a newly diagnosed seizure disorder. The nurse will implement safety measures because this patient is at an increased risk for which adverse effects with the administration of this drug?
   1. Dementia and confusion
   2. Insomnia and forgetfulness related to sleep deprivation
   3. Stroke and decreased motor function
   4. Sedation and falls

4. A 23-year-old patient has been taking gabapentin (Neurontin) for control of focal seizures with impaired awareness. He is admitted to the emergency department with slurred speech, dyspnea, reports of double vision, and sedation. The admitting nurse suspects the patient has:
   1. Not taken his drug for several days.
   2. Taken an overdose of the drug, either unintentionally or deliberately.
   3. Taken the drug with grapefruit or grapefruit juice.
   4. Continued to smoke despite prior patient education that smoking interacts with the drug.

5. The nurse, who is monitoring a patient taking phenytoin (Dilantin), has noted symptoms of nystagmus, confusion, and ataxia. Considering these findings, the nurse would suspect that the dose of the drug should be:
   1. Reduced.
   2. Increased.
   3. Maintained.
   4. Discontinued.

6. Carbamazepine (Tegretol) has been prescribed for a 24-year-old patient for the control of focal seizures with impaired awareness. The nurse will teach the patient to immediately report:
   1. Blurred vision.
   2. Leg cramps.
   3. Blister-like rash.
   4. Lethargy.

See Appendix A for answers to critical thinking questions, case study questions, and review questions.

References

Algreeshah, F. S. (2016). *Psychiatric disorders associated with epilepsy*. Medscape. http://emedicine.medscape.com/article/1186336-overview#a1

Arcot Jayagopal, L., Samson, K. K., & Taraschenko, O. (2018). Driving with drug-resistant and controlled seizures from a patient's perspective: Assessment of attitudes and practices. *Epilepsy & Behavior, 81*, 101–106. https://doi.org/10.1016/j.yebeh.2018.01.023

Baumann, L., Sullivan, S., Shirk, S., & Moo, L. (2018). Seizures in Alzheimer's disease are associated with younger onset and decreased life expectancy. *Innovation in Aging*, 2(Suppl. 1), 300. https://doi.org/10.1093/geroni/igy023.1106

Dahlin, M., & Prast-Nielsen, S. (2019). The gut microbiome and epilepsy. *EBioMedicine, 44*, 741–746. https://doi.org/10.1016/j.ebiom.2019.05.024

Epilepsy Foundation of America. (2019a). *Seizure first aid.* https://www.epilepsy.com/learn/about-epilepsy-basics/facts-about-seizures-and-epilepsy

Epilepsy Foundation of America (2019b). *State driving laws database.* https://www.epilepsy.com/driving-laws

Fan, Y., Wang, H., Liu, X., Zhang, J., & Liu, G. (2019). Crosstalk between the ketogenic diet and epilepsy: From the perspective of gut microbiota. *Mediators of Inflammation, 2019,* 8373060. https://doi.org/10.1155/2019/8373060

Haunt, S. (2016). Antiepileptic medications and breastfeeding: Better news than expected? *Epilepsy Currents, 16,* 84–86. https://doi.org/10.5698/1535–7511-16.2.84

Lambrechts, D. A., de Kinderen, R. J., Vies, H. S., de Louw, A. J., Aldenkamp, A. P., & Majole, M. J. (2015). The MCT-ketogenic diet as a treatment option in refractory childhood epilepsy: A prospective study with 2-year follow-up. *Epilepsy & Behavior, 51,* 261–266. https://doi.org/10.1016/j.yebeh.2015.07.023

Rezaei, S., Abduraham, A. A., Saghazadeh, A., Badv, R. S., & Mahmoudi, M. (2019). Short-term and long-term efficacy of classical ketogenic diet and modified Atkins diet in children and adolescents with epilepsy: A systematic review and meta-analysis. *Nutritional Neuroscience, 22,* 317–334. https://doi.org/10.1080/1028415X.2017.1387721

Vehmeijer, F. O., van der Louw, E. J., Arts, W. F., Catsman-Berrevoets, C. E., & Neuteboom, R. F. (2015). Can we predict efficacy of the ketogenic diet in children with refractory epilepsy? *European Journal of Paediatric Neurology, 19,* 701–705. https://doi.org/10.1016/j.ejpn.2015.06.004

Selected Bibliography

Abou-Khalil, B. W. (2019). Update on antiepileptic drugs 2019. *CONTINUUM: Lifelong Learning in Neurology, 25*(2), 508–536. https://doi.org/10.1212/CON.0000000000000715

Allen, B., & Vespa, P. M. (2019). Antiseizure medications in critical care: An update. *Current Opinion in Critical Care, 25*(2), 117–125. https://doi.org/10.1097/MCC.0000000000000587

Epilepsy Foundation. (2016). *New terms for seizure classification.* https://www.epilepsy.com/learn/types-seizures/new-terms-seizure-classification

Kanner, A. M., Ashman, E., Gloss, D., Harden, C., Bourgeois, B., Bautista, J. F., et al. (2018). Practice guideline update summary: Efficacy and tolerability of the new antiepileptic drugs I: treatment of new-onset epilepsy. *Epilepsy Currents, 18*(4), 260–268. https://doi.org/10.5698/1535-7597.18.4.260

Ko, D. Y. (2020). *Epilepsy and seizures.* Medscape. https://emedicine.medscape.com/article/1184846-overview

Ma, L., & McCauley, S. O. (2018). Management of pediatric febrile seizures. *Journal for Nurse Practitioners, 14*(2), 74–80. https://doi.org/10.1016/j.nurpra.2017.09.021

Ochoa, J. G. (2020). *Antiepileptic drugs.* Medscape. https://emedicine.medscape.com/article/1187334-overview#a1

Smith, G., Wagner, J. L., & Edwards, J. C. (2015). CE: Epilepsy update, part 1: Refining our understanding of a complex disease. *American Journal of Nursing, 115*(5), 40–47. https://doi.org/10.1097/01.NAJ.0000465030.89975.e8

Spiciarich, M. C., von Gaudecker, J. R., Jurasek, L., Clarke, D. F., Burneo, J., & Vidaurre, J. (2019). Global health and epilepsy: Update and future directions. *Current Neurology and Neuroscience Reports*, 19(6), 30. https://doi.org/10.1007/s11910-019-0947-6

Strozzi, I., Nolan, S. J., Sperling, M. R., Wingerchuk, D. M., & Sirven, J. (2015). Early versus late antiepileptic drug withdrawal for people with epilepsy in remission. *Cochrane Database of Systematic Reviews*, Issue 2, Article No. CD001902. https://doi.org/10.1002/14651858.CD001902.pub2

Tolaymat, A., Nayak, A., Geyer, J. D., Geyer, S. K., & Carney, P. R. (2015). Diagnosis and management of childhood epilepsy. *Current Problems in Pediatric and Adolescent Health Care, 45,* 3–17. https://doi.org/10.1016/j.cppeds.2014.12.002

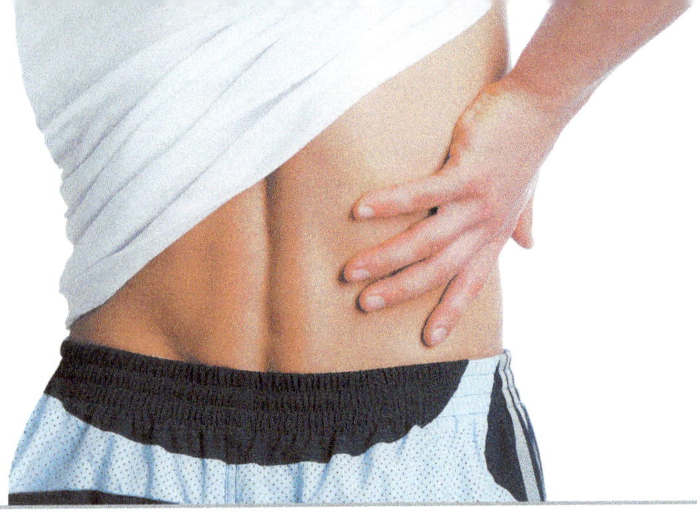

"I was lifting concrete blocks to build a landscaping wall in my front yard yesterday. When I woke up this morning, I couldn't bend down to put on my pants after my shower. My back hurts so bad I can hardly walk."
Patient "Andrew Eskew"

Chapter 23
Pharmacotherapy of Muscle Spasms and Spasticity

Chapter Outline

Learning Outcomes

After reading this chapter, the student should be able to:

1. Compare and contrast the etiology and pathophysiology of muscle spasm and muscle spasticity.
2. Describe the nonpharmacologic management of muscle spasms and muscle spasticity.
3. Identify drug classes used to treat muscle spasms and spasticity.
4. Compare and contrast the actions of the centrally acting and direct-acting skeletal muscle relaxants.
5. Explain the role of skeletal muscle relaxants as surgical adjuncts.
6. Describe the nurse's role in the pharmacologic management of muscle spasms and muscle spasticity.
7. For each of the classes shown in the chapter outline, identify the prototype and representative drugs and explain the mechanism(s) of drug action, primary indications, contraindications, significant drug interactions, pregnancy data and important adverse effects.
8. Apply clinical judgment to care for patients receiving pharmacotherapy for muscle spasms and spasticity.

Key Terms

Definitions of the terms in bold may be found in the Glossary.

Although everyone experiences muscle aches and pains from time to time, these symptoms often resolve without pharmacotherapy. There are some conditions, however, where medications may be used to relieve painful muscle pain, spasm, or spasticity. This chapter examines how these drugs produce their actions and their applications to the pharmacotherapy of muscle conditions.

Etiology and Pathophysiology of Muscle Spasms and Spasticity

23.1 Whereas muscle spasms are often caused by overuse of skeletal muscle, muscle spasticity involves damage to motor nerves.

Intense skeletal muscle contractions can cause severe pain and disability. Abnormal contractions may be classified as spasms or spasticity. Although both may occur in the same patient, the etiology, pathogenesis, and treatment strategies differ for the two conditions.

Muscle spasms: **Muscle spasms** are involuntary contractions of skeletal muscles that are usually localized to a specific muscle group. As the affected muscles strongly contract and tighten, the spasm causes sudden, intense pain, which gradually diminishes after a few minutes. Patients may refer to the condition as a charley horse or cramp. Chronic or severe spasms can impair joint mobility.

When treating a patient with muscle spasms, it is important to identify their cause. The etiology of muscle spasms may involve many body systems, including the nervous, musculoskeletal, endocrine, and cardiorespiratory systems. The most common etiology of muscle spasm is overuse of a skeletal muscle. When subjected to trauma or overexertion, the muscle may spasm. If the medical history does not reveal muscle overuse or injury, the healthcare provider will assess for possible metabolic or electrolyte imbalances such as hypocalcemia, hypokalemia, or dehydration. Poor blood circulation to the legs, known as claudication, is a common cause of muscle cramping.

Some medications, shown in Table 23.1, may cause muscle spasms, muscle weakness, and other types of myopathy as adverse effects. Signs of drug-induced myopathy usually develop slowly after several months of drug therapy. Drugs may induce spasms by causing electrolyte imbalances, generating an inflammatory or immune response, or by directly damaging muscle organelles such as mitochondria. The most important class causing this pathology is the statins, which are widely used to lower blood cholesterol levels. Statins can cause a severe form of myopathy called rhabdomyolysis that may cause significant disability and morbidity. Most drug-induced myopathies are reversible in their early stages. If a medication is suspected of causing myopathy, the dose is reduced or discontinued. Symptoms make take several weeks to resolve after the drug is discontinued.

Table 23.1 Medications That May Cause Drug-Induced Myopathy

Drug Class	Example(s)
Alzheimer's drug	donepezil
Antifungals	fluconazole, ketoconazole
Antihyperlipidemics	statins, niacin, red yeast rice, ezetimibe
Antimalarials	chloroquine, hydroxychloroquine
Antineoplastics	cisplatin, imatinib, vincristine
Antiulcer drugs: proton pump inhibitors	esomeprazole, omeprazole
Asthma drugs	albuterol, terbutaline
Calcium channel blockers	nifedipine
Diuretics	furosemide, hydrochlorothiazide
Immunosuppressants	leflunomide (Arava), tumor-necrosis factor (TNF), inhibitors (adalimumab)
Steroids	corticosteroids, dexamethasone

Muscle spasticity: Muscle spasticity has a different etiology than muscle spasm. **Muscle spasticity** is a condition caused by damage to upper motor neurons in the central nervous system (CNS), which causes certain muscle groups to remain in a continuous state of contraction. The patient may experience irritable deep tendon reflex activity, muscle spasms, involuntary jerking, and scissoring movements of the lower extremities. Patients with muscle spasticity are unable to voluntarily relax their limbs. Spasticity, also referred to as hypertonia, causes pain that is more intense than muscle spasm and produces greater impairment of mobility.

Whereas muscle spasms occur most often with overexertion, muscle spasticity is associated with neuromuscular diseases that are the result of damage to neurons in the region of the cerebral cortex that controls muscle movements. Conditions most commonly associated with muscular spasticity include severe head or spinal cord trauma, multiple sclerosis (MS), stroke, cerebral palsy (CP), trauma, and amyotrophic lateral sclerosis (ALS).

Under normal conditions a muscle receives a balance of both excitatory and inhibitory signals from motor neurons. When a muscle needs to contract, an impulse is sent from the brain or spinal cord down an excitatory motor neuron. When a muscle needs to relax, the brain sends a signal to the muscle through an inhibitory motor neuron. As a simple example, consider flexion and extension of the elbow. Forearm flexion occurs when the biceps receives an excitatory impulse; at the same time its antagonist, the triceps, receives an inhibitory impulse. On extension, the opposite occurs: The biceps receive the inhibitory message while the triceps contract after receiving the excitatory message. Proper contraction of skeletal muscle thus involves a balance of signals from the CNS through both excitatory and inhibitory motor neurons.

Muscle spasticity from a spinal cord injury occurs when there is an imbalance of excitatory and inhibitory signals. The area that is distal to the spinal cord injury or lesion becomes disassociated from the inhibitory area of the brain, and the excitatory impulses dominate at the affected muscles. The muscles may go into spastic paralysis; flexor muscles become tight, and the muscles can be extended only with great difficulty. Once extended, the muscles tend to immediately flex back. It is important to understand that although the obvious symptoms appear to be muscle related, the cause of the spasticity is actually neurologic injury.

In the advanced stages of MS, muscle spasticity is caused by destruction of the myelin sheath, which interrupts the main motor pathways from the spinal cord to the muscles. Spasticity results in a stiff, unbalanced gait and may eventually confine these patients to a wheelchair. Patients with MS are treated with a combination of medications including muscle relaxants, corticosteroids, and immunosuppressants (see Chapter 21).

Approximately 35% of patients experience spasticity following a stroke. If the brain area affected by the stroke is able to reestablish communication with the muscle, the spasticity may be reversible and voluntary movement may be restored. In many cases, however, the spasticity becomes permanent and can be recognized by a clenched fist, permanently flexed elbow, or pointed toes.

Cerebral palsy is a neurologic disorder that results in severe muscular spasticity, which can affect facial muscles; cause an unsteady, scissoring gait; and result in painful joint contractures and deformities. The primary cause of spasticity associated with CP is congenital trauma to the brain or spinal cord. Pharmacologic options for treating CP are limited. Intrathecal baclofen may be beneficial in reducing severe spasticity.

Muscle spasms, spasticity, and twitching are also characteristic of ALS, also known as Lou Gehrig's disease. ALS is caused by the degeneration and loss of lower and upper motor neurons in the CNS. The disorder is progressive and fatal. Muscle relaxants may bring some pain relief during periods of intense muscle spasticity.

Dystonia is a chronic neurologic disorder that is characterized by involuntary muscle contraction that forces body parts into abnormal, painful movements or postures. The condition may affect the entire body (generalized dystonia), or it may be localized to a single body region (focal dystonia) such as the arms, legs, trunk, neck, eyelids, face, or vocal cords. Primary dystonia is a heritable disorder, prominent among Ashkenazi Jewish people. Dystonia may also occur secondary to other neurologic disorders such as MS, Parkinson's disease, stroke, or CP. The impairment in mobility and intense pain produced by muscle spasms and spasticity inhibits the patient's ability to perform activities of daily living (ADLs). Generalized dystonias are treated with high doses of anticholinergic drugs such as benztropine, benzodiazepines, carbamazepine, antiparkinson drugs, and intrathecal baclofen. Patients with focal dystonia may obtain some relief with botulinum toxin type A.

Dupuytren's contracture is a condition of the hand in which a thick cord of connective tissue forms in the palm, causing the fingers to curl inward. Although not usually painful, the curling is progressive and can restrict motion and use of the hand. This disorder is not caused by muscles; therefore, traditional muscle relaxants and antispasmodics are ineffective. For severe cases, surgical removal of the connective tissue cord is performed. Collagenase (Xiaflex) is an enzyme medication approved to treat this disorder. The enzyme is injected multiple times into the affected cord, over a 4-week interval. The most frequently reported adverse effects are swelling of the affected hand, contusion, injection-site reaction or hemorrhage, and localized pain.

CONNECTION Checkpoint 23.1

Benzodiazepines are some of the most widely prescribed drugs. From what you learned in Chapter 18, what are the major indications for drugs in this class?

Nonpharmacologic Therapies for Muscle Spasms and Spasticity

23.2 Nonpharmacologic interventions for treating muscle spasms and spasticity are limited.

The therapeutic goals for treating muscle spasms or spasticity are to decrease discomfort and enhance mobility so that the patient is better able to perform ADLs. Nonpharmacologic complementary and alternative therapies (CATs) are sometimes implemented to achieve these goals. When the spasms or spasticity are prolonged or disabling, pharmacotherapy is initiated. A combination of CATs and drug therapy is often the most effective treatment.

Nonpharmacologic interventions that sometimes benefit patients with muscle spasm or spasticity include the application of heat or cold, massage, traction, and manipulation. The application of heat or cold to the affected site will reduce or relieve the muscle spasm and pain. If the spasm has occurred due to overexertion, application of heat to the area can reduce cramping and relieve localized pain. If the spasms persist after 3 to 5 days, the application of cold packs to the site may be used to slow the transmission of pain impulses. The application of touch, massage, and gentle pressure are sometimes effective at promoting musculoskeletal relaxation. Other nonpharmacologic techniques that may be useful include acupuncture, sensory nerve stimulation, and ankle splints for leg pain.

The implementation of physical therapy is sometimes effective for treating muscle spasticity. Routine and consistent physical therapy exercises provide the patient with increased muscle movement and decreased severity of symptoms. Effective physical therapy exercises include muscle stretching, which assists in the prevention of contractures (permanent shortening of muscles). The implementation of muscle group–strengthening and repetitive-motion exercises may allow for safer ambulation. In extreme cases, surgery may be necessary to release tendons or to sever the nerve–muscle pathway.

Herbal remedies are occasionally used to treat patients with muscle spasms, although the effectiveness of most of these treatments are based on limited studies or anecdotal evidence. One of the proven therapies uses capsaicin, a chemical derived from cayenne pepper. Capsaicin is applied topically as a cream four times per day to increase mobility and reduce muscle pain. It is important to wear gloves while applying capsaicin cream to prevent irritation of the skin on the hands and to avoid introducing the capsaicin to the eyes or other parts of the body not under treatment. A high-potency prescription drug containing 8% capsaicin (Qutenza) is approved to treat neuropathic pain associated with post-herpetic neuralgia.

A final nonpharmacologic therapy for muscle spasm is treatment with B-complex vitamins, specifically pyridoxine (B_6). In some patients, the B-complex vitamins can reduce both the intensity and duration of leg cramps.

PharmFACT

An analysis of 18 reviews of nonpharmacologic therapies for spasticity showed only two therapies with moderate evidence for effectiveness: acupuncture and neuromuscular stimulation. All other therapies were rated as having low-quality evidence (Khan et al., 2019).

Pharmacotherapy of Muscle Spasms

23.3 Nonsteroidal anti-inflammatory drugs and skeletal muscle relaxants are used to treat muscle spasms.

Muscle spasms, especially those caused by injury, are painful and sometimes associated with inflammation. Nonsteroidal anti-inflammatory drugs (NSAIDs) such as aspirin, naproxen, and ibuprofen are usually the first-line drugs for treating minor to moderate pain due to muscle overexertion. These drugs have the ability to relieve muscle pain and reduce inflammation around the injury site, which can take pressure off the surrounding nerves and enhance mobility. The pharmacology of NSAIDs is presented in Chapter 41.

For more intense muscle spasms, muscle relaxants may be prescribed. Although these drugs are not analgesics, they can promote pain relief by relaxing tight, contracted muscles without interfering with normal muscle function. When skeletal muscle relaxants are used in combination with NSAIDs, pain relief is greater than when either drug is used alone.

The centrally acting skeletal muscle relaxants relieve muscle spasms by their actions in the CNS. They do not directly affect the neuromuscular junction or muscles themselves. The precise mechanism of action of centrally acting skeletal muscle relaxants is unclear but it is believed they help to restore the balance of excitatory and inhibitory impulses from motor neurons in the CNS. Like the benzodiazepines, they can produce significant drowsiness, especially if combined with alcohol or other CNS depressants. The sedative effects may be beneficial in helping patients with muscle spasms or spasticity to obtain needed sleep. The centrally acting skeletal muscle relaxants include baclofen (Lioresal), cyclobenzaprine (Amrix), deutetrabenazine (Austedo), tetrabenazine (Xenazine), and tizanidine (Zanaflex). Some drugs in this class are used for both muscle spasms and spasticity. Mechanisms of action are shown in Pharmacotherapy Illustrated 23.1. Doses of the centrally acting muscle relaxants are listed in Table 23.2.

Drugs from a number of other classes have been used to treat and prevent muscle spasms. Calcium channel blockers including diltiazem (Cardizem, Tiazac) and verapamil (Calan) may be used off-label to prevent muscle cramps. The mechanism for this action is unknown but may be related to the drugs' ability to dilate arteries and bring additional oxygen to muscles.

Benzodiazepines such as diazepam (Valium) are occasionally prescribed to relax skeletal muscle. Diazepam may be used as an adjunct to relieve skeletal muscle spasms associated with CP, paraplegia, and tetanus. Diazepam is a featured prototype drug for seizures in Chapter 22.

Pharmacotherapy Illustrated 23.1

Mechanism of Action of Drugs Used to Treat Muscle Spasms and Spasticity

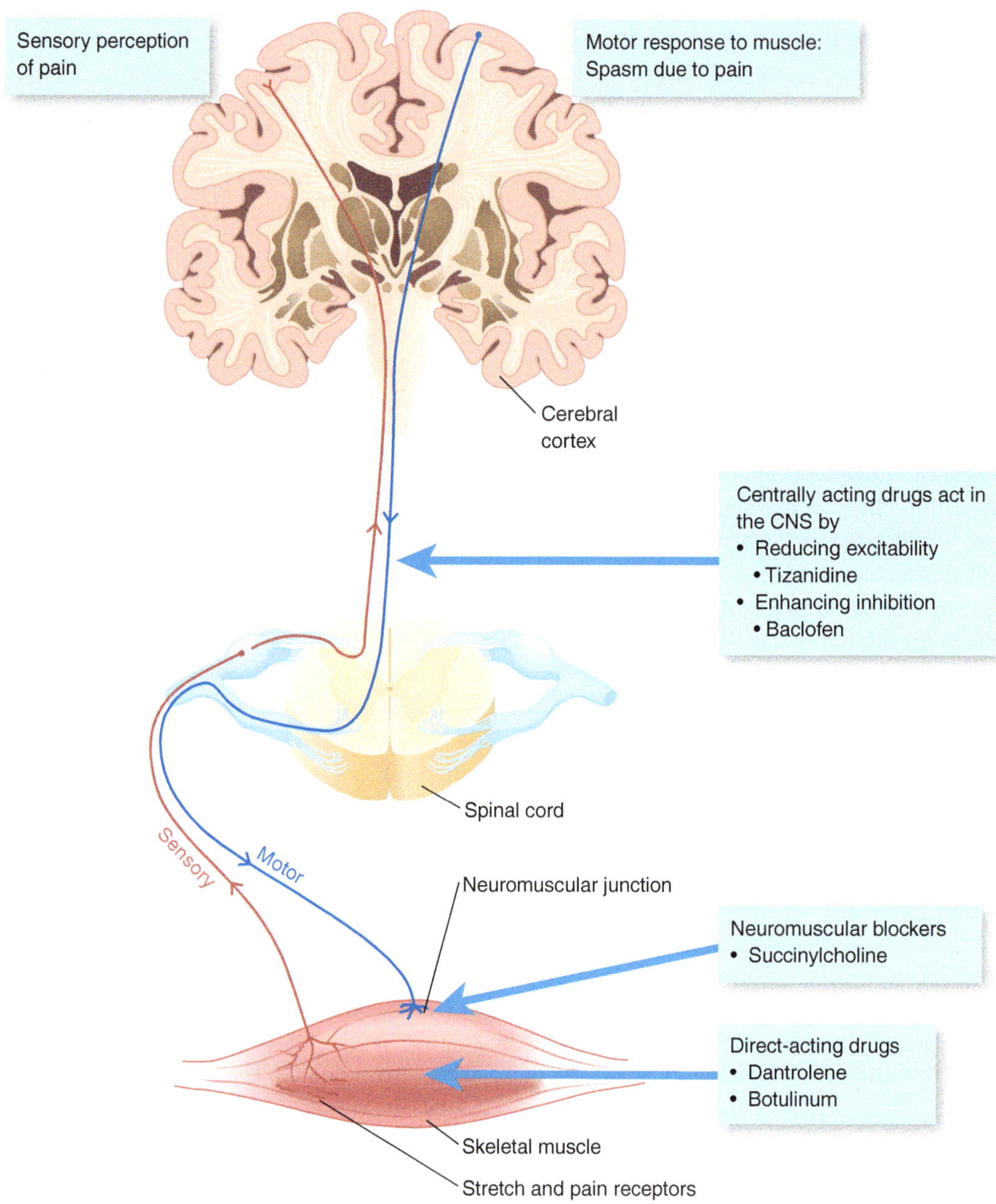

PROTOTYPE DRUG	Cyclobenzaprine (Amrix)

Classification **Therapeutic:** Skeletal muscle relaxant
Pharmacologic: Centrally acting skeletal muscle relaxant

Therapeutic Effects and Uses: Approved in 1977, cyclobenzaprine is indicated for the short-term therapy of acute musculoskeletal conditions that are unrelated to CNS disease. Cyclobenzaprine is not effective for treating muscle spasm due to spinal cord injury or CP. The drug promotes skeletal muscle relaxation, thus decreasing muscle spasms and increasing joint mobility. The manufacturer recommends that treatment not extend beyond 3 weeks. Fibromyalgia is an off-label indication for the drug.

Cyclobenzaprine is chemically related to the tricyclic antidepressants (TCAs) and it exhibits some antidepressant effects. The drug is available by immediate-release tablet or extended-release capsule. Cyclobenzaprine is occasionally abused as a recreational drug due to its sedative actions.

Table 23.2 Centrally Acting Skeletal Muscle Relaxants

Drug	Route and Adult Dose (Maximum Dose Where Indicated)	Adverse Effects
baclofen (Gablofen, Lioresal, Ozobax)	PO: 5 mg tid, increasing gradually to 40–80 mg/day (max: 80 mg/day) Intrathecal: 50-mcg bolus	*Drowsiness, dizziness, weakness, confusion, nausea, hypotonia* <u>QT prolongation, dysrhythmias, severe withdrawal symptoms if abruptly discontinued</u>
carisoprodol (Soma)	Adult: PO: 250–350 mg tid	*Drowsiness, confusion, orthostatic hypotension, nausea and vomiting, vertigo, ataxia, syncope* <u>Anaphylactic shock, physical dependence, profound sedation</u>
chlorzoxazone	PO: 250–500 mg tid–qid (max: 3 g/day)	*Drowsiness, dizziness, nausea and vomiting, diarrhea, abdominal pain, lightheadedness, overstimulation, rash, pruritus, urticaria* <u>Hepatotoxicity, anemia, neutropenia</u>
cyclobenzaprine (Amrix)	PO: 5–10 mg tid for tablets; 15 mg once daily for extended-release capsules (max: 30 mg/day)	*Drowsiness, xerostomia, dizziness, fatigue, nausea, dyspepsia* <u>Tongue edema, potential for QT prolongation, hallucinations, serotonin syndrome</u>
deutetrabenazine (Austedo) and tetrabenazine (Xenazine)	PO (Austedo): 6 mg once daily (max: 48 mg/day) PO (Xenazine): 12.5–50 mg/day in divided doses	*Sedation, fatigue, insomnia, depression, akathisia, anxiety, nausea* <u>Neurologic malignant syndrome, suicidal ideation, extrapyramidal symptoms</u>
metaxalone (Skelaxin)	PO: 800 mg tid–qid	*Nausea and vomiting, GI upset, drowsiness, dizziness, headache, anxiety* <u>Hemolytic anemia, jaundice, hepatotoxicity, anaphylaxis</u>
methocarbamol (Robaxin)	PO: 4 g/day maintenance dose IV/IM: 1–3 g once daily for 3 days	*Drowsiness, dizziness, lightheadedness, fever, rash, syncope, thrombophlebitis, pain, blurred vision, headache, tachycardia* <u>Anaphylactic shock, sloughing of skin with extravasation</u>
orphenadrine	PO: 100 mg bid IM/IV: 60 mg q12h (max: 250 mg/day)	*Dry mouth, drowsiness, weakness, dizziness, agitation, tachycardia, syncope, palpitations, increased intraocular pressure, blurred vision, nausea, urticaria* <u>Anaphylactic shock, hallucinations</u>
tizanidine (Zanaflex)	PO: 4–8 mg q6–8h (max: 36 mg/day)	*Dry mouth, somnolence, urinary tract infection, fatigue, dizziness* <u>Hepatotoxicity, hypotension, bradycardia, hallucinations</u>

Note: *Italics* indicate common adverse effects. <u>Underline</u> indicates serious adverse effects.

Mechanism of Action: The action of cyclobenzaprine is thought to occur at the brainstem and spinal cord levels. The drug increases norepinephrine activity by blocking its synaptic reuptake to produce an anticholinergic effect. Cyclobenzaprine acts centrally and thus has no direct action on skeletal muscle.

Pharmacokinetics:

Route(s)	PO
Absorption	Well absorbed in the gastrointestinal (GI) tract
Distribution	It is unknown whether the drug crosses the placenta or is secreted in breast milk; 93% bound to protein
Primary metabolism	Extensive hepatic metabolism via CYP450 enzymes to inactive metabolites
Primary excretion	Renal
Onset of action	1 h
Duration of action	12–24 h

Adverse Effects: Commonly reported adverse effects include drowsiness, dizziness, and xerostomia. Sedation can be a limiting effect with the first few doses. Other adverse effects of cyclobenzaprine include edema of the tongue and face with sweating, myalgia, hepatitis, and alopecia. Potential cardiovascular adverse events include orthostatic hypotension, tachycardia, syncope, palpitations, and vasodilation. The patient may report having an unpleasant taste, a coated tongue with discoloration, nausea and vomiting, anorexia, diarrhea with flatulence, or paralysis.

Contraindications/Precautions: Cyclobenzaprine should be used with great caution in patients older than age 65 because this population is more likely to experience confusion, hallucinations, and adverse cardiac events from the drug. Cyclobenzaprine should also be used cautiously in patients who have increased intraocular pressure, prostatic hyperplasia, urinary retention, and seizures. Patients with hypersensitivity to TCAs should not receive this drug. Like the TCAs, cyclobenzaprine can adversely affect the heart and therefore should be used with caution in patients with cardiovascular disease, including those with heart failure or dysrhythmias with heart block. It is contraindicated in patients who have QT interval prolongation on the electrocardiogram (ECG) or who are in the recovery phase of a myocardial infarction (MI). The drug is metabolized in the liver and thus should be administered cautiously to patients with hepatic impairment. Patients with a history of hyperthyroidism should not be administered cyclobenzaprine.

Drug Interactions: Cyclobenzaprine should not be administered with alcohol, opioids, barbiturates, or any other CNS depressants because significant sedation may occur. Phenothiazines and anticholinergic drugs will enhance the anticholinergic adverse effects and should be used with caution with cyclobenzaprine. Use with TCAs may result in additive CNS depression and increased anticholinergic effects. A potentially fatal hypertensive crisis can occur if cyclobenzaprine is used within 14 days of a monoamine oxidase inhibitor. Serotonin syndrome has been reported when cyclobenzaprine is coadministered with other drugs that increase serotonin such as selective serotonin reuptake inhibitors (SSRIs), serotonin–norepinephrine reuptake inhibitors (SNRIs), TCAs, tramadol, bupropion, meperidine, or verapamil. **Herbal/Food:** Additive CNS depression may occur if cyclobenzaprine is administered concurrently with valerian or kava.

Pregnancy: Animal reproduction studies did not show adverse effects on embryofetal development. Adverse effects of the drug on the breastfed neonate are unknown.

Treatment of Overdose: Signs of overdose include CNS depression and tachycardia. Physostigmine (Antilirium) may be administered to reverse serious anticholinergic adverse effects. Overdose is generally not fatal.

Clinician Responsibilities: Key clinical implications for patients receiving cyclobenzaprine are included in Applied Clinical Judgment: Patients Receiving Pharmacotherapy for Muscle Spasms and Spasticity.

Drugs Similar to Cyclobenzaprine (Amrix)

The following medications are other centrally acting skeletal muscle relaxants: baclofen, carisoprodol, chlorzoxazone, deutetrabenazine, metaxalone, methocarbamol, orphenadrine, tetrabenazine, and tizanidine.

Baclofen (Gablofen, Lioresal, Ozobax): Approved in 1977, baclofen is used to reduce muscle spasticity in patients with injury or disease of upper motor neurons associated with MS, CP, ALS, and spinal cord trauma. Off-label indications include the treatment of tardive dyskinesia related to long-term pharmacotherapy with antipsychotic drugs, and persistent hiccups and for management of neuropathic pain. The drug is an agonist of the inhibitory neurotransmitter gamma aminobutyric acid (GABA). Baclofen is usually administered PO and a new oral solution (Ozobax) was approved in 2019.

Baclofen can be administered by intrathecal injection or infusion (Gablofen, Lioresal). Delivered directly into the intrathecal space, using a small catheter and a pump, this provides a direct route for the baclofen to reach its target sites in the spinal cord and brain. The pump must be refilled every 1 to 3 months and the battery lasts 5 to 7 years. Several months of therapy may be required to achieve full therapeutic benefit from baclofen.

Adverse effects related to the administration of baclofen include drowsiness, dizziness, weakness, and fatigue. Intrathecal baclofen carries a black box warning that abrupt discontinuation may cause high fever, seizures, severe rebound muscle spasticity, altered mental status, multiple organ system failure, and death. Animal reproduction studies showed that baclofen increased fetal structural abnormalities at high doses. Baclofen is secreted in milk and withdrawal symptoms may be observed in infants when breastfeeding is stopped.

Carisoprodol (Soma): An older drug approved by the U.S. Food and Drug Administration (FDA) in 1959, carisoprodol is administered PO for the short-term therapy (up to 3 weeks) of acute, painful muscle spasms. The general sedative nature of the drug is likely responsible for its ability to relieve the pain associated with muscle spasms. The drug produces significant sedation in 40% of patients taking it and may cause CNS and respiratory depression if taken with alcohol or other CNS depressants. After many years of abuse by recreational drug users, carisoprodol was declared a Schedule IV controlled substance in 2012. The drug should be used with caution in patients with a history of substance abuse because overdose may be fatal. This medication is also available compounded with aspirin and codeine. Decades of human experience have not demonstrated increased risks for birth defects or adverse fetal outcomes. Carisoprodol is secreted in milk and breastfed infants should be observed for sedation.

Chlorzoxazone: Chlorzoxazone is a centrally acting skeletal muscle relaxant administered PO for the symptomatic treatment of discomfort associated with acute, painful musculoskeletal conditions. It is ineffective in the treatment of spasticity related to neurodegenerative disorders such as CP. The actions of the drug may be largely due to its sedative effects. It should not be combined with alcohol or other CNS depressants. Chlorzoxazone is hepatotoxic and should not be used in patients with liver impairment. Other adverse effects include anorexia, nausea and vomiting, rash, and red-orange discoloration of urine. Older adults may experience more adverse CNS effects than younger patients.

Chlorzoxazone has not been evaluated for safety during pregnancy or lactation.

Deutetrabenazine (Austedo) and Tetrabenazine (Xenazine): Deutetrabenazine (approved in 2017) and tetrabenazine (approved in 2008) have nearly identical chemical structures and are used to reduce chorea movements in patients with Huntington's chorea. They act by depleting the amounts of dopamine, serotonin, and norepinephrine at nerve terminals. The two drugs have identical actions and adverse effects except deutetrabenazine has a longer duration of action that allows once-daily dosing. Both drugs contain a black box warning regarding the risk for emergence or worsening of depression and suicidal thoughts. These drugs are contraindicated in patients who are suicidal or who have significant hepatic impairment. The drugs also prolong the QTc interval and should be used with great caution concurrently with other medications having this adverse effect. Animal reproduction studies showed that tetrabenazine increases stillbirths and postnatal mortality. Adverse effects of tetrabenazine on the breastfed neonate are unknown.

Metaxalone (Skelaxin): Approved in 1962, metaxalone is administered PO and is indicated for the symptomatic relief of muscle spasm and pain related to musculoskeletal conditions. It is ineffective in the treatment of spasticity-related neurologic disorders. The therapeutic effects of metaxalone are likely due to general CNS depression. Like chlorzoxazone, metaxalone may cause liver injury and is contraindicated in patients with significant hepatic impairment. Serotonin syndrome is possible when metaxalone is coadministered with other drugs that increase serotonin. It should not be administered to patients over age 65 due to significant anticholinergic effects. Patients should avoid concurrent use with alcohol or other CNS depressants due to additive sedative effects. Drowsiness, nausea and vomiting, and anxiety are common adverse effects. Animal reproduction studies have not indicated fetal harm or impaired fertility. Adverse effects of the drug on the breastfed neonate are unknown.

Methocarbamol (Robaxin): Approved in 1957, methocarbamol has central sedative effects that are likely responsible for its ability to induce skeletal muscle relaxation. It is used as an adjunct to physical therapy interventions. It can be administered intravenously (IV) for the treatment of tetanus or other acute musculoskeletal conditions. Methocarbamol may cause significant dizziness and sedation and should not be taken with alcohol or other CNS depressants. It is contraindicated in patients with chronic kidney disease (CKD). It should be used with caution in patients over age 65 due to significant anticholinergic effects. Animal reproduction studies have not been conducted with this drug. It is not known if methocarbamol is secreted in human milk and its effects on breastfed infants are unknown.

Orphenadrine: Orphenadrine was approved in 1959. It is administered PO or parenterally to relax skeletal muscles and reduce pain due to spasms. The drug has analgesic properties and may be administered parenterally to produce local anesthetic effects. It may be used off-label as an adjunct in the treatment of the muscular rigidity associated with Parkinson's disease. The most common side effect of orphenadrine is xerostomia. Orphenadrine is structurally very similar to diphenhydramine (Benadryl) and can cause prominent anticholinergic effects; therefore, it should not be used with other anticholinergic drugs due to the risk for additive toxicity. Although not a controlled substance, orphenadrine produces a mild to moderate euphoric effect that has led to its abuse. Animal reproduction studies have not been conducted with this drug. It is not known if orphenadrine is secreted in milk and its effects on breastfed infants are unknown.

Tizanidine (Zanaflex): Approved in 1996, tizanidine is a centrally acting alpha$_2$-adrenergic agonist that inhibits motor neurons mainly at the spinal cord level. It has no direct effect on muscle fibers. Indicated for the management of muscle spasticity, tizanidine is most effective in patients who have significantly diminished muscle tone, including spasticity related to brain or spinal cord injury or MS. Tizanidine is as effective as baclofen in treating muscle spasticity and is considered a first-line drug. One disadvantage of tizanidine is that it has a short duration of action that requires dosing every 6 to 8 hours.

The most common adverse effects of tizanidine include xerostomia, fatigue, weakness, dizziness, and drowsiness. Hypotension is common at high doses; the drug is closely related to clonidine (Catapres), which is an antihypertensive drug. Hallucinations are uncommon but patients with a history of psychosis should be carefully monitored for this adverse effect. Tizanidine is hepatotoxic and should not be used in patients with liver impairment. Older adults, especially those with CKD, may experience adverse effects such as drowsiness, dizziness, dry mouth, and asthenia. Animal studies suggest that tizanidine may cause fetal harm. It is not known if the drug is secreted in milk and its effects on breastfed infants are unknown.

CONNECTION Checkpoint 23.2

Cyclobenzaprine is very similar to the TCAs. From what you learned in Chapter 19, describe the major indications (approved and off-label) for the TCAs.

Pharmacotherapy of Muscle Spasticity

23.4 Direct-acting skeletal muscle relaxants are often used to relieve muscle spasticity.

Medications effective in the treatment of spasticity include muscle relaxants that act at the level of the CNS, neuromuscular junction, or muscle tissue. Some of the centrally acting medications used to treat muscle spasms, such as baclofen (Lioresal) and tizanidine (Zanaflex), are also effective in treating spasticity.

Dantrolene (Dantrium, Revonto) and the botulinum toxins act on skeletal muscle to relieve spasticity. These are called direct-acting muscle relaxants or antispasticity drugs. Dantrolene is the prototype for direct-acting drugs. Doses of these drugs are listed in Table 23.3. The mechanisms of action of direct-acting antispasmodics are shown in Pharmacotherapy Illustrated 23.2.

PROTOTYPE DRUG **Dantrolene (Dantrium, Revonto, Ryanodex)**

Classification **Therapeutic:** Direct-acting skeletal muscle relaxant, antispasticity drug
Pharmacologic: Calcium release blocker (skeletal muscle cells)

Therapeutic Effects and Uses: Approved in 1974, dantrolene is a direct-acting skeletal muscle relaxant indicated for spasticity, especially for spasms of the head and neck muscles following a spinal cord injury, stroke, and in cases of CP or MS. When administered PO, the drug induces relaxation of the skeletal muscles. It may be used off-label to treat malignant neuroleptic syndrome or for the treatment of pain following heavy exercise.

When administered IV, Revonto and Ryanodex are first-line drugs for treating **malignant hyperthermia**, a rare condition that is an adverse effect of succinylcholine (Anectine) and some general anesthetics. A patient with malignant hyperthermia will experience a sudden onset of tachycardia, ventricular dysrhythmia, and hypotension. This is due to the rapid release of calcium ions in muscle cells, which produces hypermetabolism and intense muscle rigidity. The muscle metabolic rate becomes so elevated that it quickly raises the body temperature to a dangerous level. There is a strong genetic predisposition to malignant hyperthermia, and patients with a family history of the disorder should not receive drugs that have the potential to cause this adverse effect. It is important for the anesthesia provider and circulating nurse to have phentolamine (Oraverse) available in the event of extravasation of dantrolene.

Mechanism of Action: Dantrolene directly relaxes spastic muscles by interfering with the release of calcium

Table 23.3 Direct-Acting Skeletal Muscle Relaxants

Drug	Route and Dose (Maximum Dose Where Indicated)	Adverse Effects
abobotulinumtoxinA (Dysport)	Cervical dystonia: IM: 500 units, in divided doses Glabellar lines: IM: 50 units given in 5 equal doses Upper-limb spasticity: IM: 100–400 units depending on muscle injected	*Injection reactions, headache, dysphagia, muscle weakness, pain, tenderness, bruising, flulike symptoms, dry mouth, ptosis of eyelids* Spread of toxin to surrounding muscles, anaphylaxis and other hypersensitivity reactions, difficulty swallowing or breathing (cervical dystonia therapy), corneal ulceration (blepharospasm therapy)
incobotulinumtoxinA (Xeomin)	Cervical dystonia: IM: 120 units Blepharospasm: IM: 10–50 units per eye in 6 injections (max: 50 units per eye) Upper-limb spasticity: IM: 5–200 units depending on muscle injected	
onabotulinumtoxinA (Botox)	Cervical dystonia: IM: 198–300 units in divided doses (max: 50 units per site) Upper-limb spasticity: IM: 75–360 units in divided doses (max: 50 units/site) Axillary hyperhidrosis: IM: 50 units per site Migraines: IM: 155 units in divided doses across specific head and neck regions (max: 5 units per site) Overactive bladder: 100–200 units across 20–30 injection sites in the detrusor muscle	
onabotulinumtoxinA (Botox Cosmetic)	Glabellar lines: IM: 20 units divided among affected muscles	
prabotulinumtoxinA (Jeuveau)	Glabellar lines: IM: 20 units divided among affected muscles	
rimabotulinumtoxinB (Myobloc)	Cervical dystonia: IM: 2500–5000 units divided among affected muscles	
dantrolene (Dantrium, Revonto, Ryanodex)	Spasticity: PO: 25 mg once daily (max: 100 mg bid–qid) Malignant hyperthermia: IV push: 1 mg/kg; repeat as needed (max: 10 mg/kg); may continue PO at 1–2 mg/kg qid for 1–3 days	*Drowsiness, dizziness, fatigue, speech disturbance, mental depression, blurred vision, photophobia, nausea and vomiting, anorexia, crystalluria, urinary retention, nocturia, enuresis, difficult erection* Hypersensitivity, muscle weakness, diarrhea, hepatitis

Note: *Italics* indicate common adverse effects. Underline indicates serious adverse effects.

Pharmacotherapy Illustrated 23.2

Mechanism of Action of Direct-Acting Antispasmodics

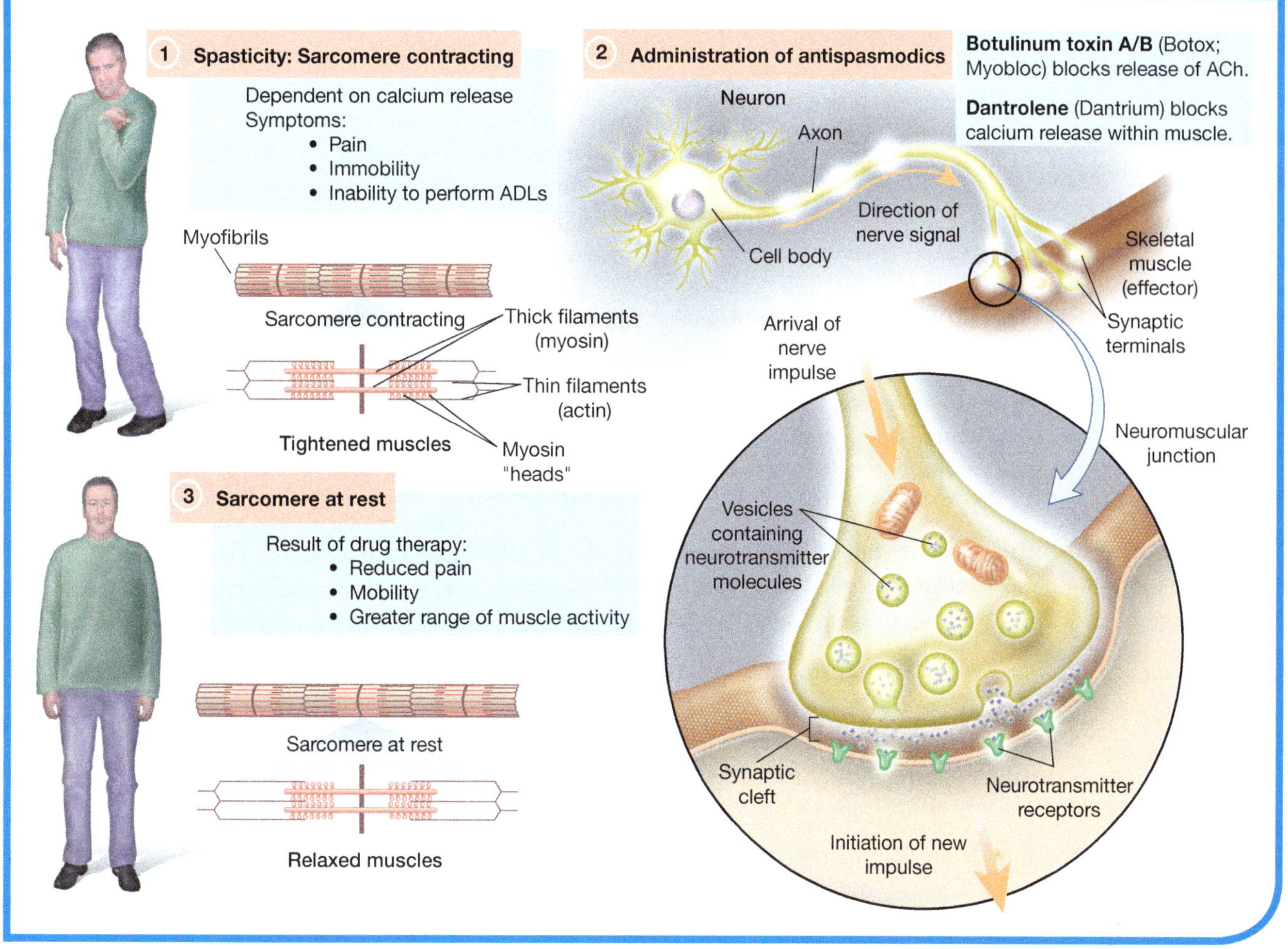

ions that have been stored in the sarcoplasmic reticulum of skeletal muscle. The relaxation of muscles results in a lowering of the core body temperature, which is critical for patients with malignant hyperthermia.

Pharmacokinetics:

Route(s)	PO, IV
Absorption	Approximately 35% is slowly and incompletely absorbed from the GI tract
Distribution	Crosses the placenta; highly bound to plasma protein
Primary metabolism	Hepatic
Primary excretion	Renal and feces
Onset of action	Peak concentration: 5 h
Duration of action	Half-life: 8.7 h (PO) or 4–8 h (IV)

Adverse Effects: Muscle weakness and drowsiness are the most common adverse effects of dantrolene therapy. Other adverse effects include xerostomia, dizziness, nausea, photosensitivity, diarrhea, tachycardia, erratic blood pressure, and urinary retention. **Black Box Warning:** Hepatitis and deaths due to liver failure have occurred in patients taking dantrolene. Baseline and periodic hepatic function tests should be conducted during therapy. The lowest possible effective dose should be used to avoid hepatotoxicity and the drug should be discontinued if no therapeutic effect is noted after 45 days of treatment.

Contraindications/Precautions: There are no contraindications to the use of dantrolene in treating malignant hyperthermia because this is a fatal condition if left untreated. For spasticity, dantrolene is contraindicated in patients with preexisting hepatic disease. Because it can cause muscle weakness, dantrolene should not be used when spasticity is necessary to sustain an upright position or balance when standing or walking. Dantrolene should be used cautiously in the presence of impaired cardiac or pulmonary function. The risk of dantrolene-induced hepatotoxicity is greatest in women over the age of 35; thus, it should be administered cautiously in these patients.

Drug Interactions: Dantrolene interacts with other CNS depressants, including alcohol, to cause additive sedation. The combination of estrogen and dantrolene in women can result in hepatotoxicity. Calcium channel blockers such as verapamil place the patient at increased risk of ventricular fibrillation and cardiovascular collapse when dantrolene sodium is administered intravenously. **Herbal/Food:** Use of kava or valerian may result in additive sedation.

Pregnancy: Animal studies suggest that dantrolene may cause fetal harm. Because this drug is secreted in milk and its effects on infants have the potential to be serious, breastfeeding is not recommended.

Treatment of Overdose: Overdose with dantrolene results in muscle weakness, lethargy, and coma. General supportive measures are administered until the effects of the drug diminish.

Clinician Responsibilities: Key clinical implications for patients receiving dantrolene are included in Applied Clinical Judgment: Patients Receiving Pharmacotherapy for Muscle Spasms and Spasticity.

Drugs Similar to Dantrolene (Dantrium)

Botulinum toxins are also direct-acting muscle relaxants.

Botulinum toxin (Botox, Botox Cosmetic, Dysport, Jeuveau, Myobloc, Xeomin): Botulinum toxin is a natural substance obtained from *Clostridium botulinum*, the gram-positive bacterium responsible for botulism. The drug blocks neuromuscular transmission by binding to motor nerve terminals and inhibiting the release of acetylcholine. Without sufficient amounts of acetylcholine, the muscle is unable to contract and flaccid paralysis occurs.

Since its initial approval by the FDA in 1989, several forms of botulinum toxin have been developed and marketed. Each of the formulations differs in potency and they may not be interchanged or substituted for each other. The botulinum products are listed in Table 23.3. Table 23.4 gives the approved indications for the products.

The first botulinum product approved was onabotulinumtoxinA (Botox, Botox Cosmetic). This formulation is approved for all indications: blepharospasm, cervical dystonia, glabellar lines (facial wrinkles; Figure 23.1), severe axillary hyperhidrosis (axillary perspiration), upper-limb spasticity, strabismus, and chronic migraines. For each of these indications, small doses are injected into the affected muscles. The dose differs for the specific indication.

One of the newer indications for Botox is for the treatment of overactive bladder or urinary incontinence in patients with an associated neurologic condition such as MS. For these indications, the drug is injected directly into the detrusor muscle of the bladder through a cystoscope. A single administration of Botox requires injections at 20 to 30 sites in the detrusor muscle, which may be repeated every 6 to 12 weeks. This therapy is approved only if therapy with an anticholinergic drug has been unsuccessful.

Because of the extreme weakness associated with botulinum, therapies may be needed to improve muscle strength. To circumvent major problems with mobility or posture, administration of botulinum toxin is often limited to the small muscle groups. Sometimes this drug is administered with centrally acting PO medications to increase the functional mobility range of muscle groups.

In general, botulinum therapy is well tolerated, and adverse effects are related to the dose injected in each muscle. The drug can cause significant pain when it is injected into the muscle. The severity of pain experienced can be blocked by the administration of a local anesthetic. The therapeutic effects of botulinum therapy are effective within 6 weeks and last for 3 to 6 months. All botulinum toxin formulations carry a black box warning that the drug may spread to distant muscles, resulting in a risk for asthenia, generalized muscle weakness, diplopia, blurred vision,

Table 23.4 Indications for Botulinum Toxin

	Axillary Hyperhidrosis	Blepharospasm	Cervical Dystonia	Chronic Migraine	Glabellar Lines	Overactive Bladder	Strabismus	Upper-Limb Spasticity
abobotulinumtoxinA (Dysport)			X		X			X
incobotulinumtoxinA (Xeomin)		X	X		X			X
onabotulinumtoxinA (Botox)	X	X	X	X		X	X	X
onabotulinumtoxinA (Botox Cosmetic)					X			
prabotulinumtoxinA (Jeuveau)					X			
rimabotulinumtoxinB (Myobloc)			X					

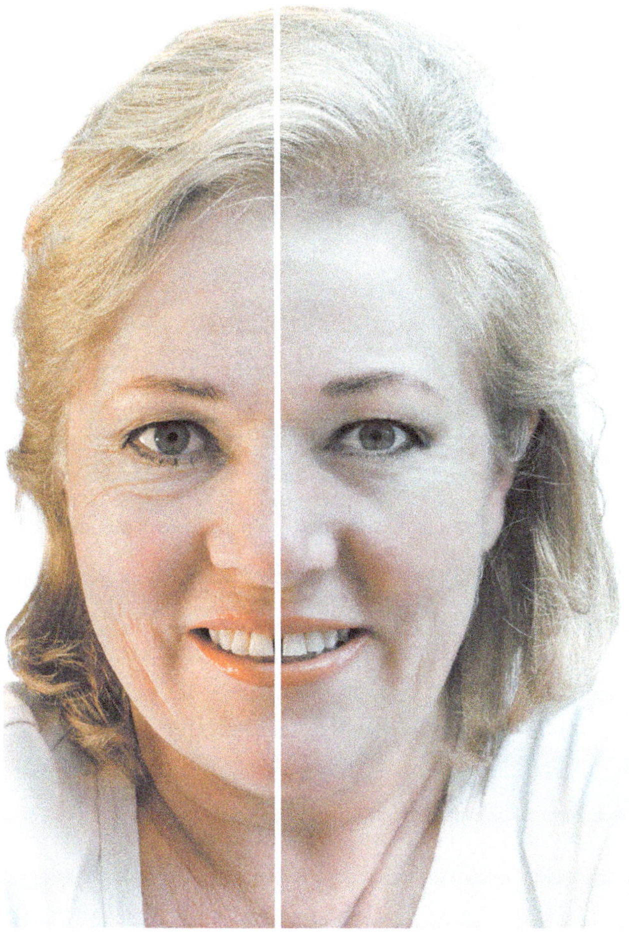

Figure 23.1 Botox therapy: (left) before treatment; (right) after treatment.
Jo Ann Snover/Shutterstock.

dysphagia, dysphonia, urinary incontinence, and breathing difficulties. Swallowing and breathing difficulties can be life-threatening. These effects may occur hours or weeks after treatment. The risk is highest for children. Animal studies suggest that botulinum toxin may cause fetal harm. It is not known if the drug is secreted in milk and its effects during lactation or on breastfed infants are unknown.

CONNECTION Checkpoint 23.3

Myasthenia gravis is a serious skeletal muscular disorder, but it does not result in spasticity. From what you learned in Chapter 13, what are the symptoms of this disorder and what is the primary pharmacotherapy?

23.5 Novel Drug Therapies Show Promise for Treating Muscular Dystrophy.

Muscular dystrophy (MD) is a rare genetic disorder in which patients (usually boys) are born with a mutation for making dystrophin. Dystrophin is a protein that protein that surrounds skeletal muscle like a skin, protecting the muscle from damage during contraction. Without a properly functioning dystrophin protein, muscle cells become damaged and eventually die.

Two new drugs "skip" over the mutation and allow dystrophin to be produced by MD patients. Golodirsen (Vyondys 53) and vitolarsen (Viltepso) were approved in 2020, and act by a process called exon skipping. There are many different dystrophin mutations and these drugs are effective only against one type. Much research remains to be done before a cure can be found for this devastating disorder.

Skeletal Muscle Relaxants as Surgical Adjuncts

23.6 Skeletal muscle relaxants are administered during surgery in combination with anesthetic agents.

During certain surgical procedures it is necessary to produce total skeletal muscle relaxation in the patient. Skeletal muscle relaxants such as succinylcholine (Anectine) and tubocurarine are administered in combination with general anesthetics

CONNECTIONS: Advanced Practice Application

Botox Administration by Nurse Practitioners

Botulinum toxins such as Botox have earned a place in the treatment of cosmetic conditions as well as more serious medical conditions such as cervical dystonia. The drug is not without risk despite its popularity and, as such, states regulate who may administer Botox and other botulinum toxins. Regulations may be defined by the state's Nurse Practice Act, the Board of Medicine, or both. Some states may allow a nurse to independently practice aesthetics after appropriate training and certification, while that practice may need to occur under a supervising physician in other states. To determine the most current regulations, the Board of Nursing and/or Medicine is the best place to begin before attending training to practice aesthetics.

States where NPs can prescribe and inject Botox without any physician involvement: AK, AZ, DC, IA, ME, MT, NH, NM, OR, UT, WA, WI, WY

States where NPs can prescribe Botox with some degree of physician involvement: AR, CA, CO, CT, DE, FL, GA, HI, ID, IL, IN, KS, MA, MI, MN, NC, ND, NE, NJ, NY, OK, PA, RI, SC, SD, TN, VT, WV

States where NPs can prescribe (excluding controlled substances) with some degree of physician involvement: AL, KY, LA, MO, MS, NV, OH, TX, VA to induce skeletal muscle relaxation, which aids in intubation and other invasive procedures. These drugs are also administered to facilitate endoscopy, to enhance the management of mechanical ventilation, and to control the severity of muscle contractions resulting from electroshock therapy.

The skeletal muscle relaxants used as surgical adjuncts have the ability to produce complete muscle paralysis; thus, mechanical ventilation may be necessary. Continuous monitoring is required. Most of these drugs have very rapid onsets of action and brief half-lives; drug effects rapidly diminish following the surgical procedure.

The skeletal muscle relaxants used as surgical adjuncts are presented in Chapter 14. A prototype feature for succinylcholine can be found in that chapter.

CONNECTIONS: APPLIED CLINICAL JUDGMENT

Patients Receiving Pharmacotherapy for Muscle Spasms and Spasticity

Key Assessment Data

- History of current condition, baseline vital signs, physical exam findings; history of cardiovascular, hepatic, or musculoskeletal disease; medication and allergy history; mental status as appropriate; pregnancy or breastfeeding status.
- Obtain a history of current symptoms, exacerbating conditions, and ability to carry out ADLs, particularly related to mobility. Note if the condition is related to a work-related injury.
- If present, assess the level of pain. Use objective screening tools when possible (e.g., FLACC [face, limbs, arms, cry, consolability] for infants or very young children, Wong-Baker FACES Pain Rating Scale for children, numerical rating scale for adults). Assess the history of pain associated with muscle spasms and what has or has not worked for the patient in the past.
- Ongoing assessment during drug therapy includes laboratory findings such as hepatic and renal function studies.
- Improvement should be observed over the first week or two of therapy. Assessment of range of motion (ROM) and drug effects on muscle tenderness and rigidity will help to determine the effectiveness of the drug therapy.

Desired Therapeutic Outcomes

Improvement is observed and measurable in decreased muscle spasm, rigidity, decreased pain, increased ROM, and increased ability to complete ADLs.

Minimizing Adverse Effects

- Drug therapy may take several days before improvement is noted. Providing support to the patient for self-care activities may be needed to prevent injury until improvement is observed.
- Muscle-relaxant drugs may cause drowsiness and dizziness, orthostatic hypotension, or impaired mental and physical abilities, increasing the risk of falls and injury. Continue to monitor vital signs, mental status, coordination, and balance periodically. Ensure patient safety; monitor ambulation until effects of the drug are known.
- Cyclobenzaprine may cause tachycardia and palpitations. Continue to monitor vital signs, particularly blood pressure and pulse. Take the blood pressure lying, sitting, and standing to detect orthostatic hypotension.
- Pain control may be supplemented by supportive nursing measures such as positional support, gentle massage, and moist heat or ice packs.
- Muscle relaxants and antispasmodic drugs may cause hepatotoxicity as an adverse effect Continue to monitor renal and hepatic function periodically if the patient is on long-term use of the drug.
- Muscle-relaxant drugs may decrease peristalsis as an adverse effect. Assess bowel sounds periodically if constipation or diarrhea is problematic. Increase fluid and dietary fiber intake to prevent GI effects and to ease dry mouth effects. Significantly diminished or absent bowel sounds should be reported to the healthcare provider.
- CNS depressants and alcohol may increase sedative properties of the drug. Antihypertensive medication may increase risk of hypotension. Avoid the use of other CNS depressants, including alcohol, and use with caution with antihypertensive medications given concurrently.
- While rare, cyclobenzaprine may cause swelling of the tongue or face and should be reported immediately.
- Muscle relaxants and antispasmodics may cause urinary retention as an adverse effect. Assess for urinary retention periodically.

Lifespan Considerations

- The older adult may be at increased risk for falls due to drowsiness, dizziness, and orthostatic hypotension. Particular care with ambulation is required because pain, spasms, or rigidity may also increase the risk of falls. Cyclobenzaprine is included in the Beers list of potentially inappropriate drugs for older adults and warrants careful monitoring.
- Women over the age of 35 taking these drugs are at greater risk for hepatotoxicity and should be monitored more frequently.
- The older adult is at increased risk of constipation due to slowed peristalsis. Additional fluids and fiber may ease constipation and prevent diarrhea, but additional medications such as MiraLAX may be needed.
- Older adult men with an enlarged prostate are at higher risk for mechanical obstruction. Assess for urinary retention periodically. Report an inability to void, increasing bladder pressure, or pain.
- Patients who are breastfeeding should talk with their provider about whether there is a need to stop nursing and pump breasts, discarding the milk, and using alternative feedings while on these drugs.

CONNECTIONS: APPLIED CLINICAL JUDGMENT *(continued)*

Patients Receiving Pharmacotherapy for Muscle Spasms and Spasticity

Patient and Caregiver Education

- Gradual improvement may be noted over several days and full therapeutic effects may take 1 week or longer. Nonpharmacologic measures and supportive measures may be needed until the full medication effect is noted.
- Rise from lying or sitting to standing slowly to avoid dizziness or falls. If dizziness occurs, sit or lie down and do not attempt to stand or walk until the sensation passes. Avoid driving or other activities requiring mental alertness or physical coordination until the effects of the drug are known.
- Call for assistance prior to getting out of bed or attempting to walk alone if pain, spasms, or rigidity are particularly severe.
- Complementary pain interventions such as positioning, gentle massage, application of heat or cold to the painful area, distraction with television or music, or guided imagery may supplement medication effects. Perform gentle ROM exercises, and exercise only to the point of mild physical discomfort but never pain, throughout the day.
- Consider the need for additional healthcare referrals if disability will require long-term physical therapy (e.g., CP) and discuss with the provider. Evaluate home safety needs.
- Increase fluids to 2 L/day and increase intake of dietary fiber such as fruits, vegetables, and whole grains to ease constipation and prevent dry mouth. Report severe constipation to the healthcare provider for additional advice on laxatives or stool softeners.
- If cyclobenzaprine is used, immediately report any swelling of the tongue, face, or throat to the provider. Seek immediate medical attention if breathing is impaired.
- Avoid alcohol and other CNS depressants while taking the drug. If other sedatives or antihypertensives are ordered, consult with the healthcare provider about dose and sequencing. Immediately report any dizziness, palpitations, or syncope.
- Report an inability to void, increasing bladder pressure, or pain.
- Pregnant or breastfeeding patients should consult the provider about recommendations to discontinue breastfeeding while on the drug, dependent on the drug used. If so, alternative feeding plans may be discussed.
- Take the drug consistently as ordered and not prn for best results, unless otherwise ordered. Maintain a medication log, noting symptoms along with dose and timing of medications, and bring the log to each healthcare visit.
- Do not open, chew, or crush extended-release tablets (e.g., cyclobenzaprine); swallow them whole with plenty of water.
- Take the drug with food or milk if stomach upset occurs.

Prescribing Considerations

- Benzodiazepines should generally be avoided in the older adult because of an increased risk of cognitive impairment, delirium, falls, and fractures.
- Starting at a low dose and titrating up slowly to the maximum daily dose is recommended to minimize side effects.
- Ongoing assessment during drug therapy includes laboratory findings such as hepatic and renal function studies.

Understanding Chapter 23

Key Concepts Summary

23.1 Whereas muscle spasms are often caused by overuse of skeletal muscle, muscle spasticity involves damage to motor nerves.

23.2 Nonpharmacologic interventions for treating muscle spasms and spasticity are limited.

23.3 Nonsteroidal anti-inflammatory drugs and skeletal muscle relaxants are used to treat muscle spasms.

23.4 Direct-acting skeletal muscle relaxants are often used to relieve muscle spasticity.

23.5 New drug therapies are used to correct mutations in muscular dystrophy.

23.6 Skeletal muscle relaxants are administered during surgery in combination with anesthetic agents.

CASE STUDY: Making the Patient Connection

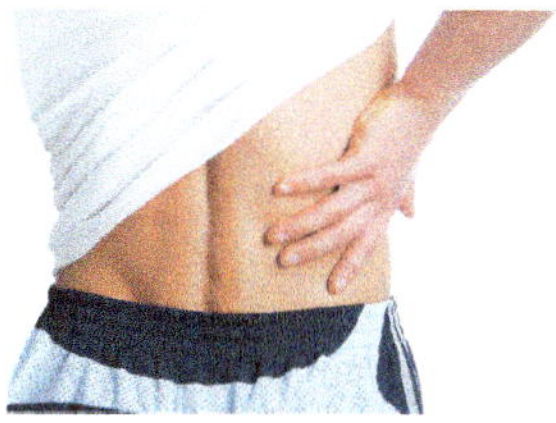

Remember the patient "Andrew Eskew" at the beginning of the chapter? Now read the remainder of the case study. Based on the information presented within this chapter, respond to the critical thinking questions that follow.

Andrew is a 27-year-old landscaper who was building a rock wall yesterday. His job requires lifting, bending, and twisting. On arising today, he stated that his back hurts and he cannot move from side to side. The nurse has performed a physical assessment on Andrew, which revealed tightened muscles in the lumbosacral region and limited mobility. The patient describes his pain as a level 7 on a scale of 1 to 10.

Critical Thinking Questions

1. What are the etiology and pathophysiology of Andrew's muscle spasms? What are other possible causes of muscle spasms?
2. Andrew has been prescribed cyclobenzaprine (Amrix) to relieve his back spasms. What is the action of this medication and why has it been prescribed?
3. What should Andrew be instructed regarding the administration of this medication?

Additional Case Study

A 46-year-old woman is diagnosed with cervical dystonia. She has difficulty maintaining normal head position and reports neck pain. She is to start on botulinum therapy.

1. What is the action of and rationale for administering onabotulinumtoxinA?
2. Create a list of adverse effects that this patient may experience due to botulinum therapy.

Chapter Review

1. A 67-year-old patient experienced a severe back strain while lifting groceries from his car. He is given a prescription for cyclobenzaprine (Amrix). The nurse will include what precautions in the teaching plan for this patient? (Select all that apply.)
   1. Report any palpitations or rapid pulse rate immediately.
   2. Take frequent walks throughout the day to relieve soreness.
   3. Rinse the mouth frequently with an alcohol-based mouthwash to relieve excess secretions.
   4. Be cautious with driving or other activities requiring alertness.
   5. Immediately report any facial or tongue swelling.
2. A patient with spastic cerebral palsy is being treated with oral baclofen (Lioresal). Which patient statement indicates the need for more teaching?
   1. "I will be cautious about activities because I may feel weak."
   2. "It may take several months before I experience the full effects of the drug."
   3. "If I experience unpleasant side effects, I can stop taking the drug."
   4. "I will be sure to get enough fluid and fiber in my diet."
3. A patient has been taught to apply capsaicin to increase mobility and relieve pain. Which instruction is most important for the nurse to give to this patient?
   1. Apply the medication liberally above and below the site of pain.
   2. Apply with a gloved hand only to the site of pain.
   3. Apply to areas of redness and inflammation.
   4. Apply liberally with a bare hand.
4. A patient has been treated for cervical dystonia with an injection of onabotulinumtoxinA (Botox). Which of the following will the nurse teach the patient to immediately report?
   1. Fever, aches, or chills
   2. Difficulty swallowing, blurred vision, or ptosis
   3. Moderate levels of muscle weakness on the affected side
   4. Continuous spasms and pain on the affected side
5. A patient has been taking cyclobenzaprine (Amrix) for muscle spasms. The patient is admitted to the emergency department with severe CNS depression. Which medication will the nurse expect to be ordered and administered?
   1. Naloxone (Narcan)
   2. Meperidine (Demerol)
   3. Diazepam (Valium)
   4. Physostigmine (Antilirium)

6. A female patient, age 45, is receiving dantrolene (Dantrium) for treatment of painful muscle spasms associated with multiple sclerosis. What will the nurse teach the patient? (Select all that apply.)

1. Increase fluid and fiber intake to prevent constipation.
2. Inform the healthcare provider if taking estrogen products.
3. Sip water or suck on ice chips or hard candy to relieve xerostomia.
4. Be sure to obtain 20 minutes of sun exposure per day to boost vitamin D levels.
5. Return periodically to the provider to monitor liver function.

See Appendix A for answers to critical thinking questions, case study questions and review questions.

References

Khan, F., Amatya, B., Bensmail, D., & Yelnik, A. (2019). Non-pharmacological interventions for spasticity in adults: An overview of systematic reviews. *Annals of Physical and Rehabilitation Medicine*, *62*(4), 265–273. https://doi.org/10.1016/j.rehab.2017.10.001

Selected Bibliography

Abel-Hamid, H. Z. (2018). *Cerebral palsy: Background.* Medscape. http://emedicine.medscape.com/article/1179555-overview#aw2aab6b2b2

Bhimani, R., Medina, F., & Carney-Anderson, L. (2018). CE: Managing movement disorders: A clinical review. *American Journal of Nursing*, *118*(12), 34–40. https://doi.org/10.1097/01.NAJ.0000549666.20957.a3

Carlson, B., & Wormuth, L. (2019). Malignant hyperthermia: An overview. *US Pharmacist*, *44*(1), HS2–HS6.

Cohen, R. I., & Warfield, C. A. (2015). Role of muscle relaxants in the treatment of pain. In T. R. Deer, M. S. Leong, & G. Vitaly (Eds.), *Treatment of chronic pain by medical approaches* (pp. 67–75). New York: Springer. https://doi.org/10.1007/978-1-4939-1818-8_7

Jabbari, B. (2018). Botulinum toxin therapy for complications of stroke. In *Botulinum toxin treatment* (pp. 63–74). Springer. https://doi.org/10.1007/978-3-319-99945-6_6

Moberg-Wolff, E. A. (2018). *Dystonias*. Medscape. http://emedicine.medscape.com/article/312648-overview#a1

Peters, C., & Sineath Jr., M. H. (2020). Do muscle relaxants improve low back pain in adults? *Evidence-Based Practice*, *23*(5), 25–26. https://doi.org/10.1097/EBP.0000000000000673

Simpson, D. M., Hallett, M., Ashman, E. J., Comella, C. L., Green, M. W., Gronseth, G. S., et al. (2019). Muscular cramp: causes and management. *European Journal of Neurology*, *26*(2), 214–221. https://doi.org/10.1111/ene.13799

Vitrikas, K., Dalton, H., & Breish, D. (2020). Cerebral palsy: An overview. *American Family Physician*, *101*(4), 213–220.

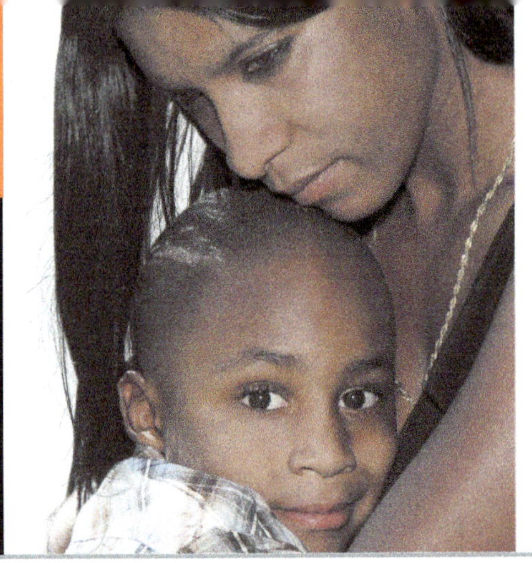

"The school nurse recommended we consider Adderall for Jonathon. He's just doing poorly in school and hates to do his homework. Why would he need a drug for that?"
—*Patient "Jonathon Hogan's" mother*

Chapter 24
Central Nervous System Stimulants and Drugs for Attention-Deficit/ Hyperactivity Disorder

Chapter Outline

Learning Outcomes

After reading the chapter, the student should be able to:

1. Describe the general actions and pharmacotherapeutic applications of central nervous system stimulants.
2. Identify the signs and symptoms of attention-deficit/hyperactivity disorder and narcolepsy.
3. Compare and contrast the central nervous system stimulants and nonstimulants in treating attention-deficit/hyperactivity disorder.
4. Describe the role of stimulant medication in the treatment of narcolepsy.
5. Describe the nurse's role in the pharmacologic management of attention-deficit/hyperactivity disorder and narcolepsy.
6. For each class shown in the chapter outline, identify the prototype and representative drugs and explain the mechanism(s) of drug action, primary indications, contraindications, significant drug interactions, pregnancy data and important adverse effects.
7. Apply clinical judgment to care for patients receiving pharmacotherapy with central nervous system stimulants.

Key Terms

Definitions of the terms in bold may be found in the Glossary.

The central nervous system (CNS) stimulants are a small group of drugs that have limited pharmacotherapeutic applications. Attention-deficit/hyperactivity disorder (ADHD) and narcolepsy are conditions that diminish mental alertness and that may benefit from treatment with these medications. Some of the CNS stimulants such as cocaine and methamphetamine are widely abused. The purpose of this chapter is to examine the actions and pharmacotherapeutic applications of the CNS stimulants.

Characteristics of Central Nervous System Stimulants

24.1 Central nervous system stimulants increase alertness, enhance the ability to concentrate, and delay the symptoms of fatigue.

The **central nervous system (CNS) stimulants** are a diverse group of pharmacologic agents that range from widely accessible substances such as caffeine to Schedule I controlled substances such as Ecstasy. All CNS stimulants have the common action of raising the general alertness level of the brain. Wakefulness and the ability to focus or concentrate are increased. Mood is often elevated, and the individual may temporarily become unaware of physical fatigue. For some of the controlled substances, mood elevation may progress to **euphoria**, an intense sense of happiness and well-being.

Because people generally view the sensations associated with CNS stimulation as desirable, many are driven to repeat the pleasurable experience. With continued use, physical and psychologic dependence occur. Because of this, many CNS stimulants are highly regulated as scheduled drugs (Table 24.1).

Not all effects of these drugs on the CNS are pleasurable. Stimulants have the potential to cause serious adverse effects due to excessive excitation. Nervousness, dizziness, and irritability are common, and convulsions may occur at higher doses. Most of the stimulants also affect the cardiovascular system and can increase heart rate and cause dysrhythmias. Loss of appetite, or anorexia, occurs with some of the CNS stimulants.

Some medications produce CNS excitation as an adverse effect. For example, antihistamines and pseudoephedrine are taken to treat allergy and cold symptoms but may cause CNS stimulation and insomnia in some patients. Albuterol (Proventil) inhalers are used for asthma, but the drug may cause nervousness, tremors, and anxiety. Drugs that normally cause CNS depression, such as antidepressants, may cause paradoxical CNS excitement, especially in the very young or very old. Occasionally, drugs are purposefully taken in large amounts for their CNS stimulation adverse effects. For example, the primary over-the-counter (OTC) drug for treating cough, dextromethorphan, is abused by teenagers and can cause dizziness, restlessness, hallucinations, and seizures when taken in very high amounts. Additional information on the substance abuse aspects of the CNS stimulants is presented in Chapter 27.

The therapeutic applications of the CNS stimulants are limited. These include the following:

- ADHD
- Narcolepsy
- Weight management
- Stimulation of respiration
- Migraines.

If CNS stimulants elevate mood, why are they not used to treat major depressive disorder? In fact, CNS stimulants

Table 24.1 Central Nervous System Stimulants That Are Scheduled Drugs

Schedule	Central Nervous System Stimulants
I	3,4-methylenedioxymethamphetamine (MDMA, Ecstasy), 4-methylaminorex (U4EUH), aminorex, cathinone (constituent of Khat plant), fenethylline (Captagon), mephedrone, methcathinone (CAT),
II	amphetamine (Adderall, Dexedrine), cocaine (Crack), lisdexamfetamine (Vyvanse), methamphetamine (Desoxyn, ICE, Speed)), methylphenidate (Concerta, Daytrana, Focalin, Methylin, Ritalin), phenmetrazine (Preludin)
III	benzphetamine (Didrex, Ineptly), chlorphentermine, clortermine (Voranil), dronabinol (Marinol, Synthetic THC), phendimetrazine (Plegine, Prelu-2)
IV	armodafinil (Nuvigil), cathine (constituent of Khat plant, norpseudoephedrine), diethylpropion (Tenuate), fencamfamine (Reactivan), fenproporex (Gacilin), mazindol (Sanorex), mefenorex, modafinil (Provigil), phentermine (Adipex, Fastin), pipradrol
V	pyrovalerone (Centroton)

From Lists of: Scheduling Actions, Controlled Substances and Regulated Chemicals, U.S. Department of Justice, Drug Enforcement Administration, 2020. Retrieved from http://www.deadiversion.usdoj.gov/schedules/orangebook/orangebook.pdf

have been used in the past to treat major depression. CNS stimulants, however, are nonselective in their CNS actions; the excitement produced by these drugs affects all parts of the brain. They produce many potentially serious adverse effects, including physical and psychologic dependence. The atypical antidepressants and the selective serotonin reuptake inhibitors (SSRIs) are more effective and safer than stimulants in the treatment of depression. These drugs are able to elevate mood without causing CNS excitation.

PharmFACT

Approximately 77% of children 4 to 17 years of age diagnosed with ADHD are receiving treatment for the disorder. About 30% are receiving medication alone, 32% receive both medication combined with behavioral therapy. About 23% of children with the disorder are not receiving either medication for ADHD or mental health counseling (Centers for Disease Control and Prevention [CDC], 2019).

Etiology and Pathophysiology of Attention-Deficit/Hyperactivity Disorder

24.2 Attention-deficit/hyperactivity disorder is characterized by inattention, hyperactivity, and impulsive behavior.

Attention-deficit/hyperactivity disorder (ADHD) is a neuropsychiatric condition that may present in early childhood and extend into adulthood. It is characterized by symptoms of impulsive behavior, lack of attention, and hyperactivity. To receive a diagnosis of ADHD, a patient must exhibit symptoms of inattention and hyperactivity, as listed in Table 24.2 (CDC, 2020).

Table 24.2 Symptoms That May Lead to a Diagnosis of Attention-Deficit/Hyperactivity Disorder

Inattention

1. Often does not give close attention to details or makes careless mistakes in schoolwork, workplace, or other activities.
2. Often has trouble keeping attention on tasks or play activities.
3. Often does not seem to listen when spoken to directly.
4. Often does not follow instructions and fails to finish schoolwork, chores, or duties in the workplace (not due to oppositional behavior or failure to understand instructions).
5. Often has trouble organizing activities.
6. Often avoids, dislikes, or does not want to do things that take a lot of mental effort for a prolonged period of time (such as schoolwork or homework).
7. Often loses things needed for tasks and activities (e.g., toys, school assignments, pencils, books, or tools).
8. Is often easily distracted.
9. Is often forgetful in daily activities.

Hyperactivity and Impulsivity

1. Often fidgets with hands or feet or squirms in seat.
2. Often gets up from seat inappropriately in school or workplace.
3. Often runs about or climbs when and where it is not appropriate (adolescents or adults may feel very restless).
4. Often has trouble playing or enjoying leisure activities quietly.
5. Is often uncomfortable or restless when standing or sitting for extended period of time.
6. Often talks excessively.
7. Often blurts out answers before questions have been finished.
8. Often has trouble waiting one's turn.
9. Often interrupts or intrudes on others (e.g., butts into conversations or games).

Symptoms of ADHD such as impulsive behavior, distractibility, lack of attention, and hyperactivity during the school-age years can lead to poor performance and lack of interest in school activities. The symptoms of inattention and hyperactivity also contribute to difficulty with peer and family relationships. Hyperactive children usually have increased motor activity with impulsivity and a tendency to interrupt at inappropriate times. This behavior can result in disciplinary action by teachers and parents. Some additional symptoms noted include difficulty remembering details and the placement of personal items, changing tasks without completing prior tasks, and disturbances in sleep.

Symptoms continue into adulthood in 35 to 55% of individuals diagnosed with childhood ADHD. Symptoms in adults include impulsiveness, restlessness, low tolerance for frustration, chronic boredom, short temper, quitting jobs abruptly, personal relationship problems, and multiple driving violations. Adults with ADHD are more likely to exhibit mood disorders such as depression, bipolar disorder, or substance abuse disorders. Adult ADHD is treated with the same therapies as childhood ADHD.

Considerable attention has focused on the causes of ADHD, and it is clear that the etiology is complex and involves multiple variables. Studies on twins have indicated that genetics is an important contributor to the development of ADHD. An identical twin has over 80% probability of presenting with ADHD if his or her twin has been diagnosed with the disorder, and about 25% of families with a member diagnosed with ADHD will have other relatives also diagnosed. This percentage is significantly higher than the general population, which is approximately 5%.

Brain injury has been studied as a contributing factor in the development of ADHD because some children who experience head trauma will exhibit symptoms of the disorder. The percentage of brain injuries that lead to a diagnosis of ADHD is small but remains relevant in assessing for the condition as the patient ages.

Environmental agents such as lead can contribute to the development of ADHD in children. Children living in buildings built prior to 1972 have a higher risk of developing lead poisoning. Other environmental agents that contribute to the development of ADHD include alcohol and cigarette smoking by the mother during pregnancy. Food additives and sugar intake by the child have been implicated as causes of ADHD, but research studies have failed to find strong links.

Differences are seen in the anatomy and physiology of children with ADHD and control participants. Children with a known diagnosis of ADHD possess a smaller brain volume in the frontal lobes, temporal gray matter, caudate nucleus, and cerebellum. These children also have a deficiency in the catecholamines dopamine and norepinephrine. The brain of a child with ADHD also has decreased development in the area of self-regulation. This factor yields the development of symptoms such as irritability, aggression, learning disability, and motor disorders when the child is stimulated.

CONNECTIONS: Treating the Diverse Patient

Attention-Deficit/Hyperactivity Disorder and Athletics

ADHD treatment within the athletic population presents a unique challenge. For the athlete with ADHD, sports are a natural outlet and help fulfill the need to be physically active. But ADHD, and the drugs used to treat the condition, may significantly affect how an athlete performs and responds to injury, as well as increasing the risk for certain conditions such as hypertension, stroke, myocardial infarction, heat illness, and mental disorders such as paranoid psychosis (Pujalte et al., 2019). It has also been noted that signs and symptoms of a concussion are not exhibited in individuals with ADHD in the same manner as a non-ADHD individual, and some concussion-like symptoms may be present even in the absence of a concussion in individuals without ADHD (Cook et al., 2019; Iverson et al., 2016; Stewman et al., 2018).

The National Collegiate Athletic Association (NCAA), World Anti-Doping Agency, and the International Olympic Committee regulate the use of psychostimulants for treatment of ADHD due to their performance-enhancing effects (NCAA, 2020; Stewman et al., 2018). Potential performance enhancements include improved concentration and attention to tasks, increased aggression, decreased pain perception, and euphoria (Pujalte et al., 2019). For these reasons, stimulant medications are considered banned substances, or may be used only tight regulations (NCAA, 2020; Stewman et al., 2018). When they are absolutely needed by the athlete, their use requires the institution to maintain documentation on file, including a medical exception request, a written report of the medical evaluation conducted to support the diagnosis of ADHD, and medical treatment notes from the prescribing provider.

ADHD is a condition recognized by the American with Disabilities Act (ADA; n.d.) and reasonable accommodations must be made when possible.

Pharmacotherapy of Attention-Deficit/Hyperactivity Disorder

24.3 Psychostimulants are central nervous system stimulants indicated for the treatment of ADHD and narcolepsy.

Medications used to treat patients with ADHD are simply classified as either stimulants or nonstimulants. Stimulants account for 70 to 80% of drugs taken for this disorder. The nonstimulants were not developed until 2003 and generally have a longer duration of action with fewer adverse effects. Successful treatment of ADHD usually requires a combination of pharmacotherapy and behavioral therapies.

The most frequently prescribed medications for ADHD are CNS stimulants: amphetamines and amphetamine-like drugs. During the 1920s, amphetamines were used to treat asthma, hay fever, and the common cold. Amphetamine use became widespread in World War II because these drugs were able to keep soldiers alert and delay fatigue during combat. Amphetamines were not listed as scheduled substances until 1970. Amphetamine sulfate has been used to make several other salts that have psychoactive properties, including methamphetamine and Ecstasy (methylenedioxymethamphetamine or MDMA), an illegal substance used to induce euphoria.

CONNECTION Checkpoint 24.1

The older adult may experience different responses to drugs related to the aging process or to adverse effects of drug therapy. From what you learned in Chapter 10, what symptoms might be anticipated in an older adult taking CNS stimulants and what action should the nurse take if they occur?

Amphetamine exists in two closely related but distinct chemical forms: d-amphetamine (dextroamphetamine) and l-amphetamine (levoamphetamine). When using the term *amphetamine*, it is understood that the drug is a combination of the d- and l-forms (called a racemic mixture). The d-form, dextroamphetamine, is marketed separately as Dexedrine. The psychostimulants approved for ADHD include methylphenidate, dextroamphetamine, dexmethylphenidate, and lisdexamfetamine. Doses of these drugs are listed in Table 24.3.

Despite the name *psychostimulant*, these drugs do not act by stimulating the brain in a patient with ADHD. Instead, they increase attention and enhance the child's ability to focus on tasks and improve learning. Significant improvement in academic performance and in peer and family relationships is common. When used appropriately for ADHD, these drugs do not cause euphoria, and dependence has not been a serious problem. Studies have demonstrated that the use of CNS stimulants in childhood does not lead to an

Table 24.3 Central Nervous System Stimulants and Drugs for Attention-Deficit/Hyperactivity Disorder and Narcolepsy

Drug	Route and Dose (Maximum Dose Where Indicated)	Adverse Effects
Amphetamines and Amphetamine-Like Drugs		
amphetamine and dextroamphetamine (Adderall, Adderall XR)	Child ages 3–5: PO: 2.5 mg 1–2 times/day (max: 40 mg/day) Child ages 6–12: PO: 5–10 mg daily to bid (max: 40 mg/day) Adult: PO (extended release): 20 mg once daily (max: 40 mg/day)	*Irritability, dizziness, palpitations, euphoria, insomnia, tachycardia, weight loss, application site reactions (Daytrana)* Sudden death, dependence, psychosis, seizures, growth suppression, priapism, psychiatric reactions including mania and psychoses
dexmethylphenidate (Focalin, Focalin XR)	PO (regular release): 2.5 mg bid (max: 20 mg/day) PO (extended release): 10 mg once daily (max: 20 mg/day)	
lisdexamfetamine (Vyvanse)	PO: 30 mg once daily (max: 70 mg/day)	
methylphenidate (Adhansia XR, Aptensio XR, Concerta, Cotempla XR-ODT, Daytrana, Jornay PM, Metadate CD, Methylin ER, Mydayis, Ritalin, QuilliChew ER, Quillivant XR)	Narcolepsy: Adult: PO: 10 mg bid–tid ADHD: Child: PO: 5–10 mg (max: 60 mg/day) Adult: 20–30 mg (max: 60 mg/day)	
serdexmethylphenidate and dexmethylphenidate (Azstarys)	PO: 39.2 mg/7.8 mg once daily (max: 52.3 mg/10.4 mg/day)	
Nonstimulants for ADHD		
atomoxetine (Strattera)	Child less than 70 kg: PO: 0.5 mg/kg/day (max: 1.4 mg/kg or 100 mg) Adult: PO: 40 mg once daily (max: 100 mg/day)	*Headache, palpitations, decreased appetite, insomnia, irritability, fatigue, somnolence, dry mouth, upper abdominal pain, nausea and vomiting, constipation, urinary retention, cough* Suicidal ideation, severe liver injury
clonidine (Kapvay)	Child ages 6–17: PO: 0.1 mg/day (max: 4 mg/day)	*Somnolence, fatigue, upper respiratory infection, irritability, sore throat, insomnia, nightmares, emotional disorder, constipation, increased body temperature* Bradycardia, syncope, serious sedation, severe hypotension
guanfacine (Intuniv)	Child ages 6–17: PO: 1 mg/day (max: 4 mg/day)	*Sedation, abdominal pain, dizziness, mild hypotension, dry mouth, constipation* Bradycardia, syncope, serious sedation, severe hypotension
Drugs for Narcolepsy		
armodafinil (Nuvigil)	PO: 150–250 mg/day given as a single dose in the morning or 1 h prior to the start of the work shift	*Dizziness, nausea, insomnia, headache, anxiety* Stevens–Johnson syndrome (SJS), hypersensitivity, mania
modafinil (Provigil)	PO: 200 mg once daily in the morning or 1 h prior to the start of the work shift	*Headache, nausea, nervousness, rhinitis, diarrhea, back pain, anxiety, insomnia, dizziness, dyspepsia* Hypersensitivity reaction, SJS
Methylxanthines		
caffeine (Cafcit)	Neonatal apnea: PO or IV: 20–30 mg/kg as a loading dose; maintenance dose: 5 mg/kg for 10–12 days Mental alertness: PO: 100–200 mg tid–qid as needed	*Tachycardia, flushing, restlessness, insomnia, irritability, tremor, palpitations* Dysrhythmias, hypotension, seizures, circulatory failure, respiratory arrest
theophylline (Theo-24)	PO: 300–600 mg/day in divided doses (max: 900 mg/day)	

Note: *Italics* indicate common adverse effects. Underline indicates serious adverse effects.

increased incidence of alcohol, tobacco, or illicit drug use in adulthood. Psychostimulants are the most effective drugs for this disorder, reducing the symptoms of ADHD in 70 to 80% of treated children.

The stimulants have actions on both the autonomic nervous system and the CNS. Amphetamines are sympathomimetics and activate alpha- and beta-adrenergic receptors by promoting the release of norepinephrine in the autonomic nervous system (see Chapter 15). Typical symptoms of sympathetic activation caused by amphetamines include vasoconstriction, hypertension (HTN), and tachycardia.

In people without ADHD, amphetamines inhibit the reuptake of dopamine in presynaptic neurons, thereby increasing the amount of this neurotransmitter. At very high doses, amphetamines enhance the release of the neurotransmitter serotonin (5-hydroxytryptamine or 5-HT) in the brain, which is responsible for psychotic behaviors. Amphetamines are also **anorexiants**, which means that they diminish the appetite. This effect is produced by direct inhibition of the appetite center in the hypothalamus. The application of the amphetamines to the pharmacotherapy of obesity is presented in Chapter 63.

Almost from the time they were discovered, amphetamines have been abused for their stimulant effects. These drugs are often abused by those who wish to delay fatigue, for example, truck drivers, students, and healthcare workers working long shifts. Athletes may take amphetamines to increase their energy level and enhance performance. Long-term amphetamine abuse may lead to tolerance, dependence, and serious adverse effects. Amphetamine and methamphetamine are Schedule II drugs. Cocaine has similar effects as amphetamine. In fact, the signs and symptoms of cocaine abuse are indistinguishable from those of amphetamine abuse. Additional details regarding cocaine dependence are included in Chapter 27.

Overall, the psychostimulant medications for ADHD have equivalent effectiveness and very similar adverse effect profiles. Thus, the choice of stimulant and the dose are largely determined individually, by therapeutic response. Therapy is always begun with a low dose, which is gradually increased until the desired therapeutic effect is attained. For children who have difficulty swallowing medications, transdermal patches and chewable forms are available. Regardless of the medication taken, it is important for the nurse and caregiver to understand that drugs are used to *manage* the disorder, not cure it. Many children with the disorder will continue to need medication into their adult years. It is also important to note that only a few of the psychostimulants are approved for very young children, ages 3 to 5; most are for those ages 6 to 17. Most, but not all, are approved for adults.

The dosing schedule for children is an important consideration when choosing a medication for ADHD. Older preparations must be taken every 4 hours, which is inconvenient for the school-age child. Extended-duration products are available that last 10 to 12 hours and provide a consistent therapeutic level throughout the day. Following are some examples of the different durations.

- *Short-acting (4–6 hours):* Adderall, Dexedrine, Focalin, Methylin, ProCentra, Ritalin
- *Intermediate-acting (8 hours):* Metadate CD, Metadate ER, Ritalin LA, Quillichew ER
- *Long-acting (10–12 hours):* Adderall XR, Concerta, Focalin XR, Mydayis, Quillivant XR, Vyvanse

PROTOTYPE DRUG Amphetamine and Dextroamphetamine (Adderall, Adderall XR)

Classification **Therapeutic:** Drug for ADHD
Pharmacologic: CNS stimulant, anorexiant, sympathomimetic

Therapeutic Effects and Uses: Adderall is a combination drug containing four different salts of amphetamine and dextroamphetamine. Amphetamine was approved in 1939 and Adderall in 1996. A short-acting form of the drug, Evekeo, was approved in 2014 to treat ADHD, as well as narcolepsy and obesity.

Adderall increases motor activity, alertness, and wakefulness and elevates the patient's mood. In children with ADHD the medication produces a paradoxical sedation effect. The mechanism of this effect is unclear. The drug affects the satiety center in the hypothalamus, causing anorexiant effects that lead to loss of appetite and weight.

Amphetamines are used to treat ADHD and narcolepsy. Although an effective appetite suppressant, amphetamine is rarely used for weight loss therapy because its inhibition of appetite is short term, and dependence results from long-term use. Illegal forms of amphetamine may be smoked, inhaled, or injected.

Mechanism of Action: Adderall produces sympathomimetic effects as well as central stimulation actions on the cerebral cortex and the reticular activating system. The actions of the medication are due to the release of norepinephrine and dopamine. The benefits of the drug in treating ADHD may also be due to its effects on the neurotransmitter serotonin in the brain.

Pharmacokinetics:

Route(s)	Oral (PO)
Absorption	Rapidly absorbed
Distribution	Widely distributed to all tissues, including the CNS; secreted in breast milk
Primary metabolism	Hepatic
Primary excretion	Renal
Onset of action	30 min–4 h, depending on formulation
Duration of action	4–12 h, depending on formulation

Adverse Effects: Symptoms of excessive CNS and peripheral stimulation by Adderall include irritability, insomnia, nervousness, palpitations, elevated blood pressure, and tachycardia. Weight loss is noted with the medication. In adults, impotence and change in libido may occur with high doses. Long-term use of amphetamines has been reported to cause growth inhibition in children; however, discontinuation of the drug often results in rebound growth. Psychiatric symptoms associated with amphetamine abuse include euphoria, hallucinations, delusions, paranoia, delirium, and depression.

Long-term users of amphetamine will experience tolerance to the mood-elevating effects of the drug. This results in abusers requiring increasingly higher doses to achieve the same stimulant effect. **Black Box Warning:** All amphetamine-containing products, including Adderall, have a high potential for abuse and administration for prolonged periods may lead to drug dependence. In addition, amphetamines may cause sudden death due to serious cardiac events. This has occurred primarily in children with preexisting cardiac abnormalities.

Contraindications/Precautions: Patients with hypersensitivity to sympathomimetic amines (e.g., epinephrine or norepinephrine) or who have a history of drug abuse should not be prescribed Adderall. Because the conditions may worsen, Adderall is contraindicated in patients with the following disorders: diabetes, glaucoma, hyperthyroidism, moderate to severe HTN, cardiac disorders, and Tourette's syndrome. Patients with bipolar disorder may exhibit signs of mania when administered amphetamines. Amphetamines should be discontinued gradually to prevent withdrawal symptoms such as severe depression, anxiety, agitation, hypersomnia, dysphoric mood, or suicidal ideation.

Drug Interactions: Alkaline drugs such as acetazolamide and sodium bicarbonate decrease the elimination of Adderall from the body and prolong its half-life. On the other hand, acidic drugs such as ammonium chloride and ascorbic acid increase the elimination of Adderall from the body. The administration of Adderall with furazolidone can cause an increase in blood pressure effects. Monoamine oxidase inhibitors such as selegiline can precipitate a hypertensive crisis; thus, they are contraindicated within 14 days of amphetamine administration. **Herbal/Food:** Foods and fluids containing caffeine can cause additive CNS stimulation and increase insomnia, nervousness, and anxiety. Melatonin should be avoided because it may enhance the CNS stimulation from Adderall.

Pregnancy: In animal studies, very high doses suggested that amphetamine caused fetal harm. Human experience with amphetamines during pregnancy do not indicate clear evidence of malformations or teratogenicity. However, neonates exposed in utero may experience signs of withdrawal after delivery, including irritability, feeding difficulties, and excessive drowsiness. Amphetamine-dependent mothers are at risk for preterm birth. Because amphetamines are secreted in human milk and may cause adverse effects in the neonate, breastfeeding is not recommended.

Treatment of Overdose: The treatment of amphetamine and amphetamine-related medication overdosage includes gastric lavage and the administration of chlorpromazine. Chlorpromazine contains strong alpha-adrenergic blocking actions that counteract the effects of amphetamine. In the event that overdosage results in severe HTN, phentolamine may be administered intravenously (IV). Acidification of the urine can speed the renal elimination of the drug.

Clinician Responsibilities: Key clinical implications for patients receiving amphetamine and dextroamphetamine are included in Applied Clinical Judgment: Patients Receiving Pharmacotherapy with Central Nervous System Stimulants.

Drugs Similar to Amphetamine and Dextroamphetamine (Adderall, Adderall XR)

Other psychostimulants for ADHD include dexmethylphenidate, lisdexamfetamine, and methylphenidate. Benzphetamine (Didrex) is an amphetamine indicated for obesity (see Chapter 63). All drugs in this class have the potential to cause the same effects on pregnancy and lactation as amphetamine-dextroamphetamine.

Dexmethylphenidate (Focalin, Focalin XR): Approved in 2001, dexmethylphenidate has effects identical to methylphenidate and the amphetamines. The drug blocks the reuptake of norepinephrine and dopamine in presynaptic neurons. It is used to manage symptoms of ADHD. A once-daily extended-release capsule (Focalin XR) is available. In 2021 Azatarys was approved, which is a combination capsule containing dexmethylphenidate with its prodrug, serdexmethylphenidate. The most common adverse effects are abdominal pain, nausea, fever, and decreased appetite. Although not common, twitching and vocal or motor tics may cause discontinuation of therapy. Inhibition of growth is a potential long-term adverse effect of the use of stimulants in children. Dexmethylphenidate should not be administered to patients who have primary psychiatric disorders because the drug may worsen these conditions. The drug has a high potential for dependence and is a Schedule II substance.

Lisdexamfetamine (Vyvanse): Approved in 2007, lisdexamfetamine is a prodrug of dextroamphetamine approved for the treatment of ADHD. Because the drug is rapidly metabolized to dextroamphetamine, the actions and adverse effects are identical to those of other psychostimulants. This drug is a Schedule II controlled substance.

Methylphenidate (Adhansia XR, Aptensio XR, Concerta, Cotempla XR-ODT, Daytrana, Jornay PM, Metadate, Methylin, Quillivant XR, Ritalin): Although structurally dissimilar to amphetamine, methylphenidate shares the same mechanism of action, pharmacologic actions, and adverse effects. Methylphenidate is approved for the treatment of ADHD and narcolepsy. Rarely, it may be used off-label for major depression refractory to more traditional therapies. In treating ADHD, it is as effective as the amphetamines. The patient's condition should be regularly assessed, and drug-free periods may be ordered during prolonged therapy. The drug is available in multiple formulations, including several extended-release forms, transdermal patches, chewable tablets, and orally disintegrating tablets. Doses and administration of these forms are not interchangeable. The extended-duration forms benefit children because they do not require the school nurse to administer a dose during the school day. It is important to note that this medication is contraindicated in children under the age of 6. Like other amphetamine-like drugs, all forms of methylphenidate are Schedule II controlled substances.

Methylphenidate is well tolerated and produces fewer peripheral adverse effects than amphetamine. Physical dependence is uncommon at therapeutic doses, although it may occur with the illicit parenteral or inhaled forms of the drug. Withdrawal symptoms are uncommon when the drug is discontinued. Nervousness, loss of appetite, and insomnia are the most common adverse effects. Methylphenidate should not be used in patients with severe anxiety, psychoses, or bipolar disorder because it may worsen these conditions. The drug may worsen tics due to Tourette's syndrome. Sudden unexplained cardiac death has occurred in some people taking this drug; therefore, all patients should be screened for preexisting cardiac disease, especially structural abnormalities or ventricular dysrhythmias. The FDA has issued safety announcements that methylphenidate may cause priapism, a prolonged and painful penile erection, and that the drug is associated with an increased risk for peripheral vasculopathy, specifically Raynaud's disease.

24.4 Several nonstimulants are effective in treating symptoms of attention-deficit/hyperactivity disorder.

The first nonstimulant for the treatment of ADHD, atomoxetine (Strattera), was approved in 2002. Clonidine and guanfacine were subsequently approved for ADHD in 2010 and 2006, respectively. The three nonstimulants do not exhibit abuse potential and are not controlled substances. These drugs offer alternatives for parents who are hesitant to place their children on CNS stimulants. The doses for these drugs are listed in Table 24.3.

Tricyclic antidepressants (TCAs) that have been used off-label for ADHD include imipramine, desipramine, and nortriptyline. The TCAs are less effective than the psychostimulants, can cause significant anticholinergic adverse effects such as dry mouth and constipation, and are cardiotoxic when taken in high doses. Bupropion, Desipramine, and venlafaxine are atypical antidepressants that have been used off-label for treating ADHD. Antidepressants are considered second-line therapy for ADHD and are usually used only when the patient has not responded adequately to psychostimulants or has a comorbid condition such as depression or anxiety.

CONNECTION Checkpoint 24.2

From what you learned in Chapter 19, what class of antidepressants contains the preferred drugs for major depressive disorder? To what antidepressant class does bupropion belong?

PROTOTYPE DRUG Atomoxetine (Strattera)

Classification **Therapeutic:** Drug for ADHD
Pharmacologic: Nonstimulant, norepinephrine reuptake inhibitor

Therapeutic Effects and Uses: Atomoxetine is administered to improve attentiveness and the ability to follow tasks in patients with ADHD. The medication decreases distraction and forgetfulness. It has the ability to diminish symptoms of ADHD in children and adults, and it is approved for patients ages 6 years and older. Unlike the stimulants that have an onset of action of 1 hour, atomoxetine can take up to 6 weeks for optimal reduction of ADHD symptoms.

Mechanism of Action: Atomoxetine is a selective norepinephrine reuptake inhibitor, which allows for increased concentration of the neurotransmitter in the prefrontal cortex. This region of the brain is associated with control of social behavior, personality expression, and short-term memory.

Pharmacokinetics:

Route(s)	PO
Absorption	Rapidly absorbed
Distribution	Distributed to most tissues; unknown if secreted in breast milk; 98% bound to protein
Primary metabolism	Hepatic, by CYP2D6
Primary excretion	Renal; small amounts in feces
Onset of action	2–4 weeks for ADHD symptoms
Duration of action	Half-life: 5.2 h

Adverse Effects: Common adverse effects with atomoxetine include xerostomia, headache, decreased appetite, and insomnia. CNS adverse effects include mood swings, irritability, and agitation. Because rare incidences of liver injury have been reported, patients with elevated hepatic enzymes or symptoms such as jaundice, nausea and vomiting, or anorexia should immediately discontinue the drug. Cardiovascular adverse effects include orthostatic hypotension, tachycardia, HTN, and palpitations. The patient may experience cough due to rhinorrhea, nasal congestion, and sinusitis. Weight loss and anorexia, along with urinary retention, urinary hesitancy, impotence, priapism, delayed menses, and menstrual irregularities, have been reported. **Black Box Warning:** Atomoxetine has been associated with a small increased risk for suicidal ideation. Caregivers should immediately report suicidal thoughts or unusual behavioral changes to their healthcare provider.

Contraindications/Precautions: If the patient has received a monoamine oxidase inhibitor in the past 14 days, the administration of atomoxetine should be delayed due to the risk of neuroleptic malignant syndrome or hypertensive crisis. Administration of the medication to any patient who has jaundice or elevated liver enzymes should be delayed until enzyme levels are in the normal range. Atomoxetine is also contraindicated in those diagnosed with closed-angle glaucoma because the drug is associated with an increased risk of mydriasis in some patients. It is important to administer atomoxetine cautiously in patients with HTN, tachycardia, moderate to severe hepatic insufficiency, and cardiovascular disease.

Drug Interactions: The elimination of atomoxetine is prolonged if it is administered with fluoxetine, paroxetine, or quinidine. Concurrent administration of albuterol with atomoxetine can result in increased heart rate and HTN. Drugs that activate the sympathetic nervous system should be used cautiously with atomoxetine due to the possibility of HTN. Some common sympathomimetics include amphetamines, pseudoephedrine, ephedrine, phenylephrine, dopamine, and norepinephrine. **Herbal/Food:** It is recommended that the patient not consume any herbal supplements while taking atomoxetine.

Pregnancy: Animal studies showed that high doses may cause fetal harm, including decreased offspring survival and skeletal malformations. It is not known if atomoxetine is secreted in human milk, and its effects on the breastfeeding infant are unknown. Pregnant or lactating women are advised to not use this drug unless the potential benefits justify the potential risks to the fetus or neonate.

Treatment of Overdose: Overdose with atomoxetine will cause agitation, abnormal behavior, and signs of sympathetic stimulation such as mydriasis, dry mouth, and tachycardia. The patient should receive supportive treatment for cardiopulmonary effects. Gastric lavage and repeated applications of activated charcoal may prevent systemic absorption.

Clinician Responsibilities: Key clinical implications for patients receiving atomoxetine are included in Applied Clinical Judgment: Patients Receiving Pharmacotherapy with Central Nervous System Stimulants.

Drugs Similar to Atomoxetine (Strattera)

Other nonstimulant drugs approved for ADHD include clonidine and guanfacine. Both medications are classified as centrally acting alpha$_2$-adrenergic agonists.

Clonidine (Kapvay): Clonidine, an older drug that was originally approved to treat HTN in 1974, was approved in 2010 to treat ADHD. In addition, it has been used off-label to treat a number of conditions, including pain, hot flashes, Tourette's syndrome, and withdrawal symptoms from alcohol, opioids, and nicotine. Clonidine is a centrally acting alpha$_2$-adrenergic agonist, but it is not known how this mechanism improves the clinical symptoms of ADHD. It is not a psychostimulant and there is no risk of physical dependence. The extended-release tablet (Kapvay) offers the advantage of once-daily dosing and optimum effects may require 4 to 8 weeks of therapy. The tablets should not be crushed, chewed, or broken. Kapvay is not interchangeable with other forms of clonidine. Kapvay can cause significant sedation and fatigue, especially during the early stages of therapy.

Blood pressure should be monitored during therapy because the drug can cause hypotension, syncope, and bradycardia. Clonidine should be discontinued gradually to prevent withdrawal effects such as tachycardia, anxiety, and headache. Caution should be used if other antihypertensives or CNS depressants are concurrently administered. Drugs that affect sinus node function may interact with clonidine to cause bradycardia and AV block. The drug is approved to treat ADHD in patients ages 6 to 17. Clonidine readily crosses the placenta, but no well-controlled studies have been performed in pregnant patients. It also enters breast milk and the manufacturer urges caution during lactation.

Guanfacine (Intuniv): Originally approved in 1986 for the treatment of HTN, guanfacine was reformulated as an extended-release tablet for ADHD in 2009. Approved for children ages 6 to 17, it may be used as monotherapy or in combination therapy with stimulant-type ADHD medications. Like clonidine, guanfacine is an alpha$_2$-adrenergic agonist. It is not a psychostimulant, and it does not cause dependence. The extended-release tablet offers the advantage of once-daily dosing. The tablets should not be crushed, chewed, or broken. Because the drug is a known antihypertensive, blood pressure should be monitored during therapy; some patients experience bradycardia and syncope due to reduced blood pressure. The drug should not be abruptly discontinued because transient rebound HTN may result. Sedation and lethargy are common, especially at the start of therapy. Caution should be used if other antihypertensives or CNS depressants are concurrently administered. Animal studies did not show evidence of fetal harm with guanfacine. It is not known if this drug is secreted in human milk, and its effects on the breastfeeding infant are unknown.

Pharmacotherapy of Narcolepsy

24.5 Narcolepsy is characterized by excessive daytime sleepiness and is treated with central nervous system stimulants and antidepressants.

Narcolepsy is a chronic neurologic disorder in which the patient experiences excessive daytime sleepiness. The disorder affects 1 in 2000 Americans and usually begins in childhood, although it may not be diagnosed until adulthood. Severe narcolepsy can be disabling and interfere with normal activities such as employment or success at school.

Narcolepsy is characterized by four symptoms: **Sleep attacks** (sudden bouts of sleep that last 10 to 30 minutes), **sleep paralysis** (extreme difficulty waking up from sleep), **cataplexy** (loss of muscle tone and emotion), and **hypnagogic hallucinations** (vivid, fearful dreams that occur at the onset of sleep). A complete discussion of narcolepsy pharmacotherapy is included in Chapter 18. This section focuses on the use of stimulants to treat this disorder.

The goal of narcolepsy pharmacotherapy is to reduce the incidence of daytime drowsiness and other symptoms associated with the disorder. Traditional therapies have focused on CNS stimulants. Dextroamphetamine and methylphenidate are approved to treat narcolepsy (see Section 24.3). The CNS stimulants are effective at reducing daytime drowsiness but may cause nervousness, insomnia, and dependence. Two other stimulants, modafinil and armodafinil, have frequently been used in the treatment of narcolepsy.

For patients who experience narcolepsy *with* cataplexy, additional drugs are necessary. These include sodium oxybate (gamma-hydroxybutyrate [GHB], Xyrem) and the off-label use of antidepressants such as selegiline (Eldepryl), imipramine (Tofranil), and fluoxetine (Prozac) have been used to treat cataplexy and provide relief for most patients.

PROTOTYPE DRUG Modafinil (Provigil)

Classification **Therapeutic:** Drug for narcolepsy
Pharmacologic: CNS stimulant

Therapeutic Effects and Uses: Approved in 1998, modafinil is a stimulant given PO to improve wakefulness in adult patients with excessive sleepiness associated with narcolepsy, shift work sleep disorder (circadian rhythm disruption), and obstructive sleep apnea syndrome. The drug increases daytime alertness and locomotor activity. Modafinil may also be prescribed off-label to treat fatigue related to Parkinson's disease and multiple sclerosis.

Similar to amphetamines, modafinil can induce euphoria and psychoactive symptoms. Although the abuse potential for modafinil is less than that of other CNS stimulants, it is still classified as a Schedule IV controlled substance. Unlike amphetamines, it does not appear to suppress appetite or promote weight loss.

Mechanism of Action: The mechanism by which modafinil exerts its wake-promoting effects is unknown. The drug increases dopamine levels in the brain by inhibiting dopamine uptake.

Pharmacokinetics:

Route(s)	PO
Absorption	Rapidly absorbed
Distribution	Distributed to most tissues; unknown if secreted in breast milk; 60% bound to protein
Primary metabolism	Hepatic by multiple CYP450 enzymes
Primary excretion	Renal
Onset of action	Peak: 2–4 h
Duration of action	Half-life: 15 h

Adverse Effects: Serious adverse effects from modafinil are infrequent. The primary CNS adverse effects are headache, nervousness, and insomnia. Cardiovascular adverse effects include blood pressure changes (either increased or decreased), vasodilation, and syncope. Nausea and vomiting, diarrhea, and dry mouth are frequent gastrointestinal (GI) adverse effects. Pulmonary effects include pharyngitis, rhinitis, and dyspnea. Modafinil has about the same abuse potential as other CNS stimulants such as methylphenidate.

Contraindications/Precautions: Modafinil should not be administered to patients who have had an acute myocardial infarction (MI) or those with valvular heart disease or a hypersensitivity to modafinil. The drug should be discontinued at the first sign of serious rash, including rare cases of SJS. The drug should be used with caution in patients with a history of psychiatric disorders because mania, delusions, hallucinations, and suicidal ideation have been reported. The drug should be used with caution in those with a history of substance abuse. Severe hepatic impairment may increase serum modafinil levels as much as 50%; doses in these patients must be reduced to prevent toxicity. This drug is not approved for use in children for any indication.

Drug Interactions: CYP450 enzymes metabolize modafinil, and the drug can inhibit and induce different isozymes. For example, modafinil inhibits CYP2C19, the primary metabolic enzyme for phenytoin, diazepam, and propranolol; levels of these drugs increase when given concurrently with modafinil. When modafinil is administered with cyclosporine, the therapeutic levels of cyclosporine decrease. Modafinil may increase the levels of clomipramine and warfarin. TCA levels increase with the drug. Modafinil may decrease the effectiveness of oral contraceptives and cause unplanned pregnancies. **Herbal/Food:** Foods and beverages containing caffeine may worsen insomnia.

Pregnancy: Aanimal studies showed modafinil may cause fetal harm, including an increased risk for spontaneous abortion. It is not known if this drug is secreted in human milk, and its effects on the breastfeeding infant are unknown.

Treatment of Overdose: Overdose causes agitation, insomnia, anxiety, aggressiveness, palpitations, and confusion. Overdoses are usually not fatal. The patient should receive supportive treatment and gastric lavage.

Clinician Responsibilities: Key clinical implications for patients receiving modafinil are included in Applied Clinical Judgment: Patients Receiving Pharmacotherapy with Central Nervous System Stimulants.

Drugs Similar to Modafinil (Provigil)

Antidepressants used to treat narcolepsy are presented in Chapter 19, and the amphetamines are discussed in Section 24.3. Armodafinil is a stimulant specifically indicated for narcolepsy.

Armodafinil (Nuvigil): Approved in 2007, armodafinil is closely related to modafinil and exhibits the same actions and adverse effects. It is approved to treat narcolepsy and shift work sleep disorder and to improve wakefulness in patients with obstructive sleep apnea who often experience daytime drowsiness. Like modafinil, serious rashes, including cases of SJS, have been reported with the use of the drug. Armodafinil is a Schedule IV controlled substance and has the same pregnancy risk as modafinil.

CONNECTION Checkpoint 24.3

From what you learned in Chapter 18, during which stage of sleep does most of an individual's active dreaming occur?

Methylxanthines

24.6 Methylxanthines are central nervous system stimulants used for their ability to increase alertness or their effects on the respiratory system.

Methylxanthines are substances similar to xanthine, a chemical produced during the breakdown of deoxyribonucleic acid (DNA). Unlike the other CNS stimulants discussed in this chapter, the methylxanthines are not used for their effects on the brain. Instead, the methylxanthines are associated with treating patients with chronic obstructive pulmonary disease, asthma, and other restrictive lung diseases due to their ability to relax bronchial smooth muscle. The methylxanthines include caffeine, theophylline, and theobromine. Caffeine is the prototype drug for the methylxanthines. The dose of caffeine is listed in Table 24.3.

Theophylline and theobromine are formed by the metabolic breakdown of caffeine in the liver. Although rarely used, theophylline is still available as a drug to treat asthma that is resistant to other therapies. Theobromine is a natural substance found in chocolate that once was used as a drug to treat HTN and other vascular disorders. Although similar to caffeine, it has very little CNS stimulant activity.

PROTOTYPE DRUG Caffeine (Cafcit)

Classification **Therapeutic:** CNS and respiratory stimulant
Pharmacologic: Methylxanthine

Therapeutic Effects and Uses: Caffeine is a methylxanthine naturally found in over 60 plant species. Most consumption in the United States is from coffee, tea, soft drinks, chocolate, and energy beverages. Caffeine has potent psychoactive properties. When taken PO it quickly restores mental alertness and aids in wakefulness. In addition to its consumption in beverages and food, caffeine is also available in OTC products designed to increase alertness and delay fatigue.

Caffeine itself has no analgesic properties. However, it enhances pain relief when administered with an analgesic. Products approved for tension headaches include caffeine combined with acetaminophen, aspirin, codeine, or butalbital (a barbiturate). Caffeine is also combined with ergotamine (Cafergot, Migergot) in the treatment of migraine headaches. It may be administered parenterally in emergency situations to treat circulatory collapse.

Caffeine is used as a respiratory stimulant in the management of apnea in premature infants. For this indication, caffeine (Cafcit) may be administered IV or PO, added to formula feedings.

Caffeine also has a number of off-label indications. In patients with asthma, orally administered caffeine will produce bronchodilation and smooth muscle relaxation. Caffeine produces a mild diuresis due to increased blood flow to the glomerulus and has been used as an OTC diuretic product. Caffeine may be administered IV to relieve headache associated with lumbar puncture.

Mechanism of Action: Caffeine is metabolized in the liver to theobromine and theophylline, both of which are active metabolites that enhance the CNS and respiratory stimulant effects of caffeine. When higher doses are administered, the medulla, respiratory center, and vagus nerve are stimulated and produce a relaxation of smooth muscle, which is particularly evident in the bronchi and coronary and systemic blood vessels.

Pharmacokinetics:

Route(s)	PO, intramuscular (IM), IV
Absorption	Rapidly absorbed
Distribution	Widely distributed; crosses the blood–brain barrier and the placenta; secreted in breast milk; 36% bound to plasma proteins
Primary metabolism	Hepatic
Primary excretion	Renal
Onset of action	15–45 min
Duration of action	Half-life: 3–5 h in adults; 36–144 h in neonates

Adverse Effects: Caffeine may cause adverse effects at therapeutic doses, many of which are extensions of its pharmacologic actions. Excessive CNS stimulation may cause nervousness, insomnia, tremors, and restlessness. The cardiovascular effects of caffeine include tingling of the face, palpitations, tachycardia, bradycardia, and ventricular ectopic beats. GI effects noted with the administration of caffeine are related to the stimulation of the vagus nerve and include nausea and vomiting, epigastric pain, hematemesis, and kernicterus in neonates. Clonic seizures can result in rare instances. Caffeine withdrawal can produce symptoms of irritability, headache, lethargy, or anxiety.

Contraindications/Precautions: Caffeine should not be administered during acute MI or to patients with cardiac dysrhythmias because the drug increases the workload of the heart. Caffeine increases the secretion of gastric acid; therefore, patients who have peptic ulcer disease should limit their caffeine intake. Patients with anxiety disorders, insomnia, or panic attacks should not be administered caffeine because it may worsen these conditions. It should be used cautiously in patients with diabetes mellitus, hiatal hernia, HTN, and heart disease. Patients with hepatic impairment or chronic kidney disease should receive lower doses because the drug may accumulate to toxic levels.

Drug Interactions: Caffeine administered with cimetidine will increase the effect of cimetidine. Beta-adrenergic agonists administered with caffeine will result in increased cardiovascular stimulation. Additive effects are likely if the drug is taken concurrently with other CNS stimulants. Patients taking drugs for insomnia or anxiety should limit their intake of caffeine. Caffeine is a substrate of hepatic cytochrome CYP1A2. Drugs that enhance or inhibit this enzyme may interact with caffeine. **Herbal/Food:** Food and fluids that contain caffeine will increase the insomnia or restlessness that is normally noted with methylxanthines.

Pregnancy: Human data does not clearly show that caffeine increases the risk for adverse pregnancy outcomes; however, some clinicians advise the mother to consume less than 300 mg/day (equivalent to 3 cups of coffee). Caution is advised during lactation because caffeine is secreted in milk and can cause irritability and poor sleeping patterns in the breastfed infant.

Treatment of Overdose: Caffeine overdose can potentially cause dysrhythmias, insomnia, delirium, and seizures. The patient is supported through symptom management. High serum levels of caffeine can be dialyzed with peritoneal dialysis or hemodialysis.

Clinician Responsibilities: Key clinical implications for patients receiving caffeine are included in Applied Clinical Judgment: Patients Receiving Pharmacotherapy with Central Nervous System Stimulants.

Drugs Similar to Caffeine

Theophylline is the only other methylxanthine used as a drug.

Theophylline (Theo-24): Available in immediate-release and extended-release forms, theophylline is administered to produce bronchodilation in patients with acute bronchospasm. It decreases wheezing and obstructed airways in asthma and bronchitis. It is important to note that the medication is a CNS stimulant that can produce restlessness, insomnia, and irritability. Close monitoring is required to prevent drug toxicity. Once widely prescribed, theophylline use has declined due to the development of safer drugs for patients with asthma. Use of theophylline is not advised during pregnancy or lactation: corticosteroids are the preferred medications for treating asthma during pregnancy.

CONNECTIONS: APPLIED CLINICAL JUDGMENT

Patients Receiving Pharmacotherapy with Central Nervous System Stimulants

Key Assessment Data

- History of current condition, baseline vital signs, physical exam findings; history of cardiovascular, hepatic, or neurologic disease, including epilepsy, and neonatal or previously existing symptoms of cardiac problems; medication and allergy history; mental status as appropriate; pregnancy or breastfeeding status.
- Obtain a social and behavioral history. Use objective screening tools when possible.
- Obtain a nutritional history and assess normal sleep patterns. Obtain height and weight, especially on pediatric or older adult patients.
- Ongoing assessment during drug therapy includes laboratory findings such as hepatic and renal function studies, CBC, electrolytes.

(continued)

CONNECTIONS: APPLIED CLINICAL JUDGMENT *(continued)*

Patients Receiving Pharmacotherapy with Central Nervous System Stimulants

Desired Therapeutic Outcomes

Improvement is observed and measurable in the ability to focus and stay on task, lessened impulsivity, and improved social interactions (ADHD) and decreased excessive sleepiness with increased daytime alertness and locomotor activity (narcolepsy).

Minimizing Adverse Effects

- Tachycardia, increased blood pressure, or HTN may occur if dose is excessive. An increased risk of dysrhythmias and sudden death has been noted with some drugs. Continue to monitor pulse and blood pressure on healthcare visits.
- Diminished appetite or anorexia from stimulating effects of the drug, or use of other stimulants, may impair normal nutrition needed for growth and development. Weigh the patient weekly and obtain height on children. Report any weight loss or failure to gain weight during expected growth periods. Assess nutrition and use of other stimulating products (e.g., energy drinks and caffeinated beverages).
- Stimulatory effects of the drug may affect normal sleeping patterns and may indicate excessive dosage. Monitor sleep patterns.
- Excessive CNS stimulation may cause seizures as an adverse effect. Assess for excessive stimulatory effects of agitation, aggression, tremors, or seizures and report immediately.
- Atomoxetine and other norepinephrine reuptake inhibitors may cause urinary retention as an adverse effect. Assess for urinary retention periodically.
- Armodafinil and methylphenidate have been associated with severe skin effects including SJS and exfoliative dermatitis. Continue to monitor for dermatologic effects including red or purplish skin rash, blisters, or sunburn.
- Dependent on the degree of behavior, drug holidays on nonschool days or vacation periods may be recommended. Assess the need for continuous medication or the need for drug holidays with the patient, family caregiver, and the healthcare provider based on social and behavioral diary findings.
- Atomoxetine has been associated with an increased risk of suicide. Modafinil and armodafinil have been associated with an increased risk of psychiatric symptoms, including paranoia and suicidal ideations. Assess for increasing depression, agitation, delusional thoughts, or expressions of suicide or self-harm. Promptly refer any of these symptoms to the provider.
- Some drugs are scheduled drugs and may not be used by any individual other than the patient. Safeguard the medication in the home to prevent overdose.

Lifespan Considerations

- Children, adolescents, and older adults are more likely to experience adverse effects related to anorexia from the drug. Monitor nutritional intake, weight, and height (pediatrics).
- Older adult men with an enlarged prostate are at higher risk for mechanical obstruction. Assess for urinary retention periodically. Report an inability to void, increasing bladder pressure, or pain.

Diversity Considerations

- Modafinil may inhibit or induce CYP450 enzymes and may interact with other drugs. Observe for less than optimal therapeutic effects, especially in ethnically diverse patients.

Patient and Caregiver Education

- To assess and monitor improvement, keep a social and behavioral diary. Involve school faculty and other caregivers (e.g., afterschool care) as needed.
- Take the pulse along with weekly height and weight, or any time symptoms warrant (e.g., child reports chest discomfort or palpitations).
- Inform the provider of disruption to sleep, increased agitation during the day (possible effect from lack of sleep), or excessive sleepiness during the day. Take the dose early in the day and before 4:00 p.m. to help alleviate insomnia unless extended-release formulation is used. Take extended release formulations in the morning.
- Report tremors or seizures to the healthcare provider immediately.
- Immediately report an inability to void, increasing bladder pressure, or pain.
- Wear sunscreen and protective clothing for sun exposure and avoid tanning beds. Immediately report any severe sunburn or rashes.
- Be alert for signs of increased depression, confusion, paranoia, or expressions of suicide. Promptly notify the provider if symptoms are noted.
- The provider may recommend the option of scheduling drug holidays. If the drug dose is at the upper range, consider tapering the dose prior to beginning the drug holiday to avoid rebound hyperactivity or agitation.
- Avoid or eliminate all foods, beverages, or OTC drugs that contain caffeine or other stimulants.
- Take the medication exactly as ordered, and in the morning to prevent insomnia. Do not take double or extra doses to increase mental focus or prevent sleepiness. The drug will not achieve these effects but will increase the adverse effects of the drug. Do not abruptly discontinue the medication without consulting the healthcare provider. Do not open, chew, or crush extended-release tablets; swallow them whole with plenty of water.
- Proper medication storage is needed, and the drug should be used by the patient only. Prescription renewal restrictions (i.e., new prescription each time, no refills, and prescription may not be called in) are applicable and school policies will direct in-school use (e.g., single dose sent each day, and secured blister pack used if multiple doses are sent).

Prescribing Considerations

- Prior to prescribing, assess for the presence of cardiac disease. Perform a careful history, family history of sudden death or ventricular arrhythmia, and physical exam and electrocardiogram.
- Hepatic and renal function, CBC, and electrolytes should be monitored.
- Schedule drug holidays and if the drug dose is at the upper range, consider tapering the dose prior to beginning the drug holiday to avoid rebound hyperactivity or agitation.
- Assess the risk of abuse prior to prescribing and monitor for signs of abuse or dependence while on therapy.
- If paradoxical reactions or aggravation of symptoms occur, reduce dosage or discontinue the drug.
- Closely monitor growth (weight and height) in pediatric patients and if patients are not growing or gaining height or weight as expected, then treatment may need to be interrupted.

Understanding Chapter 24

Key Concepts Summary

24.1 Central nervous system stimulants increase alertness, enhance the ability to concentrate, and delay the symptoms of fatigue.

24.2 Attention-deficit/hyperactivity disorder is characterized by inattention, hyperactivity, and impulsive behavior.

24.3 Psychostimulants are central nervous system stimulants indicated for the treatment of ADHD and narcolepsy.

24.4 Several nonstimulants are effective in treating symptoms of attention-deficit/hyperactivity disorder.

24.5 Narcolepsy is characterized by excessive daytime sleepiness and is treated with central nervous system stimulants and antidepressants.

24.6 Methylxanthines are central nervous system stimulants used for their ability to increase alertness or their effects on the respiratory system.

CASE STUDY: Making the Patient Connection

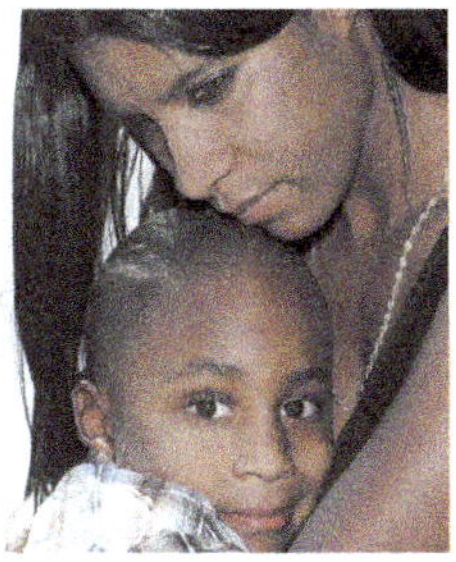

Remember the patient "Jonathon Hogan" at the beginning of the chapter? Now read the remainder of the case study. Based on the information presented within this chapter, respond to the critical thinking questions that follow.

Jonathon Hogan has had trouble at school beginning in kindergarten and for the past year. His teachers have consistently reported that he is easily distracted and wanders around the classroom, even during a lesson. Getting him to do his homework after school has been a struggle. Jonathon loves art and does well at video games. Because he is a happy-go-lucky child, his parents have assumed that Jonathon's right-brain dominance has created trouble with left-brain logical work. With more homework now in second grade, Jonathon is struggling to keep up in school. The school nurse suspects he may have ADHD. She has recommended an appointment with Jonathon's healthcare provider and told his parents that Adderall may help him focus on his schoolwork.

Critical Thinking Questions

1. What is ADHD and why would Jonathon be experiencing more difficulty as he becomes older?
2. How might amphetamine sulfate and dextroamphetamine (Adderall) help Jonathon with his ADHD?
3. What caregiver education would be appropriate regarding dextroamphetamine and amphetamine sulfate (Adderall)?
4. What are other nonpharmacologic treatments for ADHD?

Additional Case Study

Anna Steinmetz has graduated from nursing school and is working nights. She is having difficulty adjusting to her night schedule. Her healthcare provider suggested she utilize a medication to assist with her adjustment to shift work. She has been prescribed modafinil (Provigil).

1. What effect does modafinil (Provigil) have on the patient's ability to maintain alertness during shift work?
2. What teaching will you provide to the patient regarding this medication?
3. The patient reports feelings of lightheadedness with position changes. What interventions will assist in maintaining patient safety?

Chapter Review

1. An elementary school nurse is providing education to the faculty on the use of central nervous system stimulants to treat attention-deficit/hyperactivity disorder. Of the following, which is most important for the nurse to convey to the faculty?
    1. Have the child bring the drug dose in a lunch bag and come to the office to take it to avoid being teased.
    2. Request that the parents leave an extra copy of the prescription at the school in case the dose runs out.
    3. Suggest that the parents have two prescriptions filled, one for home and one to keep at school.
    4. Keep the drugs in a locked drawer, clearly labeled with the student's name and only the number of doses allowed by school policy.

2. Which therapeutic outcome would the nurse consider most significant in evaluating a patient who started atomoxetine (Strattera) 6 months ago?
    1. Decrease in attention
    2. Decrease in hyperactivity
    3. Development of mydriasis
    4. Elevated liver enzymes

3. A patient who has overdosed on amphetamine sulfate and dextroamphetamine (Adderall XR) is admitted to the emergency department. The nurse would anticipate which medications to be administered to assist in counteracting the effects of the overdosage?
    1. Chlorpromazine (Thorazine)
    2. Phenytoin (Dilantin)
    3. Propofol (Diprivan)
    4. Dexamethasone (Decadron)

4. A high school student taking atomoxetine (Strattera) for ADHD visits the school nurse's office and confides, "I am so depressed. The world would be better off without me." Which action would the nurse take for this patient?
    1. Tell the patient to stop taking atomoxetine immediately and not to take it until checking with the provider.
    2. Assure the patient that these are normal symptoms because the drug may take 3 or 4 weeks to work.
    3. Alert the family or caregiver that immediate attention and treatment are needed for these symptoms.
    4. Have the patient increase intake of caffeine by consuming cola products, coffee, or tea to counteract the depressive effect.

5. Modafinil (Provigil) has been ordered for a patient with narcolepsy. Which of the following are true statements? Select all that apply.
    1. Modafinil is a Schedule IV drug and has restrictions on ordering and renewing prescriptions.
    2. Modafinil may cause euphoria and psychoactive symptoms, similar to other stimulant drugs.
    3. Modafinil is known to suppress appetite and promote weight loss.
    4. Modafinil may cause nervousness or hyperactivity.
    5. Modafinil may be used in patients with heart disease (e.g., myocardial infarction, valvular conditions) who cannot take traditional stimulant drugs.

6. A patient who is taking methylphenidate (Concerta, Metadate, Ritalin) for attention-deficit/hyperactivity disorder reports having insomnia. Which intervention will assist in the promotion of sleep?
    1. Have a glass of wine with dinner.
    2. Eat a chocolate bar at bedtime.
    3. Take the drug before 4:00 p.m.
    4. Switch to decaffeinated coffee.

See Appendix A for answers to critical thinking questions, case study questions and review questions.

References

ADA (n.d.). *Information and technical assistance on the Americans with Disabilities Act*. https://www.ada.gov/ta-pubs-pg2.htm

Centers for Disease Control and Prevention. (2019). *Attention-deficit/hyperactivity disorder (ADHD) data and*. http://www.cdc.gov/ncbddd/adhd/data.html

Centers for Disease Control and Prevention. (2020). *Attention-deficit/hyperactivity disorder (ADHD) symptoms and diagnosis*. https://www.cdc.gov/ncbddd/adhd/diagnosis.html

Cook, N. E., Kelshaw, P. M., Caswell, S. W., & Iverson, G. L. (2019). Children with attention-deficit/hyperactivity disorder perform differently on pediatric concussion assessment. *Journal of Pediatrics*, *214*, 168–174. https://doi.org/10.106/j.peds.07.048

Iverson, J. L., Atkins, J. E., Zafonte, R., & Berkner, P. D. (2016). Concussion history in adolescent athletes with attention-deficit hyperactivity disorder. *Journal of Neurotrauma*, *33*, 2077–2080. https://doi.org/10.1089/neu.2014.3424

National Collegiate Athletic Association. (2020). *Medical exemptions procedures*. http://www.ncaa.org/sport-science-institute/medical-exceptions-procedures

Pujalte, G. G. A., Maynard, J. R., Thurston, M. J., Taylor, W. C. III, & Chauhan, M. (2019). Considerations in the care of athletes with attention deficit hyperactivity disorder. *Clinical Journal of Sports Medicine*, *29*, 245–256. https://doi.org/10.1097/JSM.0000000000000508

Stewman, C. G., Liebman, C., Fink, L., & Sandella, B. (2018). Attention deficit hyperactivity disorder: Unique considerations in athletes. *Sports Health*, *10*, 40–46. https://doi.org/10.1177/1941738117742906

U.S. Department of Justice, Drug Enforcement Administration. (2020). *Lists of: Scheduling actions, controlled substances and regulated chemicals*. http://www.deadiversion.usdoj.gov/schedules/orangebook/orangebook.pdf

Selected Bibliography

Akutagava-Martins, G. C., Rohde, L. A., & Hutz, M. H. (2016). Genetics of attention-deficit/hyperactivity disorder: An update. *Expert Review of Neurotherapeutics*, *16*, 145–156. https://doi.org/10.1586/14737175.2016.1130626

Buoli, M., Serati, M., & Cahn, W. (2016). Alternative pharmacological strategies for adult ADHD treatment: A systematic review. *Expert Review of Neurotherapeutics*, *16*, 131–144. https://doi.org/10.1586/14737175.2016.1135735

Cohen Children's Medical Center. (2020). *The ADHD medication guide*. http://www.adhdmedicationguide.com

Cunill, R., Castells, X., Tobias, A., & Capellà, D. (2016). Efficacy, safety and variability in pharmacotherapy for adults with attention deficit hyperactivity disorder: A meta-analysis and meta-regression in over 9000 patients. *Psychopharmacology*, *233*, 187–197. https://doi.org/10.1007/s00213-015-4099-3

Grimm, O., Kranz, T. M., & Reif, A. (2020). Genetics of ADHD: What should the clinician know? *Current Psychiatry Reports*, *22*(4), 18. https://doi.org/10.1007/s11920-020-1141-x

Jansen, M. (2019). NPs' use of guidelines to diagnose and treat childhood ADHD. *The Nurse Practitioner*, *44*(7), 37–42. https://doi.org/10.1097/01.NPR.0000559845.76249.48

Kooij, J. J. S., Bijlenga, D., Salerno, L., Jaeschke, R., Bitter, I., Balazs, J., et al. (2019). Updated European Consensus Statement on diagnosis and treatment of adult ADHD. *European Psychiatry*, *56*(1), 14–34. https://doi.org/10.1016/j.eurpsy.2018.11.001

Nallu, S. (2019). *Narcolepsy*. Medscape. http://emedicine.medscape.com/article/1188433-overview

National Institute of Mental Health. (2019). *Attention deficit hyperactivity disorder*. http://www.nimh.nih.gov/health/topics/attention-deficit-hyperactivity-disorder-adhd/index.shtml

Preda, A. (2018). *Stimulants*. Medscape. http://emedicine.medscape.com/article/289007-overview

Torgersen, T., Gjervan, B., Lensing, M. B., & Rasmussen, K. (2016). Optimal management of ADHD in older adults. *Neuropsychiatric Disease and Treatment*, *12*, 79–87. https://doi.org/10.2147/NDT.S59271

Wolraich, M. L., Hagan, J. F., Allan, C., Chan, E., Davison, D., Earls, M., et al. (2019). Clinical practice guideline for the diagnosis, evaluation, and treatment of attention-deficit/hyperactivity disorder in children and adolescents. *Pediatrics*, *144*(4), e20192528. https://doi.org/10.1542/peds.2019-2528

World Anti-Doping Association. (2020). *2020 list of prohibited substances and methods*. https://www.wada-ama.org/en/content/what-is-prohibited?gclid=EAIaIQobChMI_r3uu7mx6gIVE4bICh232gT2EAAYASAAEgLu4fD_BwE

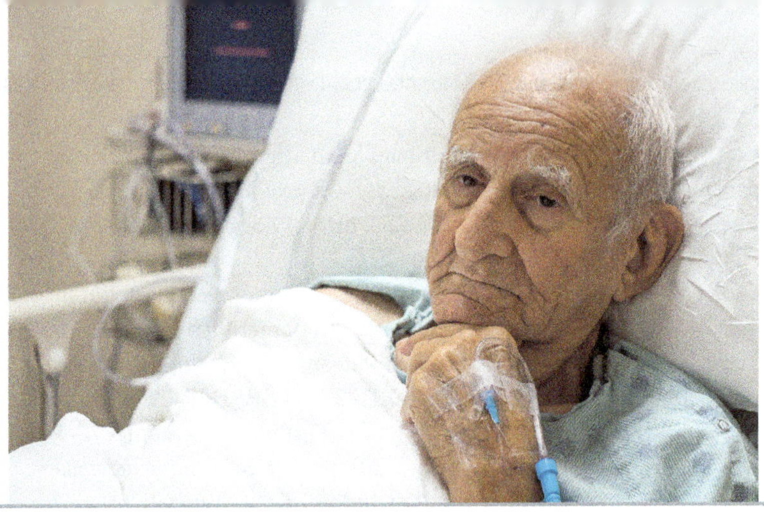

"I'm having urologic surgery tomorrow and I am worried about pain. I've taken pain medicine daily for years because of chronic pain from back problems and numerous back surgeries. Will I experience severe pain after this procedure?"

—*Patient "Larry Smith"*

Chapter 25
Pharmacotherapy of Severe Pain and Migraines

Chapter Outline

Learning Outcomes

After reading this chapter, the student should be able to:

1. Identify key principles of pain management.
2. Describe the assessment and classification of pain.
3. Refute the common pain myths, using objective evidence.
4. Explain the phases of pain physiology: transduction, transmission, perception, and modulation.
5. Describe pharmacologic and nonpharmacologic therapies used in pain management.
6. Describe the types of opioid receptors in the central nervous system.
7. Identify the classes of drugs used for minor, moderate, and severe pain.
8. Compare and contrast the actions of opioid agonists and opioid antagonists.
9. Describe the use of nonopioids and adjuvant analgesics in the treatment of pain.
10. Compare and contrast the actions and adverse effects of the opioids and nonopioids for analgesia.
11. Explain the role of opioid antagonists in the diagnosis and treatment of acute opioid toxicity.
12. Compare the types of drugs used for preventing migraines to those for terminating migraines.
13. For each of the classes shown in the chapter outline, identify the prototype and representative drugs and explain the mechanism(s) of drug action, primary indications, contraindications, significant drug interactions, pregnancy data and important adverse effects.
14. Apply clinical judgment to care for patients receiving pharmacotherapy for pain and for migraines.

Key Terms Definitions of the terms in bold may be found in the Glossary.

Pain is a subjective experience that has both physiologic and emotional components. Often associated with trauma or disease, pain may be viewed as a natural defense mechanism that helps people avoid potentially damaging situations and encourages them to seek medical help. Pain medications are some of the most frequently used drugs in medicine. This chapter examines the drug classes used in pain management and for the pharmacotherapy of migraines.

General Principles of Pain Management

25.1 The primary goal of pain management is to reduce pain to a level that allows the patient to continue normal daily activities.

Pain management is one of the most important tasks for healthcare providers. It is also one of the most difficult because the experience of pain by patients and its assessment by healthcare providers are subjective. The perception of pain is clearly influenced by comorbid conditions such as anxiety, fatigue, and depression. For example, knowing that healthcare providers and caregivers are attentive and actively engaged in pain management may lower patients' anxiety, thus reducing pain perception and increasing pain tolerance. Listening carefully, showing respect, and helping patients to understand their treatment options are important steps to attaining optimal pain relief.

The immediate goal of pain management is to reduce pain to a level that allows the patient to perform reasonable activities of daily living (ADLs) such as sleeping, eating, and normal physical activities. For some disorders, the patient should understand that the total elimination of pain may not be a realistic goal, or that the pain may require a long period of treatment. Several key principles underlie the nursing management of pain:

- The patient should be considered the expert on his or her own pain; the nurse should always believe the patient's self-assessment of pain.
- Pain management is a patient right and should be based on the patient's goals. The patient should be screened for pain during an initial assessment and periodically thereafter. If pain cannot be effectively managed, then a pain management specialist should be consulted.
- Nonpharmacologic interventions such as massage or the application of heat or cold should be encouraged in pain management. A combination of therapies is optimal because different modalities work by different mechanisms, thus improving the effectiveness of pain management.
- Dosing should be individualized and adjusted to produce the established pain management goal in each patient.
- Adverse effects from pain medications should be anticipated and prevented whenever possible. Should they appear, adverse effects should be immediately addressed.
- Around-the-clock dosing for moderate to severe pain should be implemented because it is much easier to *maintain* a pain-free level than to *eliminate* existing or escalating pain.

25.2 Proper assessment and classification of pain guides its treatment.

Pain assessment includes documenting the location, intensity, and quality (sharp, dull, burning) of the pain and any precipitating or relieving factors. For most adults, the 0-to-10 numerical rating scale is the standard for rating pain intensity, with 0 being no pain and 10 being the greatest pain imaginable. The pain rating is used as a reference point, initially as a baseline level of pain and later as an indicator of effectiveness as to how well the treatment is achieving the patient's goals.

Pain may be classified as acute or chronic. Acute pain has an abrupt onset but brief duration; it subsides as healing takes place or the pain stimulus ceases. Examples of acute pain include that associated with surgical incisions, labor and delivery, sprained joints, or myocardial infarction (MI). Although it may be severe, acute pain is often self-limiting; high doses of pain medication may be necessary, but therapy is usually of short duration. There is little risk of chronic drug adverse effects or dependence because of the relatively brief treatment period.

Chronic pain is pain that persists longer than 6 months, can interfere with ADLs, and is sometimes associated with feelings of helplessness or hopelessness. Chronic pain can be further grouped as either nonmalignant or malignant (cancer) pain. Chronic nonmalignant pain is not life-threatening and usually responds favorably to a consistent, stable dose of pain medication as part of a treatment regimen. The most common example is low back pain. Cancer pain ends with control of the disease or death. Although the majority of patients with cancer experience pain during the advanced stages of the disease, 90% of the cancer pain can be controlled with oral (PO) drugs, using around-the-clock dosing, with as-needed (prn) doses for breakthrough pain.

PharmFACT

Low Back Pain in Children

Although pediatric low back pain (LBP) is less common than in adults, its incidence has been increasing. Pediatric LBP is associated with obesity, use of heavy backpacks and lack of physical activity. Children with LBP at an early age are more likely to suffer that condition as adults (Hwang et al., 2019).

Another useful method for classifying pain is according to its source: nociceptor or neuropathic. **Nociceptors** are the sensory nerve receptors located throughout the body that initiate pain transmission when stimulated. For example, a needlestick will activate receptors in the finger, producing **nociceptor pain**. This type of pain may be further subdivided into somatic pain, which produces sharp, localized sensations usually experienced in muscles and joints, or visceral pain, which is described as a generalized dull, throbbing, or aching pain usually located in internal organs. Nociceptor pain responds quite well to **analgesics**, which are medications that relieve pain.

In contrast, **neuropathic pain** is caused by injury or irritation to nerve tissue and is typically described as burning, shooting, or numbing pain. The cause of neuropathic pain is sometimes difficult to determine. Analgesic treatment of neuropathic pain is often unsuccessful or high doses may be required. Neuropathic pain responds well to adjuvant analgesics such as antiseizure drugs and antidepressants (see Section 25.11).

25.3 Healthcare providers and patients sometimes hold myths about pain that impede optimal pain management.

Commonly held but untrue beliefs by both patients and healthcare providers may interfere with effective pain management. For example, healthcare providers may undertreat pain because of common misconceptions about pain. Furthermore, patients may not report their pain accurately or may refuse pain medications because of similar misconceptions.

A pervasive myth is that healthcare professionals can successfully recognize pain, independent of the patient's report. The nurse must understand that patients are the authorities on their own pain. Pain is whatever the patient says it is, existing whenever the patient says it does. Patient self-report of pain is sufficient for a nursing diagnosis of pain.

A closely related myth is that someone in pain must look and act like he or she is in pain. Some patients do not show or report pain accurately because they feel it is a sign of weakness. In addition, vital signs are sometimes unreliable indicators of pain. Although they may be elevated during the initial experience of acute pain owing to sympathetic arousal, vital signs return to normal as the body adapts. A related misconception is the belief that if an individual is able to sleep, he or she must not be experiencing much pain. Although it is certainly true that pain can interfere with sleep quality and quantity, social withdrawal and excessive sleep may be indicators of coping mechanisms for some people with severe or chronic pain.

Both patients and healthcare providers may share the myth that the use of potent analgesics inevitably leads to addiction. **Addiction** is the continued use of a substance despite serious health and social consequences (see Chapter 27). The incidence of addiction to opioids, which are used in the treatment of severe pain, is less than 1% in patients with no previous history of drug abuse. Related to this myth is the belief that patients experiencing chronic pain overreport pain because they are addicted to opioids.

Another contradictory myth is the belief that the more pain an individual experiences, the more he or she is likely to tolerate it. In fact, the opposite is more likely to occur. Unrelieved pain creates anxiety and fatigue, both of which increase pain perception and decrease tolerance. A related myth is that there is no physiologic basis for the moderating effects of emotions on pain perception.

25.4 Pain transmission processes allow multiple targets for pharmacologic intervention.

Pain physiology may be divided into four phases: transduction, transmission, perception, and modulation. These phases are illustrated in Figure 25.1.

Pain transduction: Pain transduction begins when nociceptor nerve endings in the peripheral nervous system are stimulated. This occurs when local tissue injury causes the release of chemical mediators of inflammation, including prostaglandins, leukotrienes, histamine, bradykinin, and substance P. These substances sensitize peripheral nociceptors, making them easier to activate.

Pain transmission: The nerve impulse signaling the pain travels from the nociceptor to the spinal cord along two types of sensory neurons called A and C fibers. A fibers are wrapped in myelin, a lipid substance that speeds nerve transmission, and carry signals for intense, well-defined pain. In contrast, C fibers are unmyelinated and thus carry information more slowly and conduct poorly localized pain, which is often perceived as burning or a dull ache.

A fibers have three subtypes: alpha (α), beta (β), and delta (Δ). Aα fibers have the fastest transmission and respond to touch and pressure on muscle; Aβ fibers are slower and respond to touch and pressure on skin. Finally, AΔ fibers are the slowest of the A fibers and respond to tissue injury, producing the sensation of sharp pain.

The sensory nerve fibers enter the dorsal horn of the spinal cord and have adjacent synapses in an area called the substantia gelatinosa. The **gate control theory** proposes a gating mechanism for the transmission of pain in the spinal

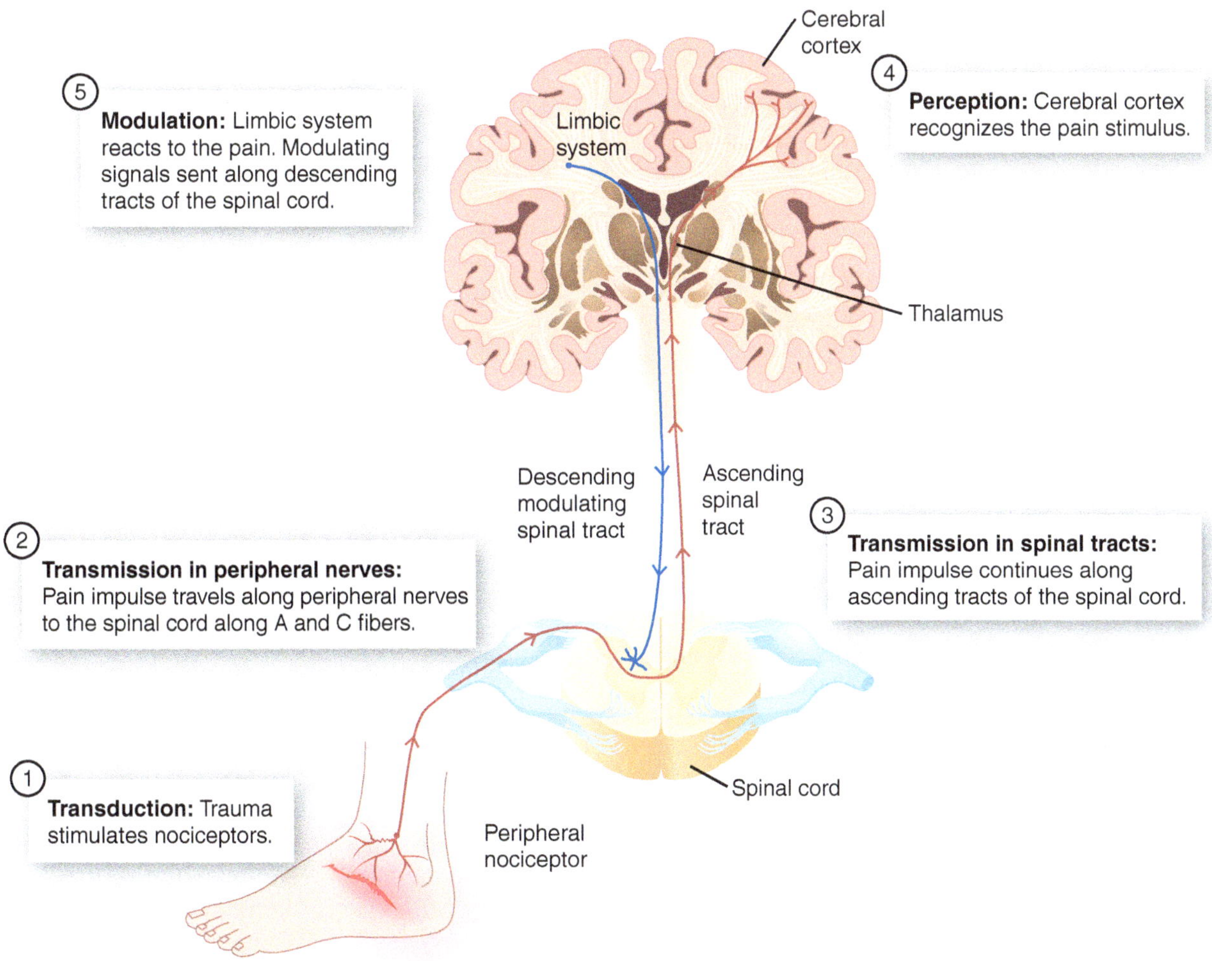

Figure 25.1 Phases of pain physiology.

cord. Signals from faster Aα or Aβ fibers reach the spinal cord and close the gate before those of C fibers reach the region (or gate), in effect blocking the transmission of these types of pain impulses. The gate control theory, proposed in 1965, has withstood the test of time and has been found to be more complex than originally proposed. The "gates" can also be closed when flooded with non-nociceptor impulses. Gate control explains the effectiveness of massage, transcutaneous electrical nerve stimulation, and, possibly, acupuncture in reducing pain.

Once a pain impulse reaches the spinal cord, neurotransmitters are responsible for passing the message along to the next neuron. At the spinal cord level, glutamate is the neurotransmitter for A fibers, whereas both glutamate and substance P are neurotransmitters for C fibers. Impulse transmission from the spinal cord to the brain is moderated by both excitatory and inhibitory neurotransmitters. The activity of substance P may be affected by other neurotransmitters released from neurons in the central nervous system (CNS). One group of neurotransmitters functions as endogenous opioids, or natural pain modifiers; these include **endorphins** and enkephalins.

Pain perception: Perception, the conscious experience of pain, occurs in the brain. Numerous cortical structures and pathways are involved in perception, including the reticular activating system, the somatosensory system, and the limbic system (see Chapter 17). When the pain impulse reaches the brain, it may respond to the sensation with a wide variety of possible actions, ranging from signaling the skeletal muscles to jerk away from a sharp object to mental depression in those experiencing chronic pain.

Pain modulation: Modulation involves descending nervous impulses traveling down the spinal cord that inhibit afferent pain transmission via a feedback mechanism. Neurotransmitters such as serotonin, norepinephrine, and endogenous opioids (endorphins and enkephalins) inhibit pain transmission.

The four phases of pain physiology allow for multiple targets for pharmacologic intervention. The two primary classes of analgesics act at different locations: The nonsteroidal anti-inflammatory drugs (NSAIDs) act at the peripheral level, whereas the opioids act on the CNS. Drugs that affect or mimic the inhibitory neurotransmitters are used as adjuvant analgesics.

25.5 Both pharmacologic and nonpharmacologic therapies are used in pain management.

Effective pain management requires a holistic approach to meet the patient's need for pain relief. In some cases, such as a headache, pain relief is easy to accomplish using over-the-counter (OTC) medications or relaxation or biofeedback therapies. In other cases, such as during cancer treatment, prescription medications must be used to reduce pain levels. For these patients, pain management requires considerable skill on the part of the healthcare provider.

Nonpharmacologic therapies: Nonpharmacologic techniques may be used to attain adequate pain relief in place of drugs, or they may serve as adjuncts to analgesics. When used concurrently with medication, nonpharmacologic techniques allow for improved comfort, lower doses, and the potential for fewer drug-related adverse events. Nondrug interventions should routinely be considered in the nursing plan of care for patients with pain. Some complementary and alternative therapies used for reducing pain include the following:

- Acupressure and acupuncture
- Application of cold or heat
- Biofeedback therapy
- Distraction, including art or music therapy, or laughter
- Electrical nerve stimulation
- Hypnosis
- Massage
- Meditation
- Physical therapy
- Yoga.

Pharmacologic therapies: Dozens of OTC and prescription pain medications are available, and the selection of a specific one depends on many factors. Foremost is the severity of the pain. The drug selected must be capable of providing adequate pain relief. Secondarily, the choice of analgesic depends on potential adverse events, drug interactions and contraindications. A key point is that every analgesic, even an OTC pain reliever, has the potential to cause serious adverse effects in susceptible patients. This reinforces the need to utilize nonpharmacologic therapies for pain relief whenever possible.

The two broad categories of analgesics are the opioids and nonopioids. A third category of drugs for the management of pain is the adjuvant analgesics. The adjuvant analgesics have no pain relief activity when used alone, but they are able to enhance the analgesic action of opioids and nonopioids.

The most effective drug class for relieving severe pain is the opioids. Minor to moderate pain is treated with nonopioids such as NSAIDs, centrally acting drugs, or acetaminophen. There are dozens of opioids and NSAIDs to choose from and it is difficult for beginning students, and even experienced healthcare providers, to learn the subtle differences of drugs within each class. Although the large number of analgesics appears overwhelming, most of them are quite similar and healthcare providers often prescribe only a few drugs in each class. The various drugs used for analgesia and the levels at which they act are shown in Pharmacotherapy Illustrated 25.1.

The pharmacologic management of acute and chronic pain is based on the analgesic ladder proposed by the World Health Organization. Pain ratings of less than 4 are treated with nonopioid analgesics, complementary and alternative therapies (CATs), or a combination of the two. When pain ratings become moderate (4 to 6), PO opioids are added to the baseline treatment. When pain is severe (7 to 10), parenteral opioids are used. If chronic pain has neuropathic qualities, adjuvant analgesics are added.

Combination drugs for pain: Healthcare providers often use opioid and nonopioid analgesics concurrently in the pharmacotherapy of pain. For convenience, these combinations are available as fixed-dose tablets or capsules. The two classes of analgesics work synergistically to relieve pain, and the dose of opioid can be lowered to avoid dependence and opioid-related adverse effects. Use of these combinations in chronic pain management has a dose ceiling due to the toxicities of the nonopioid analgesic. For example, patients taking a combination product containing acetaminophen need to be aware of the risk of acute liver failure with high doses. Liver enzyme levels should be monitored regularly, and care must be taken not to exceed the maximum daily dosages for acetaminophen. The FDA mandated that manufacturers limit the dose of acetaminophen in prescription products to a maximum of 325 mg per dosage unit. However, the maximum daily dose of acetaminophen is 4000 mg/day. Therefore, the healthcare provider can still prescribe 12 dosage units per day of the drug and remain below the maximum. Example combination analgesics include:

- Anexia (hydrocodone, 5.0–7.5 mg; acetaminophen, 325 mg)
- Norco (hydrocodone, 7.5–10 mg; acetaminophen, 325 mg)
- Oxycet (oxycodone, 5.0 mg; acetaminophen, 325 mg)
- Percocet (oxycodone, 2.5–10 mg; acetaminophen, 325 mg)
- Percodan (oxycodone, 4.8355 mg; aspirin, 325 mg)
- Reprexain (hydrocodone, 2.5–10 mg; ibuprofen, 200 mg)

Management of cancer pain: Patients with intractable cancer pain require more invasive techniques because rapidly growing tumors often press on vital tissues and nerves. Furthermore, chemotherapy and surgical treatments for cancer can cause severe pain. Radiation therapy may provide pain relief by shrinking solid tumors that may be

Pharmacotherapy Illustrated 25.1

Sites of Analgesic Action

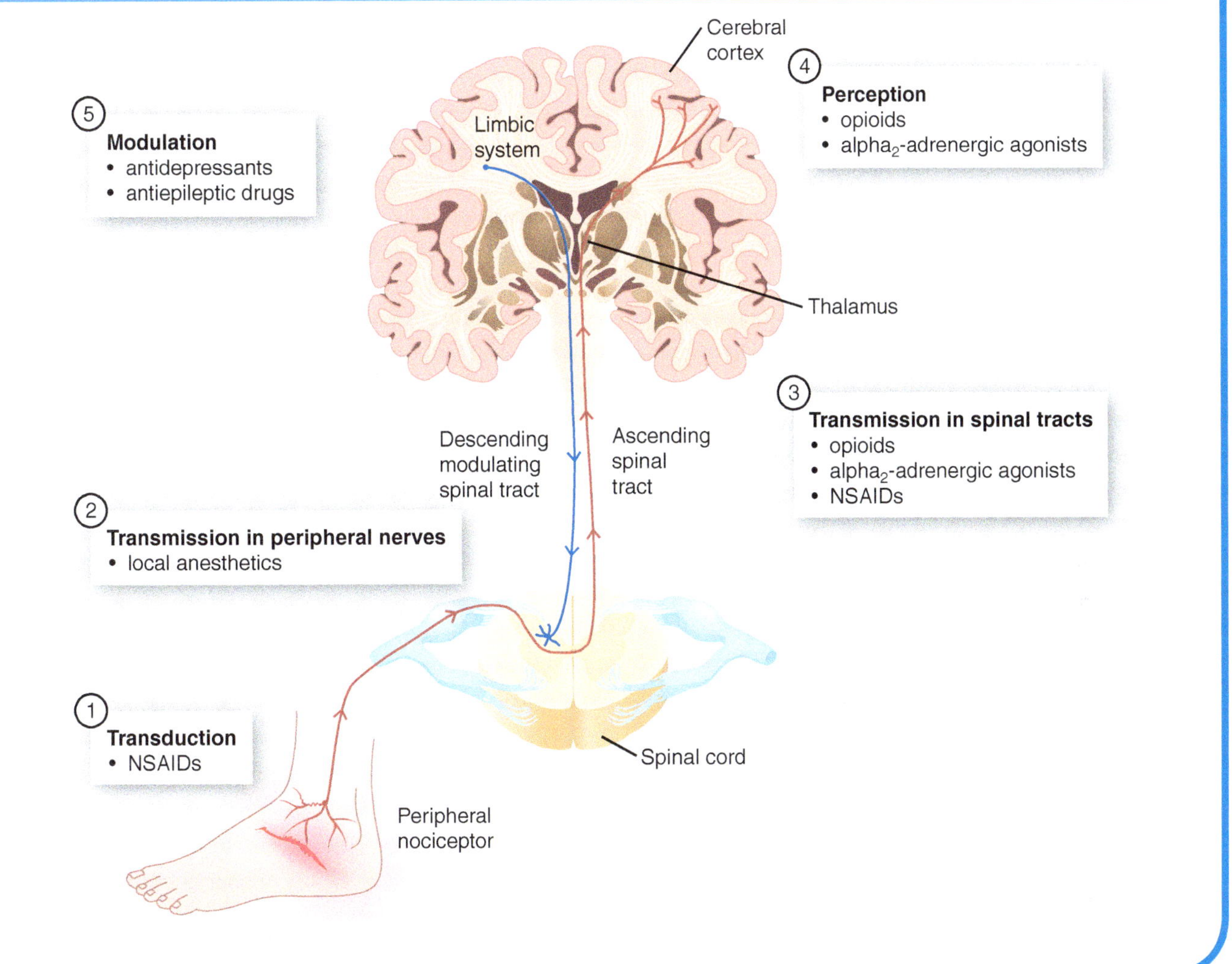

pressing on nerves. Surgery may be used to reduce pain by removing part of or the entire tumor. Injection of alcohol or another neurotoxic substance into neurons is occasionally performed to cause nerve blocks. Nerve blocks irreversibly stop impulse transmission along the treated nerves and have the potential to provide total pain relief. Injection of local anesthetics or steroid hormones as nerve blocks can provide relief for months and is used for pain resulting from pressure on spinal nerves.

Patient-controlled analgesia: Patient-controlled analgesia (PCA) is a method of drug delivery that uses an infusion pump to deliver a prescribed amount of opioid by patient self-administration. By pressing a button, the patient can self-administer the opioid, thus relieving the anxiety of waiting for a prn drug administration. The patient does not have unlimited access to the drug; the infusion pump is programmed by the nurse to deliver a prescribed amount of drug over a designated time period. If the patient attempts to self-administer the drug too often, the patient is locked out until the next dose interval. The program is adjusted depending on the patient's response to the drug. Morphine is the opioid usually used for PCA; however, fentanyl or hydromorphone may be used.

PCA allows patients to participate in their own care. Frequent, small doses of analgesics give a more consistent serum drug level than would be obtained by administering larger doses three to four times per day. PCA requires that the patient be conscious and capable of understanding the operation of the pump. Patients should be taught not to be overly concerned about activating the pump because the program is set to prevent the possibility of overdose. Nurses, family members, or visitors should not use the device to give the patient more medication but should consult with the healthcare provider if they feel that the patient's pain is not relieved.

Pain Management with Opioids

25.6 Opioid analgesics exert their effects by interacting with specific receptors in the central nervous system.

Opium is one of the oldest known natural remedies; it has been used to relieve pain for thousands of years. Extracted from the unripe seeds of the poppy plant, *Papaver somniferum*, **opium** is a milky substance that contains over 20 different chemicals having pharmacologic activity. Opium contains 9 to 14% morphine and 0.8 to 2.5% codeine. Natural substances obtained from opium (such as morphine and codeine) are called **opiates**.

In the late 1800s, scientists began to create synthetic and semisynthetic substances with morphine-like properties. More than a dozen different synthetic drugs with morphine-like activity are now available. **Opioid** is a general term referring to any of these substances, natural or synthetic, and is often used interchangeably with the term *opiate*.

Pharmacotherapy with opioids is predominantly used to relieve moderate to severe pain. With proper dosing, opioids can relieve any degree of pain; they are most effective in treating constant, dull types of pain. In large quantities opioids produce euphoria and severe CNS depression that can lead to stupor, coma, or death. When used for prolonged periods at high doses, opioids cause physical and psychologic dependence.

Narcotic is a term commonly used to describe certain medications. In the context of law enforcement, *narcotic* is used to describe a broad range of abused illegal drugs such as hallucinogens, cocaine, amphetamines, and marijuana. In medical settings, however, narcotic is more restrictively defined as a morphine-like drug used to alleviate pain. To avoid confusion, it is best to use the combined term *narcotic analgesic* rather than simply *narcotic*. In clinical practice, a narcotic analgesic is the same as an opioid, and the terms may be used interchangeably.

Opioids exert their actions by interacting with at least six types of receptors in the CNS: mu, kappa, and delta are the three major receptor types. From the perspective of pain management, the **mu receptors** and **kappa receptors** are the most important, as shown in Figure 25.2. Activation of the mu receptor is responsible for the analgesic properties of the opioids as well as some of the adverse effects such as respiratory depression and physical dependence (see Chapter 27). Drugs that activate opioid receptors are called opioid agonists; those that block these receptors are called opioid antagonists. Because there are multiple opioid receptors, three general types of drug–receptor interactions are possible:

- *Opioid agonists.* Drugs that activate both mu and kappa receptors; for example, morphine and codeine (see Section 25.7)

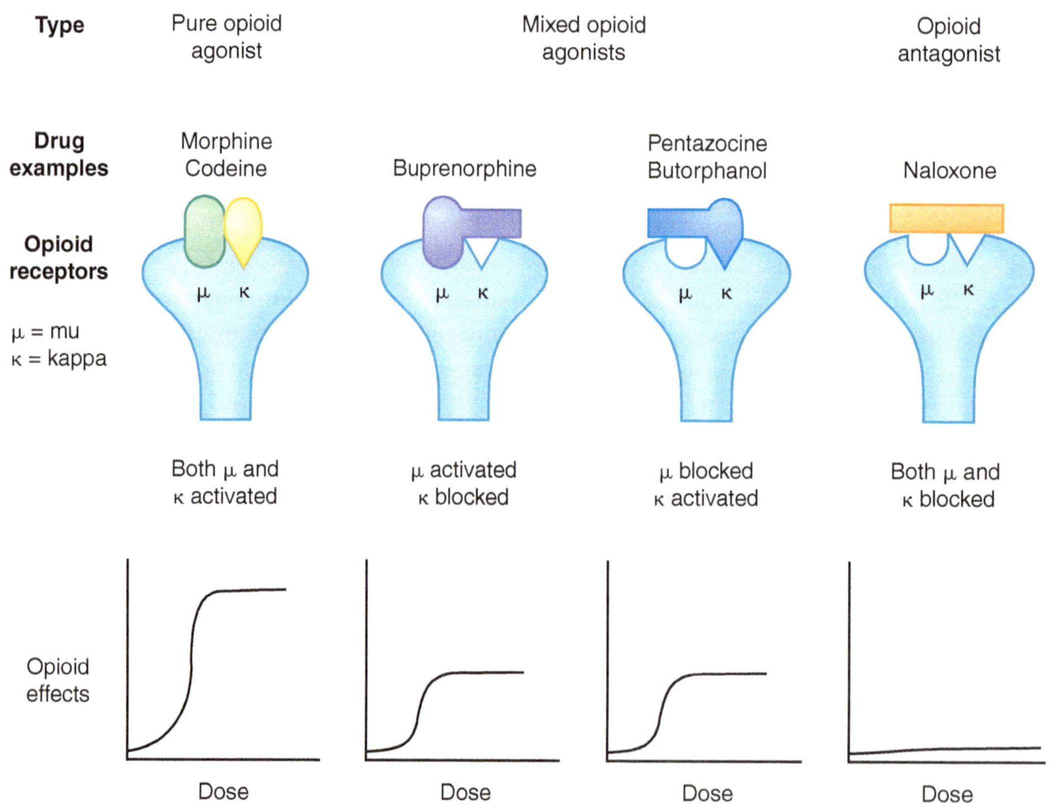

Figure 25.2 Types of opioid receptors.

- *Mixed opioid agonist–antagonists.* Drugs that occupy one receptor and block (or have no effect) on the other; for example, buprenorphine (Buprenex, Butrans) and butorphanol (see Section 25.8)
- *Opioid antagonists.* Drugs that block both mu and kappa receptors; for example, naloxone (Narcan) (see Section 25.12).

The types of agonist actions produced by activating the mu and kappa receptors are shown in Table 25.1. Analgesia is obviously the desired response in pain management. The other responses constitute adverse effects of opioid therapy and must be assessed, prevented, or managed as part of the plan of care for a patient receiving opioid therapy (see Applied Clinical Judgment for Patients Receiving Pharmacotherapy for Pain).

Opioids neither lower the threshold for pain at the nociceptor level nor slow or block the transmission of the pain impulse. It is the *perception and emotional response to pain* that is altered by these medications. Essentially the patient knows that the pain still exists, but it does not cause concern or anxiety.

Table 25.1 Responses Produced by Activation of Specific Opioid Receptors

Response	Mu Receptor	Kappa Receptor
Analgesia	Yes	Yes
Decreased GI motility	Yes	Yes
Euphoria	Yes	No
Miosis	No	Yes
Physical dependence	Yes	No
Respiratory depression	Yes	No
Sedation	Yes	Yes

25.7 Opioids are the preferred drugs for moderate to severe pain that cannot be controlled with other classes of analgesics.

Over 20 different opioids are available as medications. This large group is split into subclasses by similarities in their chemical structures, mechanisms of action, and effectiveness. Each classification is useful in explaining some of the similarities and differences among the opioids. The opioids are listed in Table 25.2. The opioids that have very short durations of action are used primarily as anesthesia adjuncts and are presented in Chapter 26.

Opioids produce many important physiologic actions in addition to analgesia. They are effective at suppressing

Table 25.2 Selected Opioid Analgesic Comparison

Drug	Route and Dose (Maximum Dose Where Indicated)	Equianalgesic Dose (Parenteral)	Equianalgesic Dose (PO)
Codeine	PO: 15–60 mg qid IM: 15–30 mg q4–6h	120 mg	200 mg
fentanyl (Sublimaze)	IM: 0.05–0.1 mg Transdermal: 25–100 mcg q72h	0.1–0.2 mg	–
hydrocodone	PO: 5–10 q4–6h	–	30 mg
hydromorphone (Dilaudid)	PO: 1–4 mg q4–6h Subcutaneous/IM/IV: 1–4 mg q4–6h	1.5 mg	7.5
levorphanol	PO: 2–3 mg tid–qid Subcutaneous/IV: 1–2 mg q6–8h	2 mg	4 mg
meperidine (Demerol)	PO: 50–150 mg q3–4h IM: 50–100 mg q3–4h IV: 1–1.5 mg/kg q3–4h	100	300 mg
methadone	PO: 20 mg q6–8h	10 mg	7.5
morphine (Duramorph RF, Kadian, Mitigo, Morphabond ER, MS Contin)	PO: 30 mg q4h IM: 10 mg q4h IV: 2–10 mg q2–4h; 0.1–1 mg/mL continuous	10 mg	30 mg
oxycodone (OxyContin)	PO: 5–10 mg qid Controlled release: 10–20 mg q12h	–	20 mg
oxymorphone	Subcutaneous: 1.0–1.5 mg q4–6h Rectal: 1 suppository (5 mg) q4–6h PO (extended release): 5–20 mg bid	1 mg	10 mg
Partial Agonists			
buprenorphine (Buprenex)	IM/IV: 0.3 mg q6h	0.3 mg	–
butorphanol	IM: 1–4 mg q3–4h IV: 0.5–2 mg IV q3–4h	2 mg	–
nalbuphine	Subcutaneous/IM/IV: 10–20 mg q3–6h	10 mg	–

the cough reflex and at slowing the motility of the gastrointestinal (GI) tract in patients with severe diarrhea. Opioids are powerful CNS depressants and can cause sedation, which may be considered a therapeutic effect or an adverse effect, depending on the patient's disease state. Some patients experience euphoria and intense relaxation, which are reasons why these drugs are frequently abused.

Opioids have the potential to produce many serious adverse effects, including respiratory depression, sedation, nausea and vomiting, and constipation. Management of opioid adverse effects is summarized in Table 25.3. Through activation of primarily the mu receptors, opioids can cause profound respiratory depression, which is the most serious adverse effect of these medications. Respiratory depression is most problematic during the initial period of drug administration and with patients who have not previously taken these drugs (opiate naive). Patients at greatest risk include those with preexisting respiratory impairment or those concurrently taking other respiratory depressant drugs. A current medication history is very important, especially alcohol use and other CNS depressants, because these drugs will cause additive respiratory depression and sedation. Tolerance to respiratory depression usually occurs within 48 to 72 hours of initiation of therapy.

Respirations should be monitored before initiating therapy and regularly throughout opioid pharmacotherapy. The drugs should be withheld if respirations fall below 12 breaths/min. Narcotic antagonists such as naloxone (Narcan) should be readily available if respirations fall below 10 breaths/min (see Section 25.12). If opioids are administered by continuous epidural or intravenous (IV) routes, interventions should be taken to reduce the risk of respiratory depression. These include frequent monitoring of vital signs, level of consciousness, and pain rating as well as proper body positioning. Airway equipment and narcotic antagonists are usually kept at the bedside.

Table 25.3 Management of Opioid Adverse Effects

Adverse Effect	Management
Constipation	Assume it will occur and initiate preventive measures: Increase dietary fiber and fluid intake; use stool softeners and mild laxatives, if needed.
Nausea	Usually transient. Antiemetics are administered, as needed.
Orthostatic hypotension	Assess blood pressure before ambulation; change positions slowly; assist with ambulation, if needed.
Respiratory depression	Monitor respiratory status frequently, especially initially and with dosage increases. Avoid other CNS depressants that could have additive effects such as alcohol, antidepressants, and barbiturates. Use coughing, deep breathing, and incentive spirometry. If the patient is unresponsive and the respiratory rate is less than 12 breaths/min, administer naloxone per protocol.
Sedation	Common with initiation of therapy or during dosage increase. Tolerance develops in several days. Use safety precautions, especially with ambulation.
Urinary retention	Monitor for bladder distention. More common in older adult men. Tolerance usually develops with long-term dosing. If receiving epidural administration, use an indwelling catheter.

Opioids can cause orthostatic hypotension by inhibiting the baroreceptor reflex and by causing peripheral vasodilation. Dizziness and fainting are possible; assistance may therefore be needed with ambulation. Hydromorphone and meperidine are especially prone to causing hypotension. Patients with hypovolemia are more sensitive to this hypotensive effect; therefore, volume deficiencies should be corrected before initiating opioid therapy.

Increased intracranial pressure (ICP) is a severe adverse reaction that can occur as an indirect result of respiratory depression. When respiration is suppressed, the CO_2 content of the blood increases. The result is vasodilation of cerebral blood vessels and rising ICP. This is of particular concern in patients with conditions that might cause elevated ICP, such as those with head injury, intracranial bleeding, or brain tumors. Narcotic analgesics are usually contraindicated in these patients.

Opioids promote urinary retention by increasing the tone in the bladder sphincter and by suppressing stimuli that normally signal bladder fullness. If the patient has not voided within 6 hours, especially after surgery, insertion of a urinary catheter may be necessary. Patients prone to urinary hesitancy, such as those with benign prostatic hyperplasia, must be carefully monitored.

Constipation and nausea and vomiting frequently occur during opioid administration. Constipation occurs because the drugs suppress intestinal peristalsis, increase the tone of the anal sphincter, and inhibit secretion of fluids into the intestine. Bowel function should be closely monitored, especially after surgery or with long-term use. The plan of care for these patients should include a bowel program to prevent or manage constipation. A baseline program would include increased dietary fiber, adequate fluid intake, and a stool softener such as docusate sodium. More active interventions are implemented if the patient does not resume or maintain normal bowel elimination. The constipation-promoting effect of the opioids is used to advantage in the treatment of severe diarrhea (see Chapter 60).

Opioids directly stimulate the chemoreceptor trigger zone in the medulla to cause intense nausea and vomiting in certain patients. An antiemetic such as promethazine (Phenergan) or ondansetron (Zofran) may be indicated. Orders for prn antiemetics should be made available whenever parenteral opioids are used.

Prolonged use of opioids results in tolerance. Typically, tolerance is noted when patients report that the duration of analgesia is decreasing or admit to taking the drug more frequently as therapy progresses. Increasingly higher doses will be needed to produce the same degree of analgesia. Tolerance does not develop equally for all opioid actions. Whereas tolerance to respiratory depression, sedation, and euphoria develops rapidly, tolerance never develops to the constipation or miosis effects. Remember that as doses of opioids are increased to more effectively manage pain, the incidence of adverse effects will also increase.

All of the narcotic analgesics have the potential to cause physical and psychologic dependence (see Chapter 27). Dependence is most likely to occur when high doses are taken for extended periods. Healthcare providers and nurses are sometimes hesitant to administer the proper amount of opioid analgesics for fear of causing patient dependence or of producing serious adverse effects such as sedation or respiratory depression. Undermedication, however, results in patients not receiving adequate pain relief. When used according to accepted medical practice, patients can, and indeed should, receive the pain relief they need without fear of dependence or serious adverse effects.

Opioids are frequently abused for nonmedical purposes. The risk of abuse is especially high in patients with a history of substance abuse. Opioids are frequently diverted from medical sources (e.g., patients, pharmacies, hospitals), either stolen or sold for criminal intent. Opioids are even stolen from family members, especially older adults. Illicit users may "doctor shop" and obtain opioids from different prescribers and then sell the pills for profit.

Many patients who experience an adverse reaction to an opioid will report that they are allergic to these drugs. For example, patients who experience nausea and vomiting or severe dizziness will often state they are allergic to narcotics. True allergic (Type I hypersensitivity) reactions to opioids, however, are actually rare. Although some of the opioids do indeed cause direct histamine release from mast cells, these types of idiosyncratic reactions do not result in the classic signs of anaphylaxis; thus, they are not true allergic reactions. Morphine, codeine, and meperidine have the highest potential for nonimmune histamine release. When a real immune hypersensitivity reaction does occur, it may extend to other drugs in the opioid class.

Table 25.2 includes a column labeled "Equianalgesic Dose." It is often necessary to change the route of a patient's pain medication or even the drug itself. One of the most frequently occurring examples that a nurse may encounter is the transition a patient makes from IV medications after surgery to PO analgesics prior to discharge. Using relative potency information (equivalent dose), the primary healthcare provider can determine the appropriate new dose. Following surgery, it is not unusual to have orders for a parenteral opioid for severe pain, an oral opioid for moderate pain, and a combination opioid and nonopioid for mild pain. The nurse can use these same equivalencies in choosing the drug and dose when a range of analgesic options is ordered. Caution should be used when using tables of equianalgesic doses because they differ widely based on formulation, route of administration, and whether the patient is opioid naive or opioid tolerant.

CONNECTION Checkpoint 25.1

A common abbreviation for morphine sulfate is MS. From what you learned in Chapter 6, why should this abbreviation be avoided and what can you do to prevent this type of medication error?

PROTOTYPE DRUG Morphine Sulfate (Duramorph RF, Kadian, Mitigo, Morphabond ER, MS Contin)

Classification **Therapeutic:** Narcotic analgesic
Pharmacologic: Opioid agonist

Therapeutic Effects and Uses: Morphine sulfate is the narcotic analgesic of choice for the management of most types of acute and severe chronic pain. The drug was in use for thousands of years prior to its approval by the FDA in 1939 and is still obtained from unripe seeds of the poppy plant.

In addition to relieving severe pain, morphine is used off-label to treat several other conditions. Its CNS depressant action may be used to provide preanesthetic sedation and to calm severely agitated patients. In patients who are terminally ill, its respiratory depressant action may be used to relieve the shortness of breath associated with end-stage cancer, heart failure, or pulmonary edema.

The advantages of morphine therapy, especially in the treatment of chronic cancer pain where dosing increases over time, are that morphine has no upper-end dose limit, and that patients develop tolerance to all the adverse effects except constipation. Extended-release tablets (MorphaBond ER, MS Contin) or capsules (Kadian) are available. Initiation of therapy is usually begun with shorter-acting drugs. Once the correct dose has been titrated, the patient may be switched to extended-release formulations.

Mechanism of Action: Morphine occupies mu and kappa receptor sites in the brain and dorsal horn of the spinal cord that alter the release of afferent neurotransmitters. The dominant effect alters the perception of and emotional response to pain, producing analgesia and euphoria. The drug mimics the actions of endogenous endorphins.

Pharmacokinetics:

Route(s)	PO, IV, subcutaneous, intramuscular (IM), rectal, epidural, intrathecal
Absorption	PO variable, 30%; subcutaneous or IM may be erratic or delayed
Distribution	Widely distributed; crosses the placenta; secreted in breast milk

Primary metabolism	Hepatic; significant first-pass metabolism
Primary excretion	Renal; 7–10% in bile and feces
Onset of action	PO: 30–60 min; IV: rapid; epidural: 15–30 min
Duration of action	PO: 4–7 h; IV: 4–5 h; epidural: 4–24 h

Adverse Effects: Morphine depresses the CNS, causing sedation, dizziness, anxiety, and a feeling of floating or disorientation. Tolerance often develops to these CNS effects after a few days of therapy. Hallucinations and seizures may occur at high doses. Morphine reduces the sensitivity of the respiratory center to CO_2, thus decreasing tidal volume and rate and producing respiratory depression. The resulting increase in CO_2 produces cerebral vasodilation and increases cerebrospinal fluid pressure. Morphine stimulates the chemoreceptor trigger zone in the medulla, producing nausea and vomiting, which may require the administration of an antiemetic drug during the first few days of therapy. The drug delays digestion, increases smooth muscle tone in the intestinal tract, and slows peristalsis in the colon, leading to constipation. Morphine also causes spasm of the sphincter of Oddi, which can result in intense pain (biliary colic) and potential obstruction of bile flow. Urinary retention may occur due to increasing bladder sphincter tone. Peripheral vasodilation may cause orthostatic hypotension. Pruritus is more common when morphine is given by the IV and epidural routes and is not considered a sign of hypersensitivity in the absence of skin rash. **Black Box Warning:** Morphine is a Schedule II controlled substance with a high potential for physical and psychologic dependence. The extended-release forms are prescribed for opioid-tolerant patients only and are not intended for prn use. The extended-release forms should never be opened, chewed, dissolved, or crushed because this can lead to fatal overdose.

Contraindications/Precautions: Morphine is contraindicated in patients with hypersensitivity to opioids. Premature infants are especially sensitive to the effects of morphine; thus, the drug should not be used during pregnancy or during the delivery of premature infants. It should be used with caution in older adults and in those with undiagnosed abdominal pain, hepatic impairment, chronic kidney disease (CKD), shock, CNS depression, head injury or increased ICP, chronic obstructive pulmonary disease, or other conditions with decreased respiratory reserve, including severe obesity. Mothers should wait 4 to 6 hours after a dose of morphine before breastfeeding; withdrawal symptoms have been noted in nursing infants whose mothers abruptly discontinue opioid use. Morphine should never be withdrawn abruptly in patients who have been on prolonged therapy because this will precipitate symptoms of acute opioid withdrawal. Discontinuation should be conducted gradually over several days.

Drug Interactions: When morphine is used with other CNS depressants, including alcohol, skeletal muscle relaxants, and monoamine oxidase inhibitors (MAOIs), increased sedation will result. Administration of an opioid antagonist such as naloxone will reverse the effects of morphine and may produce immediate withdrawal symptoms. Concurrent use with antidiarrheal drugs such as loperamide will cause additive constipation. **Herbal/Food:** Use of kava, valerian, or chamomile can increase CNS depression. St. John's wort may decrease the analgesic action of morphine.

Pregnancy: Chronic opioid use during pregnancy has been associated with poor fetal growth, stillbirths, preterm birth, and possibly birth defects. After delivery, neonates may experience neonatal abstinence syndrome (NAS) with signs of withdrawal that include tremors, irritability, seizures, poor feeding, and vomiting. The American College of Obstetricians and Gynecologists recommends that pregnant women with opioid use disorder be treated with opioid replacement medications such as methadone or buprenorphine, along with behavioral therapy and counseling (Committee on Obstetric Practice, 2017). Breastfeeding is encouraged for women on stable replacement therapy, except those who are taking street drugs or infected with human immunodeficiency virus. The small amount of methadone or buprenorphine entering milk lessens the severity of NAS and shortens the hospital stay for the infant.

Treatment of Overdose: Morphine overdose can cause coma and life-threatening respiratory depression and requires immediate treatment. Naloxone is a specific antidote for morphine intoxication (see Section 25.12).

Clinician Responsibilities: Key clinical implications for patients receiving morphine are included in Applied Clinical Judgment: Patients Receiving Pharmacotherapy for Pain.

Drugs Similar to Morphine Sulfate

Other opioids used for pain management are listed in Table 25.2. The following are descriptions of opioids with pure agonist activity. All these medications have the same actions and adverse effects as morphine. All are controlled substances.

Codeine: Approved by the FDA in 1939, codeine can be administered by the PO, subcutaneous, or IM routes. Because it has stronger antitussive action than morphine, it is often used for suppression of severe cough. At the low doses needed for cough suppression, codeine does not produce serious adverse effects in adults. When used to treat cough and other severe cold symptoms, low doses are usually combined with guaifenesin (a non-narcotic antitussive), promethazine (a phenothiazine with antihistamine action), phenylephrine (a decongestant), or brompheniramine (an antihistamine). Doses required to produce analgesia are much higher than those needed for cough suppression. When prescribed for analgesia, it is usually in combination with acetaminophen and its use is often limited by nausea and vomiting. During the metabolism of codeine in the CNS, about 10% is converted to morphine, which is partly responsible for its analgesic effects. Codeine may also be used off-label to treat serious diarrhea. In 2017, the FDA issued a contraindication that codeine should not be used for cough or pain in children younger than 12 years of age. The warning also stated that breastfeeding may cause serious adverse reactions in infants.

Fentanyl (Actiq, Duragesic, Fentora, Sublimaze, Subsys): Originally approved in 1968 as an IV anesthetic (Sublimaze) for short-term surgical procedures, fentanyl has since been introduced in multiple formulations. These include buccal tablets (Fentora), buccal film, sublingual tablets, oral transmucosal lozenges (Actiq), transmucosal spray (Subsys), nasal spray (Lazanda), and transdermal patches (Duragesic).

The nonanesthetic formulations of fentanyl are restricted to the management of breakthrough pain in patients who are already receiving and who are tolerant to around-the-clock opioid therapy for their chronic, persistent pain. This includes intractable cancer pain. Giving these formulations to patients who are opioid naive can result in serious or fatal respiratory depression. Generally, the initial dose depends on how much morphine the patient has been receiving, that is, how tolerant the patient has become to the effects of opioids. Doses are gradually increased until the breakthrough pain is relieved. The buccal, transdermal, and transmucosal forms of fentanyl have black box warnings regarding the dependence potential for this drug and the serious adverse effects that can occur if the drug is misused.

Several other opioids—for example, remifentanil (Ultiva), alfentanil (Alfenta), and sufentanil (Dsuvia, Sufenta)—are closely related to fentanyl and are used as IV anesthetics. These drugs and a prototype feature for fentanyl are presented in Chapter 26.

Hydrocodone (Hysingla ER, Zohydro ER): Approved in 1957, hydrocodone is used for analgesia, most often combined with acetaminophen, aspirin, or ibuprofen in fixed dose combinations such as Anexsia, Reprexain, and Norco. Hydrocodone is an effective antitussive and is combined with decongestants or antihistamines for severe cold and flu symptoms. Although it is slightly more effective than codeine as an antitussive, it causes more sedation. Hysingla ER is formulated using abuse-deterrent technology. If crushed, the tablet or capsule forms a viscous gel that is unusable by abusers.

Hydromorphone (Dilaudid): Approved in 1984, hydromorphone is available by the PO, rectal, and parenteral routes. Its primary application is analgesia, including PCA. Hydromorphone produces less nausea but more orthostatic hypotension than morphine. It has a more rapid onset of action and a shorter duration of activity than morphine, requiring PO dosing every 3 to 6 hours. An extended-duration formulation is available. Hydromorphone has black box warnings regarding the dependence potential for this drug and the serious adverse effects that can occur if the drug is misused.

Levorphanol: Approved in 1953, levorphanol is a pure opioid agonist available by the PO route for severe pain. At equianalgesic doses, levorphanol exhibits the same actions and adverse effects as morphine. It offers no advantages over the use of other drugs in this class.

Oliceridine (Olinvyk): In 2020 the FDA approved the use of oliceredine to manage pain that is severe enough to require an IV opioid. Oliceredine works by a unique mechanism. Conventional opioids activate the mu receptor which triggers two pathways in the cell: the G protein pathway and the beta-arrestin pathway. By bypassing the beta-arrestin pathway, oliceredine produces less respiratory depression, nausea and vomiting. The medication is given IV for short-term use in hospital settings.

Meperidine (Demerol): Approved in 1942, meperidine is available by both the PO and parenteral routes for the treatment of severe pain. Toxicity can occur due to its active metabolite, called normeperidine, which is a CNS stimulant with a half-life of 15 to 30 hours. Accumulation of this metabolite can result from doses greater than 400 to 600 mg/day or administration longer than 48 hours. Normeperidine can cause tremors and seizures, which are not reversed with narcotic antagonists. For this reason, meperidine is not recommended for use longer than 48 hours, for chronic pain, or for use in PCA. When meperidine is used in high doses or longer than 48 hours, the nurse needs to consult with the prescriber and report any incidences of tremors and irritability before giving the next dose. Because of these adverse effects, meperidine is considered a second-line medication that is used when other opioids are contraindicated. An off-label use for meperidine is for the management of shivering, a common complication in the postoperative period. The drug has a short half-life that requires dosing every 3 to 4 hours.

Methadone: Approved in 1947, methadone is an oral preparation with pharmacologic effects similar to those of morphine; adverse effects are similar with lower incidence. Methadone is frequently prescribed in the management of opiate dependency (see Chapter 27) and is increasingly used for management of chronic pain. Methadone has a long duration of action and can be dosed once daily. Oral liquid (Methadose) and dispersible tablets (Diskets) are available for treating opiate withdrawal symptoms because they offer less risk for abuse than regular tablets. IV methadone is used for the short-term therapy of hospitalized patients. A black box warning indicates that when converting from other analgesics to methadone particular diligence is necessary because deaths have been reported during the conversion period. The deaths were likely due to raising the dose of methadone too quickly, resulting in cardiac and respiratory failure.

Oxycodone (Oxaydo, OxyContin, Xtampza ER): Approved in 1976, oxycodone is an oral opioid that is often combined with acetaminophen or with aspirin for the management of moderate to severe pain. The drug is used when around-the-clock analgesia is needed for an extended period of time. It is not indicated for short-term or prn use. Oxycodone causes less nausea and vomiting and hallucinations than morphine. The immediate-release forms of this drug have a short duration of action, requiring dosing every 3 to 4 hours. The controlled release form (OxyContin) can be dosed twice a day. OxyContin has become a frequent drug of abuse (see Chapter 27). To counteract the potential for abuse, OxyContin, and Xtampza ER are formulated using dose-deterrent technology. A black box warning states that all patients receiving oxycodone should be routinely monitored for signs of misuse, abuse, and addiction.

Tapentadol (Nucynta): Tapentadol was approved in 2008 and is indicated for moderate to severe pain. The immediate-release form (Nucynta) is for acute pain, whereas the extended-release form (Nucynta ER) is for chronic pain and pain associated with diabetic neuropathy. Tapentadol acts by dual mechanisms: It is used as a mu-receptor agonist and blocks the reuptake of norepinephrine. It has the same abuse potential (Schedule II) as other drugs in this class and has the same spectrum of adverse effects. The most common adverse effects include nausea, constipation, dizziness, headache, and somnolence. The incidence of GI-related adverse effects may be lower with tapentadol than with other drugs in this class.

Tramadol (Conzip, Ultram): Tramadol was approved for the treatment of moderate pain in 1995. The immediate-release formulations are indicated for short-term (5 days or less) relief of acute pain, whereas the extended-release product (ConZip) is approved to treat moderate to moderately severe chronic pain that requires around-the-clock analgesia. Ultracet is a fixed dose combination of tramadol and acetaminophen. Off-label uses of tramadol include treatment of neuropathic pain and restless leg syndrome.

Tramadol has both opioid and nonopioid actions. The drug and one of its metabolites bind to the opioid mu receptor. This opioid agonist activity is weak: approximately 10 times weaker than that of codeine. In addition to its central opioid action, tramadol inhibits norepinephrine and serotonin reuptake in spinal neurons, which inhibits the transmission of pain impulses.

Tramadol is well tolerated, and its most common adverse effects are vertigo, dizziness, headache, nausea and vomiting, constipation, and lethargy. Seizures have been reported, especially in patients who are concurrently taking antidepressants. Although respiratory depression can occur, it is not as severe as that caused by opioids. In 2014, tramadol became a Schedule IV drug, thus physical dependence is possible. Symptoms of opioid withdrawal, such as anxiety, sweating, tremors, panic attacks, and paresthesias, may occur if the drug is abruptly discontinued. Tramadol should not be administered to patients with a history of depression or suicidal ideation because the drug can be fatal in overdose situations, especially if combined with alcohol or other CNS depressants. In 2017, the FDA issued a safety notice that tramadol is contraindicated in children younger than age 12.

25.8 Mixed agonist and antagonist opioids exhibit moderate analgesia with less risk of dependence than morphine.

The mixed agonist–antagonist opioids are narcotic analgesics that were developed with the intention of producing drugs with strong analgesia that have fewer adverse effects than morphine and other pure opioid agonists. The four drugs in this class are used to treat moderate pain but are not as effective as morphine in treating severe pain. Their advantage is that they cause less respiratory depression and have a lower potential for dependence. These drugs have some abuse potential but less so than the pure opioid agonists. The types of adverse effects, contraindications, and nursing responsibilities are similar to those of the pure opioid agonists (see Section 25.7).

With both agonist and antagonist actions, what would happen if an individual addicted to morphine or heroin took one of the drugs in this class? Blocking opioid receptors would likely cause the patient to experience opioid withdrawal symptoms. In fact, some of the mixed agonist–antagonist drugs are indicated for the induction of opioid withdrawal and the maintenance of opioid dependence (see Chapter 27).

Buprenorphine (Buprenex, Butrans, Others): Originally approved in 1981, is a partial agonist at the mu receptors and an antagonist at the kappa receptors. It is indicated in many formulations for the relief of moderate to severe pain, including tablets and the parenteral route (Buprenex). A transdermal patch system (Butrans) and an extended-release subcutaneous injection (Sublocade) are available, both of which provide 7 days of analgesia. Probuphine is a subdermal implant consisting of four, 1-inch rods inserted under the skin of the upper arm. The implant releases buprenorphine over a 6-month period, at which time the rods are removed. Buprenorphine is also available in sublingual form, as a buccal film (Belbuca). Sublingual (Suboxone) and orally disintegrating tablet (Zubsolv) forms combine buprenorphine with naloxone for the management of opioid withdrawal and dependence (see Chapter 27). Abuse

CONNECTIONS: Advanced Practice Application

Opioid Prescribing and Addiction

Case

Laura, a 36-year-old mother of three, presented to the emergency room (ER) with a 6-year history of opioid use. Laura was first prescribed an opioid following surgery after a skiing accident. Her surgeon prescribed her Oxycontin for 10 days postsurgery. Months after her injury, and long after her scars had healed, Laura still struggled with deep, biting pain. Her pain had transitioned from acute surgical pain to chronic pain and she had developed a tolerance to opioids.

As her tolerance grew, Laura found that even 15 milligrams of oxycodone no longer worked to control the pain, she no longer had a provider willing to prescribe for her, and she was buying heroin from a "friend."

By the time she arrived to the ER, Laura had a $100-a day-heroin habit and the drugs had ravaged her 5′ 2′′ frame to a mere 87 pounds. Upon presentation to the ER, she tells you that her children had been removed from her care and her ex-husband had been awarded custody 3 years ago.

Laura is admitted to the hospital for intravenous antibiotics and surgical excision and debridement of an abscess. During her hospitalization she started to detox from the heroin. Her hospitalist nurse practitioner was able to start Laura on Suboxone and helped to connect her to outpatient care prior to being discharged.

Discussion

Tragically, 80% of patients addicted to opioids don't receive the treatment they need. There are many factors that contribute to this, including healthcare access challenges, stigma, and cost. Research has shown that medication-assisted treatment (MAT), a combination of medication and therapy, can successfully treat individuals struggling with addiction and help control the intensities of the cravings. There are three drugs approved by the U.S. Food and Drug Administration (FDA) for the treatment of opioid dependence: buprenorphine, methadone, and naltrexone. All three have been shown to be safe and effective and there is no maximum recommended duration of treatment, for some patients, treatment may need to be continued indefinitely (Substance Abuse and Mental Health Service Administration, n.d.).

Nurse practitioners play a critical role in increasing access to MAT, most specifically access to Suboxone. Suboxone (buprenorphine and naloxone) has become the preferred treatment medication for opioid addiction. For nurse practitioners (NPs), physician assistants (PAs), certified nurse specialists (CNSs), certified registered nurse anesthetists (CRNAs), and certified nurse midwives (CNMs) to be eligible to apply for a buprenorphine waiver through SAMHSA, they must complete 24 hours of training that covers the following topics: opioid maintenance and detoxification; clinical use of all FDA-approved drugs for medication-assisted treatment; patient assessment; treatment planning; psychosocial services; staff roles; and diversion control. Once a practitioner has taken the required training course, they may apply for a waiver to begin treating 30 patients with buprenorphine.

of buprenorphine has been reported but is less common because the drug produces less euphoria than the pure opioid agonists. Withdrawal symptoms from buprenorphine are generally mild and its onset may be delayed 1 to 2 weeks. Buprenorphine is a Schedule III drug.

There are several black box warnings. Buprenorphine has the potential for abuse, which can lead to overdose and death. Life-threatening respiratory depression may occur at high doses. Even a single dose in children may result in death. Prolonged use during pregnancy can result in neonatal opioid withdrawal syndrome, which may be life-threatening. Concurrent use with benzodiazepines, alcohol, or other CNS depressants may result in profound sedation, coma, and death. When using the transdermal form of the drug, a dose of 20 mcg/h (the highest dose patch, worn for 7 days) should not be exceeded due to a risk of QT interval prolongation. The patch application site should not be subjected to high external temperatures because this increases drug release and can cause overdose or death. The subcutaneous form may cause severe harm or death if accidentally injected intravenously. The subdermal implant rods are associated with risk for expulsion, migration and protrusion, and rare nerve damage resulting from their insertion. This drug is pregnancy category C. A prototype drug feature for buprenorphine with naloxone (Suboxone, Zubsolv, others) can be found in Chapter 27.

Butorphanol: Approved in 1978, butorphanol is an agonist at the kappa receptors and is a weak antagonist at the mu receptors. Delivered IV, IM, or via nasal spray, it is approved for moderate to severe pain and as a preanesthetic medication that supplements general anesthesia. Drowsiness and dizziness are experienced by a large number of patients, and the intranasal form can cause nasal congestion. It is contraindicated in patients who are opioid dependent and in patients with respiratory depression. Like buprenorphine, the drug is less commonly abused and has milder withdrawal symptoms than many opioids. Butorphanol is a Schedule III drug.

Nalbuphine (Nubain): Approved in 1979, nalbuphine is an agonist at the kappa receptors and a weak antagonist at the mu receptors. Given by the IV, IM, or subcutaneous route, it is approved for moderate to severe pain and as a preanesthesia or general anesthesia adjunct. Drowsiness is the most common adverse effect. The risk for dependence is low, and nalbuphine is not a scheduled drug. Abrupt discontinuation, however, can precipitate mild opioid withdrawal symptoms. It is contraindicated in patients with serious respiratory depression or asthma. Concurrent use with benzodiazepines, alcohol, or other CNS depressants may result in profound sedation, coma, and death.

Pentazocine: Approved in 1967, pentazocine was the first of the agonist–antagonist opioids marketed. Once available as Talwin by the PO and parenteral routes, it is now only combined with naloxone to treat moderate to severe pain. The drug acts as an agonist at the kappa receptors and a weak antagonist at the mu receptors. Like other drugs in this class, drowsiness and dizziness are common adverse effects. Also like other mixed agonists–antagonists, pentazocine does not produce euphoria and has a low potential for abuse (Schedule IV). Pentazocine with naloxone comes with the same black box warnings as buprenorphine regarding the risks of addiction and abuse, severe respiratory depression, ingestion by children, neonatal opioid withdrawal, and concurrent use with other CNS depressants

Pain Management with Nonopioids

25.9 Nonsteroidal anti-inflammatory drugs are the preferred medications for mild to moderate pain.

The **nonopioid analgesics** include NSAIDs, acetaminophen, and a few centrally acting medications. NSAIDs, such as aspirin and ibuprofen, are preferred medications for relieving mild to moderate pain, especially for pain associated with inflammation. Nonopioids have significant advantages over the opioids. Acetaminophen, aspirin, and many NSAIDs are available OTC and are inexpensive. They are available in many different formulations, including those designed for pediatric patients. For most patients, they are safe when used as directed on the labels. NSAIDs have antipyretic and anti-inflammatory actions as well as analgesic properties. Indeed, some NSAIDs are used primarily for their anti-inflammatory effects. The doses and roles of NSAIDs in the treatment of inflammation and fever are discussed in Chapter 41. Prototype features for aspirin and ibuprofen are also included in Chapter 41. Nursing practice applications for the nonopioid analgesics are similar to those for the opioid analgesics and are presented in the Applied Clinical Judgment for Patients Receiving Pharmacotherapy for Pain. Additional nursing responsibilities for the nonopioids can be found with the prototype drugs and the Applied Clinical Judgment for Patients Receiving Pharmacotherapy for Inflammation and Fever in Chapter 41.

NSAIDs act at peripheral sites by inhibiting pain mediators at the nociceptor level. When tissue is damaged, chemical mediators, including histamine, potassium ion, hydrogen ion, and bradykinin, are released locally. Also released during tissue damage is arachidonic acid, which is metabolized into chemical mediators of inflammation and pain such as prostaglandins. Prostaglandins can induce pain through the formation of free radicals.

NSAIDs inhibit cyclooxygenase, an enzyme responsible for the formation of prostaglandins. Because they act by a different mechanism than opioids, NSAIDs do not produce the severe adverse effects observed with the narcotic analgesics. The most prominent effects are GI related and include nausea and vomiting, anorexia, dyspepsia, and ulceration of the GI mucosa. At high doses, the ulceration can be severe, resulting in bleeding and even perforation. A fixed dose combination of naproxen and esomeprazole (Vimovo) is approved to reduce the potential for developing NSAID-induced gastric ulcers. Other common NSAID adverse events include dizziness, headache, and rash. These drugs do not cause physical or psychologic dependence. When combined with opioids in fixed dose combinations, NSAIDs produce a synergistic analgesic effect that allows the dose of opioid to be lowered.

Acetaminophen is an important nonopioid analgesic that is not classified as an NSAID. Its effectiveness in relieving pain and reducing fever is equal to that of aspirin and ibuprofen. Acetaminophen is featured as a prototype antipyretic in Chapter 41.

CONNECTIONS: APPLIED CLINICAL JUDGMENT

Patients Receiving Pharmacotherapy for Pain

Key Assessment Data

- History of current condition, baseline vital signs, height and weight, physical exam; history of hepatic, renal, respiratory, cardiovascular, or neurologic disease, cancer, or gallbladder or urologic disease; medications, allergy, and substance use history; pregnancy or breastfeeding status. Note recent surgeries or injuries.
- Assess the level of pain. Use objective screening tools when possible (e.g., FLACC [face, limbs, arms, cry, consolability] for infants or very young children, Wong-Baker FACES scale for children, numerical rating scale for adults). Assess pain history and what has worked successfully or not for the patient in the past.
- Ongoing assessment during drug therapy includes pain assessment, appropriate laboratory findings (e.g., hepatic or renal function studies), vital signs, especially BP and respiratory rate.

Desired Therapeutic Outcomes

Improvement is observed and measurable in absent or greatly diminished pain, ability to move more easily without pain or carry out postoperative treatment care, increased ability to carry out ADLs.

CONNECTIONS: APPLIED CLINICAL JUDGMENT (*continued*)

Patients Receiving Pharmacotherapy for Pain

Minimizing Adverse Effects

- Respiratory depression is most common with the first dose of an opioid and when given in the presence of other CNS depressants, for example, postoperatively when the patient may still be experiencing the effects of general anesthesia drugs. Continue to monitor vital signs, especially respirations and pulse oximetry as ordered, postoperatively and in patients with acute pain. Contact the provider before giving if the respirations are below 12 breaths/min in the adult patient or as ordered in the child. Continue to assess the respiratory rate every 15 to 30 minutes for the first 4 hours. For terminal cancer pain, obtain instructions from the oncologist or hospice provider on any dose restrictions; the drug might not be withheld regardless of respiratory rate, dependent on the provider.
- Opioids may cause hypotension as an adverse effect and increase the risk of falls. Monitor blood pressure and pulse periodically or if symptoms warrant. Ensure patient safety; monitor ambulation until the effects of the drug are known.
- Decreased peristalsis is an adverse effect of opioid drugs. Continue to assess bowel sounds. Increase fluid and dietary fiber intake.
- Opioids may cause histamine release with itching or a sensation of itching. In severe cases, antihistamines may be required. Assess for itching as an expected side effect versus signs and symptoms of true allergy or anaphylaxis. Assess also for changes in vital signs, especially hypotension, tachycardia, dyspnea, or urticaria.
- Neurologic changes such as changes in level of consciousness, agitation, disorientation, or confusion may indicate overmedication, increased ICP, or adverse drug effects. Assess for changes in level of consciousness, disorientation or confusion, agitation, headache, sluggish or pinpoint pupils, or seizures immediately.
- Opioids may cause urinary retention. Assess for urinary retention, especially in the postoperative period.
- Nausea and vomiting are common. Administer antiemetics 30 to 60 minutes before opioid dose if nausea and vomiting occur.
- Opioids may cause hypotension and significant dizziness, especially when the drug is given IV. Keeping the patient supine will limit these effects. For IV push administration, dilute the drug with 4 to 5 mL of sterile normal saline and administer over 4 to 5 minutes unless otherwise ordered. The patient should remain supine to prevent dizziness or hypotension. Monitor blood pressure, pulse rate, and respiratory rate before and after the dose.

Lifespan Considerations

- Older adults may be at increased risk for falls due to hypotension, drowsiness, dizziness, or confusion related to drug therapy. Monitor ambulation and provide assistance as needed.
- The older adult is at increased risk of constipation due to slowed peristalsis as a result of the aging process. Significantly diminished or absent bowel sounds should be reported to the healthcare provider immediately. Additional fluids and fiber may ease constipation but additional medications such as MiraLAX or Colace may be required.
- The older male adult is at higher risk for mechanical obstruction of the urinary tract due to an enlarged prostate. Immediately report the inability to void, increasing bladder pressure, or pain.

Diversity Considerations

- Tramadol and other nonopioid analgesics metabolize through the CYP450 pathways and may interact with other drugs. Monitor for less than optimal effects of the drug.
- Opioids cross the placenta and are present in breast milk. Extra caution should be exercised when using opioids in pregnancy or breastfeeding.

Patient and Caregiver Education

- Pain relief, rather than merely control, is the goal of therapy. Take the drug consistently during the acute postoperative or postprocedure period rather than requesting only when pain is severe. Encourage the use of additional, nonmedicinal pain relief techniques. Patients with terminal cancer should take the dose consistently around the clock with prn doses as required. Advise the family or caregiver of the provider's instructions for adequate pain relief and to contact the provider if any pain remains.
- Rise from lying or sitting to standing slowly to avoid dizziness or falls. If dizziness occurs, sit or lie down and do not attempt to stand or walk until the sensation passes.
- Be cautious or avoid driving or other activities requiring mental alertness or physical coordination until the effects of the drug are known.
- Ensure for safety if disorientation is present. Immediately report increasing lethargy, disorientation, confusion, changes in behavior or mood, slurred speech, or ataxia.
- Take deep breaths in the postoperative period. Move about in bed and start early ambulation as soon as allowed postoperatively.
- Increase fluids to 2 L/day and increase intake of dietary fiber such as fruits, vegetables, and whole grains. Report severe constipation to the healthcare provider for additional advice on laxatives or stool softeners.
- Immediately report the inability to void, increasing bladder pressure, or pain.
- Report itching to the healthcare provider, especially if severe or increasing. Immediately report any itching associated with dizziness or lightheadedness, difficulty breathing, palpitations, or significant hives.
- Report nausea if it occurs. Small amounts of food intake (e.g., dry crackers) and sips of carbonated beverages (e.g., ginger ale) may help unless NPO.
- Because opioids are scheduled drugs, discuss the need for proper medication storage, need for the drug to be used by the patient only, and prescription renewal restrictions (i.e., new prescription each time, no refills, prescription may not be called in) as appropriate for the schedule of the drug.
- Do not open, chew, or crush extended-release tablets (e.g., oxycodone [OxyContin]); swallow them whole with plenty of water.

Prescribing Considerations

- Calculating the total daily dose of opioids helps identify patients who may benefit from closer monitoring and prescribing of naloxone or other measures to reduce risk of overdose.
- Morphine milligram equivalents (MME) is an opioid dosage's equivalency to morphine. To determine dose in MMEs, multiply the dose for each opioid by the conversion factor. For example, tablets containing hydrocodone 5 mg and acetaminophen 300 mg taken four times a day would contain a total of 20 mg of hydrocodone daily.
- Prescribe the lowest effective dosage below 50 MME/day.
- Use particular caution when prescribing fentanyl since it is dosed in mcg/hr instead of mg/day; its absorption is affected by heat and other factors.
- When considering opioid therapy for chronic pain, assess the risks to patient safety by conducting a physical examination and mental health screening, check the state prescription drug monitoring program, and consider routine urine drug tests.

25.10 Adjuvant analgesics have primary indications other than pain control but can enhance analgesia.

Some types of pain are not adequately relieved by analgesics alone. **Adjuvant analgesics** are a diverse group of drugs that are used to enhance analgesia for specific indications. All of these drugs have other primary classifications, such as antidepressant, antiseizure, tranquilizer, or anti-inflammatory. The use of adjuvant analgesics includes two primary indications:

- Pain that is refractory to opioids, such as intractable cancer pain
- Neuropathic pain, which is caused by damage to the nerve itself, and pain caused by swelling in the CNS, which puts pressure on nerves.

In patients with intractable cancer pain, adjuvant analgesics are used in combination with analgesics to enhance the level of pain relief. It is important to understand that these medications *supplement* pain relief; they do not substitute for proper dosing of opioid analgesics in patients with severe pain. Adjuvant analgesics are generally not necessary if the pain is well managed with opioids because these drugs have additional adverse effects and drug interactions that can complicate therapy.

Neuropathic pain is difficult to control with analgesics. The most common cause of neuropathic pain is diabetes, but herpes zoster infections, acute trauma, cancer, and certain autoimmune conditions can also cause this type of pain. Neuropathic pain is commonly described as steady burning, electric shock, or "pins and needles" sensations. Rather than treat with high doses of opioids, several adjuvant analgesics have been found to be effective at relieving neuropathic pain. These drugs may be used alone or in combination with opioids.

Adjuvant analgesics can be added at any step in the pain management ladder; they are usually dosed on a regular schedule as opposed to prn. The use of specific adjuvant analgesics and their doses are often guided by experience, rather than controlled clinical trials, and the majority of these drugs are prescribed off-label for their analgesic effects. Table 25.4 summarizes the effects and uses of selected adjuvant analgesics.

Antidepressants: Some of the most commonly prescribed adjuvant analgesics come from the antidepressant drug class. All classes of antidepressants, including tricyclic antidepressants (TCAs), selective serotonin reuptake inhibitors (SSRIs), selective norepinephrine reuptake inhibitors (SNRIs), and atypical antidepressants, have been used as adjuncts in the management of neuropathic pain. Most experience has been with the TCAs, although they tend to produce more frequent side effects than the SSRIs, SNRIs, and atypical antidepressants. Patients experiencing neuropathic pain may need trials with different antidepressants until the right combination of effectiveness and tolerable adverse effects is found. Doses of these medications are

Table 25.4 Adjuvant Analgesics

Drug Class	Examples	Effect	Use
Antiseizure drugs	carbamazepine (Tegretol) gabapentin (Gralise, Neurontin) pregabalin (Lyrica)	Decrease overactive nerve impulse transmission and spontaneous neuron firing.	Reduce peripheral nerve pain in diabetic neuropathy, post-herpetic neuralgia, and trigeminal neuralgia.
Atypical, SNRI, and SSRI antidepressants	citalopram (Celexa) duloxetine (Cymbalta) sertraline (Zoloft) trazodone venlafaxine (Effexor)	Increase concentrations of inhibitory neurotransmitters (serotonin and norepinephrine) in the CNS.	Reduce neuropathic pain.
Benzodiazepines	diazepam (Valium) lorazepam (Ativan)	Potentiate effects of gamma aminobutyric acid (GABA) and other inhibitory neurotransmitters.	Relax skeletal muscles in muscle spasm.
Bisphosphonates	pamidronate zoledronic acid (Reclast, Zometa)	Inhibit bone resorption.	Reduce cancer-related bone pain.
Corticosteroids	dexamethasone prednisone	Reduce cerebral and spinal edema via various mechanisms in prostaglandin cascade.	Reduce swelling and pain in CNS cancer, spinal cord compression, postspinal surgery.
Miscellaneous adjuvant analgesics	clonidine (Catapres, Duraclon) ziconotide (Prialt)	Activate $alpha_2$-adrenergic receptors Block N-type calcium channels	Reduce cancer pain (epidural use) Reduce cancer pain (intrathecal use)
Tricyclic antidepressants (TCAs)	amitriptyline amoxapine desipramine (Norpramin) doxepin (Silenor) imipramine (Tofranil) nortriptyline (Pamelor) protriptyline (Vivactil)	Increase concentrations of inhibitory neurotransmitters (serotonin and norepinephrine) in the CNS.	Reduce neuropathic pain.

generally lower than those used to treat depression, and the drugs act to relieve pain within 5 to 7 days. If improvement in pain relief is not noted within 1 week, an alternative drug may be substituted. Duloxetine (Cymbalta) was the first of the antidepressants to receive FDA approval for the treatment of diabetic peripheral neuropathic pain, chronic musculoskeletal pain, and fibromyalgia pain. Other drugs used for this purpose include amitriptyline, imipramine (Tofranil), doxepin (Silenor), paroxetine (Paxil), and venlafaxine (Effexor).

CONNECTION Checkpoint 25.2

Use of tricyclic antidepressants has declined in recent decades due to a higher incidence of adverse effects compared to drugs in the SSRI class, but they are useful in the treatment of neuropathic pain. From what you learned in Chapter 19, what type of adverse effects would likely be observed in patients taking TCAs for migraines?

Antiseizure drugs: Antiseizure drugs FDA-approved for neuropathic pain include gabapentin (Neurontin), pregabalin, and carbamazepine (Tegretol). The antiseizure drugs act by suppressing neuronal discharges and reducing the hyperexcitability that occurs after nerve injury. These drugs may cause nausea and vomiting, sedation, confusion, or dizziness. Gabapentin is considered a first-line drug for treating neuropathic pain, and an extended-release tablet form of the drug (Gralise) is approved to treat post-herpetic neuralgia.

Corticosteroids: Corticosteroids are used as adjuvants in pain management because they reduce inflammatory swelling and pressure on the brain, spinal cord, and spinal nerves. Dexamethasone is a preferred drug when given parenterally to reduce either cerebral or spinal cord edema; oral prednisone may follow for a period of time. Steroids can also be injected directly into joints in refractory arthritis or epidural-spinal tracts for chronic musculoskeletal pain. Their effects are discussed in Chapter 68.

Local anesthetics: Mexiletine (Mexitil) is a Class IB antidysrhythmic drug with anesthetic properties that may be given off-label for neuropathic pain refractory to other analgesics. Caution must be used when giving this drug to patients with heart disease or dysrhythmias. Short IV infusions of lidocaine (Xylocaine) may also provide temporary relief for some patients. A 5% lidocaine patch is approved for post-herpetic neuralgia.

Muscle relaxants: Muscle relaxants such as the benzodiazepines may be used effectively as adjuvant analgesics when muscle spasm is a component of the pain. Muscle spasm can be present following orthopedic injury or with musculoskeletal disease or degenerative nervous system conditions. Benzodiazepines can also be used to reduce anxiety in the terminal dyspnea of heart failure or end-stage respiratory disease. Examples include diazepam (Valium), lorazepam (Ativan), and oxazepam.

Bone-specific medications: Patients with bone cancer or metastases may experience severe pain. For palliative care, the administration of calcitonin, either subcutaneously or intranasally, may provide some relief for bone pain. The adjuvant analgesic activity of the bisphosphonates such as pamidronate and zoledronate (Reclast, Zometa) has been well established. The use of calcitonin and bisphosphonates in treating bone disorders is presented in Chapter 72.

Miscellaneous drugs: Capsaicin is a product obtained from chili peppers that is available as a cream to treat minor musculoskeletal pain. A prescription patch containing 8% capsaicin (Qutenza) was approved in 2010 for the relief of pain associated with post-herpetic neuralgia. Milnacipran (Savella) is an SNRI whose only indication is the treatment of fibromyalgia. Although the exact mechanism by which milnacipran acts is unknown, it is believed that pain relief occurs through regulation of abnormal serotonergic and noradrenergic pathways.

Two miscellaneous adjuvants are administered to treat severe, intractable cancer pain that is not relieved by opioids. Clonidine may be administered as an epidural infusion, usually in combination with opioids. Clonidine activates alpha$_2$-adrenergic receptors in the spinal cord, resulting in decreased pain signals reaching the brain. Ziconotide (Prialt) is administered by intrathecal infusion. An off-label use is for severe muscle spasticity due to spinal cord injury. The drug provides analgesia by blocking N-type calcium channels at the presynaptic nerve terminals in the spinal cord. This prevents neurotransmitter release, thus blocking pain transmission.

Pharmacotherapy with Opioid Antagonists

25.11 The primary indication for an opioid antagonist is to reverse symptoms of opioid overdose.

Opioid overdose can result from excessive doses during pain therapy or from attempted suicide or substance abuse. Any opioid may be abused for its psychoactive effects; however, morphine, oxycodone, fentanyl, and heroin are preferred by abusers due to their potency. Although heroin is currently available as a legal analgesic in many countries, it is deemed too dangerous for therapeutic use by the FDA, and it is a major drug of abuse. Once injected or inhaled, heroin rapidly crosses the blood–brain barrier to enter the brain, where it is metabolized to morphine. Thus, the effects of heroin administration are actually caused by activation of the mu and kappa receptors from its morphine metabolite. The initial effect is an intense euphoria, or rush, followed by several hours of deep relaxation.

In recent years, the FDA has strongly encouraged manufacturers of opioids to adopt **abuse-deterrent formulations** (ADFs). These formulations are resistant to two frequent means of opioid abuse: crushing tablets or capsules in order to inject or inhale the product. ADFs are not "abuse proof" but they are a significant step toward that goal. These formulations are discussed further in Chapter 27.

Acute opioid intoxication is a medical emergency, with respiratory depression being the most serious medical challenge. In a clinical setting, an intravenous infusion of the opioid antagonist naloxone (Narcan) can be used to reverse severe respiratory depression and other acute symptoms of overdose. In administering naloxone, small doses are used and repeated until the respiratory depression is reversed and the patient begins to exhibit opioid withdrawal symptoms. The patient must be monitored to ensure that the effects of the drug are sufficiently long to outlast the respiratory depression caused by the opioid overdose; IV doses of naloxone only last 1 hour. Maintenance of a patent airway is essential and resuscitation equipment should be immediately available. It is important to understand that naloxone will reverse both the toxic and therapeutic effects of opioids. Thus, if the patient was using the opioid for analgesia, naloxone will reverse this effect and pain will quickly return.

Naloxone is also available in two other formulations that can be used in nonclinical settings. Evzio is a handheld autoinjector containing naloxone. This device is designed to be used by family members or caregivers to treat someone experiencing a known or suspected opioid overdose. Once turned on, the device gives verbal instructions for injecting the drug into the anterolateral thigh, through clothing if necessary. Caregivers should seek emergency medical care for the patient immediately after Evzio use. Narcan nasal spray is a second formulation for families and caregivers to use in cases of suspected opioid overdose. The drug is sprayed into one nostril. A second dose is in the package in the event the first one is ineffective. Evzio and Narcan nasal spray are carried by emergency medical service and law enforcement personnel. Although a prescription drug, some states allow the drug to be purchased from a pharmacist without a physician prescription.

If an opioid antagonist fails to quickly reverse the acute symptoms, the overdose was likely due to a nonopioid substance. Doses for the opioid antagonists are listed in Table 25.5. The fixed dose combination of naloxone and buprenorphine (Suboxone, Zubsolv, others) has become a first-line therapy for the *maintenance treatment* of opioid dependence. Naloxone with buprenorphine is a prototype drug in Chapter 27.

When abusing an opioid, the user usually develops tolerance to the euphoric effects of the drug and quickly escalates the dose. Following therapy with an opioid antagonist, however, the patient will become much more sensitive to the effects of opioids. If the patient returns to drug-taking behavior at the same dose used prior to opioid antagonist therapy, death may result.

Another indication for opioid antagonists is for the treatment of opioid-induced constipation or postoperative ileus. Alvimopan (Entereg) and methylnaltrexone (Relistor), both approved in 2008, act at mu receptors in the GI tract. Because they do not cross the blood–brain barrier, these drugs do not interfere with the central effects of opioids such as analgesia.

CONNECTION Checkpoint 25.3

Prochlorperazine (Compro, Procomp) is an antiemetic drug in the phenothiazine class that may be prescribed to decrease the nausea and vomiting caused by opioids. From what you learned in Chapter 20, what conditions are drugs in the phenothiazine class used to treat? Considering the adverse effects of the phenothiazines, what additive effects are more likely to occur when taking a phenothiazine and an opioid analgesic together?

Pharmacotherapy of Migraines

25.12 Migraines are a severe type of headache related to specific triggers.

Headaches are some of the most common complaints of patients. The pain and inability to concentrate causes a significant number of work-related absences and can interfere with activities of daily life. When the headaches are persistent, or manifest as migraines, drug therapy is warranted.

Why does a headache hurt? Although the skull and the brain lack pain receptors, the muscles of the scalp, face, and neck are abundantly supplied with nociceptors. These receptors can be stimulated by muscle tension, dilated blood vessels, and other headache triggers.

Table 25.5 Opioid Antagonists

Drug	Route and Adult Dose (Maximum Dose Where Indicated)	Adverse Effects
naloxone (Evzio, Narcan)	IV: 0.4–2 mg; may be repeated every 2–3 min up to 10 mg, if necessary	*Muscle and joint pain, difficulty sleeping, anxiety, headache, nervousness, withdrawal symptoms, vomiting*
naltrexone (Vivitrol)	PO: 25 mg followed by another 25 mg in 1 h if no withdrawal response (max: 800 mg/day)	<u>Hepatotoxicity</u>

Note: *Italics* indicate common adverse effects. <u>Underline</u> indicates serious adverse effects.

Table 25.6 Differentiation of Major Headache Types

Characteristics	Migraine	Tension Headache	Cluster Headache
Pain quality	Pulsating or throbbing	Steady pressure or tightness	Constant and steady
Pain location	Unilateral (more often) or bilateral	Bilateral (headband or ice tongs) pattern	Always on one side, on temple or behind the eye
Pain severity	Moderate to severe	Mild to moderate	Severe
Duration	4–72 h	Usually several hours	30–90 min; recur several times a day
Precursors or triggers	Hormonal changes in women; stress or heightened emotions; bright or flickering lights; change in weather or altitude Foods: alcohol, aged cheeses, chocolate, caffeine, fermented or pickled foods, aspartame, monosodium glutamate (MSG)	Stress or anxiety, lack of sleep	Alcohol, strong smells or fumes, smoking
Associated symptoms	May be preceded by aura, nausea and vomiting, extreme sensitivity to light or sound; aggravated by physical activity	No nausea	Eyes water and nose runs or feels stuffy on side of head, restless and anxious

Of the several varieties of headaches, the most common type is the **tension headache**. This occurs when muscles of the head and neck become tight due to stress, causing a steady and lingering pain. Although quite painful, tension headaches are self-limiting and more of an annoyance than an emergency. Tension headaches can be effectively treated with OTC analgesics such as aspirin, acetaminophen, or ibuprofen. Table 25.6 differentiates the two common types of headaches.

Although relatively rare, cluster headaches can occur multiple times a day (in clusters) and cause intense, debilitating pain. Other characteristics are shown in Table 25.6. OTC analgesics are usually ineffective at terminating a cluster headache. Although it lacks portability, oxygen (100%) is one of the most effective therapies. Some of the medications used to terminate migraines, such as intranasal triptans, are more convenient.

The **migraine** headache is characterized by throbbing or pulsating pain. Three basic categories include migraine with aura, migraine without aura and chronic migraine. **Auras** are sensory warnings of an imminent migraine attack. Examples include flashing lights, visual blind spots, and arm or leg tingling. Nausea and vomiting and extreme sensitivity to light and sound accompany most migraines.

The neurotransmitter serotonin (5-hydroxytryptamine or 5-HT) appears to be a key factor (although not the only factor) in the pathogenesis and treatment of migraines. What is the connection between serotonin levels and migraines? During a migraine, the amount of serotonin in the brain declines, causing the vessels to dilate. Nerves surrounding the dilated vessels become inflamed, resulting in pain. As neurons in the brain generate additional serotonin, or serotonin agonist drugs are administered, the vessels dilate and pain diminishes.

PharmFACT

Migraine Statistics

- About 70% of patients with migraines have a first-degree relative with a history of migraine.
- Before puberty, more boys have migraines than girls; after puberty, women are three times more likely to have migraines than men.
- History of migraine is associated with an increased incidence of major cardiovascular disease, especially if the patient experiences migraines with aura.
- Migraines are rare after age 50 (Chawla, 2020).

25.13 Analgesics and triptans are the primary classes of drugs used to abort acute migraine pain.

The two primary goals of migraine pharmacotherapy are to terminate or abort an acute migraine in progress and to prevent or reduce the frequency of the disorder. With a few exceptions, drugs used to abort a migraine are different from those used for prophylaxis. The prophylactic medications are discussed in Section 25.15.

Migraine pharmacotherapy is more successful if therapy begins before the pain reaches a severe level. Drug therapy is conducted in stages based on the severity of the migraine.

- **Mild migraine (occasional headaches with no other functional impairment).** NSAIDs offer the safest and least expensive therapy; thus, they are tried initially. Acetaminophen is generally not effective alone but offers additive pain relief when combined with an NSAID and caffeine.
- **Moderate migraine (moderate pain, nausea, and some functional impairment).** Oral, intranasal, or

subcutaneous serotonin ($5\text{-}HT_1$) agonists (triptans or ergot alkaloids) are the preferred drugs. If serotonin agonists are contraindicated or ineffective, dopamine agonists such as metoclopramide (Reglan) or prochlorperazine (Compro, Procomp) may be prescribed.

- **Severe migraine (severe pain more than three times per month, marked nausea and/or vomiting, and functional impairment).** Subcutaneous, IM, or IV serotonin agonists may be indicated. A secondary choice would be a parenteral dopamine agonist, either as monotherapy or in combination with a serotonin agonist. Narcotic analgesics are effective at terminating pain from migraines that have proven to be refractory to other therapies.

The two major drug classes used to terminate migraines, the triptans and the ergot alkaloids, are both serotonin receptor agonists. At least seven serotonin receptor subtypes have been identified. In 2019, the FDA approved lasmiditan (Reyvow), the first drug for treating acute migraine to act at the serotonin subtype $5\text{-}HT_1F$. Other drugs acting at serotonin receptors include certain antianxiety medications, antidepressants, antiemetics, and various hallucinogens. Doses for the triptans and ergot alkaloids are listed in Table 25.7.

Triptans: The first of the triptans, sumatriptan (Imitrex, Onzetra, others), was marketed in the United States in 1992. This drug was quickly followed by the introduction of the

Table 25.7 Drugs Used to Terminate Acute Migraines

Drug	Route and Adult Dose (Maximum Dose Where Indicated)	Adverse Effects
Triptans		
almotriptan (Axert)	PO: 6.25–12.5 mg, may repeat in 2 h (max: 2 doses/24 h)	*Paresthesia, tingling, dry mouth, warming sensation, dizziness, vertigo*
eletriptan (Relpax)	PO: 20–40 mg, may repeat in 2 h (max: 80 mg/24 h)	Coronary artery vasospasm, MI, stroke
frovatriptan (Frova)	PO: 2.5 mg, may repeat in 2 h (max: 3 doses/24 h)	
naratriptan (Amerge)	PO: 1–2.5 mg, may repeat in 4 h (max: 5 mg/24 h)	
rizatriptan (Maxalt)	PO: 5–10 mg, may repeat in 2 h (max: 30 mg/24 h)	
sumatriptan (Imitrex, Onzetra, others)	PO: 25–100 mg, may repeat in 2 h (max: 200 mg/24 h) Intranasal (Onzetra): 22 mg, may repeat once (max: 44 mg/24 h) Subcutaneous: 6 mg, may repeat in 1 h, once in 24 h	
zolmitriptan (Zomig, Zomig ZMT)	PO: 2.5 mg or less, may repeat in 2 h (max: 10 mg/24 h) PO (orally disintegrating tablet): 1.25–2.5 mg (max: 5 mg) Intranasal: 5 mg, may repeat once after 2 h (max: 10 mg/24 h)	
Ergot Alkaloids		
dihydroergotamine (DHE 45, Migranal)	Intranasal: 1 spray (0.5 mg) each nostril, may repeat once in 15 min (max: 3 mg/24 h, 4 mg/wk) IM/subcutaneous: 1 mg, repeat at 1-h intervals for total 3 mg (max: 6 mg/wk)	*Weakness, nausea and vomiting, abnormal pulse, throat irritation, nasal irritation, or dysgeusia (distorted sense of taste)* Delirium, seizures, cerebrovascular events (hemorrhage), intermittent claudication, birth defects, inhibition of lactation or cause of infant vomiting, physical dependence, withdrawal resembles migraine
ergotamine (Ergostat; with caffeine: Cafergot; with caffeine, belladonna, pentobarbital: Cafergot P-B)	Sublingual: 2 mg, may repeat in 30 min for total 3 doses/24 h or 5 doses/wk PO: 2 tablets (2 mg), 1 additional tablet repeated every 30 min (max: 6 mg/attack or 10 mg/wk) Rectal: 2 mg, may repeat once in 1 h	
Ditan		
lasmiditan	PO: 50–200 mg/day	*Dizziness, fatigue, paresthesia* Sedation, serotonin syndrome, fetal harm
CGRP antagonists		
rimegepant (Nurtec ODT) ubrogepant (Ubrelvy)	PO: 75 mg/day (max 7.5 mg/24 h) PO: 50–100 mg/day (max: 200 mg/24 h)	*Nausea, dry mouth* Somnolence, hypersensitivity

Note: *Italics* indicate common adverse effects. Underline indicates serious adverse effects.

"second-generation" triptans with improved pharmacokinetic profiles: more thorough absorption, faster onset of action, and longer duration. Although all triptans have very similar actions and adverse effects, individual patients may respond more favorably and, with fewer adverse effects, to one triptan over another. The longer-duration triptans are believed to be better at preventing the migraine from recurring following its termination.

Triptans are selective for the 5-HT_1 receptor subtype, and they are thought to act by constricting certain intracranial vessels. They are effective in aborting migraines with or without auras. Although the PO forms of the triptans are most convenient, patients who experience nausea and vomiting during the migraine may require an alternate dosage form. Intranasal formulations are available and prefilled syringes of triptans may be used for patients who are able to self-administer the medication.

Triptans are not effective at preventing migraines. Other drugs, accompanied by lifestyle changes, must be used for prophylaxis (see Section 25.15).

Ergot alkaloids: For patients who are unresponsive to triptans, the ergot alkaloids may be used to abort migraines. They should be separated from triptan use by at least 24 hours. The first purified alkaloid, ergotamine (Ergostat), was isolated from the ergot fungus in 1920, although the actions of the ergot alkaloids had been known for thousands of years. Ergotamine is an inexpensive drug that is available in PO, sublingual, and suppository forms. Modification of the original molecule has produced a number of other pharmacologically useful drugs, such as dihydroergotamine (Migranal), which is available parenterally and as a nasal spray. Because the ergot alkaloids interact with adrenergic, dopaminergic, and serotonergic receptors, they produce multiple actions and adverse effects. The ergot alkaloids promote vasoconstriction, which terminates a migraine in progress. Adverse effects may include nausea and vomiting, weakness in the legs, myalgia, numbness and tingling in fingers and toes, angina-like pain, and tachycardia. Toxicity may be evidenced by constriction of peripheral arteries: cold, pale, numb extremities and muscle pain. Other possible adverse effects include dizziness, drowsiness, vasoconstriction, warming sensations, tingling, lightheadedness, weakness, and neck stiffness.

Ergot alkaloids, which constrict both arteries and veins, are contraindicated in peripheral vascular disease, coronary artery disease, and severe hypertension (HTN) because they decrease blood flow. Metoclopramide or prochlorperazine may be administered concurrently with ergot alkaloids to reduce or prevent nausea and vomiting. Many ergot alkaloids can cause fetal harm and should not be used by women who may become pregnant. These drugs may inhibit lactation or cause vomiting in breastfed infants. Regular daily use can cause physical dependence. Withdrawal symptoms of headache and nausea and vomiting resemble the symptoms of migraines. Dosing and duration of use need to be restricted. Dangers of overuse and dependence should be included in patient and family teaching.

PROTOTYPE DRUG Sumatriptan (Imitrex, Onzetra Xsail, Others)

Classification **Therapeutic:** Antimigraine drug
Pharmacologic: Serotonin (5-HT_1) receptor agonist

Therapeutic Effects and Uses: Available by the PO, intranasal, and subcutaneous routes, sumatriptan is used to relieve acute migraines. It was the first triptan approved by the FDA in 1992. It is not effective for long-term prophylaxis of migraines; other drugs must be used for this purpose. Two forms of sumatriptan, Zembrace SymTouch and Imitrex StatDosePen, are available in prefilled syringes for subcutaneous injection by the patient. Intranasal forms of sumatriptan include Onzetra Xsail, an intranasal powder, and Imitrex Intranasal and Tosymra, which are liquid spray formulations. Treximet is a fixed dose combination of sumatriptan and naproxen that is approved for the treatment of acute migraines

Mechanism of Action: Sumatriptan is structurally similar to serotonin. Sumatriptan activates the 5-HT_1 serotonin receptors on intracranial and extracerebral blood vessels, resulting in vasoconstriction and reduced transmission in trigeminal pain pathways. It has no intrinsic analgesic activity.

Pharmacokinetics:

Route(s)	PO, intranasal, subcutaneous
Absorption	15% PO; 97% subcutaneous
Distribution	Widely distributed; crosses the placenta; secreted in breast milk; less than 21% bound to plasma protein
Primary metabolism	Hepatic
Primary excretion	60% renal; 40% feces
Onset of action	PO: 30–60 min; intranasal: 30 min; subcutaneous: 10–15 min
Duration of action	PO: 6–8 h; intranasal: unknown; subcutaneous: 4–6 h

Adverse Effects: Sumatriptan has infrequent adverse effects that include mild and transient dizziness or nausea, diarrhea, myalgia, and inflammation and pain at the subcutaneous injection site. Headache recurrence occurs in a large percentage of patients taking sumatriptan. Although rare, serious cardiac events have been documented with sumatriptan use. These events include coronary artery vasospasm, myocardial ischemia, dysrhythmias, and MI. These serious events are more likely to occur in patients with preexisting cardiac disease.

Contraindications/Precautions: Sumatriptan is contraindicated in patients with coronary artery disease, cerebrovascular disease, or peripheral vascular disease. This drug is not recommended for patients with uncontrolled HTN, hypercholesterolemia, or those who have a strong family history of cardiovascular disease. Sumatriptan is contraindicated in patients with serious CKD or hepatic impairment. Patients with a history of epilepsy have an increased risk for seizures when taking sumatriptan. The drug is associated with fetal deformities and demise in animal studies; it should be avoided in pregnant women. Overuse of abortive therapies for migraines can lead to rebound headaches.

Drug Interactions: Sumatriptan is metabolized by monoamine oxidase and should not be used within 2 weeks of MAOIs or SSRIs. Use of sumatriptan should be avoided within 24 hours of ergot alkaloids or any other 5-HT_1 agonist due to risk of synergistic vasospasms. Serotonin syndrome is possible when giving sumatriptan with other drugs that increase serotonin levels or activity, including buspirone, other triptans, amphetamines, sibutramine, trazodone, TCAs, lithium, duloxetine, venlafaxine, or meperidine. **Herbal/Food:** St. John's wort and feverfew should be avoided during therapy with sumatriptan.

Pregnancy: Animal studies showed evidence for embryotoxicity, fetal toxicity and offspring mortality. Small levels of sumatriptan are secreted in human milk but effects on the breastfed infant are unknown. Sumatriptan should be used during pregnancy and lactation only if the potential benefits justify the risks to the fetus or neonate.

Treatment of Overdose: Few overdoses have been recorded. Treatment of overdose is supportive.

Clinician Responsibilities: Key clinical implications for patients receiving sumatriptan are included in Applied Clinical Judgment for Patients Receiving Pharmacotherapy for Migraines.

Drugs Similar to Sumatriptan

Other triptans include almotriptan, eletriptan, frovatriptan, naratriptan, rizatriptan, and zolmitriptan. All of the triptans have the same therapeutic effects and spectrum of adverse effects. All of the drugs in this class have the same pregnancy and lactation risks as sumatriptan.

Almotriptan (Axert): Almotriptan was approved as an oral antimigraine drug in 2001. The drug is well absorbed and has an onset of action of 1 to 3 hours. The drug is extensively metabolized to inactive metabolites by CYP450 enzymes, and 75% is excreted via the kidneys. Drug–drug interactions with agents metabolized in the liver may occur.

Eletriptan (Relpax): Approved in 2002, eletriptan has improved GI absorption, a more rapid onset of action, and a longer duration than sumatriptan. Less than 10% is excreted via the kidneys, making the drug safe to use in patients with CKD. The drug is extensively metabolized by CYP450 enzymes and thus has the potential for drug–drug interactions with agents metabolized in the liver.

Frovatriptan (Frova): Approved in 2001, frovatriptan has the same effects as sumatriptan but has a slow onset and a very long duration. The 26-hour half-life results in less pain recurrence with this drug. This drug is extensively metabolized by hepatic CYP450 enzymes, and the majority is eliminated in the feces.

Naratriptan (Amerge): Approved in 1998, this drug has a relatively slow onset of action (3–4 hours) but with a longer duration of action than sumatriptan. This drug is extensively metabolized to inactive metabolites by CYP450 enzymes and is excreted by the kidneys.

Rizatriptan (Maxalt): Approved in 1998, rizatriptan is absorbed more quickly than sumatriptan, with an onset of 60 to 90 minutes. It is available as PO disintegrating tablets (Maxalt-MLT), which are allowed to dissolve on the tongue and be swallowed with saliva. Hepatic CYP450 enzymes do not significantly metabolize the drug. The most common adverse effects include asthenia, fatigue, somnolence, pain or pressure sensation, and dizziness.

Zolmitriptan (Zomig, Zomig ZMT): Zolmitriptan is an oral drug that has the same effects as sumatriptan but is available in additional formulations as a nasal spray and as orally disintegrating tablets (Zomig ZMT). This drug is metabolized to an active metabolite in the liver, which is responsible for some of its antimigraine activity. The most common adverse effects include neck, throat, and jaw pain, dizziness, paresthesia, somnolence, warm or cold sensation, nausea, and dry mouth. Zolmitriptan should not be used to treat cluster headaches.

25.14 Drugs from many different classes are used for migraine prophylaxis.

Prior to initiation of drug therapy for migraine prophylaxis, patients should attempt lifestyle changes and nonpharmacologic therapies. First and foremost, the patient needs to identify personal triggers for migraines. The nurse can help by guiding the patient through the process of assessing and identifying those triggers. Foods are a common culprit, especially those containing nitrates or MSG. Omitting common migraine triggers from the diet is a first step in prophylaxis. Other lifestyle changes that may help include adopting regular sleep patterns and meals, participating in aerobic exercise (start slowly because sudden intense activity may cause headaches), avoiding alcohol (especially red wine), and smoking cessation. Other helpful self-care measures include keeping a diary that notes when headaches start, how long they last, what provides relief, what the response is to the medication, and food intake or stress in the past 24 hours. Relaxation exercises, meditation, yoga, or progressive muscle relaxation may help. Nontraditional therapies may also be useful in preventing migraines in some patients.

Drugs for migraine prophylaxis include various classes of drugs that are discussed in other chapters of this textbook. These include beta-adrenergic blockers, calcium channel blockers, antidepressants, and antiseizure drugs. Because all of these drugs have the potential to produce adverse effects, prophylaxis is only initiated if the incidence of migraines is high and the patient is unresponsive to the drugs used to abort migraines. Example prophylactic antimigraine drugs are given in Table 25.8. Doses for these drugs are found in the chapters where their primary indication is presented.

Preventive treatment is recommended for headaches that occur three or more times a month. Of the various medications, the beta-adrenergic blocker propranolol (Inderal) is one of the most commonly prescribed, although other drugs in this class have similar effectiveness. The use of beta blockers is particularly beneficial in patients with comorbid conditions such as HTN or angina.

TCAs, especially amitriptyline, have been used for decades to prevent migraines and are preferred for patients who may have a mood disorder or insomnia in addition to their migraines. The antimigraine action of these drugs is independent of their antidepressant action. SSRIs such as fluoxetine (Prozac) have been prescribed off-label for migraines because they exhibit fewer adverse effects than the TCAs.

Other classes of drugs used for migraine prevention include calcium channel blockers, certain antiseizure drugs, and estrogens for menstrual migraines. An extended-release form of valproic acid (Depakote ER) is approved for migraine prophylaxis. OnabotulinumtoxinA (Botox), a drug often used to erase facial wrinkles, is approved to treat chronic migraines (see Chapter 23).

Table 25.8 Drugs Used for Migraine Prophylaxis

Drug Class	Examples
Antiseizure drugs	gabapentin (Neurontin) topiramate (Topamax) valproic acid (Depakote ER)
Beta-adrenergic blockers	atenolol (Tenormin) metoprolol (Lopressor) propranolol (Inderal) timolol (Blocadren)
Botulinum toxin	onabotulinumtoxinA (Botox)
Calcium channel blockers	nifedipine (Procardia) nimodipine (Nimotop) verapamil (Calan, Verelan)
CGRP inhibitors	eptinezumab (Vyepti) erenumab (Aimovig) fremanezumab (Ajovy) galcanezumab (Emgality)
Tricyclic antidepressants	amitriptyline imipramine (Tofranil) protriptyline (Vivactil)

25.15 CGRP inhibitors offer a novel approach to the prevention and treatment of migraines.

In 2018 the first of a new class of antimigraine drugs was approved by the FDA, called the **calcitonin gene–related peptide (CGRP) inhibitors** or antagonists. The CGRP is a small protein found in sensory nerves that supply the head and neck. When the CGRP protein binds to its receptors, it causes a cascade of events that causes neurogenic inflammation, dilation of cerebral vessels, and enhancement of pain transmission. Levels of CGRP are elevated during acute migraine events, as well as cluster headaches. The CGRP pathway is believed to be a key step in migraine attacks. Because of their increased cost, the CGRP inhibitors are reserved for patients who continue to have migraines after trying older medications.

The CGRP inhibitors work by two separate mechanisms. The two different mechanisms determine whether the drugs are effective at *preventing* migraines or *terminating* migraines.

- Ubrogepant (Ubrelvy) and rimegepant (Nurtec ODT), sometimes called "gepants," are small molecules that rapidly enter the brain and block receptors for CGRP. They are both given PO. They are effective at terminating migraine attacks without causing vasoconstriction, an adverse effect of the triptans. Both drugs may cause fetal harm and no data are available regarding adverse effects on breastfed neonates.
- Eptinezumab (Vyepti), erenumab (Aimovig), fremanezumab (Ajovy), and galcanezumab (Emgality) are humanized monoclonal antibodies. These biologic therapies are designed to specifically bind to the CGRP protein or its receptors. Unlike the gepants, the monoclonal antibodies are given parenterally and used for migraine prophylaxis. Vyepti is given IV once monthly, whereas the others are given subcutaneously once per month. Animal reproduction studies for all four drugs did not show evidence of embryo or fetal toxicity. No data are available regarding adverse effects on breastfed neonates.

CONNECTIONS: APPLIED CLINICAL JUDGMENT

Patients Receiving Pharmacotherapy for Migraines

Key Assessment Data
- History of current condition, baseline vital signs, physical exam; history of hepatic, renal, cardiovascular, or neurologic disease; medications and allergy history; pregnancy or breastfeeding status.
- Assess the level of pain. Use objective screening tools when possible (e.g., numerical rating scale for adults). Assess pain history and what has worked successfully or not for the patient in the past and coping strategies.
- Ongoing assessment during drug therapy includes pain assessment, appropriate laboratory findings (e.g., hepatic or renal function studies), level of consciousness and neurologic symptoms (e.g., numbness or tingling), and vital signs, especially cardiovascular (e.g., chest pain or tightness, palpitations, tachycardia, HTN).

Desired Therapeutic Outcomes
Improvement is observed and measurable in decreased frequency of migraines and diminished or absent migraine pain.

Minimizing Adverse Effects
- Triptans and ergot alkaloids cause vasoconstriction. Monitor blood pressure and pulse periodically, especially in patients at risk for undiagnosed cardiovascular disease. Cardiovascular status should be monitored frequently following the first dose given.
- Sudden severe headaches of "thunderclap" quality can signal subarachnoid hemorrhage. Headaches that differ in quality and are accompanied by such signs as fever, rash, or stiff neck may herald meningitis. Observe for changes in severity, character, or duration of headache.
- Dizziness or lightheadedness may be related to headache, an adverse drug effect, or may signal cerebral ischemia. Continue to monitor neurologic status periodically.
- Some foods or beverages may trigger an acute migraine. Correlating symptoms with food or beverages assists in avoiding the cause of the headache. Monitor dietary intake of foods that contain tyramine, caffeine, alcohol, or other known food triggers.

Lifespan Considerations
- Postmenopausal women, men over age 40, smokers, and people with other known coronary artery disease risk factors may be at greatest risk for cardiovascular effects. Older adults may have undetected cardiovascular disease, placing them at greater risk for adverse effects.
- Triptans and ergot alkaloids may cause fetal harm. Women who are planning a pregnancy, pregnant, or breastfeeding should discuss the use of drug therapy and alternative treatment before using antimigraine drugs.

Patient Education
- Take the drug before a headache becomes severe, and take it consistently as ordered.
- Immediately report any chest pain or tightness or throat pain that is severe or continues following drug dosage.
- Immediately report changes in headache character or duration or if accompanied by additional symptoms such as fever, rash, or stiff neck.
- Immediately report increasing dizziness, lightheadedness, or blurred vision.
- A food diary may be helpful to correlate symptoms with specific foods or beverages. Avoid or limit foods containing tyramine, such as pickled foods, beer, wine, and aged cheeses, which are often known triggers for migraines.
- Women of childbearing age should discuss the use of antimigraine drugs before planning a pregnancy and to discontinue use if pregnant or breastfeeding unless directed otherwise by the provider.
- Take the medication at the first symptoms of a migraine, if possible, before the pain becomes severe.
  - Use the drug exactly as prescribed; overuse can lead to rebound headaches.
  - Pain or redness at the injection site is common but usually disappears within an hour after the dose is taken. Report any worsening redness or pain to the provider.
  - Appropriate intranasal dose is one spray into one nostril unless otherwise ordered by the healthcare provider.

Prescribing Considerations
- In selecting the most appropriate pharmacotherapy for the abortive management of migraine, consider the severity of the pain.
- Patients with mild-to-moderate migraine attacks can often be treated with simple analgesics or NSAIDs and the triptans or ergots reserved for moderate-to-severe pain.
- Combination therapy may be necessary for some patients.

Understanding Chapter 25

Key Concepts Summary

25.1 The primary goal of pain management is to reduce pain to a level that allows the patient to continue normal daily activities.

25.2 Proper assessment and classification of pain guides its treatment.

25.3 Healthcare providers and patients sometimes hold myths about pain that impede optimal pain management.

25.4 Pain transmission processes allow multiple targets for pharmacologic intervention.

25.5 Both pharmacologic and nonpharmacologic therapies are used in pain management.

25.6 Opioid analgesics exert their effects by interacting with specific receptors in the central nervous system.

25.7 Opioids are the preferred drugs for moderate to severe pain that cannot be controlled with other classes of analgesics.

25.8 Mixed agonist and antagonist opioids exhibit moderate analgesia with less risk of dependence than morphine.

25.9 Nonsteroidal anti-inflammatory drugs are the preferred medications for mild to moderate pain.

25.10 Adjuvant analgesics have primary indications other than pain control but can enhance analgesia.

25.11 The primary indication for an opioid antagonist is to reverse symptoms of opioid overdose.

25.12 Migraines are a severe type of headache related to specific triggers.

25.13 Analgesics and triptans are the primary classes of drugs used to abort acute migraine pain.

25.14 Drugs from many different classes are used for migraine prophylaxis.

25.15 CGRP inhibitors offer a novel approach to the prevention and treatment of migraines.

CASE STUDY: Making the Patient Connection

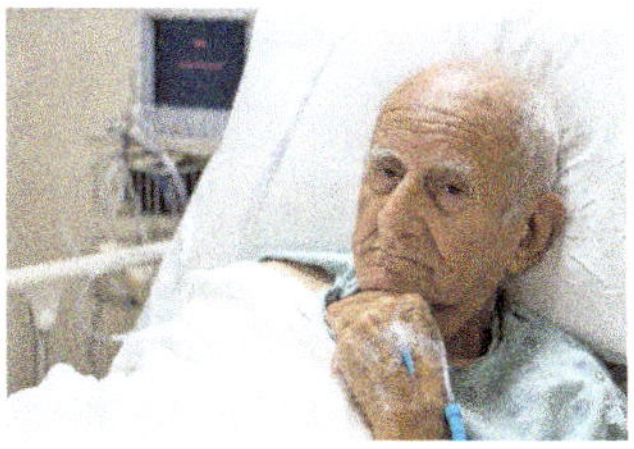

Remember the patient "Larry Smith" at the beginning of the chapter? Now read the remainder of the case study. Based on the information presented within this chapter, respond to the critical thinking questions that follow.

Larry Smith was being seen for an outpatient preoperative workup the evening before scheduled urologic surgery. The nurse conducts a thorough history and examination related to his back pain and current pain management. His anticipated hospital stay is 2 days postoperatively.

Larry Smith is a 68-year-old man. Vital signs are blood pressure, 108/64 mmHg; pulse, 88 beats/min; respirations, 16 breaths/min. He has a well-healed midline scar on his back from lumbar vertebrae surgery, with a shorter scar over his right iliac crest. Larry moves a bit slowly with some limited lumbar range of motion. He also uses a cane for ambulating any distance. He describes his pain as a constant dull ache in the lower back that increases with prolonged standing or walking. Larry also reports a feeling of "cold electricity" down both legs, with the left greater than the right, which increases with standing and walking, as well as numbness of the middle toes on his left foot. He has been using mixed opioid and nonopioid analgesics for the past 8 years and previously had used SSRI antidepressants as adjuvant for his pain. Larry's current healthcare provider weaned him off Vicodin ES about a year ago. He now takes methadone 20 mg twice a day. When the pain is not relieved, he uses Norco for breakthrough pain. His use of Norco is one to two doses per day. Constipation is an ongoing problem, requiring stool softeners and occasional laxatives.

Critical Thinking Questions

1. How should Larry's postoperative pain be managed? Is there a referral the nurse can make to facilitate effective pain management?
2. How could the nurse best communicate Larry's needs to the postoperative nursing staff?
3. What should be included in the care plan for postoperative management of analgesic adverse effects?

Additional Case Study

Rita Manson presents to the emergency department with vomiting, severe abdominal and back pain, and jaundice. Her jaundice is recent, but the pain and vomiting have continued for a couple of months. Her diagnostic workup reveals advanced pancreatic cancer with metastasis to the spine.

1. What is the preferred drug for Rita's pain management? Which route of administration would be expected initially?
2. Her prescribed pain medication is morphine sulfate 2 to 10 mg IV every 2 hours as needed for pain. Outline a nursing approach to pain management for the first 24 hours.
3. What adverse effects would the nurse expect?
4. As part of the patient's pain management, dexamethasone 5 mg IV is prescribed every 6 hours for 2 days. Explain the use of corticosteroids in pain management.

Chapter Review

1. The nurse is monitoring the patient for adverse effects associated with morphine. Which adverse effects would be expected? (Select all that apply.)
   1. Respiratory depression
   2. Hypertension
   3. Urinary retention
   4. Constipation
   5. Nausea

2. Several days postoperative bowel surgery, the patient is eating soft food, ambulating regularly, and using hydrocodone (Vicodin) for pain. What should the nursing care plan include?
   1. Monitoring vital signs for respiratory depression
   2. Inserting a urinary catheter for urinary retention
   3. Weaning pain medication to prevent addiction
   4. Increasing dietary fiber and fluids and administering a stool softener, if needed

3. A patient who has migraines self-administered sumatriptan (Imitrex) for the first time yesterday. Today, the patient informs the nurse that after taking the medication, the patient began to experience chest pain. The patient further states that the drug was effective in relieving the headache. The nurse should:
   1. Encourage the patient to continue using the drug because it was effective.
   2. Advise the patient to tell the healthcare provider about the chest pain at the next visit.
   3. Instruct the patient to contact the healthcare provider to report the chest pain today and to not use the sumatriptan until the healthcare provider has been consulted.
   4. Encourage the patient to lie down in a quiet room and use cold packs during the next migraine.

4. A patient with diabetes reports increasing pain and numbness in his legs: "It feels like pins and needles all the time, especially at night." Which drug would the nurse expect to be prescribed for this patient?
   1. Ibuprofen (Motrin)
   2. Gabapentin (Neurontin)
   3. Naloxone (Narcan, Evzio)
   4. Methadone

5. The emergency department nurse is caring for a patient with a migraine. Which drug would the nurse anticipate administering to abort the patient's migraine?
   1. Morphine
   2. Dihydroergotamine (Migranal)
   3. Propranolol (Inderal)
   4. Ibuprofen (Motrin)

6. The nurse is caring for several patients who are receiving opioids for pain relief. Which patient is at the highest risk of developing hypotension, respiratory depression, and mental confusion?
   1. A 23-year-old woman, postoperative ruptured appendix
   2. A 16-year-old adolescent, post–motorcycle injury with lacerations
   3. A 54-year-old woman, post–myocardial infarction
   4. An 86-year-old man, postoperative femur fracture

See Appendix A for answers to critical thinking questions, case study questions and review questions.

References

Chawla, J. (2020). *Migraine headache*. Medscape. http://emedicine.medscape.com/article/1142556-overview

Committee on Obstetric Practice. (2017). Committee Opinion No. 711: opioid use and opioid use disorder in pregnancy. *Obstetrics and Gynecology, 130*(2), e81. https://www.acog.org/clinical/clinical-guidance/committee-opinion/articles/2017/08/opioid-use-and-opioid-use-disorder-in-pregnancy

Hwang, J., Louie, P. K., Phillips, F. M., An, H. S., & Samartzis, D. (2019). Low back pain in children: A rising concern. European Spine Journal, 28, 211–213. https://doi.org/10.1007/s00586-018-5844-1

Substance Abuse and Mental Health Service Administration (SAMHSA). (n.d.). *Medication and counseling treatment*. https://www.samhsa.gov/medication-assisted-treatment/treatment#medications-used-in-mat

Selected Bibliography

Bhola, R., & Greenwood, F. (2018). Migraine and CGRP: an overview of current preventive treatments and new CGRP pathway monoclonal antibodies. *British Journal of Neuroscience Nursing*, *14*(5), 215–224. https://doi.org/10.12968/bjnn.2018.14.5.215

Chang, K. L., Fillingim, R., Hurley, R. W., & Schmidt, S. (2015). Chronic pain management: Nonpharmacological therapies for chronic pain. *FP Essentials*, *432*, 21–26.

Dart, R. C., Surratt, H. L., Cicero, T. J., Parrino, M. W., Severtson, S. G., Bucher-Bartelson, B., & Green, J. L. (2015). Trends in opioid analgesic abuse and mortality in the United States. *New England Journal of Medicine*, *372*, 241–248. https://doi.org/10.1056/NEJMsa1406143

Edvinsson, L. (2018). The CGRP pathway in migraine as a viable target for therapies. *Headache: Journal of Head and Face Pain*, *58*, 33–47. https://doi.org/10.1111/head.13305

Finnerup, N. B., Attal, N., Haroutounian, S., McNicol, E., Baron, R., Dworkin, R. H., et al. (2015). Pharmacotherapy for neuropathic pain in adults: A systematic review and meta-analysis. *The Lancet Neurology*, *14*, 162–173. https://doi.org/10.1016/S1474-4422(14)70251-0

Harvey, P., Shah, P., & Shipley, S. (2020). An overview of new biologics for migraine prophylaxis. *U.S. Pharmacist*, *45*(1) 21–24.

Marie, B. S., Arnstein, P., & Zimmer, P. A. (2018). Pain and opioids: Call for policy action. *Journal for Nurse Practitioners*, *14*(1), 40–44. https://doi.org/10.1016/j.nurpra.2017.10.002

McNicol, E. D., Ferguson, M. C., & Hudcova, J. (2015). Patient controlled opioid analgesia versus non-patient controlled opioid analgesia for postoperative pain (Review). *Cochrane Database of Systematic Reviews*, Issue 6, Article No. CD003348. https://doi.org/10.1002/14651858.CD003348.pub3

Moulin, D. E., Clark, A. J., Gilron, I., Ware, M. A., Watson, C. P. N., Sessle, B. J., et al. (2007). Pharmacological management of chronic neuropathic pain–consensus statement and guidelines from the Canadian Pain Society. *Pain Research and Management*, *12*(1), 13–21. https://doi.org/10.1155/2007/730785

O'Connor, A. B., & Dworkin, R. H. (2009). Treatment of neuropathic pain: an overview of recent guidelines. *American Journal of Medicine*, *122*(10), S22–S32. https://doi.org/10.1016/j.amjmed.2009.04.007

Peck, K. R., Smitherman, T. A., & Baskin, S. M. (2015). Traditional and alternative treatments for depression: Implications for migraine management. *Headache: The Journal of Head and Face Pain*, *55*, 351–355. https://doi.org/10.1111/head.12521

Schwedt, T. J. (2019). New and emerging treatments for the acute and preventive therapy of migraine and other headaches. *Headache: The Journal of Head and Face Pain*, *59*(Suppl 2), 1–2. https://doi.org/10.1111/head.13584

Volkow, N., Benveniste, H., & McLellan, A. T. (2018). Use and misuse of opioids in chronic pain. *Annual Review of Medicine*, *69*, 451–465. https://doi.org/10.1146/annurev-med-011817-044739

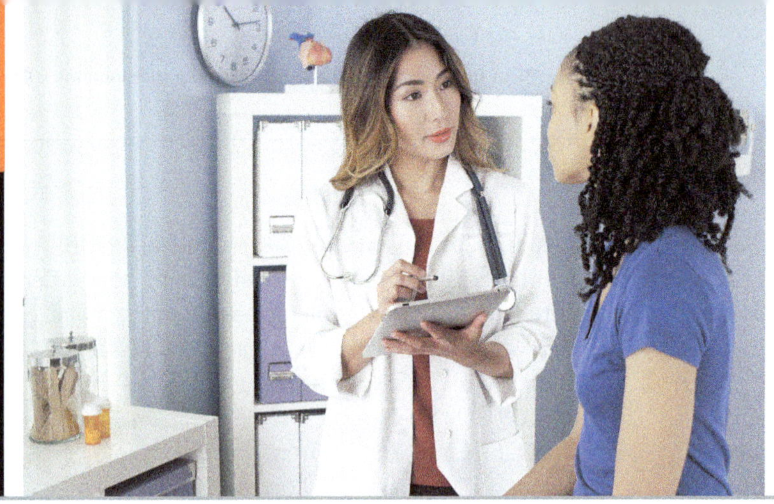

"I have never had surgery before. I'm so scared of being put to sleep."
—*Patient "Elena Moore"*

Chapter 26
Anesthetics and Anesthesia Adjuncts

Chapter Outline

Learning Outcomes

After reading this chapter, the student should be able to:

1. Compare and contrast the four basic types of anesthesia.
2. Explain the five general purposes of balanced anesthesia.
3. Compare and contrast the four stages of general anesthesia.
4. Identify drug classes used to produce general anesthesia.
5. Describe the nursing care associated with the administration of regional and general anesthesia.
6. Explain the rationale for using adjunct agents during general anesthesia.
7. For each of the classes shown in the chapter outline, identify the prototype and representative drugs and explain the mechanism(s) of drug action, primary indications, contraindications, significant drug interactions, pregnancy data and important adverse effects.
8. Apply clinical judgment to care for patients receiving local or general anesthesia.

Key Terms

Definitions of the terms in bold may be found in the Glossary.

Throughout history, the application of anesthesia has allowed patients to experience a temporary loss of sensation, resulting in comfort during surgical intervention. The use of opium as an anesthetic was recorded as far back as 4200 BC, and the ancient Chinese recorded acupuncture as a form of anesthesia. The modern implementation of anesthesia dates back to 1846 when Dr. John C. Warren performed a surgical procedure using ether. Modern anesthesia now offers safer and more effective drugs. This chapter introduces drugs used for general and local anesthesia along with the adjuvant medications administered during surgical procedures.

Types of Anesthesia

26.1 Anesthesia is used to produce a controlled loss of sensation during a diagnostic or surgical procedure.

Certain medical procedures produce a significant degree of pain and would not be possible without anesthesia. There are four types of anesthesia. The type of anesthesia selected depends on the degree of sedation and analgesia needed to conduct the procedure.

General anesthesia is the loss of sensation throughout the entire body, accompanied by loss of consciousness. General anesthesia is necessary for major surgical procedures.

The application of **local anesthesia** results in loss of sensation to a limited body region without loss of consciousness. It affects only the immediate area that surrounds where the anesthetic is administered. **Regional anesthesia** is similar, except that it encompasses a larger body area, such as an entire limb. Local and regional anesthesias produce fewer adverse effects than general anesthesia and are thus the methods of choice where applicable.

A fourth type of anesthesia is **monitored anesthesia care (MAC)**, also called conscious sedation, uses sedatives, analgesics, and other low-dose drugs that allow patients to remain responsive and breathe without assistance during a medical procedure. This type of anesthesia is used during diagnostic procedures and minor surgeries to supplement local and regional anesthesias. Subtypes of MAC are based on the degree of sedation produced:

- *Minimal sedation (anxiolysis).* Patients respond to verbal commands. Airway, ventilation, and cardiovascular functions are normal.
- *Moderate (conscious) sedation.* Patients respond to verbal or light tactile prompting. Airway, ventilation, and cardiovascular functions are usually adequate.
- *Deep sedation and analgesia.* Patients lose the ability to respond verbally but can be aroused by repeated or painful stimulation. Airway and ventilation intervention may be required. Cardiovascular functions are usually adequate.

Principles of General Anesthesia

26.2 Balanced anesthesia uses multiple drugs to provide for the safe induction and maintenance of general anesthesia.

General anesthesia is accomplished by the administration of a variety of drugs. The purposes of general anesthesia include the following:

- *Analgesia:* blocking the sensation of pain
- *Relaxation:* relieving the intense anxiety associated with medical procedures
- *Hypnosis:* producing unconsciousness to block awareness of the procedure
- *Amnesia:* blocking memory of the events associated with the procedure
- *Loss of reflexes:* blocking autonomic and other reflexes that may be affected by the procedure.

Because no single drug can safely accomplish all five purposes, a pharmacologic approach called balanced anesthesia is used. **Balanced anesthesia** is the use of a combination of medications to produce general anesthesia. Drugs administered to achieve balanced anesthesia include neuromuscular blockers, short-acting benzodiazepines, opioids, and general anesthetics. The purpose of combining these medications is to provide sedation, rapid induction of unconsciousness, muscle relaxation, and analgesia. The use of multiple drugs reduces the need for large amounts of inhaled anesthetics, which increases patient safety.

Balanced anesthesia involves the administration of intravenous (IV) medications prior to the general anesthetic. The IV medications produce muscle relaxation, diminish pain, and promote sleep. After the patient loses consciousness, inhaled general anesthetics are administered to maintain the anesthetized state. For short procedures, lower amounts of anesthesia are administered, or parenteral agents alone may be sufficient.

General anesthesia is a progressive process that occurs in distinct phases, which are described in Table 26.1. The most effective medications can quickly induce all four stages, whereas others are able to induce only stage 1. Major surgical procedures require the patient to be maintained in stage 3, which is referred to as **surgical anesthesia**. The patient should progress from stage 2 to stage 3 rapidly because stage 2 produces excitement, hyperactivity, and a feeling of panic. During stage 2 the patient is monitored closely for heart rate irregularities and increases in blood pressure. During recovery from general anesthesia, the patient moves in reverse order back up through the four stages.

Table 26.1 Stages of General Anesthesia

Stage	Characteristics
1	*Analgesia:* The patient loses general sensation but may remain awake. This stage progresses until the patient loses consciousness.
2	*Excitement and hyperactivity:* The patient may become delirious and attempt to resist treatment. The heart rate and respiratory rate may become irregular. The patient's blood pressure may increase. The administration of IV agents may calm the patient.
3	*Surgical anesthesia:* The patient's skeletal muscles become relaxed and delirium stabilizes. The cardiopulmonary effects stabilize. The patient becomes still with diminished eye movements. The surgical procedure is begun. The patient remains in stage 3 until the procedure ends.
4	*Paralysis of the medulla:* If breathing and cardiac function cease, death could result. This stage of general anesthesia is avoided.

Intravenous Anesthetics

26.3 Intravenous anesthetics include opioids, benzodiazepines, and several miscellaneous agents.

IV anesthetics are important components of balanced anesthesia. After a single IV bolus, these drugs enter the brain, allowing the patient to quickly progress through stages 1 and 2. They are occasionally used alone for minor diagnostic and surgical interventions. Concurrent administration of IV and inhaled anesthetics allows the dose of the inhaled anesthetic to be reduced. The lower dosage of inhaled anesthetic produces a better surgical outcome and lowers the risk of serious adverse effects from the anesthesia. The combined use of IV and inhaled anesthesia also allows for a greater degree of analgesia and muscle relaxation than when inhalation anesthetics are used alone.

Fewer than a dozen drugs are used as IV anesthetics. Some of these medications also have nonanesthetic indications. Drugs from the following classes are used for IV anesthesia:

- Opioids
- Benzodiazepines
- Miscellaneous agents.

PharmFACT

There are over 120 accredited nurse anesthesia programs in the United States that use over 1800 sites for clinical training (American Association of Nurse Anesthetists, 2019).

Opioid Anesthetics

26.4 Opioids are used as intravenous anesthetics to provide analgesia and to accomplish neurolept anesthesia.

As presented in Chapter 25, the opioids, or narcotic analgesics, are the most effective drugs available for pain relief, including perioperative pain management. To produce deep anesthesia, however, opioids must be combined with other anesthetics. Combinations allow lower doses to be used and provide the necessary analgesia for painful procedures.

Alfentanil (Alfenta), fentanyl (Sublimaze), remifentanil (Ultiva), and sufentanil (Sufenta) are opioids used as IV anesthetics. These medications are opioid receptor agonists that provide a rapid onset of action with a short duration of 10 to 30 minutes. Their primary disadvantage is respiratory depression. Muscle rigidity may occur, which can further impair ventilation. A complete discussion of the mechanisms, actions, and adverse effects of the opioids is included in Chapter 25. A prototype feature for morphine can also be found in that chapter. Doses for the opioid anesthetics are listed in Table 26.2.

The combination of droperidol and fentanyl produces a type of anesthesia called **neurolept analgesia**. Neurolept analgesia produces feelings of indifference to the patient's surroundings. The patient appears to be asleep but does not lose consciousness. Fentanyl is a potent opioid agonist with pharmacologic action that is similar to that of morphine. Droperidol is an antipsychotic drug related to haloperidol. It has the ability to reduce the adverse effects of nausea and vomiting of opioids and produces sedation by reducing anxiety and motor activity.

PROTOTYPE DRUG **Fentanyl (Sublimaze)**

Classification **Therapeutic:** Analgesic, anesthetic
Pharmacologic: Opioid agonist

Therapeutic Effects and Uses: Fentanyl is an opioid analgesic that is administered IV for short-duration analgesia as part of premedication, balanced anesthesia, induction and maintenance of anesthesia, and postoperative pain. When given IV, it has an immediate onset of action, and its analgesic effects last about 60 minutes. As an anesthetic it may be administered with oxygen in high-risk patients, such as those undergoing open heart surgery or certain complicated neurologic or orthopedic procedures.

Since its approval in 1968 as an IV anesthetic, fentanyl has been introduced in multiple formulations, including buccal tablets (Fentora), buccal film, sublingual tablets, oral transmucosal lozenges (Actiq), transmucosal spray (Subsys), intranasal spray (Lazanda), and transdermal patches (Duragesic). All of these nonanesthetic formulations of fentanyl are prescribed for the management of breakthrough pain in patients who are already receiving and who are tolerant to around-the-clock opioid therapy for their chronic, persistent pain. Opioids such as fentanyl will result in tolerance if taken in high drug dosages over an extended period of time. Doses need to be adjusted periodically for adequate pain management. Physical and psychologic dependence may occur with continued use. Abrupt discontinuation of the drug may cause intense withdrawal symptoms

Table 26.2 Intravenous Anesthetics

Drug	Route and Adult Dose (Maximum Dose Where Indicated)	Adverse Effects
Opioids		
alfentanil (Alfenta)	IV: 8–20 mcg/kg for surgery lasting longer than 30 min Maintenance anesthesia: 3–5 mcg/kg in incremental doses Continuous infusion: 0.5–1 mcg/kg/min Total dose: 8–40 mcg/kg	*Skeletal muscle rigidity, nausea and vomiting, postoperative drowsiness, shivering, hypertension (HTN), bradycardia, prolonged QT interval, constipation* <u>Apnea, respiratory depression, laryngospasm, bronchospasm, circulatory depression, cardiac arrest, respiratory depression, respiratory arrest, anaphylactoid reaction</u>
fentanyl (Sublimaze)	IM/IV: 2–100 mcg/kg with dosage individualized to patient and indication	
remifentanil (Ultiva)	IV: 0.5 mcg/kg/min or 1 mcg/kg IV bolus	
sufentanil (Sufenta)	IV: 1–8 mcg/kg; may give additional doses of 10–50 mcg, if needed Primary anesthetic: 1–30 mcg/kg IV administered with 100% oxygen	
Benzodiazepines		
diazepam (Valium)	IV: 5–10 mg, repeat every 10–15 min as needed	*Drowsiness, hypotension, tachycardia, retrograde amnesia* <u>Cardiovascular collapse, respiratory arrest, laryngospasm</u>
midazolam	IV (premedication): 0.15–0.25 mg/kg over 20–30 sec IV (unpremedicated patients): 0.3–0.35 mg/kg over 20–30 sec	
remimazolam (Byfavo)	IV: 2.5-5 mg followed by additional doses to achieve desired sedation	
Miscellaneous IV Anesthetics		
etomidate (Amidate)	IV: 0.2–0.6 mg/kg over a period of 30–60 sec for induction	*Pain on injection, transient skeletal muscle movements* <u>Changes in ventilation (hyper or hypo) and blood pressure (hyper or hypo)</u>
ketamine (Ketalar)	IV: 1–4 mg/kg IM: 6.5–13 mg/kg	*Respiratory depression, laryngospasm, apnea, nausea and vomiting* <u>HTN, tachycardia, vivid dreams, hallucinations, delirium</u>
methohexital (Brevital)	IV: For induction: 1–1.5 mg/kg at a rate of 1 mL every 5 sec	*Postoperative psychomotor impairment, retrograde amnesia, hypothermia, sloughing with extravasation, skeletal muscle hyperactivity* <u>Circulatory depression, respiratory depression, respiratory arrest, apnea, anaphylaxis</u>
propofol (Diprivan)	IV: 2–2.5 mg/kg every 10 sec until induction onset	*Pain at injection site, skeletal muscle movements* <u>Dysrhythmias, hypotension</u>

Note: *Italics* indicate common adverse effects. <u>Underline</u> indicates serious adverse effects.

(see Chapter 27). Fentanyl is a Schedule II controlled substance. When taken illegally, fentanyl gives the same effects as heroin.

Mechanism of Action: Fentanyl is an opioid agonist at the mu and kappa receptors. The mechanism of action is the same as that of morphine and other opioids. Fentanyl has a more rapid onset of action than morphine.

Pharmacokinetics:

Route(s)	IV, intramuscular (IM), transdermal, transmucosal, epidural
Absorption	Rapid
Distribution	Crosses the placenta; secreted in breast milk; 80% bound to protein
Primary metabolism	Hepatic (CYP3A4)
Primary excretion	Renal
Onset of action	IV: immediate; IM: 7–15 min; transdermal: 24–72 h peak; transmucosal: 20–30 min peak; epidural: 10–15 min
Duration of action	IV: 0.5–1 h; IM: 1–2 h; transdermal: 17-h half-life; transmucosal: unknown; epidural: 2–3 h

Adverse Effects: The most common adverse effects of fentanyl include respiratory depression, apnea, skeletal muscle rigidity, and bradycardia. The peak respiratory depression occurs 5 to 15 minutes after an IV dose. The respiratory depression, however, will continue postoperatively and outlast the analgesic effects of the drug. Nausea and vomiting and constipation are common adverse effects produced by most opioids. Fentanyl may cause syncope and severe bradycardia and hypotension. Transdermal patches can cause localized pain, irritation, ulceration, and bleeding.

Black Box Warning: Fentanyl carries several black box warnings. This drug has significant abuse potential and should not be prescribed to patients with a high risk for misuse, abuse, or diversion. The drug carries a high risk for death due to overdose or respiratory depression. Concurrent use with CYP3A4 inhibitors will increase fentanyl plasma concentrations and the risk of serious adverse effects. Concurrent use with other central nervous system (CNS) depressants such as benzodiazepines or alcohol may result in profound sedation, respiratory depression, coma, and death. Prolonged use during pregnancy can result in neonatal opioid withdrawal syndrome, which may be life-threatening. Accidental ingestion of even one dose by children may be fatal.

Contraindications/Precautions: Patients with respiratory impairment should be administered fentanyl with caution due to the respiratory depression caused by the drug. Patients with hepatic or chronic kidney disease should receive lower doses. The drug may worsen bradydysrhythmia. Patients with head trauma should not receive fentanyl because intracranial pressure (ICP) may increase. Fentanyl is secreted in breast milk and can cause sedation and respiratory depression in the neonate; thus, it should not be administered during lactation.

Drug Interactions: Extreme caution should be used when administering fentanyl with alcohol or other CNS depressants due to additive sedation and respiratory depression. Fentanyl is metabolized by CYP450 enzymes (CYP3A4) in the liver and intestinal mucosa and has the potential to interact with other drugs that induce or inhibit this enzyme. Cardiovascular depression may occur if nitrous oxide is used with high doses of fentanyl. **Herbal/Food:** St. John's wort may intensify or prolong the effects of fentanyl anesthesia and may induce the metabolism of fentanyl via CYP3A4. Use of valerian or kava may cause additive CNS depression.

Pregnancy: Animal studies showed fentanyl to be embryocidal. Chronic opioid use during pregnancy has been associated with poor fetal growth, stillbirths, preterm birth, and possibly birth defects. After delivery, neonates may experience neonatal abstinence syndrome with signs of withdrawal that include tremors, irritability, seizures, poor feeding, and vomiting. Studies regarding breastfeeding are inconclusive, however, short-duration use of fentanyl such as intrathecal or epidural use for anesthesia is likely safe for the breastfed neonate.

Treatment of Overdose: In the event of an overdose, the patient is supported with mechanical ventilation until the drug is metabolized and the effects diminish. The patient may be administered a narcotic antagonist such as naloxone (Narcan) to reverse serious respiratory depression.

Clinician Responsibilities: Key clinical implications for patients receiving fentanyl are included in Applied Clinical Judgment: Patients Receiving General Anesthesia in this chapter and in the Applied Clinical Judgment: Patients Receiving Pharmacotherapy for Pain in Chapter 25.

Drugs Similar to Fentanyl (Sublimaze)

Additional opioid IV general anesthetics include alfentanil, remifentanil, and sufentanil. These opioids have the same pregnancy and lactation data as fentanyl.

Alfentanil (Alfenta): Approved in 1996, alfentanil is an opioid that has a more rapid onset and a shorter duration of action than fentanyl. It is administered IV to provide analgesia as a component of balanced anesthesia. Uses include assisting in intubation, promoting the induction of anesthesia, and as an infusion for the maintenance of anesthesia. The most common adverse effects are respiratory depression, bradycardia, and muscle rigidity. Respiratory depression may be delayed; thus, the patient should be monitored for some time after surgery. Alfentanil must be used with caution with other CNS depressants. Other actions and adverse effects are the same as those for fentanyl.

Remifentanil (Ultiva): Approved in 1996, remifentanil is an IV opioid that is similar to fentanyl. It is rapidly metabolized, which allows for a shorter duration of respiratory depression than fentanyl. Recovery from anesthesia occurs 5 to 10 minutes after discontinuation of the drug. This agent is administered during the induction and maintenance of general anesthesia to provide analgesia during the postoperative period. Although it does not produce deep anesthesia, remifentanil may be used alone or in combination with midazolam in monitored anesthesia care. Hypotension is greater with remifentanil than with fentanyl. Respiratory depression, hypotension, sweating, and nausea and vomiting are other adverse effects. Other actions and adverse effects are the same as those for fentanyl.

Sufentanil (Sufenta): Approved in 1984, sufentanil is an IV opioid used as a component of balanced anesthesia or as a primary anesthetic agent. As a primary anesthetic the patient should be administered 100% oxygen. During IV use, the onset of action is immediate and recovery time is comparable to that of fentanyl. It is sometimes administered with bupivacaine as an epidural anesthesia adjunct during labor and delivery. During epidural use, the onset of action is about 10 minutes and recovery time is 1.7 hours. Sufentanil is 5 to 10 times more potent than fentanyl. The most common adverse effects are respiratory depression and muscle rigidity, and the drug must be used with caution with other CNS depressants. Dsuvia is a sublingual tablet containing sufentanil that is indicated for the management of severe pain. The most frequent adverse effects for Dsuvia are nausea and vomiting, headache, dizziness, and hypotension.

CONNECTION Checkpoint 26.1

In pain management, opioids are often available in fixed-dose combinations with nonopioids. From what you learned in Chapter 25, what is the rationale for using a nonopioid analgesic with an opioid? What specific nonopioid analgesic is most frequently found in these combination drugs?

Benzodiazepine Anesthetics

26.5 Benzodiazepines are used in anesthesia to produce relaxation, sedation, and amnesia.

The primary indication for benzodiazepines is to treat symptoms of anxiety (see Chapter 18). For anesthesia, drugs in this class are used at high doses to cause sedation and induce unconsciousness. Benzodiazepines are a component of balanced anesthesia, most often administered in combination with inhalation anesthetics to allow the patient to feel less anxiety and experience amnesia. They may be administered PO as a premedication to relax the patient prior to minor medical procedures. The most commonly utilized benzodiazepine for surgical procedures is midazolam. Diazepam (Valium) and lorazepam have a slower onset and longer duration than midazolam and are occasionally used as anesthesia adjuncts. In 2020 a new benzodiazepine, remimazolam (Byfavo), was approved for anesthesia. A detailed discussion of benzodiazepines is found in Chapter 22, along with a prototype feature for diazepam. Doses for the two benzodiazepines used as IV anesthetics are listed in Table 26.2.

PROTOTYPE DRUG Midazolam

Classification **Therapeutic:** IV anesthetic
Pharmacologic: Benzodiazepine, gamma aminobutyric acid (GABA) receptor agonist

Therapeutic Effects and Uses: Approved in 1985, midazolam is administered to reduce the anxiety and stress associated with surgery. It is approved by the U.S. Food and Drug Administration (FDA) for the induction of amnesia, induction and maintenance of general anesthesia, and sedation prior to short diagnostic procedures such as an endoscopy. It is also used to treat status epilepticus in adults and for sedation of mechanically ventilated patients. Midazolam syrup is indicated for use in children to produce sedation, anxiolysis, and amnesia prior to minor medical procedures or induction of anesthesia. Midazolam is sometimes known by its trade name, Versed, which is no longer available.

Induction of anesthesia occurs in 1 to 2 minutes following an IV bolus of midazolam. If the patient has received an opioid premedication, induction is even more rapid. Awakening and complete recovery of memory occurs in about 2 hours but may extend to 6 hours in older adults or those with heart failure or hepatic impairment.

Midazolam is a Schedule IV controlled substance. It has abuse potential similar to that of other benzodiazepines.

Mechanism of Action: Midazolam acts at the limbic, thalamic, and hypothalamic regions of the brain to produce CNS depression and skeletal muscle relaxation. This is the same mechanism of action as other benzodiazepines.

Pharmacokinetics:

Route(s)	IV, IM, PO
Absorption	Rapid absorption
Distribution	Widely distributed; crosses the blood–brain barrier and the placenta; secreted in breast milk; 97% protein bound
Primary metabolism	Hepatic
Primary excretion	Renal
Onset of action	IV: 1.5 min; IM: 5–15 min; PO: 10–30 min
Duration of action	IV/IM/PO: 2–6 h

Adverse Effects: Respiratory depression and apnea are potentially serious adverse events. CNS adverse effects include drowsiness, fatigue, ataxia, slurred speech, and tremor. Potentially serious cardiovascular effects include hypotension, tachycardia, and cardiovascular collapse. Laryngospasm is the most severe pulmonary complication noted with the administration of midazolam. Paradoxical reactions such as hyperactivity or aggressive behavior have been reported in pediatric patients and in those with preexisting psychiatric disorders. **Black Box Warning:** Respiratory depression and arrest have occurred with midazolam use. Respiratory status must be continuously monitored, and resuscitative equipment must be readily available. When used concurrently with benzodiazepines or opioids, the dosage and duration of midazolam anesthesia should be limited to the minimum required.

Contraindications/Precautions: Patients who have acute, closed-angle glaucoma should not be administered midazolam because the drug may increase intraocular pressure. Patients experiencing acute alcohol intoxication, shock, coma, or depressed vital signs should not be administered benzodiazepines because the drug may worsen these conditions.

Drug Interactions: The administration of benzodiazepines with any medication that depresses the CNS, including alcohol, increases the patient's risk for sedation. Use of benzodiazepines and phenytoin (Dilantin) will result in an increased serum phenytoin level and additive CNS depression. Midazolam is metabolized by hepatic CYP3A4 enzyme, and inhibitors or inducers of this enzyme may interact with midazolam. **Herbal/Food:** Increased sedation may occur if benzodiazepines are administered with kava or valerian. Grapefruit juice may increase the serum concentration of midazolam. Melatonin should be avoided because it may increase sedation.

Pregnancy: Benzodiazepines have the potential to cause fetal harm. Neonates born to mothers taking benzodiazepines during pregnancy or breastfeeding may experience withdrawal symptoms. Benzodiazepines should not be used during pregnancy or breastfeeding unless the potential benefits to the mother justify the potential risks to the fetus or neonate.

Treatment of Overdose: Overdose with midazolam causes sedation, confusion, diminished reflexes, and coma. General supportive measures should be taken, and the patient may be treated with flumazenil (Romazicon), which is a specific benzodiazepine antagonist. Flumazenil acts within minutes but may induce seizures with rapid reversal.

Clinician Responsibilities: Key clinical implications for patients receiving midazolam are included in Applied Clinical Judgment: Patients Receiving General Anesthesia in this chapter and in Applied Clinical Judgment: Patients Receiving Pharmacotherapy for Anxiety or Sleep Disorders in Chapter 18.

Drugs Similar to Midazolam

Diazepam and remimazolam (Byfavo) are other benzodiazepines administered to produce anesthesia.

Diazepam (Valium): Diazepam has been widely prescribed for anxiety and as an adjunct in seizure management. In the surgical suite diazepam is used as a premedication (by the IM route) for relief of anxiety associated with the surgical procedure. It is used by the IV route prior to cardioversion for the relief of anxiety and tension and to produce amnesia. When administered parenterally, it has an onset of action of 1 to 5 minutes and produces short-acting effects. Diazepam decreases the patient's anxiety and relaxes the skeletal muscles. Diazepam impairs the patient's ability to remember the perioperative events. A prototype feature for diazepam is found in Chapter 22.

Remimazolam (Byfavo): In 2020 remimazolam was approved for the induction and maintenance of sedation for procedures lasting 30 minutes or less such as colonoscopy or bronchoscopy. Given by the IV route, induction and recovery are very rapid. Benzodiazepines may produce respiratory depression in neonates. Remimazolam is likely secreted in milk and the manufacturer recommends discarding breast milk for 5 hours following treatment.

CONNECTION Checkpoint 26.2

Benzodiazepines are sometimes used for seizure control. From what you learned in Chapter 22, what are the indications for lorazepam and diazepam in treating seizures?

Miscellaneous Intravenous Anesthetics

26.6 Propofol and ketamine are widely used intravenous drugs for inducing and maintaining anesthesia.

Several miscellaneous drugs are used as parenteral anesthetics. Propofol (Diprivan) and ketamine (Ketalar) are two widely used IV anesthetics. The two drugs are not related chemically, but both have short durations and can induce anesthesia rapidly. Etomidate (Amidate) and methohexital (Brevital) are much less frequently used in balanced anesthesia. Doses for these drugs are listed in Table 26.2.

PROTOTYPE DRUG **Propofol (Diprivan)**

Classification **Therapeutic:** IV anesthetic, sedative–hypnotic drug
Pharmacologic: N-methyl-D-aspartate (NMDA) receptor agonist

Therapeutic Effects and Uses: Approved in 1989, propofol has become the most widely used IV anesthetic due to its effectiveness and relative safety profile. It is indicated for the induction and maintenance of general anesthesia. In the intensive care unit (ICU), the drug may be administered to intubated, mechanically ventilated adult patients to provide continuous sedation and control of stress responses. It has an almost immediate onset of action and is used effectively for conscious sedation. Emergence from anesthesia is rapid, and few adverse effects occur during recovery. Unlike other anesthetics that cause nausea and vomiting, propofol has an antiemetic effect that can prevent nausea and vomiting in patients receiving chemotherapy. Off-label uses include refractory migraines, refractory status epilepticus, and the treatment of agitation associated with alcohol withdrawal.

Mechanism of Action: The exact mechanism by which propofol produces anesthesia is not clear. It is believed to act by activating GABA receptors, which causes a general inhibition of CNS activity.

Pharmacokinetics:

Route(s)	IV
Absorption	Rapid
Distribution	Widely distributed to body tissues; highly protein bound
Primary metabolism	Hepatic
Primary excretion	Renal
Onset of action	Immediate
Duration of action	IV: 10–15 min

Adverse Effects: Injection-site pain, apnea, respiratory depression, and hypotension are common adverse effects. Propofol has been associated with a collection of metabolic abnormalities and organ system failures, referred to as propofol infusion syndrome (PRIS). The syndrome is characterized by severe metabolic acidosis, hyperkalemia, lipemia, rhabdomyolysis, hepatomegaly, and cardiac and kidney failure. PRIS is usually associated with prolonged, high-dose infusions of the drug. Deaths have resulted from this syndrome.

Contraindications/Precautions: Propofol is contraindicated in patients who have a known hypersensitivity reaction to the medication or its emulsion, which contains soybean and egg products. The emulsion supports rapid microorganism growth; unused portions must be discarded. Obstetric patients and those with increased ICP should not be administered propofol. The drug should be used with caution in patients with cardiac or respiratory impairment. It is not recommended for induction of anesthesia in children younger than 3 years. Although not a controlled substance, incidences of propofol abuse have occurred, including the high-profile case of musician Michael Jackson, who used this medication (among others) to induce sleep.

Drug Interactions: The dose of propofol should be reduced in patients receiving preanesthetic medications such as opioids or benzodiazepines. Use with other CNS depressants can cause additive CNS and respiratory depression. **Herbal/Food:** Unknown.

Pregnancy: Animal studies showed no evidence of fetal harm. Propofol is not recommended during breastfeeding because the drug is secreted in milk and has the potential to cause adverse effects on the neonate.

Treatment of Overdose: Overdose will produce cardiac and respiratory depression. The treatment includes mechanical ventilation of the patient, increasing the flow rate of IV fluids, and administering vasopressor agents as needed to maintain blood pressure.

Clinician Responsibilities: Key clinical implications for patients receiving propofol are included in Applied Clinical Judgment: Patients Receiving General Anesthesia.

Drugs Similar to Propofol

Other miscellaneous IV anesthetics include etomidate, ketamine, and methohexital.

Etomidate (Amidate): Approved in 2007, etomidate is a hypnotic drug indicated for the IV induction of general anesthesia for short medical–surgical procedures such as cardioversion, endotracheal intubation, or reduction of dislocations. It is also approved to supplement anesthesia produced by low-potency drugs such as nitrous oxide. It has a very rapid onset of action and hypotension is uncommon. It provides only 5 to 10 minutes of anesthesia. A major adverse effect is that it suppresses corticosteroid synthesis and can cause dangerous adrenal insufficiency if used for long periods. Concurrent use of opioids or benzodiazepines can worsen this suppression. Animal reproduction studies showed increased stillbirths and lowered offspring survival. It is not known if etomidate is secreted in milk or if it has adverse effects on the breastfed neonate.

Ketamine (Ketalar): Approved in 1970, ketamine is an IV anesthetic that produces a trancelike feeling of being separated from the environment called **dissociative anesthesia**. When used alone, ketamine is indicated during surgeries and brief diagnostic procedures that do not require skeletal muscle relaxation. It is also used prior to the administration of other general anesthetic agents. Ketamine is used with pediatric patients due to its rapid induction of general anesthesia and the fact that it lasts up to 25 minutes. Ketamine has strong analgesic actions and immediately increases blood pressure and skeletal muscle tone. The patient's eyes may be open during the surgical procedure. Potentially serious cardiovascular adverse effects of ketamine include HTN and tachycardia. Respiratory depression occurs with the administration of IV ketamine. The most serious neurologic adverse effect is emergence phenomena in adult patients, which can occur for 24 hours postoperatively. Emergence phenomena include delirium, hallucinations, confusion, excitement, and irrational behavior. Ketamine is a Schedule III drug. Ketamine may cause fetal harm and the drug is secreted in milk. Use of ketamine is not recommended during pregnancy or lactation unless the potential benefits justify the potential risks to the fetus or neonate.

Ketamine is a common drug of abuse that is known by the names jet, super acid, Special K, green K, and cat Valium. It is a club drug that is similar to phencyclidine (PCP), which is popular among teens and young adults. It is easily added to drinks or administered through injection to cause temporary amnesia and is sometimes referred to as a date-rape drug (see Chapter 27).

Methohexital (Brevital): Approved in 2001, methohexital is an ultrashort-acting barbiturate that can be used to induce general anesthesia or administered as a continuous IV infusion. It is also approved to supplement anesthesia produced by low-potency drugs such as nitrous oxide. Like other IV anesthetics, it has a rapid onset, a short duration of action, and a relatively fast recovery period. IM and rectal forms are available for use in children. Severe adverse reactions include respiratory depression, laryngospasm, and hypotension. Adverse CNS effects may persist for 24 hours and include confusion, delirium, somnolence, anxiety, and seizures. Other adverse events include shivering, nausea and vomiting, and anaphylaxis. Methohexital is a Schedule IV controlled substance. Details on the mechanisms of action of barbiturates and their applications as sedatives may be found in Chapter 18. Animal reproduction studies showed no evidence of fetal harm. Methohexital is secreted in milk but its effect on the breastfed neonate are unknown.

Inhalation Anesthetics

26.7 Inhalation anesthetics used to produce loss of consciousness are classified as gases or volatile liquids.

Following the administration of IV agents, inhalation anesthetics are given to rapidly produce unconsciousness and total analgesia. Inhalation anesthetics are supplied as gases or volatile liquids. These drugs produce their effects on the CNS by inhibiting the flow of sodium into neurons, which delays the nerve impulses and dramatically reduces the activity of the neurons. Although the mechanism of action is incompletely understood, inhibitory GABA receptors in the brain become active and are thought to be responsible for the anesthetic action. This action is similar to that of the antiepileptic medications described in Chapter 22. Other CNS neurotransmitters likely contribute to the sedative effects of the inhalation anesthetics.

The first general anesthetic was the gas diethyl ether, which was discovered in the 1840s. Although popular for over 100 years, gaseous anesthetics were explosive and presented a danger to the surgical team members, who were exposed to fumes from the drugs. Furthermore, the gases produced a very high incidence of nausea and vomiting following the procedure. The only gaseous anesthetic in use today is nitrous oxide.

The potency of inhalation anesthetics is described by the **minimum alveolar concentration**: the concentration of drug vapor in the alveoli that prevents a motor response in 50% of patients when exposed to a painful stimulus. A low value of minimum alveolar concentration indicates that a very small amount of anesthetic is needed to immobilize the patient. Inhalation anesthetics have low minimum alveolar concentrations and are thus very potent. The exception is nitrous oxide, which is a low-potency anesthetic with a high minimum alveolar concentration value. The minimum alveolar concentration changes with the age of the patient. It is lowest in newborns, peaks in infants, and gradually declines with age.

Inhalation anesthetics are rapidly absorbed from the alveoli into the general circulation. The anesthesiologist controls the length and depth of anesthesia by delivering the exact concentration of drug needed to maintain a desirable degree of immobility. These drugs are very lipid soluble and quickly cross the blood–brain barrier to produce sedating effects. Metabolism of inhalation anesthetics is minimal, and elimination of the drug is mostly by exhalation. Modern anesthetics are designed to have a fast recovery time so that the patient regains consciousness soon after the infusion is stopped. Because anesthetics are lipid soluble, they are stored in fat and slowly released, which explains why patients with obesity may take longer to recover from anesthesia.

CONNECTIONS: Using Research in Practice

Malignant Hyperthermia and Anesthetic Agents

Malignant hyperthermia (MH) is a rare and potentially fatal condition that occurs when a susceptible individual receives certain triggering medications (e.g., succinylcholine) during anesthesia. A genetic predisposition to malignant hyperthermia has been discovered, but it is not yet possible to predict whether genetic predisposition will necessarily result in its occurrence (Shaw & Hopkins, 2019). Patients with other preexisting musculoskeletal conditions, especially those that are genetically linked, may be at greater risk, even if the true incidence of malignant hyperthermia occurring in these populations is unknown. With a greater number of surgeries occurring in an outpatient setting, including dental offices, it is recommended that dantrolene, a treatment for MH, be available whenever drugs known to trigger MH are used (e.g., succinylcholine) (Larach, Riazi, & Rosenberg, 2019).

The nurse plays a key role in assessing a patient for possible malignant hyperthermia risk during the preoperative period. Existing myopathies, unusual heat-associated illnesses in a child or adult, or previous history of statin-associated myopathy should be noted and the anesthesiologist or anesthetist alerted. A personal or immediate-family history of problems with previous anesthetic use should also be noted. Symptoms of malignant hyperthermia often begin with unexplained tachycardia. Jaw muscle spasms and rigidity may occur, followed by a dramatic increase in body temperature, rhabdomyolysis indicated by dark brown–colored urine, dysrhythmias, and potential death. Any patient experiencing mild spasms in the jaw muscles must be observed more closely for development of malignant hyperthermia for at least 10 hours postprocedure. Patients with darkened urine or with severe jaw rigidity should be hospitalized overnight postoperatively to observe for the development of malignant hyperthermia.

PROTOTYPE DRUG Nitrous Oxide

Classification **Therapeutic:** Gaseous general anesthetic
Pharmacologic: GABA-receptor agonist, opioid agonist

Therapeutic Effects and Uses: Nitrous oxide is an odorless, nonirritating, inorganic gas used for a large number of medical and surgical procedures. When administered alone it is one of the least potent anesthetics and is unable to induce deep anesthesia at therapeutic doses. Because of its low potency, the use of nitrous oxide is either limited to minor surgical procedures or combined with the IV anesthetic agents for more complex procedures. The majority of patients requiring sedation for dental, diagnostic, and surgical procedures are administered nitrous oxide.

One major advantage of nitrous oxide is that it has strong analgesic properties. At a concentration of 20%, nitrous oxide delivers analgesic efficiency equaling that of morphine. This agent has a low potency and does not produce loss of consciousness or profound skeletal muscle relaxation.

Nitrous oxide is always combined with oxygen (25–30%) and is administered in a semiclosed method. The patient may be administered an IV anesthetic to produce sedation. When drowsy or asleep, the patient inhales the nitrous oxide through a tube or by mask. Nitrous oxide is also used for dental procedures in which the mask is placed over the nose. Other procedures in which nitrous oxide is administered include those related to obstetrics and surgery. Nitrous oxide lowers the minimum alveolar concentration of other anesthetics, essentially making them more potent. This permits a decrease in the dosages required for IV and inhalation anesthetics.

Nitrous oxide has been used illegally to produce relaxation, euphoria, and hallucinations. Abusers may steal the nitrous oxide tanks from medical facilities. The gas has also been used as a propellant in whipped cream canisters and cooking sprays, and abusers can obtain small amounts from those sources. Long-term abuse can lead to anemia, depletion of vitamin B_{12}, tinnitus, and peripheral neuropathy.

Mechanism of Action: The mechanism of action of nitrous oxide is not fully known. Its analgesic effects are believed to be due to activation of opioid receptors in the midbrain. The relaxation properties of the drug are likely due to activation of GABA receptors, which inhibits neuronal firing.

Pharmacokinetics:

Route(s)	Inhalation
Absorption	Rapid
Distribution	Crosses the blood–brain barrier to concentrate in the nerve cells
Primary metabolism	Not metabolized
Primary excretion	100% through the lungs, unchanged
Onset of action	2–5 min
Duration of action	Half-life is variable; peak effect: less than 10 min

Adverse Effects: When administered in low to moderate doses, nitrous oxide produces few adverse effects. When administered in higher doses, patients exhibit some adverse effects of stage 2 anesthesia such as anxiety, excitement, and combativeness. Lowering the inhaled dose quickly reverses these adverse effects. Because nitrous oxide is exhaled, the patient may temporarily have some difficulty breathing at the end of the procedure.

Rapid diffusion of the gas from the bloodstream back into the lungs causes alveolar hypoxia, with symptoms that include nausea and vomiting, lethargy, and dizziness. Some patients describe these symptoms as equivalent to a "hangover" from too much alcohol consumption. Alveolar hypoxia can be prevented by breathing 100% oxygen for several minutes following the conclusion of nitrous oxide therapy.

Contraindications/Precautions: When patients must be awake and follow the instructions of the physician or dentist, nitrous oxide is contraindicated in those with an impaired level of consciousness or an inability to comply with instructions. Because the diffusion of nitrous oxide may lead to expansion of closed spaces, its use in patients with conditions such as undiagnosed abdominal pain, abdominal distention, bowel obstruction, head injury, or pneumothorax is contraindicated. Patients who have hypotension, shock, chronic obstructive pulmonary disease, cyanosis, or chest pain should not be administered nitrous oxide.

Drug Interaction: The administration of adrenergic agonists (such as epinephrine) or caffeine with nitrous oxide may exacerbate dysrhythmias. Use with CNS depressants may cause additive sedation and respiratory depression. Excessive hypotension may result if amiodarone or antihypertensive drugs are used concurrently with nitrous oxide. **Herbal/Food:** Milk thistle taken before and after anesthesia may lower the potential risk of liver damage. St. John's wort should be discontinued 2 to 3 weeks prior to administration of general anesthetics due to possible hypotension risk.

Pregnancy: Short-duration anesthesia using nitrous oxide are not associated with fetal risk. With a short half-life of 3 minutes, nitrous oxide is not predicted to have adverse effects on the breastfed infant.

Treatment of Overdose: Effects of the drug usually diminish quickly after the gas is discontinued. Metoclopramide (Reglan) or another antiemetic agent may be administered to reduce the nausea and vomiting associated with nitrous oxide.

Clinician Responsibilities: Key clinical implications for patients receiving nitrous oxide are included in Applied Clinical Judgment: Patients Receiving General Anesthesia.

Drugs Similar to Nitrous Oxide

Nitrous oxide is the sole gaseous general anesthetic.

PharmFACT

Nitrous oxide is being examined as a therapy for treatment-resistant depression. Clinical studies have demonstrated the drug to be effective in enhancing mood and reducing anxiety and suicidal ideation (Kalmoe et al., 2020).

Volatile Liquid Anesthetics

26.8 Volatile liquid general anesthetics are used to induce and maintain deep anesthesia.

The volatile liquids form a second class of inhalation anesthetics. The volatile liquid drugs have a low vapor pressure that allows them to vaporize (form a gas) at low temperatures and pressures. An anesthesia machine is used to vaporize the liquid, mix the vapors with oxygen and air, and deliver them to patients in precisely controlled amounts. The anesthesia machine also establishes a partial pressure gradient that ensures the anesthetic will continue to flow from the machine to the alveoli, to the blood, and eventually to the brain. Like the gases, the volatile liquid anesthetics are lipid soluble and rapidly cross the blood–brain barrier to cause sedation. All of these drugs have a rapid onset of action. The gaseous and volatile liquid anesthetics are listed in Table 26.3.

The minimum alveolar concentrations of the volatile liquid anesthetics are very low, making them very potent. This factor contributes to the ability of these drugs to rapidly produce unconsciousness at low doses. Although they have the ability to produce deep anesthesia, they produce little analgesia and are usually used in combination with nitrous oxide and opioids as part of balanced anesthesia.

Some volatile liquid anesthetics sensitize the heart to the action of catecholamines such as epinephrine, norepinephrine, and dopamine and can cause serious dysrhythmias. These drugs also depress cardiovascular and pulmonary function, placing the patient at risk for laryngospasm or respiratory arrest.

PROTOTYPE DRUG Isoflurane (Forane)

Classification **Therapeutic:** Inhaled general anesthetic
Pharmacologic: GABA and glutamate receptor agonist

Therapeutic Effects and Uses: Approved in 1979, isoflurane is a first-line inhalation anesthetic due to its effectiveness and favorable safety profile. Isoflurane provides smooth and rapid induction of general anesthesia with a low degree of metabolism by the body. It is almost entirely eliminated through respirations. The drug provides excellent muscle relaxation. It is FDA approved for the induction and maintenance of general anesthesia and may be used off-label as adjuvant therapy in the treatment of status asthmaticus.

Isoflurane does not sensitize the myocardium for dysrhythmias, and it produces fewer cardiovascular effects than other general anesthetics. Isoflurane does not cause the hepatotoxicity observed with halothane.

Mechanism of Action: The exact mechanism of action of isoflurane is unknown. It interacts with multiple receptors in the brain, including glutamate and GABA receptors.

Pharmacokinetics:

Route(s)	Inhalation
Absorption	Rapidly absorbed by the lungs
Distribution	Crosses the blood–brain barrier to concentrate in neurons; unknown if it is secreted in breast milk
Primary metabolism	Minimal metabolism
Primary excretion	95% pulmonary
Onset of action	7–10 min for surgical anesthesia
Duration of action	Patient begins to regain consciousness less than 1 h after drug is discontinued

Table 26.3 Inhalation Anesthetics

Drug	Adult Concentration	Adverse Effects
Gas		
nitrous oxide	70% with 30% oxygen	*Anxiety, nausea and vomiting* <u>Hypoxia, hallucinations, disorientation</u>
Volatile Liquids		
desflurane (Suprane)	7.3% concentration	*Nausea and vomiting, shivering* <u>Laryngospasm, hypotension, apnea, increased secretions, vasodilation, respiratory depression, tachycardia, malignant hyperthermia,</u>
isoflurane (Forane)	0.1–2% concentration	
sevoflurane (Sojourn, Ultane)	0.5–3% concentration	

Note: *Italics* indicate common adverse effects. <u>Underline</u> indicates serious adverse effects.

Adverse Effects: Mild nausea and vomiting and tremor are common adverse effects. The drug produces a dose-dependent respiratory depression and a reduction in blood pressure. Malignant hyperthermia with elevated temperature and unstable blood pressure has been reported, although the incidence is rare.

Contraindications/Precautions: Patients with a known history or genetic predisposition to malignant hyperthermia should not use isoflurane. Caution should be used when treating patients with head trauma or brain neoplasms due to possible increases in ICP. Safety has not been established in patients under age 18. Older adult patients are more susceptible to the cardiovascular effects of the drug. Patients with a prolonged QT interval should be administered isoflurane with caution.

Drug Interactions: Coughing, breath holding, or laryngospasm may occur when used concurrently with nitrous oxide. Skeletal muscle weakness, respiratory depression, or apnea may occur if isoflurane is administered concurrently with systemic polymyxin or aminoglycosides. Additive effects can occur if isoflurane is administered with other skeletal muscle relaxants. Additive hypotension may result if used concurrently with antihypertensive medications such as beta-adrenergic blockers. Epinephrine, norepinephrine, dopamine, and other adrenergic agonists should be administered with caution because of the possibility of dysrhythmias. Levodopa should be discontinued 6 to 8 hours before isoflurane administration. Isoflurane should be administered with caution with other drugs that prolong the QT interval, such as amiodarone, ibutilide, droperidol, and phenothiazines. **Herbal/Food:** St. John's wort should be discontinued 2 to 3 weeks prior to administration of general anesthetics due to possible hypotension risk.

Pregnancy: Animal studies suggest that isoflurane may be embryocidal and lengthy surgeries (3 hours or more) may have negative effects on fetal brain development during the third trimester. Effects on the breastfed infant are unknown.

Treatment of Overdose: Isoflurane causes profound respiratory depression. The patient is treated symptomatically until the effects of the drug diminish.

Clinician Responsibilities: Key clinical implications for patients receiving isoflurane are included in Applied Clinical Judgment: Patients Receiving General Anesthesia.

Drugs Similar to Isoflurane (Forane)

Volatile liquid anesthetics similar to isoflurane include desflurane and sevoflurane. Halothane (Fluothane), the historical prototype for this drug class, was voluntarily removed from the market due to a small incidence of fatal hepatitis associated with the drug.

Desflurane (Suprane): Desflurane, approved in the 1990s, produces a rapid induction of general anesthesia. It is administered to induce and maintain anesthesia in adults. When administered to children it is used to maintain anesthesia. Adverse effects of desflurane are laryngospasm, apnea, and increased pulmonary secretions. The drug produces a dose-dependent reduction in blood pressure, and malignant hyperthermia has been reported. Desflurane must be used with IV anesthetics because it may cause coughing and excitation during induction. It does not sensitize the myocardium for dysrhythmias. In laboratory animals, desflurane showed embryofetal toxicity.

Sevoflurane (Sojourn, Ultane): Approved in 1995, sevoflurane is a volatile liquid general anesthetic agent that is administered to induce and maintain sedation. It has a faster uptake, distribution, and elimination than isoflurane. It also does not cause the cardiovascular reactions commonly encountered with some of the other general anesthetics, and it is safer to use in patients with coronary artery disease. Sevoflurane does not cause respiratory irritation and is safe for administration with children. Furthermore, this drug does not cause coughing and excitation during induction and can thus be used without IV anesthetics. Sevoflurane produces a dose-dependent reduction in blood pressure, and malignant hyperthermia has been reported. In laboratory animals, sevoflurane showed embryofetal toxicity.

CONNECTIONS: APPLIED CLINICAL JUDGMENT

Patients Receiving General Anesthesia

Key Assessment Data

- History of current condition, baseline vital signs, height and weight, physical exam; history of cardiovascular, respiratory, hepatic, renal, or neurologic disease, pregnancy, or breastfeeding; medications and allergy, and testing appropriate to the procedure (e.g., MRI or CT scan results).
- Note previous history of anesthesia and note any significant reactions. Obtain family history of anesthesia problems, particularly related to use of neuromuscular blockers (e.g., succinylcholine), or any unusual effects related to surgery.
- Note time and type of last oral intake.
- Ongoing assessment during anesthesia includes level of consciousness; vital signs, especially BP and pulse; urine output; and laboratory or pathology results as appropriate to the procedure.

Desired Therapeutic Outcomes

Drug effect is observed and measurable in a diminished level of consciousness appropriate to the type and duration of the procedure, absent of adverse drug effects (e.g., bradycardia, hypotension).

(continued)

CONNECTIONS: APPLIED CLINICAL JUDGMENT *(continued)*

Patients Receiving General Anesthesia

Minimizing Adverse Effects

- CNS depression will cause decreases in all vital signs but significant bradycardia, hypotension, decreased respiratory rate, or dyspnea should be reported promptly. Immediately report any jaw muscle rigidity or brown-colored urine and fever, which may indicate malignant hyperthermia.
- General anesthetics do not necessarily provide analgesia, dependent on the drug used. Assess for nonverbal signs of pain such as restlessness or grimacing as the patient regains consciousness. Provide adequate pain relief in the postoperative period.
- Begin passive and active range-of-motion exercises in the postoperative period to reduce the risk of venous thrombosis and complications.
- Begin deep-breathing exercises and early ambulation to clear inhaled anesthetic from the lungs.
- During the period of anesthesia, consciousness is lost along with the ability to orient to day, time, and person. Confusion related to these effects in the postoperative period is common. Use of safety measures such as side rails may be necessary until the patient regains consciousness and reorient the patient frequently.
- General anesthetics depress the CNS and some autonomic activity. As autonomic activity returns, shivering is common. Provide warm blankets for comfort during this period.
- During recovery from neurolept analgesia drugs such as ketamine, confusion and misinterpretation of sensory stimulation may cause extreme anxiety, fear, or paranoia. Keep all stimuli to a minimum until the patient regains full consciousness.

Lifespan Considerations

- The older adult is more sensitive to the effects of anesthesia and may be more likely to experience adverse effects such as hypotension and delirium.
- Normal physiologic changes related to aging may increase the risk of toxicity in the older adult requiring drugs with hepatic metabolism. Monitor hepatic function pre- and postoperatively.
- For pediatric patients, allow the parents or caregiver to stay with the child as long as agency policy permits to decrease patient anxiety. Provide a simple explanation of the procedure appropriate for the age of the child.
- When working with older adults, note assistive devices (e.g., glasses, hearing aids) and remove only when necessary. Give to the family or caregiver or provide for safekeeping. Ensure that devices are available in the postoperative period.

Diversity Considerations

- Drugs such as fentanyl and midazolam are metabolized through the CYP450 system. Monitor for less than optimal results and adverse effects.

Patient and Caregiver Education

- Reinforce preoperative teaching, including deep-breathing exercises. Provide the family or caregiver with information on the anticipated length of the procedure, the waiting-room area, and cafeteria or food availability.
- Immediately report any fever, jaw muscle rigidity, or brown-colored urine to the provider.

Prescribing Considerations

- For patients with hepatic or renal insufficiency, anesthesia may precipitate acute failure.

Local Anesthetics

Classification of Local Anesthetics

26.9 Local anesthetic agents block pain transmission in peripheral nerves and are grouped in two major classes.

Local anesthesia results in the loss of sensation to a small, limited area of the body. The primary advantage of local anesthesia is that pain relief can be provided without causing generalized depression of the CNS and respiratory systems. The nausea and vomiting, tremors, and anxiety associated with general anesthetic recovery are avoided. The types of adverse events associated with local anesthesia are relatively minor relative to the potential risks of general anesthesia.

Several techniques are used to deliver local and regional anesthesia. The method employed is dependent on the location and extent of the desired anesthesia (Figure 26.1):

- *Topical (surface) anesthesia.* The drug is applied or sprayed directly on the surface of the skin or mucous membrane. The anesthesia does not penetrate into deeper skin layers. This is used to provide relief for minor skin irritations or prior to needlesticks.
- *Nerve block.* The drug is injected surrounding a peripheral nerve and all regions innervated by the nerve lose sensation. This is used for dental procedures or for regional anesthesia.
- *Infiltration anesthesia.* The drug is injected into deeper skin layers and travels to surrounding regions. This provides pain relief during minor skin surgeries or dental procedures or prior to deep needlesticks.
- *Spinal anesthesia.* The drug is injected into the cerebrospinal fluid, usually in the lumbar region. This procedure is used to block sensation to larger areas of the lower abdomen or pelvis.
- *Epidural anesthesia.* The drug is injected into the epidural space surrounding the spinal cord. The anesthetic blocks sensation to multiple nerve roots supplying limited regions of the chest, pelvis, abdomen, or limbs. It is used for urologic and obstetric procedures.

Although safer than general anesthetics, the healthcare provider has less control over the onset and duration of drug action with local anesthetics. The onset of local anesthesia is dependent on the drug's ability to diffuse from the application site to the surrounding nerves. In general, local anesthetics are small, lipid-soluble molecules that can move quickly through tissues and spaces to enter neurons. Local anesthetics are nonselective; they will block transmission at all types of sensory nerves. The sense of sharp pain is usually affected first, followed by other senses such as warmth,

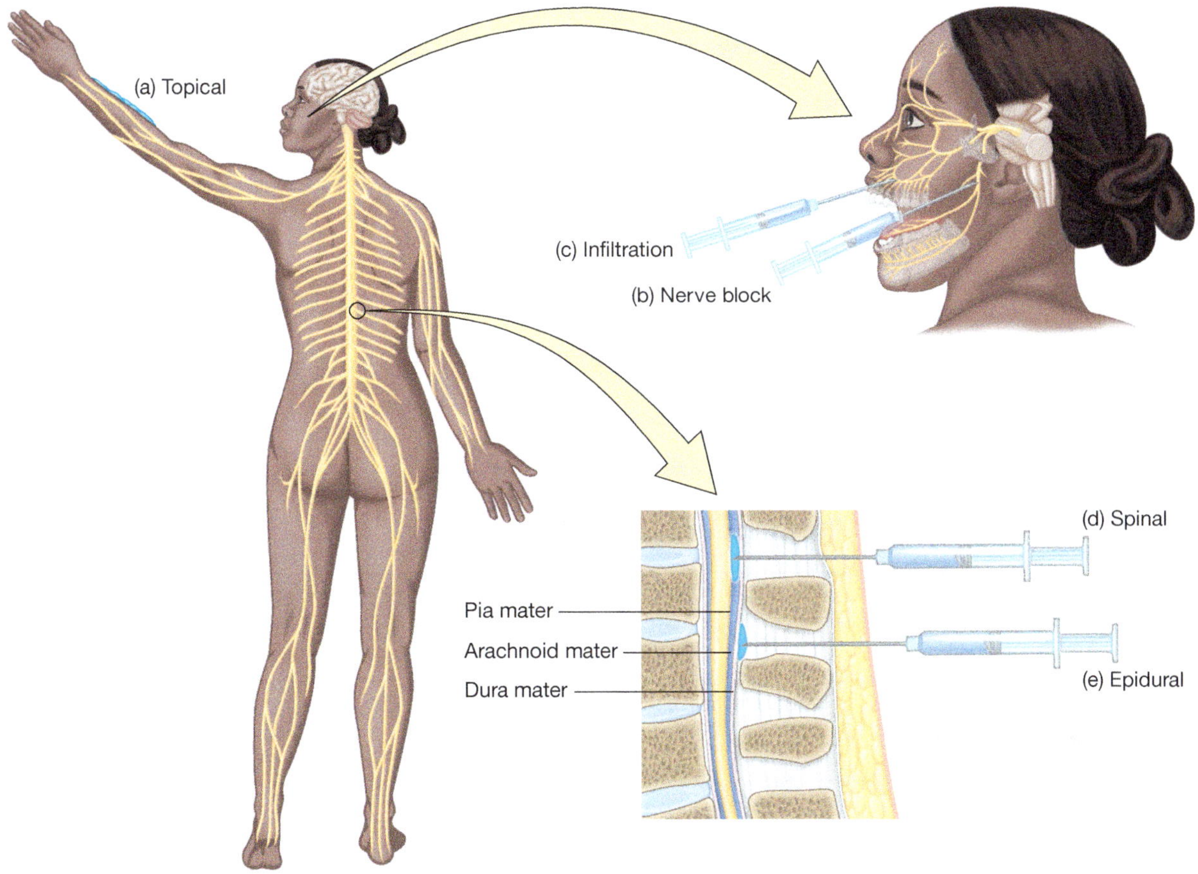

Figure 26.1 Techniques for applying local anesthesia: (a) topical, (b) nerve block, (c) infiltration, (d) spinal, (e) epidural.

cold, touch, and pressure. Motor fibers are also affected by local anesthetics.

Termination of local anesthetic action depends on blood flow to the region. Local blood vessels carry the drug away from the application site to the systemic circulation, where it is metabolized and excreted. Usually only minimal systemic effects are observed because absorption into the general circulation is slow and the drug is sufficiently diluted by the blood.

The duration of anesthetic action may be extended by injecting a vasoconstrictor such as epinephrine in combination with the local anesthetic. The epinephrine reduces blood flow to the region and slows absorption of the anesthetic. This not only extends the duration of anesthesia, it also prevents the anesthetic from reaching the circulation too quickly, which could result in systemic toxicity. The amount of epinephrine used in local anesthesia is very small and it is released very slowly into the systemic circulation; therefore, adverse effects from the epinephrine are rare.

The two major classes of local anesthetics are named by their chemical structures: esters and the amides. The two classes differ primarily by their incidence of allergic reactions, with the amide type having the lower incidence. Although they vary in time of onset and duration of action,

CONNECTIONS: Lifespan Considerations

Postoperative Delirium in the Older Adult

Postoperative delirium (POD) has been noted after surgery in the older adult population. Symptoms include transient confusion and declines in cognitive skills such as word recall, word learning, and memory. Adults with a higher risk include those over the age of 70, those with a history of dementia or cognitive dysfunction, and those with a history of alcohol abuse or use of preoperative opioids (Murthy et al., 2015). It has also been noted that emergence delirium, delirium that occurs as a patient comes out of anesthesia, is associated with a higher risk of developing POD (Zhang et al., 2020). Risk factors for emergence delirium are similar to that for POD and include old age, preexisting conditions, substance misuse, and cognitive impairment.

The American Geriatrics Society and the American College of Surgeons have published best practice guidelines for managing the perioperative course of older adults (American Geriatrics Society Expert Panel on Perioperative Delirium in Older Adults, 2015; Mohanty et al., 2016). To reduce the risk of postoperative delirium, it is recommended that benzodiazepines, meperidine, and drugs with anticholinergic side effects such as antihistamines (H_1 blockers) be avoided.

Table 26.4 Local Anesthetics

Drug	Route and Adult Dose (Maximum Dose Where Indicated)	Adverse Effects
Ester Type		
benzocaine (Americaine, Anbesol, others)	Topical: 5–8% spray, cream, ointment 20% spray, ointment, gel, liquid, otic solution	**Topical applications:** *Erythema, dermatitis, burning* Anaphylaxis **Infiltration, nerve block, epidural applications:** *Postspinal headache, sedation, paresthesia, blurred vision, urinary retention* Myocardial depression, anaphylactic reactions, cardiac arrest, respiratory arrest, seizures, fetal bradycardia
chloroprocaine (Nesacaine)	Infiltration and nerve block: 1–2% solution (max: 800 mg without epinephrine, 1 g with epinephrine) Caudal and epidural block: 2–3% solution (max: 800 mg without epinephrine, 1 g with epinephrine)	
procaine	Spinal: 10% solution diluted in normal saline at 1 mL/5 sec subcutaneous Infiltration or peripheral nerve block: 0.25–0.5% solution subcutaneous	
tetracaine	Ophthalmic: 1–2 drops of 0.5% into affected eye Spinal: 1% solution diluted with dextrose injected in the subarachnoid space	
Amide Type		
articaine (Orabloc, Septocaine)	Infiltration: 0.5–2.5 mL (20–100 mg) Nerve block: 0.5–3.4 mL (20–136 mg) Oral surgery: 1–5.1 mL (40–204 mg)	**Topical applications:** *Erythema, dermatitis, burning* **Infiltration, nerve block, epidural applications:** *Hypersensitivity, dizziness, drowsiness, urinary retention, fecal incontinence, slowing of labor, numbness of lips or tongue, hypotension, blurred or double vision* Laryngeal edema, bradycardia, anaphylactoid reaction, respiratory arrest, seizures, rectal bleeding (dibucaine)
bupivacaine (Exparel, Marcaine, Sensorcaine)	Local infiltration, sympathetic block: 0.25% solution Epidural, caudal, or retrobulbar block: 0.25–0.75% solutions Liposomal (Exparel): 8–20 mL of 1.3% solution	
dibucaine (Nupercainal)	Topical: Apply to skin 1 oz q24h	
lidocaine (Xylocaine, Zingo, others)	Infiltration: 0.5–1% solution Nerve block or epidural: 1–2% solution Caudal: 1–1.5% solution Spinal: 5% solution with dextrose Topical: 2.5–5% jelly, ointment, cream, or solution	
mepivacaine (Carbocaine, Polocaine)	Subcutaneous: 1–5 cartridges, each containing approximately 1.8 mL (54 mg) of a 3% solution	
prilocaine (Citanest Forte Dental)	Infiltration: 1–2 mL (40–80 mg) of 4% solution for local dental anesthesia	
ropivacaine (Naropin)	Surgical anesthesia: Intrathecal administration: Epidural or nerve block: 5–250 mg (0.5–1% solution) Labor pain: 20–40 mg (0.2% solution) Postoperative pain management: Epidural: 12–20 mg/h (0.2% solution) Infiltration: 2–200 mg (0.2–0.5% solution)	

Note: *Italics* indicate common adverse effects. Underline indicates serious adverse effects.

most local anesthetics have equivalent effectiveness. The local anesthetics are listed in Table 26.4.

Ester-Type Anesthetics

26.10 Ester-type local anesthetics have been widely used for topical and spinal anesthesia.

Cocaine was the first local anesthetic to be widely used for medical procedures. Cocaine is a natural ester found in the leaves of *Erythroxylum coca*, a plant native to the Andes Mountains in Peru. Cocaine was discovered by a German chemist in 1855 and ultimately used in 1884 as a topical eye anesthetic. Although still approved by the FDA as a local anesthetic, cocaine is a Schedule II controlled substance and is rarely used because of its high potential for abuse. In 1904 a German chemist named Einhorn discovered procaine, which soon came into widespread use, especially in dental offices.

Esters act by decreasing the amount of sodium that enters the neuron, thereby depressing depolarization and preventing conduction of the pain impulse. Esters may be administered with epinephrine as a vasoconstrictor to limit blood loss at the surgical site and to decrease the amount of anesthetic absorbed systemically. The local anesthetic effect of an ester is rapid, occurring in 1 to 8 minutes. The duration ranges from 15 to 60 minutes.

Ester-type anesthetics are generally safe when applied as directed. All can cause serious CNS and cardiac toxicity, however, if they reach the blood in high concentrations. The first CNS symptoms may be stimulatory: anxiety, nervousness, dizziness, tremor, or seizures. Subsequent CNS depression may cause the patient to become drowsy, experience respiratory depression, and enter a coma. High amounts can cause dysrhythmias, QT prolongation, hypotension, and cardiac arrest. Care must be taken that the drug is administered correctly to prevent serious adverse effects.

PROTOTYPE DRUG Procaine

Classification **Therapeutic:** Local anesthetic
Pharmacologic: Ester, sodium channel blocker

Therapeutic Effects and Uses: Procaine is used for spinal, epidural, and peripheral nerve blocks through injection or infiltration. It produces local anesthesia with loss of sensation close to the injection or application site. It has a short duration of action. An off-label use is for the treatment of severe pain due to cancer, herpes, or burns. Once used widely in dentistry, it has largely been replaced by other local anesthetics. Procaine was widely known as Novocain, its trade name, but this proprietary product is no longer available.

Procaine causes vasodilation, which could potentially increase its rate of absorption from tissues and cause systemic toxicity. Some procaine solutions contain small amounts of epinephrine, which constricts arteries to keep the procaine localized and prolong the anesthetic effect. The drug is rapidly metabolized to inactive metabolites by esterase, an enzyme found in the plasma. Once it reaches the plasma, the half-life of procaine is only 40 seconds.

Mechanism of Action: Procaine decreases the influx of sodium into the neuron, which increases the threshold for depolarization and prevents the conduction of the nerve impulse.

Pharmacokinetics:

Route(s)	Subcutaneous
Absorption	Rapid
Distribution	Not distributed; highly bound to plasma proteins
Primary metabolism	Metabolized by plasma esterase
Primary excretion	Renal: 80% as metabolites
Onset of action	2–5 min
Duration of action	1 h

Adverse Effects: With therapeutic doses, adverse effects are rare. Adverse events may occur, however, if multiple doses of procaine are administered or if it is injected intravascularly. The most severe adverse effects include respiratory arrest and anaphylaxis. A patient who has experienced an allergic reaction to procaine will likely be allergic to other esters. Myocardial depression may result in atrioventricular (AV) block dysrhythmias or cardiac arrest. CNS effects are stimulatory and usually transient; nervousness, dizziness, confusion, and tremor may occur. Spinal anesthesia with procaine can cause headache, palsies, spinal nerve paralysis, and meningism (nuchal rigidity, photophobia, and headache). Cutaneous lesions can occur in a delayed time frame. The caudal or epidural administration of procaine in the obstetric patient can result in urinary incontinence, loss of perineal sensation, slowing of labor, and increased incidence of forceps delivery.

Contraindications/Precautions: Patients who have experienced hypersensitivity to any ester anesthetic or agent containing para-aminobenzoic acid (PABA) should not receive procaine. Patients with generalized septicemia, inflammation, or sepsis should not be injected with procaine. It is also contraindicated in patients with heart block, hypotension, HTN, or altered coagulation. It should be used cautiously in older and acutely ill patients. Patients who have increased abdominal pressure should be administered procaine cautiously.

Drug Interactions: Ester anesthetics such as procaine may antagonize the antimicrobial effects of sulfonamides. Risk of hypotension increases when administered with antihypertensives. Procaine is incompatible with aminophylline, chlorothiazide, magnesium sulfate, phenobarbital, phenytoin, secobarbital, and sodium bicarbonate. **Herbal/Food:** Unknown.

Pregnancy: Animal studies have not been conducted to determine the effects of procaine during pregnancy or lactation. The potential adverse effects on the fetus likely depend on the procedure performed and the amount of drug used.

Treatment of Overdose: The effects of procaine overdosage are treated symptomatically. Rapid systemic absorption will affect the cardiovascular system and could require cardiopulmonary resuscitation.

Clinician Responsibilities: Key clinical implications for patients receiving procaine are included in Applied Clinical Judgment: Patients Receiving Local Anesthesia.

Drugs Similar to Procaine

Other local anesthetic esters include benzocaine, chloroprocaine, and tetracaine.

Benzocaine (Americaine, Anbesol, others): Approved in 1938, benzocaine is an over-the-counter (OTC) local anesthetic ester applied topically as a lotion, cream, ointment, spray, gel, or otic solution. Chemically it is almost identical to procaine, but it has a prolonged duration of anesthetic action. It provides temporary relief of pain and discomfort due to sunburn, minor wounds, pruritus, serous otitis media, swimmer's ear, otitis externa, canker sores, sore throat, hemorrhoids, and anal fissures. It can be applied to the penis as a male desensitizer to slow the onset of ejaculation. Benzocaine preparations are commonly used as an anesthetic for the passage of catheters and endoscopic tubes. Onset of anesthetic action occurs in less than a minute, and because absorption of benzocaine is minimal, systemic effects are rare. Contact dermatitis can occur and is more common with benzocaine than with some of the other topical anesthetics. Although rare, benzocaine sprays have been associated with serious methemoglobinemia, a condition in which hemoglobin is unable to bind sufficient oxygen. Animal studies have not been conducted to determine the effects of benzocaine during pregnancy or lactation. It is unlikely that topical benzocaine would have any adverse effects during pregnancy or lactation.

Chloroprocaine (Nesacaine): Approved in 1957, chloroprocaine is a short-acting local anesthetic ester that is used for infiltration, epidural, and caudal anesthesia. It is not effective as a topical agent. Anesthesia occurs in 6 to 12 minutes and can last up to 90 minutes if epinephrine is added to the injection. A test dose is given before epidural use to assess for intravascular or subarachnoid injection. In the event of intravascular injection, the patient would experience an epinephrine response with tachycardia, circumoral pallor, palpitations, and nervousness. Signs of subarachnoid injection include motor paralysis and extensive sensory anesthesia. Like other ester anesthetics, allergic reactions such as rash, pruritus, and anaphylaxis are possible. Animal studies have not been conducted to determine the effects of chloroprocaine during pregnancy or lactation. The potential adverse effects on the fetus likely depend on the procedure performed and the amount of drug used.

Tetracaine (Pontocaine): Tetracaine is a local anesthetic ester that is used in spinal anesthesia and topically to anesthetize the conjunctiva during eye surgery. Tetracaine and lidocaine are combined as a transdermal patch (Synera) or cream (Pliaglis) to provide local anesthesia for superficial dermatological procedures. An intranasal form (Kovanaze) combines tetracaine with oxymetazoline for dental anesthesia. It is administered on the skin to relieve pruritus, pain, and burning. Onset of action is rapid for topical use (3–10 minutes) but longer following spinal administration (15 minutes). Of the topical anesthetics, tetracaine is the most likely to cause skin sensitivity, including rash, erythema, pruritus, burning, and edema. Systemic absorption can cause significant CNS and cardiac toxicity. Tetracaine is contraindicated in patients who are hypersensitive to ester-type anesthetics, sulfites, or PABA. Animal studies showed no evidence of fetal harm. It is not known if tetracaine is secreted in milk or if it affects the breastfed neonate.

Amide-Type Anesthetics

26.11 Local anesthetics from the amide class have a lower incidence of adverse effects than those from the ester class.

Amide-type local anesthetics have largely replaced the administration of drugs from the ester class. The amides produce less effect on myocardial contractility, and the incidence of allergic reactions is lower. Amides and esters have the same mechanism of action: decreasing the sodium flux into the neuron, thus inhibiting the initial depolarization and conduction of the nerve impulse. Whereas the esters are inactivated by the enzyme esterase in the plasma, the amides are metabolized by hepatic CYP450 enzymes. Caution should be exercised when administering large amounts of amide anesthetics to patients with hepatic impairment.

PROTOTYPE DRUG **Lidocaine (Xylocaine, Zingo, Others)**

Classification **Therapeutic:** Local anesthetic
Pharmacologic: Amide, sodium channel blocker

Therapeutic Effects and Uses: Lidocaine is a local anesthetic that has a prompt onset of action of 2 to 5 minutes. It has a longer duration of action than procaine, lasting 10 to 90 minutes, depending on its route of administration. It may be administered as a surface and infiltration anesthetic agent to block the nerve. It is also used in caudal and spinal block anesthesia to relieve local discomfort of the skin and mucous membranes. Lidocaine patches are administered to relieve pain related to post-herpetic neuralgia (Lidoderm) or dental procedures (DentiPatch). Parenteral lidocaine is administered to treat life-threatening ventricular dysrhythmias (see Chapter 37). Zingo (lidocaine hydrochloride monohydrate) is a needle-free intradermal injection system. Zingo is indicated for rapid local anesthesia for procedures such as IV insertions or blood draws.

Mechanism of Action: Lidocaine blocks the conduction of action potentials by reducing the sodium permeability, thus decreasing the action potential and slowing nerve conduction.

Pharmacokinetics:

Route(s)	Subcutaneous, IM, IV, IV bolus; topical
Absorption	Topical absorption: 3% through intact skin
Distribution	Crosses the blood–brain barrier and the placenta; secreted in breast milk
Primary metabolism	Hepatic via CYP3A4 and 2D6

Primary excretion	Renal
Onset of action	IV: 45–90 sec; IM: 5–15 min; topical: 2–5 min
Duration of action	IV: 10–20 min; IM: 60–90 min; topical: 30–60 min Half-life: 1.5–2 h

Adverse Effects: When used topically, adverse reactions to lidocaine are uncommon. Mild and transient reactions at the site of application include erythema, pruritus, dermatitis, and burning. The transoral DentiPatch may cause alterations in taste, headache, and gingivitis. Should the drug be unintentionally injected intravascularly, CNS adverse effects will be those of stimulation (anxiety, tremors, shivering, and seizures) followed by depression (drowsiness, respiratory depression, and coma). Cardiovascular effects include hypotension, dysrhythmias, cardiovascular collapse, and cardiac arrest. **Black Box Warning:** Significant systemic absorption may occur with topical use.

Contraindications/Precautions: Patients who have experienced a hypersensitivity reaction to amide-type local anesthetics should not be administered lidocaine. Topical lidocaine should not be applied to skin seriously damaged by trauma, burns, or eczema.

Other precautions apply to patients receiving parenteral lidocaine, although these also apply to situations in which the drug is unintentionally injected intravascularly. Patients who have been diagnosed with Stokes–Adams syndrome, untreated sinus bradycardia, or sinoatrial, AV, or intraventricular heart block should not be administered lidocaine. The medication should be used cautiously in the presence of liver or kidney disease, myasthenia gravis, and hypovolemia as well as in debilitated patients and older patients or when there is a family history of malignant hyperthermia.

Drug Interactions: Lidocaine patches can cause toxic effects with tocainide and mexiletine. Barbiturates decrease lidocaine activity. Increased pharmacologic effects of lidocaine will be noted if it is administered with cimetidine, beta blockers, or quinidine. **Herbal/Food:** After receiving transoral lidocaine, patients should not eat or drink until the effects of the anesthesia have worn off.

Pregnancy: Animal studies showed no evidence of fetal harm. It is not known if lidocaine is secreted in milk or if it affects the breastfed neonate. It is unlikely that topical lidocaine would have any adverse effects during pregnancy or lactation. Studies have shown that the second trimester is the safest time for dental procedures during pregnancy. Small anounts of lidocaine enter breast milk but is not expected to cause any adverse affects in the breastfed neonate.

Treatment of Overdose: Overdose may occur if the drug is injected intravascularly. The patient is treated through symptom management.

Clinician Responsibilities: Key clinical implications for patients receiving lidocaine are included in Applied Clinical Judgment: Patients Receiving Local Anesthesia.

Drugs Similar to Lidocaine (Xylocaine, Zingo, Others)

Other local anesthetic amides include articaine, bupivacaine, dibucaine, mepivacaine, prilocaine, and ropivacaine.

Articaine (Orabloc, Septocaine): Approved in 2000, articaine is approved for administration by infiltration or by nerve block for dental procedures. It is unique because it has both an amide and an ester group. Anesthesia is rapid, occurring in 1 to 6 minutes, and lasts up to an hour. Articaine appears to diffuse through soft tissue and bone better than other local anesthetics. It is always combined with epinephrine, which provides vasoconstriction and prolongs the duration of action. The adverse effects are the same as those of other amide anesthetics. Animal reproduction studies showed that articaine may cause fetal harm. It is not known if this drug is secreted in milk or if it affects the breastfed neonate. Articaine should be used during pregnancy or lactation only if the potential benefit to the mother justifies the potential risk to the fetus or neonate.

Bupivacaine (Exparel, Marcaine, Sensorcaine): Approved in 1972, bupivacaine is an amide local anesthetic that is used for infiltration anesthesia, peripheral sympathetic nerve block, and epidural block. Bupivacaine in dextrose solution is administered for spinal anesthesia. Its 3- to 9-hour duration of action is one of the longest of any local anesthetic. A liposomal form (Exparel) provides analgesia for up to 72 hours. The anesthetic is injected into the surgical area for procedures such as bunionectomy and hemorrhoidectomy. In 2020 a surgical implant of bupivacaine (Xaracoll) was approved. Xaracoll is a collagen-based, resorbable implant that is inserted at the site of surgical repair of hernias, to give immediate pain relief and reduce the need for systemic opioids. Adverse effects of bupivacaine are similar to those of other amide anesthetics. Animal reproduction studies showed that bupivacaine may cause fetal harm. This drug is secreted in milk and has the potential to cause adverse effects on the breastfed neonate. Bupivacaine should be used during pregnancy or lactation only if the potential benefit to the mother justifies the potential risk to the fetus or neonate.

Dibucaine (Nupercainal): Approved in 1947, dibucaine is administered OTC to relieve pain and itching related to hemorrhoids and other anorectal disorders. It is also administered to relieve discomfort from insect bites, sunburn, minor burns, cuts, and scratches. It is a long-acting amide anesthetic that inhibits the initiation and conduction of nerve impulses by reducing the permeability of nerve cells to sodium ions. It is unlikely that topical dibucaine causes adverse effects during pregnancy or lactation.

Mepivacaine (Carbocaine, Polocaine): Approved in 1960, mepivacaine is an amide anesthetic used for infiltration, transtracheal anesthesia, and epidural nerve blocks in surgical and dental procedures. Onset of action is very rapid—less than a minute for the upper and lower jaws. Epidural onset is 7 to 15 minutes. This drug has an intermediate duration of action of 60 to 100 minutes for soft tissue and 115 to 150 minutes for epidural. Mepivacaine is sometimes combined with levonordefrin, a vasoconstrictor that prolongs the duration of action of the local anesthetic. The adverse effects are the same as those of other amide anesthetics. Animal studies have not been conducted to determine the effects of mepivacaine during pregnancy or lactation. This drug should be used during pregnancy or lactation only if the potential benefit to the mother justifies the potential risk to the fetus or neonate.

Prilocaine (Citanest Forte Dental): Approved in 1965, prilocaine is used for dental anesthesia via infiltration. Onset of action is 2 minutes and its duration is 1 to 2 hours. The adverse effects are the same as those of other amide anesthetics. Animal studies showed no evidence of fetal harm. It is not known if prilocaine is secreted in milk or if it affects the breastfed neonate.

Ropivacaine (Naropin): Ropivacaine is a local anesthetic agent approved in 1996 that is used in epidural anesthesia and postoperative pain management. It has an onset of action of 1 to 30 minutes and a duration of anesthetic action of 2 to 6 hours. It is important that disinfecting agents with heavy metal content not be used to disinfect the skin prior to the insertion of the epidural catheter because these have been associated with swelling and edema. Also, the container of ropivacaine should not be cleaned with a heavy metal disinfecting agent. Unlike most local anesthetics, the presence of epinephrine does not affect the systemic absorption of ropivacaine. Like other amide anesthetics, high serum concentrations may cause serious CNS and cardiac toxicity; care must be taken not to inject the drug intravascularly or intrathecally. Animal studies showed no evidence of fetal harm. It is not known if prilocaine is secreted in milk or if it affects the breastfed neonate.

Adjuncts to Anesthesia

26.12 Adjunctive agents are used during the perioperative phase to enhance anesthesia or to treat the potential adverse effects of anesthetics.

Surgery is often a stressful and painful procedure for patients. In addition, anesthetics dampen vital reflexes, which can lead to aspiration pneumonia. Diminished autonomic function can have serious adverse effects on the cardiovascular and gastrointestinal (GI) systems. Adjunctive medications are those used to enhance anesthesia or to make the procedure safer and less unpleasant for patients.

Preoperative medications. The most common preoperative symptom is anxiety. Oral benzodiazepines may be given for several days prior to a major procedure to lessen anxiety. Just prior to surgery, midazolam may be administered parenterally to sedate the patient and to cause perioperative amnesia (see Section 26.5).

Aspiration pneumonia is a potentially serious problem during a surgical procedure because the patient may lose protective airway reflexes. Histamine (H_2) receptor antagonists such as famotidine (Pepcid) can reduce the possibility of aspiration pneumonia by decreasing gastric fluid volume and reducing acidity. For aspiration prophylaxis, the H_2 receptor antagonist may be given PO the night prior to surgery and by IV infusion an hour before the procedure. A drug prototype feature for ranitidine is found in Chapter 59.

Anticholinergics such as atropine may be administered prior to surgery to reduce salivary and airway secretions. Atropine also blocks the bradycardia caused by some anesthetics. The drug is given by the IM route 45 to 60 minutes prior to anesthesia. A prototype feature for atropine is presented in Chapter 14.

Pain management. Pain reduction is an important component of preanesthesia and postanesthesia care. Opioids are used when the pain is expected to be severe, but these drugs can cause significant respiratory depression. If the pain level is moderate or mild, nonsteroidal anti-inflammatory drugs (NSAIDs) are administered because they cause fewer serious adverse reactions than the opioids. Clonidine (Catapres, Duraclon) is a centrally acting alpha$_2$-adrenergic agonist that has been used to reduce severe pain associated with surgery. When administered epidurally Duraclon allows the dosages of the anesthetic and opioids to be reduced. The primary indication of clonidine is HTN (Catapres), but it has largely been replaced by safer antihypertensives (see Chapter 34).

Neuromuscular blockers. Skeletal muscle relaxation is an important component of general anesthesia. Insertion of an endotracheal tube would be difficult and painful without muscle relaxation, and contraction or spasticity of muscles during a surgical procedure could render some operations impossible. Complete paralysis of muscle is necessary for major surgical procedures. Although some of the general anesthetics do have mild to moderate ability to relax skeletal muscles, most are incapable of causing the degree of relaxation necessary for surgery.

It is important to note that neuromuscular blockers do not enter the CNS. Although these drugs cause muscle paralysis, they do not induce unconsciousness or provide analgesia. The patient is still able to feel pain and is aware of his or her surroundings.

Nondepolarizing neuromuscular blocking agents such as atracurium and cisatracurium (Nimbex) bind competitively with acetylcholine to produce skeletal muscle relaxation that lasts 30 to 45 minutes. The depolarizing neuromuscular blocking agent succinylcholine (Anectine, Quelicin) produces muscular paralysis in less than a minute when given IV, but its effects only last 2 to 3 minutes after the infusion is stopped.

The neuromuscular blocking agents are very dangerous; the diaphragm and intercostal muscles are paralyzed and breathing requires a mechanical ventilator. Serious cardiovascular adverse effects are possible. Details of the actions, indications, and adverse effects of the neuromuscular blockers are included in Chapter 14. A prototype feature for succinylcholine is also included in that chapter.

Postoperative medications. Because many anesthetics induce severe nausea and vomiting in the postanesthesia phase, the administration of antiemetic drugs is indicated for prophylaxis in high-risk patients or for treatment. Several drugs have been used as antiemetics. Promethazine is an older antiemetic that may be administered pre- or postoperatively. It has the advantage of also being a sedative; thus, it can be used in the induction phase of anesthesia. Also an older medication, metoclopramide (Reglan) may be administered near the end of the surgical procedure for prophylaxis of postanesthetic nausea and vomiting. A newer and very effective antiemetic is ondansetron (Zofran), a 5-HT_3 antagonist. Commonly used to prevent the acute nausea and vomiting caused by cancer chemotherapeutic agents, ondansetron may be injected just prior to chemotherapy or 30 minutes before the end of the surgical procedure.

CONNECTION Checkpoint 26.3

Atropine and succinylcholine are both cholinergic blockers, but they produce very different effects. From what you learned in Chapter 14, explain the mechanisms for the differences in pharmacologic actions. (*Hint:* One drug affects the muscarinic receptor and the other the nicotinic receptor.)

CONNECTIONS: APPLIED CLINICAL JUDGMENT

Patients Receiving Local Anesthesia

Key Assessment Data

- History of current condition, baseline vital signs, height and weight, physical exam; history of cardiovascular, respiratory, hepatic, renal, or neurologic disease, pregnancy, or breastfeeding; medications and allergy, especially to "caine" drugs.
- Assess for areas of broken skin, abrasions, burns, or other wounds in the area to be treated with a local anesthetic.
- Ongoing assessment during anesthesia includes level of consciousness and vital signs, especially BP and pulse, if a large regional block is used.
- Assess the local or regional area blocked; expect blanching in the localized area if the local anesthetic contained epinephrine. If a regional area was blocked, periodically assess the patient's ability to move limbs distal to the block.

Desired Therapeutic Outcomes

Drug effect is observed and measurable in diminished or absent sensation in the area under anesthesia.

Minimizing Adverse Effects

- Adverse effects of local anesthesia are rare. Regional blocks may cause hypotension with the possibility of reflex tachycardia. Bradycardia, hypotension, decreased level of consciousness, decreased respiratory rate, and dyspnea may signal that the anesthesia has entered the systemic circulation and is acting as a general anesthetic. Report blood pressure below 90/60 mmHg or per the parameters as ordered by the healthcare provider, tachycardia, bradycardia, changes in level of consciousness, dyspnea, or decrease in respiratory rate immediately.
- Duration of anesthetic action will depend on the solution used and whether it contains epinephrine. If a large regional area is blocked (e.g., epidural), the patient may regain some motor ability before sensation returns and the return of motor activity signals decreasing levels of anesthesia. Epinephrine in the anesthetic solution will constrict localized blood vessels and result in blanching of the area. Assess the localized area for numbness and blanching if the local anesthetic included epinephrine. Assess the patient's ability to move limbs distal to the regional anesthetic.
- Local anesthetics are effective for up to 3 h or more. Biting injuries to oral mucous membranes may occur while tissue is numb. Aspiration of food or liquids is possible until swallowing sensation and gag reflex return. If throat anesthesia is used, assess gag reflex before eating.
- Large open or denuded areas may increase the amount of drug absorption into the general circulation. Use sterile technique to apply the drug to open areas. Assess areas of abrasion, burns, or open wounds if a local anesthetic is applied to area.
- Pain sensation will increase as the regional block wears off. Monitor pain relief in patients post-regional block (e.g., epidural); additional pain relief may be required.
- Solutions containing epinephrine must *never* be used IV or for local anesthesia in areas of decreased circulation [e.g., fingertips, toes, earlobes, tip of nose, penile tissue] due to vasoconstrictive effects. Read all labels carefully before using parenteral solutions.

Lifespan Considerations

- The older adult is more sensitive to the effects of anesthesia and is at increased risk for hypotension due to physiologic changes related to aging or concurrent vasoactive drug use.
- Numbness or effects on motor ability postregional anesthetic may impair movement and increase the risk of falls or injuries. Be particularly cautious with older adults who are at increased risk for falls.

Diversity Considerations

- Amide anesthetics such as lidocaine are metabolized through the CYP450 system and may result in less than optimal results based on differences in enzymes. Continue to monitor hepatic function and drug effects.

(continued)

CONNECTIONS: APPLIED CLINICAL JUDGMENT *(continued)*

Patients Receiving Local Anesthesia

Patient and Caregiver Education

- It is normal that a slight pressure sensation may remain during anesthesia (e.g., sensation of "tugging" during suturing) but that no pain should be felt. Alert the healthcare provider if more than slight pressure sensation or any pain is noticed during anesthesia.
- The anesthetized area may be numb for several hours after the procedure is completed and it is normal to regain some ability to move limbs (e.g., after epidural anesthetic); movement may return before the ability to feel the movement.
- Report any increasing nausea, drowsiness, dizziness, lightheadedness, confusion, or anxiety immediately. If dizziness occurs, the patient should sit or lie down and not attempt to stand or walk until the sensation passes.
- Refrain from eating or drinking for 1 h or more postanesthesia, or until sensation has completely returned to the oral cavity or throat.
- Call for assistance prior to getting out of bed or attempting to walk alone post–epidural block and to avoid driving or other activities requiring physical coordination (e.g., regional upper limb block) until residual effects of the drug are known.
- Report increased redness, swelling, or drainage from open areas under treatment.
- Take oral medication (e.g., lidocaine viscous) by swishing and spitting if used for oral cavity, or by gargling, and do not swallow unless directed by the healthcare provider. Apply topical medication in a thin layer to the skin area as directed.

Prescribing Considerations

- Local anesthetic agents can affect the cardiovascular system, especially at higher doses.
- The use of vasoconstrictor-containing local anesthetic is not recommended for patients with HTN or existing cardiac dysrhythmia.
- For patients with known kidney function impairment, drugs metabolized by the kidneys should be avoided, if possible, or the dosage at least decreased.
- For patients with known liver function impairment, drugs metabolized by the liver should be avoided, if possible, or the dosage at least decreased.

Understanding Chapter 26

Key Concepts Summary

26.1 Anesthesia is used to produce a controlled loss of sensation during a diagnostic or surgical procedure.

26.2 Balanced anesthesia uses multiple drugs to provide for the safe induction and maintenance of general anesthesia.

26.3 Intravenous anesthetics include opioids, benzodiazepines, and several miscellaneous agents.

26.4 Opioids are used as intravenous anesthetics to provide analgesia and to accomplish neurolept anesthesia.

26.5 Benzodiazepines are used in anesthesia to produce relaxation, sedation, and amnesia.

26.6 Propofol and ketamine are widely used intravenous drugs for inducing and maintaining anesthesia.

26.7 Inhalation anesthetics used to produce loss of consciousness are classified as gases or volatile liquids.

26.8 Volatile liquid general anesthetics are used to induce and maintain deep anesthesia.

26.9 Local anesthetic agents block pain transmission in peripheral nerves and are grouped in two major classes.

26.10 Ester-type local anesthetics have been widely used for topical and spinal anesthesia.

26.11 Local anesthetics from the amide class have a lower incidence of adverse effects than those from the ester class.

26.12 Adjunctive agents are used during the perioperative phase to enhance anesthesia or to treat the potential adverse effects of anesthetics.

CASE STUDY: Making the Patient Connection

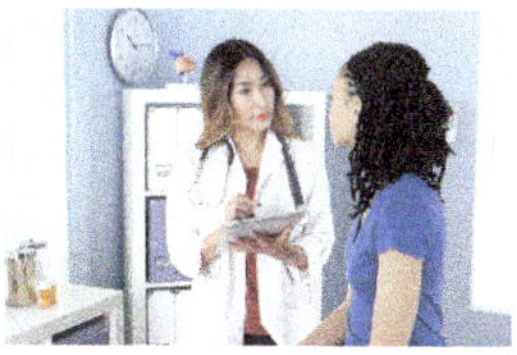

Remember the patient "Elena Moore" at the beginning of the chapter? Now read the remainder of the case study. Based on the information presented within this chapter, respond to the critical thinking questions that follow.

Elena is a 37-year-old woman who is scheduled for a vaginal hysterectomy after a positive Pap smear returned with results suggestive of cancer. While in the holding area of the operating room suite, she states that she is fearful of general anesthesia. The preoperative nurse caring for Elena notices that she is very anxious. Upon further assessment and conversation, she states that her mother died of breast cancer when she was young.

Elena's vital signs are as follows: blood pressure, 138/88 mmHg; temperature, 36.3°C (97.4°F); pulse, 94 beats/min; and respiration, 20 breaths/min. She denies pain and states that she is concerned she will wake up during the surgery. She is to receive balanced anesthesia.

Critical Thinking Questions

1. In your own words, how would you describe balanced anesthesia to Elena?
2. How does nitrous oxide differ from IV anesthetic agents?
3. How should the nurse educate a patient regarding the use of IV propofol?

Additional Case Study

Anthony Holiday is a 28-year-old steelworker for a heating and cooling company. While on the job he cut his right hand on a piece of steel from an air-conditioning vent. He is admitted to the emergency department for sutures to the right middle finger and palm. The laceration will be anesthetized with lidocaine prior to suturing.

1. What is the action of lidocaine?
2. Why is lidocaine preferred over procaine?

Chapter Review

1. The surgical nurse becomes alerted that the patient who is receiving general anesthesia has become excitable and hyperactive with irregular heart and respiratory rates. The nurse knows that the patient has entered which stage of general anesthesia?
   1. Stage 1
   2. Stage 2
   3. Stage 3
   4. Stage 4

2. The nurse should question the administration of propofol (Diprivan) for which patient? An individual with:
   1. Allergy to eggs or soy products.
   2. Allergy to iodine.
   3. Kidney disease.
   4. Addison's disease.

3. During the administration of nitrous oxide, the patient develops anxiety, excitement, and combativeness. The nurse would anticipate what change in the patient's anesthesia is needed?
   1. The nitrous oxide dose will be increased.
   2. Propofol (Diprivan) will be given along with the nitrous oxide.
   3. Succinylcholine (Anectine) will be given to the patient.
   4. The nitrous oxide dose will be decreased.

4. The nurse is providing the patient, who will be receiving ketamine (Ketalar), with preoperative instructions. Which statement, if made by the patient, indicates that teaching is successful?
   1. "The medication will decrease anxiety during surgery."
   2. "I will experience increased energy due to this drug."
   3. "I may experience a feeling of being separated from the environment."
   4. "The drug will cause me to have dry mouth after the operation."

5. The patient who is having a scalp laceration sutured will be receiving local anesthesia with lidocaine (Xylocaine) that contains epinephrine. The nurse knows that the purpose of this drug combination is to:
   1. Increase the duration of the anesthetic action.
   2. Increase vasodilation at the site of the laceration.
   3. Decrease blood pressure in individuals who are hypertensive.
   4. Ensure that infection at the wound site will not occur.

6. Identify the general anesthetic agents that are parenteral opioid agents. (Select all that apply.)
   1. Nitrous oxide
   2. Alfentanil (Alfenta)
   3. Sufentanil (Sufenta)
   4. Remifentanil (Ultiva)
   5. Succinylcholine (Anectine)

See Appendix A for answers to critical thinking questions, case study questions and review questions.

References

American Association of Nurse Anesthetists. (2019). *Education of nurse anesthetists in the United States—at a glance.* https://www.aana.com/membership/become-a-crna/education-of-nurse-anesthetists-in-the-u.s

American Geriatrics Society Expert Panel on Perioperative Delirium in Older Adults. (2015). Postoperative delirium in older adults: Best practice statement from the American Geriatrics Society. *Journal of the American College of Surgeons, 220*, 136–148. https://doi.org/10.1016/j.jamcollsurg.2014.10.019

Larach, M. G., Riazi, S., & Rosenberg, H. (2019). Dantrolene should be readily available wherever malignant hyperthermia triggering drugs are stocked. *Anesthesia and Analgesia, 129*, e175–e176. https://doi.org/10.1213/ANE.0000000000004399

Kalmoe, M. C., Janski, A. M., Zorumski, C. F., Nagele, P., Palanca, B. J., & Conway, C. R. (2020). Ketamine and nitrous oxide: The evolution of NMDA receptor antagonists as antidepressant agents. *Journal of the Neurological Sciences, 412*, 116778. https://doi.org/10.1016/j.jns.2020.116778

Mohanty, S., Rosenthal, R. A., Russell, M. M., Neuman, M. D., Ko, C. Y., & Esnaola, N. A. (2016). Optimal perioperative management of the geriatric patient: A best practices guideline from the American College of Surgeons NSQIP and the American Geriatrics Society. *Journal of the American College of Surgeons, 222*, 930–947. https://doi.org/10.1016/j.jamcollsurg.2015.12.026

Murthy, S., Hepner, D. L., Cooper, Z., Bader, A. M., & Neuman, M. D. (2015). Controversies in anaesthesia for noncardiac surgery in older adults. *British Journal of Anaesthesia, 115*(Suppl. 2), ii15–ii25. https://doi.org/10.1093/bja/aev396

Shaw, M. A., & Hopkins, P. M. (2019). Mission impossible or mission futile: Estimating penetrance for malignant hyperthermia. *Anesthesiology, 131*, 957–959. https://doi.org/10.1097/ALN.0000000000002884

Zhang, Y., He, S. T., Nie, B., Li, X. Y., & Wang, D. X. (2020). Emergence delirium is associated with increased postoperative delirium in elderly: A prospective observational study. *Journal of Anesthesia.* https://doi.org/10.1007/s00540-020-02805-8

Selected Bibliography

Adler, A. C. (2018). *General anesthesia.* Medscape. http://emedicine.medscape.com/article/1271543-overview

Alai, A. N. (2017). *Nitrous oxide administration.* Medscape. http://emedicine.medscape.com/article/1413427-overview

El-Boghdadly, K., Pawa, A., & Chin, K. J. (2018). Local anesthetic systemic toxicity: current perspectives. *Local and Regional Anesthesia, 11*, 35. https://dx.doi.org/10.2147%2FLRA.S154512

Gan, T. J., Belani, K. G., Bergese, S., Chung, F., Diemunsch, P., Habib, A. S., et al. (2020). Fourth Consensus Guidelines for the Management of Postoperative Nausea and Vomiting. Anesthesia & Analgesia, *131*(2), 411–448. https://doi.org/10.1213/ANE.0000000000004833

Kapitanyan, R. (2019). *Local anesthetic toxicity.* Medscape. http://emedicine.medscape.com/article/1844551-overview

Prabhakar, A., Lambert, T., Kaye, R. J., Gaignard, S. M., Ragusa, J., Wheat, S., et al. (2019). Adjuvants in clinical regional anesthesia practice: A comprehensive review. Best Practice & *Research Clinical Anaesthesiology, 33*(4), 415–423. https://doi.org/10.1016/j.bpa.2019.06.001

Tateosian, V. S., Champagne, K., & Gan, T. J. (2018). What is new in the battle against postoperative nausea and vomiting? *Best Practice & Research Clinical Anaesthesiology*, *32*(2), 137–148. https://doi.org/10.1016/j.bpa.2018.06.005

Tóth, B., Lantos, T., Hegyi, P., Viola, R., Vasas, A., Benkő, R., et al. (2018). Ginger (Zingiber officinale): An alternative for the prevention of postoperative nausea and vomiting. A meta-analysis. *Phytomedicine*, *50*, 8–18. https://doi.org/10.1016/j.phymed.2018.09.007

U.S. Drug Enforcement Administration. (2019). *Ketamine.* http://www.deadiversion.usdoj.gov/drug_chem_info/ketamine.pdf

Waldinger, R., Weinberg, G., & Gitman, M. (2020). Local anesthetic toxicity in the geriatric population. *Drugs & Aging*, *37*(1), 1–9. https://doi.org/10.1007/s40266-019-00718-0

Ware, M. R., Feller, D. B., & Hall, K. L. (2018). Neuroleptic malignant syndrome: Diagnosis and management. *Primary Care Companion for CNS Disorders*, *20*(1), 17r02185. https://doi.org/10.4088/pcc.17r02185

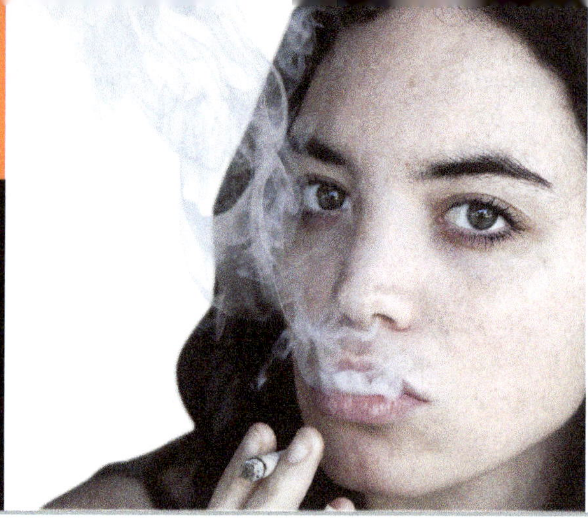

"I have been getting high
since I was 14 years old.
Do I need to stop just because
I am pregnant?"
—*Patient "Jamie Wilkins"*

Chapter 27
Pharmacology of Substance Abuse

Chapter Outline

Learning Outcomes

After reading this chapter, the student should be able to:

1. Describe the types of substances abused by individuals.
2. Identify the five drug schedules of controlled substances and give examples of drugs in each schedule.
3. Explain major legislation regulating controlled substances in the United States.
4. Identify factors contributing to addiction.
5. Compare and contrast physical and psychologic dependence.
6. Compare and contrast withdrawal syndromes for the different classes of abused substances.
7. Discuss the significance of drug tolerance to pharmacology.
8. Explain the major characteristics of abuse, dependence, and tolerance resulting from use of the following substances: antianxiety drugs, sedatives, opioids, alcohol, marijuana, hallucinogens, club drugs, amphetamines, methylphenidate, cocaine, caffeine, nicotine, inhalants, and anabolic steroids.

Key Terms

Definitions of the terms in bold may be found in the Glossary.

Throughout history individuals have consumed substances to increase performance, assist with relaxation, induce spiritual visions, or simply fit in with their peer group. **Substance abuse** is the self-administration of a drug in a manner that does not conform to the norms within the individual's given culture or society. The term *substance abuse* is preferred over the term *drug abuse* because some of these agents are not considered to be drugs by users. The fifth edition of the *Diagnostic and Statistical Manual of Mental Disorders* (DSM-5) no longer uses the terms *substance abuse* or *substance dependence*; rather, it refers to the term *substance use disorder* (American Psychiatric Association, 2013). Both substance abuse and substance use disorder will be used in this chapter.

This chapter introduces the types of drugs commonly abused by patients, focusing on the pharmacologic management of withdrawal syndromes.

Fundamental Concepts of Substance Abuse

27.1 A wide variety of substances may be abused by patients.

Characteristics of substance abuse vary widely from drug to drug and person to person. Diagnosis of this disorder is often difficult, even for experienced healthcare providers. Recognition of abuse is relatively easy for substances such as heroin, cocaine, or hallucinogens. However, what about legal substances such as alcohol, tobacco, or marijuana (in some states)? How many beers must one drink or cigarettes must one smoke before it is labeled as substance abuse? And with legal prescription drugs, is it considered substance abuse if a patient continues to refill prescriptions, such as oxycodone, even after symptoms have resolved? It is apparent that, with the exception of certain illegal substances, the distinction among proper use, misuse, and substance abuse is often not clear.

Certain characteristics, however, assist in the proper diagnosis of substance abuse. Nurses should be aware of these characteristics because they may be the first to recognize the following when obtaining a patient history:

- Craving for a specific substance despite an understanding that the substance is lowering the patient's quality of life (physical dependence)
- Failure to maintain normal work or home relationships because a substance is being used repeatedly
- Recognition that, over time, increased amounts of the substance are needed to produce the desired effect (tolerance)
- Repeated, unsuccessful attempts have been made to discontinue using the substance
- Recognition that behavioral changes occur when the substance is discontinued, such as agitation, drowsiness, anxiety, or pain (withdrawal syndrome)
- Increased amount of time is devoted to obtaining or using the substance, which reduces time available for work, home, or leisure activities.

Abused substances belong to a large number of diverse chemical classes. Although they have few structural similarities, most have in common the ability to affect the brain. Some illicit drugs are taken to stimulate the brain, whereas others are used to sedate the brain or dull the sensation of pain. Still other substances are used to provide alternative psychoactive experiences such as visions or hallucinations. An important exception is the anabolic steroids, which are used for their effects on the muscular system rather than the nervous system.

Although the public associates substance abuse with illegal drugs, this is not necessarily the case. Alcohol and nicotine are the two most commonly abused substances, and both are legal for adults. In addition, legal prescription drugs, such as oxycodone (OxyContin), methylphenidate (Adderall), and alprazolam (Xanax), are frequent drugs of abuse.

Several drugs that were once used therapeutically are now illegal due to their high potential for abuse. Cocaine was once used as a local anesthetic, but today all the cocaine acquired by users is obtained illegally. Lysergic acid diethylamide (LSD) is now illegal, although it was briefly used in psychotherapy in the 1940s and 1950s. Phencyclidine (PCP) was popular back in the early 1960s as an anesthetic but was withdrawn from the market due to patients reporting serious adverse effects while recovering from anesthesia. Many amphetamines once used for bronchodilation were discontinued in the 1980s after psychotic episodes were reported.

Legislation of Controlled Substances

27.2 Drugs with a potential for abuse are restricted by the Controlled Substances Act and are categorized into schedules.

It is not surprising that drugs and other substances with abuse potential are highly regulated. Many of these substances can cause significant harm to the user and members of the public when memory or performance becomes impaired. A significant percentage of motor-vehicle crashes and other injuries result from substance abuse. The government clearly has a role in protecting the public from such dangerous drugs. The Controlled Substances Act (CSA), the primary legislation establishing scheduled drugs, was discussed in Chapter 2.

Diversion from medical use is a major source of some of the abused drugs. Because of this, legislation has been enacted to closely track potential drugs of abuse from manufacturer to consumer. Prescription drugs may be stolen from pharmacies, healthcare provider offices, or patients and sold illegally, sometimes at a high profit. In some cases, healthcare workers who have the responsibility of dispensing or administering the medications conduct the theft.

Patients contribute to the diversion by faking or exaggerating their symptoms to obtain prescriptions for pain medication or sedatives. Some patients obtain the same prescription from several healthcare providers, commonly referred to as "doctor shopping," and sell their pills to substance abusers. Because of the multitude of ways that legal drugs can be diverted to abusers, the tracking of drugs with abuse potential must be closely monitored.

In the United States, controlled substances are classified according to their potential for abuse and toxicity. This classification uses five schedules, with Schedule I drugs having the highest potential for abuse (see Chapter 2). In recent years, a few exceptions have been made to the placement of drugs in the schedules. For example, gamma hydroxybutyrate is used illegally as a club drug as a stimulant or aphrodisiac and is classified as a Schedule I drug that has "no therapeutic use." However, this same substance is approved to treat narcolepsy as the drug Xyrem, a Schedule III drug. As another example, marijuana is a Schedule I agent, yet some states have legalized its use for specific medical indications and recreational use.

CONNECTION Checkpoint 27.1

Prior to the CSA, other attempts were made to legislate narcotics. From what you learned in Chapter 2, name the first major law in the United States that was passed in 1914 to control narcotic use and explain its major provisions.

27.3 Addiction is an overwhelming compulsion to continue repeated drug use.

Addiction is an overwhelming compulsion that drives someone to repeat drug-taking behavior, despite serious health and social consequences. Why do people continue to abuse drugs even when they are aware of its compelling negative consequences? The drug experience is highly personal for each user, and it is difficult to generalize reasons for continued substance abuse. Simply stated, the drug experience brings some degree of pleasure or satisfaction to the user. Whether it be euphoria, sedation, hallucinations, or feelings of well-being or excitement, the substance abuser finds the drug experience reinforcing and worth repeating. In many cases, use continues not to bring pleasure but simply to avoid severe withdrawal symptoms.

Addiction depends on multiple, complex, and interacting variables. These variables focus on the following categories:

- **Agent or drug factors.** Cost, availability, dose, mode of administration (e.g., oral [PO], intravenous [IV], inhalation), speed of onset, duration of drug action, length of drug use
- **User factors.** Genetic factors (e.g., metabolic enzymes, innate tolerance), risk-taking behavior, prior experiences with drugs, pathologic state (such as severe pain) that may indicate a drug with abuse potential
- **Environmental factors.** Social and community norms, role models, peer influences, educational opportunities.

In the case of prescription drugs, addiction may begin with a legitimate need for pharmacotherapy. For example, narcotic analgesics may be indicated for pain relief or sedatives for a sleep disorder. These drugs may result in a favorable experience, such as pain relief or sleep, and patients will want to repeat these positive experiences. If pharmacotherapy is not carefully monitored, patients may take these drugs at high doses for prolonged periods, thus increasing the risk of addiction.

When used according to accepted medical protocols, prescription drugs can be used safely and effectively. The risk of addiction for prescription medications is primarily a function of the dose and the length of therapy. Because of this, medications having a potential for abuse are prescribed at the lowest effective dose and for the shortest time necessary to treat the medical problem. Nurses should administer these medications as prescribed for the relief of patient symptoms without undue fear of producing dependency.

PharmFACT

In 2018, almost 20% (53.2 million) of Americans age 12 years or older used illicit drugs in the past year. The top three substances were marijuana, pain relievers, and sedatives (Substance Abuse and Mental Health Services Administration, 2019).

Addiction and Dependence

27.4 Physical and psychologic dependence lead to continued drug-seeking behavior despite negative health and social consequences.

Whether or not a drug is addictive is related to how easily someone can stop taking the substance on a repetitive basis. Substance dependence occurs when an individual has an overwhelming craving to take a drug and cannot stop. Dependence is classified by two distinct categories: physical dependence and psychologic dependence.

Physical dependence occurs when the body adapts to repeated use of the substance by altering normal physiology.

Essentially, the cells adapt and view the medication-altered environment as normal. These changes in physiology are reversible and when the agent is discontinued, uncomfortable symptoms known as withdrawal result (see Section 27.5). Opioids, such as morphine and heroin, produce physical dependence relatively quickly with repeated doses, particularly when taken IV. Alcohol, central nervous system (CNS) depressants, some stimulants, and nicotine are other examples of substances that may produce physical dependence relatively easily with chronic use.

It is important to understand that physical dependence is not the same as addiction. Physical dependence may occur during the normal course of therapy, such as in patients receiving high doses of narcotic analgesics during cancer treatment. A patient with cancer may be physically dependent, that is, withdrawal symptoms may occur on discontinuing the drug. However, withdrawal from a medication taken under medical supervision such as analgesics, antidepressants, or antianxiety drugs should not be considered as evidence that the patient has a substance use disorder. Addiction implies destructive, compulsive substance use. Although physical dependence does indeed occur in patients who are addicted, it is important to understand that the two terms have different meanings.

In contrast, **psychologic dependence** produces no signs of physical discomfort after the agent is discontinued. The user, however, has an intense *emotional* desire to continue and this intense craving becomes worse if the person has an unsupportive home environment or social contacts who also have substance use disorders. Strong psychologic craving for a substance is responsible for relapses during substance abuse therapy and often causes a return to drug-seeking behavior. The development of psychologic dependence usually requires the use of relatively high doses for a prolonged time; however, psychologic dependence may also develop quickly, perhaps after only one use, with crack cocaine. Whereas physical dependence is often overcome within a few days or weeks after discontinuing the drug, psychologic dependence may persist for months, years, or even an entire lifetime.

27.5 A withdrawal syndrome is a set of characteristic symptoms that occurs when an abused substance is discontinued.

Once a patient becomes physically dependent and the substance is abruptly discontinued, a **withdrawal syndrome** will occur. Some substances exhibit severe and prolonged withdrawal symptoms, whereas others produce barely noticeable symptoms. Because the withdrawal syndrome may be particularly acute for patients dependent on alcohol and sedatives, the process of withdrawal from these agents is best accomplished in a substance abuse treatment facility. Examples of the types of withdrawal syndromes experienced with the different abused substances are shown in Table 27.1. In a medical setting a withdrawal syndrome may be induced by a rapid dosage reduction or by the administration of an antagonist drug.

Table 27.1 Withdrawal Symptoms and Treatment for Select Drugs of Abuse

Drug Class	Symptoms	Pharmacologic Treatment
Alcohol	Tremors, fatigue, anxiety, abdominal cramping, hallucinations, confusion, seizures, delirium	Benzodiazepines such as lorazepam, antiseizure drugs; agitated patients may require an antipsychotic; disulfiram and naltrexone to prevent relapses after withdrawal is over
Anabolic steroids	Mood swings, fatigue, restlessness, anorexia, insomnia, reduced sex drive, depression, psychologic craving for steroids	Symptomatic treatment such as antidepressants
Barbiturates and other sedative–hypnotics	Insomnia, anxiety, weakness, abdominal cramps, tremor, anorexia, seizures, hallucinations, delirium	Place patient on a long-acting benzodiazepine and gradually reduce dose
Benzodiazepines	Insomnia, irritability, abdominal pain, nausea, sensitivity to light and sound, headache, fatigue, tremors	Gradual tapering of dosage over several weeks or months; for acute benzodiazepine intoxication, flumazenil is administered by rapid IV infusion (15–20 sec)
Cocaine and amphetamines	Mental depression, anxiety, agitation, irritability, extreme fatigue, hunger, disturbed sleep, psychologic craving	No specific pharmacologic treatment available
Hallucinogens	Dependent on the specific drug; may include anxiety, mental depression, insomnia, paranoid delusions, panic attacks, lethargy	Treatment is usually not necessary; symptoms resolve in about 12 h; PCP excretion is pH dependent and acidification of the urine increases the clearance rate of PCP by about 100-fold
Marijuana	Irritability, restlessness, insomnia, tremor, chills, weight loss	No pharmacologic treatment
Nicotine	Irritability, anxiety, restlessness, headaches, increased appetite, insomnia, inability to concentrate, decrease in heart rate and blood pressure	Nicotine replacement therapy, varenicline (Chantix) or bupropion (Zyban)
Opioids	Excessive sweating, restlessness, dilated pupils, agitation, goose bumps, tremor, violent yawning, increased heart rate and blood pressure, nausea and vomiting, abdominal cramps and pain, muscle spasms with kicking movements, weight loss	Methadone maintenance; buprenorphine therapy; clonidine or a benzodiazepine reduces anxiety, agitation, cramping, and sweating; oxazepam reduces muscle spasms and insomnia; antiemetics such as ondansetron for nausea and vomiting; detoxification can be completed in 2–3 days; withdrawal may be done more rapidly using naltrexone in combination with propofol anesthetic

In general, symptoms of withdrawal are opposite to those of the drug's effects. For example, an individual may use alprazolam to *reduce* anxiety, but withdrawal will *cause* symptoms of intense anxiety. People who abuse methamphetamine as a stimulant to stay awake will experience lethargy and fatigue upon withdrawal. Once these **rebound effects** become intense, people are driven to take additional doses of the abused substance because that will eliminate the withdrawal symptoms. For some patients, avoidance of withdrawal symptoms is the *primary* motivator for continuing drug use. Thus, the cycle of continued substance abuse is perpetuated.

Prescription drugs may be used to reduce the severity of withdrawal symptoms. For example, alcohol withdrawal can be treated with a short-acting benzodiazepine such as oxazepam, and opioid withdrawal can be treated with methadone. Symptoms of nicotine withdrawal may be relieved by nicotine replacement therapy in the form of patches or chewing gum. No specific pharmacologic intervention is indicated for withdrawal from CNS stimulants, hallucinogens, marijuana, or inhalants.

With chronic substance abuse, patients will often associate the drug use with their surroundings, including social contacts with other users. Users tend to revert back to drug-seeking behavior when they return to the company of other substance abusers. Counselors often encourage users to refrain from associating with past social contacts or relationships with other substance abusers to lessen the possibility for relapse. The formation of new social contacts, including association with self-help groups such as Alcoholics Anonymous, helps some patients transition to a drug-free lifestyle.

Addiction and Tolerance

27.6 Tolerance occurs when the body adapts to a drug and larger doses are needed to produce a therapeutic effect.

Tolerance is a biological condition that occurs when the body adapts to a substance after repeated administration. Over time, larger doses of the drug are required to produce the same initial effect. For example, at the start of pharmacotherapy, a patient may find that 2 mg of a sedative is effective at inducing sleep. After taking the medication for several months, the patient may require 4 or perhaps 6 mg to fall asleep. Development of drug tolerance is common for drugs that affect the nervous system. Tolerance should be considered a natural consequence of continued drug use: Development of tolerance is not evidence of a substance use disorder. Indeed, tolerance is an expression of natural homeostasis—the body's attempt to return systems to normal.

Tolerance does not develop at the same rate for all actions of a drug. For example, patients usually develop tolerance to the nausea and vomiting produced by opioids after only a few doses. Tolerance to the mood-altering effects of these drugs and to their ability to reduce pain develops more slowly but eventually may be complete. Tolerance to the drug's ability to constrict the pupils never develops. Patients will often endure annoying side effects of drugs, such as the sedation caused by antihistamines, if they know that tolerance to these effects will develop quickly. Thus, knowing details regarding the development of tolerance helps the nurse to deliver essential patient information that may enhance adherence.

Tolerance may lead to serious consequences. As a patient self-administers higher and higher doses to obtain a desired effect such as euphoria or sedation, the risk of overdose escalates. In some cases, the drug abuser may reach a daily dose that would be lethal for a nonaddicted individual. Tolerance fades after the patient discontinues the abused drug, often after 10 to 14 days. If the patient should return to drug-taking behavior with the *same* high dose, the results can be fatal.

The rapid development of tolerance after only a couple of doses, called **tachyphylaxis**, occurs with drugs such as cocaine, LSD, and amphetamines but is not unique to abused substances. For example, patients with coronary artery disease will exhibit acute tachyphylaxis to the therapeutic effects of nitroglycerin. Tachyphylaxis can occur to virtually any action of a drug, adverse effects as well as therapeutic effects. Tachyphylaxis is beneficial when it occurs to an adverse effect of a drug, such as nausea and/or vomiting or dizziness.

Cross-tolerance occurs between closely related drugs. The more two drugs are similar chemically, the greater the possibility of cross-tolerance between them. This occurs frequently between drugs in the same class, such as among different barbiturates or among various opioids. It sometimes occurs between dissimilar drugs that have the same pharmacologic action. For example, patients who are physically dependent on ethanol exhibit cross-tolerance to other CNS depressant drugs such as benzodiazepines and barbiturates. Ethanol-dependent patients will require higher doses of these drugs to produce a therapeutic effect. Ethanol does not exhibit cross-tolerance to drugs in very different pharmacologic classes, such as amphetamines or LSD.

The term *resistance* is often confused with tolerance. Resistance, however, refers to microorganisms and infections and should not be used interchangeably with tolerance. For example, microorganisms may become resistant to the effects of an antibiotic; they do not become tolerant. Patients may become tolerant to the effects of pain relievers; they do not become resistant.

Central Nervous System Depressants

27.7 Depressants, which include sedatives, opioids, and alcohol, decrease the activity of the central nervous system.

CNS depressants form a diverse group of drugs that cause patients to feel sedated or relaxed (see Chapters 18 and 25). Drugs in this group include sedatives, antianxiety drugs, opioids, and alcohol. Although the majority are legal substances, these classes of drugs are strictly controlled due to their abuse potential.

Antianxiety Drugs and Sedatives

Antianxiety drugs are the most widely prescribed CNS depressants having abuse potential. The two primary classes are the benzodiazepines and nonbenzodiazepine anxiolytics.

Although their primary indication is anxiety, benzodiazepines may be used to treat seizures, insomnia, and muscle spasms. Benzodiazepines that are frequently abused include alprazolam (Xanax), clonazepam (Klonopin), diazepam (Valium), temazepam (Restoril), triazolam (Halcion), and lorazepam. Chronic benzodiazepine abuse is much more serious, and can be fatal when combined with other CNS depressants such as opioids or alcohol.

Flunitrazepam (Rohypnol) is an infamous benzodiazepine of abuse because it causes **anterograde amnesia**, a type of short-term memory loss in which the user cannot remember events that occur while under the influence of the drug. Effects begin 30 minutes after PO administration and last for 8 hours or longer. The abuser is conscious during this time but is unable to transfer thoughts from short-term to long-term memory. Flunitrazepam is called a "date-rape" drug because sexual predators can expose an unknowing individual to the drug and perform a physical assault with the likelihood that the victim will not remember the event. Flunitrazepam is not approved by the U.S. Food and Drug Administration (FDA) for any medical condition.

The nonbenzodiazepine anxiolytics such as zolpidem (Ambien), zaleplon (Sonata), and eszopiclone (Lunesta) also have abuse potential. Symptoms of abuse are similar to those of the benzodiazepines.

Sedatives, also known as sedative–hypnotics and tranquilizers, are primarily prescribed for sleep disorders. The primary, older class of sedative–hypnotics is the barbiturates. Physical and psychologic dependence develop when high doses of barbiturates are taken for extended periods. Doses may be three or more times above normal due to the development of tolerance. Addicts often alternate between amphetamines (uppers), which keep them awake for several days, and sedatives (downers), which are needed to relax and fall asleep.

Sedative users appear dull or apathetic and exhibit signs similar to alcohol intoxication such as slurred speech and motor incoordination. The medical use of barbiturates has declined markedly over the past two decades because safer alternatives such as the benzodiazepines are available. With the decline in therapeutic use, fewer cases of illicit barbiturate use have been reported. Overdose of barbiturates is extremely dangerous because they suppress the respiratory centers in the brain; very high doses are often fatal. In the 1960s and 1970s, barbiturates were the drugs most commonly used to commit suicide. The withdrawal syndrome from these drugs resembles that of alcohol and may be life-threatening.

Another popular abused CNS depressant is a substance that occurs naturally in the body called *gamma-hydroxybutyric acid (GHB)*. The drug is approved by the FDA as sodium oxybate (Xyrem) to treat patients with narcolepsy who experience excessive daytime sleepiness or cataplexy (weak or paralyzed muscles). Although Xyrem is regulated as a Schedule III drug, its active ingredient, GHB, is classified as Schedule I. It is very unusual for the FDA to classify a drug in two schedules.

Once sold in health food stores as a dietary supplement to enhance athletic performance, GHB is now abused by recreational users for its ability to produce euphoria at low doses. Like flunitrazepam, GHB is called a date-rape drug because it induces retrograde amnesia in the user and has been used in sexual assaults. Most illegal GHB is obtained through home laboratories in the United States, with batches varying widely in purity and potency. The drug is usually dissolved in liquid and doses are difficult to estimate. The same enzyme that metabolizes ethanol also metabolizes GHB; concurrent use, which is common, leads to prolonged effects of GHB and an increased risk of overdose. Overdose causes severe respiratory depression, seizures, and coma. There is no antidote for overdose with GHB.

Opioids

Opioids are substances naturally found in the poppy plant or made synthetically in the laboratory that are prescribed for chronic pain, anesthesia, persistent cough, and severe diarrhea. The opioid class includes morphine, codeine, meperidine (Demerol), oxycodone (OxyContin), fentanyl (Sublimaze), methadone, and heroin. The therapeutic effects of the opioids are discussed in detail in Chapter 25. Dependence on opioids is called **opioid use disorder** (formerly called *opioid addiction*).

PharmFACT

Among adolescents ages 12 to 17, 14% have taken prescription pain medicine without a doctor's prescription. The highest rates (19.3%) were in Louisiana and Arkansas and the lowest rate (7.8%) was in Vermont (Kann et al., 2018).

The effects of oral opioids begin within 30 minutes and may last over a day. Injecting or smoking opium produces immediate effects, including the brief, intense rush of euphoria sought by heroin addicts. Individuals experience a range of emotions, from extreme pleasure to slowed body activities and profound sedation. Other symptoms include slurred speech, constricted pupils (miosis), an increase in the pain threshold, and respiratory depression. Tolerance develops rapidly to most effects of opioids, and a patient who is addicted may eventually require 10 times the initial dose to achieve the desired effects.

Opioid dependence can occur rapidly, and withdrawal produces very intense and unpleasant symptoms that start within a few hours after discontinuation of parenteral agents and within 3 to 5 days for those dependent on oral opiates. Withdrawal symptoms include dysphoria, diaphoresis, violent yawning, lacrimation, rhinorrhea, pupil dilation (mydriasis), fever, diarrhea, goose bumps, and muscle cramping and tremor. Although extremely unpleasant, withdrawal from opioids is not life-threatening. The withdrawal syndrome is self-limiting, peaking within 36 to 72 hours after discontinuation of parenteral opioids, and individual symptoms are treated as necessary. For patients dependent on low to moderate doses, withdrawal symptoms are relatively mild and resemble a case of the flu. Babies born to pregnant opioid users will experience opioid withdrawal symptoms following birth.

Abuse-Deterrent Formulations: In the 1990s, pharmaceutical companies developed extended-release (ER) opioids that offered around-the-clock pain control. Abusers soon discovered, however, that ER opioids such as oxycodone (OxyContin) could be crushed and snorted or dissolved and injected for an intense high. Oxycodone soon became the world's most commonly abused prescription drug, which signaled the start of a serious opioid epidemic.

The FDA has responded to this public health crisis by encouraging pharmaceutical companies to reformulate ER opioids to make them less susceptible to abuse (FDA, 2021). The result has been the development of opioid products with *abuse-deterrent formulations (ADFs)*. The ADFs use chemical and physical barriers to make it more difficult to misuse the drug by crushing, snorting, or dissolving it for injection. Hydrocodone (Hysingla ER) and oxycodone (Oxycontin, Xtampza ER) are examples of opioids with abuse-deterrent properties listed on the medication labels. A significant number of other ADFs were approved by the FDA but never marketed or were discontinued. These include morphine (Arymo ER, Embeda), hydrocodone (Vantrela), oxymorphone (Opana ER), and oxycodone (Targiniq, Troxyca).

To claim that a product has abuse-deterrent properties, the manufacturer must meet FDA standards for testing ADFs. The manufacturer must also conduct postmarketing studies to determine if their ADF actually resulted in a meaningful decrease in misuse and abuse of their product.

While they are a significant advance, the ADFs have important limitations. The ADF products are not "abuse proof" and misuse can still occur. It is important to understand that the most common way that opioids are abused is by the oral route, and none of the deterrent technologies impact that route of administration. At this time, most of the ADFs only exist for extended-release opioids. Immediate-release forms and generic forms of extended-release opioids are not included, although the FDA is encouraging ADFs for those products. The ADF medications are more expensive than their generic equivalents (without abuse deterrence) and may not be covered by insurance companies.

Medication-Assisted Treatment: For treatment of opioid use disorder, the two basic choices for the chronic user are to simply stop taking the drug ("cold turkey") or to participate in a *medication-assisted treatment (MAT)* program. While suddenly stopping opioid use results in very uncomfortable physical withdrawal symptoms, they last for a few days and are not considered life-threatening. The more difficult problem, however, is that the majority of users (90%) quickly return to drug-seeking behavior. Going cold turkey is largely unsuccessful at solving the user's long-term opioid addiction problem.

MAT for opioid use disorder has proven to be more successful at reducing long-term addictive behaviors. There are three types of MAT. The first two, methadone and a combination of buprenorphine plus naloxone, involve substituting a safer opioid for the abused opioid (usually heroin). The third MAT uses monotherapy with naltrexone, a non-narcotic medication.

MAT eliminates the need for needle-sharing and other associated destructive health effects such as transmission of human immunodeficiency virus or hepatitis. The patient receives their daily medication legally, without participating in criminal activity to obtain it. The MAT allows those addicted to opioids to prevent unpleasant withdrawal symptoms. MAT improves patient survival and increases the patient's retention in treatment programs and the ability to obtain employment. The patient may continue the MAT treatment indefinitely, or he or she may eventually decide to undergo medical-supervised detoxification, tapering the doses of the medication over several months or years.

Methadone maintenance therapy (MMT) has been the standard treatment for opioid addiction for decades. Although methadone has addictive properties of its own, it does not produce the same degree of euphoria as other opioids; it may be taken PO and its effects last 24 hours. If the patient does decide to take heroin during methadone therapy, most of the euphoric rush will be blocked because the opiate receptors are already occupied by methadone. During MMT, patients must report to the methadone clinic daily for their dose and to receive counseling. Patients who have remained heroin-free may be trusted with several doses for home administration.

Buprenorphine has become an important alternative to methadone for MAT. As monotherapy, buprenorphine is a partial opioid agonist given parenterally (Buprenex), transdermally (Butrans), or buccally for the treatment of moderate to severe pain. In the treatment of opioid use disorder, buprenorphine has a wider margin of safety than methadone and is combined with naloxone (see prototype feature in this chapter).

The third option for MAT is naltrexone (Vivitrol), which is a nonopioid and can be prescribed by any physician or nurse practitioner. Naltrexone blocks the euphoric and sedative effects of opioids and suppresses drug cravings.

PROTOTYPE DRUG Buprenorphine with Naloxone (Suboxone, Zubsolv)

Classification **Therapeutic:** Drug for treating opioid addiction, narcotic analgesic
Pharmacologic: Opioid agonist-antagonist

Therapeutic Effects and Uses: Approved in 2002, buprenorphine is a Schedule III narcotic analgesic that is part of an opioid use treatment plan. The combination of buprenorphine with naloxone, a narcotic antagonist, is given by the oral, sublingual (Suboxone, Zubsolv), or buccal routes for the maintenance treatment of opioid dependence. When taken as directed, the combination drug reduces craving in opioid-dependent patients and prevents the unpleasant symptoms of withdrawal. When starting therapy, the patient must abstain from opioid use for at least 12 to 24 hours and be in the early stages of withdrawal. This is because patients with opioids in their system may experience acute withdrawal symptoms from the naloxone. Once stabilized on buprenorphine-naloxone, patients may be switched to long-term preparations of buprenorphine only, such as a 6-month subdermal implant (Probuphine) or a once-monthly subcutaneous injection (Sublocade). Buprenorphine plus naloxone therapy may be continued indefinitely or, under medical guidance, the dose may be slowly tapered over several months to avoid withdrawal symptoms and relapse.

Buprenorphine with naloxone offers certain advantages over MMT. It is unlikely that the combination drug will be abused by injection because the presence of naloxone would cause unpleasant withdrawal symptoms. Detoxification can be more rapid, and the maintenance can be conducted by qualified practitioners through office environments, rather than a daily visit to a methadone clinic. Naloxone is also used alone for the emergency treatment of severe opioid-induced respiratory depression (see Chapter 25).

Mechanism of Action: Buprenorphine produces its analgesic effects by occupying mu receptors in the brain and dorsal horn of the spinal cord in a manner similar to that of other opioid agonists. Because buprenorphine exhibits some opioid antagonist activity at the kappa receptor, it is considered a mixed opioid agonist-antagonist. Naloxone competes with opioid agonists for the mu and kappa receptors, thus antagonizing the effects of morphine and other opioids.

Pharmacokinetics:

Route(s)	Sublingual tablets or film
Absorption	Variable (buprenorphine well absorbed; naloxone poorly absorbed)
Distribution	Bound to plasma protein (96% buprenorphine, 45% naloxone); crosses the placenta; secreted in breast milk
Primary metabolism	Hepatic
Primary excretion	Renal (30%) and feces (69%)
Onset of action	Approximately 45 min
Duration of action	8–12 h (may be as long as 72 h at high doses)

Adverse Effects: Buprenorphine with naloxone is a relatively safe drug that produces mild and transient side effects. The most frequently reported adverse events include headache, nausea and vomiting, hyperhidrosis, constipation, insomnia, pain, and peripheral edema. Abrupt discontinuation will precipitate immediate opioid withdrawal symptoms. Respiratory depression and death have occurred with high doses, although these have been with the IV route.

Buprenorphine is an opioid and thus can produce dependence when taken on a chronic basis. Although Suboxone and Zubsolv are both sublingual forms of the drug, they are not dose equivalent and care must be taken when switching between products.

Contraindications/Precautions: Buprenorphine with naloxone is contraindicated in patients with hypersensitivity to either drug. This combination may induce withdrawal in patients who have chronic physical dependence on opioids. Naloxone should be used with caution in patients with cardiovascular disease. It may precipitate seizures in patients with seizure disorders.

Drug Interactions: Caution should be used when taking buprenorphine with other opioids and CNS depressants because additive sedation will occur. Deaths have occurred when taking very high doses of buprenorphine concomitantly with benzodiazepines. The use of buprenorphine is contraindicated with alvimopan (Entereg).

Pregnancy: Animal studies with naloxone did not show teratogenicity and human data has not shown evidence of adverse neonatal outcomes. Because buprenorphine is secreted in milk, the newborn may experience neonatal opioid withdrawal symptoms following delivery.

Treatment of Overdose: Buprenorphine overdose can cause coma, hypotension, and life-threatening respiratory depression, and requires immediate treatment. Additional naloxone doses are indicated to reverse the opioid intoxication.

Clinician Responsibilities: Key clinical implications for patients receiving buprenorphine are included in Applied Clinical Judgment: Patients Receiving Pharmacotherapy for Substance Abuse Disorders.

Drugs Similar to Buprenorphine with Naloxone (Suboxone, Zubsolv, Others)

Naltrexone is an opioid antagonist that exhibits actions similar to those of naloxone. It is presented later in this chapter as a treatment for alcohol dependence.

Alcohol (Ethanol)

One of the most commonly abused drugs is alcohol, the pharmacologically active agent in beer, wine, and liquor. Although there are many types of alcohol, the only one having widespread medical significance is ethanol or ethyl alcohol. Therefore, in this text, the terms *ethanol* and *alcohol* are used interchangeably. The economic, social, and health consequences of alcohol abuse are staggering. The chronic consumption of alcohol such that it impairs normal interpersonal relationships and job performance or causes injury or harm to self or others is called **alcohol use disorder**.

PharmFACT

In a large nationwide survey of high school students, about 60% had drunk alcohol and almost 16% had their first drink before age 13. Almost 6% reported that they had driven a car while drinking 30 days before the survey (Kan et al., 2018).

Alcohol is readily absorbed across the gastrointestinal (GI) tract, primarily from the small intestine. Food slows the absorption of alcohol by prolonging gastric emptying time and diluting the alcohol, thus delaying its onset of action. Once it has entered the blood, alcohol is immediately distributed to the tissues. The drug easily crosses the blood–brain barrier so its effects on the brain are observed quickly, within 5 to 30 minutes after consumption.

Alcohol is metabolized and excreted at a constant rate, depending on the activity of two hepatic enzymes, alcohol

CONNECTIONS: Community-Oriented Practice

Naloxone Use in the Community

Treating an opioid overdose as quickly as possible is a crucial lifesaving measure. Hesitancy of bystanders to call 911 for fear of law enforcement involvement, or delayed response times such as may occur in rural communities, lengthens the time from overdose to treatment with possible devastating consequences. Naloxone kits are available for community use and, as noted in Chapter 25, are available as autoinjectors and nasal sprays. State laws vary as to whether a pharmacist or community organization may dispense the drug without a provider's prescription and whether the drug may be dispensed to a third party (i.e., not the intended user of the drug; SAFE Project, 2020).

Naloxone by nasal spray has been shown to be effective in reversing the effects of an opioid overdose and may be an easier method to administer the drug by community bystanders (Aventian et al., 2018). Many opportunities exist to provide naloxone to those who may need it, including to friends or relatives of a substance user, but research suggests these opportunities are sometimes missed or not used to full advantage (Dunne, 2018). Members of the nursing profession may advocate for expanded treatment or prescribe the drug to those who may be able to act quickly in the case of an overdose. The results may be significant. States that have adopted a naloxone access law demonstrated a 9–10% decrease in opioid fatalities (Rees, Sabia, Argys, Dave, & Latshaw, 2019).

dehydrogenase and aldehyde dehydrogenase. Metabolism is a two-step process, first yielding acetaldehyde and then acetic acid, or acetate, as shown in Pharmacotherapy Illustrated 27.1. Wide genetic variability is seen in the amounts and activity of these enzymes. For example, a significant number of Asians have a deficiency of aldehyde dehydrogenase, resulting in an accumulation of acetaldehyde and severe flushing and other uncomfortable symptoms when consuming alcohol. Patients who are alcohol dependent and those who drink alcoholic beverages regularly have higher amounts of these enzymes and thus are able to drink greater quantities of alcohol without becoming intoxicated.

The elimination of alcohol from tissues occurs at a constant rate, which is independent of the concentration of alcohol in the blood. The blood alcohol level declines at about 15 mg/h; no food or drug can speed up the rate of alcohol excretion once it has reached the blood. Eating pizza or drinking strong coffee following an alcohol binge does nothing to speed up excretion of the drug. It is a simple fact that if an individual drinks alcohol at a faster rate than it can be metabolized, intoxication will occur and will continue until the body eventually metabolizes the alcohol that has accumulated in the blood. The average rate of metabolism is one alcoholic drink per hour. Because alcohol is vaporized

Pharmacotherapy Illustrated 27.1

Metabolism of Alcohol

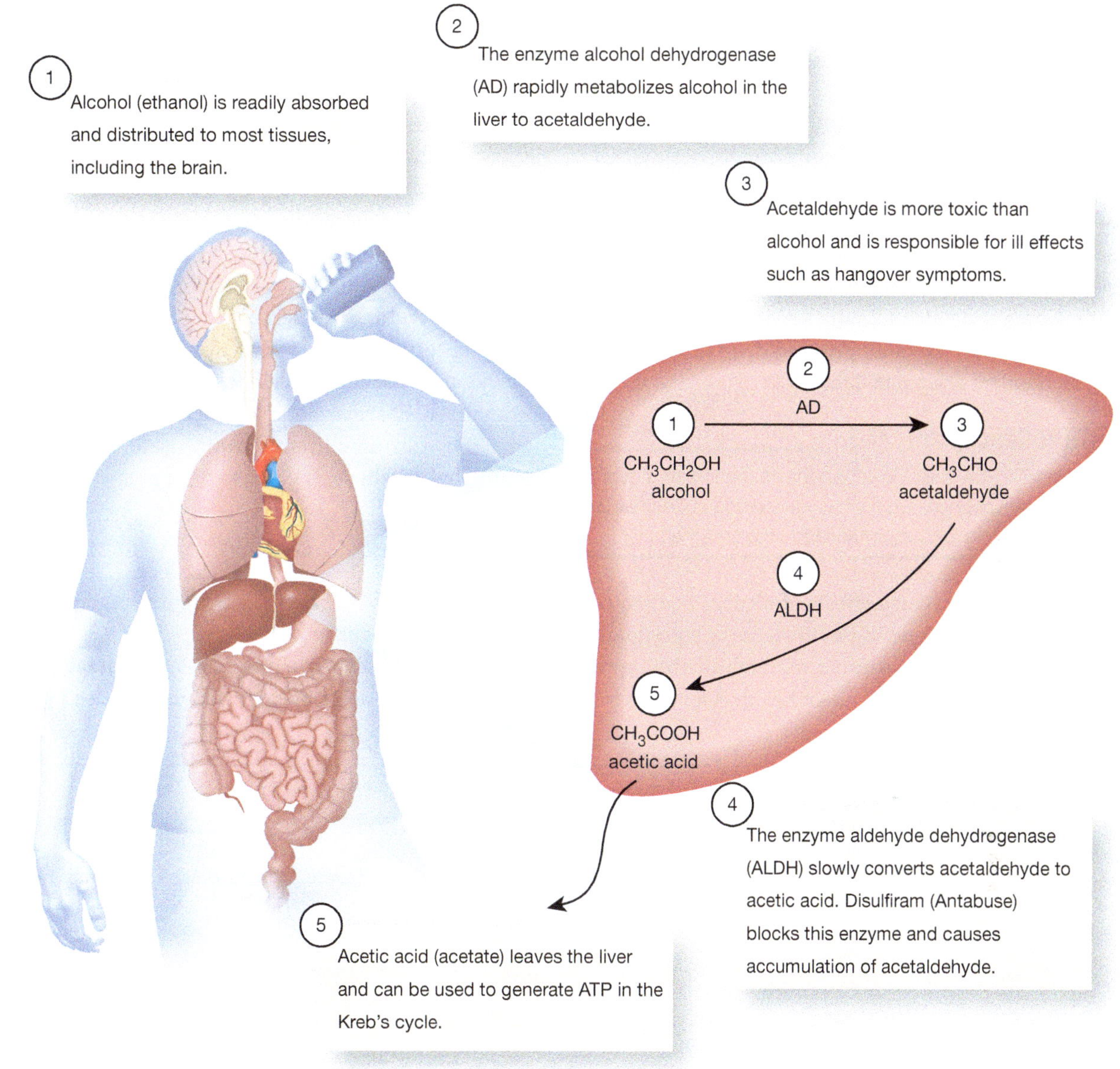

and excreted by the lungs, breath testing can be used to estimate the amount of alcohol in the blood, a common practice in law enforcement.

Classified as a CNS depressant, alcohol has the ability to slow the region of the brain controlling alertness and wakefulness. Effects of alcohol include sedation, relaxation, loss of motor coordination, reduced judgment, and decreased inhibition. Alcohol intoxication may cause partial or total amnesia, resulting in an inability to remember details that occurred during an alcohol binge. Alcohol also increases blood flow in certain areas of the skin, causing a flushed face, pink cheeks, or red nose. Like most drugs, the effects of alcohol are directly related to the amount consumed. Acute overdoses of alcohol produce vomiting, severe hypotension, respiratory failure, and coma. Death due to alcohol poisoning is not uncommon.

Chronic alcohol consumption produces both psychologic and physiologic dependence and leads directly to a large number of adverse health effects. Not surprisingly, the organ most affected by alcohol use disorder is the liver, which is responsible for metabolizing and detoxifying alcohol. Hepatitis occurs in up to 90% of heavy users. Alcoholism is a common cause of cirrhosis, a debilitating and often fatal failure of the liver to perform its vital functions.

Liver impairment results in abnormalities in blood clotting and nutritional deficiencies and makes the patient very sensitive to the effects of medications. Chronic alcohol use also damages the brain, impairing memory and cognitive function.

Drug doses for patients with alcoholism should be decreased to avoid toxicity because such patients are more susceptible to adverse drug effects and drug interactions. Combining alcohol with nonsteroidal anti-inflammatory drugs (NSAIDs) such as aspirin can promote serious GI bleeding. Combining alcohol with acetaminophen can increase the risk of fatal hepatic injury. Alcohol should never be combined with other CNS depressants because their effects are cumulative and profound sedation or coma may result. Combining alcohol with sedatives, benzodiazepines, or opioids may be fatal. Selected drug interactions involving alcohol are shown in Table 27.2.

CONNECTION Checkpoint 27.2

Alcohol induces CYP3A and increases the formation of a toxic metabolite of acetaminophen. From what you learned in Chapter 3, what is CYP3A and what is its importance to pharmacotherapy?

One of the major adverse effects of alcohol consumption occurs not in the patient, but in the fetus of a pregnant alcohol user. These effects, known as fetal alcohol syndrome, include birth defects and major health challenges for the child. There is no safe "dose" for alcohol consumption during pregnancy; thus, use of this drug must be strictly avoided. Additional details on alcohol as a teratogen are presented in Chapter 8.

Alcohol withdrawal symptoms can be severe and even life-threatening. About 5–10% of patients proceed to **delirium tremens**, a syndrome of intense agitation, confusion, terrifying hallucinations, uncontrollable tremors, panic attacks, and paranoia. Without treatment, 35% of the patients with delirium tremens will die. Prevention of seizures and delirium tremens is a top priority and may be accomplished by administering a benzodiazepine such as lorazepam (Ativan) or diazepam (Valium). Hallucinations may require the administration of an antipsychotic drug such as risperidone (Risperdal).

Long-term therapy for alcohol dependence includes behavioral counseling and self-help groups such as Alcoholics Anonymous. Pharmacologic management of alcohol dependence includes disulfiram, acamprosate, and naltrexone. Disulfiram (Antabuse) is given to discourage relapses.

PROTOTYPE DRUG Disulfiram (Antabuse)

Classification **Therapeutic:** Drug for treating alcohol abuse
Pharmacologic: Alcohol antagonist; acetaldehyde dehydrogenase inhibitor

Table 27.2 Drug–Drug Interactions with Alcohol

Class	Example Drug(s)	Interaction	Consequences
Analgesic	acetaminophen	Increased acetaminophen metabolism to toxic metabolites	Severe, possibly fatal liver damage
Anesthetics	propofol	Cross-tolerance	Larger anesthetic doses needed to induce anesthesia
		Additive hepatic toxicity	Increased risk of liver damage
Antianginal medications	nitroglycerin, isosorbide dinitrate	Additive effects on blood pressure	Hypotension, dizziness, possible fainting
Antianxiety drugs	diazepam, lorazepam, alprazolam	Additive CNS depression and sedation	Drowsiness, lethargy
Anticoagulants	warfarin	Acute consumption enhances warfarin bioavailability; chronic consumption reduces its availability	Modification of coagulation: bleeding disorders, hemorrhage
Antidepressants	amitriptyline, paroxetine, sertraline, fluoxetine	Additive CNS depression or sedation	Drowsiness, lethargy
Antihistamines	diphenhydramine, loratadine, cetirizine	Additive CNS depression	Drowsiness, lethargy, dizziness
Antipsychotics	chlorpromazine	Additive CNS depression	Drowsiness, lethargy
		Additive hepatotoxicity	Increased risk of liver damage
Antiseizure medications	phenytoin	Chronic alcohol use may decrease phenytoin bioavailability	Increased risk of seizures
Antituberculars	rifampin	Decreased bioavailability	Decreased effectiveness in eliminating tuberculosis
Beta blockers	propranolol	Additive effects on blood pressure	Hypotension, dizziness, possible fainting
HMG-CoA reductase inhibitors (statins)	atorvastatin, simvastatin	Additive hepatotoxicity	Liver damage
NSAIDs	aspirin, ibuprofen, naproxen, others	Additive GI toxicity	Increased risk of GI bleeding
Opioids	morphine, codeine, meperidine	Additive CNS depression and sedation	Drowsiness, lethargy

Therapeutic Effects and Uses: By itself, disulfiram produces few effects. If alcohol is consumed while taking disulfiram, however, the patient becomes violently ill in a syndrome called the disulfiram–alcohol reaction. Approved in 1951, the only indication for disulfiram is the management of alcohol use disorder. The use of disulfiram does not cure alcohol abuse; it only prevents impulsive drinking as long as the patient chooses to take it. The protective action of disulfiram may last for 2 weeks after it is discontinued. Disulfiram should only be administered to patients who are fully informed of its effects and who are motivated to maintain sobriety.

Mechanism of Action: Disulfiram irreversibly inhibits the enzyme acetaldehyde dehydrogenase, causing toxic acetaldehyde to build up in the blood. Acetaldehyde is sometimes called the "hangover" chemical because it is responsible for causing miserable symptoms following a night of high alcohol consumption.

Pharmacokinetics:

Route(s)	PO
Absorption	Rapidly absorbed
Distribution	Crosses the placenta; may be secreted in breast milk
Primary metabolism	Hepatic
Primary excretion	Lung and feces
Onset of action	12 h
Duration of action	1–2 weeks

Adverse Effects: At therapeutic doses, disulfiram produces few adverse effects, unless ingested with alcohol. At extreme doses, the drug itself can cause neurologic toxicity, psychosis, hepatotoxicity, and blood dyscrasias.

Because the disulfiram–alcohol reaction can be serious and even fatal, disulfiram therapy should not be initiated in patients at high risk for returning to alcohol abuse. Disulfiram is contraindicated in patients who are receiving metronidazole because acute psychosis may occur. All products containing alcohol must be strictly avoided, including cough syrups, mouthwashes, or liquid vitamins. Even topical products containing alcohol should be avoided because the alcohol may be absorbed across the skin. Disulfiram is also contraindicated in patients with severe heart disease and psychoses. **Black Box Warning:** Disulfiram should never be administered to a patient in a state of alcohol intoxication or without the patient's full knowledge.

Drug Interactions: Ingestion of even small amounts of alcohol will immediately result in headache, palpitations, chest pain, dyspnea, nausea and violent vomiting, and, sometimes, bizarre behaviors. Severe respiratory depression may occur. Symptoms begin within 5 to 10 minutes after alcohol consumption and may continue for several hours.

Pregnancy: Limited human data suggest that disulfiram may cause various abnormalities, including microcephaly, cleft palate, and club feet. Pregnancy outcomes attributed to disulfiram are difficult to assess due to the patient's possible use of ethanol and other drugs during pregnancy. It is not known if this drug is secreted in milk. Disulfiram should be used during pregnancy and lactation only if the potential benefits justify the potential risks to the fetus and neonate.

Treatment of Overdose: No specific treatment for disulfiram overdose is available.

Nursing Responsibilities: Key nursing implications for patients receiving disulfiram are included in Applied Clinical Judgment: Patients Receiving Pharmacotherapy for Substance Abuse Disorders.

Drugs Similar to Disulfiram (Antabuse)

Acamprosate and naltrexone are two additional medications for treating alcohol use disorder

Acamprosate: Acamprosate is an enteric-coated tablet approved in 2004 to maintain alcohol abstinence following a detoxification program. The drug reduces alcohol intake and does not cause a disulfiram-type reaction if the patient ingests alcohol. The mechanism of action of acamprosate is not well understood. The drug is well tolerated, with diarrhea being the most common side effect. It is contraindicated in patients with severe renal impairment. Animal studies showed teratogenicity and increased stillbirths and malformations. The drug is secreted in animal milk but adverse effects on the breastfed neonate are unknown.

Naltrexone (Vivitrol): Approved in 1984, naltrexone is an opioid antagonist that reduces cravings for alcohol and is associated with fewer drinking days and reduced likelihood of returning to drinking. Why does a drug that blocks opiate receptors have an effect on alcohol dependence? Although the mechanism is unclear, endogenous opioids appear to be involved in "reward pathways" for alcohol. Blocking the reward pathways with naltrexone affects the psychologic experience or craving characteristic of alcohol dependence. Naltrexone does not produce a "hangover" reaction when an individual consumes alcohol, as does disulfiram. Oral naltrexone may be given once daily for several months up to a year. An intramuscular (IM) suspension of naltrexone (Vivitrol) offers the convenience of once-a-month injections. Vivitrol is approved to treat opioid dependence as part of MAT. Successful use of naltrexone in alcohol or opioid rehabilitation programs is entirely dependent on patient adherence; if the patient stops taking naltrexone, the CNS effects of alcohol or opioids will return. Severe opioid withdrawal may occur if the drug is administered to a patient who has received opioids within 5 to 7 days prior to naltrexone dosing; thus, the drug is contraindicated in these patients. In addition, patients who relapse on naltrexone MAT will have a substantially reduced tolerance to opioids. Taking even small doses of opioids may cause life-threatening symptoms.

Naltrexone with bupropion (Contrave) is approved as an adjunct in the treatment of obesity. Naltrexone may be used off-label to treat nicotine withdrawal. Patients with serious hepatic impairment should not receive naltrexone. Animal studies did not show teratogenicity. The drug is secreted in human milk but adverse effects on the breastfed neonate are unknown.

Marijuana and Related Substances

27.8 Marijuana is the most frequently abused illicit substance.

Cannabinoids are natural products obtained from the hemp plant *Cannabis sativa*, which thrives in tropical climates. Cannabinoids include marijuana, hashish, and hash oil. Hashish is a solid, dried resin of the plant that is extremely potent. Hash oil is made by dissolving hashish or marijuana in a solvent such as alcohol, then allowing the liquid to evaporate to form a thick, oily concentrated form of cannabis.

Although more than 60 natural cannabinoid substances have been identified, the ingredient responsible for most of the psychoactive properties is **tetrahydrocannabinol (THC)**. Selective breeding and cultivation of *Cannabis* has produced varieties of the plant that produce much higher concentrations of THC than in previous decades. The THC content of marijuana varies from 12 to 30%; hashish from 20 to 60%; and hash oil from 30 to 80%.

Humans, as well as many other mammals, fish, and birds, produce small amounts of endogenous cannabinoids. These substances, known as endocannabinoids, are types of internal messengers that allow for intercellular communication. The exact purpose of the endocannabinoids has yet to be discovered, although they have some of the same characteristics as neurotransmitters and can modulate neuronal function. The endocannabinoids have some structural similarities to THC and bind to the same receptors, known as CB1 and CB2 receptors. Agonists and antagonists to CB1 and CB2 have been discovered, with the hope that the research may lead to new pharmacologic agents.

Marijuana is usually smoked as cigarettes (joints), but it may be used in pipes, brewed as teas, or added to food. When inhaled, marijuana produces effects that occur within minutes and last 1 to 3 hours. Oral absorption results in a lower serum blood level of the drug than does inhalation.

Use of marijuana slows motor activity, decreases coordination, and causes disconnected thoughts and euphoria. The experience is usually pleasant and involves laughter and an increase in the subjective perception of sounds, colors, and thoughts. Positive, friendly surroundings produce a more favorable drug experience than taking the drug alone. Time appears to pass more slowly. It increases thirst and a craving for food, particularly chocolate and other sweets. One hallmark symptom of marijuana use is red or bloodshot eyes, caused by dilation of blood vessels.

Following feelings of euphoria, the individual may become sleepy or depressed or experience paranoia. Driving is sometimes impaired, particularly when the drug is combined with alcohol. Because marijuana smoke is inhaled more deeply and held within the lungs for a longer period than cigarette smoke, marijuana smoke introduces four times more particulates (tar) into the lungs than does tobacco smoke. Smoking marijuana on a daily basis may increase the risk of respiratory disorders. Chronic use is associated with apathy and a lack of motivation in achieving or pursuing life goals, and very high doses may cause hallucinations.

The chronic use of marijuana such that it impairs normal interpersonal relationships, job performance or continuing to use the drug despite psychological or physical problems is called **cannabis use disorder**. Withdrawal symptoms from cannabis last 1 to 3 days and include continued cravings for the drug, anxiety, irritability, depression, headaches, and sleep disorders. Metabolites of THC remain in the body for months to years, allowing laboratory specialists to determine whether someone has used marijuana. For 3 to 5 days after a single use, THC can be detected in the urine.

Medical marijuana is a controversial topic; many healthcare providers and politicians are reluctant to endorse a drug that impairs judgment and may harm users. THC appears to reduce the pressure in the eyeball (glaucoma). Patients receiving antineoplastic drugs have reported that THC reduces severe nausea and vomiting. The ability of THC to reduce muscle spasticity may lead to applications for patients with multiple sclerosis and other spasticity disorders. In most cases, however, current drugs for these conditions have been demonstrated to be more effective and safer. Several states allow the medical and recreational use of marijuana, despite its being a Schedule I drug.

Also obtained from *Cannabis sativa*, cannabidiol (CBD) has no psychoactive effects, no abuse potential, and is readily available without a prescription (depending on state laws). Users claim that CBD reduces anxiety, improves sleep, and reduces chronic pain. Because CBD is marketed as a dietary supplement, the FDA does not regulate its safety, effectiveness, or purity. Because CBD has side effects and can potentially interact with medications such as warfarin (Coumadin), individuals should check with their healthcare provider before taking this substance.

Hallucinogens

27.9 Hallucinogens and club drugs cause an altered state of thought and perception.

Hallucinogens are a diverse class of chemicals that have in common the ability to produce an altered, dreamlike state of consciousness. These drugs sometimes produce a profound emotional experience, allowing the user to feel enhanced interconnectedness with others and experience a higher, spiritual plane of consciousness. Sometimes called *psychedelics*, the prototype drug for this class is LSD. More recently, some drugs in this class have become closely associated with the nightclub scene and are abused by those seeking a drug-induced experience from the music, dancing, and social contact, thus the name "club drugs."

For nearly all drugs of abuse, predictable symptoms occur in every user. Effects from hallucinogens, however, are highly variable and depend on the mood and expectations of the user and the surrounding environment in which the substance is used. Two people taking the same drug will report completely different experiences, and the same person may report different symptoms with each use. All hallucinogens are Schedule I drugs: They have no medical use.

LSD and Similar Hallucinogens

LSD, also called acid, the beast, blotter acid, and California sunshine, is derived from a fungus that grows on rye and other grains. LSD is nearly always administered PO and can be manufactured in capsule, tablet, or liquid form. A common and inexpensive method for distributing LSD is to place drops of the drug on paper, often containing the images of cartoon characters or graphics related to the drug culture, as shown in Figure 27.1. After drying, the paper is then cut into small squares to be ingested, with each square representing a "dose." The drug is extremely potent, with doses as low as 25 mcg producing an effect.

Immediately after use, LSD is widely distributed throughout the body, including the brain. Effects begin within an hour and may last from 6 to 12 hours. Although the exact mechanism of action of the drug is unclear, it affects the central and autonomic nervous systems, increasing blood pressure, elevating body temperature, dilating pupils, causing dry mouth, and increasing the heart rate.

LSD and other hallucinogens are used for their psychoactive, rather than their physical, effects. LSD users may experience symptoms such as laughter, visions, religious revelations, or deep personal insights. Common occurrences are hallucinations and after-images being projected onto people as they move. Users also report extremely bright lights and vivid colors. Some users hear voices; others report seeing sounds and hearing colors. Many experience a profound sense of truth and deep directed thoughts. The user's sense of time is altered.

Unpleasant experiences with LSD, known as "bad trips," can be terrifying and may include acute anxiety, panic attacks, confusion, severe depression, and paranoia. Repeated use may impair memory and the ability to reason. In extreme cases, patients may develop psychoses. One common adverse effect is flashbacks, in which the user experiences the effects of the drug again, sometimes weeks, months, or years after the drug was initially taken. Flashbacks may occur without warning.

LSD is considered a recreational drug: Users rarely become dependent on the drug, and there are no withdrawal symptoms. Continuous users will experience tolerance very quickly, sometimes after only 2 to 3 days.

The following drugs are considered similar to LSD and produce equivalent psychoactive effects:

- *Psilocybin.* The primary psychoactive substance in over 100 species of psilocybin mushrooms found in Mexico and Central America (see Figure 27.2). Known as "magic mushrooms" or "shrooms," psilocybin is a prodrug that is metabolized to its active metabolite psilocin. Possession of these mushroom species is illegal.

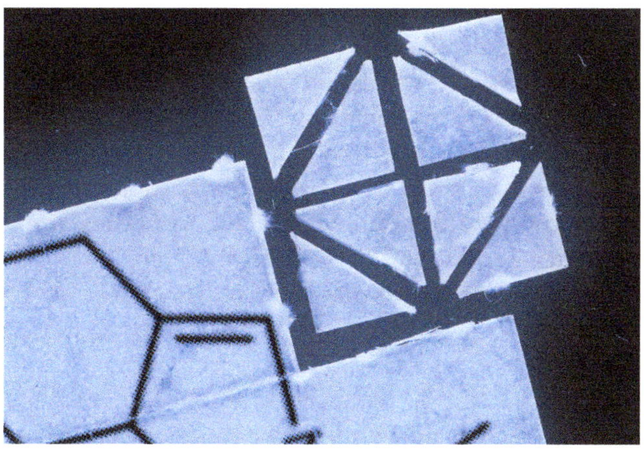

Figure 27.1 Liquid LSD is dropped on paper, dried and then separated by squares for dosing.
yurok/123RF.

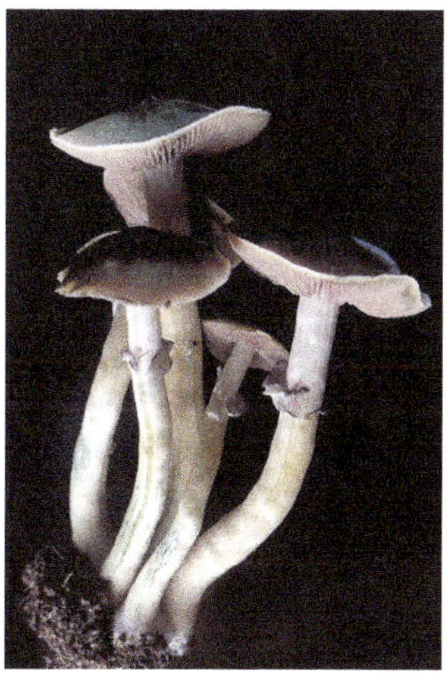

Figure 27.2 Fresh mushrooms containing the hallucinogen psilocybin.
Eric Limon/123RF.

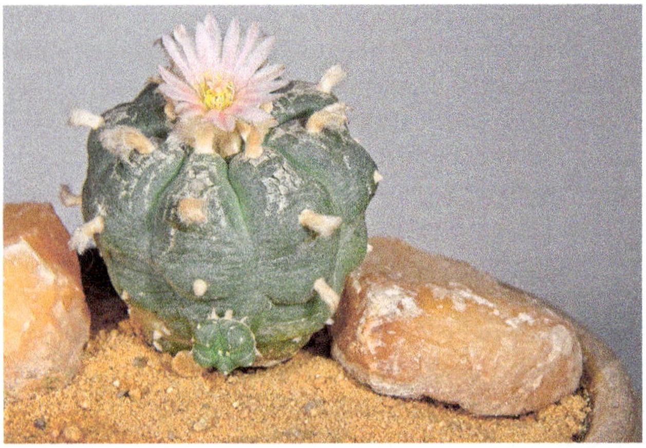

Figure 27.3 Peyote cactus containing the hallucinogen mescaline.
janfries/123RF.

Psilocybin and psilocin are listed as Schedule I drugs. The drug is taken by eating fresh psilocybin mushrooms or by ingesting dried extracts.

- *Mescaline.* Found in the peyote cactus and several other cacti species of Mexico and Central America, as shown in Figure 27.3. The drug is usually taken in capsules consisting of dried cactus. The cactus, which grows very slowly, has become rare due to overharvesting. In the United States, peyote use is illegal for all but members of the Native American Church, who use the drug in religious ceremonies.
- *Dimethyltryptamine (DMT).* A natural substance found in many species of plants in Central and South America and the Caribbean Islands. Like some of the other hallucinogens, DMT was used by native cultures in their spiritual ceremonies to induce visions. The drug is usually smoked but may be snuffed (snorted through the nostrils), injected, or taken PO.

Club Drugs and Miscellaneous Hallucinogens

Club drug refers to substances taken by people at festivals, dance clubs, all-night parties, and raves. It is a vague term that refers to a diverse group of abused substances that includes Ecstasy, GHB, methamphetamine, Rohypnol, ketamine, and other agents, usually ingested with alcohol. Not all club drugs are hallucinogens, and some of these are covered in other sections of this chapter. The following are descriptions of several major club drugs and some miscellaneous hallucinogens:

- *MDMA (3, 4-methylenedioxymethamphetamine, XTC, or Ecstasy).* An amphetamine originally synthesized for research purposes that has since become popular among teens and young adults. Taken PO, its effects last 3 to 6 hours. The drug is unique because it produces both stimulant and hallucinogenic effects simultaneously. MDMA enhances emotions and awareness, increases social and extroversion behaviors, and allows the user to stay awake and physically active for long periods. Chronic users exhibit behavioral disorders such as depression, anxiety, sleeplessness, and hostility. It has a narrow therapeutic index and overdoses may be fatal.
- *MDA (3, 4-methylenedioxyamphetamine).* Called the "love drug" due to a belief that it enhances sexual desire. This drug is sometimes a component of Ecstasy.
- *DOM (2, 5 dimethoxy-4-methylamphetamine).* A recreational drug popular at rave parties; also called STP, the drug has effects similar to LSD but with a longer duration.
- *Phencyclidine (PCP, crystal, angel dust).* Produces a trancelike state without loss of consciousness that may last for days. Once available as an anesthetic, the substance was removed from the market because patients experienced delirium and panic attacks as they recovered from anesthesia. The powdered drug is sometimes sprinkled on marijuana and smoked or it may be snorted or taken as tablets. Typical effects include slurred speech, detachment from reality, time distortion, and a sensation of floating in space. Phencyclidine is probably the most dangerous of the hallucinogens because high doses can cause severe and violent panic attacks, seizures, coma, and death.
- *Ketamine (K, kitkat, or special K).* Closely related to phencyclidine, ketamine has been used as an IV anesthetic to produce dissociative anesthesia. Liquid ketamine may be added to drinks, injected, or evaporated to a solid form, which is snorted or taken as pills. Effects are similar to those of phencyclidine, although they only last 35 to 40 minutes. Unconsciousness and amnesia may occur at high doses, and psychoses can be induced with continued use.

  Ketamine infusions are used off-label for patients with chronic pain, severe depression, bipolar disorder, or personality disorders that have not responded to first-line therapies. In 2019, the FDA approved a form of ketamine, esketamine (Spravato), as a nasal spray for treatment-resistant depression. Ketamine and esketamine are Schedule III controlled substances.
- *Dextromethorphan (DXM, robo).* A substance included in over-the-counter (OTC) cold remedies for its cough-suppressant properties. Abusers will purchase extra-strength remedies and consume large quantities to achieve dissociative effects similar to those of phencyclidine and ketamine. Effects include slurred speech, dizziness, drowsiness, euphoria, and lack of motor coordination. Overdose can cause brain damage, seizures, stroke, hypothermia, and death. Because cold medicines often contain multiple drugs, abusers of dextromethorphan may experience toxicity due to

overdoses of antihistamines, aspirin, or acetaminophen. Pure dextromethorphan is also available on the black market in high-dosage tablet form.

Central Nervous System Stimulants

27.10 Stimulants such as amphetamines and cocaine increase the activity of the central nervous system.

The stimulants include a diverse family of drugs with the ability to excite the CNS. Some are prescription drugs used to treat narcolepsy and attention-deficit/hyperactivity disorder (ADHD). As drugs of abuse, stimulants are taken to produce a sense of exhilaration, improve mental and physical performance, reduce appetite, or prolong wakefulness. Stimulants include the amphetamines, methylphenidate, and cocaine. Some CNS stimulants are club drugs. Caffeine is also included as a CNS stimulant, although it does not have the same type of negative health characteristics as the other drugs in this group.

Amphetamines and Methylphenidate

Amphetamines and methylphenidate are first-line drugs for ADHD, and their actions, uses, and adverse effects were detailed in Chapter 24. The discussion below is limited to their abuse potential.

Amphetamines produce their effects by increasing the activity of the endogenous neurotransmitters norepinephrine, serotonin (5-HT), and dopamine. High doses give the user a feeling of self-confidence, elevated mood, euphoria, and empowerment. Fatigue is diminished and the individual can perform at a high level of alertness for an extended time. Appetite is suppressed.

Many physiologic actions of amphetamines resemble those of sympathetic nervous system activation (see Chapter 15). Cardiovascular and respiratory activities are significantly affected, resulting in increased heart rate, high blood pressure, and increased breathing rate. Other symptoms include dilated pupils, sweating, and tremors. Overdoses of some stimulants lead to seizures, dysrhythmias, stroke, and cardiac arrest.

Although short-term use of amphetamines induces pleasurable feelings, long-term use causes restlessness, anxiety, defensiveness, and fits of rage, especially when the user is coming down from a prolonged drug experience. Chronic use can lead to a psychosis that closely resembles paranoid schizophrenia, although this condition usually resolves within several days after discontinuation of the drug. Tolerance to the pleasurable effects of amphetamines occurs very quickly, especially if the drugs are injected.

Current therapeutic applications of amphetamines are extremely limited. Most substance abusers obtain these drugs from illegal laboratories, which can produce some of the amphetamines using readily available chemicals. Physical dependence to amphetamines is unusual and withdrawal symptoms are not life-threatening. The only potentially serious symptom of amphetamine withdrawal is depression.

Methamphetamine, commonly called *ice*, is often used as a recreational drug for users who like the rush of euphoria that it gives them. It is usually administered in powder or crystal form (crystal meth) but it may also be smoked. Methamphetamine is a Schedule II drug marketed under the trade name Desoxyn, although most abusers obtain it from illegal methamphetamine laboratories. Methamphetamine can be easily synthesized from pseudoephedrine, an OTC decongestant. This has led to states placing pseudoephedrine behind the pharmacy counter and has motivated pharmaceutical manufacturers to find a replacement drug for pseudoephedrine in cold and flu remedies. A structural analog of methamphetamine, methcathinone (street name Cat), is made illegally and snorted, taken PO, or injected IV. Methcathinone is a Schedule I agent.

Methylphenidate is a Schedule II drug that has many of the same pharmacologic actions as cocaine and amphetamines. It is sometimes abused by adolescents and adults seeking euphoria, increased alertness, or appetite suppression. Tablets are crushed and snorted or dissolved in liquid and injected IV. Ritalin is sometimes mixed with heroin, a combination called a "speedball." Most Ritalin used illegally is obtained by diversion from legal prescriptions, by theft, or by patients selling or sharing their drugs.

Cocaine

Cocaine is a natural substance obtained from leaves of the coca plant, which grows in the Andes Mountains of South America. Natives in this region chew the coca leaves or make teas of the substance. Much of the cocaine entering the United States comes from Colombia and other South American countries. It was once used as an anesthetic for eye, nose, and throat surgery but is no longer used for this purpose.

Cocaine is a Schedule II drug that produces psychoactive and physiologic actions similar to the amphetamines, although its effects can be much more rapid and intense. Routes of administration include snorting, smoking, inhaling vapors, and injecting. In small doses, cocaine produces feelings of intense euphoria, a decrease in hunger and pain, illusions of physical strength, and increased sensory perception. Larger doses will increase these effects and cause rapid heartbeat, dysrhythmias, sweating, dilation of the pupils, and an elevated body temperature. The half-life of cocaine is short, 60 to 90 minutes when injected, and tolerance rapidly develops to the pleasurable aspects of the drug. Because of the short half-life, addicts may take cocaine at intervals of

10 to 45 minutes, sometimes for several consecutive days. As the abuser escalates the doses to produce a desired level of euphoria, cardiovascular damage may be progressive.

Cocaine readily crosses the placenta to produce marked effects on the fetus. Because the fetus does not have the hepatic enzymes necessary to metabolize cocaine, drug effects are prolonged. Reports of cocaine-related changes include increased risk of miscarriage, preterm labor, low birth weight, and, possibly, birth defects. Newborns have increased irritability, feeding difficulties, and are easily startled.

The adverse effects of cocaine use are essentially the same as those for amphetamines. Metabolism by the liver forms an active metabolite that is more toxic than cocaine itself. After the feelings of euphoria diminish, the cocaine user may be left with a sense of irritability, exhaustion, insomnia, depression, and extreme distrust. Some users report the sensation that insects are crawling under the skin. Users who snort cocaine develop a runny nose, a crusty redness around the nostrils, and deterioration of the nasal cartilage. Overdose can result in dysrhythmias, seizures, stroke, or death due to respiratory arrest. Psychologic dependence often leads to intense craving for the drug.

Caffeine

Caffeine is a natural substance found in the seeds, leaves, or fruits of more than 63 plant species throughout the world. Significant amounts of caffeine are consumed in chocolate, coffee, tea, soft drinks, and ice cream. Caffeine is sometimes added to OTC pain relievers and stimulants because it has been shown to increase the effectiveness of these medications. Caffeine is rapidly distributed throughout the body after ingestion, and several hours are needed to metabolize and eliminate the drug. Caffeine has a pronounced diuretic effect.

Caffeine is considered a CNS stimulant because it produces increased mental alertness, restlessness, nervousness, irritability, and insomnia. The physical effects of caffeine include dilation of the respiratory passages, increased blood pressure, increased production of stomach acid, and changes in blood glucose levels. Repeated use of caffeine may result in physical dependence and tolerance. Withdrawal symptoms include severe headaches, fatigue, depression, and impaired performance of daily activities. A drug prototype feature for caffeine is included in Chapter 24.

Nicotine

27.11 Nicotine is a powerful and highly addictive cardiovascular and central nervous system stimulant.

Although nicotine is sometimes considered a CNS stimulant because it enhances alertness, its actions and long-term consequences place it in a class by itself. Nicotine is unique among abused substances in that it is legal, strongly addictive, and highly carcinogenic. Furthermore, tobacco use can cause harmful effects to those in the immediate area due to secondhand smoke. Patients often do not consider tobacco use disorder to be a type of substance abuse. It is the most common form of chemical dependence in the United States. Tobacco use among all age groups has been declining.

The most common method by which nicotine enters the body is through the inhalation of cigarette, pipe, or cigar smoke. Tobacco smoke contains several thousand chemicals, a significant number of which are carcinogens. The primary addictive drug present in cigarette smoke is nicotine, which reaches the brain in only 15 seconds, with effects that last from 30 minutes to several hours. Although nicotine has a half-life of only 2 to 3 hours, it accumulates in the body and is slowly released from the tissues, giving the patient virtually 24-hour exposure to the drug.

Nicotine affects many body systems, including the nervous, cardiovascular, and endocrine systems. Nicotine promotes the release of epinephrine and has a direct stimulatory effect on the reticular activating system of the brain, causing symptoms that range from increased alertness and ability to focus to feelings of relaxation or lightheadedness. The psychoactive effects of smoking are generally described as pleasurable. The cardiovascular effects of nicotine include an accelerated heart rate and increased blood pressure, caused by activation of nicotinic receptors located throughout the autonomic nervous system (see Chapter 12). The cardiovascular effects of nicotine are particularly serious in smokers who are taking oral contraceptives—their risk of a fatal heart attack is five times greater than that of nonsmokers. Muscular tremors may occur with moderate doses of nicotine, and convulsions result from very high doses. Nicotine produces lower body weight by reducing appetite and increasing body metabolism. Chronic use leads to emphysema, heart disease, and lung cancer. Smokers are much more likely to be infertile, and tobacco use during pregnancy can cause birth defects and lower birth weight.

Both psychologic and physical dependence occur relatively quickly with nicotine. Patients tend to continue their drug use for many years, despite overwhelming medical evidence that the quality of their life will be adversely affected and their lifespan shortened. Furthermore, a large majority of smokers try to quit each year and are unsuccessful and state that they wish they had never started the habit.

Discontinuation of tobacco results in a withdrawal syndrome that includes extreme craving, agitation, impaired concentration, weight gain, anxiety, and headache. The syndrome peaks at 24 to 48 hours after the last dose and may continue over several weeks. Symptoms vary in intensity among patients and are not related to dose or duration of use; those who are light smokers or who have smoked for a shorter length of time do not necessarily have less intense withdrawal symptoms. Approximately 90% of individuals who successfully stop smoking do so without any treatment.

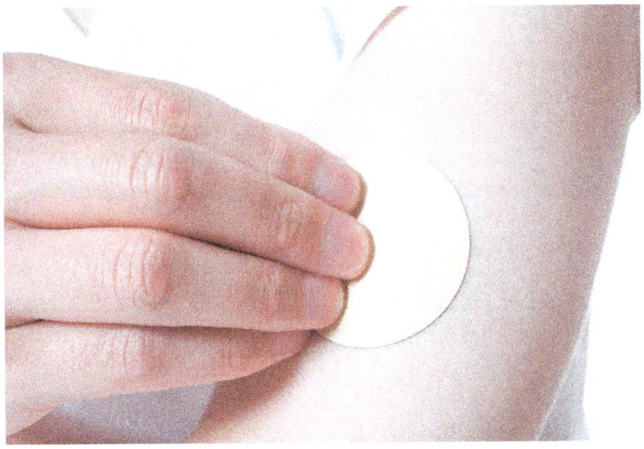

Figure 27.4 Transdermal patch being applied as part of a nicotine replacement program.
PaylessImages/123rf.com.

Nicotine replacement therapy (NRT) is based on the assumption that the blood level of nicotine is what drives people to continue smoking. When blood nicotine levels fall, the individual begins to experience early symptoms of withdrawal, which are quickly eliminated by smoking another cigarette. Indeed, blood nicotine levels have clearly been shown to influence smoking behavior. For example, if a smoker switches to low-nicotine cigarettes, he or she will take longer and more frequent puffs. NRT delivery systems include transdermal patches (Figure 27.4), nasal sprays, and chewing gum that raise serum nicotine levels and help patients to deal with the unpleasant withdrawal symptoms. Tobacco use, however, has a strong psychologic component and simply replacing nicotine with patches or gum is ineffective for a large number of patients.

Two prescription medications are used to promote smoking cessation. Bupropion, classified as an antidepressant, reduces cravings for nicotine and has been found to double the likelihood of becoming tobacco-free if it is taken for 3 to 6 months. Therapy generally begins 1 to 2 weeks before smoking cessation to lessen the severity of withdrawal symptoms. Bupropion is sometimes given concurrently with NRT. Common side effects include insomnia, agitation, headache, and dry mouth.

Varenicline (Chantix) is approved to manage nicotine withdrawal in patients seeking smoking cessation. Both bupropion and varenicline carry a warning that advises patients of serious neuropsychiatric events such as hostility or suicidal thoughts that can occur during therapy or shortly after discontinuation of the drug.

PROTOTYPE DRUG | Varenicline (Chantix)

Classification **Therapeutic:** Drug for smoking cessation
Pharmacologic: Nicotinic receptor agonist

Therapeutic Effects and Uses: Approved in 2006, the only indication for varenicline is smoking cessation treatment. Doses are gradually increased over an 8-day period and maintained for 12 to 24 weeks to reduce withdrawal symptoms and cravings for smoking. Therapy with varenicline may begin after smoking has been discontinued, or the dose may be gradually increased while tobacco use declines. The goal is often to reach complete smoking cessation by 12 weeks, and then continue varenicline for another 12 weeks to improve the chances for long-term abstinence.

Mechanism of Action: Varenicline activates nicotinic acetylcholine receptors in the brain and blocks nicotine from reaching the brain's receptors. It blocks some of the pleasurable sensations of tobacco use, should the patient relapse and start smoking again.

Pharmacokinetics:

Route(s)	PO
Absorption	Completely absorbed
Distribution	Bound to plasma protein (20%)
Primary metabolism	Mostly unmetabolized
Primary excretion	Renal
Onset of action	3–4 h
Duration of action	24 h

Adverse Effects: Nausea and vomiting, vivid or unusual dreams, and constipation are the most common side effects. Rare adverse events include angioedema, serious skin reactions, and myocardial infarction. Varenicline contains a warning that serious neuropsychiatric events can occur during therapy or shortly after discontinuation of the drug. Patients experiencing unusual changes in behavior such as agitation, hostility, depressed mood, paranoia or thoughts of suicide should contact their healthcare provider immediately. Some patients experience an increase in the effects of alcohol.

Contraindications/Precautions: The only contraindication is a history of serious skin reactions with varenicline.

Drug Interactions: When used in combination with NRT, varenicline causes an increased incidence of nausea and vomiting, headache, dizziness, and fatigue, which may result in premature termination of therapy. Concurrent use with alcohol has been reported to cause aggressive behavior.

Pregnancy: Animal studies did not show teratogenicity. It is not known if varenicline is secreted in milk or if it has adverse effects on the breastfed neonate. Large human epidemiological studies have not shown an increased risk for major birth defects in women taking varenicline compared with women who smoke.

Treatment of Overdose: No specific treatment for varenicline overdose is available.

Clinician Responsibilities: Key clinical implications for patients receiving varenicline are included in Applied Clinical Judgment: Patients Receiving Pharmacotherapy for Substance Abuse Disorders.

Drugs Similar to Varenicline (Chantix)

There are no drugs for smoking cessation that are similar to varenicline.

Inhalants

27.12 Inhalant abuse occurs when patients breathe the fumes of vaporized substances.

Inhalants are a diverse group of substances that have in common the ability to vaporize or form a gas at room temperature. Some are already in gaseous form, whereas others are liquids that have the property of volatility—rapid evaporation when exposed to air. Sometimes the liquids are heated to increase the speed or extent of vaporization. Most drugs in this class are placed in a paper or plastic bag or soaked on a cloth and deeply inhaled. Inhaling the fumes is known as huffing.

Inhalants differ greatly in their chemical structures and include nearly any chemical that can be vaporized. These products are readily available and include adhesives and glues, aerosols, cleaning agents, solvents, and fuels. The highest use of inhalants is found among teens and preteens, probably because these agents can be found in every household (see Table 27.3). Legal anesthetics such as nitrous oxide that are sometimes abused by medical personnel are also classified as inhalants and are discussed in Chapter 26.

The inhalation route affords almost instantaneous drug action and, because most of the inhalants are lipid soluble, the substances quickly enter the brain. The specific psychoactive effects depend on the inhalant used but generally include lightheadedness, drowsiness, exhilaration, and euphoria. Hallucinations are common. Symptoms of inhalant abuse often resemble alcohol intoxication. Because most psychoactive effects of inhalants are transient and disappear within minutes, the user may repeat the drug use multiple times over a period of several hours. Coma and death are possible with repeated exposure or high doses.

Because most inhalant abuse is sporadic, physical dependence is not observed. Some of the inhalants cause hangover-like symptoms after the psychoactive effects wear off. Chronic effects can be serious and permanent, with the most obvious effects on the nervous system. Cognitive impairment, tremors, loss of coordination, hallucinations, psychosis, and dementia may be observed. Nephrotoxicity is common with certain inhalants.

Treatment for inhalant use disorder is symptomatic. Long-term behavioral therapy may be needed to reinforce to the patient that permanent damage will result from chronic, continued abuse.

Table 27.3 Monitoring the Future Study: Trends in Prevalence of Inhalants for 8th Graders, 10th Graders, and 12th Graders; 2019 (in percent)*

Drug	Time Period	8th Graders	10th Graders	12th Graders
Inhalants	Lifetime	9.5	6.80	5.30
	Past Year	4.7	2.80	1.90
	Past Month	2.10	1.10	0.89

Source: From Inhalants: How Many Teens Use Inhalants? National Institute on Drug Abuse for Teens, 2019. Retrieved from https://teens.drugabuse.gov/drug-facts/inhalants.

CONNECTIONS: APPLIED CLINICAL JUDGMENT

Patients Receiving Pharmacotherapy for Substance Use Disorders

Key Assessment Data

- History of current condition, baseline vital signs, weight, physical exam; history of hepatic, renal, respiratory, cardiovascular, or neurologic disease; medications, allergy, and substance use history; pregnancy or breastfeeding status. Obtain a dietary history, especially noting possible vitamin deficiencies.
- Assess for the presence and level of pain. Use objective screening tools when possible.
- Ongoing assessment during drug therapy includes pain assessment, appropriate laboratory findings (e.g., hepatic or renal function studies), vital signs, and adherence to medication therapy.

Desired Therapeutic Outcomes

Improvement is observed and measurable in decreased use or abstinence from the substance.

Minimizing Adverse Effects

- As an opioid, buprenorphine may cause opioid-related adverse effects in higher dosages. Disulfiram may cause intense reactions when alcohol is ingested or absorbed through the skin and may cause cardiovascular effects such as dysrhythmias, chest pain, and respiratory depression. Continue to monitor vital signs, including respiratory rate, pulse, and blood pressure, as ordered in patients receiving buprenorphine and disulfiram. As an opioid, buprenorphine may cause opioid-related adverse effects in higher dosages. Disulfiram may cause intense reactions when alcohol is ingested or absorbed through the skin and may cause cardiovascular effects such as dysrhythmias, chest pain, and respiratory depression.
- The sublingual form of buprenorphine should be taken by placing the tablet under the tongue and allowing it to dissolve. Do not chew or swallow the tablet. If more than one tablet is used, place all tablets under the tongue at the same time.
- Varenicline may cause serious neuropsychiatric effects. Monitor for changes in behavior, including depression, hostility, agitation, or thoughts of suicide.
- Serious dermatologic reactions including angioedema have been noted in patients taking varenicline. Monitor for skin rashes and facial or throat edema.
- Additional NRT should not be used during smoking cessation therapy with varenicline as it may increase the incidence of adverse drug effects and may lead to early cessation of therapy.

CONNECTIONS: APPLIED CLINICAL JUDGMENT *(continued)*

Patients Receiving Pharmacotherapy for Substance Use Disorders

Patient and Caregiver Education

- Maintaining consistency of treatment to decrease substance use and eventual abstinence is the goal of therapy. Nonpharmacologic measures such as supportive therapy (e.g., Alcoholics Anonymous, Narcotics Anonymous, or smoking cessation groups) may be beneficial during therapy and assist in maintaining a substance-free state after treatment.
- Maintain the buprenorphine dosage as prescribed and do not increase the dose.
- All forms of alcohol must be avoided when taking disulfiram, including skin preparations and mouth rinses that contain alcohol. Adverse reactions may occur up to 14 days after the last dose of disulfiram.
- Additional NRT should not be used during smoking cessation therapy.
- While taking varenicline, immediately report any unusual changes in mood or behavior to the provider.
- While taking varenicline, immediately report any unusual rashes, changes in skin condition, or swelling of the tongue, face, or throat to the provider.
- Other NRT, including OTC patches and gum, should not be used while taking varenicline.

Prescribing Considerations

- Patients should not receive more than a 7-day supply of MAT medication at the time of initiation.
- The state Prescription Monitoring Program database must be checked at 3-month intervals for the first 6 months of MAT treatment.
- Urine drug screens must be performed during the first month of MAT.
- Naltrexone should not be prescribed for clients who have used or have shown signs of acute opioid withdrawal in the last 3 days, who are pregnant, or who have decompensated liver disease.
- Buprenorphine is only indicated for women who are pregnant and meet DSM-IV criteria for opioid dependence or DSM-5 criteria for moderate or severe opioid use disorder.
- Use caution in prescribing acamprosate and ensure patients have a creatinine clearance greater than 30ml/min.

Anabolic Steroids

27.13 Anabolic steroids are abused for their ability to increase muscle strength.

All of the drugs presented thus far in this chapter have in common the ability to affect the CNS and produce psychoactive effects. Many produce euphoria, some induce relaxation, and yet others enhance alertness. In most cases, the user views the drug experience as pleasurable and the drug effects are experienced soon after it is taken, sometimes within seconds. Anabolic steroids, however, are not taken for their CNS actions, and their desirable effects may be delayed for weeks or months.

Anabolic steroids are similar to testosterone, the primary male sex hormone or androgen. The term *anabolic* means "growth" or "building up." Because these substances can add to skeletal muscle mass and increase strength, they are usually abused in an attempt to enhance athletic performance. Do these drugs actually boost performance? The answer is a qualified yes. The most important aspects of athletic performance are skill, training, and confidence. If these factors are equal among performers, anabolic steroids may indeed provide an extra boost in performance, which is all-important in a competitive sport such as track, downhill skiing, or swimming where a few hundredths of a second can mean the difference between first and sixth place. On the other hand, no amount of steroid is able to overcome lack of athletic skill or inadequate training. Amateur and professional sports organizations have banned the use of these drugs and athletes may be eliminated from competition if they test positive for anabolic steroids. Some abusers take anabolic steroids to enhance their appearance and self-confidence, rather than for athletic competition.

Anabolic steroids have legitimate medical uses as replacement therapy for men who secrete insufficient quantities of testosterone and they are used to treat certain cancers. Doses used by abusers, however, are 10 to 100 times higher than those required for therapeutic use.

Anabolic steroids may be taken as tablets, as IM injections, or applied as ointments or as a transdermal patch. Abusers may take two or more different types of steroids concurrently, sometimes by different routes, a practice called "stacking." The drugs may be taken in a cyclic pattern called "pyramiding" in which the dose is progressively increased over 6 to 12 weeks, then slowly decreased to zero. Abusers believe that this is a safer and more effective way to obtain benefits from the drugs.

One of the ironies of steroid abuse is that the very drug that is being taken to enhance appearance and performance eventually produces serious consequences that have the opposite effect. Men may believe that anabolic steroids make them appear more masculine, but the drugs can cause infertility, impotence, testicular atrophy, and breast enlargement (gynecomastia). Women taking anabolic steroids will develop masculine characteristics, excessive growth of body hair (hirsutism), shrinking of breast size, menstrual irregularities, and deepening of the voice. The most serious adverse effects, in both men and women, include hepatic cysts, elevated cholesterol, myocardial infarction, and stroke. Personality changes include aggression, violent behavior, depression, insomnia, anorexia, and decreased libido.

Anabolic steroids are classified as Schedule II drugs due to their abuse potential. In an attempt to stem the rising abuse of these drugs, Congress passed the Anabolic Steroid Control Act of 2004 to control 26 different steroid precursors, such as androstenedione (Andro). Some companies were legally selling these precursors as dietary supplements, despite the fact that these agents are metabolized to steroids in the body and essentially carry the same risks. It is interesting to note that one of the most popular supplements, dehydroepiandrosterone (DHEA), was specifically and intentionally omitted from that list and remains legal. DHEA is a natural steroid precursor secreted by the adrenal gland that is claimed to have antiaging and performance-enhancing properties.

Understanding Chapter 27

Key Concepts Summary

27.1 A wide variety of substances may be abused by patients.

27.2 Drugs with a potential for abuse are restricted by the Controlled Substances Act and are categorized into schedules.

27.3 Addiction is an overwhelming compulsion to continue repeated drug use.

27.4 Physical and psychologic dependence lead to continued drug-seeking behavior despite negative health and social consequences.

27.5 A withdrawal syndrome is a set of characteristic symptoms that occurs when an abused substance is discontinued.

27.6 Tolerance occurs when the body adapts to a drug and larger doses are needed to produce a therapeutic effect.

27.7 Depressants, which include sedatives, opioids, and alcohol, decrease the activity of the central nervous system.

27.8 Marijuana is the most frequently abused illicit substance.

27.9 Hallucinogens and club drugs cause an altered state of thought and perception.

27.10 Stimulants such as amphetamines and cocaine increase the activity of the central nervous system.

27.11 Nicotine is a powerful and highly addictive cardiovascular and central nervous system stimulant.

27.12 Inhalant abuse occurs when patients breathe the fumes of vaporized substances.

27.13 Anabolic steroids are abused for their ability to increase muscle strength.

CASE STUDY: Making the Patient Connection

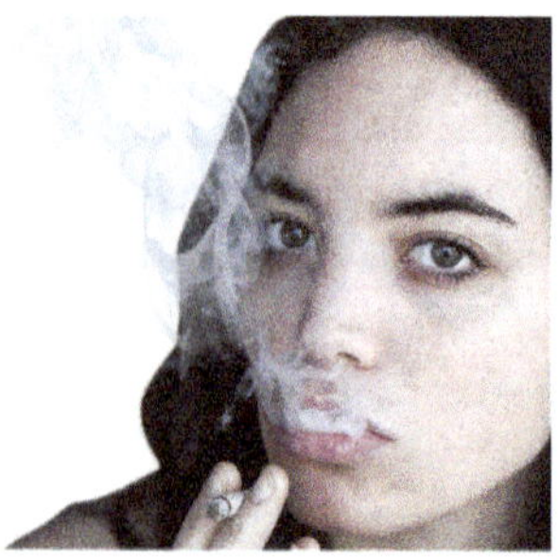

Remember the patient "Jamie Wilkins" at the beginning of the chapter? Now read the remainder of the case study. Based on the information presented within this chapter, respond to the critical thinking questions that follow.

Jamie Wilkins has come to the counseling clinic to get information and advice about her pregnancy and drug use. She is a 19-year-old woman who has been living with her boyfriend for the past 18 months. Since she moved in, she has been a daily user of heroin.

Jamie has a long history of substance abuse. When she was 14 years old, her stepfather sexually abused her on a regular basis. To cope with the guilt and shame, she began using alcohol and marijuana. On her 16th birthday, Jamie ran away from home and never returned. Since then she has done anything and everything possible to survive, including selling herself for sex.

To support herself and her heroin addiction, Jamie has become a prostitute. She states that she usually drinks at least four to five beers before she walks the streets at night. If she cannot score enough heroin, she will smoke crack or take Valium just to "mellow out." Jamie says that her drug abuse is only to calm her nerves and get her through the night. In periods when she was not able to obtain drugs, she states she felt sick with trembling and perfuse sweating.

However, she is convinced that she can stop anytime she wishes.

Jamie reports that she has not had a menstrual period in 2 months and her breasts are swollen and tender. She is certain she is pregnant, although she has not been tested, and is confused about what to do. She is hopeful that her unemployed boyfriend is the father but is not totally sure. She believes that if she stops working, he will abandon her, and there will be no means to support herself or a baby.

Critical Thinking Questions

1. How would you classify Jamie's substance abuse: physical dependence or psychologic dependence, or both? Explain.
2. Create a list of abused substances reported by Jamie. What symptoms of withdrawal would you expect with each?
3. What effect will Jamie's substance abuse have on her unborn baby? Should Jamie stop using drugs while pregnant? Why or why not?
4. As the nurse, describe your approach in dealing with this patient. What is one evidence-based intervention you should consider when speaking with Jamie?
5. Addiction depends on multiple variables such as drug, user, and environmental factors. Based on the case study, describe how each variable contributes to Jamie's substance abuse.

Additional Case Study

A neighbor reports that patient Martin Thomas was discovered wandering the halls in his apartment building in a confused state. The neighbor states that Martin called him by the wrong name even though they have known each other for several years. Martin was agitated about not being able to find the bus stop. In the emergency department, Martin appears apprehensive, diaphoretic, and trembling. His nose and cheeks are red with spider veins, and his abdomen is noticeably distended. He tells you that up until 3 days ago, he consumed alcohol daily. However, because he has no money, he cannot buy any liquor and has not been drinking.

1. Define *delirium tremens*. What is the treatment priority for this condition?
2. Discuss how food or beverages can increase the excretion rate of alcohol.
3. Describe the effects of alcohol on the central nervous system. Is alcohol a stimulant or a depressant?

Chapter Review

1. The patient returned from major surgery 3 hours ago and requests medication for pain. In considering the best action for this patient, the nurse knows that:

1. Prescription drugs rarely cause addiction when used according to accepted medical protocol for the limited time prescribed.
2. All drugs should be withheld until the patient's past substance abuse history is evaluated.
3. It is best to wait until the patient can no longer tolerate the pain to avoid addiction problems.
4. Patients often request analgesia when it is not really needed.

2. Which of the following statements made by the patient recovering from a substance use disorder would indicate high potential for relapse?

1. "I need the help of a support system to stop using."
2. "After I stop using, I will no longer have a desire to use drugs."
3. "Whom I hang out with doesn't make any difference in whether or not I use drugs."
4. "Talking with other recovering addicts will help me cope."

3. A nurse is teaching a patient who will begin varenicline (Chantix) for smoking cessation. Which of the following instructions will the nurse give the patient? (Select all that apply.)

1. Doses will be increased over a week's period and the drug used for up to 6 months.
2. Smoking may continue because the drug blocks the harmful effects of nicotine.
3. The drug is not known to cause any adverse effects and has an excellent safety profile.
4. Any unusual rashes, skin reactions, or facial edema should be reported immediately.
5. Any unusual changes in behavior including depression, hostility, or thoughts of suicide should be reported immediately.

4. Which parameter is most critical when a nurse is assessing a patient with an overdose of sedatives?
   1. Cardiac stimulation
   2. Respiratory suppression
   3. Hepatic dysfunction
   4. Depression of consciousness

5. A 22-year-old heroin addict is exhibiting withdrawal symptoms. Which symptoms of withdrawal does the nurse expect?
   1. Somnolence, lethargy, and fatigue
   2. Dry skin, rash, and itching
   3. Paranoia, hallucinations, and delusions
   4. Chills, runny nose, and muscle spasms

6. While teaching the patient about disulfiram (Antabuse), which of the following should the nurse instruct the patient to avoid?
   1. Mouthwash, alcoholic beverages, and over-the-counter cold medications
   2. Dairy products such as milk, cream, and yogurt
   3. Foods high in iron such as green leafy vegetables
   4. Driving or operating machinery while taking this medication

See Appendix A for answers to critical thinking questions, case study questions, and review questions.

References

American Psychiatric Association. (2013). *Diagnostic and statistical manual of mental disorders* (5th ed.). Author.

Aventian, G. K., Fluty, P., Mazzella, S., Koppa, D., Heye, V., & Hebbar, P. (2018). Use of naloxone nasal spray 4 mg in the community setting: A survey of use by community organizations. *Current Medical Research and Opinion*, *34*, 573–576. https://doi.org/10.1080/03007995.2017.1334637

Dunne, R. B. (2018). Prescribing naloxone for opioid overdose intervention. *Pain Management*, *8*, 197–208. https://doi.org/10.2217./pmt-2017-0065

Kann, L., McManus, T., Harris, W. A., Shanklin, S. L., Flint, K. H., Queen, B., et al. (2018). Youth risk behavior surveillance—United States, 2017. *MMWR Surveillance Summaries*, *67*(8), 1. https://doi.org/10.15585/mmwr.ss6708a1

National Institute on Drug Abuse for Teens. (2019). *Inhalants: How many teens use inhalants?* https://teens.drugabuse.gov/drug-facts/inhalants

Rees, D. I., Sabia, J. J., Argys, L. M., Dave, D., & Latshaw, J. (2019). With a little help from my friends: The effects of Good Samaritan and naloxone access laws on opioid-related deaths. *Journal of Law & Ethics*, *62*. https://doi.org/10.1086/700703

SAFE Project. (2020). *State naloxone access rules and resources.* https://www.safeproject.us/naloxone-awareness-project/state-rules/

Substance Abuse and Mental Health Services Administration. (2019). *Key substance use and mental health indicators in the United States: Results from the 2018 National Survey on Drug Use and Health* (HHS Publication No. PEP19-5068, NSDUH Series H-54). https://www.samhsa.gov/data/sites/default/files/cbhsq-reports/NSDUHNationalFindingsReport2018/NSDUHNationalFindingsReport2018.pdf

U.S. Food and Drug Administration. (2021). *FDA facts: Abuse-deterrent opioid medications.* https://www.fda.gov/drugs/postmarket-drug-safety-information-patients-and-providers/abuse-deterrent-opioid-analgesics

Selected Bibliography

Carinci, A. J. (2020). Abuse-deterrent opioid analgesics: a guide for clinicians. *Pain Management*, *10*(1), 55–62. https://doi.org/10.2217/pmt-2019-0052

Chan, B., Kondo, K., Ayers, C., Freeman, M., Montgomery, J., Paynter, R., & Kansagara, D. (2018). *Pharmacotherapy for stimulant use disorders: A systematic review.* U.S. Department of Veterans Affairs. https://pubmed.ncbi.nlm.nih.gov/30715830/

Claire, R., Chamberlain, C., Davey, M. A., Cooper, S. E., Berlin, I., Leonardi-Bee, J., & Coleman, T. (2020). Pharmacological interventions for promoting smoking cessation during pregnancy. *Cochrane Database of Systematic Reviews*, Issue 3, Article No. CD010078. https://doi.org/10.1002/14651858.CD010078.pub3

Dixon, D. W. (2020). *Opioid abuse and treatment.* Medscape. https://emedicine.medscape.com/article/287790-overview

Grinspoon, P. (2018). *Cannabadiol (CBD)—what we know and what we don't.* https://www.health.harvard.edu/blog/cannabidiol-cbd-what-we-know-and-what-we-dont-2018082414476

Hyland, A., Kasza, K. A., Borek, N., Kimmel, H. L., Taylor, K. A., Compton, W. M., et al. (2020). Overview of tobacco use transitions for population health. *Tobacco Control, 29*(Suppl. 3), s134–s138. http://dx.doi.org/10.1136/tobaccocontrol-2019-055367

Khan, M., & Thomas, A. (2020). Steroids, dissociatives, club drugs, inhalants, and hallucinogens. *Absolute Addiction Psychiatry Review*, pp. 205–230. https://doi.org/10.1007/978-3-030-33404-8_13

Klein, J. W. (2016). Pharmacotherapy for substance use disorders. *Medical Clinics of North America, 100*, 891–910. https://doi.org/10.1016/j.mcna.2016.03.011

Kranzler, H. R., & Soyka, M. (2018). Diagnosis and pharmacotherapy of alcohol use disorder: A review. *Journal of the American Medical Association, 320*(8), 815–824. https://doi.org/10.1001/jama.2018.11406

Kreek, M. J., Reed, B., & Butelman, E. R. (2019). Current status of opioid addiction treatment and related preclinical research. *Science Advances, 5*(10), eaax9140. https://doi.org/10.1126/sciadv.aax9140

Lee, N. K., Jenner, L., Harney, A., & Cameron, J. (2018). Pharmacotherapy for amphetamine dependence: A systematic review. *Drug and Alcohol Dependence, 191*, 309–337. https://doi.org/10.1016/j.drugalcdep.2018.06.038

McKeown, N. (2020). *Withdrawal syndromes*. Medscape. https://emedicine.medscape.com/article/819502-overview#a1

Nielsen, S., Gowing, L., Sabioni, P., & Le Foll, B. (2019). Pharmacotherapies for cannabis dependence. *Cochrane Database of Systematic Reviews*, Issue 1, Article No. CD008940. https://doi.org/10.1002/14651858.CD008940.pub3

Pourmand, A., Mazer-Amirshahi, M., Chistov, S., Li, A., & Park, M. (2018). Designer drugs: Review and implications for emergency management. *Human & Experimental Toxicology, 37*(1), 94–101. https://doi.org/10.1177/0960327117698542

Reus, V. I., Fochtmann, L. J., Bukstein, O., Eyler, A. E., Hilty, D. M., Horvitz-Lennon, M., et al. (2018). The American Psychiatric Association practice guideline for the pharmacological treatment of patients with alcohol use disorder. *American Journal of Psychiatry, 175*(1), 86–90. https://doi.org/10.1176/appi.ajp.2017.1750101

Ronsley, C., Nolan, S., Knight, R., Hayashi, K., Klimas, J., Walley, A., et al. (2020). Treatment of stimulant use disorder: A systematic review of reviews. *PloS One, 15*(6), e0234809. https://doi.org/10.1371/journal.pone.0234809

Soghoian, S. (2019). *Disulfiram toxicity*. Medscape. http://emedicine.medscape.com/article/814525-overview

Substance Abuse and Mental Health Services Administration. (2020). *Medication-assisted treatment*. https://www.samhsa.gov/medication-assisted-treatment

Unit 5

Pharmacology of the Cardiovascular System

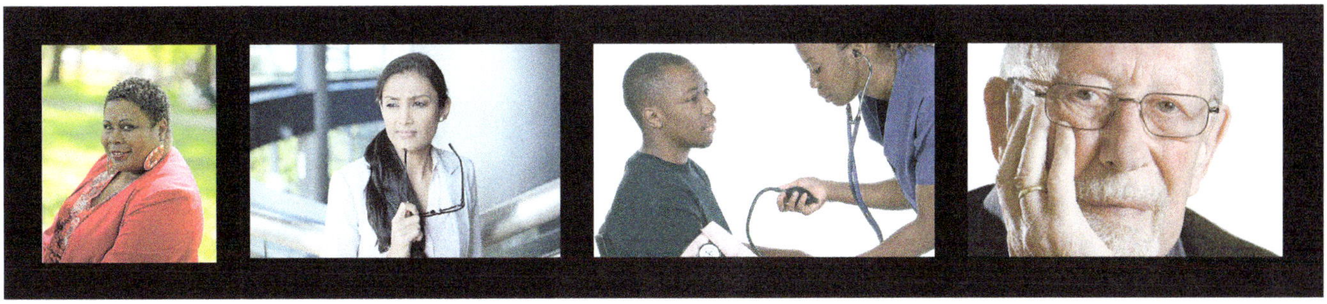

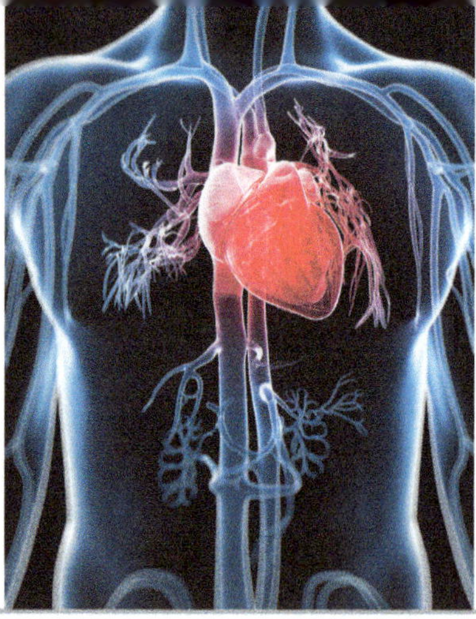

Chapter 28
Review of the Cardiovascular System

Chapter Outline

- Structure and Function of the Cardiovascular System
- Functions and Properties of Blood
  - Components of Blood
  - Hemostasis
- Cardiac Structure and Function
  - Cardiac Muscle
  - Coronary Arteries
  - Cardiac Conduction System
  - Cardiac Output
- Hemodynamics and Blood Pressure
  - Hemodynamic Factors Affecting Blood Pressure
  - Neural Regulation of Blood Pressure
  - Hormonal Influences on Blood Pressure

Learning Outcomes

After reading this chapter, the student should be able to:

1. Describe the major structures of the cardiovascular system.
2. Identify the components of blood and their functions.
3. Construct a flowchart diagramming the primary steps of hemostasis.
4. Describe the structure of the heart and the function of the myocardium.
5. Describe the role of the coronary arteries in supplying the myocardium with oxygen.
6. Illustrate the flow of electrical impulses through the normal heart.
7. Explain the major factors affecting cardiac output.
8. Explain the effects of cardiac output, peripheral resistance, and blood volume on hemodynamics.
9. Discuss how the vasomotor center, baroreceptors, chemoreceptors, and hormones regulate blood pressure.

Key Terms

Definitions of the terms in bold may be found in the Glossary.

It is likely that the nurse will administer more cardiovascular drugs than any other class of medications. Why is this the case? First, healthcare providers have discovered the huge benefits of keeping blood pressure and blood lipid values within normal limits to prevent heart attack and stroke. Second, the heart and vessels weaken over time and, as the average lifespan of the population increases, pharmacotherapy will be needed to treat the chronic cardiovascular diseases of older adults.

A comprehensive knowledge of cardiovascular anatomy and physiology is essential to understanding cardiovascular pharmacology, which encompasses the next 11 chapters of this text. The purpose of this chapter is to offer a brief review of the components of the structure and function of the cardiovascular system that will be important to understand for pharmacotherapy. For more comprehensive treatments of these topics, the student should refer to an anatomy and physiology textbook.

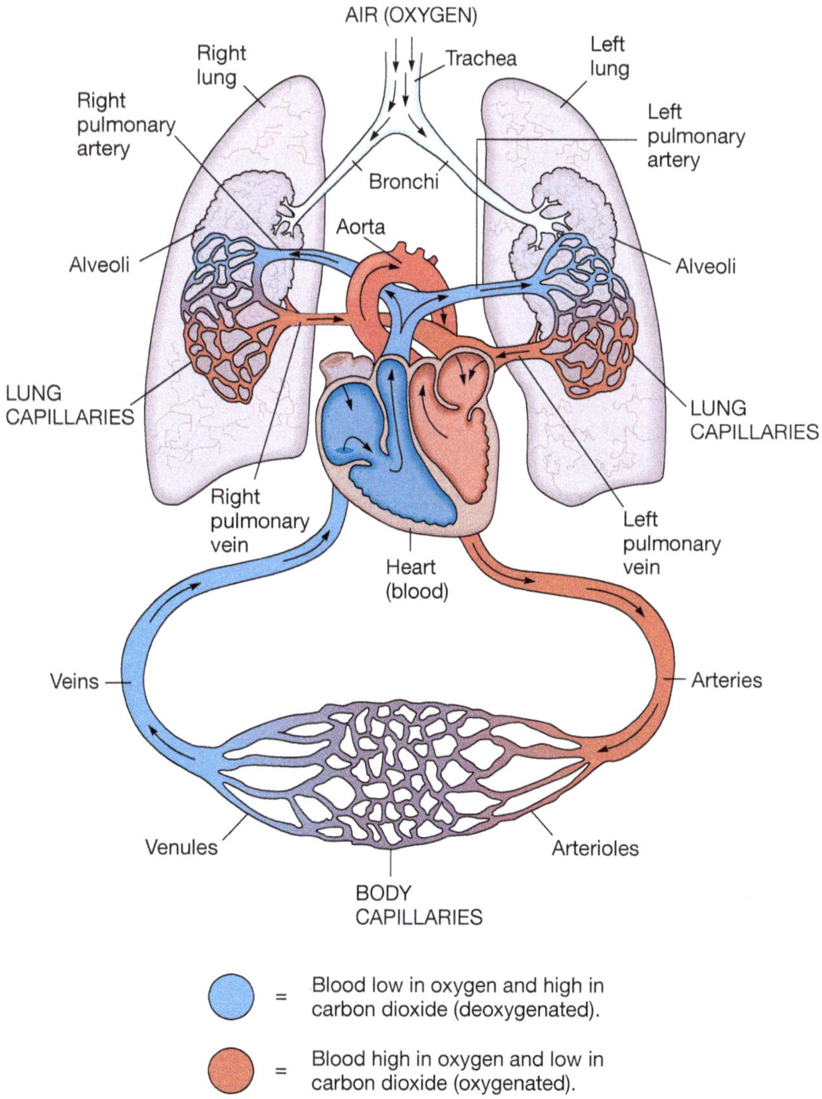

Figure 28.1 The cardiovascular system.

Structure and Function of the Cardiovascular System

28.1 The cardiovascular system consists of the blood, heart, and blood vessels.

The three major components of the cardiovascular system are the blood, heart, and blood vessels, as shown in Figure 28.1. These three components work as an integrated whole to transport the essential oxygen, nutrients, and other substances that keep the body in homeostasis. Disruption of this flow for even brief periods can have serious, if not lethal, consequences. The functions of the cardiovascular system are diverse and include the following:

- Transport of nutrients and wastes
- Pumping of blood
- Regulation of blood pressure
- Regulation of acid–base balance
- Regulation of fluid balance
- Regulation of body temperature
- Protection against invasion by microbes.

The cardiovascular system can function only with the cooperation of other body systems. For example, the role of the autonomic nervous system in controlling heart rate and blood vessel diameter is presented in Chapter 12. The kidneys are intimately involved in assisting the cardiovascular system with fluid and acid–base balance, as discussed in Chapter 33. The respiratory system must bring oxygen to the blood and remove carbon dioxide from it. The student should view the cardiovascular system as an important part of the body's ability to maintain overall homeostasis.

Functions and Properties of Blood

28.2 Blood consists of formed elements and plasma.

Blood is a liquid connective tissue that consists of formed elements suspended in plasma. The solid, formed elements of the blood are the erythrocytes, leukocytes, and platelets. When combined, the formed elements comprise about 45% of the composition of blood.

The most numerous blood cells are erythrocytes, which comprise 99.9% of the formed elements. Carrying the iron-containing protein hemoglobin, the erythrocytes are responsible for transporting oxygen to the tissues and carbon dioxide from the tissues to the lungs. Erythrocyte homeostasis is controlled by **erythropoietin**, a hormone secreted by the kidney in response to low oxygen levels in the blood. Once secreted, erythropoietin stimulates the body's production of erythrocytes. Insufficient numbers of erythrocytes or structural defects such as sickle shapes lead to anemia, which is a common indication for pharmacotherapy (see Chapter 39).

Although small in number, leukocytes serve an essential role in the body's defense against infection. Unlike erythrocytes, which are all structurally identical, there are several types of leukocytes, each serving a different function. For example, neutrophils are the most common leukocyte and they respond to bacterial infections through phagocytosis of the microbes. The second most common leukocyte, the lymphocyte, is the key cell in the immune response that responds by secreting antibodies (B lymphocytes) or secreting cytokines (T lymphocytes) that rid the body of the microbe. A review of body defenses and the immune system is presented in Chapter 40.

The final formed elements of the blood are thrombocytes or platelets, which are actually fragments of larger cells called megakaryocytes. Platelets stick to the walls of damaged blood vessels to begin the process of blood coagulation, which prevents excessive bleeding from sites of injury. Abnormally low numbers of platelets, or thrombocytopenia, can result in serious delays in blood clotting. Platelet homeostasis is controlled by the hormone **thrombopoietin**, which promotes the formation of additional platelets. The role of platelets and thrombopoietin in blood coagulation is a major topic in Chapter 38, which discusses the pharmacotherapy of blood coagulation.

The production and maturation of blood cells, called **hemopoiesis** or hematopoiesis, occurs in red bone marrow. It is here that primitive stem cells of the blood become committed to forming erythrocytes, leukocytes, or platelets. This process occurs continuously throughout the lifespan and is subject to various homeostatic controls as well as certain drugs and physical agents. For example, ionizing radiation and a large number of drugs have the potential to adversely affect bone marrow and cause myelosuppression. Myelosuppression is a very serious adverse effect that reduces the number of erythrocytes, leukocytes, and thrombocytes, leaving patients susceptible to anemia, infection, and bleeding. Many drugs used to treat cancer and those given to reduce the possibility of transplant rejection can produce profound myelosuppression as a dose-limiting adverse effect.

Plasma is the fluid portion of blood that consists of water, proteins, electrolytes, lipoproteins, carbohydrates, and other regulatory substances. The primary proteins in plasma are albumins, globulins, and fibrinogen. Albumin is the primary regulator of blood osmotic pressure, which determines the movement of fluids among the vascular, interstitial, and cellular compartments or spaces. Globulins, also called immunoglobulins or antibodies, protect the body from foreign pathogens such as bacteria or viruses. Fibrinogen is a critical protein in the coagulation of blood. The liver synthesizes over 90% of the plasma proteins; therefore, patients with serious hepatic impairment will have deficiencies in coagulation and in maintaining body defenses.

Serum is a term closely related to plasma. Serum contains all the components of plasma, except clotting factors such as fibrinogen have been removed. Serum is often used for blood typing and for determining blood levels of substances such as cholesterol, glucose, and hormones.

Fluid balance in the body is achieved by maintaining the proper amount of plasma in the blood. Too little water in plasma results in dehydration, whereas too much causes edema and hypertension (HTN). Various organs help to maintain normal fluid balance, including the kidneys, gastrointestinal tract, and skin. The pharmacotherapy of fluid and electrolyte imbalances is an important topic in pharmacology and is discussed in Chapter 33.

CONNECTION Checkpoint 28.1

From what you learned in Chapter 3, what role does plasma protein play in the distribution of drugs?

28.3 Hemostasis is a complex process involving multiple steps and a large number of enzymes and factors.

The process of **hemostasis** is complex, involving at least 13 different clotting factors that contribute to the slowdown and ultimate stoppage of blood flow. Hemostasis occurs in a series of sequential steps and is an essential mechanism that the body uses to prevent excessive bleeding following injury. Medications can be used to modify several of these steps, either to speed up or delay the clotting process (see Chapter 38).

Injury to a blood vessel exposes collagen at the site of vessel injury. The vessel spasms, causing constriction, which slows blood flow to the injured area. Chemicals released by the damaged endothelium activate platelets, which become sticky and adhere to each other and to the endothelium. These form a platelet plug, which further reduces blood loss. The clumping of platelets, or aggregation, is facilitated by adenosine diphosphate (ADP), the enzyme thrombin, and thromboxane A_2. Platelet receptor sites and von Willebrand's factor make adhesion possible. The basic steps of hemostasis are shown in Figure 28.2.

Coagulation, or blood clotting, occurs in a multistep process, or cascade. During the cascade, various plasma

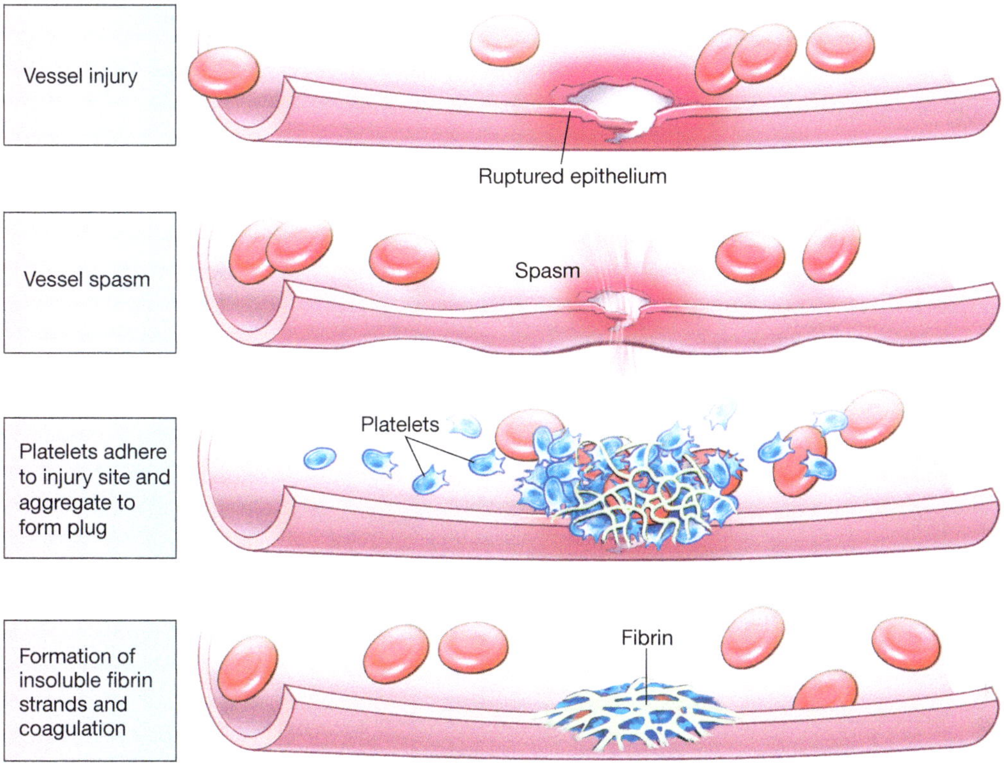

Figure 28.2 The basic steps in hemostasis.

proteins that are circulating in an inactive state are converted to their active forms. Two separate pathways, along with numerous biochemical processes, lead to coagulation. The **intrinsic pathway** is activated in response to injury and takes several minutes to complete. The **extrinsic pathway** is activated when blood leaks out of a vessel and enters tissue spaces. The extrinsic pathway is less complex and is completed within seconds. The two pathways share some common steps and the outcome is the same—the formation of a fibrin clot. The steps in each pathway are shown in Figure 28.3.

Near the end of the common pathway, a chemical called prothrombin activator (see Active X in Figure 28.3) is formed. The prothrombin activator converts the clotting factor **prothrombin** to an enzyme called **thrombin**. Thrombin then converts **fibrinogen**, a plasma protein, to long strands of **fibrin**. The fibrin strands provide a framework to anchor the clot. Thus, two of the factors essential to clotting, thrombin and fibrin, are only formed after injury to the vessels. The fibrin strands form an insoluble web over the injured area to stop blood loss. Normal blood clotting occurs in about 6 minutes.

It is important to note that several clotting factors, including thromboplastin and fibrinogen, are proteins made by the liver that are constantly circulating through the blood in an inactive form. Vitamin K, which is made by bacteria residing in the large intestine, is required for the liver to make four of the clotting factors. Because of the crucial importance of the liver in creating these clotting factors, patients with serious hepatic impairment often have abnormal coagulation.

Cardiac Structure and Function

28.4 The heart is responsible for pumping blood throughout the circulatory system.

The heart is the hardest working organ in the body, pumping blood from before birth to the last minute of life. With the continuous workload, it is not surprising that this organ eventually weakens and that heart disease is the leading cause of death in the United States. The heart is a frequent target for pharmacotherapy.

The heart may be thought of as a thick, specialized muscle. The muscular layer, or myocardium, is the thickest of the heart layers and is responsible for the physical pumping action of the heart. The thickness of the myocardium is greatest in the left ventricle because this chamber performs the greatest amount of work. Cardiac muscle contains extensive branching networks of cellular structures that connect cardiac muscle cells to each other, allowing the entire myocardium to contract as a coordinated whole.

When myocardial cells (myocytes) die, the body is unable to replace them because cardiac muscle cells do not undergo mitosis. If a large area of cardiac muscle becomes

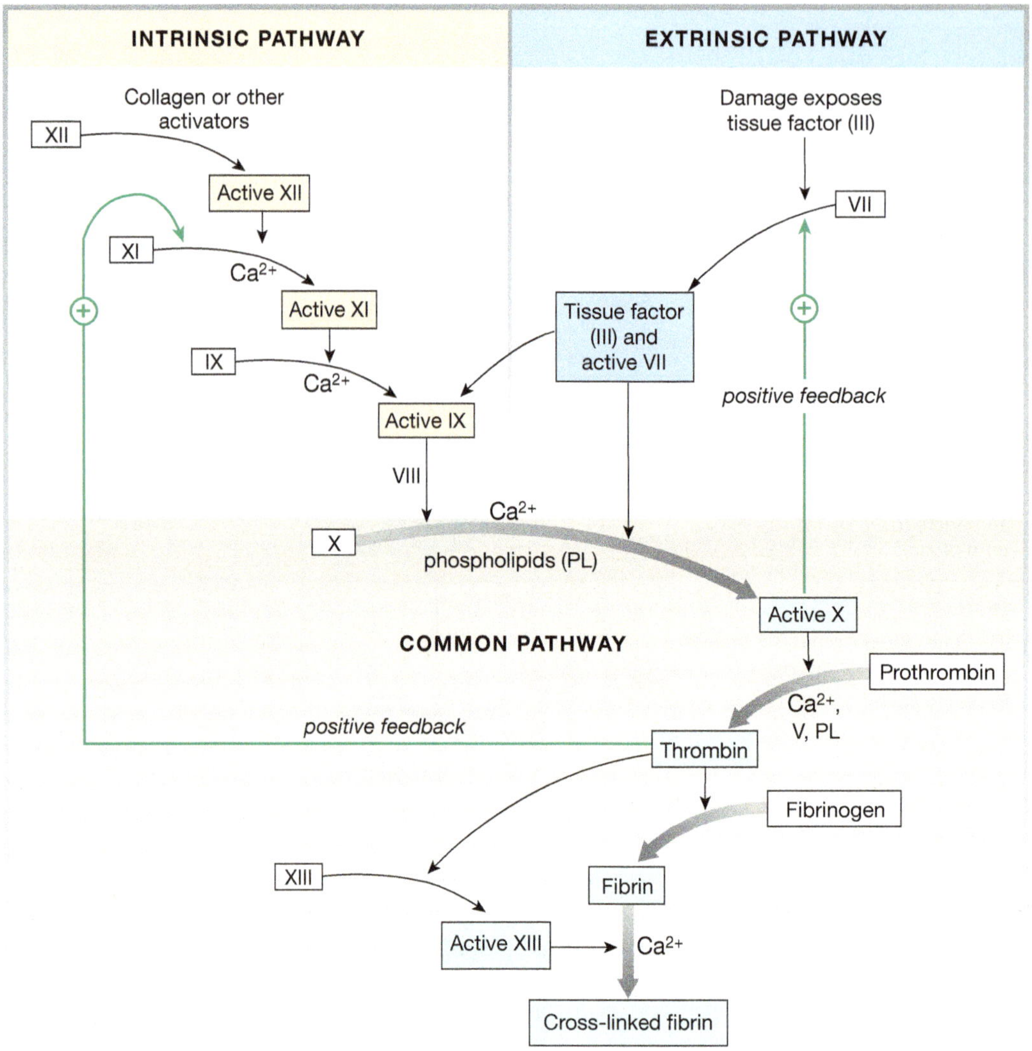

Figure 28.3 The coagulation cascade. Both the intrinsic pathway and extrinsic pathway lead to a common pathway and eventually a dense fibrin clot.

From *Human Physiology: An Integrated Approach*, 5th ed., by D. U. Silverthorn, 2010. Reprinted and electronically reproduced by permission of Pearson Education, Inc., Upper Saddle River, New Jersey.

deprived of oxygen and undergoes necrosis, the myocytes are replaced by fibrotic scar tissue and heart function becomes impaired. The different regions of the heart may not contract in a coordinated manner because conduction of the electrical potential may skip over areas of necrosis on the myocardium. This can result in heart failure or dysrhythmias, which are frequent indications for pharmacotherapy (see Chapters 36 and 37).

The heart has four chambers that receive blood prior to being pumped, as illustrated in Figure 28.4b. These chambers differ in size, depending on their function. The left ventricle is the largest and most powerful chamber because it must hold and pump enough blood to all body tissues. During heart failure, the size of the left ventricle and the thickness of the myocardium in this chamber can increase in size, a condition known as left-ventricular hypertrophy.

28.5 The coronary arteries bring essential nutrients to the myocardium.

Working continuously around the clock, the heart requires a bountiful supply of oxygen and other nutrients. These are provided by the right and left coronary arteries and their branches, as shown in Figure 28.4a. The coronary arteries have the ability to adapt rapidly to the heart's needs for oxygen. For example, during exercise the heart rate and strength of contraction markedly increase, and healthy coronary arteries dilate quickly to provide oxygen to meet this increased workload on the myocardium.

The coronary arteries are subject to atherosclerosis, a buildup of fatty plaque, which narrows the lumen and restricts the blood supply reaching myocytes. If allowed to progress, the narrowing results in chest pain, a condition known as angina pectoris. The first sign of angina is pain

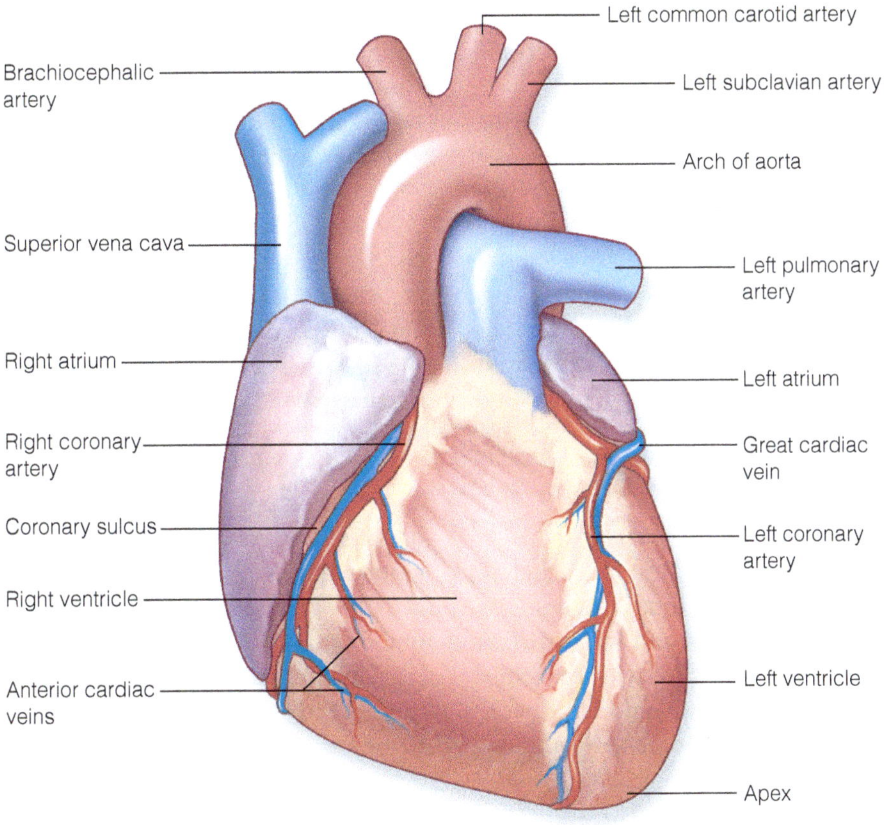

(a)

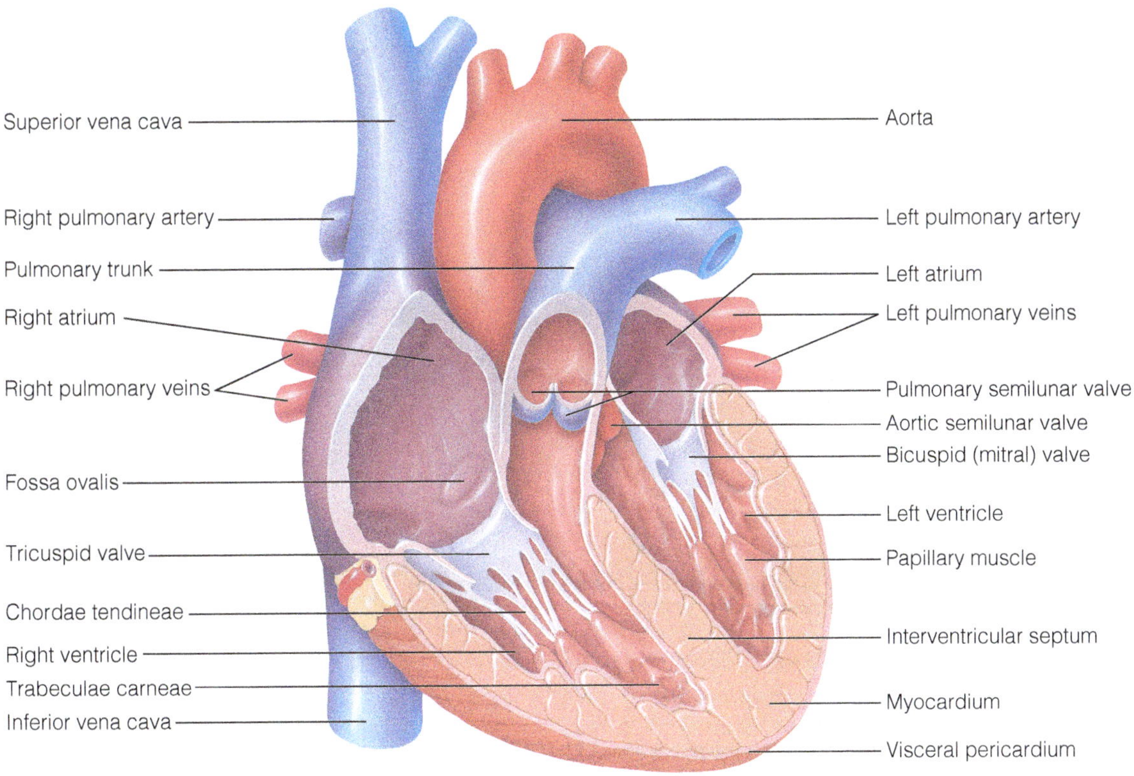

(b)

Figure 28.4 The heart: (a) coronary arteries and veins and (b) chambers and valves.

upon exercise or exertion, since this is when the workload on the heart is increased. Continued narrowing increases the risk of a myocardial infarction.

The coronary arteries are important targets for pharmacotherapy. Chapter 29 explains how reducing lipid levels in the blood can decrease the risk of atherosclerosis in these and other arteries. Chapter 35 discusses how drugs can be used to reduce angina pain and decrease the risk of mortality following a heart attack. Chapter 36 introduces drugs that reduce the cardiac workload in patients with heart failure so that the heart does not require as much oxygen from the coronary arteries.

28.6 The cardiac conduction system keeps the heart beating in a synchronized manner.

For the heart to function properly, the atria must contract simultaneously, sending their blood into the ventricles. Following atrial contraction, the right and left ventricles then must contract simultaneously. Lack of synchronization of the atria and ventricles or of the right and left sides of the heart may have profound consequences. Proper timing of chamber contractions is made possible by the cardiac conduction system, a branching network of specialized cardiac muscle cells that sends a synchronized, electrical signal across the myocardium. These electrical impulses, or action potentials, carry the signal for the cardiac muscle cells to contract and must be coordinated precisely for the chambers to beat in a synchronized manner. The cardiac conduction system is illustrated in Figure 28.5.

Control of the cardiac conduction system begins in a small area of tissue in the wall of the right atrium known as the sinoatrial (SA) node or cardiac pacemaker. Cells in the SA node have the property of **automaticity**, the ability to spontaneously generate action potentials without an outside signal from the nervous system. The SA node generates a new action potential approximately 75 times per minute under resting conditions. This is referred to as the normal **sinus rhythm**. The SA node is greatly influenced by the activity of the sympathetic and parasympathetic divisions of the autonomic nervous system.

Upon leaving the SA node, the action potential travels quickly across both atria and through internodal pathways to the atrioventricular (AV) node. Myocytes in the AV node

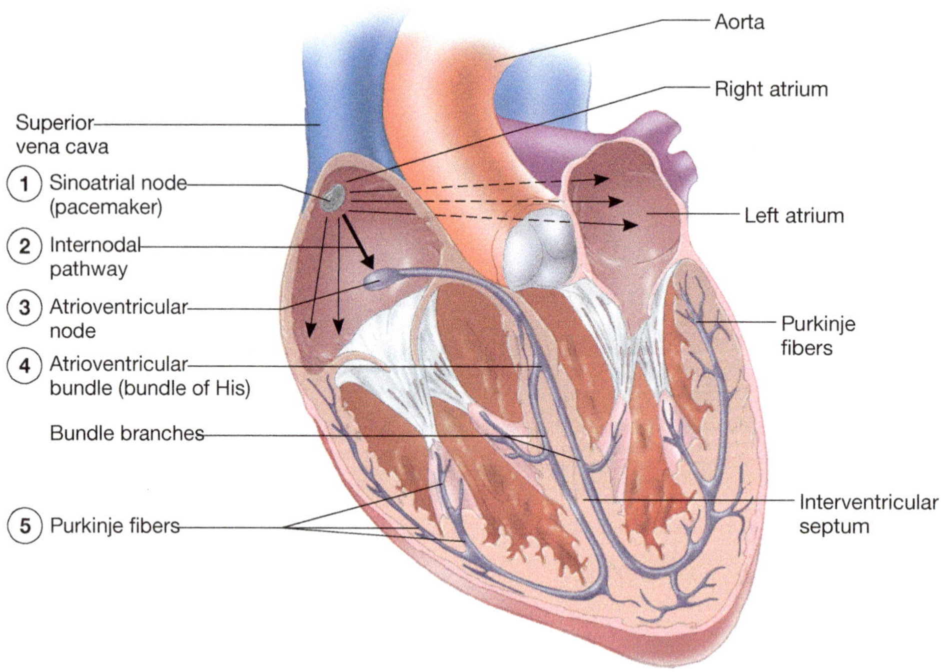

Figure 28.5 The cardiac conduction system.

also have the property of automaticity, although less so than the SA node. Should the SA node malfunction, the AV node has the ability to spontaneously generate action potentials and continue the heart's contraction at a rate of 40 to 60 beats/min. Compared to other areas in the heart, impulse conduction through the AV node is slow. This allows the atria sufficient time to completely contract and empty their blood before the ventricles receive their signal to contract.

As the action potential leaves the AV node, it travels rapidly to the AV bundle or bundle of His. The pathway between the AV node and the bundle of His is the only electrical connection between the atria and the ventricles. The impulse is conducted down the right and left bundle branches to the Purkinje fibers, which rapidly carry the action potential to all regions of the ventricles almost simultaneously. Should the SA and AV nodes become nonfunctional, cells in the AV bundle and Purkinje fibers can continue to generate myocardial contractions at a rate of about 30 beats/min.

Although action potentials normally begin at the SA node and spread across the myocardium in a coordinated manner, other regions of the heart may also initiate beats. These **ectopic foci**, or ectopic pacemakers, may send waves of depolarization across the myocardium that compete with those from the normal conduction pathway. The timing and synchronization of atrial and ventricular contractions may be affected. Although healthy hearts occasionally experience an extra beat without incident, ectopic foci in diseased hearts have the potential to cause dysrhythmias, or disorders of cardiac rhythm. The events associated with the cardiac conduction system are recorded on an electrocardiogram (ECG or EKG).

The underlying purpose of the cardiac conduction system is to keep the heart beating in a regular, synchronized manner so that cardiac output can be maintained. Dysrhythmias that profoundly affect cardiac output have the potential to produce serious, if not mortal, consequences. These types of dysrhythmias require pharmacologic intervention, as discussed in Chapter 37.

28.7 Cardiac output is determined by stroke volume and heart rate.

To understand how medications act on the heart and to predict the consequences of pharmacotherapy, it is essential to have a comprehensive knowledge of normal cardiac physiology. This includes a thorough understanding of factors that determine the amount of blood pumped by the heart and the forces acting on the chambers.

The amount of blood pumped by each ventricle per minute is the **cardiac output (CO)**. The CO is essentially a measure of how effectively the heart is performing as a pump. The average CO is 5 L/min. CO can be calculated by multiplying stroke volume by the heart rate:

$$\text{CO} = \text{stroke volume (mL/beat)} \times \text{heart rate (beats/min)}$$

Stroke volume is the amount of blood pumped by a ventricle in a single contraction. What types of factors might cause a ventricle to eject more blood during a contraction? To understand these factors, a simple comparison to a rubber band is useful. If you stretch a small rubber band 2 inches, it will snap back with a certain force. Stretching the band 4 inches will cause it to snap back with greater force. The force of the snap will continue to increase up to a certain limit, after which the rubber band has been stretched as far as possible and has reached maximum force (or it breaks!).

Cardiac muscle fibers are analogous to rubber bands. If you fill the chambers with more blood, the fibers will have more stretch and will "snap back" with greater force. This is known as Starling's law of the heart: The strength (force) of contraction, or **contractility**, is proportional to the muscle fiber length (stretch). The contractility determines the amount of blood ejected per beat, or the stroke volume. The degree to which the ventricles are filled with blood and the myocardial fibers are stretched just prior to contraction is called **preload**. Up to a physiologic limit, drugs that increase preload and contractility will increase the CO. In addition to preload, the force of contraction can be increased by activation of beta$_1$-adrenergic receptors in the autonomic nervous system.

What causes the chambers to fill up with more blood, become stretched (more preload), and contract with greater force? Although several factors affect preload, the most important is **venous return**: the volume of blood returning to the heart from the veins. Giving a drug that constricts veins will increase venous return to the heart, as will simply increasing the total amount of blood in the vascular system (increased blood volume). Drugs or other mechanisms that constrict veins or increase blood volume will therefore increase stroke volume and CO. Conversely, drugs that dilate veins or reduce blood volume will lower CO.

Medications that increase cardiac contractility are called positive inotropic drugs and include epinephrine, norepinephrine, thyroid hormone, and dopamine. Factors that decrease cardiac contractility are called negative inotropic drugs. Examples include quinidine and beta-adrenergic antagonists such as propranolol.

A second primary factor affecting stroke volume is afterload. In order for the left ventricle to pump blood out of the heart, it must overcome a substantial "back pressure" in the aorta. **Afterload** is the systolic pressure in the aorta that must be overcome for blood to be ejected from the left ventricle. As afterload increases, the heart pumps less blood, and stroke volume (and thus CO) decreases. The most common cause of increased afterload is an increase in systemic blood pressure, or HTN. HTN creates an increased workload on the heart, which explains why patients with chronic HTN are more likely to experience heart failure. Antihypertensive drugs create less afterload, increase stroke volume, and result in less workload for the heart. Preload and afterload are illustrated in Figure 28.6.

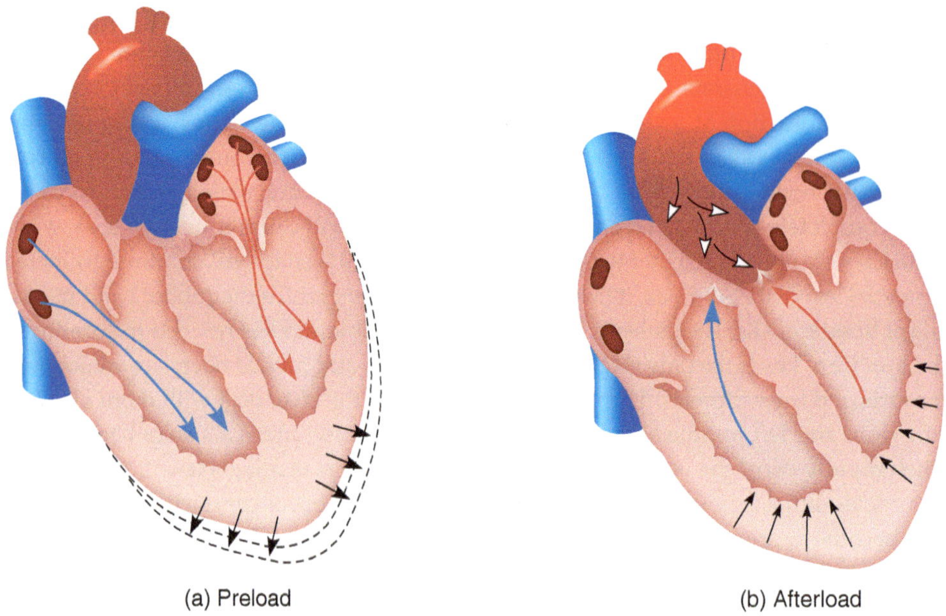

Figure 28.6 (a) Preload is the degree to which the ventricles are filled with blood and the myocardial fibers are stretched just prior to contraction. (b) Afterload is the systolic pressure in the aorta that must be overcome for blood to be ejected from the left ventricle.

Heart rate is the second primary factor determining CO. Heart rate is generally controlled by the autonomic nervous system, which makes the minute-by-minute adjustments demanded by the circulatory system. Both sympathetic and parasympathetic fibers are found in the SA node, and heart rate is determined by which fibers are firing at a greater rate at any given moment. Circulating hormones such as epinephrine and thyroid hormone also affect heart rate. In theory, drugs that increase heart rate will increase CO, although compensatory mechanisms may prevent this effect (see Section 28.8). In addition, a very rapid heart rate may not give the chambers sufficient time to completely fill, thus reducing CO.

CONNECTION Checkpoint 28.2

From what you learned in Chapter 12, predict what effect the following would have on heart rate: sympathomimetics, parasympathomimetics, adrenergic agonists, and anticholinergics.

Hemodynamics and Blood Pressure

28.8 The primary factors responsible for blood pressure are cardiac output, peripheral resistance, and blood volume.

The homeostatic regulation of blood pressure is a key topic in pharmacology because HTN is so prevalent in the population. Regulation of blood pressure is complex with many diverse factors, both local and systemic, interacting to maintain adequate blood flow to the tissues. The three primary factors that regulate arterial blood pressure—CO, peripheral resistance, and blood volume—are shown in Figure 28.7. The following simple formula should be memorized (as well as understood) because it will help in predicting the actions and adverse effects of many classes of cardiovascular medications:

$$\text{Blood pressure} = \text{CO} \times \text{peripheral resistance}$$

CO is determined by heart rate and stroke volume, as discussed in Section 28.7. From the preceding equation, it is easy to see that as CO increases, blood pressure also increases. This is important to pharmacology because medications that change the CO, stroke volume, or heart rate have the potential to influence a patient's blood pressure.

As blood speeds through the vascular system, it exerts force against the walls of the vessels. Although the endothelium is extremely smooth, friction reduces the velocity of the blood. Further friction is encountered as the stream of fast-moving blood narrows to enter smaller vessels, divides into two channels (arteries), or encounters fatty deposits on the vessel walls (plaque). Blood flow may exhibit turbulence, a chaotic, tumbling motion that greatly increases friction. The friction that blood encounters in the arteries is called **peripheral resistance**. Arteries have smooth muscle in their walls, which controls the total peripheral resistance. For example, if the smooth muscle constricts, the inside diameter or lumen of the arteries will become smaller and create more resistance and higher blood pressure. A large number of medications affect vascular smooth muscle. Some of these drugs cause vessels to constrict, thus raising blood pressure,

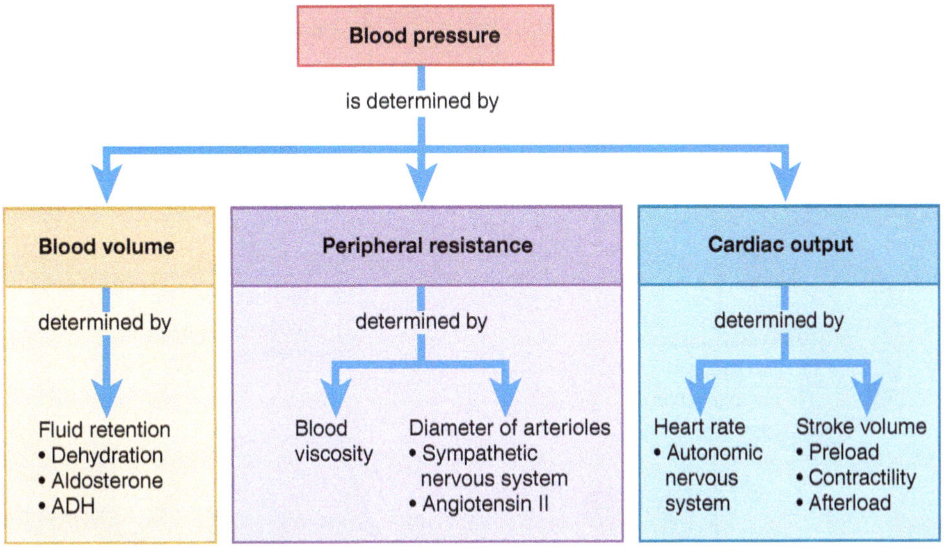

Figure 28.7 The primary factors affecting blood pressure.

whereas others relax smooth muscle, thereby opening the lumen and lowering blood pressure.

An additional factor responsible for blood pressure is the total amount of blood in the vascular system, or blood volume. Although the average person maintains a relatively constant blood volume of approximately 5 L, this can be changed by endogenous regulatory factors, certain disease states, and pharmacotherapy. More fluid in the vascular system increases venous pressure and venous return to the heart, thus increasing CO and arterial blood pressure. Drugs are frequently used to adjust blood volume. For example, infusion of intravenous (IV) fluids quickly increases blood volume and raises blood pressure. This is used to advantage when treating hypotension due to shock. On the other hand, diuretics cause fluid loss through urination, thus decreasing blood volume and lowering blood pressure.

28.9 Neural regulation of blood pressure includes baroreceptor and chemoreceptor reflexes.

It is critical for the body to maintain a normal range of blood pressure and for it to be able to safely and rapidly change pressure as it proceeds through daily activities such as sleep and exercise. Hypotension can cause dizziness and lack of adequate urine formation, whereas extreme HTN can cause vessels to rupture, resulting in ischemia of critical organs. Figure 28.8 illustrates how the body maintains homeostasis during periods of blood pressure change.

The central and autonomic nervous systems are intimately involved in regulating blood pressure. On a minute-to-minute basis, blood pressure is regulated by a cluster of neurons in the medulla oblongata called the **vasomotor center**. Sensory receptors in the aorta and the internal carotid artery provide the vasomotor center with vital information on conditions in the vascular system. **Baroreceptors** have the ability to sense pressure within large vessels, whereas **chemoreceptors** recognize levels of oxygen, carbon dioxide, and the acidity or pH in the blood. The vasomotor center reacts to information from baroreceptors and chemoreceptors by raising or lowering blood pressure accordingly. Nerve fibers travel from the vasomotor center to the arteries, where the smooth muscle is directed to either constrict (raise blood pressure) or relax (lower blood pressure). As discussed in Chapter 16, sympathetic outflow from the vasomotor center stimulates alpha$_1$-adrenergic receptors on arterioles, causing vasoconstriction. Alpha$_2$-adrenergic agonists can also decrease blood pressure by their central effects on the vasomotor center.

The baroreceptor reflex is an important mechanism used by the body for making rapid adjustments to blood pressure. If pressure in the vascular system increases, the baroreceptors in the aortic arch and carotid sinus trigger reflexes that constrict the arterioles and veins and accelerate the heart rate. Together, these actions return blood pressure to normal levels within seconds.

Drugs that raise or lower blood pressure can trigger the baroreceptor reflex. For example, antihypertensives administered by the IV route cause an immediate reduction in blood pressure that is recognized by the baroreceptors. The baroreceptors respond by attempting to return blood pressure back to the original levels. The resulting accelerated heart rate, or reflex tachycardia, may cause the patient to experience palpitations. The baroreceptors are not able to offer a continuous or sustained reduction in blood pressure. Continued administration of an antihypertensive drug will "overcome" the reflex. In addition, with aging or certain disease states such as diabetes, the baroreceptor response may be diminished.

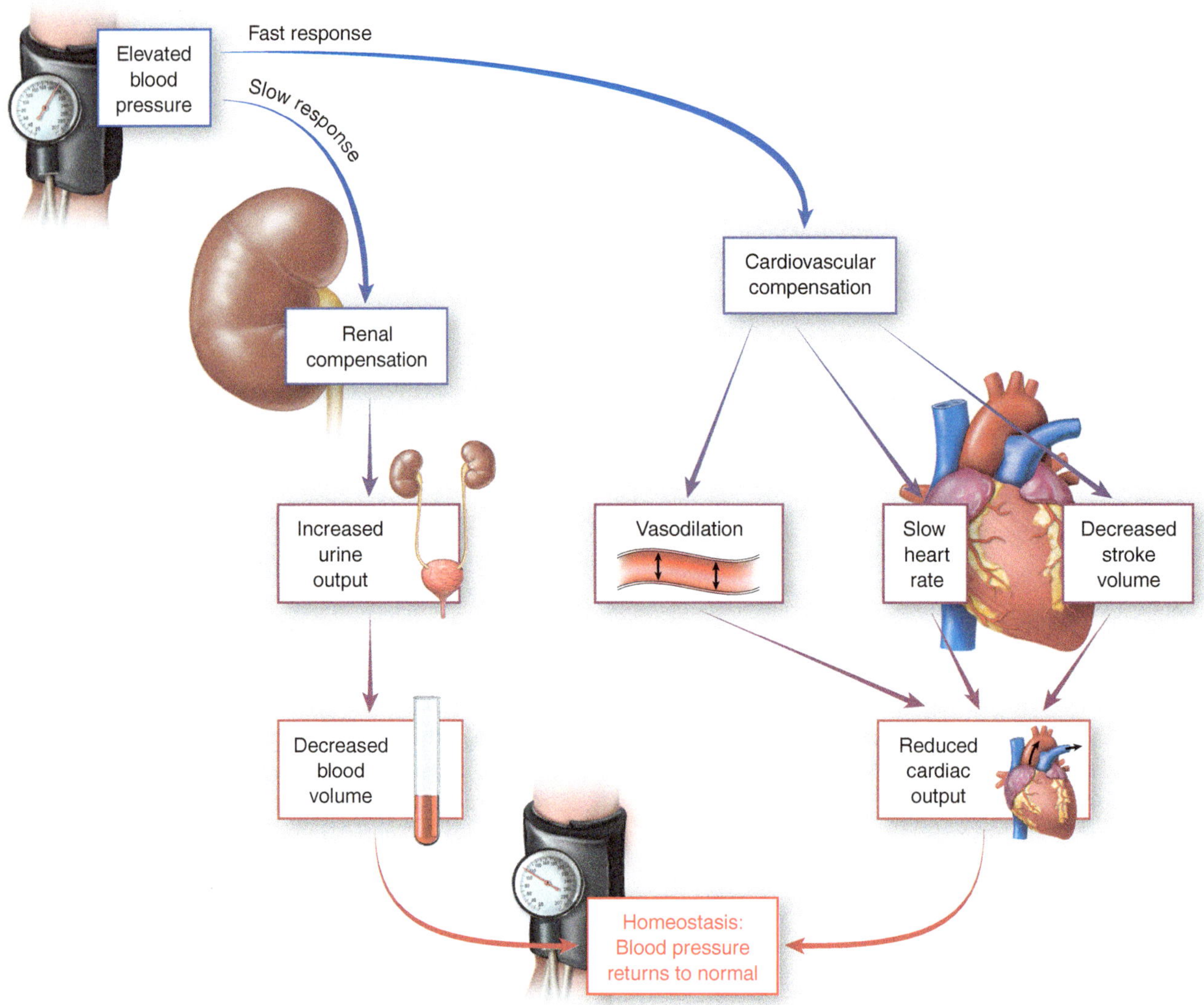

Figure 28.8 Cardiovascular and renal control of blood pressure.

Another example of the baroreceptor reflex occurs when baroreceptors in the right atrium are triggered. These receptors recognize excess stretching of the right atrium, such as might occur when large amounts of IV fluids are rapidly administered. The **atrial reflex** causes the heart rate and CO to increase until the backlog of venous blood (or IV fluid) is distributed throughout the body.

The chemoreceptor reflex can also significantly affect blood pressure. Sensors in the carotid sinus and near the aortic arch recognize levels of oxygen and carbon dioxide and the acidity (pH) in the blood. Triggering these chemoreceptors activates the sympathetic nervous system and causes heart rate and CO to increase. The purpose of this reflex is to circulate blood faster so that the respiratory system can remove excess carbon dioxide (which returns pH to normal levels) and add more oxygen to the blood.

CONNECTION Checkpoint 28.3

Many autonomic drugs dilate or constrict blood vessels. From what you learned in Chapter 12, which class of autonomic drugs is most commonly prescribed for HTN?

28.10 Hormones may have profound effects on blood pressure.

Several hormones affect blood pressure, and certain classes of medications are given to either enhance or block the actions of these hormones. For example, injection of the catecholamines epinephrine or norepinephrine will immediately raise blood pressure, which is essential for patients experiencing shock.

Antidiuretic hormone (ADH) is a hormone released by the posterior pituitary gland when blood pressure falls or when the osmotic pressure of the blood increases.

ADH, also known as vasopressin, is a potent peripheral vasoconstrictor that quickly increases blood pressure. The hormone also acts on the kidneys to conserve water and increase blood volume, thereby causing blood pressure to increase. The pharmacotherapy of ADH and related hormones is discussed in Chapter 65.

The **renin-angiotensin-aldosterone system (RAAS)** is particularly important in the drug therapy of HTN. As blood pressure falls, the enzyme renin is released by the kidneys. Through a two-step pathway, angiotensin II is formed, which subsequently increases CO and constricts arterioles to return blood pressure to original levels. Angiotensin II also promotes the release of aldosterone from the adrenal gland, which causes sodium and water retention. Drugs that block the RAAS are key drugs in the treatment of HTN and heart failure (see Chapter 31).

Atrial natriuretic peptide (ANP) is a hormone that is secreted by specialized cells in the right atrium when large increases in blood volume produce excessive stretch on the atrial wall. ANP has multiple effects, all of which attempt to return blood pressure to original levels. Sodium ion transport in the kidney is affected, resulting in enhanced sodium and water excretion. The release of ADH and aldosterone is suppressed by ANP. In addition, ANP reduces sympathetic outflow from the central nervous system, resulting in dilation of peripheral arteries. A summary of the various nervous and hormone factors influencing blood pressure is shown in Figure 28.9.

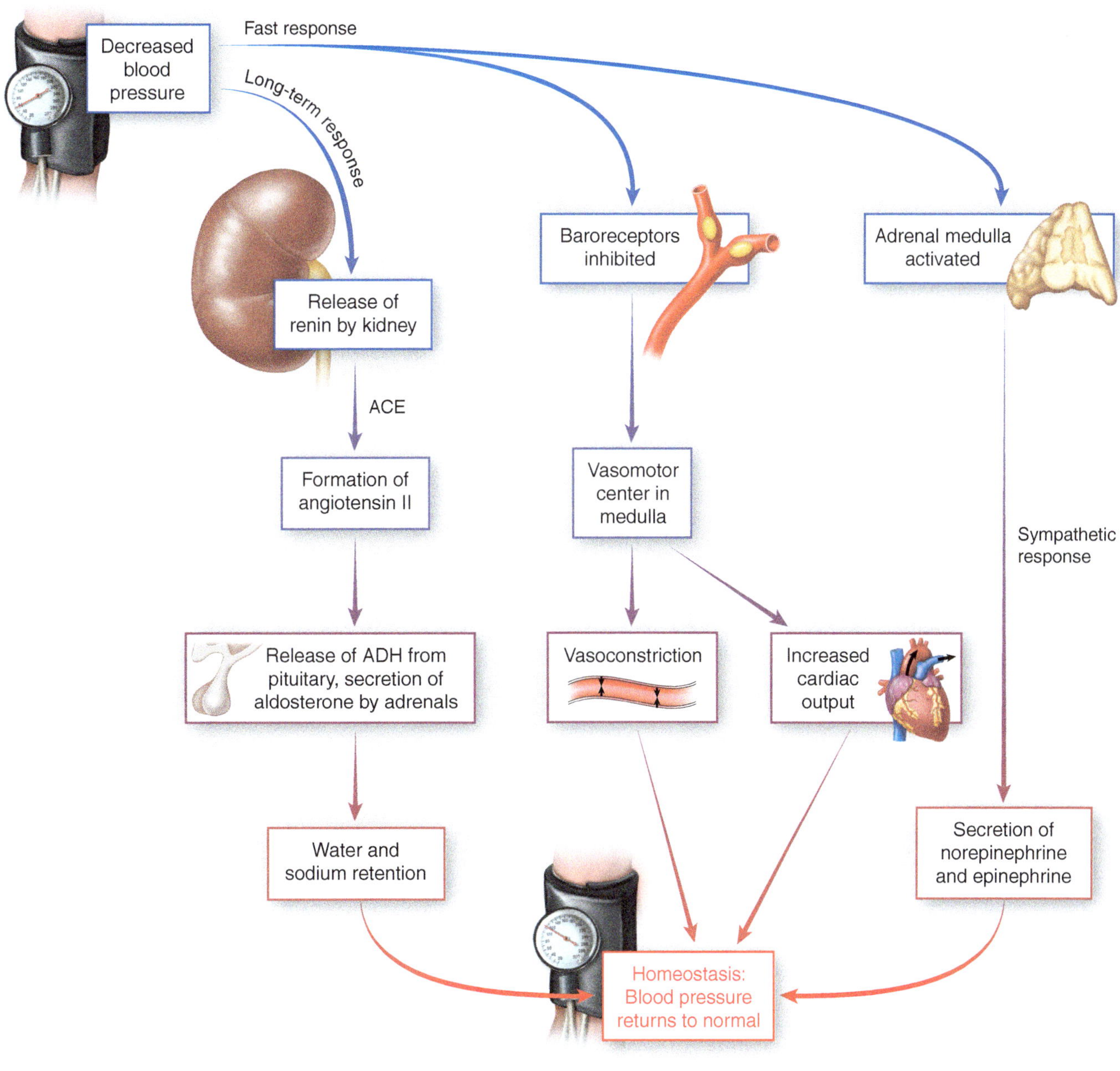

Figure 28.9 Endocrine and nervous control of blood pressure.

Understanding Chapter 28

Key Concepts Summary

28.1 The cardiovascular system consists of the blood, heart, and blood vessels.

28.2 Blood consists of formed elements and plasma.

28.3 Hemostasis is a complex process involving multiple steps and a large number of enzymes and factors.

28.4 The heart is responsible for pumping blood throughout the circulatory system.

28.5 The coronary arteries bring essential nutrients to the myocardium.

28.6 The cardiac conduction system keeps the heart beating in a synchronized manner.

28.7 Cardiac output is determined by stroke volume and heart rate.

28.8 The primary factors responsible for blood pressure are cardiac output, peripheral resistance, and blood volume.

28.9 Neural regulation of blood pressure includes baroreceptor and chemoreceptor reflexes.

28.10 Hormones may have profound effects on blood pressure.

Selected Bibliography

Hall, J. E. (2020). *Guyton & Hall textbook of medical physiology* (14th ed.). Elsevier.

Krogh, D. (2014). *Biology: A guide to the natural world, technology update* (5th ed.). Benjamin Cummings.

Marieb, E. N., & Hoehn, K. N. (2019). *Human anatomy and physiology* (10th ed.). Pearson.

Martini, F. H., Nath, J. L., & Bartholomew, E. F. (2018). *Fundamentals of human anatomy and physiology* (11th ed.). Benjamin Cummings.

Silverthorn, D. U. (2019). *Human physiology: An integrated approach* (8th ed.). Pearson.

"My mother had it and my grandmother had it too. Now, I'm told that I have it. My doctor says my cholesterol level is too high."

—Patient "Belinda Cummings"

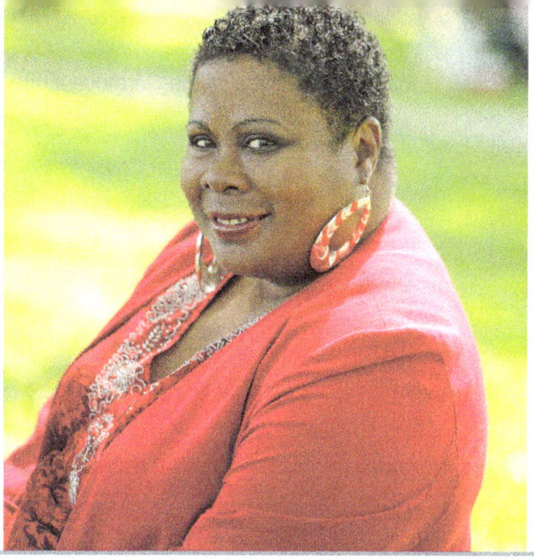

Chapter 29
Pharmacotherapy of Atherosclerotic Cardiovascular Disease

Chapter Outline

Learning Outcomes

After reading this chapter, the student should be able to:

1. Summarize the link between high blood cholesterol, low-density lipoprotein levels, and atherosclerotic cardiovascular disease.
2. Explain the different types of lipids and how they are transported through the body.
3. Illustrate how lipids are transported through the blood.
4. Compare and contrast the clinical importance of the different types of lipoproteins.
5. Give examples of how cholesterol and low-density lipoprotein levels can be managed with nonpharmacologic means.
6. Categorize drugs for atherosclerotic cardiovascular disease based on their classification and mechanism of action.
7. Explain the nurse's role in the safe administration of drugs for atherosclerotic cardiovascular disease.
8. For each of the classes shown in the chapter outline, identify the prototype and representative drugs and explain the mechanism(s) of drug action, primary indications, contraindications, significant drug interactions, pregnancy data, and important adverse effects.
9. Apply clinical judgment to care for patients receiving pharmacotherapy for atherosclerotic cardiovascular disease.

Key Terms

Definitions of the terms in bold may be found in the Glossary.

Research during the 1970s and 1980s brought about a nutritional revolution as new knowledge about lipids and their relationships to obesity and cardiovascular disease allowed people to make more responsible lifestyle choices. Since then advances in the diagnosis of lipid disorders have helped to identify those people at greatest risk for cardiovascular disease and those most likely to benefit from pharmacologic intervention. As a result of this knowledge and from advancements in pharmacology, the incidence of death due to most cardiovascular diseases has been declining, although they remain a leading cause of death in the United States.

Types of Lipids and Lipoproteins

29.1 Lipids are classified as triglycerides, phospholipids, or sterols.

Three types of lipids are important to human physiology, as illustrated in Figure 29.1. The most common types are **triglycerides** or neutral fats, which consist of three fatty acids attached to a chemical backbone of glycerol. Triglycerides are the major storage form of fat in the body and the only type of lipid that serves as an important energy source. They account for 90% of the total lipids in the body.

A second class, the **phospholipids**, is formed when a phosphorous group replaces one of the fatty acids in a triglyceride. This type of lipid comprises the majority of the lipid bilayer that forms plasma membranes. Phospholipids also form spherical sacs called liposomes, which have been used to develop unique drug delivery systems. Once enclosed in a liposome, drugs such as amphotericin B and doxorubicin are able to overcome certain obstacles to absorption and distribution.

The third class of lipids, the **steroids**, is a diverse group of substances having a common sterol nucleus or ring structure. Cholesterol is the most widely known of the steroids, and its role in promoting **atherosclerosis** has been clearly demonstrated. Atherosclerosis is the presence of plaque—a fatty, fibrous material within the walls of the arteries. Unlike the triglycerides that provide fuel for the body, cholesterol is a vital component of plasma membranes and serves as a building block for essential biochemicals, including vitamin D, bile acids, cortisol, estrogen, and testosterone. Although clearly essential for life, the body needs only minute amounts of cholesterol because the liver is able to synthesize adequate amounts from other chemicals. It is not necessary, nor desirable, to provide excess cholesterol in the diet. The dietary sources of cholesterol are obtained solely from animal products; humans do not absorb the sterols produced by plants.

29.2 Lipoproteins are important predictors of cardiovascular disease.

Because lipid molecules are not soluble in plasma, they must be specially packaged for transport through the blood. To accomplish this, the body forms **lipoproteins**, which consist of various amounts of cholesterol, triglycerides, and phospholipids bound to carrier proteins. The protein component is called an **apoprotein** (*apo-* means "separated from" or "derived from").

Lipoproteins are classified according to their composition, size, and weight or density, which come primarily from the amount of apoprotein present in the complex. Each type varies in lipid and apoprotein makeup and serves a different function in transporting lipids from the sites of synthesis and absorption to the sites of utilization or excretion. For example, **high-density lipoprotein cholesterol (HDL-C)** contains the most apoprotein, up to 50% by weight. The highest amount of cholesterol is carried by **low-density lipoprotein cholesterol (LDL-C)**. Figure 29.2 illustrates the three basic lipoproteins and their compositions.

To understand the pharmacotherapy of lipid disorders, it is important to know the functions of the major lipoproteins and their roles in transporting cholesterol. LDL-C transports cholesterol from the liver to the tissues and organs, where it is used to build plasma membranes or to synthesize other steroids. Once in the tissues it can also be stored for later use. Storage of cholesterol in the lining of blood vessels, however, is not desirable because it contributes to plaque buildup. LDL-C is often called "bad" cholesterol because this lipoprotein contributes significantly to plaque deposits. Sixty to 70% of the cholesterol circulating in the blood is found in LDL-C. Lowering the amount of LDL-C in the blood through a heart-healthy lifestyle or by pharmacotherapy significantly reduces the risk for developing atherosclerotic cardiovascular disease (ASCVD).

Very low-density lipoprotein cholesterol (VLDL-C) is the primary carrier of triglycerides in the blood. VLDL-C accounts for virtually all triglycerides being transported from the liver to storage in adipose tissue. Through a series of steps, VLDL-C is reduced in size to become LDL-C, therefore VLDL-C also contributes to plaque formation.

HDL-C assists in the transport of excess cholesterol to the liver for metabolism in a process known as **reverse cholesterol transport**. The cholesterol component of the HDL-C is then broken down and unites with bile, which is subsequently excreted in the feces. Because HDL-C transports cholesterol for destruction and removes it from the body, it is considered "good" cholesterol. Patients with very

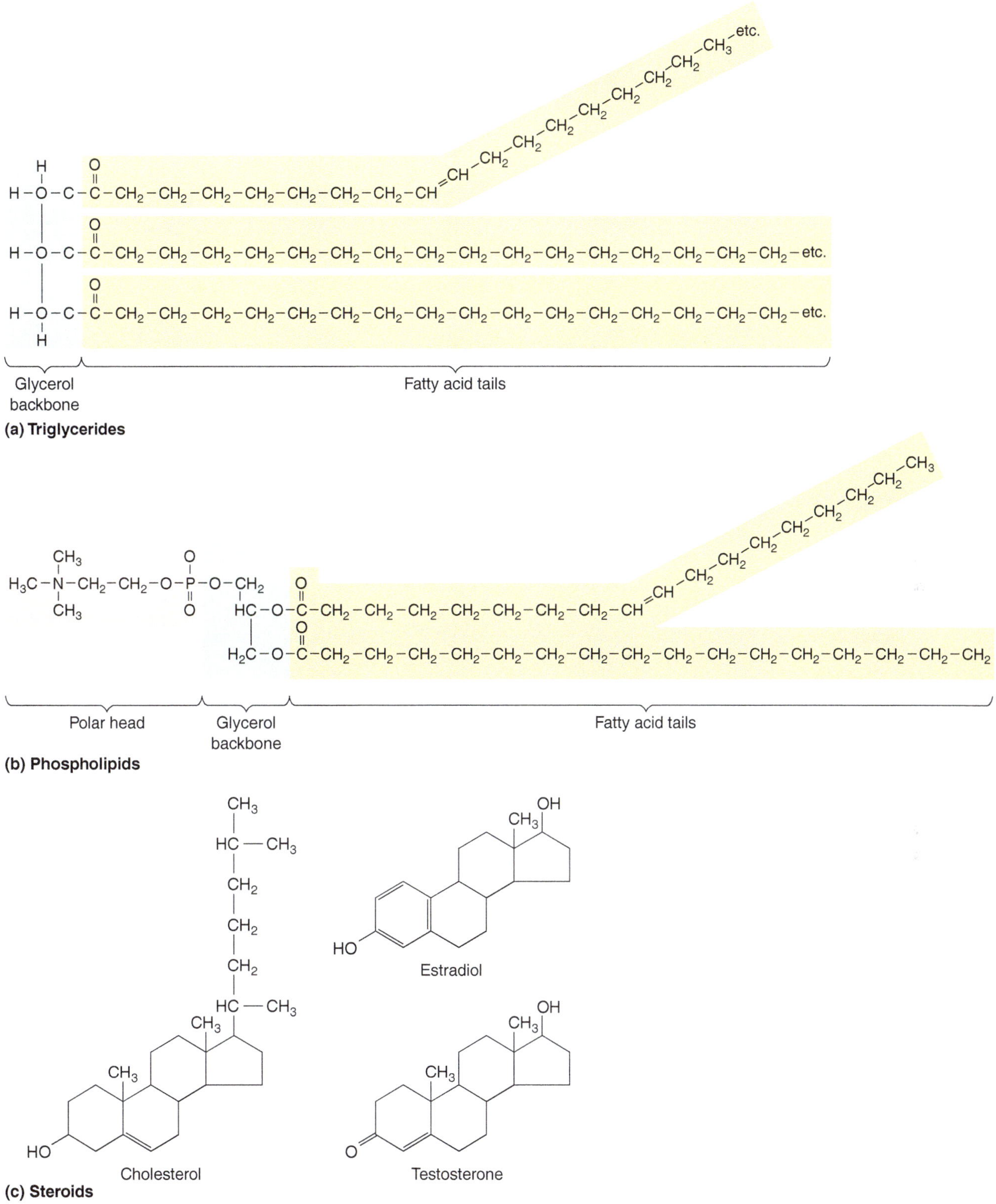

Figure 29.1 Chemical structure of lipids.

low amounts of HDL-C are at risk for ASCVD, even if their total cholesterol levels are normal.

Several terms are used to describe lipid disorders. **Dyslipidemia** is a general term that refers to abnormal amounts of lipids in the body. The most common type of dyslipidemia is **hyperlipidemia**, meaning elevated levels of lipids in the blood. The term *hyperlipidemia*, however, does not specify which lipid is elevated (cholesterol, triglyceride, or phospholipid). Elevated blood cholesterol, or **hypercholesterolemia**, is the type of hyperlipidemia most familiar to the public. Some patients exhibit an increase in triglyceride levels known as **hypertriglyceridemia**.

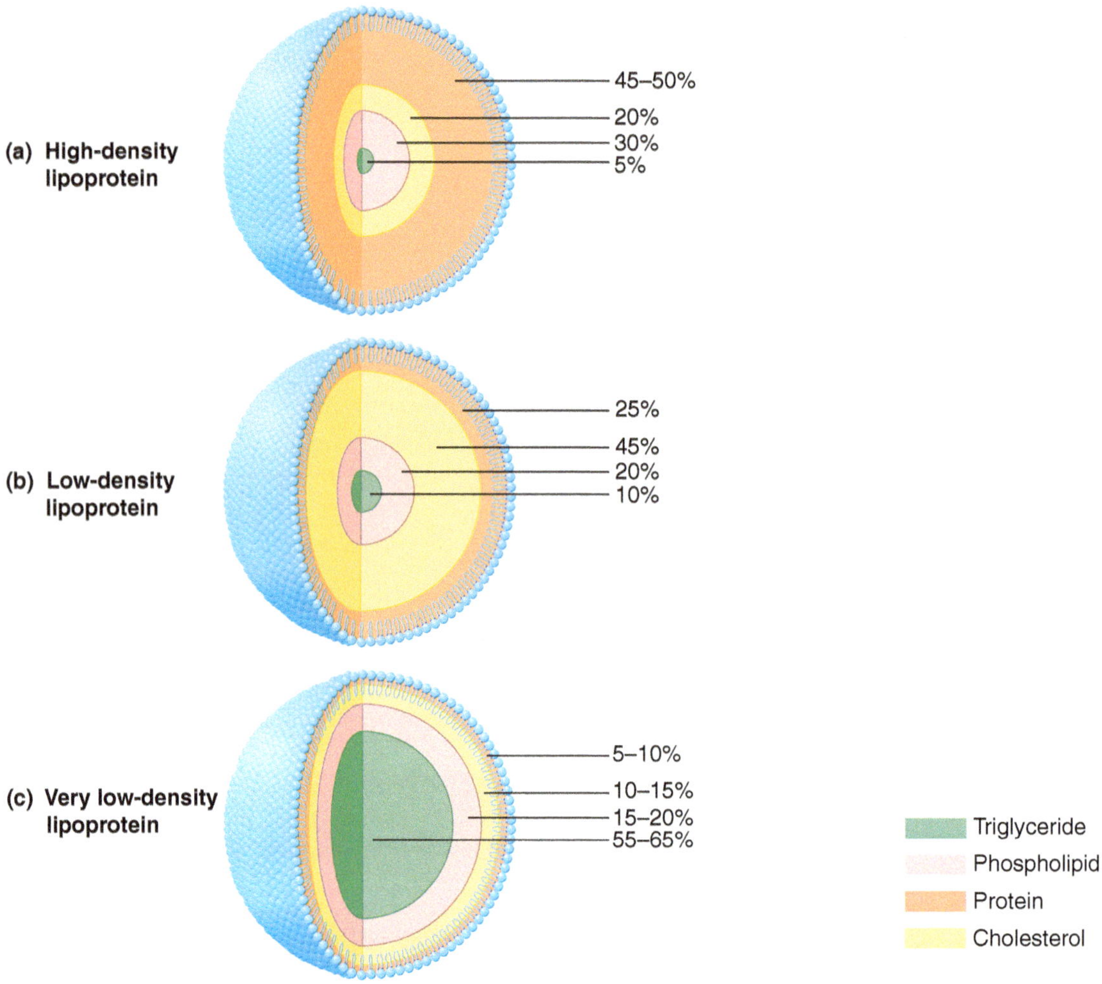

Figure 29.2 Composition of lipoproteins: (a) HDL-C, (b) LDL-C, (c) VLDL-C.

The deposition of plaque in vessels (atherogenesis) is a slow, continuous process that occurs throughout adult life. In some patients, it begins much earlier, in childhood or adolescence. Patients with lipid disorders are asymptomatic and often do not seek medical intervention until an **ASCVD event** has occurred. Serious ASCVD events include acute coronary syndrome, transient ischemic attack, angina pectoris, myocardial infarction, ischemic stroke, or peripheral artery disease. It is estimated that about 124 million people over age 20 in the United States have elevated cholesterol levels; only half of those who could benefit from pharmacotherapy are being treated for hyperlipidemia (Centers for Disease Control and Prevention, 2020). Screening for these disorders and consistent teaching about the long-term benefits of appropriate preventive lifestyle choices or pharmacotherapy is essential for the reduction in mortality and disability in these patients.

Hyperlipidemia may be inherited or acquired. Certainly, diets high in saturated fats and lack of exercise contribute greatly to the development of hyperlipidemia and resulting ASCVD. However, genetics determines one's ability to metabolize lipids and contributes to high lipid levels in substantial numbers of patients. Some genetic dyslipidemias can be so severe as to cause death due to myocardial infarction (MI) in patients as young as 1 or 2 years (Mose, 2020). For most patients, dyslipidemias are the result of a combination of genetic and environmental (lifestyle) factors.

Measurement of Serum Lipids

29.3 Serum lipid panels are important diagnostic tools in guiding the therapy of dyslipidemias.

To properly diagnose a patient's lipid disorder and plan appropriate therapy, a lipid panel must be obtained. These lab data typically include values for total cholesterol, LDL-C, HDL-C, and triglycerides. Research has clearly shown that high levels of LDL-C promote plaque formation and the development of ASCVD; therefore, keeping LDL-C within normal limits is an essential treatment goal. On the other hand, high levels of HDL-C have a protective effect. Table 29.1 gives the desirable, borderline, and high laboratory values for each of the major lipids and lipoproteins. As discussed below, treatment goals for LDL-C can be accomplished through a combination of a heart-healthy lifestyle and appropriate pharmacotherapy.

Table 29.1 Standard Laboratory Lipid Profiles

Type of Lipid	Laboratory Value (mg/dL)	Standard
Total cholesterol	Less than 200	Desirable
	200–239	Borderline high risk
	240 or higher	High risk
Low-density lipoprotein (LDL-C)	Less than 100	Optimal
	100–129	Near or above optimal
	130–159	Borderline high risk
	160–189	High risk
	190 or higher	Very high risk
High-density lipoprotein (HDL-C)	Less than 40 (men) or 50 (women)	Low risk
	Greater than 60	Desirable
Serum triglycerides	Less than 150	Normal
	150–199	Borderline high risk
	200–499	High risk
	500 or higher	Very high risk

Source: Data from Expert Panel on Detection, E. (2001). Executive summary of the third report of the National Cholesterol Education Program (NCEP) expert panel on detection, evaluation, and treatment of high blood cholesterol in adults (Adult Treatment Panel III). JAMA, 285(19), 2486.

Several additional laboratory values are important in the diagnosis of lipid disorders. While not routinely screened in every patient, the following are used by the healthcare provider to better understand and treat the specific cause of the lipid disorder.

- Apolipoprotein A1 (apo A1) is the primary protein found in HDL-C. High levels of apo A1 (50 g/dL or higher) *lower* the risk for ASCVD.
- Apolipoprotein B (apo B) is the main protein component of VLDL-C and LDL-C. High levels of apo B (130 mg/dL) promote the uptake of cholesterol into arterial walls and *increase* the risk of ASCVD.
- High-sensitivity C-reactive protein (hs-CRP) increases with inflammation, infection and following a myocardial infarction. Because having a persistent, low level of inflammation promotes atherosclerosis, abnormal levels of hs-CRP (3.0 mg/L or higher) in an otherwise healthy person may be a biomarker for development for ASCVD.

Guidelines for the Management of Atherosclerotic Cardiovascular Disease

29.4 Management of ASCVD has evolved from targeting specific lipid values to a more comprehensive approach.

Establishing treatment guidelines for preventing ASCVD has been challenging because the condition has no symptoms and the progression to cardiovascular disease may take decades. Until 2013, treatment guidelines focused on determining target levels of LDL-C and HDL-C that could prevent the development of ASCVD. Essentially, if a patient exhibited laboratory values shown to be at high risk (see Table 29.1), pharmacotherapy was initiated and continued until these values returned to the normal range. This treatment goal was the same regardless of age, gender, race, or other compelling conditions such as diabetes or chronic kidney disease (CKD).

Major revisions were made to these guidelines by the American College of Cardiology (ACC) and the American Heart Association (AHA) in 2013 and again in 2018 (Grundy et al., 2019). The ACC/AHA guidelines no longer stress identical target goals for LDL-C levels for all patients. The approach to preventing and treating ASCVD is now more comprehensive and individualized.

For each patient, the 2018 guidelines are used to estimate the lifetime risk of ASCVD *if the high cholesterol level is left untreated* and recommends strategies to reduce the risk of future disease. The question of who should be treated for abnormal lipid levels is no longer simply based on a laboratory number. For example, not all patients with a blood cholesterol of 200 mg/dL need pharmacotherapy. Some patients should be treated at a much lower value, others at a higher value. Some patients will benefit from aggressive therapy at 200 mg/dL while others may require low-intensity therapy. Levels of therapy are now established for the different treatment categories, as shown in Table 29.2.

The 2018 Guidelines recommend that a detailed risk assessment be conducted by the healthcare provider (AHA/ACC, 2020). The purpose of the risk calculation is to *estimate a patient's 10-year risk of developing ASCVD*, using information such as age, race, sex, total cholesterol, HDL-C, blood pressure, use of aspirin and blood pressure medication, diabetes status and smoking status. Results of the risk assessment are used by the healthcare provider and patient to determine whether to initiate pharmacotherapy and, if so, at what level of intensity.

Following the calculation of risk assessment, the healthcare provider considers *additional risk-enhancing factors*

Table 29.2 Categories of Interventions for Preventing and Treating ASCVD

Categories	Intervention
Clinical ASCVD	High-intensity statins
Very high risk for ASCVD Severe primary hypercholesterolemia (LDL-C greater than 190 mg/dL)	High-intensity statins plus a nonstatin
Patients with diabetes, ages 40–75 years with LDL-C levels between 70 and 189 mg/dL	Moderate-intensity statins
Patients ages 40–75 years without ASCVD or diabetes but who have LDL-C levels 70–189 mg/dL and a 5–19.9% 10-year risk of ASCVD	Moderate-intensity statins
Patients ages 40–75 years without ASCVD or diabetes and with LDL-C levels 70–189 mg/dL and 7.5% or greater 10-year risk of ASCVD	Moderate- to high-intensity statins

that could influence the treatment decision. Some of the risk-enhancing factors that favor higher-intensity statin therapy include family history of premature ASCVD, persistently high LCL-C or triglyceride levels, metabolic syndrome, CKD, chronic inflammatory disorders, high-risk ethnic groups, history of preeclampsia, or premature menopause

The calculation of risk gives heavy emphasis on age, which places individuals age 65 or older at very high risk for an ASCVD event. This means that nearly everyone in that age group should be considered for statin therapy. To support this data, subsequent research has confirmed that reduction in LDL-C does indeed significantly reduce the incidence of major ASCVD events in older adults, especially in those at high risk for an occlusive event (Armitage et al., 2019).

29.5 Lipid levels can often be managed through therapeutic lifestyle changes.

The 2018 ACC/AHA Guidelines emphasize the importance of adopting a heart-healthy lifestyle throughout the lifespan for lowering the risk for ASCVD in all patients. Preventing ASCVD from developing is called *primary* prevention. After an ASCVD event has been identified, such as a stroke or myocardial infarction, *secondary* prevention is the process of reducing the risk of a subsequent cardiovascular event, usually with the help of medications to lower serum cholesterol. Heart-healthy lifestyle changes should always be included in both primary and secondary prevention treatment plans.

Following are the important heart-healthy lifestyle interventions:

- Monitor serum lipid levels regularly and take medications, as recommended by the healthcare provider.
- Maintain weight at an optimal level.
- Implement an exercise plan that includes at least 150 minutes of aerobic activity each week and muscle-strengthening exercises twice a week.
- Reduce consumption of sodium, saturated fats, cholesterol, and sugary drinks. Eliminate trans fats.
- Consume a diet containing plenty of fruits, vegetables, whole grains, lean meats, and low-fat dairy products
- Eliminate tobacco use and limit alcohol consumption.

The single most important lifestyle factor contributing to high levels of LDL-C is a high amount of saturated fat in the diet. Nutritionists recommend that the intake of dietary fat be limited to *less* than 30% of the total caloric intake and that cholesterol intake be reduced as much as possible. It is interesting to note that restriction of dietary cholesterol alone does not result in a significant reduction in blood cholesterol levels. In fact, cutting back on cholesterol consumption may actually increase the amount of circulating cholesterol. How is this possible? The liver reacts to a low-cholesterol diet by making more cholesterol and by inhibiting its excretion whenever saturated fats are present. Saturated fats are the building blocks that the liver uses for making cholesterol. However, replacing saturated fats from meats and dairy products with polyunsaturated fats from vegetable oils has been shown to reduce LDL-C and the risk for ASCVD. Saturated fats in the diet should be reduced to 5 to 6% of total daily calories. In addition, trans fatty acids from meat, dairy products, and processed snacks and bakery items should be eliminated from the diet.

CONNECTIONS: Lifespan Considerations

Pediatric Dyslipidemias and Lipid-Lowering Drugs

Many people consider dyslipidemia to be a condition that occurs with advancing age. Dyslipidemias are also a concern for pediatric patients, and multiple research studies have demonstrated that the early stages of atherosclerosis begin in childhood. Many cases of pediatric dyslipidemia occur for reasons other than a hereditary metabolic disorder, and causes include hypothyroidism, uncontrolled diabetes, medications (e.g., oral contraceptives, corticosteroids), renal and hepatic disease, and obesity (Elkins et al., 2019). With the increasing childhood obesity epidemic, there is concern that dyslipidemias, ASCVD, and metabolic syndrome will occur at younger and younger ages. The 2011 National Heart, Lung, and Blood Institute Integrated Guidelines for Cardiovascular Health and Risk Reduction in Children and Adolescents recommended targeted screening of lipid levels for children ages 2 and older with a positive or unknown family history of dyslipidemia-related ASCVD or other major risk factor and universal screening in those ages 9 to 11 years and again between 17 and 21 years (Expert Panel, 2011). Additionally, they recommended pharmacologic treatment with statins for children with LDL-C levels above 190 mg/dL, or for those with levels above 160 mg/dL with the presence of two or more cardiovascular risk factors before age 50.

Modifications such as healthy dietary changes, increased exercise and physical activity, adequate sleep periods, and weight loss for children who are already obese should be started when LDL-C levels are 130 mg/dL or above (Elkins et al., 2019). For children whose LDL-C levels remain elevated, a statin should be considered to decrease levels to 130 mg/dL or lower (Elkins & Friedrich, 2018). The role of exercise cannot be overstated, and researchers have found that over one-third of healthy adolescents don't reach the recommended 60 minutes of physical activity each day (Connolly & Ward, 2018). As research progresses into the amount and type of exercise that will achieve the best results, providing the patient with a specific exercise "prescription," particularly in an activity or activities they find enjoyable, may help to increase the overall amount of exercise achieved.

Drugs for Atherosclerotic Cardiovascular Disease

29.6 The statins are the most effective drugs for reducing serum lipid levels.

In the late 1970s substances were isolated from various species of fungi that inhibited cholesterol production in human cells in the laboratory. This class of drugs, known as the statins, has revolutionized the treatment of lipid disorders. Statins can produce a dramatic reduction in LDL-C levels, lower triglyceride and VLDL-C levels, and raise the levels of "good" HDL-C.

Cholesterol is manufactured in the liver by a series of more than 25 metabolic steps, beginning with acetyl CoA, a two-carbon unit that is produced from the breakdown of fatty acids (Figure 29.3). Of the many enzymes involved in this complex pathway, **HMG-CoA reductase** (3-hydroxy-3-methylglutaryl coenzyme A reductase) serves as the primary regulatory enzyme for the biosynthesis of cholesterol. Under normal conditions, this enzyme is regulated through negative feedback. High levels of LDL-C in the blood will shut down production of HMG-CoA reductase, thus turning off the cholesterol synthesis pathway. Pharmacotherapy Illustrated 29.1 shows some of the steps in the biosynthesis of cholesterol and the importance of HMG-CoA reductase.

The statins act by inhibiting HMG-CoA reductase, which reduces cholesterol biosynthesis. As the liver makes less cholesterol, it responds by making more LDL-C receptors on the surface of liver cells. The greater number of LDL-C receptors on liver cells removes *additional* LDL-C from the blood. Blood levels of both LDL-C and cholesterol are reduced. The reduction in serious ASCVD events from the statins is especially high in those patients who have diabetes as a comorbid condition with hyperlipidemia. The reduction of LDL-C is not permanent, however, so patients must continue these drugs for the remainder of their lives or until their dyslipidemia can be controlled through lifestyle changes.

Large clinical research studies over more than two decades have confirmed that statins clearly prevent serious ASCVD events and reduce mortality in patients when used as either primary or secondary prevention. Currently,

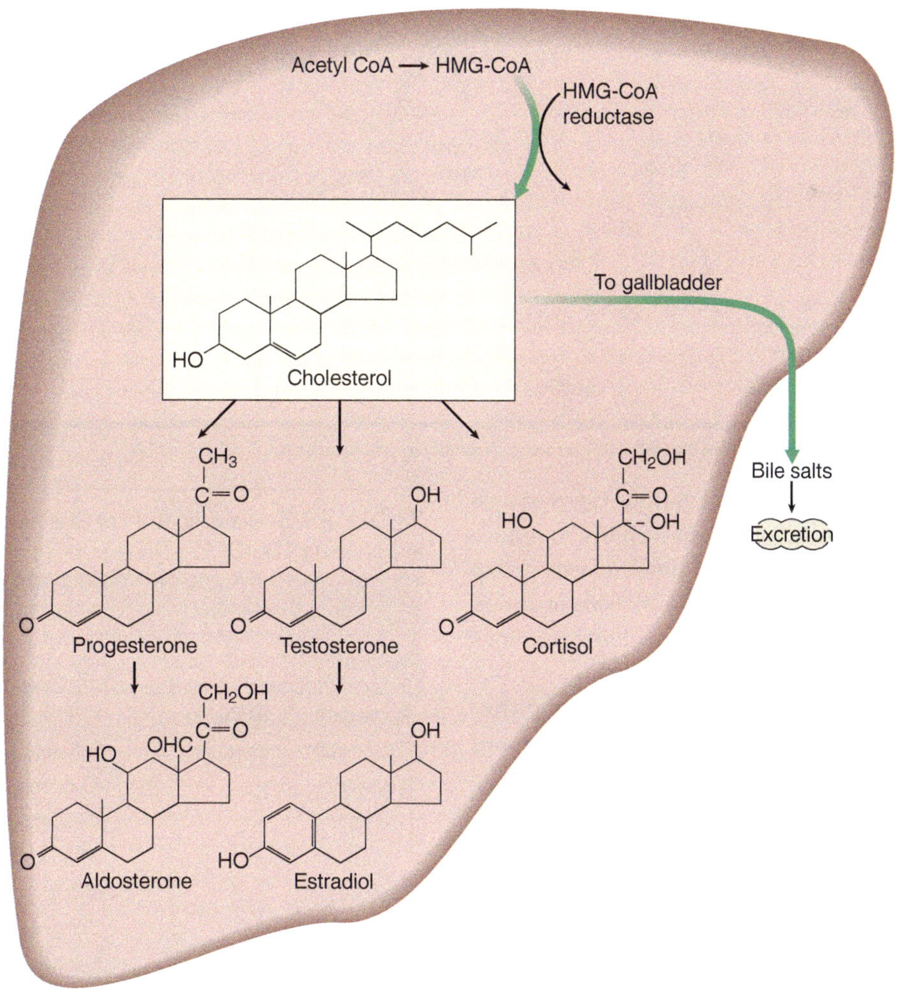

Figure 29.3 Cholesterol biosynthesis and excretion.

Pharmacotherapy Illustrated 29.1

Mechanisms of Action of Lipid-Lowering Drugs

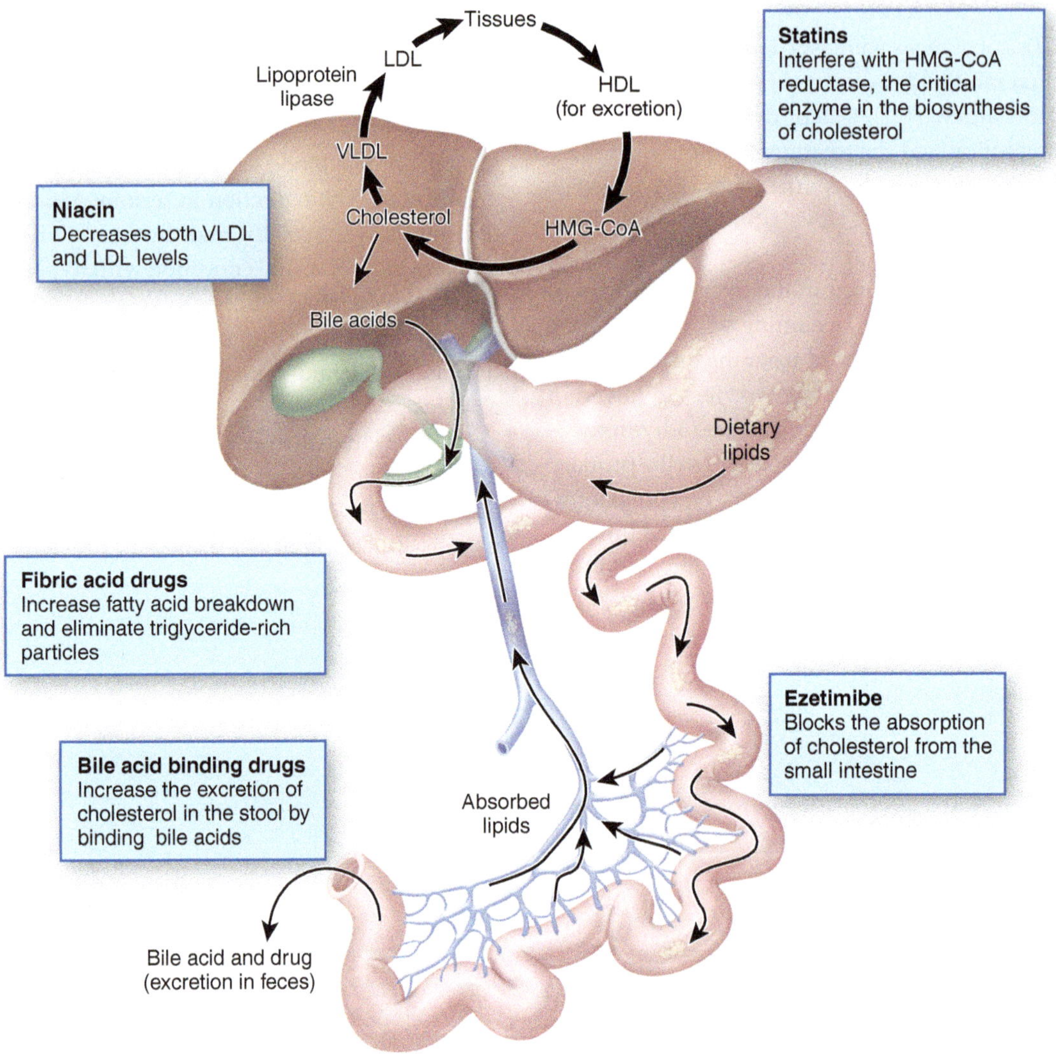

Based on Leland Norman Holland, Michael Adams, & Jeanine Brice (2018) Core concepts in pharmacology. New York: Pearson, p. 267, Figure 17.3.

seven statins are available for treating various types of dyslipidemias and they are classified by their ability to reduce LDL levels, as shown in Table 29.3. The high-intensity group includes statins that can reduce LDL-C by 50% or more. The intensity levels are used for the different interventions shown in Table 29.3.

In addition to intensity level, there are other differences among the statins. Lovastatin, pravastatin, and simvastatin are natural substances derived from fungi and have a different chemical structure than the synthetic statins. There are differences in potency among the drugs. For example, the maximum daily dose for pitavastatin is only 4 mg, whereas the maximum dose is 80 mg for atorvastatin. The half-lives of the statins vary from 20 hours (rosuvastatin) to less than an hour (fluvastatin). Whereas pravastatin is eliminated by the kidneys, the other statins are metabolized by hepatic CYP450 enzymes. In patients

Table 29.3 Classification of Statins by Their Effectiveness at Lowering LDL-C.

Statin	High Intensity Reduce LDL-C by 50% or more	Moderate Intensity Reduce LDL-C by 30–49%	Low Intensity Reduce LDL-C by less than 30%
Atorvastatin	40–80 mg	10–20 mg	–
Rosuvastatin	20–40 mg	5–10 mg	–
Pravastatin	–	40–80 mg	10–20 mg
Lovastatin	–	40–80 mg	20 mg
Simvastatin	–	20–40 mg	10 mg
Fluvastatin XL	–	80 mg	–
Fluvastatin	–	40 mg bid	20–40 mg
Pitavastatin	–	1–4 mg	–

Source: Grundy, S. M., et. al. (2019). 2018 AHA/ACC/AACVPR/AAPA/ABC/ACPM/ADA/AGS/APhA/ASPC/NLA/PCNA guideline on the management of blood cholesterol: executive summary: a report of the American College of Cardiology/American Heart Association Task Force on Clinical Practice Guidelines. Journal of the American College of Cardiology, 73(24), 3168-3209.

with renal disease, dosage adjustment is required for lovastatin, pravastatin, simvastatin, and rosuvastatin but not for fluvastatin or atorvastatin. Research evidence for cardiovascular adverse event prevention is greatest for atorvastatin and rosuvastatin. Doses for the statins are listed in Table 29.4.

All the statins are given orally (PO) and are tolerated well by most patients. Minor adverse effects include headache, abdominal cramping, diarrhea, muscle or joint pain, and heartburn.

Although rare, myopathy and rhabdomyolysis are serious, potential adverse effects of the statins. **Rhabdomyolysis** is a breakdown of muscle fibers usually due to muscle trauma or ischemia. The mechanism by which statins cause this disorder is unknown. During rhabdomyolysis, the contents of muscle cells spill into the systemic circulation,

Table 29.4 Drugs for Dyslipidemias

Drug	Route and Adult Dose (Maximum Dose Where Indicated)	Adverse Effects
HMG-CoA Reductase Inhibitors		
atorvastatin (Lipitor)	PO: 10–20 mg once daily (max: 80 mg/day)	*Headache, dyspepsia, abdominal cramping, myalgia, back pain, rash, pruritus* Rhabdomyolysis, severe myositis, elevated hepatic enzymes
fluvastatin (Lescol XL)	PO (immediate release): 20 mg daily (max: 80 mg/day) PO (extended release): 80 mg once daily	
lovastatin (Altoprev, Zypitamag)	PO (immediate release): 10–80 mg once daily (max: 80 mg/day) PO (extended release): 20–60 mg/day	
pitavastatin (Livalo)	PO: 1–4 mg daily (max: 4 mg/day)	
pravastatin (Pravachol)	PO: 10–40 mg daily (max: 80 mg/day)	
rosuvastatin (Crestor, Ezallor)	PO: 5–40 mg daily (max: 40 mg/day)	
simvastatin (Flolipid, Zocor)	PO: 5–40 mg daily (max: 80 mg/day)	
Bile Acid Sequestrants		
cholestyramine (Prevalite)	PO: 4–8 g bid–qid (max: 32 g/day)	*Constipation, nausea and vomiting, abdominal pain, bloating, dyspepsia* Gastrointestinal (GI) tract obstruction, vitamin deficiencies due to poor absorption
colesevelam (Welchol)	PO: 1.875 g bid (max: 3.75 g/day)	
colestipol (Colestid)	PO: 5–20 g/day in divided doses (30 g/day granules or 16 g/day tablets)	
Fibric Acid Drugs		
fenofibrate (Fenoglide, Triglide, others)	PO: Initial dosing 50–160 mg/day depending on trade name	*Myalgia, flulike symptoms, nausea and vomiting, increased serum transaminase and creatinine levels* Rhabdomyolysis, cholelithiasis, pancreatitis
fenofibric acid (Fibricor, Trilipix)	PO (Fibricor: regular release): 35–105 mg once daily PO (Trilipix: delayed release): 45–135 mg once daily	
gemfibrozil (Lopid)	PO: 600 mg bid (max: 1500 mg/day)	
Other Drugs for Dyslipidemia		
alirocumab (Praluent)	Subcutaneous: 75–150 mg q2wk	*Nasopharyngitis, injection-site reactions, influenza* Serious hypersensitivity reactions
evolocumab (Repatha)	Subcutaneous: 140 mg q2wk or 420 mg once monthly	*Nasopharyngitis, injection-site reactions, influenza, back pain* Serious hypersensitivity reactions
ezetimibe (Zetia)	PO: 10 mg daily (max: 10 mg/day)	*Nasopharyngitis, myalgia, upper respiratory infection, arthralgia, diarrhea* Anaphylaxis, rhabdomyolysis
icosapent (Vascepa)	PO: 4 g/day	*Arthralgia* Hypersensitivity
lomitapide (Juxtapid)	PO: 5–60 mg once daily	*Abdominal pain, diarrhea, nausea and vomiting, dyspepsia, reduced absorption of fat-soluble vitamins and fatty acids* Fetal toxicity, hepatotoxicity
mipomersen (Kynamro)	Subcutaneous: 200 mg once weekly	*Injection-site reactions, flulike symptoms, nausea, headache, and elevations in serum transaminases*
niacin (Niaspan)	Hyperlipidemia: PO: 250 mg regular release or 500 mg extended release daily (max: 6 g/day regular release or 1–2 g/day extended release)	*Flushing, nausea, pruritus, headache, bloating, diarrhea* Dysrhythmias
omega-3-acid ethyl esters (Lovaza)	PO: 4 g/day	*Belching, dyspepsia, fishy taste* Hypersensitivity

Note: *Italics* indicate common adverse effects. Underline indicates serious adverse effects.

causing potentially fatal acute kidney injury. Macrolide antibiotics such as erythromycin, azole antifungals, fibric acid drugs, and certain immunosuppressants should be avoided during statin therapy because these interfere with statin metabolism and increase the risk of severe myopathy. Levels of creatine kinase (CK), an enzyme released during muscle injury, should be obtained if myopathy is suspected. If CK levels become elevated during therapy, the drug should be immediately discontinued. Statins may be discontinued if muscle weakness persists even without CK elevation. Nurses should urge all patients who develop unexplained muscle or joint pain during statin therapy to immediately report this to the prescriber.

All the statins are contraindicated during pregnancy because teratogenic effects have been reported in laboratory animals exposed to these drugs. Females of reproductive potential should be advised to use contraception during therapy and discontinue the statin immediately if pregnancy is suspected. Breastfeeding is not recommended during treatment.

Because cholesterol biosynthesis in the liver is higher at night, statins with short half-lives such as lovastatin should be administered in the evening. The other statins have longer half-lives and are effective regardless of the time of day they are taken.

PROTOTYPE DRUG Atorvastatin (Lipitor)

Classification **Therapeutic:** Antihyperlipidemic
Pharmacologic: HMG-CoA reductase inhibitor, statin

Therapeutic Effects and Uses: Approved in 1996, atorvastatin was initially approved to treat hypercholesterolemia. Following several years of use, it became evident that the drug also prevents adverse cardiovascular events in high-risk patients. After 2 to 4 weeks of therapy, atorvastatin lowers LDL-C and VLDL-C as well as triglycerides. It appears to lower LDL-C levels greater than most other statins—50% or more. Atorvastatin may also be prescribed for the treatment of familial hypercholesterolemia. All patients receiving this drug should be placed on a cholesterol-lowering diet because this will enhance the drug's therapeutic effects. The primary goal in atorvastatin therapy is to reduce the risk of serious ASCVD events. Caduet is a combination of atorvastatin with amlodipine, a medication for hypertension.

To decrease GI discomfort, atorvastatin may be administered with food. It produces the same degree of LDL-C reduction regardless of the time of day it is taken. Because atorvastatin is not excreted by the kidneys, no adjustment in dosage is necessary in patients with CKD. Extensive metabolism to active metabolites gives atorvastatin a long duration of action.

Mechanism of Action: Atorvastatin acts by inhibiting HMG-CoA reductase, the primary regulatory enzyme in cholesterol biosynthesis. As the liver makes less cholesterol, it responds by making more LDL-C receptors, removing LDL-C from the blood. Blood levels of both LDL-C and total cholesterol are reduced.

Pharmacokinetics:

Route(s)	PO
Absorption	Rapidly absorbed but only 30% reaches the circulation; food reduces absorption
Distribution	Widely distributed; crosses the placenta and is secreted in breast milk; 98% bound to plasma proteins
Primary metabolism	Hepatic; extensively metabolized to active metabolites
Primary excretion	Biliary
Onset of action	2 weeks for lipid-lowering effect; peak plasma level: 1–2 h
Duration of action	Half-life: 14 h (20–30 h for active metabolites)

Adverse Effects: Most patients tolerate atorvastatin well and only 2% or fewer discontinue the drug due to adverse effects. Common adverse effects include headache, intestinal cramping, diarrhea, and constipation. The most serious adverse effect is rhabdomyolysis. Therapy is generally discontinued in patients reporting unexplained muscle pain, weakness, fever, or fatigue due to the potential for rhabdomyolysis.

Contraindications/Precautions: Patients with hepatic impairment should be monitored carefully because the liver extensively metabolizes atorvastatin and the drug has been associated with a small risk of liver failure. Liver enzyme tests may become elevated during therapy, although this does not necessarily indicate liver damage.

Drug Interactions: Because atorvastatin is a substrate for hepatic CYP3A4, it has the potential to interact with many other drugs. For example, it may increase digoxin levels by 20% as well as increase levels of norethindrone and ethinyl estradiol (oral contraceptives). Erythromycin may increase atorvastatin levels by as much as 40%. Risk of rhabdomyolysis increases with concurrent administration of atorvastatin with macrolide antibiotics, cyclosporine, and azole antifungals. The risk of myopathy increases when atorvastatin is administered concurrently with fibric acid drugs or niacin. Atorvastatin may increase serum transaminases and CK levels. **Herbal/Food:** Grapefruit juice inhibits the metabolism of statins, allowing them to reach high serum levels. Because HMG-CoA reductase inhibitors decrease the synthesis of Coenzyme Q10 (CoQ10), patients may benefit from CoQ10 supplements. Red rice yeast should not be taken with statins because it increases their toxicity.

Pregnancy: Atorvastatin is contraindicated during pregnancy and breastfeeding is not recommended during treatment.

Treatment of Overdose: No specific therapy is available; patients are treated symptomatically.

Clinician Responsibilities: Key clinical implications for patients receiving atorvastatin are included in Applied Clinical Judgment: Patients Receiving Pharmacotherapy for Hyperlipidemia.

Drugs Similar to Atorvastatin (Lipitor)

Other statins include fluvastatin, lovastatin, pitavastatin, pravastatin, rosuvastatin, and simvastatin.

Fluvastatin (Lescol XL): Approved in 1993, fluvastatin is a synthetic statin that has the shortest half-life of all the drugs in this class. Because the kidneys excrete less than 5% of a PO dose, dosage adjustment for patients with CKD is not necessary. Fewer drug interactions are expected with fluvastatin because it is not metabolized through the hepatic CYP450 system. It is approved for hypercholesterolemia and several other types of dyslipidemia. In 2003, the indications were expanded to include prevention of major ASCVD events. An extended-release formulation, Lescol-XL, is available. The drug may be administered without regard to meals. Fluvastatin is well tolerated and its adverse effects are similar to those of atorvastatin. It is contraindicated in patients with severe hepatic impairment and in patients who are pregnant.

Lovastatin (Altoprev): Approved in 1987, lovastatin, a natural substance derived from fungi, was the first HMG-CoA reductase inhibitor marketed. Lovastatin is a prodrug that the liver converts to several active metabolites. This drug may achieve a 20 to 40% reduction in LDL-C. Lovastatin is more effective if administered in the evening and should be taken on an empty stomach to maximize absorption. Although only 10% of this drug is excreted by the kidneys, dosage adjustment for patients with CKD is recommended. Lovastatin was originally approved for hypercholesterolemia; however, its indications have been expanded to include prevention and treatment of ASCVD. Altoprev is an extended-release form of the drug. Adverse effects are the same as those of other drugs in this class. It is contraindicated in patients with severe hepatic impairment.

Pitavastatin (Livalo, Zypitamag): Approved in 2009, pitavastatin is one of the newer drugs in the statin class. It is indicated for patients with primary hyperlipidemia and mixed dyslipidemia as an adjunctive therapy to diet to reduce elevated total cholesterol, LDL-C, apolipoprotein B, and triglycerides and to increase HDL-C. It may be administered with or without food and without regard to the time of day. It has similar effectiveness and adverse effects as other statins. Livalo is a calcium salt of lovastatin and Zypitamag is a magnesium salt. Because it is only minimally metabolized by CYP450 enzymes, it may exhibit fewer drug–drug interactions than some of the other statins. However, like other drugs in this class, hepatic enzymes should be evaluated regularly and there is a small risk of myopathy.

Pravastatin (Pravachol): Like lovastatin, pravastatin is a natural substance derived from fungi. Twenty percent of the drug is excreted by the kidneys, and dosage adjustment for patients with CKD is recommended. Like fluvastatin, it is not metabolized through the hepatic CYP450 system, thus fewer drug interactions are expected. The drug may be taken without regard to meals and is slightly more effective if administered in the evening. Approved in 1991, pravastatin is approved for primary hypercholesterolemia and prevention and treatment of ASCVD. Off-label uses include other types of dyslipidemias. Adverse effects are the same as those of other drugs in this class. It is contraindicated in patients with hepatic impairment.

Rosuvastatin (Crestor, Ezallor): Approved in 2003, rosuvastatin is a second-generation statin that contains a sulfur group. This drug is the most potent, has the longest half-life in its class (20 hours), and is capable of lowering LDL-C by as much as 65%. Rosuvastatin is not a prodrug and it undergoes minimal hepatic metabolism. This drug may be administered with or without food and without regard to time of day. Ezallor is a capsule that may be swallowed whole or opened and sprinkled on food for patients who have difficulty swallowing. Rosuvastatin is approved for hypercholesterolemia and hypertriglyceridemia and for the prevention and treatment of ASCVD. Adverse effects are the same as those of other drugs in this class.

Simvastatin (Flolipid, Zocor): Approved in 1991, simvastatin is a natural substance derived from fungi. Like lovastatin, simvastatin is a prodrug that is changed to active metabolites by the liver. The drug can lower LDL-C levels by as much as 47%. Although the kidneys excrete only 13% of the drug, dosage adjustment for patients with significant CKD is recommended. Flolipid is a suspension form of the drug. The drug may be taken with or without food but should be administered in the evening for maximum effectiveness. It is approved for hypercholesterolemia and hypertriglyceridemia and for the prevention and treatment of ASCVD. Adverse effects are the same as those of other drugs in this class. Vytorin is a combination tablet of simvastatin with ezetimibe. Simvastatin is contraindicated in patients with hepatic impairment.

CONNECTION Checkpoint 29.1

Several of the statins are prodrugs. From what you learned in Chapter 4, what type of dosage adjustment should be made if these statin prodrugs are prescribed for a patient with hepatic cirrhosis? If a dosage adjustment is not made, what types of adverse effects might you observe?

29.7 Bile acid sequestrants may be combined with statins to reduce LDL-C levels.

Bile acids contain a high concentration of cholesterol and are secreted by the liver to emulsify fats in the small intestine. After performing their digestive function, bile acids are reabsorbed in the ileum and sent back to the liver to again become part of bile through enterohepatic circulation. In effect, the cholesterol in bile acids is recycled, with only small amounts leaving the body in the feces.

Prior to the discovery of the statins, the primary means of lowering serum cholesterol was through the use of bile acid sequestrants or resins. The bile acid sequestrants bind to bile acids, forming a large complex that cannot be reabsorbed from the small intestine. The enterohepatic circulation of cholesterol is interrupted and the bound bile acids and cholesterol are eliminated in the feces. The liver responds to the loss of cholesterol by making more LDL-C receptors, which removes LDL-C from the blood in a mechanism similar to that of the statins.

The bile acid resins are capable of producing a 20% drop in LDL-C, which is less response than can be obtained from the statins. They are no longer considered first-line drugs for dyslipidemia, although they are sometimes combined with statins for patients who have contraindications or intolerance to statins.

The bile acid sequestrants cause more adverse effects than statins. Because they are not absorbed into the systemic circulation, adverse effects are limited to the GI tract, causing symptoms such as abdominal pain, bloating, diarrhea, steatorrhea, and constipation. In addition to binding bile acids, these agents can bind drugs such as digoxin and warfarin and increase the potential for drug–drug interactions. Bile acid sequestrants also interfere with the absorption of vitamins and minerals, and nutritional deficiencies may occur with extended use. Other medications and vitamins should be taken at least 1 hour before or 4 hours after taking a bile acid sequestrant to avoid drug interactions.

Bile acid sequestrants may cause a transient increase in triglyceride levels. This effect is particularly prominent and often sustained in patients with preexisting hypertriglyceridemia. Because of this, the bile acid sequestrants are generally not prescribed for patients with elevated triglycerides. Doses for the bile acid sequestrants are listed in Table 29.4.

CONNECTIONS: Complementary and Alternative Therapies

Coenzyme Q10

Description

Coenzyme Q10 (CoQ10) is a lipid-soluble vitamin-like substance found in most animal cells. It is an essential component in the cell's mitochondria for producing adenosine triphosphate (ATP) energy. Because the heart requires high levels of ATP, a sufficient level of CoQ10 is especially important to that organ.

History and Claims

The applications of CoQ10 to treating disease are relatively recent, with the agent being claimed to be an antioxidant and having benefited patients with heart failure in the mid-1960s. Subsequent reports have claimed that CoQ10 may be beneficial in angina pectoris, dysrhythmias, periodontal disease, immune disorders, neurologic disease, obesity, diabetes mellitus, and cancers.

Standardization

The dose of CoQ10 varies widely. Typical doses range from 100 to 200 mg/day.

Evidence

As with most dietary supplements, controlled research studies with CoQ10 are often lacking and give conflicting results. Supplementation with CoQ10 may be important to patients taking the HMG-CoA reductase inhibitors (statins) because these drugs significantly lower blood levels of CoQ10. Coenzyme Q10 and cholesterol share the same metabolic pathways. Inhibition of the enzyme HMG-CoA reductase by statins decreases CoQ10 levels. Many of the adverse effects of statins, including muscle weakness and rhabdomyolysis, may be due to the decrease in CoQ10 levels; supplementation with CoQ10 may improve myopathy symptoms, although these claims have not been verified by research (National Center for Complementary and Integrative Health, 2019).

Foods richest in this substance are pork, sardines, beef heart, salmon, broccoli, spinach, and nuts. Older adults appear to have an increased need for CoQ10. Although CoQ10 can be synthesized by the body, many amino acids and other substances are required for this synthesis; thus, patients with nutritional deficiencies may need supplementation.

PROTOTYPE DRUG Cholestyramine (Prevalite)

Classification **Therapeutic:** Antihyperlipidemic
Pharmacologic: Bile acid sequestrant

Therapeutic Effects and Uses: Approved in 1966, cholestyramine is indicated for the reduction of elevated serum cholesterol in patients with primary hypercholesterolemia (elevated LDL-C) who do not respond adequately to dietary modifications alone. When combined with statins, cholestyramine reduces LDL-C and helps to prevent ASCVD events. A secondary indication is to relieve pruritus associated with partial biliary obstruction. It is available as a powder that is mixed with fluid before being taken once or twice daily. The drug should be mixed with 60 to 180 mL of water, noncarbonated beverages, highly liquid soups, or pulpy fruits (applesauce, crushed pineapple) to prevent esophageal irritation. The medication should be swallowed immediately after stirring. If taken with too small a fluid volume or if not completely swallowed, the drug can swell in the throat or esophagus and cause an obstruction.

It may take 30 days or longer for cholestyramine to produce its maximum effect. To avoid interference with absorption, cholestyramine should not be taken at the same time as vitamins or other medications.

Mechanism of Action: Cholestyramine binds to bile acids, forming an insoluble complex containing cholesterol that is excreted in the feces. Cholestyramine lowers LDL-C levels by increasing LDL-C receptors on hepatocytes.

Pharmacokinetics:

Route(s)	PO
Absorption	Not absorbed
Distribution	Not distributed; acts locally in the alimentary canal
Primary metabolism	Not metabolized
Primary excretion	Feces
Onset of action	1–2 days
Duration of action	2–4 weeks

Adverse Effects: Cholestyramine is not absorbed or metabolized once it enters the intestine; thus, it does not produce systemic adverse effects. Common GI-related adverse effects include constipation, bloating, belching, and nausea. Serious adverse effects include obstruction of the GI tract, hyperchloremic acidosis, and malabsorption syndrome. Chronic use may cause increased bleeding due to hypoprothrombinemia associated with vitamin K deficiency.

Contraindications/Precautions: Cholestyramine should be used cautiously in patients with GI disorders such as peptic ulcer disease, hemorrhoids, inflammatory bowel diseases, or chronic constipation because bile acid sequestrants may worsen or aggravate these conditions. This drug should not be used in patients with complete biliary obstruction. Bile acid resins should be used with caution in patients with hypertriglyceridemia because they may increase serum triglyceride concentrations. They are absolutely contraindicated if serum triglycerides rise above 400 mg/dL. Although cholestyramine use is safe during pregnancy because it is not absorbed, precautions must be taken to ensure that this drug is not interfering with vitamin absorption, especially folic acid.

Drug Interactions: Cholestyramine can bind to other drugs and interfere with their absorption, causing reduced effects. This interaction has been reported for digoxin, penicillins, iron supplements, thyroid hormone, and thiazide diuretics, although it has the potential to occur with any drug administered PO. Cholestyramine may indirectly increase the effects of warfarin by binding to vitamin K, decreasing its absorption and lowering the levels of vitamin K in the body. The absorption of raloxifene can be reduced as much as 60% if coadministered with cholestyramine. To reduce the possibility of absorption interference, cholestyramine should be administered 1 hour before or 4 hours after other PO medications. **Herbal/Food:** Cholestyramine may block the absorption of iron and fat-soluble vitamins in food.

Pregnancy: Cholestyramine is not absorbed therefore no fetal harm would be expected. This drug does not enter breast milk; use with caution during pregnancy due to potential vitamin loss in the mother.

Treatment of Overdose: No specific therapy is available; patients are treated symptomatically.

Clinician Responsibilities: Key clinical implications for patients receiving cholestyramine are included in Applied Clinical Judgment: Patients Receiving Pharmacotherapy for Hyperlipidemia.

Drugs Similar to Cholestyramine (Prevalite)

Other bile acid sequestrants include colesevelam and colestipol.

Colesevelam (Welchol): Approved in 2000, colesevelam is a bile acid–binding drug that has the capacity to reduce LDL-C by as much as 20%. It may be administered as monotherapy or concurrently with statins to achieve greater efficacy at reducing serious ASCVD events. At least 2 weeks of therapy may be necessary before maximum therapeutic response is achieved. Colesevelam is also approved as an adjunct to diet, exercise, and antidiabetic drugs to improve glycemic control in patients with type 2 diabetes. It is not approved for patients with type 1 diabetes. The most common adverse reactions with colesevelam are constipation, dyspepsia, and nausea. Colesevelam can interfere with the absorption of other medications and should be administered 4 hours after other PO drugs. Like cholestyramine, colesevelam can increase serum triglyceride levels and is contraindicated in patients with triglyceride levels greater than 500 mg/dL. The large tablets can cause dysphagia or esophageal obstruction; thus, this drug should be used with caution in patients with swallowing disorders. An oral suspension, dissolved in 4 to 8 ounces of water, is available for patients who have difficulty swallowing the tablets. Animal reproduction studies showed no evidence of either maternal or fetal toxicity.

Colestipol (Colestid): Approved in 1977, colestipol acts by the same mechanism as cholestyramine, has similar effectiveness in lowering LDL-C, and exhibits the same adverse effects. Other drugs should be administered at least 1 hour before or 4 to 6 hours after a dose of colestipol to prevent interference with absorption. Maximum therapeutic effects may take as long as a month to appear. Because the drug can increase serum triglycerides, it should not be administered to patients with hypertriglyceridemia. Colestipol is rarely used as monotherapy. In addition to its use in treating elevated HDL-C, colestipol may be used off-label to treat digoxin overdose, diarrhea, and pruritus associated with biliary obstruction. During breastfeeding colestipol taken by the mother may interfere with vitamin absorption in the infant.

PharmFACT

Familial hypercholesterolemia affects 1 in 200 people and is a genetic disease that predisposes people to premature ASCVD (Gidding, 2016).

29.8 Niacin can reduce triglycerides and LDL-C levels, but adverse effects limit its usefulness.

Niacin, also called nicotinic acid, is a B-complex vitamin (B_3). Its ability to lower serum lipid levels, however, is unrelated to its role as a vitamin because much higher doses are needed to produce its antihyperlipidemic effects. For lowering cholesterol, the usual dose is 2 to 3 g/day. When taken as a vitamin, the dose is only 25 mg/day.

The primary action of niacin (Niaspan) is to decrease the production of VLDL-C, which lowers serum triglyceride levels. Because LDL-C is synthesized from VLDL-C, the patient also experiences a reduction in LDL-C levels. Niacin also has the desirable effect of increasing HDL-C levels, although this effect does not appear to be significant in reducing mortality from cardiovascular disease. As with other lipid-lowering drugs, maximum therapeutic effects may take a month or longer to achieve.

Although effective at reducing LDL-C by 20%, niacin produces more adverse effects than the statins. Intense flushing and hot flashes occur in most patients. Taking one aspirin tablet 30 minutes prior to niacin administration can reduce uncomfortable flushing in many patients. In addition, a variety of uncomfortable GI effects such as nausea, excess gas, and diarrhea are commonly reported. Paresthesias, such as tingling in the extremities, may also occur. No animal studies have been conducted to determine the safety of niacin during pregnancy or lactation.

More serious adverse effects such as hepatotoxicity and gout are possible but uncommon. Patients with elevated liver enzymes or a history of liver disease should use an alternate drug to lower lipids. In patients predisposed to gout, niacin may increase uric acid levels and precipitate acute gout.

Niacin is not usually prescribed for patients with diabetes mellitus because the drug can raise fasting glucose levels. When beginning therapy, patients with diabetes should monitor their blood glucose levels more frequently until the effect of niacin is determined.

Because of the high incidence of adverse effects, niacin is most often used in low doses in combination with a bile acid sequestrant; the beneficial effects of these drugs are additive. Niacin was formerly combined with statins; however, the U.S. Food and Drug Administration (FDA) determined that the combination did not offer any reduction in cardiovascular mortality over simply using a statin as monotherapy.

Because supplemental niacin is available without a prescription, patients should be instructed not to attempt self-medication with this drug. One form of niacin that is available over-the-counter (OTC) as a vitamin supplement, called nicotinamide, has no lipid-lowering effects. If niacin is to be used to lower cholesterol, it should be done under medical supervision.

29.9 Fibric acid drugs lower triglyceride levels but have little effect on LDL-C.

Three fibric acid drugs are sometimes used for patients with high triglyceride levels: fenofibrate (Fenoglide, TriCor, Triglide), fenofibric acid (Fibricor, Trilipix), and gemfibrozil (Lopid). They are preferred drugs for treating severe hypertriglyceridemia, although they have little effect on LDL-C. Fibric acid drugs activate the enzyme lipoprotein lipase, which increases the breakdown and elimination of triglyceride-rich particles from the plasma. The FDA does not recommend combining a fibric acid drug with a statin because combination therapy is not more effective at reducing ASCVD events than using a statin as monotherapy. Doses for the fibric acid drugs are listed in Table 29.4.

The most common adverse effects of the fibrates relate to the GI system: dyspepsia, diarrhea, abdominal pain and nausea and vomiting. Taking these medications with meals usually diminishes GI distress. Drugs in this class are generally not used in patients with hepatic impairment or gallbladder disease.

PROTOTYPE DRUG **Gemfibrozil (Lopid)**

Classification **Therapeutic:** Antihyperlipidemic
Pharmacologic: Fibric acid drug (fibrate)

Therapeutic Effects and Uses: Approved in 1981, gemfibrozil lowers serum triglycerides and LDL-C. It is most effective in patients who present with hypertriglyceridemia and VLDL-C. Effects of gemfibrozil include up to a 50% reduction in VLDL-C with an increase in HDL-C. It is less effective than the statins at lowering LDL-C, thus it is not used as monotherapy. It is considered a second-line therapy that is used when statins are ineffective or not well tolerated.

Mechanism of Action: The exact mechanism of action of gemfibrozil is unknown. The drug inhibits the breakdown of stored fat, or lipolysis, in adipose tissue. By inhibiting the uptake of free fatty acids by the liver, hepatic production of triglycerides is decreased. The drug may also increase the excretion of cholesterol in the feces.

Pharmacokinetics:

Route(s)	PO
Absorption	Well absorbed
Distribution	Unknown; distribution across the placenta or secretion in breast milk is unknown; 99% bound to plasma protein
Primary metabolism	Hepatic; undergoes enterohepatic recirculation
Primary excretion	Primarily renal, 6% in feces
Onset of action	1–2 h
Duration of action	Half-life: 1.5 h

Adverse Effects: The most common adverse effects of gemfibrozil are GI related, such as abdominal cramping, diarrhea, nausea, and dyspepsia. Nervous system effects include headache, dizziness, peripheral neuropathy, and diminished libido. Serious adverse effects include cholelithiasis, anemia, and eosinophilia.

Contraindications/Precautions: Gemfibrozil may worsen or cause biliary disease; thus, it is contraindicated in patients with preexisting gallbladder disease or serious liver impairment. Because it is excreted by the kidneys, the drug should be used cautiously in patients with CKD.

Drug Interactions: Although antihyperlipidemic drugs from different classes are sometimes combined to produce an enhanced effect, the use of gemfibrozil with statins increases the risk of myositis and rhabdomyolysis. CK levels should be regularly monitored during combined therapy and the combination immediately discontinued if myopathy is suspected. In most cases the risk of rhabdomyolysis, which may be fatal, outweighs the potential benefits of combined statin and gemfibrozil therapy.

Concurrent use of gemfibrozil with PO anticoagulants may increase the risk of bleeding because the fibrate displaces warfarin from its plasma protein binding sites. If a patient is taking warfarin, dosages should be lowered. More frequent monitoring of prothrombin time (PT) and international normalized ratio (INR) is necessary until stabilization occurs.

Gemfibrozil may enhance the hypoglycemic effects of antidiabetic drugs. Serum glucose levels must be carefully monitored because the dosage of the antidiabetic drug may require adjustment. **Herbal/Food:** No significant interactions.

Pregnancy: Animal studies showed adverse fetal effects such as increased stillborn and skeletal variations. It is not known if gemfibrozil is secreted in milk. This drug is not recommended during pregnancy or lactation unless the potential benefits to the mother justify the potential risks to the fetus or neonate.

Treatment of Overdose: No specific therapy is available; patients are treated symptomatically.

Clinician Responsibilities: Key clinical implications for patients receiving gemfibrozil are included in Applied Clinical Judgment: Patients Receiving Pharmacotherapy for Hyperlipidemia.

Drugs Similar to Gemfibrozil (Lopid)

Drugs similar to gemfibrozil include fenofibrate and fenofibric acid.

Fenofibrate (Fenoglide, TriCor, Triglide, Others) and fenofibric acid (Fibricor, Trilipix): Once absorbed, fenofibrate is quickly converted to fenofibric acid, its active metabolite. Thus, the actions and adverse effects of the two drugs are the same. Fenofibrate is indicated as supplemental therapy to diet to reduce elevated LDL-C, total cholesterol, triglycerides, and apo B and to increase HDL-C in patients with primary hypercholesterolemia, hypertriglyceridemia, and mixed dyslipidemia. Approved in 1993, fenofibrate may reduce serum triglycerides by as much as 30%. One advantage of the fenofibrate formulations over gemfibrozil is that they may be taken once daily rather than twice a day. The different formulations of fenofibrate and fenofibric acid vary in strength, bioavailability, and whether the drug should be administered with or without food. These forms are not interchangeable. One of the forms, Trilipix, is approved for concurrent therapy with statins, although this combination has not been found to be any more effective than statin monotherapy. The most frequent adverse effects are GI related, such as nausea and vomiting, dyspepsia, constipation, flatulence, and abdominal pain. Liver function tests should be performed periodically to monitor for elevated serum transaminases. Myopathy and rhabdomyolysis have been reported, and the risks for these adverse effects are increased when coadministered with a statin. Rash and photosensitivity are other adverse effects. Animal studies showed no evidence of embryofetal toxicity. Fenofibrate is contraindicated during breastfeeding because of possible adverse effects on infant lipid metabolism.

Miscellaneous Drugs for Dyslipidemias

29.10 Newer strategies have been developed to treat dyslipidemias.

Although the effectiveness of the statins at reducing serious ASCVD events is strongly supported by research, there are limitations. Some patients are unable to tolerate the adverse effects of statins. In some cases, maximum doses of statins are not effective at lowering LDL-C to sufficiently reduce the incidence of ASCVD events. The search for more effective antilipidemics has resulted in several new drugs for this condition.

Ezetimibe (Zetia): Ezetimibe (Zetia) is the only drug in a class called the cholesterol absorption inhibitors. Cholesterol is absorbed from the intestinal lumen by cells in the jejunum. Ezetimibe blocks this absorption by as much as 50%, causing less cholesterol to enter the blood. When given as monotherapy, ezetimibe produces a slight drop in serum triglycerides and a modest reduction in LDL-C of about 20%. Ezetimibe is usually prescribed when maximally tolerated statin therapy has been unable to lower LDL-C to target levels in patients at high risk for an ASCVD event.

Ezetimibe is available as a single tablet with a once-daily dosing regimen. Vytorin is a fixed-dose combination tablet containing ezetimibe and simvastatin, and Nexlizet combines ezetimibe with bempedoic acid. Bempedoic acid is a new medication that blocks cholesterol synthesis in the liver by a different mechanism than the statins. It is approved as an adjunct to maximally tolerated statins in lowering LDL-C levels. The combination of bempedoic acid with ezetimibe may cause fetal harm and is not recommended during breastfeeding.

Nasopharyngitis, myalgia, upper respiratory infection, arthralgia, and diarrhea are the most common adverse effects of ezetimibe, although these rarely require discontinuation of therapy. Because bile acid sequestrants inhibit the absorption of ezetimibe, these drugs should not be taken together. In addition, ezetimibe and statins should not be given concurrently to patients with serious hepatic impairment or with elevated serum transaminase levels.

Omega-3 fatty acids: Nutritionists have long reported the benefits of eating fish rich in omega-3 fatty acids such as tuna, salmon, and halibut. The two principal omega-3 fatty acids are eicosapentaenoic acid (EPA) and docosahexaenoic acid (DHA). Vegetarian sources of omega-3 fatty acids include flaxseed oil, soybeans, walnuts, and pumpkin seeds.

The role of omega-3 fatty acids in preventing cardiovascular disease is well established. When taken as dietary supplements, the omega-3 fatty acids are usually marketed as fish oil. Fish oil supplementation has been shown to decrease mortality due to MI and stroke. A typical dose of omega-3 fatty acids in fish oil capsules is 180 mg of EPA and 120 mg of DHA.

Two prescription formulations of omega-3 fatty acids are available: omega-3-acid ethyl esters (Lovaza) and icosapent (Vascepa). Both drugs are approved as an adjunct to diet in the treatment of severe hypertriglyceridemia (500mg/dL or greater). The indications for icosapent were recently expanded to include being an adjunct to maximally treated statin therapy inpatients at very high risk for ASCVD events. Adverse effects are minor and include belching, fishy taste, and arthralgia. The drugs should be used with caution in patients who are allergic to seafood, especially shellfish. Vascazen is another a prescription drug containing omega-3 fatty acids, however, it is classified as a *medical food* and only indicated for the dietary management of omega-3 deficiency in patients with cardiovascular disease. The safety of the omega-3 fatty acid medications during pregnancy and lactation have not been evaluated.

Drugs for familial hypercholesterolemia: Two drugs were approved in 2013 for a very narrow indication: as an adjunct to lowering LDL-C in patients with homozygous familial hypercholesterolemia (HoFH). HoFH is a genetic disorder in which the body has such high levels of cholesterol and LDL-C that cardiovascular disease begins in childhood and results in death by the mid-30s. Many of these patients have a diminished response to therapy with statins and other antihyperlipidemics. The two new drugs, lomitapide (Juxtapid) and mipomersen (Kynamro), act by very different and unique mechanisms. Therapy is costly and will likely limit their widespread use.

The primary protein that composes particles of LDL-C is apo B. When assembling the lipoprotein, lipid molecules are transported and loaded onto the apo B. Upon completion, the lipoprotein is assembled and leaves the intestine or liver as chylomicrons or VLDL-C, which eventually raises blood LDL-C levels. Lomitapide and mipomersen interfere with different aspects of this genesis of lipoprotein.

Lomitapide is classified as a microsomal triglyceride transfer protein (MTP) inhibitor. Inhibition of MTP interferes with the transfer of lipids to apo B, thus lowering plasma levels of LDL-C. The drug is given PO and is indicated only for HoFH. GI adverse effects such as diarrhea, nausea and vomiting, dyspepsia, and abdominal pain occur in almost all patients. Drug interactions may be serious with medications that inhibit hepatic CYP3A4, including ketoconazole, clarithromycin, lopinavir/ritonavir, or telithromycin. These drugs will markedly increase levels of lomitapide. Lomitapide is teratogenic in animals and is secreted in human milk. Use during pregnancy is contraindicated.

Mipomersen is classified as an inhibitor of apo B synthesis. The message for making apo B leaves the DNA as a strip of messenger RNA (mRNA). Mipomersen is a huge molecule that has mRNA complementary to apo B (called an antisense message). The antisense message binds to the apo B strip of RNA, preventing the synthesis of the apo B protein. Mipomersen is given as a once-weekly subcutaneous injection. Animal studies showed no fetal harm. It is not known if this drug is secreted in human milk or if it has adverse effects on the breastfed neonate. Females of childbearing potential are advised to use contraception during therapy.

Mipomersen and lomitapide carry identical black box warnings that the drugs can cause elevations in transaminases and may increase hepatic fat (hepatic steatosis). The drugs are contraindicated in patients with active hepatic disease, and alanine transaminases (ALT) and aspartate aminotransferase (AST) must be measured prior to and during therapy. The drugs are only available in restricted-use programs that require prescribers and pharmacists to be certified through special training.

PCSK9 inhibitors: A new strategy to manage increased cholesterol levels is to inhibit PCSK9 (proprotein convertase subtilisin kexin type 9), a protein that *degrades* receptors for LDL-C in the liver. Binding of the drug to PCSK9 increases the number of receptors available to clear LDL-C, thus lowering the level of LDL-C in the blood. Alirocumab (Praluent) and evolocumab (Repatha), both approved in 2015, are monoclonal antibodies given by the subcutaneous route that inhibit PCSK9. They are indicated as adjuncts to diet and LDL-C-lowering therapies such as statins and ezetimibe to reduce the risk for serious ASCVD events. They are also indicated for patients with heterozygous familial hypercholesterolemia (HeFH) or HoFH who need additional lowering of LDL-C than can be attained with other therapies. The two PCSK9 inhibitors are much more expensive than statins and some have recommended their use be reserved for very high-risk patients. The most common adverse effects of the PCSK9 inhibitors include allergic reactions, injection site reactions, nasopharyngitis, and upper respiratory infections. Animal studies have not identified major risks during pregnancy or lactation.

CONNECTIONS: APPLIED CLINICAL JUDGMENT

Patients Receiving Pharmacotherapy for Hyperlipidemia

Key Assessment Data

- History of current condition, baseline vital signs, physical exam findings; history of cardiovascular, musculoskeletal (preexisting conditions that might result in muscle or joint pain), GI (peptic ulcer disease, hemorrhoids, inflammatory bowel disease, chronic constipation, gallbladder disease, dysphagia, or esophageal strictures); drug history including allergies, current prescription and OTC drugs, herbal preparations, and alcohol use; pregnancy status.
- Ongoing assessment during drug therapy includes laboratory findings, especially liver function studies, lipid profiles, and CK.

Desired Therapeutic Outcomes

Improvement is observed and measurable in improved lipid profile levels (lowered total cholesterol and LDL-C levels, increased HDL-C levels).

Minimizing Adverse Effects

- Abnormal liver function tests or increased CK levels may indicate drug-induced adverse hepatic effects or myopathy and should be reported.
- Lipid-lowering drugs often adversely affect the liver but may also cause drug-specific adverse effects, especially musculoskeletal, hepatic, and GI. Lipid-lowering drugs given in combination increase this risk.
- If statins are used, report unusual or unexplained muscle tenderness, increasing muscle pain, numbness or tingling of extremities, or effects that hinder normal ADLs.
- If bile acid resins are used, report severe nausea, heartburn, constipation, or straining with passing stools. Any tarry stools or yellowing of the sclera or skin should also be reported.
- If fibric acid drugs are used, report unusual bleeding or bruising, right upper quadrant pain, muscle cramping, or changes in the color of the stool. Patients with diabetes on PO medications may need a change in their dosage and should monitor their glucose more frequently in early therapy.

Lifespan Considerations

- Monitor liver function and CK tests more frequently in the older adult because age-related physiologic changes may affect the drug's metabolism or excretion.
- Statins should not be used during pregnancy, if pregnancy is suspected, or while breastfeeding.
- If fibric acid drugs are used, the older adult is at increased risk for dizziness and may require assistance with ambulation to prevent falls.

Diversity Considerations

- Because statins metabolize through the CYP450 system, they may interact with other drugs. Observe for less-than-optimal therapeutic effects, especially in ethnically diverse patients.

Patient and Caregiver Education

- Adopt appropriate lifestyle changes: lowered fat intake, increased exercise, limited alcohol intake, and smoking cessation. Increase intake of foods rich in omega-3 and Coenzyme Q10: fish such as salmon and sardines, nuts, extra-virgin olive and canola oils, beef, chicken, and pork. Supplementation may be needed but seek the advice of a healthcare provider before taking supplements. A dietitian consultation may be helpful.
- Take the drug following appropriate guidelines:
  - **Statins:** Most are taken with the evening meal; avoid grapefruit and grapefruit juice, which could inhibit the drug's metabolism, leading to toxic levels.
  - **Bile acid resins:** Take before meals with plenty of fluids, mixing powders or granules thoroughly with liquid. Take other medications 1 h before or 4 h after the bile acid resin is taken.
  - **Niacin:** Take with cold water to decrease the sensation of flushing associated with the drug. Take one adult-strength (325-mg) aspirin 30 min before the niacin dose.
  - **Fibric acid drugs:** Take with a meal.

Prescribing Considerations

- Obtain baseline laboratory tests of renal and liver function before prescribing.
- Combining lipid-lowering agents requires close monitoring of liver function tests and CK levels; discontinue if serum transaminase (ALT) is more than three times the normal level, in the presence of elevated CPK levels, if myopathy occurs, or if there is a predisposition to renal failure.
- Niacin should be started at a low dose, and any increases in dosage should be made very slowly in order to minimize adverse effects.
- When combining niacin with a statin, a smaller dose of niacin should be used in order to lower patients' risk of developing hepatotoxicity, myopathy, and rhabdomyolysis.
- For patients on statins, asses for myopathy and tendonopathy at each clinical visit. These adverse effects will often resolve by lowering the dose or switching to a different statin.

Understanding Chapter 29

Key Concepts Summary

29.1 Lipids are classified as triglycerides, phospholipids, or sterols.

29.2 Lipoproteins are important predictors of cardiovascular disease.

29.3 Serum lipid panels are important diagnostic tools in guiding the therapy of dyslipidemias.

29.4 Management of ASCVD has evolved from targeting specific lipid values to a more comprehensive approach.

29.5 Lipid levels can often be managed through therapeutic lifestyle changes.

29.6 The statins are the most effective drugs for reducing serum lipid levels.

29.7 Bile acid sequestrants may be combined with statins to reduce LDL-C levels.

29.8 Niacin can reduce triglycerides and LDL-C levels, but adverse effects limit its usefulness.

29.9 Fibric acid drugs lower triglyceride levels but have little effect on LDL-C.

29.10 Newer strategies have been developed to treat dyslipidemias.

CASE STUDY: Making the Patient Connection

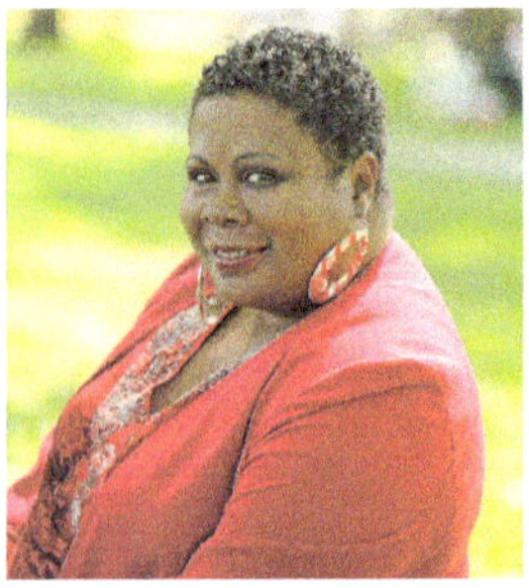

Remember the patient "Belinda Cummings" at the beginning of the chapter? Now read the remainder of the case study. Based on the information presented within this chapter, respond to the critical thinking questions that follow.

Belinda Cummings is a 39-year-old woman who feels fine. However, she recently had her cholesterol level checked at her church's health fair where she was told that it exceeded the normal value. As directed, she made an appointment and saw her healthcare provider for a checkup.

During the office visit, the nurse collects Belinda's social and health history. Belinda's vital signs are within normal limits, except her blood pressure is elevated (142/90 mmHg). She is also slightly overweight and has been on a low-carbohydrate diet for 1 week. Her favorite foods are potato chips and all dairy products, especially cheese. She admits to smoking less than a pack of cigarettes per day and occasionally drinks a glass of wine with dinner. Belinda is divorced and has one teenage son.

A series of laboratory tests is completed during the visit. Belinda's physical examination is normal, and there are no ECG abnormalities. The blood tests are unremarkable with the exception of the lipid profile.

	Patient Value	Normal Range
Total Cholesterol	240 mg/dL	Less than 200
Triglycerides	199 mg/dL	Less than 150
HDL-C	30 mg/dL	Greater than 60
LDL-C	184	Less than 100
Cholesterol-to-HDL-C Ratio	6.6	Less than 4.5

The patient is placed on a standard cholesterol-lowering diet and prescribed atorvastatin (Lipitor), 10 mg daily. Belinda is instructed to return to the office in 1 month for a follow-up visit.

Critical Thinking Questions

1. How would you respond to Belinda when she asks you, "Is high cholesterol due to heredity or what I eat?"
2. What health teaching should you provide the patient about ways to reduce high blood lipid levels?
3. Create a list of potential adverse effects that this patient should be taught to watch for related to the medication.

Additional Case Study

David Hamilton has been taking cholestyramine (Questran) for elevated blood lipid levels for 2 years. He presents today in your clinic for a routine follow-up visit that will include a lipid profile test. He states that he has been somewhat consistent with his cholesterol-lowering diet and attempting to get "a little more" exercise. You are the nurse caring for David.

1. Outline key concepts related to health promotion activities that you would want to be sure David understands.
2. What adverse effects related to Questran should David watch for?
3. If David's triglyceride levels increase or remain consistently high, what drug group(s) might be prescribed?

Chapter Review

1. The patient taking atorvastatin (Lipitor) reports weakness and fatigue, pain in the shoulders, and aching joints. The nurse initially assesses the patient for which condition?

1. Rhabdomyolysis
2. Renal failure
3. Rheumatoid arthritis
4. Hepatic insufficiency

2. A patient is receiving cholestyramine (Questran) for elevated low-density lipoprotein levels. Which adverse effect should the nurse include in the care plan to monitor the patient?

1. Orange-colored urine
2. Abdominal pain
3. Sore throat and fever
4. Decreased capillary refill

3. The provider orders colestipol (Colestid) in combination with atorvastatin (Lipitor) for a patient with elevated low-density lipoprotein levels. The nurse collaborates with the prescriber about which data related to the patient?

1. Past history of peptic ulcer disease
2. Recent myocardial infarction
3. Laboratory value for serum sodium of 136 mEq/L
4. Allergies to foods high in tyramine

4. Which assessment findings discovered by the nurse would be an expected adverse effect associated with niacin therapy? (Select all that apply.)

1. Fever and chills
2. Intense flushing and hot flashes
3. Tingling of the fingers and toes
4. Dry mucous membranes
5. Hypoglycemia

5. The community health nurse visits a patient who has been prescribed lovastatin (Mevacor). Which statement, if made by the patient, indicates that further teaching is necessary concerning this drug therapy?

1. "I should try to maintain my body weight at an optimal level."
2. "Most patients with lipid disorders don't have any symptoms."
3. "The best time for me to take this medication is before I go to bed."
4. "I will take my drug with beverages that contain grapefruit juice."

6. The nurse is caring for a patient receiving gemfibrozil (Lopid) for hyperlipidemia. The nurse would validate the order with the prescriber if the patient reported a history of which of the following? (Select all that apply.)

1. Gallbladder disease
2. Angina
3. Hypertension
4. Diabetes
5. Chronic kidney disease

See Appendix A for answers to critical thinking questions, case study questions, and review questions.

References

American Heart Association & American College of Cariology. (2020). *2018 Prevention Guidelines Tool CV Risk Calculator.* https://ccccalculator.ccctracker.com/

Armitage, J., Baigent, C., Barnes, E., Betteridge, D. J., Blackwell, L., Blazing, M., et al. (2019). Efficacy and safety of statin therapy in older people: a meta-analysis of individual participant data from 28 randomised controlled trials. *The Lancet*, *393*(10170), 407–415. https://doi.org/10.1016/S0140-6736(18)31942-1

Centers for Disease Control and Prevention. (2020). *High cholesterol facts.* http://www.cdc.gov/cholesterol/facts.htm

Connolly, S. D., & Ward, K. M. (2018). The role of exercise prescription in pediatric preventive cardiology programs. *Pediatric Annals*, *47*, e494–e498. https://doi.org/10.3928/19382359-20181114-01

Elkins, C., & Friedrich, D. (2018). Hypertriglyceridemia: A review of the evidence. *The Nurse Practitioner*, *43*, 22–29. https://doi.org/10.1097/01.NPR.0000544997.22887.0b

Elkins, C., Fruh, S., Jones, L., & Bydalek, K. (2019). Clinical practice recommendations for pediatric dyslipidemia. *Journal of Pediatric Health Care*, *33*, 494–504. https://doi.org/10.1016/j.pedhc.2019.02.009

Expert Panel on Integrated Guidelines for Cardiovascular Health and Risk Reduction in Children and Adolescents; National Heart, Lung, and Blood Institute. (2011). Expert Panel on Integrated Guidelines for Cardiovascular Health and Risk Reduction in Children and Adolescents: Summary report. *Pediatrics*, *128*(Suppl. 5), S213–256. https://doi.org/10.1542/peds.2009-2107C

Gidding, S. S. (2016). Familial hypercholesterolemia: Now part of cardiovascular disease genetic epidemiology research. *Journal of the American College of Cardiology*, *67*, 2590–2592. https://doi.org/10.1016/j.jacc.2016.03.567

Grundy, S. M., Stone, N. J., Bailey, A. L., Beam, C., Birtcher, K. K., Blumenthal, R. S., et al. (2019). 2018 AHA/ACC/AACVPR/AAPA/ABC/ACPM/ADA/AGS/APhA/ASPC/NLA/PCNA guideline on the management of blood cholesterol: Executive summary: A report of the American College of Cardiology/American Heart Association Task Force on Clinical Practice Guidelines. *Journal of the American College of Cardiology*, *73*(24), 3168–3209. https://doi.org/10.1016/j.jacc.2018.11.002

Mose, J. (2020). *Familial hypercholesterolemia.* Medscape. http://emedicine.medscape.com/article/121298-overview

National Center for Complementary and Integrative Health. (2019). *Coenzyme Q10.* https://www.nccih.nih.gov/health/coenzyme-q10

Selected Bibliography

Ahmed, S. S. (2020). An update on pharmacotherapy of dyslipidemia for adults. *Journal of Advances in Medicine and Medical Research*, *32*(8), 86–109. https://doi.org/10.9734/jammr/2020/v32i830469

American Heart Association. (2020). *2020 heart disease & stroke statistical update fact sheet: Children & cardiovascular diseases.* https://www.heart.org/-/media/files/about-us/statistics/children-ucm_505481.pdf?la=en

Elkins, C., Fruh, S., Jones, L., & Bydalek, K. (2019). Clinical Practice Recommendations for Pediatric Dyslipidemia. *Journal of Pediatric Health Care*, *33*(4), 494–504. https://doi.org/10.1016/j.pedhc.2019.02.009

Ferri, N., & Corsini, A. (2020). Clinical pharmacology of statins: An update. *Current Atherosclerosis Reports*, *22*(7), 26. https://doi.org/10.1007/s11883-020-00844-w

Himmelfarb, C. R. D., & Coke, L. (2019). New 2018 cholesterol guideline: Enhanced risk estimation and therapeutic options drive shared decision making. *Journal of Cardiovascular Nursing*, *34*(2), 103–105. https://doi.org/10.1097/JCN.0000000000000563

Kluger, A. Y., Tecson, K. M., Sudhakaran, S., Zhang, J., & McCullough, P. A. (2019). Statin update: Intolerance, benefit, and beyond. *Hypertension*, *5*(1), 3. https://doi.org/10.15713/ins.johtn.0141

Lavecchia, A., & Cerchia, C. (2019). Recent advances in developing PCSK9 inhibitors for lipid-lowering therapy. *Future Medicinal Chemistry*, *11*(5), 423–441. https://doi.org/10.4155/fmc-2018-0294

Palmer, C. (2019). New directions in managing dyslipidemia. *Journal for Nurse Practitioners*, *15*(1), 73–79. https://doi.org/10.1016/j.nurpra.2018.08.033

Rosenberg, K. (2019). Healthy lifestyle most important for prevention of ASCVD. *American Journal of Nursing*, *119*(6), 68. https://doi.org/10.1097/01.NAJ.0000559810.44553.e9

Rubenfire, M., & Lloyd-Jones, D. M. (2016). *Expert consensus on role of non-statin therapies for LDL-C lowering for management of ASASCVD risk.* American College of Cardiology. http://www.acc.org/latest-in-cardiology/ten-points-to-remember/2016/03/30/11/58/2016-acc-expert-consensus-decision-pathway-on-the-role-of-nonstatin

Steffens, D., Bramlage, P., Scheeff, C., Kasner, M., Hassanein, A., Friebel, J., & Rauch-Kröhnert, U. (2020). PCSK9 inhibitors and cardiovascular outcomes. *Expert Opinion on Biological Therapy*, *20*(1), 35–47. https://doi.org/10.1080/14712598.2020.1677604

Ward, N. C., Watts, G. F., & Eckel, R. H. (2019). Statin toxicity: mechanistic insights and clinical implications. *Circulation Research*, *124*(2), 328–350. https://doi.org/10.1161/CIRCRESAHA.118.312782

"My friends all take diuretics for their hypertension, but my provider is giving me something called a 'calcium channel blocker.' Would someone please tell me what calcium has to do with high blood pressure?"

—*Patient "Angela Rivera"*

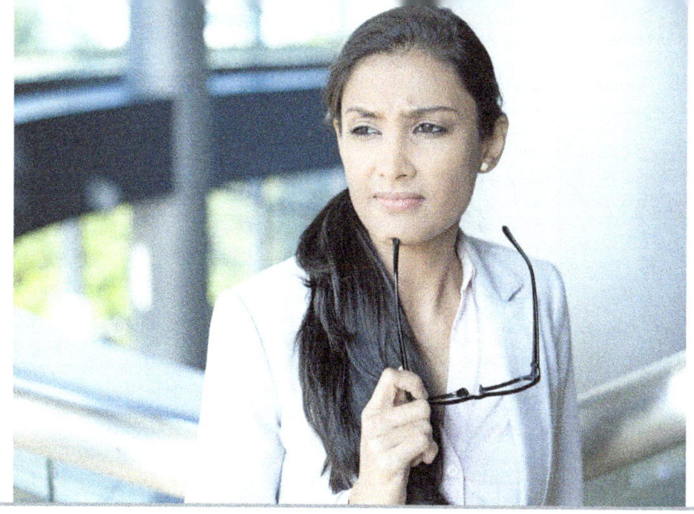

Chapter 30 Pharmacotherapy with Calcium Channel Blockers

Chapter Outline

Learning Outcomes

After reading this chapter, the student should be able to:

1. Describe the role of calcium ions in the contraction of smooth and cardiac muscle.
2. Explain why the actions of the $beta_1$-adrenergic antagonists are similar to those of the calcium channel blockers.
3. Describe how calcium channel blockers interact with the L-type calcium channel.
4. Identify the physiologic effects of calcium channel blockers on arterial smooth muscle and cardiac muscle.
5. Explain the classification of calcium channel blockers.
6. Compare and contrast the actions of dihydropyridine versus nondihydropyridine calcium channel blockers.
7. For each of the classes shown in the chapter outline, identify the prototype and representative drugs and explain the mechanism(s) of drug action, primary indications, contraindications, significant drug interactions, pregnancy data and important adverse effects.
8. Apply clinical judgment to care for patients receiving pharmacotherapy with calcium channel blockers.

Key Terms

Definitions of the terms in bold may be found in the Glossary.

Since the approval of the first calcium channel blocker (CCB) over 50 years ago, this class of drugs has become one of the most widely prescribed in cardiovascular medicine. One reason for their widespread use is that these drugs treat two chronic diseases that affect millions of people: hypertension (HTN) and coronary artery disease (CAD). Their success is also related to their effectiveness and a favorable safety profile.

CCBs are also known as calcium channel antagonists. These drugs do not physically block calcium channels; therefore, *antagonist* is a more accurate term than *blocker*. Because both terms are used interchangeably in clinical practice, they are used as synonyms throughout this text.

Physiologic Role of Calcium Channels in Muscle Contraction

30.1 Calcium channels facilitate contraction in cardiac and smooth muscles.

Recall from muscle physiology that the signal for contraction is an action potential traveling across the muscle plasma membrane, or **sarcolemma**. The action potential causes a depolarization that opens voltage-gated channels in the sarcolemma, allowing ions to enter and leave the muscle cell. In skeletal muscle, as in nervous tissue, the primary ion channels facilitate Na^+ and K^+ movement. However, in cardiac and smooth muscle, a third type of voltage-gated channel, the **calcium channel**, is of particular importance to cardiovascular physiology and pharmacotherapy. Contraction of these muscle types requires the movement of calcium ions (Ca^{2+}).

Under resting conditions, the concentration of free Ca^{2+} in the cytoplasm of a muscle cell is very low. Depolarization of the sarcolemma, however, changes the amount of free Ca^{2+} in two ways. First, calcium channels in the sarcolemma open, allowing extracellular calcium to rush into the cell. Secondly, depolarization releases large amounts of calcium ions stored in cellular structures called **sarcoplasmic reticula**. This huge increase in cytoplasmic Ca^{2+} removes the inhibition of actin and myosin filaments by the proteins calmodulin (smooth muscle) or troponin C (cardiac muscle) through a cascade of complex reactions. Actin and myosin are then free to slide, and muscle contraction occurs. This process is illustrated in Figure 30.1.

Muscle contraction is terminated when the amount of free cytoplasmic Ca^{2+} is reduced, by either pumping to the outside of the cell or by returning the Ca^{2+} to storage in the sarcoplasmic reticulum.

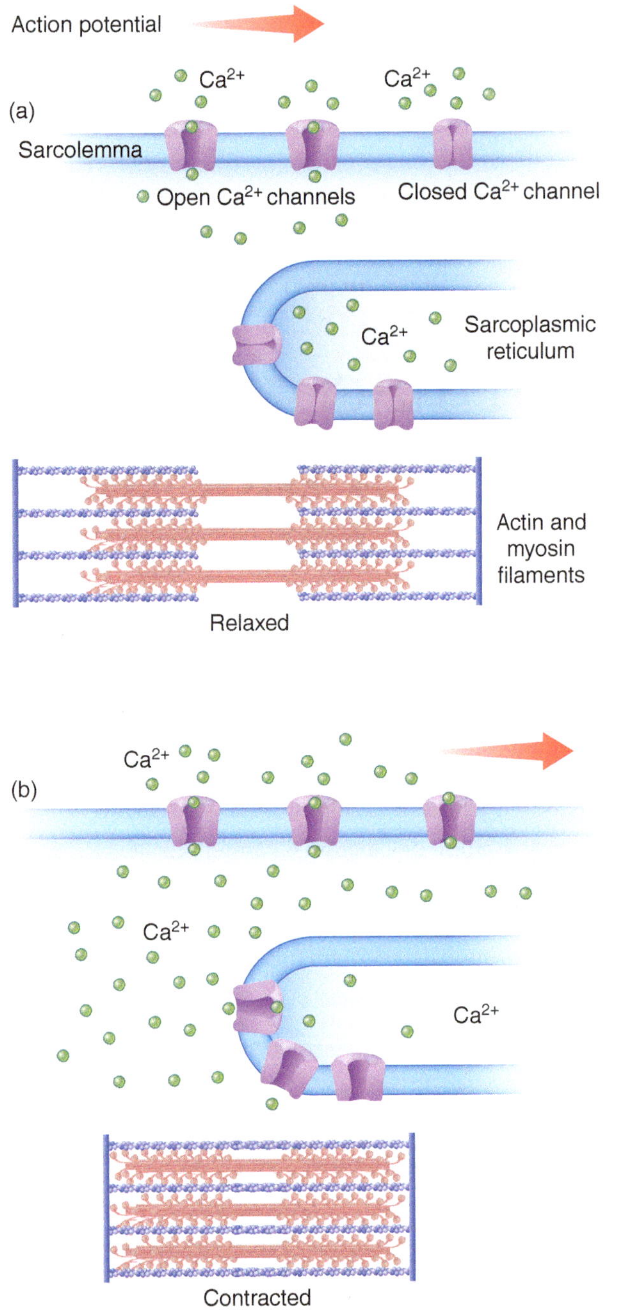

Figure 30.1 Calcium channels and muscle contraction: (a) Calcium channels open as the action potential travels along the sarcolemma. (b) Large amounts of calcium are released from storage in the sarcoplasmic reticula, causing actin and myosin filaments to slide and muscle contraction to occur.

Recall from Chapter 15 that activation of beta$_1$-adrenergic receptors in cardiac muscle increases heart rate and contractility. This is because, in myocardial cells, the signal for opening calcium channels is linked to activation of the sympathetic nervous system. In effect, calcium channels open when the sympathetic nervous system supplies the action potential, depolarizing the sarcolemma. This has important implications to pharmacology. Blocking cardiac beta$_1$ receptors with adrenergic antagonists will *prevent* the opening of calcium channels. Thus, the cardiac effects of beta$_1$-adrenergic blockers, and their pharmacotherapeutic indications and adverse effects, are similar to those of CCBs.

CONNECTION Checkpoint 30.1

From what you learned in Chapters 15 and 16, what type of drug–drug interaction would you expect between a CCB and (a) a beta-adrenergic antagonist such as propranolol (Inderal) and (b) a sympathomimetic such as epinephrine?

Types of Calcium Channels

30.2 The calcium channel consists of multiple subunits and is present in many tissues.

Research has identified different types of calcium ion channels, which are named by the letters *L*, *T*, and *N*. Differences in the structures and locations of the channels are important to drug action.

Pharmacologically, the most important calcium channels are the L type because they are the ones that bind CCBs. L-type calcium channels are found on the sarcolemma of cardiac and smooth muscles. The channel spans across the membrane and consists of three main parts. An extracellular portion serves as a receptor to bind CCBs. A central portion serves as a pore through which calcium ions travel. An intracellular portion serves as a second messenger capable of initiating a cascade of events that signal the cell to perform specific functions.

The L-type calcium channel is regulated by voltage changes across the sarcolemma. When an action potential depolarizes the membrane, the channel opens, allowing Ca^{2+} to rush in. The L-type channels are relatively slow, which allows for a sustained flow of Ca^{2+} into the cell. When a CCB medication is present, the channel changes shape. Although the drug does not physically block the opening, the change in shape of the channel is enough to prevent Ca^{2+} from entering the muscle cell. The L-type calcium channel is illustrated in Figure 30.2.

L-type calcium channels are widespread in the cardiovascular system, and these channels bind all current CCBs. L-type calcium channels are also present in other tissues, particularly in neurons and endocrine and sensory cells. This leads to other potential uses of these drugs, a topic discussed later in this chapter.

T-type calcium channels are present in vascular smooth muscle as well as the sinoatrial (SA) node where they are involved in pacemaker functions of the heart. Like the L-type channels, they are also located in other tissues, including the central nervous system (CNS). At this time, the only medication that acts by blocking T-type channels is ethosuximide (Zarontin), which is used to treat seizures. Other potential indications for T-type CCBs include pain, obesity, insomnia, and anxiety.

N-type calcium channels are found throughout the brain and peripheral nervous systems. Their primary role appears to be to control neurotransmitter release at synapses. They are also involved in the transmission of pain impulses in the spinal cord. At this time ziconotide (Prialt)

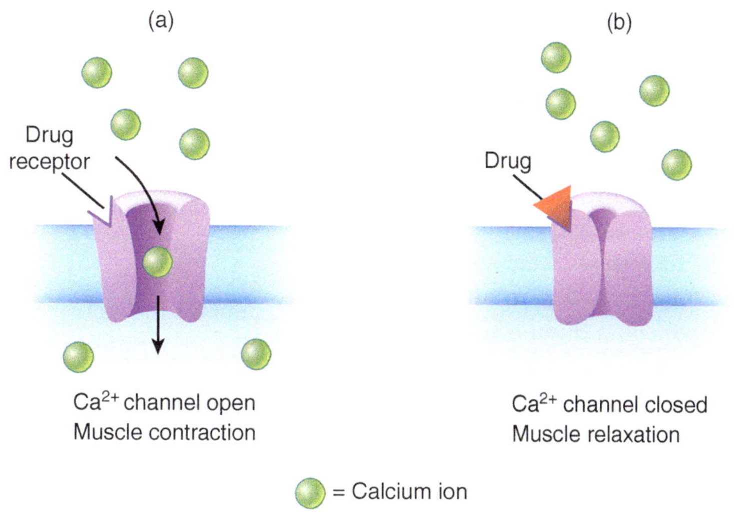

Figure 30.2 L-type calcium channel: (a) Calcium channel opens when an action potential passes across the sarcolemma. Calcium enters the cell and muscle contraction occurs. (b) Calcium channel antagonist binds to the receptor, changing its shape; channel closes and muscle relaxation occurs.

is the only approved drug that directly blocks N-type calcium channels. When delivered intrathecally, ziconotide blocks N-type channels in the spinal cord to ease severe, chronic pain. Although the drug has limited applications, in the future other medications may be developed that target the neuronal N-type calcium channels to achieve pain relief.

Consequences of Calcium Channel Blockade

30.3 Blocking calcium channels has significant physiologic effects on the heart and vascular smooth muscle.

The therapeutic applications of CCBs are the result of actions of the drugs on vascular smooth muscle, cardiac muscle, and the conduction system in the heart. Some CCBs have greater actions on the heart, whereas others have more effect on arteriolar smooth muscle. None of the CCBs affects serum calcium levels.

Effects on vascular smooth muscle: The influx of calcium ions into smooth muscle cells is essential for contraction. Because the degree of contraction of arterioles controls peripheral resistance, the blockade of calcium channels has significant physiologic effects on blood pressure. All CCBs dilate peripheral arterioles, causing systemic blood pressure to decrease. Afterload is reduced, resulting in lower myocardial oxygen demand and less workload for the heart. This is particularly important for patients with angina, who will experience less chest pain due to the decrease in cardiac workload (see Chapter 35).

Another important group of vessels affected by CCBs is the coronary arteries. Dilation of the coronary arteries by the CCBs brings more blood to the myocardium, which is beneficial for patients with myocardial ischemia. Veins and cardiac preload are not affected by drugs in this class.

Effects on the myocardium: Most CCBs reduce the force of myocardial contraction. This **negative inotropic effect** occurs because these drugs reduce the inward movement of Ca^{2+} during the plateau phase of the action potential. This delayed entry of Ca^{2+} prevents the release of Ca^{2+} from its storage depots in the sarcoplasmic reticulum, resulting in fewer actin–myosin cross bridges and a diminished force of contraction.

For verapamil and diltiazem, the negative inotropic effect is clearly apparent at therapeutic doses. The remainder of the CCBs will only exhibit this effect at higher doses or in overdose situations.

Effects on cardiac conduction: In general, CCBs exhibit a **negative chronotropic effect**: the property of slowing the speed of electrical conduction across the myocardium. Under normal conditions, the SA node automatically generates an action potential because of an inward movement of Ca^{2+} through calcium channels. Blocking calcium entry causes the SA node to generate fewer action potentials, thus decreasing automaticity and slowing heart rate. Similarly, some of the CCBs block calcium channels in the atrioventricular (AV) node, reducing conduction velocity through this region of the heart and further slowing the spread of the action potential across the myocardium. Because of these actions on the cardiac conduction system, the CCBs are sometimes used to correct certain rhythm abnormalities of the heart (see Chapter 37).

Not all CCBs affect cardiac conduction to the same degree. Verapamil and diltiazem exhibit this effect at therapeutic doses, whereas the remainder of the CCBs exhibit a negative chronotropic effect only at high doses, or not at all.

CONNECTION Checkpoint 30.2

From what you learned in Chapter 28, define *afterload*. If a drug increases afterload, what effect would this likely have on cardiac output?

Classification of Calcium Channel Blockers

30.4 Calcium channel blockers are classified by their chemical structures as dihydropyridines or nondihydropyridines.

Despite the fact that all CCBs affect L-type calcium channels, there are differences in actions and adverse effects among the specific drugs. This is because the drugs interact with different subunits of the calcium channel. This gives rise to a classification of calcium channel antagonists based on their chemical structures.

The **dihydropyridines** are the largest class of CCBs. They include amlodipine (Norvasc), clevidipine (Cleviprex), felodipine, isradipine, nicardipine (Cardene), nifedipine (Adalat CC, Procardia XL), nimodipine (Nymalize), and nisoldipine (Sular). The dihydropyridines bind reversibly to *closed-type* (inactivated) calcium channels, changing the channels' structure and making them unresponsive to depolarization. Because closed-type channels are found in greater numbers in vascular smooth muscle than in cardiac muscle, dihydropyridines are primarily used for their vasodilation effect on arterial smooth muscle.

The remaining CCBs are chemically dissimilar to the dihydropyridines and bind to different subunits of the L-type calcium channel. Although they are chemically different from each other, diltiazem (Cardizem, Cartia XT, Dilacor, Taztia XT, Tiazac, others) and verapamil (Calan SR, Verelan) have quite similar pharmacologic properties and may be grouped together as **nondihydropyridines**. These drugs bind to *open-type* calcium channels, causing them to revert

Table 30.1 FDA-Approved Indications for Calcium Channel Blockers

Drug	Hypertension	Chronic Stable Angina	Vasospastic Angina	Unstable Angina	Dysrhythmias	Subarachnoid Hemorrhage
Dihydropyridines						
amlodipine (Norvasc)	X	X	X			
clevidipine (Cleviprex)	X					
felodipine	X					
isradipine	X					
nicardipine: PO	X	X				
nicardipine (Cardene injectable)	X					
nifedipine (Adalat, Procardia XL)	X	X	X			
nimodipine (Nymalize)						X
nisoldipine (Sular)	X					
Nondihydropyridines						
diltiazem (Cardizem, Dilacor)		X	X			
diltiazem extended release (Cardizem CD)	X	X	X			
diltiazem extended release (Cardizem LA, Cartia XT, Dilacor XR, Taztia XT, Tiazac)	X	X				
diltiazem injection (Cardizem)					X	
verapamil (Calan SR, Verelan)	X	X	X	X	X	
verapamil injection					X	

to their inactivated or closed state. These drugs also delay reactivation of the calcium channel, thus slowing repolarization of the muscle cell membrane. This effect is particularly noticeable in cardiac muscle, where the nondihydropyridines slow the speed of myocardial conduction. Like the dihydropyridines, the nondihydropyridines have a vasodilation effect on vascular smooth muscle. Indications for the various CCBs that have been approved by the U.S. Food and Drug Administration (FDA) are shown in Table 30.1.

Dihydropyridines

30.5 The dihydropyridines are selective for vascular smooth muscle and are used to treat hypertension and angina pectoris.

All dihydropyridines have similar actions and adverse effects. All except clevidipine are well absorbed after oral (PO) administration, and most are highly protein bound, excreted by the liver, and undergo extensive first-pass metabolism. Because of this, dosage adjustments are necessary in patients with significant hepatic impairment.

Drugs in this class are highly selective for calcium channels located in vascular smooth muscle. At high doses, however, the dihydropyridines lose their selectivity and also affect calcium channels in the heart. All dihydropyridines are equivalent in effectiveness for treating HTN and angina. Some are available in extended-release formulations that allow for once-daily dosing. Doses for the dihydropyridines are listed in Table 30.2.

The dihydropyridines are well tolerated in most patients. Common adverse effects include flushed skin, headache, dizziness, hypotension, peripheral edema, lightheadedness, nausea, and diarrhea, although these are usually not severe enough to discontinue therapy. The vasodilation caused by the blockade of calcium channels in vascular smooth muscle may cause reflex tachycardia. This is generally transient and clinically important only in patients with preexisting myocardial ischemia or dysrhythmias. If a CCB must be used for these patients, extended-release formulations are selected because they produce a more gradual change in blood pressure with less reflex tachycardia.

PROTOTYPE DRUG **Nifedipine (Adalat CC, Procardia XL)**

Classification **Therapeutic:** Antihypertensive
Pharmacologic: Calcium channel blocker, dihydropyridine type

Therapeutic Effects and Uses: Approved in 1981, nifedipine is a CCB with several indications. For HTN it may be given alone or in combination with drugs from other antihypertensive classes. Its ability to dilate the coronary arteries makes it an important drug in the treatment of chronic stable or variant angina (see Chapter 35). When used as an antianginal, a beta-adrenergic blocker may be administered concurrently to prevent reflex tachycardia. Nifedipine may be used off-label to treat hypertensive

Table 30.2 Calcium Channel Blockers

Drug	Route and Adult Dose (Maximum Dose Where Indicated)	Adverse Effects
Dihydropyridines		
amlodipine (Norvasc)	PO: 5–10 mg once daily (max: 10 mg/day)	*Flushed skin, hypotension, headache, dizziness, peripheral edema, lightheadedness, nausea, diarrhea, constipation* Hepatotoxicity, MI, HF, confusion, mood changes, gingival hyperplasia
clevidipine (Cleviprex)	IV: 1–2 mg/h initial dose, gradually increased until blood pressure goal is reached (max: 16 mg/h)	
felodipine	PO: 2.5–10 mg once daily (max: 10 mg/day)	
isradipine	PO: 2.5 mg bid (max: 20 mg/day)	
nicardipine (Cardene)	PO: 20–40 mg tid (max: 120 mg/day) IV (Cardene): 5 mg/hr by slow infusion (max: 15 mg/hr)	
nifedipine (Adalat CC, Procardia XL)	PO (extended release): 30–60 mg once daily (max: 120 mg/day)	
nimodipine (Nymalize)	PO: 30-60 mg qid for 21 consecutive days	
nisoldipine (Sular)	PO (extended release): 17–34 mg once daily (max: 34 mg/day)	
Nondihydropyridines		
diltiazem (Cardizem, Cartia XT, Dilacor, Taztia XT, Tiazac, others)	PO: 30 mg qid (max: 480 mg/day) Extended release: 120–240 mg once daily	
verapamil (Calan SR, Verelan)	PO: 80–160 mg tid (max: 480 mg/day) PO (Verelan, Calan SR): 120–480 mg once daily	

Note: *Italics* indicate common adverse effects. Underline indicates serious adverse effects.

emergency, persistent hiccups, or premature labor contractions or to prevent migraines.

Nifedipine is usually prescribed as extended-release tablets because this allows for once-daily dosing. At high doses, the immediate-release form of nifedipine should be used with great caution because its use has been associated with an increased risk for myocardial infarction (MI).

Mechanism of Action: Nifedipine acts by selectively blocking calcium channels in vascular smooth muscle, including those in the coronary arteries, causing a decrease in the amount of intracellular calcium available for muscle contraction. This results in a fall in blood pressure and a diminished myocardial oxygen demand due to the reduced afterload. Nifedipine has no effect on myocardial conduction except at toxic doses.

Pharmacokinetics:

Route(s)	PO
Absorption	Well absorbed (90%)
Distribution	Widely distributed; secreted in breast milk; 92–98% bound to plasma protein
Primary metabolism	Hepatic; extensive first-pass metabolism
Primary excretion	Renal (80%) with small amounts in feces (15%)
Onset of action	30–60 min (immediate-release capsules); 6 h (extended-release tablet)
Duration of action	4–8 h (24 h for extended release); half-life: 2–5 h

Adverse Effects: Nifedipine is well tolerated and serious adverse effects are not common. Most adverse effects such as hypotension, dizziness, headache, and flushing are related to the vasodilation action of the drug. The most common cardiovascular-related adverse effect is peripheral edema, which occurs more frequently with nifedipine than with other CCBs. Other severe, though rare, adverse effects include hepatotoxicity, MI, heart failure (HF), severe hypotension, and confusion.

Contraindications/Precautions: The only contraindication is hypersensitivity to nifedipine or other dihydropyridines. Caution must be observed when using nifedipine in patients with bradycardia or HF because this drug has negative inotropic effects that can worsen these conditions. The immediate-release form is contraindicated in patients with acute MI or cardiogenic shock. Because nifedipine causes blood pressure to fall, it should be used cautiously in patients with preexisting hypotension. Any signs of worsening pulmonary edema call for discontinuation of the drug. Patients with significant hepatic impairment are at risk for drug accumulation and toxicity. Older adults are at much greater risk of nifedipine toxicity and experience a higher overall mortality when treated with this drug.

Drug Interactions: Nifedipine is a substrate for hepatic CYP3A4 and may interact with drugs that induce or inhibit this enzyme. When given concurrently with nifedipine, other antihypertensive drugs have additive effects on blood pressure. These additive hypotensive effects are used to advantage in the pharmacotherapy of HTN (see Chapter 34). Concurrent use of nifedipine with a beta-adrenergic blocker increases the risk of HF due to additive negative inotropic and chronotropic effects. Nifedipine may increase the serum levels of digoxin by as much as 45%, leading to bradycardia and digoxin toxicity. Alcohol potentiates the vasodilation action of nifedipine and could lead to syncope caused by a rapid drop in blood pressure. **Herbal/Food:** Grapefruit juice may enhance the absorption of nifedipine. Melatonin may reduce the effectiveness of nifedipine by increasing blood pressure and heart rate. St. John's wort can induce CYP3A4 and increase the metabolism of nifedipine and reduce the plasma level of this drug.

Pregnancy: Animal studies showed nifedipine is embryotoxic, fetotoxic, and teratogenic. Because nifedipine is secreted in human milk and has the potential to produce serious adverse effects, breastfeeding is not recommended during therapy.

Treatment of Overdose: Overdosage may result in pronounced hypotension, which is treated with rapid-acting vasopressors such as dopamine or dobutamine. Calcium infusions may also be indicated.

Clinician Responsibilities: Key clinical implications for patients receiving nifedipine are included in Applied Clinical Judgment: Patients Receiving Pharmacotherapy with Calcium Channel Blockers.

Drugs Similar to Nifedipine (Adalat CC, Procardia XL)

Other dihydropyridines include amlodipine, clevidipine, felodipine, isradipine, nicardipine, nimodipine, and nisoldipine.

Amlodipine (Norvasc): Amlodipine is indicated for the treatment of HTN, chronic stable angina, and Prinzmetal's variant angina. Approved in 1992, amlodipine has the longest half-life (35 hours) of the dihydropyridines, which allows for once-daily dosing. Like other dihydropyridines, amlodipine affects mainly arteriolar smooth muscle, including that in the coronary arteries, and has no significant effect on cardiac conduction. The drug is well tolerated, with headache, dizziness, and dose-dependent peripheral edema being frequent adverse effects. Reflex tachycardia rarely occurs because the drug has a very gradual onset. In the treatment of HTN, several weeks may be required to achieve optimal outcomes. Amlodipine is used in many fixed-dose combination products with valsartan (Exforge), valsartan and hydrochlorothiazide (Exforge HCT), atorvastatin (Caduet), perindopril (Prestalia), olmesartan (Azor), olmesartan and hydrochlorothiazide (Tribenzor), benazepril (Lotrel), and telmisartan (Twynsta). Animals studies showed no evidence of embryotoxicity or fetal toxicity. This drug is secreted in milk but adverse effects on the breastfed neonate are unknown.

Clevidipine (Cleviprex): Approved in 2008, clevidipine is an injectable emulsion that is approved for the treatment of HTN when rapid control of blood pressure is desirable. The dose is doubled every 90 seconds until the blood pressure approaches the goal, then the infusion is slowed, with dose adjustments every 5 to 10 minutes. Blood pressure falls within minutes and must be monitored continuously during the infusion. With such rapid titration, hypotension and reflex tachycardia may occur. The most common adverse effects are nausea and vomiting and headache. Patients with HF must be monitored carefully because clevidipine may worsen this condition. Animal studies showed increased fetal mortality. It is not known if this drug is secreted in milk or if it has adverse effects in breastfed neonates.

Felodipine: Approved in 1991, felodipine is a dihydropyridine that has greater selectivity for vascular smooth muscle than nifedipine and is approved only for the pharmacotherapy of HTN. It exerts no significant effects on the heart. Its elimination half-life of 11 to 16 hours allows for once-daily dosing. Typical adverse effects are facial flushing, headache, peripheral edema, and reflex tachycardia. Animal studies showed increased fetal anomalies and mortality. It is not known if this drug is secreted in milk, but breastfeeding is not recommended because of potential adverse effects on the neonate.

Isradipine: Approved in 1990, isradipine is the most potent of the dihydropyridines and is approved for the pharmacotherapy of HTN, either alone or in combination with a thiazide diuretic. Chronic stable angina is an off-label indication for the drug. The physiologic actions of isradipine are selective to arterioles, and the drug has no appreciable effect on the heart. Reflex tachycardia is usually not significant. Optimal response may require 2 to 4 weeks of therapy. Headache, facial flushing, and dizziness are the most common adverse effects. Animal studies showed evidence of increased fetal resorption and reduced offspring survival. It is not known if this drug is secreted in milk, but breastfeeding is not recommended because of potential adverse effects on the neonate.

Nicardipine (Cardene): Approved in 1988, nicardipine is indicated for the pharmacotherapy of chronic stable angina and HTN. Beta-adrenergic blockers or sublingual nitrates may be administered concurrently to reduce the possibility of reflex tachycardia in patients with angina pectoris. An intravenous (IV) form (Cardene) is available for initiation of therapy in patients with severe HTN. An off-label use of nicardipine is for migraines. The actions, contraindications, and adverse effects are similar to those of nifedipine. Peripheral edema, dizziness, headache, and facial flushing are the most common adverse effects. Animal studies showed that nicardipine is embryocidal and decreased offspring survival. This drug is secreted in animal milk and is not recommended during lactation.

Nimodipine (Nymalize): Approved in 1988, nimodipine is an oral CCB with one very specific indication: to reduce the incidence and severity of ischemic deficits in patients with subarachnoid hemorrhage from ruptured intracranial berry aneurysms. The drug prevents vasospasm of the injured vessel and reduces the severity of the resulting neurologic deficit. Nimodipine appears to have a greater smooth muscle relaxation effect on cerebral arteries than arteries in other areas of the body. The most frequent adverse effects are hypotension, edema, and headache. This drug carries a black box warning that it should never be given by the parenteral route because life-threatening adverse events have occurred when administered by this route. Animal studies showed embryofetal mortality, fetal structural abnormalities, and decreased fetal growth. Because nimodipine is secreted in human breast milk, using this drug during lactation is not recommended.

PharmFACT

It is estimated that 10 to 20% of patients taking calcium channel antagonists will develop gingival hyperplasia. This condition can be successfully managed by professional dental care and oral antiseptic rinses such as chlorhexidine (Peridex) (Mejia, 2019).

Nisoldipine (Sular): Approved in 1995, nisoldipine is selective for vascular smooth muscle and has no significant effect on the myocardium. It is approved only for HTN but may be used off-label for angina. The extended-release form allows for once-daily dosing. Peripheral edema and headache are relatively common in patients taking this drug. Reflex tachycardia may cause angina pain in patients with myocardial ischemia. Like other CCBs, it should be used with caution in patients with hypotension, peripheral edema, or HF. Animal studies suggested that nisoldipine may increase fetal mortality. Breastfeeding is not advised because nisoldipine is likely to enter milk and may cause adverse effects in the breastfed neonate.

Nondihydropyridines

30.6 The nondihydropyridines act on both vascular smooth muscle and the myocardium.

The nondihydropyridine group of CCBs consists of two drugs, verapamil (Calan SR, Verelan) and diltiazem (Cardizem, Cartia XT, Dilacor, Taztia XT, Tiazac, others). Although the two drugs are chemically dissimilar, they share common physiologic actions, adverse effects, and indications.

Like the dihydropyridines, drugs in this class block L-type calcium channels in vascular smooth muscle, causing vasodilation. As expected from this physiologic action, the nondihydropyridines are used in the pharmacotherapy of HTN and angina. Thus, the dihydropyridines and nondihydropyridines share these two indications. Doses for the nondihydropyridines are listed in Table 30.2.

It is important to note that verapamil and diltiazem have actions on the heart that the dihydropyridines do not possess. These drugs block calcium channels in the myocardium, causing a negative inotropic effect. In addition, the nondihydropyridines decrease the speed of myocardial conduction, resulting in a slower heart rate.

These cardiac effects of the nondihydropyridines may be viewed as therapeutic or adverse, depending on the patient and the reasons for administering the drugs. For example, by slowing conduction across the heart, verapamil and diltiazem can suppress abnormal cardiac rhythms. They are indicated for specific types of dysrhythmias, such as atrial flutter or fibrillation (see Chapter 37). In certain patients, however, slowing the speed of conduction may result in serious adverse effects. For example, slowing the heart rate can diminish cardiac output in patients with moderate or severe HF and worsen this condition. Slowing impulse conduction may cause partial or complete heart block in patients with bradycardia or second-degree or third-degree AV block. Concurrent treatment with a beta-adrenergic agonist may be necessary to counteract these adverse cardiac effects.

Other adverse effects from the nondihydropyridines include constipation, flushed skin, headache, dizziness, edema of the ankles and feet, and lightheadedness. Gingival hyperplasia is an uncommon adverse effect that occurs with long-term therapy and usually reverses after the drugs are discontinued. Most patients tolerate the nondihydropyridine CCBs well and experience few serious adverse effects.

PROTOTYPE DRUG **Verapamil (Calan SR, Verelan)**

Classification **Therapeutic:** Antihypertensive, antianginal, antidysrhythmic
Pharmacologic: Calcium channel blocker; phenylalkylamine type

Therapeutic Effects and Uses: Verapamil was the first CCB approved by the FDA in 1981. The drug is a class IV antidysrhythmic (see Chapter 37) because it slows myocardial conduction velocity, especially through the AV node, and stabilizes certain types of abnormal heart rhythms. In the vasculature, calcium channel blockade causes vasodilation of arterioles, which lowers blood pressure and reduces cardiac workload. Verapamil also dilates the coronary arteries, an action that is important when the drug is used to treat angina. It is approved to treat variant, unstable, and chronic angina (see Chapter 35). Off-label indications include cluster headache and migraine prophylaxis.

Verapamil is available in PO, oral extended-release, and IV formulations. Verelan PM is a unique formulation that delays the release of verapamil until 4 to 5 hours after ingestion and then releases it slowly. Verelan PM should be taken at night so that the drug is in the bloodstream on awakening. The therapeutic serum level of verapamil is 0.08 to 0.3 mcg/mL. Tarka is a fixed-dose combination of verapamil with trandolapril for HTN.

Mechanism of Action: Verapamil acts by inhibiting the flow of calcium ions into both cardiac muscle cells and vascular smooth muscle cells. Blocking calcium entry causes vasodilation of peripheral arterioles and reduced contractility of the myocardium.

Pharmacokinetics:

Route(s)	PO and IV
Absorption	Well absorbed
Distribution	Widely distributed; crosses the placenta; secreted in breast milk
Primary metabolism	Hepatic; extensive first-pass metabolism
Primary excretion	Renal (70%) with small amounts in feces (16%)
Onset of action	PO: 1–2 h; IV: 1–5 min
Duration of action	PO: 3–7 h (extended release: 24 h); IV: 2 h Half-life: 2–8 h

Adverse Effects: Most adverse effects of verapamil are extensions of its actions on the cardiovascular system. Peripheral vasodilation may cause flushed skin, headache, dizziness, lightheadedness, and peripheral edema. High doses and IV administration may cause serious hypotension. The most serious adverse effects of verapamil are cardiac related, including worsening of HF, bradycardia, reflex tachycardia, and AV block. Constipation is relatively common. CNS effects such as confusion, drowsiness, and mood changes have been reported, though they are uncommon. Elevated hepatic enzymes and rare cases of liver damage have been reported.

Contraindications/Precautions: Verapamil is contraindicated in patients with AV heart block, sick sinus syndrome, severe hypotension, bleeding aneurysm, or those undergoing intracranial surgery. Because verapamil can cause bradycardia and pulmonary edema, patients with HF should be carefully monitored, especially when the drug is administered IV. The drug should be used with caution in patients with chronic kidney disease or hepatic impairment because this can delay clearance of verapamil and its metabolites.

Drug Interactions: Verapamil is metabolized by hepatic CYP450 enzymes and exhibits many drug–drug interactions. Verapamil has the ability to elevate blood levels of digoxin. Because digoxin and verapamil both slow conduction through the AV node, their concurrent use must be carefully monitored to avoid bradycardia. Use with other antihypertensive drugs, including ACE inhibitors or beta-adrenergic blockers, may cause additive hypotension or bradycardia. Concurrent administration of verapamil with buspirone can triple the plasma concentration of buspirone. Verapamil should not be administered with statins because the risk of myopathy increases significantly. Carbamazepine serum concentration may increase during concurrent therapy with verapamil, causing adverse effects such as diplopia, ataxia, or dizziness. Use with alcohol can raise serum levels of the CCB and prolong its effects. **Herbal/Food:** Grapefruit juice may increase verapamil levels. Use with caution with herbal supplements, such as hawthorn, which may have additive hypotensive effects. High doses of calcium supplements may diminish the effects of CCBs and should not be used without consulting the healthcare provider.

Pregnancy: Animal studies suggest verapamil is embryocidal and that it retarded fetal growth and development. Because this drug is secreted in human milk and has the potential to produce adverse effects, breastfeeding is not recommended.

Treatment of Overdose: Treatment of overdose is aimed at reversing hypotension with vasopressors such as dopamine or norepinephrine. Atropine, levarterenol, or isoproterenol may be administered to treat bradycardia. Calcium salts may be administered to increase calcium available to the myocardium and arterioles.

Clinician Responsibilities: Key clinical implications for patients receiving verapamil are included in Applied Clinical Judgment: Patients Receiving Pharmacotherapy with Calcium Channel Blockers.

CONNECTIONS: Lifespan Considerations

Calcium Channel Blockers and Dementia

Dementia, particularly when associated with Alzheimer's disease, is a devastating degenerative illness affecting over 5 million people (Alzheimer's Association, 2020). Although drug therapy can ease symptoms, there are no known cures at this time. Drugs such as cholinesterase inhibitors and N-methyl-D-aspartate (NMDA) antagonist drugs may be used to delay symptoms, but do not alter the disease's progression (see Chapter 21). Past studies have indicated that antihypertensive drugs may give some protection against the progression of symptoms from mild cognitive impairment to dementia. Research has shown that calcium channel blockers in the dihydropyridine class are associated with a significant reduction in the risk of developing dementia in older adults (Hussain et al., 2018). However, other studies suggest that this risk reduction may not occur with all classes of these drugs and further study is needed (Lawlor et al., 2018). Given mixed results from studies thus far with positive results occurring from some CCB classes but not others, the older adult with HTN and at higher risk for dementia may find additional benefit from the use of a dihydropyridine class of CCBs over other antihypertensive drugs.

Drugs Similar to Verapamil (Calan SR, Verelan)

The only other nondihydropyridine is diltiazem.

Diltiazem (Cardizem, Cartia XT, Dilacor, Taztia XT, Tiazac, others): Like other nondihydropyridines, diltiazem has the ability to relax both coronary and peripheral blood vessels. Approved in 1982, diltiazem reduces heart rate, blood pressure, and cardiac workload. The drug slows electrical conduction through the AV node. It is useful in the treatment of atrial dysrhythmias and HTN as well as stable and vasospastic angina. Migraine prophylaxis is an off-label indication. When given as extended-release capsules (Cardizem LA, Dilacor XR, Taztia XT), it is administered once daily. An IV formulation is available to treat atrial fibrillation. The drug is well tolerated and serious adverse effects are uncommon and similar to those of verapamil. Like verapamil, diltiazem should be used cautiously in patients with bradycardia, AV block, HF, or serious hypotension.

There are several formulations of diltiazem and not all are approved for the same indications (see Table 30.1). The doses among the forms are not always equivalent. Even more confusing is that generics are labeled as "diltiazem extended release," which does not tell the prescriber which trade-name product the generic is equivalent to. Caution must always be used when administering this drug to ensure that the patient is receiving the correct dose and form of diltiazem. Animal reproduction studies showed an increase in embryo and fetal death, skeletal abnormalities, and increased stillbirths. Because this drug is secreted in human milk and has the potential to produce adverse effects, breastfeeding is not recommended.

CONNECTIONS: APPLIED CLINICAL JUDGMENT

Patients Receiving Pharmacotherapy with Calcium Channel Blockers

Key Assessment Data

- History of current condition, baseline vital signs, physical exam findings; history of cardiovascular disease, including MI and HF, musculoskeletal (preexisting conditions that might cause fatigue or weakness), hepatic and renal disease; drug history including allergies, current prescription and OTC drugs, herbal preparations, and alcohol use; pregnancy status.
- Ongoing assessment during drug therapy includes laboratory findings including electrolytes, especially potassium, liver and renal function studies, lipid profiles, cardiac monitoring (e.g., electrocardiogram [ECG], cardiac output), if appropriate. Assess for location, character, and amount of edema, if present.

Desired Therapeutic Outcomes

Improvement is observed and measurable in lowered blood pressure and pulse rate within established limits; lessened or absent angina; normal cardiac rhythm or lessening of dysrhythmias, if present.

Minimizing Adverse Effects

- Monitor for orthostatic hypotension. Notify the provider if BP or pulse decreases beyond the established parameters. Severe hypotension may cause a paradoxical increase in chest pain or angina symptoms and may indicate blood pressure has decreased too quickly or too substantially.
- Continue cardiac monitoring as ordered for dysrhythmias in the hospitalized patient, promptly reporting dysrhythmias, palpitations, or angina.
- Weigh daily and report weight gain over 1 kg (2 lbs) in a 24-hour period or increasing edema.
- Hypokalemia may increase the risk for dysrhythmias. Continue to monitor periodic electrolyte levels, especially potassium, ECG as appropriate, and hepatic and renal function laboratory values.
- Monitor for increasing dyspnea or postural nocturnal dyspnea, rales or crackles in the lungs, and frothy pink-tinged sputum, which may signal HF due to negative inotropic effects of the drug.
- Observe for hypersensitivity reaction or angioedema, especially of the facial area.
- While uncommon, monitor for gingival hyperplasia or signs of gingivitis.

Lifespan Considerations

- Orthostatic hypotension may increase the risk of falls and injury. Be particularly cautious with older adults who are at increased risk for hypotension. Ensure patient safety.
- The older adult is at increased risk of constipation due to slowed peristalsis.
- The drug should not be taken during pregnancy, if pregnancy is suspected, or while breastfeeding.

Diversity Considerations

- Because CCBs metabolize through the CYP450 system, they may interact with other drugs. Observe for less than optimal therapeutic effects, especially in ethnically diverse patients.

Patient and Caregiver Education

- Monitor pulse, BP, and daily weight using a diary or log and bring these to each provider visit. Promptly report any weight gain over 1 kg in a 24-hour period or increasing edema to the provider.
- Immediately report any severe shortness of breath, frothy sputum, profound fatigue, or swelling of extremities because these are possible signs of HF.
- Rise slowly from lying or sitting to standing, pausing between changes if dizziness occurs. Don't take the medication if dizziness continues or the BP is below 90/60 or per parameters set by the provider and contact the provider for further instruction.
- Immediately seek medical attention for difficulty breathing, throat tightness, hives or rash, muscle cramps, or tremors. Promptly report any angioedema around the facial area.
- Increase fluid and fiber to prevent constipation. If constipation persists, consider use of stool softener or laxative as recommended by the provider.
- Maintain good oral hygiene and regular dental appointments.
- Avoid alcohol and melatonin use, which may increase risk for hypotension, drowsiness, and dizziness. Grapefruit juice may increase drug levels with increased adverse effects and should also be avoided.
- Carry a wallet identification card or wear medical identification jewelry indicating CCB therapy.

CONNECTIONS: APPLIED CLINICAL JUDGMENT *(continued)*

Patients Receiving Pharmacotherapy with Calcium Channel Blockers

Prescribing Considerations

- Use with caution in patients with hepatic impairment; may require starting with a low dose and titrating up slowly.
- Consider lower initial doses for older adults and titrate at no less than 2-week intervals to response.
- Use caution when prescribing calcium channel blockers to women of childbearing potential due to possible fetal harm.

Understanding Chapter 30

Key Concepts Summary

30.1 Calcium channels facilitate contraction in cardiac and smooth muscles.

30.2 The calcium channel consists of multiple subunits and is present in many tissues.

30.3 Blocking calcium channels has significant physiologic effects on the heart and vascular smooth muscle.

30.4 Calcium channel blockers are classified by their chemical structures as dihydropyridines or nondihydropyridines.

30.5 The dihydropyridines are selective for vascular smooth muscle and are used to treat hypertension and angina pectoris.

30.6 The nondihydropyridines act on both vascular smooth muscle and the myocardium.

CASE STUDY: Making the Patient Connection

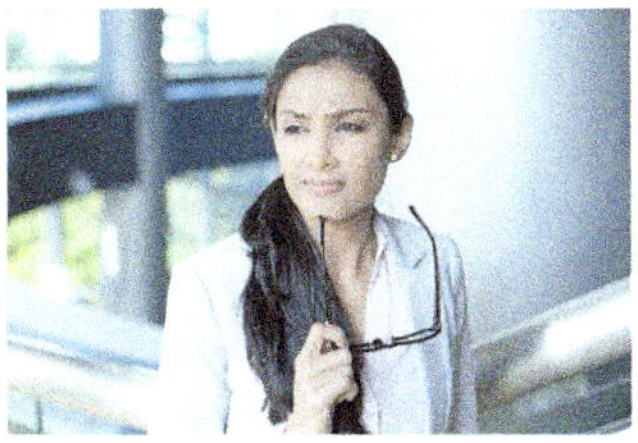

Remember the patient "Angela Rivera" at the beginning of the chapter? Now read the remainder of the case study. Based on the information presented within this chapter, respond to the critical thinking questions that follow.

Angela Rivera, a 40-year-old interior designer, had no idea that her blood pressure was elevated. One day at the shopping mall she saw an automatic blood pressure machine and thought she would try it. Angela could hardly believe the machine's reading when it revealed her blood pressure was 150/92 mmHg. She was certain that there must be something wrong with the machine. After all, she felt fine. In fact, Angela is rarely ill and never misses work due to illness.

Just to be certain, Angela made an appointment with her doctor for a checkup. During her first clinic visit, her blood pressure was 146/90 mmHg, heart rate was 78 beats/min, respiratory rate was 16 breaths/min, and temperature was 36.8°C (98.2°F). Angela was instructed on lifestyle modifications for HTN and told to return to the clinic in 1 month. The next month, Angela's blood pressure remained elevated. Multiple diagnostic studies, which included an ECG and blood chemistry levels, were completed. Her healthcare provider prescribed felodipine and instructed her to return in 1 week.

All of this has caused Angela to be concerned and worried about her health. She has accessed the internet to learn as much about HTN as possible and felodipine in particular. With all the information about high blood pressure, she is even more confused and anxious.

Critical Thinking Questions

1. Describe how calcium channel blockers control HTN.
2. Angela asks you, the nurse, if calcium channel blockers can cure HTN. How would you respond?
3. What adverse effects are associated with CCBs?

Additional Case Study

Mabel Hillside was prescribed amlodipine (Norvasc) 5 mg once daily. However, Mabel's health insurance does not cover prescription drug costs and she will be required to self-pay for the drug. As you are talking with this patient, she says, "Why should I take this medicine? After all, I feel just fine and it is very expensive. Plus, I keep forgetting to take it."

1. How would you respond to Mabel's remark about feeling "just fine"?
2. What adverse effects related to amlodipine might cause the patient to stop taking the medication?
3. List strategies that Mabel can use to remember to take her HTN medication.

Chapter Review

1. Nifedipine (Procardia) is being initiated for a patient with elevated blood pressure. What health teaching would be most appropriate? The patient should:
    1. Weigh daily at the same time each day.
    2. Avoid crowds while taking this medication.
    3. Increase intake of calcium-containing foods.
    4. Take this medication only when feeling that blood pressure is elevated.
2. A patient is receiving felodipine for hypertension. In the care plan the nurse includes the need to monitor the patient for which adverse effect?
    1. Rash and chills
    2. Increased urinary output
    3. Weight loss
    4. Reflex tachycardia
3. A patient with primary hypertension has started therapy with verapamil (Calan SR). The nurse performs what important intervention during the initial course of this treatment?
    1. Uses an electric razor to shave the patient
    2. Monitors the patient for increased thrombocyte levels
    3. Administers the medication only during waking hours
    4. Measures intake and output ratio and daily weight
4. The nurse determines that the patient understands an important principle in self-administration of nifedipine (Procardia) when the patient makes which statement?
    1. "The use of antacids when taking the medication will enhance absorption."
    2. "Grapefruit juice may enhance the absorption of nifedipine."
    3. "If I miss a dose, I should take two nifedipine capsules when I remember."
    4. "This drug will make my birth control pills ineffective."
5. What health teaching should the nurse provide for a patient receiving diltiazem (Cardizem)? (Select all that apply.)
    1. Avoid driving or performing other activities requiring mental alertness until the effects of the drug are known.
    2. Maintain adequate fluid and fiber intake to facilitate stool passage.
    3. Report weight gain of 2 kg (5 lb) per week.
    4. Rise slowly from prolonged periods of sitting or lying down.
    5. Immediately stop taking the medication if sexual dysfunction is noted.
6. A healthcare provider has ordered nifedipine (Procardia XL) for each of the following patients. A nurse will most closely monitor which patient for drug-related problems?
    1. A patient who is admitted for an appendectomy in the morning
    2. A patient who is receiving renal dialysis three times per week
    3. A patient who develops pulmonary edema in the intensive care unit
    4. A patient who receives psychotropic drugs for bipolar disease

See Appendix A for answers to critical thinking questions, case study questions, and review questions.

References

Alzheimer's Association. (2020). *2016 Alzheimer's and dementia facts and figures.* https://www.alz.org/alzheimers-dementia/facts-figures

Hussain, S., Singh, A., Rahman, S. O., Habib, A. & Najmi, A. K. (2018). Calcium channel blocker use reduces incident dementia risk in elderly hypertensive patients: A meta-analysis of prospective studies. *Neuroscience Letters, 671*, 120–127. https://doi.org/10.1016/j.neulet.2018.02.027

Lawlor, B., Segurado, R., Kennelly, S., Olde Rikkert, M. G. M., Howard, R., Pasquier, F., et al. (2018). Nilvadipine in mild to moderate Alzheimer disease: A randomised controlled trial. *PLoS Medicine, 15*, e1002660. https://doi.org/10.1371/journal.pmed.1002660

Mejia, L. M. (2019). *Drug-induced gingival hyperplasia.* Medscape. https://emedicine.medscape.com/article/1076264-overview#a6

Selected Bibliography

Ghosh, D., Syed, A. U., Prada, M. P., Nystoriak, M. A., Santana, L. F., Nieves-Cintrón, M., & Navedo, M. F. (2017). Calcium channels in vascular smooth muscle. *Advances in Pharmacology, 78*, 49–87. https://doi.org/10.1016/bs.apha.2016.08.002

Godfraind, T. (2017). Discovery and development of calcium channel blockers. *Frontiers in Pharmacology, 8*, 286. https://doi.org/10.3389/fphar.2017.00286

Graudins, A., Lee, H. M., & Druda, D. (2016). Calcium channel antagonist and beta-blocker overdose: Antidotes and adjunct therapies. *British Journal of Clinical Pharmacology, 81*(3), 453–461. https://doi.org/10.1111/bcp.12763

Lefler, L. L., Hadley, M., Tackett, J., & Thomason, A. P. (2015). New cardiovascular guidelines: Clinical practice evidence for the nurse practitioner. *Journal of the American Association of Nurse Practitioners, 28*, 241–248. https://doi.org/10.1002/2327-6924.12262

Patel, R., Montagut-Bordas, C., & Dickenson, A. H. (2018). Calcium channel modulation as a target in chronic pain control. *British journal of pharmacology, 175*(12), 2173–2184. https://doi.org/10.1111/bph.13789

Shoulders, B., & Powell, L. (2019). Reaching for goal: Incorporating the latest hypertension guidelines into practice. *Journal for Nurse Practitioners, 15*(1), 102–109. https://doi.org/10.1016/j.nurpra.2018.09.011

Sueta, D., Tabata, N., & Hokimoto, S. (2017). Clinical roles of calcium channel blockers in ischemic heart diseases. *Hypertension Research, 40*(5), 423–428. https://doi.org/10.1038/hr.2016.183

Wang, A. L., Iadecola, C., & Wang, G. (2017). New generations of dihydropyridines for treatment of hypertension. *Journal of Geriatric Cardiology, 14*(1), 67. https://doi.org/10.11909/j.issn.1671-5411.2017.01.006

Wang, D., Ragnarsson, L., & Lewis, R. J. (2020). T-type calcium channels in health and disease. *Current Medicinal Chemistry, 27*(19), 3098–3122. https://doi.org/10.2174/0929867325666181001112821

Zamponi, G. W. (2016). Targeting voltage-gated calcium channels in neurological and psychiatric diseases. *Nature Reviews Drug Discovery, 15*, 19–34. https://doi.org/10.1038/nrd.2015.5

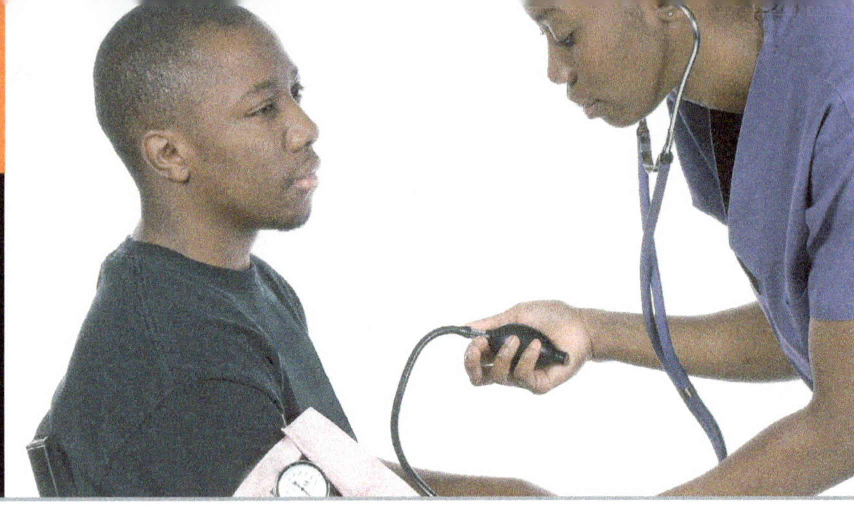

"When I saw my doctor, she said my blood pressure was still high. I'm taking my medicine as directed. So what's the problem?"
—*Patient "Carlos Avaya"*

Chapter 31
Drugs Affecting the Renin-Angiotensin-Aldosterone System

Chapter Outline

Learning Outcomes

After reading this chapter, the student should be able to:

1. Illustrate the steps in the renin-angiotensin-aldosterone pathway.
2. Identify the primary physiologic factors that control renin secretion.
3. Explain the two primary functions of angiotensin-converting enzyme.
4. Describe multiple mechanisms by which angiotensin II raises blood pressure.
5. Explain how the actions of aldosterone can lead to high blood pressure.
6. Identify the specific steps in the renin-angiotensin-aldosterone system that can be blocked by medications.
7. For each of the classes shown in the chapter outline, identify the prototype and representative drugs and explain the mechanism(s) of drug action, primary indications, contraindications, significant drug interactions, pregnancy data and important adverse effects.
8. Apply clinical judgment to care for patients receiving pharmacotherapy with angiotensin-converting enzyme inhibitors and angiotensin receptor blockers.

Key Terms

Definitions of the terms in bold may be found in the Glossary.

The renin-angiotensin-aldosterone system (RAAS) is a key homeostatic mechanism regulating blood pressure and fluid balance. The RAAS is presented early in the study of cardiovascular pharmacology because the drugs affecting this pathway are frequently used to treat hypertension (HTN) and heart failure (HF). This chapter examines components of the RAAS and describes how drugs affecting this system are used for therapeutic benefit.

Components of the Renin-Angiotensin-Aldosterone System

31.1 The formation of angiotensin II requires two enzymatic steps.

In the mid-1900s, scientists discovered a peptide circulating in the blood that caused profound vasoconstriction. Named angiotensin (*angio* = blood vessel; *tensin* = pressure), high levels of this substance were found in people with HTN. Thus began the search for components of what is now called the renin-angiotensin-aldosterone system.

We now know that there are several forms of angiotensin. **Angiotensin II** is the vasopressor substance originally isolated by scientists in the 1900s. The formation of angiotensin II requires two key enzymatic steps, which are critical to learning the pharmacology of drugs affecting the RAAS. The RAAS is illustrated in Figure 31.1.

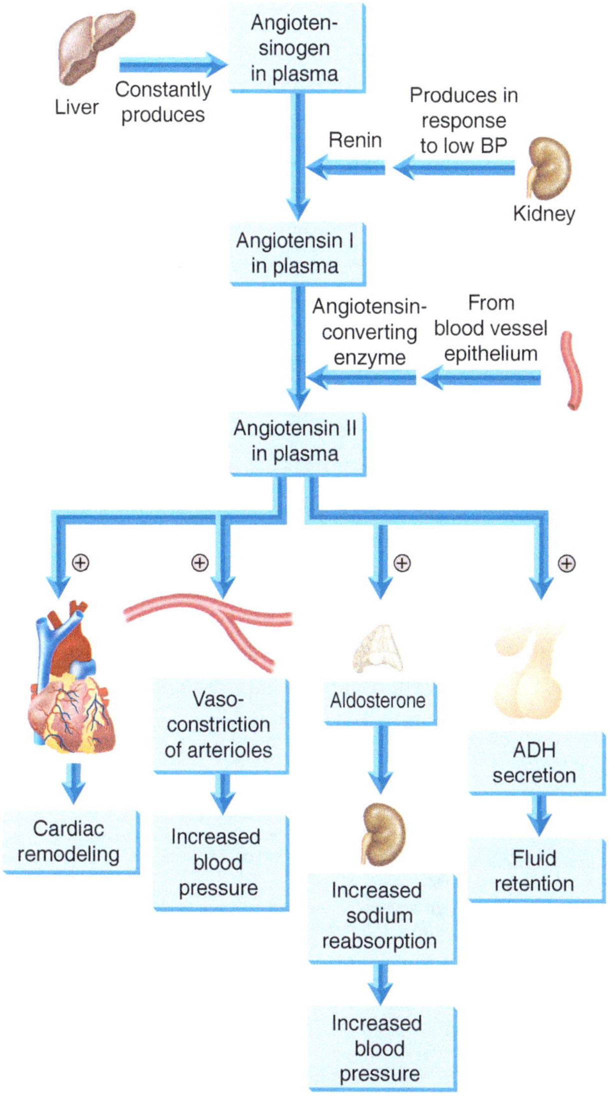

Figure 31.1 The renin-angiotensin-aldosterone pathway.

Step 1—Formation of angiotensin I. **Angiotensinogen** is a protein synthesized by the liver that is continuously circulating in the bloodstream. In the blood, angiotensinogen is split by the enzyme renin to form **angiotensin I**. Neither angiotensinogen nor angiotensin I has any significant physiologic actions; they simply serve as precursors to angiotensin II.

Step 2—Formation of angiotensin II. Angiotensin I travels through the circulation until it encounters *angiotensin-converting enzyme (ACE)*, which cleaves two amino acids to form angiotensin II. ACE is located on the membrane surface of the blood vessel endothelium. Because the lung possesses such an extensive number of capillaries, it is the primary organ responsible for converting angiotensin I to angiotensin II. Angiotensin II is one of the most potent natural vasoconstrictors known; it is approximately 40 times more potent at raising blood pressure than norepinephrine.

31.2 Renin secretion is controlled by the juxtaglomerular cells of the kidney and the sympathetic nervous system.

Because renin is responsible for the first step in the RAAS pathway, it is a major factor in determining the amount of angiotensin II produced in the body. Therefore, factors affecting the secretion of renin are important to understanding the pharmacotherapy associated with this system.

Renin is an enzyme that is synthesized, stored, and secreted by specialized cells in the kidney known as **juxtaglomerular (JG) cells** (also called *granular cells*). Found in the afferent arteriole that supplies blood to the glomerulus, JG cells are specialized smooth muscle cells that act as pressure sensors. As blood pressure falls, there is less pressure on the JG cells, which respond by releasing renin to the circulation. The increase in renin ultimately leads to larger amounts of circulating angiotensin II, which returns blood pressure to normal. The release of renin is caused by factors that lower blood pressure, such as a loss of blood volume due to dehydration or hemorrhage. Through negative feedback, increased blood pressure is sensed by the JG cells, which then turn off renin secretion.

Several other important factors influence the release of renin. Adjacent to the JG cells in the distal convoluted tubule of the nephron is a specialized cluster of cells called the **macula densa**. The macula densa is in a perfect location to sense the flow rate and the concentration of sodium ions (osmolality) in the urinary filtrate. As blood pressure falls, blood flow through the kidney diminishes and the flow of renal tubular filtrate slows. The macula densa recognizes the decreased flow rate (and less sodium) and sends a chemical message to the JG cells to release more renin. The renin release forms more angiotensin II and blood pressure rises.

Anatomically, the JG cells and the macula densa are in proximity, as shown in Figure 31.2. The JG cells and the macula densa are sometimes considered a single anatomic unit called the juxtaglomerular complex.

CONNECTION Checkpoint 31.1

Substances that lower blood pressure may trigger reflex tachycardia. From what you learned in Chapter 28, explain the mechanism involved in this reflex.

A third mechanism for controlling the release of renin is more direct: activation of the sympathetic nervous system (SNS). JG cells contain beta$_1$-adrenergic receptors, which are activated by the classic fight-or-flight response of the SNS (see Chapter 12). The release of renin helps to raise blood pressure when dealing with a stressful or harmful situation.

To summarize, factors that promote the release of renin by JG cells will raise blood pressure. The three primary factors causing an increase are decreased pressure in blood flowing through the kidney, decreased tubular flow rate (or fewer sodium ions) sensed by the macula densa, and activation of the SNS. Conversely, the factors that decrease renin secretion lower blood pressure. These factors are illustrated in Figure 31.3.

Increasing renin secretion will not always cause an increase in blood pressure. Remember that RAAS is a two-step pathway, and both steps are essential to produce a physiologic response. Section 31.3 examines this second step.

CONNECTION Checkpoint 31.2

From what you learned in Chapter 12, other than JG cells, in what organ are beta$_1$-adrenergic receptors predominantly located? What is the response of that organ when these receptors are activated?

31.3 Angiotensin-converting enzyme is responsible for the formation of angiotensin II.

Once angiotensin I is formed, its conversion to angiotensin II by ACE is almost instantaneous. A single pass of the blood

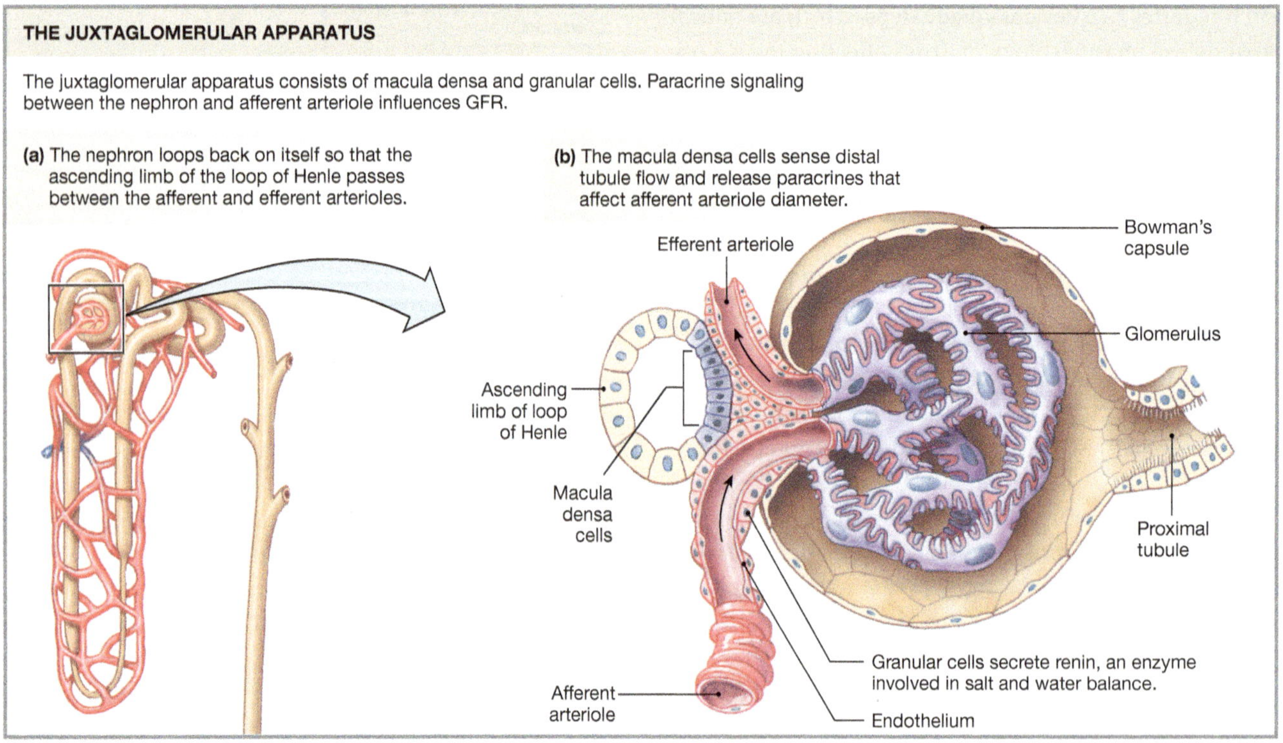

Figure 31.2 The macula densa and the juxtaglomerular (JG) cells. Osmoreceptors in the macula densa sense low sodium levels, which signals the JG cells to release renin.

From *Human Physiology: An Integrated Approach* (6th ed., p. 639), by D. U. Silverthorn, © 2013. Reprinted and electronically reproduced by permission of Pearson Education, Inc., Upper Saddle River, New Jersey.

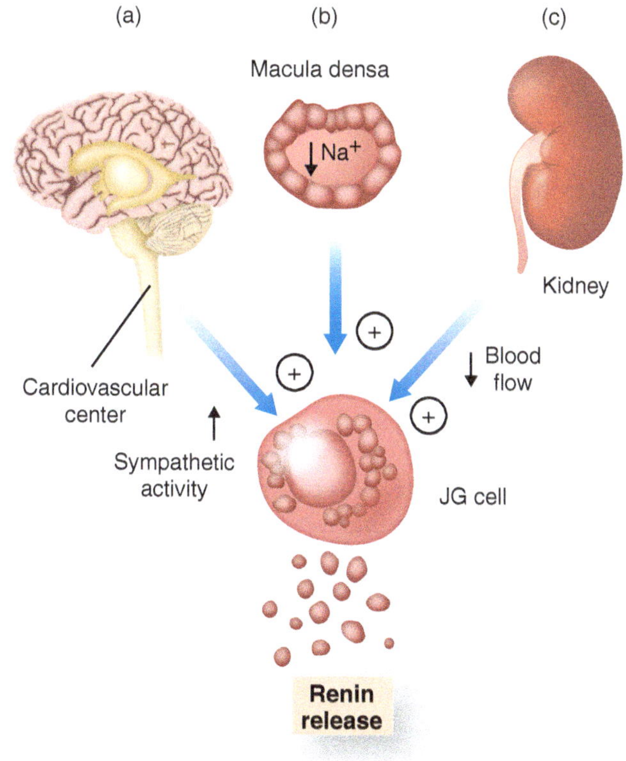

Figure 31.3 Overview of factors affecting renin release: (a) activation of the sympathetic nervous system, (b) low osmolarity in the macula densa, (c) low blood flow through the kidney.

through lung capillaries converts most of the circulating angiotensin I to angiotensin II.

In addition to its role in the formation of angiotensin II, ACE has a second, lesser known function important to homeostasis and pharmacotherapy. ACE is one of several enzymes that degrade **bradykinin**, a natural mediator of inflammation and pain. Bradykinin has many of the same effects as histamine (see Chapter 44), including increasing arteriolar vasodilation and vascular permeability. Interestingly, at the same time ACE is generating a vasoconstrictor (angiotensin II), it is also breaking down a vasodilator (bradykinin). When referring to its actions on bradykinin, ACE is sometimes called kininase II; *kininase* is the general term for an enzyme that breaks down kinins. ACE and kininase II refer to the identical enzyme.

Pharmacologically, ACE is an important enzyme in the RAAS because it serves as a target molecule for drugs in the ACE inhibitor class of medications. Inhibition of ACE will prevent the formation of angiotensin II, thus interrupting the RAAS pathway. In addition, these medications also inhibit ACE (kininase II), thus preventing the breakdown of bradykinin. Accumulation of bradykinin in certain tissues can cause several adverse effects of ACE inhibitors, such as angioedema and cough.

Physiologic Actions of the Renin-Angiotensin-Aldosterone System

31.4 Angiotensin II has multiple effects on the cardiovascular system that raise blood pressure and affect cardiac function.

The final product of the two-step renin-angiotensin pathway is angiotensin II. Angiotensin II has several physiologic effects important to homeostasis and to pharmacotherapy.

Direct vasoconstriction. Angiotensin II acts directly on vascular smooth muscle to cause vasoconstriction and increased systemic blood pressure. This effect is rapid; formation of angiotensin II results in a nearly instantaneous increase in blood pressure. This vasopressor action of angiotensin II is much greater on arterioles compared to veins; arterioles serving the kidneys are especially sensitive to this vasopressor action.

Increased sympathetic nervous system activity. Angiotensin II activates the SNS by causing the release of norepinephrine from sympathetic nerve terminals. The adrenal medulla is also affected by angiotensin II, which responds by releasing additional epinephrine to the circulation. Furthermore, through largely unknown mechanisms, angiotensin II increases sympathetic outflow from the brain. All three of these actions increase peripheral resistance and raise blood pressure.

Alteration of cardiovascular structure. The long-term presence of angiotensin II can also cause hypertrophy of myocardial cells (myocytes) and promote collagen deposits in the cardiac matrix, essentially forming scarlike tissue in the heart. These changes are known as **cardiac remodeling**. The hypertrophy, fibrosis, and remodeling of cardiac structure have been correlated with increased morbidity and mortality associated with HF. In blood vessels, angiotensin II causes the release of multiple chemical mediators of atherosclerosis, accelerating the deposition of fatty plaque on the walls of the vessels. Increased plaque deposits lead to an increased risk for myocardial infarction (MI) and stroke.

Release of aldosterone and effects on the renal tubule. Angiotensin II has two primary effects on the kidney that promote an increase in blood pressure. First, angiotensin II has a direct effect on the nephron that increases Na^+ and Cl^- reabsorption in the proximal tubule. Second, angiotensin II indirectly affects sodium reabsorption by stimulating the adrenal cortex to synthesize and secrete additional amounts of the mineralocorticoid aldosterone. The principal site of aldosterone action is on the distal and collecting tubules of the nephron, although mineralocorticoid receptors (MR) are found in other body sites, including the heart. Once occupying the MR in the kidney, aldosterone increases Na^+ reabsorption and K^+ and H^+ excretion. The enhanced sodium reabsorption from both direct and indirect actions of angiotensin II causes the body to retain water, thus increasing blood volume and raising blood pressure. Aldosterone is a key component of the RAAS.

Unlike its immediate and direct effects on sympathetic nerves, the actions of angiotensin II on the kidney develop more slowly. This slow vasopressor response on renal vessels is believed to be responsible for producing a sustained elevation of blood pressure and a gradual decline of renal function.

Students often think of angiotensin II as a "bad actor" because it can create HTN and cause the damaging effects of cardiac remodeling. Remember, however, that the cardiovascular and renal effects of angiotensin II serve an essential homeostatic function. Should blood pressure fall, the increased synthesis and production of angiotensin II help return blood pressure to normal levels to maintain blood flow to vital organs. When the body is subjected to chronically elevated levels of angiotensin II, however, the once vital reflex pathway becomes a detriment to the body.

CONNECTION Checkpoint 31.3

From what you learned in Chapter 28, what effect would you expect angiotensin II formation to have on cardiac output and afterload?

31.5 The renin-angiotensin-aldosterone pathway offers multiple points for drug intervention.

Having learned details of the different components in the short pathway leading from angiotensinogen to angiotensin II, the student should recognize several potential mechanisms by which drugs could intervene:

- **ACE inhibitors.** This is the largest and most important class of drugs modifying the RAAS. ACE inhibitors block the conversion of angiotensin I to angiotensin II.
- **Angiotensin receptor blockers.** After angiotensin II is formed, it must interact with its receptors on target cells to cause its biologic actions. There are two primary receptor subtypes, known as *AT_1* and *AT_2 receptors*. Blocking AT_1 receptors prevents angiotensin from raising blood pressure and from causing cardiac remodeling. Angiotensin receptor blockers are medications that intervene at this step in the RAAS by blocking the AT_1 receptor. The role of AT_2 receptors, which are found in greatest abundance in the fetus, is largely unknown but is an area of active research.
- **Aldosterone antagonists.** Much of the blood pressure increase resulting from the formation of angiotensin II is caused by its stimulation of aldosterone secretion. Two drugs are available that block receptors for aldosterone in the kidney, thus preventing the aldosterone-induced increase in blood pressure.
- **Renin inhibitors.** In 2007, the U.S. Food and Drug Administration (FDA) approved the first renin inhibitor. Aliskiren (Tekturna) is approved to treat HTN as monotherapy or in combination with other antihypertensives.

Drugs Affecting the Renin-Angiotensin-Aldosterone System

31.6 ACE inhibitors are key drugs in the pharmacotherapy of hypertension and heart failure.

First detected in the venom of pit vipers in the 1960s, inhibitors of ACE have been approved for HTN since the 1980s. Drugs in this class have become first-line medications in the treatment of HTN and HF. Doses for the ACE inhibitors are listed in Table 31.1.

ACE inhibitors block the conversion of angiotensin I to angiotensin II. The decline in angiotensin II levels causes blood pressure to decrease because there is less sympathetic activation and, thus, lower peripheral resistance. In addition, the decreased aldosterone secretion reduces blood volume, which also contributes to blood pressure reduction.

Therapy with ACE inhibitors slows the progression of HF and reduces mortality from this disease. This is likely due to both the reduction in systemic blood pressure and a reversal of the angiotensin II–induced structural changes in the heart. Because of their relative safety, they have replaced digoxin (Lanoxin) as the first-line drugs for the treatment of chronic HF. Indeed, unless specifically contraindicated, all patients with HF usually receive an ACE inhibitor, as discussed in Chapter 36.

Research has also indicated a clear benefit for administering ACE inhibitors to patients who have experienced a recent MI. If therapy is begun immediately after the infarction and continued for several weeks, these drugs lower the cardiovascular mortality associated with an acute MI. The mechanism by which these drugs improve the outcome following an acute MI involves reduced peripheral vascular resistance, improved perfusion, and a direct action on the myocardium that reduces the cardiac workload.

ACE inhibitors may also be prescribed as prophylaxis therapy in patients at high risk for an adverse cardiovascular event. ACE inhibitors can reduce the incidence of a stroke or MI in these high-risk patients. They may also prevent or delay the progression of renal disease and retinopathy in patients with diabetes.

All ACE inhibitors have very similar indications and adverse effect profiles. All drugs in this class are approved to treat HTN, and some are approved for HF and acute MI and for prophylaxis of cardiovascular disease. Almost all ACE inhibitors are administered orally (PO) and offer the convenience of once-daily dosing. Many of the ACE inhibitors are prodrugs, which are converted to active metabolites by hepatic enzymes. Most ACE inhibitors are excreted by the kidneys; thus, dose reductions may be required in patients with advanced chronic kidney disease (CKD).

The low incidence of serious adverse effects is a major contributing factor to the widespread use of the ACE inhibitors.

Table 31.1 ACE Inhibitors

Drug	Route and Adult Dose (Maximum Dose Where Indicated)	Adverse Effects
benazepril (Lotensin)	PO: 10–40 mg in 1–2 divided doses (max: 80 mg/day)	*Headache, dry cough, dizziness, orthostatic hypotension, rash* <u>Angioedema, acute renal failure, first-dose phenomenon, fetal toxicity</u>
captopril	PO: 6.25–25 mg tid (max: 450 mg/day)	
enalapril (Vasotec)	PO: 5–40 mg in 1–2 divided doses (max: 40 mg/day PO; 20 mg/day IV))	
fosinopril	PO: 5–40 mg once daily (max: 40 mg/day for HF; 80 mg/day for HTN)	
lisinopril (Prinivil, Zestril)	PO: 5–40 mg daily (max: 80 mg/day)	
moexipril	PO: 7.5–30 mg once daily (max: 30 mg/day)	
perindopril	PO: 4–8 mg once daily (max: 16 mg/day for HTN; 4–8 mg/day for coronary artery disease)	
quinapril (Accupril)	PO: 10–20 mg once daily (max: 40 mg/day for HF; 80 mg/day for HTN)	
ramipril (Altace)	PO: 2.5–20 mg daily (max: 20 mg/day)	
trandolapril	PO: 1–4 mg once daily (max: 8 mg/day)	

Note: Italics indicate common adverse effects. <u>Underline</u> indicates serious adverse effects.

Orthostatic hypotension following the first few doses of the drug can be severe in patients who are on low-sodium diets or who have HF. Drug therapy is sometimes begun with very low doses and increased gradually to avoid orthostatic hypotension. Hyperkalemia may occur during ACE inhibitor therapy; however, this is predominantly a major concern only for patients with diabetes or CKD and those who are taking potassium supplements or potassium-sparing diuretics. Persistent, dry cough is an annoying adverse effect that occurs in 5 to 20% of patients taking ACE inhibitors. This adverse effect is likely due to a buildup of bradykinin in the lungs. Drugs in this class have minimal or no effect on serum glucose or uric acid levels.

Though rare, the most serious adverse effect of ACE inhibitors is the development of **angioedema**, a rapid swelling of the throat, face, larynx, and tongue that can lead to airway obstruction and death. When it does occur, angioedema most often develops within a few hours after the first dose, although it may occur after several days of ACE inhibitor therapy. Accumulation of bradykinin is thought to be responsible. Treatment of angioedema is to discontinue the drug immediately and maintain the airway until the effects of the drug wear off.

A second type of ACE, ACE2, is present in most organs. Like ACE, ACE2 is attached to the cell membrane of lung cells and has the same functions as ACE, as described above. However, there is one critical difference, relating to the novel coronavirus (COVID-19) that created a global pandemic in 2020 that appeared quickly and killed hundreds of thousands of people. COVID-19 attaches to ACE2 and both the enzyme and the virus enter the human cell through endocytosis, where it replicates. Thus, ACE2 serves as the entry point for COVID-19. Several pharmaceutical companies are working on ACE2-related drugs that are able to block the entry of COVID-19 into lung cells.

Do the ACE inhibitors used in pharmacotherapy have any effect on the entry of COVID-19? Research is evolving; however, several medical groups have strongly urged healthcare providers to continue usual treatment with ACE inhibitors and angiotensin II receptor blockers (Tucker, 2020a, 2020b).

CONNECTIONS: Community-Oriented Practice

Angiotensin-Converting Enzyme Inhibitors and Angioedema

Angioedema is the development of edema of the mouth, lips, tongue, pharynx, larynx, and epiglottis that can be fatal if respiratory distress occurs secondary to the swelling of the upper airway. Less commonly, intestinal edema may also occur, causing a sudden onset of abdominal pain, vomiting, and diarrhea. Angioedema is associated with ACE inhibitors and appears to be related to the increase in bradykinin levels when ACE is no longer available to break down circulating bradykinin. Although angioedema occurs in less than about 1% of patients taking ACE inhibitors, it is more common in African Americans, particularly those of Caribbean descent, and in older adults.

In 50% of patients, angioedema occurs after the first dose of an ACE inhibitor, although it may occur anytime during therapy. Patients who have had a previous episode of angioedema after taking an ACE inhibitor are at greater risk for developing angioedema from other ACE inhibitors. It may also be caused by angiotensin receptor blockers, although less commonly. Itching and urticaria may occur prior to the development of angioedema but are not good predictors as to whether or not angioedema will develop. Immediate treatment may include administration of epinephrine, antihistamines (both H_1 and H_2 blockers), corticosteroids, and fresh frozen plasma. The ACE in fresh plasma accelerates the breakdown of bradykinin. The patient should be observed closely after the first dose, and any subsequent swelling of the facial, oral, or pharynx areas should be immediately reported to the provider.

All the ACE inhibitors carry a black box warning regarding the risk for major congenital malformations and mortality if the drugs are taken during pregnancy, especially during the second and third trimesters. The risk for other congenital defects such as heart and neural tube defects during the first trimester is not as clear. Most healthcare providers will discontinue ACE inhibitors as soon as pregnancy is determined. Women with HTN should be advised not to discontinue these drugs during pregnancy without healthcare provider knowledge because HTN itself is a risk factor for congenital defects.

PROTOTYPE DRUG Lisinopril (Prinivil, Zestril)

Classification **Therapeutic:** Antihypertensive
Pharmacologic: ACE inhibitor

Therapeutic Effects and Uses: Approved for the treatment of HF, HTN, and acute MI, lisinopril is one of the most frequently prescribed medications. Approved in 1987, it may be used as monotherapy or combined with other drugs. Qbrelis is an oral solution of lisinopril. Zestoretic is a fixed-dose combination of lisinopril and hydrochlorothiazide (a diuretic) marketed for HTN. Unlike many drugs in this class, lisinopril is active itself; it is not a prodrug. Treatment of migraines and diabetic nephropathy are off-label indications for lisinopril.

Although captopril was the first drug that was marketed in this class, lisinopril is more widely prescribed because it has a longer duration of action that allows for once-daily dosing. Like other ACE inhibitors, 2 to 3 weeks of therapy may be required to achieve maximum therapeutic outcomes.

Mechanism of Action: Lisinopril binds to and inhibits the action of ACE, thus preventing the conversion of angiotensin I to angiotensin II. The decrease in serum angiotensin II reduces aldosterone secretion, which results in less sodium and water retention. In patients with HTN, blood pressure is reduced with minimal effect on heart rate, stroke volume, or cardiac output.

Pharmacokinetics:

Route(s)	PO
Absorption	25–30% absorbed from the gastrointestinal (GI) tract
Distribution	Small amount crosses the blood–brain barrier; crosses the placenta; limited amounts are secreted in breast milk; not bound to plasma protein
Primary metabolism	Not metabolized
Primary excretion	Renal
Onset of action	1 h; peak effect: 6–8 h
Duration of action	24 h; half-life: 12 h

Adverse Effects: Lisinopril is well tolerated and adverse effects are uncommon and transient. The most common adverse effects are cough, headache, dizziness, orthostatic hypotension, and rash. Hyperkalemia occurs in about 2 to 5% of patients taking ACE inhibitors, although this usually resolves during therapy. Patients with HF or CKD or who are taking potassium supplements or potassium-sparing diuretics are at highest risk for hyperkalemia. Rare, though serious, adverse effects include angioedema, agranulocytosis, and hepatotoxicity. **Black Box Warning:** Fetal injury and death may occur when ACE inhibitors are taken during pregnancy. When pregnancy is detected, they should be discontinued as soon as possible.

Contraindications/Precautions: Lisinopril should be used with extreme caution in patients with hyperkalemia because they may experience serious and even fatal dysrhythmias. Patients with a history of angioedema should not receive lisinopril. Caution should be used when treating patients with advanced CKD, thus dosage should be reduced. Lisinopril is contraindicated during pregnancy.

Drug Interactions: Indomethacin and other nonsteroidal anti-inflammatory drugs (NSAIDs) interact with lisinopril to decrease antihypertensive activity. The combination of lisinopril and NSAIDs may also worsen preexisting renal disease. Because of synergistic hypotensive action, concurrent therapy with diuretics and other antihypertensives such as ACE inhibitors should be carefully monitored. When taken with potassium supplements or potassium-sparing diuretics, hyperkalemia may result. Lisinopril may increase lithium levels and toxicity. **Herbal/Food:** Hawthorn should not be taken concurrently with lisinopril due to the possibility of additive hypotensive action.

Pregnancy: ACE inhibitors can cause injury, birth defects, and even death to a developing fetus. Due to the potential for serious adverse effects in the neonate, breastfeeding should be discontinued during lisinopril therapy.

Treatment of Overdose: Overdose will cause hypotension, which may be treated with normal saline or a vasopressor. The drug may also be removed by hemodialysis.

Clinician Responsibilities: Key clinical implications for patients receiving lisinopril are included in Applied Clinical Judgment: Patients Receiving Pharmacotherapy with Angiotensin-Converting Enzyme Inhibitors and Angiotensin Receptor Blockers.

Drugs Similar to Lisinopril (Prinivil, Zestril)

In addition to lisinopril, there are nine other ACE inhibitors on the market. All have very similar actions and adverse effects. All ACE inhibitors carry a black box warning regarding the potential for fetal harm and are contraindicated during pregnancy, and breastfeeding is not advised during therapy.

Benazepril (Lotensin): Approved in 1991, benazepril is approved only for HTN, although an off-label indication is HF. It is a prodrug that is metabolized by hepatic enzymes to its active form, benazeprilat. It has a long duration of action that allows for once-daily dosing and is excreted by the kidneys. Orthostatic hypotension is the most common adverse effect, especially after the first dose. Other adverse effects, contraindications, and indications are the same as those of lisinopril. Lotensin HCT is a fixed-dose combination of benazepril and hydrochlorothiazide and Lotrel is a combination of benazepril with amlodipine.

Captopril: Captopril, the first ACE inhibitor marketed in 1981, is approved for HTN, HF, left-ventricular dysfunction after an acute MI, and diabetic nephropathy. It has a short half-life, which requires multiple daily doses for some patients. The drug should be taken on an empty stomach because food reduces its bioavailability. Neutropenia and agranulocytosis have occurred during captopril use. Other adverse effects, contraindications, and indications are the same as those of lisinopril.

Enalapril (Vasotec): Approved in 1985, enalapril is indicated for HTN, HF, and asymptomatic left-ventricular dysfunction in post-MI patients. It has a shorter half-life than some other ACE inhibitors and may require twice-daily dosing. Enalapril is a prodrug, being converted by hepatic enzymes to enalaprilat, which is its active form. The most frequent adverse effect is hypotension, which can be especially troublesome in patients with HF. Adverse effects, contraindications, and indications are the same as those of lisinopril. Enalaprilat (Vasotec IV) is available as a drug for severe HTN and is the only ACE inhibitor administered parenterally. Vaseretic is a fixed-dose combination of enalapril and hydrochlorothiazide.

Fosinopril: Approved in 1991, fosinopril is used to treat HTN and HF. It is a prodrug that is metabolized by hepatic enzymes to its active form, fosinoprilat. An extended half-life allows for once-daily dosing, and it may be taken without regard to meals. It is excreted by both the liver and kidneys and does not require a dosage adjustment in patients with hepatic impairment or CKD. The most common adverse effects of fosinopril are orthostatic hypotension, dizziness, and headache. A fixed-dose combination of fosinopril and hydrochlorothiazide is available to treat HTN.

Moexipril: Approved in 1995, moexipril is indicated only for HTN. It is a prodrug that is metabolized to its active form, moexiprilat, by hepatic enzymes. An extended half-life allows for once-daily dosing. This drug should be taken on an empty stomach because food reduces its bioavailability by 40 to 50%. It is excreted by the kidneys, and dosage should be reduced in patients with CKD. Dizziness is one of the most common adverse effects. Adverse effects, contraindications, and indications are the same as those of lisinopril. A fixed-dose combination of moexipril and hydrochlorothiazide is available to treat HTN.

Perindopril: Approved in 1993, perindopril is indicated for HTN and to reduce the risk of cardiovascular events such as MI in patients with coronary artery disease. HF is an off-label use. It is a prodrug that is metabolized by hepatic enzymes to its active form, perindoprilat. It is excreted by the kidneys, and its long half-life allows for once- or twice-daily dosing. Food may reduce the bioavailability of the drug by as much as 35%. Cough and dizziness are the most frequent adverse effects of perindopril. Other adverse effects, contraindications, and indications are the same as those of lisinopril. Prestalia is a fixed-dose combination of perindopril and amlodipine is available to treat HTN.

Quinapril (Accupril): Approved in 1991, quinapril is indicated for HTN and HF. It is a prodrug that is metabolized by hepatic enzymes to its active form, quinaprilat, and may be dosed either once or twice daily. Because the kidney contributes to about 96% of the excretion of the drug, doses should be reduced in patients with CKD. Adverse effects are generally mild and transient and include dizziness, cough, and diarrhea. Other adverse effects, contraindications, and indications are the same as those of lisinopril. Accuretic is a fixed-dose combination of quinapril and hydrochlorothiazide.

Ramipril (Altace): Approved in 1991, ramipril is indicated for HTN, HF following an MI, and to reduce the risk for mortality and stroke in high-risk patients with left-ventricular dysfunction. It is a prodrug that is metabolized by hepatic enzymes to its active form, ramiprilat. Excretion is predominantly renal, and dosage should be reduced in patients with advanced CKD. It may be administered without regard to meals. The most common adverse effects are orthostatic hypotension, dizziness, and headache. Other adverse effects, contraindications, and indications are the same as those of lisinopril.

Trandolapril: Approved in 1996, trandolapril is indicated for HTN and HF following an MI and to reduce the mortality in high-risk patients with left-ventricular dysfunction. It is a prodrug that is metabolized by hepatic enzymes to trandolaprilat, its active form. It has an extended half-life that permits once-daily dosing and may be administered without regard to meals. Unlike other ACE inhibitors, a large amount of trandolapril (66%) is excreted in the feces. Dosages should be lowered in patients with CKD or hepatic impairment. The most common adverse effects are cough, dizziness, and fatigue. Other adverse effects, contraindications, and indications are the same as those of lisinopril. Tarka is a fixed-dose combination of trandolapril and the calcium channel blocker verapamil SR, which is prescribed for HTN.

CONNECTION Checkpoint 31.4

ACE inhibitors decrease sympathetic activation. From what you learned in Chapters 15 and 16, what type of interactions (additive or antagonistic) would you expect from the autonomic drugs epinephrine and propranolol?

31.7 Angiotensin II receptor blockers act by inhibiting the AT_1 receptor and are used for hypertension and heart failure.

While pharmacologists were examining the mechanism of action of the ACE inhibitors in the 1980s and developing new drugs in this class, research continued on the other enzymes and components of the RAAS. The receptors for angiotensin II in smooth muscle, known as AT_1 and AT_2, were discovered, and a new class of drugs, the angiotensin II receptor blockers (ARBs), was developed. The ARBs are selective for AT_1-type receptors. Unlike the ACE inhibitors, ARBs do not prevent the formation of angiotensin II, but they do effectively block it from activating their target receptors. Doses for the ARBs are listed in Table 31.2.

The ARBs cause vasodilation, with a resultant reduction in peripheral resistance and fall in blood pressure, by blocking angiotensin II receptors in arteriolar smooth muscle. The blockade of AT_1 receptors in the adrenal gland prevents secretion of aldosterone and promotes increased Na^+ and excretion of water by the kidneys. Blockade of AT_1 receptors in the heart prevents the destructive effects of angiotensin-induced cardiac remodeling. Although they act by a different mechanism, ARBs essentially produce the same pharmacologic actions as the ACE inhibitors.

The indications for ARBs are the same as those for the ACE inhibitors. All are approved to treat HTN, and they are often combined with drugs from other classes. Valsartan (Diovan) and candesartan (Atacand) were subsequently approved to treat HF. Some are approved to treat MI and are used for the prophylaxis of stroke. All are administered orally and have prolonged half-lives that permit once-daily dosing. A few are prodrugs, and most are extensively bound to plasma proteins. Like the ACE inhibitors, ARBs may cause fetal harm and are contraindicated during pregnancy.

Are the ARBs identical to the ACE inhibitors? Not exactly. Unlike the ACE inhibitors, they do not cause cough and the incidence of angioedema lower. This is because ARBs do not promote the accumulation of bradykinin, as do the ACE inhibitors. ARBs can, however, cause dizziness, hypotension, and hyperkalemia, especially in patients with CKD or who are concurrently taking potassium supplements or potassium-sparing diuretics. Caution should be used with concurrent administration of ARBs and ACE inhibitors due to an increased risk for hypotension, hyperkalemia, and diminished renal function.

If ARBs have the same pharmacologic actions and an improved safety profile, why have they not replaced the ACE inhibitors? Because the ACE inhibitors are generally less expensive, and healthcare providers have 15 to 20 more years of clinical experience prescribing them. Because of this, the ARBs have generally been reserved for patients unable to tolerate the adverse effects of ACE inhibitors, such as angioedema and persistent cough. Recent guidelines, however, are giving equal emphasis to both classes in the treatment of HTN and HF.

Table 31.2 Angiotensin II Receptor Blockers, Aldosterone Antagonists, and Renin Inhibitors

Drug	Route and Adult Dose (Maximum Dose Where Indicated)	Adverse Effects
Angiotensin II Receptor Blockers		
azilsartan (Edarbi)	PO: 40–80 mg once daily	*Headache, dizziness, orthostatic hypotension, fatigue, diarrhea, upper respiratory infection* Angioedema, acute renal failure, first-dose phenomenon, hyperkalemia, fetal toxicity, neonatal mortality
candesartan (Atacand)	PO: 16–32 mg/day for HTN and 4–32 mg/day for HF (max: 32 mg/day)	
irbesartan (Avapro)	PO: 150–300 mg/day (max: 300 mg/day)	
losartan (Cozaar)	PO: 25–50 mg once daily (max: 100 mg/day)	
olmesartan medoxomil (Benicar)	PO: 20–40 mg/day	
telmisartan (Micardis)	PO: 40–80 mg once daily	
valsartan (Diovan)	PO: 80 mg/day (max: 320 mg/day)	
Aldosterone Antagonists		
eplerenone (Inspra)	PO: 25–100 mg/day (max: 100 mg/day for HTN; 50 mg/day for HF)	*Minor hyperkalemia, headache, fatigue, gynecomastia (spironolactone)* Dysrhythmias (from hyperkalemia), dehydration, hyponatremia, agranulocytosis and other blood dyscrasias
spironolactone (Aldactone)	PO: 50–100 mg/day in single or divided doses (max: 400 mg/day)	
Renin Inhibitor		
aliskiren (Tekturna)	PO: 150 mg/day (max: 300 mg/day)	*Diarrhea, hypotension, cough* Angioedema

Note: Italics indicate common adverse effects. Underline indicates serious adverse effects.

PROTOTYPE DRUG **Losartan (Cozaar)**

Classification **Therapeutic:** Antihypertensive
Pharmacologic: Angiotensin II receptor blocker

Therapeutic Effects and Uses: Approved for the treatment of HTN, stroke prophylaxis in patients with left-ventricular hypertrophy, and the prevention of type 2 diabetic nephropathy, losartan was the first ARB marketed in 1995. An off-label use is for HF. Although losartan undergoes extensive first-pass metabolism and has a short half-life, it is metabolized to an active intermediate that prolongs the drug's action, allowing for once-daily dosing. Two daily doses may be necessary in some patients. Its actions include vasodilation and reduced blood volume, due to the drug blocking the release of aldosterone by angiotensin II. Hyzaar is a fixed-dose combination of losartan and hydrochlorothiazide. Concurrent use of these two drugs has an additive effect on blood pressure reduction.

Mechanism of Action: Losartan and its active metabolite selectively block angiotensin AT_1 receptors, resulting in a decline in blood pressure. The blockade of angiotensin II receptors prevents cardiac remodeling and deterioration of renal function in patients with diabetes.

Pharmacokinetics:

Route(s)	PO
Absorption	Well absorbed from the GI tract
Distribution	Does not appear to cross the blood–brain barrier or the placenta or to be secreted in breast milk; approximately 99% bound to protein
Primary metabolism	Hepatic: extensive first-pass metabolism; converted to active metabolite
Primary excretion	35% renal, 60% in feces
Onset of action	6 h
Duration of action	Half-life: 1.5–2 h (losartan), 6–9 h (highly active metabolite)

Adverse Effects: The incidence of adverse effects of losartan is very low. The most common adverse effects are headache, dizziness, nasal congestion, fatigue, and insomnia. Serious adverse effects include angioedema and acute renal failure. **Black Box Warning:** Fetal injury and death may occur when ARBs are taken during pregnancy. When pregnancy is detected, they should be discontinued as soon as possible.

Contraindications/Precautions: Losartan is contraindicated in patients with prior hypersensitivity to the drug. Because ARBs exhibit the same teratogenic effects as ACE inhibitors, they should not be used during pregnancy and lactation. Caution should be used in treating patients with serious hepatic impairment or advanced CKD; dosage may need to be reduced. Patients with a history of angioedema should be monitored carefully. Patients with hypovolemia are at high risk of symptomatic hypotension during therapy. Hypovolemia should be corrected prior to administration of losartan.

Drug Interactions: The drug interactions of losartan and other ARBs are similar to those of the ACE inhibitors. Indomethacin and other NSAIDs may decrease the antihypertensive activity of losartan. When taken concurrently with potassium supplements or potassium-sparing diuretics, care must be taken to avoid hyperkalemia. Concurrent use of losartan with diuretics and other antihypertensives may cause additive hypotensive effects. Use with alcohol may also add to the hypotensive effects of losartan. Losartan may increase lithium levels and toxicity. In patients with diabetes, losartan should not be administered concurrently with aliskiren. **Herbal/Food:** Hawthorn should not be taken concurrently with losartan due to the possibility of additive hypotensive action.

Pregnancy: ARBs can cause injury, birth defects, and even death to a developing fetus. Breastfeeding should be discontinued during losartan therapy.

Treatment of Overdose: Overdose will cause hypotension, which may be treated with an infusion of normal saline or a vasopressor. The drug is not removed by hemodialysis.

Clinician Responsibilities: Key clinical implications for patients receiving losartan are included in Applied Clinical Judgment: Patients Receiving Pharmacotherapy with Angiotensin-Converting Enzyme Inhibitors and Angiotensin Receptor Blockers.

Drugs Similar to Losartan (Cozaar)

In addition to losartan, six other ARBs are available. They all have similar indications, actions, and adverse effects. All ARBs can cause injury, birth defects and even death to a developing fetus. Breastfeeding should be discontinued during ARB therapy.

Azilsartan medoxomil (Edarbi): Azilsartan was approved in 2011 for the treatment of HTN, either as monotherapy or in combination with other antihypertensives. The drug is sometimes listed by its potassium salt, azilsartan kamedoxomil. Both the medoxomil and kamedoxomil salts are prodrugs that are converted to their active form (azilsartan) when absorbed across the GI tract. Azilsartan appears to lower blood pressure faster than other drugs in its class. The drug is well tolerated, with diarrhea being the most frequent adverse effect. Caution should be used in treating volume or salt-depleted patients because transient hypotension may occur. Edarbyclor is a fixed-dose combination of azilsartan kamedoxomil with chlorthalidone approved to treat HTN.

Candesartan (Atacand): Approved in 1998, candesartan is indicated for HTN and HF in patients with left-ventricular dysfunction. It is a prodrug that is metabolized to its active form during its absorption from the GI tract. Optimal therapeutic effects may take up to 4 weeks. The drug is 99% protein bound and is primarily excreted in the bile (66%). Adverse effects are generally mild and include headache and dizziness. Other adverse effects, contraindications, and indications are the same as those of losartan. Atacand HCT is a fixed-dose combination of candesartan and hydrochlorothiazide to treat HTN.

Irbesartan (Avapro): Approved in 1997, irbesartan is indicated for HTN and type 2 diabetic nephropathy. The drug is 90% protein bound and is primarily excreted in the feces (80%). Adverse effects are generally mild and include dizziness, upper respiratory infection, orthostatic hypotension, diarrhea, dyspepsia, and fatigue. Hyperkalemia may occur in 19% of patients taking this medication. Other adverse effects, contraindications, and indications are the same as those of losartan. Avalide is a fixed-dose combination of irbesartan and hydrochlorothiazide to treat HTN.

Olmesartan medoxomil (Benicar): Approved in 2002, olmesartan is indicated only for HTN. Olmesartan medoxomil is a prodrug that is metabolized to its active form (olmesartan) during its absorption from the GI tract. Olmesartan is 99% protein bound and excreted equally in urine and the feces. The drug is administered once daily, and optimal blood pressure reduction may require 2 weeks of therapy. The drug exhibits few adverse effects, with dizziness being the most common complaint. Other adverse effects, contraindications, and indications are the same as those of losartan. There are three fixed-dose combinations of olmesartan: Benicar HCT (with hydrochlorothiazide), Azor (with amlodipine), and Tribenzor (with amlodipine and hydrochlorothiazide).

Telmisartan (Micardis): Approved in 1998, telmisartan is indicated for HTN and for cardiovascular risk reduction in patients unable to take ACE inhibitors. An off-label use is for the treatment of renal dysfunction in patients with diabetic nephropathy. It is mostly unmetabolized, 99% protein bound, and excreted primarily in the feces. Initial doses should be reduced in patients with hepatic impairment. The drug is well tolerated and serious adverse effects are uncommon. Adverse effects, contraindications, and indications are the same as those of losartan. Fixed-dose combinations include Micardis HCT (with hydrochlorothiazide) and Twynsta (with amlodipine).

Valsartan (Diovan): Approved in 1996, valsartan is indicated for HTN, HF, and post MI to reduce the risk of cardiovascular death. It undergoes hepatic metabolism, is 95% protein bound, and is eliminated in the feces. Because food can reduce drug absorption by as much as 40%, the drug should be given on an empty stomach. Headache and dizziness are common adverse effects. Other adverse effects, contraindications, and indications are the same as those of losartan. Fixed-dose combinations include Diovan HCT (with hydrochlorothiazide), Exforge (with amlodipine). and Exforge HCT (with hydrochlorothiazide and amlodipine). Entresto is a fixed-dose combination of valsartan with sacubitril, a neprilysin inhibitor, to treat HF and pediatric patients older than 1 year. The most common adverse effects with Entresto are hypotension and hyperkalemia.

31.8 Aldosterone antagonists block the biological effects of aldosterone in the renal tubule.

As described in Section 31.3, angiotensin II causes the release of aldosterone, which subsequently contributes to increased blood pressure due to sodium and water retention. Mineralocorticoid receptors (MR) for aldosterone

CONNECTIONS: Treating the Diverse Patient

Reduced Efficacy of ACE Inhibitors and ARBs in Black Patients

When treating hypertension, different drugs may have different effects depending on the genetic makeup of the patient. It has been noted that ACE inhibitors and ARBs do not have the same efficacy in Black patients as they do in white patients, although the addition of a CCB or thiazide diuretic to the ACE inhibitor or ARB treatment regimen increases the antihypertensive effects (Helmer et al., 2018). Black and Hispanic patients have also been observed to have a higher incidence of ACE inhibitor– and ARB-related angioedema than do whites (Montinaro & Cicardi, 2020).

Researchers are learning more about precision medicine based on genetic makeup and prescribing drugs based on a patient's genes. Iniesta et al. (2019) studied specific alleles associated with hypertension and differences in the frequency of those genes in Black patients in comparison to white patients. They found that the frequency of how often those genes occur, might explain the different responses. The study noted that while Black patients' response to beta blockers, ACE inhibitors, and ARBs was lower than that of white patients, the response to hydrochlorothiazide was greater in Black patients compared to white patients. Using genomics rather than an individual's self-identified race or ethnicity will likely lead to much more precise treatment of hypertension across populations and ethnicities.

are located in the distal tubule and collecting ducts of the nephron. Two drugs are available that block the MR receptors in the kidney, thus inhibiting the physiologic actions of aldosterone. Both spironolactone (Aldactone) and eplerenone (Inspra) are used to treat edema and HTN. Doses for these drugs are listed in Table 31.2.

Spironolactone is an aldosterone antagonist that has been used for its diuretic action for many decades. By binding to aldosterone receptors, spironolactone produces a mild diuresis by promoting Na^+ and Cl^- excretion. Because it has little or no effect on the excretion of potassium, spironolactone is also classified as a potassium-sparing diuretic and is featured as a prototype diuretic in Chapter 32. Because spironolactone produces only a mild diuresis, it is often combined with drugs from other diuretic classes when used for HTN. It is also useful in treating primary aldosteronism, a condition in which the body produces an overabundance of aldosterone, usually due to a tumor of the adrenal gland. Spironolactone has been shown to reduce morbidity, mortality, and dysrhythmias associated with HF. CaroSpir is an oral suspension of spironolactone approved for patients who have difficulty swallowing tablets. Aldactazide is a combination drug containing spironolactone and hydrochlorothiazide.

The primary concern with spironolactone is potassium retention, which can result in serious hyperkalemia. Some patients experience GI-related adverse effects such as nausea and vomiting and diarrhea. Because spironolactone has a chemical structure similar to that of steroid hormones, it sometimes causes endocrine adverse effects in men, such as gynecomastia and erectile dysfunction. Women may experience menstrual irregularities and breast tenderness.

Eplerenone (Inspra) is a second aldosterone receptor antagonist that has a very different chemical structure than spironolactone. It is more selective for aldosterone receptors and has a very low incidence of endocrine-related adverse effects. Like spironolactone, hyperkalemia is a potentially serious adverse effect. Headache and dizziness are common adverse effects. Eplerenone is approved to treat HTN and HF and to reduce morbidity and mortality associated with post-MI in patients with left-ventricular dysfunction. It is not considered a first-line drug for treatment of HTN. For additional information on aldosterone antagonists, see Chapter 32.

CONNECTIONS: APPPLIED CLINICAL JUDGMENT

Patients Receiving Pharmacotherapy with Angiotensin-Converting Enzyme Inhibitors and Angiotensin Receptor Blockers

Key Assessment Data

- History of current condition, baseline vital signs, physical exam findings; history of cardiovascular disease, CKD, diabetes; drug history including allergies, current prescription and over-the-counter (OTC) drugs, herbal preparations; pregnancy status.
- Ongoing assessment during drug therapy includes laboratory findings including electrolytes, especially potassium, liver, and renal function studies, and lipid profiles. Assess for location, character, and amount of edema, if present.

Desired Therapeutic Outcomes

Improvement is observed and measurable in lowered blood pressure within established limits.

Minimizing Adverse Effects

- Monitor for orthostatic hypotension. A first-dose effect may occur with a significant drop in blood pressure with the first few doses.
- Weigh daily and report weight gain over 1 kg (2 lbs) in a 24-hour period or increasing edema.
- Reduced aldosterone levels may cause hyperkalemia, especially in patients with diabetes or impaired kidney function. Continue to monitor periodic electrolyte levels, especially potassium, and hepatic and renal function laboratory values.
- ACE inhibitors increase bradykinin levels, which results in a dry cough. A change in the severity of the cough may indicate another disease process or may result in the need to consider other medications.
- Observe for angioedema, especially of the facial area.
- While uncommon, monitor for gingival hyperplasia or signs of gingivitis.

Lifespan Considerations

- Orthostatic hypotension may increase the risk of falls and injury. Be particularly cautious with older adults who are at increased risk for hypotension. Ensure patient safety.
- The older adult may be at greater risk for hyperkalemia related to renal effects of aging.
- The drug should not be taken during pregnancy, if pregnancy is suspected, or while breastfeeding.

Diversity Considerations

- The older adult and patients of African American heritage are at higher risk for the development of angioedema.

Patient and Caregiver Education

- Monitor pulse, BP, and daily weight using a diary or log and bring these to each provider visit. Promptly report any weight gain over 1 kg in a 24-hour period or increasing edema to the provider.
- Rise slowly from lying or sitting to standing, pausing between changes if dizziness occurs. Don't take the medication if dizziness continues or the BP is below 90/60 or per parameters set by the provider and contact the provider for further instruction. Taking the first dose at night may help alleviate the first-dose effect.
- Immediately seek medical attention for difficulty breathing, throat tightness, hives or rash, muscle cramps, or tremors. Promptly report any angioedema around the facial area.

(continued)

CONNECTIONS: APPLIED CLINICAL JUDGMENT *(continued)*

Patients Receiving Pharmacotherapy with Angiotensin-Converting Enzyme Inhibitors and Angiotensin Receptor Blockers

- A dry cough may occur and may persist if ACE inhibitors are taken. Use nonmedicinal measures to treat (e.g., OTC cough lozenges, hard candy, or increased fluid intake). If the cough persists, consult with the healthcare provider about the use of antihistamines. Promptly report any change in the severity or frequency of a cough. Any cough accompanied by shortness of breath, fever, or chest pain should be reported immediately because it may indicate more severe pathologic conditions.
- Be aware of the signs of hyperkalemia (nausea, irregular heartbeat, profound fatigue or muscle weakness, and slow or faint pulse) and immediately report them to the healthcare provider.
- Avoid salt substitutes containing potassium chloride, consuming snacks advertised as "electrolyte-fortified," specialized sports drinks that contain high levels of potassium, or excessive intake of foods high in potassium different from the normal diet.
- Carry a wallet identification card or wear medical identification jewelry indicating ACE inhibitor or ARB therapy.

Prescribing Considerations

- When prescribing to patients who are on diuretics, start with a lower dose.
- Consider using a lower dose in geriatric patients.
- Consider every 12-hour dosing in patients who experience diminished blood pressure response toward the end of a 24-hour dosing interval.
- Use caution when prescribing ACE inhibitors or ARBS to women of childbearing potential due to possible fetal harm.

Understanding Chapter 31

Key Concepts Summary

31.1 The formation of angiotensin II requires two enzymatic steps.

31.2 Renin secretion is controlled by the juxtaglomerular cells of the kidney and the sympathetic nervous system.

31.3 Angiotensin-converting enzyme is responsible for the formation of angiotensin II.

31.4 Angiotensin II has multiple effects on the cardiovascular system that raise blood pressure and affect cardiac function.

31.5 The renin-angiotensin-aldosterone pathway offers multiple points for drug intervention.

31.6 ACE inhibitors are key drugs in the pharmacotherapy of hypertension and heart failure.

31.7 Angiotensin II receptor blockers act by inhibiting the AT_1 receptor and are used for hypertension and heart failure.

31.8 Aldosterone antagonists block the biological effects of aldosterone in the renal tubule.

CASE STUDY: Making the Patient Connection

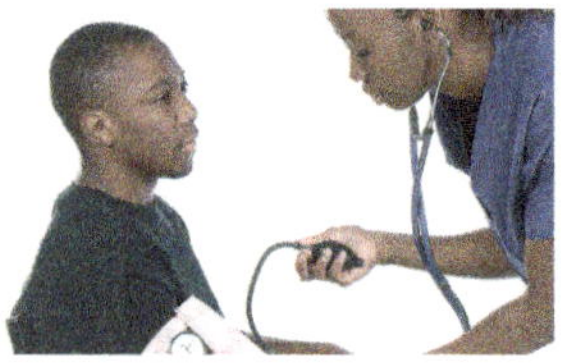

Remember the patient "Carlos Avaya" at the beginning of the chapter? Now read the remainder of the case study. Based on the information presented within this chapter, respond to the critical thinking questions that follow.

Carlos Avaya is a 26-year-old single man who was diagnosed with primary HTN 4 months ago. Carlos has been taking losartan (Cozaar) 50 mg daily PO and has been faithful in taking the medication as prescribed. When Carlos was told that his blood pressure was still elevated during this clinic visit, he was obviously distressed and concerned.

The healthcare team begins to investigate external factors that may be causing his blood pressure to remain elevated. Carlos has never smoked or used alcohol. He does not like to exercise but participates in a weekly game of soccer at the nearby community center. He denies being overly stressed with work or home life. Furthermore, he claims that he rarely salts his food.

The nurse asks Carlos to describe a typical day. During the description the nurse notices a concerning pattern.

Because Carlos lives alone, he frequently cooks for himself. He admits that he enjoys salty foods such as pretzels and popcorn. He denies having consumed either prior to the visit to the clinic. However, to Carlos, cooking a meal involves preparing canned processed foods and frozen dinners. He never reads food labels. Without recording a complete dietary history, the nurse is able to determine that Carlos's intake of sodium-rich foods is quite extensive.

Critical Thinking Questions

1. How does losartan (Cozaar) work to reduce blood pressure?
2. Considering the adverse effects of losartan (Cozaar), when would you instruct Carlos to notify the prescriber?
3. In addition to teaching Carlos about losartan (Cozaar), what additional health teaching should he receive?

Additional Case Study

Ella Daniels, a middle-aged accountant for a computer firm, takes spironolactone (Aldactone) for HTN. As the nurse responsible for providing health information, you plan to talk about what to expect when taking this drug.

1. How does the mechanism of action of spironolactone differ from that of lisinopril (Prinivil, Zestril)?
2. What are the main precautions specific to spironolactone that should be included in the teaching plan?

Chapter Review

1. The community health nurse teaches a patient at home. Lisinopril (Prinivil) has been prescribed for the patient. Which statement, if made by the patient, indicates that further teaching is necessary?

1. "I should notify my healthcare provider of symptoms of hypotension such as dizziness or fainting."
2. "I should avoid the use of salt substitutes containing potassium."
3. "If a dose is missed, I will take it as soon as possible but not too close to the next dose."
4. "Too much calcium in my diet will elevate my blood pressure."

2. The patient states, "I always keep my lisinopril on my kitchen windowsill. It helps me to remember to take it." The nurse's response would be based on which pharmacologic concept about heat and moisture?

1. They cause the medicine to break down.
2. They enhance the strength of the drug.
3. They crystallize the medication.
4. They convert the medicine to toxic metabolites.

3. A patient is hospitalized for uncontrolled HTN and is receiving enalapril (Vasotec). The nurse should notify the healthcare provider if the patient exhibits:

1. Dry mucous membranes.
2. A decline in systolic blood pressure.
3. Nonproductive cough.
4. A reduction of diastolic blood pressure.

4. The nurse is caring for a patient with chronic HTN. The patient is receiving losartan (Cozaar) daily. Which patient manifestations would the nurse conclude is an adverse effect of this medication?

1. Irritability and tremors
2. Headache and dizziness
3. Sleepiness and slurred speech
4. Pruritus and rash

5. Irbesartan (Avapro) is prescribed for each of the following patients. A nurse should question the order for a patient who has:

1. Severe dehydration from diuretic therapy.
2. Long-term diabetes mellitus.
3. A systolic blood pressure of 162.
4. A 5-year history of heart failure.

6. The nurse determines that the patient does not understand an important principle in self-administration of benazepril (Lotensin) when the patient makes which statement?

1. "I will learn to monitor my own blood pressure and write down all my daily measurements."
2. "While taking this medication, I should avoid over-the-counter medications for colds, sinus, or appetite control."
3. "This drug will not impair thinking and reaction time. I don't need to wait to start driving my car."
4. "Drinking alcohol while on this medication can lower my blood pressure and lead to dizziness and faintness."

See Appendix A for answers to critical thinking questions, case study questions, and review questions.

References

Helmer, A., Slater, N., & Smithgall, S. (2018). A review of ACE inhibitors and ARBs in Black patients with hypertension. *Annals of Pharmacotherapy, 52,* 1143–1151. https://doi.org/10.1177/1060028018779082

Iniesta, R., Venturini, C., Faconti, L., Singh, S., Irvin, M. R., Cooper-DeHoff, R. M., et al. (2019). Gene variants at loci related to blood pressure account for variation in response to antihypertensive drugs between Black and white individuals. *Hypertension, 74,* 614–622. https://doi.org/10.1161/HYPERTENSIONAHA.118.12177

Montinaro, V., & Cicardi, M. (2020). ACE inhibitor-mediated angioedema. *International Immunopharmacology, 78,* 106081. https://doi.org/10.1016/j.intimp.2019.106081

Silverthorn, D. U. (2016). *Human physiology: An integrated approach* (7th ed.). Pearson.

Tucker, M. E. (2020a). *ESC says continue hypertension meds despite COVID-19 concerns.* Medscape. https://www.medscape.com/viewarticle/926838

Tucker, M. E. (2020b). *US cardio societies: Continue antihypertensives amid COVID-19.* Medscape. https://www.medscape.com/viewarticle/926956

Selected Bibliography

Benenson, I., Waldron, F., Bradshaw, M., & Vitale, T. (2019). Endocrine hypertension: A primer for primary care nurse practitioners. *Journal for Nurse Practitioners, 15*(10), 782–786. https://doi.org/10.1016/j.nurpra.2019.08.028

Davis, L. L. (2019). Hypertension: How low to go when treating older adults. *Journal for Nurse Practitioners, 15*(1), 1–6. https://doi.org/10.1016/j.nurpra.2018.10.010

Gorini, S., Kim, S. K., Infante, M., Mammi, C., La Vignera, S., Fabbri, A., et al. (2019). Role of aldosterone and mineralocorticoid receptor in cardiovascular aging. *Frontiers in Endocrinology, 10,* 584. https://doi.org/10.3389/fendo.2019.00584

Khashkhusha, T. R., Chan, J. S. K., & Harky, A. (2020). ACE inhibitors and COVID-19: We don't know yet. *Journal of Cardiac Surgery, 35*(6), 1172–1173. https://doi.org/10.1111/jocs.14582

Lefler, L. L., Hadley, M., Tackett, J., & Thomason, A. P. (2015). New cardiovascular guidelines: Clinical practice evidence for the nurse practitioner. *Journal of the American Association of Nurse Practitioners, 28*(5), 241–248. https://doi.org/10.1002/2327-6924.12262

Lepelley, M., Bernardeau, C., Defendi, F., Crochet, J., Mallaret, M., & Bouillet, L. (2020). Update on bradykinin-mediated angioedema in 2020. *Therapies, 75*(2), 195–205. https://doi.org/10.1016/j.therap.2020.02.011

O'Donovan, K. (2018). The role of ACE inhibitors in cardiovascular disease. *British Journal of Cardiac Nursing, 13*(12), 600–608. https://doi.org/10.12968/bjca.2018.13.12.600

Palla, M., Ando, T., Androulakis, E., Telila, T., & Briasoulis, A. (2017). Renin-angiotensin system inhibitors vs other antihypertensives in hypertensive Blacks: A meta-analysis. *Journal of Clinical Hypertension, 19,* 344–350. https://doi.org/10.1111/jch.12867

Pirahanchi, Y., & Sharma, S. (2019). *Physiology, bradykinin.* StatPearls. https://pubmed.ncbi.nlm.nih.gov/30725872/

Real, J., Cowles, E., & Wierzbicki, A. S. (2018). Chronic heart failure in adults: Summary of updated NICE guidance. *British Medical Journal, 362,* k3646. https://doi.org/10.1136/bmj.k3646

Shoulders, B., & Powell, L. (2019). Reaching for goal: Incorporating the latest hypertension guidelines into practice. *Journal for Nurse Practitioners, 15*(1), 102–109. https://doi.org/10.1016/j.nurpra.2018.09.011

Silverthorn, D. U. (2016). *Human physiology: An integrated approach* (7th ed.). Pearson.

"I feel terrible. I have no energy and I feel as weak as a kitten. Lately, I don't even feel like getting out of bed in the mornings. I try to take my medications just as I was told to do."
—*Patient "Katherine Crosland"*

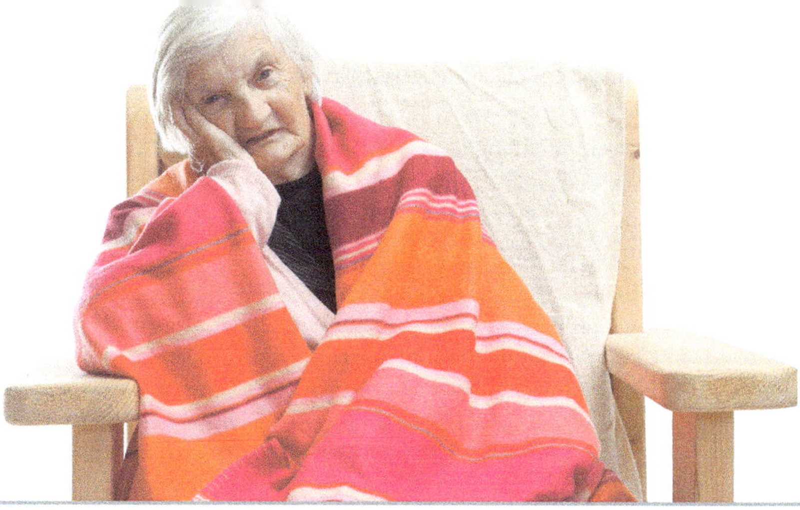

Chapter 32
Diuretic Therapy and the Pharmacotherapy of Chronic Kidney Disease

Chapter Outline

Learning Outcomes

After reading this chapter, the student should be able to:

1. Explain the role of the urinary system in maintaining fluid, electrolyte, and acid–base homeostasis.
2. Explain the physiologic processes that change the composition of filtrate as it travels through the nephrons.
3. Explain how pharmacotherapy is modified in patients with chronic kidney disease.
4. Identify indications for diuretics.
5. Compare and contrast the loop, thiazide, potassium-sparing, osmotic, and carbonic anhydrase inhibitor diuretics.
6. Describe the nurse's role in the pharmacologic management of chronic kidney disease and in diuretic therapy.
7. For each of the classes shown in the chapter outline, identify the prototype and representative drugs and explain the mechanism(s) of drug action, primary indications, contraindications, significant drug interactions, pregnancy data, and important adverse effects.
8. Apply clinical judgment to care for patients who are receiving pharmacotherapy with diuretics.

Key Terms

Definitions of the terms in bold may be found in the Glossary.

The kidneys serve an amazing role in maintaining homeostasis. By filtering a volume equivalent to the body's entire extracellular fluid every 100 minutes, the kidneys are able to make immediate adjustments to fluid volume, electrolyte composition, and acid–base balance. Failure of the kidneys to adjust to changing internal conditions of the body can result in dire consequences, and pharmacotherapy is often used to correct these imbalances. This chapter examines diuretics, drugs that increase urine output, and other medications used to treat patients with renal dysfunction.

PharmFACT

More than 23,000 kidney transplants were performed in 2019. Over 100,000 people are on the waiting list for kidney transplants (Organ Procurement and Transplantation Network, 2020).

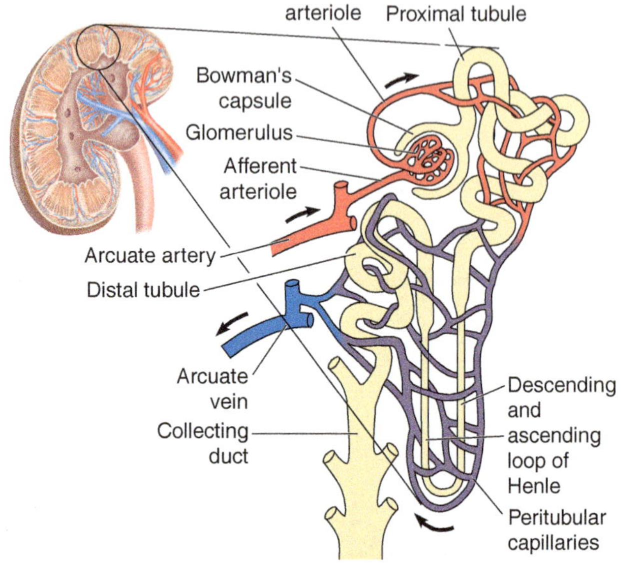

Figure 32.1 The nephron.

Review of Renal Physiology

32.1 The kidneys are major organs of excretion and body homeostasis.

When most people think of the kidneys, they think of excretion. Although this is certainly true, the kidneys have many other essential homeostatic functions. The kidneys are the primary organs for regulating fluid balance, electrolyte composition, and the pH of body fluids. They also secrete the enzyme renin, which helps to regulate blood pressure (see Chapter 31), and erythropoietin, a hormone that stimulates red blood cell production (see Chapter 39). In addition, the kidneys are responsible for the production of calcitriol, the active form of vitamin D, which helps maintain bone homeostasis (see Chapter 72). It is not surprising that our overall health is strongly dependent on the proper functioning of the kidneys.

The urinary system consists of two kidneys, two ureters, one urinary bladder, and a urethra. Blood enters the kidneys through the large renal arteries, bringing 25% of the total cardiac output to the kidneys each minute. After a series of branches, blood enters the **nephrons**, the functional units of the kidney. Each kidney contains over 1 million nephrons.

In the nephron, blood travels at high pressure through the **glomerulus**, a specialized capillary containing pores. The fluid portion of the blood is filtered through the glomerular pores and collected by the glomerular (Bowman's) capsule, the first portion of the collecting system of the nephron. Together, the glomerulus and glomerular capsule are called the renal corpuscle. During filtration, not all substances in the blood reach the glomerular capsule. Plasma proteins and the formed elements of the blood—the erythrocytes, leukocytes, and platelets—are too large to pass through the pores of the glomerulus and thus continue circulating through the bloodstream. Water and other small molecules in plasma, however, readily pass through the glomerular pores and enter the next section of the nephron.

The fluid filtered into the glomerular capsule is called **filtrate**. Essentially, the initial composition of filtrate may be thought of as plasma minus proteins. After leaving the glomerular capsule, the filtrate enters the proximal tubule, travels through the nephron loop (loop of Henle), and, subsequently, the distal tubule. The proximal and distal tubules are twisted and highly convoluted, which greatly increases the length of the nephron, allowing for enhanced processing of substances in the filtrate. The filtrate eventually reaches common collecting ducts, which empty into increasingly larger collecting structures inside the kidney. Fluid leaving the collecting ducts and entering subsequent portions of the kidney is called urine. Approximately 1 mL of urine is produced each minute. Parts of the nephron and their functions are illustrated in Figure 32.1.

Many drugs are small enough to pass through the glomerulus and enter the filtrate. If the drug is bound to a plasma protein, however, the drug–protein complex will be too large to be filtered and will continue circulating in the blood. Plasma proteins such as albumin are also too large to pass through the filter and will not be present in the filtrate or in the urine of healthy individuals. The appearance of excess plasma proteins in urine (proteinuria or albuminuria) is a sign of kidney pathology. For example, during glomerulonephritis the glomeruli become inflamed and the size of the pores increases, allowing larger substances such as proteins to enter the filtrate.

CONNECTION Checkpoint 32.1

From what you learned in Chapter 3, explain how plasma protein binding markedly affects the excretion of a drug.

32.2 The composition of filtrate changes dramatically as a result of the processes of reabsorption and secretion.

The filtrate's composition changes as it makes its long journey through the nephron. Some substances in the filtrate cross the tubule walls to reenter the blood, a process known as tubular **reabsorption**. Water is the most important molecule reabsorbed in the tubule. For every 180 L of water entering the filtrate each day, approximately 178.5 L are reabsorbed, leaving only 1.5 L to be excreted in the urine. Over 65% of the filtered sodium is reabsorbed in the proximal tubule and 25% in the loop of Henle. Glucose, amino acids, and essential ions such as chloride, calcium, and bicarbonate are also reabsorbed.

Hormones can markedly affect the degree of reabsorption in the renal tubule. Aldosterone, for example, exerts a major effect on the tubule by stimulating sodium reabsorption in the distal portions of the nephron. Under the influence of aldosterone, potassium excretion is increased because this ion is exchanged for sodium ions, which are reabsorbed. Antidiuretic hormone also affects kidney function, increasing water reabsorption by making the collecting ducts become more permeable to water. The formation of urine is indeed a dynamic process that undergoes continuous modification as the filtrate travels down the tubule. Many drugs have the ability to either enhance or block the effects of hormones on tubular processes.

Certain ions and molecules too large to pass through the glomerular capsule may still enter the urine by crossing from the blood to the filtrate using a process known as tubular **secretion**. The tubule contains molecular pumps for organic acids and bases. Acidic drugs secreted in the proximal tubule include penicillin G, ampicillin, sulfisoxazole, nonsteroidal anti-inflammatory drugs (NSAIDs), and furosemide. Basic drugs include epinephrine, dopamine, neostigmine, and trimethoprim. Potassium, phosphate, hydrogen, and ammonium ions also enter the filtrate through active secretion. The amounts of selected substances filtered, reabsorbed, and excreted are shown in Table 32.1.

Reabsorption and secretion are critical to the pharmacokinetics of medications. Some drugs are reabsorbed, whereas others are secreted into the filtrate. For example, approximately 90% of a dose of penicillin G enters the urine through tubular secretion. When the kidney is diseased, reabsorption and secretion mechanisms are impaired and serum drug levels may be dramatically affected. Figure 32.2 illustrates the possible fates of drugs entering the glomerulus.

CONNECTION Checkpoint 32.2

From what you learned in Chapter 31, explain the relationship between angiotensin II and the release of aldosterone by the adrenal gland and its significance to pharmacology.

Table 32.1 Substances Filtered, Reabsorbed, and Excreted by the Kidneys

Substance	Filtered	Reabsorbed	Excreted
Water	180 L	178–179 L	1–2 L
Glucose	162 g	162 g	0 g
Proteins	2 g	1.9 g	0.1 g
Ions			
Sodium	579 g	575 g	4 g
Potassium	29.6 g	29.6 g	2 g
Bicarbonate	275 g	274.97 g	0.03 g
Metabolic Waste Products			
Creatine	1.6 g	0 g	1.6 g
Urea	54 g	24 g	30 g
Uric acid	8.5 g	7.7 g	0.8 g

Pharmacotherapy for Patients with Chronic Kidney Disease

32.3 Chronic kidney disease may significantly impact the success of pharmacotherapy.

Chronic kidney disease (CKD), sometimes called *renal failure*, is a condition characterized by a gradual loss of kidney function, usually over a period of months or years. The kidneys lose their ability to maintain electrolyte and fluid balance and excrete waste products. Due to its prolonged, gradual development and its nonspecific symptoms, CKD may go undetected for many years. By the time the disease is diagnosed, the loss of renal function may be irreversible. The leading causes of CKD are diabetes and uncontrolled hypertension (HTN).

Pharmacotherapy with nephrotoxic drugs can lead to either CKD or acute renal failure. It is good practice for the nurse to remember common nephrotoxic drugs, which are listed in Table 32.2, so that kidney function may be continuously monitored during therapy with these medications.

The last stage of CKD, which requires dialysis or a transplant for survival, is called *end-stage renal disease*. The primary treatment goal for a patient with CKD is to maintain blood flow through the kidneys and adequate urine output so that metabolic wastes can be removed from the body.

PharmFACT

More than 37 million Americans have CKD—about 15% of the adult population. Blacks have a three times greater risk for developing end-stage renal disease than whites (National Kidney Foundation, 2020).

The most basic diagnostic test of kidney function is a urinalysis, which examines urine for the presence of blood

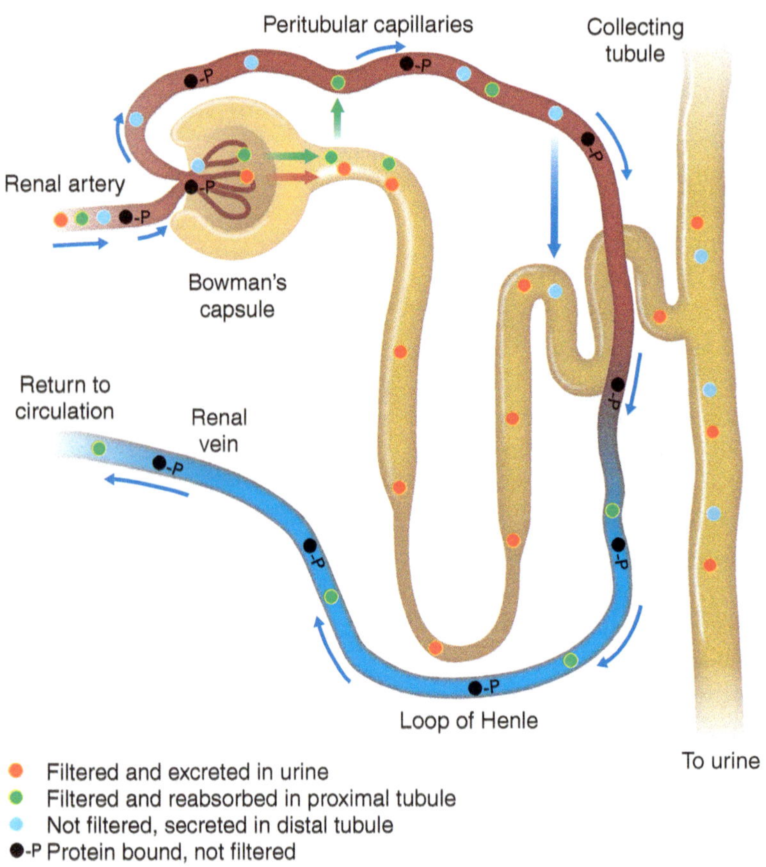

Figure 32.2 Fates of drugs entering the glomerulus: filtration, reabsorption, secretion, and excretion.

Table 32.2 Selected Nephrotoxic Drugs

Drug or Class	Indication/Classification
aminoglycosides	Antibiotics
amphotericin B	Systemic antifungal
angiotensin-converting enzyme (ACE) inhibitors and angiotensin receptor blockers (ARBs)	HTN, HF
cisplatin, carboplatin, methotrexate	Antineoplastics
cyclosporine (Neoral, Sandimmune), tacrolimus (Prograf)	Immunosuppressants
foscarnet (Foscavir)	Antiviral
nonsteroidal anti-inflammatory drugs (NSAIDs), including aspirin	Inflammation and pain
pentamidine (NebuPent, Pentam)	Anti-infective (*Pneumocystis*)
radiographic intravenous contrast agents	Diagnosis of kidney and vascular disorders

cells, proteins, pH, specific gravity, ketones, glucose, and microorganisms. The urinalysis can detect proteinuria and albuminuria, which are the primary measures of structural kidney damage. Although easy to perform, the urinalysis is nonspecific: Many diverse diseases and conditions can cause abnormal urinalysis values. Serum creatinine and blood urea nitrogen (BUN) are additional laboratory measures for detecting kidney disease. To provide a more definitive diagnosis, diagnostic imaging such as computed tomography, sonography, or magnetic resonance imaging may be necessary. Renal biopsy may be performed to obtain a more specific diagnosis.

The best marker for estimating kidney function is the **glomerular filtration rate (GFR)**, which is the volume of water filtered through the glomerular capsules per minute. The GFR can be used to predict the onset and progression of CKD and it is a measure of the kidneys' ability to excrete drugs from the body. With normal values ranging from 90 to 120 mL/min, a progressive decline in GFR indicates a reduction in the number of functioning nephrons. As nephrons "die," however, the remaining healthy ones have the ability to compensate by increasing their filtration capacity. Because of this, patients with significant kidney damage may be asymptomatic until 50% or more of the nephrons have become nonfunctional and the GFR has fallen to less than half its normal value.

Kidney disease may also be acute. *Acute kidney injury (AKI)*, also called *acute renal failure*, requires immediate treatment because retention of nitrogenous waste products in the body such as urea and creatinine can result in death if left untreated. The most common cause of AKI is renal hypoperfusion, the lack of sufficient blood flow through the kidneys, which can lead to permanent destruction of nephrons. To prevent AKI, the cause of the hypoperfusion must

Table 32.3 Pharmacologic Management of Chronic Kidney Disease

Complication	Pathogenesis	Selected Therapies
Anemia	Kidneys are unable to synthesize sufficient erythropoietin for red blood cell production.	Epoetin alfa (Epogen, Procrit)
Hyperkalemia	Kidneys are unable to adequately excrete potassium.	Dietary restriction of potassium; polystyrene sulfate (Kayexalate) with sorbitol
Hyperphosphatemia	Kidneys are unable to adequately excrete phosphate.	Dietary restriction of phosphate; phosphate binders such as calcium carbonate (Os-Cal 500, others), calcium acetate (Calphron, PhosLo), lanthanum carbonate (Fosrenol), sucroferric oxyhydroxide (Velphoro), or sevelamer (Renagel, Renvela)
Hypervolemia	Kidneys are unable to excrete sufficient sodium and water, leading to water retention.	Dietary restriction of sodium; loop diuretics in acute conditions, thiazide diuretics in mild conditions
Hypocalcemia	Hyperphosphatemia leads to loss of calcium.	Usually corrected by reversing the hyperphosphatemia, but additional calcium supplements may be necessary
Metabolic acidosis	Kidneys are unable to adequately excrete metabolic acids.	Sodium bicarbonate or sodium citrate

be quickly identified and corrected. Potential causes include heart failure (HF), dysrhythmias, hemorrhage, toxins, and dehydration.

Pharmacotherapy of CKD attempts to find and correct the cause of the dysfunction. Diuretics are given to increase urine output, and cardiovascular drugs are administered to treat underlying HTN or HF. Dietary management is often necessary to prevent worsening of CKD. Depending on the stage of the disease, dietary management may include restriction of protein and reduction of sodium, potassium, phosphorous, and magnesium intake. For patients with diabetes, management of blood glucose through intensive insulin therapy is required to reduce the risk of renal damage. See Table 32.3 for a summary of selected medications used to prevent and treat the complications of CKD.

The nurse serves a key role in assessing and providing interventions for patients with CKD. Once a diagnosis has been established, all nephrotoxic medications should be either discontinued or used with extreme caution. Because the kidneys excrete most drugs or their metabolites, many medications will require a significant dosage reduction in patients with moderate to severe renal disease. The importance of this cannot be overemphasized: Administering the "average" dose to a patient with severe kidney disease can have fatal consequences.

Diuretic Therapy

32.4 Diuretics are used to treat hypertension, heart failure, accumulation of edema fluid, and chronic kidney disease.

The primary function of a **diuretic** is to increase the formation of urine by the body. However, diuretics do more than increase urine flow; they also change the rate of excretion of specific electrolytes, most importantly sodium and potassium. The goal of most diuretic therapy is to reduce extracellular fluid volume, so that abnormal fluid retention (edema) by the body may be reversed. Excretion of excess fluid in the body is particularly important in the management of HTN, HF, CKF, hepatic failure or pulmonary edema.

The most common mechanism by which diuretics act is by blocking sodium ion (Na^+) reabsorption in the nephron, thus sending more Na^+ to the urine (**natriuresis**). The human body is particularly sensitive to sodium imbalances; dietary intake must be balanced with excretion mechanisms. For example, a 1% increase in sodium reabsorption (retention) could potentially cause a 1.8-L net gain of water each day, which is equivalent to 4 lb of body weight. On the other hand, even small decreases in sodium reabsorption can cause net losses of sodium, resulting in volume depletion and circulatory collapse. These examples illustrate the need for patients to monitor their weight daily when taking diuretics.

Natriuresis results in two other important effects. Chloride ions (Cl^-) follow sodium, potentially causing hypochloremia, a net loss of chloride from the body. In addition, because water molecules travel passively with sodium ions, blocking the reabsorption of Na^+ increases the total volume of urination, or diuresis. The amount of diuresis produced by a diuretic is directly related to the amount of sodium reabsorption that is blocked: Those that block the most sodium are the most effective at increasing urine output. Diuretics also affect the renal excretion of ions such as magnesium, potassium, phosphate, calcium, and bicarbonate. It is important to remember that imbalances may occur in virtually any electrolyte during diuretic therapy.

Diuretics are classified into five major groups, based on differences in their chemical nature and mechanism of action. The sites in the nephron at which the various diuretics act are shown in Pharmacotherapy Illustrated 32.1.

- **Loop or high-ceiling.** These drugs prevent the reabsorption of Na^+ in the loop of Henle; thus, they are

Pharmacotherapy Illustrated 32.1

Sites of Action of the Diuretics

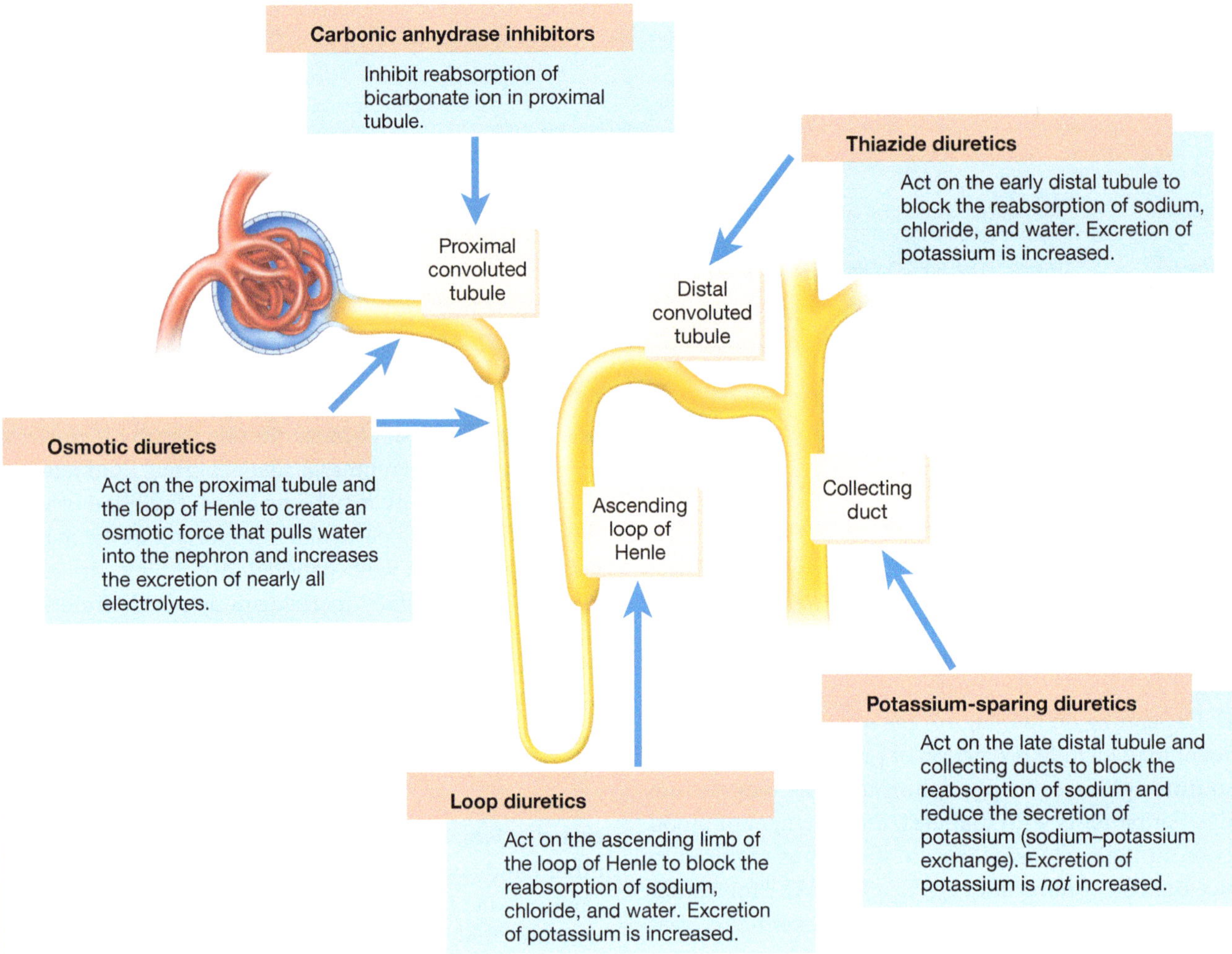

called loop diuretics. Because there is an abundance of Na^+ in the filtrate within the nephron loop, drugs in this class are capable of producing large increases in urine output.

- **Thiazides.** The largest diuretic class, the thiazides act by blocking Na^+ in the distal tubule. Because most Na^+ has already been reabsorbed from the filtrate by the time it reaches this part of the nephron, the thiazides produce a less intense diuresis than loop diuretics.
- **Potassium-sparing.** The third major class is named potassium-sparing diuretics because they have minimal effect on potassium ion (K^+) excretion. These drugs produce a mild diuresis.
- **Osmotic.** These drugs are relatively inert drugs that change the osmolality of filtrate, causing water to remain in the nephron for excretion. These drugs are very effective but are rarely prescribed because they can produce potentially serious adverse effects.
- **Carbonic anhydrase inhibitors.** These drugs block the enzyme in the nephron responsible for bicarbonate reabsorption. They produce a weak diuresis and are rarely used.

It is common practice to combine two or more drugs in the pharmacotherapy of HTN and fluid retention disorders. Diuretics are often a component of fixed-dose combinations with drugs from other classes. The primary rationales for combination therapy are that the incidence of adverse effects is decreased and the pharmacologic effects (such as diuresis or blood pressure reduction) may be enhanced. For patient convenience, some of these drugs are available in single-tablet formulations. Examples of single-tablet diuretic combinations include the following:

- **Aldactazide.** Hydrochlorothiazide and spironolactone
- **Apresazide.** Hydrochlorothiazide and hydralazine
- **Dyazide.** Hydrochlorothiazide and triamterene

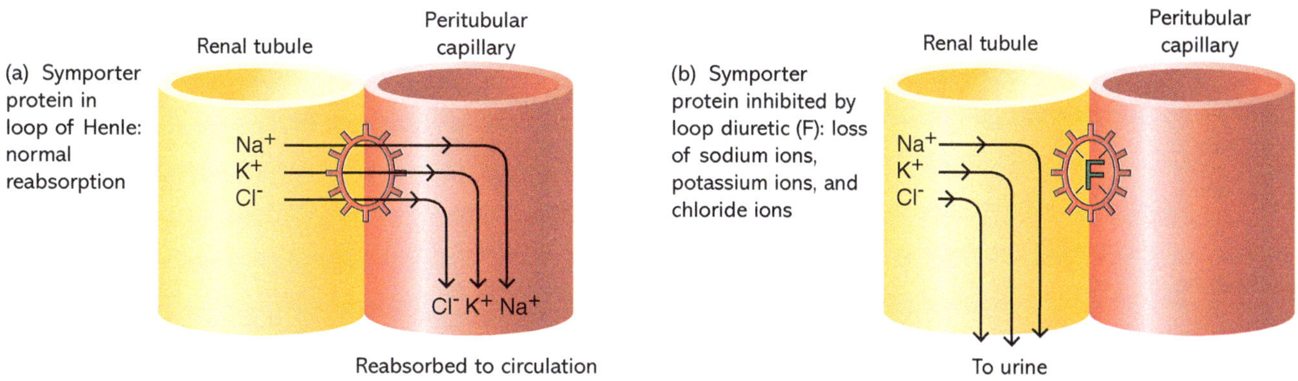

Figure 32.3 Symporter protein in the loop of Henle: (a) normal reabsorption of the Na^+, K^+, and Cl^- ions; (b) inhibition of symporter by furosemide causes excretion of Na^+, K^+, and Cl^- ions.

- Hydrochlorothiazide and amiloride
- Tekturna HCT: Hydrochlorothiazide and aliskiren
- Tribenzor: Hydrochlorothiazide, amlodipine, and Olmesartan
- Exforge HCT: Hydrochlorothiazide, amlodipine, and Valsartan
- Lotensin HCT: Hydrochlorothiazide and benazepril

Loop (High-Ceiling) Diuretics

32.5 The most effective diuretics are the loop diuretics that block sodium reabsorption in the loop of Henle.

The most effective diuretics, the loop or high-ceiling diuretics, act by blocking the reabsorption of sodium and chloride in the nephron loop. This occurs when the drug inhibits the molecule responsible for transporting sodium and chloride from the filtrate to the blood, known as the $Na^+–K^+–2Cl^-$ symporter. A **symporter** is a membrane protein that transports two molecules at the same time. When the loop diuretics block this symporter, sodium and chloride are prevented from being reabsorbed, and diuresis is increased. All loop diuretics have an additional action that is responsible for a major adverse effect of drugs in this class: increasing potassium excretion. An illustration showing the effects caused when this symporter is inhibited is shown in Figure 32.3.

Loop diuretics are available for either oral (PO) or parenteral administration and are extensively bound to plasma proteins. They have relatively short half-lives and extended-release preparations are not available. When given intravenously (IV), loop diuretics have the ability to cause large amounts of fluid to be excreted by the kidney in a very short time. Loop diuretics are used to reduce the edema associated with HF, hepatic cirrhosis, or CKD. Furosemide and torsemide are also approved for HTN, although their short half-lives make them less suitable for this indication than thiazide diuretics. Occasionally, loop diuretics are given to speed the renal excretion of a drug that has been overdosed or a toxin that has been unintentionally ingested. Doses of the loop diuretics are listed in Table 32.4.

The rapid excretion of large amounts of fluid has the potential to produce serious adverse effects, including dehydration and electrolyte imbalances. Signs of dehydration include thirst, dry mouth, weight loss, and headache. Dizziness and fainting can result from the fall in blood pressure caused by the rapid fluid loss. Potassium depletion can be serious and result in dysrhythmias. Potassium supplements are often prescribed concurrently with these diuretics to prevent hypokalemia. Potassium loss is of particular concern to those concurrently taking digoxin (Lanoxin) because hypokalemia predisposes these patients to dysrhythmias. With large doses, significant loss of sodium, magnesium, and calcium is possible. Continuous use of loop diuretics in

Table 32.4 Loop Diuretics

Drug	Route and Adult Dose (Maximum Dose Where Indicated)	Adverse Effects
bumetanide (Bumex)	PO: 0.5–2 mg/day (max: 10 mg/day) IV/IM: 0.5–1 mg over 1–2 min, repeated q2–3h prn (max: 10 mg/day)	*Minor hypokalemia, orthostatic hypotension, tinnitus, nausea, diarrhea, dizziness, fatigue* <u>Serious hypokalemia, blood dyscrasias, dehydration, ototoxicity, electrolyte imbalances, circulatory collapse</u>
ethacrynic acid (Edecrin)	PO: 50–100 mg/day (max: 400 mg/day) IV: 0.5–1 mg/kg or 50 mg (max: 100 mg/dose)	
furosemide (Lasix)	PO: 20–80 mg in one or more divided doses (max: 600 mg/day) IV/IM: 20–40 mg in one or more divided doses (max: 600 mg/day)	
torsemide (Demadex)	PO: 5–20 mg/day (max: 200 mg/day)	

Note: *Italics* indicate common adverse effects. <u>Underline</u> indicates serious adverse effects.

CONNECTIONS: Advanced Practice Application

Chronic Kidney Disease and Prescribing Considerations

Case

Nolan is a 71-year-old man who was admitted to the hospital for altered mental status. His daughter Renee reported that her father had become progressively confused and had been having visual and auditory hallucinations. In the past 24 hours, Nolan's symptoms had become more persistent and she became more concerned. Nolan has a 9-year history of heart failure and type 2 diabetes and was diagnosed 10 months ago with stage V CKD.

On admission, the nurse practitioner hospitalist, his bedside nurse, and the unit's pharmacist. reviewed his medications with Renee. Nolan was taking aspirin, atenolol, metformin, atorvastatin, and gabapentin for the diabetes neuropathy. On physical examination, he was sleepy but arousable. His blood pressure was 136/86 mmHg; pulse was 72 beats/min (regular); respiratory rate was 14 breaths/min; and oxygen saturation 96%. What pharmacologic factors should the team be considering for Nolan?

Discussion

Kidney disease, both AKI and CKD, affects every organ system in the body. The number of patients with AKI and CKD has increased due to the aging population and medical advancements. With the significant increase in polypharmacy over the last decade, it is increasingly important to understand potentially inappropriate medication use by patients with CKD. For prescribing purposes, CKD is divided into three grades:

- Mild: GFR 20–50 mL/min; serum creatinine 150–300 µmol/L
- Moderate: GFR 10–20 mL/min; serum creatinine 300–700 µmol/L
- Severe: GFR less than 10 mL/min; serum creatinine more than 700 µmol/L (GFR above 50 mL/min does not usually require any dosage adjustment.)

Drugs to which particular attention should be given include histamine H_2-receptor antagonists, specific antibiotics, anticonvulsants, digoxin, and NSAIDs. Prescribing any medication that increases potassium levels, such as potassium supplements and potassium-sparing diuretics, is potentially very dangerous. Additionally, methotrexate, enoxaparin, and metformin should no longer be prescribed even with a mild grade of CKD. With cardiovascular (e.g., atenolol) antidiabetic (e.g., metformin) or anticonvulsive (e.g., gabapentin) drugs, the recommendation is to use alternative medications, such as lisinopril, glyburide, or carbamazepine. Drug dose adjustments should be considered with antimicrobial (e.g., ampicillin), antiviral (e.g., acyclovir), and some chemotherapeutic and cytotoxic drugs (e.g., cisplatin). Products with a high sodium content (e.g., antacids) should be avoided because they may cause sodium and water retention in patients with CKD (Kurani et al., 2019).

postmenopausal women may affect bone metabolism due to excessive calcium loss. Loop diuretics can cause gout in some patients due to hyperuricemia, the accumulation of uric acid in the blood.

Although rare, loop diuretics may cause ototoxicity, which may manifest as tinnitus, vertigo, or deafness. Use of other ototoxic drugs such as the aminoglycoside antibiotics should be avoided during loop diuretic therapy due to the potential for additive hearing impairment. Because of the risk for serious adverse effects, loop diuretics are normally prescribed for patients with moderate to severe fluid retention, such as acute pulmonary edema, or when thiazide diuretics have failed to achieve therapeutic goals.

PROTOTYPE DRUG | **Furosemide (Lasix)**

Classification **Therapeutic:** Antihypertensive drug for heart failure and edema
Pharmacologic: Loop- or high-ceiling-type diuretic

Therapeutic Effects and Uses: An established diuretic since it was approved in 1966, furosemide is frequently used in the treatment of acute edema associated with liver cirrhosis, CKD, or HF because it has the ability to remove large amounts of edema fluid from the patient in a short time. When given IV, diuresis begins within 5 minutes, providing rapid relief from distressing symptoms such as dyspnea. Unlike the thiazide diuretics, furosemide is able to increase urine output even when blood flow to the kidneys is diminished, which makes it of particular value in patients with low cardiac output or CKD. It is also approved for HTN, although it is not a first-line drug for long-term use because of its short half-life and potential for serious adverse effects.

Mechanism of Action: Furosemide prevents the reabsorption of sodium and chloride by blocking the Na^-–K^-–$2Cl^-$ symporter in the nephron loop. Because this is the region of the nephron that normally filters the bulk of sodium, furosemide can cause a profound diuresis. The extensive diuresis results in the increased urinary excretion of sodium, chloride, potassium, and hydrogen ions.

Pharmacokinetics:

Route(s)	PO, IV, intramuscular (IM)
Absorption	60% absorbed PO

Distribution	Distributed to most tissues; crosses the placenta; secreted in breast milk; 95% bound to plasma protein
Primary metabolism	Hepatic (small amounts)
Primary excretion	Renal
Onset of action	PO: 30–60 min; IV: 5 min; IM: 10–30 min
Duration of action	PO: 6–8 h; IV: 2 h; IM: 4–8 h

Adverse Effects: The greatest concerns during furosemide therapy are excessive fluid loss and electrolyte imbalances. Hypovolemia may cause orthostatic hypotension and syncope. Imbalances may occur in any or all electrolytes, causing symptoms such as tachycardia, dysrhythmias, and nausea and vomiting. Ototoxicity is rare but may result in permanent hearing deficit. Hyperuricemia caused by the drug may cause exacerbations of gout. In patients with hypokalemia and hypochloremia, furosemide may induce metabolic alkalosis. **Black Box Warning:** Furosemide is a potent diuretic that, if given in excessive amounts, may lead to profound diuresis with water and electrolyte depletion. Careful medical supervision is required.

Contraindications/Precautions: Contraindications include hypersensitivity to furosemide or sulfonamide antibiotics, anuria, hepatic coma, or severe fluid or electrolyte depletion. Due to its high potency, fluid loss must be carefully monitored to avoid possible dehydration and hypotension. Any preexisting hypovolemia or hypotension should be corrected before furosemide therapy is initiated. Because loop diuretics can increase blood glucose, serum glucose levels should be assessed in patients with diabetes mellitus.

Drug Interactions: Hypokalemia from the use of furosemide may cause dysrhythmias in patients taking digoxin; therefore, combination therapy with furosemide and digoxin should be avoided or carefully monitored. Concurrent use with corticosteroids, amphotericin B, or other potassium-depleting drugs can result in hypokalemia. When given with lithium, elimination of lithium is decreased, causing a higher risk of toxicity. Furosemide may diminish the hypoglycemic effects of sulfonylureas and insulin. Concurrent use with NSAIDs can result in a diminished diuretic effect. Additive hypotension will occur if furosemide is given concurrently with antihypertensives, including other diuretics. Use of ethanol should be restricted because it may add to the hypotensive and diuretic actions of furosemide. Furosemide should not be used concurrently with aminoglycoside antibiotics due to the possibility of additive nephrotoxicity and ototoxicity. **Herbal/Food:** Oral aloe can decrease the levels of potassium and should not be used concurrently with loop diuretics. Use with hawthorn could result in additive hypotensive effects. Ginseng may decrease the effectiveness of loop diuretics. High sodium intake can reduce the effectiveness of diuretics; patients should be placed on a sodium-restricted intake of 1500 to 2300 mg/day.

Treatment of Overdose: Overdose with furosemide can result in serious hypotension, fluid loss, and electrolyte imbalances. Treatment is supportive with replacement of fluids and electrolytes and the possible administration of a vasopressor.

Pregnancy: Furosemide may cause higher birth weights and has been shown to increase mortality in laboratory animals. This drug enters human milk and may suppress lactation.

Clinician Responsibilities: Key clinical implications for patients receiving furosemide are included in Applied Clinical Judgment: Patients Receiving Pharmacotherapy with Diuretics.

Drugs Similar to Furosemide (Lasix)

Furosemide is the most commonly prescribed drug in this class. Other loop diuretics include bumetanide, ethacrynic acid, and torsemide.

Bumetanide (Bumex): Approved in 1983, bumetanide is indicated for edema usually associated with HF or CKD. This drug is available by the PO, IV, and IM routes and is 40 times more potent than furosemide but has a shorter duration of action. It may be used in acute clinical situations when furosemide has proved ineffective in patients with severe CKD. Like furosemide, bumetanide can cause electrolyte imbalances (especially hypokalemia), hypotension, and dehydration. Unlike furosemide and torsemide, bumetanide is not approved for HTN, although it may be used off-label for that indication. Bumetanide carries a black box warning that, if given in excessive amounts, may lead to profound diuresis with water and electrolyte depletion. Animal studies showed no teratogenicity, but the drug does enter human milk and may suppress lactation.

Ethacrynic acid (Edecrin): Approved in 1967, ethacrynic acid is indicated for the treatment of severe edema, usually associated with HF, hepatic cirrhosis, or CKD. Given by either the oral or IV route, ethacrynic acid is the only loop diuretic that does not contain a sulfur group in its structure; thus, it can safely be used in patients allergic to sulfonamides. Of the loop diuretics, ethacrynic acid has the highest risk for severe hearing loss, which may be irreversible. The patient must be carefully monitored to prevent excessive electrolyte and fluid losses. Although ethacrynic acid is not approved for HTN, it may be prescribed off-label for this indication. Animal studies showed reduced fetal birth weights. It is not known if the drug is excreted in human milk.

CONNECTIONS: Community-Oriented Practice

Diuretics: A Banned Substance?

Diuretics are included in the banned substance list by the International Olympic Committee and the World Anti-Doping Agency (2020), except under highly regulated use for clinical conditions. Elite athletes seeking a competitive edge may use diuretics to achieve rapid weight loss to meet specific weight categories in some sports. Diuretics have also been used illicitly to mask the presence of other banned substances by reducing their concentration in urine (by increasing urine volume) or increasing their excretion (by altering urine pH). Hydrochlorothiazide and furosemide are the most commonly detected diuretics, although all classifications have been detected. Not all drugs are able to be detected, however, and until better drug detection techniques are developed, drug use in athletics for competitive advantage, including the use of diuretics, will continue.

Torsemide (Demadex): Approved in 1993, torsemide is indicated for the treatment of HTN and edema that is associated with HF, hepatic cirrhosis, or CKD. Given orally, torsemide is twice as potent as furosemide and has a longer half-life, which offers the advantage of once-a-day dosing. The incidence of ototoxicity with torsemide is low, and the risk of hypokalemia is less than that of other drugs in this class. At higher doses, however, torsemide carries the same potential risks as furosemide and other loop diuretics, including electrolyte imbalances and hypovolemia. Torsemide is contraindicated in patients with sensitivity to sulfonylureas. Animal studies showed decreased body weight, fetal resorption, and delayed fetal ossification at high doses. No data are available regarding safety during lactation.

Thiazide and Thiazide-Like Diuretics

32.6 The thiazides are the most commonly prescribed class of diuretics.

The thiazides comprise the largest and most commonly prescribed class of diuretics. Like the loop diuretics, the thiazides block a symport protein in the renal tubule wall that is responsible for reabsorbing sodium and chloride ions from the filtrate. However, the thiazides block a different symport protein and in a different location than the loop diuretics. The thiazides act on the Na^+Cl^- symporter in the distal tubule to block Na^+ reabsorption and increase K^+ and water excretion. The thiazides are less effective than the loop diuretics because over 90% of the Na^+ has already been reabsorbed by the time the filtrate reaches the distal tubule. There are simply fewer Na^+ to block; thus, the maximum diuresis produced by thiazides is less than the loop diuretics.

The primary indication for thiazide diuretics is mild to moderate HTN. Mild HTN can often be managed with only a thiazide diuretic, whereas moderate to severe HTN often requires two or more antihypertensive drugs. Thiazides are also indicated for mild to moderate edema due to HF, hepatic cirrhosis, or CKD. They are not effective in patients with severe organ impairment because their ability to produce a diuresis diminishes as blood flow through the kidneys is reduced. Doses of the thiazide diuretics are listed in Table 32.5.

Table 32.5 Thiazide and Thiazide-Like Diuretics

Drug	Route and Adult Dose (Maximum Dose Where Indicated)	Adverse Effects
Short Acting		
chlorothiazide (Diuril)	PO: 250 mg–1 g/day in 1–2 divided doses IV: 250 mg–1 g/day in 1–2 divided doses (max: 2 g/day)	*Minor hypokalemia, fatigue* <u>Serious hypokalemia, electrolyte depletion, dehydration, hypotension, hyponatremia, hyperglycemia, coma, blood dyscrasias</u>
hydrochlorothiazide (Microzide)	PO: 25–100 mg/day as a single or divided dose (max: 200 mg/day)	
Intermediate Acting		
bendroflumethiazide and nadolol (Corzide)	PO: 1 tablet/day (40–80 mg nadolol and 5 mg bendroflumethiazide)	
metolazone (Zaroxolyn)	PO: 2.5–10 mg once daily (max: 20 mg/day)	
Long Acting		
chlorthalidone	PO: 50–100 mg/day (max: 50 mg/day for HTN; 200 mg/day for edema)	
indapamide	PO: 1.25–2.5 mg once daily (max: 5 mg/day)	
methyclothiazide (Enduron)	PO: 2.5–5 mg once daily (max: 5 mg/day for HTN; 10 mg/day for edema)	

Note: *Italics* indicate common adverse effects. <u>Underline</u> indicates serious adverse effects.

Thiazides are available only by the PO route with the exception of chlorothiazide (Diuril), which may be administered PO or parenterally. All the thiazide diuretics have equivalent effectiveness and safety profiles. They differ, however, in their potency and duration of action. For example, metolazone (Zaroxolyn) is 10 times more potent than hydrochlorothiazide (Microzide). At therapeutic doses all thiazides produce the same level of diuresis.

Three drugs in Table 32.5—chlorthalidone, indapamide, and metolazone—are not true thiazides because they do not contain the two-ring structure that chemically defines a thiazide. However, these drugs block the same symport protein and have the same pharmacologic effects as thiazides. They are sometimes called "thiazide-like" and are always considered along with the true thiazides because of their similar mechanism of action, indications, and adverse effects.

The adverse effects of thiazides are similar to those of the loop diuretics, though their frequency is less and they do not cause ototoxicity. Dehydration and excessive loss of sodium, potassium, or chloride ions may occur with overtreatment: Hypokalemia and hypochloremia can cause metabolic alkalosis. Concurrent therapy with digoxin requires careful monitoring to avoid dysrhythmias caused by excessive potassium loss. Potassium supplements are sometimes prescribed during thiazide therapy to prevent hypokalemia. Patients with diabetes should be aware that thiazide diuretics sometimes increase blood glucose levels. Like the loop diuretics, thiazides can increase serum levels of uric acid, although this is only clinically significant in patients with a history of gout.

PROTOTYPE DRUG Hydrochlorothiazide (Microzide)

Classification **Therapeutic:** Antihypertensive
Pharmacologic: Thiazide diuretic

Therapeutic Effects and Uses: Approved in 1959, hydrochlorothiazide (often abbreviated HCTZ) is the most widely prescribed diuretic for HTN. Like many diuretics, it produces few adverse effects and is effective at producing a 10- to 20-mmHg reduction in blood pressure. Patients with severe HTN or a compelling condition such as HF, post–myocardial infarction (post-MI), high risk for coronary artery disease, diabetes, CKD, or recurrent stroke prevention may require the addition of a second drug from a different class to control the disease.

Hydrochlorothiazide is approved to treat ascites, edema, HF, HTN, and nephrotic syndrome. Off-label indications include premenstrual syndrome (PMS), diabetes insipidus, hypercalciuria, and nephrolithiasis. Hydrochlorothiazide is the most common medication found in fixed-dose combination drugs for HTN.

Mechanism of Action: Hydrochlorothiazide acts on the distal tubule to decrease the reabsorption of Na^+. This results in less water reabsorption, increased diuresis, and removal of edema fluid. Blood volume decreases and blood pressure falls. Increasing the amount of sodium in the distal tubule also increases potassium excretion via a sodium–potassium exchange mechanism.

Pharmacokinetics:

Route(s)	PO
Absorption	Variable; incompletely absorbed
Distribution	Distributed to most tissues; crosses the placenta and is secreted in breast milk
Primary metabolism	Not metabolized
Primary excretion	Renal
Onset of action	2 h; peak effect: 4 h
Duration of action	6–12 h; half-life: 45–120 min

Adverse Effects: Hydrochlorothiazide is generally well tolerated and exhibits few serious adverse effects. Hypotension may cause dizziness or headache. Electrolyte imbalances such as hypochloremia, hypomagnesemia, hypokalemia, and hyponatremia may occur. Dysrhythmias due to hypokalemia may be serious if not prevented by maintaining normal serum potassium levels, usually by the administration of potassium supplements during therapy. Hydrochlorothiazide may precipitate gout attacks due to its tendency to cause hyperuricemia. Blood dyscrasias such as leukopenia, agranulocytosis, and aplastic anemia are rare, though serious, adverse effects.

Contraindications/Precautions: Contraindications include anuria and prior hypersensitivity to thiazide diuretics or sulfonamide antibiotics. Because hydrochlorothiazide can cause glycosuria and hyperglycemia, serum glucose levels must be carefully monitored in patients with diabetes. Preexisting hypovolemia or hypotension should be corrected before thiazide therapy is initiated because diuretics can worsen these conditions. Hydrochlorothiazide should not be used in neonates with jaundice because it can cause hyperbilirubinemia.

Drug Interactions: When given concurrently with other antihypertensives, an additive reduction in blood pressure will occur. Thiazides may reduce the effectiveness of anticoagulants, sulfonylureas, and antidiabetic drugs, including insulin. Cholestyramine and colestipol bind to and decrease the absorption of HCTZ, thus reducing its effectiveness. Hydrochlorothiazide increases the risk of renal toxicity from NSAIDs. Corticosteroids and amphotericin B increase potassium loss when given with HCTZ. Hypokalemia caused by HCTZ may increase digoxin toxicity and the possibility of dysrhythmias. Hydrochlorothiazide decreases the excretion of lithium and can lead to lithium toxicity. Because thiazides decrease the renal excretion of calcium, concurrent administration with calcium supplements may lead to hypercalcemia. **Herbal/Food:** Ginkgo biloba may produce a paradoxical increase in blood pressure. Use with hawthorn could result in additive hypotensive effects. High sodium intake can reduce the effectiveness of diuretics; patients should be placed on a sodium-restricted diet of 1500 to 2300 mg/day.

Treatment of Overdose: Overdose is manifested as electrolyte depletion, which is treated with infusions of fluids containing electrolytes. Infusion of fluids also prevents dehydration and hypotension.

Pregnancy: Animal studies showed no evidence of fetal harm. Small amounts of this drug are secreted in milk, although it is usually considered compatible with breastfeeding.

Clinician Responsibilities: Key clinical implications for patients receiving hydrochlorothiazide are included in Applied Clinical Judgment: Patients Receiving Pharmacotherapy with Diuretics.

Drugs Similar to Hydrochlorothiazide (Microzide)

Many thiazide and thiazide-like diuretics are available. All are used to treat HTN and edema. All have the same general actions and adverse effect profile as HCTZ. They may be grouped into subclasses based on their relative duration of action.

Short-Acting Thiazides: This group includes chlorothiazide (Diuril) and hydrochlorothiazide (Microzide). These drugs have a rapid onset of 1 to 2 hours with a duration of action of 6 to 12 hours. Chlorothiazide is available by the IV route for patients who are unable to take PO thiazides.

Intermediate-Acting Thiazides: This group includes metolazone (Zaroxolyn) and Corzide, a fixed-dose combination of bendroflumethiazide (a thiazide) with nadolol (a beta-adrenergic blocker). These drugs have an onset time of about 2 hours with a duration of action of 12 to 24 hours.

Long-Acting Thiazides: This group includes chlorthalidone, indapamide, and methyclothiazide (Enduron). These drugs have a 2-hour onset with a duration of action ranging from 24 to 72 hours.

CONNECTION Checkpoint 32.3

The use of lithium is often contraindicated when a patient is taking diuretics. From what you learned in Chapter 19, identify the indications for lithium and explain how the use of a diuretic can lead to lithium toxicity.

Potassium-Sparing Diuretics

32.7 Potassium-sparing diuretics have low effectiveness but can help prevent hypokalemia.

As discussed in Sections 32.5 and 32.6, hypokalemia is a potentially serious adverse effect of the loop and thiazide diuretics. The therapeutic advantage of the potassium-sparing diuretics is that increased diuresis can be obtained without lowering blood potassium levels. The potassium-sparing diuretics are listed in Table 32.6. There are two subclasses of potassium-sparing diuretics: sodium ion channel inhibitors and aldosterone antagonists.

Sodium Ion Channel Inhibitors: In the distal tubule, Na^+ is reabsorbed from the filtrate through sodium ion channels. As the sodium ion in the filtrate travels across the renal tubule cell and returns to the bloodstream, potassium ion moves in the opposite direction. In other words, as sodium ion is reabsorbed, potassium ion is secreted.

Triamterene (Dyrenium) and amiloride (Midamor) block the Na^+ channel, causing sodium to stay in the filtrate. Because water always follows sodium ions, additional water is retained in the filtrate and ultimately leaves in the urine. When the sodium ion channel is blocked, another important action occurs: The potassium ion is no longer secreted to the filtrate. The body, therefore, does not lose potassium, as is the case with the thiazide and loop diuretics. Because most of the sodium ion has already been removed before the filtrate reaches the distal tubule, these potassium-sparing diuretics produce only a mild diuresis.

Table 32.6 Potassium-Sparing Diuretics

<table>
<tr><th>Drug</th><th>Route and Adult Dose (Maximum Dose Where Indicated)</th><th>Adverse Effects</th></tr>
<tr><td colspan="2">Sodium Ion Channel Inhibitors</td><td></td></tr>
<tr><td>amiloride (Midamor)</td><td>PO: 5–10 mg/day (max: 20 mg/day)</td><td rowspan="5">Minor hyperkalemia, headache, fatigue, gynecomastia (spironolactone)
Dysrhythmias (from hyperkalemia), dehydration, hyponatremia, agranulocytosis, and other blood dyscrasias</td></tr>
<tr><td>triamterene (Dyrenium)</td><td>PO: 50–300 mg/day in divided doses (max: 300 mg/day)</td></tr>
<tr><td colspan="2">Aldosterone Antagonists</td></tr>
<tr><td>eplerenone (Inspra)</td><td>PO: 25–50 mg once daily (max: 100 mg/day for HTN; 50 mg/day for HF)</td></tr>
<tr><td>spironolactone (Aldactone)</td><td>PO: 25–100 mg 1–2 times/day (max: 400 mg/day)</td></tr>
</table>

Note: *Italics* indicate common adverse effects. Underline indicates serious adverse effects.

Drugs in this class are rarely prescribed alone, but they may be used in combination with thiazide or loop diuretics to minimize loss of potassium ions in the pharmacotherapy of HTN or edema.

Aldosterone Antagonists: Aldosterone is the primary mineralocorticoid hormone secreted by the adrenal gland. The physiologic targets, or mineralocorticoid receptors (MRs), for aldosterone are located in the distal tubule and collecting ducts of the nephron. Once bound to its receptors, the MR–aldosterone complex causes the renal tubule cells to synthesize more Na^+ channels, thereby allowing for more reabsorption of Na^+ from the filtrate. Simply stated, aldosterone increases sodium reabsorption.

Spironolactone and eplerenone prevent the formation of the MR–aldosterone complex and are called *aldosterone antagonists*. By blocking the actions of aldosterone, these drugs enhance the excretion of sodium and the retention of potassium. Like the sodium ion channel inhibitors, spironolactone and eplerenone produce only a weak diuresis, and they are normally combined with drugs from other classes when treating HTN or edema. Spironolactone has also been found to significantly reduce mortality in patients with HF and, because of this important beneficial effect, its use has increased. The aldosterone antagonists are also used to treat hyperaldosteronism, a rare disorder in which a tumor of the adrenal gland secretes large amounts of aldosterone.

Using potassium supplements or adding potassium-rich foods to the diet when taking these medications may lead to life-threatening hyperkalemia. Signs and symptoms of hyperkalemia include muscle weakness, ventricular tachycardia, or fibrillation. Minor adverse effects of the drugs include headache, dizziness, and nausea and vomiting. Spironolactone binds to progesterone and androgen receptors, resulting in a small incidence of gynecomastia, menstrual abnormalities, and impotence. Gynecomastia, abnormal enlargement of the breasts in men, appears to be related to dosage level and duration of therapy; it may persist after the drug is discontinued. The incidence of adverse reproductive system effects is lower with eplerenone.

PROTOTYPE DRUG Spironolactone (Aldactone)

Classification **Therapeutic:** Antihypertensive
Pharmacologic: Potassium-sparing diuretic/aldosterone antagonist

Therapeutic Effects and Uses: Approved in 1960, spironolactone is the most frequently prescribed potassium-sparing diuretic. The most common indication for spironolactone is mild HTN. Because it does not cause potassium depletion, the drug is particularly useful in patients who are at high risk for hypokalemia. However, spironolactone does such an efficient job of retaining potassium that hyperkalemia may develop, especially if the patient is taking potassium supplements or is receiving angiotensin-converting enzyme (ACE) inhibitors. When serum potassium levels are monitored carefully and maintained within normal values, serious adverse effects from spironolactone are uncommon.

Spironolactone is approved for the management of edema associated with hepatic cirrhosis, HF, or nephrotic syndrome. It is particularly useful in treating edema or ascites in patients with hepatic cirrhosis because it counteracts the large amount of aldosterone secreted by these patients. Spironolactone may also be used for the short-term, preoperative treatment of primary hyperaldosteronism. An off-label indication is to improve survival and reduce hospitalizations in patients with severe HF. Other off-label indications include treatment of minor edema associated with PMS, polycystic ovary syndrome, acne, and hirsutism in females. Aldactazide is a fixed-dose combination of spironolactone with hydrochlorothiazide.

Mechanism of Action: Spironolactone acts by inhibiting the actions of aldosterone in the distal tubule and collecting ducts of the nephron. When the actions of aldosterone are blocked by spironolactone, sodium, chloride, and water excretion are increased and the body retains potassium.

Pharmacokinetics:

Route(s)	PO
Absorption	Rapid absorption; 73% absorbed
Distribution	Distributed to most tissues; crosses the placenta; secreted in breast milk; more than 90% bound to plasma protein
Primary metabolism	Hepatic and renal; converted to active metabolites
Primary excretion	Renal (40–57%) and feces (35–40%)
Onset of action	2–3 days; may take 2 weeks for maximum effect
Duration of action	2–3 days; half-life: 1.3–2.4 h for parent compound, and 18–23 h for active metabolites

Adverse Effects: Hyperkalemia induced by spironolactone can cause life-threatening cardiac dysrhythmias. Signs and symptoms associated with spironolactone-induced hyperkalemia include muscle weakness, paresthesia, fatigue, bradycardia, flaccid paralysis of the extremities, and shock. In men, spironolactone can cause gynecomastia, impotence, and diminished libido. Women may experience menstrual irregularities, and breast tenderness. Fertility may decrease during therapy. Agranulocytosis and other blood dyscrasias are rare adverse effects. **Black Box Warning:** Spironolactone produces tumors in laboratory animals; unnecessary use of the drug should be avoided.

Contraindications/Precautions: Contraindications include anuria, severe CKD, pregnancy, and hyperkalemia. Older patients and those with renal insufficiency or diabetes mellitus are at greatest risk for hyperkalemia. At high doses, spironolactone produces teratogenic effects in laboratory animals; thus, it should not be used during pregnancy. A major metabolite of spironolactone is secreted in breast milk; thus, this drug should not be given during lactation.

Drug Interactions: Spironolactone should not be administered concurrently with eplerenone due to the potential for hyperkalemia. Aspirin and other salicylates may decrease the diuretic effect of the medication. Concurrent use with digoxin may decrease the effects of digoxin. When taken with potassium supplements, ACE inhibitors, angiotensin receptor blockers (ARBs), or the potassium salts of other drugs (such as penicillin G potassium), severe hyperkalemia and possible dysrhythmias may result. Concurrent use with other antihypertensives will result in an additive hypotensive effect. **Herbal/Food:** Licorice extract contains a substance with aldosterone-like actions and should be avoided. Use with hawthorn may result in hypotension.

Treatment of Overdose: Acute overdoses produce drowsiness, mental confusion, rash, nausea, vomiting, dizziness, or diarrhea. The most serious symptoms of spironolactone overdose are related to hyperkalemia. If severe, therapies are administered to counteract the hyperkalemia. These include IV calcium chloride, calcium gluconate, sodium bicarbonate, or the administration of glucose with rapid-acting insulin. Cationic exchange resins such as sodium polystyrene sulfonate (Kayexalate) may be administered.

Pregnancy: Animal studies showed increased resorption and reduced numbers of live fetuses. This drug exhibits an antiandrogen effect that can affect sex differentiation of the male during embryogenesis. Small amounts are secreted in milk, although adverse effects in breastfed neonates are unknown.

Clinician Responsibilities: Key clinical implications for patients receiving spironolactone are included in Applied Clinical Judgment: Patients Receiving Pharmacotherapy with Diuretics.

Drugs Similar to Spironolactone (Aldactone)

The three other potassium-sparing diuretics include amiloride, eplerenone, and triamterene.

Amiloride (Midamor): Approved in 1981, amiloride is an oral Na^+ channel inhibitor with weak diuretic activity whose major indication is HTN. It is also used to treat peripheral edema due to HF and to reverse thiazide-induced hypokalemia. When combined with a thiazide diuretic, additive blood pressure reduction is achieved and potassium balance is maintained. It should not be used as monotherapy or in combination with other potassium-sparing diuretics because hyperkalemia may develop. Contraindications and adverse effects are similar to those of spironolactone, including a black box warning for the risk of severe hyperkalemia in patients receiving other potassium-containing drugs. Moduretic is a fixed-dose combination of amiloride and hydrochlorothiazide. Animal studies did not show evidence of teratogenicity. It is not known if the drug is excreted in human milk.

Eplerenone (Inspra): Approved in 2002, eplerenone is an aldosterone antagonist administered by the oral route that is approved for HTN and the post-MI management of HF. Two to 4 weeks of therapy are required to achieve maximum therapeutic effects. Eplerenone is more selective for the MR receptor than spironolactone, and it has the advantage of producing a lower incidence of endocrine-related adverse effects such as gynecomastia, impotence, or menstrual irregularities. Like other drugs in this class, however, the development of hyperkalemia is a potentially serious adverse effect, especially if the drug is used concurrently with ACE inhibitors. Eplerenone is sometimes referred to as a selective aldosterone receptor antagonist. Animal studies showed no evidence of fetal harm. At high doses, the drug was found to impair male fertility. It is likely the drug is excreted in human milk, although effects in breastfed neonates are unknown.

Triamterene (Dyrenium): Approved in 1964, triamterene is an oral drug that acts by the same mechanism as amiloride and has the same indications and adverse effects. It is a relatively weak diuretic and is sometimes used to manage hypokalemia in patients who are unable to tolerate potassium supplements. Triamterene is rarely prescribed as monotherapy and should not be used concurrently with other potassium-sparing diuretics due to the potential for hyperkalemia. Dyazide and Maxzide are fixed-dose combinations of triamterene and hydrochlorothiazide. Animal studies did not show evidence of fetal harm. The drug is secreted in animal milk, although adverse effects in breastfed neonates are unknown.

CONNECTION Checkpoint 32.4

From what you learned in Chapter 31, explain why patients who are taking an ACE inhibitor should probably not receive an aldosterone antagonist.

Osmotic Diuretics

32.8 Osmotic diuretics cause diuresis by increasing the osmolality of the filtrate.

The osmotic diuretics, shown in Table 32.7, are a small class of drugs that are reserved for very specific indications. Unlike the thiazides and loop diuretics that block transport proteins, osmotic diuretics are mostly inert and act by raising the osmolality, which is a measure of the amount

Table 32.7 Miscellaneous Diuretics

Drug	Route and Adult Dose (Maximum Dose Where Indicated)	Adverse Effects
Carbonic Anhydrase Inhibitors		
acetazolamide	PO: 250–375 mg/day (max: 1500 mg/day) IM/IV: 250–375 mg/day	*Electrolyte imbalances, fatigue, nausea and vomiting, dizziness* Dehydration, blood dyscrasias, pancytopenia, flaccid paralysis, hemolytic anemia, aplastic anemia
methazolamide	PO: 50–100 mg bid–tid (max: 300 mg/day)	
Osmotic Diuretics		
glycerin	PO: 1–1.8 g/kg, 1–2 h before ocular surgery	*Electrolyte imbalances, fatigue, nausea and vomiting, dizziness* Hyponatremia, edema, convulsions, tachycardia
mannitol (Osmitrol)	IV: 100 g infused over 2–6 h	

Note: *Italics* indicate common adverse effects. Underline indicates serious adverse effects.

of dissolved particles, or solutes in a solution (**osmotic pressure**). Osmotic diuretics cause water to shift compartments by creating a difference in osmotic pressure across a membrane or between two body compartments.

When given IV, osmotic diuretics are filtered at the glomerulus and readily enter the renal filtrate. Once in the tubule, they remain unchanged. As normal sodium and water reabsorption progresses in the proximal tubule, the diuretic remains behind, and its concentration in the tubule begins to increase. The osmolality of the filtrate increases due to the presence of the osmotic diuretic in the tubule. This osmotic force draws water into the filtrate, resulting in increased diuresis. The influence of osmotic pressure on water movement is presented in greater detail in Chapter 33.

A second action of osmotic diuretics is their ability to raise the osmolality of the plasma. This creates an osmotic force that moves water from the intracellular and extravascular spaces to the plasma. The increased volume of water in the plasma is filtered by the kidney, resulting in enhanced diuresis. This action is used to advantage in the treatment of two conditions where fluid has accumulated in extravascular spaces. For example, following a traumatic head injury, fluid accumulates in the brain, causing dangerously high intracranial pressure. Osmotic diuretics create an osmotic force that promotes the fluid to leave the brain and enter the blood, thus reducing cerebral edema. A second example is high intraocular pressure caused by excess fluid accumulation in the eye (glaucoma). Osmotic diuretics can cause the fluid to leave the eye and enter the blood, thus relieving the high intraocular pressure.

Osmotic diuretics are rarely used due to their potential toxicity and they are contraindicated in patients with serious kidney disease. The rapid movement of water from the extravascular spaces to the blood can result in severe dehydration in the tissues and cause a serious fluid overload in patients with severe HF. Electrolyte imbalances, especially hyponatremia, may occur with these drugs.

PROTOTYPE DRUG Mannitol (Osmitrol)

Classification **Therapeutic:** Drug for acute kidney injury
Pharmacologic: Osmotic diuretic

Therapeutic Effects and Uses: Approved in 1944, mannitol is a parenteral diuretic primarily used to prevent or treat AKI in patients experiencing oliguria before the loss of renal function becomes irreversible. In addition, by its ability to increase the osmolality of plasma, this drug is able to "pull" fluid out of extravascular spaces; thus, it is used to reduce intracranial pressure following head trauma and to lower intraocular pressure in patients with acute glaucoma. Reduction in the amount and pressure of cerebrospinal fluid can occur as quickly as 15 minutes after initiating the infusion; intraocular pressure reduction may take up to an hour. Mannitol may be administered concurrently with nephrotoxic drugs such as cisplatin (an antineoplastic drug) to speed them through the kidney and reduce damage to the walls of the renal tubules.

Mannitol has nondrug uses as a sweetener and food stabilizer. When taken PO, it is absorbed so slowly that it has no effect on insulin levels, making it an alternative sweetener in foods for patients with diabetes. The drug has a laxative effect when taken in large quantities.

Mechanism of Action: Administered by the IV route, mannitol is filtered by the glomerulus of the kidney but is incapable of being reabsorbed from the renal tubule. This creates an osmotic gradient, resulting in decreased water and Na^+ reabsorption and increased diuresis.

Pharmacokinetics:

Route(s)	IV
Absorption	Does not cross biological membranes
Distribution	Remains in extracellular space; does not cross the blood–brain barrier
Primary metabolism	Hepatic (small amounts)
Primary excretion	Renal
Onset of action	1–3 h
Duration of action	4–6 h; half-life: 100 min

Adverse Effects: Electrolyte imbalances, either deficiencies or excesses, can occur during mannitol therapy. For example, as mannitol draws fluid from the intravascular spaces, hyperkalemia or hypernatremia may occur. However, mannitol also increases the excretion of sodium and potassium ions, which can result in hypokalemia or hyponatremia. The same holds true for fluid balance. As mannitol draws fluid into the extracellular spaces, peripheral edema, HF, or pulmonary edema may occur. As diuresis progresses, the patient may become hypovolemic and dehydrated. Other adverse effects include fatigue, nausea and vomiting, dizziness, convulsions, and tachycardia.

Contraindications/Precautions: Contraindications include anuria, severe HF, organic central nervous system (CNS) disease or intracranial bleeding, severe dehydration, and shock. A test dose may be given to patients with oliguria to determine renal function. Function is considered satisfactory if urine flow is at least 30 to 50 mL/h over 2 to 3 hours following an IV test dose of 0.2 g/kg. If this response is not achieved, the kidneys are too impaired to administer a full dose of mannitol.

There is evidence that high doses of mannitol may open the blood–brain barrier by temporarily shrinking the endothelial cells that line the barrier. Should this happen, mannitol will enter the brain (bringing water with it) and increase intracranial pressure. Extreme precautions must be taken when treating patients with high intracranial pressure.

Drug Interactions: Because of its intense diuretic effect, mannitol can increase the excretion of many drugs. This results in a decreased effect for drugs such as lithium, imipramine, salicylates, barbiturates, and potassium supplements. **Herbal/Food:** Unknown.

Pregnancy: Animal studies showed no evidence of fetal harm. Mannitol crosses the placenta and may cause fluid shifts in the fetus. It is not known if the drug is excreted in human milk.

Treatment of Overdose: Overdose will result in a shift of fluid to the vascular compartment, resulting in HF and pulmonary edema. Intense diuresis may cause significant electrolyte imbalances, especially hyponatremia. No specific antidote is available, and treatment is supportive to the presenting symptoms.

Clinician Responsibilities: Key clinical implications for patients receiving mannitol are included in Applied Clinical Judgment: Patients Receiving Pharmacotherapy with Diuretics.

Drugs Similar to Mannitol (Osmitrol)

The only other osmotic diuretic is glycerin.

Glycerin: Also known as glycerol, glycerin is given for a large number of indications. When given by the oral route, glycerin creates an osmotic gradient like mannitol that can reduce intraocular and intracranial pressure. As a laxative suppository, glycerin draws water into the colon, creating more bulk and promoting defecation. It is used in a variety of over-the-counter (OTC) products as an emollient or lubricant, including toothpaste, shaving cream, hair products, soaps, and artificial tears. Like mannitol, it tastes sweet and is used as a food additive to sweeten and keep products moist.

Carbonic Anhydrase Inhibitors

32.9 Carbonic anhydrase inhibitors are weak diuretics that have specific indications.

Carbonic anhydrase is an essential enzyme that helps regulate acid–base balance in the body. Carbonic anhydrase converts CO_2 to carbonic acid (H_2CO_3), which immediately dissociates to bicarbonate ion (HCO_3^-). Note that these reactions are reversible:

$$CO_2 + H_2O \longleftrightarrow H_2CO_3 \longleftrightarrow HCO_3^- + H^+$$

In the kidney tubules, carbonic anhydrase is necessary for the formation and reabsorption of bicarbonate ion, which is essential for maintaining proper acid–base balance. Sodium ions are reabsorbed with bicarbonate ion in the proximal tubule using a symporter protein.

Several drugs that inhibit carbonic anhydrase are available, as shown in Table 32.7. Blocking carbonic anhydrase prevents bicarbonate formation and reabsorption in the renal tubule. Without bicarbonate ion, sodium reabsorption does not occur, more water remains in the filtrate, and diuresis is promoted. The reduction in plasma bicarbonate eventually causes metabolic acidosis, which tends to reverse the diuretic action of this drug.

The carbonic anhydrase inhibitors are rarely prescribed as diuretics because they produce only a weak, short-lived diuresis and can contribute to metabolic acidosis. Carbonic anhydrase inhibitors that are given by the oral route include acetazolamide and methazolamide. Methazolamide is approved only for reducing intraocular pressure in patients with open-angle glaucoma. Acetazolamide also used to decrease intraocular fluid pressure, has several other indications. Two drugs in this class, dorzolamide (Trusopt) and brinzolamide (Azopt), are administered topically to the eye for open-angle glaucoma. The antiglaucoma drugs in this class are discussed in Chapter 74.

PROTOTYPE DRUG | **Acetazolamide**

Classification **Therapeutic:** Drug for edema, antiglaucoma drug
Pharmacologic: Carbonic anhydrase inhibitor

Therapeutic Effects and Uses: Given by either the oral or parenteral route, acetazolamide produces a mild diuresis and is occasionally used to reduce edema fluid in patients with HF. An older drug approved in 1953, it has largely been replaced by thiazide diuretics.

Acetazolamide also has applications for treating absence seizures and in relieving motion sickness. It has been used to acclimatize people to high altitudes to prevent or treat acute mountain sickness. It accomplishes this by increasing the renal excretion of bicarbonate, which accumulates in the body because of the hyperventilation that occurs at high altitude. Acetazolamide is effective in treating open-angle glaucoma and for preoperative treatment of acute closed-angle glaucoma, although it is not a first-line drug for either disorder.

Mechanism of Action: Acetazolamide produces its diuretic effect by inhibiting carbonic anhydrase activity in the proximal renal tubule, causing increased excretion of sodium and bicarbonate. In the eye, the inhibition of carbonic anhydrase reduces the rate of aqueous humor formation and consequently lowers intraocular pressure.

Pharmacokinetics:

Route(s)	PO, IV
Absorption	75% absorbed when given with food
Distribution	Distributed to most tissues; crosses the placenta and is secreted in breast milk
Primary metabolism	Not metabolized
Primary excretion	Renal
Onset of action	PO: 90 min; IV: 2 min
Duration of action	PO: 8–12 h; PO extended release: 18–24 h; IV: 15 min; half-life: 2.4–5.8 h

Adverse Effects: Acetazolamide can cause various electrolyte imbalances, including hyperchloremia and hypokalemia. Gastrointestinal adverse effects include nausea and vomiting, diarrhea, and anorexia. CNS effects may occur, such as dizziness, fatigue, and numbness in the extremities, lips, or facial muscles. Metabolic acidosis may result from excess bicarbonate loss.

Contraindications/Precautions: Acetazolamide is contraindicated in patients who have hypersensitivity to sulfonamides and similar drugs such as thiazide diuretics. Other contraindications include severe renal or hepatic impairment and adrenocortical insufficiency. Patients with preexisting electrolyte imbalances such as hyponatremia, hypokalemia, or hypochloremic acidosis should be treated with caution because acetazolamide may worsen these conditions.

Drug Interactions: The potential for hypokalemia is greatest early in the course of acetazolamide therapy and is accelerated by amphotericin B and corticosteroids. Because acetazolamide alkalinizes the urine, the renal excretion of many drugs may be decreased, including tricyclic antidepressants, procainamide, amphetamines, ephedrine, and quinidine. Renal excretion of lithium and phenobarbital may be increased. High-dose aspirin therapy can compete with tubular secretory mechanisms with acetazolamide, causing the carbonic anhydrase inhibitor to accumulate to toxic levels. **Herbal/Food:** Unknown.

Pregnancy: At high doses, this drug showed embryofetal toxicity in laboratory animals. The drug is excreted in human milk, although adverse effects in breastfed neonates are unknown.

Treatment of Overdose: Overdose with acetazolamide results in metabolic acidosis, which may be treated by administering sodium bicarbonate. Electrolyte depletion and dehydration are treated with infusions of fluids containing electrolytes.

Clinician Responsibilities: Key clinical implications for patients receiving acetazolamide are included in Applied Clinical Judgment: Patients Receiving Pharmacotherapy with Diuretics.

Drugs Similar to Acetazolamide

The other oral carbonic anhydrase inhibitor is methazolamide, which is used as a systemic antiglaucoma drug (see Chapter 74) rather than a diuretic.

CONNECTIONS: APPLIED CLINICAL JUDGMENT

Patients Receiving Pharmacotherapy with Diuretics

Key Assessment Data

- History of current condition, baseline vital signs, physical exam findings; history of cardiovascular disease, CKD, diabetes; drug history including allergies, current prescription and OTC drugs, herbal preparations, and use of digoxin, lithium, or antihypertensive drugs; pregnancy status.
- Ongoing assessment during drug therapy includes laboratory findings including electrolytes, especially potassium, creatinine, glucose, complete blood count (CBC), liver and renal function studies, uric acid, lipid profiles. Assess for location, character, and amount of edema, if present.
- Obtain baseline weight, vital signs, breath sounds, and cardiac monitoring (e.g., electrocardiogram [ECG], cardiac output), if appropriate. Assess for location, character, and amount of edema, if present. Assess baseline hearing and balance.

Desired Therapeutic Outcomes

Improvement is observed and measurable in adequate urine output, decreased edema, or lowered blood pressure if given for HTN.

(continued)

CONNECTIONS: APPLIED CLINICAL JUDGMENT *(continued)*

Patients Receiving Pharmacotherapy with Diuretics

Minimizing Adverse Effects

- Diuretics reduce circulating blood volume, resulting in lowered blood pressure. Monitor for orthostatic hypotension.
- Weigh daily. An increase in weight over 1 kg [2 lb] per day may indicate excessive fluid gain. A decrease of over 1 kg per day may indicate excessive diuresis and dehydration. Measure intake and output in the hospitalized patient.
- Most diuretics cause loss of Na^+ and K^+ and may increase lipid, glucose, and uric acid levels. Continue periodic monitoring of laboratory values including electrolytes, glucose, CBC, lipid profiles, liver function studies, creatinine, and uric acid levels.
- Ototoxicity of cranial nerve VIII may occur, especially with loop diuretics. Continue to monitor hearing and balance.
- Observe for signs of hypokalemia or hyperkalemia. Use with caution in patients taking corticosteroids, ACE inhibitors, ARBs, digoxin, or lithium. Report symptoms to the healthcare provider promptly. Concurrent use with corticosteroids may increase the risk of hypokalemia. Concurrent use with ACE inhibitors or ARBs may increase the risk of hyperkalemia. Concurrent use with digoxin increases the risk of serious dysrhythmias and with lithium may cause toxic levels of the drug.
- Thiazide, thiazide-like, and loop diuretics may cause hyperglycemia, especially in patients with diabetes. Use with caution in patients with diabetes and monitor blood glucose more frequently, especially early in therapy.
- Diuretics may cause hyperuricemia, which may result in gout symptoms such as warmth, pain, tenderness, swelling, and redness around the joints, especially the great toes, hand joints, elbows, and around ears; tophi [nodules]; arthritis-like symptoms; and limited movement in affected joints.
- Many diuretics cause photosensitivity and an increased risk of sunburn.
- Some diuretics may decrease white blood cell counts and the ability to fight infection. Agranulocytosis is a possible adverse effect of diuretic therapy.

Lifespan Considerations

- Orthostatic hypotension may increase the risk of falls and injury. Be particularly cautious with older adults who are at increased risk for hypotension. Ensure patient safety.
- The older adult may be at greater risk for hypokalemia related to renal effects of aging.
- Because of pharmacokinetic differences, exercise additional caution when administering diuretics to infants and very young children. Audiology and additional monitoring may be ordered.
- Monitor electrolyte levels frequently in older adults, who are at greater risk for abnormalities related to age-related physiologic changes.
- Not all diuretics should be used in pregnancy or in the breastfeeding mother. Assess for the possibility of pregnancy or breastfeeding before starting therapy.

Patient and Caregiver Education

- Monitor pulse, BP, and daily weight, using a diary or log, and bring these to each provider visit. Promptly report any weight gain over 1 kg in a 24-hour period or increasing edema to the provider.
- Rise slowly from lying or sitting to standing, pausing between changes if dizziness occurs. Don't take the medication if dizziness continues, or BP is below 90/60 or per parameters set by the provider and contact the provider for further instruction.
- Continue to consume enough liquids to remain adequately, but not overly, hydrated. Drinking when thirsty, avoiding alcoholic beverages, and ensuring adequate but not excessive salt intake will assist in maintaining normal fluid balance.
- High heat conditions contribute to excessive sweating and fluid and electrolyte loss. Extra caution is warranted in these conditions.
- If potassium-wasting diuretics are used, be aware of signs of hypokalemia (muscle weakness or cramping and palpitations) and immediately report them to a healthcare provider. Increase intake of foods high in potassium: fresh fruits such as strawberries and bananas; dried fruits such as apricots and prunes; vegetables and legumes such as tomatoes, beets, and dried beans; juices such as orange, grapefruit, or prune; and fresh meats.
- If potassium-sparing diuretics are used, be aware of the signs of hyperkalemia (nausea, irregular heartbeat, profound fatigue or muscle weakness, and slow or faint pulse) and immediately report them to the healthcare provider. Avoid foods high in potassium; do not use salt substitutes, which often contain potassium salts; and consult with a healthcare provider before taking vitamin and mineral supplements or specialized sports beverages. Typical OTC sports beverages (e.g., Gatorade and Powerade) may have lesser amounts of potassium but have high carbohydrate amounts that may lead to increased diuresis, diarrhea, and the potential for dehydration from the hyperosmolarity.
- Immediately report persistent tinnitus, difficulty hearing, or balance or coordination problems.
- For patients without diabetes, report signs and symptoms of diabetes mellitus (e.g., polydipsia, polyphagia) to the healthcare provider. For patients with diabetes, monitor blood glucose levels more frequently until the effects of the diuretic are known.
- Report signs and symptoms of gout promptly to the healthcare provider. Increase fluid intake and avoid shellfish, organ meats (e.g., liver, kidneys), alcohol, and high-fructose beverages.
- Wear sunscreen and protective clothing if prolonged sun exposure is anticipated.
- Promptly report any flulike symptoms to the healthcare provider: shortness of breath, fever, sore throat, malaise, joint pain, or profound fatigue.
- Women considering pregnancy, or who are pregnant or breastfeeding, should notify their provider before starting the drug.
- Carry an identification card or wear medical identification jewelry indicating diuretic therapy.

Prescribing Considerations

- Lab Test Considerations: Monitor electrolytes (especially potassium), blood glucose, BUN, and serum uric acid levels before and periodically throughout the course of therapy.
- Patients with heart failure and concomitant severely impaired renal function often require large doses of diuretics; specialized consultation is recommended.
- Adjust the dose according to renal function.
- Thiazides are ineffective with increasing severity of renal impairment.
- Thiazides and loop diuretics should be used with extreme caution with liver failure.
- Use lower initial doses in older adults, as they are particularly susceptible to diuretic side effects.
- Monitor for persistent or increased eye pain or decreased visual acuity.

Understanding Chapter 32

Key Concepts Summary

32.1 The kidneys are major organs of excretion and body homeostasis.

32.2 The composition of filtrate changes dramatically as a result of the processes of reabsorption and secretion.

32.3 Chronic kidney disease may significantly impact the success of pharmacotherapy.

32.4 Diuretics are used to treat hypertension, heart failure, accumulation of edema fluid, and chronic kidney disease.

32.5 The most effective diuretics are the loop diuretics that block sodium reabsorption in the loop of Henle.

32.6 The thiazides are the most commonly prescribed class of diuretics.

32.7 Potassium-sparing diuretics have low effectiveness but can help prevent hypokalemia.

32.8 Osmotic diuretics cause diuresis by increasing the osmolality of the filtrate.

32.9 Carbonic anhydrase inhibitors are weak diuretics that have specific indications.

CASE STUDY: Making the Patient Connection

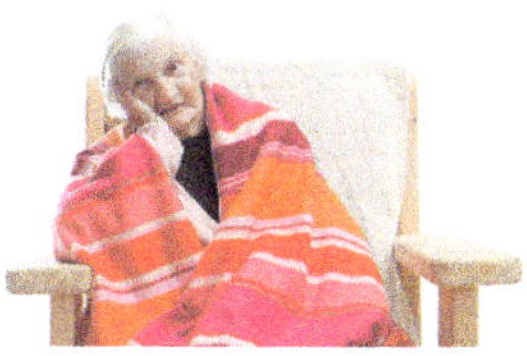

Remember the patient "Katherine Crosland" at the beginning of the chapter? Now read the remainder of the case study. Based on the information presented within this chapter, respond to the critical thinking questions that follow.

Katherine Crosland, a 79-year-old widow, has lived alone for the past 5 years. Although her son and daughters all reside in distant locations, they check on her at least weekly by telephoning. Katherine is fairly independent; however, she does not drive and is dependent on a neighbor to get her groceries and medications.

Three years ago, Katherine was hospitalized for an MI, which resulted in heart failure. She is adherent with her medications, which include digoxin 0.125 mg daily, furosemide (Lasix) 20 mg/day, and potassium supplements (K-Dur) 20 mEq daily.

Recently Katherine's neighbor went on an extended, out-of-town trip. Katherine was certain that she had enough of her medicine to last through that time. However, before the neighbor returned, Katherine discovered she had miscalculated her potassium supplement and only had enough for 10 days. Katherine figured that because the potassium was only a "supplement," she would be able to wait until her neighbor returned to get the medication refilled.

Today, she presents to the clinic with generalized weakness and fatigue. She has lost 3.6 kg (8 lb) since her last clinic visit 6 weeks ago. Her blood pressure is 104/62 mmHg, her heart rate is 98 beats/min, and she has a slightly irregular respiratory rate of 20 breaths/min. Body temperature is 97.2°F (36.2°C). The blood specimen collected for diagnostic studies showed several outstanding findings such as a serum sodium level of 150 mEq/L and potassium level of 3.2 mEq/L. Katherine is diagnosed with dehydration and hypokalemia induced by diuretic therapy.

Critical Thinking Questions

1. Discuss fluid and electrolyte imbalances related to the following diuretic therapies:
   a. Loop diuretics
   b. Thiazide diuretics
   c. Potassium-sparing diuretics
   d. Osmotic diuretics
2. What relationship exists between this patient's diuretic therapy, digoxin therapy, and hypokalemia?
3. What patient education should the nurse provide about diuretic therapy?

Additional Case Study

During a recent visit to the clinic, Miles Davenport learned that his antihypertensive medication was not maintaining his blood pressure at the desired level. The nurse practitioner prescribed spironolactone (Aldactone) 50 mg twice daily in addition to his regular antihypertensive medications.

1. Discuss the mechanism of action for spironolactone.
2. Prepare a list of foods that should be eaten sparingly while taking spironolactone.
3. List the symptoms of hyperkalemia that Miles needs to know to manage his disease and medications.

Chapter Review

1. The nurse is teaching a group of patients with cardiac conditions who are taking diuretic therapy. The nurse explains that individuals prescribed furosemide (Lasix) should:
   1. Avoid consuming large amounts of cabbage, cauliflower, and kale.
   2. Rise slowly from sitting or lying positions.
   3. Count their pulse for 1 full minute before taking the medication.
   4. Restrict fluid intake to no more than 1000 mL in a 24-hour period.
2. The patient who is receiving bumetanide (Bumex) is instructed to watch for symptoms associated with electrolyte imbalances. Which condition would the patient most likely experience?
   1. Hypernatremia
   2. Hypokalemia
   3. Hyperkalemia
   4. Hypocalcemia
3. While preparing a patient for discharge, which of the following statements should the nurse include in the instructions regarding the patient's new prescription of hydrochlorothiazide (Microzide)?
   1. "There are no limitations on the amount of salt and fluid intake."
   2. "Ingest vitamin K–rich foods daily, such as green, leafy vegetables and broccoli."
   3. "Report muscle cramps or weakness to the healthcare provider."
   4. "Antihypertensive drugs taken concurrently may produce sleepiness."
4. Patients prescribed spironolactone (Aldactone) are often at risk for electrolyte imbalance. The nurse assesses for this adverse effect because this drug may cause the body to:
   1. Retain potassium.
   2. Release magnesium.
   3. Excrete potassium.
   4. Bind calcium.
5. Which nursing measures should be a nursing priority for a patient when first beginning mannitol (Osmitrol)?
   1. Keep the urinal or bedpan available for patients with limited mobility.
   2. Assess for hypokalemia and encourage foods high in potassium.
   3. Monitor intake and output ratio and weigh the patient daily.
   4. Monitor blood pressure and assess for level of consciousness.
6. The nurse is monitoring a patient receiving acetazolamide. Which acid–base imbalance is a potential risk for this patient?
   1. Metabolic acidosis
   2. Metabolic alkalosis
   3. Respiratory acidosis
   4. Respiratory alkalosis

See Appendix A for answers to critical thinking questions, case study questions, and review questions.

References

Kurani, S., Jeffery, M., Thorsteinsdottir, B., Hickson, L., Barreto, E., Haag, J., et al. (2019). Use of potentially nephrotoxic medications by U.S. adults with chronic kidney disease: NHANES, 2011–2016. *Journal of General Internal Medicine, 35*(4), 1092–1101. https://doi.org/10.1007/s11606-019-05557-8

National Institute of Diabetes and Digestive and Kidney Diseases. (2016). *Kidney disease statistics for the United States*. http://www.niddk.nih.gov/health-information/health-statistics/Pages/kidney-disease-statistics-united-states.aspx

National Kidney Foundation. (2020). *Kidney disease: The basics*. https://www.kidney.org/news/newsroom/factsheets/KidneyDiseaseBasics

Organ Procurement and Transplantation Network. (2020). *National data*. https://optn.transplant.hrsa.gov/data/view-data-reports/national-data/

World Anti-Doping Agency. (2020). *The world anti-doping code international standard: Prohibited list January 2020*. https://www.wada-ama.org/sites/default/files/wada_2020_english_prohibited_list_0.pdf

Selected Bibliography

Barbieri, M. A., Rottura, M., Cicala, G., Mandraffino, R., Marino, S., Irrera, N., et al. (2020). Chronic kidney disease management in general practice: A focus on inappropriate drugs prescriptions. *Journal of Clinical Medicine, 9*(5), 1346. https://doi.org/10.3390/jcm9051346

Blue, L. (2015). Delivering intravenous diuretics in the community. *Journal of Community Nursing, 29*(6), 41–44.

Lefler, L. L., Hadley, M., Tackett, J., & Thomason, A. P. (2016). New cardiovascular guidelines: Clinical practice evidence for the nurse practitioner. *Journal of the American Association of Nurse Practitioners, 28*, 241–248. https://doi.org/10.1002/2327-6924.12262

Maurya, N. K. (2019). Nephrotoxic effect of herbal medicine and supplements: A review. *Research & Reviews: A Journal of Toxicology, 9*(2), 28–35.

McCrory, G., Patton, D., Moore, Z., O'Connor, T., & Nugent, L. (2018). The impact of advanced nurse practitioners on patient outcomes in chronic kidney disease: a systematic review. *Journal of Renal Care, 44*(4), 197–209. https://doi.org/10.1111/jorc.12245

National Kidney Foundation. (2019). *Herbal supplements and kidney disease*. http://www.kidney.org/atoz/content/herbalsupp.cfm

Okoro, R. N., & Farate, V. T. (2019). The use of nephrotoxic drugs in patients with chronic kidney disease. *International Journal of Clinical Pharmacy, 41*(3), 767–775. https://doi.org/10.1007/s11096-019-00811-9

Patel, J. B., & Sapra, A. (2020). *Nephrotoxic medications*. StatPearls. Retrieved from https://www.ncbi.nlm.nih.gov/books/NBK553144/

Pham, D., & Grodin, J. L. (2017). Dilemmas in the dosing of heart failure drugs: titrating diuretics in chronic heart failure. *Cardiac Failure Review, 3*(2), 108. https://doi.org/10.15420/cfr.2017:10:1

Roush, G. C., & Sica, D. A. (2016). Diuretics for hypertension: A review and update. *American Journal of Hypertension, 29*(10), 1130–1137. https://doi.org/10.1093/ajh/hpw030

Shahrbaf, F. G., & Assadi, F. (2015). Drug-induced renal disorders. *Journal of Renal Injury Prevention, 4*, 57–60. https://doi.org/10.12861/jrip.2015.12

Simonavičius, J., Knackstedt, C., & Brunner-La Rocca, H. P. (2019). Loop diuretics in chronic heart failure: how to manage congestion? *Heart Failure Reviews, 24*(1), 17–30. https://doi.org/10.1007/s10741-018-9735-7

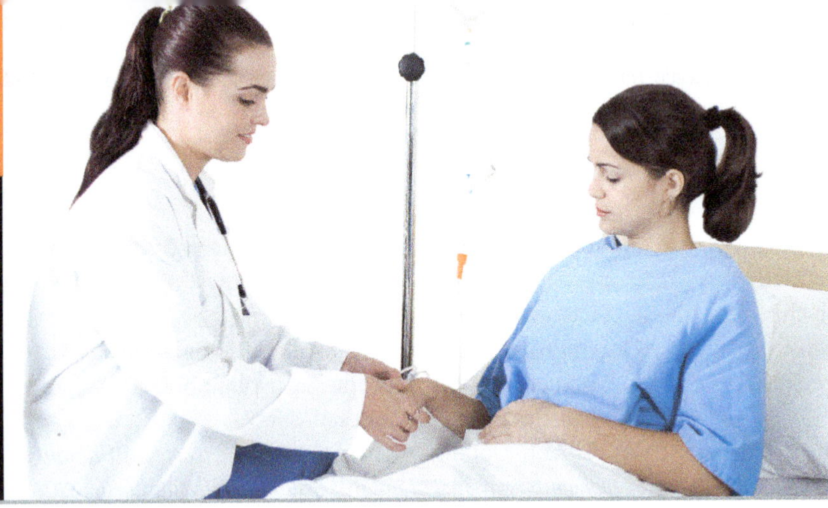

"I don't understand why I need an IV. I was told this was going to be a quick procedure."
—*Patient "Peggy Hoover"*

Chapter 33
Pharmacotherapy of Fluid Imbalance, Electrolyte, and Acid–Base Disorders

Chapter Outline

Learning Outcomes

After reading this chapter, the student should be able to:

1. Describe the exchange of fluids that occurs among the different fluid compartments in the body.
2. Identify conditions for which intravenous fluid therapy may be indicated.
3. Explain how changes in the osmolality or tonicity of a fluid can cause water to move to a different compartment.
4. Compare and contrast the use of blood products, crystalloids, and colloids in intravenous therapy.
5. Explain the pharmacotherapy of sodium, potassium, and magnesium imbalances.
6. Discuss medications used to treat acidosis and alkalosis.
7. Describe the nurse's role in the pharmacologic management of fluid imbalance, electrolyte, and acid–base disorders.
8. For each of the classes shown in the chapter outline, identify the prototype and representative drugs and explain the mechanism(s) of drug action, primary indications, contraindications, significant drug interactions, pregnancy data, and important adverse effects.
9. Apply clinical judgment to care for patients receiving pharmacotherapy for fluid imbalance, electrolyte, and acid–base disorders.

Key Terms

Definitions of the terms in bold may be found in the Glossary.

Can too much pure, sparkling water hurt you? As often as people hear "drink plenty of fluids," too much (or too little) can definitely be harmful. The volume and composition of fluids in the body must be maintained within narrow limits. Excess fluid volume can lead to hypertension (HTN), heart failure, or peripheral edema, while depletion results in dehydration.

Body fluids must also contain specific amounts of essential ions or electrolytes and be maintained at particular pH values. Imbalances in electrolytes or changes in the pH of body fluids may have fatal consequences if left untreated. This chapter examines drugs used to reverse fluid imbalance, electrolyte, or acid–base disorders.

Principles of Fluid Balance

33.1 Body fluids are exchanged between intracellular and extracellular compartments.

Body fluids travel between compartments separated by semipermeable membranes. Control of water balance in the various compartments is essential to homeostasis. Fluid imbalances are frequent indications for pharmacotherapy.

Not surprisingly, the greatest bulk of body fluid consists of water, which serves as the universal solvent in which electrolytes, minerals, and most nutrients are dissolved. Water alone is responsible for about 60% of the total body weight in a young adult. A newborn may contain 80% water, while an older adult may contain only 40%.

In a simple model, water in the body can be located in one of two places, or compartments. The **intracellular fluid (ICF) compartment**, which contains water that is inside cells, accounts for about two-thirds of total body water. The remaining one-third of body fluid resides outside cells in the **extracellular fluid (ECF) compartment**. The ECF compartment is further divided into two parts: fluid in the plasma, or intravascular space, and fluid in the interstitial spaces between cells. The relationship between these fluid compartments is illustrated in Figure 33.1.

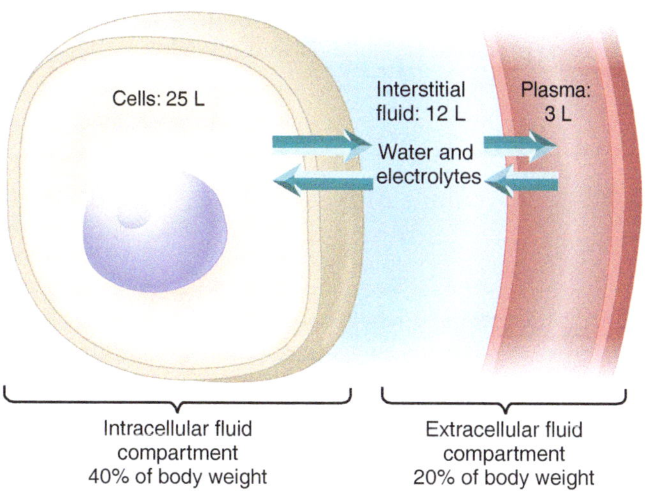

Figure 33.1 Major fluid compartments in the body.

Once contained in a compartment, water and minerals do not stay there for very long. There is a continuous exchange, turnover, and mixing of fluids between compartments, as molecules travel across the membranes that separate them. For example, the plasma membranes of cells separate the ICF from the ECF. The capillary membranes separate plasma from the interstitial fluid. Although water travels freely among the compartments, processes of diffusion and active transport govern the movement of large molecules and those with electrical charges. Movement of ions and drugs across membranes is a primary topic of pharmacokinetics (see Chapter 3).

CONNECTION Checkpoint 33.1

From what you learned in Chapter 3, what barriers does an oral drug face in moving from the gastrointestinal tract to the extracellular fluid compartment (plasma)?

33.2 Osmolality or tonicity determines the movement of body fluids.

Osmolality and *tonicity* are two related terms central to understanding the pharmacotherapy of fluid imbalance disorders. Abnormalities in the osmolality or tonicity of a body fluid can cause significant shifts in water balance between compartments. The nurse will often administer intravenous (IV) fluids to compensate for these changes.

The **osmolality** is a measure of the number of dissolved particles, or solutes, in 1 kg (1 L) of water. In most body fluids, three solutes determine the osmolality: sodium, glucose, and urea. Sodium is the greatest contributor to osmolality due to its abundance in most body fluids. The normal osmolality of body fluids ranges from 275 to 295 milliosmoles per kilogram (mOsm/kg).

The term **tonicity** is sometimes used interchangeably with osmolality, although they are somewhat different. Tonicity is the ability of a solution to cause a change in water movement across a membrane due to osmotic forces. Whereas osmolality is a laboratory value that can be precisely measured, *tonicity* is a general term used to describe the *relative* concentration of IV fluids. The tonicity of normal plasma is considered isotonic and is used as the reference point when administering IV solutions. Solutions that are isotonic have the same concentration of solutes (same osmolality) as plasma. Hypertonic solutions contain a greater concentration of solutes than plasma, whereas hypotonic solutions have a lesser concentration of solutes than plasma.

Through **osmosis**, water moves from areas of low solute concentration (low osmolality) to areas of high solute concentration (high osmolality). If a hypertonic (hyperosmolar) IV solution is administered, water will move, by osmosis, from the cells, to the interstitial fluid compartment, to the plasma compartment. If a hypotonic solution is administered, water will move in the opposite direction, from plasma to the interstitial fluid, and eventually into cells. Isotonic solutions produce no net fluid shift. From a pharmacologic perspective, water movement between compartments following an IV infusion can be either a therapeutic effect or an adverse effect depending on the patient's condition and the expected outcomes of the drug administration.

33.3 Overall fluid balance is regulated primarily by hormones acting on the kidneys.

The average adult has a water intake of approximately 2500 mL per day, most of which comes from ingested food and beverages. Water output occurs through the kidneys, lungs, skin, feces, and sweat. To maintain water balance, water intake must equal water output. Net gains or losses of water can be estimated by changes in total body weight.

The most important physiologic mechanism regulating fluid intake is thirst. The sensation of thirst occurs when osmoreceptors in the hypothalamus sense that the ECF has become hypertonic. Saliva secretion diminishes and the mouth dries, motivating the individual to drink fluids. As the ingested water is absorbed, the osmolality of the ECF falls and the thirst center in the hypothalamus is no longer stimulated.

In addition to triggering thirst, the hypothalamus also directs the pituitary gland to release antidiuretic hormone (ADH) when plasma osmolality rises. ADH acts directly on the distal tubules of the kidney to increase water reabsorption. This increased water in the intravascular space dilutes the plasma, thus lowering its osmolality. In high concentrations ADH, also called vasopressin, can cause vasoconstriction, which serves as an important compensatory mechanism during hypovolemic shock.

A second set of hormones assists in the maintenance of fluid balance. Through the renin-angiotensin-aldosterone system (RAAS) (see Chapter 31), the hormone aldosterone is secreted by the adrenal cortex. Aldosterone causes the kidneys to retain sodium and water in the body, thus increasing the osmolality of the ECF.

Failure to maintain adequate intake or output can lead to fluid imbalance disorders that are indications for pharmacologic intervention. Fluid *deficit* disorders can cause dehydration or shock, which are treated by administering oral (PO) or IV fluids. Fluid *excess* disorders are treated with diuretics (see Chapter 32). When treating fluid imbalances, the ultimate goal is to diagnose and correct the underlying cause of the disorder, while administering supporting fluids and medications to stabilize the patient.

CONNECTION Checkpoint 33.2

From what you learned in Chapter 31, name the two aldosterone antagonists and provide their indications.

Fluid Replacement Agents

33.4 Dehydration may be treated with fluid volume expanders.

When fluid output exceeds fluid intake, volume deficits may result in shock, dehydration, or electrolyte loss. Left untreated, large-volume deficits may turn fatal. The following are common causes of fluid depletion:

- Loss of gastrointestinal (GI) fluids due to vomiting, diarrhea, chronic laxative use, or GI suctioning
- Excessive sweating during hot weather, athletic activity, or prolonged fever
- Severe burns
- Hemorrhage
- Excessive diuresis due to diuretic therapy or uncontrolled diabetic ketoacidosis.

The immediate goal in treating a volume deficit disorder is to replace the depleted fluid so that blood volume and blood pressure can be maintained. In nonacute circumstances, this may be achieved by drinking more liquids or by administering fluids via a feeding tube. In acute situations, IV fluid therapy is indicated.

Choice of IV fluid therapy depends on the nature of the volume deficit. Careful attention must be paid to restoring normal levels of blood elements (erythrocytes, leukocytes, and thrombocytes) and electrolytes as well as total fluid volume. If significant blood loss has occurred, blood products may be indicated. Loss of substantial sodium and other salts involves replacement therapy with hypertonic fluids. Excessive sweating can result in water loss that requires hypotonic IV fluids. Treating dehydration with an IV fluid with the incorrect tonicity may worsen the condition.

Fluid replacement should always be conducted in a controlled, stepwise manner. Rapid infusions can cause fluid overload, pulmonary edema, and cardiovascular stress. Vital signs and plasma electrolytes should be carefully monitored during therapy. Therapy for dehydration is summarized in Table 33.1. The three basic classes of fluid replacement agents are blood products, crystalloids, and colloids.

Blood Products

33.5 Transfusions of blood products are used to treat serious conditions that cannot be managed effectively by other means.

Blood products include whole blood, packed red cells, fresh frozen plasma, cryoprecipitate, immune globulins, and platelet infusions. A single unit of whole blood can be separated into its specific constituents (erythrocytes, leukocytes, platelets, plasma proteins, fresh frozen plasma, and globulins), which can be used to treat multiple patients. Indications for the various blood products are shown in Table 33.2.

Table 33.1 Types of Dehydration Disorders and Their Treatment

Type	Isotonic Contraction	Hypotonic Contraction	Hypertonic Contraction
Fluid lost	Water and sodium in equal proportions	Sodium, without a corresponding loss of water	Water, without a corresponding loss of sodium
Pathophysiology	ECF remains isotonic; no net fluid shift	ECF becomes hypotonic; fluid shifts from ECF to ICF, lowering plasma fluid volume	ECF becomes hypertonic; fluid shifts from ICF to ECF, causing cellular dehydration
Causes	Vomiting, diarrhea, renal disease, diuretics	Diuretics, renal disease	Excessive sweating without replenishment, osmotic diuresis, burns
Treatment	Administer isotonic fluids; e.g., isotonic saline (0.9%)	Administer hypertonic fluids; e.g., hypertonic saline (3%)	Administer hypotonic fluids; e.g., hypotonic saline or 5% dextrose

Blood products may be administered to restore deficient numbers of blood cells or proteins or to increase fluid volume depending on the clinical situation. Whole blood is indicated for the treatment of acute, massive blood loss (depletion of more than 30% of the total volume) when there is a need to replace plasma volume and to supply erythrocytes to increase the blood's oxygen-carrying capacity.

PharmFACT

In the United States, over 13 million units of whole blood and red blood cells are donated each year. About 36,000 units of red blood cells are needed every day (American Red Cross, 2020).

The administration of whole blood has been largely replaced by the use of blood components. Whole blood is rarely administered for several reasons. If the patient needs only one specific component in blood, there is no need to expose the patient to unnecessary components that could potentially trigger an adverse effect. The supply of blood products depends on human donors and requires careful crossmatching to ensure compatibility between the donor and the recipient.

The most common complications of whole blood transfusion include febrile nonhemolytic and chill-rigor reactions. The patient experiences symptoms of an allergic reaction that include back pain and low-grade fever and chills. Dizziness, urticaria, and headache may occur during

Table 33.2 Indications for Blood Products

Product	Description	Indication(s)
Whole blood	Contains all blood components	Rapid, massive blood loss when safer agents are not available
Packed RBCs	One unit of packed RBCs increases hemoglobin by about 1 g/dL and hematocrit by about 3% Washed RBCs are nearly free of plasma, white blood cells, and platelets and are reserved for patients who have severe reactions to plasma components	Preferred product to increase serum hemoglobin level
Fresh frozen plasma (FFP)	An unconcentrated source of all clotting factors, without platelets	Correction of bleeding secondary to factor deficiencies for which specific factor replacements are unavailable, multifactor deficiency states, and rapid warfarin reversal FFP should not be used for simple volume expansion
Cryoprecipitate	A concentrate prepared from FFP Each concentrate contains about 80 units each of Factor VIII and von Willebrand's factor and about 250 mg of fibrinogen It also contains fibronectin and Factor XIII	Originally used for hemophilia and von Willebrand's disease, it is also used as a source of fibrinogen in acute disseminated intravascular coagulation with bleeding, treatment of uremic bleeding, cardiothoracic surgery, and obstetric emergencies such as abruptio placentae
Immune globulins	Antibody preparations used to provide an immediate boost to the immune system	Rho(D) immune globulin (RhoGAM) prevents development of maternal Rh antibodies that can result from fetomaternal hemorrhage Other immune globulins are available for postexposure prophylaxis for patients exposed to certain infectious diseases, including cytomegalovirus, hepatitis A and B, measles, rabies, respiratory syncytial virus, rubella, tetanus, smallpox, and varicella
Platelets	One unit of platelet concentrate increases the platelet count by about 10,000/mcL	Used to prevent bleeding in asymptomatic severe thrombocytopenia, for bleeding patients with less severe thrombocytopenia or with platelet dysfunction due to antiplatelet drugs but with normal platelet count, for patients receiving a massive transfusion that causes dilutional thrombocytopenia, and before invasive surgery

or immediately after the transfusion. Symptoms are generally mild and are treated with acetaminophen (Tylenol) and diphenhydramine (Benadryl) as needed.

The most serious adverse effect from administration of whole blood is an acute hemolytic transfusion reaction. This occurs when the patient receiving the transfusion develops antibodies against donor red blood cell (RBC) antigens. ABO blood type incompatibility is the most common cause of this rare, though sometimes fatal, disorder. Another uncommon, though serious, adverse effect from whole blood is transfusion-related acute lung injury. This injury occurs when the patient receives donor antibodies that attack normal granulocytes in the lung. Acute respiratory symptoms develop and may be fatal.

Whole blood, despite being carefully screened, also has the potential to transmit serious infections such as hepatitis, cytomegalovirus, malaria, or HIV. In addition, platelet concentrates are stored at room temperature, which may promote the growth of bacteria in the sample. Although disease transmission from donor to recipient is possible, the risk is very low.

PROTOTYPE DRUG **Normal Serum Albumin (Albuminar, Plasbumin, Others)**

Classification **Therapeutic:** Fluid replacement agent
Pharmacologic: Blood product, colloid

Therapeutic Effects and Uses: Normal serum albumin is a protein extracted from whole human blood, plasma, or placental plasma that contains 96% albumin and 4% globulins and other proteins. Albumin is sterilized to remove possible contamination by hepatitis viruses or HIV. Plasma protein fraction (Plasmanate) is another albumin product that contains 83% albumin and 17% plasma globulins. Albumin is classified as both a blood product and a colloid.

The functions of endogenous albumin are to maintain plasma osmotic pressure and to bind certain substances traveling through the blood, including fatty acids, hormones, enzymes, and a substantial number of drug molecules. Binding to albumin renders these substances inactive until they become unbound.

Normal serum albumin may be administered to restore plasma volume and maintain cardiac output in patients with hypovolemic shock. It may also be administered to restore the level of blood proteins in patients with hypoproteinemia, which occurs with hepatic cirrhosis. Albumin is occasionally administered to bind and remove toxic bilirubin in hemolytic disease of the newborn. It may also offer protection against kernicterus, a toxic accumulation of bilirubin in infants that causes brain injury. It has an immediate onset of action and is available in concentrations of 5% and 25%.

Mechanism of Action: Administered IV, normal serum albumin rapidly increases the osmotic pressure of the blood and causes fluid to move from the tissues to the general circulation.

Pharmacokinetics: Albumin has a half-life of 17 to 19 days.

Adverse Effects: Hypervolemia may occur if the dosage and rate of infusion are not carefully adjusted to the patient's volume status. Signs of fluid overload include headache, dyspnea, rising blood pressure, and pulmonary edema. Normal serum albumin is a natural blood product, and the patient may have antibodies to the donor's albumin that cause allergic reactions. Because coagulation factors, antibodies, and most other blood proteins have been removed, such allergic reactions from albumin are rare. Signs of allergy include fever, chills, urticaria, rash, dyspnea, and possibly hypotension.

Contraindications/Precautions: The drug is contraindicated in patients with severe anemia or cardiac failure in the presence of normal or increased intravascular volume and in those with known allergy to albumin.

Drug Interactions: There are no clinically significant interactions. **Herbal/Food:** Unknown.

Pregnancy: No data are available on the use of this drug during pregnancy or lactation.

Treatment of Overdose: Protein overload may occur if excessive albumin is infused. There is no treatment for overdose.

Clinician Responsibilities: Key clinical implications for patients receiving normal serum albumin are included in Applied Clinical Judgment: Patients Receiving Pharmacotherapy for Fluid and Electrolyte Imbalances.

Drugs Similar to Normal Serum Albumin (Albuminar, Plasbumin, Others)

Other blood products are described in Table 33.2 and include whole blood, packed RBCs, fresh frozen plasma, cryoprecipitate, immune globulins, and platelet infusions.

Crystalloids

33.6 Crystalloids are intravenous solutions that closely resemble the composition of extracellular fluid.

Crystalloids are IV solutions that contain electrolytes and other substances in concentrations that closely mimic the body's extracellular fluid. They are used to replace depleted fluids and to promote urine output. Crystalloid solutions are capable of quickly diffusing across membranes, leaving the plasma, and entering the interstitial fluid and ICF. Isotonic, hypotonic, and hypertonic solutions are available. Sodium is the most common crystalloid added to solutions,

Table 33.3 Selected Crystalloid IV Solutions

Drug	Tonicity
normal saline (0.9% NaCl)	Isotonic
hypertonic saline (3% NaCl)	Hypertonic
hypotonic saline (0.45% NaCl)	Hypotonic
lactated Ringer	Isotonic
Plasma-Lyte 148	Isotonic
Plasma-Lyte 56	Hypotonic
Dextrose Solutions	
5% dextrose in water (D_5W)	Isotonic*
5% dextrose in normal saline	Hypertonic
5% dextrose in 0.2% saline	Isotonic
5% dextrose in lactated Ringer	Hypertonic
5% dextrose in Plasma-Lyte 56	Hypertonic

*Because dextrose is metabolized quickly, the solution is sometimes considered hypotonic.

although some crystalloids contain dextrose, a form of glucose. Common crystalloids used to treat shock include normal saline, lactated Ringer's, Plasma-Lyte, and hypertonic saline. Selected crystalloids are listed in Table 33.3. Infusion of crystalloids will increase the total fluid volume in the body, but the compartment that is most expanded depends on the solute concentration of the fluid administered.

Isotonic Crystalloids Isotonic crystalloids expand the circulating intravascular (plasma) fluid volume, *without* causing major fluid shifts between compartments. This is because the osmotic pressures of the intravascular and extravascular compartments are equal. Isotonic crystalloids such as normal saline are often used to treat fluid loss due to vomiting, diarrhea, or surgical procedures, especially when blood pressure is low. The isotonic saline solutions may also be used to treat sodium deficiency (hyponatremia) because they contain sodium chloride. Because isotonic crystalloids can rapidly expand circulating blood volume, care must be taken not to cause fluid overload in the patient.

Hypertonic Crystalloids Infusion of hypertonic crystalloids raises the osmolality of the plasma and expands plasma volume by drawing water away from the cells and tissues. These drugs may be used to relieve cellular edema, especially cerebral edema. When patients are dehydrated and have hypertonic plasma, hypertonic solutions match the tonicity of the plasma as it is infused, but the dextrose in the IV solution is subsequently metabolized and the solution becomes hypotonic. This hypotonic solution then causes water to shift into the intracellular space, relieving the dehydration within the cells. Overtreatment with hypertonic crystalloids such as 3% normal saline can lead to excessive expansion of the intravascular (plasma) compartment, fluid overload, and HTN.

Hypotonic Crystalloids Hypotonic crystalloid infusions lower the serum osmolality. This causes water to move out of the plasma to the tissues and cells in the intracellular compartment; thus, these solutions are not plasma volume expanders. Hypotonic crystalloids are indicated for patients with hypernatremia and cellular dehydration. Care must be taken not to cause depletion of the intravascular compartment, which can result in hypotension, or too much expansion of the extracellular compartment, which can cause peripheral edema. Patients who are dehydrated with low blood pressure should be given normal saline; the isotonic saline will expand plasma volume and increase blood pressure while hydrating the patient. Patients who are dehydrated with normal blood pressure should be given a hypotonic solution; this infusion will hydrate cells without expanding plasma volume.

PROTOTYPE DRUG 5% Dextrose in Water (D_5W)

Classification **Therapeutic:** Fluid expander
Pharmacologic: Crystalloid

Therapeutic Effects and Uses: Commonly found in concentrations of 2.5%, 5%, or 10%, dextrose solutions are infused to replace lost water and to enhance renal function. Being a form of glucose, dextrose provides nutritional value: 1 L of 5% dextrose supplies 170 calories. In addition, water is formed during the metabolism of dextrose, adding to the rehydration of the patient. D_5W is also used as a diluent for mixing other medications for IV delivery. Dextrose 50% is indicated for the emergency treatment of insulin hypoglycemia to restore blood glucose levels.

D_5W is isotonic in the container. When infused, however, the dextrose is quickly metabolized in the body, leaving only water, and the solution becomes hypotonic. Water may then move from the plasma to the intracellular spaces, relieving cellular dehydration. Essentially, the infusion of D_5W has the same effect as administration of water. Because this may result in a lower plasma volume, patients needing fluid replacement for hypovolemia should receive lactated Ringer or normal saline rather than D_5W.

Dextrose is added to other IV solutions, as shown in Table 33.3. It is also available in other concentrations. In all cases, the dextrose is simply added as a source of calories and nutrition.

Mechanism of Action: There are two forms of glucose in nature: L-glucose and D-glucose. Only D-glucose, also called dextrose, can be used by the human body for energy. If insulin is present, glucose (dextrose) enters cells and is converted into adenosine triphosphate, CO_2, and water.

Pharmacokinetics: Because dextrose and water are natural substances, it is not possible to obtain accurate pharmacokinetic values.

Adverse Effects: Infusion of too much D_5W may cause fluid overload, thus worsening peripheral edema, pulmonary edema, and heart failure. Hyperglycemia is possible, especially in patients with deficient insulin secretion. Pain may occur at the injection site. As D_5W dilutes the plasma, the concentration of sodium in the plasma may fall, resulting in hyponatremia. Hyponatremia in children is especially dangerous because it can lead to encephalopathy as the brain swells.

Contraindications/Precautions: Caution must be used when using D_5W in patients with heart failure or who are hyperglycemic. Patients with increased intracranial pressure should not receive hypotonic agents such as D_5W because they may worsen this condition. Dextrose is obtained from corn and patients allergic to this food may be hypersensitive to the drug.

Drug Interactions: There are no significant drug interactions with D_5W. **Herbal/Food:** Unknown.

Pregnancy: No data are available on the use of this drug during pregnancy or lactation.

Treatment of Overdose: Overdose is uncommon, but diuretics may be indicated in cases of fluid overload.

Clinician Responsibilities: Key clinical implications for patients receiving 5% dextrose in water are included in Applied Clinical Judgment: Patients Receiving Pharmacotherapy for Fluid and Electrolyte Imbalances.

Drugs Similar to 5% Dextrose in Water (D5W)

Other crystalloids include Ringer solution and Plasma-Lyte.

Ringer and lactated Ringer: Ringer solution is named after pharmacologist Sydney Ringer, who created the drug in the mid-1800s. Ringer solution is an isotonic fluid that contains sodium, chloride, potassium, and calcium ions in concentrations similar to those found in plasma. Lactated Ringer solution also contains lactate, which serves as a chemical buffer in the blood to prevent acidosis. Lactated Ringer is also available with 5% dextrose. Ringer solutions are widely administered IV for fluid resuscitation following hemorrhage caused by trauma, surgery, or burns.

Plasma-Lyte: Plasma-Lyte solutions are electrolyte solutions used to correct volume and electrolyte deficiencies. The solutions also contain buffers such as lactate, acetate, or gluconate, which help to correct or prevent acidosis. Several formulations are available that differ in electrolyte composition and osmolarity. These include Plasma-Lyte-R, Plasma-Lyte-A, Plasma-Lyte 56, and Plasma-Lyte 148.

Colloids

33.7 Colloids are intravenous solutions containing large molecules that remain in the blood.

Colloids are proteins, starches, or other large molecules that remain in the blood for a long time because they are too large to easily cross capillary membranes. While circulating, they have the same effect as hypertonic solutions, drawing water molecules from the cells and tissues into the plasma through their ability to increase plasma osmolality and osmotic pressure. These drugs are sometimes called plasma volume expanders. Blood product colloids include normal serum albumin, plasma protein fraction, and serum globulins. The non–blood product colloids are dextran (40, 70, and high molecular weight) and hetastarch (Hespan). These medications are administered to provide life-sustaining support following massive hemorrhage and to treat shock, burns, acute liver failure, and neonatal hemolytic disease. Selected colloid solutions are given in Table 33.4.

Table 33.4 Selected Colloid IV Solutions

Drug	Tonicity
5% albumin	Isotonic
dextran 40 in D_5W	Isotonic
dextran 40 in normal saline	Isotonic
dextran 70 in normal saline	Isotonic
hetastarch (Hespan) 6% in normal saline	Isotonic
plasma protein fraction	Isotonic

PROTOTYPE DRUG **Dextran 40 (Gentran 40, Others)**

Classification **Therapeutic:** Plasma volume expander
Pharmacologic: Colloid

Therapeutic Effects and Uses: Dextran 40 is a synthetic polysaccharide that is too large to pass through capillary walls. It is similar to dextran 70, except dextran 40 has a lower molecular weight. Given as an IV infusion, it has the capability of doubling plasma volume within a few minutes after administration, although its effects last only about 12 hours. Cardiovascular responses include increased blood pressure, increased cardiac output, and improved venous return to the heart. Indications include fluid replacement for patients experiencing hypovolemic shock due to hemorrhage, surgery, or severe burns. When given for acute shock, it is infused as rapidly as possible until blood volume is restored.

Dextran 40 also reduces platelet adhesiveness and improves blood flow through capillaries by its ability to reduce blood viscosity. These antithrombotic properties have led to its use in preventing deep vein thrombosis and postoperative pulmonary emboli. Dextran, however, is less effective than heparin or low-molecular-weight heparin in preventing thromboembolism (see Chapter 38).

Mechanism of Action: Dextran 40 acts by raising the osmotic pressure of the blood, thereby causing fluid to move from the interstitial spaces of the tissues to the blood. The larger blood volume increases cardiac output, stroke volume, blood pressure, and urinary output. Heart rate and blood viscosity decrease.

Pharmacokinetics:

Route(s)	IV
Absorption	Not absorbed
Distribution	Does not leave the vascular system
Primary metabolism	Unknown
Primary excretion	Renal
Onset of action	Several minutes
Duration of action	12–24 h

Adverse Effects: Vital signs should be monitored continuously during dextran 40 infusions to prevent HTN resulting from plasma volume expansion. Signs of fluid overload include tachycardia, peripheral edema, distended neck veins, dyspnea, or cough. A small percentage of patients are allergic to dextran 40, with urticaria being the most common sign. Anaphylaxis is possible.

Contraindications/Precautions: Dextran 40 is contraindicated in patients with severe chronic kidney disease (CKD) because fluid overload may result. Adequate fluid intake should be ensured in patients with severe dehydration who receive dextran to prevent renal failure due to high urine viscosity. Other contraindications include severe heart failure and hypervolemic disorders.

Drug Interactions: There are no clinically significant interactions. **Herbal/Food:** Unknown.

Pregnancy: No data are available on the use of this drug during pregnancy or lactation.

Treatment of Overdose: For patients with normal renal function, discontinuing the infusion will reduce adverse effects. Patients with CKD may benefit from an osmotic diuretic.

Clinician Responsibilities: Key clinical implications for patients receiving dextran 40 are included in Applied Clinical Judgment: Patients Receiving Pharmacotherapy for Fluid and Electrolyte Imbalances.

Drugs Similar to Dextran 40 (Gentran 40, Others)

The only solution similar to dextran is hetastarch.

Hetastarch (Hespan): Hetastarch is a complex mixture of a nonprotein polymer of the starch amylopectin. It is a synthetic colloid with properties similar to those of 5% albumin, but with an extended duration of action. Hetastarch has a half-life of about 17 days and provides volume expansion for 24 to 36 hours. It is indicated for the treatment and prophylaxis of shock and acute edematous conditions. Hetastarch provides the same physiologic actions as albumin. This drug is embryocidal in laboratory animals and should be used during pregnancy only if the potential benefits to the mother justify the potential risks to the fetus.

Physiology of Electrolytes

33.8 Electrolytes are charged substances that are essential to homeostasis.

Minerals are inorganic substances needed in very small amounts to maintain homeostasis (see Chapter 61). Minerals are held together by ionic bonds and dissociate or ionize when placed in water. The resulting ions have positive or negative charges and are able to conduct electricity, hence the name **electrolyte**. Positively charged electrolytes are called cations; those with a negative charge are anions. Electrolyte levels are measured in units of milliequivalents per liter (mEq/L).

Electrolytes are essential to many body functions, including nerve conduction, membrane permeability, muscle contraction, water balance, and bone growth and remodeling. Levels of electrolytes in body fluids are maintained within very narrow ranges, primarily by the kidneys and GI tract. Because electrolytes are lost due to normal excretory functions, they must be replaced by adequate intake; otherwise, electrolyte imbalances will result, as shown in Table 33.5. Although imbalances can occur with any ion, sodium,

Table 33.5 Electrolyte Imbalances

Ion	Condition	Abnormal Serum Value (mEq/L)	Supportive Treatment*
Calcium	Hypercalcemia Hypocalcemia	Greater than 11 Less than 4	Hypotonic fluid or calcitonin Calcium supplements or vitamin D
Chloride	Hyperchloremia Hypochloremia	Greater than 112 Less than 95	Hypotonic fluid Hypertonic salt solution
Magnesium	Hypermagnesemia Hypomagnesemia	Greater than 4 Less than 0.8	Hypotonic fluid Magnesium supplements
Phosphate	Hyperphosphatemia Hypophosphatemia	Greater than 6 Less than 1	Dietary phosphate restriction Phosphate supplements
Potassium	Hyperkalemia Hypokalemia	Greater than 5 Less than 3.5	Hypotonic fluid, buffers, or dietary restriction Potassium supplements
Sodium	Hypernatremia Hyponatremia	Greater than 145 Less than 135	Hypotonic fluid or dietary restriction Hypertonic salt solution or sodium supplement

*For all electrolyte imbalances, the primary therapeutic goal is to identify and correct the cause of the imbalance.

potassium, and calcium are of greatest importance. The role of calcium in bone homeostasis is presented in Chapter 72.

An electrolyte imbalance is a sign of an underlying medical condition that needs attention. Imbalances are associated with a wide variety of acute and chronic disorders, with CKD being the most common cause. In some cases, drug therapy itself can cause the electrolyte imbalance. A classic example is the diuretic furosemide (Lasix), which can cause serious potassium depletion. In all cases, the therapeutic goal is to quickly correct the electrolyte imbalance while the underlying condition is being diagnosed and treated. Treatments for electrolyte imbalances depend on the severity of the problem and range from simple changes in dietary intake to rapid electrolyte infusions. In acute cases, serum electrolyte levels must be carefully monitored to prevent imbalances in the opposite direction; levels can change rapidly from hypoconcentrations to hyperconcentrations.

Pharmacotherapy of Electrolyte Imbalances

33.9 Sodium balance is closely associated with water balance.

Sodium is the major electrolyte in extracellular fluid. Due to its central roles in neuromuscular physiology, acid–base balance, and overall fluid distribution, sodium imbalances can have serious consequences. The normal range of serum sodium is 135 to 145 mEq/L of plasma.

Sodium balance and water balance are intimately connected. As sodium levels increase in a body fluid, solute particles accumulate and osmolality increases. Water will move toward this area of relatively high osmolality. In simplest terms, water travels toward or with sodium. The physiologic consequences of this relationship cannot be overstated: As the sodium and water content of plasma increases, so do blood volume and blood pressure. Thus, sodium movement provides an important link between water retention, blood volume, and blood pressure.

In healthy individuals, sodium intake is equal to sodium output, which is regulated by the kidneys. High levels of aldosterone secreted by the adrenal cortex promote sodium and water retention by the kidneys as well as potassium excretion. Inhibition of aldosterone promotes sodium and water excretion. When a patient ingests high amounts of sodium, aldosterone secretion decreases, thus sending the excess sodium to the urine. This relationship is illustrated in Figure 33.2.

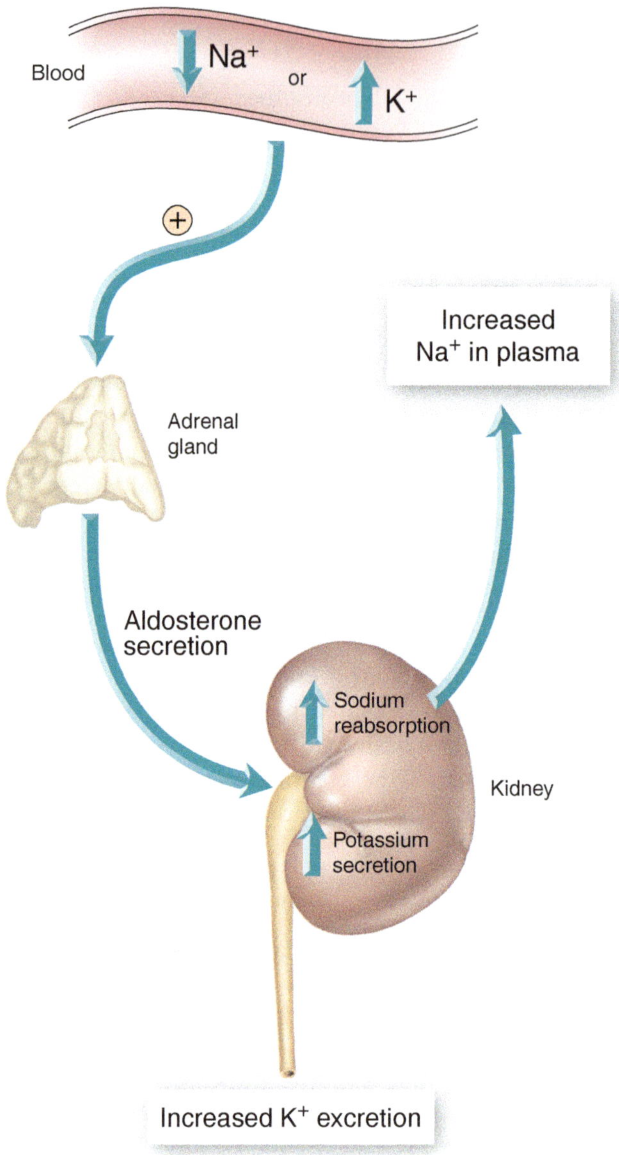

Figure 33.2 Renal regulation of sodium and potassium balance.

Hypernatremia: Sodium excess, or **hypernatremia**, occurs when the serum sodium level rises above 145 mEq/L. The most common cause of hypernatremia is decreased sodium excretion due to kidney pathology. Hypernatremia may also be caused by excessive intake of sodium, either through dietary consumption or by overtreatment with IV fluids containing sodium chloride or sodium bicarbonate. Overconsumption of table salt (NaCl) or processed foods with high sodium content will quickly exceed the daily amount needed by the body. Drinking too little water can cause hypernatremia due to the development of hypertonic plasma. Another cause of hypernatremia is high net water losses, such as that occurring from watery diarrhea, fever, or burns. High doses of glucocorticoids or estrogens also promote sodium retention.

A high serum sodium level increases the osmolality of the plasma, making the intravascular space hypertonic and drawing fluid from interstitial spaces and cells, thus causing cellular dehydration. Ordinarily, a small increase in serum sodium will trigger thirst. Other manifestations of hypernatremia include fatigue, weakness, muscle twitching, convulsions, altered mental status, and a decreased level of consciousness (LOC). For minor hypernatremia, a low-salt diet combined with adequate water intake may be effective in returning serum sodium to normal levels. In patients with acute hypernatremia, however, the treatment goal is to rapidly return the osmolality of the plasma to normal. If the patient is hypovolemic, infusing hypotonic fluids such as 5% dextrose or 0.45% NaCl will increase plasma volume and at the same time reduce osmolality by diluting the plasma. For the patient who is hypervolemic, diuretics may be used to remove sodium and excess water from the body.

Hyponatremia: **Hyponatremia** is the most common electrolyte abnormality in hospitalized patients and is defined as a serum sodium level of less than 135 mEq/L. Hyponatremia may occur through excessive dilution of the plasma caused by administration of hypotonic IV solutions or by high ADH secretion. Hyponatremia may also result from increased sodium loss due to disorders of the skin, GI tract, or kidneys. Significant loss of sodium by the skin may occur in burn patients and in those experiencing excessive sweating or prolonged fever. GI sodium losses may occur from vomiting, diarrhea, or GI suctioning, and renal sodium loss may occur with diuretic use and in certain advanced kidney disorders.

Early symptoms of hyponatremia include nausea and vomiting, anorexia, and abdominal cramping. Later signs include altered neurologic function such as confusion, lethargy, convulsions, coma, and muscle twitching or tremors. Hyponatremia caused by excessive dilution is treated with loop diuretics, which will remove the fluid overload that caused the hyponatremia (see Chapter 32). Hyponatremia caused by sodium loss may be treated with the administration of oral or parenteral sodium chloride, or with IV fluids containing salt, such as normal saline or lactated Ringer solution.

Tolvaptan (Jynarque, Samsca) is approved to quickly raise serum sodium levels in hospitalized patients experiencing symptoms of hyponatremia. Tolvaptan is a vasopressin (antidiuretic hormone) antagonist that enhances water excretion. As the amount of water in the blood is reduced, the serum sodium concentration is increased. Tolvaptan carries several black box warnings. Therapy with the drug should only be conducted in a hospital where serum sodium levels can be monitored closely because too-rapid correction of hyponatremia can result in seizures, coma, and death. In patients with advanced liver disease, severe malnutrition, or alcoholism, hyponatremia should be corrected especially slowly. Treatment should be limited to 30 days due to the risk for liver injury.

CONNECTIONS: Community-Oriented Practice

Maintaining Fluid Balance During Exercise

Hyponatremia from excessive fluid intake has been noted as a growing problem in athletes, particularly novice athletes who may have heard that they need to "keep drinking" to maintain hydration. Many sports drinks contain some electrolytes but are also high in fructose or other sugars. This creates a hypertonic solution that may paradoxically cause increased water loss. Unless exercise is extreme or prolonged, athletes, especially children, should be encouraged to drink when thirsty and maintain urine at a color of clear yellow, not dark yellow or colorless. Adequate fluid intake to match thirst will help ensure normal hydration and sodium levels and prevent complications such as exercise-associated hyponatremia.

PROTOTYPE DRUG Sodium Chloride (NaCl)

Classification **Therapeutic:** Drug for hyponatremia
Pharmacologic: Electrolyte, sodium supplement

Therapeutic Effects and Uses: Sodium chloride may be administered for hyponatremia when serum levels fall below 135 mEq/L. The drug is available in several concentrations; the decision on which NaCl concentration to administer is driven by the severity of the sodium deficiency. Normal saline consists of 0.9% NaCl and is used to treat mild hyponatremia. When serum sodium falls below 115 mEq/L, a highly concentrated 3% NaCl solution may be infused. Other concentrations include 0.45% and 0.22%, and both hypotonic and isotonic solutions are available. For less severe hyponatremia, 1-g tablets are available.

Ophthalmic solutions of NaCl may be used to treat corneal edema, and an over-the-counter nasal spray is available to relieve dry, inflamed nasal membranes. In conjunction with oxytocin, 20% NaCl may be used as an abortifacient late in pregnancy when instilled into the amniotic sac.

Mechanism of Action: Sodium chloride is a replacement solution for lost sodium.

Pharmacokinetics: Because sodium ions form natural electrolytes, it is not possible to obtain accurate pharmacokinetic values. The sodium ions in the drug are widely distributed and excreted by the kidneys in the same manner as endogenous sodium ions.

Adverse Effects: Patients receiving NaCl infusions must be monitored frequently to avoid symptoms of hypernatremia, which include lethargy, confusion, muscle tremor or rigidity, hypotension, and restlessness. Because some of these symptoms are also common to hyponatremia, periodic laboratory assessments must be taken to be certain that sodium values are moving toward the normal range. When infusing 3% NaCl solutions, the nurse should continuously check for signs of pulmonary edema.

Contraindications/Precautions: This drug should not be administered to patients with hypernatremia, heart failure, or impaired renal function.

Drug Interactions: There are no clinically significant drug interactions. **Herbal/Food:** Unknown.

Pregnancy: No data are available on the use of this drug during pregnancy or lactation.

Treatment of Overdose: There is no specific treatment for overdose. If excess fluid accumulation has occurred, diuretics may be administered to remove excess sodium ion and water to reduce pulmonary or peripheral edema.

Clinician Responsibilities: Key clinical implications for patients receiving sodium chloride are included in Applied Clinical Judgment: Patients Receiving Pharmacotherapy for Fluid and Electrolyte Imbalances.

Drugs Similar to Sodium Chloride (NaCl)

There are no drugs similar to sodium chloride.

33.10 Potassium imbalances must be quickly corrected to prevent serious cardiac consequences.

Potassium is the most abundant intracellular cation; 98% of the potassium present in the body is found inside cells, with the majority found in skeletal muscle. Potassium serves critical roles in muscular contraction and the conduction of nerve impulses.

To prevent imbalances, adequate dietary intake of potassium must be carefully balanced to potassium excretion. Patients with normal diets consume plenty of potassium for bodily functions because the mineral is abundant in fruits, vegetables, and meats.

Insulin is a key hormone for the regulation of potassium homeostasis. The uptake of potassium ion into cells is mediated by insulin. As serum potassium levels rise, the pancreas secretes additional insulin, which causes the ion to move out of the plasma and into cells, thus preventing hyperkalemia. In a typical feedback loop, as serum potassium levels fall, insulin secretion is diminished.

Acid–base imbalances may also affect potassium homeostasis. As the blood becomes acidic, the body attempts to raise plasma pH by pumping hydrogen ions (H^+) into cells. To maintain electrical neutrality, each H^+ entering the cell is exchanged for a K^+ leaving the cell. This can raise the serum potassium level, resulting in hyperkalemia. This is sometimes called a false hyperkalemia because the total body potassium is not actually increased; it has just shifted from intracellular to extracellular spaces.

Potassium ion is freely filtered at the glomerulus but is entirely reabsorbed as it travels along the kidney tubule. In the distal tubule, however, potassium is secreted back into the renal tubule and exits in the urine. Like sodium, potassium excretion is influenced by the actions of aldosterone on the kidney. In fact, the renal excretion of sodium and potassium ions is closely linked. For every sodium ion that is reabsorbed, one potassium ion is secreted into the renal tubules.

Potassium levels must be maintained within narrow limits. Both hyper- and hypokalemia are associated with fatal dysrhythmias and serious neuromuscular disorders. Because over 98% of potassium is intracellular, serum potassium may not be an accurate reflection of total body potassium. Normal adult values for serum potassium range from 3.5 to 5 mEq/L.

Hyperkalemia: **Hyperkalemia** occurs when the serum potassium level rises above 5 mEq/L. This condition may be caused by excessive consumption of potassium-rich foods or dietary supplements, particularly when patients are taking potassium-sparing diuretics such as spironolactone (see Chapter 32). In fact, overtreatment with potassium supplements is the most common cause of hyperkalemia. Excess potassium may also accumulate when renal excretion is diminished due to kidney pathology. The most serious consequences of hyperkalemia are related to cardiac function: dysrhythmias and heart block. Other symptoms are muscle twitching, fatigue, paresthesias, dyspnea, cramping, and diarrhea. Hyperkalemia is much less common than hypokalemia.

In mild cases of hyperkalemia, potassium levels may be returned to normal by restricting primary dietary sources of potassium such as bananas, citrus and dried fruits, peanut butter, broccoli, and green leafy vegetables. All potassium supplements and the use of salt substitutes containing potassium should be discontinued. If the patient is taking a potassium-sparing diuretic, the dose must be lowered, or a thiazide or loop diuretic substituted.

Several options are available for patients with severe hyperkalemia. Administration of the diuretic furosemide (Lasix) can significantly increase the urinary excretion of potassium within 5 to 15 minutes. Administering glucose or dextrose concurrently with insulin temporarily lowers serum potassium levels by causing potassium to leave the extracellular fluid and enter cells. In all patients who are symptomatic, calcium gluconate or calcium chloride is administered to prevent or treat potassium-induced cardiotoxicity. Sodium bicarbonate is sometimes infused to correct any acidosis that may be concurrent with the hyperkalemia.

Three potassium-binding drugs are available for treating hyperkalemia. Sodium polystyrene sulfonate (Kayexalate), given orally or rectally, exchanges Na^+ for K^+ as the drug travels through the intestine. The onset of action is 1 hour, and the dose may be repeated every 4 hours as needed. The drug is given concurrently with a laxative such as sorbitol to promote rapid evacuation of the potassium. The primary adverse effects are hypernatremia, diarrhea, and nausea and vomiting. A black box warning states that life-threatening colonic necrosis has been reported with this medication.

A second potassium binder, patiromer (Veltassa), was approved in 2015. Like polystyrene sulfonate, it binds potassium in the GI tract and eliminates it in the feces. Adverse effects include constipation, diarrhea, hypomagnesemia, and hypokalemia. This oral drug is slow-acting and is not for emergency control of hyperkalemia.

The newest of the potassium binders is sodium zirconium cyclosilicate (Lokelma), which was approved in 2018. Like the other potassium binders, it increases the fecal excretion of potassium by binding potassium in the GI tract. This oral drug is slow-acting and is not for emergency control of hyperkalemia. Adverse effects include edema and hypokalemia.

None of the potassium binders are absorbed from the GI tract. Because of this, no adverse effects on pregnancy or lactation are expected.

Hypokalemia: **Hypokalemia** is one of the most common electrolyte imbalances and occurs when the serum potassium level falls below 3.5 mEq/L. The most frequent cause of hypokalemia is pharmacotherapy with loop and thiazide diuretics. In addition, strenuous muscular activity and severe vomiting or diarrhea can lead to significant potassium loss. Because the body does not have large stores of potassium, adequate daily dietary intake is necessary. Neurons and muscle fibers are most sensitive to potassium loss, and muscle weakness, lethargy, anorexia, dysrhythmias, and cardiac arrest are possible consequences.

Mild hypokalemia is treated by increasing the dietary intake of potassium-rich foods. The foods highest in potassium content include dried fruit, nuts, molasses, avocados, lima beans, and bran cereals. If increasing dietary intake is not possible, a large number of potassium products are available for oral supplementation. The most common supplements are the chloride salts because they supply both potassium and chloride, which are lost during diuretic therapy. Liquid preparations are very effective, although many must be diluted with water or fruit juices prior to administration. Extended-release (K-Dur 20, Slow-K, Micro-K) forms and powders (Klor-Con) are also available.

Severe hypokalemia may require parenteral potassium supplements. Caution must always be used when using IV potassium because rapid administration of the drug can be fatal, especially for patients with CKD. Cardiac function should be closely monitored during IV potassium therapy.

PROTOTYPE DRUG | Potassium Chloride (KCl)

Classification **Therapeutic:** Drug for hypokalemia
Pharmacologic: Electrolyte, potassium supplement

Therapeutic Effects and Uses: Potassium chloride is a preferred drug for preventing or treating hypokalemia because potassium and chloride depletion usually occur concurrently. It is also used to treat mild forms of alkalosis. Oral formulations of potassium chloride include tablets, powders, and liquids, usually heavily flavored due to its unpleasant taste. Because potassium supplements can cause peptic ulcers, the drug should be diluted with plenty of water. When given IV, potassium must be administered slowly because bolus injections can overload the heart and cause cardiac arrest. Because pharmacotherapy with loop or thiazide diuretics is the most common cause of potassium depletion, patients taking these drugs are usually prescribed PO potassium supplements to prevent hypokalemia.

Mechanism of Action: Potassium chloride is a replacement solution for lost potassium.

Pharmacokinetics: Because potassium chloride is a natural electrolyte, it is not possible to obtain accurate pharmacokinetic values. The potassium ions in the drug are widely distributed and excreted by the kidneys in the same manner as endogenous potassium ions.

Adverse Effects: Nausea and vomiting, diarrhea, and abdominal pain are common because potassium chloride irritates the GI mucosa. The drug may be taken with meals or antacids to lessen gastric distress. The most serious adverse effects of potassium chloride are related to the possible accumulation of excess potassium. Hyperkalemia may occur if the patient takes potassium supplements concurrently with potassium-sparing diuretics. Because the kidneys perform over 90% of the body's potassium excretion functions, reduced renal function can rapidly lead to hyperkalemia, particularly in patients taking potassium supplements.

Contraindications/Precautions: Potassium chloride is contraindicated in patients with hyperkalemia, systemic acidosis, severe dehydration, extensive tissue breakdown as in severe burns, or adrenal insufficiency. Oral potassium supplements are contraindicated in any condition for which transit through the GI tract is delayed because prolonged contact may damage the GI mucosa. The drug should be used with extreme caution in patients with CKD or acute kidney injury (AKI) because the drug may accumulate to high levels.

Drug Interactions: Potassium supplements should not be administered to patients who are taking potassium-sparing diuretics because hyperkalemia may result. Angiotensin-converting enzyme (ACE) inhibitors prevent aldosterone secretion and cause potassium retention, thus increasing the risk for hyperkalemia if administered with potassium supplements. Drugs that slow GI transit time, such as anticholinergics, may increase the GI toxicity of potassium supplements. **Herbal/Food:** Unknown.

Pregnancy: No data are available on the use of this drug during pregnancy or lactation.

Treatment of Overdose: Potassium-sparing diuretics and all foods and medications containing potassium should be withheld. Treatment includes IV administration of 10% dextrose solution containing 10 to 20 units of crystalline insulin. Sodium bicarbonate may be infused to correct acidosis. Polystyrene sulfonate may be administered to enhance potassium elimination.

Clinician Responsibilities: Key clinical implications for patients receiving potassium chloride are included in Applied Clinical Judgment: Patients Receiving Pharmacotherapy for Fluid and Electrolyte Imbalances.

Drugs Similar to Potassium Chloride (KCl)

Other potassium drugs include acetate, bicarbonate, citrate, and gluconate salts. Potassium acetate is used as an IV alternative to potassium chloride. Potassium bicarbonate supplies bicarbonate ion, which is alkaline and may be useful in treating acidosis. Potassium citrate makes the urine less acidic and is primarily used to reduce the formation of kidney stones. Potassium gluconate is commonly available in tablet form and dissociates to potassium ion and gluconate ion, a form of glucose.

33.11 Magnesium imbalances significantly affect cardiovascular and neuromuscular function.

Magnesium is the second most abundant intracellular cation and, like potassium, it is essential for proper neuromuscular function. Magnesium also serves a metabolic role in activating certain enzymes in the breakdown of carbohydrates and proteins; it is a cofactor in over 300 biochemical reactions. Patients with disorders of magnesium homeostasis generally present with cardiovascular and neuromuscular symptoms. Because the majority of magnesium is stored in bone, serum magnesium levels are not accurate indicators of total body magnesium.

Magnesium levels are primarily controlled by the kidney. The ion is freely filtered and reabsorbed in the loop of Henle and loop diuretics such as furosemide can cause significant magnesium loss. Magnesium imbalances may occur in individuals with CKD. Magnesium is absorbed by the small intestine and small amounts are secreted in intestinal fluid.

Hypomagnesemia: Because it produces few symptoms until serum levels fall below 1 mEq/L, hypomagnesemia is sometimes called the most common undiagnosed electrolyte abnormality. Although the overall incidence for magnesium deficiency is 6 to 12%, the majority of critically ill patients present with this condition. Renal causes of hypomagnesemia include kidney failure and therapy with loop diuretics. GI causes include malabsorption disorders and loss of significant amounts of body fluids due to diarrhea, chronic laxative abuse, or nasogastric suctioning. Hypomagnesemia may also present in people with alcoholism and in those receiving prolonged parenteral feeding with magnesium-free solutions. Patients may experience general weakness, dysrhythmias, HTN, loss of deep tendon reflexes, and respiratory depression—signs and symptoms that are sometimes mistaken for hypokalemia. Additional signs include muscle twitches, tetany, or seizures. Pharmacotherapy with magnesium sulfate can quickly reverse symptoms of hypomagnesemia (see Prototype feature).

> ### CONNECTIONS: Patient Safety
> **Control of Concentrated Electrolyte Solutions**
>
> While working with a clinical nurse preceptor, a student nurse asks the preceptor, "I've noticed that we have to wait for the pharmacy to deliver some medications and IVs. For example, we're supposed to hang that IV with potassium for the patient in room 318. Wouldn't it just be faster if nurses could mix the IV themselves on the unit?" How should the nurse respond?

Hypermagnesemia: Advanced CKD is the major cause of hypermagnesemia, although overtreatment with magnesium supplements may also lead to excessive serum magnesium levels. Clinical signs include central nervous system (CNS) depression, respiratory depression, hypotension, dysrhythmias, bradycardia, complete heart block, and coma. Infusions of calcium salts will immediately reverse the neuromuscular and cardiovascular signs. If the magnesium elevation is minor, treatment with furosemide to increase urinary excretion may be sufficient to reverse the hypermagnesemia.

PROTOTYPE DRUG Magnesium Sulfate ($MgSO_4$)

Classification **Therapeutic:** Drug for hypomagnesemia and seizures associated with eclampsia
Pharmacologic: Electrolyte, magnesium supplement

Therapeutic Effects and Uses: Magnesium supplements are available for both PO and parenteral routes. Severe hypomagnesemia can be rapidly reversed by the administration of intramuscular (IM) or IV magnesium sulfate. Because IM preparations produce significant pain at the injection site, severe cases of hypomagnesemia are normally treated using the IV route. Parenteral formulations include 4%, 8%, 12.5%, and 50% solutions. After administration, magnesium sulfate is distributed throughout the body, and therapeutic effects are observed within 30 to 60 minutes. Plasma magnesium levels should be monitored frequently during therapy.

Oral forms of magnesium sulfate (Epsom salt) are used as cathartics, when complete evacuation of the colon is desired. Epsom salt is sometimes used in bath water to ease aching muscles, although the scientific basis for this use is lacking. Its action as a CNS depressant has led to its occasional use as an anticonvulsant in patients with preeclampsia or eclampsia (see Chapter 22). Magnesium sulfate has been used off-label to slow uterine contractions during preterm labor (see Chapter 69).

Mechanism of Action: Magnesium sulfate is a replacement solution for lost magnesium.

Pharmacokinetics:

Route(s)	PO, IM, IV
Absorption	Not absorbed
Distribution	Widely distributed; crosses the placenta; secreted in breast milk
Primary metabolism	Not metabolized
Primary excretion	Renal
Onset of action	PO: 1–2 h; IM: 1 h; IV: immediate
Duration of action	PO and IM: 3–4 h; IV: 30 min; half-life: unknown

Adverse Effects: Patients receiving IV infusions of magnesium sulfate require careful observation to prevent toxicity. Early signs of magnesium overdose include flushing of the skin, sedation, confusion, intense thirst, and muscle weakness. Extreme levels cause neuromuscular blockade with resultant respiratory paralysis, heart block, and circulatory collapse. Because of these potentially fatal adverse effects, the use of magnesium sulfate is restricted to patients with severe magnesium deficiency. Mild to moderate hypomagnesemia is treated with oral forms of magnesium such as magnesium gluconate or magnesium hydroxide. Oral magnesium sulfate often causes diarrhea.

Contraindications/Precautions: Magnesium is contraindicated in patients with serious cardiac disease. Oral administration is contraindicated in those with undiagnosed abdominal pain, intestinal obstruction, or fecal impaction. The drug should be used cautiously in patients with CKD because the drug may rise to toxic levels rapidly.

Drug Interactions: Use with neuromuscular blockers may increase respiratory depression and apnea. Because magnesium sulfate has CNS depression effects, patients receiving other CNS depressants may experience increased sedation. **Herbal/Food:** Magnesium salts may decrease the absorption of certain anti-infectives such as tetracycline.

Pregnancy: Continuous use during pregnancy for longer than 5 to 7 days may result in neonates with skeletal abnormalities. The drug is considered safe during lactation.

Treatment of Overdose: Serious respiratory and cardiac suppression may result from overdose. Calcium gluconate or gluceptate may be administered IV as an antidote.

Clinician Responsibilities: Key clinical implications for patients receiving magnesium sulfate are included in Applied Clinical Judgment: Patients Receiving Pharmacotherapy for Fluid and Electrolyte Imbalances.

Drugs Similar to Magnesium Sulfate ($MgSO_4$)

Several oral magnesium salts are available OTC. Magnesium citrate (citrate of magnesia) and magnesium hydroxide (milk of magnesia) are classified as laxatives or cathartics. Magnesium oxide (Mag-Ox) is an antacid, and magnesium salicylate (Doan's Pills) is used as an analgesic.

PharmFACT

Although the recommended dietary allowance for magnesium is 420 mg/day in men and 320 mg/day in women, certain patients need higher levels to maintain health. These include people with Crohn's disease, type 2 diabetes, pregnant or lactating women, older adults, and people with alcohol dependence (Office of Dietary Supplements, 2020).

Pharmacotherapy of Acid–Base Imbalances

33.12 The pH of body fluids must be maintained between very narrow limits.

The degree of acidity or alkalinity of a solution is measured by its pH. A pH of 7.0 is defined as neutral, above 7.0 as basic or alkaline, and below 7.0 as acidic. To maintain homeostasis, the pH of plasma and most body fluids must be kept within the narrow range of 7.35 to 7.45 because nearly all proteins and enzymes in the body function optimally within this range. A few enzymes, most notably those in the digestive tract, require pH values outside the 7.35 to 7.45 range to function properly.

The body generates significant amounts of acids during normal metabolic processes. Without an effective means of neutralizing these metabolic acids, the overall pH of body fluids would quickly fall below the normal range. **Buffers** are chemicals that help maintain normal body pH by neutralizing strong acids and bases. The two primary buffers in the body are bicarbonate ions and phosphate ions.

The body uses two mechanisms to remove acid. The acidic carbon dioxide (CO_2) produced during body metabolism is efficiently removed by the lungs during exhalation. The kidneys remove excess acid in the form of hydrogen ion (H^+) by excreting it in the urine. If retained in the body, either CO_2 or H^+ will lower body pH. Normal acid–base balance is maintained by the lungs and kidneys. Impairment of these organs commonly leads to change in pH.

Acidosis (excess acid) and alkalosis (excess base) are not diseases but are symptoms of an underlying medical disorder. Acidic drugs and basic drugs are administered to rapidly correct pH imbalances in body fluids, supporting the patient's vital functions while the underlying disease is being treated. The correction of acid–base imbalance is illustrated in Figure 33.3.

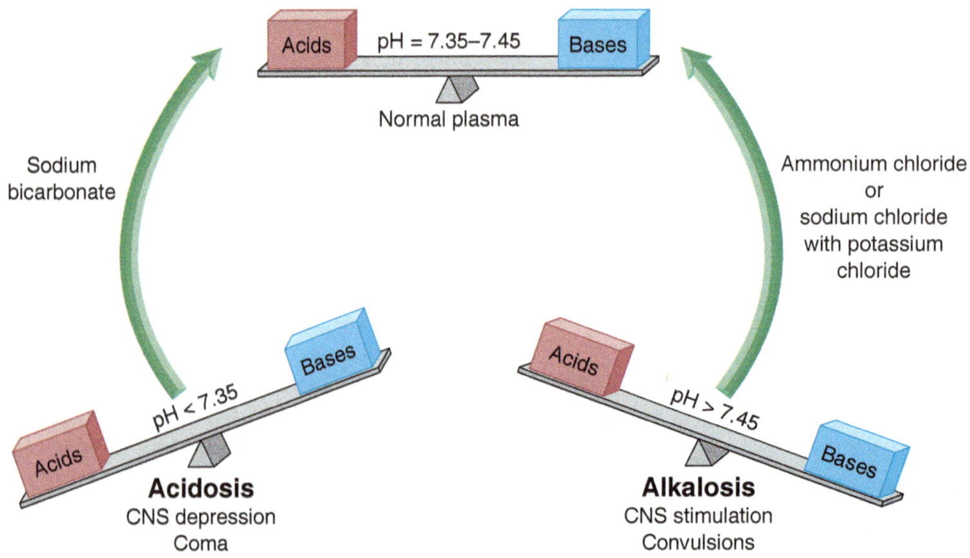

Figure 33.3 Acid–base imbalances.

Acidosis

33.13 The pharmacotherapy of acidosis includes the administration of alkaline drugs.

Acidosis occurs when the pH of the plasma falls below 7.35, which is confirmed by measuring arterial pH, partial pressure of carbon dioxide (P_{CO2}), and plasma bicarbonate levels. For proper pharmacotherapy, the diagnosis must differentiate between respiratory etiology and metabolic (renal) etiology. Occasionally, the cause has mixed respiratory and metabolic components.

The most profound symptoms of acidosis affect the CNS and include lethargy, confusion, and CNS depression leading to coma. A deep, rapid respiration rate indicates an attempt by the lungs to rid the body of excess acid. Common causes of acidosis are shown in Table 33.6.

In patients with acidosis, the therapeutic goal is to quickly reverse the adverse effects caused by excess acids in the blood. Mild acidosis may be treated with oral bicarbonate or citrate salts or other basic substances. For acute acidosis the preferred treatment is to administer infusions of sodium bicarbonate. Bicarbonate ion is a base that can quickly neutralize acids in the blood and other body fluids. The patient must be carefully monitored during infusions because this drug can overcorrect the acidosis, causing blood pH to turn alkaline. Sodium citrate, sodium lactate, and sodium acetate are alternative alkaline drugs that may be used in place of bicarbonate.

Alkalinizing drugs are also used to aid in the renal excretion of toxic substances through a phenomenon called **ion trapping**. Whenever a large pH gradient exists across a membrane, drug molecules will accumulate on the side where the opportunity for ionization is greatest. Recall from Chapter 3 that acids ionize in a basic environment; bases ionize in acidic solutions. The infusion of an alkalinizing drug will create an alkaline filtrate in the kidney tubule, a perfect environment for ionization of an acidic drug like aspirin. Rather than being absorbed back into the body, the ionized aspirin remains trapped in the filtrate and is excreted in the urine. Thus, through ion trapping, the alkalinizing drug was able to move aspirin from the blood to the urine.

Table 33.6 Causes of Acidosis and Alkalosis

Acidosis	Alkalosis
Respiratory Origins of Acidosis	**Respiratory Origin of Alkalosis**
Hypoventilation or shallow breathing Airway constriction Damage to respiratory center in medulla	Hyperventilation due to asthma, anxiety, or high altitude
Metabolic Origins of Acidosis	**Metabolic Origins of Alkalosis**
Severe diarrhea Kidney failure Diabetes mellitus Excess alcohol ingestion Starvation	Constipation for prolonged periods Ingestion of or treatment with excess sodium bicarbonate Diuretics that cause potassium depletion Severe vomiting

PROTOTYPE DRUG **Sodium Bicarbonate**

Classification **Therapeutic:** Drug to treat acidosis or bicarbonate deficiency
Pharmacologic: Electrolyte, sodium, and bicarbonate supplement

Therapeutic Effects and Uses: Sodium bicarbonate is a preferred drug for correcting metabolic acidosis. After dissociation, the bicarbonate ion directly raises the pH of body fluids. Sodium bicarbonate may be given PO if acidosis is mild or IV in cases of acute disease. IV concentrations range from 4.2% to 8.4%. Although sodium bicarbonate also neutralizes gastric acid, it is rarely used to treat peptic ulcers due to its tendency to cause uncomfortable gastric distention. The PO form of sodium bicarbonate is commonly known as baking soda.

Sodium bicarbonate may also be used to alkalinize the urine to speed the excretion of acidic medications such as aspirin and phenobarbital and as adjunctive therapy for certain chemotherapeutic drugs such as methotrexate. Sodium bicarbonate is also used in individuals with CKD to neutralize the metabolic acidosis that occurs when the kidneys cannot excrete hydrogen ion. When IV sodium bicarbonate is given, it causes the urine to become more alkaline. Less acid is reabsorbed, so more acid and acidic medicine are excreted. This process is known as ion trapping.

Mechanism of Action: The bicarbonate ion in sodium bicarbonate buffers excess acid (H^+) to raise the pH of body fluids.

Pharmacokinetics:

Route(s)	IV, PO
Absorption	Rapidly absorbed
Distribution	Widely distributed in body fluids
Primary metabolism	Not metabolized
Primary excretion	Renal
Onset of action	PO: 15 min; IV: immediate
Duration of action	PO: 1–3 h; IV: 8–10 min

Adverse Effects: Most of the adverse effects of sodium bicarbonate therapy are the result of metabolic alkalosis created by receiving too much bicarbonate ion. Symptoms may include confusion, irritability, slow respiration rate, and vomiting. Discontinuing the sodium bicarbonate infusion often reverses these symptoms; however, potassium chloride or ammonium chloride may be administered to reverse acute alkalosis. During sodium bicarbonate infusions, serum electrolytes should be carefully monitored because sodium levels may lead to hypernatremia and fluid retention. In addition, high levels of bicarbonate ion passing through the kidney tubules increase potassium secretion, which could lead to hypokalemia.

Contraindications/Precautions: Patients who are vomiting, have severe diarrhea, or have continuous GI suctioning will lose acid and chloride and may be in a state of metabolic alkalosis; therefore, they should not receive sodium bicarbonate because it may worsen alkalosis. Due to the sodium content of this drug, it should be used cautiously in patients with cardiac disease, HTN, or CKD.

Drug Interactions: Sodium bicarbonate may decrease the absorption of ketoconazole and may decrease elimination of dextroamphetamine, ephedrine, pseudoephedrine, and quinidine. The elimination of lithium, salicylates, and tetracyclines may be increased. **Herbal/Food:** Chronic use with milk or calcium supplements may cause milk-alkali syndrome, a condition characterized by serious hypercalcemia and possible kidney failure.

Pregnancy: No data are available on the use of this drug during pregnancy or lactation.

Treatment of Overdose: Overdose results in metabolic alkalosis, which is treated by administering acidic drugs (see Section 33.14).

Clinician Responsibilities: Key clinical implications for patients receiving sodium bicarbonate are included in Applied Clinical Judgment: Patients Receiving Pharmacotherapy for Fluid and Electrolyte Imbalances.

Drugs Similar to Sodium Bicarbonate

There are no drugs similar to sodium bicarbonate.

Alkalosis

33.14 The pharmacotherapy of alkalosis includes the administration of acidic drugs.

At plasma pH values above 7.45, **alkalosis** develops. Mortality can reach as high as 80% if the pH rises above 7.65. Like acidosis, alkalosis may have either respiratory or metabolic causes, as shown in Table 33.6. Also like acidosis, the CNS is greatly affected. Symptoms of CNS stimulation occur and include nervousness, hyperactive reflexes, and convulsions. In metabolic alkalosis, slow, shallow breathing indicates that the body is attempting to compensate by retaining acid and lowering internal pH. Life-threatening dysrhythmias are the most serious adverse effects of alkalosis.

In mild cases, metabolic alkalosis may be corrected by administering sodium chloride combined with potassium chloride. This combination increases the renal excretion of bicarbonate ion, which indirectly increases the acidity of the blood. More severe alkalosis may be treated with infusions of an acidic drug such as ammonium chloride or hydrochloric acid.

PROTOTYPE DRUG | **Ammonium Chloride**

Classification **Therapeutic:** Drug for treating metabolic alkalosis and hypochloremia
Pharmacologic: Acidic drug

Therapeutic Effects and Uses: Ammonium chloride is an acidic substance that has been available as a drug to treat severe metabolic alkalosis for over 80 years. Ammonium chloride acidifies the urine, which is beneficial in treating certain urinary tract infections. Historically, it has been used as a mild diuretic, though safer and more effective agents have made its use obsolete. By acidifying the urine, ammonium chloride promotes the excretion of alkaline drugs such as amphetamines through ion trapping. Oral and IV forms are available; when given for alkalosis, the IV route is preferred. Because of the potential for causing acidosis, injection-site reactions, and ammonia toxicity, the drug is infused slowly.

Mechanism of Action: During the hepatic conversion of ammonium chloride to urea, Cl^- and H^+ are formed. The H^+ combines with bicarbonate to form the weak acid carbonic acid, which dissociates to water and carbon dioxide. By removing bicarbonate, ammonium chloride decreases the pH of body fluids. The chloride ion also combines with bases to reduce the alkalinity of extracellular fluids.

Pharmacokinetics:

Route(s)	IV, PO
Absorption	Rapidly absorbed
Distribution	Unknown
Primary metabolism	Hepatic
Primary excretion	Renal
Onset of action	Unknown
Duration of action	Unknown

Adverse Effects: Aggressive treatment with ammonium chloride can cause acidosis. Characteristic symptoms of acidosis include CNS depression, drowsiness, confusion, and coma. Periods of CNS excitement may alternate with coma. Oral forms of the drug are irritating to the gastric mucosa and may cause nausea and vomiting.

Contraindications/Precautions: Ammonium chloride should not be administered to patients with serious hepatic impairment or severe CKD because the drug will accumulate to toxic levels. It should not be administered to patients with either metabolic or respiratory acidosis.

Drug Interactions: Ammonium chloride may cause crystalluria when taken with aminosalicylic acid. Antacids should not be administered concurrently because they are alkaline and will antagonize the acidifying effects of ammonium chloride. Ammonium chloride reduces levels of amphetamines, flecainide, mexiletine, methadone, ephedrine, and pseudoephedrine. Urinary excretion of sulfonylureas and salicylates is decreased. Serum magnesium values may decrease. **Herbal/Food:** Unknown.

Pregnancy: No data are available on the use of this drug during pregnancy or lactation.

Treatment of Overdose: Overdose results in metabolic acidosis, which is treated by administering alkaline drugs (see Section 33.13).

Clinician Responsibilities: Key clinical implications for patients receiving ammonium chloride are included in Applied Clinical Judgment: Patients Receiving Pharmacotherapy for Fluid and Electrolyte Imbalances.

Drugs Similar to Ammonium Chloride

The only similar drug is hydrochloric acid.

Hydrochloric acid: Hydrochloric acid may be administered IV in severe cases of metabolic acidosis. A central venous catheter must be used to administer the drug. Hydrochloric acid is only used when sodium or potassium chloride cannot be administered due to volume overload or advanced CKD. This drug can cause severe tissue necrosis if it extravasates into the tissues.

CONNECTIONS: APPLIED CLINICAL JUDGMENT

Patients Receiving Pharmacotherapy for Fluid and Electrolyte Imbalances

Key Assessment Data

- History of current condition, baseline vital signs, LOC, breath sounds, and urinary output as appropriate, physical exam findings; history of cardiovascular (including HTN, myocardial infarction [MI]), neurologic (including stroke or head injury), burns, endocrine, hepatic, or renal disease; drug history including allergies, current prescriptions and OTC drugs, herbal preparations; pregnancy status.
- Ongoing assessment during drug therapy includes laboratory findings, for example, electrolytes, complete blood count (CBC), urine specific gravity and urinalysis, blood urea nitrogen (BUN) and creatinine, total protein and albumin levels, activated partial thromboplastin time (aPTT), activated prothrombin time (aPT) or international normalized ratio (INR), renal and liver function studies. Assess for location, character, and amount of edema, if present.
- Obtain baseline weight and continue to monitor daily weight.

Desired Therapeutic Outcomes

Improvement is observed and measurable in normalization of electrolyte values, blood pressure and pulse within normal limits, adequate urine output.

CONNECTIONS: APPLIED CLINICAL JUDGMENT *(continued)*

Patients Receiving Pharmacotherapy for Fluid and Electrolyte Imbalances

Minimizing Adverse Effects

- Monitor for signs of fluid volume excess or deficit, for example, HTN (excess) or hypotension (deficit), tachycardia, or changes in the quality of pulse (bounding or thready).
- Monitor for signs of potential electrolyte imbalance including nausea and vomiting, GI cramping, diarrhea, muscle weakness, cramping, twitching, paresthesia, and irritability. Immediately report any confusion, decreasing LOC, or increasing hypotension or HTN, especially if associated with tachycardia, decreased urine output, or seizures.
- Crystalloid solutions may cause electrolyte imbalances. Colloid solutions may reduce normal blood coagulation. Frequent monitoring of electrolyte levels while on replacement therapy may be needed. Frequently monitor CBC, electrolytes, aPTT, aPT, or INR levels.
- Dehydration and electrolyte imbalances may cause dizziness and hypotension. Orthostatic hypotension may increase the risk of falls and injury.
- Weigh daily. An increase in weight over 1 kg [2 lb] per day may indicate excessive fluid gain. A decrease of over 1 kg per day may indicate dehydration. Measure intake and output in the hospitalized patient.
- Potassium and ammonium are irritating to the vessel and phlebitis may result. Potassium is a "high-alert" medication. Double-check doses with another nurse before administration to prevent medication errors. Closely monitor IV sites when infusing potassium or ammonium. Assess swallowing ability before administering potassium chloride or ammonium chloride orally; they may cause mouth, esophageal, or gastric irritation. Liquid forms should always be diluted with water or fruit juice and tablets swallowed whole.
- Colloids such as plasma protein fraction, dextran, and hetastarch may cause allergic and anaphylactic reactions. Closely monitor for signs and symptoms of allergy if colloids are used.
- Adverse effects from hypermagnesemia include respiratory and cardiac arrest and neuromuscular depression. Monitor LOC, deep tendon reflexes, urinary output, respiratory rate, and laboratory values frequently in patients receiving parenteral magnesium sulfate. Keep calcium gluconate available as an antidote to magnesium toxicity.

Lifespan Considerations

- Older adults, infants, and patients who cannot access fluids or eat by themselves (e.g., post-stroke) are at increased risk for fluid and electrolyte imbalance.
- Orthostatic hypotension may increase the risk of falls and injury. Be particularly cautious with older adults who are at increased risk for hypotension. Ensure patient safety.
- Monitor LOC, deep tendon reflexes, urinary output, respiratory rate, and laboratory values frequently in the newborn if the mother has received the drug.

Patient and Caregiver Education

- Continue to consume enough liquids to remain adequately, but not overly, hydrated. Drinking when thirsty, avoiding alcoholic beverages, maintaining a healthy diet, and ensuring adequate but not excessive salt intake will assist in maintaining normal fluid and electrolyte balance. Assist those who cannot maintain adequate hydration (e.g., post-stroke).
- Weigh daily, ideally at the same time of day, and record weight along with blood pressure and pulse measurements as appropriate. Promptly report any weight gain over 1 kg in a 24-hour period or increasing edema to the provider.
- Rise slowly from lying or sitting to standing, pausing between changes if dizziness occurs.
- Promptly report changes in muscle strength or function; numbness and tingling in the lips, fingers, arms, or legs; palpitations; dizziness; nausea and/or vomiting; GI cramping; or decreased urination.
- Be aware of signs of hypokalemia (muscle weakness or cramping and palpitations) and immediately report them to your healthcare provider. Increase intake of foods high in potassium: fresh fruits such as strawberries and bananas; dried fruits such as apricots and prunes; vegetables and legumes such as tomatoes, beets, and dried beans; juices such as orange, grapefruit, or prune; and fresh meats. Licorice should be avoided because it causes potassium loss and sodium retention.
- Be aware of the signs of hyperkalemia (nausea, irregular heartbeat, profound fatigue or muscle weakness, and slow or faint pulse) and immediately report them to the healthcare provider. Avoid foods high in potassium; do not use salt substitutes, which often contain potassium salts; and consult with a healthcare provider before taking vitamin and mineral supplements or specialized sports beverages. Typical OTC sports beverages (e.g., Gatorade and Powerade) may have lesser amounts of potassium but have high carbohydrate amounts that may lead to diarrhea and the potential for dehydration from the hyperosmolarity.
- Assess swallowing ability before giving or taking potassium chloride or ammonium chloride; they may cause mouth, esophageal, or gastric irritation. Liquid forms should always be diluted with water or fruit juice and tablets swallowed whole.
- Excessive heat conditions contribute to excessive sweating and fluid and electrolyte loss, and extra caution is warranted in these conditions.
- If hypomagnesemia is present, consume foods high in magnesium—green leafy vegetables and legumes such as peas, beans, nuts, and whole grains—and increase fluid intake.
- If colloids are administered, report dyspnea, itching, feelings of throat tightness, palpitations, chest pain or tightening, or headache immediately.
- Consult with a healthcare provider before taking vitamin and mineral supplements.

Prescribing Considerations

- Prescribe fluids by adding or subtracting any deficits or excesses from routine fluid maintenance, in addition to adjusting for all other sources of fluids and electrolytes (e.g., oral, enteral, and medications).
- Lab Test Considerations: Monitor electrolytes, blood glucose, BUN, and hemoglobin levels before and periodically throughout course of therapy.
- Use a cautious approach to fluid prescribing for older adults.
- For patients with liver failure, excess Na^+ may cause ascites, so use 5% dextrose. If patient is hyponatremic, seek specialist input.
- For patients with AKI, avoid potassium supplementation.
- For patients with CKD, avoid excess fluids, sodium, and potassium.

Understanding Chapter 33

Key Concepts Summary

33.1 Body fluids are exchanged between intracellular and extracellular compartments.

33.2 Osmolality or tonicity determines the movement of body fluids.

33.3 Overall fluid balance is regulated primarily by hormones acting on the kidneys.

33.4 Dehydration may be treated with fluid volume expanders.

33.5 Transfusions of blood products are used to treat serious conditions that cannot be managed effectively by other means.

33.6 Crystalloids are intravenous solutions that closely resemble the composition of extracellular fluid.

33.7 Colloids are intravenous solutions containing large molecules that remain in the blood.

33.8 Electrolytes are charged substances that are essential to homeostasis.

33.9 Sodium balance is closely associated with water balance.

33.10 Potassium imbalances must be quickly corrected to prevent serious cardiac consequences.

33.11 Magnesium imbalances significantly affect cardiovascular and neuromuscular function.

33.12 The pH of body fluids must be maintained between very narrow limits.

33.13 The pharmacotherapy of acidosis includes the administration of alkaline drugs.

33.14 The pharmacotherapy of alkalosis includes the administration of acidic drugs.

CASE STUDY: Making the Patient Connection

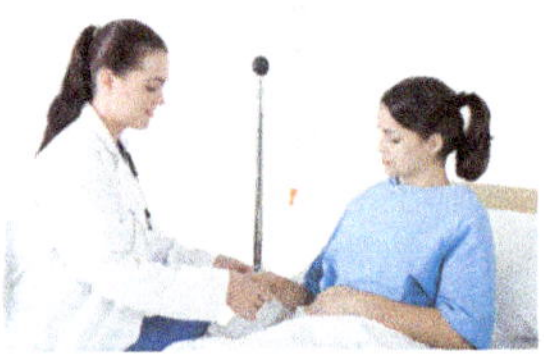

Remember the patient "Peggy Hoover" at the beginning of the chapter? Now read the remainder of the case study. Based on the information presented within this chapter, respond to the critical thinking questions that follow.

Peggy Hoover is 26 years old and has been admitted to the short-stay surgical unit for an elective laparoscopic cholecystectomy. She has been in good health except for repeated bouts of cholecystitis. It is anticipated that she will be able to go home this afternoon after the surgery is completed.

As the nurse admitting Peggy, you have orders to start a D_5W infusion prior to surgery, to run at 15 mL/h. You have started the IV in her right hand. Peggy asks you why she needs it, especially since she will be returning home that afternoon.

Critical Thinking Questions

1. Why do you think an IV was ordered for Peggy, and what will you explain to her?
2. What are the two main categories of IV solutions? Which category was ordered for Peggy?
3. Dextrose 5% in water (D_5W) is a common solution. What precautions should be taken with this fluid type?

Additional Case Study

Marvin Fields has been prescribed a loop diuretic, furosemide (Lasix), 40 mg daily, and a potassium supplement tablet, 40 mEq daily. As you are preparing to discharge this patient, he states, "I understand why I need the diuretic, but why do I have to take this potassium?"

1. How would you respond to his question?
2. What adverse effect related to potassium supplementation would you advise him to watch for?
3. What advice would you give Marvin about his dietary consumption of potassium-rich foods?

Chapter Review

1. The patient with a disorder causing metabolic acidosis is being treated with intravenous sodium bicarbonate. The nurse monitors for therapeutic effectiveness by noting which laboratory values?

1. Serum pH
2. Red blood cell count
3. Liver function test
4. Blood urea nitrogen

2. The nurse is teaching the patient about a liquid potassium chloride supplement. Which statement, if made by the patient, indicates that further teaching is necessary?

1. "I should avoid salt substitutes unless approved by my healthcare provider."
2. "Liquid preparations should not be diluted with other fluids."
3. "I should report signs of potassium deficit such as weakness and fatigue."
4. "Persistent vomiting will result in significant losses of potassium."

3. The nurse is administering dextran 40 (Gentran 40) to a patient with multiple traumatic injuries following a motor-vehicle crash. The nurse knows that which adverse effect of this medication is toxic?

1. Dehydration
2. Increased urinary output
3. Hypovolemic shock
4. Bleeding

4. The patient will be receiving 5% dextrose in water (D_5W) intravenous infusion. Which statement is correct about this therapy?

1. D_5W can cause hypoglycemia in the patient who has diabetes.
2. D_5W may be used to dilute mixed intravenous drugs.
3. D_5W is considered a colloid solution.
4. D_5W has a sufficient number of calories to supply metabolic needs.

5. The healthcare provider orders intravenous magnesium sulfate for a pregnant patient with preeclampsia. The nurse should consult with the prescriber about which patient assessment finding that may affect the drug therapy?

1. Pupil constriction to direct light
2. Chest congestion and coughing
3. Elevated blood pressure
4. Decreased patellar deep tendon reflexes

6. Which of the following nursing actions should be included in the care plan for a patient receiving normal serum albumin (Albuminar)? (Select all that apply.)

1. Document past history of blood transfusion reactions.
2. Restrict dietary intake of food high in potassium.
3. Monitor blood pressure and pulse rate.
4. Measure urinary output hourly.
5. Observe for signs related to potassium deficit.

See Appendix A for answers to critical thinking questions, case study questions, and review questions.

References

American Red Cross. (2020). *Blood needs and blood supply.* https://www.redcrossblood.org/donate-blood/how-to-donate/how-blood-donations-help/blood-needs-blood-supply.html

Office of Dietary Supplements. (2020). *Magnesium: Fact sheet for health professionals.* National Institutes of Health. http://ods.od.nih.gov/factsheets/Magnesium-HealthProfessional

Selected Bibliography

Aznar-Lou, I., Carbonell-Duacastella, C., Rodriguez, A., Mera, I., & Rubio-Valera, M. (2019). Prevalence of medication–dietary supplement combined use and associated factors. *Nutrients, 11*(10), 2466.

Coutrot, M., Dépret, F., & Legrand, M. (2019). Tailoring treatment of hyperkalemia. *Nephrology Dialysis Transplantation, 34*(Suppl. 3), iii62–iii68. https://doi.org/10.1093/ndt/gfz220

Earl, G. (2020). A new look at managing hyperkalemia in high-risk patients. *Nursing2020 Critical Care, 15*(3), 25–34. https://doi.org/10.1097/01.CCN.0000660380.54808.53

Hammond, D. A., Lam, S. W., Rech, M. A., Smith, M. N., Westrick, J., Trivedi, A. P., & Balk, R. A. (2020). Balanced crystalloids versus saline in critically ill adults: A systematic review and meta-analysis. *Annals of Pharmacotherapy, 54*(1), 5–13. https://doi.org/10.1177/1060028019866420

Huang, L. H. (2018). *Dehydration*. Medscape. http://emedicine.medscape.com/article/906999-overview

Jameson, R. A., & Bernstein, H. B. (2019). Magnesium sulfate and novel therapies to promote neuroprotection. *Clinics in Perinatology, 46*(2), 187–201. https://doi.org/10.1016/j.clp.2019.02.008

Martin, C., Cortegiani, A., Gregoretti, C., Martin-Loeches, I., Ichai, C., Leone, M., et al. (2018). Choice of fluids in critically ill patients. *BMC anesthesiology, 18*(1), 200. https://doi.org/10.1186/s12871-018-0669-3

Martin, G. S., & Bassett, P. (2019). Crystalloids vs. colloids for fluid resuscitation in the intensive care unit: A systematic review and meta-analysis. *Journal of Critical Care, 50*, 144–154. https://doi.org/10.1016/j.jcrc.2018.11.031

Morales, A., & Danziger, J. (2020). Management consideration in drug-induced lactic acidosis. *Clinical Journal of the American Society of Nephrology, 15*(10), 1511–1512. https://doi.org/10.2215/CJN.14781219

Simon, A. E. (2019. *Hyponatremia*. Medscape. https://emedicine.medscape.com/article/242166-overview

Thomas, C. P. (2018). *Metabolic alkalosis*. Medscape. http://emedicine.medscape.com/article/243160-overview

"I'm doing everything my doctor has advised me to do to control my hypertension. My doctor has prescribed several different types of drugs over the past few months. My blood pressure is still elevated. What else can I do?"

—*Patient "Elmer Foley"*

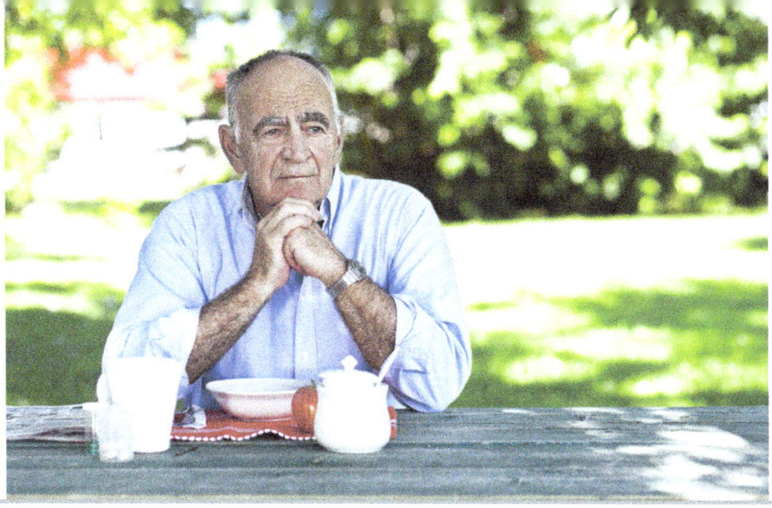

Chapter 34
Pharmacotherapy of Hypertension

Chapter Outline

- Etiology and Pathogenesis of Hypertension
- Nonpharmacologic Management of Hypertension
- General Principles of Antihypertensive Pharmacotherapy
- Drug Classes for Hypertension
  - Diuretics
  - Calcium Channel Blockers
  - Drugs Affecting the Renin-Angiotensin-Aldosterone System
  - Adrenergic Antagonists
  - Direct Vasodilators
  - **PROTOTYPE** *Hydralazine, p. 578*
- Management of Hypertensive Emergency
  - **PROTOTYPE** *Nitroprusside Sodium (Nitropress), p. 580*

Learning Outcomes

After reading this chapter, the student should be able to:

1. Summarize the long-term consequences of untreated hypertension.
2. Compare and contrast the roles of nonpharmacologic and pharmacologic methods in the management of hypertension.
3. Describe general principles guiding the pharmacotherapy of hypertension.
4. Identify first- and second-line drug classes used in the management of hypertension.
5. Describe the pharmacologic management of hypertensive emergencies.
6. For each of the classes shown in the chapter outline, identify the prototype and representative drugs and explain the mechanism(s) of drug action, primary indications, contraindications, significant drug interactions, pregnancy data, and important adverse effects.
7. Apply clinical judgment to care for patients receiving antihypertensive drugs.

Key Terms

Definitions of the terms in bold may be found in the Glossary.

Diseases affecting the heart and blood vessels are the most frequent causes of death in the United States. Hypertension (HTN) or high blood pressure is the most common of the cardiovascular diseases. Chronic HTN affects 45% of Americans and contributes to about 500,000 deaths in the United States each year (Centers for Disease Control and Prevention, 2020). Although mild HTN can be controlled with lifestyle modifications, moderate to severe HTN requires pharmacotherapy.

Because nurses encounter so many patients with this disease, it is critical for them to understand the underlying principles of antihypertensive therapy. By improving public awareness of HTN and teaching the importance of early intervention, the nurse can contribute significantly to reducing cardiovascular mortality.

Etiology and Pathogenesis of Hypertension

34.1 Failure to properly manage hypertension can lead to stroke, heart failure, or myocardial infarction.

Hypertension (HTN) is defined as the consistent elevation of arterial blood pressure. When most people use the word *hypertension*, they are referring to systemic HTN, which is measured routinely by a conventional blood pressure cuff on the upper arm over the brachial artery. Systemic HTN is a general measurement of arterial blood pressure in the body. Localized HTN may also occur. For example, patients with cirrhosis of the liver often develop portal HTN, which occurs in the portal vein and its branches serving the liver. Pulmonary HTN occurs in the pulmonary artery and its branches and is most often observed in patients with left-sided HF. These localized types of HTN respond to many of the same antihypertensive drugs used for systemic HTN.

Hypertension is a complex disease that is caused by a combination of factors. Approximately 4% of HTN cases are believed to involve genetic factors. Scientists have discovered specific genes that predispose a patient to HTN. These genes control critical activities such as renal sodium and water transport and the renin-angiotensin-aldosterone system. Environmental factors related to diet and exercise also play an important role in the development of HTN.

For the large majority of patients with HTN, no specific cause can be identified. HTN having no identifiable cause is called idiopathic, essential, or **primary hypertension** and accounts for 90% of all cases. Although patients with primary HTN cannot be cured with medication, the disease can be managed such that the risk of serious, long-term consequences can be reduced.

In some cases, a specific cause of the HTN can be identified. This type, called **secondary hypertension**, accounts for 10% of all patients with the disease. Certain diseases, such as Cushing's syndrome, primary aldosteronism, hyperthyroidism, chronic kidney disease (CKD), pheochromocytoma, and obstructive sleep apnea, are associated with elevated blood pressure. Some drugs are also associated with HTN, including alcohol, nicotine, decongestants, caffeine, amphetamines, corticosteroids, oral contraceptives, estrogen, erythropoietin, and nonsteroidal anti-inflammatory drugs (NSAIDs). The therapeutic goal for secondary HTN is to treat or remove the condition that is causing the blood pressure elevation. In many cases, correcting the comorbid underlying condition will cure the associated HTN.

Research clearly shows that failure to control HTN can have serious consequences. Prolonged or improperly controlled HTN damages blood vessels, particularly small arteries and arterioles. As it progresses, the walls of the arteries gradually thicken in an attempt to protect the vessels against injury from the increased pressure. The injured vessel walls become inflamed, increasing the permeability of the vessels and causing additional thickening of their walls. Eventually, the lumen of the artery permanently narrows, reducing blood flow to vital tissues. Chronic HTN accelerates the development of atherosclerotic cardiovascular disease.

Hypertension may exist for years, indeed decades, before becoming symptomatic. As the disease progresses, however, the risk of target-organ damage increases. Because sustained HTN may affect any artery in the body, damage may be widespread and symptoms vary greatly according to which vessels are affected.

The heart is a primary organ damaged by chronic HTN. Hypertension increases afterload, forcing the heart to work harder to pump blood to the tissues. The heart is subjected to chronic pressure overload, resulting in left-ventricular hypertrophy. If untreated, this excessive workload eventually causes the heart to fail and the lungs to fill with fluid, a condition known as heart failure (HF) (see Chapter 36). Further damaging the heart is the effect of HTN on the coronary vessels. Hypertension accelerates the deposition of atherosclerotic plaque, creating or worsening coronary artery disease (CAD). This places the patient at greater risk of dysrhythmias, angina pectoris, and myocardial infarction (MI). Heart failure and MI are the most common causes of death in patients with HTN.

The brain is also a major target organ for hypertensive damage. Occlusion of the small vessels supplying blood and oxygen to the brain can cause transient ischemic attacks and stroke. These neurologic events are common in patients with HTN and are a major cause of disability.

Because a large percentage of blood pumped per minute circulates through the kidneys, chronic HTN creates major stress on these organs. As the small arteries supplying the kidney become injured, inflamed, and atherosclerotic, renal function gradually declines. Poorly managed HTN is an important contributor to CKD and end-stage kidney disease.

Hypertension is a major cause of visual impairment. Although patients may remain asymptomatic for many years, hemorrhages that affect vision may occur, producing symptoms of retinal damage ranging from blurred vision to complete blindness. Retinopathy is particularly serious in patients who present with diabetes mellitus (DM) as a comorbid condition with HTN.

The importance of treating this disorder in its early stage cannot be overstated. The long-term damage to target organs caused by HTN will become irreversible if the disease is allowed to progress unchecked. This is especially critical in people with DM and those with CKD, as these patients are particularly susceptible to the long-term consequences of HTN.

Nonpharmacologic Management of Hypertension

34.2 Therapeutic lifestyle changes can reduce blood pressure and lessen the need for antihypertensive medications.

When a patient is first diagnosed with HTN, a comprehensive medical history is necessary to determine if the disease can be managed by nonpharmacologic means. Therapeutic lifestyle changes should be recommended for all patients with HTN or at risk for the development of HTN. Of great importance is maintaining optimal weight because obesity is closely associated with hyperlipidemia and HTN. A 5- to 9-kg (11- to 20-lb) weight loss often produces a measurable decrease in blood pressure, even in patients who are obese. Combining a medically supervised weight loss program with proper nutrition can delay the progression of HTN.

In some cases, implementing healthy lifestyle changes may eliminate the need for pharmacotherapy altogether. Even if medication is required to manage the HTN, positive lifestyle changes may allow dosages to be minimized, thus lowering the potential for drug adverse effects. The nurse plays a vital role in educating patients about controlling their HTN. Because all blood pressure medications have potential adverse effects, it is important for patients to attempt to control their disease through nonpharmacologic means, to the greatest extent possible. Nonpharmacologic methods for controlling HTN include the following:

- Limit intake of alcohol (men less than two drinks/day, women less than one drink/day)
- Restrict dietary sodium consumption to less than 1500 mg/day.
- Increase dietary potassium to 3500 to 5000 mg/day.
- Reduce intake of saturated and total fat and increase consumption of fruits, vegetables, whole grains, and low-fat dairy products.
- Establish an exercise program that includes aerobic, dynamic-resistance, and isometric-resistance physical activity.
- Discontinue use of all tobacco products.
- Maintain optimal weight.

General Principles of Antihypertensive Pharmacotherapy

34.3 The choice of antihypertensive medication is determined by the degree of hypertension and the presence of other medical conditions.

The goal of antihypertensive therapy is to reduce the morbidity and mortality associated with chronic HTN. Research has confirmed that keeping blood pressure within normal limits reduces the risk of hypertension-related target-organ damage.

To develop guidelines for treatment, many attempts have been made to define HTN and to determine which medical interventions are most effective at reducing mortality. Guidelines published in 2017 by the American College of Cardiology and the American Heart Association, lowered the cut-off value that had previously defined HTN (Whelton et al., 2018). The current guideline for Stage 1 HTN is 130–139/80–89, as shown in Table 34.1. Given these cut-off values, 48% of men and 43% of women in the United States now have HTN. The percentages are lower for younger individuals and higher for older adults.

The pharmacologic management of HTN is individualized to the patient's risk factors, comorbid medical conditions, and degree of blood pressure elevation. Patient responses to antihypertensive medications vary widely because of the many complex genetic and environmental factors affecting blood pressure.

The multiple drug classes used to treat HTN are shown in Table 34.2. Each class has specific benefits and characteristic adverse effects. The mechanisms of action of the major classes of antihypertensive drugs are summarized in Pharmacotherapy Illustrated 34.1. Although many effective drugs are available, and the data supporting the benefits of therapy are strong, HTN remains a challenging disorder to treat successfully. Choice of therapy is often based on the

Table 34.1 Blood Pressure Categories

Blood Pressure Category	Systemic (mmHg)	Diastolic (mmHg)
Normal	Less than 120	Less than 80
Elevated	120–129	Less than 80
Hypertension Stage 1	130–139	80–89
Hypertension Stage 2	140 and above	90 and above

Pharmacotherapy Illustrated 34.1

Mechanism of Action of Antihypertensive Drugs

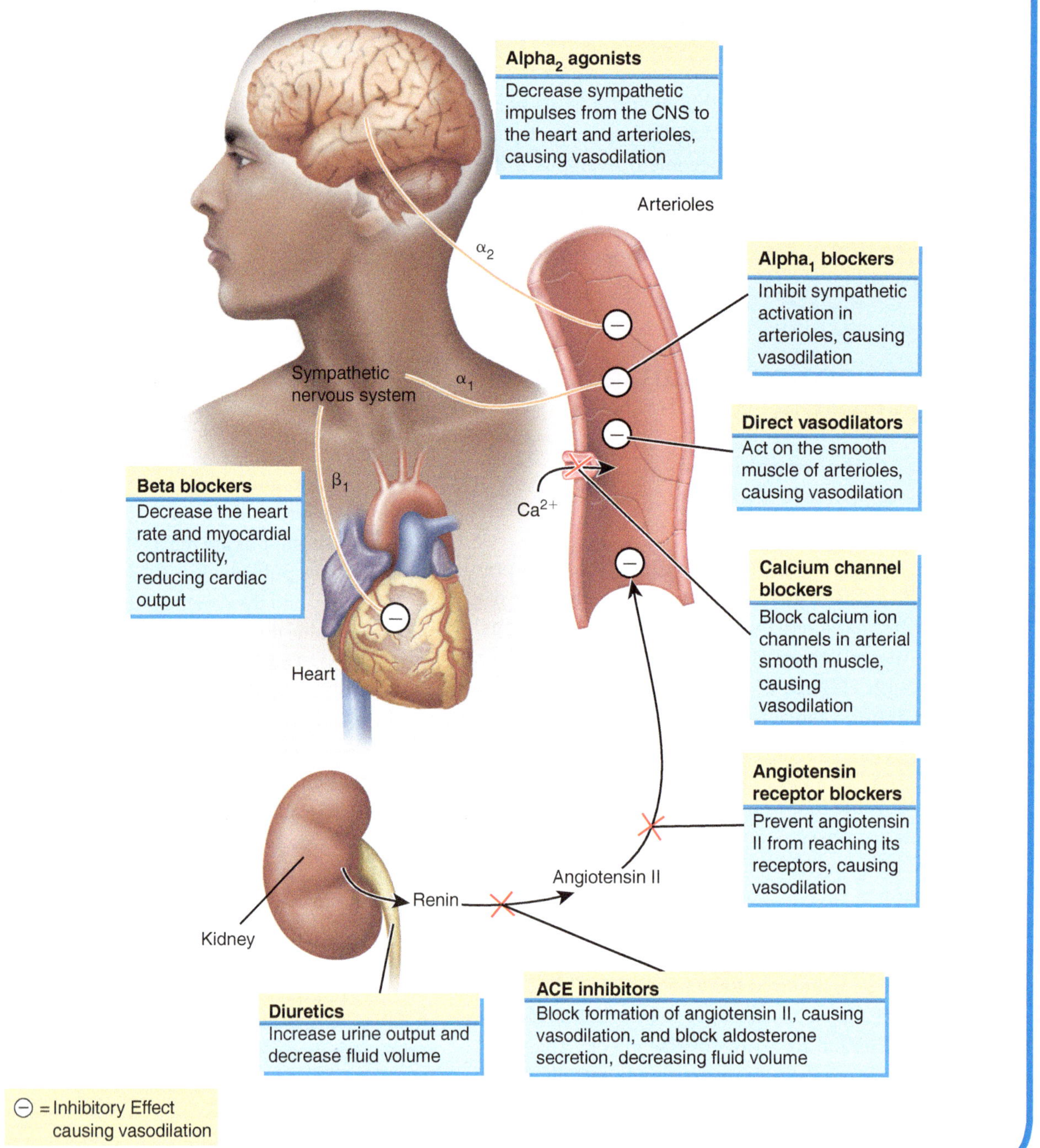

clinician's experience. Although antihypertensive treatment varies, several principles guide pharmacotherapy.

Drugs for Initial Hypertension Therapy

The current recommendation is to begin therapy with thiazide diuretics, angiotensin-converting enzyme inhibitors, angiotensin receptor blockers, or calcium channel blockers for most patients. Research has clearly demonstrated that these four primary drug classes reduce HTN-related morbidity and mortality. Treatment of stage 1 HTN is begun with a low dose of a single medication. The patient is reevaluated after an appropriate time period, and dosage is adjusted as needed to meet the target goal, usually a blood pressure of less than 130/80mm Hg.

Table 34.2 Drug Classes for Hypertension

Type	Class
First-line drugs	Angiotensin-converting enzyme (ACE) inhibitors Angiotensin receptor blockers (ARBs) Calcium channel blockers (CCBs) Diuretics: thiazide or thiazide-like
Second-line drugs	Alpha$_1$-adrenergic blockers Alpha$_2$-adrenergic agonists Beta-adrenergic blockers Centrally acting alpha$_2$ blockers Direct-acting vasodilators Direct renin inhibitors Diuretics: loop and potassium-sparing

Adding Drugs to the Antihypertensive Regimen

Additional antihypertensive medications are necessary for patients with stage 2 HTN or if the initial monotherapy for stage 1 HTN did not achieve target goals. The second medication is always from a different antihypertensive class. Prescribing two antihypertensives concurrently results in additive or synergistic blood pressure reduction and is common practice when managing resistant HTN. The use of two drugs allows lower doses, resulting in fewer adverse effects and better patient adherence. Drug manufacturers offer choices that combine two drugs into a single pill or capsule for dosing convenience. The majority of these combinations include a thiazide diuretic, usually hydrochlorothiazide, sometimes abbreviated as HCTZ, combined with an ACE inhibitor or ARB. ACE inhibitors and ARBs are not used in combination with each other because they act by very similar mechanisms. Selected combination antihypertensives are shown in Table 34.3.

Certain antihypertensive classes exhibit a higher incidence of adverse effects and are generally prescribed when drugs from the four primary classes do not produce a satisfactory response. In some cases, research studies have not demonstrated a firm link between drug use and lowered morbidity or mortality. The alternative antihypertensive drug classes are shown in Table 34.2.

Treating Hypertension in Patients with Comorbidities

Guidelines for treating hypertensive patients who present with certain comorbidities have more specific recommendations for managing HTN. In general, the target blood pressure for these patients should be less than 130/80 mm Hg. For example, beta adrenergic blockers are recommended as a first-line therapy in patients with stable ischemic heart disease. ACE inhibitors are recommended for patients with CKD because these medications have been shown to slow the progression of kidney disease. Patients with atrial fibrillation are recommended to take ARBs for their HTN.

Table 34.3 Selected Combination Medications for Hypertension

Thiazide Diuretic with ACE Inhibitor	
Accuretic	HCTZ and quinapril
Lotensin HCT	HCTZ and benazepril
Vaseretic	HCTZ and enalapril
Zestoretic	HCTZ and lisinopril
Thiazide Diuretic with Angiotensin II Blocker	
Atacand HCT	HCTZ and candesartan
Avalide	HCTZ and irbesartan
Benicar HCT	HCTZ and olmesartan
Diovan HCT	HCTZ and valsartan
Edarbyclor	chlorthalidone and azilsartan
Hyzaar	HCTZ and losartan
Micardis HCT	HCTZ and telmisartan
Thiazide Diuretic with a Beta Blocker	
Corzide	HCTZ with bendroflumethiazide and nadolol
Lopressor HCT	HCTZ and metoprolol
Tenoretic	chlorthalidone and atenolol
Ziac	HCTZ and bisoprolol
Thiazide Diuretic with Potassium-Sparing Diuretic	
Aldactazide	HCTZ and spironolactone
Dyazide	HCTZ and triamterene
Other Combinations	
Apresazide	HCTZ and hydralazine (direct vasodilator)
Azor	olmesartan and amlodipine
Exforge HCT	HCTZ with valsartan and amlodipine
Lotrel	benazepril and amlodipine
Prestalia	perindopril and amlodipine
Tarka	trandolapril and verapamil (CCB)
Tekturna HCT	HCTZ and aliskiren
Tribenzor	HCTZ with olmesartan and amlodipine

Enhancing Patient Adherence

Because chronic HTN may produce no identifiable symptoms for as long as 10 to 20 years, many people are not aware of their condition. Convincing patients to change established lifestyle habits, spend money on medication, and take drugs on a regular basis when they are feeling healthy can be a challenging task for the nurse. Patients with limited income or who do not have health insurance are at high risk for not purchasing the drugs after receiving a prescription. The prescriber should consider generic forms of these drugs to reduce costs and increase adherence. Furthermore, adherence improves when the medication is taken once daily as a single dose (or a combination pill), rather than in multiple doses.

Further reducing adherence to the regimen is the occurrence of adverse drug effects. Some of the antihypertensive drugs cause embarrassing adverse effects such as impotence, which may go unreported. Others cause fatigue and generally make patients feel sicker than they were before therapy was initiated. The nurse should teach the patient the importance of treating the disease to avoid serious long-term consequences. Furthermore, the nurse should teach patients to report adverse effects so that dosage can be adjusted, or the drug changed, so the treatment can continue without interruption. Simple adjustments to the dosage or changing the selected drug can often eliminate the causes of nonadherence.

Antihypertensive Therapy in the Black Population

The incidence of HTN is significantly higher in Blacks than in non-Blacks. As expected from this high incidence, Blacks experience greater target-organ damage than other populations. In an effort to reduce the high morbidity and mortality risks, aggressive antihypertensive therapy with two or more medications may be necessary to overcome resistant HTN. Reducing blood pressure to less than 130/80 mm Hg is optimal.

Some research suggests that certain antihypertensive drug classes are more effective than others in this population. Monotherapy with ACE inhibitors, ARBs, or beta-adrenergic antagonists does not reduce blood pressure as effectively in Blacks. Thiazide diuretics and CCBs provide the greatest blood pressure reduction and are recommended as first-line drugs for this population.

Drug Classes for Hypertension

34.4 Diuretics are often preferred drugs for treating mild to moderate hypertension.

Diuretics were the first class of medications used to treat HTN in the 1950s. Despite the many advances in drug therapy, thiazide diuretics are still considered first-line drugs for this disease because they are very effective at controlling mild to moderate HTN with few serious adverse effects. Although sometimes used as monotherapy, diuretics are frequently prescribed with other antihypertensive medications to enhance their effectiveness. Because this class of drugs was presented in detail in Chapter 32, this section is a summary of their application to the treatment of HTN.

Although dozens of diuretics are available for the treatment of HTN, all produce a similar result: the reduction of blood volume through the urinary excretion of water and electrolytes. Reducing blood volume places less pressure on the arterial walls, thereby decreasing peripheral resistance and lowering systemic blood pressure. The mechanism by which diuretics increase the excretion of water and electrolytes, specifically where and how the kidney is affected, differs among the various classes of diuretics.

Thiazide and thiazide-like diuretics: Thiazide and thiazide-like diuretics have been the mainstay for the pharmacotherapy of HTN for decades. The thiazide diuretics are inexpensive, and most are available in generic formulations. They are safe drugs, with excessive urinary potassium loss being the primary adverse effect. Because hypokalemia can induce serious dysrhythmias in susceptible patients, regular laboratory monitoring of serum potassium is necessary. Patients should increase their amount of dietary potassium, and potassium supplements may be prescribed. These diuretics may also cause hyperglycemia; therefore, blood glucose levels should be monitored in patients with diabetes. The thiazides are described in Chapter 32, with hydrochlorothiazide, or HCTZ (Microzide), featured as the prototype drug in this class.

Potassium-sparing diuretics: Although potassium-sparing diuretics such as spironolactone (Aldactone) and triamterene (Dyrenium) produce only a modest diuresis, their primary advantage is they do not cause potassium depletion. They are especially beneficial when the patient is at risk of developing hypokalemia due to a medical condition or from the use of thiazide or loop diuretics. The primary concern when using potassium-sparing diuretics is the possibility of retaining too much potassium, which can cause serious dysrhythmias. Patients with diabetes and those with CKD are particularly susceptible to hyperkalemia. Patients should be instructed to avoid excess potassium in their diet, including salt substitutes containing KCl, and not to use potassium supplements during therapy. Drugs in this class are not considered first-line drugs for the treatment of HTN. The potassium-sparing diuretics are described in Chapter 32, with spironolactone presented as the prototype drug for this class.

Loop diuretics: The loop diuretics such as furosemide (Lasix) cause greater diuresis and have the potential to produce a higher reduction in blood pressure than the thiazides or potassium-sparing diuretics. The risk of adverse effects such as hypokalemia and dehydration is great because of their ability to remove large amounts of fluid from the body in a short time period. Loop diuretics are ototoxic, an effect more likely to occur in patients with CKD or when high doses are administered. Because of their greater toxicity, loop diuretics are usually not recommended as first-line drugs for HTN but may be prescribed for patients with resistant HTN. The loop diuretics are presented in Chapter 32, with furosemide as the prototype drug in this class.

34.5 Calcium channel blockers have emerged as important drugs in the treatment of hypertension.

Calcium channel blockers are widely used in the treatment of HTN, angina pectoris, and dysrhythmias, as presented in Chapter 30. This section summarizes their application to the treatment of HTN.

CCBs exert beneficial effects on the heart and blood vessels by blocking calcium ion channels in cardiac and arteriolar smooth muscle. The flow of calcium ions into muscle cells is inhibited, limiting the degree of muscular contraction. At low doses, CCBs relax arterial smooth muscle, thus decreasing peripheral resistance and lowering blood pressure. Some CCBs such as nifedipine (Adalat CC, Procardia XL) are selective for arterioles, whereas others such as verapamil (Calan, Isoptin, Verelan) affect channels in both arterioles and the myocardium.

Due to their potent vasodilating effects, CCBs can cause reflex tachycardia, especially with those CCBs that are selective for arterioles. Because CCBs can slow myocardial conduction, they are contraindicated in patients with certain types of heart conditions such as sick sinus syndrome or third-degree atrioventricular (AV) block without the presence of a pacemaker.

CCBs are usually not used as monotherapy for chronic HTN, although they are recommended as first-line drugs for the disorder. They are useful in combination therapy for treating certain populations such as older adults and Black patients who are sometimes less responsive to drugs in other antihypertensive classes. Nifedipine is recommended as a first-line drug for HTN during pregnancy. The CCBs are presented in Chapter 30, with nifedipine and verapamil as prototype drugs in this class.

CONNECTION Checkpoint 34.1

Verapamil and nifedipine are both calcium channel blockers used for HTN. From what you learned in Chapter 30, why would a beta blocker be used concurrently with nifedipine but be contraindicated with verapamil?

34.6 Blocking the renin-angiotensin-aldosterone system leads to a decrease in blood pressure and improved kidney function.

As discussed in Chapter 31, the renin-angiotensin-aldosterone system (RAAS) is one of the primary homeostatic mechanisms controlling blood pressure and fluid balance. Drugs inhibiting the RAAS are widely used in the treatment of cardiovascular disease and are recommended as first-line drugs in the pharmacotherapy of HTN. The following sections summarize their applications to HTN pharmacotherapy.

Angiotensin-converting enzyme inhibitors: **Angiotensin-converting enzyme (ACE) inhibitors** block the formation of angiotensin II, decreasing blood pressure through two mechanisms. First, ACE inhibitors block the intense vasoconstriction of arterioles caused by angiotensin II, which decreases blood pressure due to diminished peripheral resistance. Second, these drugs block the effects of angiotensin II on the secretion of aldosterone, which lowers blood pressure by decreasing blood volume. Through their inhibition of aldosterone secretion, ACE inhibitors enhance the effects of the thiazide diuretics; thus, drugs from these two classes may be used concurrently in the management of HTN. The ACE inhibitors are presented in Chapter 31, with lisinopril as the prototype drug in this class.

Adverse effects of ACE inhibitors are usually minor and include persistent cough and orthostatic hypotension. Hyperkalemia may occur and can be a major concern for patients with DM, those with CKD, and patients taking potassium-sparing diuretics. Though rare, the most serious adverse effect of ACE inhibitors is the development of angioedema. Cough and angioedema arise more frequently in Blacks than in other ethnic groups.

Angiotensin receptor blockers and direct renin inhibitors: The ARBs afford a second method for altering the RAAS pathway. ARBs such as losartan (Cozaar) block receptors for angiotensin II in arteriolar smooth muscle and in the adrenal gland, thus causing blood pressure to fall. Their actions are similar to those of the ACE inhibitors.

Angiotensin II receptor blockers have the lowest incidence of serious adverse effects of any of the antihypertensive classes. Most ARB adverse effects are related to hypotension. Unlike the ACE inhibitors, they do not cause cough, and angioedema is rare. Medications in this class are often combined with drugs from other classes in the management of HTN. The ARBs are presented in Chapter 31, with losartan (Cozaar) as the prototype drug in this class.

Aliskiren (Tekturna) was the first in a class of antihypertensives called direct renin inhibitors. They act by interfering with part of the RAAS system. The combination of aliskiren with HCTZ (Tekturna HCT) is approved for treating HTN. The most common adverse effects of aliskiren are diarrhea, cough, flulike symptoms, and rash. The direct renin inhibitors are not considered first-line medications for HTN.

34.7 Adrenergic antagonists are commonly used to treat hypertension.

The adrenergic antagonists, or blockers, are used for a wide variety of cardiovascular disorders, including HTN, angina pectoris, dysrhythmias, and MI prophylaxis. Blocking adrenergic receptors in the sympathetic nervous system has a number of beneficial effects on the heart and blood vessels, for example, by blocking the "fight-or-flight" responses, heart rate slows, blood pressure declines, and the bronchi dilate.

Adrenergic blockers affect the sympathetic division through several distinct mechanisms, although all have in common the effect of lowering blood pressure. These mechanisms include the following:

- Blockade of beta_1-adrenergic receptors
- Blockade of alpha_1-adrenergic receptors

- Blockade of both $alpha_1$- and beta-adrenergic receptors
- Stimulation of centrally acting $alpha_2$-adrenergic receptors in the brainstem

The earliest drugs for HTN were drugs that blocked nerve transmission at the ganglia or at both alpha- and beta-adrenergic receptors. Although the nonselective medications revolutionized the treatment of HTN, they caused a high incidence of adverse effects. These drugs are rarely used today because safer and more effective alternatives are available. Of the five subclasses of adrenergic antagonists, the beta-adrenergic blockers are the most widely used group. All of the adrenergic inhibitors are considered second-line drugs for HTN.

Beta-adrenergic antagonists: In this section, the discussion of beta-adrenergic antagonists is limited to their use in treating HTN. The student should refer to Chapter 16 for a detailed discussion of the basic pharmacology of this drug class. Other important therapeutic applications of the beta blockers include angina pectoris and MI, dysrhythmias, HF, and migraines.

Beta-adrenergic antagonists may be cardioselective ($beta_1$) or nonselective ($beta_1$ and $beta_2$). Cardioselective beta blockers decrease heart rate, myocardial contractility, and cardiac conduction velocity. Nonselective beta blockers produce the same effects but also act on the respiratory system to cause bronchoconstriction. Decreasing the heart rate and contractility also reduces cardiac output and lowers systemic blood pressure. Some of their antihypertensive effect is also caused by the blockade of $beta_1$ receptors in the juxtaglomerular apparatus, which inhibits the secretion of renin and the formation of angiotensin II. Although they are usually not recommended as first-line drugs for HTN, the beta-adrenergic antagonists are still widely used for this condition.

At low doses, beta blockers are well tolerated and serious adverse events are uncommon. As the dosage is increased, however, adverse effects can become numerous and potentially serious in certain patients. Because nonselective beta blockers will slow the heart rate and cause bronchoconstriction, they should be used with caution in patients with asthma or HF. Heart rate and rhythm should be monitored regularly during beta-blocker therapy. Many patients report fatigue and activity intolerance at higher doses because the reduction in heart rate causes the heart to become less responsive to exertion. Abrupt cessation of beta-blocker therapy can result in rebound HTN, angina, MI, and even death in patients with CAD.

Prototype features for beta-adrenergic antagonists can be found for propranolol (Inderal, InnoPran XL) and metoprolol (Lopressor, Toprol XL) in Chapter 16, atenolol (Tenormin) in Chapter 35, and timolol in Chapter 74.

CONNECTION Checkpoint 34.2

From what you learned in Chapter 16, should a patient with hypertension and asthma receive a selective $beta_1$ blocker or a nonselective beta blocker for HTN?

$Alpha_1$-adrenergic antagonists: The $alpha_1$-adrenergic antagonists have several clinical applications, which were presented in Chapter 16. In addition to their use in HTN, they are prescribed for benign prostatic hyperplasia because their ability to relax smooth muscle in the prostate and bladder neck reduces urethral resistance.

The $alpha_1$-adrenergic antagonists lower blood pressure directly by blocking sympathetic receptors in arterioles, causing the vessels to dilate. They also dilate veins, which lowers blood pressure indirectly by decreasing venous return to the heart and reducing cardiac output. The alpha blockers are not first-line drugs for HTN. They are less effective at reducing the incidence of serious HTN-related cardiovascular events than diuretics. When used to treat HTN, the alpha blockers are used concurrently with other classes of antihypertensives, such as diuretics.

The $alpha_1$-adrenergic blockers may cause significant orthostatic hypotension. It is particularly serious with the initial doses of these medications and is referred to as the first-dose phenomenon, although orthostatic hypotension may persist throughout treatment. In severe cases, syncope can occur. Other common adverse effects include weakness, dizziness, dry mouth, headache, and gastrointestinal complaints such as nausea and vomiting. The $alpha_1$-adrenergic antagonists are presented in Chapter 16, with prazosin (Minipress) as the prototype drug for this class.

Combination $alpha_1$- and beta-adrenergic antagonists: Carvedilol (Coreg) and labetalol (Trandate) are unique in that they block both $alpha_1$- and beta-adrenergic receptors. These drugs act by a combination of effects: They reduce cardiac output, inhibit renin secretion, and block vasoconstriction of arterioles and veins. As expected, their adverse effects are a combination of alpha and beta blockade and include orthostatic hypotension, bradycardia, and bronchoconstriction. Labetalol is recommended as a first-line drug for HTN during pregnancy. The applications of carvedilol in treating HF are presented in Chapter 36.

$Alpha_2$-adrenergic agonists: If an alpha antagonist such as prazosin lowers blood pressure, it might be predicted that the administration of an $alpha_2$-adrenergic agonist would raise blood pressure. This is not the case. The answer to this contradiction lies in the different locations of the two subtypes of alpha receptors. The $alpha_1$ receptors blocked by prazosin lie in the peripheral nervous system (PNS) at arterioles. The $alpha_2$ receptors reside in the central nervous system (CNS).

When alpha$_2$ receptors are activated, the outflow of sympathetic nerve impulses from the CNS to the heart and arterioles is inhibited. In effect, this produces the same responses as inhibition of the alpha$_1$ receptor: slowing the heart rate and conduction velocity and dilating the arterioles. Thus, activating alpha$_2$ receptors (in the CNS) produces similar actions as inhibiting alpha$_1$ receptors (in the PNS).

The alpha$_2$ agonists may cause excessive sedation, dizziness, and orthostatic hypotension, which can be especially troublesome in older adults. Extended use results in sodium and water retention, which increases blood volume and counteracts the antihypertensive action of these drugs. Alpha$_2$ agonists are usually reserved for treating resistant HTN that cannot be managed by safer medications. The two drugs in this class are methyldopa and clonidine (Catapres, Duraclon, Kapvay, Nexiclon XR).

Methyldopa is an older drug approved in 1962. Its only indication is HTN that has not responded adequately to safer antihypertensives. The drug is normally administered by the oral (PO) route.

Because methyldopa is a centrally acting drug, CNS effects such as drowsiness, depression, headache, sedation, and bizarre dreams are relatively common. Orthostatic hypotension may occur, but it is less severe than that produced by the alpha$_1$ antagonists. Peripheral edema due to sodium retention may occur, which can be managed by administration of a thiazide diuretic. A significant number of patients develop a positive Coombs' test, which detects antibodies against the patient's own red blood cells. Because tolerance develops after 3 to 4 months of therapy, a dosage increase may be required to manage HTN. Methyldopa has been used to treat HTN during pregnancy because it maintains stable blood flow to the uterus, and its safety to the fetus has been demonstrated in long-term studies. Small amounts of the drug enter breast milk and no significant adverse events have been reported during breastfeeding.

Approved in 1974, clonidine (Catapres, Duraclon) activates alpha$_2$-adrenergic receptors in the cardiovascular control centers in the brainstem. The reduced sympathetic outflow causes vasodilation and slows the heart rate. As an antihypertensive, it is available as regular oral tablets, extended-release tablets, or a transdermal patch (Catapres) that releases the drug at a constant rate over 7 days. A second approved indication for clonidine (Duraclon) is intractable pain in patients with cancer that is not relieved by opiates. Pain control is achieved by a continuous epidural infusion of the drug. To assist in pain management, transdermal clonidine may be used to provide some degree of analgesia so that the dose of opiate can be reduced. An extended-release form of clonidine (Kapvay) is approved to treat attention-deficit/hyperactivity disorder.

Clonidine has many off-label indications. These include dysmenorrhea, menopausal flushing, migraine prophylaxis, smoking cessation, opiate and benzodiazepine withdrawal, and Tourette's syndrome.

The most common adverse effect of clonidine is dry mouth. Like methyldopa, CNS adverse effects such as sedation, fatigue, drowsiness, and dizziness are common. Transdermal clonidine produces fewer serious adverse effects, although the patches can cause skin irritation and itching. The patient should be warned not to abruptly discontinue the drug, as severe rebound HTN, agitation, nervousness, and anxiety may result. Clonidine readily crosses the placenta, but no well-controlled studies have been performed in pregnant patients. Because it readily enters milk, caution is urged if breastfeeding.

34.8 Direct-acting vasodilators lower blood pressure by relaxing arteriolar smooth muscle.

The ability to cause vasodilation is a property shared by many different classes of drugs, as shown in Pharmacotherapy Illustrated 34.1. Most vasodilators are used to treat HTN, and some are also used for the pharmacotherapy of HF, angina pectoris, and MI. Some of the drugs presented in previous sections of this chapter produce vasodilation indirectly by affecting autonomic nerves or by influencing the renin-angiotensin-aldosterone pathway. The drugs presented in this section affect the vascular smooth muscle itself; thus, they are called direct vasodilators.

Direct relaxation of arteriolar smooth muscle is an effective way to reduce blood pressure. Indeed, the direct vasodilator sodium nitroprusside (Nitropress) is used in hypertensive emergencies to lower blood pressure almost instantaneously (see Section 34.9). Unfortunately, the medications in this class have the potential to produce serious adverse effects. In the pharmacotherapy of HTN, these drugs are generally reserved for hypertensive emergencies and for HTN that has not been successfully managed with medications from safer drug classes.

All direct vasodilators cause reflex tachycardia, a compensatory increase in heart rate due to the sudden decrease in blood pressure. The baroreceptor reflex is an essential component of the normal physiologic control of blood pressure. However, when reflex tachycardia occurs as the result of vasodilator drugs, the heart is forced to work harder and the resultant blood pressure increase counteracts the effect of the antihypertensive drug. Patients with CAD may experience an acute angina attack due to the sudden increase in cardiac workload. Fortunately, reflex tachycardia can be prevented by administering a beta-adrenergic blocker, such as propranolol (Inderal). Beta blockers are sometimes administered concurrently with direct vasodilators for this reason.

A second potentially serious adverse effect of direct vasodilator therapy is salt and water retention. The reduction in blood pressure from the vasodilator causes a compensatory increase in aldosterone secretion by the adrenal gland. The increased aldosterone level signals the kidney to retain more sodium and water. Blood volume increases, thus raising blood pressure and canceling the antihypertensive action of the vasodilator. A diuretic may be administered concurrently with a direct vasodilator in order to prevent fluid retention.

PROTOTYPE DRUG Hydralazine

Classification **Therapeutic:** Antihypertensive
Pharmacologic: Direct vasodilator

Therapeutic Effects and Uses: In 1952, hydralazine was one of the first oral antihypertensive medications marketed in the United States. It is most commonly administered in tablet form for moderate to severe HTN, usually in combination with other antihypertensives. Apresazide is a fixed-dose combination of hydralazine with HCTZ. When given PO, hydralazine is administered two to four times per day, usually with food because this increases its bioavailability. Therapy is generally begun with low doses, which are gradually increased until the desired therapeutic response is obtained. After several months of therapy, tolerance to the drug develops and a dosage increase may be necessary. Although it produces an effective reduction in blood pressure, drugs in other antihypertensive classes have largely replaced hydralazine.

Hydralazine is also available by the intramuscular (IM) and IV routes for hypertensive emergencies, especially those associated with preeclampsia, although it is not a preferred drug for this indication. It is sometimes administered to patients with acute HF because the drug reduces the workload on the heart due to its antihypertensive action. ACE inhibitors have largely replaced hydralazine for patients with HF. A fixed-dose combination therapy of isosorbide dinitrate and hydralazine (BiDil) is available for the treatment of HF in Black patients.

Mechanism of Action: By causing peripheral vasodilation, hydralazine acts directly to relax arterial smooth muscle. The decreased peripheral resistance is accompanied by an increase in heart rate and cardiac output. The overall result is a reduction in afterload. Because the drug is selective for arterioles and does not cause dilation of veins, orthostatic hypotension is not a major adverse effect.

Pharmacokinetics:

Route(s)	PO, IM, IV
Absorption	Rapidly absorbed PO and well absorbed IM
Distribution	Widely distributed; crosses the placenta and is secreted in breast milk; 87% bound to plasma protein
Primary metabolism	GI mucosa and liver; extensive first-pass metabolism
Primary excretion	90% renal, 10% feces
Onset of action	PO: 20–30 min; IM: 10–30 min; IV: 5–20 min
Duration of action	3–8 h (PO); 1–4 h (IV)

Adverse Effects: Hydralazine may cause several adverse effects that have the potential to prompt discontinuation of therapy. Headache, tachycardia, palpitations, flushing, nausea, and diarrhea are common but may resolve as therapy progresses. Orthostatic hypotension, fluid retention, and peripheral edema may also occur. Patients who are slow acetylators and those with CKD or who are receiving high doses of hydralazine are susceptible to experiencing a lupus-like syndrome characterized by myalgia, arthralgia, fever, and the presence of antinuclear antibodies. Although rare, symptoms may persist for 6 months or longer and antinuclear antibodies may be present for 9 years. The occurrence of this lupus-like syndrome is more common in whites who are slow acetylators (see Chapter 11). Blood dyscrasias such as agranulocytosis and leukopenia are rare, though potentially serious, adverse effects.

Contraindications/Precautions: Patients with lupus should not receive hydralazine, as the drug can worsen symptoms. The drug is contraindicated in patients with cerebrovascular disease or rheumatic heart disease. Patients should discontinue hydralazine gradually because abrupt withdrawal may cause severe rebound HTN and anxiety. Because it is excreted primarily by the kidneys, the drug should be used with caution in patients with CKD. Caution must be used when administering hydralazine to patients who are known slow acetylators because plasma drug levels will be significantly higher in these patients. Caution should be used when treating patients with CAD because hydralazine can precipitate angina attacks and an acute MI.

Drug Interactions: Administering hydralazine with other antihypertensives or monoamine oxidase inhibitors may cause severe hypotension. This includes all drug classes used as antihypertensives. NSAIDs may decrease the antihypertensive action of hydralazine. Beta blockers are usually used concurrently with hydralazine to block reflex tachycardia, and heart rate should be carefully monitored to avoid bradycardia. Hydralazine may produce false-positive Coombs' tests. **Herbal/Food:** Hawthorn should be avoided because it may cause additive hypotensive effects.

Pregnancy: Hydralazine showed fetal harm in laboratory animals. Small amounts of the drug are secreted in milk but adverse effects on the breastfed neonate are not known.

Treatment of Overdose: Treatment includes gastric lavage, activated charcoal, and administration of a plasma volume expander to raise blood pressure. Tachycardia may require treatment with a beta blocker.

Clinician Responsibilities: Key clinical implications for patients receiving hydralazine are included in Applied Clinical Judgment: Patients Receiving Pharmacotherapy with Direct Vasodilators.

Drugs Similar to Hydralazine

Other direct vasodilators used for HTN include minoxidil and nitroprusside. Nitroprusside is a drug for hypertensive emergencies and is presented in Section 34.9.

Minoxidil (Loniten): Minoxidil is a direct vasodilator with profound vasodilation activity that is selective for arterioles: It does not dilate veins. It is administered PO for severe HTN that is unresponsive to drugs from other classes. Because of its efficacy and the potential for serious effects on the cardiovascular system, initial doses are very low, and the amount is increased gradually. Studies on laboratory animals showed a reduced ability to conceive and reduced survival of offspring. The manufacturer recommends that minoxidil not be given to nursing mothers.

Minoxidil is considerably more toxic than hydralazine. The most serious adverse effects are cardiovascular in nature, including reflex tachycardia and plasma volume expansion due to sodium and water retention. Beta blockers are usually administered concurrently to minimize tachycardia and diuretics to prevent fluid retention. Although rare, pericardial effusion has been reported with minoxidil use. Minoxidil causes **hypertrichosis**, the elongation, thickening, and increased pigmentation of body hair. This is normal and will reverse when the drug is discontinued. The drug's effect on hair growth is used to the patient's advantage in Rogaine, a topical form of minoxidil used to stimulate hair growth in patients with male-pattern baldness. The topical form of the drug is not absorbed into the systemic circulation; thus, Rogaine produces none of the serious cardiovascular effects observed with oral minoxidil.

Management of Hypertensive Emergency

34.9 Hypertensive crisis is a medical emergency that is treated by the intravenous administration of antihypertensive medications.

A **hypertensive emergency (HTN-E)**, also called *hypertensive crisis*, is defined as a diastolic pressure of greater than 180/110 mmHg, with evidence of target-organ system damage. HTN-E requires aggressive treatment, usually within

CONNECTIONS: Advanced Practice Application

Hypertension and the Geriatric Patient

Case

Mr. Balewa is an 86-year-old black man with a 24-year history of HTN and a new diagnosis of heart failure. He is being seen in the outpatient department today for a blood pressure check and laboratory follow-up. He was last seen 6 weeks ago and has not been hospitalized or treated in an emergency department since his last visit. On assessment Mr. Balewa states that his breathing and energy level are similar to his last visit and he can climb one flight of stairs before becoming dyspneic. He has two-pillow orthopnea but no nocturnal dyspnea. He denies chest pain, palpitations, lightheadedness or dizziness, nausea, or edema. Mr. Balewa follows a low-sodium diet and has no difficulty eating. On physical examination he is alert, cooperative, has no jugular venous distension, and no peripheral edema. His lungs are clear, abdomen is soft and nontender without hepatosplenomegaly. Heart rate and rhythm are regular; he has a 2/6 systolic murmur at the left lower sternal border. Mr. Balewa's blood pressure was 148/72 mm Hg; pulse, 72 bpm; weight, 182 lb (unchanged since last visit).

Serum laboratory history: sodium 138 mmol/L; potassium 4.0 mmol/L; BUN 24 mg/dL; creatinine 1.4 mg/dL; total cholesterol 184 mg/dL; HDL 72 mg/dL; LDL 93 mg/dL; triglycerides 106 mg/dL.

Medications: Losartan 100 mg/day; hydrochlorothiazide 25 mg/day.

What are some of the things that the nurse practitioner needs to consider for this patient?

Discussion

Hypertension is a common problem in older adults, reaching a prevalence as high as 70 to 80%. In the United States, it was observed in 76% of adults aged 65 to 74 years and 82% of adults aged 75 years or older (Muntner et al., 2018).

When caring for patients over the age of 80, healthcare providers should be aware that it differs from a standard medical evaluation. Due to the complexity of older patients' health conditions and multiple comorbidities, history taking and physical examination might take additional time. A decline in blood pressure over time in older adults with HTN is common and the requirements for antihypertensive treatment may decrease. Antihypertensive treatment requires frequent and longer follow-up appointments, close attention to side effects, and more frequent laboratory monitoring.

Because polypharmacy is common in this age group, starting with monotherapy should be the rule. In older hypertensive patients with DM or HF, ARBs are considered first-line treatment and an alternative to ACE inhibitors. Starting two drugs at the same time should be avoided and caution is needed if prescribing more than three antihypertensive drugs in those over 80 years of age.

minutes to hours, to prevent further organ damage. **Hypertensive urgency** is when a patient presents with a similar acute level of blood pressure but has no evidence of target-organ damage.

Target-organ damage from extreme HTN most often occurs in the cardiovascular system, the kidneys, or the CNS. In the cardiovascular system, the increased workload on the heart leads to acute left HF with pulmonary edema, sometimes accompanied by myocardial ischemia or infarction. Chest pain and dyspnea are the most common symptoms in patients with HTN-E. Renal function is diminished, as evidenced by oliguria, hematuria, and proteinuria. Acute renal failure may occur, or preexisting CKD may worsen. In the brain, thrombotic or hemorrhagic stroke may occur. The capillaries in the brain become leaky, producing hypertensive encephalopathy, with resulting headache, paralysis, seizures, or coma. In addition, retinal hemorrhages and edema of the retina (papilledema) are signs of severe HTN.

The most common cause of HTN-E is untreated or poorly controlled primary HTN. In some cases, the patient has abruptly discontinued use of the antihypertensive medication. There are, however, a large number of possible secondary causes of HTN-E, including the following conditions:

- Renovascular hypertension
- Pheochromocytoma
- Cocaine use
- Eclampsia or preeclampsia
- Head injuries
- Primary hyperaldosteronism
- Coarctation of the aorta
- Hyperthyroidism or thyroid storm.

In the management of HTN-E, the therapeutic goal is to rapidly lower blood pressure. Care must be taken, however, to not decrease blood pressure too quickly because rapid and intense vasodilation can result in serious hypoperfusion of the cerebral, coronary, or renal vascular capillaries. This can cause ischemia or infarction and worsening target-organ damage to the brain, heart, kidneys, or retina. It is recommended that the pretreatment blood pressure be progressively reduced by 20 to 25%, over 30 to 60 minutes. Additional, gradual reductions are made over a 12- to 48-hour period until blood pressure is reduced to a value within the normal range. Parenteral antihypertensives are preferred over PO medications due to their rapid onset of action and because infusions offer more precise control during the gradual pressure reduction.

In patients with hypertensive urgencies, target-organ damage has not yet developed. These patients are treated more conservatively by increasing the dose of their current antihypertensive drug or by adding a second drug to the regimen. Oral medications are used to lower blood pressure because these drugs are less toxic than parenteral antihypertensives. Oral drugs with a relatively rapid onset of action that may be used for hypertensive urgency include clonidine (Catapres), captopril, or labetalol (Trandate). The patient should be monitored for several hours, and doses may be repeated at frequent intervals, as needed, to lower pressure to acceptable levels. All patients with hypertensive urgency should receive follow-up assessments after 1 to 3 days on the new regimen.

PROTOTYPE DRUG **Nitroprusside Sodium (Nitropress)**

Classification **Therapeutic:** Drug for hypertensive emergency
Pharmacologic: Direct vasodilator

Therapeutic Effects and Uses: Nitroprusside is a first-line drug for patients with aggressive, life-threatening HTN because it has the ability to lower blood pressure almost instantaneously upon IV administration. Indications include hypertensive crisis, acute HF, and promotion of controlled hypotension to reduce bleeding during surgery. The drug has a short half-life, and the hypotensive effects disappear approximately 3 minutes after the infusion is discontinued. Unlike most direct vasodilators, nitroprusside causes very little reflex tachycardia. Although discovered in 1850, the drug was not approved by the U.S. Food and Drug Administration until 1974.

Patients must be continuously monitored while receiving nitroprusside to prevent hypotension due to overtreatment. Therapy is limited to 72 hours because the drug is metabolized to toxic *thiocyanate* and cyanide compounds. This is of special concern to patients with CKD who are unable to excrete the cyanide. If serum thiocyanate exceeds 12 mg/dL, the nitroprusside infusion should be discontinued. As a general rule, patients are switched from nitroprusside to an oral antihypertensive as soon as blood pressure has stabilized.

Mechanism of Action: Nitroprusside dilates both arteries and veins; therefore, the hypotensive action of nitroprusside is due to direct relaxation of arteriolar smooth muscle and to blood pooling in the veins. In most patients, heart rate is mildly increased, whereas cardiac output is decreased. In patients with severe left-ventricular hypertrophy, however, cardiac output may increase.

Pharmacokinetics:

Route(s)	IV
Absorption	N/A
Distribution	Unknown
Primary metabolism	Metabolized to thiocyanates in erythrocytes and other tissues
Primary excretion	Renal
Onset of action	1–2 min
Duration of action	1–10 min

Adverse Effects: Signs and symptoms of vasodilation such as hypotension, headache, dizziness, and flushing of the skin are expected adverse effects. With extended therapy, thiocyanate toxicity may manifest. Thiocyanate poisoning is characterized by hypotension, lethargy, blurred vision, metabolic acidosis, faint heart sounds, and loss of consciousness. Irritation may occur at the infusion site. **Black Box Warning:** Nitroprusside requires dilution prior to infusion and is not suitable for direct injection. The drug can cause irreversible ischemic injury and death due to significant drops in blood pressure. Accumulation of cyanide ion may occur.

Contraindications/Precautions: Patients with inadequate cerebral circulation or who have compensatory HTN should not receive nitroprusside. Because the kidneys excrete the toxic thiocyanate metabolite of the drug, patients with serious CKD should be treated cautiously. Nitroprusside is contraindicated in patients with high intracranial pressure because the drug may worsen this condition.

Drug Interactions: Antihypertensive drugs, ethanol, general anesthetics, and ganglionic blockers should be used with caution with nitroprusside because additive hypotension could result. Sympathomimetics such as epinephrine will block the antihypertensive actions of nitroprusside. Dobutamine (Dobutrex) and nitroprusside are sometimes administered concurrently because this interaction results in a beneficial synergistic increase in cardiac output and decrease in pulmonary capillary wedge pressure. **Herbal/Food:** Hawthorn may cause additive hypotensive effects.

Pregnancy: Prolonged use of high doses during pregnancy may lead to fatal cyanide toxicity in the fetus. Breastfeeding is not recommended because thiocyanate is secreted in milk.

Treatment of Overdose: Extreme hypotension may be treated with a vasopressor. Cyanide toxicity caused by the overdose may require the use of a cyanide antidote kit, which contains amyl nitrate, sodium nitrite, and sodium thiosulfate. The purpose of these drugs is to convert toxic cyanide into nontoxic thiocyanate.

Clinician Responsibilities: Key clinical implications for patients receiving nitroprusside are included in Applied Clinical Judgment: Patients Receiving Pharmacotherapy with Direct Vasodilators.

Drugs Similar to Nitroprusside Sodium (Nitropress)

Other medications for HTN-E are shown in Table 34.4, which summarizes their applications to the pharmacotherapy of hypertensive crisis. Diazoxide is a rapid-acting vasodilator that is no longer marketed for blood pressure control. An oral form of diazoxide (Proglycem) is available to treat various hypoglycemic states, usually caused by the presence of excessive insulin (hyperinsulinism).

PharmFACT

Hypertensive crisis is a common condition, affecting 1% of the patients with primary HTN. The most common presentation, occurring in 25% of patients, is stroke. The 1-year survival rate for a patient presenting with a HTN crisis has improved from only 20% prior to 1950 to more than 90% with current medical treatment (Hopkins, 2018).

Table 34.4 Drugs for Hypertensive Emergency

Drug	Class	Applications
clevidipine (Cleviprex)	Calcium channel blocker	Onset of action is 2–4 min with a short duration, allowing for rapid blood pressure reduction
enalaprilat	ACE inhibitor	Onset of action is 15–30 min; useful in HTN-E associated with HF or high plasma levels of angiotensin II
esmolol (Brevibloc)	Beta-adrenergic antagonist	Onset of action is 1–5 min; useful for patients with severe left-ventricular dysfunction or with peripheral vascular disease
fenoldopam (Corlopam)	Dopamine agonist	Onset of action is 10–15 min; useful for patients with CKD because the drug increases renal blood flow
hydralazine	Direct vasodilator	Onset of action is 5–20 min; useful in HTN-E due to eclampsia and preeclampsia because it increases uterine blood flow
labetalol (Trandate)	Alpha- and beta-adrenergic antagonist	Onset of action is 2–5 min; reduces incidences of MI and death
nicardipine (Cardene IV)	Calcium channel blocker	Onset of action is 1 min; rapid and effective for most HTN-E, with fewer adverse effects than some other HTN-E drugs
nitroprusside sodium (Nitropress)	Direct vasodilator	Onset of action is less than 1 min; preferred drug for many HTN-E
phentolamine (Oraverse)	Alpha-adrenergic antagonist	Onset of action is 1–5 min; rarely used due to high incidence of reflex tachycardia and myocardial ischemia; useful for HTN-E due to pheochromocytoma

CONNECTIONS: APPLIED CLINICAL JUDGMENT

Patients Receiving Pharmacotherapy with Direct Vasodilators

Key Assessment Data

- History of current condition, baseline vital signs, weight, physical exam findings; history of cardiovascular, cerebrovascular, respiratory disease, diabetes; medication history; pregnancy status. Baseline ECG, cardiac output, and urinary output should be assessed, depending on the drug classification being used.
- Ongoing assessment during drug therapy should include monitoring for bradycardia, hypotension, reflex tachycardia, dysrhythmias, bronchospasm, decreased urinary output, edema or weight gain over 1 kg (2 lb) per day.

Desired Therapeutic Outcomes

Improvement is observed and measurable when patient's BP is within acceptable parameters.

Minimizing Adverse Effects:

- Monitor for orthostatic hypotension. Notify the provider if BP decreases beyond the established parameters or if hypotension is accompanied by reflex tachycardia. Blood pressure and pulse should be monitored every 5 minutes or as ordered while on IV infusions of antihypertensives. Direct-acting vasodilators cause significant vasodilation, resulting in the potential for dramatically and rapidly lowered blood pressure accompanied by reflex tachycardia. Reflex tachycardia may require treatment with beta-blocking drugs.
- Patients with a preexisting history of cardiac or cerebrovascular ischemia, patients with dehydration, and patients with lupus erythematosus may experience additional adverse effects from hypotension. Immediately notify the healthcare provider if blood pressure or pulse decrease beyond established parameters or if hypotension is accompanied by reflex tachycardia.
- Weigh daily and report weight gain over 1 kg in a 24-hour period or edema. These may signal that the BP has lowered too quickly, stimulating renin release, or is an adverse effect.
- Observe for signs and symptoms of lupus in patients taking vasodilators, particularly hydralazine, which has been linked to drug-induced lupus. Other direct vasodilators are used with caution for this reason.
- Direct-acting vasodilators may cause tissue damage if the drug extravasates. Continue to monitor IV infusion sites frequently.
- Monitor for the development of priapism and notify the healthcare provider. Priapism may result in tissue damage if unrelieved and is considered a medical emergency.
- A first-dose response may result in a greater initial drop in blood pressure than subsequent doses. For oral drug therapy, give the first dose of the drug at bedtime.

Lifespan Considerations

- Older adults may be more sensitive to the effects of adrenergic antagonist drugs and dizziness may increase the risk of falls.

Diversity Considerations

- Differences exist in the response to antihypertensive therapy among various populations and ongoing assessment is needed to ensure response to drug therapy is adequate.
- Hydralazine is known to metabolize in patients who are slow acetylators, and because this cannot always be predicted, ensure that frequent monitoring continues, especially in the early stages of drug therapy.

Patient Education

- Monitor pulse, BP, and daily weight, using a diary or log, and bring these to each provider visit. Promptly report any weight gain over 1 kg in a 24-hour period, increasing or severe shortness of breath, palpitations, or chest pain to the provider.
- Immediately report changes in mental status or level of consciousness, palpitations, dizziness, dyspnea, increasing productive cough, especially if frothy sputum is present, and seek medical attention.
- Take the first dose of an antihypertensive at bedtime, if possible, to avoid excessive dizziness and first-dose hypotension.
- Rise slowly from lying or sitting to standing, pausing between changes if dizziness occurs. Don't take the medication if dizziness continues, or the BP is below 90/60 or per parameters set by the provider, and contact the provider for further instruction.
- Report symptoms such as a butterfly-shaped rash over the nose and cheeks, muscle aches, and fatigue when taking oral vasodilators, particularly hydralazine.
- Immediately report a sustained erection that lasts more than 4 h if on vasodilator therapy at home and seek immediate medical care.
- The drug should not be stopped abruptly to avoid rebound HTN. If unable to take medication for more than one day due to illness, the provider should be contacted.
- Be cautious about sudden increases in activity level. Report dizziness, palpitations, or shortness of breath that occurs while exercising.
- Take the drug at the same time(s) every day when possible.

Prescribing Considerations

- If pregnancy occurs, ensure the patient is receiving an antihypertensive that is recommended for pregnant patients. Change medication or adjust dose as necessary.
- In patients at risk for excessive hypotension, therapy should be started under close medical supervision and should be followed closely for the first 2 weeks of treatment and whenever the dose is increased.
- Periodic monitoring of white blood cell counts in patients with vascular disease and renal disease should be considered.

Understanding Chapter 34

Key Concepts Summary

34.1 Failure to properly manage hypertension can lead to stroke, heart failure, or myocardial infarction.

34.2 Therapeutic lifestyle changes can reduce blood pressure and lessen the need for antihypertensive medications.

34.3 The choice of antihypertensive medication is determined by the degree of hypertension and the presence of other medical conditions.

34.4 Diuretics are often preferred drugs for treating mild to moderate hypertension.

34.5 Calcium channel blockers have emerged as important drugs in the treatment of hypertension.

34.6 Blocking the renin-angiotensin-aldosterone system leads to a decrease in blood pressure and improved kidney function.

34.7 Adrenergic antagonists are commonly used to treat hypertension.

34.8 Direct-acting vasodilators lower blood pressure by relaxing arteriolar smooth muscle.

34.9 Hypertensive crisis is a medical emergency that is treated by the intravenous administration of antihypertensive medications.

CASE STUDY: Making the Patient Connection

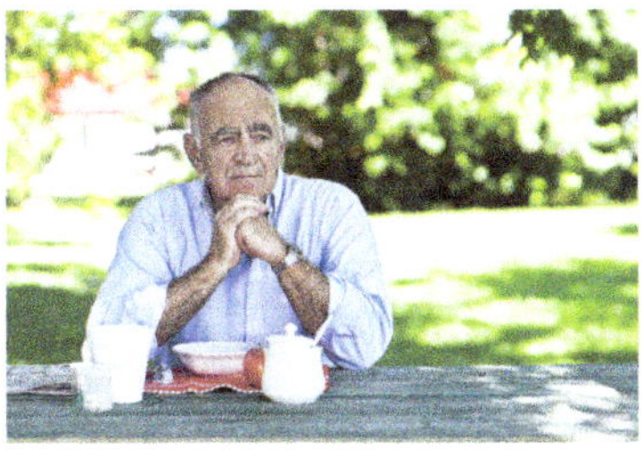

Remember the patient "Elmer Foley" at the beginning of the chapter? Now read the remainder of the case study. Based on the information presented within this chapter, respond to the critical thinking questions that follow.

Elmer Foley is a 72-year-old man with a 10-month history of poorly managed HTN. Initially, he was prescribed the thiazide diuretic HCTZ (Microzide). However, after 1 week of therapy, his blood pressure remained at 168/102 mmHg. Next, Elmer's healthcare provider added an ACE inhibitor, captopril (Capoten), to the regimen. Still, his blood pressure remained above normal limits. Lastly, the healthcare provider discontinued the captopril and started him on PO hydralazine. With this visit, his blood pressure is 146/90 mmHg.

When Elmer was first told he had HTN, he began many of the suggested lifestyle changes encouraged by his healthcare provider. He has lost a total of 15 kg (33 lb) since starting his diet 10 months ago. Elmer started walking daily for exercise and can now walk up to 1 mile without fatigue. He avoids all salty foods and diligently checks food labels for fat and salt content. Elmer occasionally drinks a glass of wine, although never more than one to two glasses per month. Although it was difficult for Elmer to stop smoking, he proudly claims he has not smoked for 8 months.

Critical Thinking Questions

1. How would you respond to Elmer's question, "What else can I do?" Is there anything else he can do to reduce his blood pressure?
2. Elmer wants to know why the previous therapies were unsuccessful. What would you say as his nurse?
3. As the nurse, how can you support Elmer before he leaves the clinic?

Additional Case Study

Helen Edwards is a 44-year-old Black female who presents to the emergency department (ED) with headache and shortness of breath. She has a long-standing history of HTN. She has never consistently adhered to any HTN management strategies and has been nonadherent with her medication regimen for the past 8 months. On arrival at the ED Helen's blood pressure is 192/126 mmHg.

When you assess the patient, you note that she is approximately 1.7 m (5′6″) in height and the self-reported weight is 107 kg (235 lb). She is slightly lethargic and reports having left arm numbness and tingling. Other physical assessment parameters are normal.

Helen is started on an infusion of nitroprusside (Nitropress) 50 mg in 250 mL in D_5W. The dose will be titrated between 0.5 and 10 mcg/kg/min to maintain the patient's diastolic pressure at less than 100 mmHg.

1. Describe the mechanism of action related to nitroprusside (Nitropress).
2. For what adverse effects should you monitor in patients receiving this drug therapy?
3. What factors does this patient have that predispose her to hypertensive crises?

Chapter Review

1. A 35-year-old Black man is given a prescription for nifedipine (Procardia XL). He asks why he can't "take a beta-blocker, like my work colleague does, and it's cheaper, too." What is the best explanation for this prescription?
   1. Different racial and ethnic groups respond differently to different classes of antihypertensives. This drug has been shown to have better results based on this patient's race/ethnicity.
   2. An extended-release drug is being given to enhance adherence since it will not interfere with his work schedule.
   3. Cost is not a determining factor for ensuring drug response.
   4. Beta-blockers are known to cause profound hypotension in Black patients.

2. A patient is receiving hydralazine for elevated blood pressure levels. The nurse would include in the care plan to monitor the patient for which adverse effects?
   1. Atelectasis
   2. Crystalluria
   3. Photosensitivity
   4. Orthostatic hypotension

3. The nurse is preparing to administer the first dose of enalapril (Vasotec). Identify the potential adverse effects of this medication. (Select all that apply.)
   1. Reflex hypertension
   2. Hyperkalemia
   3. Persistent cough
   4. Angioedema
   5. Hypotension

4. A patient with hypertensive crisis is started on nitroprusside (Nitropress) therapy. The nurse would perform what priority intervention during the course of this treatment?
   1. Monitor for the presence or absence of bowel sounds.
   2. Obtain urine samples for specific gravity measurements and glucose levels.
   3. Observe skin pressure points for turgor and integrity.
   4. Titrate intravenous infusion rate according to the blood pressure response.

5. A 65-year-old patient has been newly diagnosed with hypertension, with an average blood pressure of 164/92 mmHg. Which of the following drug groups will potentially be ordered initially? (Select all that apply.)
   1. Beta blockers
   2. Calcium channel blockers
   3. Thiazide diuretics
   4. Angiotensin-converting enzyme inhibitors or angiotensin receptor blockers
   5. Direct-acting vasodilators

6. A patient is receiving nitroprusside (Nitropress) and is being monitored in the intensive care unit. Because of toxic cyanide metabolites that develop, which of the following should the nurse evaluate in the patient? (Select all that apply.)
   1. Cardiac status and cardiac output
   2. Renal function and creatinine levels
   3. Past history of alcohol use
   4. Level of consciousness
   5. Skin color and turgor

See Appendix A for answers to critical thinking questions, case study questions, and review questions.

References

Centers for Disease Control and Prevention. (2020). *High blood pressure: Facts about hypertension fact sheet*. https://www.cdc.gov/bloodpressure/facts.htm

Hopkins, C. (2018). *Hypertensive emergencies*. Medscape. https://emedicine.medscape.com/article/1952052-overview#a2

Muntner, P., Carey, R. M., Gidding, S., Jones, D. W., Taler, S. J., Wright, J. T., Jr, & Whelton, P. K. (2018). Potential U.S. population impact of the 2017 ACC/AHA High Blood Pressure Guideline. *Journal of the American College of Cardiology*, *71*(2), 109–118. https://doi.org/10.1016/j.jacc.2017.10.073

Whelton, P. K., Carey, R. M., Aronow, W. S., Casey, D. E., Collins, K. J., Dennison Himmelfarb, et al. (2018). 2017 ACC/AHA/AAPA/ABC/ACPM/AGS/APhA/ASH/ASPC/NMA/PCNA guideline for the prevention, detection, evaluation, and management of high blood pressure in adults: Executive Summary: A report of the American College of Cardiology/American Heart Association Task Force on Clinical Practice Guidelines. *Hypertension*, *71*(6), 1269–1324. https://doi.org/10.1161/HYP.0000000000000066

Selected Bibliography

Adebayo, O., & Rogers, R. L. (2015). Hypertensive emergencies in the emergency department. *Emergency Medicine Clinics of North America*, *33*(3), 539–551. https://doi.org/10.1016/j.emc.2015.04.005

Burnier, M., & Egan, B. M. (2019). Adherence in hypertension: A review of prevalence, risk factors, impact, and management. *Circulation Research*, *124*(7), 1124–1140. https://doi.org/10.1161/CIRCRESAHA.118.313220

Davis, L. L. (2019). Hypertension: How low to go when treating older adults. *Journal for Nurse Practitioners*, *15*(1), 1–6. https://doi.org/10.1016/j.nurpra.2018.10.010

Del Pinto, R., & Ferri, C. (2019). Hypertension management at older age: An update. *High Blood Pressure and Cardiovascular Prevention*, *26*(1), 27–36. https://doi.org/10.1007/s40292-018-0290-z

Divens, L. L., & Chatmon, B. N. (2019). Cardiovascular Disease Management in Minority Women: Special Considerations. *Critical Care Nursing Clinics of North America*, *31*(1), 39–47. https://doi.org/10.1016/j.cnc.2018.11.004

Magvanjav, O., Cooper-DeHoff, R. M., McDonough, C. W., Gong, Y., Hogan, W. R., & Johnson, J. A. (2020). Combination antihypertensive therapy prescribing and blood pressure control in a real-world setting. *American Journal of Hypertension*, *33*(4), 316–324. https://doi.org/10.1093/ajh/hpz196

Muiesan, M. L., Salvetti, M., Amadoro, V., Di Somma, S., Perlini, S., Semplicini, A., et al. (2015). An update on hypertensive emergencies and urgencies. *Journal of Cardiovascular Medicine*, *16*, 372–382. https://doi.org/10.2459/JCM.0000000000000223

Oliveira-Paula, G. H., Pereira, S. C., Tanus-Santos, J. E., & Lacchini, R. (2019). Pharmacogenomics and hypertension: Current insights. *Pharmacogenomics and Personalized Medicine*, *12*, 341–359. https://doi.org/10.2147/PGPM.S230201

Qaseem, A., Wilt, T. J., Rich, R., Humphrey, L. L., Frost, J., & Forciea, M. A. (2017). Pharmacologic treatment of hypertension in adults aged 60 years or older to higher versus lower blood pressure targets: A clinical practice guideline from the American College of Physicians and the American Academy of Family Physicians. *Annals of Internal Medicine*, *166*, 430–437. https://doi.org/10.7326/M16-1785

Rivera, S. L., Martin, J., & Landry, J. (2019). Acute and chronic hypertension: What clinicians need to know for diagnosis and management. *Critical Care Nursing Clinics*, *31*(1), 97–108. https://doi.org/10.1016/j.cnc.2018.11.008

Shoulders, B., & Powell, L. (2019). Reaching for goal: Incorporating the latest hypertension guidelines into practice. *Journal for Nurse Practitioners*, *15*(1), 102–109. https://doi.org/10.1016/j.nurpra.2018.09.011

Watson, K., Broscious, R., Devabhakthuni, S., & Noel, Z. R. (2018). Focused update on pharmacologic management of hypertensive emergencies. *Current Hypertension Reports*, *20*(7), 56. https://doi.org/10.1007/s11906-018-0854-2

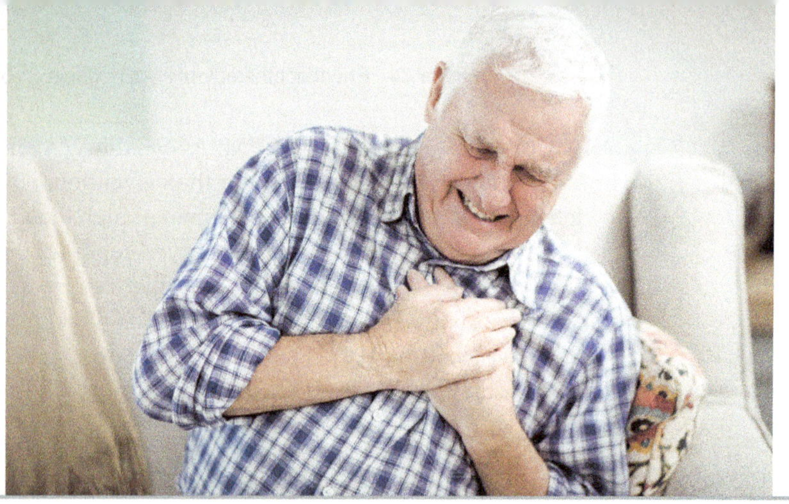

"I was simply sitting and reading the newspaper, when suddenly my chest felt tight, I felt weak, and I had difficulty breathing."
—*Patient "Michael Graff"*

Chapter 35
Pharmacotherapy of Angina Pectoris and Myocardial Infarction

Chapter Outline

Learning Outcomes

After reading this chapter, the student should be able to:

1. Describe factors that affect myocardial oxygen supply and demand.
2. Explain the relationship between atherosclerosis and coronary artery disease.
3. Explain the pathophysiology of angina pectoris and myocardial infarction.
4. Discuss the role of therapeutic lifestyle changes in the management of coronary artery disease.
5. Describe the pharmacologic management of the different types of angina.
6. Describe the pharmacologic management of myocardial infarction.
7. For each of the classes shown in the chapter outline, identify the prototype and representative drugs and explain the mechanism(s) of drug action, primary indications, contraindications, significant drug interactions, pregnancy data, and important adverse effects.
8. Apply clinical judgment to care for patients receiving pharmacotherapy for angina and myocardial infarction.

Key Terms

Definitions of the terms in bold may be found in the Glossary.

The tissues of the body depend on a continuous supply of oxygen and vital nutrients to support life and health. The heart is particularly demanding of a steady source of oxygen. Insufficient arterial blood supply to cardiac muscle may result in angina pectoris, acute myocardial infarction (heart attack), and possibly death. This chapter focuses on the pharmacologic interventions related to angina pectoris and myocardial infarction (MI).

Pathophysiology of Myocardial Ischemia

35.1 Myocardial ischemia develops when there is inadequate blood supply to meet the metabolic demands of cardiac muscle.

Myocardial ischemia is a condition in which the heart is receiving an insufficient amount of oxygen to meet its metabolic demands. This occurs when there is an imbalance between oxygen supply and oxygen demand in myocardial cells. Knowledge of factors affecting myocardial oxygen supply and demand is necessary for understanding the pharmacotherapy of the diseases associated with myocardial ischemia.

Myocardial Oxygen Supply

The heart, from the moment it begins to function *in utero* until death, works to distribute oxygen and nutrients by means of its nonstop pumping action. It is the hardest working organ in the body, functioning continuously during both activity and rest. Because the heart is a muscle, it needs a steady supply of nourishment to sustain itself and maintain the systemic circulation in a state of equilibrium. Any disturbance in blood flow to the myocardium—even for brief episodes—can result in life-threatening consequences. A review of basic coronary circulation is provided in Chapter 28.

As with other arteries in the body, the amount of blood flow through the coronary arteries is dependent on a number of hemodynamic factors. Of these, blood pressure is the most important. When systolic blood pressure falls, the quantity of blood flowing to the coronary arteries is diminished. If this occurs suddenly, such as in acute shock, it could be life-threatening. Immediate restoration of blood pressure is required to reestablish an adequate oxygen supply to the myocardium as well as to other vital tissues. Other hemodynamic factors contributing to the myocardial oxygen supply include changes in blood volume (e.g., hemorrhage) and disorders that reduce the oxygen content or carrying capacity of the blood (e.g., anemia).

The narrowing of a coronary artery resulting from atherosclerosis or coronary artery disease (CAD) deprives cells of needed oxygen and nutrients. If the narrowing develops over a long period of time, the heart compensates for its inadequate blood supply and the patient may be asymptomatic. Indeed, coronary arteries may be occluded as much as 50% or more and cause no symptoms.

Myocardial Oxygen Demand

As CAD progresses, cardiac muscle does not receive enough oxygen to meet the body's metabolic demands. The physiologic demands on the heart are highly variable and depend on a large number of hemodynamic and lifestyle factors.

Basically, anything that increases the workload of the heart will increase myocardial oxygen demand. It is not difficult to think of the many daily activities that increase cardiac workload. Exercise, for example, will cause the heart to beat faster in order to pump more blood to muscles. This physical activity need not be extreme: Simply walking at a normal pace will increase cardiac workload.

In some patients, the increased cardiac workload can be the result of mental, rather than physical, stressors. Think of the first time (or last time) you had to give a speech in front of a group or became angry with a child, spouse, or coworker. These activities resulted in your heart pumping harder or faster, even though there was no physical activity involved. What factors do physical exercise and mental stress have in common that produced the increased cardiac workload?

The answer is simple. Anything that increases heart rate, contractility, or tension on the ventricular walls causes the heart to work harder and affect cardiac oxygen consumption. For example, if heart rate increases due to exercise or hyperthyroidism, it is easy to understand why the heart needs more oxygen because it must beat more times per minute. Similarly, the heart will need more oxygen if it beats more forcefully (increased contractility). A patient with heart failure (HF) has a thickened myocardium (increased tension) that will require more work to contract. The heart of a patient with hypertension (HTN) will have to work harder to overcome resistance and eject blood. It is important to remember that anything that makes the heartbeat faster or contract with more force will increase myocardial oxygen demand. Drugs that diminish these factors are of value in the treatment of angina, MI, and HF.

Etiology of Coronary Artery Disease

35.2 Coronary artery disease is the major cause of myocardial ischemia.

Coronary artery disease (CAD) is one of the leading causes of mortality in the United States. The primary defining characteristic of CAD is narrowing or occlusion of one or more coronary arteries. Narrowing can result in symptoms of angina pectoris, whereas occlusion results in MI. The two disorders are closely related, as most patients who experience an MI have narrowing of the coronary vessels.

The most common etiology of CAD in adults is atherosclerosis, the presence of **plaque**—a fatty, fibrous material—within the walls of the coronary arteries (see Figure 35.1). Plaque develops progressively over time, producing varying degrees of intravascular narrowing that results in partial or total blockage of the vessel. During periods of rest, demands on the heart are reduced and a partially occluded artery may be able to provide adequate oxygen. During exercise (or a pharmacology test), however, workload on the heart increases, the cardiac muscle distal to the obstruction receives insufficient oxygen supply, and ischemia results.

A healthy heart responds to stress by changing the diameter of the coronary arteries. When the oxygen demands of the heart increase, the vessels will immediately dilate to bring more oxygen to the myocardium. Plaque impairs normal elasticity, and the coronary vessels are unable to dilate properly when the myocardium demands additional oxygen. Myocardial ischemia occurs when cardiac demands exceed the amount of oxygen that can be supplied through the narrowed, inelastic vessels characteristic of CAD.

CONNECTION Checkpoint 35.1

From what you learned in Chapter 28, predict what would happen to the cardiac workload when plasma volume is increased by a rapid infusion of normal saline. What effect might this have on a patient with CAD?

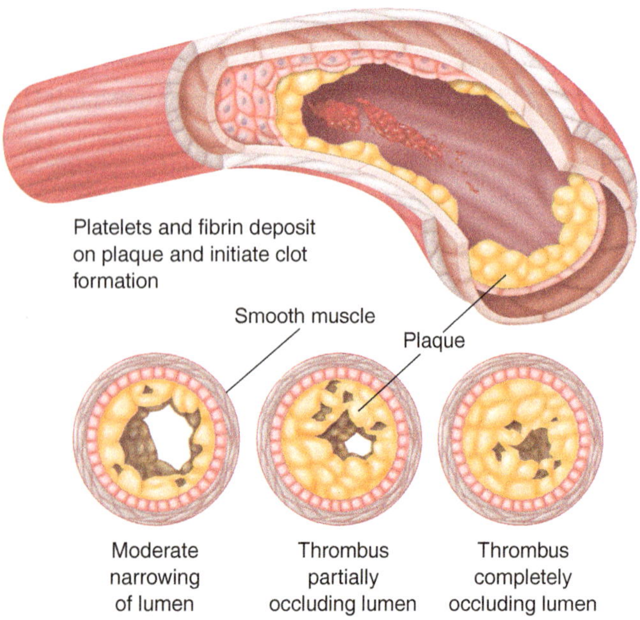

Figure 35.1 Atherosclerosis in the coronary arteries.

Primary Prevention of Coronary Artery Disease

This chapter examines two disorders that are intimately associated with CAD. The two disorders, however, may be visualized as one continuous progression starting with minimal (or no) atherosclerosis and leading to complete occlusion of a coronary vessel. Not all patients proceed through this entire process; indeed, it is the goal of healthcare providers to prevent this from occurring by the use of teaching, medications, and interventions.

35.3 Therapeutic lifestyle changes can reduce the risk of coronary artery disease.

A combination of variables influences the development and progression of CAD, including dietary patterns and lifestyle choices. The nurse is instrumental in teaching patients the means of preventing CAD by the formulation of a comprehensive plan of care that incorporates psychosocial support and an individualized teaching plan. The patient needs to understand the causes of CAD, identify the progressive nature of the disorder, and acquire the motivation to modify behaviors associated with the disease.

Listing therapeutic lifestyle changes that modify the development and progression of atherosclerotic cardiovascular disease (ASCVD) may seem repetitious, as these same factors have been included in chapters on HTN and heart disease. However, the importance of prevention and management of ASCVD through nonpharmacologic means cannot be overemphasized. Making healthy lifestyle choices can *prevent* CAD and *slow the progression* of the disease in those who have existing plaque. The following factors reduce the risk of subsequent adverse ASCVD events and mortality.

- Limit alcohol consumption to small or moderate amounts.
- Eliminate foods high in cholesterol or saturated fats.
- Keep blood lipid indicators within the normal ranges.
- Keep blood pressure within the normal range.
- Maintain blood glucose levels within the normal range.
- Exercise regularly and maintain optimal weight.
- Do not use tobacco.
- Limit sodium intake.

Primary prevention of angina and MI usually involves medications. Based on the clinical findings, statins are essential at reducing the risk for ASCVD (see Chapter 29). Medications for the management of HTN and diabetes are essential. Proper medication management clearly reduces the risk for serious adverse ASCVD events such as MI and stroke.

Pathophysiology of Angina Pectoris

35.4 Angina pectoris is characterized by severe chest pain brought on by physical exertion or emotional stress.

Angina pectoris is acute chest pain caused by myocardial ischemia. The classic presentation of angina pectoris is steady, intense retrosternal pain. Typically, the discomfort radiates to the left shoulder and proceeds down the left arm. It may also extend to the posterior thoracic region or move upward to the jaw, and in some patients the pain is experienced in the epigastrium. Accompanying the discomfort is severe emotional distress—a feeling of panic with fear of impending death. There is usually pallor, dyspnea with cyanosis, diaphoresis, tachycardia, and elevated blood pressure.

Anginal pain is usually precipitated by physical exertion or emotional excitement—events associated with increased myocardial oxygen demand. Angina pectoris episodes are of short duration. With physical rest and mental relaxation, the workload demands on the heart diminish and the discomfort subsides within 5 to 15 minutes. Descriptions of the four basic types of angina follow.

When angina occurrences are fairly predictable in frequency, intensity, and duration, the condition is described as *classic* or **stable angina**. Rest usually relieves the pain associated with stable angina in about 5 minutes or less.

Variant (Prinzmetal's) angina occurs when the decreased myocardial blood flow is caused by spasms of the coronary arteries. This type is sometimes called *vasospastic angina*. The vessels undergoing spasms may or may not contain atherosclerotic plaque. Thus, the primary cause of the narrowing and subsequent angina pain is vasoconstriction of the artery, rather than plaque buildup. Variant angina pain occurs most often during periods of rest, such as during the nighttime, although it may occur unpredictably, unrelated to rest or activity.

Although most people equate angina with chest pain, this is not always the case. When myocardial ischemia occurs in the absence of pain, it is called **silent ischemia**. Although one or more coronary arteries are partially occluded, the patient is asymptomatic. Some patients diagnosed with stable angina also experience silent ischemia. Although the mechanisms underlying silent ischemia are not completely understood, the condition is associated with a high risk for acute MI and sudden death.

Unstable angina occurs when episodes of angina happen suddenly, have added intensity, and occur during periods of rest. Unstable angina is a type of acute coronary syndrome in which plaque within a coronary artery ruptures. A thrombus quickly builds on the displaced plaque, and the artery becomes at serious risk of occlusion. This condition is a medical emergency requiring aggressive intervention because of the associated increased risk for MI.

Anginal pain often parallels the signs and symptomatology of MI. It is extremely important for the nurse to be able to accurately identify the characteristics that differentiate the two conditions, since the pharmacologic interventions related to angina differ considerably from those of MI. Angina, while aggravating and uncomfortable, rarely leads to a fatal outcome and the chest pain is usually immediately relieved by nitroglycerin. MI, however, carries with it a high mortality rate if appropriate treatment is delayed (see Section 35.9). In the event of MI, pharmacologic intervention must be initiated immediately and systematically maintained. When a patient presents with chest pain, the foremost objective for the healthcare provider is to quickly determine the cause of the pain so that proper, effective interventions can be delivered.

PharmFACT

About 9.8 million Americans experience angina each year. The risk of angina increases with age and is more common in women. Only 18% of coronary attacks are preceded by angina (Alaeddini, 2018).

Pharmacologic Management of Angina Pectoris

35.5 The pharmacologic management of angina includes organic nitrates, beta-adrenergic antagonists, and calcium channel blockers.

Once a patient develops angina, CAD has progressed to a moderate stage and treatment goals are twofold. First, a primary goal is to reduce the frequency and intensity of angina episodes. Successful pharmacotherapy should improve exercise tolerance and allow the patient to actively engage in activities of daily living. Second, the long-term goal is to prevent the progression of ASCVD and serious consequences such as dysrhythmias, HF, and MI. Treatment of angina is usually begun conservatively, through the use of medications and implementing therapeutic lifestyle changes that promote a healthy heart. These are summarized in Figure 35.2.

Medications for angina can be placed into two categories: those that *terminate* an acute angina episode in progress and those that *decrease the frequency* of angina episodes. The primary means by which antianginal medications act is by reducing the myocardial demand for oxygen. This may be accomplished by the following mechanisms:

- Slowing the heart rate
- Dilating veins so that the heart receives less blood (reduced preload)
- Causing the heart to contract with less force (reduced contractility)
- Lowering blood pressure (reduced afterload).

Overview of Stable Coronary Artery Disease Pharmacotherapy

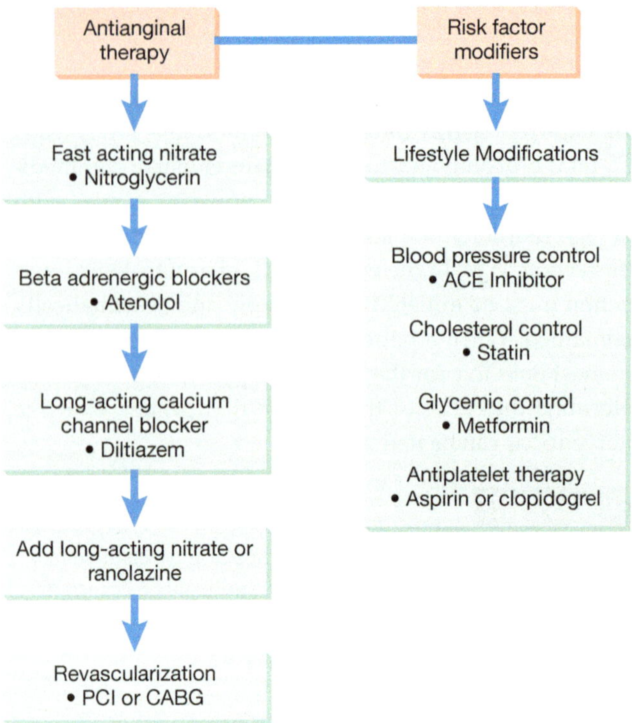

Figure 35.2 Overview of the treatment of stable coronary artery disease illustrating the dual role of antianginal medications and risk factor modification.

The pharmacotherapy of angina uses three primary classes of drugs: organic nitrates, beta-adrenergic antagonists, and calcium channel blockers (CCBs). Rapid-acting organic nitrates are preferred drugs for *terminating* an acute angina episode. Beta-adrenergic antagonists or blockers are first-line drugs for *prophylactic* treatment. CCBs are used when beta blockers are not tolerated well by a patient. Long-acting nitrates, given by the oral (PO) or transdermal routes, are alternatives for prophylaxis. Persistent angina requires drugs from two or more classes, such as a beta blocker combined with a long-acting nitrate or a CCB. Pharmacotherapy Illustrated 35.1 shows the mechanisms of action of medications used to prevent and treat angina.

Should the patient be unable to tolerate beta blockers or CCBs, ranolazine may be considered as another option. Ranolazine (Ranexa) is the only medication in a class called **partial fatty-acid oxidation inhibitors**. Ranolazine reduces the flow of sodium and calcium ions into the myocardium, which decreases the metabolic rate and oxygen demands of myocardial cells. Thus, it is the only antianginal that acts through its metabolic effects, rather than hemodynamic effects; effects on heart rate and blood pressure are minimal. The drug is approved only for chronic angina that has not responded to other medications.

It is important to understand that medications for angina do not cure the underlying disorder; the coronary vessels are still occluded. If a patient with angina begins to experience more frequent or severe acute episodes, aggressive treatment becomes necessary. This includes percutaneous coronary intervention (PCI) in which stents are placed in the affected vessels. Drug-eluting stents contain a medication such as zotarolimus, everolimus, or ridaforolimus that keep the vessel open by limiting tissue growth on the stent. If stenting is unsuccessful, coronary artery bypass graft surgery may be needed. Failure to reopen severely occluded coronary arteries presents a high risk for MI.

CONNECTION Checkpoint 35.2

Many patients take HMG-CoA reductase inhibitors (statins) concurrently with antianginal medications. From what you learned in Chapter 29, what is the rationale for prescribing drugs from this class for a patient with CAD?

Drug Classes for Angina Pectoris

35.6 Organic nitrates may be used to terminate or prevent angina episodes.

After their medicinal properties were discovered in 1879, the organic nitrates became the mainstay for the treatment of angina for over 100 years. The mechanism of action results from the formation of **nitric oxide** in vascular smooth muscle. Nitric oxide is an important cell-signaling molecule and a potent vasodilator, causing relaxation of both arterial and venous smooth muscle. Dilation of veins reduces the amount of blood returning to the heart (preload), and the chambers contain a smaller volume. With less blood for the ventricles to pump, cardiac output is reduced and the workload on the heart is decreased, thereby lowering myocardial oxygen demand. The therapeutic outcome is that chest pain is alleviated and episodes of angina become less frequent.

Organic nitrates also have the ability to dilate coronary arteries, which was once thought to be their primary mechanism of action. It seems logical that dilating a partially occluded coronary vessel would allow more oxygen to reach ischemic tissue. Although this effect does indeed occur, it is no longer considered the primary mechanism of nitrate action in the treatment of stable angina. Coronary artery vasodilation, however, is crucial in treating variant angina, in which the chest pain is caused by coronary artery spasm. The organic nitrates relax these spasms, allowing more oxygen to reach the myocardium, thereby terminating the pain.

Organic nitrates are classified by their onset and duration of action. The short-acting nitrates, such as nitroglycerin, may be taken sublingually (SL) or as an oral spray or buccal tablet to quickly terminate an acute anginal episode. Long-acting nitrates, such as isosorbide dinitrate (Isordil), are taken orally or are absorbed slowly through a transdermal patch to decrease the frequency and severity of angina episodes.

Pharmacotherapy Illustrated 35.1

Mechanisms of Action of Drugs Used to Treat Angina Pectoris

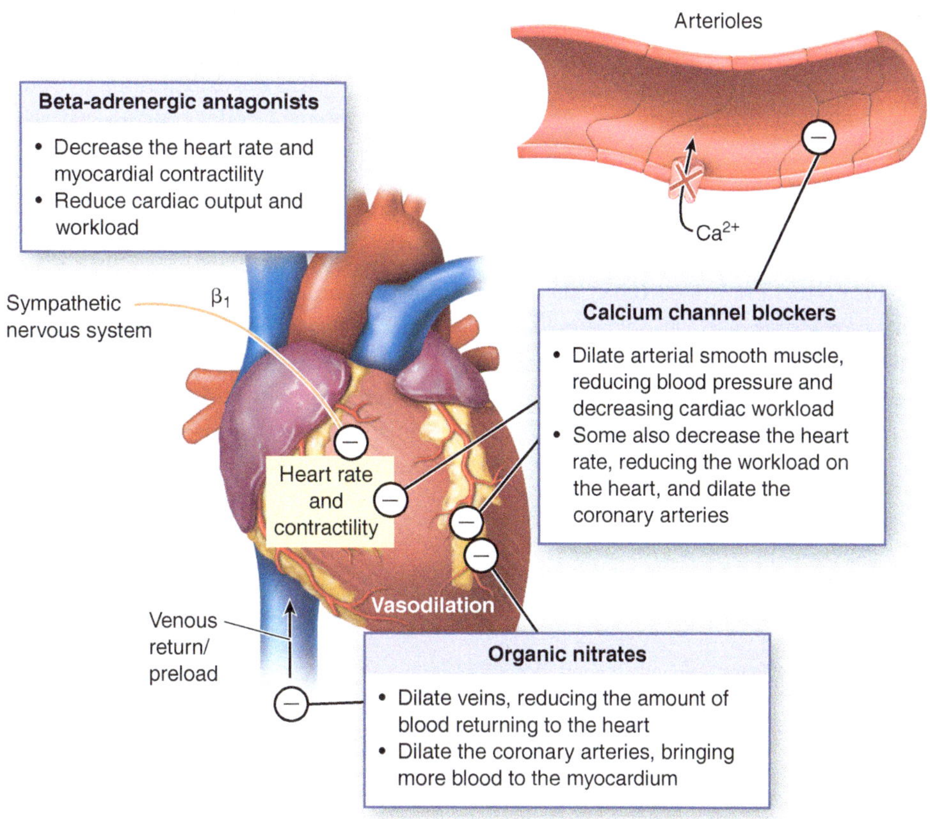

CONNECTIONS: Advanced Practice Application

Stable Angina

Case

Mrs. Sanchez, a 76-year-old female, presents to a community hospital emergency department complaining of new-onset chest pain. She is describing her chest pain as "pressure and tightness" that radiates down her left arm. She reports her pain level as 5/10. Mrs. Sanchez has had a few episodes over the past week while out walking but once she stopped walking and rested the pain eased. She did not seek medical help at the time. She denies any trouble breathing, fever, vomiting, cough, or any other complaints. Mrs. Sanchez's current medications include hydrochlorothiazide 25 mg PO daily, levothyroxine 175 mcg PO daily, metformin 500 mg PO twice per day, aspirin 81 mg PO daily, and atorvastatin 40 mg PO daily. On physical examination, her vital signs are stable with a blood pressure of 128/72 mm Hg; pulse, 76 bpm; respirations, 16 per minute; saturation of oxygen, 97% on room air. Her skin is warm and dry. Her head and neck and heart and lung sounds are also normal, as is the rest of the physical exam. Her resting ECG and chest x-ray are both normal. You suspect Mrs. Sanchez is suffering from stable angina. What are the general principles for treating stable angina? What medications should be used?

Discussion

Anginal pain is constricting discomfort in the front of the chest, neck, shoulders, jaw, or arms that is precipitated by physical exertion and is relieved by rest. Stable angina is the presenting symptom in approximately half of patients with CAD (Kloner & Chaitman, 2017). Most patients with stable angina can be managed with lifestyle changes, especially smoking cessation and regular exercise, and antianginal medication treatment. Optimal drug treatment consists of one or two antianginal drugs as necessary plus drugs for secondary prevention of cardiovascular disease. Do not offer a third antianginal drug to people whose stable angina is controlled with two antianginal drugs. Additionally, providers should avoid recommending vitamin or fish oil supplements to treat stable angina as there is no evidence supporting symptom or outcome improvement.

Long-acting organic nitrates are occasionally used to treat symptoms of HF; their role in the treatment of that disease is presented in Chapter 36. The various routes of administration are listed in Table 35.1. Doses for the organic nitrates, along with other medications for treating angina and MI, are also listed in Table 35.1.

Tolerance is a common and potentially serious problem with the long-acting organic nitrates. The magnitude of the tolerance depends on the dosage and frequency of drug administration. Although tolerance develops rapidly—as quickly as 24 hours after the initiation of therapy in some patients—it also disappears rapidly when the drug is withheld. Patients are often instructed to remove the transdermal patch for 6 to 12 hours each day or withhold a nighttime dose of the oral medications in order to delay the development of tolerance. Because the oxygen demands during sleep are diminished, the patient with stable angina experiences few angina episodes during this drug-free interval.

Most adverse effects of organic nitrates are extensions of their hypotensive action. Flushing of the face and headache are common effects related to vasodilation. Orthostatic hypotension is a frequent adverse effect of this drug class, and patients should be advised to change positions gradually to prevent lightheadedness. Blood pressure should be carefully monitored, and the nurse should hold nitrates and remove topical forms if serious hypotension is discovered. Taking organic nitrates concurrently with alcohol may cause severe hypotension and even cardiovascular collapse.

An additional adverse effect that can be limiting in some patients is reflex tachycardia. When the organic nitrates dilate vessels and blood pressure falls, the baroreceptor reflex is triggered. Sympathetic stimulation of the heart increases heart rate and contractility, which are undesirable effects in a patient with angina. This adverse effect is often transient and asymptomatic. Patients who report significant palpitations may be administered a beta blocker, which will prevent the reflex cardiac stimulation.

Table 35.1 Selected Drugs for Angina and Myocardial Infarction

Drug	Route and Adult Dose (Maximum Dose Where Indicated)	Adverse Effects
Organic Nitrates		
isosorbide dinitrate (Dilatrate SR, Isordil)	PO (regular release): 2.5–30 mg qid (max: 480 mg/day) PO (sustained release): 40 mg bid–qid (max: 160 mg/day) SL: 2.5–5 mg taken 15 min before exercise	*Headache, orthostatic hypotension, flushing of the face, dizziness, rash (transdermal patch), tolerance* Anaphylaxis, circulatory collapse due to hypotension, syncope due to orthostatic hypotension
isosorbide mononitrate (Monoket)	PO (regular release: Ismo, Monoket): 20 mg bid (max: 40 mg/day) PO (extended release: Imdur): 30–60 mg each morning (max: 240 mg/day)	
nitroglycerin (Nitrostat, Nitro-Dur, others)	SL: 1 tablet (0.3–0.6 mg) or 1 spray (0.4–0.8 mg) every 3–5 min (max: 3 doses in 15 min)	
Beta-Adrenergic Antagonists		
atenolol (Tenormin)	PO: 25–50 mg daily (max: 100 mg/day)	*Fatigue, insomnia, drowsiness, impotence or decreased libido, depression, bradycardia, confusion* Agranulocytosis, laryngospasm, Stevens–Johnson syndrome, anaphylaxis; if the drug is abruptly withdrawn, palpitations, rebound HTN, life-threatening dysrhythmias or myocardial ischemia may occur
metoprolol (Lopressor, Toprol XL)	PO (for HTN or angina): 100 mg/day (max: 400 mg/day)	
propranolol (Inderal LA, InnoPran XL)	PO (extended release): 80–120 mg once daily (max: 120 mg/day for InnoPran XL; 640 mg/day for Inderal LA)	
timolol	PO (for MI): 10 mg bid (max: 60 mg/day)	
Calcium Channel Blockers		
amlodipine (Norvasc)	PO: 5–10 mg daily (max: 10 mg/day)	*Flushed skin, headache, dizziness, peripheral edema, lightheadedness, nausea, constipation* Hepatotoxicity, MI, HF, confusion, mood changes
diltiazem (Cardizem, Cartia XT, Dilacor, others)	PO (regular release): 30 mg tid–qid (max: 480 mg/day) PO (extended release): 120–240 mg bid (max: 540 mg/day)	
nicardipine (Cardene)	PO (regular release): 20–40 mg tid PO (sustained release): 30–60 mg bid (max: 120 mg/day)	
nifedipine (Adalat CC, Procardia XL, others)	PO (regular release): 10–20 mg tid (max: 180 mg/day) PO (extended release): 30–60 mg once daily (max: 120 mg/day)	
verapamil (Calan SR, Verelan)	PO: 80–160 mg tid (max: 480 mg/day) PO (Calan SR, Verelan): 120–480 mg once daily	
Miscellaneous Drug		
ranolazine (Ranexa)	PO: 500–1000 mg bid (max: 2000 mg/day)	*Dizziness, constipation, headache, nausea* QT interval prolongation, bradycardia

Note: *Italics* indicate common adverse effects. Underline indicates serious adverse effects.

PROTOTYPE DRUG Nitroglycerin (Nitrostat, Nitro-Dur, Others)

Classification **Therapeutic:** Antianginal drug
Pharmacologic: Organic nitrate, vasodilator

Therapeutic Effects and Uses: Nitroglycerin, the oldest and most widely used organic nitrate, can be delivered by a number of different routes: sublingual, lingual spray, PO, intravenous (IV), transmucosal, transdermal, topical, and extended-release forms. The rapid-acting forms may be taken while an acute angina episode is in progress or just prior to physical activity. When given sublingually, it reaches peak plasma levels within minutes, thus quickly terminating angina pain. Chest pain that does not resolve within 5 minutes after a dose of SL nitroglycerin may indicate MI, and emergency medical services (EMS) should be contacted. The transdermal and oral sustained-release forms are for prophylaxis only, since they have a relatively slow onset of action. The long-acting forms should be discontinued gradually because vasospasm may result if they are abruptly withheld.

Nitroglycerin is also used for indications other than angina. When administered by the IV route, the drug is approved for controlled hypotension induction during anesthesia and the treatment of HF, acute pulmonary edema, acute MI, severe HTN, or hypertensive emergency. Off-label indications include use as a uterine relaxant to aid in the extraction of a retained placenta and for pain associated with anal fissures or hemorrhoids.

Mechanism of Action: Upon reaching vascular smooth muscle, nitroglycerin forms nitric oxide, which triggers a cascade resulting in the release of calcium ions in smooth muscle. Nitroglycerin relaxes both arterial and venous smooth muscle. The venous dilation decreases the amount of blood returning to the heart, reducing preload. With less blood for the ventricles to pump, myocardial oxygen demand is decreased. In addition, direct vasodilation of coronary arteries enhances the blood supply to the myocardium and is partially responsible for its therapeutic effects.

Pharmacokinetics:

Route(s)	PO: SL tablets, SL spray, buccal tablets; transdermal patch; topical ointment
Absorption	Rapid
Distribution	Widely distributed; 60% bound to plasma protein
Primary metabolism	Hepatic; extensive first-pass metabolism
Primary excretion	Renal
Onset of action	SL: 1–3 min; buccal: 2–5 min; transdermal patch: 40–60 min; topical ointment: 20–60 min
Duration of action	SL: 30–60 min; buccal: 2 h; transdermal patch: 18–24 h; topical ointment: 12 h

Adverse Effects: Most patients experience flushing of the face and a throbbing, transient headache, which result from the drug's vasodilation action. Orthostatic hypotension and syncope may occur. Stinging and rash may occur with ointments and transdermal patches. Methemoglobinemia is a rare adverse effect that can cause shock and coma. Anaphylaxis leading to circulatory collapse due to severe hypotension is rare. Tolerance develops with continuous therapy or large doses of the drug.

Contraindications/Precautions: Nitrates are contraindicated in patients with preexisting hypotension, shock, head injury with increased intracranial pressure, or head trauma because additive vasodilation would worsen these conditions. Drugs in this class are contraindicated in pericardial tamponade and constrictive pericarditis because the heart is unable to increase cardiac output to maintain blood pressure when the drug causes vasodilation. Sustained-release forms of the medicine should not be given to patients with glaucoma because the drug may increase intraocular pressure. Nitroglycerin should be used cautiously in patients with severe liver or renal disease, as the drug could build to toxic levels. Dehydration or hypovolemia should be corrected before nitroglycerin is administered, otherwise serious hypotension may result.

Drug Interactions: Concurrent use with sildenafil (Viagra) or other phosphodiesterase-5 inhibitors may cause life-threatening hypotension and cardiovascular collapse. Nitrates should not be taken within 24 hours before or after taking these drugs. Concurrent use with ethanol, CCBs, antidepressants, phenothiazines, or antihypertensive drugs may cause additive hypotension. Sympathomimetics such as epinephrine will antagonize the vasodilation effects of nitroglycerin. **Herbal/Food:** Use with hawthorn may result in additive hypotension.

Pregnancy: Administration to pregnant laboratory animals did not show adverse developmental effects. It is not known if the drug is secreted in milk or if it has adverse effects of the breastfed neonate.

Treatment of Overdose: During overdose, hypotension may be reversed with the IV administration of normal saline. If methemoglobinemia is suspected, methylene blue may be administered.

Clinician Responsibilities: Key clinical implications for patients receiving nitroglycerin are included in Applied Clinical Judgment: Patients Receiving Pharmacotherapy with Organic Nitrates for Angina and Myocardial Infarction.

Drugs Similar to Nitroglycerin (Nitrostat, Nitro-Dur, Others)

Other organic nitrates include isosorbide dinitrate and isosorbide mononitrate.

Isosorbide dinitrate (Dilatrate SR, Isordil): Approved in 1961, isosorbide dinitrate is an organic nitrate used to terminate anginal attacks (SL route) and for the prophylaxis of angina (extended-release tablets). It is occasionally used to treat HF. The dosing schedule must allow for a drug-free period of at least 14 hours to prevent tolerance to the drug's effects. The PO forms of the drug should not be used to terminate acute angina attacks because it takes as long as 60 minutes to reach therapeutic drug levels. The SL dosage forms may be taken 15 minutes prior to activities likely to precipitate angina. Adverse effects are similar to those of nitroglycerin. Like other nitrates, isosorbide dinitrate should not be administered within 24 hours of taking erectile dysfunction medications such as sildenafil. A fixed-dose combination of isosorbide dinitrate with hydralazine (BiDil) is available to reduce morbidity and mortality associated with HF. At high doses, isosorbide dinitrate is embryotoxic in laboratory animals. It is not known if the drug is secreted into milk or if it has adverse effects of the breastfed neonate.

Isosorbide mononitrate (Monoket): Approved in 1991, isosorbide mononitrate is an active, long-acting metabolite of isosorbide dinitrate. The mononitrate is only used for prophylaxis: Its 30- to 60-minute onset of action makes it unacceptable for termination of acute anginal pain. The dosing schedule must allow for a drug-free period of at least 7 hours to prevent the development of tolerance to the drug's effects. It is available as regular-release or extended-release tablets, which should be taken on an empty stomach at least 30 minutes before a meal. Adverse effects are the same as the other organic nitrates. It is not known if the drug has adverse effects during pregnancy or lactation.

Beta-Adrenergic Antagonists

35.7 Beta-adrenergic antagonists are first-line drugs for stable angina.

Beta-adrenergic antagonists decrease cardiac workload by lowering blood pressure, slowing heart rate, and reducing contractility. These actions on the heart are particularly beneficial during exercise. Beta blockers are as effective as the organic nitrates in decreasing the frequency and severity of anginal episodes caused by exertion. For the pharmacotherapy of CAD, cardioselective beta$_1$ antagonists are preferred over nonselective beta antagonists because they are less likely to cause bronchoconstriction (a beta$_2$ response). Beta-adrenergic antagonists are not effective for treating variant angina and may, in fact, worsen this condition.

Beta-adrenergic antagonists offer several advantages over the organic nitrates. Tolerance does not develop to the antianginal effects of the beta blockers during prolonged therapy. They possess antidysrhythmic properties, which help prevent cardiac conduction abnormalities that are common complications of patients with ischemic heart disease. Beta blockers are ideal for patients who have both HTN and CAD due to their antihypertensive action. They have also been shown to reduce the incidence of MI. Because of these cardioprotective actions, beta blockers are considered first-line drugs for the prophylaxis of chronic angina. The beta blockers used for angina are listed in Table 35.1. Beta blockers have a variety of indications and additional details may be found in chapters on adrenergic antagonists (see Chapter 16), HTN (see Chapter 34), HF (see Chapter 36), and dysrhythmias (see Chapter 37). An Applied Clinical Judgment feature for patients receiving beta blockers is included in Chapter 16.

Beta-adrenergic antagonists are well tolerated by most patients. In some patients, fatigue, lethargy, and depression are reasons for discontinuation of beta-blocker therapy. Nonselective beta blockers such as propranolol can cause shortness of breath and respiratory distress due to bronchoconstriction and should be used cautiously in patients with asthma or chronic obstructive pulmonary disease. Because beta blockers slow the heart rate and myocardial conduction velocity, they are contraindicated in patients with bradycardia and greater than first-degree heart block. Heart rate should be closely monitored so that it does not fall below 50 to 60 beats/min at rest or 100 beats/min during exercise. Beta blockers are also contraindicated in cardiogenic shock and overt cardiac failure.

Patients with diabetes who are prescribed beta blockers should be aware that the actions of beta blockers can obscure the initial symptoms of hypoglycemia (palpitations, diaphoresis, and nervousness). Because of this, blood glucose levels should be monitored more frequently, and insulin doses may need to be adjusted accordingly.

Beta-adrenergic antagonists should never be abruptly discontinued. With long-term beta-blocker use, the heart becomes more sensitive to catecholamines, which are blocked by these medications. When withdrawn abruptly, adrenergic receptors are activated and rebound excitation occurs. In patients with CAD, this can exacerbate angina, precipitate tachycardia, or cause an MI.

PROTOTYPE DRUG **Atenolol (Tenormin)**

Classification **Therapeutic:** Antianginal drug
Pharmacologic: Beta-adrenergic antagonist

Therapeutic Effects and Uses: Atenolol is one of the most frequently prescribed drugs in the United States, due to its relative safety and effectiveness in treating a number of chronic disorders, including HF, HTN, stable angina, and post-acute MI. Approved in 1981, it is given by the PO route and has a long duration of action that allows for once-daily dosing. Tenoretic combines atenolol with chlorthalidone and is approved to treat HTN. Off-label indications for atenolol include ethanol withdrawal, migraine prophylaxis, and unstable angina.

Mechanism of Action: Atenolol selectively blocks beta$_1$-adrenergic receptors in the heart. Its effectiveness in angina is attributed to its ability to slow the heart rate and reduce contractility, both of which lower myocardial oxygen demand.

Pharmacokinetics:

Route(s)	PO, IV
Absorption	50% absorbed from the gastrointestinal (GI) tract
Distribution	Distributed to most tissues including the placenta; secreted in breast milk; does not readily cross the blood–brain barrier; 5–15% bound to protein
Primary metabolism	Not metabolized
Primary excretion	Renal (50%), feces (50%)
Onset of action	PO: 1 h; IV: immediate
Duration of action	PO/IV: 24 h; half-life: 6–7 h

Adverse Effects: Oral atenolol is well tolerated by most patients. Beta-blocking effects can result in bradycardia and hypotension. Fatigue, weakness, and dizziness are other potential adverse effects. Nausea and vomiting occur in some patients. **Black Box Warning:** Abrupt discontinuation should be avoided in patients with ischemic heart disease because this may worsen angina or cause an MI. Doses should be gradually reduced over a 1- to 2-week period, if possible. If angina worsens during the withdrawal period, the drug should be reinstituted, at least temporarily.

Contraindications/Precautions: Because atenolol slows heart rate, it should not be used by patients with severe bradycardia, advanced atrioventricular (AV) heart block, cardiogenic shock, or decompensated HF. Due to its vasodilation effects, it is contraindicated in patients with severe hypotension. Patients with severe chronic kidney disease should receive reduced doses or have longer time intervals between doses to prevent drug accumulation. Because atenolol reduces cardiac output, patients with stroke or low cerebrovascular blood flow should not receive this drug. Patients with major depression should not receive beta blockers because these drugs can worsen this condition.

Drug Interactions: Anticholinergics may decrease the absorption of atenolol from the GI tract. Use with digoxin or other antidysrhythmic drugs that depress myocardial conduction may cause AV heart block. Concurrent use of atenolol with other antihypertensives may result in additive hypotension. Although CCBs are often used concurrently with beta blockers for their additive therapeutic actions, patients must be monitored carefully due to the possibility of excessive cardiac suppression. **Herbal/Food:** Use with hawthorn may result in additive hypotension.

Pregnancy: Atenolol may cause fetal harm during the 2nd and 3rd trimesters and its use during pregnancy is not recommended. Breastfeeding is not recommended because the drug enters milk and may cause hypoglycemia and bradycardia in the infant.

Treatment of Overdose: The most serious symptoms of atenolol overdose are hypotension and bradycardia. Atropine or isoproterenol may be used to reverse bradycardia, or a cardiac pacemaker may be used to stabilize cardiac rhythm. Atenolol can be removed from the systemic circulation by hemodialysis.

Clinician Responsibilities: Key clinical implications for patients receiving atenolol are included in the Applied Clinical Judgment: Patients Receiving Pharmacotherapy with Adrenergic Antagonists in Chapter 16.

Drugs Similar to Atenolol (Tenormin)

Atenolol, metoprolol, propranolol, and timolol are equally effective in preventing acute angina episodes. Information on these beta-adrenergic antagonists is presented in other chapters. The student should review the general information on beta blockers in Chapter 16. Several are featured as prototype drugs: metoprolol (Lopressor, Toprol XL) and propranolol (Inderal LA, InnoPran XL) in Chapter 16 and timolol is featured as an antiglaucoma medication in Chapter 74.

Calcium Channel Blockers

35.8 Calcium channel blockers are effective at reducing myocardial oxygen demand and treating stable and variant angina.

Calcium channel blockers are first-line drugs for the prevention of acute angina attacks. They may be prescribed concurrently with a beta blocker or as monotherapy. Blockade of calcium channels has a number of effects on the heart, most of which are similar to those of beta blockers. Although the first approved indication for CCBs was for the treatment of angina, these medications are also used for HTN and dysrhythmias. The mechanisms of calcium channel blockade by drugs in this class are presented in detail in Chapter 30. The CCBs used for angina are listed in Table 35.1.

CCBs have several actions on the cardiovascular system that benefit a patient with angina. Most importantly, CCBs relax arteriolar smooth muscle, thus reducing blood pressure. This reduction in afterload decreases myocardial oxygen demand. Some of the CCBs also slow cardiac conduction velocity through the AV node, thereby decreasing heart rate and contributing to the reduced cardiac workload. An additional effect of the CCBs is their ability to dilate the coronary arteries, bringing more oxygen to the myocardium. This vasodilation is especially important in patients with variant angina. CCBs are considered preferred drugs for that condition. For stable, exertional angina, they may be used as monotherapy in patients unable to tolerate beta blockers. In patients with persistent symptoms, CCBs may be administered concurrently with organic nitrates or beta blockers.

Adverse effects of CCBs are generally not serious and are related to vasodilation: headache, dizziness, and edema of the ankles and feet. CCBs should be used with caution in patients taking other cardiovascular medications that slow conduction through the AV node, particularly digoxin or beta-adrenergic antagonists. The combined effects of these drugs may cause partial or complete AV heart block, HF, or dysrhythmias. Some CCBs worsen HF by reducing myocardial contractility.

CONNECTION Checkpoint 35.3

For patients with asthma, calcium channel blockers are generally the preferred antianginal drugs, rather than beta-adrenergic antagonists. From what you learned in Chapter 16, why would calcium channel blockers be preferred for patients with this comorbid condition?

Pathophysiology of Myocardial Infarction

35.9 Early diagnosis and pharmacotherapy of myocardial infarction increase chances of survival.

Myocardial infarctions (MIs), blood clots that block coronary arteries, are responsible for a substantial number of deaths each year. Many patients die before reaching a medical facility for treatment, or within 48 hours following the initial MI, due to complications of the disorder. Clearly, MI is serious and frightening and is responsible for a large percentage of sudden deaths.

The primary cause of MI is advanced CAD: atherosclerotic plaque accumulation in the endothelial wall of one or more branches of the coronary arteries. An MI may be preceded by a history of angina, or it may occur without warning. Pieces of unstable plaque can ulcerate or rupture and lodge in a small vessel serving a portion of the myocardium. Exposed plaque activates the coagulation cascade, resulting in rapid platelet aggregation. A new clot quickly builds on the existing plaque, making obstruction of the vessel imminent. A detailed discussion of coagulation and clot formation is included in Chapter 38.

Deprived of adequate oxygen supply, the obstructed region of the myocardium becomes ischemic. The myocytes shift to anaerobic metabolism after only 8 to 10 seconds of oxygen loss. Anaerobic metabolism, however, is inefficient and cannot produce enough adenosine triphosphate to keep the heart beating efficiently for prolonged periods. Lactic acid accumulates, causing acidosis, which affects contractility and suppresses normal conduction across the myocardium. As contractility diminishes, the patient may experience HF. Myocytes will begin to die in about 20 minutes unless the blood supply is quickly restored. The necrosis of myocardial tissue, which may be irreversible, releases certain "marker" enzymes, such as creatine kinase (CK) or cardiac-specific troponin (cTn), which can be measured in the blood to confirm the patient has experienced an MI.

Extreme chest pain is often the first symptom of MI and the one that drives most patients to seek medical attention. An electrocardiogram (ECG) can give important clues as to the extent and location of the MI because the infarcted region of the myocardium is nonconducting, producing abnormal Q waves, T waves, and ST segments. Patients showing elevation of the ST segment on the ECG are at highest risk for death and require immediate treatment. An ST-elevation MI (STEMI) suggests an abrupt disruption of flow, potentially caused by a complete occlusion of a coronary artery. Laboratory test results are used to aid in diagnosis and monitor progress after an MI. Table 35.2 describes some of these important laboratory values.

Early diagnosis and prompt pharmacotherapy of MI can significantly reduce its associated mortality and long-term disability. The pharmacologic goals for treating a patient with an acute MI are as follows:

- If cardiac arrest has occurred, restart the heart and restore normal blood pressure with vasopressors.
- Restore blood supply (reperfusion) to the damaged myocardium as quickly as possible through the use of PCI or fibrinolytics.
- Reduce myocardial oxygen demand with organic nitrates, beta blockers, or CCBs to lower the risk of additional infarctions.

Table 35.2 Changes in Blood Test Values with Acute Myocardial Infarction

Blood Test	Initial Elevation After MI	Peak Elevation After MI	Duration of Elevation	Normal Range
CK: total creatine kinase (also called creatine phosphokinase)	3–8 h	12–24 h	2–4 days	Males: 5–35 mcg/L Females: 5–25 mcg/L
CK-MB	4–6 h	10–24 h	3–4 days	0–3% of CK
ESR (erythrocyte sedimentation rate)	2–3 days	4–5 days	Several weeks	Males: 15–20 mm/h Females: 20–30 mm/h
LDH: total (lactate dehydrogenase)	12–24 h	2–5 days	6–12 days	70–250 units/L
Myoglobin	2–6 h	8–12 h	1–2 days	12–90 ng/mL
Troponin I	1–3 h	24–36 h	5–9 days	0.1–0.5 mcg/L
Troponin T	1–3 h	24–36 h	10–14 days	Less than 0.2 mcg/L

- Reduce post-MI mortality with antiplatelet drugs, anticoagulants, beta blockers, and ACE inhibitors.
- Manage severe MI pain and associated anxiety with narcotic analgesics.

Pharmacologic Management of Myocardial Infarction

35.10 Fibrinolytic drugs can restore perfusion to ischemic regions of the myocardium if administered soon after a myocardial infarction.

After a STEMI has been identified the most immediate concern is restoration of blood flow to the affected artery. The preferred method is PCI, if it is available at the facility of first medical contact. If not available, reperfusion can be accomplished through the administration of fibrinolytic medications.

Fibrinolytic therapy is administered to dissolve clots obstructing the coronary arteries in order to restore circulation to the ischemic region of the myocardium. Clinical research has confirmed that quick restoration of coronary circulation reduces mortality following an acute MI. After the clot is successfully dissolved, anticoagulant or antiplatelet therapy is initiated to prevent additional thrombus formation. Dosages and descriptions of the various fibrinolytics are listed in Chapter 38 where alteplase (Activase) is presented as a drug prototype for this class. An Applied Clinical Judgment feature for fibrinolytics is also included in Chapter 38.

Fibrinolytics are most effective when administered from 20 minutes to 12 hours after the onset of MI symptoms. Ideally, the time from presentation in the emergency department to administration of the fibrinolytic should be 30 minutes or less. Research has demonstrated little or no therapeutic benefit if the drugs are administered 24 hours or more after the MI onset. In addition, research suggests that patients over age 75 do not experience reduced mortality from these drugs. Because fibrinolytic therapy is expensive and has the potential to produce serious adverse effects, it is important to identify circumstances that contribute to successful therapy. The development of clinical practice guidelines for fibrinolytic therapy remains an area of active research. Pharmacotherapy Illustrated 35.2 illustrates this reperfusion process.

Fibrinolytics exhibit a narrow margin of safety between dissolving clots and producing serious adverse effects. Although therapy is usually targeted to a single thrombus in a specific artery, once infused in the blood the drugs travel to all vessels and may cause adverse effects anywhere in the body. The primary risk of fibrinolytics is excessive bleeding from interference with the clotting process. Vital signs must be monitored continuously and signs of bleeding call for discontinuation of therapy. Because these medications have a brief half-life and are rapidly destroyed in the blood, stopping the infusion normally results in the rapid termination of adverse effects. Physical and laboratory assessment for the possibility of abnormal bleeding should continue for 2 to 4 days after therapy is discontinued.

Fibrinolytic therapy is contraindicated for many conditions, including recent trauma or surgery, internal bleeding (other than menses), active peptic ulcer, postpartum (within 10 days), history of intracranial hemorrhage, suspected ischemic stroke within the past 3 months, bleeding disorders, severe liver disease, or thrombocytopenia. Caution should be used when administering fibrinolytics to patients taking anticoagulants or antiplatelet drugs.

35.11 Drugs are used to treat the symptoms and complications of acute myocardial infarction.

In addition to restoring perfusion to the myocardium, drugs from other classes are administered soon after the onset of symptoms to prevent reinfarction and following discharge from the medical facility.

Pharmacotherapy Illustrated 35.2

Fibrinolytic Pharmacotherapy

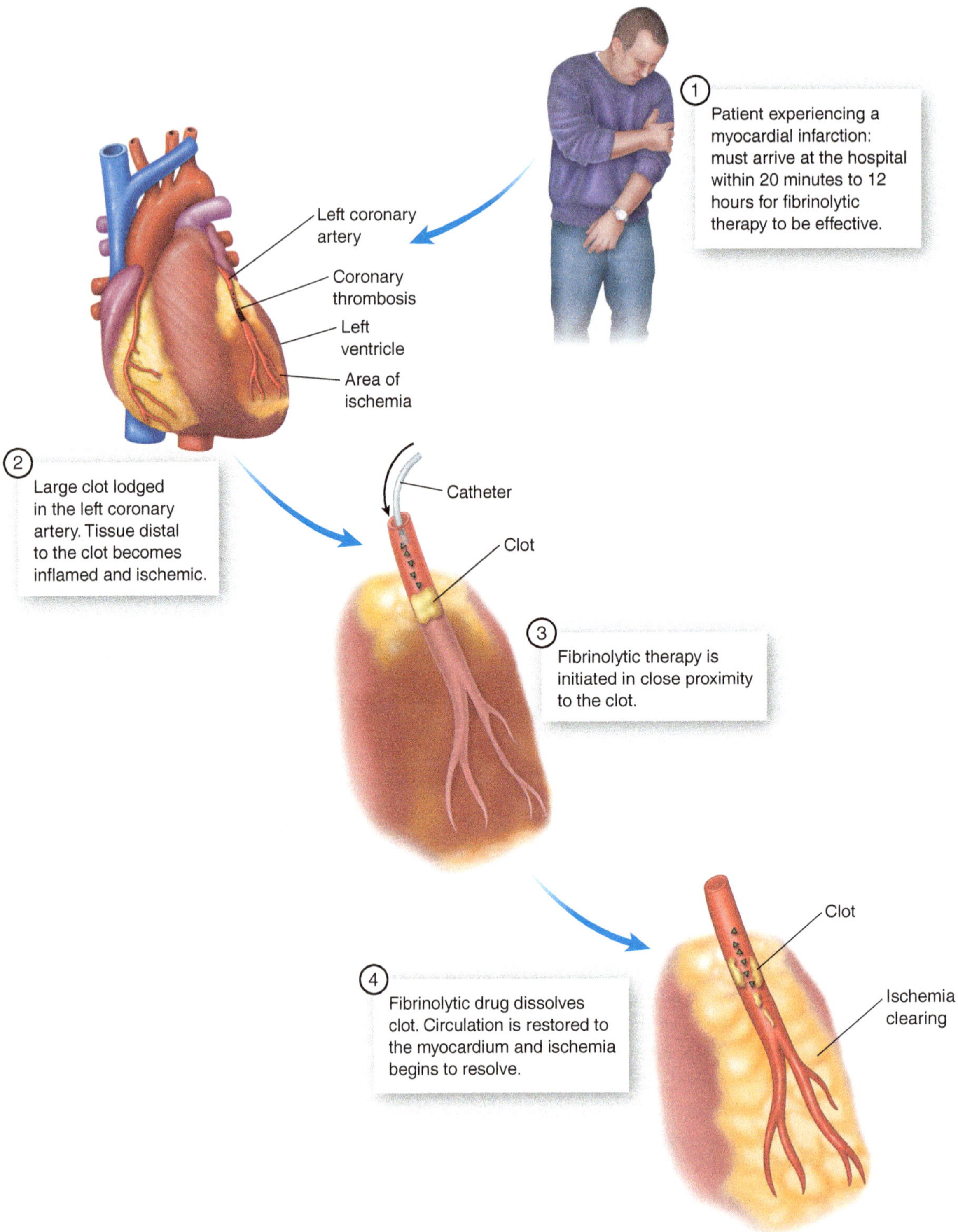

CONNECTIONS: Treating the Diverse Patient

The Effect of the CYP2C19 Genotype on Therapeutic Treatment Outcomes for Cardiovascular Patients

Recall from Chapter 11 that genetic polymorphisms in the CYP450 enzyme system have an effect on the metabolism of drugs, potentially rendering them less useful due to slowed metabolism. Genetic CYP450 variations also have other effects, such as on platelet activity. People of Asian descent and some Blacks are known to carry the CYP2C19 genotype variant.

In several recent studies, patients with the CYP2C19 genotype were found to have higher platelet activity and less response to clopidogrel and similar drugs after stenting procedures for coronary and carotid artery blockage (Cavallari et al., 2018; Xi et al., 2019). The risk for additional cardiovascular events was noted to be higher in those with the variation, especially in the acute stage.

Studies are ongoing to determine which patients with other genotypes would benefit from higher doses of clopidogrel or similar drugs or whether combining those drugs with aspirin would be beneficial. At this time, routine screening for CYP2C19 for at-risk patients who may be carriers of the genotype may be beneficial to direct antiplatelet therapy (Xi et al., 2019).

Antiplatelet Drugs

Unless contraindicated, 162 to 325 mg of chewable, nonenteric aspirin is given as soon as an MI is suspected followed by a lifelong maintenance dose of 75 to 81 mg/day. Aspirin use reduces platelet aggregation and thus the formation or enlargement of thrombi. Additionally, its anti-inflammatory properties decrease the formation of C-reactive protein, which is associated with an increased risk of MI.

A major concern over aspirin use is its tendency to promote GI bleeding, especially considering that most post-MI patients receive anticoagulants. However, the benefits of taking aspirin following an acute MI has been shown to justify the risks for most patients. Aspirin maintenance therapy can cut the risk of death due to a subsequent MI by as much as 50% in some populations. Furthermore, the low doses used in maintenance therapy rarely cause GI bleeding. Additional discussion of aspirin may be found in Chapter 41, where it is featured as a prototype drug.

In addition to aspirin, patients undergoing PCI or fibrinolytic therapy receive a second antiplatelet drug from a class called the adenosine diphosphate receptor blockers (also called $P2y_{12}$ receptor inhibitors). Medications in this class include clopidogrel (Plavix), ticlopidine (Ticlid), ticagrelor (Brilinta), and prasugrel (Effient). These drugs are approved for the prevention of thrombotic stroke and MI. Clopidogrel is one of the most frequently used drugs for prevention of MI and is featured as a prototype in Chapter 38. Patients with stent placement are given clopidogrel at the time of PCI and maintenance therapy for 12 months. Patients undergoing fibrinolytic therapy receive clopidogrel for at least 2 weeks and up to 1 year. Drugs in this class are sometimes considered aspirin alternatives for patients who are allergic to aspirin or at high risk for GI bleeding from aspirin. Some protocols call for combination therapy with clopidogrel and aspirin.

Glycoprotein IIb/IIIa inhibitors are antiplatelet medications indicated to prevent thrombi from forming in patients with unstable angina or MI or for those undergoing PCI. The drugs in this class, eptifibatide (Integrilin) and tirofiban (Aggrastat), are given only by the IV route and are usually infused at the time of PCI and continued for 12 hours after the procedure is completed to prevent reinfarction. These drugs may be used in combination therapy with aspirin and heparin, thus increasing the need for careful monitoring for bleeding. The glycoprotein IIb/IIIa inhibitors are considered second-line antiplatelet drugs and their doses are found in Chapter 38.

In 2014 the U.S. Food and Drug Administration approved the first in a new class of antiplatelet drugs called the protease-activated receptor-1 antagonists. Vorapaxar (Zontivity) is administered to reduce the incidence of thrombotic events in patients with a history of MI or other clotting disorders. It is given PO, in combination with aspirin or clopidogrel.

Anticoagulant Drugs

Upon diagnosis of MI in the ED, patients may be started on anticoagulant therapy. Unfractionated heparin is a first-line medication during PCI or fibrinolytic therapy because a therapeutic level of anticoagulation can be obtained very rapidly. Heparin therapy is sometimes continued for 48 hours at which time patients are switched to warfarin (Coumadin) or an antiplatelet drug. Alternatives to unfractionated heparin include a low-molecular-weight heparin, such as enoxaparin (Lovenox) or bivalirudin (Angiomax), a direct thrombin inhibitor. A comparison of these different anticoagulants is presented in Chapter 38, along with prototype drug features for heparin and warfarin.

Patients at high risk for thromboembolic disease and those with chronic atrial fibrillation may remain on anticoagulant therapy after hospital discharge. Research has not shown that the use of warfarin lowers mortality in post-MI patients; however, it does increase the risk of bleeding. For most patients, anticoagulation with aspirin or antiplatelet drugs is sufficient for protection from thromboembolic events.

One additional anticoagulant is occasionally used to prevent deep vein thrombosis in patients at high risk for MI. Fondaparinux (Arixtra) inhibits Factor X in the coagulation cascade. It is administered as a once-daily subcutaneous injection during hospitalization or until PCI is performed.

Nitrates

The value of nitrates in treating myocardial ischemia was presented in Section 35.6. Nitrates have additional uses in the patient with a suspected MI. At the initial onset of chest pain, sublingual nitroglycerin is administered to assist in the diagnosis, and three doses may be taken 5 minutes apart. Pain that persists 5 to 10 minutes after the initial dose may indicate an MI, and the patient should seek medical assistance. Thus, nitrates serve a diagnostic role for MI patients.

Patients with persistent pain, HF, or severe HTN may receive IV nitrates for 24 hours following the onset of pain. The arterial and venous dilation produced by the drug reduces myocardial oxygen demand. Organic nitrates also relieve coronary artery vasospasm, which may be present during the acute stage of MI. On patient discharge from the hospital, organic nitrates are discontinued, unless the patient needs them for relief of stable anginal pain.

Beta-Adrenergic Antagonists

Beta blockers have the ability to slow heart rate, decrease contractility, and reduce blood pressure. These three factors reduce myocardial oxygen demand, which is critical for patients experiencing a recent MI. In addition, they slow impulse conduction through the heart, suppressing dysrhythmias, which are serious and sometimes fatal complications following an MI. Research has demonstrated that beta blockers can reduce MI-associated mortality if administered within 8 hours of MI onset. These drugs may be initially administered IV, and then switched to oral dosing for chronic therapy. Unless contraindicated, beta-blocker therapy continues for the remainder of the patient's life. For patients unable to tolerate beta blockers, CCBs are an alternative. Selected beta blockers used for MI are listed in Table 35.1.

Angiotensin-Converting Enzyme Inhibitors

Clinical research has demonstrated increased survival for patients administered the angiotensin-converting enzyme (ACE) inhibitors captopril (Capoten) or lisinopril (Prinivil, Zestoretic) following an acute MI. These drugs are most effective when therapy is started within 24 hours after the onset of symptoms. Oral doses are normally begun after fibrinolytic therapy is completed and the patient's condition has stabilized. IV therapy may be used during the early stages of MI pharmacotherapy.

The benefit of ACE inhibitors is believed to be due to their ability to prevent cardiac remodeling and their ability to suppress dysrhythmias. Unless otherwise contraindicated, post-MI patients should receive an ACE inhibitor indefinitely to prevent HF and future ischemic development. The mechanisms of action and prototype features for several ACE inhibitors may be found in Chapter 31.

Pain Management

The pain associated with an MI can be debilitating and stressful, creating an increased workload for the myocardium. Pain control is essential in order to ensure patient comfort and to reduce stress. Narcotic analgesics such as morphine sulfate or meperidine (Demerol) are given to ease extreme pain, sedate the anxious patient, and decrease the workload of the heart. Pharmacology of the analgesics was presented in Chapter 25.

PharmFACT

About 1.5 million Americans experience a new or recurrent MI each year. About one-third of the patients experiencing an MI will die within 24 hours of the onset of the attack (Zafari, 2017).

35.12 Vasopressors are used following cardiopulmonary arrest to reestablish coronary and cerebral blood flow.

Cardiopulmonary arrest is a complete stoppage of heart and lung activity, usually resulting from a dysrhythmia such as ventricular fibrillation or pulseless ventricular tachycardia. Cardiopulmonary resuscitation (CPR) must be initiated as quickly as possible to restore ventilation and blood circulation to avoid hypoxic injury to the tissues. Defibrillation is used to restore normal cardiac rhythm.

The primary drug used in resuscitation is epinephrine. Sympathomimetics such as epinephrine cause vasoconstriction, immediately raising cerebral, coronary, and systemic blood pressure. In past years, vasopressin was considered an alternative therapy, however epinephrine is now considered more effective.

It is recommended that epinephrine be administered as soon as feasible for patients exhibiting nonshockable rhythms such as asystole and pulseless electrical activity. For patients with shockable rhythms such as ventricular tachycardia and ventricular fibrillation, epinephrine administration is recommended after defibrillation has proven unsuccessful (Panchal et al., 2019).

Use of epinephrine in cardiac arrest has been shown to improve outcomes, including survival to hospital admission, survival to hospital discharge and 30-day survival.

CONNECTIONS: APPLIED CLINICAL JUDGMENT

Patients Receiving Pharmacotherapy with Organic Nitrates for Angina and Myocardial Infarction

Key Assessment Data

- History of current condition, baseline vital signs, physical exam findings; history of cardiovascular (including previous MI, HF, valvular disease), cerebrovascular (including level of consciousness, history of stroke, head injury, increased intracranial pressure), respiratory disease, hepatic or renal disease; medication history, including use of erectile dysfunction drugs (e.g., sildenafil); pregnancy status; baseline ECG, electrolytes, troponin and/or CK-MB laboratory values, renal function studies, and lipid profiles.
- Ongoing assessment during drug therapy should include ECG monitoring for dysrhythmias, frequent BP evaluation and assessment for hypotension with reflex tachycardia,

Desired Therapeutic Outcomes

Improvement is observed and measurable when chest pain has subsided or has significantly lessened, heart rate and blood pressure remain within normal limits, ECG remains within normal limits without signs of ischemia or infarction.

Minimizing Adverse Effects

- Nitrates may cause significant vasodilation, resulting in the potential for hypotension accompanied by reflex tachycardia. Reflex tachycardia increases myocardial oxygen demand, worsening angina. Monitor for orthostatic hypotension, especially accompanied by reflex tachycardia.
- Continue cardiac monitoring (e.g., ECG) as ordered for dysrhythmias in the hospitalized patient, promptly reporting dysrhythmias or angina.
- Nitrate therapy may worsen preexisting neurologic, cardiac, or respiratory conditions as blood pressure drops and perfusion to vital organs diminishes.
- Lung congestion may signal impending HF. Evaluate breath sounds frequently and weigh daily, reporting weight gain over 1 kg (2 lb) in a 24-hour period or edema.
- Evaluate the need for adjunctive treatment with the healthcare provider for angina prevention and treatment (e.g., pain control, beta blockers, aspirin therapy) or further cardiac studies.

Lifespan Considerations

- Older adults may be at increased risk for hypotension, and dizziness may increase the risk of falls.

Diversity Considerations

- Due to differences in reporting pain, use subjective and objective data in evaluating pain relief in ethnically diverse or older adult patients.

Patient Education

- If SL nitroglycerin is prescribed, unless ordered otherwise by provider:
  - Take one nitroglycerin tablet, under the tongue, for chest pain. Remain seated or lie down to avoid dizziness or falls.
  - If chest pain continues, repeat one nitroglycerin tablet, under the tongue, in 5 min. Remain seated or lying down.
  - If chest pain continues, repeat nitroglycerin, under the tongue, in 5 min.
  - If chest pain continues, even if reduced, do not take further nitroglycerin unless specifically directed by the healthcare provider. Call EMS (e.g., 911) for assistance.
- If transdermal nitroglycerin patches are used, remove patch for 6–12 h at night, or as directed by the healthcare provider, to prevent or delay the development of tolerance to nitrates.
- Monitor BP as directed and daily weight, using a diary or log, and bring these to each provider visit. Promptly report any weight gain over 1 kg in a 24-hour period, increasing or severe chest pain, shortness of breath, or palpitations to the provider.
- Rise from lying to sitting or standing slowly to avoid dizziness or falls, especially if taking SL nitrates. If dizziness occurs, sit or lie down and do not attempt to stand or walk until the sensation passes.
- Do not take daily aspirin without discussing with the provider first. The drug may be contraindicated depending on other conditions or medications.
- Erectile dysfunction drugs lower blood pressure and, when combined with nitrates, can result in severe and prolonged hypotension. Do not take these drugs concurrently without first consulting the provider.

Prescribing Considerations

- Nitrates should not be used in conjunction with the use of phosphodiesterase inhibitors such as sildenafil (inquire if the patients have erectile dysfunction and if they are taking medications for it).
- Nitrates should not be prescribed to patients with right-ventricular infarction or patients with hypertrophic cardiomyopathy.
- Patients on diuretic therapy can become volume depleted and develop hypotension.
- Patients who have low systolic blood pressure can develop severe hypotension.
- Nitrates have not been evaluated fully in pregnancy and breastfeeding, so they should be avoided.

Understanding Chapter 35

Key Concepts Summary

35.1 Myocardial ischemia develops when there is inadequate blood supply to meet the metabolic demands of cardiac muscle.

35.2 Coronary artery disease is the major cause of myocardial ischemia.

35.3 Therapeutic lifestyle changes can decrease the risk of coronary artery disease.

35.4 Angina pectoris is characterized by severe chest pain brought on by physical exertion or emotional stress.

35.5 The pharmacologic management of angina includes organic nitrates, beta-adrenergic antagonists, and calcium channel blockers.

35.6 Organic nitrates may be used to terminate or prevent angina episodes.

35.7 Beta-adrenergic antagonists are first-line drugs for stable angina.

35.8 Calcium channel blockers are effective at reducing myocardial oxygen demand and treating stable and variant angina.

35.9 Early diagnosis and pharmacotherapy of myocardial infarction increase chances of survival.

35.10 Fibrinolytic drugs can restore perfusion to ischemic regions of the myocardium if administered soon after a myocardial infarction.

35.11 Drugs are used to treat the symptoms and complications of acute myocardial infarction.

35.12 Vasopressors are used following cardiopulmonary arrest to reestablish coronary and cerebral blood flow.

CASE STUDY: Making the Patient Connection

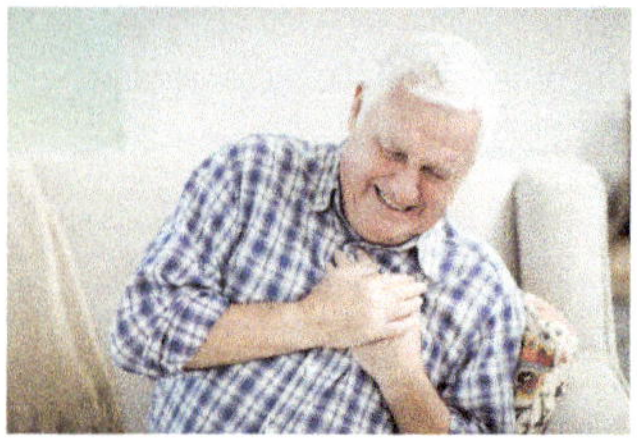

Remember the patient "Michael Graff" at the beginning of the chapter? Now read the remainder of the case study. Based on the information presented within this chapter, respond to the critical thinking questions that follow.

Early one morning, 60-year-old Michael Graff began to feel severe anterior crushing chest pain that lasted for 35 minutes. He experienced dizziness, cold sweats, and nausea. Although he considered driving to the local ED, his family insisted on calling an ambulance for emergency transport to the hospital.

Michael, a general contractor, is a two-pack-per-day smoker and consumes alcohol (beer) two to three times per week. He has a family history of CAD, diabetes mellitus, and hyperlipidemia. It has been at least 10 years since his last physical examination.

On arrival at the ED, Michael presents with symptoms of anxiety, moderate chest pain, and cold extremities. Auscultation of the thorax revealed tachycardia and clear lung fields. Blood pressure was slightly above normal at 156/90 mmHg. He had no neck venous distention. His white blood cell count was 7600/mm^3; hematocrit, 43.8%; platelets, 256,000/mm^3; CK, 87 international units/L; and troponin-I, less than 4.1 mcg/L. An ECG showed ST-segment elevation.

Once stabilized, Michael is transported to the coronary care unit with the admission diagnosis of unstable angina and to rule out MI. In the coronary care unit, he receives IV nitroglycerin 50 mg in D$_5$W 25 mL. The nurse begins the infusion at 10 mcg/min and titrates the rate based on his report of chest pain every 5 to 10 min (5–10 mcg/min).

Critical Thinking Questions

1. Michael and his family ask you to explain what is occurring with his heart. How would you describe the pathophysiology of Michael's condition to them?
2. Discuss the reason Michael is receiving nitroglycerin.
3. What adverse effects should the nurse monitor with patients receiving IV nitroglycerin?
4. How do nitroglycerin infusions differ from other IV infusions?

Additional Case Study

Bill Shackley, a 52-year-old man, is prescribed nifedipine (Procardia XL) for treatment of variant angina. While discussing his medications, Bill shares several of his concerns. How would you respond to the following questions?

1. "I have a friend who takes nitroglycerin for his chest pain. Why can't I just take that?"
2. "My friend says that he can't take drugs like Viagra. Sometimes I have some problems in the bedroom. Is it OK if I take it since I'm not taking nitroglycerin?"

Chapter Review

1. A patient with chest pain is receiving sublingual nitroglycerin. The nurse would include in the care plan to monitor the patient for which adverse effect?
   1. Photosensitivity
   2. Elevated blood pressure
   3. Vomiting and diarrhea
   4. Decreased blood pressure

2. The patient states, "I always put my nitroglycerin patch in the same place so I do not forget to take it off." The nurse's response would be based on which of the following physiologic concepts?
   1. Patients are more likely to remember to apply the patch if the same site is used daily.
   2. Repeated use of the same application site will enhance medication absorption.
   3. Rebound phenomenon is likely to occur when the same site is used more than once.
   4. Skin irritation can occur if the same site is used repeatedly.

3. The nurse is caring for a patient with chronic angina pectoris. The patient is receiving isosorbide dinitrate (Isordil) oral tablets. Which patient manifestations would the nurse conclude are common adverse effects of this medication?
   1. Flushing and headache
   2. Tremors and anxiety
   3. Lightheadedness and dizziness
   4. Sleepiness and lethargy

4. The patient asks how atenolol (Tenormin) helps angina. The response provided by the nurse is based on which concept? This medication:
   1. Slows the heart rate and reduces contractility.
   2. Increases the heart rate and diminishes contractility.
   3. Blocks sodium channels and elevates depolarization.
   4. Decreases blood pressure and blocks the $alpha_2$ receptors.

5. Which of the following assessment findings, if discovered in a patient receiving verapamil (Calan) for angina, would be cause for the nurse to withhold the medication? (Select all that apply.)
   1. Bradycardia: heart rate of 40 beats/min
   2. Tachycardia: heart rate of 126 beats/min
   3. Hypotension: blood pressure 76/46 mmHg
   4. Tinnitus with hearing loss
   5. Hypertension: blood pressure 156/92 mmHg

6. A patient experiencing an MI is brought to the emergency room. Which of the following is true about the use of fibrinolytics in treating an MI? (Select all that apply.)
   1. They are most effective when administered within the first 12 hours after the onset of MI symptoms, and ideally less than 30 minutes.
   2. The chance for extreme bleeding is possible and physical and laboratory assessments for bleeding parameters should continue for up to 4 days after therapy.
   3. Before initiating therapy, an assessment should be made for bleeding disorders, stroke within the past 3 months, or severe liver disease as these are contraindications for the drug.
   4. Anticoagulants or antiplatelet drugs are often used post-fibrinolytic therapy.
   5. Administration of a calcium channel blocker to cause vasodilation may be given before initiating fibrinolytic therapy.

See Appendix A for answers to critical thinking questions, case study questions, and review questions.

References

Alaeddini, J. (2018). *Angina pectoris*. Medscape. http://emedicine.medscape.com/article/150215-overview

Cavallari, L. H., Lee, C. R., Beitelshees A. L., Cooper-DeHoff, R. M., Duarte, J. D., Voora, D., et al. (2018). Multisite investigation of outcomes with implementation of CYP2C19 genotype-guided antiplatelet therapy after percutaneous coronary intervention. *Journal of the American College of Cardiology: Cardiovascular Interventions, 11*, 181–191. https://doi.org/10.1016/j.jcin.2017.07.022

Kloner, R. A., & Chaitman, B. (2017). Angina and its management. *Journal of Cardiovascular Pharmacology and Therapeutics, 22*(3), 199–209. https://doi.org/10.1177/1074248416679733

Panchal, A. R., Berg, K. M., Hirsch, K. G., Kudenchuk, P. J., Del Rios, M., Cabañas, J. G., et al. (2019). 2019 American

Heart Association focused update on advanced cardiovascular life support: Use of advanced airways, vasopressors, and extracorporeal cardiopulmonary resuscitation during cardiac arrest: An update to the American Heart Association guidelines for cardiopulmonary resuscitation and emergency cardiovascular care. *Circulation, 140*(24), e881–e894. https://doi.org/10.1161/CIR.0000000000000732

Xi, Z., Fang, F., Wang, J., AlHelal, J., Zhou, Y., & Liu, W. (2019). CYP2C19 genotype and adverse cardiovascular outcomes after stent implantation in clopidogrel-treated Asian populations: A systematic review and meta-analysis. *Platelets, 30*, 229–240. https://doi.org/10.1080/09537104.2017.1413178

Zafari, A. M. (2017). *Myocardial infarction*. Medscape. http://emedicine.medscape.com/article/155919-overview

Selected Bibliography

Andersen, L. W., Holmberg, M. J., Berg, K. M., Donnino, M. W., & Granfeldt, A. (2019). In-hospital cardiac arrest: A review. *Journal of the American Medical Association*, 321(12), 1200–1210. https://doi.org/10.1001/jama.2019.1696

Aves, T., Chopra, A., Patel, M., & Lin, S. (2020). Epinephrine for out-of-hospital cardiac arrest: An updated systematic review and meta-analysis. *Critical Care Medicine, 48*(2), 225–229. https://doi.org/10.1097/CCM.0000000000004130

Braun, M. M., Stevens, W. A., & Barstow, C. H. (2018). Stable coronary artery disease: Treatment. *American Family Physician, 97*(6), 376–384.

Giannopoulos, A. A., Giannoglou, G. D., & Chatzizisis, Y. S. (2016). Pharmacological approaches of refractory angina. *Pharmacology & Therapeutics, 163*, 118–131. https://doi.org/10.1016/j.pharmthera.2016.03.008

Harris, J. R., Hale, G. M., Dasari, T. W., & Schwier, N. C. (2016). Pharmacotherapy of vasospastic angina. *Journal of Cardiovascular Pharmacology and Therapeutics, 21*, 439–451. https://doi.org/10.1177/1074248416640161

Mozaffarian, D., Benjamin, E. J., Go, A. S., Arnett, D. K., Blaha, M. J., Cushman, M., et al. (2015). Executive summary: Heart disease and stroke statistics—2015 update. *Circulation, 131*, 434–441. https://doi.org/10.1161/CIR.0000000000000157

Ohman, E. M. (2016). Chronic stable angina. *New England Journal of Medicine, 374*, 1167–1176. https://doi.org/10.1056/NEJMcp1502240

Picard, F., Sayah, N., Spagnoli, V., Adjedj, J., & Varenne, O. (2019). Vasospastic angina: A literature review of current evidence. *Archives of Cardiovascular Diseases, 112*(1), 44–55. https://doi.org/10.1016/j.acvd.2018.08.002

Rogers, J., & Baker, M. (2020). Understanding the most commonly billed diagnoses in primary care: Atherosclerotic cardiovascular disease. *The Nurse Practitioner, 45*(7), 35–41. https://doi.org/10.1097/01.NPR.0000669136.88720.65

Rousan, T. A., & Thadani, U. (2019). Stable angina medical therapy management guidelines: A critical review of guidelines from the European Society of Cardiology and National Institute for Health and Care Excellence. *European Cardiology Review, 14*(1), 18–22. https://doi.org/10.15420/ecr.2018.26.1

Switaj, T. L., Christensen, S., & Brewer, D. M. (2017). Acute coronary syndrome: Current treatment. *American Family Physician, 95*(4), 232–240.

Virani, S. S., Alonso, A., Benjamin, E. J., Bittencourt, M. S., Callaway, C. W., Carson, A. P., et al. (2020). Heart disease and stroke statistics—2020 update: A report from the American Heart Association. *Circulation, 141*(9), E139–E596. https://doi.org/10.1161/CIR.0000000000000757

Winchester, D. E., & Pepine, C. J. (2015). Angina treatments and prevention of cardiac events: An appraisal of the evidence. *European Heart Journal Supplements, 17*(Suppl. G), G10–G18. https://doi.org/10.1093/eurheartj/suv054

"It seems that over the past 2 weeks, I have become more short of breath just walking around my apartment. Walking around the market and unloading my groceries has become almost impossible."
—*Patient "Thelma Walters"*

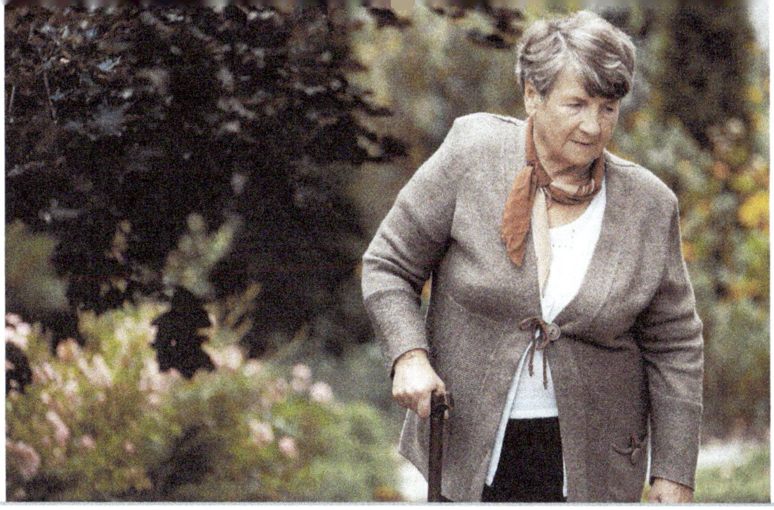

Chapter 36
Pharmacotherapy of Heart Failure

Chapter Outline

Learning Outcomes

After reading this chapter, the student should be able to:

1. Identify the major diseases associated with heart failure.
2. Relate how the symptoms associated with heart failure may be caused by a weakened heart muscle and diminished cardiac output.
3. Identify compensatory mechanisms used by the body to maintain cardiac output in patients with heart failure.
4. Describe how heart failure is classified.
5. Describe the nurse's role in the pharmacologic management of heart failure.
6. For each of the classes shown in the chapter outline, identify the prototype and representative drugs and explain the mechanism(s) of drug action, primary indications, contraindications, significant drug interactions, pregnancy data, and important adverse effects.
7. Apply clinical judgment to care for patients receiving pharmacotherapy for heart failure.

Key Terms

Definitions of the terms in bold may be found in the Glossary.

Heart failure (HF) is one of the most common and fatal of the cardiovascular diseases, and its incidence is increasing as the population ages. Although improved treatment of myocardial infarction and hypertension has led to declines in mortality due to HF, approximately one in five patients still dies within a year of diagnosis of HF, and 50% die within 5 years. Historically, this condition was called *congestive heart failure*; however, because not all incidences of this disease are associated with congestion, the more appropriate name is *heart failure*.

PharmFACT

Each year, about 960,000 new cases of heart failure are diagnosed and about 309,000 deaths are attributed to HF in the United States. Although the incidence is equal in men and women, women develop HF later in life and survive longer with the disease (Dumitru, 2018).

Etiology of Heart Failure

36.1 Heart failure is closely associated with disorders such as chronic hypertension, coronary artery disease, and diabetes.

Heart failure (HF) is the inability of the heart to pump enough blood to meet the metabolic demands of the body. HF can be caused by any disorder that affects the heart's ability to receive or eject blood. While weakening of cardiac muscle is a natural consequence of aging, the process can be caused or accelerated by the following:

- Atherosclerotic cardiovascular disease (ASCVD)
- Mitral stenosis
- Myocardial infarction (MI)
- Chronic hypertension (HTN)
- Diabetes mellitus (DM).

The student should detect a common theme throughout the chapters on cardiovascular pharmacology. That theme is the ability to prevent major causes of morbidity and mortality through the selection of healthy lifestyle choices. Controlling blood lipid levels, implementing a regular exercise program, maintaining optimal body weight, and keeping blood pressure within recommended limits reduce the incidences of ASCVD and MI. Maintaining blood glucose within the normal range reduces the consequences of uncontrolled DM. Thus, for many patients, HF is a preventable condition; controlling associated diseases will greatly reduce the risk of development and progression of HF.

Because there is no cure for HF, the treatment goals are to prevent, treat, or remove the underlying causes whenever possible and manage its symptoms, so that the patient's quality of life can be improved. Advances in understanding the pathophysiology of HF during the past several decades have led to a change in pharmacotherapeutic goals. No longer is therapy of HF focused on end stages of the disorder. Pharmacotherapy is now targeted at prevention and slowing the progression of HF. This change in emphasis has led to significant improvements in survival and quality of life in patients with HF.

Pathophysiology of Heart Failure

36.2 The body attempts to compensate for heart failure by increasing cardiac output.

Heart failure is a general term used to describe several different types of cardiac dysfunction. The dysfunction may occur on the left side, the right side, or on both sides of the heart.

Left-sided HF is sometimes called congestive heart failure because it is characterized by an accumulation of fluid causing congestion in the pulmonary capillary beds. Although left-sided HF is more common, the right side of the heart can also become weak, either simultaneously with the left side or independently from the left side. In right-sided HF, the blood pools in the veins, resulting in peripheral edema and engorgement of organs such as the liver.

Left-sided HF is further subdivided into two types. Systolic HF occurs when cardiac output (CO) is diminished due to decreased contractility of the myocardium. Approximately 60 to 80% of left-sided HF is the systolic type. Diastolic HF occurs when the lungs become congested even though CO is normal. Diastolic HF is caused by a restriction in ventricular filling, resulting in higher-than-normal pressure in the ventricle. Although CO is normal, the increased pressure in the ventricle creates higher pressure in the pulmonary capillaries, resulting in pulmonary edema. A patient may have both systolic and diastolic HF. Pharmacotherapy of the two types differs somewhat.

HF may progress slowly over many years, or it may have an acute onset. Once HF reaches the stage where CO is affected, tissues receive inadequate perfusion and organ failure is possible. The body has developed a complex series of actions to compensate for HF. Knowledge of these compensatory mechanisms is important to understanding the pharmacotherapy of HF. Prior to continuing in this chapter, factors affecting CO, stroke volume, afterload, and preload, discussed in Chapter 28, should be reviewed. The pathophysiology of HF is illustrated in Figure 36.1.

Ventricular Hypertrophy

In left HF, the left ventricle must work harder due to the increased preload or afterload. Over time, the wall of the left ventricle thickens and enlarges (ventricular hypertrophy) in an attempt to compensate for the increased workload. Changes in the size, shape, and structure of the myocardial

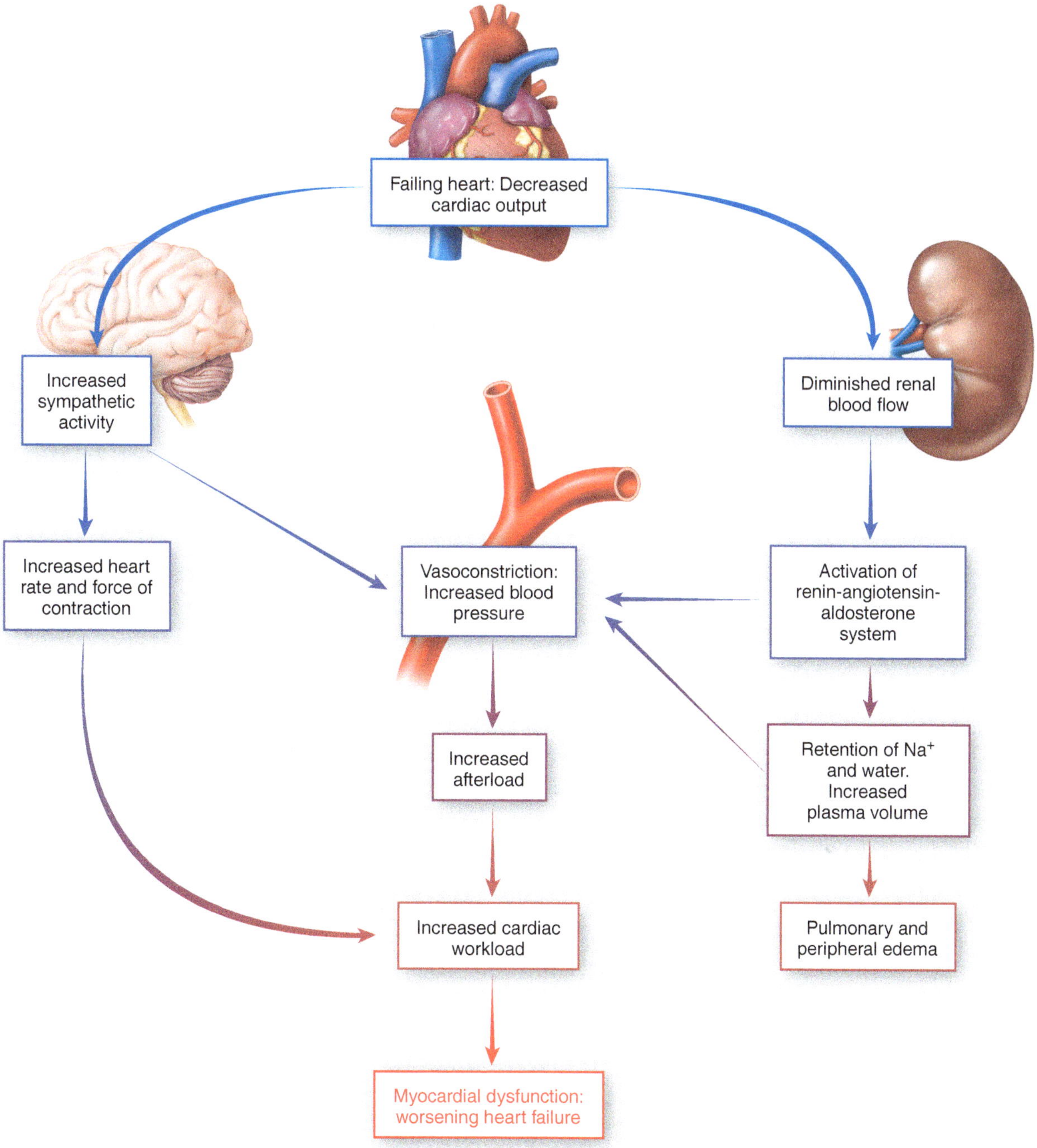

Figure 36.1 Pathophysiology of heart failure.

cells (myocytes) occur. These compensatory changes in structure benefit the heart by allowing it to better maintain adequate stroke volume and CO. The term **cardiac remodeling** is sometimes used to describe these changes to myocyte structure and function.

The benefits of cardiac remodeling as a compensatory mechanism, however, are limited. Myocytes continually die, likely due to workload injury, and fibrotic tissue fills the spaces between them. These tissue changes stiffen the myocardium, causing diminished contractility and reduced CO. The heart responds with even more remodeling, continuing the destructive cycle. Without intervention, the abnormal structural changes can result in irreversible cardiac impairment.

Activation of the Sympathetic Nervous System

One of the fastest homeostatic responses to diminished CO is activation of the sympathetic nervous system (SNS). The increased heart rate resulting from sympathetic activation is a normal compensatory mechanism that serves to increase CO.

The SNS, however, also constricts arteries and activates the renin-angiotensin-aldosterone system (RAAS). Higher angiotensin II levels raise blood pressure and afterload, causing the heart to work harder. The stressed myocardium, which already has reduced contractility and difficulty maintaining CO, is faced with even greater challenges by this additional workload. The diminished CO caused by the high afterload produces an ongoing activation of the SNS. Patients with preexisting coronary artery disease (CAD) may experience acute angina from the increased SNS activity. Again, although there are certain compensatory benefits to activating the SNS to maintain CO, a destructive cycle is created that can lead to or worsen HF.

CONNECTION Checkpoint 36.1

Propranolol (Inderal) is an example of a negative inotropic drug. From what you learned in Chapter 16, explain why this type of drug should be administered with caution to a patient with heart failure who also has asthma.

Increased Plasma Volume and Preload

When CO in a patient with HF is diminished, blood flow to the kidneys is reduced. The kidneys respond to the decreased perfusion by secreting renin and activating the RAAS. As a result of the action of angiotensin II, aldosterone secretion is increased and the body retains sodium and water. This has the beneficial effects of increasing preload, stretching the myocardial fibers, and increasing contractility, thus returning CO to normal levels. This is an important compensatory mechanism in the normal heart.

However, the heart has a limit to its ability to increase contractility. In a diseased heart, the increased preload leads to volume overload and pulmonary congestion. In addition, the increased plasma volume increases blood pressure, which further adds to afterload and to the burden of an already weak heart.

Research has discovered additional detrimental effects related to activation of the RAAS. Angiotensin II has been found to promote ventricular hypertrophy, myocyte death, and fibrosis formation in the myocardium. Aldosterone also has direct effects on the myocardium, promoting fibrosis and stiffening of the ventricular wall. Angiotensin-converting enzyme (ACE) inhibitors have become preferred drugs for HF, in part because they are able to block these detrimental effects of angiotensin II and aldosterone on cardiac remodeling.

Biomarkers for Heart Failure: Natriuretic Peptides

Beta-natriuretic peptides are substances secreted in response to increased pressure in the heart. BNP (B-type natriuretic peptide) and NT-proBNP (N-terminal pro B-type natriuretic peptides) are used as biomarkers to assess for the presence and severity of HF. In general, low values of these biomarkers exclude the presence of HF, whereas higher values are predictive for worsening HF. Evidence suggests that BNP screening with early intervention may prevent HF.

BNP biomarkers are also being used to estimate patient prognosis; for example, high levels of biomarkers on admission are associated with poorer clinical outcomes. Furthermore, patients who do not experience a reduction in natriuretic peptide biomarkers during hospitalization for HF have a higher risk for readmission and death.

Several other substances have been identified as potential biomarkers in the progression of HF. The high-sensitivity cardiac troponin test (hs-cTnT) is predictive of poor clinical outcomes. Two proinflammatory substances, tumor necrosis factor and interleukin, are found in high levels in patients with HF and are associated with a poor prognosis.

36.3 Symptoms of heart failure occur when compensatory mechanisms fail to maintain adequate cardiac output.

The classic symptoms of HF are dyspnea on exertion, fatigue, pulmonary congestion, and peripheral edema. Lung congestion causes a cough and orthopnea (difficulty breathing when recumbent). If pulmonary edema occurs, the patient feels as if he or she is suffocating and extreme anxiety may result. The condition often worsens at night.

Through pharmacotherapy and lifestyle modifications, many patients with HF can maintain a symptom-free,

CONNECTIONS: Patient Safety

Misunderstood Instructions

A patient has been taking enalapril (Vasotec) and carvedilol (Coreg CR) for stage B heart failure with a history of prior MI. The patient is brought to the emergency department due to episodes of syncope at home whenever rising from lying or sitting to standing. When questioned, the patient reports taking "all medicines as directed" and that he has been "counting my pulse rate before I take the Coreg. I am not to take it if my heartbeat is less than 60 in a minute." On assessing the patient's heart rate, the nurse notes a pulse of 42. When asked to demonstrate how he is taking his pulse, the patient requests the nurse's stethoscope and replies, "I've been using my daughter's stethoscope. She's a nurse. I count my heartbeats. It's easier than trying to find my pulse," and proceeds to demonstrate. He obtains a pulse rate of 84.

What is one possible underlying reason for the discrepancy in heart rate between the nurse's and the patient's values? What should the nurse do to correct the patient's technique?

Table 36.1 Drugs That May Worsen Heart Failure

Mechanism	Example Drugs and Classes
Negative inotropic effect: slow heart rate or reduce contractility	Antidysrhythmics Beta-adrenergic antagonists Calcium channel blockers Itraconazole (antifungal)
Cardiotoxicity: damage to the myocardium	Cyclophosphamide (antineoplastic) Daunomycin (antineoplastic) Doxorubicin (antineoplastic)
Increase blood volume: cause sodium and water retention and fluid overload	Androgens Estrogens Glucocorticoids NSAIDs Rosiglitazone and pioglitazone (antidiabetics)

compensated state for years. The most common reason patients experience decompensation is fluid overload due to nonadherence to sodium and water restrictions. The second most common reason is nonadherence to the pharmacotherapeutic regimen. The nurse must stress to patients the importance of sodium restriction and treatment adherence to promote a healthier heart. Cardiac events such as myocardial ischemia, MI, or dysrhythmias can also precipitate acute HF. Certain medications can worsen HF, and the nurse should use these drugs with caution. A list of selected drugs that may worsen HF is shown in Table 36.1.

Principles of Pharmacologic Management of Heart Failure

36.4 The specific therapy for heart failure depends on the clinical stage of the disease.

Two primary models are available to guide the pharmacologic management of HF. The New York Heart Association (NYHA) classification has been widely used in clinical practice for the staging of HF. This model classifies symptomatic HF into four functional classes:

- I: Patients with cardiac disease but with no symptoms during physical activity
- II: Patients with cardiac disease who have slight limitations on physical activity, with symptoms such as fatigue, palpitations, dyspnea, or angina
- III: Patients with cardiac disease who have marked limitations during physical activity
- IV: Patients with cardiac disease who are unable to perform physical activity and who have symptoms at rest.

A more recent model, proposed by the American College of Cardiology (ACC) and the American Heart Association (AHA), categorizes HF into four stages, as listed in Table 36.2. Although similar to the NYHA model, the ACC/AHA model better illustrates the progressive nature of the disease and the role of risk factor modification (Yancy et al., 2016).

Pharmacotherapy of HF focuses on three primary physiologic goals:

1. Reduction of preload
2. Reduction of systemic vascular resistance (reduction of afterload)
3. Inhibition of both the RAAS and vasoconstrictor mechanisms of the SNS.

The first two goals provide symptomatic relief but do not reverse the progression of the disease. In addition to reducing symptoms, inhibition of the RAAS and reduced vasoconstriction by the sympathetic nervous system also result in a significant reduction in morbidity and mortality from HF. These mechanisms are illustrated in Pharmacotherapy Illustrated 36.1.

Table 36.2 Stages for Treating Heart Failure

Stage	Description	Treatment Examples
A	At high risk of developing HF but without structural heart disease or symptoms.	Make lifestyle modifications. Manage associated conditions: HTN, dyslipidemia, obesity, and DM. If hypertensive, use ACE inhibitor or angiotensin receptor blocker (ARB).
B	Structural evidence of heart disease, such as a previous MI or valvular disease, but no symptoms of HF. (Includes NYHA Class I patients.)	Continue treatments for stage A. Treat with ACE inhibitor or ARB. Beta blockers are added for those with prior HF symptoms or history of MI.
C	Structural evidence of heart disease with current symptoms of HF such as fatigue, fluid retention, or dyspnea. (Includes NYHA Class II and III patients.)	Continue lifestyle modifications and treatment with ACE inhibitor, ARB, or beta blocker. If needed to control symptoms, add diuretic or combination of isosorbide dinitrate with hydralazine (in Blacks). Consider use of aldosterone antagonists (e.g., spironolactone) to decrease hospitalizations. Management of patients with a history of atrial fibrillation or thromboembolic event should be implemented per clinical practice guidelines.
D	Symptoms at rest or minimal exertion despite optimal medical therapy. (Includes NYHA Class IV patients.)	Continue lifestyle modifications. Consider fluid and sodium restrictions. Treatment with inotropic drugs (e.g., dopamine, dobutamine, or phosphodiesterase inhibitors) for palliative care or patients awaiting cardiac transplant.

Source: From Yancy et al. (2013).

Pharmacotherapy Illustrated 36.1

Mechanisms of Action of Drugs Used for Heart Failure

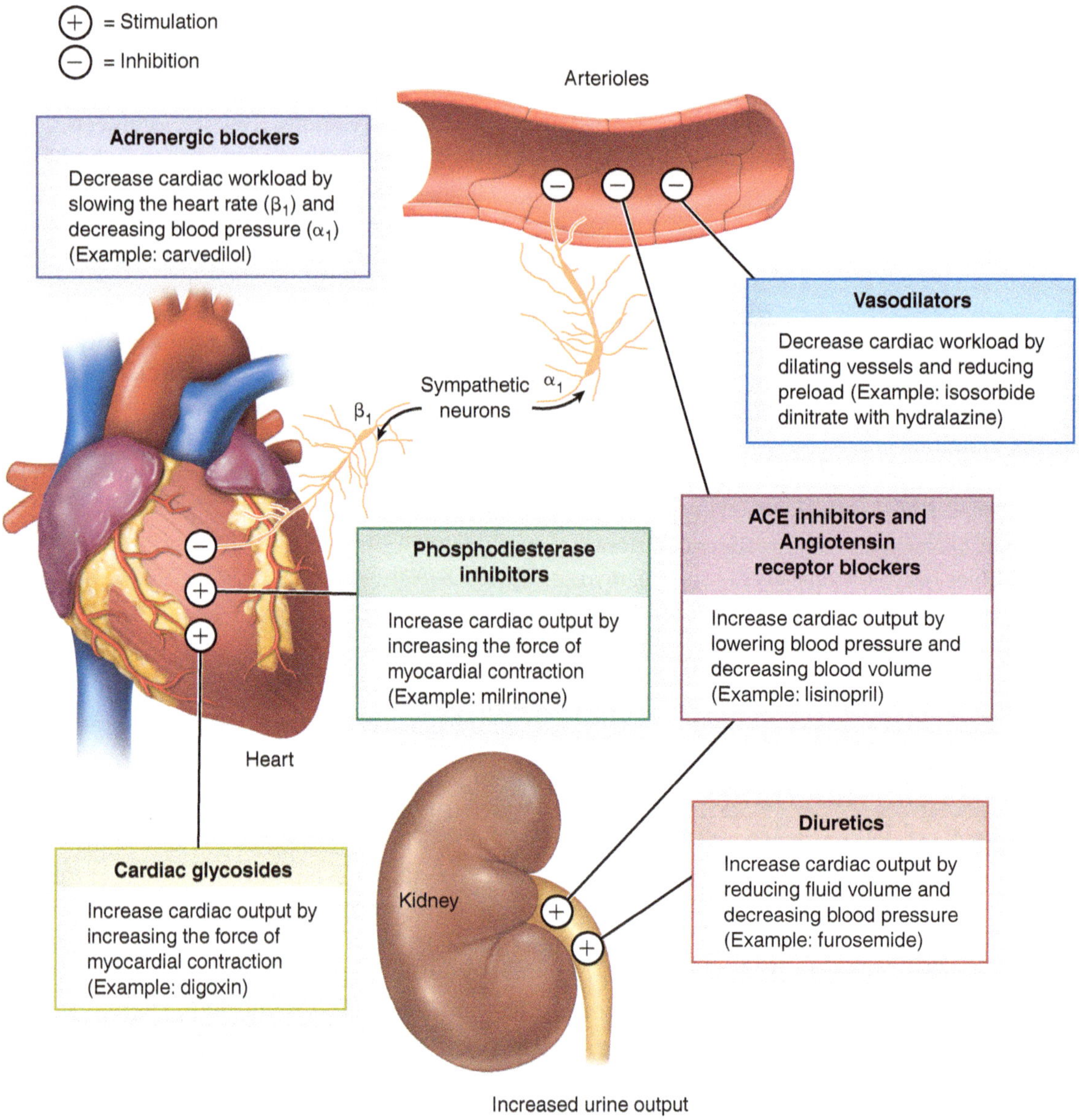

Drugs for Heart Failure

36.5 Angiotensin-converting enzyme inhibitors are first-line drugs for heart failure.

Due to their effectiveness and relative safety, the angiotensin-converting enzyme inhibitors have become first-line drugs for the treatment of chronic HF. Indeed, unless contraindicated, all patients with HF and those at high risk of HF should receive an ACE inhibitor. The student should refer to Chapter 31 for details on the pharmacology of the drugs in this class. The following section focuses on the benefits of these drugs for patients with HF.

Clinical research has clearly demonstrated that ACE inhibitors slow the progression of HF and reduce mortality from this disease. Research also suggests that there are no substantive differences among the available ACE inhibitors in their effects of HF symptoms or survival. Doses for the ACE inhibitors indicated for HF are listed in Table 36.3.

The two primary actions of the ACE inhibitors are to lower peripheral resistance through the inhibition of angiotensin II formation and to reduce blood volume through inhibition of aldosterone secretion. The resultant reduction of arterial blood pressure diminishes afterload and increases CO. An additional effect of the ACE inhibitors is dilation of veins. This action, which is probably not directly related to their inhibition of angiotensin, lowers preload and reduces pulmonary congestion and peripheral edema. The combined reductions in preload, afterload, and blood volume from the ACE inhibitors substantially decrease the workload on the heart and allow it to work more efficiently for patients with cardiac impairment. Patients taking ACE inhibitors experience fewer HF-related symptoms and hospitalizations. Exercise tolerance is improved.

Therapy with ACE inhibitors is begun at low doses, and the amount is gradually increased until the desired therapeutic level is reached. Higher doses reduce HF symptoms more effectively. Symptomatic relief from HF symptoms

Table 36.3 Selected Drugs for Early and Moderate Heart Failure

Drug	Route and Adult Dose (Maximum Dose Where Indicated)	Adverse Effects
ACE Inhibitors and Angiotensin Receptor Blockers		
candesartan (Atacand)	PO: Start at 4 mg/day and increase gradually (max: 32 mg/day)	*Headache, dizziness, orthostatic hypotension, dry cough* Severe hypotension (first-dose phenomenon), syncope, angioedema, blood dyscrasias, fetal toxicity
captopril	PO: 6.25–12.5 mg tid (max: 450 mg/day)	
enalapril (Vasotec)	PO: 2.5 mg qid–bid (max: 40 mg/day)	
fosinopril	PO: 5–40 mg/day (max: 40 mg/day)	
lisinopril (Prinivil, Zestril)	PO: 10 mg/day (max: 80 mg/day)	
losartan (Cozaar)	PO: 25–50 mg once daily (max: 100 mg/day)	
quinapril (Accupril)	PO: 10–20 mg/day (max: 40 mg/day)	
ramipril (Altace)	PO: 2.5–5 mg bid (max: 10 mg/day)	
valsartan (Diovan)	PO: 80 mg/day (max: 320 mg/day)	
Beta-Adrenergic Antagonists		
bisoprolol	PO: 2.5–5 mg once daily (max: 20 mg/day)	*Fatigue, insomnia, drowsiness, weight gain, bradycardia, dizziness* Agranulocytosis, laryngospasm, Stevens–Johnson syndrome, anaphylaxis; if the drug is abruptly withdrawn, palpitations, rebound HTN, life-threatening dysrhythmias, or myocardial ischemia may occur
carvedilol (Coreg CR)	PO (extended release): 10–20 mg/day (max: 80 mg/day)	
metoprolol (Toprol XL)	PO (extended release): 12.5–25 mg/day initial dose (max: 200 mg/day)	
Diuretics		
Loop or High-Ceiling		Loop and thiazides: *Electrolyte imbalances, fatigue, orthostatic hypotension* Severe hypotension, dehydration, serious hypokalemia, hyponatremia, hyperglycemia (thiazides), ototoxicity (loop diuretics) Potassium-sparing: *Hyperkalemia, gynecomastia in men, fatigue* Dysrhythmias due to hyperkalemia
bumetanide (Bumex)	PO: 0.5–2 mg/day (max: 10 mg/day)	
furosemide (Lasix)	PO: 20–80 mg in 1 or more divided doses (max: 600 mg/day)	
torsemide (Demadex)	PO/IV: 5–20 mg/day (max: 200 mg/day)	
Thiazide and Thiazide-Like		
hydrochlorothiazide (Microzide)	PO: 25–200 mg in 1–3 divided doses (max: 200 mg/day)	
Potassium-Sparing (Aldosterone Antagonist)		
eplerenone (Inspra)	PO: 25–50 mg once daily (max: 50 mg/day)	
spironolactone (Aldactone)	PO: 25–100 mg in divided doses (max: 400 mg/day)	
Miscellaneous Drugs		
digoxin (Lanoxin, Lanoxicaps)	PO: 0.125–0.5 mg/day	*Nausea and vomiting, headache, and visual disturbances such as seeing halos, a yellow or green tinge, or blurring* Dysrhythmias, AV block
hydralazine with isosorbide dinitrate (BiDil)	PO: 1 tablet tid (max: 2 tablets tid); each tablet contains 37.5 mg of hydralazine and 20 mg of isosorbide dinitrate	*Headache, flushing of face, orthostatic hypotension, dizziness, reflex tachycardia* Fainting, severe headache, severe hypotension with overdose, lupus-like reaction (hydralazine)
ivabradine (Corlanor)	PO: 5 mg bid initial dose (max: 7.5 mg bid)	*Bradycardia, HTN* Atrial fibrillation, fetal toxicity
sacubitril with valsartan (Entresto)	PO: 97 mg (sacubitril)/103 mg (valsartan) bid maintenance dose	*Hypotension, hyperkalemia, cough, dizziness* Renal failure, fetal toxicity, angioedema

Note: *Italics* indicate common adverse effects. Underline indicates serious adverse effects.

occurs within days of initiating therapy and maximum benefits may take several weeks.

The ACE inhibitors are well tolerated by most patients with HF. Hypotension is the most common adverse effect, and the risk is increased when the patient is receiving other drugs that lower blood pressure such as diuretics and beta blockers. Hypotension is generally worse at the beginning of therapy or when the dosage is increased. Multidrug therapy is common in these patients, and the nurse serves a key role in teaching patients how to space drug administration times to minimize hypotensive adverse effects.

An additional concern during ACE inhibitor therapy is functional renal insufficiency. Patients with severe HF have high circulating levels of angiotensin II, which helps to maintain renal blood flow by constricting efferent arterioles in the kidney. When ACE inhibitors are administered, the level of angiotensin II declines rapidly, leading to reduced blood flow through the kidneys. During therapy with ACE inhibitors, renal insufficiency may also result from sodium depletion, often secondary to the concurrent use of diuretics. To avoid this potentially serious adverse effect, kidney function should be monitored during therapy. Should an assessment discover signs of renal impairment, the dose should be immediately decreased or the drug discontinued. Other adverse effects of ACE inhibitors are angioedema, cough, and hyperkalemia. The student should refer to Chapter 31 for additional information on the adverse effects of ACE inhibitors and for a drug prototype feature for lisinopril (Prinivil, Zestril).

Another class of medications that blocks the effects of angiotensin II are the angiotensin receptor blockers. Pharmacologically, the effects of the ARBs are very similar to those of the ACE inhibitors, as would be expected, because drugs from both classes inhibit the actions of angiotensin II. In patients with HF, ARBs have equivalent efficacy to the ACE inhibitors and exhibit a much lower incidence of cough and angioedema. Patients with HF who are unable to tolerate side effects of ACE inhibitors or who are at risk for angioedema are candidates for ARB therapy. Clinical studies suggest that combining ARBs with ACE inhibitors does not improve patient survival but does increase the risk of adverse effects. The ARB losartan (Cozaar) is featured as a prototype drug in Chapter 31.

In 2015, Entresto, a combination of sacubitril (a neprilysin inhibitor) and valsartan (an ARB), was approved. This drug represents a new class called angiotensin receptor neprilysin inhibitors (ARNIs). Neprilysin is an enzyme normally present in the body that breaks down natriuretic peptides and other substances that affect fluid balance. By blocking neprilysin, the concentration of natriuretic peptides in the blood increases and cardiac efficiency improves. The most significant finding of this new class of drugs is that they are able to reduce mortality and the number of hospitalizations in patients with HF. Indeed, ARNIs are now recommended for the pharmacotherapy of HF for many patients. Concurrent use of ARNIs with ACE inhibitors is contraindicated due to an increased risk for angioedema. ARNIs are contraindicated in patients with a history of angioedema.

36.6 Beta-adrenergic antagonists can reduce hospitalizations and increase the survival of patients with heart failure.

Unless otherwise contraindicated, beta-blockers are recommended for all patients with HF. These drugs have been shown to slow disease progression, reduce hospitalizations, and lower the incidence of sudden death. They are beneficial even in patients without CAD who have minimal HF symptoms.

In patients with HF, high levels of endogenous norepinephrine and other catecholamines cause excessive activation of the SNS and are associated with cardiac remodeling and progression of the disease. Beta-adrenergic antagonists block the actions of these catecholamines, slowing the heart rate and reducing blood pressure, thus decreasing the cardiac workload. After several months of therapy, heart size, shape, and function return to normal in some patients, in essence producing a **reverse remodeling** of the heart. Doses for selected beta-adrenergic antagonists are listed in Table 36.3.

To benefit patients with HF, beta-adrenergic antagonists are administered in a very specific manner. Initial doses must be 1/10 to 1/20 of the target dose. If tolerated, the doses are doubled every 2 weeks until the target dose is reached. If therapy is begun with a high dose, or if the dose is increased too rapidly, beta blockers can worsen HF. Carvedilol, bisoprolol, and metoprolol succinate are the beta-adrenergic antagonists approved for HF. When treating HF, beta blockers are always combined with other drugs such as ACE inhibitors, ARBs, and diuretics.

Adherence to beta-blocker therapy can be a major clinical challenge for some patients. The patient may not report symptomatic improvement with the drug and, in fact, may feel worse at the initiation of therapy. To achieve maximum patient adherence, the nurse must teach the patient the important long-term benefits of beta blockers.

Four types of adverse effects may require close monitoring: fluid retention, bradycardia or heart block, fatigue, and hypotension. Beta-adrenergic antagonists are contraindicated in patients with chronic obstructive pulmonary disease and should be used with caution in patients with DM, peripheral vascular disease, and hepatic impairment. Hepatic function tests should be performed periodically.

A drug was introduced in 2015 for patients in whom beta blockers are contraindicated or when the maximum dose of the beta blocker fails to achieve therapeutic goals. Ivabradine (Corlanor) acts by a unique mechanism that slows ion (*If*) currents across the sinoatrial (SA) node, which slows the heart rate and reduces myocardial oxygen demand. The subscript *f* stands for "funny," so named because the original research determined this current had unusual properties, distinct from sodium, calcium, or potassium currents. Adverse effects include possible bradycardia, hypotension, and atrial fibrillation.

The basic pharmacology of the beta-adrenergic antagonists is presented in Chapter 16, where metoprolol is featured as a prototype for this class. Other applications of the beta-adrenergic antagonists are discussed elsewhere in this text: HTN is discussed in Chapter 34, angina and MI in Chapter 35, and dysrhythmias in Chapter 37.

36.7 Diuretics relieve symptoms of heart failure by reducing fluid overload and decreasing blood pressure.

Diuretics are commonly prescribed for the treatment of patients with HF because they are effective at reducing peripheral edema and pulmonary congestion and produce few adverse effects. By reducing blood volume and lowering blood pressure, the workload on the heart is reduced and CO increases. Diuretics are rarely used alone for HF but are prescribed in combination with other HF medications. Doses for selected diuretics are listed in Table 36.3. The student should refer to Chapter 32 for more detailed information on diuretics.

Although diuretics are effective at relieving HF symptoms, clinical research has not demonstrated their effectiveness in slowing the progression of HF or in decreasing the mortality rate associated with the disease. Because of this, diuretics are only indicated when there is evidence of fluid retention. In patients presenting with fluid retention, especially with symptoms of severe pulmonary congestion or peripheral edema, diuretics are essential medications.

Of the diuretic classes, the loop diuretics are most commonly prescribed for HF, due to their effectiveness in removing fluid from the body. Loop diuretics are also able to function in patients with chronic kidney disease (CKD), an advantage for many patients with decompensated HF. Another major advantage in treating acute HF is that loop diuretics act quickly, within minutes for intravenous (IV) formulations. For chronic HF, therapy is begun with low doses and gradually increased until the desired volume reduction is obtained.

Thiazide diuretics are also used in the pharmacotherapy of HF, sometimes combined with loop diuretics to achieve a more effective diuresis in patients with acute HF. Because they are less effective than the loop diuretics, thiazides are generally reserved for patients with mild-to-moderate HF.

In addition to being a potassium-sparing diuretic, spironolactone is also classified as an aldosterone antagonist. As a diuretic, spironolactone has a limited role in HF, due to its low efficacy at reducing volume overload. Clinical research, however, has demonstrated that the drug is able to block the deleterious effects of aldosterone on the heart. High levels of aldosterone promote cardiac remodeling and the deposition of fibrotic tissue in the myocardium of patients with HF. By blocking these cardiac effects, spironolactone may decrease mortality due to sudden death as well as progression to advanced HF. The patient must be carefully monitored for hyperkalemia caused by the potassium-sparing action of the drugs.

Diuretic use in HF patients should be routinely monitored to avoid dehydration or electrolyte imbalances. These adverse effects are more likely to occur in HF patients who have CKD. Frequent laboratory tests for blood electrolyte levels are obtained to prevent the development of hypokalemia during loop or thiazide diuretic therapy. This is especially important in patients who are also taking digoxin (Lanoxin) because hypokalemia may induce fatal dysrhythmias. Hydrochlorothiazide, furosemide, and spironolactone are featured as drug prototypes in Chapter 32.

CONNECTION Checkpoint 36.2

Conn's syndrome is characterized by excess secretion of aldosterone. From what you learned in Chapter 31, what effect would you predict this syndrome would have on the heart, and what medication might be a preferred drug?

36.8 Vasodilators reduce symptoms of heart failure by reducing preload or afterload.

Vasodilators relax blood vessels and lower blood pressure, creating less workload on the heart. They serve a limited role in the pharmacotherapy of HF.

Hydralazine combined with isosorbide dinitrate (BiDil) is approved as an adjunct to standard therapy for HF. The combination appears to be particularly effective in treating Black patients, who are sometimes resistant to therapy for HTN and HF.

Hydralazine acts on arterioles to decrease peripheral resistance, reduce afterload, and increase CO. It is an effective antihypertensive drug, although it is not a preferred drug for this indication because hypotension and reflex tachycardia are common and may limit therapy. Hydralazine is presented as a prototype vasodilator for HTN in Chapter 34.

Isosorbide dinitrate (Isordil) is a long-acting organic nitrate that reduces preload by directly dilating veins. The drug is not very effective as monotherapy, and tolerance develops to its actions with continued use. Isosorbide dinitrate is usually combined with hydralazine (BiDil) because the two drugs act synergistically when used in patients with HF. The high incidence of adverse effects, such as reflex tachycardia and orthostatic hypotension, limits their use in some patients. The use of isosorbide dinitrate in the pharmacotherapy of angina pectoris is presented in Chapter 35.

CONNECTION Checkpoint 36.3

Isosorbide dinitrate is also used for angina. From what you learned in Chapter 35, why is nitroglycerin a preferred drug for acute angina, rather than isosorbide dinitrate?

36.9 Cardiac glycosides increase the force of myocardial contraction and were once preferred drugs for heart failure.

Once used as arrow poisons by African tribes and as medicines by the ancient Egyptians and Romans, the value of the cardiac glycosides in treating heart disorders has been known for over 2000 years. Originally extracted from the beautiful flowering plants *Digitalis purpura* (purple foxglove) and *Digitalis lanata* (white foxglove), the cardiac glycosides were the mainstay of HF treatment until the discovery of the ACE inhibitors. During the past 20 years, the role of the cardiac glycosides in the pharmacotherapy of HF has become more limited. The dose for digoxin, the sole available drug in this class, is listed in Table 36.3.

Because of its long historical use, the effectiveness of digoxin in the pharmacotherapy of HF remained unquestioned until the late 1980s. With the development of safer and more effective drug classes, digoxin is now limited to late-stage HF, in combination with other drugs. Digoxin remains an important therapy in HF patients with supraventricular tachyarrhythmias because the drug has antidysrhythmic activity that can stabilize these types of cardiac conduction abnormalities.

The margin of safety between a therapeutic dose and a toxic dose of cardiac glycosides is very narrow, and severe adverse effects may result from poorly managed therapy. **Digitalization** refers to the procedure by which the dose of digoxin is gradually increased until tissues become saturated with the medication and the symptoms of HF diminish. If the patient is critically ill, digitalization can be done rapidly with IV doses in a controlled clinical environment, where adverse effects may be carefully monitored. Using oral (PO) dosing, digitalization may be completed over a period of 7 days. In either case, the goal is to determine the proper dose of medication to be administered, without undue adverse effects.

PROTOTYPE DRUG Digoxin (Lanoxin, Lanoxicaps)

Classification **Therapeutic:** Drug for heart failure
Pharmacologic: Cardiac glycoside, inotropic drug

Therapeutic Effects and Uses: The primary benefit of digoxin is its ability to increase the strength of myocardial contraction, a positive inotropic action. By increasing myocardial contractility, digoxin directly increases CO, which alleviates symptoms of HF and improves exercise tolerance. The higher CO increases urine production and results in a desirable reduction in blood volume, relieving the distressing symptoms of pulmonary congestion and peripheral edema. In current clinical practice, digoxin use is usually limited to patients who are not responding adequately to ACE inhibitor therapy or to HF patients with atrial fibrillation.

In addition to its positive inotropic effect, digoxin also affects the speed of myocardial conduction. Through a mechanism not fully understood, digoxin decreases SNS activity and increases parasympathetic activity. This helps attenuate the excessive sympathetic activation that causes tachycardia and worsens HF (see Section 36.2). Digoxin has the ability to suppress the SA node and slow electrical conduction through the atrioventricular node. The heart rate decreases, allowing greater diastolic filling of the ventricles. Because the heart rate may decline too much, healthcare providers establish parameters for each patient. As a general rule, if the apical pulse falls below 60 beats/min, the medication is withheld and the healthcare provider notified. Digoxin is sometimes used to treat dysrhythmias, as discussed in Chapter 37.

Digoxin is available by the PO or IV route. Because differences in bioavailability of digoxin formulations can potentially affect drug action and the potential for adverse effects, patients are advised to continue with the same trade name, unless otherwise changed by the prescriber.

Mechanism of Action: Digoxin inhibits Na^+–K^+–ATPase, the critical enzyme responsible for pumping sodium ions out of the myocardial cells in exchange for potassium ions. As sodium ions accumulate in myocytes, calcium ions are released from their storage areas in the cell to activate contractile elements. The release of calcium ions produces a more forceful contraction of myocardial fibers.

Pharmacokinetics:

Route(s)	PO, IV
Absorption	70–90% absorbed from the gastrointestinal tract
Distribution	Widely distributed; crosses the placenta; secreted in breast milk; 20–25% bound to protein
Primary metabolism	Hepatic, 14%
Primary excretion	Renal
Onset of action	PO: 30–90 min; IV: 5–30 min
Duration of action	Half-life: 3–4 days

Adverse Effects: Adverse effects of digoxin involve multiple body systems and can be severe. The most dangerous adverse effect is ventricular dysrhythmias, which may result in sudden cardiac death. The most common cause of digoxin-induced dysrhythmias is hypokalemia due to diuretic use. Other factors placing patients at risk for digoxin-induced dysrhythmias include hypomagnesemia, hypercalcemia, and impaired renal function. Additional serious adverse cardiac effects include atrioventricular (AV) block, atrial dysrhythmias, and sinus bradycardia. Frequent electrocardiograms (ECGs) should be obtained to assess for cardiotoxicity.

Noncardiac adverse effects include general malaise, dizziness, headache, anorexia, and nausea and vomiting. The drug may produce unusual visual effects such as halos, changes in color perception, and photophobia.

Frequent serum digoxin levels should be obtained during therapy, and the dosage adjusted based on the laboratory results and the patient's clinical response. Digoxin levels from 0.5 to 2 ng/mL give the most therapeutic benefit, with an acceptable risk of adverse effects for most patients. For each patient, the healthcare provider should establish acceptable parameters for serum digoxin levels, and the drug should be discontinued should the level rise above the maximum. Digoxin levels greater than 2.0 ng/mL are considered toxic. However, the nurse should remember that toxicity should be based on patient symptoms rather than serum level.

Contraindications/Precautions: Patients with AV block or ventricular dysrhythmias unrelated to HF should not receive digoxin because the drug may worsen these conditions. Digoxin should be administered with caution to older adults because these patients experience a higher incidence of adverse effects. Patients with CKD should receive lower doses of digoxin because the drug is excreted by this route. The drug should be used with caution in patients with MI, cor pulmonale, or hypothyroidism.

Drug Interactions: Digoxin interacts with many drugs. Concurrent use of digoxin with diuretics must be carefully monitored, since diuretics can cause hypokalemia and increase the risk of dysrhythmias. Use with ACE inhibitors, spironolactone, or potassium supplements can lead to hyperkalemia and reduce the therapeutic action of digoxin. Administration of digoxin with other positive inotropic drugs can cause additive effects on myocardial contractility. Concurrent use with beta blockers may result in additive bradycardia. Antacids and cholesterol-lowering drugs can decrease the absorption of digoxin. If calcium is administered intravenously together with digoxin, it can increase the risk of dysrhythmias. Quinidine, verapamil, amiodarone, and alprazolam will decrease the distribution and excretion of digoxin, thus increasing the risk of digoxin toxicity. **Herbal/Food:** The drug should be used with caution with ginseng, which may increase the risk of digoxin toxicity.

Pregnancy: Digoxin crosses the placenta and neonates of mothers taking the drug should be observed for vomiting and dysrhythmias. Small amounts enter milk, although data are not available regarding adverse effects on the breastfed neonate.

Treatment of Overdose: Digoxin overdose can be fatal, and the nurse should be prepared to administer digoxin immune Fab (Digibind). Digoxin immune Fab consists of digoxin-specific antibodies, which form a complex with digoxin that prevents the drug from reaching the tissues, and is removed through renal excretion. Reversal of adverse effects occurs quickly: 90% of patients respond within an hour after IV administration. As digoxin is removed from the body, the inotropic effects of the drug will diminish, and the patient may be at risk of HF. The patient must be monitored continuously during the infusion.

Clinician Responsibilities: Key clinical implications for patients receiving digoxin are included in Applied Clinical Judgment: Patients Receiving Pharmacotherapy for Heart Failure.

Drugs Similar to Digoxin (Lanoxin, Lanoxicaps)

Digoxin is the only cardiac glycoside available in the United States.

CONNECTION Checkpoint 36.4

Cholestyramine reduces the bioavailability of digoxin, thus potentially decreasing the actions of the cardiac glycoside. From what you learned in Chapter 29, what is the primary indication for cholestyramine and what is the likely reason this drug causes a decrease in digoxin bioavailability?

36.10 Beta-adrenergic antagonists, phosphodiesterase III inhibitors, and other positive inotropic drugs may be used for advanced heart failure.

Advanced or decompensated HF can be a medical emergency, and prompt, effective treatment is necessary to avoid organ failure or death. In addition to high doses of loop diuretics, positive inotropic drugs may be necessary. The two primary classes of inotropic drugs used for acute advanced HF are beta-adrenergic agonists and phosphodiesterase inhibitors. Doses for these drugs are listed in Table 36.4.

Beta-adrenergic agonists (sympathomimetics): Beta-adrenergic agonists used for HF include isoproterenol (Isuprel), epinephrine, norepinephrine, dopamine, and dobutamine. Dobutamine has been a traditional preferred drug in this class because it has the ability to rapidly increase myocardial contractility, with minimal changes to heart rate or blood pressure. This is important because increases in heart rate or blood pressure will create greater oxygen demands on the heart and possibly worsen HF. Therapy with dobutamine is usually limited to 72 hours, as continuous infusion of the drug causes the heart to become tolerant to beta-adrenergic activation, making the drug less effective. Long-term, continuous sympathomimetic therapy is usually recommended only for palliative purposes or for patients awaiting cardiac transplantation. The two most

Table 36.4 Drugs for Advanced Heart Failure

Drug	Route and Adult Dose (Maximum Dose Where Indicated)	Adverse Effects
Beta-Adrenergic Agonists		
dobutamine (Dobutrex)	IV: Infused at a rate of 2.5–40 mcg/kg/min for a max of 72 h	*Headache, palpitations, nausea and vomiting, changes in blood pressure (hypo- or hypertension)* Dysrhythmias, gangrene, severe HTN
dopamine (Dopastat, Intropin)	IV: 2–5 mcg/kg/min initial dose; may be increased to 20–50 mcg/kg/min (max: 50 mcg/kg/min)	
epinephrine (Adrenalin)	Subcutaneous: 0.1–0.5 mL of 1:1000 every 10–15 min prn IV: 0.1–0.25 mL of 1:1000 every 10–15 min	
isoproterenol (Isuprel)	IV infusion: 0.5–5 mcg/min	
norepinephrine (Levophed)	IV: Initially, 0.5–1 mcg/min until pressure stabilizes, then 2–4 mcg/min for maintenance (max: 30 mcg/min)	
Phosphodiesterase Inhibitor		
milrinone	IV: 50 mcg/kg over 10 min; then 0.375–0.75 mcg/kg/min	*Headache, hypotension* Dysrhythmias

Note: *Italics* indicate common adverse effects. Underline indicates serious adverse effects.

common adverse effects with beta agonists are tachycardia and dysrhythmias.

Patients who have both HF and hypotension benefit from dopamine, which not only increases myocardial contractility but also activates alpha-adrenergic receptors to increase blood pressure. However, tachycardia is more prominent with dopamine than with dobutamine. Patients who have been receiving a beta-adrenergic antagonist for their HF may require a higher initial dose of beta agonist. The basic pharmacology of the beta-adrenergic agonists was presented in Chapter 15, where epinephrine and isoproterenol were featured as prototypes for this drug class.

Phosphodiesterase III inhibitors: In the 1980s, two medications became available that block the enzyme **phosphodiesterase III** in cardiac and smooth muscle, which leads to increases in the amount of calcium available for myocardial contraction. The enzyme inhibition results in two main actions that benefit patients with HF: a positive inotropic action and vasodilation. Cardiac output is increased due to the increase in contractility and the decrease in left-ventricular afterload. There is little effect on heart rate. Arterial pressure is either decreased or, in some patients, it remains unchanged. Inamrinone was discontinued in 2011, leaving milrinone the only drug in this class.

Although the actions of milrinone are very similar to those of dobutamine, it has a much longer half-life. This makes it more difficult to make rapid changes in dose when controlling acute HF. In addition, if adverse effects do occur, they are more prolonged than with dobutamine.

PROTOTYPE DRUG Milrinone

Classification **Therapeutic:** Drug for heart failure
Pharmacologic: Phosphodiesterase III inhibitor; inotropic drug

Therapeutic Effects and Uses: Approved in 1987, milrinone is indicated for the short-term treatment of patients with acute advanced heart failure. It is only given intravenously, and peak effects occur in 2 minutes. Immediate effects of milrinone include an increased force of contraction (positive inotropic effect) and a resulting increase in CO. Research has not demonstrated any decrease in mortality or morbidity with the use of milrinone infusions. Drug therapy with milrinone is generally limited to 48 hours.

Mechanism of Action: Milrinone inhibits phosphodiesterase III, the enzyme responsible for the breakdown of cAMP to AMP, in cardiac and vascular smooth muscle. The rise in cAMP levels increases intracellular calcium, resulting in greater contractility. Cardiac output is increased and pulmonary capillary wedge pressure is decreased.

Pharmacokinetics:

Route(s)	IV
Absorption	N/A
Distribution	Unknown; 70% bound to plasma protein
Primary metabolism	83% is excreted unchanged; small amounts metabolized by liver
Primary excretion	Renal
Onset of action	2–10 min
Duration of action	Half-life: 3–6 h

Adverse Effects: Milrinone has serious toxicity that limits its use in patients with resistant HF. The most serious adverse effect of milrinone is ventricular dysrhythmia, which can occur in more than 10% of patients taking the drug. The ECG is monitored continuously during infusion of the drug to prevent serious dysrhythmias. Blood pressure is also continuously monitored during the infusion to prevent hypotension. Patients with NYHA Class IV HF are at high risk for life-threatening cardiovascular reactions. Less serious adverse effects include headache and nausea and vomiting.

Contraindications/Precautions: Milrinone is contraindicated in patients with severe obstructive valvular heart disease. The drug should be used with caution in patients with preexisting dysrhythmias. Hypovolemia, hypokalemia, and other electrolyte imbalances should be corrected before starting the infusion, and the dose should be reduced in patients with CKD.

Drug Interactions: Caution should be used when administering milrinone with digoxin, dobutamine, or other inotropic drugs, since their cardiac effects may be additive. Use with antihypertensive drugs may cause additive hypotension. **Herbal/Food:** Ginger may contribute to the cardiac actions of milrinone.

Pregnancy: Milrinone is not teratogenic in laboratory animals. It is unknown whether the drug enters milk.

Treatment of Overdose: Overdose of milrinone causes hypotension, which may be treated with the administration of normal saline or a vasopressor.

Clinician Responsibilities: Key clinical implications for patients receiving milrinone are included in Applied Clinical Judgment: Patients Receiving Pharmacotherapy for Heart Failure.

Drugs Similar to Milrinone

Milrinone is the only drug in the phosphodiesterase inhibitor class.

CONNECTIONS: APPLIED CLINICAL JUDGMENT

Patients Receiving Pharmacotherapy for Heart Failure

Assessment

Key Assessment Data

- History of current condition, baseline vital signs, physical exam findings; history including previous MI, HF, valvular disease, dysrhythmias (especially heart block), renal dysfunction; medication history; pregnancy status. Obtain baseline ECG, electrolytes, and renal function studies.
- Ongoing assessment during drug therapy should include ECG monitoring for dysrhythmias, electrolytes, especially potassium, BP, and assessment of lung sounds and for presence of edema.

Desired Therapeutic Outcomes

Improvement is observed and measurable when heart rate and blood pressure return to within normal limits; urine output returns to within normal limits; respiratory congestion is improved; peripheral edema is improved; level of consciousness (LOC), skin color, capillary refill, and other signs of adequate perfusion are within normal limits; fatigue lessens.

Minimizing Adverse Effects

- Monitor for orthostatic hypotension with ACE inhibitors and ARBs. A first-dose effect may occur with a significant drop in blood pressure with the first few doses.
- Weigh daily and report weight gain over 1 kg (2 lb) in a 24-hour period or increasing edema.
- Reduced aldosterone levels from ACE inhibitors or ARBs may cause hyperkalemia, especially in patients with DM or impaired kidney function. Continue to monitor periodic electrolyte levels, especially potassium, and hepatic and renal function laboratory values.
- ACE inhibitors increase bradykinin levels, which results in a dry cough. A change in the severity of the cough may indicate another disease process or may result in the need to consider other medications.
- If ACE inhibitors are used, observe for angioedema.
- Drugs that are positive inotropes increase myocardial contractility but may affect cardiac conduction. Milrinone is associated with serious and potentially life-threatening dysrhythmias. Digoxin slows the heart rate and may cause bradycardia. Monitor apical pulse and continue cardiac monitoring (e.g., ECG) as ordered for dysrhythmias in the hospitalized patient, promptly reporting dysrhythmias or angina.
- Hypokalemia increases the risk of dysrhythmias from drugs used to treat HF. Continue to monitor electrolyte levels periodically, especially potassium, renal function laboratory values, drug levels, and ECG.
- Lung congestion may signal impending HF. Monitor for signs of worsening HF (e.g., increasing dyspnea or postural nocturnal dyspnea; rales or crackles in lungs; frothy, pink-tinged sputum) and report immediately. Weigh daily, reporting weight gain over 1 kg in a 24-hour period, or edema.
- Decreased excretion of digoxin and phosphodiesterase inhibitors due to age-related changes may increase the risk of adverse effects. Digoxin levels should remain less than 1.8 mg/mL. Signs and symptoms such as bradycardia, nausea and vomiting, anorexia, visual changes, depression, changes in LOC, fatigue, dizziness, or syncope should be reported.

Lifespan Considerations

- Orthostatic hypotension may increase the risk of falls and injury. Be cautious with older adults who are at increased risk for hypotension. Ensure patient safety.
- The older adult taking ACE inhibitors or ARBs may be at greater risk for hyperkalemia related to renal effects of aging.
- Use extra caution when giving digoxin to older adults, pediatric patients, or patients with CKD. Immature renal function or declines in renal function make these populations more susceptible to adverse effects. Digoxin is on the Beers list of potentially inappropriate drugs for the older adult and warrants careful monitoring.
- For drugs such as digoxin with a long half-life and duration, toxic levels may result with only small amounts of additional drug. Use extra caution when measuring the precise dose of medication ordered, and use extreme caution when measuring liquid doses, especially for pediatric patients.
- Some drugs for HF may cause fetal harm and should be used with caution during pregnancy or breastfeeding. Assess for the possibility of pregnancy before beginning the drug.

Diversity Considerations

- Older adult and Black patients are at higher risk for the development of angioedema with ACE inhibitors or ARBs.

(continued)

CONNECTIONS: APPLIED CLINICAL JUDGMENT *(continued)*

Patients Receiving Pharmacotherapy for Heart Failure

Assessment

Patient Education

- Monitor pulse, BP, and daily weight, using a diary or log, and bring these to each provider visit. Promptly report any weight gain over 1 kg in a 24-hour period or increasing edema to the provider.
- Rise slowly from lying or sitting to standing, pausing between changes if dizziness occurs. Don't take the medication if dizziness continues, or the BP is below 90/60 or per parameters set by the provider, and contact the provider for further instruction. Taking the first dose at night may help alleviate the first-dose effect.
- If ACE inhibitors or ARBs are used, immediately seek medical attention for difficulty breathing, throat tightness, hives or rash, muscle cramps, or tremors. Promptly report any angioedema around the facial area.
- A dry cough may occur and may persist if ACE inhibitors are taken. Use nonmedicinal measures to treat (e.g., OTC cough lozenges, hard candy, or increased fluid intake). If the cough persists, consult with the healthcare provider about the use of antihistamines. Promptly report any change in the severity or frequency of a cough. Any cough accompanied by shortness of breath, fever, or chest pain should be reported immediately because it may indicate more severe conditions.
- Be aware of the signs of hyperkalemia (nausea, irregular heartbeat, profound fatigue or muscle weakness, and slow or faint pulse) and immediately report them to the healthcare provider.
- Avoid salt substitutes containing potassium chloride, consuming snacks advertised as "electrolyte-fortified," specialized sports drinks that contain high levels of potassium, or excessive intake of foods high in potassium different from the normal diet.
- Take a peripheral pulse for 1 full minute before taking the drug. Record daily pulse rates and bring the record to each healthcare visit. Do not take the drug if pulse is below 60 or above 100 beats/min and contact the provider for further direction. If the patient or caregiver choose to buy a stethoscope to take the pulse, ensure proper understanding of heart sounds (i.e., the "lub-dub" sound of a heartbeat is one heartbeat) and appropriate stethoscope placement.
- Weigh self daily, ideally at the same time of day, and record weight along with pulse measurements. Instruct the patient to report a weight loss or gain of more than 1 kg in a 24-hour period.
- Immediately report any severe shortness of breath, frothy sputum, profound fatigue, or swelling of extremities as possible signs of HF.
- Take the precise dose of medication ordered, not doubling the dose if a dose is missed, and use extreme caution when measuring liquid doses, especially for pediatric patients.
- Take the drug at the same time each day, and doses should not be skipped or doubled. The brand of the drug prescribed should not be switched without consultation with the provider to ensure consistent effects. Unless extended-release formulations are used, the drug should not be stopped abruptly. Consult with the provider if unable to take the drug.
- Carry a wallet identification card or wear medical identification jewelry indicating drug therapy for HF.

Prescribing Considerations

- ACE inhibitors should be initiated at a low dose; double the dose every 1 to 2 weeks as tolerated up to the target dose. Monitor patients for hypotension, potassium levels, and decreased renal function during the titration period to assess tolerability.
- Baseline renal function and serum potassium should be established prior to initiating ARB therapy.
- Beta blockers should be initiated at low doses and titrated slowly to target doses as tolerated. Patients should be monitored closely for changes in vital signs and symptoms during this titration period. If the target doses are not tolerated, the highest tolerated dose should be continued.
- Diuretic therapy is initiated at low doses and titrated up as needed and as tolerated.
- The initial dose of digoxin is typically 0.125 mg to 0.250 mg daily with no need for a loading dose. Patients who are elderly, have poor renal function, or who have a low lean body mass should start with 0.125 mg daily or every other day. Serum trough levels may be monitored to minimize adverse effects.

Understanding Chapter 36

Key Concepts Summary

36.1 Heart failure is closely associated with disorders such as chronic hypertension, coronary artery disease, and diabetes.

36.2 The body attempts to compensate for heart failure by increasing cardiac output.

36.3 Symptoms of heart failure occur when compensatory mechanisms fail to maintain adequate cardiac output.

36.4 The specific therapy for heart failure depends on the clinical stage of the disease.

36.5 Angiotensin-converting enzyme inhibitors are first-line drugs for heart failure.

36.6 Beta-adrenergic antagonists can reduce hospitalizations and increase the survival of patients with heart failure.

36.7 Diuretics relieve symptoms of heart failure by reducing fluid overload and decreasing blood pressure.

36.8 Vasodilators reduce symptoms of heart failure by reducing preload or afterload.

36.9 Cardiac glycosides increase the force of myocardial contraction and were once preferred drugs for heart failure.

36.10 Beta-adrenergic antagonists, phosphodiesterase III inhibitors, and other positive inotropic drugs may be used for advanced heart failure.

CASE STUDY: Making the Patient Connection

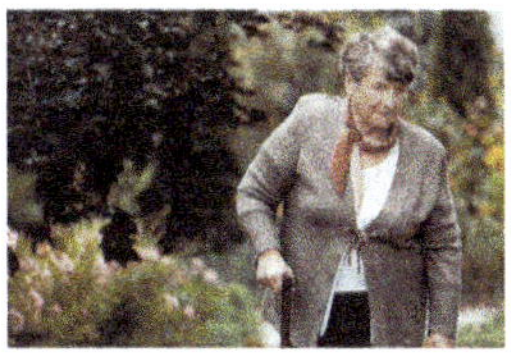

Remember the patient "Thelma Walters" at the beginning of the chapter? Now read the remainder of the case study. Based on the information presented within this chapter, respond to the critical thinking questions that follow.

Thelma Walters is a 72-year-old woman who arrives via EMS at the emergency department (ED) after experiencing increasing dyspnea for the past 2 days. She has also noticed swelling in her feet and ankles. Due to her onset of shortness of breath, she has had to sleep in a recliner and is unable to lie flat in bed at night. Thelma's past medical history includes a mild stroke occurring 8 years ago with mild residual weakness on her right side, MI 3 years ago, and an episode of HF 1 year ago. The HF was treated with captopril (Capoten) and furosemide (Lasix), which she has been taking since that time. Her surgical history includes a hysterectomy 20 years ago. She has never used tobacco or alcohol.

As the nurse performs the initial physical assessment, the following relevant findings are discovered. The patient is 1.7 m (5′6″) tall and weighs 82 kg (180 lb). She uses a walker or a cane to feel more secure and avoid falls, due to the mild residual weakness on her right side. The patient's blood pressure is 162/92 mmHg, her heart rate is 148 beats/min and irregular, and her respiratory rate is 38 breaths/min and labored. The neck veins of the patient are distended when she is placed at a 45-degree incline. She is orthopneic and cannot tolerate the head of the bed being lowered below 45 degrees. The nurse notes scattered crackles bilaterally throughout the lung fields. The patient has a productive cough with frothy, pink-tinged sputum; 4+ pitting edema of both hands and legs is noted with the nail beds moderately cyanotic. Circumoral cyanosis is also noted.

Immediately upon arrival at the ED, Thelma received oxygen therapy and an IV line was started. Blood was collected for initial laboratory data with the following results: serum sodium 136 mEq/L (normal: 135 to 147 mEq/L), serum potassium 3.1 mEq/L (normal 3.5 to 5.2 mEq/L), and arterial blood gases on room air: pH 7.32, PaO_2 54, $PaCO_2$ 48, SpO_2 68%, indicating overall hypoxemia. Thelma is in acute distress and admitted to the intensive care unit (ICU) with a diagnosis of HF. She is given a dose of furosemide (Lasix) 20 mg IV and she will receive dobutamine (Dobutrex) by IV infusion after admission to the ICU.

Critical Thinking Questions

1. Describe how dobutamine (Dobutrex) aids in treating HF.
2. Thelma's pulse and blood pressure will be monitored closely and the dobutamine stopped once her vital signs stabilize and CO improves. She will be started on sacubitril with valsartan (Entresto) in preparation for discharge. How does this drug improve heart failure?
3. Because Thelma has been taking furosemide (Lasix) at home and has received an additional dose, what additional monitoring is required? Once she is taking the sacubitril/valsartan, what ongoing monitoring is needed?

Additional Case Study

Jim Mabry, a 77-year-old man, currently takes the following medications daily: carvedilol (Coreg CR) 10 mg; furosemide (Lasix) 20 mg daily; and potassium supplementation (K-Dur) 20 mEq. As his nurse, you will be discussing Jim's medication regimen at his next healthcare provider office visit after discharge from the hospital.

1. Discuss the relationship among the three medications.
2. Considering this drug combination, what are the most common adverse effects that might be anticipated?
3. Prepare a list of foods that are rich in potassium as requested by Jim.

Chapter Review

1. A patient newly diagnosed with heart failure following an acute myocardial infarction has a prescription for enalapril (Vasotec). This drug class is frequently used in early heart failure because of what clinical improvement?
    1. It strengthens the force of myocardial contraction to improve CO.
    2. It decreases peripheral resistance, increasing CO.
    3. It slows the heart rate, improving filling time and increasing CO.
    4. It has diuretic effects, decreasing peripheral edema and pulmonary congestion.

2. In providing the patient with heart failure information prior to discharge, the nurse will discuss digoxin (Lanoxin) therapy. Which point would the nurse include in the patient's teaching?
    1. Take the drug in the morning before rising.
    2. Monitor the pulse daily prior to taking the drug.
    3. Discontinue the drug if the pulse rate is 70 beats per minute.
    4. Eat a diet high in bran fiber and calcium.

3. The nurse is performing a medication reconciliation on a new patient who has just moved to the area. Previously, the patient had an order for lisinopril (Zestril) from her general practitioner and received an order for sacubitril with valsartan (Entresto) from her previous cardiologist. The patient has been taking both medications. The nurse flags this for discussion with the cardiologist. What potential adverse effect may occur from taking both drugs together?
    1. There is an antagonist effect between the two drugs and they will be ineffective.
    2. The combination significantly increases the chance for hypokalemia.
    3. Rebound hypertension is more likely to occur.
    4. The combination increases the risk for angioedema.

4. The patient is receiving hydralazine with isosorbide (BiDil) for heart failure. The nurse should monitor this patient for:
    1. Confusion and agitation.
    2. Bleeding.
    3. Tingling or cramping in the legs.
    4. Dizziness and rapid heart rate.

5. A patient will begin taking carvedilol (Coreg) for heart failure. Before teaching the patient about this drug, the nurse will discuss the strategy for drug dosage with the healthcare provider because of which recommended routine for beta-adrenergic antagonists in heart failure?
    1. Significantly lower dosages are used first and gradually increased to a target dose.
    2. A loading dose that is higher than the subsequent daily dose must be given.
    3. The beta-adrenergic antagonist dosage must be lowered if the patient is also on ACE inhibitors.
    4. Beta-adrenergic antagonists are almost never used in HF and the order must be confirmed.

6. When planning patient education, the nurse knows that patient adherence to beta-adrenergic antagonist therapy in heart failure may be difficult to achieve despite the usefulness of these drugs. What will the nurse need to address in the teaching plan? (Select all that apply.)
    1. The dosage must be gradually adjusted over time to a beneficial dose.
    2. The patient may not notice significant improvement during early therapy.
    3. The drug may require changes to many other medications the patient is taking.
    4. The drug has significant benefit in reducing mortality from heart failure.
    5. The drug will require extensive lifestyle changes.

See Appendix A for answers to critical thinking questions, case study questions, and review questions.

References

Dumitru, I. (2018). *Heart failure*. Medscape. http://emedicine.medscape.com/article/163062-overview

Yancy, C. W., Jessup, M., Bozkurt, B., Butler, J., Casey, D. E., Colvin, M. M., et al. (2016). 2016 ACC/AHA/HFSA focused update on new pharmacological therapy for heart failure: An update of the 2013 ACCF/AHA guideline for the management of heart failure: A report of the American College of Cardiology/American Heart Association Task Force on Clinical Practice Guidelines and the Heart Failure Society of America. *Journal of the American College of Cardiology, 68*, 1476–1488. https://doi.org/10.1016/j.jacc.2016.05.011

Yancy, C. W., Jessup, M., Bozkurt, B., Butler, J., Casey, D. E. Jr., Drazner, M. H., et al. (2013). 2013 ACCF/AHA guideline for the management of heart failure: A report of the American College of Cardiology Foundation/American Heart Association Task Force on Practice Guidelines. *Circulation*, *128*, e240–e327. https://doi.org/10.1161/CIR.0b013e31829e8776

Selected Bibliography

Aggarwal, M., Bozkurt, B., Panjrath, G., Aggarwal, B., Ostfeld, R. J., Barnard, N. D., et al. (2018). Lifestyle modifications for preventing and treating heart failure. *Journal of the American College of Cardiology*, *72*(19), 2391–2405. https://doi.org/10.1016/j.jacc.2018.08.2160

Bots, S. H., Groepenhoff, F., Eikendal, A. L., Tannenbaum, C., Rochon, P. A., Regitz-Zagrosek, V., et al. (2019). Adverse drug reactions to guideline-recommended heart failure drugs in women: a systematic review of the literature. *Journal of the American College of Cardiology: Heart Failure*, *7*(3), 258–266. https://doi.org/10.1016/j.jchf.2019.01.009

Chalikias, G., & Tziakas, D. (2020). Angiotensin receptor neprilysin inhibitors—2019 update. *Cardiovascular Drugs and Therapy*, *34*, 707–722. https://doi.org/10.1007/s10557-020-07015-8

Grassi, G., Quarti-Trevano, F., & Esler, M. D. (2019). Sympathetic activation in congestive heart failure: An updated overview. *Heart Failure Reviews*. https://doi.org/10.1007/s10741-019-09901-2

Messerli, F. H., Bangalore, S., Bavishi, C., & Rimoldi, S. F. (2018). Angiotensin-converting enzyme inhibitors in hypertension: To use or not to use? *Journal of the American College of Cardiology*, *71*(13), 1474–1482. https://doi.org/10.1016/j.jacc.2018.01.058

Omar, W., Pandey, A., Haykowsky, M. J., Berry, J. D., & Lavie, C. J. (2018). The evolving role of cardiorespiratory fitness and exercise in prevention and management of heart failure. *Current Heart Failure Reports*, *15*(2), 75–80. https://doi.org/10.1007/s11897-018-0382-z

Rossignol, P., Hernandez, A. F., Solomon, S. D., & Zannad, F. (2019). Heart failure drug treatment. *The Lancet*, *393*(10175), 1034–1044. https://doi.org/10.1016/S0140-6736(18)31808-7

Sarhene, M., Wang, Y., Wei, J., Huang, Y., Li, M., Li, L., et al. (2019). Biomarkers in heart failure: the past, current and future. *Heart Failure Reviews*, *24*(6), 867–903. https://doi.org/10.1007/s10741-019-09807-z

Thygesen, K., Mair, J., Mueller, C., Huber, K., Weber, M., Plebani, M., et al. (2012). Recommendations for the use of natriuretic peptides in acute cardiac care: A position statement from the Study Group on Biomarkers in Cardiology of the ESC Working Group on Acute Cardiac Care. *European Heart Journal*, *33*(16), 2001–2006. https://doi.org/10.1093/eurheartj/ehq509

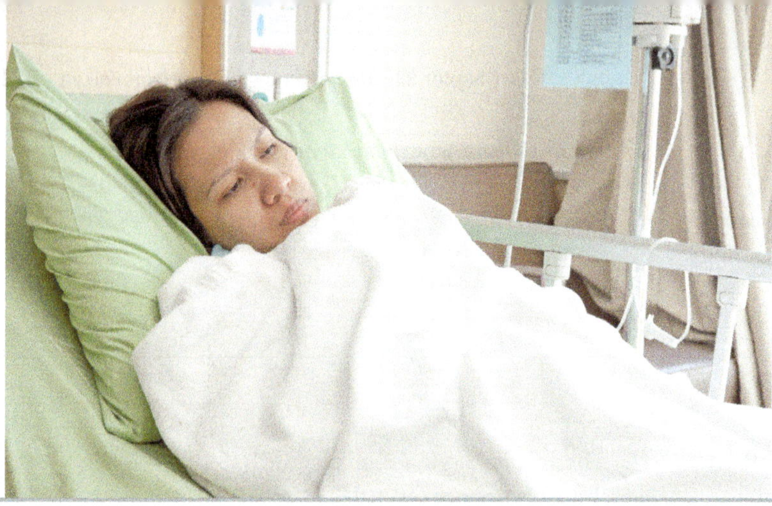

"I will never forget the fear that overwhelmed me as I woke up in the emergency department. I had no idea what had happened. I only remember a strange sensation in my chest. It was like my heart was fluttering. Then I must have passed out."
—*Patient "Jada Chinn Nguyen"*

Chapter 37
Pharmacotherapy of Dysrhythmias

Chapter Outline

Learning Outcomes

After reading this chapter, the student should be able to:

1. Identify disorders associated with an increased risk of dysrhythmias.
2. Explain how rhythm abnormalities can affect cardiac function.
3. Sketch a typical cardiac action potential and label the flow of potassium, sodium, and calcium ions during each phase.
4. Design a table that indicates the classification of dysrhythmias and the types of drugs used to treat them.
5. Describe general principles guiding the management of dysrhythmias.
6. Identify the primary mechanisms of action of antidysrhythmic drugs.
7. For each of the classes shown in the chapter outline, identify the prototype and representative drugs and explain the mechanism(s) of drug action, primary indications, contraindications, significant drug interactions, pregnancy data, and important adverse effects.
8. Apply clinical judgment to care for patients receiving pharmacotherapy for dysrhythmias.

Key Terms

Definitions of the terms in bold may be found in the Glossary.

Dysrhythmias are disorders of cardiac rhythm characterized by abnormal heart rate or irregular contractions. Also called *arrhythmias*, they encompass a number of different disorders that range from harmless to life-threatening. Dysrhythmias are diagnosed based on medical and family histories, a physical exam, and the results from tests and procedures. To diagnose the exact type of rhythm disorder, patients must be connected to an electrocardiogram (ECG) when they are experiencing symptoms. Proper diagnosis and optimal pharmacotherapy can significantly affect the frequency of dysrhythmias and their consequences.

Etiology of Dysrhythmias

37.1 Some dysrhythmias produce no patient symptoms, whereas others may be life-threatening.

Some dysrhythmias are asymptomatic and have no effect on cardiac function, whereas others require immediate treatment. Typical symptoms of dysrhythmias include dizziness, weakness, fatigue, decreased exercise tolerance, palpitations, dyspnea, and syncope. It is difficult to estimate the frequency of the disease, although it is likely that dysrhythmias are quite common in the population. Patients often wait until these symptoms occur more frequently or become acute before seeking medical intervention.

Dysrhythmias occur in all age groups and in both healthy and diseased hearts. While the actual cause of most dysrhythmias is elusive, the majority are closely associated with certain conditions, primarily heart disease and myocardial infarction: 90% of patients experiencing an MI will develop a dysrhythmia. Persistent dysrhythmias are associated with increased risk of stroke and heart failure, and severe dysrhythmias may result in sudden death. Conditions that promote the formation of cardiac rhythm abnormalities are called **prodysrhythmics**. Some of the diseases and conditions associated with dysrhythmias are as follows:

- Hypertension (HTN)
- Cardiac valve disease such as mitral stenosis
- Coronary artery disease (CAD)
- Low or high potassium levels in the blood
- Myocardial infarction (MI)
- Stroke
- Diabetes mellitus
- Heart failure (HF).

In addition to the preceding list, a number of medications have been found to *cause* new dysrhythmias or *worsen* existing ones. Caution must be used when administering prodysrhythmic drugs to patients with preexisting cardiac impairment or who may have any of the above conditions. Table 37.1 lists selected drugs known to have prodysrhythmic properties.

Table 37.1 Selected Prodysrhythmic Drugs

Class of Medication	Example Drugs
Antidysrhythmic drugs	amiodarone, disopyramide, dofetilide, flecainide, ibutilide, procainamide, propafenone, quinidine, sotalol
Autonomic drugs	atenolol, clonidine, methyldopa, nadolol, propranolol
Calcium channel blockers	diltiazem, nifedipine, verapamil
Cardiac glycosides	digoxin
Miscellaneous drugs	amitriptyline, chloroquine, cimetidine, haloperidol, lithium carbonate, phenothiazines

Phases and Measurement of the Cardiac Action Potential

37.2 The phases of cardiac action potential include rapid depolarization, a long plateau, and repolarization.

Dysrhythmias alter the normal generation or conduction of electrical impulses, or action potentials, across the myocardium. Because antidysrhythmic drugs act by correcting or modifying impulse conduction, a firm grasp of cardiac electrical properties is essential to understanding drug mechanisms. Before proceeding, the student should review the normal pathway of impulse conduction in the heart presented in Chapter 28.

Action potentials occur in neurons and cardiac muscle cells (myocytes) due to the changes in the concentration of specific ions found inside and outside the cell. Under resting conditions, sodium ions (Na^+) and calcium ions (Ca^{2+}) are in higher concentrations *outside* of myocytes, whereas potassium ions (K^+) are found in higher concentration *inside* these cells. These imbalances are, in part, responsible for the inside of a myocyte plasma membrane having a slightly negative charge (80–90 mV), relative to the outside of the membrane. A cell having this negative membrane potential is **polarized**.

An action potential illustrating the steps in electrical conduction is shown in Figure 37.1. The changes in ions, or fluxes, occurring during an action potential may be grouped into five phases.

Phase 4: It is easiest to begin with phase 4 because this is the period during which the myocyte is "resting" and the action potential has not yet started. Note in Figure 37.1, however, that during phase 4 the membrane potential is slowly increasing toward a potential that will trigger an action potential: the **threshold potential**. Sodium is slowly leaking into the cell during this period, causing the change in potential, which gives certain regions such as the sinoatrial (SA) node the property of automaticity, the ability to depolarize spontaneously, without input from the nervous system.

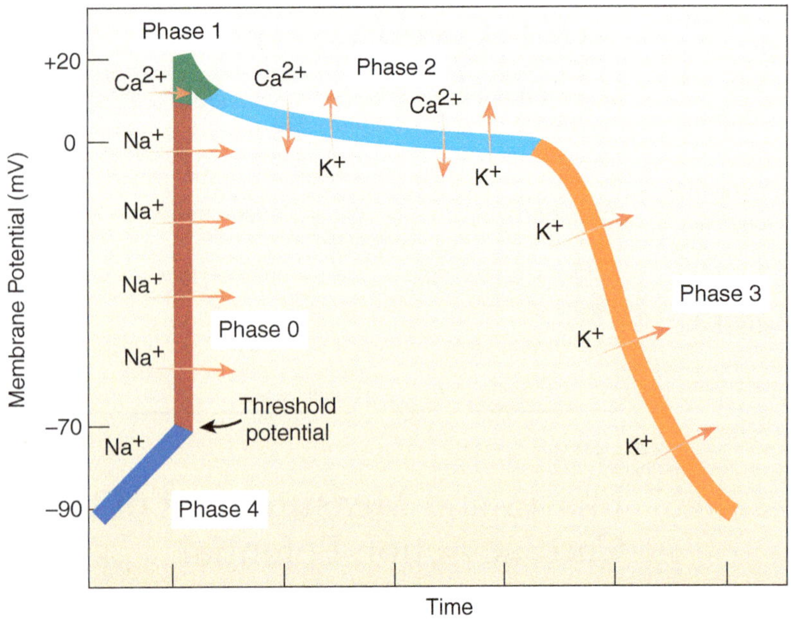

Figure 37.1 Phases of the myocardial action potential. Ion movements during each phase are shown.

Phase 0: An action potential begins when the threshold potential is reached and gated sodium ion channels in the plasma membrane become activated and open. Sodium ions rush into the cell, producing a rapid **depolarization**, or loss of membrane potential. Because they open and close rapidly, these sodium channels are sometimes referred to as fast channels. During this period, Ca^{2+} also enters the cell through calcium ion channels, although the influx is slower than that of sodium. *In myocytes located in the SA and atrioventricular (AV) nodes, it is the influx of Ca^{2+}, rather than Na^+, that generates the rapid depolarization of the membrane.*

Phase 1: During depolarization, the inside of the plasma membrane temporarily reverses its charge, becoming positive. This is a brief, transient phase.

Phase 2: During this phase, a plateau is reached in which depolarization is maintained. The entry of $Ca2^+$ into the cells in this phase is due to the release of additional calcium ions that had been held in storage inside the sarcoplasmic reticula. *This large and sudden increase in intracellular Ca^{2+} is responsible for the contraction of cardiac muscle.* Gated potassium ion channels open, causing an efflux of K^+ from the cells. The plateau is maintained as long as the positive Ca^{2+} entering the myocytes are balanced by the positive K^+ leaving the cell. Action potentials in skeletal muscle lack this plateau phase.

Phase 3: During phase 3, the calcium channels close and additional potassium channels open, thus causing a net loss of positive ions from the cell. This **repolarization** restores the negative resting membrane potential to the cell.

The synchronized pumping action of the heart requires alternating periods of contraction and relaxation. There is a brief period of time following depolarization and most of repolarization during which the cell cannot initiate a subsequent action potential. This **refractory period** ensures that the myocardial cell finishes contracting before a second action potential begins.

Although learning the different ion movements in an action potential may seem complicated, they are very important to cardiac pharmacology. Blocking potassium, sodium, or calcium ion channels are primary pharmacologic strategies used to terminate or prevent dysrhythmias. In addition, the therapeutic effect of some antidysrhythmic drugs is due to their prolongation of the refractory period. It is not possible to understand drug mechanisms without knowledge of the normal electrical conduction properties of the heart. In general, most cardiac drugs:

- Increase impulse formation (or automaticity).
- Increase conduction velocity.
- Increase both impulse formation and conduction velocity.

OR

- Decrease impulse formation or automaticity.
- Decrease conduction velocity.
- Decrease both impulse formation or automaticity and conduction.

CONNECTION Checkpoint 37.1

From what you learned in Chapter 30, what are the three types of calcium channels? Which type is blocked by calcium channel blocker medications?

37.3 The electrocardiogram is used to measure electrical conduction across the myocardium.

The **electrocardiogram (ECG)** is a graphic recording of the wave of electrical conduction across the myocardium. The ECG is a primary tool in the diagnosis of dysrhythmias, MI, and other heart diseases. A normal ECG and its relationship to impulse conduction in the heart are shown in Figure 37.2.

Three distinct waves are produced during a normal ECG: the P wave, the QRS complex, and the T wave. Changes to the wave patterns or in their timing are associated with certain pathologies. The different classes of antidysrhythmic drugs also affect the ECG in characteristic manners. A summary of the different waves, segments, and intervals and their importance to cardiac physiology is given in Table 37.2.

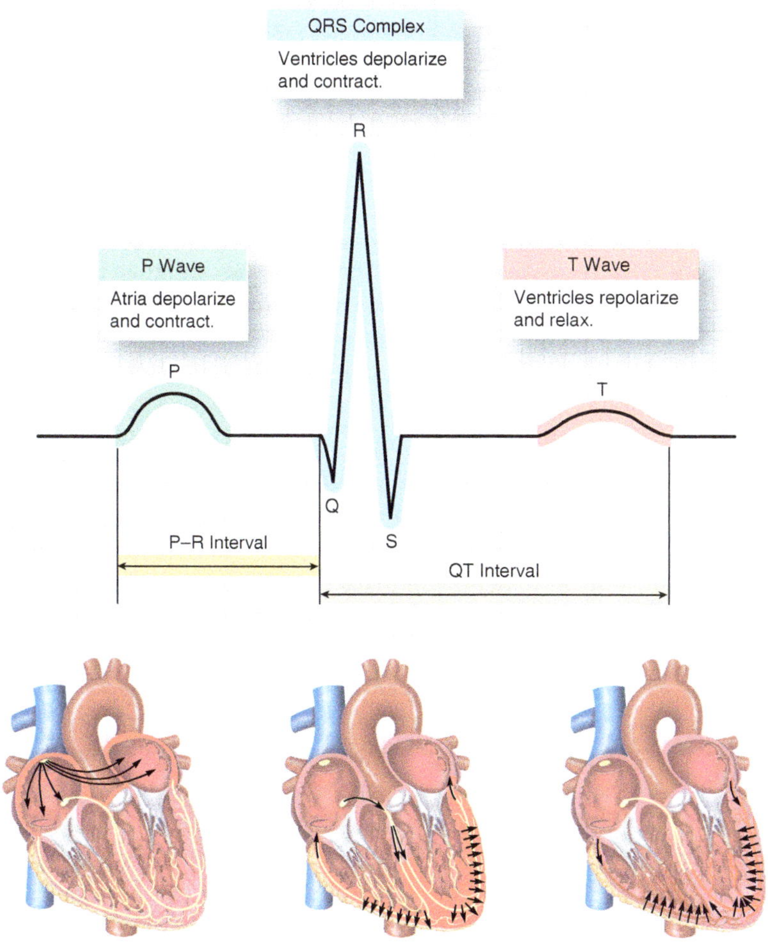

Figure 37.2 Relationship of the electrocardiogram to electrical conduction in the heart.

PharmFACT

Long QT syndrome (LQTS) is a congenital dysrhythmia that causes about 4000 sudden deaths in children and young adults each year. It is usually diagnosed during childhood and 60 to 70% of the patients are females. The first-line treatment for LQTS is beta-adrenergic blockers (Sovari, 2017).

Classification of Dysrhythmias

37.4 Dysrhythmias are classified by the impulse origin and type of rhythm abnormality produced.

There are many types of dysrhythmias and they are classified by a number of different methods. The two broad categories of rhythm abnormalities are those that affect impulse *formation* and those that affect impulse *conduction*. Although a correct diagnosis of the type of dysrhythmia is sometimes difficult, it is essential for effective treatment.

Bradydysrhythmias are disorders characterized by a heart rate of less than 60 beats/min. Bradydysrhythmias are very common in older adults because the number of cells in the SA node declines progressively such that by age 75 about 90% of the cells are nonfunctional. Similar age-related changes occur in the AV node, where normal cells

Table 37.2 ECG Waves and Intervals

Wave or Interval	Physiologic Significance	Importance
P wave	Atrial depolarization	A large P wave (voltage greater than 2.5 mm) suggests the atria may be enlarged.
PQ segment	Delay at the AV node; sometimes referred to as the PR segment	This delay is vital so the ventricles can fill with blood. Prolonged PQ segments suggest slow or nonconducting fibrotic areas in the myocardium.
PQ interval	All electrical activity prior to the impulse reaching the ventricles and contains the P wave and the PQ segment; sometimes referred to as the PR interval	Slightly prolonged PQ intervals are common and considered harmless. More prolonged PQ intervals suggest a first-degree heart block.
QRS complex	Ventricular depolarization and atrial repolarization	An exaggerated R wave suggests enlargement of the ventricles. Patients experiencing an MI may show QRS complexes that are abnormally high or that have extended durations.
T wave	Ventricular repolarization	A flat T wave suggests ischemia to the myocardium; an elevated T wave indicates hyperkalemia.
ST segment	Plateau phase of the action potential when the ventricles are depolarized	An ST elevation myocardial infarction (STEMI) is the most serious type of heart attack.
QT interval	Time from the start of ventricular depolarization to the completion of ventricular repolarization	Drugs that lengthen the QT interval have been linked to cardiac dysrhythmias, cardiac arrest, and sudden death. At the same time, prolongation of the action potential duration is a primary antidysrhythmic mechanism.

die and are replaced by fibrotic tissue. Bradydysrhythmias are the major indication for pacemaker implantation. Common bradydysrhythmias include the following:

- **Sinus bradycardia.** This is the most common slow heart rhythm. Sinus bradycardia generally does not require treatment unless the patient is experiencing syncope or dizziness due to lack of sufficient blood flow to the brain or if the heart rate fails to increase during periods of exertion.
- **Sinoatrial node dysfunction (sick sinus syndrome).** The SA node fails to generate or transmit sufficient electrical impulses. Patients with this condition may experience severe bradycardia (less than 40 beats/min resting), failure of the heart rate to increase with exercise, or significant sinus pauses. Severe episodes of bradycardia may alternate with periods of abnormally rapid heart rates.
- **Atrioventricular conduction block.** The AV node fails to conduct impulses to the rest of the myocardium. AV blocks are classified by degree. In first-degree AV block, the AV node conducts the impulse slowly, and conduction is delayed. In second-degree AV block, some, but not all, impulses are prevented (blocked) from leaving the AV node. Second-degree AV block results in nonconducted P waves. A third-degree AV block results in total stoppage of impulses through the AV node. None of the impulses originating in the atria can make their way through the block into the ventricles. Second- and third-degree blocks require pharmacotherapy or the insertion of a temporary or permanent pacemaker. Some AV blocks are temporary in origin and can be due to cardiac drug toxicity. Any drug that slows AV conduction can cause a temporary form of AV block.

Tachydysrhythmias are disorders exhibiting a heart rate greater than 100 beats/min. The incidence of tachydysrhythmias increases in older adults and in patients with preexisting cardiovascular disease. The simplest method for categorizing tachydysrhythmias is according to the type of rhythm abnormality produced and its location. Dysrhythmias that originate in the atria are sometimes referred to as supraventricular. Those that originate in the ventricles are generally more serious because they are more likely to interfere with the normal cardiac function. Common tachydysrhythmias include the following:

- **Atrial tachycardia.** This may be caused by a rapidly firing SA node or by an ectopic focus in the atria that suppresses the SA node and establishes a rapid heart rate, often between 160 and 200 beats/min. When these episodes alternate with periods of normal rhythm, it is called *paroxysmal atrial tachycardia (PAT)* or **paroxysmal supraventricular tachycardia (PSVT).**
- **Atrial flutter.** This is a rapid, regular heartbeat in which the atria may beat 250 to 350 times per minute. During atrial flutter, the job of the AV node is to selectively block some of the impulses coming from the atria, so the ventricular rate (pulse) is 125 to 175 beats/min (usually two, three, or four atrial beats for each ventricular beat).
- **Atrial fibrillation.** A complete disorganization of rhythm, this is the most common type of dysrhythmia. It is caused by multiple ectopic foci in the atria, all firing in a chaotic fashion. The atrial rate can range from 300 to 600 beats/min, causing an irregular ventricular rate ranging from 50 to 200 beats/min. The rapid atrial rate causes a loss of organized atrial contraction and results in quivering (fibrillation). This lack of contraction causes blood to lie dormant in parts of the atria and leads to the development of a thrombus. Potential dislodgement or fragmentation of the clot makes atrial fibrillation a leading risk factor for stroke. For prevention of stroke, most patients are placed on anticoagulation therapy with warfarin, Factor Xa inhibitors, or direct thrombin inhibitors (January et al., 2019) (see Chapter 38).
- **Ventricular tachycardia.** This is usually recognized by regular, rapid, wide beats with a ventricular rate of 100 to 200 beats/min. Patients with sustained or symptomatic ventricular tachycardia must be treated immediately because this condition is associated with a high risk of sudden death. **Torsades de pointes** is a specific type of ventricular tachycardia that is characterized by rates between 200 and 250 beats/min and "twisting of the points" of the QRS complex on the ECG.
- **Ventricular fibrillation.** This is a complete disorganization of rhythm in which the ventricles pump little or no blood, quickly starving the tissues of oxygen. Ventricular fibrillation is considered cardiac arrest.

General Principles of Dysrhythmia Management

37.5 Antidysrhythmic drugs are only used when there is a clear benefit to the patient.

Most antidysrhythmic drugs have the potential to produce serious adverse effects. The very drugs used to treat dysrhythmias may actually worsen or create new dysrhythmias and increase mortality. The following guidelines are used in the management of the patient with dysrhythmias.

Asymptomatic dysrhythmias: Research has shown little or no benefit to the patient in treating asymptomatic dysrhythmias with medications. Antidysrhythmic drugs are normally reserved for patients experiencing overt symptoms or for those whose condition cannot be controlled by other means.

Acute dysrhythmias: Some types of dysrhythmias are serious and may be life-threatening. In these cases, pharmacotherapy or cardioversion is warranted. For example, ventricular dysrhythmias often interfere with cardiac output and have greater potential for harm than atrial dysrhythmias. Dysrhythmias that are sustained may worsen and affect cardiac function. Several antidysrhythmics available by the intravenous (IV) route have an immediate onset of action to terminate life-threatening dysrhythmias.

Prophylaxis of dysrhythmias: Patients who are afflicted with recurring dysrhythmias or who have a comorbid condition, such as preexisting heart disease, may benefit from prophylactic therapy with antidysrhythmics. These patients should be monitored regularly to assess for prodysrhythmic effects from the drugs. Drug combinations that have the potential to prolong the QT interval are avoided and doses are kept as low as possible to minimize risk. Prophylactic therapy is initiated only for high-risk patients.

Nonpharmacologic treatment: Serious types of dysrhythmias are corrected through electrical stimulation of the heart, a treatment called **cardioversion** or **defibrillation**. The electrical shock momentarily stops all electrical impulses in the heart, both normal and abnormal. Under ideal conditions, the temporary cessation of electrical activity will allow the SA node to automatically return conduction to a normal sinus rhythm.

Other types of nonpharmacologic treatment include identification and destruction of the myocardial cells responsible for the abnormal conduction through a surgical procedure called catheter ablation. Cardiac pacemakers are sometimes inserted to correct the types of dysrhythmias that cause bradycardia. Implantable cardioverter defibrillators (ICDs) are placed in a patient to restore normal rhythm by either pacing the heart or giving it an electric shock when dysrhythmias occur. In addition, the ICD is capable of storing information regarding the heart rhythm for the healthcare provider to evaluate.

Drugs for Dysrhythmias

37.6 Antidysrhythmic drugs are classified by their mechanism of action.

The therapeutic goals of antidysrhythmic pharmacotherapy are to terminate existing dysrhythmias or to prevent abnormal rhythms for the purpose of reducing the risks of sudden death, stroke, or other complications resulting from the disease. Antidysrhythmic drugs act by altering specific electrophysiologic properties of the heart. They do this through two basic mechanisms: blocking flow through ion channels (conduction) or altering autonomic activity (automaticity).

In use since 1985, the most common method of classifying antidysrhythmic drugs is the Vaughan Williams classification. This classification scheme groups drugs as Classes I, II, III, and IV based on the stage at which they affect the action potential. A fifth group includes miscellaneous drugs not acting by one of the first four mechanisms. Although widely used, the Vaughan Williams classification method is simplistic because some of these drugs act by more than one mechanism, and the drugs within each class have unique properties that distinguish them from each other. For example, the Class I drugs have three subclasses. The categories of antidysrhythmics and their mechanisms are shown in Table 37.3.

The use of antidysrhythmic drugs has significantly declined because research has determined that the use of these medications for prophylaxis may actually increase patient mortality. Drugs affecting cardiac electrophysiology have a narrow margin of safety between a therapeutic effect and a toxic effect. While they have the ability to correct dysrhythmias, they can also worsen or even create new dysrhythmias. These prodysrhythmic effects have resulted in less use of these drugs, especially those medications in Class I.

Another reason for the decline in antidysrhythmic drug use is the success of nonpharmacologic techniques. Catheter

Table 37.3 Classification of Antidysrhythmics

Class	Actions	Primary Indications
I: Sodium Channel Blockers		
IA	Delays repolarization; slows conduction velocity; increases duration of the action potential.	Atrial fibrillation, premature atrial contractions, premature ventricular contractions, tachycardia
IB	Accelerates repolarization; slows conduction velocity; decreases duration of action potential.	Severe ventricular dysrhythmias
IC	No significant effect on repolarization; slows conduction velocity.	Severe ventricular dysrhythmias
II: Beta-Adrenergic Antagonists	Slows conduction velocity; decreases automaticity; prolongs refractory period.	Atrial flutter and fibrillation, tachydysrhythmias, ventricular dysrhythmias
III: Potassium Channel Blockers	Slows repolarization; increases duration of action potential; prolongs refractory period.	Severe atrial and ventricular dysrhythmias
IV: Calcium Channel Blockers	Slows conduction velocity; decreases contractility; prolongs refractory period.	Paroxysmal supraventricular tachycardia, supraventricular tachydysrhythmias

ablation and implantable defibrillators are more successful in managing many types of dysrhythmias than is the prophylactic use of medications.

Sodium Channel Blockers: Class I

37.7 Class I antidysrhythmics act by blocking ion channels in myocardial cells.

Sodium channel blockers, the Class I drugs, are the largest group of antidysrhythmics. They are further divided into three subgroups (IA, IB, and IC) based on subtle differences in their mechanisms of action. Because initiation of the action potential is dependent on the opening of gated sodium ion channels, a blockade of these channels will prevent depolarization of the myocardium. The spread of the action potential will slow, and areas of ectopic pacemaker activity will be suppressed. The sodium channel blockers are shown in Table 37.4 and Figure 37.3.

The sodium channel blockers are similar in structure and action to local anesthetics. In fact, the Class I antidysrhythmic lidocaine is a prototype local anesthetic in Chapter 26. This anesthetic-like action slows impulse conduction across the heart. Some, such as quinidine and procainamide, are effective against many types of dysrhythmias. The remaining Class I drugs are more specific and indicated only for life-threatening ventricular dysrhythmias.

The adverse effects of the sodium blockers vary with each individual drug. All these medications can cause new dysrhythmias or worsen existing ones. The slowing of the heart rate can cause hypotension, dizziness, and fainting. During pharmacotherapy, the ECG should be monitored for signs of cardiotoxicity, such as increases in the PR and QT intervals and widening of the QRS complex. Some Class I drugs have significant anticholinergic adverse effects such as dry mouth, constipation, and urinary retention. Special precautions should be taken with older adults because adverse effects may worsen urinary hesitancy in men with prostate enlargement.

Class IA: The Class IA antidysrhythmics include quinidine, disopyramide (Norpace), and procainamide. Although quinidine is the oldest and best-known Class IA drug, procainamide is the prototype because it has been more widely used than quinidine in recent decades. All are available by the oral (PO) route and act by blocking sodium ion channels during phase 0 of the action potential.

The primary action responsible for the antidysrhythmic effects of the Class IA drugs is a slowing of conduction velocity. These drugs also inhibit potassium channels, which delays repolarization and increases the refractory period. Subsequent action potentials must wait slightly longer before triggering the next electrical impulse. These actions allow the Class IA drugs to inhibit the formation of ectopic foci in both the atria and ventricles.

The actions of Class IA medications can be recognized on the ECG. The QRS complex widens, owing to the slowed depolarization of the ventricles. The QT interval is increased due to the delay in repolarization of the ventricles.

PROTOTYPE DRUG **Procainamide**

Classification **Therapeutic:** Antidysrhythmic, Class IA
Pharmacologic: Sodium channel blocker

Therapeutic Effects and Uses: Approved in 1950, procainamide is a broad-spectrum antidysrhythmic chemically related to the local anesthetic procaine that has the ability to correct many different types of atrial and ventricular dysrhythmias. Indications include ventricular tachycardia during cardiopulmonary resuscitation (CPR); refractory ventricular fibrillation or pulseless ventricular tachycardia during CPR; conversion to sinus rhythm in patients with paroxysmal atrial tachycardia, atrial flutter, or atrial fibrillation; and treatment or prophylaxis of PSVT. Procainamide is now considered a drug of last choice for advanced cardiac life support due to its toxicity; it is used when other drugs have failed to reverse a severe dysrhythmia. The major hepatic metabolite of the drug, N-acetyl procainamide, also has antidysrhythmic activity. Because the rate of acetylation to the active metabolite is genetically determined, "slow acetylators" and "fast acetylators" will require adjustments in dosages to obtain optimal therapeutic results.

Procainamide is available in IV and intramuscular (IM) formulations: PO forms of procainamide have been discontinued. Dosage is guided by periodic serum drug levels, which are maintained between 4 and 8 mcg/mL. The supine position should be used during IV administration because severe hypotension may occur during the infusion. Use of procainamide must be terminated if the QRS widens more than 50% of its original width.

Mechanism of Action: Procainamide blocks sodium ion channels in myocardial cells, thus reducing automaticity and slowing the velocity of the action potential across the myocardium. This slight delay in conduction velocity prolongs the refractory period and can suppress dysrhythmias.

Pharmacokinetics:

Route(s)	IV, IM
Absorption	Readily absorbed
Distribution	Widely distributed; crosses the placenta; secreted in breast milk; 15% bound to plasma protein
Primary metabolism	Hepatic; metabolized to active metabolite
Primary excretion	Renal, 50–70% unchanged
Onset of action	IV: immediate; IM: 10–30 min
Duration of action	IM/IV: 3–4 h

Table 37.4 Antidysrhythmic Drugs

Drug	Route and Adult Dose (Maximum Dose Where Indicated)	Adverse Effects
Class IA: Sodium Channel Blockers		
disopyramide (Norpace)	PO (immediate release): 400–800 mg in divided doses PO (extended release): 300 mg bid	*Nausea and vomiting, diarrhea, dry mouth, urinary retention, cinchonism (quinidine), anorexia, rash, photosensitivity* May produce new dysrhythmias or worsen existing ones; hypotension, torsades de pointes, blood dyscrasias, hepatotoxicity (quinidine), lupus (procainamide)
procainamide	IV: 100 mg q5min at a rate of 25–50 mg/min (max: 1 g)	
quinidine gluconate ER	PO: 324–648 mg tid–qid (max: 3–4 g/day)	
quinidine sulfate	PO: 200–400 mg tid–qid (max: 3–4 g/day); therapeutic serum drug level is 2–5 mcg/mL	
Class IB: Sodium Channel Blockers		
lidocaine (Xylocaine)	IV: 1–4 mg/min infusion (max: 3 mg/kg per 5–10 min)	*Nausea and vomiting, drowsiness, dizziness, lethargy, confusion (phenytoin)* May produce new dysrhythmias or worsen existing ones; hypotension, bradycardia, central nervous system (CNS) toxicity (lidocaine), malignant hyperthermia (lidocaine), cardiac arrest (lidocaine), blood dyscrasias (phenytoin), teratogenicity (phenytoin)
mexiletine	PO: 200–300 mg tid (max: 1200 mg/day)	
phenytoin (Dilantin)	IV: 50–100 mg q10–15min until dysrhythmia is terminated (max: 1 g/day)	
Class IC: Sodium Channel Blockers		
flecainide (Tambocor)	PO: 50 mg bid (max: 400 mg/day)	*Nausea and vomiting, fatigue, dizziness, headache, visual disturbances (flecainide)* May produce new dysrhythmias or worsen existing ones; hypotension, bradycardia, cardiac arrest (flecainide), blood dyscrasias, lupus (propafenone), HF (propafenone), acute liver injury (propafenone)
propafenone (Rythmol SR)	PO (extended release): 225 mg bid (max: 425 mg bid)	
Class II: Beta-Adrenergic Antagonists		
acebutolol	PO: 200–600 mg bid–tid (max: 1200 mg/day)	*Fatigue, insomnia, drowsiness, impotence, decreased libido, dizziness, bradycardia, confusion* Agranulocytosis, HF, bronchospasm, hypotension, Stevens–Johnson syndrome, anaphylaxis, fetal harm; if the drug is abruptly withdrawn, palpitations, rebound HTN, life-threatening dysrhythmias, or myocardial ischemia may occur
esmolol (Brevibloc)	IV: 50–300 mcg/kg/min (maintenance dose)	
propranolol (Inderal, InnoPran XL)	PO: 10–30 mg tid–qid (max: 480 mg/day) IV: 0.5–3.1 mg q4h or prn	
Class III: Potassium Channel Blockers		
amiodarone (Nexterone, Pacerone)	PO: 400–600 mg/day in 1–2 divided doses (max: 1600 mg/day as loading dose)	*Blurred vision (amiodarone), photosensitivity, nausea and vomiting, anorexia* May produce new dysrhythmias or worsen existing ones; hypotension, HF, heart block, bradycardia, pneumonia-like syndrome (amiodarone, dronedarone), angioedema (dofetilide), CNS toxicity (ibutilide), fetal harm
dofetilide (Tikosyn)	PO: 125–500 mcg bid based on creatinine clearance	
dronedarone (Multaq)	PO: 400 mg bid	
ibutilide (Corvert)	IV: 1 mg infused over 10 min (for patients over 60 kg) (max: 2 mg infused over at least 20 min)	
sotalol* (Betapace, Betapace AF, Sorine)	PO: 80 mg bid (max: 320 mg/day)	
Class IV: Calcium Channel Blockers		
diltiazem (Cardizem, Cartia XT, Dilacor, Taztia XT, Tiazac, others)	IV: 5–10 mg/h continuous infusion for a maximum of 24 h (max: 15 mg/h)	*Flushed skin, headache, dizziness, peripheral edema, lightheadedness, nausea, diarrhea, syncope* Hepatotoxicity, MI, HF, confusion, mood changes, hypotension, fetal harm
verapamil (Calan SR, Verelan)	PO: 240–480 mg/day in divided doses IV: 5–10 mg direct; may repeat in 15–30 min	
Miscellaneous Antidysrhythmics		
adenosine	IV: 6–12 mg given as a bolus injection every 1–2 min as needed (max: 12 mg/dose)	*Facial flushing, dyspnea, headache* May produce new dysrhythmias or worsen existing ones, AV block
digoxin (Lanoxicaps, Lanoxin)	PO: 0.125–0.5 mg qid Therapeutic serum drug level: 0.8–2 ng/mL	*Nausea and vomiting, headache, diarrhea, visual disturbances* May produce new dysrhythmias or worsen existing ones

Note: *Italics* indicate common adverse effects. Underline indicates serious adverse effects.

* Sotalol is a beta blocker, but because its cardiac effects are more similar to amiodarone, it is in Class III. Adverse effects are those of Class II and Class III.

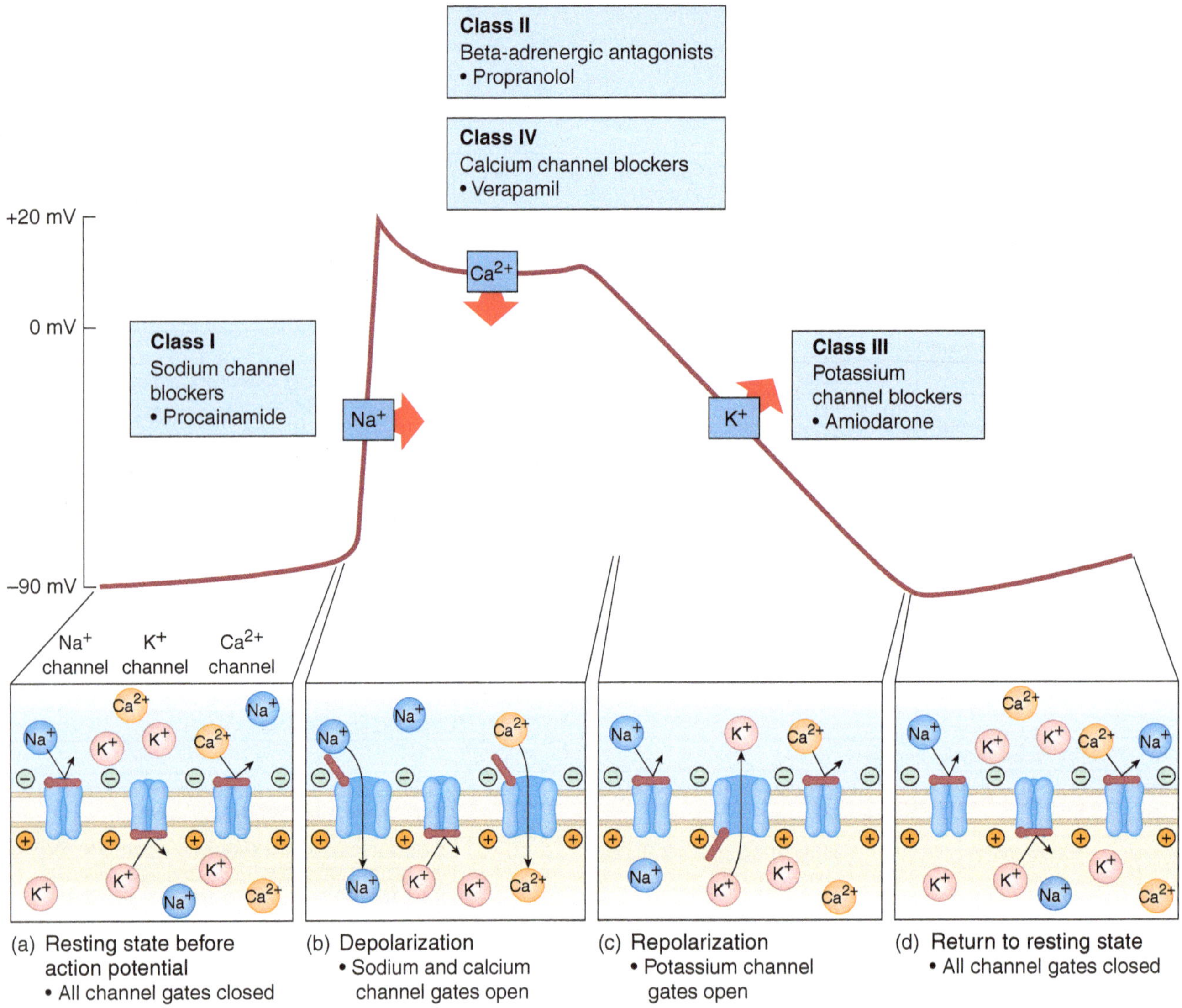

Figure 37.3 Ion channels in myocardial cells: (a) resting state before action potential (all channel gates closed); (b) depolarization (sodium and calcium channel gates open); (c) repolarization (potassium channel gates open); (d) return to resting state (all channel gates closed).

Adverse Effects: Procainamide has a narrow therapeutic index and dosage must be monitored carefully to avoid serious adverse effects. Nausea and vomiting, abdominal pain, and headache are common during therapy. The drug can cause fever, accompanied by anorexia, weakness, nausea, and vomiting. High doses may produce CNS effects such as confusion or psychosis. Rapid IV administration of procainamide can cause severe hypotension. **Black Box Warnings:** Chronic administration may result in an increased titer of antinuclear antibodies. A lupus-like syndrome may occur in 30 to 50% of patients taking the drug for more than a year. Procainamide should be reserved for life-threatening dysrhythmias because it has the ability to produce new dysrhythmias or worsen existing ones. Agranulocytosis, bone marrow depression, neutropenia, hypoplastic anemia, and thrombocytopenia have been reported, usually within the first 3 months of therapy. Complete blood counts should be monitored carefully and the drug discontinued at the first sign of potential blood dyscrasia.

Contraindications/Precautions: Procainamide is contraindicated in patients with second- or third-degree AV block (unless controlled by a pacemaker), severe HF, peripheral neuropathy, and myasthenia gravis. Because procainamide may activate or worsen lupus, the drug is only used in these patients when there is no safer alternative. Doses must be lowered in patients with chronic kidney disease (CKD) due to possible accumulation of the drug. Patients in shock or with severe hypotension should not receive this drug due to additive hypotension. Procainamide may worsen blood dyscrasias; thus, it should be used with caution in patients with preexisting bone marrow suppression.

Drug Interactions: Additive cardiac depressant effects may occur if procainamide is administered with other antidysrhythmics. Additive anticholinergic adverse effects will occur if procainamide is used concurrently with anticholinergic drugs. Procainamide may increase plasma levels of amiodarone or quinidine. Use with antihypertensives may result in hypotension. **Herbal/Food:** The use of herbal products or supplements should be avoided unless approved by the healthcare provider due to the toxicity of the drug.

Pregnancy: No data are available regarding the effects of this drug during pregnancy. Procainamide enters milk and has the potential to cause adverse effects on the breastfed neonate.

Treatment of Overdose: No specific therapy is available for overdose. Supportive treatment is targeted to reversing hypotension with vasopressors and preventing or treating procainamide-induced dysrhythmias.

Clinician Responsibilities: Key clinical implications for patients receiving procainamide are included in Applied Clinical Judgment: Patients Receiving Pharmacotherapy for Dysrhythmias.

Drugs Similar to Procainamide

Class IA: The Class IA antidysrhythmics similar to procainamide include disopyramide and quinidine.

Disopyramide (Norpace): Approved in 1977, disopyramide has actions and indications similar to those of other Class IA drugs. Available only by the PO route, the drug is used infrequently due to a high incidence of anticholinergic effects such as xerostomia (dry mouth) and urinary retention in patients with benign prostatic hyperplasia. The anticholinergic effects cause an increase in heart rate, which may directly cancel out the therapeutic cardiac depressant effects of the drug. Off-label uses include maintenance of, or conversion to, sinus rhythm in patients with atrial flutter or atrial fibrillation. Disopyramide has a black box warning that the drug should be restricted to patients with life-threatening ventricular dysrhythmias. Disopyramide has been shown to cause fetal harm in laboratory animals. The drug enters milk and has the potential to cause adverse effects in the breastfed neonate.

Quinidine: Approved in 1938, quinidine is the oldest antidysrhythmic drug, originally obtained as a natural substance from the bark of the South American cinchona tree. Like procainamide, quinidine is a broad-spectrum drug having the ability to correct many different types of atrial and ventricular dysrhythmias. The two salts of quinidine are sulfate, which is given PO, and gluconate, which is given as an extended release tablet. Like other drugs in this class, quinidine blocks sodium ion channels in myocardial cells, thus reducing automaticity and slowing the velocity of the action potential across the myocardium. In addition to dysrhythmias, quinidine gluconate has been used to treat malaria but has been largely replaced by more effective drugs. The most common adverse effect of quinidine is diarrhea, which occurs in about one-third of patients and may be intense. The drug can induce various types of dysrhythmias when serum levels rise above normal. High doses result in a syndrome called **cinchonism** with symptoms such as tinnitus, headache, blurred vision, hearing loss, and dysrhythmias. These symptoms are reversible once the drug is discontinued. Quinidine is contraindicated in patients with incomplete AV block because it can induce total blockage of conduction. Quinidine carries a black box warning that the drug has resulted in increased mortality when used for non-life-threatening dysrhythmias. Extensive human data have not shown evidence for an increase in adverse pregnancy outcomes or teratogenicity above the baseline rate. Small amounts of this drug are secreted in human milk although adverse effects on the breastfed neonate are unknown.

Class IB: The Class IB antidysrhythmics include lidocaine, mexiletine, and phenytoin. Like other Class I drugs, these agents act by blocking gated sodium ion channels in cardiac muscle cells. Unlike the Class IA drugs, the Class IB agents shorten the refractory period and have little effect on conduction velocity. The Class IB drugs have minimal effects on the ECG and their primary indication is ventricular dysrhythmias.

Lidocaine (Xylocaine): Lidocaine, the most frequently prescribed Class IB antidysrhythmic, was featured as a prototype local anesthetic in Chapter 26. It is an important treatment for life-threatening ventricular dysrhythmia, although amiodarone is considered a preferred drug for this indication. It is not effective in preventing or treating atrial dysrhythmias. Lidocaine decreases the refractory period of the action potential, especially in ischemic myocardial tissue. For acute conditions, lidocaine is administered by IV bolus or infusion; it is rarely given by the IM or subcutaneous routes. Serum lidocaine levels may be monitored and should be between 2 and 6 mcg/mL. The first signs of lidocaine toxicity usually involve the CNS and include confusion, anxiety, tremors, and paresthesias. As doses increase, the patient may become comatose and experience seizures or respiratory arrest. The correct lidocaine formulation must be used for IV infusions: Local anesthetic lidocaine preparations may contain preservatives and epinephrine and should not be given IV. Lidocaine crosses the placenta. The drug enters milk and has the potential to cause adverse effects in the breastfed neonate.

Mexiletine: Approved in 1985, mexiletine is chemically similar to lidocaine, has local anesthetic properties, and is used only for serious ventricular dysrhythmias. Mexiletine is well absorbed orally and may be used off-label for the treatment of neuropathic pain. The most common adverse effects are nausea and vomiting. CNS effects such as dizziness, tremor, and ataxia are common. Less common, though potentially serious, adverse effects include blood dyscrasias, pulmonary fibrosis, and worsening of HF. A black box warning informs of the possibility of acute liver damage in patients taking mexiletine. The target range for serum mexiletine concentration is 0.5 to 2 mcg/mL. Studies in pregnant laboratory animals showed an increase in fetal absorption but no teratogenicity. Mexiletine enters milk and has the potential to cause adverse effects in the breastfed neonate.

Phenytoin (Dilantin): The primary use for phenytoin is to treat seizures, and it was presented in Chapter 22 as a prototype antiseizure medication. Phenytoin is rarely used for its antidysrhythmic properties and is not approved by the U.S. Food and Drug Administration (FDA) for this purpose. Historically, it has been used off-label to treat dysrhythmias secondary to digoxin (Lanoxin) toxicity. Phenytoin is a known teratogen in humans and is contraindicated during pregnancy. Breastfeeding is not recommended.

Class IC: The Class IC antidysrhythmics include two drugs: flecainide and propafenone. Like other Class I drugs, these medications block gated sodium ion channels in cardiac muscle cells. The Class IC antidysrhythmics profoundly decrease conduction velocity. Thus, the PR, QRS, and QT intervals are often prolonged. The refractory period may be shortened slightly but is mostly unchanged by the Class IC drugs. Their primary indication is for life-threatening atrial dysrhythmias, although they can also prevent ventricular dysrhythmias. These drugs have a pronounced prodysrhythmic effect that has the potential to increase mortality in patients who have experienced a recent MI.

Flecainide (Tambocor): Flecainide is an oral drug used primarily to treat or prevent paroxysmal atrial fibrillation or atrial flutter due to its ability to markedly decrease conduction velocity. It is approved for the prophylaxis of life-threatening ventricular dysrhythmias, although it is rarely used for this purpose. The FDA has issued several black box warnings regarding flecainide. The prodysrhythmic effects of the drug may generate new ventricular dysrhythmias in about 10% of patients. Due to an excessive mortality rate, the drug is contraindicated in patients with left-ventricular dysfunction who have experienced a recent MI. Serum flecainide levels should be monitored, especially in patients with CKD or hepatic impairment, and maintained between 0.2 and 1 mcg/mL. Pulmonary fibrosis and bone marrow suppression are potentially serious adverse effects. Other adverse effects include dizziness, headache, asthenia, tremor, and malaise. Flecainide causes fetal harm in laboratory animals. The drug enters milk and has the potential to cause adverse effects in the breastfed neonate.

Propafenone (Rythmol SR): Approved in 1989, propafenone is an oral drug similar to flecainide that is used primarily for atrial fibrillation and the prophylaxis of PSVT. Its prodysrhythmic activity limits its use in treating ventricular dysrhythmias. Unlike flecainide, propafenone exhibits clinically significant beta-adrenergic antagonist activity. This beta-blocker action may cause a negative inotropic effect that can worsen symptoms of HF. Furthermore, the beta-blocking actions may cause bronchospasm in patients with asthma or chronic obstructive pulmonary disease (COPD). Propafenone is metabolized to active metabolites, which account for much of the drug's effects. In addition to exacerbating or creating new dysrhythmias, propafenone may cause dizziness and dysgeusia (altered sense of taste). Like some of the other antidysrhythmics, propafenone has a black box warning that it should be restricted to patients with life-threatening ventricular dysrhythmias. Because propafenone crosses the placenta, the fetus and neonate should be monitored for dysrhythmias. Small amounts of drug enter milk, but there are no data regarding adverse effects on the breastfed neonate.

Beta-Adrenergic Antagonists: Class II

37.8 Beta-adrenergic antagonists reduce automaticity and slow conduction velocity in the heart.

Beta-adrenergic antagonists, or blockers, are used to treat HTN, MI, HF, and dysrhythmias. The basic pharmacology of beta-adrenergic antagonists was explained in Chapter 16; the student should refer to that chapter for additional details. Only the actions of these drugs that relate to dysrhythmias are discussed in this section.

As expected from their effects on the autonomic nervous system, beta-adrenergic antagonists slow the heart rate (negative chronotropic effect) and decrease conduction velocity. These effects are primarily caused by the blockade of calcium ion channels in the SA and AV nodes, although these drugs also block gated sodium ion channels in the atria and ventricles. The reduction in myocardial automaticity stabilizes many types of dysrhythmias. The main value of beta blockers as antidysrhythmic drugs is to treat atrial dysrhythmias associated with HF. When administered to post-MI patients, beta blockers decrease the likelihood of sudden death due to fatal dysrhythmias. Tachydysrhythmias respond well to beta blockers, including those that are induced by exercise.

Only a few beta blockers are approved for dysrhythmias, due to potential adverse effects, and these are listed in Table 37.4. Unless a functioning pacemaker is present, these drugs are contraindicated in patients with severe bradycardia, sick sinus syndrome, or advanced AV block because they depress conduction through the AV node. Blockade of beta-adrenergic receptors in the heart causes bradycardia, which may not be well tolerated in patients with preexisting cardiac disease, and hypotension, which may cause dizziness and fainting. Nonselective beta blockers may affect $beta_2$ receptors in the lung, causing bronchospasm in patients with asthma or COPD. Higher doses may produce depression, as well as hallucinations and psychosis, especially in older adults. Abrupt discontinuation of beta blockers can lead to dysrhythmias and HTN.

Acebutolol: Approved in 1984, acebutolol is a cardioselective $beta_1$-adrenergic antagonist available only by the oral route. Like other beta blockers, acebutolol reduces sympathetic activity to the heart, thus lowering heart rate. It also has a negative inotropic effect. As an antidysrhythmic, it is used to treat premature ventricular contractions and reduce exercise-induced tachycardia. Other indications include chronic, stable angina and HTN. Adverse effects such as hypotension and bradycardia are extensions of its beta-blocking action. At high doses, the selectivity for $beta_1$ receptors diminishes and the drug may cause bronchoconstriction ($beta_2$ receptors). Because the negative inotropic effects of the drug may worsen symptoms of HF, it is usually contraindicated in these patients. Neonates of mothers taking this drug during pregnancy showed reduced birth weight, reduced blood pressure, and decreased heart rate. It is not known if acebutolol enters milk or causes adverse effects, so breastfeeding is not recommended.

Esmolol (Brevibloc): Approved in 1986, esmolol differs from the other antidysrhythmic beta blockers in that it has a very short half-life of 9 minutes and is only given by IV infusion. As an antidysrhythmic, esmolol is used for the immediate termination of atrial tachyarrhythmias and noncompensatory sinus tachycardia and to control ventricular rate in patients with atrial flutter or fibrillation. When a loading dose is administered, peak plasma levels can be reached in 5 minutes. Off-label indications include treatment of hypertensive emergencies, acute MI, and unstable angina. Hypotension and bradycardia are common adverse effects, but they quickly resolve once the infusion is discontinued. At therapeutic doses, the drug is selective for $beta_1$-adrenergic receptors. No data are available regarding the effects of this drug during pregnancy. It is not known if esmolol enters milk.

Propranolol (Inderal, InnoPran XL): Propranolol is a nonselective beta-adrenergic antagonist. Because it slows automaticity, propranolol is indicated for many types of dysrhythmias including suppression of exercise-induced tachycardia, atrial dysrhythmias, ventricular dysrhythmias, premature ventricular contractions, and digoxin-induced tachydysrhythmias. Propranolol exhibits few serious adverse effects at therapeutic doses. At high doses, patients may experience bradycardia, hypotension, HF, and bronchospasm. Propranolol is featured as a prototype beta-adrenergic antagonist in Chapter 16. Propranolol use during pregnancy has been shown to produce congenital malformations, small placentas, and intrauterine growth retardation. Small amounts enter human milk.

CONNECTION Checkpoint 37.2

Both $alpha_1$ blockers and $beta_1$ blockers are used to treat HTN but only the $beta_1$ blockers are antidysrhythmics. From what you learned in Chapter 16, explain why the selective $alpha_1$ blockers are not used to treat dysrhythmias.

CONNECTIONS: Treating the Diverse Patient

Sensitivity of Asian Patients to Propranolol

Research studies have shown a differential drug response to propranolol among patients of Chinese ancestry (Zhou et al., 1993). Some populations of these individuals typically lack a specific enzyme (mephenytoin hydroxylase) that is needed to metabolize propranolol. Because of this sensitivity, propranolol has a significantly greater effect on heart rate. In other words, individuals of Chinese descent will develop signs of toxicity more quickly than Whites. The nurse should assess this population for signs and symptoms of early drug toxicity, possible overdosage, and adverse reactions due to high drug levels. Assessing for unique cultural sensitivity to drug therapies is necessary for safe drug administration.

Potassium Channel Blockers: Class III

37.9 Potassium channel blockers prolong the refractory period of the heart.

The potassium channel blockers are a small but diverse class of drugs that have very important applications to the treatment of dysrhythmias. After the action potential has passed and the myocardial cell is in a depolarized state, repolarization depends on removal of potassium from the cell. The drugs in Class III exert their actions by blocking potassium ion channels in myocardial cells. Although there are significant differences among the drugs, all have in common the ability to delay repolarization and prolong the refractory period. This action is reflected by an increase in the QT interval on the ECG. Automaticity is also reduced.

Most drugs in this class have multiple actions on the heart and also affect adrenergic receptors or sodium channels. For example, in addition to blocking potassium channels, sotalol (Betapace, Betapace AF, Sorine) is considered a beta-adrenergic antagonist. The potassium channel blockers are listed in Table 37.4.

Drugs in this class have limited uses due to potentially serious toxicity. Like other antidysrhythmics, potassium channel blockers slow the heart rate, resulting in bradycardia and possible hypotension in a significant percentage of patients. These drugs can create or worsen dysrhythmias, especially during the first few doses. Older adults with preexisting HF must be carefully monitored because these patients are at higher risk for the cardiac adverse effects of potassium channel blockers.

PROTOTYPE DRUG Amiodarone (Nexterone, Pacerone)

Classification **Therapeutic:** Antidysrhythmic, Class III
Pharmacologic: Potassium channel blocker

Therapeutic Effects and Uses: Approved in 1985, amiodarone is the most frequently prescribed Class III antidysrhythmic. It is considered a broad-spectrum antidysrhythmic because it is effective in terminating both atrial and ventricular dysrhythmias. It is approved for the treatment of resistant ventricular tachycardia and recurrent fibrillation that may prove life-threatening, and it has become a preferred medication for the treatment of atrial dysrhythmias in patients with HF.

Amiodarone is available as PO tablets and as an IV infusion. IV infusions are limited to short-term therapy (2 to 4 days). Although its onset of action may take several weeks when the medication is given PO, its effects can last 4 to 8 weeks after the drug is discontinued because it has an extended half-life that may exceed 100 days. Amiodarone is a structural analog of thyroid hormone. The therapeutic serum level for amiodarone is 1 to 2.5 mcg/mL.

Mechanism of Action: Amiodarone exerts multiple, complex actions on the heart and its exact mechanism of action is not completely known. In addition to blocking potassium ion channels, some of this drug's actions relate to its blockade of sodium ion channels and inhibiting sympathetic activity to the heart. Repolarization is delayed, the refractory period prolonged, and automaticity reduced. In addition to prolonging the QT interval, amiodarone increases the PR interval and widens the QRS complex on the ECG.

Pharmacokinetics:

Route(s)	PO, IV
Absorption	Completely absorbed by the gastrointestinal tract
Distribution	Widely distributed; crosses the placenta; secreted in breast milk; concentrated in the lung, kidneys, spleen, and adipose tissue
Primary metabolism	Hepatic to active metabolites; some enterohepatic recirculation; inhibits some CYP450 enzymes
Primary excretion	Primarily biliary; some feces
Onset of action	PO: 2–3 days; IV: 2 h
Duration of action	PO/IV: 10–150 days

Adverse Effects: Potentially serious adverse effects limit the use of amiodarone. This drug may cause nausea and vomiting, anorexia, fatigue, dizziness, and hypotension. Visual disturbances are common in patients taking amiodarone for extended periods and include blurred vision due to cornea deposits, photophobia, xerostomia, cataracts, and macular degeneration. Rashes, photosensitivity, and other skin reactions occur in 10 to 15% of patients taking the drug. Certain tissues concentrate this medication; thus, adverse effects may be slow to resolve, persisting long after the drug has been discontinued. **Black Box Warnings:** Amiodarone has been associated with severe and sometimes fatal pulmonary toxicity. It has prodysrhythmic action and may cause bradycardia, cardiogenic shock, or AV block. Liver injury is frequent with amiodarone.

Contraindications/Precautions: Amiodarone is contraindicated in patients with severe bradycardia, cardiogenic shock, sick sinus syndrome, severe sinus node dysfunction, or third-degree AV block. Because amiodarone contains iodine in its chemical structure, patients who have hypersensitivity to this element should not receive the drug. It should be used with caution in patients with HF because it has a negative inotropic effect that can worsen symptoms. Electrolyte imbalances, especially hypokalemia and hypomagnesemia, should be corrected before administering amiodarone because these conditions predispose the patient to the development of dysrhythmias. Due to the drug's pulmonary toxicity, it is contraindicated in patients with COPD or respiratory insufficiency. Breastfeeding during amiodarone therapy may cause infant hypothyroidism; thus, the drug is contraindicated during lactation.

Drug Interactions: Amiodarone is metabolized by the cytochrome CYP450 enzymes and markedly inhibits the metabolism of many other drugs. This can raise the serum levels of these drugs and cause toxicity. For example, amiodarone can increase serum digoxin levels by as much as 70%. Amiodarone greatly enhances the actions of anticoagulants; thus, the dose of warfarin must be cut by as much as half. Use with beta-adrenergic antagonists or calcium channel blockers may potentiate sinus bradycardia, sinus arrest, or AV block. Amiodarone may increase phenytoin levels two- to threefold. Caution must be used during therapy with loop diuretics because hypokalemia can enhance the prodysrhythmic properties of amiodarone. Because of the large number of potential drug interactions, the nurse should regularly check current reference sources when patients are taking amiodarone concurrently with other medications. **Herbal/Food:** Use with echinacea may increase the risk of hepatotoxicity. Aloe may increase the effect of amiodarone. When the drug is administered PO, grapefruit juice can increase serum amiodarone levels by over 80%.

Pregnancy: Amiodarone can cause fetal harm and is contraindicated during pregnancy. Because the drug enters milk in high amounts, breastfeeding is not recommended.

Treatment of Overdose: Overdose will cause bradycardia, hypotension, and life-threatening dysrhythmias. Supportive treatment is targeted to reversing hypotension with vasopressors and bradycardia with atropine or isoproterenol.

Clinician Responsibilities: Key clinical implications for patients receiving amiodarone are included in Applied Clinical Judgment: Patients Receiving Pharmacotherapy for Dysrhythmias.

Drugs Similar to Amiodarone (Nexterone, Pacerone)

Other Class III antidysrhythmics include dofetilide, dronedarone, ibutilide, and sotalol.

Dofetilide (Tikosyn): Approved in 1999, dofetilide is an oral drug indicated for conversion of symptomatic atrial flutter or fibrillation to normal sinus rhythm. Like other potassium channel blockers, dofetilide prolongs the refractory period and action potential duration, thus increasing the QT interval. Dofetilide does not exhibit a negative inotropic effect, as do amiodarone and sotalol. The drug has no effect on the PR interval, and it does not widen the QRS complex. Dofetilide has many potentially serious adverse effects, and a black box warning states that therapy should begin in a clinical setting under continuous monitoring for a minimum of 3 days. The drug exhibits significant dose-related prodysrhythmic effects, including heart block, ventricular tachycardia, and torsades de pointes. The risk for drug-induced dysrhythmias is increased when dofetilide is administered concurrently with other medications that prolong the QT interval, including Class I and Class III antidysrhythmics. Because dofetilide may accumulate to toxic levels in patients with CKD, serum creatinine levels are monitored frequently during therapy. Electrolyte imbalances, especially hypokalemia or hypomagnesemia, should be corrected before administering dofetilide because these conditions predispose the patient to developing dysrhythmias. Studies in pregnant laboratory animals showed adverse effects on intrauterine growth and survival. It is not known if dofetilide enters human milk.

Dronedarone (Multaq): Approved in 2009, dronedarone is given PO to reduce the risk of hospitalization in patients with atrial dysrhythmias and associated cardiovascular risk factors such as HTN, diabetes, or previous stroke. The drug has a black box warning that it is contraindicated in patients with advanced HF with recent decompensation. It is also contraindicated in patients with bradycardia (less than 50 beats/min), prolonged QT interval, and severe hepatic impairment. The most common adverse effects are diarrhea, nausea and vomiting, abdominal pain, and asthenia. Dronedarone inhibits CYP450 enzymes and can participate in multiple drug–drug interactions with other cardiovascular medications. Dronedarone can cause fetal harm and is contraindicated during pregnancy. The drug enters animal milk and has the potential to cause adverse effects in a breastfed infant.

Ibutilide (Corvert): Approved in 1995, ibutilide is only administered as an IV infusion. Continuous ECG monitoring should be conducted for at least 4 hours following the infusion to identify any development of new or worsening dysrhythmias. Administered over 10 minutes, ibutilide is a first-line drug for rapidly converting atrial flutter or fibrillation to normal sinus rhythm. The drug prolongs the duration of the cardiac action potential without affecting the PR interval or QRS complex. The infusion is stopped as soon as the dysrhythmia is terminated. Ibutilide is generally well tolerated, although it does have prodysrhythmic effects, including induction of ventricular tachycardia and torsades de pointes. Like other Class III drugs, precautions must be taken when administering this drug concurrently with other medications that prolong the QT interval or if given to patients with hypokalemia or hypomagnesemia, as these conditions increase the risk of dysrhythmias. Studies in pregnant laboratory animals showed embryocidal and teratogenic effects. It is not known if ibutilide enters milk, but breastfeeding is not recommended.

Sotalol (Betapace, Betapace AF, Sorine): Approved in 1992, sotalol is unique in that the medication has both Class II and Class III antidysrhythmic properties. As a Class II drug, it is a nonselective beta blocker that slows conduction through the AV node. Its Class III actions delay repolarization and prolong the refractory period, thus widening the QT interval. Its mixed mechanisms are reflected in the diversity of indications for the drug.

Betapace and its generic equivalents are indicated for sustained ventricular fibrillation that is deemed to be life-threatening. Betapace AF converts atrial fibrillation to normal sinus rhythm and is indicated for highly symptomatic atrial dysrhythmias. The drugs contain a black box warning stating that they are not interchangeable.

Because of its prodysrhythmic activity, the first 3 days of therapy with sotalol are usually conducted in a controlled clinical setting with continuous monitoring. The drug should be used with caution when taken concurrently with other medications that prolong the QT interval or if given to patients with hypokalemia or hypomagnesemia, as these conditions increase the risk of dysrhythmias. Other adverse effects and contraindications for beta-adrenergic antagonists are given in Chapter 16. Sotalol can cause fetal harm in laboratory animals. Because sotalol enters breast milk in high amounts, breastfeeding is not recommended.

Calcium Channel Blockers: Class IV

37.10 Calcium channel blockers are used to treat atrial dysrhythmias.

Although about 10 calcium channel blockers (CCBs) are available to treat cardiovascular disease, only a limited number are approved for dysrhythmias. Review Chapter 30 for details regarding the mechanism of actions, indications, and clinician responsibilities for this drug class. Only actions relevant to dysrhythmias are discussed in this section. The antidysrhythmic CCBs are listed in Table 37.4.

Blockade of calcium ion channels has a number of effects on the heart that are very similar to those of beta-adrenergic antagonists. Effects include reduced automaticity in the SA node and slowed impulse conduction through the AV node. These effects are predictable because nodal tissues are more dependent on calcium channels than other areas of the myocardium. This slows the heart rate and prolongs the refractory period. On an ECG, the most prominent effect of CCBs is prolongation of the PR interval. Indications include the control of ventricular rate in cases of atrial flutter or fibrillation and prophylaxis of PSVT. CCBs are effective only against atrial dysrhythmias.

CCBs are well tolerated by most patients. As with many other antidysrhythmics, patients should be carefully monitored for bradycardia and hypotension. Because their cardiac effects are almost identical to those of beta-adrenergic antagonists, patients concurrently taking drugs from both classes are especially at risk for bradycardia and possible HF. Because older adults often have multiple cardiovascular disorders, such as HTN, HF, and dysrhythmias, it is not unusual to find older patients taking drugs from multiple classes.

Diltiazem (Cardizem, Cartia XT, Dilacor, Taztia XT, Tiazac, others): Like other CCBs, diltiazem inhibits the transport of calcium into myocardial cells. The actions and indications for diltiazem are the same as those of verapamil. The IV form of the drug is indicated for the management of acute atrial dysrhythmias, including paroxysmal supraventricular tachycardia. In addition to its use in treating and preventing atrial dysrhythmias, the oral forms are indicated for HTN as well as stable and vasospastic angina. Adverse effects of diltiazem are generally not serious and are related to vasodilation: headache, dizziness, and edema of the ankles and feet. Because of its profound depressant effects on nodal tissue, diltiazem is contraindicated in patients with severe bradycardia, AV block, or sick sinus syndrome. Concurrent use of diltiazem with digoxin or beta-adrenergic antagonists may cause partial or complete heart block, HF, or dysrhythmias. Diltiazem caused fetal harm in laboratory animals. Because this drug is secreted in human milk and has the potential to produce adverse effects, Breastfeeding is not recommended.

Verapamil (Calan, Isoptin SR, Verelan): Verapamil was the first CCB approved by the FDA. In the heart, verapamil slows conduction velocity and stabilizes dysrhythmias. The IV form of the drug is indicated for the rapid control of acute atrial dysrhythmias. Because verapamil can cause bradycardia and AV block, patients with HF should be carefully monitored. Because the drug may produce profound bradycardia, patients should notify their healthcare provider if their heart rate falls below 60 beats/min or if systolic blood pressure falls below 90 mmHg. The therapeutic serum level is 0.08 to 0.3 mcg/mL. A prototype drug feature that describes other indications for verapamil is presented in Chapter 30. Verapamil caused fetal harm in laboratory animals. Breastfeeding is not recommended during therapy.

CONNECTION Checkpoint 37.3

Nifedipine (Procardia) is a prototype CCB discussed in Chapter 30. From what you learned in Chapter 30, why is this drug (and other dihydropyridines) not effective in treating dysrhythmias?

Miscellaneous Antidysrhythmics

37.11 Adenosine and digoxin are used for specific dysrhythmias.

Two other medications, adenosine and digoxin, are occasionally used to treat specific dysrhythmias, but they do not act by the mechanisms described previously. Doses for these miscellaneous drugs are listed in Table 37.4.

Adenosine (Adenocard, Adenoscan): Adenosine is a naturally occurring nucleoside that activates potassium channels in the SA and AV nodes, causing the potassium to leave cardiac muscle cells. When given as a rapid 1- to 2-second IV bolus, adenosine blocks reentry pathways in the AV node and terminates the tachycardia. It is usually followed by a 1- to 5-second period of asystole. Patients should be laid supine prior to adenosine use and warned that they may feel faint. The IV site used to give adenosine should be antecubital or above, and an 18-gauge angiocatheter or larger should be used. A rapid saline flush immediately after instillation of the medication is necessary due to its short half-life. Immediate medical assistance must be nearby during the procedure. If the tachycardia has not been eliminated in 1 to 2 minutes, a second rapid bolus may be given. The primary indication for adenosine is PSVT, for which adenosine is a preferred drug. It is also used to assist in the diagnosis of CAD of dysrhythmias in patients who are unable to undergo a cardiac exercise stress test. It is not effective in treating ventricular dysrhythmias. Although the drug has prodysrhythmic effects and dyspnea is common, adverse effects are generally self-limiting because of its 10-second half-life. In 2013, the FDA issued a safety alert that the use of adenosine may be associated with an increased risk of heart attack and death. It is not known if adenosine causes fetal harm if administered during pregnancy or produces adverse effects in the breastfed neonate.

Digoxin (Lanoxicaps, Lanoxin): Although digoxin is primarily used to treat HF, it is also prescribed for atrial flutter or fibrillation and PSVT because of its ability to decrease automaticity of the SA node and slow conduction through the AV node. The drug is not effective against ventricular dysrhythmias. Because excessive levels of digoxin can produce serious dysrhythmias and interactions with other medications are common, patients must be carefully monitored during therapy. Additional information on the mechanism of action, adverse effects, and clinician responsibilities for digoxin may be found in Chapter 36, where the drug is featured as a prototype.

CONNECTIONS: APPLIED CLINICAL JUDGMENT

Patients Receiving Pharmacotherapy for Dysrhythmias

Key Assessment Data

- History of current condition, baseline vital signs, physical exam findings; history of cardiovascular disease, including HTN, MI, and HF, musculoskeletal (preexisting conditions that might cause fatigue or weakness), hepatic and renal disease; drug history including allergies, current prescription and over-the-counter (OTC) drugs, herbal preparations, and alcohol use; pregnancy status.
- Ongoing assessment during drug therapy includes laboratory findings including electrolytes, especially potassium, liver and renal function studies; lipid profiles; cardiac monitoring. Assess for location, character, and amount of edema, if present.

Desired Therapeutic Outcomes

- Improvement is observed and measurable by diminished or absence of dysrhythmias. Blood pressure and pulse remain within normal limits.

Minimizing Adverse Effects

- Not all dysrhythmias are symptomatic. Assess apical pulse rate for 1 full minute. Correlate symptoms with an ECG to assist in determining the need for further symptom management.
- A first-dose effect may occur with a significant drop in blood pressure with the first few doses. Orthostatic hypotension may increase the risk of falls and injury.
- Hypokalemia, hypocalcemia, and hypomagnesemia increase the risk of dysrhythmias. Inadequate or high levels of antidysrhythmic drugs may lead to increased or more lethal dysrhythmias. Continue to monitor periodic electrolyte levels, especially potassium, ECG as appropriate, and hepatic and renal function laboratory values.
- Weigh daily and report weight gain over 1 kg (2 lb) in a 24-hour period or increasing edema. Weight gain or edema may indicate adverse drug effects or worsening cardiovascular disease processes.
- Monitor for increasing dyspnea or postural nocturnal dyspnea, rales or crackles in the lungs, and frothy, pink-tinged sputum, which may signal HF due to negative inotropic effects of the drug. Potassium channel blockers are associated with pulmonary toxicity.
- Observe for hypersensitivity reaction or angioedema, especially of the facial area, which may occur with calcium channel blockers. Potassium channel blockers may cause photosensitivity, skin rashes, and blurred vision
- While uncommon, monitor for gingival hyperplasia or signs of gingivitis if calcium channel blockers or phenytoin is used.

Lifespan Considerations

- Orthostatic hypotension may increase the risk of falls and injury. Be particularly cautious with older adults who are at increased risk for hypotension. Ensure patient safety.
- Many antidysrhythmic drugs should not be taken during pregnancy, if pregnancy is suspected, or while breastfeeding.
- Lower dosages are required for older patients than would be used for younger patients.

Diversity Considerations

- Because of differences in acetylation and because some antidysrhythmics metabolize through the CYP450 pathways, monitor ethnically diverse patients more frequently to ensure optimal therapeutic effects and to minimize adverse effects.

Patient and Caregiver Education

- Monitor pulse, BP, and daily weight, using a diary or log, and bring these to each provider visit. Promptly report any weight gain over 1 kg in a 24-hour period or increasing edema to the provider.
- Immediately report any severe shortness of breath, frothy sputum, profound fatigue, or swelling of extremities.
- Rise slowly from lying or sitting to standing, pausing between changes if dizziness occurs. Don't take the medication if dizziness continues, or the BP is below 90/60 or per parameters set by the provider, and contact the provider for further instructions.
- Immediately seek medical attention for difficulty breathing, throat tightness, hives or rash, muscle cramps, or tremors. Promptly report any angioedema around the facial area.
- Maintain good oral hygiene and regular dental appointments.
- Avoid alcohol and melatonin use, which may increase risk for hypotension, drowsiness, and dizziness. Grapefruit juice may increase drug levels with increased adverse effects and should also be avoided.
- Carry a wallet identification card or wear medical identification jewelry indicating the type of antidysrhythmic therapy taken.

Prescribing Considerations

- Before prescribing, visit www.drug-interactions.com to ensure no interactions with other medications.
- Routine laboratory testing at least every 6 months should include at a minimum assessment of electrolytes, thyroid, liver, and kidney function tests.

Understanding Chapter 37

Key Concepts Summary

37.1 Some dysrhythmias produce no patient symptoms, whereas others may be life-threatening.

37.2 The phases of cardiac action potential include rapid depolarization, a long plateau, and repolarization.

37.3 The electrocardiogram is used to measure electrical conduction across the myocardium.

37.4 Dysrhythmias are classified by the impulse origin and type of rhythm abnormality produced.

37.5 Antidysrhythmic drugs are only used when there is a clear benefit to the patient.

37.6 Antidysrhythmic drugs are classified by their mechanism of action.

37.7 Class I antidysrhythmics act by blocking ion channels in myocardial cells.

37.8 Beta-adrenergic antagonists reduce automaticity and slow conduction velocity in the heart.

37.9 Potassium channel blockers prolong the refractory period of the heart.

37.10 Calcium channel blockers are used to treat atrial dysrhythmias.

37.11 Adenosine and digoxin are used for specific dysrhythmias.

CASE STUDY: Making the Patient Connection

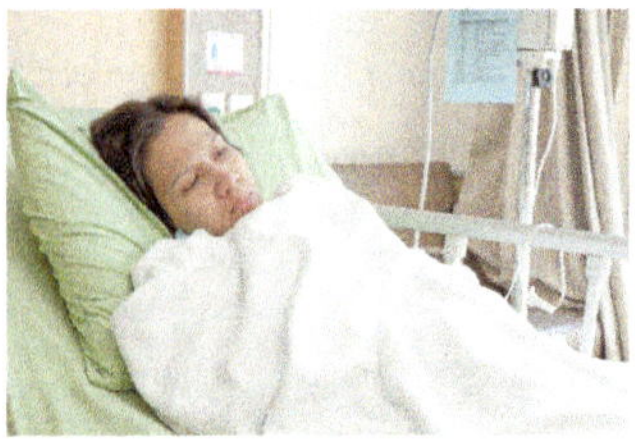

Remember the patient "Jada Chinn Nguyen" at the beginning of the chapter? Now read the remainder of the case study. Based on the information presented within this chapter, respond to the critical thinking questions that follow.

The day had been busy as Jada prepared for her daughter's upcoming wedding. There were so many arrangements to be made, and she felt overwhelmed. During the day Jada experienced heaviness in her chest, but she attributed it to the stress of the wedding and perhaps a touch of bronchitis. Nonetheless, she knew there was no time to stop and rest; there was too much to do.

Later that afternoon, Jada realized that she had to take it easy. Then she experienced that strange sensation once again. As she sat in a chair, Jada suddenly felt dizzy with extreme weakness and difficulty breathing. Her family members report that she became pale and unexpectedly collapsed. Emergency personnel were called to the scene, and Jada was taken to the nearest hospital.

In the emergency department, Jada's physical examination revealed the following findings: weak, middle-aged Asian woman; vital signs: blood pressure, 102/68 mmHg; heart rate, 116 beats/min; respiratory rate, 18 breaths/min, afebrile; weight 53 kg (116 lb). She has clear bilateral breath sounds and active bowel sounds heard in all four quadrants. Her ECG reveals atrial fibrillation with a ventricular rate of 116 beats/min. She is admitted to the coronary care unit for further testing and observation.

Critical Thinking Questions

1. Jada's ECG shows atrial fibrillation. Trace the electrical conduction system through the heart. What part of the ECG complex would be most affected by this patient's medical diagnosis?
2. While in the coronary care unit, Jada will receive amiodarone IV infusion. She wants to know how long she will need to receive the IV medication and how it works. How would you respond to this patient's questions?
3. Because the lack of atrial contraction in atrial fibrillation may lead to the development of a thrombus, increasing stroke risk, what additional drug therapy would be anticipated for this patient?
4. The patient is being discharged on amiodarone 400 mg twice daily. What instructions should this patient receive?

Additional Case Study

Malcolm Hibbert is a 56-year-old man who was diagnosed with a rapid atrial dysrhythmia and placed on diltiazem (Cardizem) to control the condition. He has been surfing the internet to find out more about his condition and drug therapy. When he returns to the clinic, he has multiple questions to ask you. How would you respond to each of the following?

1. "My neighbor had a fast heartbeat and now he's on something called digoxin. Why didn't they use that for me?"
2. "If I'm on a calcium channel blocker, does that mean my bones might get weak?"
3. "Might any of my medications cause an increase in dysrhythmias?"

Chapter Review

1. A healthcare provider has ordered procainamide for each of four patients. A nurse should question the order for a patient with which condition?
   1. Ventricular tachycardia
   2. Paroxysmal atrial tachycardia
   3. Atrial fibrillation
   4. Severe heart failure

2. A patient is receiving intravenous lidocaine for ventricular dysrhythmias. Which nursing intervention is appropriate for this therapy?
   1. Monitor the patient for decreased platelet levels.
   2. Place the patient in a supine position during administration.
   3. Monitor for paresthesias, drowsiness, or confusion.
   4. Encourage coughing and deep breathing to remove secretions.

3. The patient with a rapid atrial dysrhythmia is being treated with verapamil (Calan). The nurse would monitor for therapeutic effectiveness by noting which of the following?
   1. Change in blood pressure
   2. Increase in serum potassium level
   3. Changes in cardiac rhythm
   4. Reduction in urine output

4. A patient is to receive adenosine for rapid supraventricular tachycardia. This drug must be administered:
   1. Over a 24-hour period by IV drip.
   2. Along with potassium chloride to prevent electrolyte imbalance.
   3. Over 20 to 30 minutes IV.
   4. By a rapid IV bolus injection over 1 to 2 seconds.

5. The patient is prescribed propranolol (Inderal) for the treatment of atrial dysrhythmias associated with heart failure. The nurse knows this drug is used cautiously in patients with HF because of which effect?
   1. It causes sodium retention, worsening congestion.
   2. Its adverse effects include HTN, worsening HF.
   3. It is a negative inotropic drug and will decrease myocardial contractility and cardiac output.
   4. It may cause bronchoconstriction.

6. A patient is being discharged with a diagnosis of dysrhythmias. The nurse is teaching the patient about amiodarone. What patient teaching is needed related to this medication?
   1. Avoid crowds while taking this medication.
   2. Avoid birth control pills and use an alternate form of birth control.
   3. Wear protective clothing and adequate sunscreen.
   4. Use an electric razor to shave.

See Appendix A for answers to critical thinking questions, case study questions, and review questions.

References

January, C. T., Wann, L. S., Calkins, H., Chen, L. Y., Cigarroa, J. E., Cleveland, J. C., et al. (2019). 2019 AHA/ACC/HRS focused update of the 2014 AHA/ACC/HRS guideline for the management of patients with atrial fibrillation: A report of the American College of Cardiology/American Heart Association Task Force on Clinical Practice Guidelines and the Heart Rhythm Society. *Journal of the American College of Cardiology, 74*(1), 104–132. https://doi.org/10.1016/j.jacc.2019.01.011

Sovari, A. A. (2017). *Long QT syndrome*. Medscape. https://emedicine.medscape.com/article/157826-overview

Zhou, H. H., Shay, S. D., & Wood, A. J. (1993). Contribution of differences in plasma binding of propranolol to ethnic differences in sensitivity. Comparisons between Chinese and Caucasians. *Chinese Medical Journal, 106 (12)*, 898–902.

Selected Bibliography

American Heart Association. (2016). *About arrhythmia*. http://www.heart.org/HEARTORG/Conditions/Arrhythmia/AboutArrhythmia/About-Arrhythmia_UCM_002010_Article.jsp#.V_RSkijt4RY

Atwood, S., Stanton, C., & Storey-Davenport, J. (2018). *Introduction to basic cardiac dysrhythmias* (5th ed.). Jones & Bartlett.

Carlisle, M. A., Fudim, M., DeVore, A. D., & Piccini, J. P. (2019). Heart failure and atrial fibrillation, like fire and fury. *JACC: Heart Failure, 7*(6), 447–456.

Ferdinand, K. C., & Puckrein, G. A. (2015). Race/ ethnicity in atrial fibrillation stroke: Epidemiology and pharmacotherapy. *Journal of the National Medical Association, 107*(1), 59–67. https://doi.org/10.1016/S0027-9684(15)30010-9

Ferreira, J. P., & Santos, M. (2015). Heart failure and atrial fibrillation: From basic science to clinical practice. *International Journal of Molecular Sciences, 16*, 3133–3147. https://doi.org/10.3390/ijms16023133

Halpern, D. G., Weinberg, C. R., Pinnelas, R., Mehta-Lee, S., Economy, K. E., & Valente, A. M. (2019). Use of medication for cardiovascular disease during pregnancy: JACC state-of-the-art review. *Journal of the American College of Cardiology, 73*(4), 457–476. https://doi.org/10.1016/j.jacc.2018.10.075

Huang, C. L. H., Wu, L., Jeevaratnam, K., & Lei, M. (2020). Update on antiarrhythmic drug pharmacology. *Journal of Cardiovascular Electrophysiology, 31*(2), 579–592. https://doi.org/10.1111/jce.14347

Sasi, N. (2019). *Antidysrhythmic toxicity*. Medscape. https://emedicine.medscape.com/article/813046-overview

Tse, G. (2016). Mechanisms of cardiac arrhythmias. *Journal of Arrhythmia, 32*, 75–81. https://doi.org/10.1016/j.joa.2015.11.003

Turagam, M. K., Flaker, G. C., Velagapudi, P., Vadali, S., & Alpert, M. A. (2015). Atrial fibrillation in athletes: Pathophysiology, clinical presentation, evaluation and management. *Journal of Atrial Fibrillation, 8*(4), 1309. https://doi.org/10.4022/jafib.1309

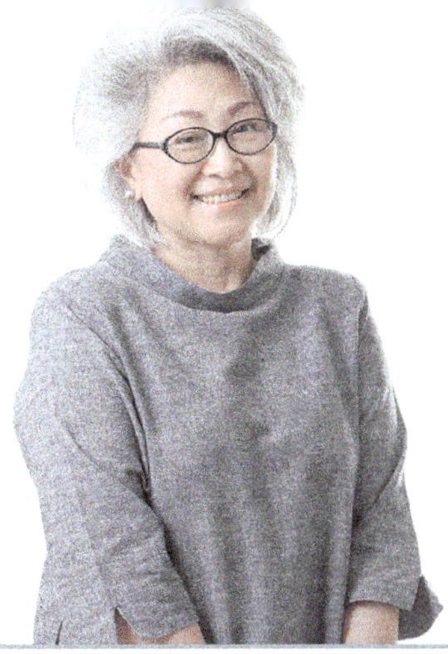

"Ever since I returned from my trip to Bangkok, my right calf has really hurt. I first thought my arthritis was flaring up again, especially after sitting on the plane for so long."
—*Patient "Jihyo Yun"*

Chapter 38
Pharmacotherapy of Coagulation Disorders

Chapter Outline

Learning Outcomes

After reading this chapter, the student should be able to:

1. Describe primary risk factors for thromboembolic disorders.
2. Explain the etiology and symptoms of coagulation disorders.
3. Identify the primary mechanisms by which coagulation-modifying drugs act.
4. Explain how laboratory testing of coagulation parameters is used to monitor anticoagulant pharmacotherapy.
5. Describe the nurse's role in the pharmacologic management of patients with coagulation disorders.
6. For each of the classes shown in the chapter outline, identify the prototype and representative drugs and explain the mechanism(s) of drug action, primary indications, contraindications, significant drug interactions, pregnancy data, and important adverse effects.
7. Apply clinical judgment to care for patients receiving pharmacotherapy for coagulation disorders.

Key Terms

Definitions of the terms in bold may be found in the Glossary.

Everyone is familiar with the bleeding associated with simple cuts and scrapes, and we take for granted that bleeding will stop in a few minutes. The stoppage of blood flow, or hemostasis, is complex and essential to our well-being. The underlying mechanisms of hemostasis promote blood clotting that protects us from injuries that could lead to shock and perhaps death. Too much clotting, however, can be just as dangerous. The physiologic processes of hemostasis must maintain a delicate balance between blood fluidity and coagulation.

Many common diseases and conditions affect hemostasis, including myocardial infarction (MI), stroke, venous or arterial thrombosis, sepsis, and cancer. Because these conditions are prevalent in clinical practice, nurses will have frequent occasions to administer and monitor the effects of coagulation-modifying medications. Drugs may be used to enhance coagulation, inhibit coagulation, or dissolve existing clots to restore blood flow.

Disorders of Hemostasis

38.1 Thromboembolic disorders are abnormalities of hemostasis that include deep vein thrombosis and pulmonary embolism.

Coagulation is regulated by a large number of natural substances circulating in the blood. Some of these are **procoagulants**, which favor the formation of clots, while others are **anticoagulants**, which inhibit clot formation. Coagulation, then, can be thought of as a delicate balance between procoagulants and anticoagulants. For example, injuries to blood vessels release procoagulants that tip the balance in favor of initiating coagulation. The student should review the coagulation cascade presented in Chapter 28 before proceeding.

Once a stationary clot, or thrombus, forms in a vessel, it often grows larger as more fibrin is added. Pieces of the thrombus may break off and travel in the bloodstream to block other vessels. A traveling clot is called an *embolus*. Because these two conditions often occur concurrently in patients, the term **thromboembolic disorder** is used to describe conditions in which the body forms undesirable clots. Thromboembolic disorders may be classified as either venous or arterial.

Venous thromboembolism (VTE) is a common condition that occurs when blood flow through a vein is very slow (stasis). Venous stasis allows procoagulation factors to accumulate and overcome the natural anticoagulant substances in the blood. There are two primary manifestations of VTE: deep vein thrombosis and pulmonary embolism.

When thrombosis occurs in the legs it is called **deep vein thrombosis (DVT)**. Because blood flow is slowest in the deep veins of the lower limbs, these vessels are the most common sites for VTE. Conditions associated with venous stasis and DVT include the following:

- **Extended immobility.** During major illness or following surgery, patients may be immobile for extended periods. Because the movement of blood through the deep veins is entirely dependent on the squeezing action from skeletal muscular contraction, blood in the deep veins of these patients has difficulty returning to the heart.
- **Major trauma.** Trauma that causes serious bleeding activates procoagulation factors. In addition, stasis will likely occur surrounding the injured area, promoting the development of DVT. Trauma involving the lower extremities places the patient at high risk for DVT.
- **Major surgery.** Surgery of the lower extremities, especially knee and hip replacements, are common causes of DVT for the same reasons as trauma; bleeding activates procoagulation factors and stasis occurs around the surgical site.
- **Hypercoagulability states.** Malignancy, lupus, and pregnancy are examples of conditions associated with an increased risk of coagulation and DVT. Certain genetic disorders also produce hypercoagulability, the most common being a genetic deficiency of protein C, a natural anticoagulant.
- **Drug therapy.** High amounts of estrogen, prescribed as replacement therapy or as a component of oral contraceptives, have been associated with DVT in numerous studies. Selective estrogen receptor modulators, such as raloxifene (Evista), are also associated with a higher risk of DVT.

The second major thromboembolic disorder is **pulmonary embolism**, which occurs when a venous clot dislodges, migrates to the pulmonary vessels, and blocks arterial circulation to the lungs. Pulmonary emboli are the most serious consequence of VTE because death may occur within minutes after the onset of symptoms. The factors associated with an increased risk of pulmonary embolism are the same as those for patients with DVT: prolonged immobility, major trauma, lower-extremity surgery, hypercoagulability states, and estrogen therapy. Prevention of pulmonary embolism is a primary goal for all patients with VTE and a major indication for pharmacotherapy.

Patients with DVT are sometimes asymptomatic, or report nonspecific symptoms such as pain, swelling, or warmth of the legs. The disorder may be present for years, causing progressive damage to venous valves, thus worsening blood flow in the region and increasing the risk of an acute episode. A pulmonary embolism, however, produces a sudden onset of cough, chest pain, tachypnea, dyspnea, tachycardia, and hemoptysis. Symptoms of pulmonary embolism resemble an MI, and rapid diagnosis and treatment are essential.

PharmFACT

Up to 30% of patients presenting with DVT have a malignancy. This is because about 90% of patients with cancer have some abnormal clotting factors (Patel, 2019).

Arterial thromboembolism may deprive an area of blood flow and is a medical emergency because tissue hypoxia and cellular death will result soon after blood stoppage. The most serious arterial thromboembolism disorders are MI and stroke.

Arterial thrombi and emboli commonly result from procedures involving arterial punctures such as angiography and stent placement. They may also originate from the heart. Emboli are common complications of mitral valve disease, prosthetic heart valves, and atrial dysrhythmias. Emboli originating from the left side of the heart may lodge in any organ in the body.

CONNECTION Checkpoint 38.1

Coagulation occurs by intrinsic and extrinsic pathways. From what you learned in Chapter 28, which pathway is activated when blood leaks from a vessel? Which is more complex and takes several minutes? Which results in the formation of fibrin?

38.2 Coagulation disorders are caused by decreased numbers of platelets or by deficiencies in specific clotting factors.

Whereas thromboembolic disorders are caused by too much clotting, coagulation disorders result from too little clotting. Serious consequences result if the body does not form clots in a timely manner. The two most common etiologies of coagulation disorders are decreased numbers of platelets and deficiencies in one or more clotting factors.

Platelets are central to the process of coagulation. Recognizing a site of vessel injury, activated platelets release von Willebrand's factor, which causes platelets to become "sticky" and adhere to the site. Following adhesion, platelets secrete substances such as adenosine diphosphate (ADP) and thromboxane A_2 that promote platelet aggregation and the formation of a platelet plug at the site. Procoagulation factors become activated on the platelets, resulting in a fibrin mesh clot. Nearly every step of this pathway requires sufficient numbers of properly functioning platelets.

The most common coagulation disorder is a deficiency of platelets, or **thrombocytopenia**, which occurs when platelet counts fall below 150,000 mm^3. Thrombocytopenia is the result of either decreased platelet production or increased platelet destruction. Any condition or disease that suppresses bone marrow function has the potential to cause decreased platelet production. Other common causes of decreased platelet production are folic acid or vitamin B_{12} deficiencies and decreased production of thrombopoietin by the liver during hepatic failure. Increased destruction of platelets may occur in patients with thrombocytopenic purpura, disseminated intravascular coagulation (DIC), or lupus.

Of special concern is thrombocytopenia caused by drug therapy. A significant number of drugs have the potential to increase platelet destruction, either by direct toxic effects on bone marrow or by inducing the immune system to destroy them. When caring for patients receiving these drugs, the nurse must be vigilant in assessing the results of blood laboratory tests and observing for signs of thrombocytopenia such as bleeding gums, nosebleeds, and extensive bruising. Selected drugs that cause thrombocytopenia are listed in Table 38.1. Heparin-induced thrombocytopenia, a particularly serious form of this disorder, is discussed in Section 38.4.

Deficiencies in specific clotting factors may prolong coagulation and lead to excess bleeding. Deficiencies in multiple coagulation factors occur frequently in patients with serious hepatic impairment because the liver synthesizes most clotting factors. Deficiency in a single coagulation factor suggests **hemophilia**, a series of coagulation disorders caused by genetic deficiencies in specific clotting factors. Hemophilia disorders are typified by prolonged coagulation times, resulting in persistent bleeding that can

Table 38.1 Selected Drugs That Cause Thrombocytopenia

Class	Examples
Analgesics	acetaminophen, aspirin, diclofenac, ibuprofen, indomethacin, morphine, naproxen
Anticoagulants and antiplatelets	clopidogrel, glycoprotein IIb/IIIa inhibitors, heparin
Anti-infectives	acyclovir, amphotericin B, ampicillin, clarithromycin, ethambutol, fluconazole, indinavir, isoniazid, itraconazole, linezolid, oxacillin, piperacillin, rifampin, sulfonamides, trimethoprim, vancomycin
Antineoplastic and immunotherapy drugs	carboplatin, interferon-alfa, methotrexate
Cardiovascular drugs	amiodarone, atorvastatin, captopril, digoxin, hydrochlorothiazide, nitroglycerin, procainamide, quinidine, simvastatin
Central nervous system drugs	carbamazepine, chlorpromazine, diazepam, haloperidol, lithium, phenobarbital, phenytoin, valproic acid
Other drug classes	cimetidine, isotretinoin, measles–mumps–rubella vaccine, octreotide, sirolimus

be acute or chronic. Patients may experience various forms of the disease, with symptoms ranging from mild to severe. Approximately two-thirds of patients with hemophilia will report a family history of the disease. The pharmacotherapy of hemophilia is described in Section 38.14.

To diagnose coagulation and thromboembolic disorders, a thorough medical history and physical examination are necessary. Laboratory tests measuring coagulation must be obtained. These usually include a whole-blood clotting time, **prothrombin time (PT)**, thrombin time, **activated partial thromboplastin time (aPTT)**, liver function tests, platelet count, and, in some instances, a bleeding time. Another test frequently ordered to assess hemostatic function is the D-dimer. D-dimer tests are used to help rule out the presence of a thrombus, DVT, and pulmonary embolism. Additional tests, such as serum levels of specific clotting factors, may be indicated.

Overview of Coagulation Modifiers

38.3 The normal coagulation process can be modified by a number of different mechanisms.

Medications can be used to modify hemostasis in a number of ways. An overview of the basic mechanisms of coagulation-modifying drugs is presented in Table 38.2. These mechanisms are illustrated in Figure 38.1.

The most commonly prescribed coagulation modifiers are the anticoagulants and antiplatelet drugs. Although they work by different mechanisms, both of these drug classes have the ability to prevent clot formation or enlargement. Some basic differences between the two are as follows:

- **Anticoagulant drugs** inhibit specific clotting factors in the coagulation cascade. Patients usually call these drugs "blood thinners," but that is an inaccurate description because they do not change the viscosity or thickness of the blood. Examples include heparin and warfarin (Coumadin).
- **Antiplatelet drugs** inhibit the clotting action of platelets. Examples include aspirin and clopidogrel (Plavix).

Compared to antiplatelets, anticoagulants are considered more aggressive therapy for those at high risk for strokes. However, anticoagulants carry a higher risk of serious adverse effects, participate in more drug interactions, and require more extensive follow-up (American Stroke Association, 2018). Anticoagulants and antiplatelets are widely used for thromboembolic disease and are discussed in Sections 38.4 through 38.6.

Once an abnormal clot has formed, it may block blood vessels that serve critical tissues; it must be quickly removed to restore normal function. This is particularly important for vessels serving the heart, lungs, and brain. A specific class of drugs, the fibrinolytics, has been developed to dissolve life-threatening clots. These drugs are presented in Section 38.12.

Coagulation modifiers are also used to promote the formation of clots. Drugs called hemostatics inhibit the normal removal of fibrin, thus keeping the clot in place for a longer period of time. These drugs are primarily used to speed clot formation to limit bleeding from a surgical site; they are discussed in Section 38.13. For patients with hemophilia, clotting factors may be administered to promote clotting by providing a missing or deficient component in the coagulation cascade, as presented in Section 38.14.

Because hemostasis involves a fine balance of factors favoring clotting versus those inhibiting clotting, pharmacotherapy with coagulation modifiers is individualized to each patient. Serious adverse effects may occur if the drugs are not used properly; therefore, these patients will require frequent assessment and monitoring to ensure that the goal of normal coagulation is being achieved without serious adverse events.

Table 38.2 Overview of Coagulation Modifiers

Type of Modification	Mechanism	Drug Classification
Prevention of clot formation	Inhibition of specific clotting factors	Anticoagulants
	Inhibition of platelet actions	Antiplatelet drugs
Removal of an existing clot	Clot dissolved by the drug	Fibrinolytics
Promotion of clot formation	Inhibition of fibrin destruction	Hemostatics
	Administration of missing clotting factors	Clotting factor concentrates

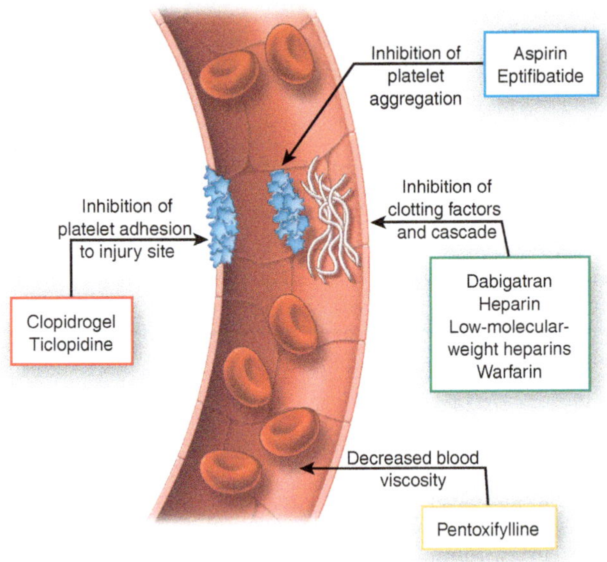

Figure 38.1 Mechanisms of action of coagulation modifiers.

Anticoagulants

38.4 Heparin is the traditional drug for rapid anticoagulation.

Extensively used in the treatment of thromboembolic disease, anticoagulants lengthen clotting time and prevent thrombi from forming or growing larger. Since thromboembolic disease can be life-threatening, therapy is often begun by administering anticoagulants parenterally to achieve the most rapid onset of action. As the disease stabilizes and the desired degree of anticoagulation has been achieved, the patient is gradually switched to oral anticoagulants, with careful monitoring of appropriate coagulation laboratory values. Traditionally, the most frequently prescribed parenteral anticoagulant has been heparin; warfarin is the prototype oral anticoagulant (see Section 38.5). The anticoagulants are listed in Table 38.3.

Heparin is a natural chemical found in the liver and the lining of blood vessels. As a drug, heparin has been used for many decades and is one of the few drugs still obtained from animal tissue, usually beef lung or pig intestine. Chemically, heparin is a special type of carbohydrate called a glycosaminoglycan that consists of repeated disaccharide units of differing lengths. Thus, heparin is actually a mixture of different molecules, varying in size. This drug is also called *unfractionated* heparin because it contains a mixture of different molecular pieces or "fractions." This mixture affects protein binding and drug bioavailability and is partially responsible for the wide variation in patient responses to heparin.

Heparin produces its anticoagulant effects by binding to **antithrombin III (AT-III)**. As its name implies, antithrombin inactivates thrombin (as well as several other clotting factors). The binding to heparin produces a structural change in AT-III that makes it 1000 times more active in inhibiting thrombin, Factor Xa, Factor IXa, and other substances involved in coagulation. Within minutes after intravenous (IV) administration, the loss of these activated clotting factors prevents the formation of fibrin clots.

Because responses to heparin anticoagulation vary considerably among patients, regular monitoring of laboratory values during heparin therapy is essential to patient safety. The aPTT value is the conventional measurement that guides heparin therapy, with normal values ranging from 25 to 40 seconds. For therapeutic anticoagulation, the aPTT should be between 1.5 and 2 times the patient's baseline, or

Table 38.3 Anticoagulants

Drug	Route and Adult Dose (Maximum Dose Where Indicated)	Adverse Effects
antithrombin, recombinant (ATryn)	IV infusion: Dose is individualized based on pretreatment antithrombin level and body weight	*Minor bleeding, nausea and vomiting, transient thrombocytopenia (heparin), anemia (fondaparinux)* Hemorrhage, anaphylaxis, heparin-induced thrombocytopenia
fondaparinux (Arixtra)	Subcutaneous: 2.5 mg/day starting at least 6 h postop for 5–9 days (max: 10 mg/day)	
heparin	IV: 5000-unit bolus dose, then 20,000–40,000 units infused over 24 h (use agency-specific heparin nomogram) Subcutaneous: 10,000–20,000 units followed by 8000–20,000 units q8–12h	
warfarin (Coumadin)	PO: Dose varies based on target international normalized ratio (INR), which is usually within the range of 2–3	
Low-Molecular-Weight Heparins		
dalteparin (Fragmin)	Subcutaneous (DVT prophylaxis): 2500–5000 units/day for 5–10 days (max: 18,000 international units/day) Subcutaneous (DVT treatment): 120 international units/kg bid	*Minor bleeding, nausea and vomiting, hematoma, local pain, fever* Hemorrhage, thrombocytopenia, pancytopenia, anaphylaxis, local site reactions
enoxaparin (Lovenox)	Subcutaneous (DVT prophylaxis): 30 mg bid Subcutaneous (DVT treatment): 1 mg/kg q12h or 1.5 mg/kg/day IV (acute STEMI): 30-mg bolus followed by subcutaneous doses	
Direct Thrombin Inhibitors		
argatroban (Acova, Novastan)	IV: 2 mcg/kg/min (max: 10 mcg/kg/min)	*Fever, nausea, allergic skin reactions, hepatic impairment, pneumonia, fever, minor bleeding, back pain (bivalirudin)* Serious internal hemorrhage, hemoptysis, hematuria, sepsis, heart failure (HF)
bivalirudin (Angiomax)	IV: 0.75 mg/kg initial bolus followed by 1.75 mg/kg/h for 4 h	
dabigatran (Pradaxa)	PO: 75–150 mg bid	
Factor Xa Inhibitors		
apixaban (Eliquis)	PO: 5 mg bid	*Minor bleeding, rash* Major bleeding, including stroke; anemia; hypersensitivity reactions
betrixaban (Bevyxxa)	PO: Single dose of 160 mg followed by 80 mg once daily	
edoxaban (Savaysa)	PO: 30–60 mg once daily	
rivaroxaban (Xarelto)	PO: 10–20 mg once daily	

Note: *Italics* indicate common adverse effects. Underline indicates serious adverse effects.

60 to 80 seconds. Elevated aPTT values indicate the patient is at high risk for bleeding and that a reduction in heparin dose is necessary. aPTT values of less than 60 seconds indicate the need for higher heparin doses. During continuous IV heparin therapy, the aPTT is measured daily and 6 to 8 hours after any changes in dosage.

The heparin molecule has been shortened and modified to create a different class of drugs called *low-molecular-weight heparins (LMWHs)*. Given subcutaneously, the mechanism of action of these drugs is very similar to that of heparin, except the shorter heparin molecules are unable to bind thrombin, making them more selective for Factor Xa inhibition. For some applications, the LMWHs have begun to replace traditional heparin anticoagulation.

LMWHs possess the same anticoagulant activity as heparin but have several advantages. They produce a more predictable anticoagulant response than heparin because there is less binding of the drug to proteins and macrophages; therefore, less frequent laboratory monitoring is required. They are about 10 times less likely to cause thrombocytopenia, a potentially serious adverse effect of heparin. They also exhibit a half-life that is two to four times longer than heparin that permits once-daily dosing, and family members or the patient can be trained to give the necessary subcutaneous injections at home. Like heparin, the LMWHs do not cross the placenta. LMWHs have become first-line drugs for a number of clotting disorders, including the prevention of DVT following surgery.

When using LMWHs, the aPTT laboratory value does not reflect the anticoagulant effects of the drugs because aPTT is insensitive to changes in Factor Xa. Instead, dosage calculations with LMWHs are fixed and based on the patient's weight. A given amount of subcutaneous LMWH results in a predictable plasma drug level. This is a major advantage over heparin, for which levels continually fluctuate and doses must be adjusted based on aPTT levels. In highly unstable patients or those with chronic kidney disease (CKD), measurement of anti–factor Xa activity may be used to gauge therapeutic response. Acceptable target values for anti–factor Xa range from 0.5 to 1 unit/mL.

PROTOTYPE DRUG Heparin

Classification **Therapeutic:** Anticoagulant
Pharmacologic: Indirect thrombin inhibitor

Therapeutic Effects and Uses: Heparin is the traditional standard to which other parenteral anticoagulants are compared. Because it has an immediate onset of action when administered IV, heparin is a first-line drug for acute thromboembolic disorders where rapid anticoagulation is necessary. Subcutaneous heparin is injected into the deep fatty layers of the abdomen and may take up to 1 hour to achieve a therapeutic effect. A continuous IV infusion allows for better titration and finer management of aPTT values. Indications include DVT, pulmonary embolism, unstable angina, evolving MI, and prevention of thrombosis in high-risk patients. Heparin and LMWHs are preferred anticoagulants during pregnancy because heparin molecules are too large to cross the placenta. Heparin is also used to maintain the patency of peripheral catheters (heparin locks) and arterial lines.

Heparin prolongs coagulation time, thereby inhibiting excessive clotting within blood vessels. As a result, it prevents the enlargement of existing clots and the formation of new ones. It has no ability to dissolve existing clots. Clotting time is prolonged, although bleeding time is only affected at high doses.

Mechanism of Action: Heparin activates the enzyme antithrombin III, which in turn inhibits thrombin. To a lesser extent, and by a separate mechanism, heparin also inactivates Factor Xa. Other clotting factors are affected by heparin, but these have less clinical significance. High doses interfere with platelet aggregation.

Pharmacokinetics:

Route(s)	Subcutaneous, IV bolus injection, or continuous infusion
Absorption	Heparin is poorly absorbed by the gastrointestinal (GI) mucosa because of rapid metabolism by the hepatic enzyme heparinase
Distribution	Unknown; does not cross the placenta and is not secreted in breast milk
Primary metabolism	Hepatic and by reticuloendothelial system
Primary excretion	Reticuloendothelial system
Onset of action	Subcutaneous: 30–60 min; IV: immediate
Duration of action	8–12 h; half-life: 90 min

Adverse Effects: Abnormal bleeding occurs in about 10% of patients and is the most serious adverse effect. Bleeding may be major or minor and may involve any system in the body. The risk of bleeding is dose dependent; the higher the dose, the greater the risk. Should the aPTT become excessively prolonged or bleeding be observed, discontinuation of the drug will result in loss of anticoagulant activity within hours. **Black Box Warning:** Epidural or spinal hematomas may occur when heparin or LMWHs are used in patients receiving spinal anesthesia or lumbar puncture. Because these can result in long-term or permanent paralysis, frequent monitoring for neurologic impairment is essential.

Heparin-induced thrombocytopenia (HIT) is a serious complication that occurs in up to 30% of patients taking the drug. Symptoms range from mild to severe. More severe symptoms usually appear after 5 to 10 days of therapy; thus, frequent blood laboratory testing should be conducted during this period. Although thrombocytopenia usually leads to excessive bleeding, HIT causes the opposite effect: an increase in adverse thrombotic events. HIT markedly increases platelet aggregation and the patient may experience serious and even life-threatening thrombosis. Although the half-life of heparin is brief, it may take a week after the drug is discontinued for platelets to recover. In addition, HIT may not even become evident until several weeks after the drug is discontinued.

Because heparin is derived from animal sources, hypersensitivity reactions are possible. Mild allergic symptoms include fever, chills, and urticaria. Anaphylaxis is rare. Osteoporosis has been reported in patients taking the drug longer than 30 days and may be severe enough to cause bone fractures. Skin lesions may develop, especially at the site of parenteral injections.

Contraindications/Precautions: Heparin should not be administered to patients with active internal bleeding, serious bleeding pathologies, severe hypertension (HTN), recent trauma, intracranial hemorrhage, or bacterial endocarditis. Some heparin products may contain sulfites and should not be administered to patients with sulfite sensitivity. Patients with severe thrombocytopenia or HIT should not be given heparin. Whenever possible, intramuscular (IM) injections of other medications should be avoided because they may cause serious bruising, bleeding, or hematomas. Although relatively safe during pregnancy, the drug should be used with caution during the peripartum period due to the risk of maternal hemorrhage. Caution must be used when administering heparin to patients with serious CKD or hepatic impairment because the drug may rise to toxic levels.

Drug Interactions: Oral anticoagulants, including warfarin, potentiate heparin activity. Drugs that inhibit platelet aggregation (such as aspirin, indomethacin, and ibuprofen) may induce bleeding. Nicotine, digoxin, tetracyclines, or antihistamines may inhibit anticoagulation. **Herbal/Food:** Herbal supplements that may affect coagulation such as ginger, garlic, green tea, feverfew, or ginkgo should be avoided because they may increase the risk of bleeding.

Pregnancy: Heparin does not cross the placenta and animal studies showed no teratogenicity. It is unlikely that any heparin secreted in breast milk is absorbed by the breastfed neonate.

Treatment of Overdose: If serious hemorrhage occurs, a specific antagonist, protamine sulfate, may be administered IV (1 mg for every 100 units of heparin) to neutralize the anticoagulant activity of heparin. Protamine sulfate has an onset of action of 5 minutes and a duration of 2 hours. Multiple doses may be necessary to control extensive hemorrhaging. Protamine is also an antagonist to the LMWHs.

Clinician Responsibilities: Key clinical implications for patients receiving heparin are included in Applied Clinical Judgment: Patients Receiving Pharmacotherapy with Anticoagulants.

Drugs Similar to Heparin

The LMWHs include dalteparin and enoxaparin. A third LMWH, tinzaparin, is no longer marketed in the United States. Antithrombin (recombinant) and fondaparinux are parenteral anticoagulants that act by unique mechanisms.

Antithrombin, recombinant (ATryn): ATryn is a unique coagulation modifier approved in 2009 to treat patients who have a congenital deficiency of antithrombin III. These patients have a high incidence of blood clots, especially DVT. The drug is indicated for the *prevention* of thrombosis during surgical or obstetrical procedures in antithrombin-deficient patients. Antithrombin (ATryn) is unusual because it is obtained from genetically engineered goats. The goats are engineered through recombinant deoxyribonucleic acid (DNA) technology to secrete human antithrombin in their milk. The drug is then purified and powdered for reconstitution as an IV infusion.

Levels of antithrombin activity in the blood must be monitored before, during, and immediately following IV infusions of the drug. The initial and subsequent drug doses are based on the level of antithrombin activity. The treatment goal is to maintain blood antithrombin activity between 80 and 120% of normal. The most common adverse effects are hemorrhage and infusion site reaction. ATryn enhances the anticoagulant effect of heparin and LMWHs. Observational data from pregnant women have not demonstrated a risk for fetal abnormalities if administered during the third trimester. Because this drug is secreted in milk, breastfeeding is not recommended.

Dalteparin (Fragmin): As an LMWH, dalteparin has smaller glycosaminoglycan chains than unfractionated heparin. Approved in 1994, dalteparin is given by the subcutaneous route for the treatment and prophylaxis of DVT or pulmonary embolism in patients having abdominal surgery or hip replacement surgery or those with severely restricted movement during acute illness. Other approved indications include thrombosis prophylaxis in patients at increased risk due to unstable angina, an acute MI, or cancer. In 2019, dalteparin became the first drug ever approved to treat venous thromboembolism in pediatric patients one month or older. The usual time of therapy is 5 to 10 days after surgery, and aspirin is usually administered concurrently. Dalteparin has a longer half-life than heparin, which allows for less frequent dosing. Like other LMWHs, bleeding is the most serious adverse effect, and the drug should not be administered to patients with active bleeding. Dalteparin contains the same black box warning as heparin regarding the risk for spinal and epidural hematomas. Animal reproduction studies did not show evidence of fetal harm. Dalteparin enters milk but its effects on the breastfed neonate are unknown.

Enoxaparin (Lovenox): Enoxaparin was the first LMWH approved by the U.S. Food and Drug Administration (FDA) in 1993. Indications include treatment and prophylaxis of DVT and pulmonary embolism in patients having abdominal surgery or hip or knee replacement surgery or those with severely restricted movement during acute illness. The usual time of therapy is 12 to 14 days after surgery, and aspirin is usually administered concurrently. Some orthopedic procedures such as repair of hip fractures require more prolonged therapy. Enoxaparin may also be administered for the prophylaxis of coronary artery thrombosis and the prevention of ischemic complications in patients with acute coronary syndrome, for patients with unstable angina, and for patients having percutaneous coronary intervention (PCI). Bleeding is the most serious adverse effect, and the drug should not be administered to patients with active bleeding. Enoxaparin contains the same black box warning as heparin and dalteparin regarding the risk for spinal and epidural hematomas. Animal reproduction studies did not show evidence of significant fetal harm. Enoxaparin enters milk but its effects on the breastfed neonate are unknown.

Fondaparinux (Arixtra): Approved in 2001, fondaparinux is an anticoagulant used for many of the same indications as heparin and the LMWHs, but it has certain differences that make it unique. Fondaparinux is a synthetic drug that consists of only five saccharide units (a pentasaccharide) that is structurally identical to the region of the heparin molecule that binds AT-III. The pentasaccharide unit is able to selectively inhibit Factor Xa without directly affecting thrombin. Fondaparinux is only given by the subcutaneous route and is approved for the prophylaxis of VTE following orthopedic or abdominal surgery and for the treatment of acute DVT or pulmonary embolism in conjunction with warfarin. The usual time of therapy is 5 to 9 days after surgery. Like other anticoagulants, the most frequent adverse effects of fondaparinux are bleeding complications. Like the LMWHs, fondaparinux is administered as fixed doses based on the patient's weight, and routine laboratory monitoring is not required because aPTT and PT are not accurate measures of drug activity. Doses of fondaparinux are not interchangeable with heparin or the LMWHs. There is no specific antidote for overdose; administration of protamine is ineffective. Fondaparinux contains a similar black box warning as heparin regarding the risk for spinal and epidural hematomas. Animal reproduction studies with high doses did not show evidence of significant fetal harm. Fondaparinux enters milk but its effects on a breastfed neonate are unknown.

38.5 Warfarin is a widely used drug for oral anticoagulant therapy.

Although parenteral anticoagulants have the advantage of an almost immediate onset of action, drugs given by this route require close medical supervision because adverse effects such as bleeding can rapidly ensue. When the patient's condition allows, oral anticoagulants are used due to their convenience and greater safety.

Warfarin (Coumadin) has been available as an anticoagulant for over 50 years and is the historical prototype for oral anticoagulants. In acute situations, patients begin anticoagulation therapy with heparin and are switched to warfarin when their condition stabilizes. When transitioning, the two drugs must be administered concurrently for 2 to 3 days. This is because heparin has a brief half-life (90 minutes), and aPTT returns to normal within 2 to 3 hours following discontinuation of heparin. Warfarin, on the other hand, takes 1 to 3 days of therapy to achieve optimal anticoagulation. Thus, concomitant pharmacotherapy is necessary to ensure continuous anticoagulation. During this transition, risk of bleeding increases, due to the additive anticoagulant action of the two drugs.

Whereas heparin is monitored with aPTT values, the standard laboratory test used to monitor the effectiveness of warfarin is the PT value. The normal PT range is 12 to 15 seconds. During therapeutic anticoagulation, PT should increase to 1.5 to 2 times the patient's baseline. Because laboratory testing methods for PT vary, however, PT time

CONNECTIONS: Lifespan Considerations

Miscarriage Prevention with Anticoagulants

Miscarriage in pregnancy is devastating, and recurrent miscarriage even more so. Autoimmune diseases are related to poorer obstetric outcomes than that of the general population, especially in mothers with undiagnosed thrombophilia (genetic hypercoagulability disorders) such as antiphospholipid syndrome. In a study of women who had experienced recurrent miscarriages, after controlling for other potential causes of miscarriage (e.g., metabolic, anatomical, or chromosomal), the prevalence of thrombophilia was found to be higher in women with recurrent miscarriages, compared to the general population (Nahas et al., 2018).

Research on treatment recommendations for the use of heparin, LMWH, or aspirin for recurrent miscarriage before 10 weeks of pregnancy is ongoing and the use of anticoagulant therapy has shown mixed results for prevention of such miscarriages (Lin et al., 2019). It is recommended that a woman experiencing such loss discuss the situation with her provider and whether genetic testing should be conducted. If genetic coagulation abnormalities are found, heparin, LMWH, or aspirin may be considered an option.

is also reported as an INR value; INR values averaging 2.5 are considered therapeutic for most indications. PT is measured daily until the desired level of therapeutic anticoagulation is achieved. Then, the frequency of laboratory testing is decreased to weekly or monthly as the patient's condition stabilizes. Home monitoring devices are available to provide convenient and reliable INR values, which can guide patients to adjust their own medication amounts. Self-monitoring has its limitations, however. The devices are expensive and the patient or their caregiver must be capable of understanding how to properly adjust the dosage.

Several newer drugs have emerged as significant alternatives to warfarin for stroke prevention. While warfarin affects coagulation *indirectly* by inhibiting vitamin K, these newer drugs *directly* inhibit an aspect of the coagulation cascade. Thus, these drugs are referred to as direct oral anticoagulants (DOACs). The DOACs include three drugs that directly inhibit Factor Xa and one that directly inhibits thrombin. The Factor Xa inhibitors include rivaroxaban (Xarelto), apixaban (Eliquis), and edoxaban (Savaysa). The fourth DOAC is dabigatran (Pradaxa), which is a prototype thrombin inhibitor discussed in Section 38.6.

PROTOTYPE DRUG Warfarin (Coumadin)

Classification **Therapeutic:** Anticoagulant
Pharmacologic: Vitamin K antagonist

Therapeutic Effects and Uses: Indications for warfarin therapy include the long-term prophylaxis of arterial thromboembolism, including prevention of stroke and MI. Other uses include the prophylaxis and treatment of DVT or pulmonary embolism in patients undergoing hip or knee surgery, or in those with long-term indwelling central venous catheters or prosthetic heart valves. The drug may be given to prevent thromboembolic events in high-risk patients following an MI or an atrial fibrillation episode.

Warfarin is well absorbed after PO administration but takes several days to produce an optimal therapeutic effect. Ninety-nine percent of absorbed warfarin is bound to plasma proteins and is not immediately available to produce its effect. This high level of protein binding is also responsible for some of the many drug–drug interactions that occur with warfarin.

Patient responses to warfarin therapy vary widely. Dosage levels must be determined individually for each patient and carefully monitored. Patients stabilized on warfarin should not switch brands of the drug unless recommended by the healthcare provider, due to differences in bioavailability. For most indications, the therapeutic range of serum warfarin levels varies from 1 to 10 mcg/mL to achieve a target INR value of 2 to 3.

Mechanism of Action: Warfarin inhibits two enzymes involved in the formation of activated vitamin K, which is required for the synthesis of clotting Factors II, VII, IX, and X. Warfarin inhibits the synthesis of new clotting factors but does not affect clotting factors that are already circulating in the blood. It takes 3 to 4 days for the plasma levels of existing clotting factors to fall and for the anticoagulant effect of warfarin to appear. After discontinuing the drug, 3 to 4 days are needed for the body to make new clotting factors and return coagulation to baseline levels.

Pharmacokinetics:

Route(s)	PO
Absorption	Well absorbed
Distribution	Widely distributed; crosses the placenta; small amounts may be secreted in breast milk; 99% bound to plasma protein
Primary metabolism	Hepatic
Primary excretion	Renal; small amounts in bile
Onset of action	2–7 days
Duration of action	3–5 days; half-life: 0.5–3 days

Adverse Effects: Like all anticoagulants, the most serious adverse effect of warfarin is abnormal bleeding, which may occur in any body system. Warfarin may release pieces of atheromatous plaque from vessel walls, resulting in systemic cholesterol microembolization that may occlude small vessels. For example, "purple-toe syndrome" is caused by cholesterol microembolization and severe cases may lead to gangrene or amputation. Long-term use of warfarin may increase the risk of osteoporosis and bone fractures. **Black Box Warning:** Warfarin can cause major or fatal bleeding, and regular monitoring of INR is required. Patients should be instructed about prevention measures to minimize bleeding risk and to immediately notify healthcare providers of signs and symptoms of bleeding.

Contraindications/Precautions: Patients with recent trauma, active internal bleeding, serious bleeding disorders, intracranial hemorrhage, severe HTN, bacterial endocarditis, severe CKD, or hepatic impairment should not take warfarin. When possible, warfarin should be discontinued or the dosage lowered before dental or elective surgical procedures. Patients with HF may exhibit excessive anticoagulation with warfarin, which requires lower doses. Whenever possible, IM injections of other medications should be avoided because they may cause bruising, bleeding, or hematomas.

Drug Interactions: Drug–drug interactions with warfarin are numerous. Because the therapeutic index of warfarin is very low, drugs that interact with warfarin have the potential to affect coagulation time and cause harm. Concurrent use with other drugs with anticoagulant activity, including aspirin, heparin, and antiplatelet drugs, may produce additive effects and excessive bleeding.

Table 38.4 Drug–Drug Interactions with Warfarin

Interaction	Drug or Drug Class
Increased anticoagulant effect	acetaminophen, amiodarone, anabolic steroids, aspirin, azole antifungals, cephalosporins, cimetidine, clopidogrel, danazol, disulfiram, heparin, isoniazid, macrolides, metronidazole, nonsteroidal anti-inflammatory drugs (NSAIDs), omeprazole, paroxetine, penicillin, propafenone, quinidine, statins, tamoxifen, tetracyclines, thyroid hormone, trimethoprim-sulfisoxazole
Decreased anticoagulant effect	barbiturates, bile-acid sequestrants, carbamazepine, cyclosporine, dicloxacillin, oral contraceptives, rifampin
Mixed effect	allopurinol, corticosteroids, ethanol, phenytoin
Supplements and food	American ginseng, cranberry, feverfew, ginkgo, green tea, vitamin E, vitamin K

Extensive protein binding is responsible for numerous drug–drug interactions, some of which include NSAIDs, diuretics, selective serotonin reuptake inhibitors and other antidepressants, steroids, antibiotics, vaccines, and vitamins (e.g., vitamin K). NSAIDs increase bleeding risk. During warfarin therapy, the patient should not take any other prescription or over-the-counter (OTC) drugs or herbal products unless approved by the healthcare provider. A listing of selected drugs and supplements affecting warfarin therapy is given in Table 38.4. **Herbal/Food:** Herbal supplements such as green tea, ginkgo, feverfew, garlic, cranberry, chamomile, and ginger may increase the risk of bleeding.

Pregnancy: Warfarin is contraindicated during pregnancy due to multiple serious adverse effects on the embryo and fetus. Contraception should be used during therapy. Warfarin is believed to be safe for lactating women who are at risk for postpartum DVT because very little of the drug enters milk. Studies have shown no change in the INR values of lactating infants whose mothers are receiving warfarin. Breastfed neonates should be monitored for bruising or bleeding.

Treatment of Overdose: The specific treatment for warfarin overdose is PO or parenteral administration of vitamin K_1. When administered IV, vitamin K_1 can begin to reverse the anticoagulant effects of warfarin within 6 hours, but full reversal may take 48 hours. For urgent reversal of anticoagulation in patients with acute bleeding, prothrombin complex concentrate (Kcentra) is used. Kcentra contains vitamin K–dependent coagulation Factors II, VII, IX, and X and the antithrombotic proteins C and protein S.

Clinician Responsibilities: Key clinical implications for patients receiving warfarin are included in Applied Clinical Judgment: Patients Receiving Pharmacotherapy with Anticoagulants.

Drugs Similar to Warfarin (Coumadin)

Warfarin is the only vitamin K antagonist prescribed for anticoagulation.

38.6 The direct thrombin inhibitors and Factor Xa inhibitors have become important drugs in the prevention and treatment of venous thromboembolism.

The direct thrombin inhibitors and Factor Xa inhibitors, listed in Table 38.3, are relatively new drugs in the prevention and treatment of VTE and pulmonary embolism. They offer several advantages over warfarin and heparin.

The direct thrombin inhibitors have an interesting history; they were originally derived from chemicals found in leeches. Leeches are wormlike animals that survive by sucking and digesting blood from mammals. Medical leeches are an ancient treatment that dates back to early Egyptian and Greek civilizations. They were applied to the skin as a type of bloodletting, which was thought to remove harmful substances from the body. Known as hirudotherapy, the use of leeches was largely discontinued with the advent of modern medicine in the early 1900s. However, leeches are still an approved therapy for relieving venous congestion in transplanted or reattached fingers or limbs. While studying leeches, scientists isolated a potent chemical called hirudin, which prevented blood from coagulating in the leech.

The direct thrombin inhibitors bind reversibly to thrombin, preventing the formation of fibrin. They are highly specific for thrombin and do not require AT-III as an intermediate in promoting anticoagulation as does heparin. They bind to circulating thrombin as well as thrombin attached to fibrin clots. These drugs exhibit typical anticoagulant actions and are used for the same types of indications as heparin and the LMWHs. The only drug in this class given by the PO route is dabigatran.

The Factor Xa inhibitors bind to activated Factor Xa, which blocks the formation of thrombin from both the intrinsic and extrinsic pathways of the coagulation cascade. They block Factor Xa in both plasma and in clots and have no effects on platelets. They are well absorbed by the PO route and do not require routine laboratory monitoring. The number of adverse bleeding events is the same, or less, than that of warfarin. Peak concentrations can be reached in 3 hours. The American College of Chest Physicians (ACCP) recommends 3 months of therapy with dabigatran (Pradaxa), rivaroxaban (Xarelto), apixaban (Eliquis), or edoxaban (Savaysa) as initial choices for DVT or pulmonary embolus prevention (Kearon et al., 2016). The drugs are well tolerated, with the most common adverse effects being diarrhea, dizziness, and peripheral edema.

The Factor Xa inhibitors offer significant advantages over warfarin. The Factor Xa inhibitors require no laboratory monitoring to determine their anticoagulant effect—the same dose is used for most patients. They exhibit fewer drug–drug and drug–food interactions than warfarin. Their anticoagulant effect clears in 1 to 2 days after discontinuation, versus 5 to 7 days for warfarin.

The most serious adverse effect for Factor Xa inhibitors is excessive bleeding. In 2019, an antidote, coagulation Factor Xa (recombinant), inactivated-zhzo (Andexxa), was approved by the FDA to reverse the anticoagulation effects of rivaroxaban and apixaban. A less expensive option for anticoagulation reversal of DOACs is the use of plasma complex concentrate (Kcentra), although this is an off-label indication.

The three Factor Xa inhibitors carry a black box warning that abrupt discontinuation can increase the risk of thromboembolism. Unless discontinued for a pathologic reason (excessive bleeding), another drug should be immediately substituted so that continuous anticoagulation is obtained. A second black box warning is that spinal or epidural hematomas may occur in anticoagulated patients receiving epidural or spinal anesthesia or who are undergoing spinal puncture.

PROTOTYPE DRUG Dabigatran (Pradaxa)

Classification **Therapeutic:** Anticoagulant
Pharmacologic: Direct thrombin inhibitor

Therapeutic Effects and Uses: Dabigatran is a direct thrombin inhibitor that was approved in 2010 for stroke prophylaxis in patients with nonvalvular atrial fibrillation. Indications have been extended to include treatment of DVT and pulmonary embolus in patients who have been treated with a parenteral anticoagulant for 5 to 10 days, and prophylaxis of DVT and pulmonary embolism in patients who have undergone hip replacement surgery. Administered PO, dabigatran is an alternative to both heparin and warfarin. Although more expensive, dabigatran has equal efficacy to warfarin and does not require the same degree of laboratory monitoring as does warfarin or heparin.

Mechanism of Action: Dabigatran directly inhibits the action of thrombin without requiring the intermediate step of AT-III inhibition.

Pharmacokinetics:

Route(s)	PO
Absorption	3–7% absorbed
Distribution	35% bound to plasma proteins; unknown if it crosses the placenta or is secreted in breast milk
Primary metabolism	Hepatic to active metabolites
Primary excretion	Renal 80%
Onset of action	30–90 min
Duration of action	Half-life: 12–17 h

Adverse Effects: Like other anticoagulants, the most serious adverse effect of dabigatran is bleeding. Symptoms may include bleeding from puncture or wound sites, epistaxis, hematuria, vaginal bleeding, or GI bleeding. Hypersensitivity reactions, including anaphylaxis, have been reported. Dyspepsia and gastritis are common during therapy. **Black Box Warnings:** Premature discontinuation of dabigatran increases the risk of thrombotic events. Epidural or spinal hematomas may occur when administering this drug to patients who are receiving neuraxial anesthesia or spinal puncture.

Contraindications/Precautions: Dabigatran should not be administered to patients with active bleeding or those with impaired hemostasis. Patients with mechanical heart valves should not receive this drug due to an increased risk of thrombotic events. Patients with severe CKD or on hemodialysis should not receive dabigatran. The drug should be used with caution in patients with recent hemorrhage, recent surgery, intracranial hemorrhage, ulcerative GI disease, or symptoms of gastritis.

Drug Interactions: Additive risk for bleeding may occur if dabigatran is administered concurrently with other coagulation modifiers, including warfarin, heparin, aspirin, and fibrinolytic drugs. **Herbal/Food:** Herbal supplements that affect coagulation such as ginger, garlic, green tea, feverfew, St. John's wort, or ginkgo should be avoided because they may increase the risk of bleeding.

Pregnancy: Animal reproduction studies showed an adverse effect on reproductive capacity and increased uterine bleeding close to parturition. Breastfeeding is not recommended during therapy.

Treatment of Overdose: Administration of protamine and vitamin K are not effective. In 2015, idarucizumab (Praxbind) was approved for emergency use to reverse the anticoagulant action of dabigatran. When given IV, idarucizumab binds to free dabigatran and fully reverses anticoagulation after 4 hours in most patients.

Clinician Responsibilities: Key clinical implications for patients receiving dabigatran are included in Applied Clinical Judgment: Patients Receiving Pharmacotherapy with Anticoagulants.

CONNECTIONS: APPLIED CLINICAL JUDGMENT

Patients Receiving Pharmacotherapy with Anticoagulants

Key Assessment Data

- History of current condition, baseline vital signs, physical exam findings; history of cardiovascular disease (HTN, MI, HF), peripheral vascular disease (including thrombophlebitis), respiratory (including previous pulmonary embolism), neurologic (including recent head injury or stroke), hepatic disease, CKD, diabetes, peptic ulcer disease, hypercholesterolemia; assess for the possibility of alcoholism, pregnancy status; drug history including allergies, current prescription and OTC drugs, and herbal preparations. Ask women of menstrual age about length and heaviness of usual menstrual flow.
- Ongoing assessment during drug therapy includes laboratory findings (e.g., aPTT, PT/INR), complete blood count (CBC), renal and liver function studies, arterial blood gases (ABGs) as appropriate, lipid profiles, liver and renal function studies. Assess for presence, quality, location of angina, and for presence of dyspnea or chest pain. Assess extremities for symptoms of thrombophlebitis (e.g., warmth, swelling, tenderness in calf) and for location, character, and amount of edema, if present.

Desired Therapeutic Outcomes

Improvement is observed and measurable in improvement in phlebitis with no symptoms of thrombosis formation; signs and symptoms of existing thrombosis show gradual improvement (e.g., previous anginal or peripheral extremity pain has diminished or is eliminated); peripheral pulses are improving in quality and volume.

Minimizing Adverse Effects

- Bleeding is the most common adverse effect of anticoagulant therapy. Frequent assessment for both visible and occult bleeding is necessary to prevent hemorrhage and to start early corrective treatment as appropriate.
- Therapeutic aPTT levels are usually 1.5 to 2.5 times the normal control value. INR is usually 2 to 3.5 or 4. Values below the norm indicate less than optimal therapeutic levels of the drug; values above the norm indicate a high potential for bleeding and hemorrhage. Continue to monitor CBC, especially red blood cells (RBCs), Hgb and Hct, and platelet levels. Decreasing values on CBC may indicate excessive bleeding and the need to assess for location of bleeding.
- Minimize opportunities for injury or bleeding where possible: Avoid IM injections, and be cautious when providing care, especially with older adults who have more fragile skin.
- Many drugs interact with anticoagulants, enhancing the action and increasing the risk for bleeding. All OTC medications containing salicylates (e.g., aspirin and NSAIDs) are contraindicated. Closely evaluate all new prescriptions or use of OTC medications for drug interactions.
- Sudden changes in dietary intake of vitamin K–rich foods may increase or decrease the effectiveness of anticoagulants, particularly oral anticoagulant therapy. Excessive intake of alcohol, more than two drinks in men or one in women per day, may alter the effectiveness of oral anticoagulants. Encourage the use of a food diary if coagulation panels do not remain stable.
- Drug-induced hepatitis is a possible adverse effect of oral anticoagulant therapy. Evaluate hepatic labs and assess for signs and symptoms of hepatitis.

Lifespan Considerations

- Be especially cautious with the older adult as age-related hepatic changes may increase the risk of bleeding.
- The drug should not be taken during pregnancy, if pregnancy is suspected, or while breastfeeding.
- Women of menstrual age should report excessively heavy or prolonged menstrual bleeding and should keep a pad count and report to the healthcare provider.

Diversity Considerations

- Because some drugs such as clopidogrel metabolize through the CYP450 system pathways, monitor ethnically diverse patients to ensure optimal therapeutic effects and to minimize adverse effects.

Patient and Caregiver Education

- Monitor for signs and symptoms of excessive bleeding, including occult. If external bleeding occurs, pressure over the site should be held up to 15 min. If bleeding continues, is severe, or is accompanied by dizziness or syncope, immediate medical attention (e.g., 911) should be obtained.
- Utilize ways to minimize opportunities for injury or bleeding, including:
  - Switch to a soft-bristle toothbrush and inspect gums after brushing.
  - Use an electric razor, or be extra cautious with a safety razor, holding prolonged pressure over small nicks.
  - Be cautious with food preparation, especially when cutting food.
  - Avoid contact sports, amusement park rides, or other physical activities that may cause intense or violent bumping, jostling, or injury.
- During travel: stretch periodically, ambulate for short periods, avoid sitting for prolonged periods, and increase fluid intake.
- Avoid increases or decreases in vitamin K–rich foods and limit or eliminate alcohol intake. Vitamin K supplements and protein supplement drinks (e.g., Ensure or Boost), which often have vitamin K added, should also be avoided.
- Carry a wallet identification card or wear medical identification jewelry indicating anticoagulant therapy.

Prescribing Considerations

- Whenever an oral anticoagulant is prescribed, a baseline coagulation profile and renal function should be obtained.
- A patient's INR should be checked and be at a safe level before oral anticoagulation is given.
- Levels of INR do not change rapidly; ordering INR levels more than every 24 hours is not recommended.
- To assist with anticoagulation with warfarin, a template should be made to help the prescriber know the therapeutic INR for different conditions

Drugs Similar to Dabigatran (Pradaxa)

Other direct thrombin inhibitors include argatroban, and bivalirudin. Desirudin and lepirudin have been withdrawn from the market.

Argatroban (Acova, Novastan): Approved in 2000, argatroban is a synthetic thrombin inhibitor that is given by the IV route for prophylaxis of thrombosis in patients with HIT and to treat or prevent thrombotic events associated with PCI. Unlike dabigatran, which is excreted by the kidneys, argatroban is metabolized and eliminated by the liver and therefore may be used in patients with CKD. Caution must be observed, however, when administering the drug to patients with hepatic impairment. Allergic reactions occur in up to 10% of patients receiving argatroban. Bleeding is the most serious adverse effect, and the drug should not be administered to patients with active bleeding. Animal reproduction studies revealed no significant impairment in fertility or harm to the fetus. It is not known if argatroban is secreted in human milk or if it causes harm in breastfed neonates.

Bivalirudin (Angiomax): Approved in 2000, bivalirudin is a direct throm bin inhibitor that is available only by the IV route. Bivalirudin is given concurrently with aspirin to reduce the incidence of thromboembolic events associated with HIT and to provide anticoagulation in patients undergoing PCI. Back pain is a common adverse effect of the drug, occurring in about 40% of patients. Nausea and vomiting, hypotension, and headache also occur in a significant number of patients. Bleeding is the most serious adverse effect, and the drug should not be administered to patients with active bleeding. Bivalirudin is as effective as heparin and produces a lower incidence of serious bleeding, although it is very expensive. Animal reproduction studies revealed no fertility impairment or fetal harm. It is not known if bivalirudin is excreted in human milk or if it causes harm in breastfeeding neonates.

Factor Xa inhibitors: Factor Xa inhibitors include betrixaban (Bevyxxa), rivaroxaban (Xarelto), apixaban (Eliquis), and edoxaban (Savaysa). The four differ somewhat in their pharmacokinetics but have similar actions and adverse effects. Animal reproduction studies have shown fetal toxicity and death, bleeding complications, and pregnancy loss with some drugs in this class. Although it is unknown if these medications are secreted in human milk, they have the potential for adverse reactions in nursing infants. Indications for the Factor Xa inhibitors include the following:

- **betrixaban (Bevyxxa):** indicated for prevention of VTE in patients with prolonged hospitalization or restricted mobility
- **rivaroxaban (Xarelto):** indicated for prevention of VTE and pulmonary emboli in patients undergoing knee or hip replacement; also used to reduce the risk of stroke or embolism in patients with nonvalvular atrial fibrillation
- **apixaban (Eliquis):** used to reduce the risk of stroke or embolism in patients with nonvalvular atrial fibrillation
- **edoxaban (Savaysa):** used to reduce the risk of stroke or embolism in patients with nonvalvular atrial fibrillation; also indicated for treatment of DVT and pulmonary embolism following 5 to 10 days of initial therapy with a parenteral anticoagulant.

Antiplatelet Drugs

38.7 Antiplatelet drugs provide anticoagulation by reducing the aggregation properties of platelets.

Antiplatelet drugs modify coagulation primarily by interfering with platelet aggregation. Unlike the anticoagulants, which are used primarily to prevent thrombosis in veins, the primary indications for antiplatelet drugs are to prevent clot formation in arteries. The antiplatelet medications are listed in Table 38.5.

Table 38.5 Antiplatelet Drugs

Drug	Route and Adult Dose (Maximum Dose Where Indicated)	Adverse Effects
anagrelide (Agrylin)	PO: 0.5 mg qid or 1 mg bid (max: 10 mg/day)	*Nausea and vomiting, diarrhea, abdominal pain, dizziness, headache* Increased bleeding, CNS effects (dipyridamole), anaphylaxis (aspirin), interstitial lung disease (anagrelide)
aspirin (ASA, acetylsalicylic acid)	PO: 80 mg daily to 650 mg bid	
dipyridamole (Persantine)	PO: 75–100 mg qid as adjunct to warfarin therapy	
vorapaxar (Zontivity)	PO: 2.08 mg/day	
ADP Receptor Blockers		
cangrelor (Kengreal)	IV: 30 mcg/kg single dose followed immediately by 4 mcg/kg/minute continuous infusion	*Minor bleeding* Serious bleeding, hypersensitivity, dyspnea
clopidogrel (Plavix)	PO: 75 mg/day (max: 300 mg/day for life-threatening cases)	*Minor bleeding, dyspepsia, abdominal pain, headache, rash, diarrhea* Increased clotting time, GI bleeding, blood dyscrasias, angina
prasugrel (Effient)	PO: 60-mg loading dose followed by 10 mg/day	
ticagrelor (Brilinta)	PO: 180-mg loading dose followed by 90 mg bid	
Glycoprotein IIb/IIIa Receptor Antagonists		
eptifibatide (Integrilin)	IV: 180 mcg/kg initial bolus over 1–2 min, then 2 mcg/kg/min for 24–72 h (max: 180 mcg/kg bolus, 2 mcg/kg/min infusion)	*Dyspepsia, dizziness, pain at injection site, hypotension, bradycardia, minor bleeding* Major hemorrhage, thrombocytopenia
tirofiban (Aggrastat)	IV: 0.4 mcg/kg/min for 30 min, then 0.1 mcg/kg/min for 12–24 h	
Drugs for Intermittent Claudication		
cilostazol	PO: 100 mg bid	*Dyspepsia, nausea and vomiting, dizziness, myalgia, headache* Tachycardia and palpitations (cilostazol), CNS effects (pentoxifylline), HF, MI
pentoxifylline (Trental)	PO: 400 mg tid (max: 1200 mg/day)	

Note: *Italics* indicate common adverse effects. Underline indicates serious adverse effects.

Because platelets are a central component of blood hemostasis, reducing the number of platelets or their function can profoundly increase bleeding time. Three groups of drugs are classified as antiplatelet drugs:

- Aspirin
- ADP receptor blockers
- Glycoprotein IIb/IIIa receptor blockers.

Aspirin deserves special mention as an antiplatelet drug. Because it is available OTC, patients may not consider aspirin a potent medication; however, its anticoagulant activity is well documented. Aspirin acts by binding irreversibly to the enzyme cyclooxygenase in platelets. This binding inhibits the formation of thromboxane A_2, a powerful inducer of platelet aggregation. The anticoagulant effect of a single dose of aspirin may persist for as long as 1 week. Concurrent use of aspirin with other coagulation modifiers should be avoided, unless medically approved. Nursing responsibilities and a prototype feature for aspirin are given in Chapter 41.

38.8 The adenosine diphosphate receptor blockers are antiplatelet drugs prescribed for the prevention and treatment of arterial thrombosis.

Although platelets are simply fragments of cells that have no nucleus, they contain many receptors on their plasma membranes and their functions are complex. Chemicals such as epinephrine, thromboxane A_2, thrombin, serotonin, and fibrinogen can bind to these receptors and modify coagulation through their interaction with the platelets.

Following vessel injury, platelets become "sticky," bind to exposed collagen, and release substances that recruit additional platelets to the site. One of these chemicals is ADP, which binds to the platelet to cause aggregation or clumping . The ADP receptor on the platelet is known as $P2Y_{12}$. Drugs in the ADP receptor blocker class bind to $P2Y_{12}$, thus blocking the platelet aggregation and slowing the clotting process. For the remainder of their lifespan, the affected platelets are unable to recognize the chemical signals required for them to aggregate. In the medical literature, drugs in this class are sometimes called $P2Y_{12}$ antagonists.

Ticagrelor (Brilinta), clopidogrel (Plavix), and prasugrel (Effient) are ADP receptor blockers given PO to prevent thrombi formation in patients who have experienced a recent thromboembolic event such as stroke or MI. The newer drugs in this class, ticagrelor and prasugrel, act more rapidly than clopidogrel and achieve a more consistent and effective antithrombotic effect. Cangrelor (Kengreal) is the only parenteral drug in this class. Adverse effects among the three drugs are similar.

Drugs affecting platelet aggregation increase the risk of bleeding should the patient sustain trauma or undergo dental or surgical procedures. These drugs are sometimes given concurrently with anticoagulants, which can further increase bleeding risk. Prolonged direct pressure over injection or venipuncture sites may be required to control bleeding. Bleeding lasting more than 10 minutes may require special medical or nursing interventions, such as suturing or applying a sandbag to a venipuncture site that does not stop bleeding.

CONNECTIONS: Complementary and Alternative Therapies

Garlic

Description

Garlic (*Allium sativum*) is a perennial plant in the onion family that can be grown and cultivated worldwide.

History and Claims

Garlic has been used for centuries by most cultures as a flavoring and as a medicine. Historical uses have included curing deafness and earaches and treating leprosy and scurvy. Modern claims have focused on cardiovascular uses: treatment of high blood lipid levels, atherosclerosis, and HTN. Other modern claims are that garlic reduces blood glucose levels and has antibacterial and antineoplastic activity.

Standardization

Substances called alliaceous oils have been isolated from garlic and shown to have pharmacologic activity. Dosage forms include eating prepared garlic oil or the fresh bulbs (cloves) from the plant. In tablet or capsule form, doses range from 1 to 4 g/day. Extracts may be standardized by percent allicin.

Evidence

Garlic is one of the best-studied herbs. Like most other herbal products, garlic likely has some health benefits, but controlled, scientific studies are lacking and the results are mixed. Research has found associations between garlic consumption and lowered cholesterol, decreased blood pressure, and a reduced incidence of cancer, but that correlation has not been proven in controlled studies (National Center for Complementary and Integrative Health, 2016).

Garlic is safe for consumption in small and moderate amounts. Patients taking anticoagulant medications should limit their intake of garlic to avoid bleeding complications. Patients with diabetes should monitor their blood glucose levels closely if taking high doses of garlic.

PROTOTYPE DRUG Clopidogrel (Plavix)

Classification **Therapeutic:** Antiplatelet drug
Pharmacologic: ADP receptor blocker

Therapeutic Effects and Uses: Approved in 1997, clopidogrel is used for the prophylaxis of arterial thromboembolism to reduce the risk of stroke, MI, and death in patients with acute coronary syndrome. For patients with ST-elevation MI (STEMI), this drug has been shown to reduce the risk of death, reinfarction, or stroke. For some indications, clopidogrel is given concurrently with a low dose of aspirin.

Clopidogrel is given PO and has the advantage of once-daily dosing. Inhibition of platelet function may persist for 7 to 10 days after the drug is discontinued. When possible, clopidogrel should be discontinued at least 5 days prior to surgery to avoid excessive bleeding.

Many patients are resistant to the antiplatelet actions of clopidogrel due to a mutation in the *CYP2C19* gene. This gene is responsible for producing an enzyme that converts clopidogrel to its active metabolite. About half of all people with Asian ancestry and 30% of those of European ancestry are at risk to having reduced effect or no effect when given the medication.

Mechanism of Action: Clopidogrel inhibits ADP $P2Y_{12}$ receptors on platelets and prolongs bleeding time by irreversibly inhibiting platelet aggregation. Clopidogrel itself has little activity; however, it is changed to a highly active metabolite in the liver through extensive first-pass metabolism.

Pharmacokinetics:

Route(s)	PO
Absorption	Rapidly absorbed
Distribution	Unknown; unknown if it crosses the placenta or is secreted in breast milk; 94–98% bound to plasma protein
Primary metabolism	Hepatic; metabolized to active metabolite
Primary excretion	Renal 50%; feces 50%
Onset of action	1–2 h
Duration of action	5 days

Adverse Effects: Clopidogrel has approximately the same tolerability as aspirin and adverse effects are rarely severe enough to cause discontinuation of therapy. Although excessive bleeding is a potential adverse effect, it occurs in only about 1% of patients. Older adults are more susceptible to bleeding during therapy and should be carefully monitored. The incidence of GI bleeding is less than that of aspirin. Common adverse effects are flulike syndrome, headache, diarrhea, dizziness, bruising, upper respiratory infection, and rash or pruritus. **Black Box Warning:** Because the effectiveness of clopidogrel is dependent on its metabolic activation by CYP450 enzymes, poor metabolizers will exhibit less therapeutic effect and more adverse cardiovascular events. Genetic tests are available to identify poor metabolizers.

Contraindications/Precautions: Clopidogrel is contraindicated in patients with active bleeding and should be used with caution in patients at high risk for bleeding, including those with peptic ulcer disease. Severe hepatic disease may impair the ability of the liver to convert the drug to its active metabolite. The drug should be discontinued at least 5 days prior to elective surgery

Drug Interactions: Use with anticoagulants, other antiplatelet drugs, fibrinolytics, or NSAIDs, including aspirin, will increase the risk of bleeding. Drugs that inhibit hepatic metabolic enzymes—such as the azole antifungals, protease inhibitors, erythromycin, verapamil, or zafirlukast—may diminish the antiplatelet actions of clopidogrel. Drugs that increase hepatic metabolic enzyme activity, such as barbiturates, rifampin, or carbamazepine, may increase the anticoagulant activity of clopidogrel. **Herbal/Food:** Herbal supplements that affect coagulation such as feverfew, green tea, ginkgo, fish oil, ginger, or garlic may increase the risk of bleeding.

Treatment of Overdose: There is no specific therapy for clopidogrel overdose. Platelet transfusions may be beneficial in preventing hemorrhage.

Pregnancy: Animal reproduction studies showed no evidence of significant impaired fertility or fetal harm. It is not known if clopidogrel is secreted in human milk or if it has adverse effects on the breastfed neonate.

Clinician Responsibilities: Key clinical implications for patients receiving clopidogrel are included in Applied Clinical Judgment: Patients Receiving Pharmacotherapy with Anticoagulants. Although nursing responsibilities are similar to those for the anticoagulant drugs, bleeding risk is lessened with the antiplatelet drugs.

Drugs Similar to Clopidogrel (Plavix)

Other antiplatelet drugs include anagrelide, cangrelor, dipyridamole, prasugrel, ticagrelor, and vorapaxar. Aspirin also provides anticoagulation by this mechanism and is discussed in Section 38.7.

Anagrelide (Agrylin): Approved in 1977, anagrelide is an antiplatelet medication used for one very specific indication: to reduce elevated platelet counts in patients with myeloproliferative neoplasms. Elevated platelet levels in patients with these disorders can increase the risk of thrombosis. Unlike other antiplatelet drugs that reduce platelet aggregation, anagrelide reduces the production of platelets. Use with other antiplatelet drugs such as aspirin increases the risk of bleeding. Common adverse effects included headache, palpitations, diarrhea, and asthenia. Animal reproduction studies showed no evidence of impaired fertility or fetal harm. It is not known if anagrelide is secreted in human milk or if it has adverse effects on the breastfed neonate.

Cangrelor (Kengreal): Approved in 2015, cangrelor is the only ADP $P2Y_{12}$ receptor blocker given IV. It is used to reduce the risk of MI, repeat coronary revascularization, or stent thrombosis during PCI. It is administered as a single-bolus dose prior to PCI, immediately followed by an infusion for at least 2 hours or the duration of PCI, whichever is longer. It has an onset of action of only 2 minutes, with a half-life of 3 to 6 minutes. After the infusion is completed, the patient is switched to an oral ADP receptor blocker to continue antiplatelet action. Bleeding is the most frequent adverse effect. Animal reproduction data did not show significant fetal harm. Due to its very brief half-life, adverse effects on the breastfed neonate are not expected.

Dipyridamole (Persantine): Approved in 1961, the only approved use of dipyridamole is in combination with warfarin to prevent thromboembolism in patients following cardiac valve replacement. Dipyridamole acts by a different mechanism than clopidogrel. Rather than blocking ADP receptors, dipyridamole elevates levels of cyclic AMP (cAMP), which is a potent inhibitor of platelet aggregation. Adverse effects are generally minimal and transient and include dizziness, abdominal pain, and headache. Animal reproduction studies showed no significant evidence of fetal harm. Dipyridamole is secreted in human milk, although it is unknown if this has adverse effects on the breastfed neonate.

Prasugrel (Effient): Prasugrel is an ADP receptor blocker that was approved in 2009 to reduce the risk for thrombotic events in patients with acute coronary syndrome who undergo PCI. Prasugrel is a prodrug that is rapidly metabolized to its active form as it crosses the intestinal mucosa. Antiplatelet effects begin to occur within 30 minutes. Prasugrel is usually concurrently taken with aspirin. Compared to clopidogrel, prasugrel is associated with a reduced risk of adverse cardiovascular events, such as stroke and MI, and it is less prone to interact with other medications. The drug carries a black box warning that it can cause serious and life-threatening bleeding. It should not be used in patients with active bleeding or a history of transient ischemic attack or stroke. Prasugrel should not be started in acute patients likely to undergo coronary artery bypass grafts and should be discontinued at least 7 days prior to expected surgery. Animal reproduction studies showed no significant evidence of fetal harm. Prasugrel is secreted in human milk, although it is unknown if this has adverse effects on the breastfed neonate.

Ticagrelor (Brilinta): Approved in 2011, ticagrelor is indicated to reduce the risk of cardiovascular death, MI, and stroke in patients with acute coronary syndrome or a history of MI. In patients with PCI, the drug reduces the risk of stent thrombosis. Like clopidogrel and prasugrel, ticagrelor acts by blocking the ADP receptor on platelets. The most frequent adverse effects are dyspnea and bleeding. Ticagrelor carries a black box warning that the drug can cause serious or fatal bleeding, that it is contraindicated in patients with a history of intracranial hemorrhage or pathologic bleeding, and that it should be discontinued at least 5 days prior to surgery. The black box warning also states that maintenance doses of aspirin should not exceed 100 mg/day because aspirin decreases the effectiveness of ticagrelor. In animal reproduction studies ticagrelor caused structural abnormalities and fetal death; it should not be used during pregnancy unless potential benefits to the mother justify the potential risks to the fetus. This drug is secreted in human milk, although adverse effects on the breastfed neonate are unknown.

Vorapaxar (Zontivity): In 2014 the FDA approved vorapaxar, a new type of antiplatelet drug, to reduce the risk for blood clots in patients with a history of MI or with peripheral arterial disease. Given PO, it is the first medication to cause anticoagulation by blocking the protease-activated receptor (PAR-1) on platelets. It may be used concurrently with aspirin or clopidogrel. Like other anticoagulants, its primary adverse effect is increased bleeding risk. Vorapaxar carries a black box warning that it is contraindicated for patients with a history of stroke, transient ischemic attack, or intracranial hemorrhage because it may increase the risk for serious and fatal bleeding. Based on animal reproduction studies, vorapaxar is predicted to have a low probability of adverse developmental effects. It is not known if vorapaxar is secreted in human milk or if it has adverse effects on the breastfed neonate.

38.9 The glycoprotein IIb/IIIa receptor inhibitors are effective antiplatelet drugs for preventing coagulation.

Glycoprotein IIb/IIIa is a receptor found on the surface of platelets. The receptor contains two distinct protein chains, designated IIb and IIIa. Platelets contain a huge number of glycoprotein IIb/IIIa receptors: approximately 50,000 to 80,000 per cell. These receptors serve as docking stations, waiting for signals from chemical messengers that indicate injury may have occurred.

Substances that normally bind to and activate glycoprotein IIb/IIIa receptors include thrombin, von Willebrand's factor (vWF), ADP, and thromboxane A_2. Following activation of the surface glycoprotein, the platelets change shape, bind fibrinogen, and become sticky. Essentially, the platelets develop an enhanced ability to bind to each other, to fibrinogen, and to the exposed collagen of damaged vessels. This process is illustrated in Figure 38.2.

Inhibition of the glycoprotein IIb/IIIa receptor prevents platelet activation and thrombus formation in patients with a recent MI, stroke, and PCI, with or without stent placement. Although these medications are effective antiplatelet drugs, they are expensive. Another major disadvantage is that they are given only by the IV route. PO forms of these drugs recently entered clinical trials but proved less effective than aspirin in reducing thromboembolic events.

There are only two drugs in the glycoprotein IIb/IIIa inhibitor class: eptifibatide and tirofiban. The first drug approved in this class, abciximab, was the most widely used until it was withdrawn from the U.S. market in 2019. Because the remaining two medications are so similar, no prototype exists for the class. Eptifibatide and tirofiban are given in cardiac emergencies, and data on pregnancy or lactation is not available. Because of their short half-lives, adverse effects during pregnancy or lactation are not predicted.

Eptifibatide (Integrilin): Approved in 1998, eptifibatide is a synthetic drug administered by the IV route that is highly specific to binding the glycoprotein IIa/IIIb receptor. The binding of eptifibatide is rapidly reversible and a large amount of unbound drug may circulate in the plasma. In overdose situations, platelet infusions may be of little benefit because the unbound drug will quickly occupy glycoprotein IIb/IIIa receptors on the new platelets to prevent their activation by procoagulants. The drug is indicated for the prevention of thromboembolic events in patients undergoing PCI, including those with acute coronary syndrome and those having stent placements. Eptifibatide is given in an IV bolus, followed by a continuous infusion for at least 12 hours. Aspirin and heparin are usually administered concurrently with eptifibatide. Should platelet count decrease to less than 100,000/mm^3, the aspirin or heparin is discontinued. The kidneys primarily excrete the drug; thus, caution should be used in patients with CKD. Bleeding at the arterial access site is the most common adverse effect.

Tirofiban (Aggrastat): Like eptifibatide, tirofiban is an IV synthetic drug highly selective for binding the glycoprotein IIb/IIIa receptor in a rapid, reversible manner. The drug is indicated for the prevention of thromboembolic events in patients with acute coronary syndrome and those undergoing PCI. Tirofiban is given in an IV bolus, followed by a continuous infusion for at least 12 hours. Aspirin and heparin are usually administered concurrently. Its duration of action (4 to 8 hours) is longer than that of eptifibatide. The kidneys primarily excrete the drug; thus, caution should be used in

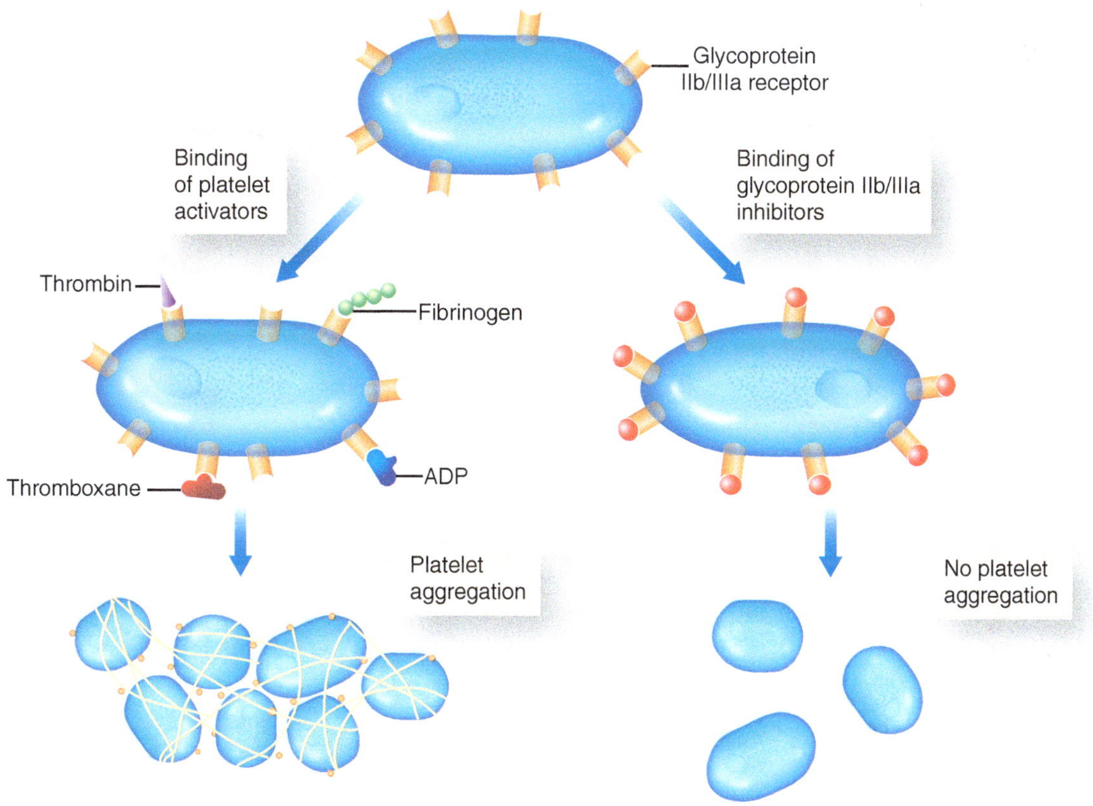

Figure 38.2 Glycoprotein IIb/IIIa receptor activation of platelet function.

patients with CKD. Tirofiban is contraindicated in patients with a history of stroke in the past 30 days or with platelet counts less than 100,000/mm^3. Bleeding secondary to the drug's antiplatelet effect is the most common adverse effect.

Drugs for Intermittent Claudication

38.10 Coagulation modifiers can be used to treat symptoms of intermittent claudication.

Intermittent claudication (IC) is pain or cramping in the lower legs that worsens with walking or exercise. IC is the primary symptom of peripheral vascular disease (PVD), in which progressive atherosclerosis of vessels causes a lack of oxygen to major muscles of the leg. Factors that cause angina pectoris are those that also worsen PVD: diabetes, smoking, and HTN. Exercise, smoking cessation, reduction of blood pressure, and blood glucose management are important nonpharmacologic therapies for IC. Medications are used to reduce symptoms and increase pain-free walking time, although none are able to reverse the underlying cause of PVD.

Pentoxifylline (Pentoxil)) and cilostazol are specifically approved for IC, although statins, aspirin, and clopidogrel may also be used in managing the condition. Pentoxifylline is a unique drug with anticoagulation properties that acts on RBCs to reduce their viscosity and increase their flexibility, allowing them to enter vessels that are partially occluded and prevent thrombi formation. It also inhibits platelet aggregation. It is given PO to increase the microcirculation in patients with IC. Two to 3 months of therapy with pentoxifylline may be necessary before improvement in IC symptoms is noted.

Cilostazol is indicated to improve walking distance before the onset of IC pain. Given PO, the drug has antiplatelet and antithrombotic activity. The antiplatelet action of cilostazol is 10 to 30 times more potent than that of aspirin. Onset of therapeutic effects takes 2 to 12 weeks. It should be used with caution if the patient is taking anticoagulant or antiplatelet medications because this enhances the risk of hemorrhage. Cilostazol has a black box warning that it is contraindicated in patients with congestive heart failure of any severity because it has been shown to decrease survival.

38.11 Fibrinolysis is a process that removes thrombi.

The goal of hemostasis has been achieved once a blood clot is formed and the body is protected from excessive hemorrhage. The process of hemostasis, however, is a positive feedback mechanism in which small amounts of clotting lead to additional clotting. Without an effective means of controlling the process, clotting would spread far beyond the zone of injury and, indeed, occur throughout the vascular system until existing clotting factors were used up. Furthermore, fibrin clots can prevent blood flow to the surrounding area. Circulation must eventually be restored so that the tissue can resume normal activities.

Fibrinolysis is the physiologic process that limits clot formation and removes existing clots. During the time a fibrin clot is forming, the surrounding damaged tissue secretes anticoagulant chemicals that limit the spread of the clot to the area of injury. Removal of the clot begins about 24 to 48 hours following clot formation and continues until it is dissolved.

Like hemostasis, fibrinolysis involves several cascading steps. The process is initiated by plasminogen activators. The two best-studied plasminogen activators are tissue-plasminogen activator (tPA), which is secreted by the endothelium of blood vessels, and urokinase-plasminogen activator (uPA), secreted by the kidney. The function of tPA and uPA is to convert the inactive protein **plasminogen**, which is present in the fibrin clot, to its active form called plasmin. Plasmin is an enzyme that attacks the fibrin strands, breaking them into small fragments that are soluble and no longer able to hold the clot together. The procoagulation factors fibrinogen, prothrombin, and clotting Factors V and XII are also inactivated by plasmin. The body normally regulates fibrinolysis such that unwanted fibrin clots are removed, while fibrin present in wounds is left to maintain hemostasis. The steps of fibrinolysis are shown in Figure 38.3.

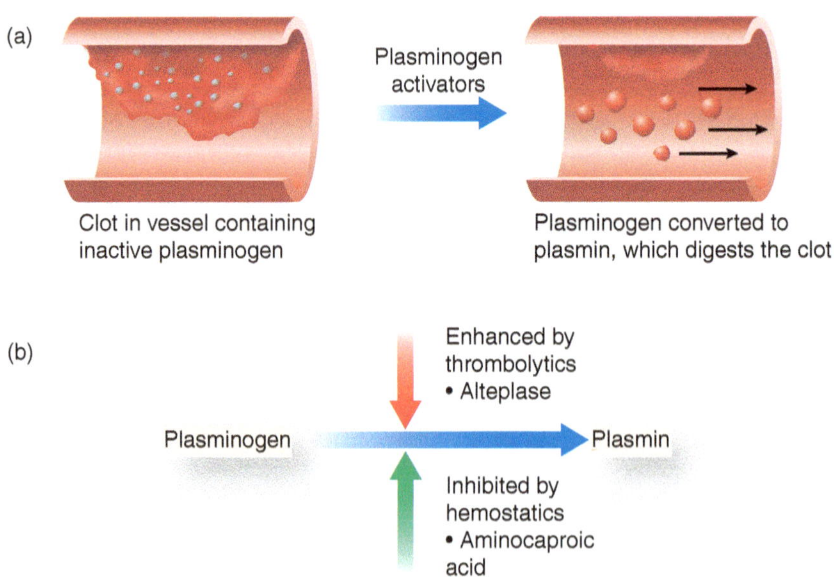

Figure 38.3 Steps in fibrinolysis: (a) Clot dissolves when plasminogen is converted to plasmin. (b) Fibrinolytics enhance fibrinolysis; hemostatics inhibit fibrinolysis.

Fibrinolytics

38.12 Fibrinolytics are used to dissolve existing intravascular clots in patients with myocardial infarction and stroke.

It is often mistakenly believed that the purpose of anticoagulants such as heparin or warfarin is to digest clots. This is not the case. A totally different type of drug is needed for this goal. The fibrinolytics, listed in Table 38.6, are administered very differently from the anticoagulants and antiplatelet drugs, and they produce their effects by different mechanisms. Fibrinolytics are prescribed for disorders in which an intravascular clot has already formed, such as acute MI, pulmonary embolism, acute ischemic stroke, and DVT.

These medications promote fibrinolysis by converting plasminogen to plasmin. The enzyme plasmin then digests fibrin, breaking it into small soluble fragments. In essence, the fibrinolytics simply accelerate the normal process of clot removal in the body. The fibrinolytics are also called thrombolytics, owing to their destructive effects on thrombin. The therapeutic outcomes of fibrinolytic therapy are strongly dependent on the time frame in which they are administered. They are considerably more effective when given as soon as possible after the clot has formed—preferably within 4 hours. The mechanism of action of the fibrinolytics is shown in a Pharmacotherapy Illustrated feature in Chapter 35.

Fibrinolytics are nonspecific and have a very narrow margin of safety between dissolving "normal" and "abnormal" clots. Vital signs must be monitored continuously, and any signs of bleeding may call for discontinuation of therapy. Patients with recent trauma, active bleeding, or surgery may have "fresh" clots that could be disrupted by the action of these drugs. Thus, they may not be candidates for fibrinolytic therapy due to the risk of bleeding.

The use of fibrinolytics in older patients is controversial. Research has shown that fibrinolytic therapy in patients older than age 75 does not decrease mortality from the MI or stroke the patient has experienced. The risks of serious bleeding following drug administration may outweigh the therapeutic benefits. Patients older than age 75 must be carefully screened for contraindicated conditions, such as uncontrolled HTN, recent ischemic stroke, or current use of anticoagulants.

Because these medications are rapidly destroyed in the bloodstream, discontinuing the infusion will quickly terminate fibrinolytic activity. After the clot is successfully dissolved with the fibrinolytic, anticoagulant therapy is initiated to prevent the reformation of clots. Since the discovery of streptokinase, the first drug in this class, there have been several subsequent generations of fibrinolytics. The remaining drugs are more fibrin specific and have fewer adverse effects than streptokinase.

The FDA recommends that TNK and tPA not be used as abbreviations for fibrinolytics because this has led to numerous medication errors. Instead, the full generic or trade name should be used on all prescriptions (FDA, 2015).

PROTOTYPE DRUG Alteplase (Activase)

Classification **Therapeutic:** Drug for dissolving blood clots
Pharmacologic: Fibrinolytic (Thrombolytic)

Therapeutic Effects and Uses: Produced through recombinant DNA technology, alteplase is identical to human tPA. Approved in 1987, alteplase is a first-line drug for the treatment of thrombotic stroke, acute MI, and acute massive pulmonary embolism. Activase (Cathflo Activase) is approved to restore function to central venous access devices. Although not routinely indicated for treating venous clots, the drug may be used in cases where a limb is at risk of gangrene and possible amputation due to vessel occlusion. Like other drugs in this class, it is administered by the IV route.

To achieve maximum effect, alteplase therapy should begin within 6 hours of onset of MI symptoms and within 3 hours of thrombotic stroke. Therapy should be initiated only after intracranial hemorrhage has been ruled out. Alteplase elicits fewer allergic reactions than streptokinase.

Mechanism of Action: The primary action of alteplase is to convert plasminogen to plasmin, which then dissolves fibrin clots. Alteplase is more fibrin specific than streptokinase but less so than some of the other fibrinolytics. The drug also degrades the procoagulant Factors V and VIII and lowers the circulating amounts of fibrinogen and plasminogen.

Table 38.6 Fibrinolytics (Thrombolytics)

Drug	Route and Adult Dose (Maximum Dose Where Indicated)	Adverse Effects
alteplase (Activase)	IV: Begin with 60 mg and then infuse 20 mg/h over next 2 h	*Superficial bleeding at injection sites, allergic reactions* Serious internal bleeding, intracranial hemorrhage, HTN
reteplase (Retavase)	IV: 10 units over 2 min; repeat dose in 30 min	
tenecteplase (TNKase)	IV: 30–50 mg infused over 5 sec	

Note: *Italics* indicate common adverse effects. Underline indicates serious adverse effects.

Pharmacokinetics:

Route(s)	IV
Absorption	NA
Distribution	Unknown; unknown if the drug crosses the placenta or is secreted in breast milk
Primary metabolism	Hepatic
Primary excretion	Renal
Onset of action	Immediate
Duration of action	3 h; half-life: less than 10 min

Adverse Effects: The most common adverse effect of alteplase is bleeding, which may occur superficially at catheter access or needle puncture sites or internally. Signs of bleeding such as spontaneous ecchymoses, hematomas, or epistaxis should be reported to the healthcare provider immediately. Fibrinolysis of clots in the coronary arteries may cause transient dysrhythmias. Angioedema and intracranial bleeding are rare, though serious, adverse effects.

Contraindications/Precautions: History of stroke within the past 3 months, recent trauma or surgery, active bleeding, severe uncontrolled HTN, intracranial neoplasm, and arteriovenous malformation are contraindications to the use of alteplase. Whenever possible, parenteral injections of other drugs should be avoided during alteplase therapy to avoid an increased risk of bleeding at the injection site. Alteplase should not be administered if the patient is on warfarin and INR is greater than 1.7 or PT is greater than 15 seconds.

Drug Interactions: Concurrent use with anticoagulants, antiplatelet drugs, or NSAIDs, including aspirin, will increase the risk of bleeding. Intravenous nitroglycerin enhances the hepatic degradation of alteplase, reducing its ability to dissolve clots. **Herbal/Food:** Use with supplements that affect coagulation such as feverfew, green tea, ginkgo, fish oil, ginger, or garlic should be avoided because they may increase the risk of bleeding.

Pregnancy: Alteplase was embryocidal in some laboratory species but did not show fetal harm in others. It is not known if alteplase is secreted in human milk or if it has adverse effects on the breastfed neonate.

Treatment of Overdose: There is no specific treatment for overdose. Excessive bleeding may require the administration of blood, blood products, or hemostatics.

Clinician Responsibilities: Key clinical implications for patients receiving alteplase are included in Applied Clinical Judgment: Patients Receiving Pharmacotherapy with Fibrinolytics.

Drugs Similar to Alteplase (Activase)

Other fibrinolytics include reteplase and tenecteplase. Streptokinase, the first FDA-approved fibrinolytic, is no longer available in the United States.

Reteplase (Retavase): Approved in 1996, reteplase is used to treat acute MI with ST elevation due to coronary artery thrombosis and also acute peripheral arterial thromboembolism. The drug is a modified form of human tPA produced through recombinant DNA technology. Reteplase has the same adverse effects and contraindications as alteplase. It has a more rapid onset of action than alteplase, perhaps because reteplase is better able to reach the inside of clots. Like alteplase, it is selective for lysing fibrin and the most serious adverse effect is bleeding. There are no data available to predict adverse effects during human pregnancy or lactation.

Tenecteplase (TNKase): Approved in 2000 for the treatment of acute MI with ST elevation with coronary artery thrombosis, tenecteplase is a modified form of human tPA. The drug has similar indications, contraindications, and adverse effects to alteplase but has greater fibrin specificity and a longer half-life. This may be responsible for a slightly lower incidence of noncerebral bleeding with tenecteplase. Another advantage is that it can be administered using a single, 5-second bolus injection. Allergic reactions are rare. At high doses, tenecteplase was embryocidal in laboratory animals. There are no data available to predict adverse effects on the breastfed neonate.

CONNECTIONS: APPLIED CLINICAL JUDGMENT

Patients Receiving Pharmacotherapy with Fibrinolytics

Key Assessment Data

- History of current condition, baseline vital signs; cardiovascular, peripheral vascular disease, respiratory, neurologic (including recent head injury), recent surgeries or injuries, hepatic disease, CKD, diabetes, peptic ulcer disease, recent childbirth (within 10 days), or the possibility of pregnancy; drug history including allergies, current prescription and OTC drugs, and herbal preparations.
- Obtain ECG and breath sounds. Assess presence, quality, and location of angina; for presence of dyspnea or chest pain; and neurologic status.
- Evaluate laboratory findings (aPTT, PT/INR, bleeding time), CBC and platelets, renal and liver function studies, ABGs as appropriate, and lipid profiles. Support the patient during other required tests (e.g., CT or MRI prior to thrombolytic therapy for stroke).
- Establish all monitoring equipment and necessary lines or arrange for their insertion (e.g., ECG monitoring, IV, Foley catheter, arterial line).
- Ongoing assessment during drug therapy includes laboratory findings (e.g., aPTT, PT/INR, Hgb, Hct, platelets, RBCs, urinalysis, ABGs), CBC, renal and liver function studies.
- Monitor vital signs and ECG every 15 min during the first hour of infusion, and then every 30 minutes during the remainder of the infusion. Continue to monitor vital signs every 30 minutes to 1 hour for the first 8 hours following the infusion.

CONNECTIONS: APPLIED CLINICAL JUDGMENT *(continued)*

Patients Receiving Pharmacotherapy with Fibrinolytics

Desired Therapeutic Outcomes

Improvement is observed and measurable by angina has diminished significantly or is eliminated, ECG findings within normal limits, respiratory effort and ABGs significantly improved.

Minimizing Adverse Effects

- Bleeding is the most common adverse effect of fibrinolytic therapy. Frequent assessment for both visible and occult bleeding is necessary to prevent extensive hemorrhage and to start early corrective treatment as appropriate. Bleeding risk is elevated up to 2 to 4 days post-treatment and if the patient is maintained on anticoagulant or antiplatelet therapy after treatment.
- Dysrhythmias may occur postperfusion of the coronary arteries or may be associated with adverse effects. Further treatment with antidysrhythmic drugs may be necessary.
- A sudden change in neurologic status or sudden severe headache is a possible sign of an intracranial bleed with increased intracranial pressure. Monitor neurologic status frequently, especially if fibrinolytics are used for stroke.
- Avoid invasive procedures during infusion and up to 8 hours post-infusion when possible. Any puncture site or site of invasive procedure will create an additional site for bleeding. Whenever an invasive procedure must be used (e.g., ABGs), the site must be maintained under pressure for 30 minutes or longer to prevent hemorrhage.
- Limited physical activity and bedrest during the infusion decrease the chance for bruising, injury, and bleeding.

Patient and Caregiver Education

- Report any palpitations, dyspnea, or angina post-infusion.
- Immediately any change in mental status or LOC during the post-infusion period.
- Activities will be restricted and frequent monitoring will occur throughout the infusion and for a period during the post-infusion time.
- If anticoagulants are prescribed after fibrinolytic therapy, carry a wallet identification card or wear medical identification jewelry indicating anticoagulant therapy.

Prescribing Considerations

- Prior to administration check for current anticoagulant or antiplatelet use, as well as for any dietary supplements that affect coagulation.
- Following administration, advise patient not to take aspirin or other antiplatelets medications or supplements unless approved by the healthcare provider.

Hemostatics

38.13 Hemostatics are used to promote the formation of clots.

The hemostatics, or antifibrinolytics, have an action opposite to that of anticoagulants: to shorten bleeding time. Although their mechanisms differ, all drugs in this class prevent fibrin from dissolving, thus enhancing the stability of the clot and preventing excessive bleeding. The hemostatics, listed in Table 38.7, have very specific indications.

Aminocaproic acid (Amicar) and tranexamic acid (Cyklokapron, Lysteda) are hemostatics that are administered IV. Injection sites should be monitored frequently for thrombophlebitis and extravasation. These drugs may affect muscles, causing wasting and weakness. High doses can promote the formation of abnormal clots. Chest pain and shortness of breath may indicate pulmonary thrombus or embolus. Use is contraindicated in patients with DIC or severe CKD.

PROTOTYPE DRUG **Aminocaproic Acid (Amicar)**

Classification **Therapeutic:** Drug for shortening bleeding time
Pharmacologic: Hemostatic, antifibrinolytic

Therapeutic Effects and Uses: Approved in 1982, aminocaproic acid is prescribed for conditions where there

Table 38.7 Hemostatics

Drug	Route and Adult Dose (Maximum Dose Where Indicated)	Adverse Effects
aminocaproic acid (Amicar)	IV: 4–5 g for 1 h, then 1–1.25 g/h until bleeding is controlled	*Allergic skin reactions, nausea, sinus and nasal symptoms, headache* Anaphylaxis, thrombosis, bronchospasm, nephrotoxicity
desmopressin (DDAVP, Stimate)	IV: 0.3 mcg/kg infused over 15–30 min Intranasal: 300 mg (1 spray per nostril)	*Headache, dizziness, flushing, nosebleed, mild abdominal pain* Hyponatremia, thrombosis
thrombin (Evithrom, Recothrom, Thrombinar)	Topical: Amount varies based on the size of the treated area	*Incision-site complications, pruritus, nausea* Antibody development, anaphylaxis, atrial fibrillation
tranexamic acid (Cyklokapron, Lysteda)	PO: Two 650-mg tablets tid for a maximum of 5 days IV: 10 mg/kg, tid or qid, for 2–8 days	*Headache, nasal and sinus symptoms, back and abdominal pain* Anaphylaxis, thromboembolic events

Note: Italics indicate common adverse effects. Underline indicates serious adverse effects.

is excessive hemorrhage due to clots being dissolved rapidly or prematurely. Excessive fibrinolysis is associated with conditions such as aplastic anemia, hepatic cirrhosis, postoperative cardiac surgery, and in certain carcinomas. It is most commonly prescribed following surgery to reduce postoperative bleeding. Patients with hemophilia A (see Section 38.14) may receive aminocaproic acid immediately following dental procedures to control bleeding. The combination of aminocaproic acid with desmopressin (DDAVP) has been used to reduce postoperative bleeding in patients undergoing cardiopulmonary bypass.

During acute hemorrhage, aminocaproic acid can be given IV to reduce bleeding in 1 to 2 hours. It is also available in tablet form. The therapeutic serum level is 100 to 400 mcg/mL.

Mechanism of Action: Aminocaproic acid occupies binding sites on plasminogen and plasmin. This effectively prevents digestion of the fibrin clot by plasmin.

Pharmacokinetics:

Route(s)	PO, IV
Absorption	Rapidly absorbed from GI tract
Distribution	Widely distributed; unknown if it crosses the placenta or is secreted in breast milk
Primary metabolism	Unknown
Primary excretion	Renal
Onset of action	1–2 h
Duration of action	3–4 h

Adverse Effects: Aminocaproic acid is well tolerated and adverse effects are generally mild. By inhibiting fibrinolysis, the incidence of thrombosis may increase. Myopathy is an uncommon adverse effect that requires monitoring because the drug may lead to rhabdomyolysis. Rapid IV administration may cause hypotension or bradycardia. The IV site should be checked frequently for extravasation or thrombophlebitis.

Contraindications/Precautions: Since aminocaproic acid tends to stabilize clots, it should be used cautiously in patients with a recent history of thromboembolic disease, including those with DIC. Aminocaproic acid is contraindicated in patients with urinary tract bleeding because the drug promotes the formation of clots in the renal pelvis or ureters that may cause obstruction. Caution must be used when administering the drug to patients with serious CKD because the drug may accumulate to toxic serum levels. Renal function laboratory tests should be monitored frequently, especially in older adults.

Drug Interactions: Aminocaproic acid antagonizes the action of fibrinolytic drugs. Hypercoagulation may occur with concurrent use of estrogens and oral contraceptives. In individuals with hemophilia, concurrent administration of aminocaproic acid with Factor IX increases the risk of thrombosis and acute MI. **Herbal/Food:** Unknown.

Pregnancy: There are no data available regarding safety or adverse effects during pregnancy or lactation.

Treatment of Overdose: Overdose may lead to hypotension and renal failure. No treatment for overdose is known, although hemodialysis or peritoneal dialysis may be used to remove the drug.

Drugs Similar to Aminocaproic Acid (Amicar)

Other hemostatics include desmopressin, thrombin (recombinant), and tranexamic acid.

Desmopressin (DDAVP, Stimate): Approved in 1978, DDAVP differs from other hemostatics in being a hormone similar to vasopressin (antidiuretic hormone), a drug that promotes the renal conservation of water. As a hemostatic, it is approved for the treatment of spontaneous bleeding, trauma-induced hemorrhage, or bleeding prophylaxis in patients with hemophilia A or von Willebrand's disease type 1 with Factor VIII activity. The drug may be given parenterally in acute care scenarios or by the nasal route (Stimate) for prophylaxis. Because desmopressin inhibits diuresis, caution must be used to prevent water intoxication. Headache and facial flushing are common adverse effects of the intranasal formulation. Tolerance rapidly develops to the actions of desmopressin, although this is usually not a problem when the drug is used to treat hemorrhage because only one to two doses are needed. Desmopressin has uses other than hemostasis that include the control of excessive or nocturnal urination (enuresis) and polydipsia in patients with diabetes insipidus. Reproduction studies in laboratory animals showed no significant evidence of fetal harm. Only small amounts are secreted in milk and it is poorly absorbed by the infant.

Thrombin, topical (Evithrom, Recothrom, Thrombinar): Topical thrombin is applied with a spray or gelatin sponge to areas that are oozing blood and for minor bleeding from capillaries. The drug is not to be used for serious arterial bleeding or bleeding over large areas. Care must be taken not to inject this drug or to allow systemic absorption due to the risk of thrombi formation.

Approved by the FDA in 2007, human thrombin (Evithrom) is prepared from human plasma. Although screened and treated to inactivate viruses, products obtained from human plasma carry a small risk for transmission of infectious agents, such as viruses and the Creutzfeldt–Jakob disease agent. In 2008 the FDA approved recombinant thrombin (Recothrom), the first recombinant formulation of thrombin. It is unknown if topical thrombin has any adverse effects during pregnancy or lactation.

Tranexamic acid (Cyklokapron, Lysteda): Like aminocaproic acid, tranexamic acid produces an antifibrinolytic effect by inhibiting plasminogen and plasmin activity. The drug was first approved in 1986 as an IV medication to reduce or prevent bleeding in patients with hemophilia who are undergoing dental procedures. In 2009, the PO form of the drug (Lysteda) was approved for the treatment of excessive menstrual bleeding. Because the drug inhibits clot removal, patients must be monitored carefully for signs and symptoms of thromboembolism. Taking Lysteda concurrently with estrogen contraceptives increases the risk of thromboembolic adverse effects. The drug is 8 to 10 times more potent and has a longer half-life than aminocaproic acid. Adverse effects are similar to those of aminocaproic acid. Reproduction studies in laboratory animals showed no significant evidence of fetal harm. Small amounts are secreted in human milk.

Drugs for Hemophilia

38.14 Hemophilia is treated by replacing the missing clotting factor(s) or by inhibiting coagulation.

Hereditary disorders of coagulation are relatively rare and may be caused by deficiency in any blood factor in the coagulation cascade. Symptoms of congenital coagulation disorders manifest as bleeding in muscles or weight-bearing joints, ecchymoses, epistaxis, gingival bleeding, and abnormally long bleeding times following trauma or surgery. Joint bleeding causes chronic inflammation and may result in permanent deformity and loss of mobility.

Some patients have mild forms of hemophilia, exhibiting no symptoms of excessive bleeding until they experience major trauma or surgery. The most severe forms of these disorders, however, are diagnosed shortly after birth and require a lifetime of lifestyle adjustment and pharmacotherapy. Because symptoms associated with the different clotting disorders are nonspecific, diagnosis requires laboratory assays for each of the clotting factors to determine which deficiency is causing the disorder.

The pharmacotherapy of hereditary coagulation disorders has resulted in a remarkable change in the lifespans of afflicted patients. Prior to 1960, the average lifespan of a male with severe hemophilia A was 11 years; the lifespan is now 50 to 60 years.

PharmFACT

Hemophilia A is the most common X-linked genetic disease. Of the 20,000 people with hemophilia A in the United States, about 50 to 60% have the most severe form of the disease (Zaiden, 2020).

Hemophilia A: Lack of clotting Factor VIII results in hemophilia A, which accounts for approximately 80% of all hemophilia. Adequate amounts of Factor VIII are necessary to activate Factor X in the intrinsic coagulation pathway. Because the gene for Factor VIII is carried on the X chromosome, hemophilia A is a sex-linked disease with nearly all cases occurring in males. Females are asymptomatic carriers. Remarkably, patients may have a 75% reduction in the amount of Factor VIII in the blood and yet have no major symptoms. Those with 1% or less of Factor VIII have severe forms of the disease.

The traditional treatment for hemophilia A is administration of fresh frozen plasma. Plasma obtained from blood donors contains all the necessary components to replace the missing clotting factor(s). Unfortunately, there is a small risk of transmitting blood-borne diseases, therefore fresh frozen plasma is no longer used to treat hemophilia.

Hemophilia A is now treated with the administration of a concentrated solution of Factor VIII. A large number of Factor VIII products are available, all essentially having the same actions and indications. More recently, the FDA has approved longer-duration products such as Jivi and Esperoct, which allow for less frequent dosing. These products are indicated for on-demand control of bleeding episodes, perioperative management and routine prophylaxis.

Adverse reactions to Factor VIII administration are uncommon. Flushing, headache, dyspnea, and urticaria may signal an allergic reaction. Anaphylaxis is possible, though rare.

Patients with severe hemophilia A may receive Factor VIII with the goal of *preventing* chronic joint damage and disability. To be most effective, therapy should begin before joint damage has occurred, usually prior to age 2. Prophylactic therapy is expensive and must be continued throughout the patient's lifespan. A central venous access device may be installed to allow more convenient dosing.

Although Factor VIII therapy revolutionized the treatment of hemophilia A, it was noted that some patients did not respond well to this replacement therapy. Subsequent research identified the cause: 30 to 50% of the patients produced *inhibitors* to the Factor VIII concentrate. These inhibitors essentially inactivated the Factor VIII molecule and the patient again experienced excessive bleeding.

In 2019 emicizumab-kxwh (Hemlibra), a monoclonal antibody, was approved. This drug serves the same role as Factor VIII in the coagulation cascade but is not affected by the Factor VIII inhibitor. Emicizumab is given subcutaneously every 1 to 4 weeks and is approved for patients with or without Factor VIII inhibitors.

Desmopressin is an alternative therapy for treating minor bleeding episodes in patients with mild hemophilia A. Available by infusion or intranasal spray, desmopressin causes the release of Factor VIII and vWF from storage sites within the body. The drug can cause a two- to fourfold increase in Factor VIII levels. Desmopressin therapy is usually limited to 2 to 3 days because repeated administration results in a diminished response. If desmopressin is used for a minor surgical procedure, a test dose is usually administered 1 week prior to surgery to determine if the patient is responsive to the drug. In adults with hemophilia, 10 to 20% of patients will not respond to desmopressin therapy. Those with severe forms of the disease have no internal storage depots of Factor VIII or vWF; thus, the drug will be ineffective in these patients.

Other therapies for hemophilia A include the hemostatic drugs aminocaproic acid and tranexamic acid. These drugs are primarily used for short-term therapy to reduce bleeding related to dental procedures.

Hemophilia B: Hemophilia B, or Christmas disease, is caused by a deficiency of Factor IX and comprises about 20% of those with hemophilia. Factor IX, in conjunction with activated Factor VIII, is required for the activation of Factor X in the coagulation cascade. Like Factor VIII, the gene for Factor IX is on the X chromosome, thus this disease occurs predominantly in males. The disease is much less common than hemophilia A, but symptoms of excessive bleeding are the same. Laboratory testing is necessary to distinguish between the two diagnoses.

Treatment of hemophilia B is through replacement therapy with recombinant Factor IX concentrates. The drug is administered for treating and preventing excessive bleeding events such as acute trauma or surgery. Numerous products containing recombinant Factor IX are available. A typical regimen for acute bleeding includes an initial dose of 20 to 80 international units/kg, followed by repeat doses every 24 hours until the target level of Factor IX is obtained. Target levels can sometimes be achieved after a single dose and maintained with lower doses. Factor IX is also administered to prevent spontaneous bleeding. Hemostatic drugs such as aminocaproic acid and tranexamic acid may be used for short-term therapy to reduce bleeding related to dental procedures in patients with hemophilia B.

Hemophilia C: Factor XI deficiency, or hemophilia C, occurs in equal numbers of males and females and is a milder form of hemophilia. In the general population, hemophilia C occurs at a rate of 1 per million births, but it affects up to 13% of those with Ashkenazi Jewish heritage. No therapy is generally indicated unless the patient is undergoing a medical, surgical, or dental procedure. Administration of fresh frozen plasma supplies adequate amounts of Factor XI to prevent or slow bleeding during these procedures. Hemostatics such as desmopressin (DDVAP) may be used.

von Willebrand's Disease: The most common inherited coagulation disorder, **von Willebrand's disease (vWD)**, affects 1 in every 100 to 500 people. This disorder results in a decrease in quantity or quality of vWF, which is required for platelet adhesion to injured blood vessel endothelium. vWF is also a carrier molecule for Factor VIII, protecting it from destruction as it circulates through the blood. Thus, a deficiency in vWF will decrease levels of Factor VIII and affect coagulation. Like hemophilia, the disease has mild and severe forms, both characterized by abnormal bleeding. The disease affects males and females equally, and life expectancy is usually normal.

This type of bleeding disorder is treated with Factor VIII concentrate as well as desmopressin, which promotes the release of stored vWF. For the most severely affected patients, plasma products containing vWF may be required.

Understanding Chapter 38

Key Concepts Summary

38.1 Thromboembolic disorders are abnormalities of hemostasis that include deep vein thrombosis and pulmonary embolism.

38.2 Coagulation disorders are caused by decreased numbers of platelets or by deficiencies in specific clotting factors.

38.3 The normal coagulation process can be modified by a number of different mechanisms.

38.4 Heparin is the traditional drug for rapid anticoagulation.

38.5 Warfarin is a widely used drug for oral anticoagulant therapy.

38.6 The direct thrombin inhibitors and Factor Xa inhibitors have become important drugs in the prevention and treatment of venous thromboembolism.

38.7 Antiplatelet drugs provide anticoagulation by reducing the aggregation properties of platelets.

38.8 The adenosine diphosphate receptor blockers are antiplatelet drugs prescribed for the prevention and treatment of arterial thrombosis.

38.9 The glycoprotein IIb/IIIa receptor inhibitors are effective antiplatelet drugs for preventing coagulation.

38.10 Coagulation modifiers can be used to treat symptoms of intermittent claudication.

38.11 Fibrinolysis is a process that removes thrombi.

38.12 Fibrinolytics are used to dissolve existing intravascular clots in patients with myocardial infarction and stroke.

38.13 Hemostatics are used to promote the formation of clots.

38.14 Hemophilia is treated by replacing the missing clotting factor(s) or by inhibiting coagulation.

CASE STUDY: Making the Patient Connection

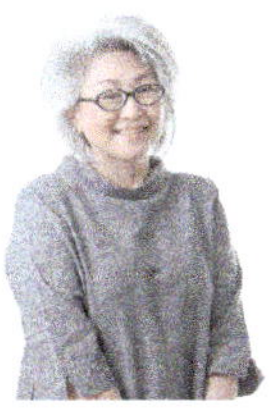

Remember the patient "Jihyo Yun" at the beginning of the chapter? Now read the remainder of the case study. Based on the information presented within this chapter, respond to the critical thinking questions that follow.

Jihyo Yun had looked forward to the trip and was anxious to see her grandchildren. When her son accepted an executive position with his company, she had no idea that he would be relocated to Bangkok. The trip would be long but certainly worth the effort. Jihyo never dreamed in her 74 years that she would be flying out of the United States, much less to Thailand. When the opportunity came to see her son and his family, she jumped at the chance. After all, it had been 5 years since he had left their home in Chicago.

When Jiyho returned from her trip, she noticed some pain in her right leg. Although she sees herself as a healthy older woman, she does experience occasional arthritis pain. Considering that she was on a commercial airliner for more than 20 hours, she did not think much about the leg discomfort. However, after a few days, Jihyo's leg became increasingly more painful and swollen. She could not imagine what was causing this problem. Finally, after 3 days, Jihyo became worried about what seemed to be increasing leg swelling and pain.

Jiyho is seen in her healthcare provider's office. The following health information is documented in her medical record:

> Jihyo Yun, 74-year-old Asian American woman. Her physical examination revealed the following findings: alert, oriented 74-year-old woman with chief complaint of swelling, painful right lower extremity × 3 days. Cardio: Heart rate regular without murmurs; blood pressure, 118/74 mmHg; all pulses present equal and strong in all extremities; no respiratory distress—regular, clear, breath sounds; audible bowel sounds in all four quadrants. Her right mid-calf area has 3–4+ pitting edema and is hot and painful to touch, and she has a moderate amount of varicosities in lower extremities bilaterally.
>
> Jihyo had a hysterectomy 15 years ago and does not drink alcohol or use tobacco. She takes occasional aspirin for muscle aches and has no known allergies. Her family history indicates that her father died from a stroke and her mother died of "old age." She has one sister who has diabetes.

Jihyo was diagnosed with DVT in her right leg. The treatment plan was to admit her into the hospital for anticoagulant therapy and pain control. In the hospital setting, Jihyo will receive heparin therapy. You are the nurse caring for this patient.

Critical Thinking Questions

1. Jihyo asks, "How soon will the heparin dissolve my blood clot?" How would you respond to this question?
2. What patient education should you provide Jihyo about anticoagulation therapy?
3. What is an aPTT? How will this test be used to direct heparin therapy?
4. What factors predisposed this patient to DVT?
5. What should Jihyo be taught about taking aspirin for arthritis pain?

Additional Case Study

You are attending your annual family reunion and begin talking to your favorite uncle, Lewis, about his recent hospitalization. Lewis Kinard, a 55-year-old man, was recently discharged from the hospital following an episode of atrial fibrillation. He returned home with instructions to take warfarin (Coumadin) 10 mg daily. He has many questions for you, his favorite relative.

1. Why would someone with atrial fibrillation be prescribed Coumadin?
2. What special precautions should Lewis take while on this drug?
3. Are there any foods that he should avoid or limit in his diet?
4. What laboratory testing will be done to determine this drug's effectiveness?

Chapter Review

1. A patient with deep vein thrombosis is being treated with a heparin infusion. The nurse would monitor for therapeutic effectiveness by noting which of the following?

1. Activated partial thromboplastin time
2. Prothrombin time
3. Platelet counts
4. International normalized ratio

2. Which of the following should the nurse include in the teaching plan for a patient receiving subcutaneous heparin? (Select all that apply.)

1. Inject medication in the deep fatty layer of the abdomen.
2. When brushing your teeth, use a soft-bristle toothbrush.
3. Hold direct pressure on any puncture sites for 15 minutes.
4. Use dental floss daily after brushing.
5. Take a daily aspirin tablet, 325 mg, to prevent inflammation at the injection site.

3. A patient who is taking warfarin (Coumadin) states, "I wake up every morning with arthritis pain and I always take aspirin or ibuprofen." The nurse's response would be based on which physiologic concepts?

1. Aspirin and ibuprofen (Motrin) will counteract the therapeutic effects of many anticoagulants.
2. Anticoagulants will reduce the half-life of drugs such as aspirin and ibuprofen.
3. Many substances such as aspirin and ibuprofen will increase the risk of bleeding.
4. The combination of aspirin products with anticoagulants will worsen arthritis pain.

4. What should the nurse teach the patient who is to receive alteplase (Activase) as part of the treatment for myocardial infarction?

1. The drug will be given IV, and the patient should be able to go home later today.
2. The patient should remain quiet and lying down during drug administration and for up to 8 hours after infusion.
3. The risk of bleeding returns to normal within 24 hours after the drug has been infused.
4. An increase in vitamin K–rich foods or a supplement will be needed for the week following the treatment.

5. A patient who is taking clopidogrel (Plavix) to prevent a stroke asks the nurse how the medication works. The nurse's response should be based on an understanding that Plavix:

1. Inhibits platelet aggregation to prevent clot formation.
2. Activates antithrombin III and subsequently inhibits thrombin.
3. Inhibits enzymes involved in the formation of vitamin K.
4. Converts plasminogen to plasmin to dissolve fibrin clots.

6. A patient will be receiving dabigatran (Pradaxa). Which of the following is true concerning this drug therapy? (Select all that apply.)

1. Ginger, garlic, and green tea may increase the risk of bleeding.
2. Vitamin B^{12} is used to augment this drug's response.
3. Pradaxa is used for deep vein thrombosis.
4. Activated partial thromboplastin time may be monitored to determine effectiveness.
5. This drug is contraindicated for patients with gastritis.

See Appendix A for answers to critical thinking questions, case study questions, and review questions.

References

American Stroke Association. (2018). *Anti-clotting agents explained.* http://www.strokeassociation.org/STROKEORG/LifeAfterStroke/HealthyLivingAfterStroke/ManagingMedicines/Anti-Clotting-Agents-Explained_UCM_310452_Article.jsp#.V_VoKyjt4RY

Kearon, C., Akl, E. A., Ornelas, J., Blaivas, A., Jimenez, D., Bounameaux, H., et al. (2016). Antithrombotic therapy for VTE disease: CHEST guideline and expert panel report. *CHEST Journal, 149*(2), 315–352. https://doi.org/10.1016/j.chest.2015.11.026

Lin, T., Chen, Y., Cheng, X., Li, N., & Sheng, X. (2019). Enoxaparin (or plus aspirin) for the prevention of recurrent miscarriage: A meta-analysis of randomized controlled studies. *European Journal of Obstetrics,*

Gynecology, and Reproductive Biology, *234*, 53–57. https://doi.org/10.1016/j.ejogrb.2018.12.023

Nahas, R., Saliba, W., Elias, A., & Elias, M. (2018). The prevalence of thrombophilia in women with recurrent fetal loss and outcome of anticoagulation therapy for the prevention of miscarriages. *Clinical and Applied Thrombosis*, *24*, 122–128. https://doi.org/10.1177/1076029616675967

National Center for Complementary and Integrative Health. (2016). *Garlic*. https://www.nccih.nih.gov/health/garlic

Patel, K. (2019). *Deep venous thrombosis*. http://emedicine.medscape.com/article/1911303-overview

U.S. Food and Drug Administration. (2015). *FDA information in medication errors involving activase and TNKase*. https://www.fda.gov/downloads/ForHealthProfessionals/LearningActivities/UCM464193.pdf

Zaiden, R. A. (2020). *Hemophilia A*. http://emedicine.medscape.com/article/779322-overview#a2

Selected Bibliography

Agarwal, S. K., & Agarwal, S. (2019). Role of intracoronary fibrinolytic therapy in contemporary PCI practice. *Cardiovascular Revascularization Medicine*, *20*(12), 1165–1171. https://doi.org/10.1016/j.carrev.2018.11.021

Capodanno, D., Huber, K., Mehran, R., Lip, G. Y., Faxon, D. P., Granger, C. B., et al. (2019). Management of antithrombotic therapy in atrial fibrillation patients undergoing PCI: JACC state-of-the-art review. *Journal of the American College of Cardiology*, *74*(1), 83–99. https://doi.org/10.1016/j.jacc.2019.05.016

Dominguez, J. A. (2019). *Peripheral arterial occlusive disease treatment & management*. Medscape. https://emedicine.medscape.com/article/460178-treatment

Drelich, D. A. (2020). *Hemophilia A treatment and management*. Medscape. https://emedicine.medscape.com/article/779322-treatment#d12

Franchini, M., Marano, G., Pati, I., Candura, F., Profili, S., Veropalumbo, E., et al. (2019). Emicizumab for the treatment of haemophilia A: A narrative review. *Blood Transfusion*, *17*(3), 223–228. https://doi.org/10.2450/2019.0026-19

Giordano, A., Musumeci, G., D'Angelillo, A., Rossini, R., Biondi Zoccai, G., Messina, S., et al. (2016). Effects of glycoprotein IIb/IIIa antagonists: Anti platelet aggregation and beyond. *Current Drug Metabolism*, *17*, 194–203. https://doi.org/10.2174/1389200217666151211121112

Khoshmohabat, H., Paydar, S., Kazemi, H. M., & Dalfardi, B. (2016). Overview of agents used for emergency hemostasis. *Trauma Monthly*, *21*(1), e26023. https://doi.org/10.5812/traumamon.26023

Lier, H., Maegele, M., & Shander, A. (2019). Tranexamic acid for acute hemorrhage: A narrative review of landmark studies and a critical reappraisal of its use over the last decade. *Anesthesia and Analgesia*, *129*(6), 1574-1584. https://doi.org/10.1213/ANE.0000000000004389

National Hemophilia Foundation. (2020). *Recommendation on the use and management of emicizumab-kxwh (Hemlibra) for hemophilia A with and without inhibitors*. https://www.hemophilia.org/Researchers-Healthcare-Providers/Medical-and-Scientific-Advisory-Council-MASAC/MASAC-Recommendations

Paul, J. D., & Cifu, A. S. (2019). Prevention and management of venous thromboembolism. *Journal of the American Medical Association*, *322*(16), 1602–1603. https://doi.org/10.1001/jama.2019.13853

Roberts, S. H., & Lawrence, S. M. (2017). CE: Venous thromboembolism: Updated management guidelines. *American Journal of Nursing*, *117*(5), 38–47. https://doi.org/10.1097/01.NAJ.0000516249.54064.53

Schweickert, P. A., Gaughen, J. R., Kreitel, E. M., Shephard, T. J., Solenski, N. J., & Jensen, M. E. (2016). An overview of antithrombotics in ischemic stroke. *The Nurse Practitioner*, *41*(6), 48–55. https://doi.org/10.1097/01.NPR.0000483077.47966.6e

Shahjouei, S., Tsivgoulis, G., Goyal, N., Sadighi, A., Mowla, A., Wang, M., et al. (2020). Safety of intravenous thrombolysis among patients taking direct oral anticoagulants: A systematic review and meta-analysis. *Stroke*, *51*(2), 533–541. https://doi.org/10.1161/STROKEAHA.119.026426

Weitz, J. I., & Chan, N. C. (2019). Advances in antithrombotic therapy. *Arteriosclerosis, Thrombosis, and Vascular Biology*, *39*(1), 7–12. https://doi.org/10.1161/ATVBAHA.118.310960

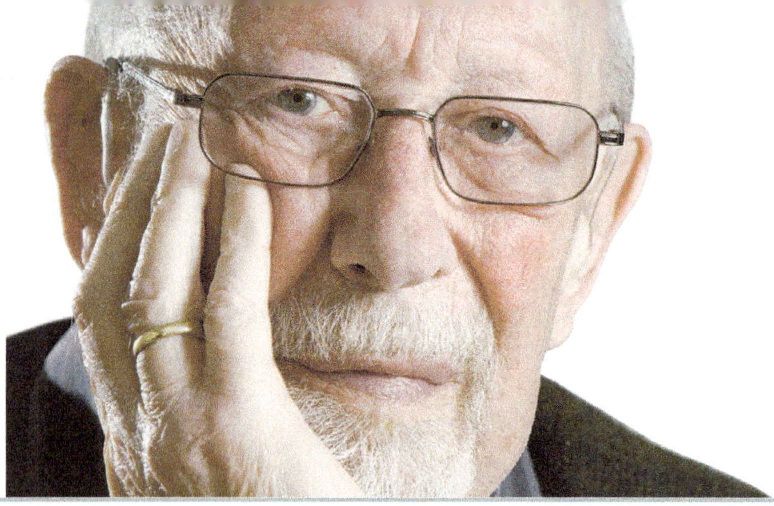

"For me, the worst part is the isolation from people. It's almost unbearable. I feel so lonely. If I could just be with people, I know I would feel better."
—*Patient "Carl Guenther"*

Chapter 39
Pharmacotherapy of Hematopoietic Disorders

Chapter Outline

Learning Outcomes

After reading this chapter, the student should be able to:

1. Describe the physiology of hematopoiesis.
2. Describe how aspects of hematopoiesis can be modified by the administration of medications.
3. Explain the functions of erythropoietin.
4. Explain the functions of colony-stimulating factors.
5. Classify types of anemia based on their causes.
6. Illustrate the metabolism, storage, and transfer of iron in the body.
7. Identify the role of intrinsic factor in the absorption of vitamin B_{12}.
8. Compare and contrast anemias caused by vitamin B_{12} and folate deficiency.
9. Describe the nurse's role in the pharmacologic management of hematopoietic disorders.
10. For each of the classes shown in the chapter outline, identify the prototype and representative drugs and explain the mechanism(s) of drug action, primary indications, contraindications, significant drug interactions, pregnancy data, and important adverse effects.
11. Apply clinical judgment to care for patients receiving pharmacotherapy for hematopoietic disorders.

Key Terms

Definitions of the terms in bold may be found in the Glossary.

The blood serves all other cells in the body and is the only fluid tissue. Because of its diverse functions, diseases affecting blood constituents have widespread effects on the body. This chapter examines medications used to enhance the functions of erythrocytes, leukocytes, and platelets. Pharmacology of the hematopoietic system is a small, though emerging, branch of medicine.

Physiology of Hematopoiesis

39.1 Hematopoiesis is a dynamic process that is responsive to the changing demands of the body.

Blood is a highly dynamic tissue; over 200 billion new blood cells are formed every day. The process of blood cell formation is called **hematopoiesis**, or hemopoiesis. In adults, hematopoiesis occurs primarily in red bone marrow and requires B vitamins, vitamin C, copper, iron, and other nutrients. Before proceeding, the student should read the brief review of blood found in Chapter 28.

Hematopoiesis responds to internal and external challenges faced by the body. For example, the production of white blood cells (WBCs) can increase tenfold in response to infection. The number of red blood cells (RBCs) can increase as much as fivefold in response to anemia or hypoxia. Homeostatic control of hematopoiesis is influenced by a number of hormones and growth factors, which allow for points for pharmacologic intervention. The process of hematopoiesis is illustrated in Figure 39.1.

The process of hematopoiesis begins in bone marrow with **pluripotent stem cells (hemocytoblasts)**, which are capable of maturing (differentiating) into any blood cell type.

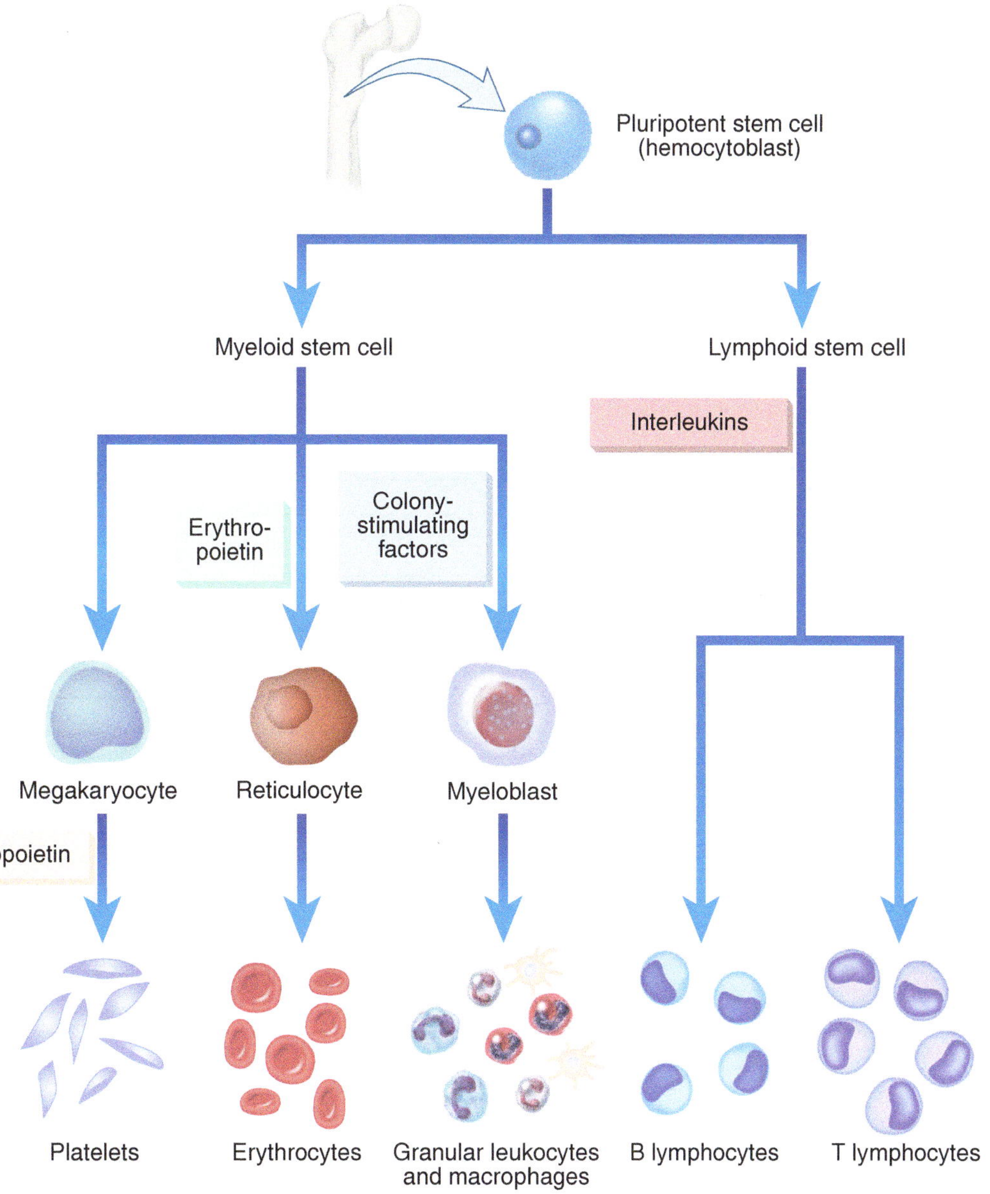

Figure 39.1 Hematopoiesis: Blood cells are formed from stem cells under the influence of hormones such as thrombopoietin, colony-stimulating factors, and erythropoietin.

What determines whether the stem cell produces RBCs, macrophages, lymphocytes, or perhaps platelets? The specific path taken by the pluripotent stem cell depends on the internal needs of the body. These needs are transmitted to pluripotent stem cells by regulatory substances that include various hormones and proteins. For example, high amounts of the hormone erythropoietin circulating through the blood signal the stem cells to differentiate into erythrocytes. Many types of cells secrete cytokines (interferons and interleukins) that signal the stem cells to increase or decrease the production of specific WBCs. Through recombinant deoxyribonucleic acid (DNA) technology, some of these regulatory agents, shown in Figure 39.1, are now available in sufficient quantities to be used as medications.

PharmFACT

Iron deficiency is common during pregnancy and affects about 7% of women in their first trimester, 14% in the second trimester, and 30% in the third trimester (Office of Dietary Supplements, 2020a).

The pharmacologic management of hematopoietic disorders often involves simply replacing a deficient substance that is essential to hematopoiesis. In some cases, the drug is identical to, or very closely resembles, the deficient endogenous factor. For example, the drug epoetin alfa (Epogen, Procrit) is identical to the natural hormone erythropoietin and stimulates the production of RBCs in the same manner. Administration of antianemia medications such as ferrous sulfate or vitamin B_{12} supplies the patient with essential factors that may be deficient.

Some of the hematopoietic drugs have become important adjunct medications in the pharmacotherapy of malignancies. Antineoplastic drugs are often toxic to bone marrow and cause neutropenia, a reduced number of WBCs. Neutropenia is a primary cause of patient morbidity and mortality in the treatment of cancer. Hematopoietic drugs can be used to boost the WBC counts in these patients.

Natural hormones that regulate some aspect of blood formation are called hematopoietic growth factors. These drugs and their doses are listed in Table 39.1.

Table 39.1 Hematopoietic Growth Factors

Drug	Route and Adult Dose (Maximum Dose Where Indicated)	Adverse Effects
Erythropoietic Growth Factors		
darbepoetin alfa (Aranesp)	Subcutaneous/IV: 0.45 mcg/kg once per wk (max: 74 mg/kg)	*Headache, fever, nausea and vomiting, diarrhea, insomnia, cough, upper respiratory infection, edema, pyrexia, rash* HTN, seizures, HF, MI, stroke
epoetin alfa (Epogen, Procrit)	Subcutaneous/IV: Start with 50–100 units/kg/dose and adjust to target Hct range of 30–33% (max: 36%); Hct should not increase by more than 4 points in any 2-wk period	
Colony-Stimulating Factors		
filgrastim (Granix, Neupogen, Zarxio): granulocyte-CSF	IV: 5–10 mcg/kg by 30-min infusion or as a subcutaneous single-bolus dose	*Flulike syndrome, fever, dyspnea, nausea and vomiting, weakness, alopecia, peripheral edema, arthralgia, bone pain* Thrombocytopenia, cutaneous vasculitis, pericardial effusion (sargramostim), tachycardia (sargramostim), acute respiratory distress syndrome, splenic rupture
pegfilgrastim (Neulasta)	Subcutaneous: 6 mg once per chemotherapy cycle	
sargramostim (Leukine): GM-CSF	IV: 250 mcg/m^2/day infused for 14 days, begin 2–4 h after bone marrow transfusion and not less than 24 h after last dose of chemotherapy	
Platelet Enhancers		
avatrombopag (Doptelet)	PO: 40–60 mg (begin dosing 10–13 days prior to a medical procedure)	*Pyrexia, abdominal pain, nausea, headache, fatigue, peripheral edema* Fetal toxicity, thromboembolic complications
eltrombopag (Promacta)	PO: 25–50 mg once daily (max: 75 mg/day)	*Arthralgia, myalgia, paresthesia, insomnia* Bone marrow fibrosis, thromboembolism, hematologic malignancy, hepatotoxicity
fostamatinib (Tavalisse)	PO: 100–150 mg bid	*Hypertension (HTN), diarrhea, nausea, respiratory infection* Hepatotoxicity, neutropenia, embryofetal toxicity
lusutrombopag (Mulpleta)	PO: 3 mg once daily for 7 days (given 8–14 days prior to a medical procedure)	*Headache* Thromboembolic complications in patients with chronic liver disease
romiplostim (Nplate)	Subcutaneous: 1 mcg/kg/wk (max mcg/kg/wk)	*Arthralgia, dizziness, insomnia, myalgia, confusion, fatigue* Thromboembolism, bone marrow fibrosis

Note: *Italics* indicate common adverse effects. Underline indicates serious adverse effects.

Hematopoietic Growth Factors

39.2 Erythropoietin stimulates production of red blood cells and is used to treat anemia.

The process of RBC formation, or erythropoiesis, is regulated by the hormone erythropoietin. In adults, 90% of erythropoietin is secreted by the kidneys and 10% is secreted by the liver.

The primary signal to increase the renal secretion of erythropoietin is hypoxia, a reduction in oxygen reaching the proximal tubule cells in the kidney. Once secreted, erythropoietin travels to the bone marrow where it interacts with receptors on stem cells and delivers the message to increase erythrocyte production. Just as important, erythropoietin also stimulates the production of hemoglobin (Hgb), which is required for a functional erythrocyte. Hemorrhage, chronic obstructive pulmonary disease, anemia, or high altitudes may increase serum levels of erythropoietin as much as 1000-fold in response to severe hypoxia. Erythropoietin is marketed as the drug epoetin alfa (Epogen, Procrit). Darbepoetin alfa (Aranesp) is closely related to epoetin alfa but has a duration of action that is two to three times longer. These drugs are sometimes called erythropoietic growth factors.

PROTOTYPE DRUG **Epoetin Alfa (Epogen, Procrit)**

Classification **Therapeutic:** Hematopoietic growth factor, drug for anemia
Pharmacologic: Erythropoietin

Therapeutic Effects and Uses: Approved in 1989 by the U.S. Food and Drug Administration (FDA), epoetin alfa is made through recombinant DNA technology and is functionally identical to human erythropoietin. Although the drug may be administered intravenously (IV), the subcutaneous route is generally preferred because lower doses are needed, absorption is slower, and a more sustained response can be achieved. Epoetin is not used for the emergency correction of severe anemia or as a substitute for transfusion because it has a gradual onset of action. The hematocrit (Hct) increases 2% per week during the initial weeks of epoetin therapy and some patients require 2 to 6 weeks for a change in Hct to occur. Most patients on epoetin therapy also receive iron supplements to meet the increased demands caused by the elevated erythrocyte production. Although epoetin alfa does not cure any primary disease, it reduces anemia symptoms and dramatically improves the patient's ability to perform activities of daily living (ADLs). A typical initial regimen for epoetin alfa requires 50 to 100 units/kg three times per week until a target Hgb level of 10 to 12 g/dL is achieved.

Epoetin is indicated for the treatment of anemia associated with chronic kidney disease (CKD). Patients with CKD often experience anemia because they are unable to secrete sufficient endogenous erythropoietin. The drug is occasionally prescribed to reduce the need for transfusions in patients with anemia prior to elective surgery, if a significant blood loss is expected. Patients with HIV infection who are receiving zidovudine may receive epoetin alfa to treat anemia caused by antiretroviral drugs.

Epoetin alfa is given to patients undergoing chemotherapy for nonmyeloid malignancies to counteract the anemia commonly caused by antineoplastic drugs. It should be carefully noted that the anemia must be secondary to the chemotherapy, not to the cancer itself. Research has shown that the administration of epoetin alfa does not benefit patients when the anemia is caused by the malignancy; in fact, mortality is increased in these patients by the administration of the drug. Care must be taken not to administer epoetin alfa to patients with myeloid malignancies such as myelogenous leukemia because the drug may increase tumor growth.

In 2018 the FDA approved epoetin alfa-epbx (Retacrit), a biosimilar to Epogen and Procrit. As a biosimilar, Retacrit has the same indications and adverse effects as epoetin alfa. It is expected to cost less than the brand name products Epogen and Procrit.

Mechanism of Action: Epoetin alfa stimulates the division and differentiation of stem cells in the bone marrow to become erythrocytes. Erythropoietin also promotes the synthesis of Hgb and causes a shift of marrow reticulocytes into the circulation.

Pharmacokinetics:

Route(s)	IV, subcutaneous
Absorption	Readily absorbed (subcutaneous)
Distribution	Unknown if the drug crosses the placenta or is secreted in breast milk
Primary metabolism	Plasma
Primary excretion	Mostly feces; 10% renal
Onset of action	7–14 days
Duration of action	2 weeks; half-life: 4–13 h

Adverse Effects: The most serious adverse effect of epoetin alfa is HTN, which occurs in up to 27% of patients receiving the drug. An antihypertensive drug may be indicated. Some patients with CKD develop neutralizing antibodies to subcutaneous epoetin alfa, which can lead to a rapidly developing severe anemia known as pure red cell aplasia. Seizures may occur during the first 90 days of therapy, especially if blood pressure and Hct rise rapidly. Common adverse effects include headache, fever, nausea and vomiting, diarrhea, cough, and edema. **Black Box Warning:** The risk of serious cardiovascular and thromboembolic events is increased with epoetin alfa therapy. Transient ischemic attack (TIA), myocardial infarction (MI), and stroke have occurred in patients with CKD who are on dialysis and being treated with epoetin alfa. Epoetin increased the rate of deep vein thrombosis (DVT) in patients not receiving concurrent anticoagulation. The lowest dose possible should be used in patients with cancer because the drug can promote tumor progression and shorten overall survival in some patients.

Contraindications/Precautions: The drug should not be given to patients with uncontrolled HTN because epoetin alfa may increase blood pressure. The risk of thromboembolic events, stroke, and MI greatly increases when Hgb level rises above 12 g/dL. Patients with known hypersensitivity to products derived from mammal cells, such as albumin, should not receive this drug.

Drug Interactions: Androgens can increase blood viscosity, resulting in an increased response from epoetin alfa. The effectiveness of epoetin alfa will be greatly reduced in patients with iron deficiency or other vitamin-depleted states. Whenever possible, such deficiencies should be corrected prior to initiating epoetin alfa therapy. Hemodialysis patients with preexisting heart disease who are taking epoetin may require increased doses of heparin. **Herbal/Food:** Unknown.

Pregnancy: Eepoetin alfa caused embryofetal death, skeletal anomalies, and growth defects in laboratory animals. Data is not available on the amount of epoetin alfa in human milk or its effects on nursing infants.

Treatment of Overdose: Overdose may lead to polycythemia (too many erythrocytes), which can be corrected by phlebotomy.

Clinician Responsibilities: Key clinical implications for patients receiving epoetin alfa are included in Applied Clinical Judgment: Patients Receiving Pharmacotherapy with Erythropoietin.

Drugs Similar to Epoetin Alfa (Epogen, Procrit)

The only other erythropoietic growth factor is darbepoetin alfa.

Darbepoetin alfa (Aranesp): Approved in 2001, darbepoetin alfa has a chemical structure that closely resembles that of epoetin alfa. It has the same mechanism of action, efficacy, and safety profile as epoetin alfa. It is administered by the subcutaneous or IV route and has an extended duration of action that allows it to be administered once weekly. Maximum response occurs in 2 to 4 weeks. Darbepoetin alfa is approved for the treatment of anemia associated with cancer chemotherapy or CKD. Like epoetin alfa, darbepoetin should be administered only to patients with anemia secondary to the chemotherapy and not caused by the malignancy itself. In addition, Hgb levels should be maintained below 12 g/dL to reduce the risks of serious cardiovascular adverse events. Darbepoetin has similar adverse effects and the same black box warning as epoetin alfa. Animal reproduction studies showed no placental transfer of darbepoetin alfa during pregnancy. No data are available on adverse effects of the drug during breastfeeding.

CONNECTIONS: APPLIED CLINICAL JUDGMENT

Patients Receiving Pharmacotherapy with Erythropoietin

Key Assessment Data

- History of current condition, baseline vital signs, physical exam findings; history of cardiovascular disease (HTN, MI), peripheral vascular disease, respiratory (including previous pulmonary embolism), neurologic (including stroke), hepatic disease, CKD, and pregnancy status; assess drug history including allergies, current prescription and over-the-counter (OTC) drugs, and herbal preparations. Obtain baseline vital signs, especially blood pressure. Assess level of fatigue.
- Ongoing assessment during drug therapy includes laboratory findings (e.g., CBC, activated partial thromboplastin time [aPTT], international normalized ratio [INR], transferrin and serum ferritin levels, renal and liver function studies). Continue to monitor vital signs and blood pressure, especially during the first 2 weeks of therapy.

Desired Therapeutic Outcomes

Improvement is observed and measurable by increase in Hct, RBC count significantly improved, patient's activity level and ability to carry out ADLs has improved.

Minimizing Adverse Effects

- Because Hct rapidly increases during the first 2 weeks of therapy, HTN or seizures may occur and should be reported immediately. Peripheral thrombosis, including coronary or cerebral, may also occur.
- Response to epoetin alfa may be decreased if blood levels of iron, folic acid, and vitamin B_{12} are deficient. Continue to monitor laboratory values and dietary intake.
- Adequate fluid intake with water or nonhyperosmolar beverages will help to maintain adequate fluid balance as Hct levels rise.
- For patients receiving hemodialysis, the heparin dose during dialysis may need to be increased as Hct increases.

Lifespan Considerations

- The older adult is at greater risk for thromboembolic events due to age-related vascular changes.
- The drug should not be taken during pregnancy, if pregnancy is suspected, or while breastfeeding unless ordered by the provider.
- Epoetin alfa may contain preservatives such as benzyl alcohol. Benzyl alcohol may cause fetal gasping syndrome. Use preservative-free formulations.

CONNECTIONS: APPLIED CLINICAL JUDGMENT *(continued)*

Patients Receiving Pharmacotherapy with Erythropoietin

Patient and Caregiver Education

- Immediately report sudden onset or severe headache, changes in LOC, weakness or numbness in extremities, or premonitory signs and symptoms of seizure activity (e.g., aura), angina, or symptoms of peripheral thrombosis (e.g., leg pain, pale extremity, diminished peripheral pulses).
- Rest when fatigued and space activities throughout the day to allow for adequate rest periods during early therapy and until RBC counts are within normal limits.
- Maintain a healthy diet with adequate amounts of iron, folic acid, and vitamin B_{12} such as is found in meats, dairy, eggs, fortified cereals and breads, leafy green vegetables, citrus fruits, beans, and peas.
- Proper injection technique includes:
  - The vial should be gently rotated, never shaken, to mix the content. Vials are kept under refrigeration and should be gently warmed in the hand.
  - All vials are for one-time use only and any remaining amount should be discarded.
  - If an indwelling subcutaneous soft catheter (e.g., Insuflon) is left in place, follow appropriate site care and insertion technique as appropriate and rotate sites weekly.

Prescribing Considerations

- Evaluate patient's iron status before and during treatment.
- Correct or exclude other causes of anemia (vitamin deficiency, metabolic or chronic inflammatory conditions, bleeding) before initiating therapy.
- Individualize patient dosing and use the lowest dose that will maintain hemoglobin levels sufficiently to reduce the need for RBC transfusions.

39.3 Colony-stimulating factors increase the production of leukocytes.

Regulation of WBC production, or leukopoiesis, is more complicated than erythropoiesis because the blood has different types of leukocytes. Adding to the complication is that a large number of substances modify the synthesis and activation of leukocytes and the processes of leukopoiesis regulation are incompletely understood. Pharmacologically, the most important substances are **colony-stimulating factors (CSFs)**. CSFs are hormones that stimulate the growth and differentiation of one or more types of leukocytes.

CSFs are produced by a diverse group of cells including endothelial cells, fibroblasts, macrophages, and T lymphocytes. Normally present at minute levels in the blood, the production of CSFs rapidly increases when the body receives a bacterial challenge. Although the leukopoietic growth factors are active at very low concentrations, each stem cell stimulated by these growth factors is capable of producing as many as 1000 mature leukocytes. CSFs not only increase the production of new leukocytes, but they also activate existing WBCs. Examples of enhanced functions include increased migration of leukocytes to antigens, increased antibody toxicity, and increased phagocytosis.

CSFs are named according to the types of blood cells that they stimulate. For example, granulocyte colony-stimulating factor (G-CSF) increases the production of neutrophils, the most common type of granulocyte. Granulocyte-macrophage colony-stimulating factor (GM-CSF) stimulates both neutrophil and macrophage production. The process of identifying the many endogenous CSFs, determining their normal functions, and discovering their potential value as therapeutic agents is an emerging area of pharmacology.

Through recombinant DNA technology, several CSFs are now available as medications (see Table 39.1). The goal of CSF therapy is to produce a rapid increase in the number of neutrophils in patients who have suppressed immune systems (neutropenia). CSF therapy shortens the length of time patients are neutropenic and susceptible to life-threatening bacterial and fungal infections. Severe neutropenia may also cause chemotherapy schedules to be delayed or abandoned. By raising neutrophil counts, CSFs can assist in keeping antineoplastic dosing regimens on schedule and more effective. The degree of increase in circulating neutrophils is dose related. Indications for CSF therapy include the following:

- To decrease the incidence of infections in patients with nonmyeloid malignancies who are receiving myelosuppressive antineoplastic drugs.
- To reduce the time to neutrophil recovery and the duration of fever in patients receiving chemotherapy for acute myeloid leukemia.
- To reduce the duration of neutropenia in patients receiving myeloablative chemotherapy followed by bone marrow transplantation.
- To reduce the incidence of infections and fever in patients with severe, chronic neutropenia (such as those with AIDS).
- To mobilize hematopoietic progenitor cells into the peripheral blood for collection by leukapheresis (collection of WBCs from a blood sample).

It is often difficult to assess the adverse effects of CSF medications because the same types of patient symptoms may be caused by the condition or disease being treated. Nonspecific adverse effects include nausea and vomiting, fatigue, fever, and flushing. Therapy requires careful laboratory monitoring to avoid producing too many neutrophils. Several recent research studies have suggested that the risk of developing acute myeloid leukemia or myelodysplastic syndrome may be doubled when CSFs are administered to patients undergoing chemotherapy for breast cancer.

PROTOTYPE DRUG **Filgrastim (Granix, Neupogen, Zarxio)**

Classification **Therapeutic:** Drug for increasing neutrophil production
Pharmacologic: Colony-stimulating factor

Therapeutic Effects and Uses: Produced through recombinant DNA technology, filgrastim is nearly identical in structure to human G-CSF and has the same biologic activity. Approved in 1991, its primary actions are to increase neutrophil production in the bone marrow and to enhance the phagocytic and cytotoxic functions of existing neutrophils. The subcutaneous route is preferred, although filgrastim may also be administered by slow IV infusion. A typical regimen is 5 to 10 mcg/kg given once or twice daily. Continued therapy is based on absolute neutrophil counts (ANCs): Therapy is usually discontinued once laboratory results indicate 10,000 cells/mm^3 or greater.

Two biosimilar medications are available, which have identical indications, effectiveness, and adverse reactions to filgrastim, the reference molecule. In 2015, filgrastim-sndz (Zarxio) was the first biosimilar product approved in the United States. In 2018, filgrastim-aafi (Nivestym) was approved. It is predicted that the biosimilars will reduce the cost of filgrastim therapy. TBO-filgrastim (Granix) was approved in 2012 as a self-administration kit that allows the drug to be injected at home. Granix is technically not a biosimilar because it was approved prior to the FDA initiating the biosimilar pathway. Unlike the others, it only has one indication: to reduce the duration of neutropenia in patients with nonmyeloid malignancies who are receiving myelosuppressive antineoplastic drugs.

Mechanism of Action: Filgrastim acts by the same mechanism as endogenous G-CSF. The drug causes an increase in neutrophil production in the bone marrow, resulting in higher levels of circulating neutrophils.

Pharmacokinetics:

Route(s)	IV, subcutaneous
Absorption	Rapidly absorbed (subcutaneous)
Distribution	Unknown if it crosses the placenta or is secreted in breast milk
Primary metabolism	Unknown
Primary excretion	Renal
Onset of action	4 h
Duration of action	4 days

Adverse Effects: Although filgrastim is well tolerated, the drug is associated with potentially serious adverse effects and close monitoring is required. Nausea and vomiting occur in the majority of patients. Bone pain may occur in up to 33% of patients receiving filgrastim. The pain may be diffuse or localized to bones with the greatest amount of bone marrow: long bones, sternum, ribs, and pelvis. The degree of pain is dose dependent and can usually be managed with nonopioid analgesics. Frequent laboratory tests are conducted to ensure that excessive numbers of neutrophils (leukocytosis) do not occur. Leukocyte counts higher than 100,000 cells/mm^3 increase the risk of serious adverse effects such as respiratory failure, intracranial hemorrhage or infarction, retinal hemorrhage, and MI. Hyperuricemia and elevated lactate dehydrogenase and alkaline phosphatase levels occur in a significant number of patients. Splenomegaly may occur in 30% of patients receiving long-term therapy with filgrastim. Other common adverse effects include fatigue, rash, epistaxis, decreased platelet counts, neutropenic fever, alopecia, and diarrhea. Allergic reactions, including anaphylaxis, are rare.

Contraindications/Precautions: Patients with hypersensitivity to *Escherichia coli* (*E. coli*) proteins should not receive filgrastim because this microbe is used to produce the recombinant drug. Patients with sickle cell disease should be treated with caution because filgrastim may worsen this condition. Filgrastim should not be administered to patients with myeloid cancers.

Drug Interactions: Because antineoplastic drugs and CSFs produce opposite effects, filgrastim is not administered until at least 24 hours after a chemotherapy session. Lithium causes the release of neutrophils and may contribute to filgrastim-induced leukocytosis. **Herbal/Food:** Unknown.

Pregnancy: Filgrastim reduced embryofetal survival and increased fetal abortion in laboratory animals. Small amounts of filgrastim are secreted in breast milk; however, the drug is not orally absorbed in neonates.

Treatment of Overdose: Overdose can lead to leukocytosis and should be prevented by discontinuing the drug when ANC rises above 10,000 cells/mm^3. There is no specific therapy for overdose.

Clinician Responsibilities: Key clinical implications for patients receiving filgrastim are included in Applied Clinical Judgment: Patients Receiving Pharmacotherapy with Colony-Stimulating Factors.

Drugs Similar to Filgrastim (Granix, Neupogen, Zarxio)

The two other CSFs are pegfilgrastim and sargramostim. Both showed fetal harm in laboratory animals. It is not known if they cause adverse effects in the breastfed neonate.

Pegfilgrastim (Neulasta): Approved in 2002, pegfilgrastim is a form of filgrastim bonded to a molecule of polyethylene glycol. This delays the renal excretion of the molecule, allowing the drug to remain in the body with a sustained duration of action. Its only approved indications are to decrease the incidence of infections in patients with nonmyeloid malignancies who are receiving myelosuppressive antineoplastic drugs or as prophylaxis of chemotherapy-induced neutropenia. The drug is available as a single-use prefilled syringe given by the subcutaneous route, once per chemotherapy cycle. It should not be administered 14 days before or 24 hours after the administration of cytotoxic chemotherapy. Adverse effects, interactions, and contraindications are the same as those of filgrastim.

Biosimilars that have been approved include pegfilgrastim-jmdb (Fulphila), pegfilgrastim-cbqv (Udenyca), pegfilgrastim-bmez (Ziextenzo), and pegfilgrastim-apgf (Nyvepria). The biosimilars have the same effectiveness, and adverse effects as pegfilgrastim (Neulasta), the reference product.

Sargramostim (Leukine): Sargramostim is structurally very similar to natural GM-CSF and has the same biologic activity. It may be administered IV, but subcutaneous is the preferred route. The drug has multiple effects that include increasing the number of circulating neutrophils, eosinophils, and monocytes; activating macrophages; increasing the cytotoxic activity of monocytes; and enhancing the bactericidal activity of other cells of the immune system. Indications are essentially the same as filgrastim. Typically, therapy with sargramostim is initiated when ANC is less than 500 cells/mm^3 and continues until an ANC of 1500 cells/mm^3 for 3 consecutive days is achieved. To prevent leukocytosis, sargramostim should be discontinued if the ANC rises above 10,000 cells/mm^3.

Like filgrastim, bone pain is a common adverse effect. A serious adverse effect of sargramostim is respiratory distress that occurs during the IV infusion the first time the drug is administered, which appears to be related to the trapping of granulocytes in the pulmonary circulation. The patient develops difficulty breathing, tachycardia, low blood pressure, and lightheadedness. These symptoms usually call for discontinuing sargramostim therapy. Other common adverse effects include abdominal pain, diarrhea, and fever.

CONNECTION Checkpoint 39.1

Zarxio is a biosimilar drug to filgrastim (Neupogen). From Chapter 1, define the term *biosimilar* and describe how a biosimilar drug compares to its reference product.

CONNECTIONS: APPLIED CLINICAL JUDGMENT

Patients Receiving Pharmacotherapy with Colony-Stimulating Factors

Key Assessment Data

- History of recent or current infections, especially viral or fungal; recent surgeries, injuries, or wounds; yeast infections (e.g., thrush); vaccination history; cardiac conditions (e.g., dysrhythmias, heart failure [HF]); respiratory, renal, and hepatic conditions; pregnancy status; assess drug history including allergies, current prescription and OTC drugs, and herbal preparations. Obtain baseline vital signs.
- Ongoing assessment during drug therapy includes laboratory findings of CBC, WBC, or ANC (total WBC multiplied by total percentage of neutrophils [segmented plus bands]), renal and liver function studies, uric acid levels, and electrocardiogram (ECG).

Desired Therapeutic Outcomes

Improvement is observed and measurable by CBC, WBC, or ANC has increased and there are no signs or symptoms of infection.

Minimizing Adverse Effects

- Rise in WBC or ANC counts will depend on the condition treated (e.g., depth and length of nadir from cytotoxic chemotherapy). Counts are usually monitored twice per week or as ordered.
- Bone pain tends to occur 2 to 3 days prior to rise in circulating WBCs due to the production of WBCs in bone marrow. Continue to monitor for bone pain, especially lower back, posterior iliac crests, and sternum.
- The risk for infections continues until WBC or ANC levels rise. Opportunistic infections, such as yeast, and viruses, such as herpes simplex, may occur. Maintain meticulous infection control measures and immediately report any signs and symptoms of fever or infections, especially viral or fungal. Parameters should be set for reporting fever (e.g., any temperature over 38°C [100.5°F]), dependent on the underlying disease condition and drug therapy.
- Sargramostim may cause significant ST-segment depression with potential for serious dysrhythmias, especially in patients with previous cardiac conditions. Monitor ECG periodically for ST-segment depression or dysrhythmias.
- Sargramostim may cause respiratory distress as granulocyte counts rise, especially in patients with preexisting respiratory disorders. Monitor for signs of dyspnea or respiratory distress, especially when accompanied by tachycardia and hypotension.
- Hypersensitive to proteins used in the drug development process may occur. Monitor for signs and symptoms of allergic-type reactions.
- Filgrastim may cause an elevation in liver enzymes. Monitor hepatic status during drug administration.
- Filgrastim has been associated with rare but potentially fatal cases of splenomegaly and rupture. Assess for spleen enlargement periodically.
- Hyperuricemia may cause gout attacks. Increase fluid intake, especially in gout-prone patients.
- Filgrastim may be stopped when neutrophil counts reach 10,000/mm^3, sargramostim when neutrophil counts reach 20,000/mm^3, or unless otherwise ordered.

Lifespan Considerations

- Pediatric patients with forms of congenital neutropenia (e.g., congenital agranulocytosis) are at greater risk for developing acute myelogenous leukemia and myelodysplastic neutropenia related to drug therapy.
- The drug should not be taken during pregnancy, if pregnancy is suspected, or while breastfeeding unless ordered by the provider.

(continued)

CONNECTIONS: APPLIED CLINICAL JUDGMENT *(continued)*

Patients Receiving Pharmacotherapy with Colony-Stimulating Factors

Patient and Caregiver Education

- Report any fever per the parameters set by the healthcare provider, or symptoms of infection such as wounds with redness or drainage, increasing cough, increasing fatigue, white patches on oral mucous membranes, white and itchy vaginal discharge, or itchy blister-like vesicles on the skin.
- Report any severe bone pain not relieved by non-narcotic analgesics.
- Immediately report any palpitations, dizziness, angina, dyspnea, respiratory distress, or symptoms of allergic reaction such as rash, urticaria, wheezing, and dyspnea immediately.
- Gout-prone patients should report signs and symptoms of gout and increase fluid intake to enhance renal elimination of uric acid.
- Report any significant itching, yellowing of the sclera or skin, darkened urine, or light or clay-colored stools.
- Report any symptoms of left upper abdominal pain or left shoulder pain, which may indicate spleen enlargement or rupture.
- Rest when fatigued and to space activities throughout the day to allow for adequate rest periods during early therapy and until WBC counts are within normal limits.
- Practice general infection control measures, such as:
  - Wash hands frequently and avoid crowded indoor places.
  - Avoid people with known infections or young children because they have a higher risk of having an infection.
  - Cook food thoroughly and do not consume raw fruits or vegetables. Allow the caregiver to prepare raw meats or fish and to clean up.
- Proper injection technique includes:
  - The vial should be gently rotated, never shaken, to mix the content. Vials are kept under refrigeration and should be gently warmed in the hand.
  - All vials are for one-time use only and any remaining amount should be discarded.
  - If an indwelling subcutaneous soft catheter (e.g., Insuflon) is left in place, follow appropriate site care and insertion technique as appropriate and rotate sites weekly.

Prescribing Considerations

- Do not give in the period 24 hours prior to the administration of chemotherapy, no earlier than 24 hours after chemotherapy, or for 24 hours after a RBC infusion.
- A CBC and platelet count should be obtained before instituting therapy and monitored twice weekly during therapy.
- Should be used during pregnancy only if the potential benefit to the mother justifies the potential risk to the fetus.
- Doses may be increased in increments for each chemotherapy treatment and should be administered daily for up to 2 weeks until the ANC has reached 10,000 mm^3 following the expected chemotherapy-induced neutrophil nadir.

CONNECTIONS: Using Research in Practice

Colony-Stimulating Factors in the Treatment of COVID-19

Because SARS-CoV-2, the cause of COVID-19, is a novel virus not seen before, research into potential treatments is ongoing and is continuing even after vaccine availability. It is known that the virus causes an extraordinary inflammatory response, and drug therapies are in part targeting that overreaction by the immune system. Corticosteroids, immune modulators, and convalescent plasma are part of the arsenal that may be used.

The colony-stimulating factor GM-CSF (sargramostim) may also be beneficial by encouraging pulmonary repair in cases of the acute respiratory distress syndrome caused by COVID-19. Unlike its usual subcutaneous administration, sargramostim is administered by inhalation in this treatment, and it appears to improve bronchoalveolar epithelial cells, exerting a lung-protective effect (Rizk et al., 2020).

39.4 Platelet enhancers may be used to treat thrombocytopenia.

The production of platelets, or thrombocytopoiesis, begins when megakaryocytes in the bone marrow start shedding membrane-bound packets. These packets enter the bloodstream and become platelets. A single megakaryocyte can produce thousands of platelets. A normal platelet count ranges from 150,000 to 450,000 platelets per microliter of blood. Megakaryocyte activity is controlled by the hormone thrombopoietin, which is produced by the liver and bone marrow. Thrombopoietin is not available as a medication, although several medications have been developed to boost platelet production.

Thrombocytopenia can be a serious condition because a deficiency in the number of platelets can result in bleeding. There are many possible causes of thrombocytopenia. One common cause is immune thrombocytopenia or ITP (formerly called idiopathic thrombocytopenic purpura). ITP is an autoimmune disorder in which platelets are destroyed in the spleen by macrophages. Secondary thrombocytopenia can be caused by medications, leukemia, or systemic lupus erythematosus. In 2021 a newly described type of thrombocytopenia was discovered to be associated with administration of several Covid-19 vaccines. Vaccine-induced immune thrombotic thrombocytopenia (VITT) occurs 4 to 30 days after vaccination and is extremely rare. The causes and treatment of this disorder are rapidly evolving.

First-Line Options for Thrombocytopenia

The American Society of Hematology Guidelines (Neunert et al., 2019) recommend oral corticosteroids such as prednisone or dexamethasone as the initial treatment of ITP with a platelet count less than 30,000/microliter for asymptomatic patients or those with minor bleeding. Corticosteroids decrease the production of antiplatelet antibodies and increase the platelet count in 2 to 4 weeks. Therapy is recommended for only 6 weeks because long-term corticosteroid therapy may result in significant adverse effects (see Chapter 68).

Two blood products have been used as a supplement to corticosteroids to treat ITP for many years. Intravenous immune globulin (IVIG) (Carimune, Gammagard, others) contains pooled antibodies obtained from donor plasma. The product contains concentrated IgG antibodies. Through multiple, complex actions, the infused IgG suppresses the macrophage phagocytosis of antibody-coated platelets, thus dampening the autoimmune hyperresponse that is causing the thrombocytopenia. The patient may experience temporary headache, fever, and nausea or vomiting. IVIG is used to treat dozens of infections and immunodeficiencies (see Chapter 43). IVIG is administered over 3 to 6 hours.

Intravenous RhIg (RhoGam, WinRho SDF) is a specialized IgG solution containing concentrated antibodies to the Rh protein. In blood typing, the Rh factor is called the D protein, therefore intravenous RhIg is called Anti-D. When given to Rh-positive patients, the anti-D antibodies from the medication will attach to the patient's RBCs. The splenic macrophages, which were attacking platelets, now begin removing the anti-D-coated RBCs, allowing the number of platelets to increase. Platelet counts rise within 1 to 2 days and peak at 14 days. Common side effects include headaches, chills, and fever and a small number may develop mild anemia. RhIg is infused in a significantly shorter time (3 to 5 minutes) with a smaller volume than IVIG. This treatment is only effective in patients who are Rh positive.

Second-Line Options for Thrombocytopenia

If the patient is unresponsive to corticosteroid and immunoglobulin treatments, thrombopoietin receptor agonists and a few other second-line medications are available. Thrombopoietin receptor agonists (TPO-RAs) are medications that activate the natural thrombopoietin receptor, thus inducing megakaryocyte division and differentiation. Each of the second-line medications are presented separately.

Avatrombopag (Doptelet): Approved in 2018, avatrombopag is a TPO-RA indicated for the treatment of thrombocytopenia in adults with chronic liver disease who are scheduled to undergo a medical procedure. The drug stimulates megakaryocytes in the bone marrow to increase platelet production. The medication is taken for 5 consecutive days, and the medical procedure must be done within 5 to 8 days after the last dose. Peak effects occur at 10 to 13 days. The most common adverse reactions are pyrexia, abdominal pain, nausea, headache, fatigue, and peripheral edema. The most serious potential adverse effects are thromboembolic complications. Avatrombopag showed fetal harm and spontaneous abortion in laboratory animals. Breastfeeding is not recommended during therapy and for at least 2 weeks after the last dose.

Eltrombopag (Promacta): Approved in 2008, eltrombopag is an oral medication that increases the number of platelets in the blood by activating thrombopoietin receptors. It is indicated for the treatment of thrombocytopenia in patients with chronic ITP who have not responded to corticosteroids, immunoglobulins, or splenectomy. Platelet increases may take 10 to 15 days to appear. The drug carries a black box warning that it may cause hepatotoxicity. Liver laboratory values (alanine aminotransferase [ALT], aspartate aminotransferase [AST], and bilirubin) must be closely monitored and the drug discontinued if abnormal values persist. The most common adverse effects include nausea and vomiting, diarrhea, upper respiratory infection, increased ALT, myalgia, urinary tract infection, oropharyngeal pain, increased AST, pharyngitis, back pain, influenza, paresthesia, and rash. Because of the potential for serious adverse effects, the drug is available through a restricted distribution program. There are no data regarding the use of eltrombopag during pregnancy or lactation. Due to the potential for serious adverse effects, the drug is not recommended during breastfeeding. Sexually active females of reproductive potential should use effective contraception during eltrombopag therapy and for at least 7 days after stopping treatment.

Fostamatinib (Tavalisse): Approved in 2018, fostamatinib is given orally to treat thrombocytopenia in patients with ITP who have not responded to first-line therapies. Fostamatinib acts by a mechanism very different from the TPO-RAs. This medication inhibits the enzyme tyrosine kinase in the spleen. Its primary metabolite reduces the antibody-mediated destruction of platelets. The most common adverse effects are diarrhea, hypertension, nausea, respiratory infection, and dizziness. Blood pressure, liver enzymes, and CBCs should be monitored regularly. Fostamatinib showed fetal harm in laboratory animals. Sexually active females of reproductive potential should use effective contraception during therapy and for at least 30 days after stopping treatment. Breastfeeding is not recommended for at least 30 days after the last dose.

Lusutrombopag (Mulpleta): Approved in 2018, lusutrombopag is a TPO-RA that has the same indication as avatrombopag: the treatment of thrombocytopenia in adult patients with chronic liver disease who are scheduled to undergo a medical procedure. The medication is taken for 7 consecutive days, and the procedure must be done within 2 to 8 days after the last dose. Peak effects occur after about 5 days. The most common adverse reaction is headache. Like other TPO-RAs, thromboembolic complications are possible. Lusutrombopag showed developmental abnormalities in laboratory animals. Breastfeeding is not recommended during therapy and for at least 28 days after the last dose.

Romiplostim (Nplate): Like eltrombopag, romiplostim was approved in 2008 and increases platelet count by activating the thrombopoietin receptor. Also like eltrombopag, the only indication is for the treatment of thrombocytopenia in patients with chronic ITP who have not responded to corticosteroids, immunoglobulins, or splenectomy. Romiplostim is administered as a once-weekly subcutaneous injection. Platelet numbers may take 10 to 15 days to appear. Unlike eltrombopag, romiplostim does not exhibit hepatotoxicity. The most common adverse effects are arthralgia, dizziness, insomnia, myalgia, pain in extremity, abdominal pain, shoulder pain, dyspepsia, and paresthesia. This medication should not be administered to patients with thrombocytopenia caused by myelodysplastic syndrome because it may increase the risk of progression to acute myelogenous leukemia. Like other TPO-RAs, thromboembolic complications are possible. It is only administered by a restricted distribution program. Romiplostim may cause fetal harm during pregnancy. The drug is not recommended during breastfeeding due to the potential for serious adverse effects.

CONNECTION Checkpoint 39.2

Eptifibatide and tirofiban are drugs that can cause severe ITP. From what you learned in Chapter 38, to what class do these drugs belong and what is the primary indication for their use?

Classification of Anemias

39.5 Anemias may be caused by hemorrhage or a change in red blood cell production or destruction.

Anemia is a condition in which RBCs have a reduced capacity to deliver oxygen to tissues. It is estimated that over 3.4 million Americans have the disorder, which can have a major impact on the quality of life. Although there are dozens of possible causes of anemia, most fall into one of the following categories:

- Blood loss due to hemorrhage
- Increased erythrocyte destruction
- Decreased erythrocyte production.

Anemia is considered a sign of an underlying disorder rather than a distinct disease. For example, anemia is commonly associated with peptic ulcer, various malignancies, and CKD. For therapy to be successful, the underlying pathology must be identified and treated. Despite the fact it is often considered secondary to other diseases, proper treatment of anemia is necessary to improve the patient's ability to adequately perform ADLs.

Classification of anemia is generally based on a description of the erythrocyte's size and color. Sizes are described as normal (normocytic), small (microcytic), or large (macrocytic). Color is based on the amount of Hgb present and is described as normal red (normochromic) or light red (hypochromic). This classification is shown in Table 39.2. It is not unusual for patients to have more than one type of anemia concurrently.

Depending on the type of anemia, several vitamins and minerals may be given to enhance the oxygen-carrying capacity of blood. The most common antianemia drugs are iron salts, cyanocobalamin (Nascobal), and folic acid. Doses of these drugs are listed in Table 39.3.

Antianemia Drugs

39.6 Administration of iron salts can rapidly reverse symptoms of iron deficiency anemia.

Iron is a mineral essential to the function of several mitochondrial enzymes involved in metabolism and energy production in cells. It is also a component of certain antioxidant enzymes that assist in clearing the body of free radicals. Most iron in the body, 60 to 80%, is associated with Hgb inside erythrocytes. Knowledge of iron balance and homeostasis is necessary to understand the pharmacotherapy of iron deficiency anemia. Factors affecting iron balance are illustrated in Figure 39.2.

The two basic forms of iron in biological systems are ferrous (Fe^{2+}) and ferric (Fe^{3+}). Most food contains iron in the ferric state, which is not absorbed in the gastrointestinal (GI) tract. In the presence of stomach acid, however, the ferric form is converted to the ferrous form, which is readily absorbed in the duodenum. Iron absorption is dynamic; if the body senses a shortage of iron in the blood, GI absorption increases. When iron stores are plentiful, less iron is absorbed from food and the excess is excreted in the feces. Since adults only need about 8 mg of iron per day, a

Table 39.2 Classification of Anemia

Morphology	Description	Examples
Macrocytic-normochromic	Large, abnormally shaped erythrocytes with normal Hgb concentration	Pernicious anemia, folate deficiency anemia
Microcytic-hypochromic	Small, abnormally shaped erythrocytes with decreased Hgb concentration	Iron deficiency anemia, thalassemia
Normocytic-normochromic	Destruction or depletion of normal erythroblasts or mature erythrocytes	Aplastic anemia, hemorrhagic anemia, sickle cell disease, hemolytic anemia

Table 39.3 Antianemia Drugs

Drug	Route and Adult Dose (Maximum Dose Where Indicated)	Adverse Effects
cyanocobalamin (Nascobal)	IM/deep subcutaneous: 30 mcg/day for 5–10 days, then 100–200 mcg/month Intranasal: 1 spray (500 mcg) in one nostril once weekly	*Diarrhea, hypokalemia, rash* Anaphylaxis
folic acid	PO/IM/subcutaneous/IV: less than 1 mg/day	*Flushing, rash* Hypersensitivity
Iron Salts		
ferric maltol (Accrufer)**	PO: 30 mg bid	*Nausea, heartburn, constipation, dark stools* Cardiovascular collapse, aggravation of peptic ulcers or ulcerative colitis, hepatic necrosis, hypotension (ferumoxytol), anaphylaxis (iron dextran), respiratory arrest (iron dextran), seizures (iron dextran)
ferrous fumarate (Feostat, others)	PO: 200 mg tid or qid	
ferrous gluconate (Fergon, Ferralet)	PO: 325–600 mg qid; may be gradually increased to 650 mg qid as needed	
ferrous sulfate (Feosol, Feostat, others)	PO: 100–200 mg elemental iron q12h	
ferumoxytol (Feraheme)	IV: Single dose of 510 mg followed by a second 510-mg dose 3–8 days later	
iron dextran (Infed)	IM/IV: Dose is individualized and determined from a table supplied by the drug manufacturer that correlates body weight to Hgb values (max: 100 mg within 24 h)	
iron sucrose (Venofer)	IV: 100–200 mg by slow IV injection or infusion	

Note: *Italics* indicate common adverse effects. Underline indicates serious adverse effects.

** Ferric maltol is not a true iron salt but has the same actions and effects as other iron products in this table.

normal diet supplies sufficient amounts of the mineral for most people.

Other factors affect the absorption of iron. Iron in heme, which is found in meat, fish, and poultry, is three times more absorbable than the nonheme iron found in vegetables and grains. Thus, meats are considered the best natural source of absorbable iron. Calcium inhibits the absorption of iron; thus, those who drink milk with meals are at greater risk for iron deficiency. Vitamin C increases iron absorption about 30%, whereas black tea diminishes absorption.

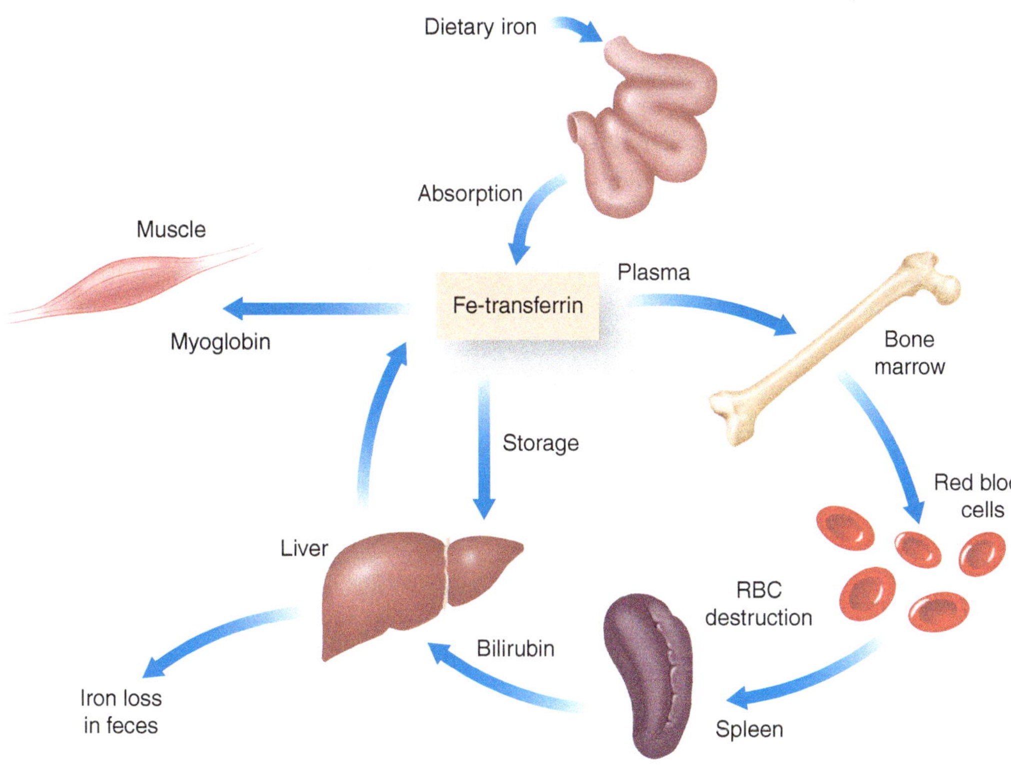

Figure 39.2 Iron metabolism.

Because free iron is toxic, the body binds the mineral to the protein complexes **ferritin**, **hemosiderin**, and **transferrin**. Ferritin and hemosiderin maintain iron stores inside cells, whereas transferrin transports iron to sites throughout the body where it is needed, such as to the bone marrow for incorporation into Hgb. Serum ferritin levels are a reliable indicator of how much iron is being stored by the body. Low serum ferritin levels (less than 12 ng/mL) are characteristic of iron deficiency anemia. In addition to Hgb, major storage depots for iron are the liver and myoglobin in skeletal muscle.

After erythrocytes die, nearly all of the iron in their Hgb is incorporated into transferrin and recycled for later use. Because of this efficient recycling, only about 1 mg of iron is excreted from the body per day, making daily dietary iron requirements in most individuals quite small. Vegetarians are at higher risk of iron deficiency anemia because of a lack of heme intake from meat and must take care to select foods rich in iron. Iron requirements may double during growth, pregnancy, and menses; thus, intake of iron must be increased to maintain proper iron balance.

Iron deficiency is the most common cause of anemia worldwide. More than 50% of patients diagnosed with iron deficiency anemia have GI bleeding, such as may occur from GI malignancies or chronic peptic ulcer disease (PUD). In the United States and Canada, iron deficiency most commonly occurs in women of childbearing age due to pregnancy and as a result of blood losses during menses. Low-dose iron supplements are recommended during pregnancy to prevent this condition. Certain individuals have an increased demand for iron, including those who are on meat-free diets or undergoing intensive athletic training. These conditions may require more than the recommended dietary allowance of iron (see Chapter 61). In undeveloped countries, the primary cause of iron deficiency anemia is the lack of meat or fresh fruits and vegetables in the diet. The most significant effect of iron deficiency is a reduction in erythropoiesis, resulting in symptoms of anemia.

Iron therapy is initiated to alleviate symptoms of anemia caused by blood loss or dietary deficiency. Once diagnosed, a primary goal is to identify the etiology of the disorder and treat the underlying pathology. Choice of therapy depends on the etiology and severity of the deficiency:

- Mild anemia may be prevented or corrected in most patients by increasing the intake of iron-rich foods, such as fish, red meat, fortified cereal, and whole-grain breads.
- Moderate anemia is corrected by oral iron supplementation.
- Severe anemia, and that caused by iron malabsorption disorders, is corrected by parenteral iron therapy.

CONNECTIONS: Patient Safety

Iron Poisoning in Children

While talking with a group of young mothers, the nurse becomes concerned about the remarks made by one of the members. The mother states, "I insist that my children take iron-fortified vitamins every day. My children really enjoy taking the cute little cartoon vitamins. They call the vitamins their 'morning candy.'" How should the nurse respond? Is this statement made by the mother concerning to the nurse?

PROTOTYPE DRUG Ferrous Sulfate (Feosol, Feostat, Others)

Classification **Therapeutic:** Drug for anemia
Pharmacologic: Iron supplement

Therapeutic Effects and Uses: Ferrous sulfate is an iron supplement containing about 20% elemental iron. Desiccated (dried) ferrous sulfate contains 30% elemental iron. It is inexpensive and available in a wide variety of dosage forms to prevent or rapidly reverse symptoms of iron deficiency anemia. Enteric-coated and extended-release forms are available. If tolerated, the drug should be taken on an empty stomach, at least 1 hour before or 2 hours after a meal.

In general, patients with iron deficiency respond rapidly to the administration of ferrous sulfate. Although a positive therapeutic response may be achieved in 48 hours, therapy may continue for several months to replenish iron storage depots and stabilize hemoglobin levels. As the deficiency is corrected, the body will absorb a smaller percentage of elemental iron in each dose until iron intake balances iron loss. This is assuming, of course, that the source of the iron imbalance, such as bleeding or dietary insufficiency, has been corrected. Laboratory evaluation of Hgb, transferrin, and Hct levels is conducted regularly to assess the progress of pharmacotherapy. Dosage is decreased as therapy progresses and the deficiency is corrected.

If rapid, symptomatic improvement is not experienced, the reasons for the treatment failure must be carefully explored. The patient may be experiencing continued bleeding or may have a malabsorption disorder that prevents the iron from being absorbed. A common reason for treatment failure is lack of adherence to pharmacotherapy. Patients may stop taking the drug due to severe nausea and vomiting, or they may take the drug with food or other drugs that inhibit iron absorption. Excellent assessment and teaching skills on the part of the nurse are key to achieving successful pharmacotherapeutic outcomes in these patients.

Mechanism of Action: After absorption, most iron is used by the body to make Hgb. Laboratory values of Hgb should increase 2 to 4 g/dL every 3 weeks until normal values are achieved. In addition, therapy is continued until serum ferritin levels return to normal, indicating that the iron storage depots are filled.

Pharmacokinetics:

Route(s)	PO
Absorption	5–30% absorbed
Distribution	Well distributed; crosses the placenta
Primary metabolism	Undergoes extensive enterohepatic recirculation
Primary excretion	Feces, urine, and skin
Onset of action	3 days to 4 weeks
Duration of action	Unknown

Adverse Effects: The most common adverse effects of ferrous sulfate are nausea and vomiting, which will occur to some degree in most patients. Taking the drug with food will diminish GI upset but can decrease the absorption of iron by 50 to 70%. The degree of nausea and vomiting is dose related and serious symptoms may require a dosage adjustment. Contact of liquid iron with teeth should be avoided because the drug can cause brown stains. Iron preparations will darken stools, but this is a harmless adverse effect. Because constipation is common, especially in older adults, an increase in dietary fiber intake is indicated. **Black Box Warning:** Unintentional overdoses of iron-containing products are a leading cause of fatal poisoning in children. Iron medication should be kept in secured locations, away from children.

Contraindications/Precautions: Iron salts should not be administered for anemia other than that caused by iron deficiency because iron will not correct these conditions and may build to toxic levels. The drug should not be administered to patients with hemochromatosis, a disease in which the patient has excess iron stores. Ferrous sulfate may irritate the stomach mucosa and increase bleeding in patients with PUD. The drug may cause diarrhea if administered to patients with regional enteritis or ulcerative colitis.

Drug Interactions: Absorption is reduced when oral iron salts are given concurrently with antacids, proton pump inhibitors, or calcium supplements. Iron decreases the absorption of tetracyclines, fluoroquinolones, levodopa, and etidronate. To prevent possible interactions, it is advisable to take iron supplements 1 to 2 hours before or after other medications. **Herbal/Food:** Food (especially dairy products), coffee, and tea will inhibit iron absorption. Vitamin C will increase absorption.

Pregnancy: It is not known if ferrous sulfate adversely affects the fetus or has adverse effects in the breastfed infant.

Treatment of Overdose: Iron is very toxic and most overdoses are unintentional, occurring in children under the age of 6 years. The antidote for acute iron intoxication is the parenteral drug deferoxamine (Desferal). This chelating drug binds iron, which is removed by the kidneys, turning the urine a reddish-brown color.

Drugs Similar to Ferrous Sulfate (Feosol, Feostat, Others)

At least eight iron salts are available for administration to patients with iron deficiency anemia. Iron salts are often classified by their route of administration, either oral (PO) or parenteral.

Oral iron salts: Oral iron salts include ferrous fumarate, ferrous gluconate, polysaccharide–iron complex, and carbonyl iron. The choice of specific drug and dose are based on iron content and degree of GI tolerability. Table 39.4 lists the amount of elemental iron in these drugs. In 2019 a new oral iron product, ferric maltol (Accrufer), was approved to treat iron deficiency. Ferric maltol is reported to cause fewer GI side effects than the other oral iron products.

A large number of iron products and formulations are available, including tablets, drops, elixirs, and suspensions. Nausea and vomiting, constipation, and diarrhea are common adverse effects with all oral iron preparations. Slow-release products, called carbonyl iron (Feosol-caps, Ferronyl), are more expensive but are less dangerous in children following unintentional ingestion because there is a longer time period for intervention before toxic effects materialize. Some products have an enteric coating so that the capsule or tablet dissolves in the intestine, thus causing less gastric irritation. Recall, however, that stomach acid is necessary to convert iron to its more absorbable form. In addition, enteric coatings are less reliable because they may dissolve after the drug has passed the duodenum, which is the primary site for iron absorption. Vitamin C is added to many oral iron supplements because it enhances iron

Table 39.4 Iron Content of Oral Iron Formulations

Preparation	Elemental Iron	Dose Needed to Provide 200 mg of Elemental Iron per Day
carbonyl iron	100%	200 mg
ferrous fumarate	33%	600 mg
ferrous gluconate	12%	720 mg
ferrous sulfate: desiccated	30%	660 mg
ferrous sulfate: regular	20%	1000 mg
polysaccharide–iron complex	100%	200 mg

absorption. Some products are formulated as multivitamins. For example, Niferex PN Forte, which is formulated specifically for pregnant or lactating women, contains a polysaccharide–iron complex and vitamins A, D, C, folic acid, B complex, calcium, iodine, magnesium, copper, and zinc. Adding extra enhancers such as additional vitamins, extended-release properties, or an enteric coating increases the cost of the drug but not necessarily its effectiveness. The amount of elemental iron in the product and adverse effects should be the primary factors guiding therapy.

Parenteral iron salts: Ferumoxytol (Feraheme), iron dextran (Infed), iron sucrose (Venofer), and ferric gluconate (Ferrlecit) are parenteral preparations reserved for patients who cannot tolerate oral iron preparations or who have a malabsorption disorder preventing iron absorption from the GI tract. Giving parenteral iron does not lead to a faster recovery for patients with iron deficiency anemia because the body is limited as to how quickly it can make Hgb and new RBCs. These drugs are clearly more toxic than the oral iron products and require careful monitoring during pharmacotherapy.

Ferumoxytol (Feraheme) is an iron salt approved to treat iron deficiency associated with CKD (with or without dialysis). The drug consists of iron oxide protected by a carbohydrate shell. The shell remains intact until the drug enters macrophages, whereby the iron is released to its storage depots. The advantage of ferumoxytol over other iron salts is that it can be administered safely by the IV route and can raise iron levels more rapidly.

All parenteral drugs are equally effective at raising iron levels. All are given IV. Iron dextran is also available by the IM route, although this is rarely used due to pain at the injection site and unreliable absorption from the muscle. Iron sucrose and iron gluconate have more limited application. They are approved only for patients with iron deficiency anemia undergoing chronic hemodialysis who are also receiving erythropoietin.

Parenteral iron salts contain a black box warning regarding the potential for anaphylaxis and other serious allergic reactions. Patients should be observed for at least 30 minutes following the completion of the infusion to assess for possible allergic reactions, which may cause respiratory arrest and circulatory collapse. Some healthcare providers order test doses prior to every administration of IV iron salts because anaphylaxis may occur on second and subsequent doses. Ferric gluconate produces a lower incidence of anaphylactic shock.

Common adverse reactions of iron dextran are hypotension, headache, muscle pain, and joint pain; these are more severe when given IV. Iron dextran appears to increase bone density in the joints, which is the probable cause of the muscle and joint pain. Frequent adverse effects with ferric gluconate include cramping, nausea and vomiting, hypotension, and rash. Iron sucrose is well tolerated, with some patients experiencing leg cramps and hypotension.

CONNECTION Checkpoint 39.3

From what you learned in Chapter 8, explain why a patient who is pregnant has a substantially higher iron requirement compared to a nonpregnant woman.

Pernicious Anemia

39.7 Pernicious anemia may be successfully treated with the administration of vitamin B_{12}.

Vitamin B_{12} and folic acid are dietary nutrients essential for rapidly dividing cells. The continuous, high rate of erythropoiesis occurring throughout the lifespan demands a continuous supply of these vitamins. Without them, the normal production of RBCs is interrupted and large, immature erythrocytes that are unable to carry the same amount of oxygen as normal RBCs are released into the blood, and anemia results.

Vitamin B_{12} is an essential component of two coenzymes required for normal cell growth and DNA replication. Neither plants nor animals synthesize vitamin B_{12}; only bacteria can make this vitamin. Because the body requires only miniscule amounts of vitamin B_{12} (3 mcg/day), deficiency of this vitamin is usually not due to insufficient dietary intake. Instead, the most common cause of vitamin B_{12} deficiency is absence of **intrinsic factor**, a protein secreted by stomach cells. Intrinsic factor forms a complex with vitamin B_{12}, which is then absorbed into the circulation. Without the formation of this complex, vitamin B_{12} is not absorbed from the intestine. Figure 39.3 illustrates the metabolism of vitamin B_{12}.

Deficiency of intrinsic factor is caused by inflammatory diseases of the stomach or by gastric resection. Inflammatory diseases of the small intestine that affect food and nutrient absorption may also cause vitamin B_{12} deficiency. Because vitamin B_{12} is found primarily in foods of animal origin, strict vegetarians may require a vitamin supplement to avoid deficiency. The center portion of the vitamin B_{12} molecule contains the metal ion cobalt, which is a micromineral essential to human nutrition.

The most profound consequence of vitamin B_{12} deficiency is a megaloblastic anemia called **pernicious anemia**, which affects both the hematologic and nervous systems. In pernicious anemia, the hematopoietic stem cells produce abnormally large erythrocytes that do not fully mature. Although RBCs are most affected, lack of maturation of all blood cell types may occur in severe disease. Symptoms of pernicious anemia are often nonspecific and develop slowly, sometimes over several years. Profound nervous system symptoms distinguish this disease from most other

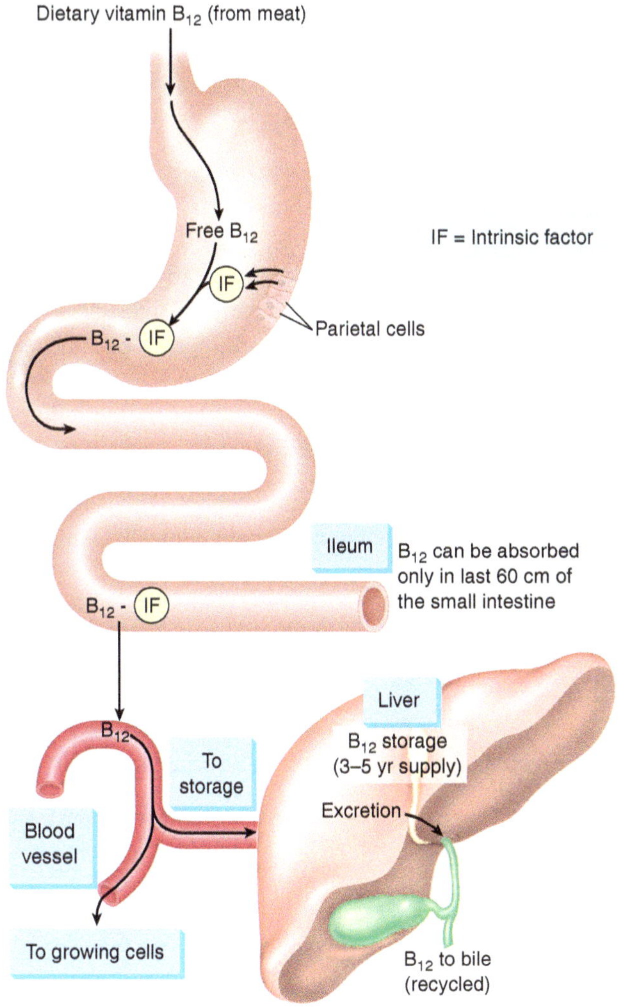

Figure 39.3 Metabolism of vitamin B_{12}.

anemias and include memory loss, confusion, unsteadiness, tingling or numbness in the limbs, delusions, mood disturbances, and even hallucinations in severe deficiencies. Permanent nervous system impairment may result if the disease remains untreated for 6 to 12 months. Pharmacotherapy includes the administration of cyanocobalamin, a form of vitamin B_{12}. Prior to administration of vitamin B_{12}, the nurse should assess for other causes of anemia including GI bleeding, GI surgery, tapeworm infestation, and gluten enteropathy.

Folic acid, or **folate**, is a B-complex vitamin that is essential for normal DNA and ribonucleic acid synthesis. Like B_{12} deficiency, insufficient folic acid levels can manifest as anemia. In fact, the metabolisms of vitamin B_{12} and folic acid are intricately linked; a B_{12} deficiency will create a lack of activated folic acid. Folate deficiency is one of the most common types of anemias in the United States.

Folic acid does not require intrinsic factor for intestinal absorption, and the most common cause of deficiency is insufficient dietary intake. This is often observed in patients with chronic alcohol use disorder because their diets are often deficient in this nutrient, and ethanol interferes with folate metabolism in the liver. Fad diets and absorption diseases of the small intestine can also lead to folate-deficiency anemia. Hematopoietic symptoms of folate deficiency are the same as those for B_{12} deficiency; however, no neurologic signs are present. Folate deficiency during pregnancy has been linked to neural birth defects such as spina bifida. Mild deficiency or prophylaxis of folate deficiency is accomplished by increasing the dietary intake of folic acid through fresh green vegetables, beans, and wheat products. In cases when adequate dietary intake cannot be achieved, therapy with folic acid is warranted. Folic acid is presented as a drug prototype for water-soluble vitamins in Chapter 61.

PharmFACT

A deficiency of vitamin B_{12}, folate, or vitamin B_6 may increase the blood level of homocysteine, an amino acid normally found in the blood. An elevated blood level of homocysteine is a risk factor for heart disease and stroke (Office of Dietary Supplements, 2020b).

PROTOTYPE DRUG Cyanocobalamin (Nascobal)

Classification **Therapeutic:** Agent for anemia
Pharmacologic: Vitamin supplement

Therapeutic Effects and Uses: Cyanocobalamin is a purified form of vitamin B_{12} that is indicated for patients with vitamin B_{12} deficiency anemia. Treatment of vitamin B_{12} deficiency is most often by weekly, biweekly, or monthly intramuscular (IM) or subcutaneous injections. A typical regimen for pernicious anemia would be 100 mcg IM or subcutaneous once daily for 1 week, followed by 100 mcg on alternate days for seven doses. Dose reduction continues, with administration every 3 to 4 days for another 2 to 3 weeks, then 100 mcg IM monthly for life. Oral vitamin B_{12} formulations are available primarily as vitamin supplementation, although they are only effective in patients who have sufficient amounts of intrinsic factor and normal absorption in the small intestine.

An intranasal spray formulation (Nascobal) is available that provides for once-weekly dosage. Nascobal is generally used for maintenance therapy after normal vitamin B_{12} levels have been restored by parenteral preparations. The intranasal form is also indicated to prevent vitamin B_{12} deficiency in people who are strict vegetarians.

Parenteral administration of cyanocobalamin rapidly reverses most signs and symptoms of B_{12} deficiency, usually within a few days or weeks. If the disease has been prolonged, symptoms may take longer to resolve, and some neurologic damage may be permanent. In most cases, treatment must often be maintained for the remainder of the patient's life. Periodic laboratory blood testing and Hgb values are used to gauge the success of pharmacotherapy.

Mechanism of Action: Administration of cyanocobalamin reverses vitamin B_{12} deficiency and results in rapid improvement of anemia symptoms. Normal RBC production resumes, with laboratory evaluation of blood and bone marrow showing continuous improvement over about 7 days. Therapy may extend to several months to restore hepatic stores of the vitamin.

Pharmacokinetics:

Route(s)	PO, IM, deep subcutaneous, intranasal
Absorption	Well absorbed; PO absorption requires intrinsic factor
Distribution	Widely distributed; crosses the placenta; secreted in breast milk
Primary metabolism	Primarily converted in tissues to coenzyme B_{12} and stored in liver; extensive enterohepatic recirculation
Primary excretion	Renal
Onset of action	Peak serum level: 8–12 h (PO), 1–2 h (intranasal), and 1 h (IM/subcutaneous)
Duration of action	Half-life: 6 days

Adverse Effects: Adverse effects from cyanocobalamin are uncommon. Because hypokalemia may occur, serum potassium levels should be monitored, especially during the first 48 hours. A small percentage of patients receiving vitamin B_{12} exhibit rashes, itching, or other signs of allergy. Anaphylaxis is possible, though rare, with parenteral administration. Sodium retention occurs in some patients, with possible worsening of HF.

Contraindications/Precautions: Patients with suspected sensitivity to cobalt should receive an intradermal test dose because they may experience allergic reactions or anaphylaxis to the drug. Monotherapy with folic acid will not improve symptoms of vitamin B_{12} deficiency anemia. Cyanocobalamin is contraindicated in patients with severe pulmonary disease and should be used cautiously in patients with heart disease because of the potential for sodium retention caused by the drug.

Drug Interactions: Drug interactions with cyanocobalamin are minor and are normally not clinically significant. **Herbal/Food:** Unknown.

Pregnancy: Animal reproduction data are not available. Human observational data have not shown fetal harm to be associated with doses recommended during pregnancy. Cyanocobalamin enters human milk, but adverse reactions in the breastfed neonate have not been associated with this drug.

Treatment of Overdose: Treatment for overdosage has not been reported.

Drugs Similar to Cyanocobalamin (Nascobal)

There are no drugs similar to cyanocobalamin.

Understanding Chapter 39

Key Concepts Summary

39.1 Hematopoiesis is a dynamic process that is responsive to the changing demands of the body.

39.2 Erythropoietin stimulates production of red blood cells and is used to treat anemia.

39.3 Colony-stimulating factors increase the production of leukocytes.

39.4 Platelet enhancers may be used to treat thrombocytopenia.

39.5 Anemias may be caused by hemorrhage or a change in red blood cell production or destruction.

39.6 Administration of iron salts can rapidly reverse symptoms of iron deficiency anemia.

39.7 Pernicious anemia may be successfully treated with the administration of vitamin B_{12}.

CASE STUDY: Making the Patient Connection

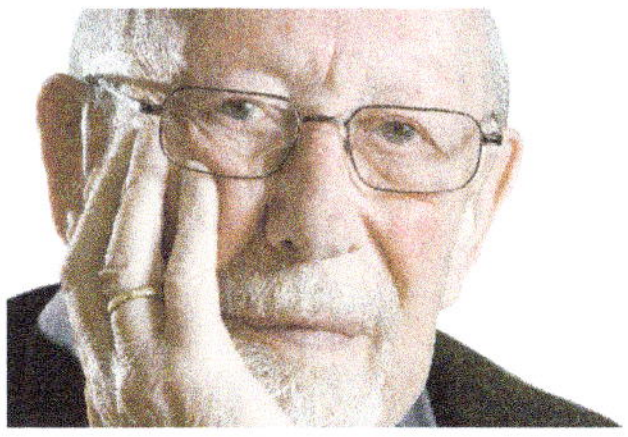

Remember the patient "Carl Guenther" at the beginning of the chapter? Now read the remainder of the case study. Based on the information presented within this chapter, respond to the critical thinking questions that follow.

"A real people-person who never met a stranger." That is how family and friends have always described Carl Guenther. His positive and outgoing personality is well known in the community. When Carl was informed about his prostate cancer, he handled the diagnosis well and with his usual optimism. He was confident that the chemotherapy would be successful. His mantra for years had been to "Live every day as if it were your last." However, the treatment for the cancer had adverse effects that he did not expect and his enthusiasm diminished.

Carl is a 72-year-old retired sales representative for a chain of department stores. His entire career was centered on interacting with all kinds of people. When he retired, his outgoing nature was an asset for the many community agencies at which he volunteered. Carl was active in the local Lions Club, his church's outreach ministry, and at the children's hospital. He had even considered working as a greeter at his neighborhood department store.

As Carl went through chemotherapy, the associated nausea and vomiting were well managed with antiemetic drugs. His physical appearance did not change much because Carl had minimal hair loss due to the chemotherapy. Now he faces an exceedingly low WBC count and has been advised to avoid potential sources of infection, including people. By far this is the worst adverse effect of the chemotherapy for Carl. He feels socially isolated and depressed. *Is this the end?*, he wonders. *Am I to die lonely?*

Critical Thinking Questions

1. The healthcare provider orders filgrastim (Neupogen) 10 mcg/kg daily for 4 days. Carl asks you, his nurse, "How does this drug work?" What is your response?
2. List interventions that should be followed during this period of chemotherapy-induced neutropenia to protect Carl from infection.
3. What adverse effects would you monitor in patients receiving filgrastim?

Additional Case Study

When the blood test returned from Betty Arnold's preemployment physical, the results indicated anemia. "No wonder I feel so exhausted all the time," she said. "I thought my fatigue was from taking care of my five children, my home, and my aging parents." When she saw her primary healthcare provider, she was diagnosed with iron deficiency anemia and prescribed ferrous sulfate (Feosol) 160-mg sustained-release tablets daily.

1. What adverse effects should Betty watch for while taking Feosol?
2. Is there a best time of the day to take this medication? Why?

Chapter Review

1. Which statement would the nurse include in the care plan for a patient receiving epoetin alfa?
    1. Avoid fresh fruit and vegetables and partially cooked meats.
    2. Encourage frequent rest periods to minimize fatigue.
    3. Limit exposure to direct sunlight and use sunscreen when outdoors.
    4. Protect tissues and mucous membranes from traumatic injury.
2. Darbepoetin (Aranesp) is prescribed for each of the following patients. A nurse should question the order for which condition?
    1. A patient with HIV who is receiving zidovudine
    2. A patient with uncontrolled hypertension
    3. A patient with chronic kidney disease
    4. A patient with chemotherapy-induced anemia

3. A patient is being treated with filgrastim (Neupogen). Which of the following would the nurse monitor to determine the effectiveness of this drug?

1. Red blood cell counts
2. Platelet counts
3. White blood cell counts
4. Reticulocyte count and mean cell volume

4. The nurse is teaching the patient with ITP about fostamatinib (Tavalisse). Which statement, if made by the patient, indicates that additional health teaching is needed?

1. "This drug prevents the body from destroying platelets."
2. "I should periodically check my blood pressure."
3. "I will notify my healthcare provider if I develop any cough or lung infection."
4. "I should be able to get pregnant since this is not an injectable drug."

5. A patient who regularly consumes significant amounts of alcohol is prescribed cyanocobalamin and states, "I don't understand why my healthcare provider has prescribed B_{12} injections." The nurse's response would be based on which physiologic concept?

1. Patients who regularly consume large amounts of alcohol are often deficient in this nutrient.
2. Alcohol facilitates folate metabolism in the liver, which destroys vitamin B_{12}.
3. Patients who regularly consume large amounts of alcohol are at high risk for neutropenia, a condition that develops from vitamin B_{12} loss.
4. Liver cirrhosis caused by large amounts of alcohol ingestion diminishes natural physiologic deposits of B_{12}.

6. What differences exist when giving parenteral iron rather than oral forms of the drug? (Select all that apply.)

1. The drug can be given to patients with malabsorption conditions or those who cannot tolerate oral iron preparations.
2. They avoid most of the common adverse effects associated with iron preparations.
3. They improve iron deficiency anemia and raise Hgb and RBC levels more quickly than oral formulations.
4. They may raise iron levels more quickly than oral preparations.
5. They may cause a severe anaphylactic reaction.

See Appendix A for answers to critical thinking questions, case study questions, and review questions.

References

Neunert, C., Terrell, D. R., Arnold, D. M., Buchanan, G., Cines, D. B., Cooper, N., et al. (2019). American Society of Hematology 2019 guidelines for immune thrombocytopenia. *Blood Advances*, *3*(23), 3829–3866. https://doi.org/10.1182/bloodadvances.2019000966

Office of Dietary Supplements. (2020a). *Iron: Dietary supplement fact sheet*. National Institutes of Health. http://ods.od.nih.gov/factsheets/Iron-Health Professional/#h2

Office of Dietary Supplements. (2020b). *Vitamin B_{12}: Dietary supplement fact sheet*. National Institutes of Health. http://ods.od.nih.gov/factsheets/VitaminB12-HealthProfessional

Rizk, J. G., Kalantar-Zadeh, K., Mehra, M. R., Lavie, C. J., Rizk, Y., & Forthal, D. N. (2020). Pharmaco-immunomodulatory therapy in COVID 19. *Drugs*, *80*, 1267–1292. https://doi.org/10.1007/s40265-020-01367-z

Selected Bibliography

Al-Samkari, H., & Kuter, D. J. (2019). Optimal use of thrombopoietin receptor agonists in immune thrombocytopenia. *Therapeutic Advances in Hematology*, *10*. https://doi.org/10.1177/2040620719841735

Camaschella, C. (2019). Iron deficiency. *Blood*, *133*(1), 30–39. https://doi.org/10.1182/blood-2018-05-815944

Chatterjee, R., Shand, A., Nassar, N., Walls, M., & Khambalia, A. Z. (2016). Iron supplement use in pregnancy–Are the right women taking the right amount? *Clinical Nutrition*, *35*, 741–747. https://doi.org/10.1016/j.clnu.2015.05.014

Clemons Bankston, P., & Al-Horani, R. A. (2019). New small molecule drugs for thrombocytopenia: Chemical, pharmacological, and therapeutic use considerations. *International Journal of Molecular Sciences*, *20*(12), 3013. https://dx.doi.org/10.3390%2Fijms20123013

Cooper, N., & Ghanima, W. (2019). Immune thrombocytopenia. *New England Journal of Medicine, 381*(10), 945–955. https://doi.org/10.1056/NEJMcp1810479

Edelsberg, J., Weycker, D., Bensink, M., Bowers, C., & Lyman, G. H. (2020). Prophylaxis of febrile neutropenia with colony-stimulating factors: The first 25 years. *Current Medical Research and Opinion, 36*(3), 483–495. https://doi.org/10.1080/03007995.2019.1703665

Juul, S. E., Derman, R. J., & Auerbach, M. (2019). Perinatal iron deficiency: Implications for mothers and infants. *Neonatology, 115*(3), 269–274. https://doi.org/10.1159/000495978

Katz, J. (2018). *Intravenous immunoglobulin*. Medscape. https://emedicine.medscape.com/article/210367-overview

Kessler, C.M. (2020). *Immune thrombocytopenia (ITP)*. Medscape. https://emedicine.medscape.com/article/202158-overview

Thiagarajan, P. (2020). *Platelet disorders*. Medscape. http://emedicine.medscape.com/article/201722-overview#a1

Walker, S. T., Grigg, S., Kirkpatrick, C., Urbancic, K., Cohen, E., Grigg, A., & Trubiano, J. (2020). Nurse-initiated pre-prescribed antibiotic orders to facilitate prompt and appropriate antibiotic administration in febrile neutropenia. *Supportive Care in Cancer, 28*(9), 4337–4343. https://doi.org/10.1007/s00520-019-05290-2

Waller, C. F., & Friganović, A. (2020). Biosimilars in oncology: key role of nurses in patient education. *Future Oncology, 16*(25), 1931–1939. https://doi.org/10.2217/fon-2020-0486

Unit 6

Pharmacology of Body Defenses

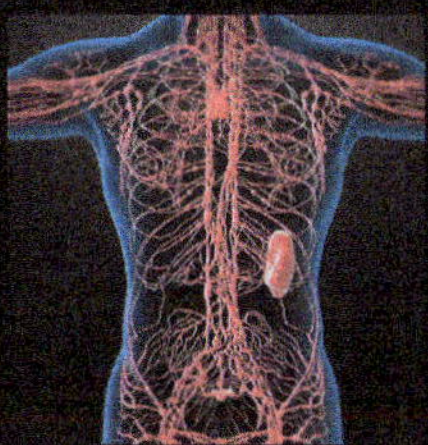

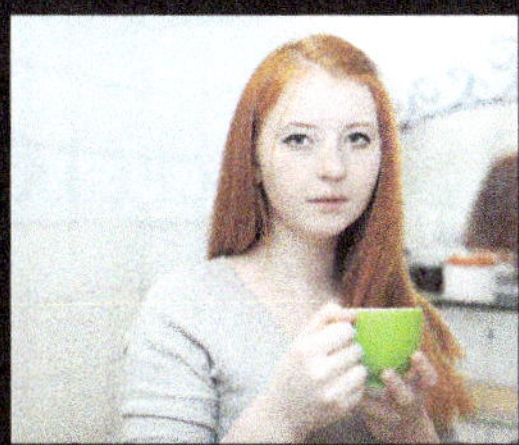

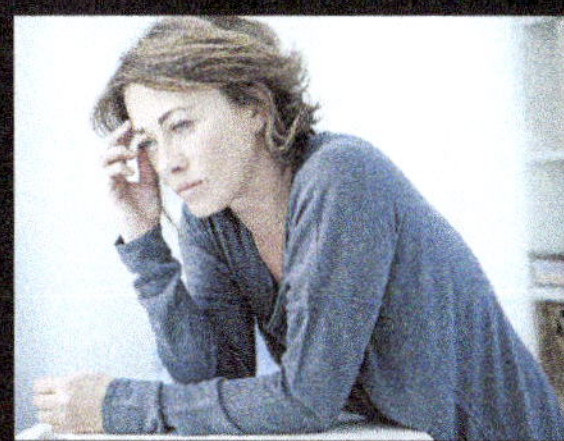

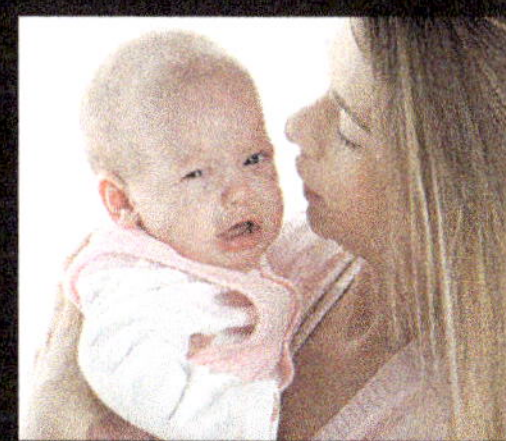

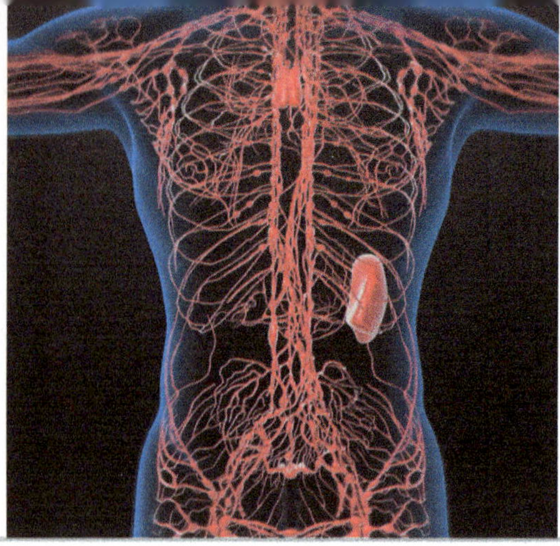

Chapter 40
Review of Body Defenses and the Immune System

Chapter Outline

- Organization of the Lymphatic System
- Innate (Nonspecific) Defenses
  - Inflammation
- Adaptive (Specific) Defenses
  - Humoral Immunity
  - Cell-Mediated Immunity

Learning Outcomes

After reading this chapter, the student should be able to:

1. Identify the major components of the lymphatic system.
2. Describe the components of the innate defense system and their functions.
3. Compare and contrast innate and adaptive defenses.
4. Identify the signs and symptoms of inflammation.
5. Outline the basic steps in the acute inflammatory response.
6. Explain the role of histamine and other chemical mediators in the inflammatory response.
7. Compare and contrast the humoral and cell-mediated immune responses.

Key Terms

Definitions of the terms in bold may be found in the Glossary.

The human body is under continuous attack from a host of foreign invaders, including viruses, bacteria, fungi, and even single-celled animals. Some of these pathogens intentionally seek out humans because it is an essential part of their lifecycle, whereas others happen to be "at the right place and time" when a cut or scrape allows entrance into the body. Fortunately, the body's extensive defenses are capable of mounting a rapid and effective response against most of these pathogens. Drugs used to modify body defenses, which include anti-inflammatory drugs, immunostimulants, immunosuppressants, and vaccines, are presented in Chapters 41 through 43. The purpose of this chapter is to review the fundamental concepts of body defenses that apply to the pharmacotherapy of the immune system and infectious disease. For a more thorough review of this topic, the student should consult an anatomy and physiology textbook.

Organization of the Lymphatic System

40.1 The lymphatic system is the primary organ system that protects the body from invasion by foreign agents.

The components of the lymphatic system provide the body with **immunity**, which is the ability to resist injury and infections. The **lymphatic system** comprises a network of cells, vessels, and tissues that provide immune surveillance. This monitoring function begins when fluid leaves the vascular system at the capillaries due to the osmotic forces and high pressure in the capillaries. This fluid, known as lymph, enters blind-ended lymphatic vessels and slowly travels on its journey through the lymphatic system. As much as 3 L of fluid per day travel through the highly branched lymphatic vessel network to eventually return to the cardiovascular circulation.

Lymphatic vessels carry more than escaped fluid. Viruses, bacteria, cellular debris, and even cancer cells can enter these vessels. Should these pathogens or cancer cells be permitted to return to the bloodstream, an infection (or cancer) could quickly spread throughout the body with potentially disastrous consequences. Fortunately, before these pathogens can return to the general circulation, they must pass through dozens of **lymph nodes**, which are the principal lymphoid organs in the body. Lymph nodes are solid, spherical bodies that are packed with macrophages and lymphocytes, which are cells specialized to recognize anything that is "nonself" or foreign to the body. Recognition of these foreign agents activates the immune response, which neutralizes or removes the pathogens before they can reach the general circulation. Each lymph node serves as a minifilter, removing up to 99% of the foreign agents entering the node. Should a pathogen be clever enough to escape surveillance in a particular lymph node, it is then faced with passing through dozens, and sometimes hundreds, more lymph nodes in the lymphatic system.

In addition to lymph vessels and nodes, lymphoid tissues line connective tissue at every potential portal of entrance into the body, including the gastrointestinal tract, respiratory tract, and genitourinary tract. Lymphoid tissue contains lymphocytes, which "patrol" the region for potential injury or exposure to microbes. Other large collections of lymphoid tissue include the tonsils, spleen, and thymus. These are considered organs of the lymphatic system.

Although the lymphatic system can be divided into individual structures and components for ease of study, it is best to think of it as an integrated whole. The various components of this system are in continuous communication and work together as a single unit to accomplish effective immune surveillance. A malfunction in a single component may affect the effectiveness of the entire lymphatic system. An overview of the primary divisions of immunity is shown in Figure 40.1.

PharmFACT

Tumors are able to create new lymphatic vessels, a process called lymphangiogenesis. The new lymphatic vessels induced by the cancer cells prime areas of the body for metastasis and signal a poorer prognosis (Yamakawa et al., 2018).

Innate (Nonspecific) Defenses

40.2 Innate defenses are the body's first line of defense against pathogens.

Innate body defenses are those that are present even before an infection has occurred and that provide the first line of protection from pathogens. These are sometimes referred to as *nonspecific defenses* because they are unable to distinguish one type of threat from another; the body's response is the same regardless of the particular pathogen. A summary of nonspecific body defenses is given in Table 40.1. A useful way of categorizing the innate defenses is to consider them as types of barriers:

- Physical barriers: skin and mucous membranes
- Cellular barriers: phagocytes and natural killer cells
- Process barriers and antimicrobial proteins: complement, fever, inflammation, and interferons.

Physical barriers: The skin and mucous membranes are considered the first line of defense against pathogen invasion. The intact skin is a formidable physical barrier to pathogens. The cells of the epidermis are packed tightly together, which discourages penetration by microbes. The outer layer of skin cells is continually shed, along with

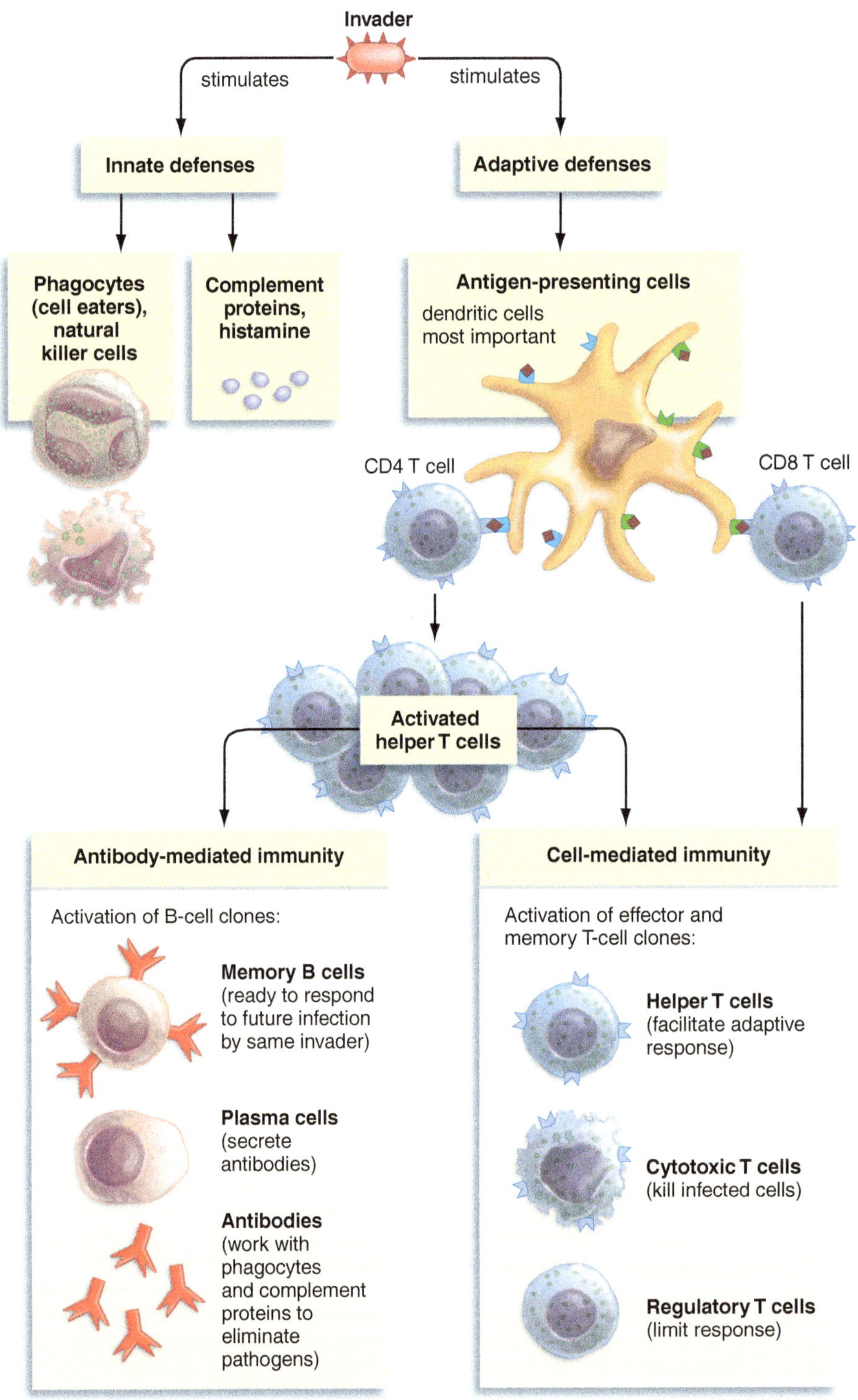

Figure 40.1 Overview of body defenses.
From Krogh (2014), p. 563.

any microbes that may be clinging to them. The accessory structures of the skin secrete sebum (oil), sweat, and antimicrobial peptides that discourage microbial growth on the surface. The skin is also colonized with a variety of bacteria and fungi that are normally harmless to the host. This microbiota (flora) competes with pathogens for space and nutrients, thus creating an unfavorable growth environment for harmful organisms. However, should the skin become broken or compromised by needlesticks or catheters, some species of normal flora may become pathogenic.

The body cavities that open to the outside environment are lined with a mucosal epithelium that not only provides

Table 40.1 Summary of Nonspecific Body Defenses

Component	Functions
Physical Barriers	
Skin	Forms a mechanical barrier to prevent pathogens and other harmful substances from entering the body. Surface contains keratin, which is resistant to water and acid.
Mucous membranes	Line the portals of entry to inhibit the entry of pathogens. Mucus inhibits microbial growth. Cilia in the respiratory tract and saliva in the mouth discourage pathogen entry.
Cellular Barriers	
Phagocytes	Ingest antigens. Specific types include neutrophils, eosinophils, and monocytes, which differentiate into macrophages. Also include dendritic cells that reside deep in the skin, in lymph nodes, and in the inner lining of the respiratory and digestive tracts.
Natural killer (NK) cells	Directly attack virus-infected and cancer cells by releasing substances that are toxic to the antigen.
Process Barriers and Antimicrobial Proteins	
Complement	Promotes inflammation and phagocytosis; lyses microbes.
Fever	Systemic response that increases body temperature to activate body defenses; inhibits the growth of some microbes.
Inflammation	Limits the spread of infection and releases substances that attract phagocytes; initiates repair of the injured area.
Interferons	Proteins secreted by cells infected by viruses. They protect uninfected cells and also stimulate the activity of phagocytes and NK cells; used as medications to treat certain types of cancer.

a physical barrier but also contains proteins, lysozymes, and other substances that discourage pathogen growth. The respiratory tract secretes a sticky mucus that traps microbes. The stomach and genitourinary tracts provide an acidic environment that kills many microbes. Like the skin, the mucosa of the mouth, colon, and vagina have a normal population of flora, which discourages pathogen growth by competing for space and nutrients.

Cellular barriers: Once physical barriers are breached, **phagocytes** are the primary cells of innate immunity. The primary job of phagocytes is to engulf pathogens and other foreign substances that enter the body. Once engulfed, the phagocytes destroy the microbe in vesicles called lysosomes, which contain powerful destructive enzymes. As expected, phagocytes are found in large numbers in the blood, in lymphatic tissues, and in locations where pathogens have the highest likelihood of entering. For example, the deeper layers of the epidermis contain specialized phagocytes called dendritic cells, which are able to remove pathogens that penetrate the superficial layers. Phagocytes have the ability to migrate to distant sites when an infection is detected, a process called *chemotaxis*.

Phagocytes have proteins on their surface that allow them to recognize cells and cellular components that are "nonself." When recognized as "nonself," the pathogen is internalized and destroyed within the phagocyte. Pieces of the microbe are sometimes displayed on the plasma membrane of the phagocyte, which serves to activate other components of the immune response. Not all pathogens can be engulfed by phagocytosis. Some, such as *Mycobacterium tuberculosis*, are not only resistant to phagocytosis but they can also multiply while residing inside macrophages.

Cancer cells or virus-infected cells attract a different type of innate cellular response: natural killer (NK) cells. Found in most lymphoid organs, NK cells are not phagocytic, but they do release toxins that kill cancer cells or virus-infected cells. NK cells also secrete chemicals that enhance inflammation and modulate the adaptive immune response.

Process barriers and antimicrobial proteins: Processes and proteins associated with innate defenses are complement activation, fever, inflammation, and interferons. The **complement system** is a cluster of 20 plasma proteins that combine in a specific sequence and order when an infection occurs. Activation of complement attracts phagocytes to the infection site, attacks and breaks down the cell walls of pathogens, and stimulates the inflammatory process.

Fever and inflammation are also key processes of the nonspecific defense system. Fever accelerates body defenses and associated repair processes by raising the temperature of the body. When excessive, however, fever can harm the body and must be treated with drugs known as antipyretics (see Chapter 41). From a pharmacologic perspective, one of the most important nonspecific defenses is inflammation. Because of its significance, inflammation is presented separately in Sections 40.3 and 40.4.

Interferons (IFNs) are antimicrobial proteins that are crucial components of the innate body defense system. Released by infected macrophages and lymphocytes, IFNs protect uninfected cells from pathogens. IFNs have been isolated and are now available as medications for the treatment of immune disorders (see Chapter 42), viral infections (see Chapter 54), and cancer (see Chapter 57).

Inflammation

40.3 Inflammation is a nonspecific defense mechanism that neutralizes or destroys foreign substances and microbes.

Inflammation occurs in response to many different stimuli, including physical injury, exposure to toxic chemicals, extreme heat, invading microorganisms, or death of cells. Inflammation is considered a nonspecific defense mechanism because it proceeds in the same manner regardless of the cause.

The central purposes of inflammation are to contain the injury, destroy the pathogen, and initiate repair of the area. The repair of the injured area can proceed at a faster pace by neutralizing the foreign agent and removing cellular debris and dead cells. Signs of inflammation include swelling, pain, warmth, and redness of the affected area.

Inflammation may be classified as acute or chronic. During acute inflammation, such as that caused by minor physical injury, 8 to 10 days are normally needed for the symptoms to resolve and for repair to begin. If the body cannot neutralize the damaging agent, inflammation may continue for long periods and become chronic. In chronic autoimmune disorders such as lupus and rheumatoid arthritis, inflammation may persist for years, with symptoms becoming progressively worse over time. Other disorders such as seasonal allergy arise at predictable times during each year, and inflammation may produce only minor, annoying symptoms.

40.4 Inflammation proceeds with the release of chemical mediators.

During inflammation, pathogens, chemicals, or physical trauma cause the damaged tissue to release chemical mediators that act as alarms to notify the surrounding area of the injury. Chemical mediators of inflammation include histamine, leukotrienes, bradykinin, complement, and prostaglandins. These inflammatory mediators, some of which are listed in Table 40.2, are called proinflammatory substances. Several inflammatory mediators are important targets for anti-inflammatory drugs. For example, aspirin and ibuprofen are prostaglandin inhibitors that are effective at treating fever, pain, and inflammation.

The rapid release of the chemical mediators of inflammation on a large scale throughout the body is responsible for anaphylaxis, a life-threatening allergic response that may result in shock and death. A number of chemicals, insect stings, foods, and some therapeutic drugs can cause this widespread release of histamine from mast cells if the individual has an allergy to these substances.

Histamine is a key chemical mediator of inflammation. It is stored primarily within mast cells located in tissue spaces under epithelial membranes such as the skin, bronchial tree, and digestive tract and along blood vessels. Mast cells detect foreign agents or injury and respond by releasing histamine, which initiates the inflammatory response within seconds. In addition to its role in inflammation, histamine also directly stimulates pain receptors and is a primary agent responsible for the symptoms of seasonal allergies.

When released at an injury site, histamine dilates nearby blood vessels, causing the capillaries to become more permeable. Plasma, complement proteins, and phagocytes can then enter the area to neutralize microbes or their toxins. The affected area may become congested with blood, which can lead to significant swelling and pain. Figure 40.2 illustrates the fundamental steps in acute inflammation.

Histamine interacts with two different receptors to elicit an inflammatory response. H_1 receptors are present in the smooth muscle of the vascular system, the respiratory passages, and the digestive tract. Stimulation of these receptors results in itching, pain, edema, vasodilation, bronchoconstriction, and the characteristic symptoms of inflammation and allergy. In contrast, H_2 receptors are present primarily in the stomach, and their stimulation results in the secretion of large amounts of hydrochloric acid.

Table 40.2 Selected Chemical Mediators of Inflammation

Mediator	Description
Bradykinin	Protein present in an inactive form in plasma and mast cells; increases vascular permeability and causes pain; effects are similar to those of histamine; broken down by angiotensin-converting enzyme (ACE).
Complement	Series of at least 20 proteins that combine in a cascade fashion to neutralize or destroy an antigen; stimulates histamine release by mast cells; causes cell lysis.
C-reactive protein	Occurs as an early response to acute inflammation; activates complement; used as a biomarker to gauge the extent of inflammation.
Cytokines	Proteins produced by macrophages, leukocytes, and dendritic cells that mediate and regulate immune and inflammatory reactions; examples include interleukins and tumor necrosis factor (TNF).
Histamine	Stored and released by mast cells; causes vasodilation, smooth muscle constriction, tissue swelling, and itching.
Leukotrienes	Lipids stored and released by mast cells; effects are similar to those of histamine; synthesized from arachidonic acid; responsible for some symptoms of asthma and allergies.
Prostaglandins	Lipid present in most tissues and stored and released by mast cells; increase capillary permeability, attract white blood cells to the site of inflammation, cause pain, and induce fever; aspirin inhibits their synthesis; some are available as medications.

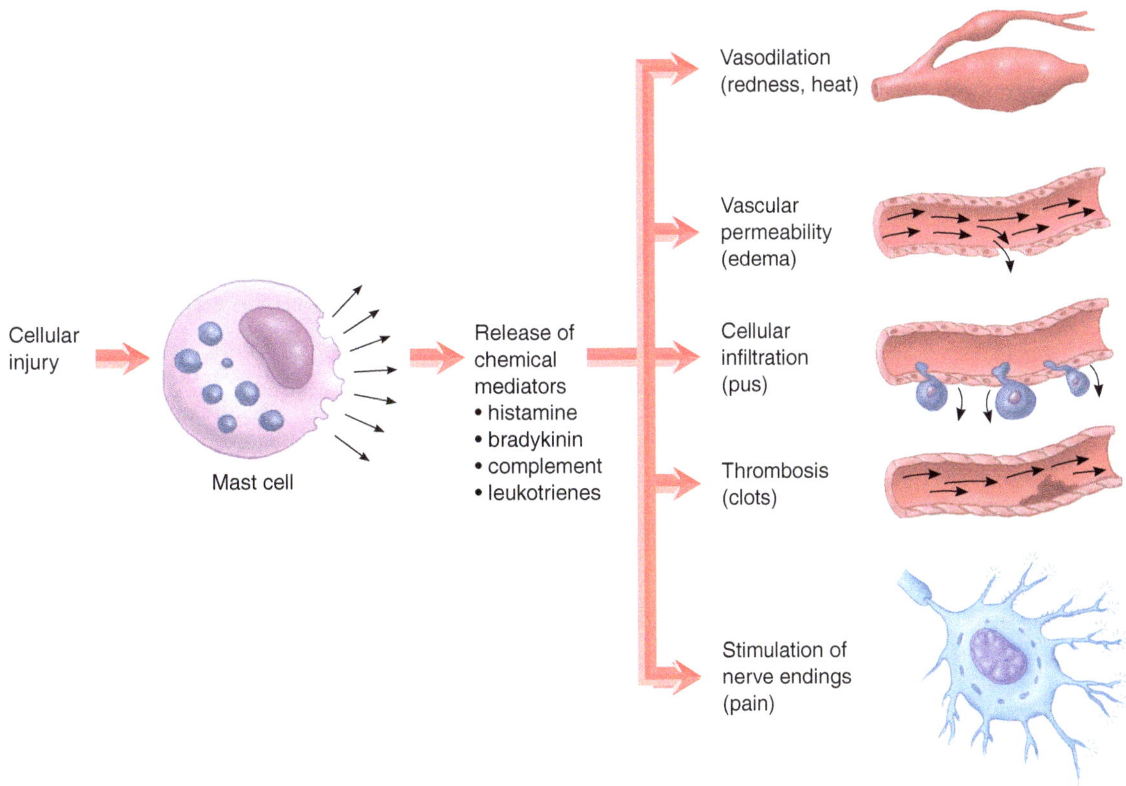

Figure 40.2 Steps in acute inflammation.

Drugs that act as specific antagonists for H_1 and H_2 receptors are in widespread therapeutic use. H_1-receptor antagonists, which are used to treat allergies and inflammation, are discussed in Chapter 45. H_2-receptor antagonists are used to treat peptic ulcers and are discussed in Chapter 59.

CONNECTION Checkpoint 40.1

In addition to being a mediator of inflammation, bradykinin is responsible for one of the most common adverse effects of ACE inhibitors. From what you learned in Chapter 31, describe this adverse effect.

Adaptive (Specific) Defenses

40.5 The adaptive defenses include the humoral and cell-mediated immune systems.

The body also has the ability to mount a third line of defense that is specific to certain threats. For example, a specific defense may act against only a single species of bacteria and be ineffective against all others. These are known as **adaptive defenses** or, more commonly, the immune response. The primary cell of the immune response is the lymphocyte.

Microbes and foreign substances that elicit an immune response are called **antigens**. Foreign proteins, such as those present on the surfaces of pollen grains, bacteria, nonhuman cells, and viruses, are the strongest antigens. Typically, only a small fragment or piece of a foreign protein is required to activate the immune system. It is estimated that the immune system is able to recognize and react to over a billion different antigens.

The immune response is extremely complex. Several important aspects of the immune response are specificity, systemic, and memory.

Specificity. Each aspect of the immune response recognizes only particular pathogens and not others. Recognition of the antigen is dependent on the immune cells interacting with specific foreign proteins. Once an immune response is mounted, it generally only affects the one specific antigen that was recognized.

Systemic. Despite being specific to a particular antigen, the immune response is systemic. Thus, antigens that exist in remote regions beyond the initial site of infection will be neutralized.

Memory. After an antigen interaction occurs, cells of the adaptive immune system remember the immune response. This is different from the components of nonspecific defenses, which have no memory. Upon subsequent exposures to the *same* antigen, the body is able to mount a stronger and more rapid response.

The basic steps of the immune response involve recognition of the antigen, communication and coordination with other defense cells, and destruction or suppression of the antigen. A large number of chemical messengers and complex interactions are involved in the immune response, many of which have yet to be discovered. The two primary divisions of the immune response are antibody-mediated (humoral) immunity and cell-mediated immunity.

Humoral Immunity

40.6 The humoral immune response is mediated by B lymphocytes and includes the secretion of antibodies.

Humoral immunity is triggered when an antigen encounters a *B lymphocyte*, more simply known as a **B cell**. The activated B cell divides to form millions of identical copies of itself in a process known as clonal division. Most cells in this clone are called **plasma cells**, and their primary function is to secrete antibodies specific to the antigen that initiated the challenge. Each plasma cell is capable of manufacturing antibodies at an astounding rate, as many as 2000 each second.

Circulating through body fluids are **antibodies**, also known as *immunoglobulins (Ig)*, which physically interact with antigens to neutralize or mark them for destruction by other cells of the immune response. The activation of complement, with subsequent inflammation and enhanced phagocytosis, is a major defense mechanism resulting from the formation of antigen–antibody complexes. Peak production of antibodies occurs about 10 days after an initial antigen challenge. The important functions of antibodies are illustrated in Figure 40.3.

After the antigen challenge, memory B cells are formed that will remember the specific antigen–antibody interaction. Should the body be exposed to the same antigen in the future, the humoral immune system will manufacture even higher levels of antibodies in a shorter period, approximately 2 to 3 days. For some antigens, such as those for measles, mumps, or chickenpox, memory can be retained for an entire lifetime. Vaccines are sometimes administered to produce these memory cells in advance of exposure to the antigen,

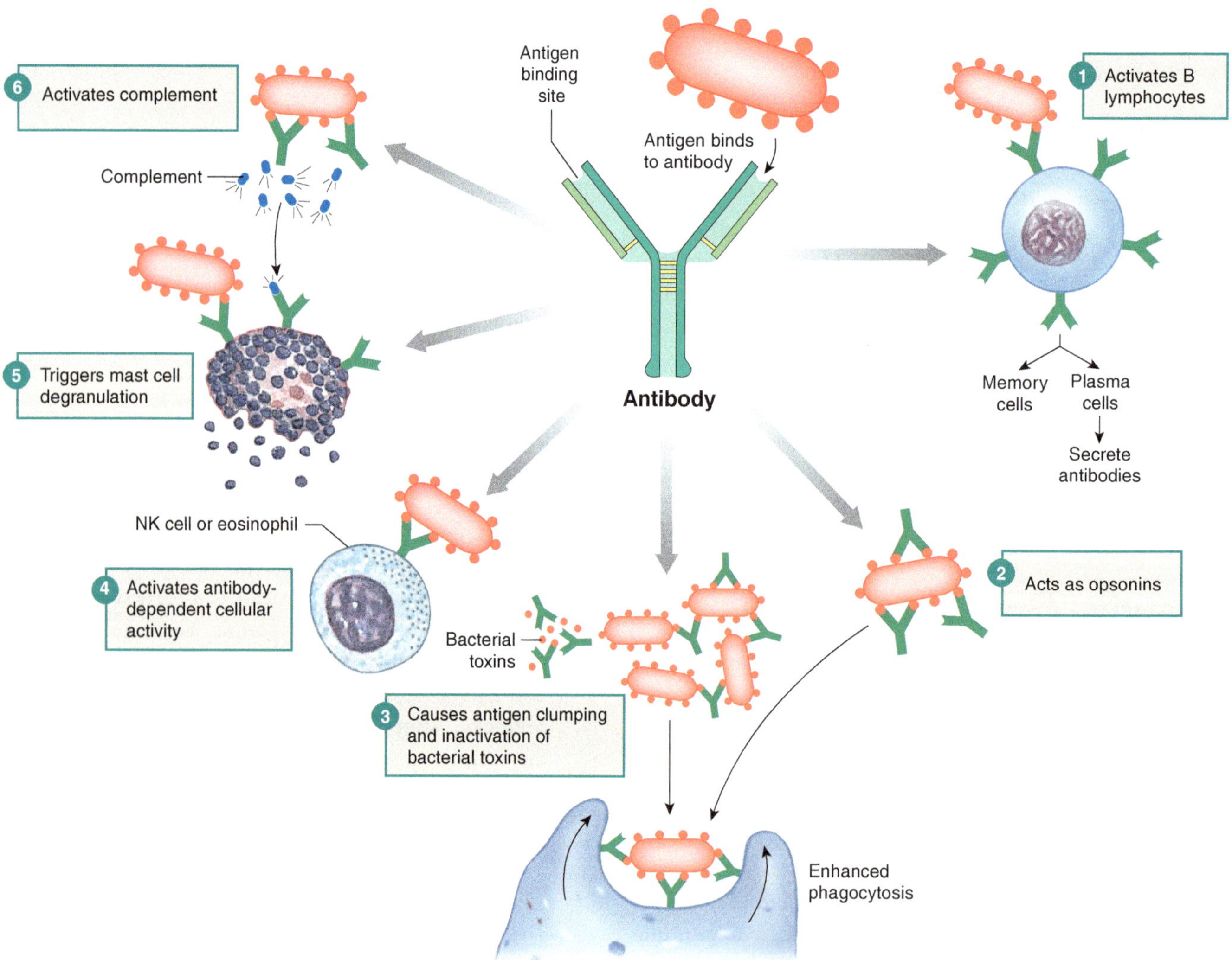

Figure 40.3 Functions of antibodies.
From Silverthorn (2019), Figure 24.24, p. 771.

so that when the body is exposed to the actual organism it can mount a fast, effective response (see Chapter 43).

It is important to remember that the body contains millions of different B cells, each programmed to react to a specific antigen. These B cells, in turn, are able to construct millions of different types of antibodies, each specific to a particular antigen. The body is preprogrammed with the genetic information to defend against millions of different antigens. Although it is unlikely that an individual will ever be infected during a lifetime with all the different antigens, the body is waiting for the challenge.

PharmFACT

Once generated, a single plasma cell is capable of manufacturing antibodies at an astounding rate, as many as 2000 antibodies each second. The cell dies after about 4 to 5 days (Marieb & Hoehn, 2019).

Cell-Mediated Immunity

40.7 The cell-mediated immune response is mediated by T lymphocytes and includes the secretion of cytokines.

A second branch of the immune response involves *T lymphocytes*, or **T cells**. Two major types of T cells are called helper T cells and cytotoxic T cells. These cells are named after a protein receptor on their plasma membrane. The helper T cells have a CD4 receptor, and the cytotoxic T cells have a CD8 receptor. The helper (CD4) T cells are particularly important because they are responsible for activating most other immune cells, including B cells and other types of T cells. Cytotoxic (CD8) T cells travel throughout the body, directly killing certain bacteria, parasites, virus-infected cells, and cancer cells.

PharmFACT

T cells move quickly throughout the body. In a typical day, a T cell may spend 30 minutes in the blood, 5 to 6 hours in the spleen, and 15 to 20 hours in a lymph node (Martini, Nath, & Bartholomew, 2018).

T cells rapidly form clones after they are activated or sensitized following an encounter with their specific antigen. Unlike B cells, however, T cells do not produce antibodies. Instead, activated T cells produce huge amounts of **cytokines**, which are hormone-like proteins that regulate the intensity and duration of the immune response and mediate cell-to-cell communication. Some cytokines kill foreign organisms directly, whereas others induce inflammation or enhance the killing power of macrophages. Specific cytokines released by activated T cells include interleukins, gamma interferon, tumor necrosis factor (TNF), and perforin. Some cytokines are used therapeutically to stimulate the immune system (see Chapter 42). Small amounts of cytokines are also secreted by certain macrophages, B lymphocytes, mast cells, endothelial cells, and the stromal cells of the spleen, thymus, and bone marrow.

Like B cells, some sensitized T cells become memory cells. If the patient encounters the same antigen in the future, the memory T cells assist in mounting a more rapid immune response.

Understanding Chapter 40

Key Concepts Summary

40.1 The lymphatic system is the primary organ system that protects the body from invasion by foreign agents.

40.2 Innate defenses are the body's first line of defense against pathogens.

40.3 Inflammation is a nonspecific defense mechanism that neutralizes or destroys foreign substances and microbes.

40.4 Inflammation proceeds with the release of chemical mediators.

40.5 The adaptive defenses include the humoral and cell-mediated immune systems.

40.6 The humoral immune response is mediated by B lymphocytes and includes the secretion of antibodies.

40.7 The cell-mediated immune response is mediated by T lymphocytes and includes the secretion of cytokines.

References

Krogh, D. (2014). *Biology: A guide to the natural world, technology update* (5th ed.). Benjamin Cummings.

Marieb, E., & Hoehn, K. N. (2019). *Human anatomy and physiology* (11th ed.). Pearson.

Martini, F. H., Nath, J. L., & Bartholomew, E. F. (2018). *Fundamentals of human anatomy and physiology* (11th ed.). Pearson.

Yamakawa, M., Doh, S. J., Santosa, S. M., Montana, M., Qin, E. C., Kong, H., et al. (2018). Potential lymphangiogenesis therapies: Learning from current antiangiogenesis therapies—A review. *Medicinal Research Reviews*, *38*(6), 1769–1798. https://doi.org/10.1002/med.21496

Silverthorn, D. U. (2019). *Human physiology: An integrated approach* (8th ed.) Pearson.

Selected Bibliography

Hall, J. E. (2020). *Guyton & Hall textbook of medical physiology* (14th ed.). Elsevier.

Katzung, B. G. (2018). *Basic and clinical pharmacology.* McGraw-Hill

"I haven't been feeling good this week. It's probably just the flu like all my friends have. I'll just take some of the aspirin my mom uses for her arthritis so I don't miss school and I'll be fine."
—*Patient "Joycee Layne"*

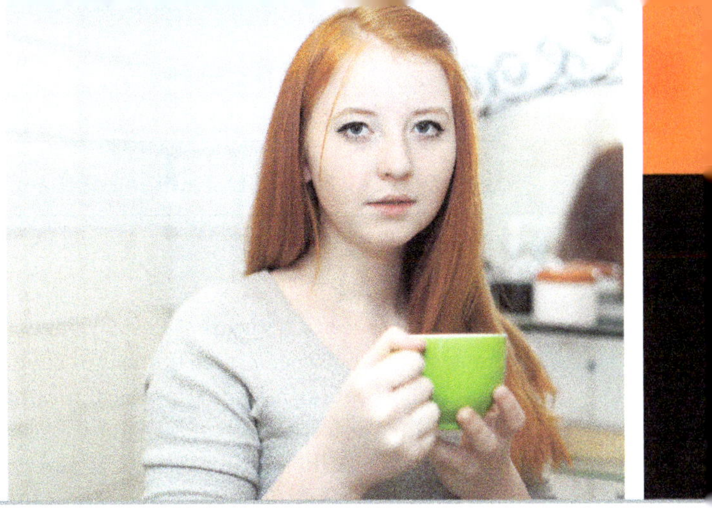

Chapter 41
Pharmacotherapy of Inflammation and Fever

Chapter Outline

Learning Outcomes

After reading this chapter, the student should be able to:

1. Explain the pathophysiology of inflammation and fever.
2. Identify drug classes used to treat inflammation and fever.
3. Explain how aspirin damages the gastrointestinal mucosa.
4. Describe the symptoms and treatment of salicylism.
5. Compare the actions and adverse effects of aspirin to ibuprofen and ibuprofen-like drugs.
6. Compare the actions and adverse effects of the cyclooxygenase-2 inhibitors to other nonsteroidal anti-inflammatory drugs.
7. Describe the nurse's role in the pharmacologic management of inflammation and fever.
8. For each of the classes shown in the chapter outline, identify the prototype and representative drugs and explain the mechanism(s) of drug action, primary indications, contraindications, significant drug interactions, pregnancy data, and important adverse effects.
9. Apply clinical judgment to care for patients receiving pharmacotherapy for fever or inflammation.

Key Terms

Definitions of the terms in bold may be found in the Glossary.

Inflammation is a response to injury that destroys agents that could damage human tissue. A large number of conditions can trigger inflammation, including physical trauma, burns, chemical injury, infections, hypersensitivity reactions, or tissue necrosis. Although it is a natural defense mechanism, excessive inflammation causes symptoms that range from minor discomfort to severe, disabling pain, fever, and limitation of mobility. This chapter examines drugs used to diminish the inflammatory response and reduce fever.

Pathophysiology of Inflammation and Fever

41.1 Inflammation is a nonspecific body response to antigens and tissue injury.

The basic process of inflammation and the proinflammatory chemical mediators involved are described in Chapter 40. The student should review that chapter before proceeding.

Acute inflammation: Acute inflammation has an immediate onset and lasts 1 to 2 weeks. The inflammatory process is initiated when the body is exposed to a foreign substance, or antigen. The antigen may be anything from ragweed pollen to a microorganism; it may even be a normal cell that has been damaged or changed. Once the inflammation process is initiated, nearby blood vessels become permeable, allowing phagocytic cells to reach and neutralize the antigen. The increased permeability causes edema of the surrounding tissue, which often leads to acute pain and, possibly, joint immobility. The greater the tissue damage from the antigen or the inflammation, the greater the edema and the greater the immobility at the site.

Occasionally, acute inflammation is initiated by a rapid, massive release of inflammatory chemical mediators throughout the entire body. This condition, known as **anaphylaxis**, is a life-threatening allergic response that may cause cardiovascular shock and death. A number of chemicals, insect stings, foods, and some therapeutic drugs can cause this widespread release of histamine from mast cells if an individual has hypersensitivity to these substances.

The resolution of acute inflammation occurs when damaged tissue begins the process of regeneration and may conclude within a matter of weeks or continue throughout the individual's life with the regeneration of new tissue. Regeneration processes may replace normal cells with scar tissue, especially in nerve, cardiac, and muscle tissues. Replacement with fibrotic tissue can impair the function of the inflamed tissue.

Chronic inflammation: Chronic inflammation has a slow onset and may lack the distinct stages characteristic of acute inflammation. Whereas acute inflammation is the result of an influx of neutrophils, chronic inflammation is caused primarily by lymphocytes and macrophages. The chronic invasion of an area by macrophages and the resultant chemical reaction at the tissue site activates fibroblasts and generates scar tissue, which may limit mobility or narrow vessel lumens. Lymphocytes sometimes surround macrophages, resulting in granulomas. For example, chronic inflammation from *Mycobacterium tuberculosis* in the lung may occur over many years and yield the development of granulomas. The granulomas serve as a means of protection, walling off the agent from the rest of the body. In the event that the host's immune response diminishes, the host is susceptible to the reemergence of inflammation and the possible onset of active infection.

When acute or chronic inflammation is caused by an infection, the patient is at risk for the development of a febrile episode, which is characterized by an increase in body temperature due to cytokine-induced changes in the hypothalamus. The systemic manifestations of inflammation associated with an infection are elevated temperature above 39°C (102°F), pulse rate greater than 90 beats/min, respirations greater than 20 breaths/min, and a white blood cell count greater than 12,000/mm^3.

Pharmacotherapy of Inflammation

41.2 Treatment of inflammation includes nonpharmacologic therapies and the administration of anti-inflammatory drugs.

Because inflammation is a nonspecific process and may be caused by a variety of physical and infectious etiologies, it may occur in virtually any tissue or organ system. When treating the patient with inflammation, the following general principles apply:

- Inflammation is not a disease but a symptom of an underlying disorder. Whenever possible, the cause of the inflammation is identified and treated.
- Inflammation is a natural process for ridding the body of antigens, and it is usually self-limiting. Nonpharmacologic treatments such as ice packs and rest should be used for mild symptoms whenever applicable.

- Topical drugs should be used when applicable because they cause few adverse effects. Inflammation of the skin and mucous membranes of the mouth, nose, rectum, and vagina are best treated with topical drugs. These include creams, ointments, patches, suppositories, and intranasal sprays. Inhalation drugs may be used for pulmonary inflammation.

The goal of pharmacotherapy with anti-inflammatory drugs is to prevent or decrease the intensity of the inflammatory response and reduce fever, if present. Most anti-inflammatory drugs are nonspecific; that is, whether the inflammation is caused by an injury, autoimmune disease, or allergy, the drug will exhibit the same inhibitory actions. Common diseases that benefit from anti-inflammatory medications include allergic rhinitis, anaphylaxis, ankylosing spondylitis, contact dermatitis, Crohn's disease, glomerulonephritis, Hashimoto's thyroiditis, peptic ulcer disease (PUD), rheumatoid arthritis (RA), systemic lupus erythematosus, and ulcerative colitis.

If fever is associated with the inflammation, medications used to reduce body temperature, or **antipyretics**, may be administered. The goal of antipyretic therapy is to lower body temperature while treating the underlying cause of the fever, which is usually an infection. Many of the drugs used for inflammation also reduce fever and relieve mild to moderate pain.

Two major drug classes are used for nonspecific inflammation: nonsteroidal anti-inflammatory drugs (NSAIDs) and the corticosteroids. For mild to moderate pain, inflammation, and fever, NSAIDs are the preferred class of drugs. Should inflammation become severe or disabling, corticosteroid therapy is begun. Due to the potential for serious long-term adverse effects, oral or parenteral corticosteroids are usually used for only 1 to 3 weeks to bring inflammation under control. The patient is then switched to NSAIDs. Corticosteroids are used for a large number of conditions, and their pharmacotherapy is presented in Chapter 68.

A few anti-inflammatory drug classes are specific to certain disorders. For example, the 5-aminosalicylic acid drugs such as sulfasalazine (Azulfidine) are specific to treating inflammatory bowel disease (see Chapter 60). Colchicine and allopurinol (Zyloprim) are used for the inflammation specifically caused by gouty arthritis (see Chapter 72). These specific anti-inflammatory drugs are less widely prescribed because they are more toxic than the NSAIDs.

PharmFACT

In the United States, approximately 70 million NSAID prescriptions are written each year. If over-the-counter (OTC) use is included, more than 30 billion NSAID doses are consumed each year (Wiegand, 2020).

Nonsteroidal Anti-Inflammatory Drugs

The NSAIDs consist of three major classes: salicylates, ibuprofen (including ibuprofen-like drugs), and cyclooxygenase-2 (COX-2) inhibitors. These drug classes are sometimes grouped as first-generation NSAIDs (salicylates and ibuprofen-like drugs) and second-generation NSAIDs (COX-2 inhibitors). This is not a particularly useful means of grouping the drugs because there are over 20 first-generation NSAIDs and only one second-generation NSAID. The ibuprofen-like NSAIDs are described in Section 41.4 and the COX-2 inhibitors are presented in Section 41.5.

Salicylates

41.3 Aspirin is an inexpensive, effective, first-generation nonsteroidal anti-inflammatory drug commonly used by adults.

The first NSAID to be discovered was originally extracted from the bark of the common willow tree. The medical uses of willow bark, especially for pain relief and fever reduction, had been known for centuries but it was not until 1828 that the active ingredient, called salicin, was identified and converted to salicylic acid. Quite toxic in concentrated amounts, salicylic acid was converted into its most useful form, known as aspirin or acetylsalicylic acid, by a scientist at the Bayer Pharmaceutical Company in 1897. The chemical family to which aspirin belongs is known as the **salicylates**. Since its discovery, aspirin has become one of the most highly used therapeutic drugs in the world. Aspirin has the following indications for use:

- *Analgesic.* The ability to relieve mild to moderate pain
- *Anti-inflammatory.* The ability to decrease mild to moderate inflammation
- *Antipyretic.* The ability to lower body temperature
- *Suppression of platelet aggregation.* The ability to prevent or treat cardiovascular conditions such as acute myocardial infarction (MI) and stroke.

Understanding the mechanism of action of aspirin is important because it explains both the therapeutic actions of the drug as well as its adverse effects. All NSAIDs act by inhibiting the synthesis of prostaglandins. **Prostaglandins** are local hormones found in virtually every tissue that have many diverse functions depending on their location. Several prostaglandins are available as drugs, including carboprost (Hemabate, prostaglandin F_2 alpha), dinoprostone (Cervidil, prostaglandin E_2), and misoprostol (Cytotec, prostaglandin E_1). The physiologic properties of prostaglandins include the following:

- *Mediation of inflammation.* Cause vasodilation and pain and increase capillary permeability
- *Gastrointestinal (GI) protection.* Increase bicarbonate and mucus production to protect the stomach mucosa from acid
- *Renal protection.* Help maintain blood flow through the kidneys
- *Smooth muscle.* Help regulate smooth muscle tone in blood vessels; increase smooth muscle tone in the uterus; may cause bronchodilation or bronchoconstriction
- *Blood clotting.* Increase platelet aggregation to promote clot formation.

Aspirin blocks the synthesis of prostaglandins by inhibiting the enzyme **cyclooxygenase (COX)**. Aspirin and the ibuprofen-like NSAIDs block both forms of the enzyme, known as COX-1 and COX-2, by changing their structures and preventing the formation of prostaglandins. This inhibition of COX is responsible for the therapeutic and adverse effects of these drugs, depending on the location and function of the prostaglandin that is being blocked. For example, the inhibition of COX in peripheral tissues will reduce the pain and inflammation caused by prostaglandins. The inhibition of COX in the stomach, however, will remove the protective effect of prostaglandins and result in damage to the GI mucosa. The mechanism by which aspirin produces its effects is illustrated in Figure 41.1.

Aspirin is a potent inhibitor of thromboxane, a substance secreted by platelets. The inhibition of thromboxane in platelets is especially prolonged and may last for the entire 8- to 11-day lifespan of the platelet. This antithrombotic action inhibits platelet aggregation and reduces the risk of adverse cardiovascular events, including MI and stroke. The antipyretic effect of aspirin results from a suppression of prostaglandin synthesis in the hypothalamus of the brain. It lowers temperature by indirectly causing centrally mediated peripheral vasodilation and sweating. The principal analgesic effect of aspirin occurs in the peripheral areas of the body and in the central nervous system (CNS). Doses for aspirin and the other salicylates are listed in Table 41.1.

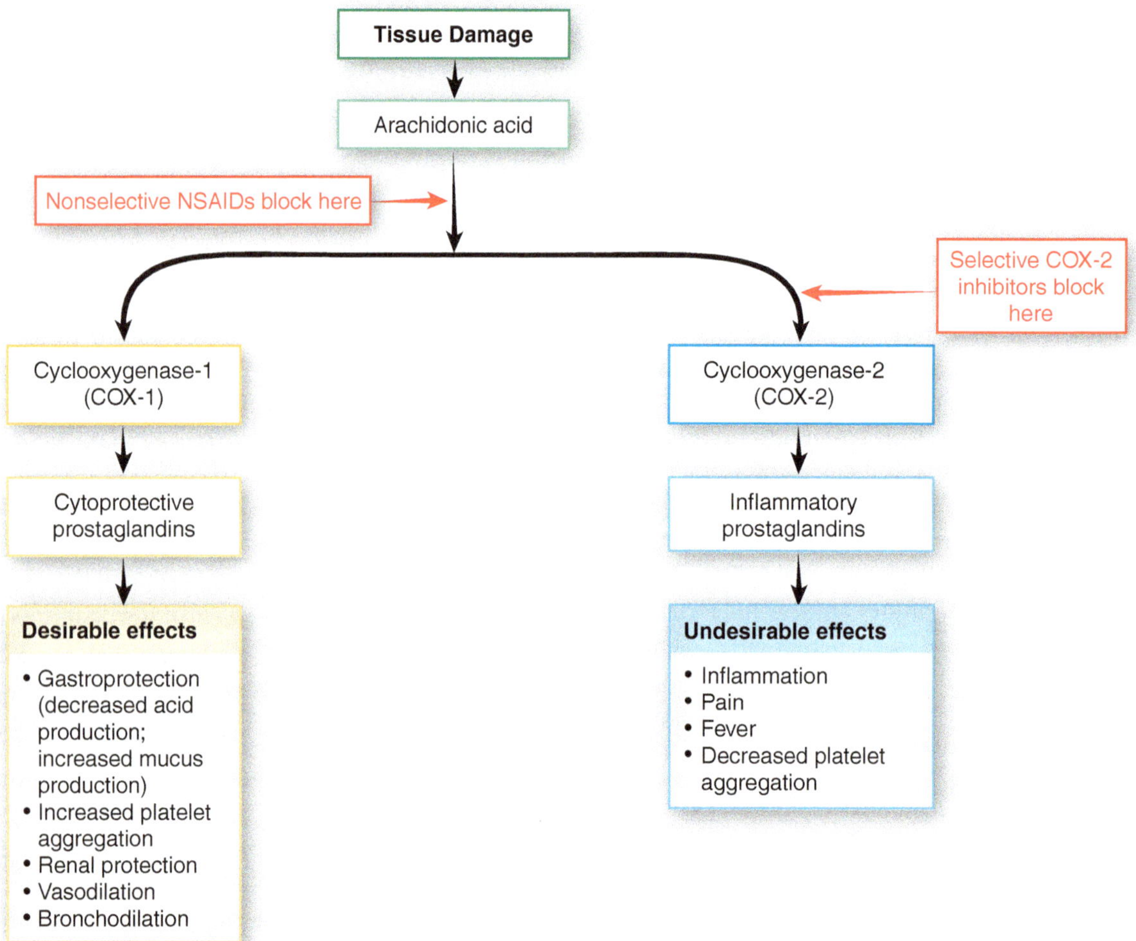

Figure 41.1 Inhibition of cyclooxygenase-1 and -2. Nonselective NSAIDs block the cytoprotective effects as well as inflammation. Selective COX-2 inhibitors block only the inflammation effects.

Table 41.1 Salicylates

Drug	Route and Adult Dose (Maximum Dose Where Indicated)	Adverse Effects
aspirin (acetylsalicylic acid, ASA)	Mild to moderate pain or fever: PO: 350–650 mg, q4h (max: 4 g/day) Arthritic conditions: PO: 3.6–5.4 g/day in 4–6 divided doses TIA prophylaxis: PO: 5–325 mg/day MI or thromboembolic disorder prophylaxis: PO: 80–325 mg/day	*Tinnitus, deafness, urticaria, nausea and vomiting, confusion, drowsiness, prolonged bleeding time, dyspepsia, stomach pain* Bronchospasm, anaphylactic shock, laryngeal edema, hemolytic anemia, salicylism, angioedema, Reye's syndrome, metabolic acidosis, severe GI bleeding, hepatotoxicity
choline magnesium trisalicylate (Trilisate)	PO: 1.0–2.5 g/day in 1–3 divided doses (max: 4.5 g/day)	
magnesium salicylate (Doan's Pills)	Analgesic/antipyretic: PO: 650 mg tid or qid Arthritic conditions: PO: 9.6 g/day in divided doses (max: 4.8 g/day)	
salsalate (Mono-Gesic, Salsitab)	PO: 325–3000 mg/day in divided doses (max: 4 g/day)	

Note: *Italics* indicate common adverse effects. Underline indicates serious adverse effects.

Aspirin is sometimes combined with prescription and OTC medications, and its presence is not always obvious unless the label is carefully inspected. This is especially important for patients with aspirin allergy, which is present in about 1% of the population. Patients with asthma or food allergies are most likely to be allergic to aspirin. Aspirin allergy symptoms include rash, urticaria, dyspnea, wheezing, rhinorrhea, and cough. To prevent aspirin allergy, the patient should be instructed to read labels carefully and avoid products containing salicylates. This is not always possible because salicylates are naturally found in certain foods and are used as preservatives in others. Patients with aspirin allergies should consult with a dietitian regarding which food sources to avoid. Allergists may be able to desensitize a patient if exposure to the drug is unavoidable or if the patient's allergy is severe. Patients who are hypersensitive to aspirin will likely be sensitive to other NSAIDs. For pain or fever relief, acetaminophen may be an option for these adult patients.

The most significant adverse effect of aspirin and other NSAIDs is GI bleeding, which is shown in Pharmacotherapy Illustrated 41.1. Although the risk is dose related, even low doses of aspirin (75–325 mg/day) may double the risk of GI bleeding. Risk factors for aspirin-induced GI bleeding include history of peptic ulcers, age greater than 60, use of anticoagulants or corticosteroids, *Helicobacter pylori* infection, smoking, and use of alcohol. Aspirin has the following adverse effects on the GI mucosa:

- As aspirin is absorbed across the stomach mucosa, it causes direct cellular injury. This topical damage to the stomach may be lessened by the use of enteric-coated formulations.
- After aspirin is absorbed systemically, it inhibits COX-1 and depletes the GI mucosa of prostaglandins. Prostaglandins normally provide a protective function in the GI mucosa by directing the secretion of mucus and bicarbonate and promoting cellular repair of mucosal damage.
- If GI damage or active ulcers are already present, the antiplatelet effects of aspirin will prolong bleeding.

In addition to GI bleeding, aspirin can cause dyspepsia, nausea, and ulcer perforation. For patients who must take high doses of aspirin, proton pump inhibitors (PPIs), such as omeprazole, may provide some degree of protection against GI damage by reducing acid secretion in the stomach. PPIs are effective and relatively safe drugs (see Chapter 59). An alternative therapy for GI protection is oral misoprostol (Cytotec), which is a prostaglandin. Misoprostol can cause fetal harm and abortion, which prohibits its use in women with childbearing potential.

The antiplatelet effects of aspirin can promote bleeding at sites other than the GI tract. Because it irreversibly inhibits COX-1 in platelets, the antiplatelet action of aspirin can be prolonged. It may take longer for minor cuts and injuries to stop bleeding. Patients undergoing surgical or dental procedures should discontinue aspirin use a week prior to the procedure. Patients with known bleeding disorders should not take aspirin at all.

Children under age 19 should never be administered products that contain aspirin when they have flu symptoms, fever, or chickenpox due to the risk of Reye's syndrome, a potentially fatal disease. It is unclear how aspirin contributes to Reye's syndrome because the condition can appear without aspirin use. The incidence of Reye's syndrome is now very rare due to public awareness of the risk associated with aspirin use.

Pharmacotherapy Illustrated 41.1

NSAID-Induced Ulcer Formation

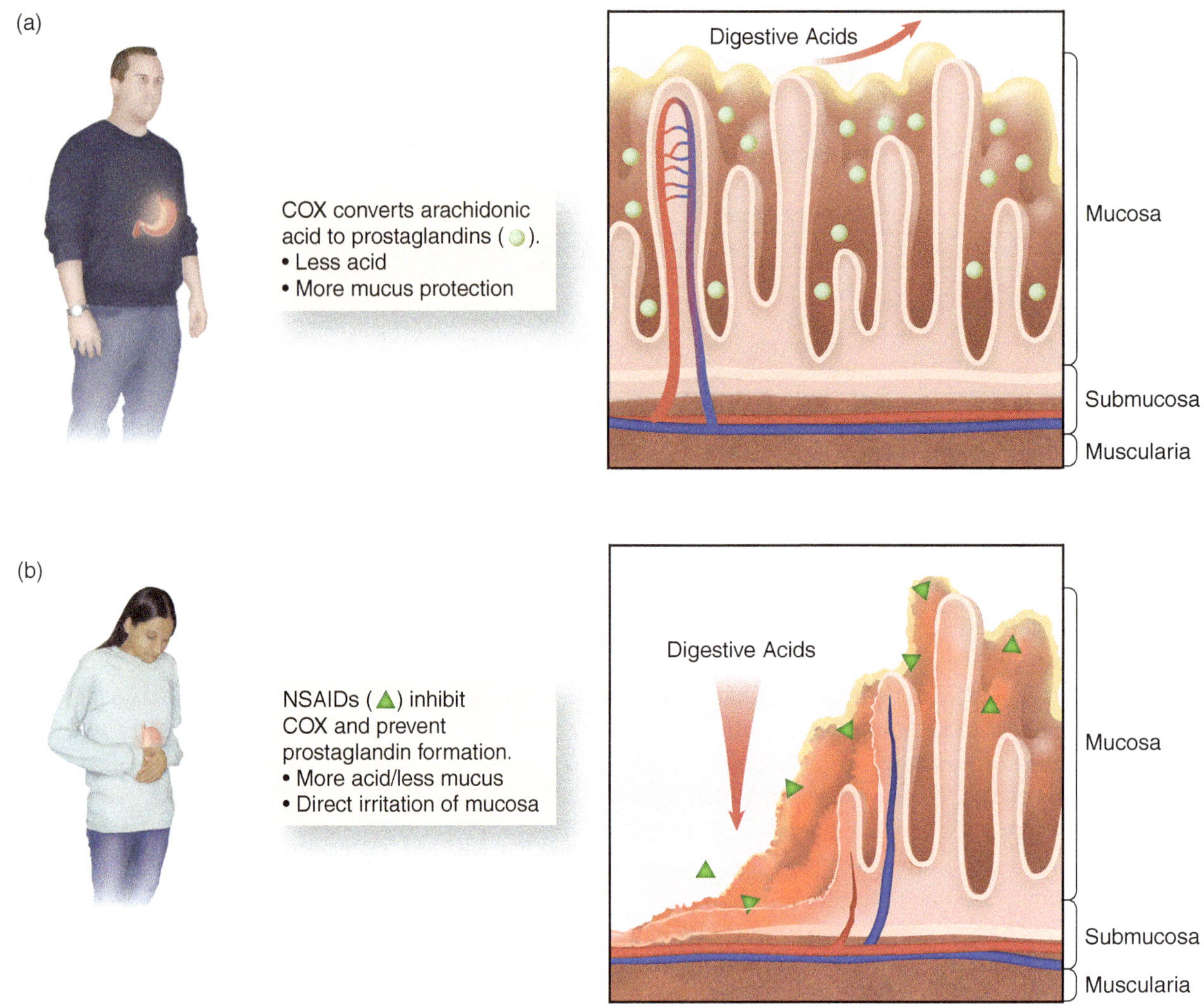

PharmFACT

More than 24,000 salicylate poisonings occur each year, of which about 5000 are intentional overdoses. Approximately 15 deaths from acute salicylate overdose occur each year (Waseem, 2020).

PROTOTYPE DRUG **Aspirin (Acetylsalicylic Acid)**

Classification **Therapeutic:** Non-narcotic analgesic, antipyretic, antiplatelet
Pharmacologic: Salicylate, NSAID

Therapeutic Effects and Uses: Approved by the U.S. Food and Drug Administration (FDA) in 1939, aspirin is one of the best-known medications. The ability of aspirin to reduce pain, inflammation, and fever makes it an extremely versatile and widely used drug. It is used to reduce pain and inflammation that is mild to moderate in intensity. The doses of aspirin needed to control severe pain or inflammation often result in a high incidence of adverse effects.

Aspirin is approved by the FDA for the prevention of thromboembolic events. Aspirin is a first-line treatment for stroke prophylaxis in patients with a history of transient ischemic attack (TIA) or who have persistent or paroxysmal atrial fibrillation. It is approved for MI prophylaxis in patients who are at risk for a cardiac event and who are not already taking warfarin or an antiplatelet drug, including those with coronary artery disease who have already experienced an MI. To lower the risk of thromboembolic events, emergency medical services professionals administer aspirin to patients with a suspected coronary thrombosis prior to hospital arrival. Patients with a high risk for arterial thromboembolism may receive low-dose aspirin therapy.

An off-label use of aspirin is to prevent colorectal cancer. Regular, long-term aspirin use has been determined to reduce the risk of colorectal cancer in certain populations (National Cancer Institute, 2017). The reduction in the incidence of colorectal cancer from the drug must be balanced against the potential risk for increased GI bleeding. The effectiveness of aspirin in preventing cancer is an area of active research.

Mechanism of Action: The anti-inflammatory action of aspirin is caused by the inhibition of COX-1 and COX-2 that leads to reduced prostaglandin synthesis. The analgesic action of aspirin occurs peripherally with limited action in the CNS on the hypothalamus. The suppression of prostaglandin synthesis in or near the hypothalamus results in the lowering of body temperature. Aspirin acts indirectly, causing centrally mediated peripheral vasodilation and sweating.

Pharmacokinetics:

Route(s)	Oral (PO), rectal
Absorption	80–100% absorbed
Distribution	Widely distributed; crosses the placenta; secreted in breast milk; 80–90% bound to plasma protein
Primary metabolism	Hepatic; metabolized to salicylic acid, an active metabolite, in the GI mucosa, plasma, and erythrocytes
Primary excretion	Renal
Onset of action	PO: 5–30 min; rectal: 1–2 h
Duration of action	PO: 1–4 h; rectal: 7 h

Adverse Effects: A major adverse effect of aspirin is the risk of a serious hypersensitivity reaction, which is noted with symptoms such as bronchospasm, laryngeal edema, and anaphylaxis. It also causes significant stomach irritation, heartburn, nausea and vomiting, diarrhea, and stomach pain in 10 to 30% of patients. The risk of GI bleeding increases with dose. The hematologic adverse effects of aspirin administration include thrombocytopenia, hemolytic anemia, and occult bleeding. Long-term administration of aspirin may produce nephrotoxic effects and hepatotoxicity. Tinnitus and hearing loss are common adverse effects with high doses.

Contraindications/Precautions: Patients who have a hypersensitivity to any salicylate (including that found in foods) should not be administered aspirin or other NSAIDs. Patients who have the "aspirin triad," which includes aspirin allergy, nasal polyps, and asthma, should not be administered aspirin. Aspirin is also contraindicated in chronic rhinitis, acute bronchospasm, agranulocytosis, head trauma, increased intracranial pressure, history of GI bleeding, hypoprothrombinemia, vitamin K deficiency, and heart failure (HF). Children and teenagers should not be administered aspirin or products containing aspirin if they have a fever or a flulike illness. Patients over age 60 are especially prone to GI ulceration and bleeding due to aspirin. It should be used cautiously in patients with hypothyroidism, immunosuppression, asthma, and gout. It should also be used cautiously in patients with chronic kidney disease (CKD), hepatic impairment, glucose-6-phosphate dehydrogenase (G6PD) deficiency, anemia, preoperatively, and in the presence of Hodgkin's disease.

Drug Interactions: Concurrent administration of aspirin with other salicylates such as the 5-aminosalicylic acid drugs used to treat inflammatory bowel disease increases the risk of salicylate toxicity. The combined use of aspirin with acetaminophen may cause additive nephrotoxicity. Ammonium chloride and other acidifying agents decrease the renal elimination of aspirin, resulting in salicylate toxicity. The administration of aspirin with anticoagulants, fibrinolytics, or antiplatelet drugs increases the patient's risk for bleeding. When oral antidiabetic drugs are administered concurrently with high doses of aspirin, hypoglycemic activity increases. Patients who consume three or more alcoholic drinks per day may experience additive GI ulceration. Corticosteroids increase the risk of gastric irritation and result in ulcerogenic effects when administered with aspirin. Methotrexate administered with aspirin results in methotrexate toxicity. Low doses of salicylates may antagonize the uricosuric effects of probenecid and sulfinpyrazone. The antihypertensive effects of beta blockers may decrease if administered concurrently with aspirin. **Herbal/Food:** The administration of feverfew, garlic, ginger, horse chestnut, and red clover will increase the patient's risk for bleeding. Taking aspirin with caffeine will increase the rate of aspirin absorption. St. John's wort may increase sedation.

Pregnancy: When taken during the first trimester, NSAIDs may increase the risk for miscarriage. When taken during the third trimester of pregnancy, aspirin may cause premature closure of the fetal ductus arteriosus and prolonged bleeding during delivery. Small doses appear to have no adverse effect on the breastfed neonate, but breastfeeding is not recommended for women taking large doses.

Treatment of Overdose: Acute or chronic overdose of aspirin is known as **salicylism**, which is defined as a serum salicylate level above 200 mcg/mL. The symptoms depend on the dose but include tinnitus, metabolic acidosis, hyperventilation, respiratory alkalosis (secondary to stimulation of the respiratory center), dehydration, agitation, CNS depression, and nausea and vomiting. Emesis, gastric lavage, and alkalinization of urine are indicated. Hemodialysis is of benefit in severe salicylate poisonings.

Clinician Responsibilities: Key clinical implications for patients receiving aspirin are included in Applied Clinical Judgment: Patients Receiving Pharmacotherapy for Inflammation and Fever.

Drugs Similar to Aspirin (Acetylsalicylic Acid)

Drugs that produce similar actions to aspirin include choline magnesium trisalicylate, magnesium salicylate, and salsalate. All the salicylates have the same potential adverse effects on pregnancy and lactation as aspirin.

Choline magnesium trisalicylate (Trilisate): Approved in 1938, this drug combines choline salicylate and magnesium salicylate. It is an oral drug approved for fever and mild to moderate pain and inflammation associated with osteoarthritis, RA, bursitis, and other muscle or joint conditions. This drug causes less GI irritation than aspirin, and it exhibits less antiplatelet activity. Choline magnesium trisalicylate should not be administered to patients with known hypersensitivity to other salicylates. Other contraindications and adverse effects are similar to those of aspirin.

Magnesium salicylate (Doan's Pills): Approved in 1938, magnesium salicylate is an oral drug approved for fever and mild to moderate pain and inflammation associated with osteoarthritis, RA, bursitis, and other muscle or joint conditions. It inhibits prostaglandin synthesis in the same manner as aspirin, but it is less potent, causes less GI irritation, and has less effect on platelet aggregation than aspirin. Magnesium salicylate should not be administered to patients with known hypersensitivity to other salicylates. Other contraindications and adverse effects are similar to those of aspirin.

Salsalate (Mono-Gesic, Salsitab): Approved in 1977, salsalate has analgesic properties similar to those of aspirin but it causes less gastric irritation. It is an oral drug approved to treat mild to moderate pain due to osteoarthritis and RA. Like other salicylates, salsalate produces its effects by inhibiting prostaglandin synthesis. It has little antipyretic activity and has less effect on platelet aggregation than aspirin. Salsalate should not be administered to patients with known hypersensitivity to other salicylates. Other contraindications and adverse effects are similar to those of aspirin.

CONNECTION Checkpoint 41.1

Aspirin is classified as an antiplatelet drug in Chapter 38. Name the other two classes of drugs that are antiplatelets and state the prototype drug for each class.

Ibuprofen-Like Drugs

41.4 Ibuprofen and similar nonsteroidal anti-inflammatory drugs are the most common medications for treating mild to moderate pain and inflammation.

In the 1950s researchers began searching for safer alternatives to aspirin or corticosteroids for treating the severe inflammation of RA. An exhaustive search of over 600 potential compounds over a 15-year period resulted in the discovery of ibuprofen, one of the safest and most widely prescribed NSAIDs in the world. The drug was introduced in the United States in 1974, and it became one of the first prescription-only drugs to be changed to OTC status in 1984.

Since the discovery of ibuprofen, over 20 other nonaspirin NSAIDs have been approved by the FDA. Although their chemical structures vary, they are grouped as "ibuprofen-like" because they share very similar actions and adverse effects with the original drug. Doses for the NSAIDs are listed in Table 41.2. When used at recommended doses, NSAIDs have the following similarities:

- All have the same mechanism of action: They inhibit both COX-1 and COX-2.
- All have analgesic properties: They are widely prescribed to treat patients with mild to moderate pain.
- All have anti-inflammatory properties: Most are specifically approved for osteoarthritis and RA.
- All have antipyretic properties, although not all of them are approved for this indication.
- Most are weak acids that are readily absorbed in the GI tract.
- Most are strongly bound to albumin in the blood.
- Most are metabolized in the liver to inactive metabolites, which are excreted by the kidneys.
- All have the ability to damage the GI mucosa, including bleeding and ulcer formation.
- Many pose an increased risk of cardiac events, such as HF and MI.
- Many are nephrotoxic at high doses.

From the preceding list, it should be clear that the available nonaspirin NSAIDs share many properties. There are, however, some differences in pharmacokinetic profiles. For example, some have longer half-lives or are available in sustained-release formulations that permit once-daily dosing. Some are available by the parenteral route, and a few are formulated for children. Some are enteric coated, which may reduce stomach pain but does not appear to be protective against the formation of ulcers. Another consideration that is important to many consumers is cost. A month's supply of generic ibuprofen 200 mg or naproxen 220 mg costs less than $25 and is available OTC. At the opposite extreme are prescription-only celecoxib (Celebrex)

Table 41.2 Nonaspirin NSAIDs and Acetaminophen

Drug	Route and Adult Dose (Maximum Dose Where Indicated)	Adverse Effects
acetaminophen (Tylenol)	PO: 325–650 mg q4–6h (max: 4 g/day for all products containing this drug) Rectal: 650 mg q4–6h	*Epigastric pain, abdominal pain* Hepatotoxicity, acute renal failure
celecoxib (Celebrex)	PO: 100–400 mg bid (max: 800 mg/day)	*Back pain, peripheral edema, abdominal pain, dyspepsia, flatulence, dizziness, headache, insomnia, hypertension (HTN)* Increased risk of cardiovascular events, acute renal failure
diclofenac (Voltaren, Zorvolex, others)	PO: 25–100 mg/day in one or more doses	*Dyspepsia, dizziness, headache, drowsiness, tinnitus, rash, pruritus, increased liver enzymes, prolonged bleeding time, edema, nausea and vomiting, occult blood loss* Peptic ulcer, GI bleeding, anaphylactic reactions with bronchospasm, blood dyscrasias, CKD, MI, HF, hepatotoxicity
diflunisal	PO: 250–500 mg bid (max: 1500 mg/day)	
etodolac	PO: 200–1200 mg/day in 2–4 divided doses (max: 1200 mg)	
fenoprofen (Nalfon)	PO: 200–600 mg tid or qid (max: 3200 mg/day)	
flurbiprofen	PO: 200–300 mg in 2–4 divided doses (max: 300 mg/day and 100 mg/dose)	
ibuprofen (Advil, Motrin, others)	PO: 400–800 mg tid to qid (max: 3200 mg/day)	
indomethacin (Indocin, Tivorbex)	PO (immediate release): 25–50 mg bid or tid PO (extended release): 75–100 once daily or bid	
ketoprofen	PO (immediate release): 25–75 mg tid or qid (max: 300 mg/day) PO (extended release): 200 mg once daily	
ketorolac (Sprix)	IM/IV: 30–60 mg qid (max: 120 mg/day) PO: 10–20 mg qid (max: 40 mg/day) Intranasal: 1 spray (15.75 mg) in each nostril q4–6h	
meclofenamate	PO: 200–400 mg/day in 3–4 divided doses (max: 400 mg/day)	
mefenamic acid (Ponstel)	PO: 500-mg loading dose followed by 250-mg maintenance dose qid (max: 1250 mg/day for no longer than 7 days)	
meloxicam (Mobic)	PO: 7.5–15 mg once daily (max: 15 mg/day)	
nabumetone	PO: 1000 mg/day as a single dose (max: 2000 mg/day)	
naproxen (Naprosyn) and naproxen sodium (Aleve, Anaprox, others)	PO: 250–500 mg bid (naproxen/naproxen controlled-release max: 1500 mg/day; naproxen sodium max: 1650/day; nonprescription max: 660 mg/day)	
oxaprozin (Daypro)	PO: 600–1200 mg daily (max: 1800 mg/day)	
piroxicam (Feldene)	PO: 10–20 mg once daily (max: 20 mg/day)	
sulindac	PO: 150–200 mg bid (max: 400 mg/day)	
tolmetin	PO: 400 mg tid (max: 1800 mg/day)	

Note: *Italics* indicate common adverse effects. Underline indicates serious adverse effects.

200 mg and tolmetin 600 mg, which may cost $60 to $300 for a monthly supply. Indications for each of the NSAIDs are listed in Table 41.3.

There are important differences between aspirin and the ibuprofen-like drugs in their effects on the blood and heart. Although ibuprofen-like drugs affect blood coagulation, their inhibitory effects on platelets are reversible and short lived. Because they have less antiplatelet effect than aspirin, the ibuprofen-like drugs are not used for the prophylaxis of adverse cardiovascular events. In fact, some of the nonaspirin NSAIDs such as indomethacin and sulindac significantly increase the risk of cardiovascular events. Caution should be used with all the nonaspirin NSAIDs when they are given for prolonged periods to patients with a history of cardiac disease.

NSAIDs are considered equivalent to aspirin in their effectiveness for treating pain, inflammation, and fever. For the occasional user who takes the medications at recommended doses and who has no risk factors, the drugs are very safe and rarely produce any significant adverse effects. For patients who must take high doses for a chronic illness, ibuprofen appears to cause less GI bleeding than aspirin, although both drugs place patients at high risk for GI adverse effects.

PROTOTYPE DRUG Ibuprofen (Advil, Motrin, Others)

Classification **Therapeutic:** Analgesic, anti-inflammatory drug, antipyretic
Pharmacologic: NSAID

Table 41.3 Indications for Selected Nonsteroidal Anti-Inflammatory Drugs

NSAID	Arthritis	Mild to Moderate Pain	Fever	Dysmenorrhea	Other Approved Indications
celecoxib	A	A		A	Acute migraine, ankylosing spondylitis; familial adenomatous polyposis
diclofenac	A	A		A	Ankylosing spondylitis; actinic keratosis (topical); ocular pain and inflammation (ophthalmic)
diflunisal	A	A			
etodolac	A	A			
fenoprofen	A	A			
flurbiprofen	A				Miosis inhibition (ophthalmic)
ibuprofen	A	A	A	A	Acute migraine
indomethacin	A	A			Ankylosing spondylitis; close patent ductus arteriosus (IV)
ketoprofen	A	A	A	A	
ketorolac		A			Allergic conjunctivitis; reduce ocular pain and inflammation (ophthalmic)
meclofenamate	A	A		A	
mefenamic acid		A		A	
meloxicam	A				
nabumetone	A				
naproxen and naproxen sodium	A	A	A	A	Ankylosing spondylitis
oxaprozin	A				
piroxicam	A				
sulindac	A				Ankylosing spondylitis; acute painful shoulder
tolmetin	A				

A, FDA approved.

Therapeutic Effects and Uses: Approved in 1974, ibuprofen was the first nonaspirin NSAID marketed in the United States. Like aspirin, it possesses analgesic, anti-inflammatory, and antipyretic properties. It is indicated for the relief of fever and mild to moderate pain associated with chronic symptomatic RA and osteoarthritis, myalgia, headache, dental pain, and dysmenorrhea. Chewable tablets, drops, and solutions are available in low doses for administration to children.

Unlike aspirin, ibuprofen is not indicated to treat or prevent any cardiovascular conditions. Ibuprofen inhibits platelet aggregation and prolongs the bleeding time without affecting the prothrombin time (PT) or whole-blood clotting times. Its effects on platelets are reversible within 24 hours after discontinuation of the drug.

Ibuprofen lysine (NeoProfen) is an intravenous (IV) form of the drug that was approved in 2006 to close patent ductus arteriosus in premature infants. The drug has a 75% success rate in infants who are no more than 32 weeks gestational age. Although the mechanism of action is not known, it is believed that prostaglandins delay closing of the ductus. By blocking prostaglandin synthesis with ibuprofen, the ductus closes.

Mechanism of Action: Ibuprofen inhibits COX-1 and COX-2, which block prostaglandin synthesis and modulate T-cell function. Ibuprofen inhibits inflammatory cell chemotaxis, decreases the release of superoxide radicals, and increases the scavenging of these products at the inflammatory sites.

Pharmacokinetics:

Route(s)	PO
Absorption	80% absorbed
Distribution	Crosses the placenta; unknown if secreted in breast milk; highly protein bound
Primary metabolism	Hepatic
Primary excretion	Renal; small amount biliary
Onset of action	1 h
Duration of action	6–8 h

Adverse Effects: In low to moderate doses, ibuprofen is well tolerated and serious adverse effects are uncommon. The most frequent adverse events are GI related and include bleeding, anorexia, heartburn, nausea and vomiting, and constipation or diarrhea. Adverse CNS effects include dizziness, headache, drowsiness, and tinnitus. Rare, though serious, adverse effects include peripheral edema, aplastic anemia, leukopenia, and anaphylaxis. Chronic use of ibuprofen may lead to polyuria, azotemia, hematuria, and increased creatinine and blood urea nitrogen (BUN) levels. **Black Box Warnings:** Ibuprofen may increase the risk of serious and potentially fatal cardiovascular thrombotic events, MI, and stroke. This risk may increase with duration of use and in patients with cardiovascular risk factors. Ibuprofen also increases the risk of serious GI adverse effects including bleeding, ulcer, and stomach or intestine perforation. These GI events may occur at any time during use and without prior warning, especially in older adults.

Contraindications/Precautions: Patients who have a known allergy to aspirin or other NSAIDs should not be administered ibuprofen. In addition, patients who have been diagnosed with PUD, bleeding abnormalities, and perioperative pain related to coronary artery bypass graft (CABG) should not receive ibuprofen. The drug should be used cautiously in patients with HTN, history of GI bleeding, diabetes mellitus, and impaired renal or hepatic function. It should also be used cautiously in patients who have HF or a history of stroke or MI. Children with asthma may experience diminished respiratory function when administered ibuprofen. Patients with severe hepatic impairment should not receive ibuprofen because the drug can accumulate to toxic levels.

Drug Interactions: Oral anticoagulants and antiplatelet drugs taken with ibuprofen increase the risk of bleeding. Ibuprofen may increase the toxicity of digoxin, lithium, or methotrexate if taken concurrently. Use with other NSAIDs, alcohol, or corticosteroids may cause serious adverse GI events. The antihypertensive action of diuretics, beta blockers, and angiotensin-converting enzyme (ACE) inhibitors may be reduced if taken with ibuprofen. **Herbal/Food:** Ibuprofen combined with feverfew, garlic, ginger, and ginkgo may result in an increased risk of bleeding.

Pregnancy: When taken during the first trimester, NSAIDs may increase the risk for miscarriage. Because NSAIDs may cause premature closure of the fetal ductus arteriosus, use in late in pregnancy should be avoided. Because only small amounts enter human milk and the drug has a short half-life, ibuprofen is considered by many clinicians to be safe during lactation.

Treatment of Overdose: Overdose may lead to acute renal failure, apnea, cyanosis, drowsiness, GI bleeding, nausea and vomiting, and sweating. Treatment is supportive and includes the administration of activated charcoal and nasogastric suction.

Clinician Responsibilities: Key clinical implications for patients receiving ibuprofen are included in Applied Clinical Judgment: Patients Receiving Pharmacotherapy for Inflammation and Fever.

Drugs Similar to Ibuprofen (Advil, Motrin, Others)

There are a number of subclasses of NSAIDs that are based on the chemical structures of the molecules. These subclasses include the propionic acids (e.g., ibuprofen), phenylacetic acids (e.g., diclofenac), indole acetic acids (e.g., indomethacin), fenamates (e.g., mefenamic acid), ketones (e.g., nabumetone), and oxicams (e.g., piroxicam). From a clinical perspective, the nonaspirin NSAIDs are remarkably similar to ibuprofen. Doses and indications for these drugs differ, as listed in Tables 41.2 and 41.3.

PharmFACT

It is estimated that NSAID use is associated with about 100,000 hospitalizations and 16,000 deaths annually in the United States, largely as a result of GI complications (Wiegand, 2020).

Cyclooxygenase-2 Inhibitors

41.5 Celecoxib is an effective second-generation nonsteroidal anti-inflammatory drug, but its use is limited due to an increased risk of myocardial infarction and stroke.

Celecoxib (Celebrex) is a second-generation NSAID that blocks COX-2 without inhibiting COX-1. The selective inhibition of COX-2 produces the analgesic, anti-inflammatory, and antipyretic effects typical of other NSAIDs, but without causing platelet aggregation or GI irritation. The primary advantage of celecoxib is that it causes less GI bleeding and ulcer formation than aspirin or ibuprofen. This medication is the newest and most controversial of the NSAIDs.

The ability to treat arthritis without adverse effects caused excitement throughout the medical field in the 1990s, and the three drugs originally in this class were widely prescribed. This elation quickly ended when postmarketing data revealed that rofecoxib (Vioxx) doubled the risk of MI and stroke in patients taking the drug for extended periods. Based on the research data, the drug manufacturer voluntarily removed rofecoxib from the market. Shortly afterward a second COX-2 inhibitor, valdecoxib (Bextra), was also voluntarily withdrawn, leaving celecoxib the sole drug in this class.

PROTOTYPE DRUG Celecoxib (Celebrex)

Classification **Therapeutic:** Anti-inflammatory
Pharmacologic: COX-2 inhibitor, NSAID

Therapeutic Effects and Uses: Initially approved in 1998, celecoxib is used to treat mild to moderate pain and inflammation associated with RA, osteoarthritis, dysmenorrhea, dental procedures, headache, and ankylosing spondylitis. It is also an effective antipyretic drug. The effectiveness of celecoxib at reducing pain and inflammation is equivalent to that of other NSAIDs. In 2020 an oral solution of celecoxib (Elyxyb) was approved for termination of acute migraine in adults. Each bottle of Elyxyb contains one full dose (120 mg).

In addition to its anti-inflammatory indications, celecoxib is also used for the prophylaxis of adenomas or colorectal polyps in adults with familial adenomatous polyposis. Patients with this condition have an inherited mutation in a gene that results in hundreds of polyps and an almost 100% risk of colon cancer. Although celecoxib reduces the number of polyps in these patients, it has not been proven to reduce the risk of malignancies.

Mechanism of Action: Celecoxib selectively inhibits the enzyme COX-2. It inhibits prostaglandin synthesis to reduce inflammation. This action relieves pain and inflammation in the joints and smooth muscle tissue.

Pharmacokinetics:

Route(s)	PO
Absorption	Well absorbed
Distribution	Widely distributed; is likely secreted in breast milk; 97% protein bound
Primary metabolism	Hepatic by CYP2C9
Primary excretion	Primarily feces (57%), with some in urine (27%)
Onset of action	Peak: 3 h
Duration of action	Half-life: 11.2 h

Adverse Effects: Common adverse effects include headache, HTN, fever, dyspepsia, upper respiratory tract infection, arthralgia, cough, vomiting, and diarrhea. CNS adverse effects include headache, dizziness, and insomnia. Adverse effects of the integumentary system are generally rare and include erythema multiforme, exfoliative dermatitis, rash, Stevens–Johnson syndrome, and toxic epidermal necrolysis. The long-term use of celecoxib may cause CKD and hepatic impairment. **Black Box Warnings:** Celecoxib carries the same warnings as the ibuprofen-like drugs. It may increase the risk of serious and potentially fatal cardiovascular thrombotic events, MI, and stroke. This risk may increase with duration of use and in patients with cardiovascular risk factors. Celecoxib also increases the risk of serious GI adverse effects including bleeding, ulcer, and stomach or intestine perforation. These GI events may occur at any time during use and without prior warning. Older adults are at greater risk for serious GI events.

Contraindications/Precautions: Celecoxib should not be administered to patients with hepatic insufficiency because the primary site of drug metabolism is the liver. It is also contraindicated in patients with CKD. This drug is contraindicated in patients with anemia or in the postoperative phase of a CABG. Celecoxib is administered cautiously in patients who are poor CYP2C9 metabolizers. This drug is contraindicated in patients with a history of GI bleeding or PUD, and it should be administered with caution to patients receiving anticoagulants. Patients with a history of asthma, bone marrow suppression, stroke, peripheral vascular disease, elevated liver function tests, HF, kidney disease, and fluid retention should be administered celecoxib cautiously.

Drug Interactions: If taken with celecoxib, oral coagulation modifiers such as clopidogrel or warfarin may cause an increased risk of bleeding. Celecoxib may increase the toxicity of lithium if taken concurrently. Use with alcohol, corticosteroids, aspirin, or other NSAIDs may cause serious adverse GI events. The antihypertensive action of diuretics or ACE inhibitors may be reduced if taken with celecoxib. Concurrent use with fluconazole may increase serum celecoxib levels. **Herbal/Food:** Feverfew, garlic, ginger, ginkgo, horse chestnut, and red clover may increase the risk of bleeding if used during celecoxib therapy.

Pregnancy: Celecoxib showed embryotoxicity and reduced fetal survival. in laboratory animals. Because NSAIDs may cause premature closure of the fetal ductus arteriosus, use should be avoided in late pregnancy. Because only small amounts are secreted in human milk, the drug is considered by some clinicians to be safe during lactation.

Treatment of Overdose: Overdose may cause acute renal failure, apnea, cyanosis, drowsiness, GI bleeding, nausea and vomiting, and sweating. Treatment is supportive and includes the administration of activated charcoal and nasogastric suction.

Clinician Responsibilities: Key clinical implications for patients receiving celecoxib are included in Applied Clinical Judgment: Patients Receiving Pharmacotherapy for Inflammation and Fever.

Drugs Similar to Celecoxib (Celebrex)

Celecoxib (Celebrex) is the sole medication in this class.

CONNECTIONS: Advanced Practice Application

Intravenous Acetaminophen—Is it Worth the Cost?

Case

Sarah is a 27-month-old who had a surgical reduction of intussusception (telescoping of the intestines). The surgery was uncomplicated and the patient has been brought into the pediatric postoperative area on IV morphine prn. Her parents are with her and she has already received 2 doses of IV morphine but continues to cry out in pain. Her parents are distraught, and they ask you, the pediatric nurse practitioner (NP) hospitalist, to evaluate Sarah for pain management. IV acetaminophen has recently become available at your institution, and you wonder if it could be added to her pain plan. Would this help minimize the potential for adverse opioid effects for this patient?

Discussion

IV acetaminophen (Ofirmev) was approved by the FDA in November 2010 for the management of mild to moderate pain, the management of moderate to severe pain (along with opioid analgesics), and the reduction of fever in patients ages 2 years and older. Ofirmev has been advertised as an opioid-sparing analgesic with a potential for reducing opioid-related side effects. Recent studies have shown mixed outcomes to using IV acetaminophen. Early research had shown benefit in the use of IV acetaminophen with a reduction in opioid administration by up to 20% (Shaffer et al., 2017); however, more recent studies have suggested that there may actually be no added benefit in the routine use of IV acetaminophen and that it increases the overall hospital costs per patient (Suarez et al., 2018; Taylor et al., 2020).

The cost of IV acetaminophen is significantly higher than that of oral or rectal acetaminophen. The clinician must weigh its benefits against the risk of increased overall healthcare costs due to adverse events related to increased opioid consumption by patients. The IV route should primarily be used for patients who cannot tolerate oral and rectal acetaminophen, such as those who are NPO (nothing by mouth) or who cannot receive NSAIDs due to risk of bleeding or opioid complications.

IV acetaminophen is administered over 15 minutes and may be given as a single or repeated dose. The maximum daily dose of acetaminophen is based on all routes of administration (IV, oral, and rectal) and all products (prescription and nonprescription) containing acetaminophen.

The recommended dosage of Ofirmev is 15 mg/kg every 6 hours or 12.5 mg/kg every 4 hours, with a maximum single dose of 15 mg/kg, a minimum dosing interval of 4 hours, and a maximum daily dose for all routes of acetaminophen of 75 mg/kg per day.

CONNECTION Checkpoint 41.2

Several NSAIDs are approved to treat mild migraines. From what you learned in Chapter 25, what non-NSAID drug classes are used to terminate severe migraine episodes?

Antipyretic and Analgesic Drugs

41.6 Acetaminophen is administered for pain relief and to reduce fever, but it has no anti-inflammatory properties.

Acetaminophen (Tylenol) is administered for pain relief and to reduce fever. Unlike aspirin, ibuprofen, and celecoxib, acetaminophen has no anti-inflammatory properties and therefore is not classified as an NSAID. Acetaminophen has equal effectiveness to the NSAIDs in reducing pain and fever, and it is often a preferred drug for treating noninflammatory pain. It is the primary alternative to NSAIDs when patients have a contraindication to taking aspirin or ibuprofen. Acetaminophen is frequently combined with other OTC drugs in treating severe flu symptoms. It is often combined with opioid analgesics; adding acetaminophen provides additive pain relief and allows for lower doses of the narcotic (see Chapter 25). Due to a safety recommendation from the FDA, drug manufacturers now limit the strength of acetaminophen in prescription combination products to 325 mg per tablet, capsule, or dosing unit to lower the potential for acetaminophen-induced hepatotoxicity.

Acetaminophen has no effect on platelet aggregation and does not exhibit cardiotoxicity. Most importantly, it does not cause GI bleeding or ulcers, as do the NSAIDs.

PROTOTYPE DRUG Acetaminophen (Tylenol)

Classification **Therapeutic:** Nonopioid analgesic, antipyretic
Pharmacologic: Para-aminophenol derivative

Therapeutic Effects and Uses: Approved in 1950, acetaminophen relieves mild to moderate pain but has no effect on inflammation. Acetaminophen is approved to treat pain associated with osteoarthritis of the hip or knee, dysmenorrhea, dental procedures, headache, and myalgia. It is a preferred drug for reducing fever. Acetaminophen is administered as a substitute for aspirin when NSAIDs are contraindicated due to age, allergy, or gastric irritation. It is not linked with Reye's syndrome, as is aspirin; thus, it is safe to administer to infants, children, and adolescents who have flulike symptoms or chickenpox.

Acetaminophen is available for the oral (suspension, tablets, chewable tablets, extended-release tablets, and oral granules) or rectal route. Childhood and infant preparations are available. Ofirmev is an IV formulation of acetaminophen.

Mechanism of Action: Acetaminophen acts centrally in the CNS by inhibiting COX. It has no effect on COX in peripheral tissues. It may also inhibit the chemical mediators of pain, but its mechanism is unclear. The reduction of fever occurs by its direct action on the heat-regulating center of the hypothalamus to produce peripheral vasodilation, sweating, and dissipation of heat.

Pharmacokinetics:

Route(s)	PO, rectal, IV
Absorption	Rapid and complete absorption
Distribution	Distributed to all body fluids; crosses the placenta; secreted in breast milk; 25% bound to plasma protein
Primary metabolism	Hepatic
Primary excretion	Renal
Onset of action	PO: 30–60 min; IV: 15 min
Duration of action	3–8 h

Adverse Effects: At recommended doses, acetaminophen is well tolerated and serious adverse effects are rare. The risk for adverse effects is dose related and increases with long-term use. Acute acetaminophen poisoning is very serious, and symptoms include anorexia, nausea and vomiting, dizziness, lethargy, diaphoresis, chills, epigastric or abdominal pain, and diarrhea. Excessive acetaminophen use is the number-one cause of acute hepatic failure in the United States. The onset of hepatotoxicity is noted with elevated transaminases (alanine aminotransferase, aspartate aminotransferase) and bilirubin. The patient may also experience hypoglycemia, hepatic coma, and acute renal failure. Chronic ingestion of acetaminophen results in neutropenia, pancytopenia, leukopenia, thrombocytopenic purpura, hepatotoxicity in alcohol-dependent patients, and CKD. In 2013, the FDA issued a safety alert that recommended the drug be immediately discontinued if skin reactions or blisters develop. These skin lesions may indicate the development of rare, though serious, disorders such as Stevens–Johnson syndrome. **Black Box Warning:** Acetaminophen has the potential to cause severe liver injury and may cause serious allergic reactions with symptoms of angioedema, difficulty breathing, itching, or rash.

Contraindications/Precautions: Patients who are allergic to acetaminophen should not be administered this medication. It should be used cautiously in patients with anemia, G6PD deficiency, or hepatic disease. Acetaminophen should be administered cautiously to patients with RA or osteoarthritis, malnutrition, bone marrow depression, and immunosuppression. Chronic administration of acetaminophen should be avoided in patients with CKD because this drug can worsen kidney function.

Drug Interactions: Acetaminophen should not be administered with alcohol or to patients who consume alcohol with regularity because this greatly increases the risk of hepatotoxicity. Alcohol-induced hepatotoxicity can occur at therapeutic doses of acetaminophen. Due to additive hepatotoxic effects, acetaminophen should not be administered with barbiturates, carbamazepine, isoniazid, and rifampin. Long-term use of acetaminophen will increase the anticoagulant actions of warfarin. Zidovudine administered with acetaminophen may increase the risk of bone marrow suppression. **Herbal/Food:** Caffeine will enhance the analgesic effects of acetaminophen. Hepatotoxicity has been reported with concurrent echinacea use.

Pregnancy: Acetaminophen showed evidence of fetal toxicity in laboratory animals. Large-scale human studies have not found an increased risk for major birth defects when taken during pregnancy. Very small amounts of this drug are secreted in human milk and many clinicians consider acetaminophen safe during lactation.

Treatment of Overdose: Acetaminophen overdose is treated with oral or IV acetylcysteine (Acetadote). For maximum effectiveness, the antidote should be administered within 8 hours of acetaminophen ingestion. The IV form (Acetadote) is administered by the "three-bag method":

- *Loading dose.* Dilute 150 mg/kg in 200 mL of 5% dextrose and administer over 60 minutes.
- *Second dose.* Dilute 50 mg/kg in 500 mL of 5% dextrose and administer over 4 hours.
- *Third dose.* Dilute 100 mg/kg in 1,000 mL of 5% dextrose and administer over 16 hours.

Clinician Responsibilities: Key clinical implications for patients receiving acetaminophen are included in Applied Clinical Judgment: Patients Receiving Pharmacotherapy for Inflammation and Fever.

Drugs Similar to Acetaminophen (Tylenol)

Acetaminophen is the only medication in this class.

CONNECTIONS: Treating the Diverse Patient

Ethnic Differences in Acetaminophen Metabolism

Patients of Asian, African American, or Middle Eastern descent, may have higher rates of an enzyme deficiency that affects how they metabolize certain drugs. More than 200 million people worldwide are believed to have a hereditary deficiency of the enzyme G6PD. Patients with G6PD deficiency are at risk for developing hemolysis after ingesting certain drugs, including acetaminophen. In patients with the deficiency, therapeutic dosages of acetaminophen may cause hemolysis. Because acetaminophen is one of the most common drugs used for fever, pain control, and in many OTC cough and cold medicines, and because patients may not know that they have the deficiency, healthcare providers should recommend that ethnically diverse patients exercise caution when using acetaminophen and report any signs or symptoms associated with anemia. Patients with known G6PD deficiency should avoid this drug. Patients receiving IV forms of acetaminophen should have frequent complete blood count (CBC) laboratory monitoring.

CONNECTIONS: APPLIED CLINICAL JUDGMENT

Patients Receiving Pharmacotherapy for Inflammation and Fever

Key Assessment Data

- History of current condition, baseline vital signs, physical exam findings; ulcers or GI bleeding, bleeding disorders, hepatic, renal, respiratory, cardiovascular, or neurologic disease; medication history; pregnancy status.
- Ongoing assessment during drug therapy should include monitoring appropriate laboratory findings (e.g., CBC, coagulation panels, bleeding time, electrolytes, glucose, lipid profile, and hepatic or renal function studies); assessment for GI bleeding (dark or tarry stools, hematemesis, coffee-ground emesis, or blood in the stool), abdominal pain, severe tinnitus, dizziness, drowsiness, lightheadedness, palpitations, tachycardia, HTN, increased respiratory rate and depth, pulmonary congestion, or edema. Weight gain over 1 kg (2 lb) in a 24-hour period or more than 2 kg (5 lb) in 1 week should be reported.

Desired Therapeutic Outcomes

Improvement is observed and measurable by temperature within normal range, decreased or absent pain, signs and symptoms of inflammation such as redness or swelling are decreased. Fever should begin to diminish within 1 to 3 hours after taking the drug.

Minimizing Adverse Effects:

- Ibuprofen and similar drugs may increase the risk for cardiovascular thrombotic events such as MI and stroke. Continue to monitor vital signs, especially temperature if fever is present, and blood pressure and pulse for patients on ibuprofen and similar drugs.
- NSAIDs may cause GI irritation and bleeding. Monitor for abdominal pain, black or tarry stools, blood in the stool, hematemesis, coffee-ground emesis, dizziness, lightheadedness, and hypotension, especially if associated with tachycardia.
- Aspirin and salicylates affect platelet aggregation. Acetaminophen may be hepatotoxic in large doses or if taken when hepatic dysfunction is present. Periodic monitoring of CBC, coagulation studies or bleeding time, hepatic and renal function tests, electrolytes, glucose, and lipid levels may be required if the drug is used long term or if excessive bleeding or bruising is noted.
- NSAIDs and salicylates may be ototoxic and cause hearing loss. Monitor for tinnitus, difficulty hearing, lightheadedness, or difficulty with balance.
- NSAIDs and salicylates may be nephrotoxic and patients on long-term or high-dose therapy should monitor urine output, edema, and have periodic renal function studies.
- NSAIDs may cause blurred or diminished vision, decreased color sense, diplopia, or scotomas. Changes in visual acuity, blurred or diminished vision, reports of spots in vision, or changes in color sense require additional evaluation.

Lifespan Considerations

- Age-related physiologic changes increase the risk of adverse renal and hepatic effects in the older adult.
- Due to age-related physiologic changes, the older adult is at increased risk for GI irritation or bleeding.
- Aspirin has been associated with an increased risk of Reye's syndrome in children under age 19, particularly associated with the flu virus and varicella infections. Avoid the use of aspirin or salicylates in children under age 19 unless explicitly ordered by the healthcare provider.
- Assess for the possibility of pregnancy before beginning drug therapy.

Diversity Considerations

- Due to the potential for undetected G6PD deficiency, ethnically diverse patients should exercise caution when using acetaminophen and report any signs or symptoms associated with anemia. Patients with known G6PD deficiency should avoid acetaminophen, even at therapeutic doses.

Patient Education

- Report a fever that does not diminish below 37.8°C (100°F) or per provider's instructions. Immediately report febrile seizures, changes in behavior or LOC, tachycardia, palpitations, or increased blood pressure.
- Immediately report any signs or symptoms of GI bleeding. Take the drug with food or milk to decrease GI irritation. Enteric-coated tablets should be swallowed whole without chewing, crushing, or breaking.
- When NSAIDs or salicylates are used, report any signs or symptoms of ringing, humming, buzzing in ears, difficulty with balance, dizziness or vertigo, or nausea to the healthcare provider.
- Men who consume more than two alcoholic beverages per day or women who consume more than one alcoholic beverage per day should consult their healthcare provider before taking acetaminophen.
- Do not take routine (daily) aspirin without discussing with the provider first. The drug may be contraindicated depending on other conditions or medications.
- When NSAIDs or salicylates are used, promptly report any changes in the quantity of urine output, darkening of urine, or edema. Increase fluid intake, especially if fever is present. When the drug is used long term, obtain a daily weight, ideally at the same time of day. Report a weight gain of more than 1 kg in a 24-hour period or more than 2 kg per week or increasing peripheral edema to the healthcare provider.
- Women who are pregnant or considering pregnancy should notify their provider before using NSAIDs.
- Do not use aspirin or salicylates in children unless ordered by the provider or within 2 to 3 weeks after the varicella vaccination has been administered. Read labels on all OTC medications and avoid formulations with aspirin or salicylate on the label.
- Liquid doses of acetaminophen or NSAIDs should be measured with the dosage cup, dropper, or spoon enclosed with the prescription. If that measuring device is no longer available, do *not* use a household spoon. Obtain another calibrated measuring cup or dropper.

(*continued*)

CONNECTIONS: APPLIED CLINICAL JUDGMENT *(continued)*

Patients Receiving Pharmacotherapy for Inflammation and Fever

Prescribing Considerations
- Use with caution and consider dosage adjustment or avoiding use, depending on degree of hepatic and renal impairment and other patient-specific factors.
- Use with caution and consider reduced initial dosage with the use of acetaminophen in patients with alcoholism or serious kidney or liver disease.
- In patients with asthma, ibuprofen and other NSAIDs that inhibit cyclooxygenase-1 can exacerbate the condition.

Understanding Chapter 41

Key Concepts Summary

41.1 Inflammation is a nonspecific body response to antigens and tissue injury.

41.2 Treatment of inflammation includes nonpharmacologic therapies and the administration of anti-inflammatory drugs.

41.3 Aspirin is an inexpensive, effective, first-generation nonsteroidal anti-inflammatory drug commonly used by adults.

41.4 Ibuprofen and similar nonsteroidal anti-inflammatory drugs are the most common medications for treating mild to moderate pain and inflammation.

41.5 Celecoxib is an effective second-generation nonsteroidal anti-inflammatory drug, but its use is limited due to an increased risk of myocardial infarction and stroke.

41.6 Acetaminophen is administered for pain relief and to reduce fever, but it has no anti-inflammatory properties.

CASE STUDY: Making the Patient Connection

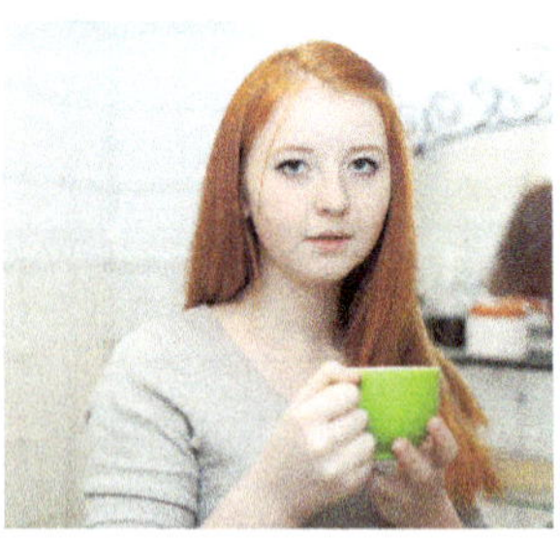

Remember the patient "Joycee Layne" at the beginning of the chapter? Now read the remainder of the case study. Based on the information presented within this chapter, respond to the critical thinking questions that follow.

Joycee Layne is a 17-year-old high school student in her senior year. She is an honors student, works hard to get good grades, and hates to miss school. For the past 3 days, she has not been feeling well. This morning her temperature is 39°C (102.2°F), and she has chills and a headache. Several of her friends at school have the flu. She has taken ibuprofen for fevers and menstrual cramps in the past, but Joycee cannot find any in the house as she prepares to leave for school. Her parents have already left for work, and they trust her to check with you, the nurse who lives next door, before taking any medication. Joycee calls you to ask, "Is it okay to take the aspirin that my mom uses for her arthritis so I can go to school?" As the nurse, this presents an opportunity for you to teach Joycee about aspirin and her fever.

Critical Thinking Questions

1. Describe the pathophysiology of fever and inflammation.
2. Why is aspirin administered for fever?
3. Should Joycee take the aspirin? Why or why not?
4. What will you teach Joycee about aspirin and the flu-like symptoms she is having? What additional patient teaching will she need?

Additional Case Study

Tameeka Jones has a postoperative infection following a vaginal hysterectomy. The infection is noted at the site of the laparoscopic incision of the lower abdomen. She has developed a fever of 38.8°C (102°F). The healthcare provider has ordered acetaminophen (Tylenol) 650 mg PO every 4 to 6 h as needed for the fever.

1. What is the action of acetaminophen (Tylenol)?
2. What pain medications should be avoided while the patient is receiving acetaminophen (Tylenol) for fever reduction?
3. What patient teaching is important for the patient who has a fever related to infection?

Chapter Review

1. A 30-year-old patient with depression has attempted suicide by overdosing on acetaminophen (Tylenol). The nurse in the emergency department will anticipate that the patient's treatment will consist of:
    1. An intravenous infusion with normal saline to infuse at 1000 mL per hour.
    2. The administration of acetylcysteine (Acetadote) by intravenous infusion.
    3. Preparation for cardioversion due to the impending arrhythmia.
    4. The assessment of liver hepatic enzymes to determine hepatotoxicity.

2. A patient has a fever and is allergic to aspirin. Which medication will the nurse anticipate administering to reduce the patient's fever?
    1. Ibuprofen (Motrin, Advil)
    2. Ketorolac
    3. Acetaminophen (Tylenol)
    4. Celecoxib (Celebrex)

3. An anti-inflammatory drug is ordered to be given intravenously to the patient for pain. Which anti-inflammatory drug is administered parenterally?
    1. Ketorolac
    2. Ketoprofen
    3. Ibuprofen (Motrin, Advil)
    4. Celecoxib (Celebrex)

4. An 80-year-old woman who is scheduled for a total knee replacement next month currently takes ibuprofen (Motrin, Advil) 600 mg three times per day. Which patient teaching intervention is most important?
    1. Continue ibuprofen (Motrin, Advil) until surgery.
    2. Stop ibuprofen (Motrin, Advil) today.
    3. Decrease ibuprofen (Motrin, Advil) to two times per day.
    4. Stop ibuprofen (Motrin, Advil) 7 to 14 days before surgery.

5. The nurse should question the order of acetaminophen (Tylenol) for which patient?
    1. A patient with cirrhosis of the liver
    2. A patient with chronic obstructive pulmonary disease
    3. A patient with breast cancer
    4. A patient who is taking warfarin (Coumadin)

6. A patient takes aspirin (acetylsalicylic acid) daily for pain in the right knee. Which toxic effects may be present with aspirin overdosage? (Select all that apply.)
    1. Tinnitus
    2. Hyperventilation
    3. GI bleeding
    4. Decreased urinary output
    5. Peripheral neuropathy

See Appendix A for answers to critical thinking questions, case study questions, and review questions.

References

National Cancer Institute (2017). *Aspirin to reduce cancer risk*. https://www.cancer.gov/about-cancer/causes-prevention/research/aspirin-cancer-risk

Shaffer, E. E., Pham, A., Woldman, R. L., Spiegelman, A., Strassels, S. A., Wan, G. J., & Zimmerman, T. (2017). Estimating the effect of intravenous acetaminophen for postoperative pain management on length of stay and inpatient hospital costs. *Advances in Therapy*, 33, 2211. https://doi.org/10.1007/s12325-016-0438-y

Suarez, J., Al-Mansoori, A., Kanwar, S., Semien, G., Villa, J., McNamara, C., & Patel, P. (2018). Effectiveness of novel adjuncts in pain management following total knee arthroplasty: A randomized clinical trial. *Journal of Arthroplasty*, *33*(7), S136–S141. https://doi.org/10.1016/j.arth.2018.02.088

Taylor, B., Chakraborty, S., Harthan, A., Tripathi, S., Wang, H., & Swayampakula, A. (2020). Effect of IV acetaminophen usage on opioid requirements, outcomes and costs of care for postoperative children in a pediatric intensive care unit. *Journal of Pediatric Pharmacology and Therapeutics*, *25*(6), 514–520. https://doi.org/10.5863/1551-6776-25.6.514

Waseem, M. (2020). *Salicylate toxicity*. Medscape. http://emedicine.medscape.com/article/1009987-overview#a0156

Wiegand, T. J. (2020). *Nonsteroidal anti-inflammatory drug (NSAID) toxicity*. Medscape. http://emedicine.medscape.com/article/816117-overview

Selected Bibliography

Bindu, S., Mazumder, S., & Bandyopadhyay, U. (2020). Non-steroidal anti-inflammatory drugs (NSAIDs) and organ damage: a current perspective. *Biochemical Pharmacology*, *180*, 114147. https://doi.org/10.1016/j.bcp.2020.114147

Farrell, S. E. (2020). *Acetaminophen toxicity*. Medscape. http://emedicine.medscape.com/article/820200-overview#aw2aab6b2b4

Fisher, E. S., & Curry, S. C. (2019). Evaluation and treatment of acetaminophen toxicity. *Advances in Pharmacology*, *85*, 263–272. https://doi.org/10.1016/bs.apha.2018.12.004

Grosser, T., Ricciotti, E., & FitzGerald, G. A. (2017). The cardiovascular pharmacology of nonsteroidal anti-inflammatory drugs. *Trends in Pharmacological Sciences*, *38*(8), 733–748. https://doi.org/10.1016/j.tips.2017.05.008

Mallick-Searle, T. (2016). Over-the-counter analgesics: What nurse practitioners need to know. *Journal for Nurse Practitioners*, *12*(3), 174–180. https://doi.org/10.1016/j.nurpra.2015.11.016

Moriarty, C., & Carroll, W. (2016). Ibuprofen in paediatrics: Pharmacology, prescribing and controversies. *Archives of Disease in Childhood-Education & Practice Edition*, *101*, 327–330. https://doi.org/10.1136/archdischild-2014-307288

Pearlman, B. L., & Gambhir, R. (2009). Salicylate intoxication: A clinical review. *Postgraduate Medicine*, *121*(4), 162–168. https://doi.org/10.3810/pgm.2009.07.2041

Purssell, E., & Collin, J. (2016). Fever phobia: The impact of time and mortality—a systematic review and meta-analysis. *International Journal of Nursing Studies*, *56*, 81–89. https://doi.org/10.1016/j.ijnurstu.2015.11.001

Walker, C., & Biasucci, L. M. (2018). Cardiovascular safety of non-steroidal anti-inflammatory drugs revisited. *Postgraduate Medicine*, *130*(1), 55–71. https://doi.org/10.1080/00325481.2018.1412799

Yuan, J. Q., Tsoi, K. K. F., Yang, M., Wang, J. Y., Threapleton, D. E., Yang, Z. Y., et al. (2016). Systematic review with network meta-analysis: Comparative effectiveness and safety of strategies for preventing NSAID-associated gastrointestinal toxicity. *Alimentary Pharmacology and Therapeutics*, *43*, 1262–1275. https://doi.org/10.1111/apt.13642

"I don't know what's worse—
the symptoms or the treatment.
I feel terrible."
Patient "Carole Banks"

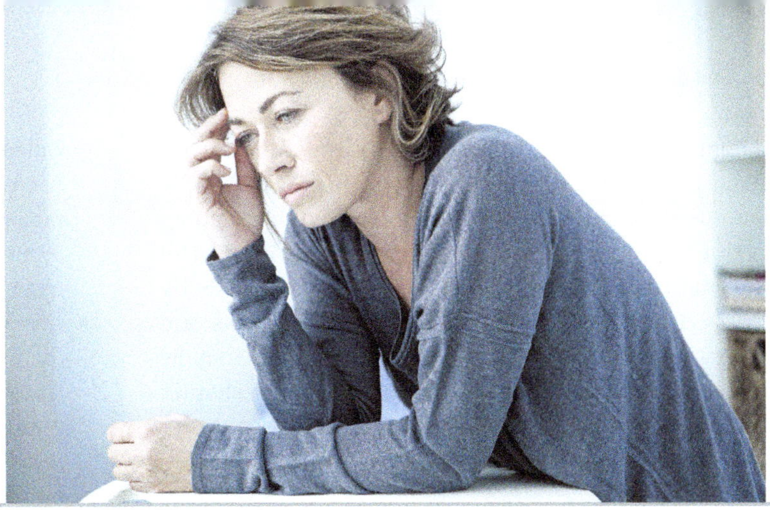

Chapter 42
Immunostimulants and Immunosuppressants

Chapter Outline

Learning Outcomes

After reading this chapter, the student should be able to:

1. Compare and contrast the therapeutic applications of the immunostimulants and immunosuppressants.
2. Describe the roles of interferons, interleukins, and other cytokines in modulating the immune response.
3. Explain how pegylation of the interferon molecule allows for less frequent dosing.
4. Explain why therapy with immunosuppressant medications is necessary following organ transplantation.
5. Identify the classes of drugs used as immunosuppressants.
6. Compare and contrast polyclonal and monoclonal antibodies.
7. For each of the classes shown in the chapter outline, identify the prototype and representative drugs and explain the mechanism(s) of drug action, primary indications, contraindications, significant drug interactions, pregnancy data, and important adverse effects.
8. Apply clinical judgment to care for patients receiving pharmacotherapy with immunostimulants and immunosuppressants.

Key Terms

Definitions of the terms in bold may be found in the Glossary.

The immune system and other body defenses are truly formidable deterrents to invading microorganisms. A healthy defense system can protect the body from life-threatening infections caused by thousands of different species of organisms, often over an entire lifetime. In addition, body defenses can protect against internal invaders such as cancer cells. In certain circumstances, however, drugs may be necessary to modulate the body's defenses. This chapter examines pharmacotherapy with drugs that either stimulate or suppress immune function.

42.1 Immunomodulators are substances that either enhance or suppress the ability of the body to fight infection and disease.

Body defenses are composed of a complex system of cells, tissues, and processes designed with a single goal: to protect the body from invasion by foreign substances, or antigens, that may cause harm. Some of these defenses are specific to a single species of microbe, whereas others are nonspecific and provide the same response or protection regardless of the invading pathogen. The student should review the components of body defenses in Chapter 43 before proceeding.

Immunomodulator is a general term referring to any drug or therapy that affects body defenses. An overview of the immunomodulators is given in Figure 42.1. Two basic types of immunomodulators are used for pharmacotherapy:

- **Immunostimulants** are drugs that enhance the ability of the immune system to fight infection and disease. Many of these drugs are used to treat patients with cancer. The use of immunostimulants to treat cancer is called *immunotherapy*. Some immunostimulants are also used to treat hepatitis. The use of colony-stimulating factors to treat neutropenia was presented in Chapter 39 and the application of vaccines to boost the immune response is presented in Chapter 43.
- **Immunosuppressants** are drugs that diminish the ability of the immune system to fight infection and disease. Immunosuppressants are used to prevent transplant rejection and to dampen hyperactive immune responses, such as those that may occur during exacerbations of systemic lupus erythematosus (SLE) or rheumatoid arthritis (RA).

Immunostimulants

42.2 Interferons are biologic response modifiers that have antiviral and antineoplastic activity.

When challenged by antigens, certain cells of the immune system secrete cytokines, which are substances that help the body mediate and intensify the immune response. Because cytokines have powerful actions on the immune system, the body generally only produces them when challenged by an antigen; their production is rapid though transient. Although cytokines are essential components of body defenses, a chronic high level of cytokines can greatly worsen symptoms of disorders such as psoriasis, Crohn's disease, or RA.

Cytokines exhibit multiple complex actions. A single cytokine can affect multiple target cells, each resulting in a different action. There is also considerable overlap or redundancy among the cytokines in that different cytokines can

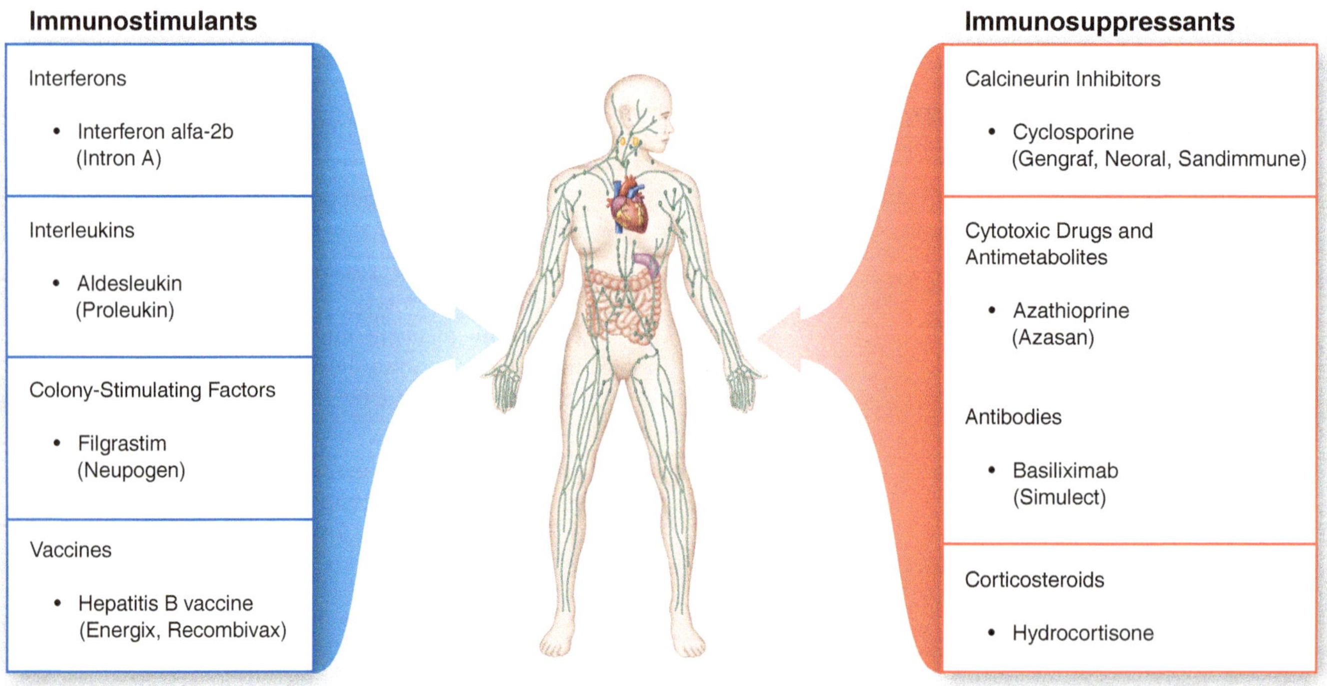

Figure 42.1 Overview of immunomodulators.

produce the same biologic actions. In addition to affecting their target cells, cytokines interact with each other by turning the synthesis of other cytokines on or off. The physiology of cytokines is complex and is an active research field.

Natural cytokines have been identified and, through recombinant deoxyribonucleic acid (DNA) technology, enough quantity has been made available to treat certain disorders. Also called **biologic response modifiers**, some of these drugs have been approved to boost specific functions of the immune system.

Interferons (IFNs) are cytokines secreted by lymphocytes and activated macrophages that have been infected with a virus. IFNs are unable to protect the infected cell, but they warn surrounding cells that a viral infection has occurred. IFNs attach to nearby uninfected cells, inducing the production of protective antiviral proteins. When the virus attempts to attack the protected cell, the pathogen is inactivated.

IFNs are part of the body's nonspecific (innate) defense system. Their actions slow the spread of viral infections, stimulate the activity of existing leukocytes, increase phagocytosis, and enhance the cytotoxic ability of T cells. Interestingly, IFNs promote apoptosis in infected cells, which is a form of programmed cell death in which the infected cell kills itself to limit the replication and spread of the virus. In addition to their antiviral actions, IFNs have antineoplastic and anti-inflammatory properties.

Many different cell types produce IFNs. Although their functions are nearly identical, each IFN has a slightly different structure, and some have different receptors. To distinguish among the different IFNs, each type is assigned numbers and a Greek letter. The most common types are IFN alfa-2b, IFN beta-1a, IFN beta-1b, and IFN gamma-1a. When the drug consists of a mixture of IFNs, the letter *n* is assigned. For example, IFN alfa-n3 is a mixture of IFN alfa subtypes. The alfa IFNs have the greatest clinical utility. The formulations available are shown in Table 42.1.

Two formulations have the molecule polyethylene glycol (PEG) bonded to the IFN. PEG is a polymer with low toxicity that can be found in skin creams, laxatives, lubricants, toothpastes, and many other products. The addition of PEG to another molecule, known as **pegylation**, increases the molecule's solubility and extends its stability. The addition of PEG to an IFN extends the half-life of the drug to allow for once-weekly dosing. Indications for IFN alfa therapy include hairy cell leukemia, non-Hodgkin's lymphoma, acquired immunodeficiency syndrome (AIDS)–related Kaposi's sarcoma, and chronic hepatitis B or C. The use of IFN alfa in the pharmacotherapy of hepatitis is presented in Chapter 54. Doses of the IFNs are listed in Table 42.1.

IFN beta consists of two different formulations, beta-1a and beta-1b, which are primarily reserved for the treatment of severe multiple sclerosis (MS) (see Chapter 21). A third drug in this class, called IFN gamma-1b, has limited clinical

Table 42.1 Immunostimulants

Drug	Route and Adult Dose (Maximum Dose Where Indicated)	Adverse Effects
aldesleukin (Proleukin)	IV: 600,000 units/kg (0.037 mg/kg) q8h by a 15-min IV infusion for a total of 14 doses	*Flulike symptoms, rash, anemia, nausea and vomiting, diarrhea, confusion, dyspnea* Cardiac arrest, hypotension, tachycardia, thrombocytopenia, oliguria, anuria, pulmonary edema, capillary leak syndrome
bacillus Calmette-Guérin (BCG) vaccine (TheraCys, Tice)	Interdermal (Tice): 0.1 mL as vaccine Intravesical (TheraCys): Bladder instillation for bladder carcinoma	*Flulike symptoms, dysuria, hematuria, anemia, lymphadenopathy* Thrombocytopenia, cystitis, urinary tract infection (UTI), disseminated mycobacteria
Interferons		
IFN alfa-2b (Intron A)	IM/Subcutaneous: Hairy cell leukemia: 2 million units/m^2 3 times/wk for up to 6 months Kaposi's sarcoma: 30 million units/m^2 3 times/wk for 16 wk Chronic hepatitis B: 30–35 million units/wk for 16 wk	*Flulike symptoms, myalgia, fatigue, headache, anorexia, diarrhea, nausea* Myelosuppression, thrombocytopenia, neutropenia, suicide ideation, severe depression, seizures (IFN beta), myocardial infarction (MI) (IFN gamma), anaphylaxis, hepatotoxicity
IFN alfa-n3 (Alferon N)	Intralesion: 0.05 mL (250,000 international units) per wart twice/wk for up to 8 wk	
IFN beta-1a (Avonex, Rebif)	IM (Avonex): 30 mcg/wk Subcutaneous (Rebif): 44 mcg 3 times/wk	
IFN beta-1b (Betaseron, Extavia)	Subcutaneous: 0.25 mg (8 million units) every other day	
IFN gamma-1b (Actimmune)	Subcutaneous: 50 mcg/m^2 3 times/wk	
pegIFN alfa-2a (Pegasys)	Subcutaneous: 180 mcg once weekly for 48 wk	
pegIFN alfa-2b (Pegintron, Sylatron)	Subcutaneous (Pegintron): 1.5 mcg/kg once weekly for 48 wk Subcutaneous (Sylatron): 6 mg/kg/wk for 8 doses followed by 3 mg/kg/wk for up to 5 years	

Note: *Italics* indicate common adverse effects. Underline indicates serious adverse effects.

application in the treatment of chronic granulomatous disease and severe osteoporosis.

PROTOTYPE DRUG **Interferon Alfa-2b (Intron A)**

Classification **Therapeutic:** Immunostimulant
Pharmacologic: Interferon, biologic response modifier

Therapeutic Effects and Uses: Approved in 1986, IFN alfa-2b is a biologic response modifier prepared by recombinant DNA technology. Indications include neoplastic including hairy cell leukemia, malignant melanoma, non-Hodgkin's lymphoma, and AIDS-related Kaposi's sarcoma as well as viral infections (chronic hepatitis virus B and C). IFN alfa-2b is also indicated for the intralesional treatment of condylomata acuminata, which are genital warts caused by human papillomavirus (HPV). Off-label indications include chronic myelogenous leukemia, bladder cancer, herpes simplex virus, multiple myeloma, renal cell carcinoma, human immunodeficiency virus (HIV), varicella-zoster virus (VZV), and West Nile virus. It is available for intravenous (IV), intramuscular (IM), and subcutaneous administration.

Mechanism of Action: IFN alfa-2b has both antiviral and antineoplastic activities. It is a nonspecific inhibitor of viral replication. It affects cancer cells by two mechanisms. First, it enhances the general functions of the immune system: IFNs increase the phagocytic activity of macrophages and monocytes, resulting in enhanced cytotoxicity against tumor cells. Second, this drug suppresses the growth of cancer cells.

Pharmacokinetics:

Route(s)	IV, IM, subcutaneous
Absorption	80% absorbed
Distribution	Unknown if secreted in breast milk
Primary metabolism	Minimal hepatic metabolism
Primary excretion	Renal
Onset of action	Peak: 3–12 h
Duration of action	Half-life: 2–3 h

Adverse Effects: The most common adverse effect of IFN therapy is a flulike syndrome of fever, chills, dizziness, weight loss, and fatigue that occurs in about 50% of patients and that usually diminishes as therapy progresses. Fatigue may be severe at higher doses. Neutropenia occurs in most patients and headache, nausea and vomiting, diarrhea, and anorexia are common. Hair loss may occur with prolonged therapy. Depression and suicidal ideation have been reported and may be severe enough to require discontinuation of the drug. The depression may persist after the drug is discontinued. With prolonged therapy, serious adverse effects such as immunosuppression, hepatotoxicity, and neurotoxicity may be observed. **Black Box Warning:** IFNs may cause or aggravate fatal or life-threatening neuropsychiatric, autoimmune, ischemic, or infectious disorders. The drug should be discontinued if these symptoms are persistent or severe.

Contraindications/Precautions: Contraindications include hypersensitivity to IFNs, autoimmune hepatitis, or hepatic decompensation. Neonates and infants should not receive this drug because it contains benzyl alcohol, which is associated with an increased incidence of neurologic and other serious complications in this age group. If infection occurs during therapy, anti-infectives should be started immediately. Hepatic enzymes may become elevated during IFN therapy and may require discontinuation of the drug. This effect is worse in patients with preexisting hepatic impairment. IFN alfa-2b should be used with caution in patients with cardiac disease, herpes zoster, and recent exposure to chickenpox. Triglycerides should be monitored during therapy because elevated levels have resulted in symptoms of pancreatitis in some patients.

Drug Interactions: IFN alfa-2b may increase theophylline levels. Zidovudine may increase hematologic toxicity and cause immunosuppression. **Herbal/Food:** Unknown.

Pregnancy: In laboratory animals, interferon alfa-2b impaired fertility and increased the risk for spontaneous abortion. When used with ribavirin, the combination is embryocidal and teratogenic and is contraindicated during pregnancy and in the male partners of women who are pregnant. It is not known if the drug is secreted in breast milk but because of the potential for serious adverse effects, breastfeeding is not recommended.

Treatment of Overdose: Overdose with IFN may cause lethargy and coma. Treatment is by general supportive measures.

Clinician Responsibilities: Key clinical implications for patients receiving IFN alfa-2b are included in Applied Clinical Judgement: Patients Receiving Pharmacotherapy with Immunomodulators.

Drugs Similar to Interferon alfa-2b (Intron A)

Other available IFNs include IFN alfa-n3, IFN beta-1a, IFN beta-1b, IFN gamma-1b, pegIFN alfa-2a, and pegIFN alfa-2b. See the IFN 2b prototype for the potential risks of use during pregnancy and lactation.

IFN alfa-n3 (Alferon N): Approved in 1989, IFN alfa-n3 is a mixture of IFN alfa subtypes purified from human leukocytes. Indications include genital warts caused by HPV. Two injections per week for 8 weeks are usually sufficient to cause warts to disappear. Unlike the other IFNs, this drug is injected directly into lesions (intralesionally). Its off-label indications include treatment of hepatitis C, herpes simplex, and other viral infections by the subcutaneous route. This product may contain egg protein and is contraindicated in patients with egg sensitivity. IFN alfa-n3 exhibits few adverse effects when administered intralesionally.

IFN beta-1a (Avonex, Rebif) and IFN beta-1b (Betaseron, Extavia): The beta interferons are first-line drugs for the pharmacotherapy of MS. These medications decrease the frequency of clinical exacerbations and slow the progression to physical disability, which is characteristic of MS. Both beta interferons are available by the subcutaneous route; beta-1b can also be administered. Adverse effects are similar to those of other IFNs, with flulike symptoms being observed in the majority of patients. Patients should be monitored for depression and suicidal ideation. Liver injury is a rare, though serious, adverse effect; thus, patients should be monitored for changes in hepatic function during therapy. Injection site necrosis is possible. Additional details on the pharmacotherapy of MS and a drug prototype feature for IFN beta-1b are presented in Chapter 21.

IFN gamma-1b (Actimmune): Approved in 1999, IFN gamma-1b is produced by recombinant DNA technology and is very similar to natural IFN gamma. IFN gamma-1b has both direct and indirect antiviral activity. This drug activates macrophages to increase the production of interleukin-12 and tumor necrosis factor (TNF), which increases the killing ability of these cells. IFN gamma-1b also promotes the recruitment of leukocytes to the sites of infection or inflammation. IFN gamma-1b is the only IFN indicated for the treatment of chronic granulomatous disease (CGD). CGD is an inherited disorder of phagocytic cells that leads to recurrent life-threatening bacterial and fungal infections. A second characteristic of CGD is the development of nodular granulomas in the skin, gastrointestinal tract, and genitourinary tract due to chronic infections at these sites. IFN gamma-1b reduces the frequency and severity of infections in patients with CGD. Off-label indications include infections by *Mycobacterium avium* complex, pulmonary fibrosis, and ovarian cancer. The most common adverse effects include flulike symptoms, nausea and vomiting, diarrhea, rash, and elevated hepatic enzymes. Because of the potential for neutropenia and thrombocytopenia, periodic complete blood counts (CBCs) are required.

PegIFN alfa-2a (Pegasys): PegIFN alfa-2a is a biologic response modifier that has a molecule of PEG attached to IFN alfa-2a, which is identical to the natural IFN produced by human lymphocytes and macrophages. Approved in 2002, it is prepared through recombinant DNA technology and is available as single-use prefilled syringes and administered by the subcutaneous route. Approved indications for pegIFN alfa-2a include chronic hepatitis B and hepatitis C virus infections when laboratory evidence suggests that the virus is replicating. Off-label uses may include renal cell carcinoma and chronic myelogenous leukemia. Patients should be monitored for serious depression and suicidal ideation. Routine monitoring of CBCs should be conducted during therapy because neutropenia and thrombocytopenia may be severe. Other potential adverse effects include colitis, pancreatitis, hyper- or hypothyroidism, hypertension (HTN), and dysrhythmias. Periodic ophthalmic exams should be conducted because pegIFN alpha-2a can cause a decrease or loss of vision, especially in patients with preexisting eye pathology. A black box warning for IFNs states that pegIFN alfa-2a may cause or aggravate fatal or life-threatening neuropsychiatric, autoimmune, ischemic, or infectious disorders. The warning also states that when combined with ribavirin, the drug may cause birth defects or fetal death.

PegIFN alfa-2b (PegIntron, Sylatron): Approved in 2001, pegIFN alfa-2b (Pegintron) is indicated for the treatment of chronic hepatitis C in patients age 3 years and older with compensated liver disease. It may be used off-label to treat chronic hepatitis B infections and neoplastic disease. Pegintron is usually given in combination with the antiviral ribavirin over a period of 24 to 48 weeks. It is important to note that ribavirin can cause fetal injury and death and is a possible carcinogen. Sylatron is approved for the adjunctive treatment of melanoma that has lymph node involvement.

PegIFN alfa-2b has a molecule of PEG attached to the IFN molecule, which gives the drug an extended half-life. Peak concentrations can be sustained for 48 to 72 hours, which results in greater antiviral activity. The most frequently reported adverse effects with pegIFN alfa-2b are injection-site reactions, fatigue, headache, rigors, fever, nausea, myalgia, and emotional lability. A black box warning for IFNs states that these drugs may cause or aggravate fatal or life-threatening neuropsychiatric, autoimmune, ischemic, or infectious disorders. The warning also states that when combined with ribavirin, pegIFN alfa-2b may cause birth defects or fetal death.

42.3 Interleukins, vaccines, and colony-stimulating factors are used to boost the immune system.

Interleukins (ILs) are a class of cytokines synthesized by lymphocytes, monocytes, macrophages, and certain other cells in response to antigen exposure. Like IFNs, ILs are signaling molecules that enable cells of the immune system to communicate with each other. The ILs, however, work by different mechanisms than the IFNs. The ILs have widespread effects on immune function that include the following:

- Stimulation of cytotoxic T-cell activity against tumor cells
- Activation and increased production of natural killer (NK) cells

- Increased B-cell and plasma cell production
- Increased neutrophil chemotaxis
- Promotion of inflammation.

More than 30 different ILs have been identified, though only one is available as an immunostimulant. IL-2, which is derived from helper T cells, promotes the proliferation of both T cells and activated B cells. Several drugs are available that block interleukin receptors and act as immunusuppressants (see Table 42.3). These medications are used to treat autoimmune disorders such as rheumatoid arthritis and plaque psoriasis in which there is an excessive amount of interleukin causing inflammation.

Bacillus Calmette-Guérin (BCG) vaccine (TheraCys, Tice) is a biologic response modifier that is available to enhance the immune system. BCG is an attenuated strain of *Mycobacterium bovis* used for the pharmacotherapy of certain types of bladder cancer.

Vaccines are types of immunostimulants that have the ability to mobilize the body against specific antigens. A small amount of an inactivated antigen is administered, and the patient develops a subclinical immune reaction. If reexposed to the antigen in future years, memory B or T cells will develop a rapid response, eliminating the antigen before it causes disease. Vaccines are presented in Chapter 43.

The final type of immunostimulant includes the colony-stimulating factors, which are drugs that promote the production of white blood cells (WBCs). For example, filgrastim (Neupogen) stimulates the production of granulocytes, and sargramostim (Leukine) activates multiple types of leukocytes. These drugs are used to shorten the length of neutropenia in patients with cancer and in those who have had a bone marrow transplant and whose bone marrow has been suppressed by drugs. Filgrastim, the prototype, and other colony-stimulating factors are presented in Chapter 39.

CONNECTION Checkpoint 42.1

From Chapter 39, why is filgrastim discontinued when ANC rises above 10,000 cell/mm^3?

PROTOTYPE DRUG Aldesleukin (Proleukin)

Classification **Therapeutic:** Immunostimulant
Pharmacologic: Interleukin, biologic response modifier

Therapeutic Effects and Uses: Approved in 1992, aldesleukin has a structure very similar to natural IL-2, and it has identical actions in the body. It is approved by the U.S. Food and Drug Administration (FDA) for the pharmacotherapy of metastatic renal cell carcinoma and metastatic malignant melanoma. It has been designated by the FDA as an orphan drug for the chemotherapy of non-Hodgkin's lymphoma and acute myelogenous leukemia. It is used off-label to treat leprosy.

Aldesleukin is a very toxic drug that should be administered only by personnel familiar with its use. It must be administered in multiple, brief IV infusions because of its short half-life.

Mechanism of Action: The mechanism of action of aldesleukin is identical to that of endogenous IL-2. It initiates a series of actions that activate IFNs, TNF, and other ILs. The drug promotes proliferation of both B cells and T cells, macrophages, and NK cells, which in turn increase the body's ability to fight cancer cells.

Pharmacokinetics:

Route(s)	IV
Absorption	N/A
Distribution	Widely distributed; unknown if secreted in breast milk
Primary metabolism	Renal
Primary excretion	Renal
Onset of action	Unknown
Duration of action	Half-life: 85 min

Adverse Effects: Aldesleukin is a toxic drug that has the potential to cause serious adverse effects in virtually any organ system. Many of the adverse effects are caused by **capillary leak syndrome**, a serious condition in which plasma proteins and other substances leave the blood and enter the interstitial spaces because of porous capillaries. If not monitored carefully, capillary leak syndrome can result in death. Over 70% of patients taking aldesleukin will experience hypotension, which can sometimes be severe enough to cause tissues and organs to receive an insufficient blood supply to function properly. Tachycardia and other dysrhythmias occur in a significant number of patients. Diarrhea or nausea and/or vomiting may occur in as many as half the patients taking the drug. Other common adverse effects include confusion, drowsiness, oliguria, stomatitis, anorexia, hyperbilirubinemia, hypothyroidism, elevated hepatic enzymes, weight gain, dyspnea, and pulmonary congestion. Common changes in blood values include thrombocytopenia, anemia, and leukopenia. Flu-like symptoms such as fever and malaise occur frequently. **Black Box Warnings:** Aldesleukin can cause severe capillary leak syndrome. Death may result from infection that can spread throughout the body because of impaired neutrophil function. If moderate to severe fatigue develops, the drug should be withheld. The drug should be used with extreme caution in patients with a history of cardiac or pulmonary disease.

Contraindications/Precautions: There are many contraindications to using aldesleukin, and a thorough baseline assessment of health status is required. If the assessment indicates a preexisting bacterial infection, this should be treated prior to initiating therapy with aldesleukin. Aldesleukin should not be administered to patients with developing moderate to severe lethargy because the drug may induce coma. Patients with significant cardiac, central nervous system, pulmonary, renal, or hepatic impairment should not receive this drug. Aldesleukin may cause seizures and should be used with caution in patients with epilepsy. This drug may worsen the condition of patients with autoimmune disease, including those with scleroderma, RA, diabetes mellitus, and thyroiditis.

Drug Interactions: Aldesleukin has the potential to interact with nearly any other drug. Given concurrently with aldesleukin, drugs that affect mental status such as many antianxiety drugs, opioids, sedatives, or antipsychotic medications may cause mood disturbances and drowsiness. Concurrent administration with drugs that are hepatotoxic or nephrotoxic may cause additive organ damage. Caution should be practiced when using drugs that modify coagulation such as aspirin, nonsteroidal anti-inflammatory drugs, or platelet inhibitors due to an increased risk of bleeding. Antihypertensive drugs may cause additive hypotension when used with aldesleukin. **Herbal/Food:** None known.

Pregnancy: In laboratory animals, high doses of aldesleukin are embryocidal. It is not known if this drug is secreted in breast milk and effects on the breastfed neonate are unknown. Sexually active men and women should use effective contraception during therapy.

Treatment of Overdose: Most adverse effects of aldesleukin stop when the medication is discontinued. Dexamethasone may be used to reverse some of the toxicities observed from an overdose of aldesleukin.

Clinician Responsibilities: Key clinical implications for patients receiving aldesleukin are included in Applied Clinical Judgment: Patients Receiving Pharmacotherapy with Immunomodulators.

Drugs Similar to Aldesleukin (Proleukin)

BCG vaccine is a miscellaneous biologic response modifier.

Bacillus Calmette-Guérin vaccine (TheraCys, Tice): BCG vaccine is a live, attenuated vaccine that is available in two distinct strains with different indications. Animal studies have not been conducted to determine the risk of these drugs during pregnancy or lactation.

TheraCys: TheraCys is approved for the prophylaxis and treatment of patients with superficial bladder cancer. This drug is instilled into the urinary bladder for 2 hours, after which the patient voids the medication. The treatment may be repeated at 3-month intervals. TheraCys produces a nonspecific immune reaction in the bladder that attracts lymphocytes, macrophages, and NK cells to the site of the cancer. Adverse effects include local reactions such as bladder irritability, hematuria, dysuria, cystitis, incontinence, and nocturia. A flulike syndrome may occur. This drug contains a black box warning that intravesical instillation may cause disseminated infections because the drug contains live attenuated mycobacteria.

Tice: Tice is used to stimulate immunity against *Mycobacterium tuberculosis*. Vaccination with BCG simulates exposure to tuberculosis and induces an immune response against the organism. This drug is used to prevent tuberculosis and is not given to treat active infections. It is the only FDA-approved treatment for tuberculosis prophylaxis. The drug is not 100% effective and its length of protection is variable. Flulike symptoms often develop 1 to 2 days after administration. Minor skin papules appear at the site of percutaneous puncture.

Immunosuppressants

42.4 Immunosuppressants are used to prevent transplant rejection and for the treatment of autoimmune disorders.

Used to inhibit the immune response, immunosuppressants are prescribed for patients who are receiving transplanted tissues or organs and to treat autoimmune disorders. Doses for these medications are listed in Table 42.2.

Transplants may include specific cells, parts of tissues, or complete organs. They may originate from the patient's own body (autografts), genetically identical donors (isografts), or genetically dissimilar donors (allografts). Most transplantation procedures use allografts.

Typing for transplanted tissues attempts to match, as closely as possible, donor and recipient human leukocyte antigen (HLA) and ABO blood-type antigens. Despite accurate tissue matching, allografts always contain certain antigens that have the potential to trigger the patient's immune defenses. This response, called **transplant rejection**, is often acute; antibodies sometimes destroy the transplanted tissue within 48 hours after a transplant. The cell-mediated branch of the immune system responds more slowly to the transplant, attacking it about 2 weeks following surgery. Chronic rejection of the transplant may occur months or even years after surgery.

Successful transplantation requires the use of immunosuppressant drugs. One or more immunosuppressants are administered at the time of transplantation and are continued for several months following surgery. In some

Table 42.2 Immunosuppressants

Drug	Route and Adult Dose (Maximum Dose Where Indicated)	Adverse Effects
Antibodies		
antithymocyte globulin (Atgam, Thymoglobulin)	IV (Atgam): 10–30 mg/kg daily IV (Thymoglobulin): 1.5 mg/kg daily infused over 4–6 h for 7–14 days	*Local reactions at the injection site (pain, erythema, myalgia), flulike symptoms (malaise, fever, chills), headache, dizziness* Anaphylaxis, HTN, serious infections, thrombocytopenia, leukopenia, kidney impairment (basiliximab), antithymocyte globulin, post-transplant lymphoproliferative disorder (PTLD) (belatacept)
basiliximab (Simulect)	IV: 20 mg times 2 doses (first dose 2 h before surgery; second dose 4 days after transplant)	
belatacept (Nulojix)	IV: 5–10 mg/kg using enclosed silicone-free disposable syringe	
Calcineurin Inhibitors		
cyclosporine (Gengraf, Neoral, Sandimmune)	Transplants: PO: 5–15 mg/kg/day Autoimmune disorders: PO: 1.25–2.5 mg/kg/day (max: 4 mg/day)	*Hirsutism, tremor, nausea and vomiting* HTN, MI, nephrotoxicity, hyperkalemia, seizures, paresthesia, hepatotoxicity
tacrolimus (Astagraf XL, Prograf, others)	PO (immediate release): 0.1–0.15 mg/kg/day in 2 divided doses q12h; give first PO dose 8–12 h after discontinuing IV therapy IV (Prograf): 0.03–0.05 mg/kg/day as continuous infusion	*Oliguria, nausea, constipation, diarrhea, headache, abdominal pain, insomnia, peripheral edema, fever* Infections, HTN, nephrotoxicity, neurotoxicity (tremors, paresthesia, psychosis), hyperkalemia, anemia, hyperglycemia, malignancy, thrombocytopenia, seizures
Cytotoxic Drugs and Antimetabolites		
anakinra (Kineret)	Subcutaneous: 100 mg (0.67 mL) once daily	*Injection-site reactions, UTI, headache, nausea, diarrhea, sinusitis, arthralgia, flulike symptoms* Leukopenia, infections, malignancy, anaphylaxis
azathioprine (Azasan)	PO/IV: 3–5 mg/kg/day initially; may be able to reduce to 1–3 mg/kg/day	*Nausea and vomiting, anorexia* Severe nausea and vomiting, bone marrow suppression, thrombocytopenia, serious infections, malignancy, hepatotoxicity
cyclophosphamide	PO: 2.5–3 mg/kg daily for a period of 60–90 days (higher doses are used for malignant disease)	*Nausea and vomiting, anorexia, neutropenia, alopecia* Anaphylaxis, leukopenia, pulmonary emboli, interstitial pulmonary fibrosis, toxic epidermal necrolysis, Stevens–Johnson syndrome, hemorrhagic cystitis, oligospermia
etanercept (Enbrel)	Subcutaneous: 50 mg once/wk	*Injection-site reactions (pain, erythema, myalgia), abdominal pain, vomiting, headache* Infections, pancytopenia, leukopenia, anemia, MI, heart failure, malignancy
ibrutinib (Imbruvica)	PO: 420 mg once daily	*Fatigue, bruising, diarrhea, muscle spasms* Hemorrhage, fetal toxicity, thrombocytopenia, anemia, infections
methotrexate (Rheumatrex, Trexall)	PO/IM/IV: 15–30 mg/day for 5 days; repeat every 12 wk for three courses	*Headache, glossitis, gingivitis, mild leukopenia, nausea, alopecia* Ulcerative stomatitis, myelosuppression, aplastic anemia, hepatic cirrhosis, nephrotoxicity, sudden death, pulmonary fibrosis, or pneumonia
mycophenolate (CellCept, Myfortic)	PO/IV: 720 mg bid in combination with corticosteroids and cyclosporine; start within 24 h of transplant	*Peripheral edema, diarrhea, headache, tremor, dyspepsia, abdominal pain* UTI, leukopenia, anemia, thrombocytopenia, sepsis, HTN
Kinase Inhibitors (Rapamycins)		
everolimus (Afinitor, Zortress)	PO (Afinitor): 10 mg once daily PO (Zortress): Begin with 0.75 mg bid and adjust to achieve a trough concentration of 3–8 ng/mL	*Peripheral edema, hyperlipidemia, nausea, HTN, UTI, asthenia, weight changes (loss or gain), elevated serum creatinine, hyperglycemia, and fever* Leukopenia, anemia, thrombocytopenia, sepsis, secondary infections, malignancy, anaphylaxis, interstitial lung disease or pneumonia, birth defects
sirolimus (Rapamune)	PO: 6–15 mg loading dose immediately after the transplant, then 2–5 mg/day maintenance dose	
temsirolimus (Torisel)	IV: 25 mg once weekly infused over 30–60 min	

Note: *Italics* indicate common adverse effects. Underline indicates serious adverse effects.

cases, they are continued indefinitely at low doses. Transplantation would be impossible without the use of effective immunosuppressant drugs. Although immunosuppressant therapies have proven very successful at preventing acute transplant rejection, they have been less successful at preventing chronic rejection.

Prior to the initiation of immunosuppressant therapy, it is critical that the patient be carefully assessed to rule

CONNECTIONS: Community-Oriented Practice

Fever in the Patient on Immunosuppressant Drugs

Immunosuppressant drugs are now given to treat a variety of conditions, and more uses are being discovered. Patients taking immunosuppressants are at greater risk for infection but may not always exhibit symptoms to the same degree that patients with competent immune systems do. The patient must be assessed for subtle signs of infection including low-grade fever (less than 37.8°C [100°F]), unusual skin lesions with or without drainage, excessive fatigue, malaise, arthralgias, cough, headache, diarrhea, or nausea. Any of these symptoms should be immediately reported to the healthcare provider so that appropriate follow-up examination can be conducted.

Before going home with an immunosuppressant drug, the patient should receive explicit instructions on when to call the provider for a fever and how often the temperature should be taken when fever is present or symptoms such as those listed above are present. Self-administration of antipyretics such as acetaminophen and ibuprofen is usually not appropriate because they can mask the symptoms of a significant infection. Fevers that fall outside of the parameters set by the healthcare provider need to be evaluated.

Many patients on immunosuppressant drugs are able to live active, normal lives. However, they should be taught measures to reduce their exposure to infections and should always receive appropriate instruction for fever management before they begin to take the medication.

out active infections. This includes screening for viruses such as cytomegalovirus (CMV), hepatitis B and C viruses, Epstein-Barr virus, VZV, HIV, and herpes simplex virus. If an active infection is discovered, it should be treated prior to transplantation. In addition, patients should be screened for the presence of cancer prior to surgery because immunosuppression will allow preexisting cancers to grow rapidly.

During immunosuppressant therapy the patient is susceptible to infection from all types of pathogens: viral, bacterial, fungal, or protozoan. Infections in immunosuppressed patients are called *opportunistic infections*. Opportunistic pulmonary infections are the leading cause of morbidity and mortality in patients receiving a transplant. Many patients receive antibiotics for the prophylaxis of opportunistic infections for 4 to 12 months following surgery. Six months following the transplant, 80% of patients will return to their baseline risk of infection, but the remainder will remain at high risk indefinitely.

Long-term survivors of transplants are also at high risk of developing cancers. These include non-Hodgkin's lymphoma, squamous and basal cell skin cancer, cervical cancer, and Kaposi's sarcoma. Regular follow-up monitoring for cancer is required in these patients.

PharmFACT

More than 109,000 people are waiting for organ transplants. About 84% of these are waiting for a kidney, 11% for a liver, and 3.2% for a heart (Organ Procurement and Transplantation Network, 2020).

Autoimmune disorders are those in which the body creates antibodies against normal tissues. The body attacks its own cells as if they were foreign, resulting in tissue injury. Examples of autoimmune disorders include RA, SLE, myasthenia gravis, and Hashimoto's thyroiditis.

Autoimmune diseases are characterized by symptomatic periods alternating with remissions. Although the remissions may last many months or even years, relapses are often progressive, with symptoms worsening as the disease progresses. During acute relapses, fever and signs of widespread inflammation may be present. Virtually any tissue or organ may be affected, depending on the specific autoimmune disease.

Unlike transplant recipients who may receive immunosuppressants indefinitely, patients with autoimmune disease are usually given these drugs for brief periods in high doses to control relapses. In some cases, however, these patients may receive low doses for longer periods for prophylaxis.

The immunosuppressant class includes drugs that block the immune response by several different mechanisms, as shown in Pharmacotherapy Illustrated 42.1. These include blocking the receptors and production of IL-2, inhibiting the proliferation of T cells, and using antibodies specific to certain receptors or cells of the immune response. The drugs may be classified into the following categories:

- Calcineurin inhibitors and similar drugs
- Cytotoxic drugs and antimetabolites
- Antibodies
- Corticosteroids (glucocorticoids).

42.5 Calcineurin inhibitors are preferred drugs for the prophylaxis of transplant rejection.

When a T cell encounters an antigen, calcineurin is activated. **Calcineurin** is an enzyme that acts as an intracellular messenger, telling the T cell to begin synthesizing IL-2. As described in Section 42.3, IL-2 is an important chemical mediator in promoting the proliferation of B cells, T cells, macrophages, and NK cells. Blocking IL-2 suppresses the immune response.

Two of the most important drugs in transplant medicine, cyclosporine (Gengraf, Neoral, Sandimmune) and tacrolimus (Astagraf XL, Prograf), are calcineurin inhibitors.

Pharmacotherapy Illustrated 42.1

Mechanism of Action of Immunosuppressants

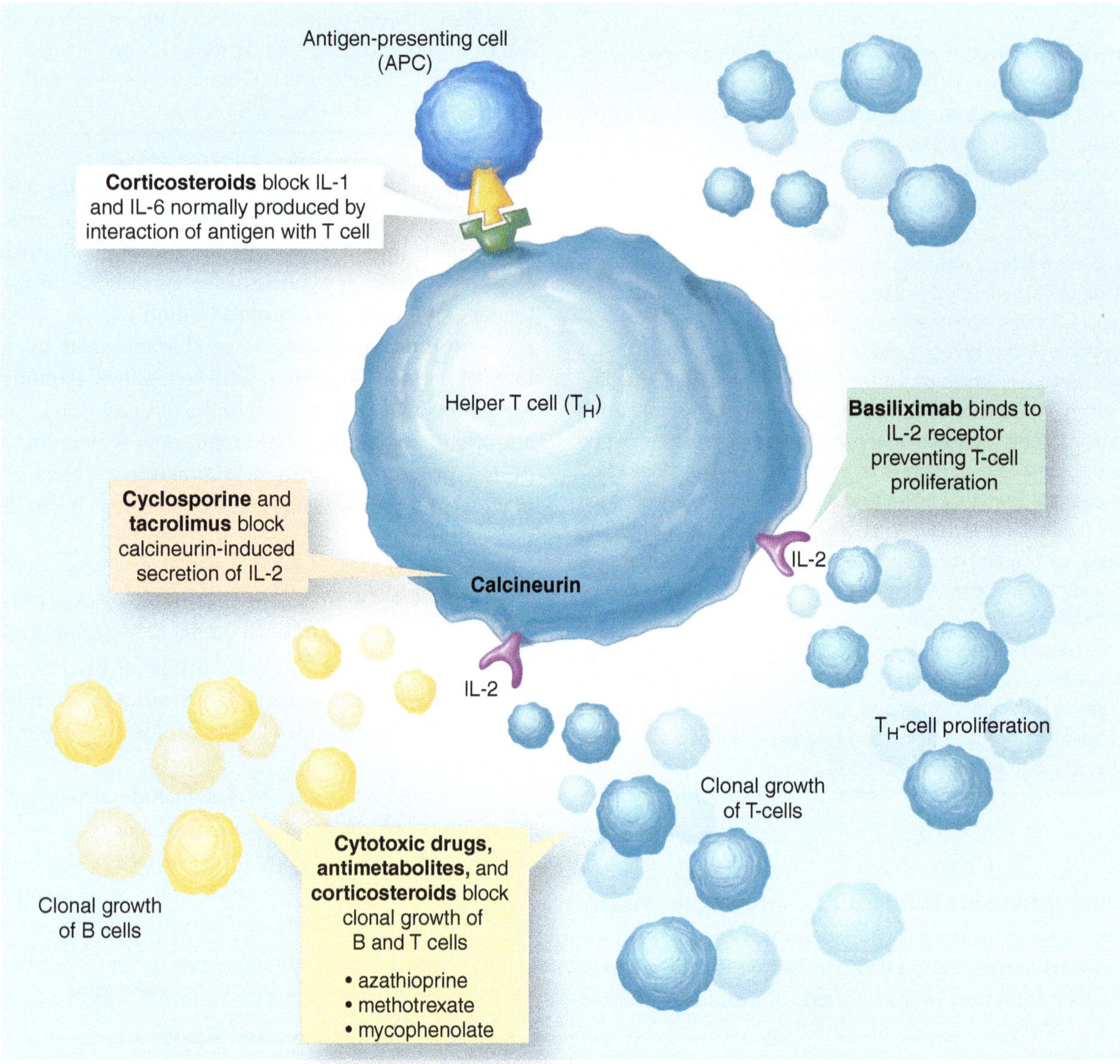

These drugs revolutionized the pharmacotherapy of transplant rejection and have been the mainstay of transplant therapy since the 1980s. Although newer medications have been developed, the calcineurin inhibitors remain critical drugs for transplant recipients. They allow the doses of corticosteroids to be lowered, thereby reducing the incidence of opportunistic infections following transplants.

Approved in 1983, cyclosporine was the first calcineurin inhibitor and remains the prototype for this class. Some data suggest that tacrolimus may be more effective in preventing transplant rejection and reducing the mortality associated with transplants. It is the most common immunosuppressant used in certain types of transplants. In addition to their use in preventing transplant rejection, the calcineurin inhibitors are also of value in treating the acute inflammation associated with RA and psoriasis, an inflammatory disorder of the skin.

Everolimus (Afinitor, Zortress), sirolimus (Rapamune), and temsirolimus (Torisel) produce immunosuppressant effects similar to the calcineurin inhibitors. They prevent the activation of T cells by inhibiting a key regulatory protein kinase called mTOR. Thus, these drugs are sometimes called mTOR inhibitors or kinase inhibitors. The kinase inhibitors used to treat cancer (see Chapter 57) inhibit a different cellular kinase than the mTOR inhibitors.

PROTOTYPE DRUG **Cyclosporine (Gengraf, Neoral, Sandimmune)**

Classification **Therapeutic:** Immunosuppressant
Pharmacologic: Calcineurin inhibitor

Therapeutic Effects and Uses: Cyclosporine is a complex chemical obtained from a soil fungus. It is FDA approved for the prophylaxis of kidney, heart, and liver transplant rejection; psoriasis; severe RA; and xerophthalmia, an eye condition of diminished tear production caused by ocular inflammation. Off-label indications include a number of autoimmune and inflammatory conditions such as ulcerative colitis, SLE, myasthenia gravis, aplastic anemia, Crohn's disease, psoriatic arthritis, and graft-versus-host disease (GVHD).

Cyclosporine may be administered as capsules, oral solution, or IV or as an ophthalmic solution (Restasis) for xerophthalmia. Due to the risk of anaphylaxis, the IV route is used only when patients are unable to take oral (PO) medications. Cyclosporine (modified) refers to the capsule, microemulsion dosage formulation of cyclosporine (Gengraf, Neoral). Cyclosporine (modified) has increased bioavailability compared to that of cyclosporine (nonmodified) and cannot be used interchangeably without close monitoring.

Unlike some of the more cytotoxic immunosuppressants, cyclosporine is less harmful to bone marrow cells. When prescribed for transplant recipients, it is often used in combination with a corticosteroid such as prednisone.

Mechanism of Action: Cyclosporine inhibits the function of calcineurin. This diminishes the activity of T cells and B cells and suppresses the immune response.

Pharmacokinetics:

Route(s)	PO, IV, ophthalmic
Absorption	Oral absorption is highly variable
Distribution	Widely distributed; crosses the placenta; secreted in breast milk; 90% bound to lipoproteins
Primary metabolism	Hepatic (CYP3A), extensive first-pass metabolism
Primary excretion	Bile and feces
Onset of action	Peak: 3–4 h
Duration of action	Half-life: 16–27 h

Adverse Effects: The primary adverse effect of cyclosporine is nephrotoxicity, with up to 75% of patients experiencing a reduction in urine flow. Over half the patients taking the drug will experience HTN and tremor. Hirsutism occurs in many patients. Other common adverse effects are elevated hepatic enzymes, mild to moderate HTN, headache, and gingival hyperplasia. Infections are common during cyclosporine therapy, including reactivation of latent herpes or varicella infections. Periodic blood counts are necessary to ensure that leukocytes do not fall below 4000 or platelets below 75,000. Anaphylaxis has been reported with IV administration. Long-term therapy increases the risk of malignancy, especially lymphomas and skin cancers. **Black Box Warning:** This drug should only be administered by healthcare providers experienced in immunosuppressive therapy. Use may result in serious infections and possible malignancies. Kidney damage may occur, thus renal function should be monitored during therapy. Patients with psoriasis who are taking cyclosporine with other psoriasis medications are at an increased risk of developing skin malignancies.

Contraindications/Precautions: Patients who are taking cyclosporine should avoid direct exposure to the sun due to an increased risk of skin cancer. Because cyclosporine is nephrotoxic, the drug is either contraindicated or should be used with extreme caution in patients with chronic kidney disease; renal laboratory function should be regularly evaluated. The drug should not be used during pregnancy or lactation. Because cyclosporine is primarily eliminated via the bile, its dose should be reduced in patients with hepatic or biliary impairment. Patients with active infections should be treated with anti-infectives prior to cyclosporine therapy. Caution should be used in patients with preexisting HTN because the drug may worsen this condition.

Drug Interactions: Cyclosporine is a major substrate of CYP3A4 and may interact with drugs that inhibit or induce this enzyme. Drugs that may decrease cyclosporine levels include phenytoin, phenobarbital, carbamazepine, and rifampin. Azole antifungal drugs, oral hypoglycemics, and macrolide antibiotics may increase cyclosporine levels. Because cyclosporine increases blood pressure, the doses of antihypertensives will require adjustment. Potassium-sparing diuretics should be avoided because their concurrent use with cyclosporine causes hyperkalemia. Cyclosporine should be given with caution with other nephrotoxic drugs due to the potential for additive kidney damage. Statins should not be used concurrently with cyclosporine due to the potential for myopathy or rhabdomyolysis. **Herbal/Food:** Food decreases the absorption of the drug. Grapefruit juice can raise cyclosporine levels by 50 to 200%. The immune-enhancing effects of astragalus and echinacea may interfere with the action of immunosuppressants.

Pregnancy: Cyclosporine is embryotoxic and fetotoxic in laboratory animals. The drug is secreted in milk and has the potential to cause serious adverse effects in the breastfed neonate. It is recommended that cyclosporine not be taken during pregnancy or lactation unless the potential benefits to the mother justify the potential risks to the fetus or neonate.

Treatment of Overdose: An overdose of cyclosporine can result in significant nephrotoxicity and hepatotoxicity. General supportive measures are indicated.

Clinician Responsibilities: Key clinical implications for patients receiving cyclosporine are included in Applied Clinical Judgment: Patients Receiving Pharmacotherapy with Immunomodulators.

Drugs Similar to Cyclosporine (Gengraf, Neoral, Sandimmune)

The only other calcineurin inhibitor is tacrolimus. Although not calcineurin inhibitors, everolimus, sirolimus, and temsirolimus are immunosuppressants similar to tacrolimus. These immunosuppressants are embryotoxic and fetotoxic in laboratory animals and have the potential to cause adverse effects on the breastfed neonate. It is recommended that these drugs not be taken during pregnancy or lactation unless the potential benefits to the mother justify the potential risks to the fetus or neonate. For some immunosuppressants, the male and female partners should both use effective contraception during and for several months following therapy.

Everolimus (Afinitor, Zortress): Everolimus was initially approved in 2009 (Afinitor) to treat advanced renal cell carcinoma, astrocytoma, and other forms of cancer. Subsequently, Zortress was approved for the prophylaxis of organ rejection in patients receiving a kidney or liver transplant. When used as an antineoplastic, the dose is much higher than that when used in transplant patients (see Table 42.2). In transplant medicine, the drug is given in combination with basiliximab and concurrently with reduced doses of cyclosporine and corticosteroids. To prevent potential toxicity, therapeutic drug monitoring is recommended.

Everolimus is functionally similar to sirolimus and temsirolimus and blocks a key kinase enzyme that activates B and T cells. Like most immunosuppressants, the drug carries a black box warning regarding its potent immunosuppressive actions and the possible development of serious infections and malignancies. In addition, the black box warning includes an increased risk of kidney damage, including renal arterial and venous thrombosis.

Sirolimus (Rapamune): Approved in 1999, sirolimus is a PO drug isolated from a soil bacterium that shares a similar structure and potent immunosuppressant properties with tacrolimus. Sirolimus, however, acts by a unique mechanism; that is, it binds to a protein known as FKBP that prevents T-cell activation and proliferation and the production of antibodies by B cells. Sirolimus does not exhibit the serious organ toxicity characteristic of tacrolimus. This drug appears to be less effective than the calcineurin inhibitors, but it does exert synergistic immunosuppression when used with other immunosuppressive drugs. Sirolimus is only approved for use in the prophylaxis of kidney transplant rejection in combination with cyclosporine and corticosteroids for the first year after transplantation. At 2 to 4 months post-transplantation, the cyclosporine may be gradually withdrawn over a 4- to 8-week period. The serum levels of sirolimus must be adjusted upward when cyclosporine is withdrawn. Adverse effects include hyperlipidemia, hypercholesterolemia, peripheral edema, tremor, azotemia, elevated serum creatinine, HTN, diarrhea, and anemia. Like most immunosuppressants, the drug carries a black box warning regarding its potent immunosuppressive actions and the possible development of serious infections and malignancies. In addition, the black box warning states that the use of this drug is not recommended in patients with liver transplants (excess mortality and graft loss) or lung transplants (bronchial rupture).

Tacrolimus (Astagraf XL, Envarsus XR, Prograf, Protopic, others): Approved by the FDA in 1994, tacrolimus is available in PO capsule or IV forms for the prophylaxis of heart and liver transplant rejection. Envarsus XR and Astagraf XL are extended-release forms approved as once-daily oral drugs to prevent rejection of kidney transplants. A topical form of tacrolimus (Protopic) is approved for the short-term treatment of eczema and atopic dermatitis. The topical form contains a black box warning of possible lymphoma and skin cancer. Tacrolimus is also used off-label for other transplants as well as for GVHD, nephritic syndrome, psoriasis, and uveitis. Tacrolimus is 100 times more potent than cyclosporine and appears to be more effective in some patients at preventing transplant rejection. Nephrotoxicity may occur in half the patients taking this drug. Neurotoxicity symptoms are common and include headache, tremor, paresthesias, insomnia, and dizziness. HTN, anemia, hyperglycemia, and GI complaints occur in a significant number of patients who are taking tacrolimus. Like cyclosporine, an increased incidence of infections and malignancies may occur with tacrolimus use.

Temsirolimus (Torisel): Approved in 2007, temsirolimus is metabolized in the liver to sirolimus. It is approved to treat patients with advanced renal cell carcinoma that has not responded to other therapies. This drug is administered only by the IV route, and the patient is pretreated with diphenhydramine 30 minutes prior to the injection to prevent a hypersensitivity reaction. Temsirolimus is toxic to the hematologic system; 94% of patients will experience anemia, 53% will experience lymphopenia, and 32% will experience leukopenia. Hyperglycemia occurs in most patients; thus, patients with diabetes require close monitoring. Most patients who are taking the drug will also experience hyperlipidemia that may be serious enough to require pharmacotherapy. Interstitial lung disease is a rare though potentially fatal adverse effect.

PharmFACT

Over 120,000 Americans are on the national transplant waiting list. Each day in the United States about 20 people die waiting for transplants (organdonor.gov, 2020).

42.6 Cytotoxic drugs and antimetabolites are used to suppress proliferating B cells and T cells.

Cytotoxic drugs are immunosuppressive medications used to kill B cells and T cells. Antimetabolites do not kill directly, but instead severely restrict the replication of B cells and T cells. Each of these medications acts by a different mechanism. Some of the drugs resemble essential chemical building blocks needed for the biosynthesis of DNA and block replication. Others inhibit protein synthesis. Most of the cytotoxic and antimetabolite immunosuppressants are nonspecific, affecting many different cells of the immune response. They have similar indications and adverse effects as the calcineurin inhibitors.

PROTOTYPE DRUG Azathioprine (Azasan)

Classification **Therapeutic:** Immunosuppressant
Pharmacologic: Cytotoxic drug

Therapeutic Effects and Uses: An older immunosuppressant approved in 1968, azathioprine is indicated for the prophylaxis of kidney transplant rejection and for the treatment of severe RA. Off-label indications include other inflammatory disorders such as Crohn's disease, autoimmune hepatitis, myasthenia gravis, SLE, and ulcerative colitis. When treating nontransplant conditions, it is generally prescribed only when standard treatments fail.

Azathioprine is usually given PO, but it may be given by the IV route to patients who are unable to take the drug by mouth. When used to prevent transplant rejection, it is usually administered in combination with other immunosuppressants.

Mechanism of Action: Azathioprine inhibits DNA synthesis, resulting in DNA damage and chromosome breakage. The drug is metabolized to mercaptopurine in the liver, an active substance marketed as an antineoplastic drug for leukemia.

Pharmacokinetics:

Route(s)	PO, IV
Absorption	Well absorbed
Distribution	Crosses the placenta; secreted in breast milk; 30% bound to plasma proteins
Primary metabolism	Hepatic; metabolized to mercaptopurine, an active metabolite
Primary excretion	Renal
Onset of action	7–14 days
Duration of action	Half-life: 3 h

Adverse Effects: Azathioprine causes bone marrow suppression that can result in pancytopenia, agranulocytosis, leukopenia, and thrombocytopenia. Serious infections may occur secondary to immunosuppression, and latent herpes or varicella infections may become reactivated during azathioprine therapy. Hepatotoxicity has been reported with this drug. Nausea and vomiting are common, especially during the first few weeks of therapy. Patients who have received a kidney transplant and who are being treated with azathioprine have an increased risk of developing skin and lymphoid malignancies. The toxicities of azathioprine are dose related and occur more frequently in patients who have received a kidney transplant compared with those who are treated for RA. **Black Box Warning:** Use may result in serious or fatal infections and possible malignancies such as lymphomas. CBCs should be monitored during therapy.

Contraindications/Precautions: Azathioprine should be used with extreme caution in patients with preexisting hematologic disease or hepatic impairment. Blood counts and hepatic enzymes must be regularly monitored.

Drug Interactions: Additive bone marrow suppression is expected if azathioprine is given concurrently with other immunosuppressants. Concurrent use of allopurinol with azathioprine can result in a large increase in azathioprine activity and hematologic toxicity. The use of angiotensin-converting enzyme (ACE) inhibitors with azathioprine may induce anemia and severe leukopenia. **Herbal/Food:** None known.

Pregnancy: Azathioprine can cause fetal harm and the drug and its metabolites are secreted in milk. It is recommended that this drug not be taken during pregnancy or lactation unless the potential benefits to the mother justify the potential risks to the fetus or neonate.

Treatment of Overdose: Hemodialysis may be of value in removing some azathioprine from the blood following an overdose. Other treatment measures are supportive.

Clinician Responsibilities: Key clinical implications for patients receiving azathioprine are included in Applied Clinical Judgment: Patients Receiving Pharmacotherapy with Immunomodulators.

Drugs Similar to Azathioprine (Azasan)

Other cytotoxic and antimetabolite drugs indicated for immunosuppression include anakinra, cyclophosphamide, etanercept, methotrexate, and mycophenolate.

Anakinra (Kineret): Approved in 2001, anakinra is an IL-1 receptor antagonist that prevents the formation of certain inflammatory cytokines. The primary indication for anakinra is for the treatment of moderate to severe RA that has not responded to first-line drugs. It is administered by the subcutaneous route, and injection-site reaction is the most frequent adverse effect. Because the drug lowers WBC counts, secondary infections occur in almost 40% of patients taking anakinra. Animal reproduction studies did not show fetal harm. It is not known if anakinra is secreted in breast milk and adverse effects on the breastfed neonate are unknown.

Cyclophosphamide: Cyclophosphamide is one of the most commonly prescribed medications for patients with malignancies. It acts by forming cross-links in DNA, which prevents cancer cell replication. It is a powerful immunosuppressant, affecting both B cells and T cells. It is used off-label for SLE, GVHD, and RA and for the transplant prophylaxis of solid organs. Hematologic toxicity (pancytopenia, leukopenia, anemia, and thrombocytopenia) is a major dose-limiting adverse effect. Cyclophosphamide is a prototype antineoplastic drug discussed in Chapter 57. Cyclophosphamide is teratogenic and may cause fetal harm in both laboratory animals and humans. The drug is secreted in milk and has the potential to cause serious adverse effects in the breastfed neonate. It is recommended that cyclophosphamide not be taken during pregnancy or lactation unless the potential benefits to the mother justify the potential risks to the fetus or neonate.

Etanercept (Enbrel): Approved in 1998, etanercept is a protein that closely resembles the natural receptor for TNF. Rather than binding to its receptors on T cells, TNF binds with the etanercept. This inhibition of TNF activity reduces the levels of damaging cytokines responsible for causing inflammation and joint destruction in patients with RA. The drug is FDA approved to treat RA, psoriatic arthritis, plaque psoriasis, and ankylosing spondylitis. It is used off-label to prevent transplant rejection. It is administered only by the subcutaneous route. The most common adverse effects are injection-site reactions and infections. Etanercept has a black box warning regarding the possibility of malignancy and serious infections during therapy, including tuberculosis and bacterial sepsis. Patients should be monitored for tuberculosis prior to and during treatment. Animal reproduction studies did not show fetal harm. It is not known if etanercept is secreted in milk or has adverse effects on the breastfed neonate.

Methotrexate (Rheumatrex, Trexall): Methotrexate is an older antimetabolite approved in 1953 that acts by inhibiting the enzyme responsible for folic acid metabolism. Like cyclophosphamide, it is indicated for various cancers as well as serious inflammatory disorders such as RA, psoriasis, SLE, and ulcerative colitis. Methotrexate is used off-label to prevent transplant rejection. The most frequently reported adverse reactions include nausea and vomiting, stomatitis, esophagitis, oral ulceration, and abdominal distress. Hematologic adverse reactions are common. The drug carries a black box warning regarding the possibility of malignancy and serious hematologic, GI, hepatic, pulmonary, and dermatologic toxicity. There is evidence that methotrexate can cause teratogenic effects or fetal death when taken during pregnancy. Effective contraception should be used if either partner is receiving this drug. Breastfeeding is contraindicated. Methotrexate is a prototype antineoplastic drug discussed in Chapter 57.

CONNECTIONS: Complementary and Alternative Therapies

Echinacea

Description

Nine species of echinacea have been identified, and all are native to the midwestern United States and central Canada. *Echinacea purpurea* (purple coneflower) and *Echinacea angustifolia* (narrow-leaf coneflower) are the two most commonly studied species. All portions of the plant contain chemicals that have potential pharmacologic activity.

History and Claims

Echinacea was used by Native Americans to treat various wounds and injuries. Until the widespread manufacture of antibiotics in the late 1940s, echinacea was commonly used as an anti-infective.

Standardization

The flowers, leaves, and stems of this plant are harvested and dried. Preparations include dried powder, tincture, fluid extracts, and teas. No single ingredient seems to be responsible for the herb's activity. A large number of potentially active chemicals have been identified from the extracts. Recommended doses include 300 mg dry powdered extract (standardized to 3.5% echinacoside) or 0.5 to 1 g dried root or tea.

Evidence

The quality and doses of echinacea used in research studies have varied widely, which makes comparisons and conclusions extremely difficult. Some evidence demonstrates that echinacea may shorten the duration of a cold, but effects on other health conditions do not have sufficient evidence to support its use. Adverse effects are rare, with GI effects such as nausea being the most common. It may cause allergic reactions in patients who are allergic to plants in the daisy family such as ragweed, marigolds, daisies, and chrysanthemums. There is insufficient evidence as to its effects in pregnancy or breastfeeding and it is not recommended that echinacea be used during either of these conditions (National Center for Complementary and Integrative Health, 2020).

Mycophenolate (CellCept, Myfortic): Approved in 1995, mycophenolate is a potent immunosuppressant that acts by inhibiting the DNA synthesis of B cells and T cells. There are two forms of mycophenolate. Mycophenolate mofetil (CellCept) is a prodrug that is converted in the body to its active form, mycophenolic acid. It is given IV or PO, usually in combination with other immunosuppressants such as cyclosporine and corticosteroids. Mycophenolate sodium (Myfortic) is a delayed-release tablet. Although the two drugs are therapeutically equivalent, they are not interchangeable.

Indications for mycophenolate include the prophylaxis of heart, kidney, or liver transplant rejection. Mycophenolate also was given orphan drug status for the treatment of patients with myasthenia gravis and pemphigus vulgaris. Off-label indications include SLE, GVHD, and atopic dermatitis. GI adverse effects such as nausea and vomiting, constipation, diarrhea, dyspepsia, and abdominal pain are common. Other relatively frequent adverse effects include tachycardia, tremor, back pain, sinusitis, increased urinary frequency, and blood dyscrasias. Weekly CBCs should be obtained and the drug withheld if the absolute neutrophil count falls below $1.3 \times (10)^3$ cells/mcL. Mycophenolate carries a black box warning regarding the possibility of malignancy, serious infections, and embryofetal toxicity. There is evidence that this drug can cause teratogenic effects and fetal death when taken during pregnancy. Women of childbearing potential should provide a negative pregnancy test before starting therapy. Effective contraception should be used during therapy and for 6 weeks following treatment. Mycophenolate may reduce the effectiveness of oral contraceptives.

42.7 Antibodies are used to prevent acute transplant rejection, autoimmune disorders, and malignancies.

Recall from Chapter 40 that antibodies are proteins that are produced following an antigen challenge. B cells become plasma cells, which subsequently produce massive amounts of antibodies that help rid the body of the antigen through multiple mechanisms. Antibodies that are produced by a plasma cell are very specific to the antigen. For example, exposure to *Streptococcus* would result in different antibodies than would *Escherichia coli*. In this example, antibodies *boost* the immune system. It may seem puzzling then to learn that certain antibodies may be administered to patients to *suppress* the immune response. How is this possible?

The answer is to create antibodies against human immune cells. A simple method is to inject animals (usually horses, rabbits, or mice) with human T cells, B cells, or thymocytes. The animal forms antibodies against the human immune cells, which can be collected and purified. When injected in humans, the animal's antibodies will attack the T cells (or T-cell receptors). These are called **polyclonal antibodies** because they contain a wide mixture of different antibodies. This polyclonal drug product, called antithymocyte globulin (Atgam, Thymoglobulin), is a potent immunosuppressant and is available for the prophylaxis of kidney transplant rejection and aplastic anemia.

In the 1980s a technique was developed to harvest antibodies produced by a single B cell. Because a single B cell produces a single antibody, it is called a **monoclonal antibody (MAB)**. A MAB is very specific, targeting a single type of target cell or receptor. This allows greater effects on the target cell or receptor at lower doses and with fewer adverse effects than using polyclonal antibodies.

The first MABs were derived from mouse cells and had short half-lives. The human immune system quickly recognized them as foreign when they were injected in patients. Through genetic engineering, scientists have been able to replace the mouse portions of the antibody with human sequences, thus allowing it to escape detection by the immune system for longer periods and extending its half-life.

Scientists have created approximately 30 different MABs to attack a diverse number of targets. The majority of the MABs are designed to attack specific types of cancer cells. Others are used to treat autoimmune or inflammatory disorders such as RA or psoriasis by attacking specific cells of the immune system that secrete proinflammatory mediators. Selected FDA-approved MABs are listed in Table 42.3. Those used exclusively for cancer are found in Chapter 57.

MAB medications are challenging to learn because many have similar names that end in *-mab* (for monoclonal antibody). There is, however, some consistency to the names—they reflect the origin of the antibody:

- MABs that have 75% human sequences are called chimeric and have *-xi* in the name (e.g., basiliximab).
- MABs that have 90% human sequences are called humanized and have *-zu* in their name (e.g., trastuzumab).
- MABs that are 100% human have *-mumab* in their name (e.g., golimumab).

PROTOTYPE DRUG **Basiliximab (Simulect)**

Classification **Therapeutic:** Immunosuppressant
Pharmacologic: Monoclonal antibody

Therapeutic Effects and Uses: Basiliximab is a monoclonal antibody approved in 1998 for the prophylaxis of acute kidney transplant rejection. The drug dampens the immune response by inhibiting CD25, a receptor on the surface of activated T cells. By binding to CD25, basiliximab stops IL-2 from activating the T cell, and the immune response is prevented. This drug does not lower the total number of circulating T cells; it does, however, lower their ability to respond to an antigen challenge.

Table 42.3 Selected Monoclonal Antibodies for Immunosuppression

Drug/Antibody	Approval Date	Target	Approved Indication(s)
adalimumab (Humira, others)	2002	TNF blocker	Ankylosing spondylitis, Crohn's disease, juvenile idiopathic arthritis, plaque psoriasis, psoriatic arthritis (PsA), RA and ulcerative colitis
basiliximab (Simulect)	1998	IL-2 receptor blocker	Prevent kidney transplant rejection
belatacept (Nulojix)	2011	Blocks CD28 costimulation of T lymphocytes	Prevent kidney transplant rejection
belimumab (Benlysta)	2011	Inhibits autoreactive B lymphocytes	SLE
certolizumab pegol (Cimzia)	2008	TNF blocker	Ankylosing spondylitis, Crohn's disease, plaque psoriasis, PsA, and RA
eculizumab (Soliris)	2007	Blocks complement protein C5	Atypical hemolytic uremic syndrome, ankylosing spondylitis, myasthenia gravis, and paroxysmal nocturnal hemoglobinuria
golimumab (Simponi)	2009	TNF blocker	PsA, RA, and ulcerative colitis
infliximab (Remicade, others)	1998	TNF blocker	Ankylosing spondylitis, Crohn's disease, plaque psoriasis, PsA, RA, and ulcerative colitis
natalizumab (Tysabri)	2006	Inhibits integrin which blocks migration of leukocytes across epithelium	Crohn's disease and MS
siltuximab (Sylvant)	2014	IL-6 receptor blocker	Castleman disease (rare blood disorder)
tocilizumab (Actemra)	2010	IL-6 receptor blocker	Cytokine release syndrome, giant cell arteritis, juvenile idiopathic arthritis, and RA

Administered by IV infusion, the standard regimen is two doses; one is given 2 hours prior to transplantation and the other is given 4 days later. Following the two infusions, the actions of basiliximab may last for 4 to 6 weeks. It is administered in combination with other immunosuppressants, usually cyclosporine and corticosteroids.

Mechanism of Action: Basiliximab inhibits the binding of IL-2 to CD25 on the surface of activated T cells. This prevents the rapid proliferation of T cells that would normally release cytokines to attack transplanted tissue.

Pharmacokinetics:

Route(s)	IV
Absorption	N/A
Distribution	Unknown
Primary metabolism	Unknown
Primary excretion	Unknown
Onset of action	30 min
Duration of action	7.2-day half-life

Adverse Effects: Basiliximab causes few adverse effects compared to the calcineurin inhibitors or the cytotoxic immunosuppressants. The most common adverse effects are GI related, such as nausea and vomiting, abdominal pain, and diarrhea. Anaphylaxis has been reported. **Black Box Warning:** Basiliximab should be administered only by healthcare providers experienced in immunosuppressive therapy.

Contraindications/Precautions: The only contraindication to the use of basiliximab is hypersensitivity to the drug. Because patients receiving this drug have suppressed immune systems, vaccinations are normally postponed until immune function returns.

Drug Interactions: Basiliximab does not interact significantly with the major drugs used in transplant medicine. However, caution must always be used when administering multiple drugs that suppress immune function. **Herbal/Food:** None known.

Pregnancy: Animal studies did not show evidence of teratogenicity or embryotoxicity. Because the effects on human pregnancy are unknown, women of childbearing potential are advised to use effective contraception during therapy and for 4 months after completion. Adverse effects on the breastfed neonate are unknown.

Treatment of Overdose: Overdose with this drug is very rare, since only two doses are administered.

Clinician Responsibilities: Key clinical implications for patients receiving basiliximab are included in Applied Clinical Judgment: Patients Receiving Pharmacotherapy with Immunomodulators.

Drugs Similar to Basiliximab (Simulect)

The other antibody drugs used in transplant medicine are antithymocyte globulin and belatacept. The MABs used for

RA such as adalimumab (Humira) and infliximab (Remicade) are discussed in Chapter 72.

Antithymocyte globulin (Atgam, Thymoglobulin): Approved in 1981, antithymocyte globulin consists of polyclonal antibodies obtained from the serum of horses (Atgam) or rabbits (Thymoglobulin) exposed to human T cells. Doses of the two are not interchangeable. The drug is a potent immunosuppressant used for the prophylaxis and management of transplant rejection and for the treatment of moderate to severe aplastic anemia in patients who are unable to have bone marrow transplantation. It is used off-label to treat GVHD and myelodysplastic syndrome. Given by the IV route, a single infusion may lower the lymphocyte count by 85 to 90%. After discontinuation of therapy, T-cell counts take several months to return to baseline levels. The most common adverse effects are fever, chills, malaise, headache, diarrhea, itching, and other flulike symptoms. Corticosteroids, antihistamines, and acetaminophen may be administered 1 hour prior to antithymocyte globulin therapy to prevent **cytokine release syndrome**, a condition in which massive amounts of cytokines are released by the lymphocytes affected by the drug. Anaphylaxis has been reported. Like other immunosuppressants, an increased incidence of infections and malignancies is expected. A black box warning states that antithymocyte globulin should be administered only by healthcare providers experienced in immunosuppressive therapy. Animal studies have not been conducted to determine if antithymocyte has adverse effects during pregnancy or lactation.

Belatacept (Nulojix): Belatacept is a MAB approved in 2011 for the prophylaxis of organ rejection in patients receiving kidney transplants. The drug blocks specific receptors on T lymphocytes, inhibiting their proliferation and stopping the production of cytokines that could damage a newly transplanted organ. The drug acts by the same mechanism as abatacept (Orencia), which is approved to treat RA. Belatacept is always used in combination with basiliximab, mycophenolate mofetil, and corticosteroids. The drug carries a black box warning that it may increase the risk for PTLD, a serious condition in which B cells proliferate unchecked and may cause B-cell tumors. Recipients who have never been exposed to the Epstein-Barr virus are especially susceptible to PTLD. The warning also states that the drug may increase the risk for malignancies and that it should not be used for liver transplants due to possible graft rejection. Common adverse effects include anemia, diarrhea, URI, and peripheral edema. Like other immunosuppressants, belatacept may increase the risk for serious infections. This drug may cause fetal harm in laboratory animals. Adverse effects on the breastfed neonate are unknown.

CONNECTION Checkpoint 42.2

Basiliximab (Simulect) binds to CD25 and an immune response is prevented. From what you learned in Chapter 40, which type of immunity—humoral or cell mediated—does this drug affect?

42.8 Corticosteroids are widely used as immunosuppressants but have significant long-term adverse effects.

The corticosteroids, or glucocorticoids, are potent inhibitors of inflammation and are discussed in detail in Chapters 41 and 68. They are often the preferred drugs for the short-term therapy of severe inflammation.

In addition to their anti-inflammatory effects, corticosteroids affect nearly every aspect of the immune response. They intervene at multiple steps in the immune response, including antigen presentation, production of cytokines, and the proliferation of lymphocytes.

- **Lymphocyte effect.** A single dose of corticosteroid reduces circulating lymphocyte counts within a few hours. This inhibits the ability of the body to react to an antigen challenge.
- **Monocyte effect.** Corticosteroids quickly deplete the body of monocytes and macrophages. Macrophages are responsible for presenting antigens to lymphocytes.
- **Neutrophil effect.** Corticosteroids cause neutrophils to move from the bone marrow into the general circulation, resulting in increased numbers of circulating neutrophils. The drug then prevents the neutrophils from migrating out of the circulation to sites of inflammation.
- **Other effects.** Corticosteroids block the production of prostaglandins and ILs. This results in T cells being unable to react to antigens and proliferate.

Two common drugs in this class, prednisone and methylprednisolone, have been widely used to prevent transplant rejection since the 1960s. When used for a few weeks, the corticosteroids are safe and effective immunosuppressants. The long-term adverse effects of corticosteroids, however, are serious and include osteoporosis, cataract formation, mental status changes, fluid and salt retention, HTN, hyperglycemia, obesity, and adrenal atrophy. Because of their long-term effects, healthcare providers have begun to look at the possibility of eliminating corticosteroids from the transplant regimen. Some regimens call for the initial use of corticosteroids, with their gradual withdrawal at some point, usually within 3 to 6 months following the transplant. The issue remains unresolved and an active area of research.

CONNECTIONS: APPLIED CLINICAL JUDGMENT

Patients Receiving Pharmacotherapy with Immunomodulators

Key Assessment Data

- History of current condition, baseline vital signs, physical exam findings; previous history or current case of cancer; fever; active infections (especially herpes, varicella, and CMV); oral and dental health; hepatic, renal, cardiovascular, neurologic, or autoimmune disease; dermatologic conditions; HIV infection; pregnancy or breastfeeding. Obtain a drug history, especially the use of corticosteroids, and usual intake of grapefruit juice.
- Ongoing assessment should include monitoring appropriate laboratory findings (e.g., CBC, platelets, electrolytes, glucose, hepatic and renal laboratory values, lipid levels); assessment for infections, especially with opportunistic infections such as herpes, varicella, CMV, and fungal infections; signs of neurologic changes.

Desired Therapeutic Outcomes

Improvement is observed and measurable by autoimmune response is suppressed with general improvement of condition (lessened pain, inflammation, improved function) and transplant organ function is maintained with no signs or symptoms of transplant rejection (e.g., maintenance of urine output).

Minimizing Adverse Effects

- Immunosuppressant drugs may increase the risk of infections, especially with opportunistic infections. Observe for signs and symptoms of infection: fever over 38.3°C (101°F), sore throat, diarrhea, malaise, white patches in the oral cavity, painful or vesicular rashes, reddened or warm areas at the site of injury, or lethargy.
- Immunosuppressant drugs may cause HTN and immunostimulants may cause hypotension. Continue to monitor vital signs, especially blood pressure.
- Neurologic changes may indicate adverse drug effects. Assess for changes in level of consciousness, disorientation, confusion, or tremors.
- Immunosuppressants may cause leukopenia, anemia, thrombocytopenia, hyperglycemia, and hyperkalemia. Continue to monitor appropriate laboratory results.
- Immunosuppression increases the risk of oral candidiasis and gingivitis. Oral antifungal rinses may be required.
- Grapefruit juice significantly increases cyclosporine levels and should be avoided or eliminated while on immunosuppressant therapy.
- Psychosis, depression, and suicidal ideations are potential adverse effects of interferon (IFN) use.
- Hirsutism and alopecia are possible adverse effects. Hirsutism related to cyclosporine is reversible when the drug is discontinued. Alopecia may indicate significant immunosuppression.

Lifespan Considerations

- Older adults may be at increased risk for hypotension, and dizziness may increase the risk of falls.
- Age-related physiologic changes increase the risk of adverse renal and hepatic effects in the older adult.
- Pregnancy should be avoided during and for up to 4 months after discontinuing immunosuppressive therapy. Women who become pregnant while on the drug should consult with their healthcare provider.

Diversity Considerations

- Because drugs such as cyclosporine metabolize through the CYP450 system pathways, monitor ethnically diverse patients more frequently for appropriate therapeutic effects.

Patient Education

- Report a fever that does not diminish below 37.8°C (100°F) or per provider's instructions.
- Report blood pressure over 140/90 mmHg or parameters set by the healthcare provider. Chest pain or pressure should be reported immediately.
- If taking immunostimulants, rise from lying to sitting or standing slowly to avoid dizziness or falls. If dizziness occurs, sit or lie down and do not attempt to stand or walk until the sensation passes.
- Immediately report signs and symptoms of infection such as wounds with redness or drainage, increasing cough, increasing fatigue, white patches on oral mucous membranes, white and itchy vaginal discharge, or itchy blister-like vesicles on the skin.
- Report increasing lethargy, disorientation, confusion, changes in behavior or mood, slurred speech, tremors, or ataxia.
- Maintain excellent oral hygiene, inspecting the oral cavity daily. Keep regular dental visits and consult the dentist about the required frequency.
- Avoid grapefruit juice while on cyclosporine. Flavored beverages without juice are permissible.
- If mixing of the medication is required:
  - Use the enclosed equipment to measure or mix the drug.
  - Use a glass, and not paper or plastic cups, unless the package directions indicate they are to be used.
  - Mix the drug with milk, chocolate milk, or orange juice, unless directed to use water and stir well. After taking the drug, rinse the cup with additional liquid and drink it to ensure the entire dose is taken.
  - Take the medication at the same time each day.
- Practice general infection control measures, including:
  - Wash hands frequently. Use lotion afterward to prevent excessive drying and cracking of the skin.
  - Wear a facial mask that covers both mouth and nose.
  - Avoid large crowds, especially indoors.
  - Avoid people with known infection or young children because they have a higher risk of having an infection.
  - Cook food thoroughly, allowing the family or caregiver to prepare raw meat or fish and clean up, and do not consume raw fruits or vegetables, which may contain bacteria on their surfaces.

Prescribing Considerations

- Early diagnosis and immediate initiation of antiinfective therapy are essential to the management of patients on immunosuppressants.
- Measure serum lipids, liver aminotransferases, serum creatinine, absolute neutrophil counts, and platelets at a minimum baseline prior to drug initiation and throughout treatment. Drug dosages may need adjustment based on results.
- Pregnancy tests and counseling on contraceptive options should be done prior to drug initiation.

Understanding Chapter 42

Key Concepts Summary

42.1 Immunomodulators are substances that either enhance or suppress the ability of the body to fight infection and disease.

42.2 Interferons are biologic response modifiers that have antiviral and antineoplastic activity.

42.3 Interleukins, vaccines, and colony-stimulating factors are used to boost the immune system.

42.4 Immunosuppressants are used to prevent transplant rejection and for the treatment of autoimmune disorders.

42.5 Calcineurin inhibitors are preferred drugs for the prophylaxis of transplant rejection.

42.6 Cytotoxic drugs and antimetabolites are used to suppress proliferating B cells and T cells.

42.7 Antibodies are used to prevent acute transplant rejection, autoimmune disorders, and malignancies.

42.8 Corticosteroids are widely used as immunosuppressants but have significant long-term adverse effects.

CASE STUDY: Making the Patient Connection

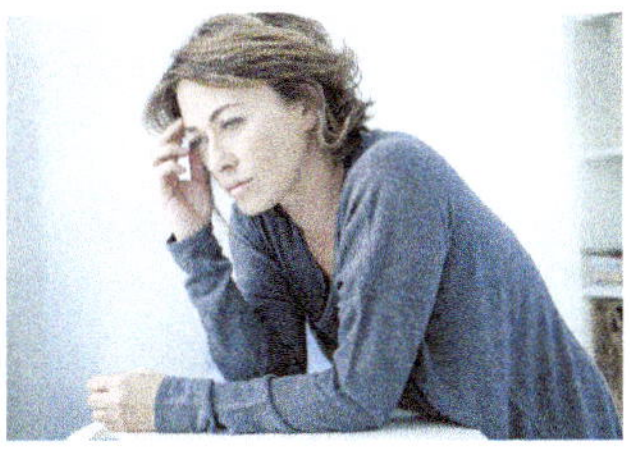

Remember the patient "Carole Banks" at the beginning of the chapter? Now read the remainder of the case study. Based on the information presented within this chapter, respond to the critical thinking questions that follow.

Carole Banks is a 42-year-old woman diagnosed with hepatitis C who was recently seen by her healthcare provider at an office visit. She reported having right upper quadrant pain, fatigue, anorexia, and nausea and vomiting. She has been feeling progressively worse for the past year but did not seek medical care for her problem. She has lost 5.4 kg (12 lb) over the past 6 months.

Carole was initially hospitalized to receive IV fluids for dehydration and to be further evaluated. Once in the hospital, a full hepatitis panel found that she was positive for hepatitis C virus.

During the initial interview with Carole, she discloses that she was addicted to illegal IV drugs for 15 years and was an alcohol abuser for 20 years. However, Carole claims that she has abstained from substance abuse for the past 5 years. She resides with her husband and three children and is employed as a clerk in a local retail convenience store.

As part of the treatment for Carole's hepatitis, she is prescribed IFN alfa-2b (Intron A). She is taught to self-administer (subcutaneously) the standard dose of IFN, 3 million units, 3 times weekly.

Critical Thinking Questions

1. Discuss the rationale for the use of IFN alfa-2b (Intron A) in the treatment of hepatitis C.
2. What adverse effects might Carole experience with this drug therapy? How can the nurse assist Carole to cope with the related adverse effects?
3. Identify the patient education that Carole will need concerning her drug therapy.

Additional Case Study

Gordon Sharp had been on kidney dialysis since his car crash 2 years ago. He sustained severe traumatic injuries and subsequently developed renal failure. Gordon has recently received a kidney transplant and is currently on cyclosporine (Sandimmune).

1. How does cyclosporine work and why is Gordon receiving the drug?
2. Describe the patient teaching that the nurse should give to Gordon concerning this drug therapy.
3. What dietary precautions would be indicated for this patient?

Chapter Review

1. The nurse is monitoring the laboratory findings of a patient who is taking interferon alfa-2b (Intron A). Which findings would indicate that the patient is experiencing common adverse effects?
   1. Flulike symptoms of fever, chills, fatigue, and weight loss
   2. Depression with thoughts of suicide
   3. Edema, hypotension, and tachycardia
   4. Fluid volume overload, HTN, and renal insufficiency

2. The patient is receiving basiliximab (Simulect) and cyclosporine (Sandimmune) after a kidney transplant to prevent organ rejection. The patient develops a high fever and chills, with a temperature of 39.4°C (103°F). The nurse interprets that the patient is most likely experiencing:
   1. Capillary leak syndrome.
   2. A significant infection related to immunosuppression.
   3. Graft-versus-host rejection.
   4. Androgen-insensitivity syndrome.

3. The nurse who is caring for a patient receiving cyclosporine (Sandimmune) will discontinue the medication immediately and call the provider if which of the following occurs?
   1. Red blood cell count above 8.5 million/mm^3
   2. White blood cell count below 4000/mm^3
   3. Platelet count above 100,000/mm^3
   4. Serum creatinine level less than 1.0 mg/100 mL

4. Azathioprine (Azasan) is prescribed to a patient who had a kidney transplant. A nurse reviews the patient's medical record and would question the medication order for the patient with a history of:
   1. Benign prostatic hyperplasia.
   2. Cataracts.
   3. Varicella zoster.
   4. RA.

5. A nurse is instructing a patient who is receiving tacrolimus (Prograf) following a liver transplant. Which point should be included in the teaching plan?
   1. Take a "baby" strength aspirin every day.
   2. Increase physical activity to avoid weight gain.
   3. Record radial pulse rate every morning in a journal.
   4. Avoid raw fruits and vegetables and eat only fully cooked meats.

6. A nurse is particularly cautious in monitoring the patient who is prescribed aldesleukin (Proleukin). To monitor for the development of capillary leak syndrome, the nurse would frequently assess:
   1. Skin condition and rashes.
   2. Laboratory values for increasing amylase and lipase.
   3. Blood pressure and urine output.
   4. Vision and hearing.

See Appendix A for answers to critical thinking questions, case study questions and review questions.

References

National Center for Complementary and Integrative Health. (2020). *Echinacea.* https://www.nccih.nih.gov/health/echinacea

Organ Procurement and Transplantation Network. (2020). *Data.* http://optn.transplant.hrsa.gov/data

organdonor.gov. (2020). *Organ donation statistics.* http://www.organdonor.gov/statistics-stories/statistics.html

Selected Bibliography

Cossart, A. R., Staatz, C. E., Campbell, S. B., Isbel, N. M., & Cottrell, W. N. (2019). Investigating barriers to immunosuppressant medication adherence in renal transplant patients. *Nephrology, 24*(1), 102–110. https://doi.org/10.1111/nep.13214

Freeman, R., Koerner, E., Clark, C., & Halabicky, K. (2016). Cardiac transplant postoperative management and care. *Critical Care Nursing Quarterly, 39*, 214–226. https://doi.org/10.1097/CNQ.0000000000000116

Jani, A. A. (2017). *Infections after solid organ transplantation*. Medscape. http://emedicine.medscape.com/article/430550-overview

Pelligrino, B. (2021). *Immunosuppression*. Medscape. http://emedicine.medscape.com/article/432316-overview#a1

Petty, M. (2016). Antibody-mediated rejection in solid organ transplant. *AACN Advanced Critical Care, 27*, 316–323. https://doi.org/10.4037/aacnacc2016366

Williams, A., Low, J. K., Manias, E., & Crawford, K. (2016). The transplant team's support of kidney transplant recipients to take their prescribed medications: A collective responsibility. *Journal of Clinical Nursing, 25*, 2251–2261. https://doi.org/10.1111/jocn.13267

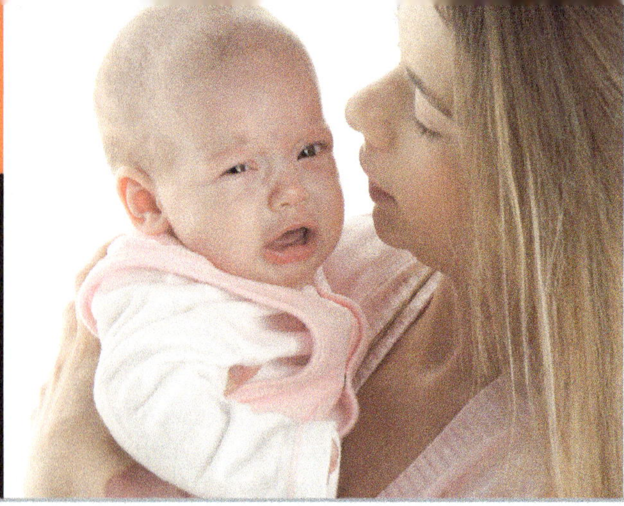

"I don't think these immunizations are necessary. They made her so sick last time!"
—*Mother of patient "Samantha Abbott"*

Chapter 43
Immunizing Agents

Chapter Outline

- Discovery of Vaccines
- Vaccines and the Immune System
- Types of Vaccines
- General Principles of Vaccine Administration
- Active Immunity: Bacterial Immunizations
- Active Immunity: Viral Immunizations

  PROTOTYPE *Hepatitis B Vaccine (Engerix-B, Recombivax HB), p. 745*
- Passive Immunity

  PROTOTYPE *Rho(D) Immune Globulin (RhoGAM), p. 751*

Learning Outcomes

After reading this chapter, the student should be able to:

1. Explain why the development of vaccines was one of the most significant discoveries of modern medicine.
2. Compare and contrast active and passive immunity.
3. Explain the immune response that leads to the development of active immunity.
4. Prepare a table listing the types of vaccines, their indications, and potential adverse effects.
5. Explain why it is important to administer childhood vaccines at specific ages.
6. Identify contraindications for vaccine administration.
7. Describe the pathogenesis and immunization of bacterial infections, including diphtheria, pertussis, tetanus, pneumococcus, and meningococcus.
8. Describe the pathogenesis and immunization of viral infections, including hepatitis A and B, influenza, rabies, measles, mumps, rubella, polio, varicella zoster, human papillomavirus, and rotavirus.
9. Explain the rationale for administering antibodies to establish passive immunity.
10. For each of the major vaccines and patient age groups, identify the schedule for the recommended dosage sequence established by the Centers for Disease Control and Prevention.
11. Apply clinical judgment to care for patients receiving immunizing agents.

Key Terms

Definitions of the terms in bold may be found in the Glossary.

The earliest attempts at treatments to prevent infection were reported in ancient Indian and Chinese literature when dried, powdered scabs from infected individuals were administered to healthy people. Vaccinations have since become one of the most important medical interventions for the prevention of serious infectious disease. Routine vaccinations for polio, pertussis, diphtheria, tetanus, and measles are estimated to prevent 3 million deaths annually. This chapter examines the role of vaccines in promoting the health of both children and adults and the potential adverse effects of these drugs.

Discovery of Vaccines

43.1 The eradication of smallpox was a great triumph in modern medicine.

In the 1790s, Dr. Edward Jenner was experimenting with the use of **inoculation**, the placement of a foreign substance on or in an individual for the purpose of disease prevention. Inoculation uses live virus particles obtained from an infected patient. Jenner used the cowpox virus, a benign pathogen in humans, because he predicted that exposure to that virus would provide immunity to smallpox, which was one of the most dreaded human diseases of that era. Case fatality rates of 30% or more were reported with smallpox infections. In the 18th century, the disease was a frequent cause of blindness and death for 400,000 people worldwide annually.

Jenner's inoculation of a single 8-year-old boy ultimately led to one of the greatest triumphs in disease prevention. On May 8, 1980, the World Health Assembly certified that global medical interventions had actually eradicated smallpox infections from the planet. Although this announcement was heralded by the scientific community as proof of the success of routine immunization, it also has presented new challenges. With the last known case of the disease, the need for smallpox immunization ceased, resulting in a growing, nonimmune population. The widespread reappearance of the pathogen in an unvaccinated population could have disastrous consequences.

Vaccines and the Immune System

43.2 Vaccines are used to activate the immune system for the purpose of disease prevention.

An immune response occurs when an antigen is recognized by the B or T lymphocytes. Antigens are microbes and foreign substances that elicit an immune response. Most microbes, nonhuman proteins, bacterial or plant toxins, and normal cells that become damaged or cancerous are considered antigens. Following the first exposure to an antigen, sufficient time is needed for the body to process the antigen and mount an effective response. It is during this time, known as the **incubation period**, that the symptoms of infection and tissue injury develop. During this first antigen exposure, memory B cells or T cells are formed. Should a second or subsequent exposure to the same antigen occur, the memory cells react quickly to produce a more rapid immune response with fewer (or no) symptoms of infection. The student should review Chapter 40 for a summary of the humoral and cell-mediated immune responses before proceeding.

Edward Jenner was the first to use the term *vaccination*. **Vaccination** is the process of introducing foreign proteins or inactive cells (vaccines) into the body to trigger immune activation *before* the patient is exposed to the real pathogen. As a result of the vaccination, memory B cells or T cells are formed. When later exposed to the real infectious organism, these cells will react quickly by producing large quantities of antibodies and cytokines that help to neutralize or destroy the antigen. Whereas some vaccinations are needed only once, most require follow-up doses, known as **boosters**, to provide prolonged protection. The type of response induced by the real pathogen, or its vaccine, is called **active immunity**. During this response the body produces its own antibodies in response to exposure. The active immunity induced by vaccines closely resembles that caused by natural exposure to the antigen, including the generation of memory cells. The term **immunization** is considered equivalent to the term *vaccination*, and either one may be used to describe this process of disease prevention.

The effectiveness of most vaccines can be assessed by measuring the amount of antibodies produced after the vaccine has been administered, a quantity called *titer*. If the titer falls below a specified, protective level over time, a booster dose is indicated. Antibodies are a product of the humoral immune system. The cell-mediated immune system is also important in producing immunity, but its cellular responses are less readily measured.

Passive immunity occurs when preformed antibodies are transferred or "donated" from one person to another. For example, maternal antibodies cross the placenta and provide protection for the fetus and newborn. Other examples of passive immunity include the administration of immune globulin following exposure to hepatitis, antivenins for snakebites, and sera to treat botulism, tetanus, and rabies. The drugs for passive immunity are administered when the patient has already been exposed to a virulent pathogen, or when the patient is at very high risk for exposure and there is not sufficient time to develop active immunity. Patients who are immunosuppressed may receive these drugs to prevent infections. Because these medications do not stimulate the patient's immune system, no memory cells are produced and protective effects last only 2 to 3 weeks. Passive immunity is presented in Section 43.7.

Most vaccines are administered with the goal of *preventing* illness. Common vaccines include those used to prevent patients from acquiring measles, influenza, diphtheria, polio, pertussis (whooping cough), tetanus, and hepatitis B (HBV). Anthrax vaccine has been used to immunize people who are at high risk for exposure to anthrax from a potential bioterrorism incident (see Chapter 75). In the case of infection by the human immunodeficiency virus (HIV), experimental HIV vaccines are given after infection has occurred for the purpose of enhancing the immune response, rather than preventing the disease. Unlike other vaccines, experimental vaccines for HIV have thus far been unable to prevent acquired immunodeficiency syndrome (AIDS).

CONNECTION Checkpoint 43.1

The humoral and cell-mediated immune responses are components of the specific (adaptive) body defenses. From what you learned in Chapter 40, compare and contrast the humoral and cell-mediated responses to an antigen.

Types of Vaccines

43.3 Five methods are used to produce vaccines.

The goal of vaccine administration is to induce long-lasting immunity to a pathogen without producing an illness in an otherwise healthy individual. Therefore, the microorganisms and other substances used as vaccines must be able to strongly activate the immune system but be modified to pose no significant risk of disease development. The vaccine must be economical to develop and be stable for storage and administration. For long-standing disease protection, the vaccine must be able to stimulate the production of memory B cells and T cells. The five methods used to produce safe and effective vaccines, as listed in Table 43.1. All four methods are capable of inducing active immunity.

Attenuated (live) vaccines: Live vaccine products contain microorganisms that are capable of replicating and causing disease. Live vaccines are very effective at inducing immunity but are not used for vaccination because of their risk. However, effective vaccines can be developed from organisms that are **attenuated** or rendered less able to cause disease through the application of heat or chemicals. Attenuated (live) vaccines cause the development of a mild or subclinical case of the disease while still inducing lasting immunity. The type of immune response obtained from the administration of a live or attenuated organism is the same as if the patient had been exposed to the natural, nonattenuated organism. There must, however, be adequate immune functioning for the vaccine to work. The use of attenuated (live) vaccines is dangerous for individuals who are immunosuppressed because the organism may retain some residual ability to replicate and cause disease. In very rare cases, the attenuated virus may mutate to an infectious form in patients who receive the vaccine. An example of a live or attenuated vaccine is the measles, mumps, and rubella (MMR) vaccine.

Inactivated (killed) vaccines: Inactivated or killed vaccines are of two types: whole agent and subunit. Whole-agent vaccines consist of microbes killed by heat or chemicals. Subunit vaccines consist of specific segments of a cell membrane, foreign proteins, or sequences of a chromosome rather than the whole microbe.

Inactivated or killed vaccines are safer than live vaccines because the organism is unable to replicate, mutate, or cause disease. Subsequent booster doses are required to maintain immunity if inactivated or killed vaccines are used. Examples of inactivated or killed vaccines include the influenza and hepatitis A (HAV) vaccines. Examples of subunit vaccines are the human papillomavirus (HPV) vaccine and the acellular pertussis vaccine.

Toxoid vaccines: Some pathogens secrete toxins, which are responsible for the symptoms of the infection. **Toxoids** are bacterial toxins that have been chemically modified to be incapable of causing disease. When injected as a type of immunization, toxoids induce the formation of antibodies

Table 43.1 Vaccine Types

Type of Vaccine	Immune System Response	Vaccine Examples	Remarks
Attenuated (live) virus	B-cell response; T-cell response	Polio (oral), measles, mumps, rubella, varicella	Risk for disease in individuals with reduced immune function
Inactivated (killed) virus	B-cell response	Salk polio (injectable), influenza, rabies, hepatitis A	Does not confer lifelong immunity
Toxoid	B-cell response	Tetanus toxoid, diphtheria toxoid	Large quantities of antigen needed
Recombinant technology vaccine	B-cell response	Hepatitis B, human papillomavirus	Contains no viral genetic material
Nucleic acid vaccine	B-cell response	Covid-19	Delivers genetic instructions for making viral protein spikes to human immune cells

that are capable of neutralizing the real toxins. Toxoids attack the bacterial toxin, not the invading pathogen itself. Examples include the diphtheria and tetanus toxoids.

Recombinant technology vaccines: Modern biologic techniques have allowed the development of vaccines that contain viral subunits or proteins that are generated in a laboratory. Two examples of the use of this form of biotechnology are immunizations for the HBV and HPV. These vaccines do not contain viral genetic material; therefore, the viruses cannot multiply or become infectious.

Nucleic acid vaccines: In 2020 the world faced a massive public health crisis: Covid-19 viral infection. Several vaccines were rapidly developed that contain genetic instructions for making the protein spikes that are present on the exterior of the Covid-19 virus. Once delivered via messenger RNA (m-RNA) or encased in a harmless adenovirus, human immune cells use the instructions to make millions of copies of the spike and create antibodies against Covid-19. Because only a tiny piece of genetic material is used, there is no possibility of acquiring a Covid-19 infection from the vaccination.

General Principles of Vaccine Administration

43.4 Vaccines should be administered by an established schedule with precautions taken for patients who are immunosuppressed or pregnant.

The effective use of vaccines requires that they be delivered according to a specified schedule at the proper dose. Childhood vaccines have a specific age range at which they should be administered. Should a child miss the recommended vaccination date, "catch-up" doses can sometimes be administered to provide adequate protection. In addition, comorbid health conditions sometimes cause the delay of vaccinations in certain patients. Although each vaccine has different indications, certain general principles apply to the administration of most immunizations.

In the United States, the Centers for Disease Control and Prevention (CDC) is the government agency that establishes immunization schedules. Immunization protocols are reviewed on a regular basis by the CDC's Advisory Committee on Immunization Practices, and revisions are frequently made based on current research. The practicing nurse should refer often to the CDC website for updates.

Many of the vaccine-preventable diseases are rare in the United States, but endemic to specific regions of the world. The nurse should advise patients traveling to these regions to check that their vaccinations are current. The CDC provides updated country-specific health information for those traveling abroad.

Dose and timing: The total dose of a vaccine is important for the development of immunity. For some vaccinations, multiple doses are required to achieve immunity. Omitting subsequent doses could result in incomplete or no disease protection.

To prevent childhood diseases, certain vaccinations should begin at birth and proceed with booster doses at specific ages according to the schedule recommended by the CDC. The timing established by the CDC allows the vaccine to be given prior to the expected exposure to the pathogen. For example, the pertussis vaccine is begun in the first few months of life because infection by *Bordetella pertussis* often occurs by age 1 or 2 years. On the other hand, vaccination for HPV is recommended at 11 to 12 years of age because this virus is spread by sexual contact, which often occurs during the teen years. Vaccination outside the guidelines of the vaccination schedule is permitted, but its effectiveness may be reduced.

Route of administration: Vaccines must be administered by the specific route indicated for each product. Failure to follow administration protocol may result in an insufficient immune response. For example, HBV vaccine elicits a satisfactory response when administered into the deltoid muscle but not the gluteus muscle. Injection into the gluteus muscle also risks injury to the sciatic nerve. Varicella vaccine is given subcutaneously.

Precautions and contraindications: There are few absolute contraindications for the use of vaccines. However, caution must be used in immunocompromised patients, such as those with cancer, recent tissue transplant recipients, or those infected with HIV. Patients receiving high-dose, systemic corticosteroid therapy may also have suppressed immune systems. Vaccinations in an immunocompromised patient should be avoided if the patient is having an exacerbation of the disorder. In some cases, only inactivated (killed) vaccines are indicated for these patients. Because it is suppressed, the patient's immune system may not be able to develop effective immunity in response to the vaccine, and subsequent laboratory results should be assessed to confirm that immunity has actually occurred.

The CDC (2016) provides guidelines for receiving vaccines during pregnancy and lactation. Inactivated (killed) vaccines may be administered to pregnant patients if the benefits of disease prevention justify the possible risk to the mother and fetus. For example, the CDC recommends vaccination for influenza (inactivated) and Tdap (tetanus, diphtheria, and pertussis booster vaccine). A woman should be vaccinated for HBV if she is at risk for HBV infection during pregnancy. Some vaccines, including those for HPV, varicella, and MMR, should not be administered during pregnancy due to the potential risk to the fetus. For other vaccines, the pregnant patient should consult with her healthcare provider.

Anaphylaxis and allergy: The most common adverse effects of vaccination are pain, swelling, and redness at the injection sites. Allergy or anaphylaxis following vaccination is extremely rare. Some preparations may contain preservatives such as gelatin or the mercury compound thimerosal, which could trigger an allergic response. Patients with confirmed vaccine anaphylaxis should not receive subsequent doses of that vaccine.

Adverse event reporting: Healthcare providers are required to report all vaccine-related adverse events requiring medical attention to the Vaccine Adverse Event Reporting System (VAERS). The VAERS is a postmarketing surveillance program conducted by the CDC and the U.S. Food and Drug Administration (FDA). Voluntary reports may be submitted to the VAERS by patients and parents as well as healthcare providers. Vaccine manufacturers are required to report any adverse effects of which they are aware.

VAERS has a number of limitations. VAERS merely collects data and reports incidences of adverse events; it does not attempt to confirm that the reported event was actually caused by the vaccine. Reports are not checked by the FDA or CDC for accuracy or completeness. Despite its limitations, VAERS serves as an important, central repository of information for identifying potential adverse effects of vaccines.

Active Immunity: Bacterial Immunizations

43.5 Active immunity can be induced to prevent bacterial infections.

Vaccinations are performed to provide protection against both viral and bacterial pathogens. However, the role of vaccines is very different for each type of infectious agent. Table 43.2 summarizes the incidence and immunizations associated with these pathogens. Immunizations against viruses are presented in Section 43.6.

Many bacterial infections cause host cellular injury by releasing toxic substances. Vaccination for bacterial infections, therefore, may be achieved by exposing the immune system to inactive bacterial toxins. When later faced with the actual bacterial infection, the immune system will remember the protein-based toxin and respond rapidly by producing antibodies to neutralize it.

Table 43.2 Disease Incidence and Immunizations

Disease	U.S. Incidence (Annually)	Immunization (Age)	Remarks
Coronavirus-19	Millions of cases since 2020	One and two dose series available. Development of vaccines is evolving	Symptoms worse in older adults and those with preexisting conditions
Diphtheria	Very rare due to high vaccination rate	2, 4, 6, and 15–18 months; 4–6 years	Under 10 reported cases
Hepatitis A	About 25,000 cases; has been increasing since 2016	Two-dose series: 12 months and 6–12 months later Adults at risk for infection	Route: oral–fecal from carriers; immune globulin available
Hepatitis B	About 22,000 cases	Three-dose series: 0, 1, and 6–18 months (Recombivax HH or Engerix-B)	Number of cases have been stable since 2011
Hepatitis C	About 50,000 cases	Not yet available	Vaccine under development
Human papilloma virus (HPV)	About 42% of population age 18–59 (genital HPV) and 7% (oral HPV) are infected	First dose at age 11–12; second 6–12 months after the first	In 2018 only 22% of women and 9% of men completed the recommended dosing schedule
Influenza (*Haemophilus influenzae* type b [Hib])	24,000–62,000 deaths	Annual vaccine, usually one dose	High risk to those over age 65 and in general ill health
Measles (rubeola)	Very rare	MMR: 12–15 months; booster: 4–6 years	Only 10 cases annually, all of which contracted the virus outside the U.S.
Meningococcus	About 350 cases; rates are highest for children under age 1	11–12 years; booster: age 16	Airborne droplet exposure; antibiotics if known exposure
Mumps	Variable	MMR: 12–15 months; booster: 4–6 years	Usually rare but large outbreaks in unvaccinated college students frequently occur
Pertussis	About 16,000 cases	2, 4, 6, and 15–18 months; 4–6 years	Increased incidence in adolescent age group
Pneumococcal disease	About 1 million cases with about 5000 deaths	All children younger than 2 years (PCV13) and all people over age 65 (PPSV23)	Most deaths occur in individuals age 65 and older
Poliomyelitis	Very rare	Inactivated virus: 2, 4, and 12 months; booster: 4–6 years	No cases in the U.S. since 1979
Rabies	Very rare	Preexposure vaccine for veterinarians; postexposure immune globulin	Only about 3 cases annually
Rubella	Very rare	MMR: 12–15 months; booster: 4–6 years	Only 10 cases annually, all of which contracted the virus outside the U.S.
Tetanus	Very rare; about 30 cases	2, 4, 6, and 15–18 months; 4–6 years	Illness usually results from inadequate or missed immunizations
Varicella (chickenpox)	About 3.5 million cases and 100 deaths	Two-dose series: 12–15 months and 4–6 years	Reoccurs as herpes zoster (shingles)

It is common practice to combine several childhood vaccines for a single administration. For example, DTaP combines diphtheria, tetanus, and pertussis into a single injection. Combining vaccines is less traumatic for the child and is more convenient and efficient for the caregiver and the healthcare provider.

Diphtheria

Pathophysiology: Diphtheria is an infection of the upper respiratory tract caused by the gram-positive bacterium *Corynebacterium diphtheriae*. The bacterium releases a potent toxin that causes a low-grade fever, malaise, and a painful oropharynx. The organism causes the formation of a thick, gray coating across the membranes of the soft palate, tonsillar areas, and uvula. The thickened membranes can partially occlude the airway and cause difficulty swallowing or a feeling of choking. The membrane softens and disappears in approximately 1 week. A majority of deaths associated with diphtheria are related to toxin escape, leading to acute systemic toxicity or myocarditis. Because of effective immunization programs, the disease has almost been entirely eradicated from the United States.

Diphtheria toxoid: Given to young children, the diphtheria toxoid triggers an immune response that produces memory cells. Currently diphtheria toxoid is available as a combination immunization with tetanus toxoid and acellular pertussis (DTaP) as well as in combination with other compatible immunizations. DTaP is part of the recommended routine immunization schedule for infants older than 6 months of age.

Pertussis (Whooping Cough)

Pathophysiology: Pertussis is a highly contagious infection by the gram-negative bacterium *Bordetella pertussis* that is transmitted via aerosolized droplets from an infected individual. Once inhaled, the bacteria attach to the ciliated respiratory epithelial cells and release a toxin. Pertussis begins with a low-grade fever and irritated cough and progresses to spasmodic coughing episodes characterized by an inspiratory "whoop," leading to the common name "whooping cough." The coughing episodes are productive and may be induced by laughing, talking, or activity in children and lead to gagging or vomiting. The cough will usually resolve at the termination of the infection in approximately 2 to 6 weeks. Active pertussis infection is treated with the antibiotic erythromycin, with the best results seen when treatment is early and aggressive.

Immunization: The current pertussis vaccine contains no bacterial cells, which is called an acellular form (aP). The acellular form of pertussis vaccine became available in 1996 and has replaced the whole-cell, original form.

Local injection-site reactions, drowsiness, persistent crying, and fever occur in 3 to 5% of patients receiving the vaccine. The vaccine is always administered concurrently with the diphtheria and tetanus toxoids. The childhood vaccine is called DTaP. Children receive five intramuscular (IM) doses of DTaP, one dose at each of the following ages: 2 months, 4 months, 6 months, 15 to 18 months, and 4 to 6 years. Because the severity of pertussis declines with age, vaccination for pertussis is not recommended for children after age 7 or for adults. Adults, however, may receive a booster vaccine (Tdap) if they are anticipating contact with patients with pertussis.

Tetanus

Pathophysiology: *Clostridium tetani* normally lives in soil as a spore but can infect humans when the gram-positive anaerobe enters an open wound. Symptoms of infection may present over a wide range of time, averaging from 3 to 21 days after exposure. *C. tetani* produces a toxin that is one of the most toxic substances known; receiving 2.5 mg (one billionth of a gram) per kilogram of body weight can be lethal. The toxin enters the peripheral nervous system and migrates to the central nervous system to cause continuous, painful muscle contractions. Symptoms range from local muscle spasm, including the muscles of the jaw (lockjaw), to neck stiffness and seizures that are sometimes unresponsive to drug therapy. Treatment includes the administration of antibiotics but is primarily supportive in advanced cases.

Immunization: Tetanus toxoid (TT) is available alone, combined with diphtheria (DT), or combined with both diphtheria and pertussis (DTaP). The initial series of recommended immunizations uses the DTaP and is given in five doses during the first 6 years of the child's life. A contaminated wound in an adult with an appropriate immunization history requires only the booster administration of TT. To retain immunity, the booster for tetanus prevention should be given to adults every 10 years. In patients with symptomatic tetanus infection, the TT injection may be coupled with passive immunization of antibodies against the toxin. The vaccine is nearly 100% effective at preventing tetanus and its widespread use has nearly eradicated this disease in the United States.

Pneumococcus

Pathophysiology: Infection by *Streptococcus pneumoniae* is the most common cause of bacterial otitis media, meningitis, and pneumonia. Pneumococcal infection begins in the nasopharynx and may spread to the middle ear, sinuses, and lower respiratory tract. It occurs with a higher incidence in the winter months, when air pollution increases, or as a secondary infection following viral disease. The immune health of the patient greatly impacts the progress of *S. pneumoniae* infection and those with decreased immune function are at greater risk for the development of serious infections. Also at risk are patients with diminished cough and gag reflexes who have difficulty clearing secretions from the upper airways, such as in cases of neuromuscular diseases or postanesthetic exposure. Smoking is a contributing factor in approximately half of the *S. pneumoniae* infections in nonelderly populations, probably due to the change in upper-airway clearance of secretions in these patients.

Immunization: The immunization for pneumococcal infection has two different formulations. The first to be approved by the FDA, called pneumococcal polysaccharide vaccine (PPSV23), is derived from the cell walls of 23 strains of *S. pneumoniae*. PPSV23 is recommended for those who are age 65 and older and for patients from age 2 to 64 who have a chronic illness, smoke cigarettes, have asthma, or live in environments where exposure risk is increased. The vaccine is also recommended in immunocompromised patients (age 2 to 64) who have HIV infection, leukemia, lymphoma, Hodgkin's disease, or multiple myeloma; patients who receive dialysis; patients who are receiving high-dose corticosteroid therapy; and transplant recipients. A booster 5 or more years following the first vaccination is recommended.

A second vaccine, called pneumococcal conjugate vaccine (PCV13), has been specially developed for routine immunization in children under the age of 5. This immunization differs from PPSV23 in that the *S. pneumoniae* polysaccharides are coupled with a protein that leads to improved immune activation in infants with immature immune function. PCV13 protects against 13 types of pneumococcal bacteria. PCV13 is used in a series of four IM injections at 2 months, 4 months, 6 months, and 12 to 15 months. PCV13 is also approved for adults 65 years or older who have had no previous pneumococcal vaccinations.

Both PPSV23 and PCV vaccines are well tolerated and contraindicated only in individuals with prior severe reactions to immunizations. The most common symptoms following the administration of either PPSV23 or PCV13 are mild fever, local redness, swelling, and pain at the injection site, which lasts from 1 to 3 days.

Meningococcus

Pathophysiology: Meningococcal infection (meningitis) is caused by *Neisseria meningitidis*, a highly virulent gram-negative, toxin-secreting organism. Although meningitis usually occurs sporadically in the United States, it sometimes causes epidemics in other nations. Early meningococcal infection is very difficult to discriminate from other viral or bacterial infections because it initially presents with nonspecific fever and rash; frequently symptoms appear less than 24 hours before individuals are hospitalized. Neurologic symptoms rapidly develop, including nuchal rigidity, headache, photophobia, and seizures. Infants present with reduced feeding, irritability or lethargy, and bulging fontanels. Early hospitalization and aggressive treatment with intravenous (IV) penicillin-based antibiotics or cephalosporins have reduced the mortality and morbidity of meningococcal infection. About 10% of patients die from the infection and up to 20% experience some degree of permanent neurologic disability.

Immunization: There are at least 12 types (serogroups) of *N. meningitidis*. Groups A, B, C, W, and Y cause most of the infections in the United States. The various types of meningococcal vaccine are indicated for different age groups.

For children, meningococcal conjugate vaccine (MenACWY or Hib-MenCY-TT) is recommended for children 2 months through 10 years of age who are at high risk for meningococcal infection. This includes children with certain medical conditions, those traveling to countries with high rates of meningococcal disease, or because of a community outbreak. Hib-MenCY-TT (MenHibrix) combines the three vaccines: meningococcus, tetanus toxoid, and *Haemophilus influenza* type b. Neither vaccine protects against meningococcus serogroup B, which is responsible for about two-thirds of all cases of meningitis in children 0 to 59 months of age.

For preteens and teens, MenACWY (Menactra, Menveo) is a two-dose regimen at ages 11 to 12 years with a booster at age 16. This vaccine protects against serogroups ACWY, but not B. Populations that should receive MenACWY include individuals traveling to regions where meningococcal infection is endemic or those living in crowded conditions, such as college residence halls. Because college freshmen living in dormitories are at increased risk for infection, some colleges now require meningococcal vaccination for these students. Serogroup B meningococcal vaccine (Bexsero, Trumenba) is available for community outbreaks of this strain.

Adults may receive MenACWY or meningococcal polysaccharide vaccine (MPSV-4) (Menomune). Adults who have already received their first MenACWY dose should receive MenACWY as their second dose. MPSV-4 is generally recommended for adults over age 55 who anticipate requiring only a single dose, such as travelers or during a community outbreak.

Active Immunity: Viral Immunizations

43.6 Effective vaccines that prevent viral infections have been developed.

Vaccinations for viral infections have a different form and function than those for bacterial infections. Viruses are nonliving and contain only a few strands of nucleic acid (deoxyribonucleic acid [DNA] or ribonucleic acid [RNA]), an outer protein coat, and a few viral enzymes. Viruses require a host cell for replication and transmission. The signs and symptoms that follow viral invasion may be caused by either the effects of the viral infection itself or by the host's immune response.

Most viral proteins are readily recognized as foreign by the immune system and will trigger an immune response. In some cases, immune cells are able to recognize that a virus has entered one of its own cells and has become infected. Recognition of infected cells takes place through the host secretion of special communication proteins called interferons (IFNs), which signal the surrounding noninfected cells of the approaching virus. The infected cells are programmed to undergo cell death, or apoptosis, when they are invaded, thus decreasing the viral spread to adjacent cells. Because viruses undergo rapid mutations that allow them to constantly change structure and evade the host's defense mechanisms, they present enormous challenges for effective vaccine development.

The term *live viral vaccine* is commonly used in clinical practice. It should be understood, however, that viruses are nonliving particles. In vaccine terminology, the term *live* refers to a virus's ability to produce symptoms in the host and does not indicate that the virus is actually alive.

CONNECTION Checkpoint 43.2

From what you learned in Chapter 42, what are the indications for pharmacotherapy with interferons?

Hepatitis B

Pathophysiology: Infection with HBV leads to symptoms that range from a self-limiting acute illness to life-threatening liver failure. Patients with HBV infection are at risk for developing a chronic carrier state, which is associated with the development of cirrhosis and hepatic cancer. Of the five viral infections known to cause hepatitis, HBV has the highest incidence worldwide.

Hepatitis B cannot be discriminated from the other forms of viral hepatitis by symptoms alone; serologic testing is required for diagnosis. The onset of symptoms ranges between 6 weeks and 6 months postexposure and includes low-grade fever, nausea and vomiting, malaise, fatigue, and anorexia. The patient may present with signs of hepatitis, including jaundice, dark urine, and clay-colored stools that appear 1 to 2 weeks following the onset of symptoms. Approximately 30% of patients are hospitalized during the acute phase of hepatitis infection. End-stage hepatitis includes encephalopathy, confusion and disorientation, and coma and carries a mortality rate of 60 to 70% without transplantation. Details on the pharmacotherapy of HBV infections are presented in Chapter 54.

Immunization: All HBV vaccines are made through recombinant technology, contain no blood products, and pose no risk of disease transmission. Current HBV vaccines contain only proteins from the viral coat, known as hepatitis B surface antigen (HBsAg). These proteins are recognized as highly antigenic by the immune system, which produces antibodies and memory cells against the virus. Single-antigen HBV vaccines include Recombivax HB, Engerix B, and Heplisav B (for adults). Combinations that include the HBV vaccine include Pediarix (hepatitis B, DTaP, and inactivated poliovirus) and Twinrix (hepatitis A and hepatitis B).

PROTOTYPE DRUG Hepatitis B Vaccine (Engerix-B, Recombivax HB)

Classification **Therapeutic:** Vaccine
Pharmacologic: Vaccine

Therapeutic Effects and Uses: The HBV vaccine is a noninfectious, highly immunogenic agent that provides immunity to HBV in 99 to 100% of patients when given in the recommended three-dose regimen. The effectiveness of the vaccine in producing immunity in adults declines with age. The vaccine is 98% effective in patients ages 20 to 29, 94% in patients ages 30 to 39, and 89% in those age 40 and older. The HBV vaccine may be administered in combination with hepatitis B immunoglobulin for post-exposure prophylaxis or to prevent the perinatal transmission of the virus from mother to infant. The vaccine is indicated for immunity against all known subtypes of HBV. Indications for the HBV vaccine include the following (CDC, 2020c):

- All infants at birth
- All children younger than age 19 who have not been vaccinated
- Healthcare and public safety workers who are at risk for exposure to blood on the job and residents and staff of facilities for people where a high proportion of clients have known risk factors for HBV infection
- People at risk for infection by sexual exposure
- People at risk for infection by percutaneous or mucosal exposure to blood
- Travelers to regions with intermediate or high rates of endemic HBV infection
- People with chronic liver disease (including those infected with the hepatitis C virus [HCV]), HIV, or diabetes.

Mechanism of Action: The HBV vaccine consists of HBsAg produced through recombinant DNA technology using yeast cells. Antibodies induced by the HBV vaccine decline over time and may require a booster dose for continued immunization.

Pharmacokinetics:

Route(s)	IM injection in the deltoid or anterolateral thigh in infants and small children
Absorption	Rapid, following IM injection
Distribution	Unknown
Primary metabolism	Unknown
Primary excretion	Unknown
Onset of action	Antibodies to HBV appear within 2 weeks
Duration of action	Immunity lasts 5–7 years

Adverse Effects: The most common adverse effects from HBV vaccination are pain at the injection site and mild to moderate fever. Approximately 15% of patients will experience systemic effects, usually fatigue, dizziness, fever, and headache. Children may experience irritability, fever, diarrhea, fatigue, weakness, diminished appetite, and rhinitis. Anaphylaxis is rare and is usually reported within a few hours after the vaccination. Guillain-Barré syndrome is a very rare adverse effect of the HBV vaccine.

Contraindications/Precautions: Known hypersensitivity to yeast or any component of the vaccine is an absolute contraindication. Patients who demonstrated severe hypersensitivity to the first dose should not receive subsequent doses. Although anaphylaxis is rare, proper emergency equipment or facilities should be available. Patients with active infections or unexplained fever should delay use of the vaccine unless the health of the patient is endangered by withholding the vaccine. Caution should be exercised when administering the vaccine to patients with severe cardiopulmonary impairment. The vaccine should be given to pregnant or lactating women only if clearly needed to protect the health of the mother or child.

Drug Interactions: Hepatitis B immunoglobulin should not be administered in the same syringe or at the same site as the vaccine because it can impair the development of immunity from the vaccine. Patients receiving immunosuppressant drugs may require a higher dose of vaccine. **Herbal/Food:** Unknown.

Pregnancy: Animal studies did not show fetal malformations or developmental abnormalities. Human epidemiological studies have not found evidence of an elevated risk of fetal harm. Secretion of the drug in milk or its effects on the breastfed neonate are unknown.

Treatment of Overdose: Overdose with this drug has not been reported.

Clinician Responsibilities: Key clinical implications for patients receiving HBV vaccination are included in Applied Clinical Judgement: Patients Receiving Immunizations.

Drugs Similar to Hepatitis B Vaccine (Engerix-B, Recombivax HB)

There are no vaccines similar to the HBV vaccine.

Hepatitis A

Pathophysiology: Unlike HBV, which is mostly bloodborne, HAV is acquired by the fecal–oral route. At highest risk for HAV infection are household contacts or sexual partners of infected individuals and travelers to regions of the world where HAV is endemic (Africa, South America, and most of Asia). Good personal hygiene and proper sanitation can prevent HAV infection. Children are at risk due to generally poor hygiene habits.

Approximately one-third of the U.S. population has lifelong immunity to HAV based on a past infection. Symptoms associated with HAV infection are age dependent. In children less than 5 years old, 50 to 90% of infections are asymptomatic, whereas 70 to 95% of adults will exhibit symptoms. Signs and symptoms include elevation in liver enzyme levels, jaundice, fatigue, anorexia, fever, dull abdominal pain, and nausea and vomiting. Symptoms are often mild, and most patients report the resolution of symptoms in several weeks. The disease is rarely fatal and normally produces no permanent hepatic impairment.

Immunization: Following the introduction of the HAV vaccine in 1995, the number of cases of HAV infection in the United States dropped dramatically. Current recommendations for HAV vaccinations include:

- All children and adolescents age 2 to 18
- Persons at increased risk for HAV infection: international travelers, men who have sex with men, illegal drug users, residents and staff of facilities for people where a high proportion of clients have known risk factors for HAV infection, persons who anticipate close personal contact with an international adoptee, and persons experiencing homelessness
- Persons at increased risk for severe disease from HAV infection: people with chronic liver disease (including those with HBV and HCV infections) and those infected with HIV
- Pregnant women at risk for HAV infection during pregnancy
- Unvaccinated persons in outbreak situations who are at severe risk for HAV infection (Nelson et al., 2020).

Vaccines to prevent HAV include Havrix and Vaqta. Twinrix is a vaccine that protects against both HAV and HBV and is administered in three doses. HAV vaccines are highly immunogenic, with 95 to 100% of vaccinated individuals developing protective antibodies. Antibody coverage may last as long as 20 years following vaccination. Adverse effects of the HAV vaccine are mild and include soreness at the injection site, headache, anorexia, and fatigue.

Influenza

Pathophysiology: Influenza, or flu, is a respiratory disease spread by the three forms of the influenza virus: types A, B, and C. Influenza type A is the most dangerous and the primary focus for the annual development of a vaccine for the prevention of epidemic outbreaks. Influenza type A causes seasonal outbreaks during the winter months that are usually self-limiting but may lead to serious health consequences in patients who are debilitated, immunosuppressed, or have chronic medical conditions. Influenza type A is also harbored in wild aquatic birds and is responsible for outbreaks of bird flu. Influenza types B and C are less common and generally do not cause epidemics or result in serious symptoms. The influenza viruses mutate at a rapid rate and change their antigenic appearance; almost every time the viral RNA replicates, a new mutant is created. Once an outbreak of influenza occurs, immunization is no longer effective and pharmacotherapy of the active infection may be initiated. Because treatment of influenza infection is minimally effective, the best approach for dealing with this infection is through prevention. The pharmacotherapy of influenza infection is presented in Chapter 54.

Immunization: The first influenza immunization took place in 1945 following a worldwide outbreak during World War II. Throughout the history of influenza immunization, the viral particles used for the inoculation have been incubated in chicken eggs, leading to an increased risk of anaphylaxis in patients with egg allergies. With the development of recombinant human DNA preparations, the risk of allergy has decreased.

The development of the annual influenza vaccine begins with a prediction on the part of scientists as to what strains of the virus are most likely to appear that year. Each year one influenza vaccine is prepared that contains portions of the most likely strains of type A and type B. If their prediction is accurate, the vaccine will prevent 70 to 90% of flu cases; however, the effectiveness of the vaccine is significantly lower in some years.

The influenza vaccines contain either three (trivalent) or four components (quadrivalent). The trivalent influenza vaccine is a formulation that contains protection against one H1N1 virus, one H3N2 virus, and one influenza B virus. The standard-dose trivalent vaccine is approved for people age 16 to 64. The high-dose trivalent vaccines contain either more flu antigen or an adjuvant substance. These vaccines are specifically developed to create a stronger immune response in those 65 years of age and older.

Most flu vaccine in the United States is quadrivalent: 99% of doses are of this type. The quadrivalent vaccine protects against two influenza type A viruses as well as two type B viruses. It comes in two forms: an intradermal form that is injected under the skin for individuals age 18 to 64, and a form containing the virus grown in culture for those age 4 and older.

In 2020, the first monovalent influenza vaccine (Audenz) to protect against the H5N1 influenza virus was approved. Audenz is not intended to be used as part of a seasonal flu vaccination program. Instead, this vaccine will be stockpiled for deployment in the event an H5N1 pandemic erupts. H5N1 is sometimes referred to as the "bird flu."

Annual influenza vaccination is recommended for all persons age 6 months and older. The following are considered high-risk groups:

- Children ages 6 through 59 months
- Persons age 50 and older
- Residents of nursing homes and long-term care facilities
- People who have extreme obesity (BMI greater than 40)
- Adults and children who have chronic conditions such as asthma, diabetes, or heart disease
- Anyone immunocompromised due to HIV infection, high-dose corticosteroid therapy, or cancer chemotherapy
- Women who are or expect to be pregnant during the influenza season
- Healthcare providers
- Household contacts (including children) and caregivers of individuals at high risk of acquiring influenza.
- Children ages 6 months to 18 years who are receiving aspirin who might be at risk of Reye's syndrome.
- American Indians and Alaska natives. (CDC, 2020a)

The most common adverse effects of the influenza vaccine are soreness and redness at the injection site. About 1% of patients may experience fever, chills, and muscle aches that last 1 to 2 days. Serious adverse effects are rare. Mercury-free and egg-free quadrivalent vaccines are available to those allergic to these substances.

Rabies

Pathophysiology: Rabies is caused by a virus that can invade the nervous system of most mammals. The rabies virus is carried in saliva and is passed to humans through animal bites from infected dogs, coyotes, wolves, foxes, raccoons, skunks, and bats. In unvaccinated individuals, the mortality rate is nearly 100%.

Following the bite of an infected animal, the incubation period for rabies infection is long, from 20 to 60 days. When possible, the biting animal is confined and examined for rabies infection. Because the infection is always fatal if untreated, therapy is immediately implemented while waiting for the results of animal testing.

Symptoms include pain or paresthesia surrounding the bite, fever, headache, malaise, irritability, anxiety, and insomnia. Short periods of agitation, aggressiveness, hyperactivity, and disorientation are followed by normal behavior. Nuchal rigidity, seizures, bizarre behavior, and hydrophobia indicate a progression of the disease;

if untreated, rabies will progress to cardiac or respiratory arrest or paralysis. Death usually occurs within 10 days of the onset of symptoms.

Immunization: preexposure and postexposure: Prevention of rabies may be accomplished through vaccination. Although effective, few people are administered preexposure immunization because of the very small risk of coming into contact with a rabid animal. However, this immunization is offered to people with potential exposure to rabid animals, such as animal handlers or veterinarians, and to travelers to countries where rabies is prevalent. Cave explorers often receive the vaccine because of their potential exposure to rabid bats, which is the common animal carrying the virus. Preexposure immunization includes three inoculations.

Once a potential exposure to rabies occurs, the patient should immediately receive postexposure vaccination. The immune response to dead or attenuated organisms in a rabies vaccine takes approximately 2 weeks to develop, which is well within the incubation period of rabies. Patients receive one dose of rabies immunoglobulin, which offers immediate protection. Five doses of rabies vaccine are then administered over a 28-day period. If instituted promptly, postexposure vaccination is successful. If the biting animal is shown not to have rabies, the sequence of vaccinations may be discontinued.

The most common adverse effects of the rabies vaccine are pain and redness at the injection site and mild, transient flulike symptoms. Pregnant women may receive the vaccine if exposure to the rabies virus is suspected.

Measles, Mumps, and Rubella

Measles (rubeola) pathophysiology: The measles virus, *Morbillivirus*, is one of the most contagious viral pathogens, being readily transmitted by airborne particles and respiratory secretions. Because humans are the only known reservoir for the virus, routine immunization has eliminated measles as a common childhood disease in the United States. Measles is still widespread in other countries and occasional outbreaks across the United States emphasize the importance of continued MMR immunizations.

Symptoms of measles infection appear 10 to 12 days following airborne exposure and begin with nonspecific cough, malaise, and low-grade fever. The fever can subsequently spike to as high as 40.6°C (105°F). A rash appears first on the oral mucosa but then develops into a reddened, raised rash on the face, hairline, ears, and neck, spreading to the trunk and extremities. The rash lasts approximately 1 week and then fades and disappears. Individuals are considered to be infectious 4 days prior to and after rash appearance. In developing countries, measles infection carries a mortality rate as high as 2 to 15%.

Mumps pathophysiology: Mumps is a viral infection in the parotid salivary glands that is transmitted by exposure to contaminated saliva. Symptoms develop 16 to 18 days after exposure, resulting in mild fever, headache, anorexia, and malaise. The fever usually lasts 1 to 6 days but the swelling in the parotid glands may continue for 10 days or more. The infection is usually self-limiting and mortality is rare. Complications of mumps include orchitis (swelling of the testes) in approximately 37% of infected, postpubescent boys and deafness in children.

Rubella (German measles) pathophysiology: Rubella, also called German measles, is a viral infection that produces mild symptoms in most people. The rubella virus is transmitted by infected aerosol droplets and symptoms include enlarged cervical lymph nodes, mild fever, and malaise, followed by a raised rash 14 to 17 days later.

The major concerns with rubella are the consequences of maternal infection during pregnancy. Infection occurring during the first 12 weeks of pregnancy carries the greatest risk of fetal defects. Rubella infection rapidly spreads to all fetal organ systems and may cause congenital cataracts and blindness, heart disease, and deafness in infants. Since the initiation of routine rubella immunization and maternal antibody screening, the incidence of rubella infection of the fetus or newborn has declined to 0.01 per 10,000 pregnancies in the United States. A single, subcutaneous rubella vaccine made from attenuated (live) virus grown in human tissue cultures is available and usually very well tolerated.

Immunization: Widespread immunization with MMR has led to a 98% decrease in the incidences of these viral infections. Current recommendations include a two-dose subcutaneous immunization, with the first given at 12 to 15 months of age and the second at 4 to 6 years of age. The overall effectiveness of the MMR vaccine is 92 to 95%. In 2005, the FDA approved the addition of varicella vaccine to the combination, which is known as MMRV (ProQuad). MMRV and MMR use the same dosing schedule.

A single dose of MMR vaccine is recommended for those individuals born after 1957 without contraindication or past history of measles infection or positive immunity. A second dose of MMR is recommended in the following situations: epidemic outbreak or exposure to measles infection, healthcare workers, those traveling internationally, and nonimmune students in postsecondary educational settings.

Although generally well tolerated, several groups are usually excluded from vaccination:

- Pregnant patients or women expecting to be pregnant.
- Patients who are immunosuppressed; however, MMR can be given to individuals living in the same setting with asymptomatic HIV disease and individuals with mild immunosuppression.
- Individuals who have received any vaccine in the previous 4 weeks
- People with a severe, life-threatening allergy to any portion of the vaccine or to neomycin.

CONNECTIONS: Patient Safety

Adequate Patient History to Avoid Adverse Effects

A nurse new to working in the outpatient clinic is preparing an MMR injection for a patient who has just moved to the United States and was not vaccinated previously. The nurse-mentor assigned to the new nurse asks if the patient's history was taken and the nurse replies, "Yes, and there is no history of vaccination." What else should be assessed in the history before administering the MMR injection?

Adverse reactions to MMR vaccination are minimal and include fever and lymphadenopathy, rare encephalitis (one occurrence per 1 million vaccinations), and arthralgia in adults. MMR is now available in an aerosolized formulation that has fewer associated adverse effects and an improved immunogenicity as compared to the injected forms.

Polio

Pathophysiology: Poliomyelitis was the leading cause of permanent disability in the era just prior to vaccines. Highly contagious polio epidemics in the 1800s and early 1900s prompted the search for, and eventual discovery of, vaccines. The virus replicates in the gastrointestinal tract and is spread by the oral–fecal route via contaminated food and water.

Over 90% of those exposed to the poliovirus are asymptomatic. Rarely (less than 1%), the virus reaches the motor tracts of the spinal cord, where it leads to the development of flaccid muscle paralysis of the infected motor cells. On rare occasions the respiratory muscles are involved, leading to the need for artificial ventilation. Global immunization has made the disease extremely rare and global eradication is possible.

Immunization: Several vaccines have been developed since 1955, but the inactivated polio vaccine (IPV) has been exclusively used in the United States for the immunization of infants since 2000. Children get four doses of IPV, at 2 months, 4 months, 12 months, and a booster dose at 4 to 6 years. IPV is available as a single suspension or in combination with DTaP, HBV, or influenza vaccines. Routine IM administration of IPV results in redness, swelling, and tenderness at the administration site. Children receiving the complete IPV regimen are provided 99 to 100% lifelong immunity. The vaccine can be given to adults who did not receive the vaccination in childhood.

Varicella Zoster

Pathophysiology: Infection by the varicella zoster virus (VZV) leads to the development of two very different diseases. The initial outbreak of VZV, known as chickenpox (varicella), generally occurs during childhood. Following the initial infection, the virus becomes dormant for 30 to 40 years in nerve roots until it reactivates to cause herpes zoster (HZ), or shingles.

The initial VZV infection is transmitted through inhaled droplets or by direct contact with infectious skin lesions. The virus replicates in the local lymph nodes for several days and then becomes bloodborne. By day 10 to 14, a blistered rash appears, with new lesions opening, draining, and crusting within 24 hours. Intense itching may lead to secondary bacterial infections and permanent scarring. General illness is common in individuals for 5 to 7 days with fever, malaise, and anorexia. Adults with chickenpox have more intense symptoms than children and have a seven times greater risk of encephalitis. Furthermore, women who acquire VZV during pregnancy have a small risk of passing the infection to the fetus, resulting in birth defects.

Following the initial infection, the virus migrates to the spinal nerves, where it may remain dormant for the life of the individual. In about 20% of patients, however, the virus becomes reactivated and causes an HZ infection, or **shingles**, usually after age 50; this increases to approximately 50% for individuals over the age of 85. Shingles often begins with a burning or tingling pain, numbness, or itch in one particular location on the surface of the body. After several days or a week, fluid-filled blisters, similar to chickenpox, appear in one area of the body. Shingles lesions can be very painful and may require up to a month for resolution. In immunocompromised individuals, the infection may be prolonged, taking 3 to 4 weeks for lesion scabbing and several months for complete resolution. Up to 30% of patients with shingles experience a serious form of the disease called **postherpetic neuralgia** in which the pain lasts for years. In about 15% of patients with shingles, the virus infects the eye and can cause blindness.

Antiviral drugs such as acyclovir (Zovirax) are sometimes administered to reduce the severity and duration of a shingles attack and postherpetic neuralgia. Other treatments for postherpetic neuralgia include corticosteroids and nonsteroidal anti-inflammatory drugs.

Immunization: An attenuated or live VZV vaccine (Varivax) has been used in the United States since 1995, and it is estimated that widespread vaccination has reduced the incidence of varicella infection by more than 70%. Current vaccination is especially important for people at high risk for exposure to varicella, including healthcare workers, teachers, childcare workers, residents and staff in nursing homes, college students, international travelers, military personnel, inmates and staff at correctional institutions, and nonpregnant women of childbearing potential.

Current recommendations include a two-dose varicella vaccination schedule for children. There are two varicella products. Varivax contains only the varicella vaccine;

ProQuad consists of the varicella vaccine with the MMR vaccine. The first dose is administered at age 12 to 15 months and the second dose at age 4 to 6 years. The effectiveness of the vaccine varies widely, and 10 to 15% of immunized individuals will still acquire the infection, which is a condition known as breakthrough varicella. Breakthrough varicella infection produces milder symptoms compared to those in nonimmunized patients.

There are two vaccines for shingles. Zostavax is a live vaccine first marketed in 2006 that is being phased out and replaced with Shingrix. The CDC recommends that all people over age 50 receive two doses of Shingrix that are spaced 2 to 6 months apart. Shingrix is 90% effective at preventing the reactivation of VZV for about 4 years. The shingles vaccine is essentially a booster of the VZV vaccine administered to prevent chickenpox. It is not effective at treating symptoms of shingles or postherpetic neuralgia once they develop.

Adverse effects associated with VZV vaccine include low-grade fever, tenderness at the injection site, and rash localized to the injection site. Finally, the administration of this vaccine in immunosuppressed patients may increase the incidence of adverse effects or cause a decrease in developed immunity.

PharmFACT

Approximately 95% of adults in the United States have antibodies to the VZV, indicating prior exposure to and reactivation of this pathogen. About 4% of patients develop a recurrent episode later in life, usually as a result of immunosuppression (Janniger, 2020).

Human Papillomavirus

Pathogenesis: Genital HPV, the most common sexually transmitted infection (STI) in the United States, is associated with a higher risk of cervical cancer, which is a significant cause of cancer deaths in women. Although there are over 100 different forms of HPV, only seven are associated with cervical cancer. HPV is also associated with an elevated risk of other cancers, including vaginal, vulvar, and anal. Some types of HPV are responsible for causing genital warts. The virus infects both males and females, and it may be transmitted from mother to child during vaginal delivery. It is estimated that HPV vaccination can prevent up to 90% of HPV-associated cancers.

Spread through sexual contact, HPV infection may be asymptomatic or lead to the development of a low-grade infection that resolves spontaneously in people with a healthy immune system. A high-grade HPV infection may lead to the development of dysplasia, a precancerous change in the cervical cells that is directly related to the viral infection.

Immunization: The HPV vaccine (Gardasil-9) was created using recombinant DNA technology. The vaccine is noninfectious and prepared from purified virus-like particles containing only proteins from the coat of the virus, rather than a complete attenuated virus. The HPV vaccine is intended to prevent cervical, vulvar, and vaginal cancer and certain precancerous lesions in women. In men and women, the HPV vaccine is indicated to prevent genital warts caused by HPV. It is not effective against existing cancers or genital diseases not caused by HPV.

The CDC (2019) recommends the routine vaccination of boys and girls at 11 to 12 years of age. The HPV vaccine is

CONNECTIONS: Advanced Practice Application

The Need for the HPV Vaccination

Case

James and Janice are 15-year-old twins who are freshmen in high school and live with their parents. They present to the community clinic for a sports physical. They are both excited to try out for their school basketball team.

While taking their health history separately, you determine that neither twin has much knowledge about STIs. They understand that engaging in sex can result in pregnancy, but do not know much more about STIs. They show very little understanding of how STIs are contracted and how they can be avoided. When asked about what they learned in high school health class or at home about HPV, both said they had never heard of it or that it could cause cancer. You individually educated the twins about HPV and the risks and the benefits of the HPV vaccine. Should both Janice and James be encouraged to get the HPV vaccine?

Discussion

The CDC recommends HPV vaccination for boys and girls at age 11 or 12. HPV is the most common STI in the United States and, according to the CDC (2019), 50% of all sexually active men and women will get it at some point in their lives. Most HPV infections do not cause any symptoms, but some may result in cervical cancer, the second-leading cause of cancer deaths among women worldwide. Men and women can contract and transmit HPV to sexual partners.

HPV is responsible for more than 90% of anal and cervical cancers, about 70% of vaginal and vulvar cancers, more than 60% of penile cancers, and about 70% of cancers of the oropharynx may be linked to HPV. The oropharynx is uniquely susceptible to HPV and HPV-related tumors, which have increased more than 300% over the last 20 years (Näsman et al., 2019).

Nurses and nurse practitioners have been identified by many young adults as approachable and informative resources regarding HPV vaccination and STIs in general (Bellia-Weiss et al., 2013). More information about teen vaccines can be found at the CDC website.

administered as a two-dose series of IM injections with the second dose given 6 to 12 months after the first. The vaccine has close to 100% effectiveness in preventing HPV infection and appears to offer long-lasting protection. For those receiving their first vaccination at age 15 years and older, a three-dose series is recommended. Vaccinations after age 26 provide less benefit because people have already been exposed to HPV prior to that age. The vaccine is not recommended during pregnancy. Mild adverse effects include pain, swelling, and redness at the injection site.

Rotavirus

Pathophysiology: Approximately 680,000 children die worldwide each year from rotavirus infection, mostly in developing countries. Although the virus rarely causes death in the United States, it is estimated that nearly every child is infected by age 5 and that most will experience gastroenteritis, resulting in severe diarrhea and dehydration. Viral replication of the rotavirus occurs only in mature red blood cells (RBCs) found in the tips of the intestinal villi, leading to a strictly oral–fecal means of viral transmission.

Immunization: There are two rotavirus vaccines, and both are administered by putting drops in the infant's mouth. RotaTeq is given in three doses, at 2, 4, and 6 months of age. Rotarix is given in two doses at 2 and 4 months of age. The CDC recommends rotavirus vaccine be administered before 15 weeks of age for the prevention of gastroenteritis. The vaccines reduce the overall incidence of gastroenteritis by 74% and of hospitalization due to the virus by 96%. Most infants experience no side effects, but a few may develop mild cases of diarrhea and vomiting.

Passive Immunity

43.7 Antibodies are administered to provide passive immunity.

Passive immunization is very different from active immunization. Whereas active immunity requires mobilization of the patient's immune response, which leads to the development of memory cells, passive immunity is the administration of preformed antibodies (immunoglobulins). During passive immunity, the immune system is not activated and memory cells are not produced.

Passive immunization is typically used to provide immediate protection against a recent infection, a potential infection, or a disease in progress. Several examples serve to illustrate the benefits of passive immunization:

- Someone has just been bitten by a potentially rabid dog. It will take several days to determine if the dog is infected with rabies.
- An individual has been in a motorcycle crash and sustained serious trauma. He has never had a tetanus vaccination.
- A student nurse has learned that she has been exposed to blood from a patient with confirmed HBV. She has not been vaccinated for HBV.

What do these three scenarios have in common? First, immediate treatment is indicated because the consequences of infection can be serious or fatal. The disease would have the opportunity to create serious illness before a vaccine activates an immune response. In these cases, antibodies against the infection can be administered to provide immediate prevention against rabies, tetanus, or HBV infection. Antibodies are sometimes given concurrently with the vaccine series to provide complete immunity against the disease. For example, following an exposure to rabies, the patient is given rabies immunoglobulin as well as the rabies vaccine.

The preceding scenarios illustrate a second message of importance to the nurse. If the patients had kept their tetanus and HBV vaccinations up to date, they would have developed active immunity to these pathogens and there would be no need to provide passive immunity.

A second indication for the use of passive immunity is for situations where the activation of the immune system and the development of memory are not desirable. In this case, the individual is given the antibodies against the foreign agent and the immune system does not mount a response. The administration of RhoGAM is an example of this type of indication.

Table 43.3 lists selected immunoglobulin preparations. Pharmacotherapy Illustrated 43.1 shows the development of immunity through vaccines or the administration of antibodies.

PROTOTYPE DRUG **Rho(D) Immune Globulin (RhoGAM)**

Classification **Therapeutic:** Immunizing agent (passive)
Pharmacologic: Antibody, immunoglobulin

Therapeutic Effects and Uses: Erythrocytes contain two types of surface antigens that are used to designate the blood type. The first identifier is ABO; the presence or absence of antigen A and antigen B will determine the blood type as A, B, AB, or O. A second identifier on the cell membrane of the RBC is the Rhesus factor, or Rh antigen. If the antigen is present, the individual is said to be Rh positive (Rh^+) and if it is missing, Rh negative (Rh^-); 85% of individuals living in North America are Rh positive.

Erythroblastosis fetalis (EF), or hemolytic disease of the newborn, is a disorder that was first described in 1940 and

Table 43.3 Immunoglobulin Preparations

Drug	Route and Adult Dose (Maximum Dose Where Indicated)	Adverse Effects
cytomegalovirus immune globulin (Cytogam)	IV: 150 mg/kg within 72 h of transplantation; then 100 mg/kg for 2, 4, 6, and 8 wk post-transplant; then 50 mg/kg for 12 and 16 wk post-transplant	*Local reactions at the injection site (pain, erythema, myalgia), flulike symptoms (malaise, fever, chills), headache, joint stiffness* Anaphylaxis, nephrotoxicity, thrombosis
hepatitis B immune globulin (HBIG)	IM: 0.06 mL/kg as soon as possible after exposure, preferably within 24 h, but no later than 7 days; repeat 28–30 days after exposure	
immune globulin infusion and hyaluronidase (HyQvia)	Subcutaneous: Start with 7.5 g and increase over 7 wk to 30 g, then 300–600 mg/kg at 3- to 4-wk intervals	
immune globulin intravenous (Carimune, Gammagard, IGIV, Octagam)	IV: 100–400 mg/kg per month IM: 1.2 mL/kg followed by 0.6 mL/kg q2–4wk	
rabies immune globulin (HyperRAB, Imogam Rabies-HT, Kedrab)	IM: 20 units/kg as a single dose with rabies vaccine	
Rho(D) immune globulin (RhoGAM)	IM/IV: 1 vial or 300 mcg at 28 wk, followed by 1 vial of mini-dose or 120 mcg within 72 h of delivery if infant is Rh^+	
tetanus immune globulin (HyperTET S/D)	IM: 250–6,000 units for prophylaxis	
varicella zoster immune globulin (VariZIG)	IM: 62.5–625 international units	

Note: *Italics* indicate common adverse effects. Underline indicates serious adverse effects.

is caused by an Rh incompatibility between the mother and her fetus. This condition can occur only if the mother is Rh^-.

EF does not occur with the first pregnancy because the two types of RBC (Rh^- mother and Rh^+ child) are separated by the placenta and the blood is not physically exchanged. At birth, however, their blood mixes and the mother's immune system reacts by producing antibodies against the foreign Rh^+ antigen. The presence of circulating antibodies against the Rh antigen creates a potential risk for an Rh incompatibility in future pregnancies. If in a subsequent

Pharmacotherapy Illustrated 43.1

Mechanisms of Active and Passive Immunity

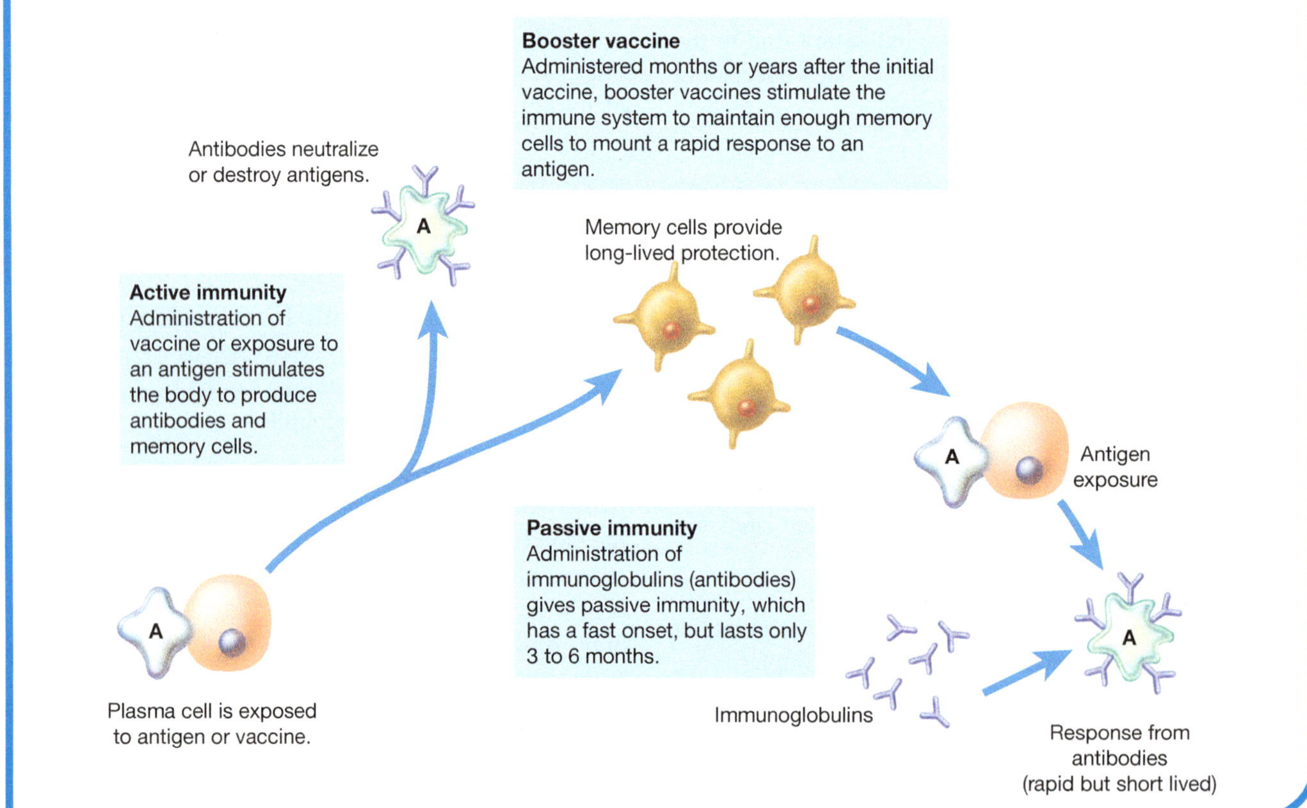

pregnancy the fetus is Rh^+, the mother's antibodies against the Rh^+ antigen will cross the placenta and destroy erythrocytes in the fetus. This may lead to severe anemia or brain damage in the developing fetus and even fetal death.

Rho immunoglobulins are obtained from filtered human serum for the prevention of Rh incompatibility in Rh^- women. This drug has been used to provide passive immunity since 1968 and has significantly reduced the incidence of EF. Administration of Rho immunoglobulins will prevent the mother from forming Rh antibodies, so that there will be no risk of incompatibility in subsequent pregnancies. Rho(D) immune globulin prophylaxis is not indicated if either the father or the fetus is Rho(D) negative.

The administration of RhoGAM is recommended:

- At 26 to 28 weeks' gestation
- An additional dose within 72 hours postpartum if baby is Rh^+
- Within 3 hours of spontaneous or induced pregnancy termination
- Following any event that could lead to transplacental hemorrhage (such as amniocentesis, chorionic villi sampling, or abdominal trauma).

Mechanism of Action: Rho(D) antibodies act by suppressing the immune response of Rh^- mothers to Rh^+ fetuses or newborns. Sensitization to Rho(D)-positive blood in future pregnancies is therefore less likely to occur.

Pharmacokinetics:

Route(s)	IM, IV
Absorption	Unknown
Distribution	Unknown
Primary metabolism	Unknown
Primary excretion	Unknown
Onset of action	Peak antibody levels: 2 h (IV) or 5–10 days (IM)
Duration of action	Half-life: 24–30 days

Adverse Effects: The most commonly reported adverse reactions include local swelling, redness, and mild pain at the injection site. A small number of patients experience low-grade fever. Hypersensitivity reactions are rare and may include hives, generalized urticaria, tightness of the chest, wheezing, hypotension, and anaphylaxis. Also rarely reported are anemia, anorexia, bruising, disseminated intravascular coagulation (DIC), dyspnea, dysuria, edema, hematuria, hemolysis, hypertension, increased risk of bleeding, lower back pain, malaise, nausea and vomiting, polydipsia, and weight gain.

Contraindications/Precautions: This drug is contraindicated in individuals with a history of hypersensitivity reaction to human immunoglobulin injection. Rho(D) antibodies are also contraindicated in patients having immunoglobulin A deficiencies or in patients with severe anemia and should be used with caution in patients who have disseminated intravascular coagulation, hemolysis, renal disease, and splenectomy.

Drug Interactions: No drug interactions have been reported. **Herbal/Food:** Unknown.

Pregnancy: Animal reproduction studies have not been conducted with this drug. No significant adverse effects have been found in breastfed infants.

Treatment of Overdose: Overdose with this drug has not been reported.

Clinician Responsibilities: Key clinical implications for patients receiving Rho(D) immune globulin are included in Applied Clinical Judgment: Patients Receiving Immunizations.

Drugs Similar to Rho(D) Immune Globulin (RhoGAM)

Other immunoglobulins include cytomegalovirus immune globulin, hepatitis B immune globulin, and IV immune globulin. For the three immunoglobulins discussed below, adverse effects on the fetus or on the breastfed infant are unknown. Other products include anthrax immune globulin (Anthrasil), botulism immune globulin (BabyBIG), and vaccinia immune globulin (Cnj-016).

Cytomegalovirus immune globulin (CytoGam): About half of the U.S. adult population has been exposed to cytomegalovirus (CMV). Few people, however, have experienced symptoms because healthy immune systems prevent symptomatic, active infections. When donating organs or tissues, CMV may be inadvertently transferred to a transplant recipient with a suppressed immune system. Cytomegalovirus immune globulin is recommended for the prevention of CMV infections in at-risk individuals receiving kidney, liver, pancreas, and heart transplants. The drug can lower the incidence of serious CMV-associated disease by 50%. Current dosage recommendations include the IV administration of seven doses, beginning within 72 hours of the receipt of the organ and ending 30 days later. The most common adverse effects are minor and include flushing, chills, muscle cramps, back pain, fever, nausea and vomiting, arthralgia, and wheezing.

Hepatitis B immune globulin (HBIG): The goal of HBIG administration is to prevent the transmission of HBV to those who have been exposed to the virus. The administration of HBIG is recommended for the following instances:

- Nonimmunized individuals who have had acute and significant exposure to HBV-infected blood. This includes unintentional needlestick, oral ingestion, or direct mucous membrane contact with infected blood or blood products. One dose is usually given immediately after exposure and another dose 1 month later. The administration of HBIG is effective in the prevention of clinical HBV infection in approximately 75% of individuals who are treated.

- Infants born to women infected with HBV. These infants should receive HBIG and start the HBV vaccine series within 12 hours of birth. This regimen is 70 to 90% effective in preventing infection in the infant.
- Sexual partners of HBV-infected patients. A single dose of HBIG is 75% effective at preventing HBV infection if the drug is administered within 2 weeks of sexual contact.
- Household exposure of infants less than 12 months of age who are born to a mother or have a primary caregiver who is infected with HBV. These infants should receive HBIG and start the HBV vaccine series before 12 months of age.

The administration of HBIG is effective in the prevention of clinical HBV infection in approximately 75% of individuals who are treated, but this immune protection is temporary, lasting approximately 2 to 3 months. HBIG is usually given concurrently (different IM site) with hepatitis immunization in infants born of HBV-infected mothers. Adverse reactions to HBIG are rare and include injection-site reactions such as tenderness, redness, and swelling. Hypersensitivity reactions have also been reported. HBIG is provided in a prefilled, single-dose syringe in either pediatric or adult preparations. It is not known if this drug causes adverse effects on the fetus or on the breastfed infant.

Immune globulin intravenous (Carimune, Gammagard, IGIV, Octagam): Immune globulin contains pooled antibodies obtained from human plasma that is used to provide passive immunity following exposure to an organism for which no active immunization exists, when there is inadequate time to develop active immunity, and as replacement therapy for those with antibody deficiencies. IGIV contains 95% or more immunoglobulin G. The passive immunity induced by IGIV is capable of attenuating or preventing a wide range of infectious diseases and adverse effects from toxins, mycoplasma, parasites, bacteria, and viruses. IGIV may be thought of as a "generic" treatment for balancing immune systems. It contains components that strengthen immune function as well as substances that can suppress overactive immune systems. Disease protection lasts for 3 weeks or longer. Because this drug contains antibodies to live viruses, active vaccinations should not be given until 3 to 5 months after IGIV has been administered. Two newer immune globulin medications indicated for primary immunodeficiency in adults include Cutaquig and Xembify.

CONNECTIONS: APPLIED CLINICAL JUDGMENT

Patients Receiving Immunizations

Key Assessment Data

- Obtain baseline vital signs, especially temperature; previous history of the actual disease (e.g., chickenpox); history of hepatic, renal, cardiovascular, neurologic, or autoimmune disease, HIV infection, fever or active infections; pregnancy or breastfeeding; previous allergic response to immunizations or allergies to products contained within immunization (e.g., sensitivity to yeast, eggs, or albumin products), previous drug history, especially the use of immunosuppressants or corticosteroids.
- Ongoing assessment during drug therapy should include monitoring appropriate laboratory findings (e.g., CBC, hepatic and renal laboratory values); patient adherence to the recommended immunization schedule (e.g., need for repeated immunizations, boosters in adults).

Desired Therapeutic Outcomes

Improvement is observed and measurable by adherence to recommended immunization schedule appropriate for age; if drawn, titers demonstrate immune levels.

Minimizing Adverse Effects

- Immunizations may cause dermatologic, cardiovascular, and neurologic adverse effects. Increase in temperature, localized ulcerations, signs of infection at the injection site, tachycardia, palpitations, dizziness, or changes in level of consciousness may indicate significant adverse effects. Report all significant adverse effects to the healthcare provider for reporting to VAERS.
- Immediately report any fever over 38°C or as instructed by the healthcare provider, changes in consciousness such as drowsiness or disorientation, dyspnea, tachycardia, or palpitations.
- Neurologic changes may indicate adverse drug effects. Assess for changes in level of consciousness, disorientation, confusion, or tremors.
- Avoid or defer immunizations in any patient with a fever or autoimmune disease or who take corticosteroids as immune response to the vaccine may result in less than the desired immunity or an increased risk of adverse effects.
- Bacillus Calmette-Guérin (BCG) stimulates immunity to the tuberculin, and recent vaccination may cause an adverse reaction to purified protein derivative (PPD) injection or result in a false-positive reaction. Other testing may be warranted. Assess patients for previous use of BCG vaccine and consult with the healthcare provider before giving PPD skin testing for TB.

Lifespan Considerations

- Pregnancy is a contraindication for vaccination with live viruses, and women who become pregnant within 3 months of immunization with a live vaccine should consult their healthcare provider.
- Pregnancy should be avoided during and for up to 4 months after discontinuing immunosuppressive therapy. Women who become pregnant while on the drug should consult with their healthcare provider.

Diversity Considerations

- For religious or other reasons, some patients may refuse to accept administration of any component derived from human blood or serum, including Rho[D] immune globulin.

CONNECTIONS: APPLIED CLINICAL JUDGMENT *(continued)*

Patients Receiving Immunizations

Patient Education

- Coordinate vaccination schedules with healthcare provider to remain current on vaccinations.
- Keep vaccination records and copy records if needed for school or work situations but retain the originals.
- Older adults should consult with their healthcare provider to arrange having titers drawn to confirm immunity and the need for booster vaccinations.
- Acetaminophen may be utilized for low-grade fevers of less than 38°C, for localized tenderness, or for minor arthralgias and malaise. Cool compresses to the injection site may help alleviate malaise, fever, or injection-site soreness.
- Immediately report any fever over 38°C or as instructed by the healthcare provider, changes in consciousness such as drowsiness or disorientation, dyspnea, tachycardia, or palpitations.
- Alert the healthcare provider to any home situation that may require deferral of live vaccinations before the vaccination is given.
- Women who are pregnant or who may become pregnant within the first 3 months after vaccination should return to the healthcare provider for follow-up.
- Previous use of BCG may result in a false-positive tuberculosis test or an unusual reaction to the PPD test. Other testing may be required to confirm or refute current infection.

Prescribing Considerations

- Severely immunocompromised persons should not receive live vaccines.
- Pregnant women should not receive live, attenuated virus vaccines.
- Persons who experienced encephalopathy within 7 days after administration of a previous dose of pertussis-containing vaccine not attributable to another identifiable cause should not receive additional doses of a vaccine that contains pertussis.
- After vaccination advise the patient to not donate blood without first checking for eligibility with the blood bank or healthcare provider.

Understanding Chapter 43

Key Concepts Summary

43.1 The eradication of smallpox was a great triumph in modern medicine.

43.2 Vaccines are used to activate the immune system for the purpose of disease prevention.

43.3 Five methods are used to produce vaccines.

43.4 Vaccines should be administered by an established schedule with precautions taken for patients who are immunosuppressed or pregnant.

43.5 Active immunity can be induced to prevent bacterial infections.

43.6 Effective vaccines that prevent viral infections have been developed.

43.7 Antibodies are administered to provide passive immunity.

CASE STUDY: Making the Patient Connection

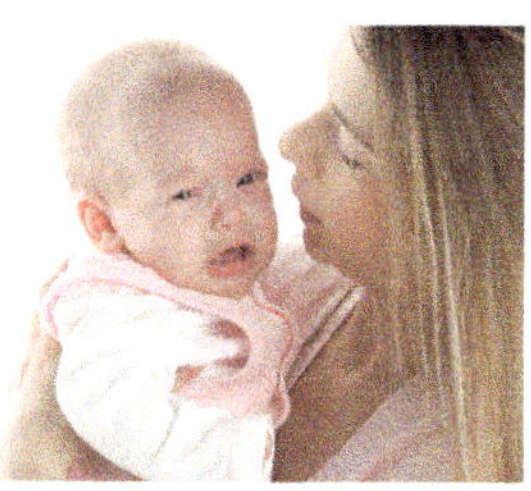

Remember the patient "Samantha Abbott" at the beginning of the chapter? Now read the remainder of the case study. Based on the information presented within this chapter, respond to the critical thinking questions that follow.

Mr. and Mrs. Abbott arrive in the office where you work with their 4-month-old infant, Samantha, for her checkup. She is scheduled to receive the following immunizations today: DTaP, Hib, PCV, and IPV. Samantha's mother states, "I don't think these immunizations are necessary. Don't these shots usually make children sick?"

As first-time parents, Mr. and Mrs. Abbott are new to the experience of childhood immunizations and require careful teaching. While obtaining her history, you find that 4-month-old Samantha has been doing well and is in the 90th percentile for height and 89th percentile for weight. She has achieved the developmental milestones for her age, is bright, and interacts well with her environment.

Critical Thinking Questions

1. What information should you obtain from the Abbotts about Samantha's first response to immunization?
2. Why is it important to discuss the potential adverse effects of vaccines with Samantha's parents?
3. What educational information should be given to the Abbotts?

Additional Case Study

As a nurse working in the intensive care unit, today you are assigned to care for a critically ill patient who is known to be HIV positive and hepatitis B and C positive. You are cleaning up after assisting a first-year resident with the insertion of a central line and, as you are putting the disposable drapes into the trash, you feel a sharp pain in your right hand. As you pull your hand away you see a needle pushed through the glove into your hand. You report the incident to your supervisor and report to the emergency department (ED) per exposure protocol.

The ED physician orders you to have antibody testing for anti-HBsAg, to have baseline HIV testing, and to receive gamma globulin and antiviral prophylaxis.

1. What is the rationale for the HBV testing?
2. What is the rationale for the HIV testing?
3. Why is gamma globulin ordered?
4. Why is antiviral prophylaxis appropriate?

Chapter Review

1. Mary is a 4-month-old infant who is brought to the clinic for her first checkup. Her mother tells the nurse that the child has never been ill. Which factor would the nurse consider most significant in assessing the baby's likelihood of receiving immunizations?
    1. Allergies to previously administered medications
    2. Mother's preconceptions and reservations relating to vaccines
    3. Maternal and paternal allergies or reactions to vaccine administration
    4. The nurse's knowledge of the recommended pediatric immunization schedule
2. The nurse is preparing to administer an MMR vaccination to a 15-month-old child. What would cause the nurse to hold the injection and recheck this order with the provider?
    1. The mother tells the nurse that the family will be going to the beach for the next few weeks.
    2. The mother states that she was told that she had a reaction to the injection when she was a child.
    3. The mother tells the nurse that her husband is having chemotherapy for Hodgkin's lymphoma.
    4. The mother tells the nurse that the child's older brother is home with a cold.
3. A 7-year-old girl, who was bitten by a stray dog, is treated in the ED. The dog has not been tested to rule out rabies. The nurse will anticipate that this patient will receive which immunizations? (Select all that apply.)
    1. Tetanus toxoid
    2. DTaP vaccine
    3. Rabies immunoglobulin
    4. Rabies vaccine
    5. Rabies toxoid
4. The nurse determines that the patient understands the teaching given for care required after receiving a tetanus toxoid injection when the patient states:
    1. "I will keep my arm still for the next 24 hours to give the vaccine time to absorb."
    2. "I will limit my fluid intake for the next 8 hours in case I have nausea."
    3. "I will avoid crowds and people with viruses for the next 7 days."
    4. "I will take some acetaminophen (Tylenol) or ibuprofen (Advil) if my arm is sore."
5. The occupational health nurse will be administering HBV vaccine to a new employee. Which assessment finding discovered by the nurse would necessitate withholding the injection? The patient is:
    1. A two-pack-per-day smoker.
    2. Known to have transient hypertension.
    3. Allergic to yeast and yeast products.
    4. Frightened by needles and injections.

6. A postpartum patient received Rho(D) immune globulin (RhoGAM) therapy after the delivery of an 8-lb baby boy. The nurse performs what important intervention during the course of this treatment?
   1. Monitors the patient for 20 minutes following the administration for hypersensitivity reaction.
   2. Evaluates the laboratory results for thrombocytopenia, anemia, and increased liver enzymes.
   3. Provides the patient with the information needed to maintain a low-saturated-fat, low-cholesterol diet.
   4. Instructs the patient to use nonmedicated sugar-free lozenges or hard candies to relieve a cough.

See Appendix A for answers to critical thinking questions, case study questions, and review questions.

References

Bellia-Weiss, T., Parsons, M., Sebach, A. M., & Rockelli, L. A. (2013). Promoting HPV prevention in the school setting. *NASN School Nurse, 28*, 86–93. https://doi.org/10.1177/1942602X12463249

Centers for Disease Control and Prevention (CDC). (2016). *Guidelines for vaccinating pregnant women.* http://www.cdc.gov/vaccines/pregnancy/hcp/guidelines.html#modalIdString_CDCTable_0

Centers for Disease Control and Prevention (CDC). (2019). *Human papilloma virus: HPV fact sheet.* http://www.cdc.gov/std/HPV/STDFact-HPV.htm#a5

Centers for Disease Control and Prevention (CDC). (2020a). *Influenza (flu) 2020-2021 ACIP summary.* https://www.cdc.gov/flu/professionals/acip/summary/summary-recommendations.htm

Centers for Disease Control and Prevention (CDC). (2020c). *Viral hepatitis: Q&As for health professionals.* https://www.cdc.gov/hepatitis/hbv/hbvfaq.htm#D4

Janniger, C. K. (2020). *Herpes zoster.* Medscape. http://emedicine.medscape.com/article/1132465-overview

Näsman, A., Du, J., & Dalianis, T. (2019). A global epidemic increase of an HPV-induced tonsil and tongue base cancer – potential benefit from a pan-gender use of HPV vaccine. *Journal of Internal Medicine, 287*(2), 134–152. https://doi.org/10.1111/joim.13010

Nelson, N. P., Weng, M. K., Hofmeister, M. G., Moore, K. L., Doshani, M., Kamili, S., et al. Prevention of hepatitis A virus infection in the United States: Recommendations of the Advisory Committee on Immunization Practices, 2020. *MMWR Recommendations and Reports, 69*(No. RR-5), 1–38. http://dx.doi.org/10.15585/mmwr.rr6905a1 external icon.

Selected Bibliography

Anderson, P., & Bryson, J. (2020). Confronting vaccine hesitancy: What nurses need to know. *Nursing2020, 50*(8), 43–46. https://doi.org/10.1097/01.NURSE.0000668436.83267.29

Ball, J. W., Bindler, R. C., Cowen, K., & Shaw, R. (2017). *Pediatric nursing: Caring for children* (7th ed.). Pearson.

Brooks, M. (2020). *HPV vaccination rates nearly double in young adults: CDC.* Medscape. https://www.medscape.com/viewarticle/923466

Centers for Disease Control and Prevention (CDC). (2015). *Parent's guide to childhood immunizations.* https://www.cdc.gov/vaccines/parents/tools/parents-guide/downloads/parents-guide-508.pdf

Centers for Disease Control and Prevention (CDC). (2017). *Smallpox.* http://www.cdc.gov/smallpox/index.html

Centers for Disease Control and Prevention (CDC). (2018). *HPV and oropharyngeal cancer.* https://www.cdc.gov/cancer/hpv/basic_info/hpv_oropharyngeal.htm

Centers for Disease Control and Prevention (CDC). (2020a). *ACIP vaccine recommendations.* http://www.cdc.gov/vaccines/hcp/acip-recs/index.html

Centers for Disease Control and Prevention (CDC). (2020b). *Travelers' health.* http://wwwnc.cdc.gov/travel

Centers for Disease Control and Prevention (CDC). (2020c). *Vaccines and immunizations.* https://www.cdc.gov/vaccines/index.html

Geoghegan, S., O'Callaghan, K. P., & Offit, P. A. (2020). Vaccine safety: Myths and misinformation. *Frontiers in Microbiology, 11*, 372. https://doi.org/10.3389/fmicb.2020.00372

Vaccine Adverse Event Reporting System (VAERS). (n.d.). *Vaccine event reporting system.* U.S. Department of Health and Human Services. https://vaers.hhs.gov/index

Williams, L. (2019). Role of the pediatric nurse practitioner in enhancing vaccination rates. *AACN Advanced Critical Care, 30*(3), 278–281. https://doi.org/10.4037/aacnacc2019992

Unit 7

Pharmacology of the Respiratory System and Allergy

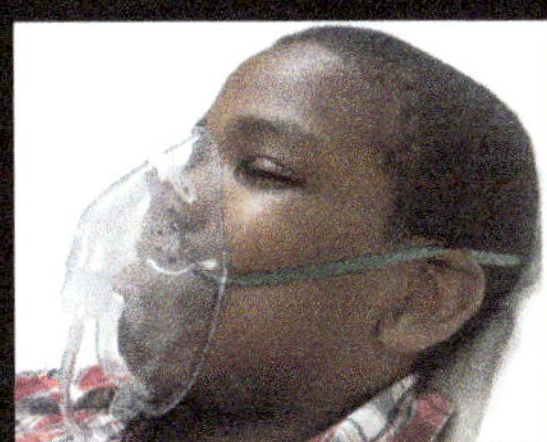

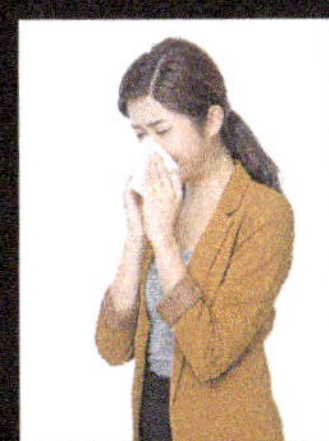

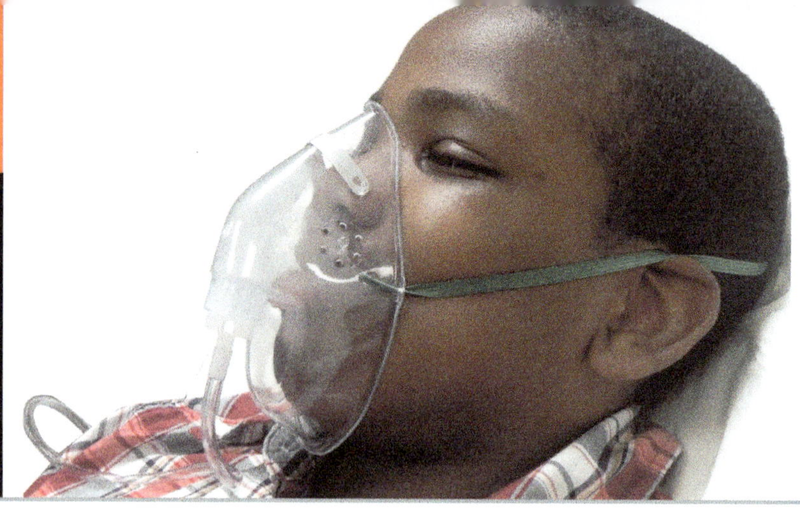

"I really hope my asthma gets under control. I want to try out for the swim team this fall."
—*Patient "Nathan Almond"*

Chapter 44
Pharmacotherapy of Asthma and Other Pulmonary Disorders

Chapter Outline

Learning Outcomes

After reading this chapter, the student should be able to:

1. Identify the anatomic structures associated with the lower respiratory tract and their functions.
2. Explain how the autonomic nervous system regulates airway diameter.
3. Explain the role of inflammation and bronchospasm in the pathogenesis of asthma.
4. Compare the advantages and disadvantages of using the inhalation route of drug administration for pulmonary drugs.
5. Describe the types of devices used to deliver aerosol therapies via the inhalation route.
6. Explain the three basic principles of asthma management recommended by the National Asthma Education and Prevention Program.
7. Compare and contrast the indications for pharmacotherapy with the short- versus long-acting beta-adrenergic agonists.
8. Describe the nurse's role in the pharmacologic management of lower respiratory tract disorders.
9. For each of the classes shown in the chapter outline, identify the prototype and representative drugs and explain the mechanism(s) of drug action, primary indications, contraindications, significant drug interactions, pregnancy data, and important adverse effects.
10. Apply clinical judgment to care for patients receiving pharmacotherapy for lower respiratory tract disorders.

Key Terms Definitions of the terms in bold may be found in the Glossary.

The flow of oxygen, carbon dioxide, and other gases in and out of the human body is in constant flux. Minute-by-minute control of the airways is necessary to bring an adequate supply of oxygen to the pulmonary capillaries and to rid the body of some of its most toxic waste products. Any restriction in this dynamic flow, even for brief periods, may result in serious consequences. This chapter examines drugs used in the pharmacotherapy of two primary pulmonary disorders: asthma and chronic obstructive pulmonary disease (COPD).

Physiology of the Lower Respiratory Tract

44.1 The physiology of the respiratory system involves two main processes: perfusion and ventilation.

The primary function of the respiratory system is to bring oxygen into the body and to remove carbon dioxide. The process by which these gases are exchanged is called *respiration*. The basic structures of the lower respiratory tract are shown in Figure 44.1.

Blood flow through the lung is called **pulmonary perfusion**. The bronchial tree ends in microscopic sacs called *alveoli*, which have no smooth muscle and inflate like balloons during inspiration. The alveoli are abundantly rich in capillaries. An extremely thin membrane in the alveoli separates the inspired air from the pulmonary capillaries, allowing gases to readily move between the internal environment of the blood and the inspired air. As oxygen crosses this membrane to enter the bloodstream, it is exchanged for carbon dioxide, which is a cellular waste product that leaves the bloodstream to enter the alveoli. The process of gas exchange is illustrated in Figure 44.1.

Ventilation is the process of moving air into and out of the lungs. As the diaphragm contracts and lowers in position, it creates a negative pressure that draws air into the lungs and inspiration occurs. During expiration the diaphragm relaxes and air leaves the lungs passively. Ventilation is a purely mechanical process that occurs approximately 12 to 18 times per minute in adults. This rate is determined by neurons in the brainstem and may be modified by a number of factors, including emotions, fever, stress, and the pH of the blood.

One of the most important factors that affect ventilation is the size of the thousands of tubes or passageways leading from the outside to the alveoli, collectively known as the airways. The nervous system controls ventilation by changing the diameter of the airways, specifically the very small and abundant bronchioles.

Bronchioles are muscular, elastic, tubular structures whose diameter, or lumen, varies with the contraction or relaxation of bronchiolar smooth muscle. Bronchodilation allows air to enter the alveoli more freely, thus increasing the supply of oxygen to the body's tissues during periods

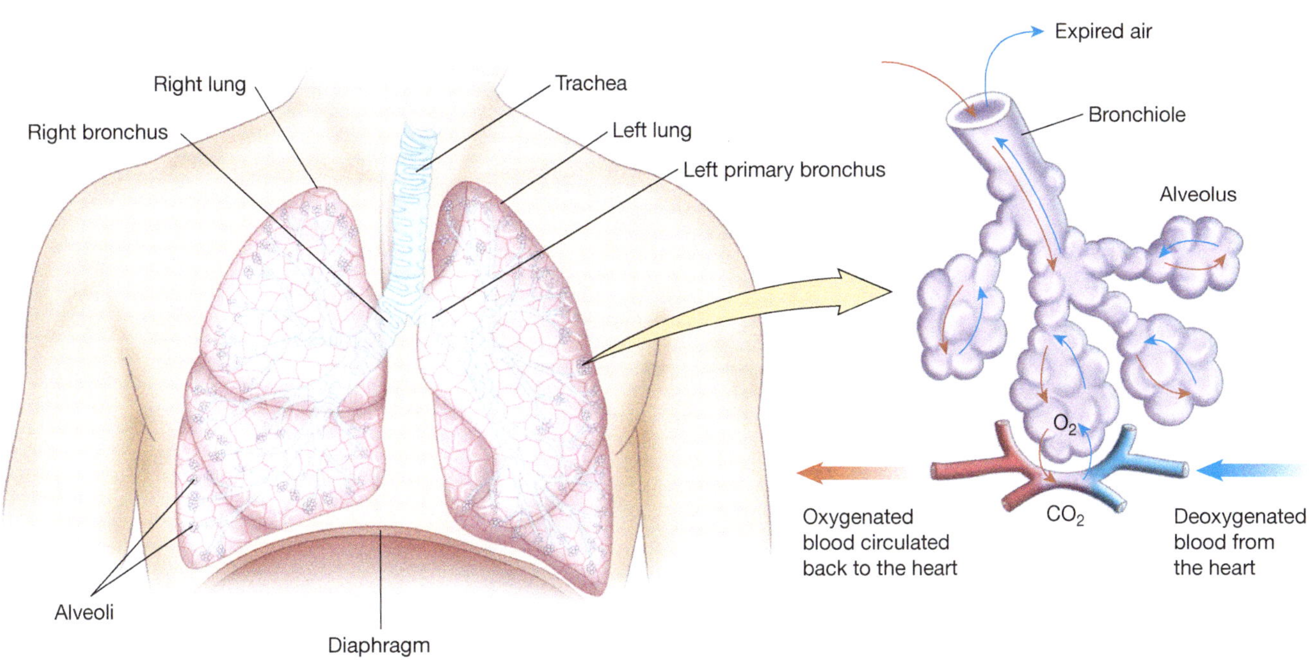

Figure 44.1 The lower respiratory tract and the process of gas exchange.

of exercise. Bronchoconstriction increases airway resistance, resulting in less airflow. Bronchodilation and bronchoconstriction are largely regulated by the two branches of the autonomic nervous system:

- The *sympathetic branch* activates $beta_2$-adrenergic receptors, causing bronchiolar smooth muscle to relax, the airway diameter to increase, and bronchodilation to occur.
- The *parasympathetic branch* causes bronchiolar smooth muscle to contract, the airway diameter to narrow, and bronchoconstriction to occur.

In practical terms, drugs that enhance bronchodilation enable the patient to breathe easier. In contrast, drugs causing bronchoconstriction result in more labored breathing and shortness of breath in the patient.

Bronchoconstriction is a common indication for pharmacotherapy. It may occur through several mechanisms, and the choice of pharmacotherapy will differ depending on the mechanism. The airways may narrow due to **bronchospasm**, a sudden contraction of the smooth muscle of the airways that causes acute dyspnea. Drug treatment for bronchospasm is targeted at immediately relaxing the smooth muscle spasm. A second mechanism of bronchoconstriction is the production of thick, viscous secretions that plug up the airways. Depending on the cause, treatment may involve antibiotics for an infection or drugs that break up viscous secretions (mucolytics). A third mechanism of bronchoconstriction is edema that is caused by engorgement of the pulmonary blood vessels. Treatment may include diuretics and drugs to enhance cardiac function.

Pathophysiology of Asthma

44.2 Asthma is a chronic disease that has both inflammatory and bronchospasm components.

Asthma is one of the most common chronic conditions in the United States, and it is increasing at an alarming rate. Asthma affects almost 25 million Americans. The prevalence of asthma is higher among non-Hispanic Blacks, compared to non-Hispanic whites, and females account for about 65% of all patients with asthma (Centers for Disease Control and Prevention, 2016). Although often considered a condition of childhood, asthma can occur at any age.

Asthma is characterized by chronic inflammation that occurs when potent mediators of the immune and inflammatory responses are released by mast cells lining the bronchial passageways. These mediators include histamine, leukotrienes, prostaglandins, and interleukins. The result of inflammation is an increase in airway edema coupled with increased mucus secretion, which narrows the airways, compromises the process of respiration, and contributes to airway obstruction. This is illustrated in Figure 44.2.

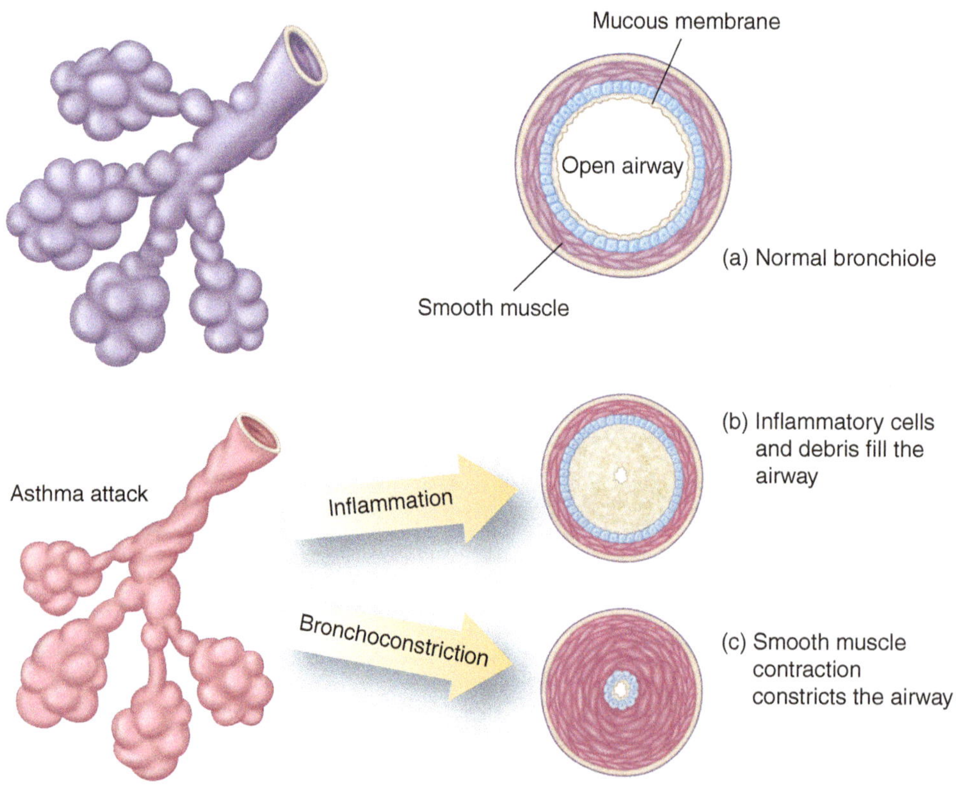

Figure 44.2 Changes in the bronchioles during an asthma attack: (a) Normal open bronchiole. (b) Inflammation plugs the airway. (c) Bronchoconstriction narrows the airway.

Table 44.1 Common Triggers of Asthma

Cause	Sources
Air pollutants	Tobacco smoke Air pollution Fumes from cleaning fluids or solvents Strong odors or sprays
Allergens	Pollen from trees, grasses, and weeds Animal dander Household dust mites Mold
Chemicals and food	Drugs, including aspirin, ibuprofen, and beta blockers Preservatives (sulfites and benzalkonium chloride) Food and condiments, including nuts, monosodium glutamate (MSG), shellfish, and dairy products
Respiratory infections	Bacterial, fungal, and viral
Stress	Emotional stress, strong emotions, anxiety, and exercise in dry, cold climates

The second component in the pathogenesis of asthma is bronchospasm. The inflammatory conditions in the airway make the smooth muscle hyperresponsive to a variety of stimuli. Stimuli such as breathing smoke, pollutants, or cold air may trigger acute bronchospasm. Specific triggers are listed in Table 44.1. Some patients experience bronchospasm on exertion, a condition called exercise-induced asthma. Gastroesophageal reflux can trigger an asthma event when acid in the esophagus induces reflex bronchoconstriction.

PharmFACT

About 1 in every 13 Americans has asthma. Asthma is an associated cause of death for over 3500 people each year (Asthma and Allergy Foundation of America, 2019).

The patient with asthma may present with a variety of symptoms, including evening cough, shortness of breath, chest tightness, and wheezing. Intervals between symptoms may vary from days to weeks to months. The severity of asthma is often graded by the frequency and intensity of acute episodes, as given in Table 44.2. **Status asthmaticus,** an emergency situation in which asthma is unresponsive to drug treatment, may lead to respiratory failure. Drugs may be given to prevent asthmatic attacks or to terminate attacks in progress.

Administration of Pulmonary Drugs Via Inhalation

44.3 Inhalation is a common route of administration for pulmonary drugs because it delivers drugs directly to their sites of action.

Many drugs that are used to treat asthma are available for administration by the inhalation route. Inhalation offers a rapid and efficient mechanism for delivering drugs directly to their site of action in the lungs. The enormous surface area of the bronchioles and alveoli and the rich blood supply to these areas result in an almost instantaneous onset of action for inhaled substances.

Medications are delivered to the respiratory system by aerosol therapy. An **aerosol** is a suspension of minute liquid droplets or fine solid particles suspended in a gas. The major advantage of aerosol therapy is that it delivers the drugs directly to the site of action. Not only does this dramatically decrease the onset of action, but it also allows for much smaller doses of a drug. The small doses of drug given by the inhalation route minimize any systemic effects that might result from absorption across pulmonary capillaries when compared to PO medications. Several devices are used to deliver drugs via the inhalation route. The most common are metered-dose inhalers, dry powder inhalers, and nebulizers.

The **metered-dose inhaler (MDI)**, often simply called an inhaler, is the most common type of aerosol delivery device. It consists of a canister that holds the medicine and a mouthpiece. To use an MDI, the patient presses the canister toward the mouthpiece to deliver a measured dose or "puff" of medication. By inhaling during drug delivery, the patient helps to ensure that the drug reaches the site of action in the lungs. Even when MDIs are used properly, however, the majority of the aerosolized drug never reaches the lungs. There are two primary reasons for this problem. One is that heavier aerosolized particles fall out by gravity and are deposited in the oropharynx. The other reason is that proper coordination of drug delivery with inhalation can be difficult for some patients. To decrease oropharyngeal deposition and to enhance drug delivery to the lungs, many healthcare providers recommend that patients use a spacer with their MDI. A spacer is a special tube that attaches to the mouthpiece that is designed to hold the cloud of aerosolized medication. This serves two

Table 44.2 Assessment of Asthma

Level	Frequency of Symptoms (Cough, Wheezing, Dyspnea, Chest Tightness)	Nocturnal Attacks	Activity Limitations
Intermittent	Less than 2 times/week	Less than 2 times/month	Normal activity between flare-ups
Mild persistent	3–6 times/week	More than 3–4 times/month	Flare-ups may limit activity
Moderate persistent	Daily	More than 5 times/month	Flare-ups affect activity
Severe persistent	Continuous	Frequent	Flare-ups limit activity

primary purposes. First, the spacer holds drops that fall out of the aerosol so that less medication is deposited on the oropharynx and in the mouth. Second, because the spacer holds the medication, the patient does not have to precisely coordinate inhalation with activation, so that more drug reaches the site of action.

A **dry powder inhaler (DPI)** delivers the medication as a fine dry powder. Whereas the MDI is activated by pressing the canister, the DPI is automatically activated when the patient inhales through the mouthpiece. Because the timing of drug delivery and inhalation does not have to be coordinated, more medication is delivered to the lung with a DPI. The DPI has no propellants in the canister (propellants can be harmful to some patients with lung problems).

A **nebulizer** (or **small-volume nebulizer**) is a machine that delivers medication as a fine mist. When using a nebulizer, the medication to be delivered is poured into a receptacle. The machine then vaporizes the liquid medication into a mist that is inhaled by using a face mask or other handheld device. These "breathing treatments" may take up to 30 minutes to administer the drug so it may not work as quickly as a drug taken from an MDI or DPI; however, medication delivered in this fashion is often more effective because it is delivered over many inhalations that occur during the period of medication delivery.

Principles of Asthma Pharmacotherapy

44.4 The goals of asthma pharmacotherapy are to terminate acute bronchospasms and to reduce the frequency of asthma attacks.

The choice of medications for asthma is determined by evidence-based guidelines coupled with the patient's response to therapy and adjusted according to each patient's situation. Treatment guidelines have been developed by experts in asthma management and are based on research findings. In the United States, the National Asthma Education and Prevention Program (NAEPP) issued guidelines for asthma treatment in 1991, which were subsequently updated. The NAEPP (2020) guidelines recommend a stepwise approach to asthma control based on the frequency and severity of symptoms, as shown in Figure 44.3.

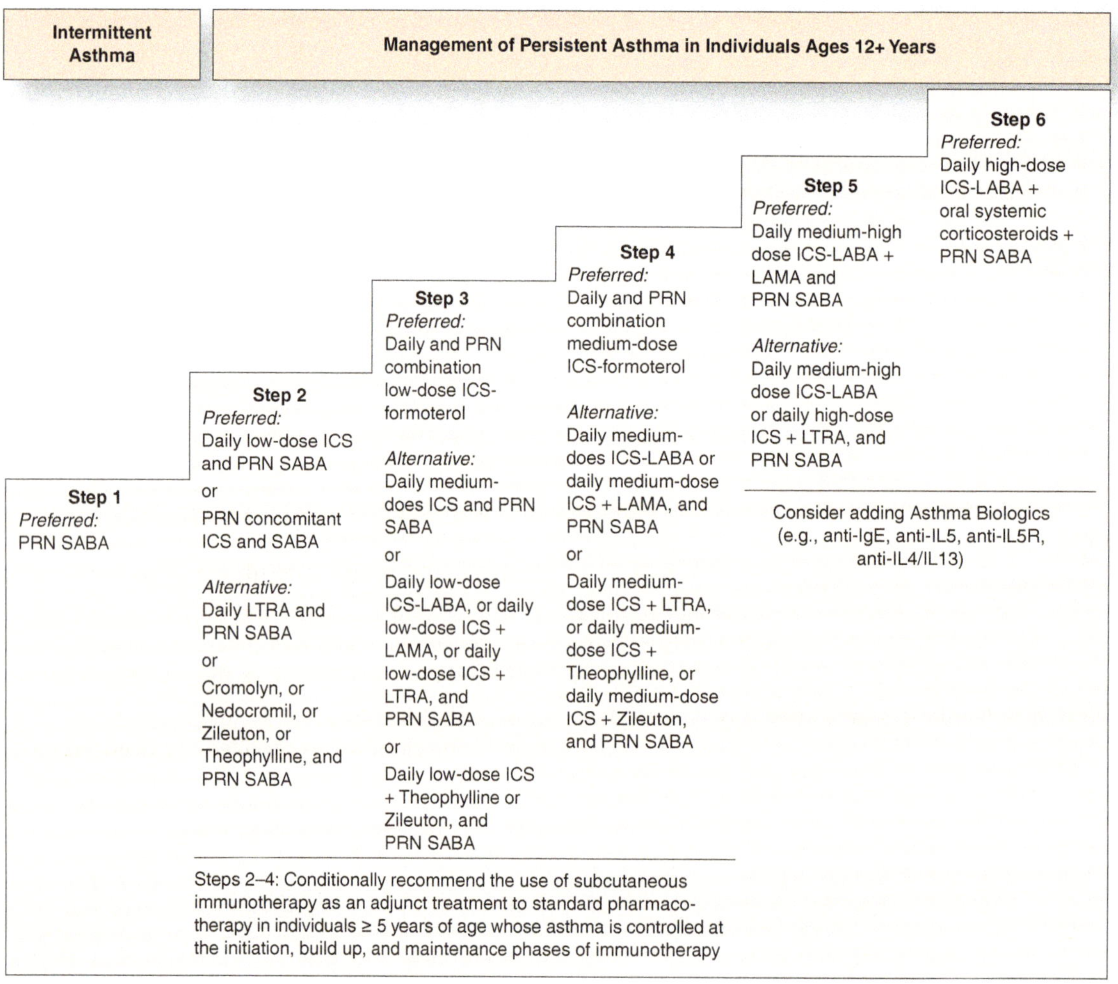

Key: ICS, inhaled corticosteroid; LABA, long-acting inhaled beta$_2$-agonist; LAMA, long-acting muscarinic antagonist; LTRA, leukotriene receptor antagonist; SABA, inhaled short-acting beta$_2$ agonist

Figure 44.3 Stepwise approach for managing asthma in patients 12 years and older.
Adapted from National Asthma Education Prevention Program (2020).

As patient symptoms worsen, the pharmacotherapy is adjusted accordingly by going to the next step. This provides a rational, evidence-based approach to asthma management. The three general strategies for asthma management from the NAEPP are as follows:

- Incorporate four components of care: medications, patient education, environmental control measures, and management of comorbidities.
- Initiate therapy based on asthma severity. Patients who have persistent asthma require daily long-term control medication.
- Adjust the therapy based on asthma control. Once therapy is initiated, monitor the level of asthma control and adjust the therapy accordingly: step up and step down, if necessary, to identify the minimum amount of medication required to maintain asthma control.

The goals of asthma pharmacotherapy are twofold: to terminate acute bronchospasms and to prevent or reduce the frequency of asthma attacks. Different medications are needed to achieve each of these goals. The NAEPP categorizes asthma drugs into two simple classes: quick-relief medications and long-term control medications. A summary of the different classes used for asthma management is given in Table 44.3.

PharmFACT

Currently, more than 7 million U.S. children (under age 18) have asthma. African American children and children from households earning less than $35,000 annually have the highest asthma rates (National Center for Health Statistics, 2020).

44.5 Beta$_2$-adrenergic agonists are the most effective drugs for relieving acute bronchospasm.

Beta-adrenergic agonists are some of the most frequently prescribed drugs for treating pulmonary disorders. Beta agonists are drugs that activate the sympathetic nervous system, which relaxes bronchial smooth muscle, resulting in bronchodilation. They are preferred drugs for the treatment of bronchoconstriction.

Beta-agonist medications may act on either beta$_1$ receptors, which are located primarily in the heart, or on beta$_2$ receptors, which are located in smooth muscle of the lung, uterus, and other organs. Beta agonists that activate both beta$_1$ and beta$_2$ receptors are called nonselective bronchodilators. Beta agonists that activate only the beta$_2$ receptors are called selective drugs. The selective beta$_2$-adrenergic agonists have largely replaced the older, nonselective drugs such as epinephrine and isoproterenol (Isuprel) for asthma pharmacotherapy because they produce fewer adverse cardiac effects. For a review of the nonselective beta agonists and prototype features for epinephrine and isoproterenol, refer to Chapter 15.

Beta$_2$-adrenergic agonists are classified by their duration of action. Short-acting beta agonists (SABAs) such as albuterol have a rapid onset of action, usually several minutes, so they are effective in terminating an acute asthma attack. SABAs are recommended by the NAEPP to abort or terminate an acute asthma attack. For this reason, they are sometimes referred to as rescue medications. Their effects, however, last only 2 to 6 hours, so the use of SABAs is limited to as-needed (prn) management of acute episodes. Doses of these drugs are listed in Table 44.4.

Long-acting beta agonists (LABAs) have a duration of 12 hours but have a relatively slow onset of action. The U.S.

Table 44.3 Overview of Drug Classes for Asthma Management

Class	Mechanism	Use
Quick-Relief Medications		
Short-acting beta$_2$-adrenergic agonists (SABAs)	Bronchodilators	Preferred drugs for relief of acute symptoms.
Anticholinergics	Bronchodilators	The long-acting types are used for persistent asthma.
Corticosteroids: systemic	Anti-inflammatory	Although not rapid acting, these PO drugs are used for short periods to reduce the frequency of acute exacerbations.
Long-Term Control		
Biologics	Monoclonal antibody	Used as adjunctive therapy for patients who have allergies and severe, persistent asthma.
Corticosteroids: inhaled	Anti-inflammatory	Preferred drugs for long-term asthma management. Oral doses may be required for severe, persistent asthma.
Mast cell stabilizers	Anti-inflammatory	Alternative drugs to control mild, persistent asthma or exercise-induced asthma.
Leukotriene modifiers	Anti-inflammatory	Alternative drugs to control mild, persistent asthma or as adjunctive therapy with inhaled corticosteroids.
Long-acting beta$_2$-adrenergic agonists (LABAs)	Bronchodilators	Used in combination with inhaled corticosteroids for prophylaxis of moderate to severe persistent asthma.
Methylxanthines	Bronchodilators	Alternative drugs used in combination with inhaled corticosteroids for prophylaxis of mild to moderate persistent asthma.

Table 44.4 Bronchodilators for Asthma and COPD

Drug	Route and Adult Dose (Maximum Dose Where Indicated)	Adverse Effects
Beta Agonists/Sympathomimetics		
albuterol (Proventil HFA, Ventolin HFA, VoSpire ER)	Metered-dose inhaler (MDI): 2 inhalations q4–6h prn PO (Vospire ER): 8 mg bid (max: 32 mg/day)	*Headache, dizziness, tremor, nervousness, throat irritation, drug tolerance*
arformoterol (Brovana)	Nebulizer (for COPD): 15 mcg bid (max: 30 mcg/day)	Tachycardia, dysrhythmia, hypokalemia, hyperglycemia, paradoxical bronchoconstriction, hypomagnesemia, maternal heart problems during pregnancy (terbutaline), increased risk for asthma-related death
formoterol (Perforomist)	Nebulizer (for COPD): 20 mcg bid (max: 40 mcg/day)	
levalbuterol (Xopenex)	Nebulizer: 0.63 mg tid–qid MDI: 2 inhalations q4–6h Inhalation (for COPD): 2–3 inhalations/day (max: 12 inhalations/day)	
metaproterenol	PO: 20 mg q6–8h	
olodaterol (Striverdi Respimat)	Inhalation (for COPD): 2 inhalations bid	
salmeterol (Serevent)	DPI (for asthma and COPD): 1 inhalation bid	
terbutaline	PO: 2.5–5 mg tid (max: 15 mg/day) Subcutaneous: 250 mcg (may be repeated in 15 min)	
Anticholinergics		
aclidinium (Tudorza Pressair)	DPI: 1–2 inhalations (400 mcg) bid	*Headache, bad taste, cough, dry mouth, blurred vision, paradoxical bronchospasm, upper respiratory infection* Pharyngitis
ipratropium (Atrovent)	MDI (for COPD): 2 inhalations (50 mcg) qid (max: 12 inhalations/day) Nebulizer (for COPD): 500 mcg q6–8h as needed	
revefenacin (Yupelri)	Nebulizer (for COPD): 1 vial (175 mcg) once daily	
tiotropium (Spiriva)	Inhalation (for COPD): 2 inhalations of 1 capsule daily with Spiriva HandiHaler device Inhalation (for asthma and COPD): 2 inhalations daily with Spiriva Respimat device	
umeclidinium (Incruse Ellipta)	DPI (for COPD): 1 inhalation/day (62.5 mcg)	
Methylxanthine		
theophylline	PO: 300–600 mg/day in divided doses (max: 900 mg/day)	*Nervousness, tremors, dizziness, headache, nausea and vomiting, anorexia* Tachycardia, dysrhythmias, hypotension, seizures, circulatory failure, respiratory arrest

Note: *Italics* indicate common adverse effects. Underline indicates serious adverse effects.

Food and Drug Administration (FDA) has published a public health advisory regarding an increase in deaths among patients who take LABAs. Because LABAs are not indicated to abort an asthma attack, taking the longer-acting drug instead of a SABA could result in unrelieved bronchospasm and subsequent death. The LABAs are also delivered via handheld inhalers and patients may assume that they have the same actions as the SABAs. Patients must be alerted to the dangers inherent in taking these during an acute episode. Although the risk of asthma-related death is small, LABAs are usually reserved for patients with persistent asthma who clearly require two medications for disease management (see Table 44.3). They are not to be used as monotherapy for this disease.

Beta$_2$-adrenergic agonists are available in PO, inhaled, and parenteral formulations. When taken for asthma and other respiratory problems, inhalation is the most common route. Inhaled beta$_2$ agonists produce minimal systemic toxicity because only small amounts of the drugs are absorbed. When given PO a longer duration of action is achieved, but systemic adverse effects are more frequently experienced. Systemic effects may include some activation of beta$_1$ receptors in the heart, which could cause an angina attack or a dysrhythmia in patients with cardiac disease. With chronic use, tolerance may develop to the bronchodilation effect and the duration of action will become shorter. Should this occur, the dose of beta$_2$ agonist may need to be increased, or a second drug may be added to the therapeutic regimen.

PROTOTYPE DRUG **Albuterol (Proventil HFA, Ventolin HFA, VoSpire ER)**

Classification **Therapeutic:** Bronchodilator
Pharmacologic: Beta$_2$-adrenergic agonist

Therapeutic Effects and Uses: Approved in 1981, albuterol is a SABA that is used to relieve and prevent the bronchospasm that is a characteristic pathophysiologic feature of asthma. Its rapid onset and excellent safety profile have made inhaled albuterol a preferred drug for the termination of acute bronchospasm. In addition to relieving bronchospasm, the drug facilitates mucus drainage and can inhibit the release of inflammatory chemicals from mast cells. When inhaled 15 to 30 minutes prior to physical activity, it can prevent exercise-induced bronchospasm for 2 to 3 hours. Inhaled albuterol is considered safe for use during pregnancy.

Oral forms of albuterol include immediate-release and extended-release tablets (VoSpire ER) and an oral solution. The PO forms have a longer onset of action and are not suitable for terminating acute asthma attacks. The NAEPP does not recommend the use of SABAs such as albuterol for asthma prophylaxis.

Mechanism of Action: Albuterol acts by selectively binding to $beta_2$-adrenergic receptors in bronchial smooth muscle to cause bronchodilation.

Pharmacokinetics:

Route(s)	Inhalation, PO
Absorption	Slow by the inhalation route; some of the inhaled drug is swallowed and absorbed by the gastrointestinal (GI) tract; rapid when given PO
Distribution	Delivered directly to the lungs (site of action); crosses the blood–brain barrier; may cross the placenta; unknown if secreted in breast milk
Primary metabolism	Hepatic (CYP450)
Primary excretion	Renal (less than 10% feces)
Onset of action	Inhalation: 5–15 min; PO: 30 min; peak effect: 0.5–2 h
Duration of action	Inhalation: 2–6 h; PO, sustained release: 8–12 h

Adverse Effects: Serious adverse effects from inhaled albuterol are uncommon when taken as directed; PO forms cause more sympathomimetic adverse effects. Some patients experience palpitations, headaches, throat irritation, tremor, nervousness, restlessness, and tachycardia. Less common adverse reactions include insomnia and dry mouth. Uncommon adverse effects include chest pain, paradoxical bronchospasm, and allergic reactions.

Contraindications/Precautions: Albuterol use is contraindicated if the patient has hypersensitivity to the drug. Because albuterol may exhibit cardiovascular effects in some patients, caution is required when administering it to patients with a history of tachyarrhythmias, prolongation of the QT interval, coronary artery disease, or hypertension.

Drug Interactions: Concurrent use with beta blockers will inhibit the bronchodilation effect of albuterol and may induce bronchospasm in patients with asthma. To prevent hypertensive crisis, patients should also avoid monoamine oxidase inhibitors within 14 days of beginning therapy. Concurrent use with thyroid hormone may produce additive stimulatory effects on the cardiovascular system. **Herbal/Food:** Products containing caffeine such as coffee and tea may cause nervousness, tremor, or palpitations.

Pregnancy: Although teratogenic in laboratory animals, human epidemiological studies do not confirm a pattern of increased birth defects or miscarriages. Adverse effects of albuterol on the breastfed neonate are unknown.

Treatment of Overdose: Overdose results in an exaggerated sympathetic activation, causing dysrhythmias, hypokalemia, and hyperglycemia. Cardiac arrest and death have been reported. In severe cases, administration of a beta antagonist may be necessary.

Clinician Responsibilities: Key clinical implications for patients receiving albuterol are included in Applied Clinical Judgment: Patients Receiving Pharmacotherapy for Asthma and COPD.

Drugs Similar to Albuterol (Proventil HFA, Ventolin HFA, VoSpire ER)

The only other SABA is levalbuterol. LABAs include arformoterol, formoterol, metaproterenol, olodaterol, salmeterol, and terbutaline. Indacaterol was withdrawn from the market in 2019. Adverse effects are the same as those of other $beta_2$ agonists and include tachycardia, nervousness, angina, and headache.

Arformoterol (Brovana): Arformoterol was approved in 2007 for the treatment of COPD, including chronic bronchitis and emphysema. This drug is an isomer of formoterol and was the first LABA available by inhalation via nebulizer. Although it begins to relax bronchi within about 7 minutes, its maximum effects take 1 to 3 hours. Thus, this drug is not suitable for relieving acute symptoms or terminating acute asthma attacks. Arformoterol is well tolerated and exhibits few serious adverse effects. The drug has a black box warning that it (and other LABAs) has been shown to increase the risk of asthma-related death; thus, it should be prescribed only when short- and intermediate-acting drugs are unable to control symptoms. The drug should be used with extreme caution if given with medications that prolong the QT interval. A combination drug (Dulera) containing arformoterol and mometasone (a corticosteroid) is available. At very high doses, arformoterol was teratogenic in animal studies. It is not known if this drug is secreted in human milk or if it has any adverse effects on the breastfed neonate

Formoterol (Perforomist): Approved in 2001, formoterol is a LABA that is administered by inhalation using a nebulizer. It is approved by the FDA for the relief of bronchospasm due to COPD. Onset of action begins in 1 to 3 minutes, although maximum effects do not occur until 1 to 3 hours. Formoterol is not suitable for relieving acute symptoms or terminating acute asthma attacks. When combined with an inhaled corticosteroid such as mometasone or budesonide, formoteral is a first-line drug for asthma that is not adequately controlled on a long-term asthma-control medication (see Figure 44.3). This drug is well tolerated and has the same adverse effect profile as that of other drugs in this class. Formoterol has a black box warning that it (and other LABAs) has been shown to increase the risk of asthma-related death; thus, it should be prescribed only when short- and intermediate-acting drugs are unable to control symptoms. At very high doses, formoterol was teratogenic in animal studies. It is not known if this drug is secreted in human milk or if it has any adverse effects on the breastfed neonate.

Levalbuterol (Xopenex): Approved in 1999, levalbuterol is an isomer of albuterol and has almost identical indications, actions, and adverse effects. This drug is administered via nebulized or aerosolized oral inhalation. It is indicated for the relief of acute bronchospasm symptoms and can be administered three to four times daily. Regular, daily use of levalbuterol is not recommended by the NAEPP as a means to prevent bronchospasm. Like other drugs in this class, levalbuterol has few serious adverse effects, with nervousness and tremor being frequently reported. Animal studies on levalbuterol did not show teratogenicity, however, studies with albuterol (which contains 50% levalbuterol) did show fetal harm. It is not known if this drug is secreted in human milk or if it has any adverse effects on the breastfed neonate

Metaproterenol: Approved in 1981 to treat bronchospasm, metaproterenol is a beta agonist available by the oral route. It has an onset of action of 30 minutes and a duration of 4 to 6 hours. The actions and adverse effects are similar to those of other drugs in this class. Effects of metaproterenol during pregnancy and lactation are unknown.

Olodaterol (Striverdi Respimat): Approved in 2014, olodaterol is a LABA used to treat airflow obstruction associated with COPD. It is available by the inhalation route and is administered once daily. This drug is not indicated for the relief of acute symptoms. Like other LABAs, olodaterol has a black box warning that it has been shown to increase the risk of asthma-related death. The warning also states that the drug is not approved to treat asthma. Common adverse effects include nasopharyngitis, upper respiratory tract infection, and bronchitis. At very high doses, olodaterol is teratogenic in laboratory animals. It is not known if this drug is secreted in human milk or if it has any adverse effects on the breastfed neonate.

Salmeterol (Serevent): Approved in 1994, salmeterol is a LABA given by DPI that is prescribed for asthma prophylaxis and the long-term therapy of bronchospasm associated with COPD. The LABAs salmeterol and formoterol are considered less effective at preventing asthma attacks than the inhaled corticosteroids. Because salmeterol has a 14-minute onset of action, it should not be used to terminate acute bronchospasm. Peak effects are observed at 3 to 4 hours. Pharyngitis and upper respiratory tract infections occur in patients who are taking the drug, and headache is a common adverse effect. Advair Diskus is a combination inhaler that combines salmeterol and fluticasone. Salmeterol has a black box warning that it (and other LABAs) has been shown to increase the risk of asthma-related death; thus, it should be prescribed only when short- and intermediate-acting drugs are unable to control symptoms. Adverse effects of salmeterol during pregnancy and lactation are unknown.

Terbutaline: An older drug approved in 1974, terbutaline is indicated for the treatment of bronchospasm associated with asthma or bronchitis. When given by the PO route, terbutaline may take 30 minutes or longer to act; thus, it is not indicated for acute conditions. The subcutaneous form can relieve bronchospasm within 15 minutes. PO terbutaline has a shorter duration of action than oral albuterol or salmeterol and it must be administered three times daily. Terbutaline is moderately selective for $beta_2$ receptors but may produce some activation of $beta_1$ receptors in the heart. Adverse effects are similar to those observed with other drugs in this class. Terbutaline has been used off-label to delay preterm labor contractions because its effects on $beta_2$ receptors in the uterus cause smooth muscle relaxation (see Chapter 69). However, in 2011 the FDA issued a black box warning that *oral* terbutaline should not be used to prevent or treat preterm

CONNECTIONS: Using Research in Practice

Allergen Exposure to Reduce Asthma Risk

Asthma is particularly challenging to treat or prevent because there is no one single causative factor in its development. While exposure to allergens accounts for a major factor in asthma development, not all patients with allergies have asthma, and not all patients with asthma have allergies. Maciag and Phipatanakul (2019) noted several strategies that can assist in controlling asthma related to allergens, including early and intensive treatment of atopic dermatitis, using inhaled corticosteroids for asthma prevention, and the use of vitamin D and probiotics in the treatment of allergic disorders in general. But none of these strategies worked across the entire population of patients with asthma, even those with allergies. Allergen immunotherapy (AIT)—the introduction of controlled amounts of allergen given subcutaneously or orally—has been a proven strategy, particularly for patients with allergic asthma not well controlled by their asthma medications (Virchow, 2019). A newer strategy is to combine allergen immunotherapy with omalizumab, a monoclonal antibody agent (Har & Lee, 2019). While stimulating tolerance to the allergen through the AIT doses, the omalizumab may help to control a systemic reaction to the allergen.

labor because it has not been shown to be effective and there is a potential for serious maternal heart problems and death. In very serious conditions, the *injectable* form of the drug may still be used, but treatment is limited to no longer than 48 to 72 hours to delay preterm labor. Terbutaline may cause fetal tachycardia and reduce labor contractions, thus it should be used cautiously, if at all, for asthma control during pregnancy. The drug enters milk but adverse effects on the breastfed neonate are unknown.

CONNECTION Checkpoint 44.1

The medications for asthma are selective for beta$_2$-adrenergic receptors. From what you learned in Chapter 15, what are the primary indications for the drugs selective for beta$_1$-adrenergic receptors?

44.6 Inhaled anticholinergics are used for preventing bronchospasm.

Although SABAs are the preferred drugs for treating acute bronchospasm, anticholinergics are alternative bronchodilators. Although anticholinergics such as atropine have been available for many decades, their adverse effect profile made them poorly suited for the management of asthma. With the delivery of the anticholinergics by inhalation, however, they have become important drugs in the arsenal of asthma pharmacotherapy. Four inhalation anticholinergics are available for the treatment of respiratory disorders. The first to be developed was ipratropium (Atrovent), which is considered a short-acting drug. Aclidinium (Tudorza Pressair), revefenacin (Yupelri), umeclidinium (Incruse Ellipta), and tiotropium (Spiriva) are newer, long-acting anticholinergics. In addition to being anticholinergics, these newer drugs are sometimes called long-acting muscarinic antagonists (LAMAs).

Anticholinergics block the parasympathetic nervous system, which results in actions similar to those of stimulating the sympathetic nervous system (see Chapter 14). It is predictable then that anticholinergic drugs would cause bronchodilation and have potential applications in the pharmacotherapy of asthma and COPD.

Anticholinergics have actions that are similar to those of beta-adrenergic agonists, and drugs from the two classes may be combined to produce a greater and more prolonged bronchodilation than either drug used separately. This additive effect is particularly useful for patients with persistent bronchospasm for whom either drug alone is inadequate to alleviate bronchoconstriction. Taking advantage of this increased effect, pharmaceutical companies have developed inhalants that combine both an anticholinergic and a beta agonist into a single canister.

The inhaled anticholinergics are relatively safe medications. The wide range of anticholinergic adverse effects that is observed when drugs in this class are administered systemically rarely occurs when administered by inhalation.

PROTOTYPE DRUG Ipratropium (Atrovent HFA)

Classification **Therapeutic:** Bronchodilator
Pharmacologic: Anticholinergic

Therapeutic Effects and Uses: Approved by the FDA in 1986, ipratropium is an anticholinergic medication that is delivered by the inhalation and intranasal routes. The inhalation form is approved to relieve and prevent the bronchospasm that is characteristic of asthma and COPD. It is a first-line drug for treating bronchospasms due to COPD (e.g., bronchitis and emphysema). Although it has not received FDA approval for the treatment of asthma, it is nevertheless prescribed off-label for the disorder. It is sometimes combined with albuterol to provide additive bronchodilation.

When administered via inhalation, ipratropium can relieve acute bronchospasm within minutes of administration, although peak effects may take 1 to 2 hours. Ipratropium is considered a maintenance therapy and is not to be used to terminate acute episodes of bronchospasm. Bronchodilation action may continue for up to 6 hours.

The nasal spray formulation of ipratropium is indicated for the symptomatic relief of rhinorrhea associated with the common cold and perennial rhinitis. The drug inhibits nasal secretions but does not have decongestant action. Treatment is limited to 3 weeks.

Mechanism of Action: Ipratropium causes bronchodilation by blocking cholinergic receptors in bronchial smooth muscle. Intranasal administration blocks parasympathetic receptors, thus reducing nasal hypersecretion characteristic of the common cold.

Pharmacokinetics:

Route(s)	Inhalation, intranasal
Absorption	Minimal systemic absorption; some of the inhaled drug is swallowed but is not absorbed by the GI tract
Distribution	Small amount is secreted in breast milk; minimally bound to plasma protein
Primary metabolism	Hepatic (CYP450)
Primary excretion	Renal and feces
Onset of action	5–15 min; peak effect: 1.5–2 h
Duration of action	3–6 h; half-life: 1.5–2 h

Adverse Effects: Because it is not readily absorbed from the lungs, ipratropium produces few systemic adverse effects. Though rare, it can worsen glaucoma with sufficient systemic absorption. Typical anticholinergic adverse effects such as dry mouth, nausea, and GI distress are among the most common adverse effects but occur in less than 3% of patients. Irritation of the upper respiratory tract may cause cough, drying of the nasal mucosa, or hoarseness. Paradoxical acute bronchospasm is a rare adverse effect that may be life-threatening. This drug produces a bitter taste that some patients find problematic. Intranasal administration may cause epistaxis and excessive drying of the nasal mucosa.

Contraindications/Precautions: Ipratropium is contraindicated in patients with hypersensitivity to soya lecithin or related food products such as soybean and peanut. Soya lecithin is used as a propellant in the inhaler. Ipratropium is contraindicated in patients who have demonstrated a hypersensitivity to ipratropium. All anticholinergics should be used with caution in patients with closed-angle glaucoma or urinary tract obstruction because they may worsen these conditions.

Drug Interactions: Because it has little systemic absorption, ipratropium interacts with very few drugs. Use with other anticholinergics such as atropine may lead to additive anticholinergic adverse effects. Ipratropium should not be used concurrently with pramlintide (Symlin) because both slow GI peristalsis and can cause nausea and/or vomiting or constipation. **Herbal/Food:** Unknown.

Pregnancy: Ipratropium did not show evidence of fetal harm in laboratory animals. Human experience has not shown adverse effects during pregnancy or lactation.

Treatment of Overdose: Overdose with ipratropium is unlikely because very little of the drug is absorbed.

Clinician Responsibilities: Key clinical implications for patients receiving ipratropium are included in Applied Clinical Judgment: Patients Receiving Pharmacotherapy for Asthma and COPD.

Drugs Similar to Ipratropium (Atrovent)

The other anticholinergics currently approved for inhalation are aclidinium, revefenacin, tiotropium, and umeclidinium. All four are long-acting (LAMAs) and used as maintenance therapy for COPD.

Aclidinium (Tudorza Pressair): Aclidinium is an anticholinergic approved in 2012 for the long-term maintenance treatment of bronchospasm associated with COPD. It is administered twice daily by DPI and is used to prevent, not terminate, bronchospasm. It has an onset of action of 60 minutes, a peak effect at 2 to 4 hours, and a sustained duration of action. It has very similar actions and adverse effects to those of the other two drugs in this class. Common side effects include headache, nasopharyngitis, and cough. Animal studies show evidence of fetal harm. The drug is secreted in animal milk and caution should be used if breastfeeding.

Revefenacin (Yupelri): Approved in 2018, revefenacin is a once-daily maintenance therapy for treating COPD. It has an onset of action of 45 minutes, a peak effect at 2 to 3 hours, and a sustained duration of action. The most frequent side effects are cough, nasopharyngitis, upper respiratory infection, and headache. Like other drugs in this class, it should not be used to treat acute bronchospasm. Animal studies with revefenacin did not show fetal harm. It is not known if this drug is secreted in human milk or if it has any adverse effects on the breastfed neonate.

Tiotropium (Spiriva): Approved in 2004, tiotropium is closely related to ipratropium and is indicated for the long-term maintenance treatment and prophylaxis of bronchospasm in patients with COPD, including chronic bronchitis and emphysema. It is not used to terminate acute bronchospasm; SABAs are more effective for this condition. An advantage of tiotropium is its long duration of action. Unlike ipratropium, which must be taken four or more times a day, tiotropium needs to be taken only once a day so patients are less likely to miss doses. Another difference between the two drugs is that ipratropium is administered by MDI, whereas tiotropium is administered by DPI (HandiHaler device). For patients with COPD who have difficulty using an MDI, tiotropium can be a viable alternative. Adverse effects are the same as those of ipratropium. Animal studies show that tiotropium may cause fetal harm. It is not known if this drug is secreted in human milk or if it has any adverse effects on the breastfed neonate.

Umeclidinium (Incruse Ellipta): Approved in 2013, umeclidinium is an inhaled anticholinergic indicated for the long-term management of airflow obstruction in patients with COPD. It offers the advantage of once-daily dosing. Like other drugs in this class, it should not be used to treat acute bronchospasm. Side effects are the same as those of other inhaled anticholinergics. Animal studies with umeclidinium did not show fetal harm. It is not known if this drug is secreted in human milk or if it has any adverse effects on the breastfed neonate.

44.7 Inhaled corticosteroids are the most effective drugs for the long-term control of asthma.

Corticosteroids are the most potent natural anti-inflammatory substances known. Because asthma has a major inflammatory component, it should not be surprising that drugs in this class play a major role in the management of this disorder. *Inhaled* corticosteroids are first-line drugs for the prevention of asthmatic attacks and for the management of chronic asthma. *Oral* corticosteroids are used for the short-term management of acute asthma attacks. The therapeutic actions of the corticosteroids have resulted in their widespread use in the pharmacotherapy of allergic rhinitis (see Chapter 45) and other inflammatory disorders. Doses for the inhaled corticosteroids are given in Table 44.5.

Table 44.5 Anti-Inflammatory Drugs for Asthma and COPD

Drug	Route and Adult Dose (Maximum Dose Where Indicated)	Adverse Effects
Inhaled Corticosteroids*		
beclomethasone (Beconase AQ, Qvar)	MDI: 1–2 inhalations bid (max: 20 inhalations/day)	*Hoarseness, dry mouth, cough, sore throat* Oropharyngeal candidiasis, hypercorticism, hypersensitivity reactions
budesonide (Pulmicort)	DPI (Pulmicort Flexhaler): 1–2 inhalations (360 mcg) bid (max: 720 mcg bid) Nebulizer (Pulmicort Respules): 0.5 mg/day either once daily or bid	
ciclesonide (Alvesco)	Inhalation: 1–2 inhalations (80–320 mcg/inhalation) bid	
flunisolide	MDI: 2–3 inhalations bid–tid (max: 12 inhalations/day)	
fluticasone (Flovent)	DPI (Flovent Diskus): 100–500 mcg bid (max: 1000 mcg bid) MDI (Flovent HFA): 88–220 mcg bid (max: 880 mcg bid)	
mometasone (Asmanex)	MDI: 1–2 inhalations bid (100–200 mcg) (max: 2 inhalations/day)	
Mast Cell Stabilizer		
cromolyn	Nebulizer: 1 inhalation qid	*Nausea, sneezing, cough, unpleasant taste* Anaphylaxis, angioedema, bronchospasm
Leukotriene Modifiers and Miscellaneous Drugs		
montelukast (Singulair)	PO: 10 mg/day in evening	*Headache, nausea, diarrhea, throat pain, weight loss (roflumilast)* Increased aspartate aminotransferase (AST), hepatotoxicity, psychiatric events including suicidality (roflumilast)
roflumilast (Daliresp)	PO (for COPD): 500 mcg once daily	
zafirlukast (Accolate)	PO: 20 mg bid 1 h before or 2 h after meals	
zileuton (Zyflo CR)	PO (extended release): 1200 mg bid (max: 2400 mg/day)	

Note: *Italics* indicate common adverse effects. Underline indicates serious adverse effects.

* For doses of systemic corticosteroids, refer to Chapter 68.

CONNECTIONS: Patient Safety

Proper Inhaler Use by Older Adults

A 73-year-old man with a history of COPD (chronic bronchitis) is brought to the emergency department of his local hospital in acute respiratory distress. On assessment, he has inspiratory and expiratory wheezing bilaterally, and his pulse oximetry value is 90%. When taking a brief drug history, the nurse notes that the patient has been managing his condition with PO roflumilast (Daliresp) and occasional low-dose corticosteroids. He tells the nurse that he has recently finished an antibiotic prescription "because I had a cold and they didn't want it to get worse." He also tells the nurse that at that time, his provider gave him a prescription for an albuterol (VoSpire ER) inhaler, which he has been using for the past 2 days, "but I've been getting worse, not better." What does the nurse suspect may be the cause of his recent respiratory distress?

Corticosteroids decrease inflammation of the airways by inhibiting the synthesis and release of inflammatory mediators, including histamine, leukotriene, cytokines, and prostaglandins. They also inhibit the number of circulating leukocytes and decrease vascular permeability. This results in diminished mucus production and edema, thus reducing airway obstruction. Although corticosteroids are not bronchodilators, they sensitize the bronchial smooth muscle to be more responsive to beta-agonist stimulation. In addition, they reduce the bronchial hyperresponsiveness to allergens, which is responsible for triggering many asthma attacks.

When inhaled on a daily schedule, corticosteroids suppress inflammation without producing major adverse effects. Although symptoms will improve in the first 1 to 2 weeks of therapy, 4 to 8 weeks may be required for maximum benefit. Because of the dangerous adverse effects of long-term therapy, systemic corticosteroids are generally reserved for short-term management of acute asthma exacerbations. For outpatient management in these instances, PO corticosteroids such as prednisone are given for the shortest length of time possible, usually 5 to 7 days. In the hospital setting, intravenous (IV) corticosteroids may be given. Regardless, at the end of the brief treatment period, patients are usually switched to inhaled corticosteroids for long-term management.

When taken long term, both PO and inhaled formulations of corticosteroids have the potential to affect bone physiology in adults and children. Adults who are at risk for osteoporosis should receive periodic bone mineral density tests and possibly pharmacotherapy with bisphosphonates to prevent fractures (see Chapter 72). In children, small decreases in linear bone growth have been documented. Although these effects are usually temporary, growth should be monitored and the prescriber should weigh the risks of growth suppression against the benefits of corticosteroid use. In all cases, effects on bone growth are dose and frequency dependent; thus, patients should be administered the lowest doses possible to maintain adequate asthma control.

PROTOTYPE DRUG **Beclomethasone (Beconase AQ, Qvar)**

Classification **Therapeutic:** Anti-inflammatory
Pharmacologic: Corticosteroid

Therapeutic Effects and Uses: Approved in 1976, beclomethasone is a corticosteroid that is available for administration by aerosol inhalation for asthma (Qvar) or as a nasal spray (Beconase AQ) for allergic rhinitis. Guidelines from the NAEPP place beclomethasone and other inhaled corticosteroids as first-line drugs for the long-term management of persistent asthma in both children and adults. Two inhalations, two to three times per day, usually provide adequate prophylaxis, although 3 to 4 weeks of therapy may be necessary before optimal benefits are achieved. A double-strength formulation of beclomethasone (Qvar) is available with smaller drug particles that is able to deliver half the usual dose and achieve the same therapeutic effect. Beclomethasone is not a bronchodilator and should not be used to terminate asthma attacks in progress.

The intranasal formulation (Beconase AQ) is effective at reducing the symptoms of allergic rhinitis. Therapeutic effects may take 2 weeks to be fully apparent. Intranasal beclomethasone is also approved to prevent recurrence of nasal polyps following surgical removal. Very little of this drug is absorbed in the systemic circulation when it is administered by this route.

Mechanism of Action: Beclomethasone acts by reducing inflammation and immune responses, thus decreasing the frequency of asthma attacks.

Pharmacokinetics:

Route(s)	Inhalation, intranasal
Absorption	Small amounts of systemic absorption
Distribution	Delivered directly to the lungs (site of action); small amount is secreted in breast milk
Primary metabolism	Liver (CYP450: 3A substrate) and lung
Primary excretion	Mostly feces with about 10% in urine
Onset of action	1–3 weeks
Duration of action	Half-life: 15 h

Adverse Effects: Inhaled beclomethasone produces few systemic adverse effects. Because small amounts may be swallowed with each dose, the patient should be observed for signs of corticosteroid toxicity (hypercorticism) when taking this drug for prolonged periods. Local effects may include hoarseness, dry mouth, and changes in taste. Inhaled corticosteroid use has been associated with the development of cataracts in adults. Some studies have shown that long-term intranasal or inhaled corticosteroids may cause growth inhibition in children.

Like all corticosteroids, the anti-inflammatory properties of beclomethasone can mask signs of infections and the drug is contraindicated if active infection is present. A large percentage of patients taking beclomethasone on a long-term basis will develop oropharyngeal candidiasis, a fungal infection in the throat, due to the constant deposits of drug in the oral cavity. Children who have not been vaccinated for varicella should receive the vaccine because of the potential for developing serious disseminated varicella infections during treatment with corticosteroids.

Contraindications/Precautions: The only contraindication to using beclomethasone is hypersensitivity to the drug.

Drug Interactions: Because very little of the drug is absorbed, no clinically significant drug interactions occur. **Herbal/Food:** None known.

Pregnancy: Large human epidemiological studies have not found evidence of congenital malformations or adverse pregnancy outcomes in women taking inhaled corticosteroids for asthma control as compared to women taking no medication for asthma.

Treatment of Overdose: Overdose does not occur when taken by the inhalation route.

Clinician Responsibilities: Key clinical implications for patients receiving beclomethasone are included in Applied Clinical Judgment: Patients Receiving Pharmacotherapy for Asthma and COPD.

Drugs Similar to Beclomethasone (Beconase AQ, Qvar)

Other corticosteroids for inhalation include budesonide, ciclesonide, flunisolide, fluticasone, and mometasone.

Budesonide (Pulmicort): Budesonide is a corticosteroid that is available by the intranasal route for allergic rhinitis (Rhinocort), oral inhalation, nebulizer for asthma prophylaxis (Pulmicort), or PO capsules for Crohn's disease (Entocort). Symbicort is a combination drug for asthma that contains budesonide with formoterol. The most common adverse effects with the inhaled use of budesonide include respiratory infections, rhinitis, cough, and otitis media. Visual impairment may occur. Growth effects should be monitored in pediatric patients.

Ciclesonide (Alvesco): Approved in 2006, ciclesonide is a corticosteroid available by the oral inhalation (Alvesco) route for asthma maintenance and prophylaxis in patients over 12 years of age or by the intranasal (Omnaris) route for allergic rhinitis. Ciclesonide is a prodrug that is converted to an active metabolite following administration. Like other drugs in this class, ciclesonide is not a bronchodilator and should not be used to treat acute bronchospasm. Actions and adverse effects are the same as those of other corticosteroids administered by inhalation.

Flunisolide: Flunisolide is a corticosteroid that is available by oral inhalation for asthma prophylaxis. The most common adverse effects with inhaled use include upper respiratory infections, dry mouth, hoarseness, nausea and vomiting, and taste changes. Like other drugs in this class, visual impairment may occur and growth effects should be monitored in pediatric patients.

Fluticasone (Flovent): Fluticasone is a corticosteroid that is available by the intranasal route for allergic rhinitis (Flonase); oral inhalation for asthma prophylaxis or COPD (Flovent); or topical cream or ointment for dermatitis, eczema, and other skin conditions (Cutivate). The most common adverse effects with the inhaled use of fluticasone include headache, throat irritation, and upper respiratory tract infections. Visual impairment may occur. Growth effects should be monitored in pediatric patients. Like other inhaled corticosteroids, fluticasone is not indicated for the relief of acute bronchospasm.

Mometasone (Asmanex): Mometasone is an inhaled corticosteroid that is available for the prevention of acute asthmatic attacks. When inhaled it may take an hour or longer to produce its effects; therefore, it is not indicated for the relief of acute bronchospasm. Actions and adverse effects are the same as those of other inhaled corticosteroids. An intranasal form is available for allergic rhinitis (Nasonex), and a topical preparation (Elocon) is used to treat various inflammatory skin conditions. Dulera is a combination of mometasone and formoterol used for asthma maintenance therapy.

CONNECTION Checkpoint 44.2

From what you learned in Chapter 42, describe strategies that could be used to limit the incidence of serious adverse effects when corticosteroids must be taken PO for prolonged periods.

44.8 Mast cell stabilizers are used for the prophylaxis of asthma and act by preventing the release of histamine.

Mast cell stabilizers serve limited, though important, roles in the prophylaxis of asthma. Mast cells are large cells that contain inflammatory granules, such as histamine, that mediate inflammatory and allergic reactions. When these cells are sensitized, they degranulate and release the inflammatory substances into the body where they initiate an inflammatory response. Mast cell stabilizers are helpful in managing asthma and COPD because they prevent degranulation of the mast cell, preventing the release of histamine and other inflammatory mediators in the airways. Cromolyn is the only mast cell stabilizer approved for respiratory indications. The dose for this drug is given in Table 44.5. A second drug in this class, nedocromil, was formerly used to treat asthma, but is now available only as an ophthalmic solution to treat allergic conjunctivitis.

PROTOTYPE DRUG Cromolyn

Classification **Therapeutic:** Anti-inflammatory
Pharmacologic: Mast cell stabilizer

Therapeutic Effects and Uses: An older drug that was approved by the FDA in 1973, cromolyn prevents the inflammation that is a characteristic pathophysiologic feature of asthma and COPD. Because it has no effect on previously released inflammatory mediators from mast cell degranulation, the effects will not be noted immediately. The NAEPP guidelines place cromolyn as an alternate drug for the treatment of mild to moderate asthma when corticosteroids are contraindicated or have not proven effective. This drug should not be used to terminate acute asthma attacks.

For asthma therapy, the drug is administered via oral inhalation. An intranasal over-the-counter (OTC) formulation (NasalCrom) is available for allergic rhinitis. An ophthalmic solution (Crolom) is used to treat various allergic disorders of the conjunctiva. Gastrocrom is a PO dosage form of cromolyn that is the only FDA-approved drug to treat systemic mastocytosis, which is a rare condition in which the patient has an excessive number of mast cells. Gastrocrom is also used off-label to treat ulcerative colitis and to prevent symptoms associated with food allergies.

Mechanism of Action: By stabilizing mast cells, cromolyn helps to prevent the inflammatory response that occurs when mast cells degranulate.

Pharmacokinetics:

Route(s)	Inhalation
Absorption	Minimal systemic absorption (less than 1%)
Distribution	Delivered directly to the lungs (site of action); small amount crosses the placenta; small amount is secreted in breast milk
Primary metabolism	Hepatic
Primary excretion	Bile (and, subsequently, feces) and renal
Onset of action	Adequate effect may not be noted until 2–4 weeks of use
Duration of action	Unknown

Adverse Effects: Adverse effects are uncommon when the drug is administered by oral inhalation. The most common effects are bronchospasm, cough, and pharyngeal irritation. Intranasal and ophthalmic administration may cause local burning and stinging.

Contraindications/Precautions: As with any drug, individuals who have demonstrated a hypersensitivity to this drug should not take it. It should be discontinued if the patient develops pulmonary eosinophilia.

Drug Interactions: No significant interactions are known. **Herbal/Food:** Unknown.

Pregnancy: Animal studies with cromolyn did not show fetal harm. Small amounts are secreted in human milk but it is unknown if this has adverse effects on the breastfed neonate.

Treatment of Overdose: There are no noted problems associated with overdosage. Toxicity is unlikely.

Clinician Responsibilities: Key clinical implications for patients receiving cromolyn are included in Applied Clinical Judgment: Patients Receiving Pharmacotherapy for Asthma and COPD.

Drugs Similar to Cromolyn

Cromolyn is the only mast cell stabilizer indicated for respiratory conditions.

44.9 The leukotriene modifiers, which are primarily used for asthma prophylaxis, act by reducing the inflammatory component of asthma.

Leukotriene modifiers are a newer drug class added to the arsenal of asthma management. They are able to ease bronchoconstriction by reducing inflammation. Because of their delayed onset, these drugs are ineffective at terminating acute asthma attacks. The NAEPP guidelines list the leukotriene modifiers as alternative drugs to be considered when inhaled corticosteroids and SABAs are unable to control asthma symptoms. Doses for these drugs are listed in Table 44.5.

Leukotrienes are mediators of the immune and inflammatory responses that are involved in allergic and asthmatic reactions. Leukotrienes are synthesized by mast cells as well as neutrophils, basophils, and eosinophils. When released in the airway, they promote edema, inflammation, and bronchoconstriction. Leukotriene modifiers reduce inflammation by either blocking the enzyme that controls leukotriene synthesis or by blocking leukotriene receptors. They are not considered bronchodilators, although they do produce some bronchodilation through indirect mechanisms. The leukotriene modifiers are only available by the PO route.

PROTOTYPE DRUG Montelukast (Singulair)

Classification **Therapeutic:** Drug for asthma prophylaxis and allergic rhinitis
Pharmacologic: Leukotriene modifier

Therapeutic Effects and Uses: First approved in 1998, montelukast is a PO drug that prevents the inflammation that is a characteristic feature of asthma. It is intended for the long-term control of asthma symptoms and not for the relief of an acute asthma attack. In addition to asthma, the drug is indicated for relief of symptoms associated with seasonal allergic and perennial rhinitis. For pediatric use it is available as chewable tablets and oral granules that may be sprinkled on soft food. In 2007, montelukast was approved for the prevention of exercise-induced bronchospasm, when taken 2 or more hours prior to the expected physical activity. It is the only drug in this class approved for this indication.

Mechanism of Action: Montelukast blocks leukotriene receptors in the airways, which prevents airway edema and inflammation.

Pharmacokinetics:

Route(s)	PO
Absorption	Rapidly absorbed
Distribution	Secreted in breast milk; more than 99% bound to plasma protein
Primary metabolism	Extensive hepatic metabolism (CYP2C9, CYP3A4)
Primary excretion	Mostly bile
Onset of action	1 week
Duration of action	Unknown; half-life: up to 5.5 h

Adverse Effects: Side effects of montelukast are generally mild, with headache being the most common complaint. Rhinitis, influenza, and abdominal pain have been reported by some patients. **Black box warning**: Although rare, neuropsychiatric events have been documented, including aggression, anxiety, depression, suicidal ideation, and memory impairment. This drug should only be used for allergic rhinitis in patients unable to tolerate safer alternatives.

Contraindications/Precautions: The only absolute contraindication is hypersensitivity to this drug. Patients with known aspirin sensitivity should avoid taking montelukast.

Drug Interactions: Montelukast is metabolized by CYP450 enzymes and has the potential to interact with substrates that inhibit this enzyme such as carbamazepine, erythromycin, and the azole antifungals. **Herbal/Food:** St. John's wort may decrease the effects of montelukast.

Pregnancy: Animal studies with montelukast did not show fetal harm. This drug is secreted in human milk but it is unknown if it has any adverse effects on the breastfed neonate.

Treatment of Overdose: Symptoms of overdose include headache, abdominal pain, and nausea and vomiting. Treatment is supportive.

Clinician Responsibilities: Key clinical implications for patients receiving montelukast are included in Applied Clinical Judgment: Patients Receiving Pharmacotherapy for Asthma and COPD.

Drugs Similar to Montelukast

Roflumilast, zafirlukast, and zileuton are other leukotriene modifiers and miscellaneous drugs.

Roflumilast (Daliresp): Roflumilast was approved in 2011 to prevent symptoms such as coughing and excess mucus production in patients with COPD. It is indicated for the chronic management of the disease and not for acute bronchospasms. It is available PO, administered once daily. Roflumilast acts by blocking the enzyme phosphodiesterase 4 (PDE4). PDE4 is the main enzyme that degrades cAMP in cells of the immune system. By inhibiting PDE4, roflumilast increases the levels of cAMP, which leads to reduced inflammatory cell activity in the lungs. The most common adverse effects are diarrhea, nausea, headache, back pain, influenza, insomnia, dizziness, and decreased appetite and weight loss. Neuropsychiatric adverse reactions such as insomnia, anxiety, depression and suicidal ideation have been reported. Animal studies suggest that roflumilast may cause fetal harm at high doses. This drug is likely secreted in milk and is not recommended during lactation.

Zafirlukast (Accolate): Zafirlukast was the first leukotriene modifier, approved in 1996 for the prophylaxis of persistent, chronic asthma. It is less effective than inhaled corticosteroids. Off-label uses include allergic rhinitis and prevention of exercise-induced bronchospasm. Its relatively long onset of action makes it unsuitable for the termination of acute bronchospasm. Zafirlukast produces few serious adverse effects. Headache is the most common complaint. Neuropsychiatric adverse reactions such as insomnia and depression have been reported. Animal studies with montelukast did not show fetal harm. This drug is likely secreted in milk and is not recommended during lactation.

Zileuton (Zyflo CR): Approved in 1996, zileuton is a PO drug that acts by inhibiting lipoxygenase, which is the first enzyme in the pathway of leukotriene synthesis. Like other leukotriene inhibitors, zileuton is considered an alternate drug in the prophylaxis of persistent, chronic asthma. An extended-release formulation (Zyflo CR) allows for twice-daily dosing. Zileuton should not be used to treat acute asthma attacks. This drug is generally well tolerated, with sinusitis, nausea, and throat pain being the most common adverse effects. The most serious concern with zileuton is the potential for liver damage. Zileuton raises liver enzymes, and cases of jaundice and severe hepatic injury have been reported. This drug is contraindicated in patients with hepatic impairment, and liver function tests should be conducted on a regular basis during therapy. Because zileuton can increase serum warfarin levels, prothrombin time should be regularly monitored. Animal studies suggest that zileuton may cause fetal harm. This drug is likely secreted in milk and is not recommended during lactation.

44.10 Methylxanthines were once the mainstay of asthma pharmacotherapy but are now rarely prescribed for the disorder.

The **methylxanthines** were preferred drugs for treating asthma 30 years ago. Now they are reserved for the long-term management of persistent asthma that is unresponsive to beta agonists or inhaled corticosteroids. One reason methylxanthines are used less often now is because their narrow therapeutic index increases the risk of toxicity, especially with prolonged use. These drugs also have significant interactions with numerous other drugs. Doses for the methylxanthines are listed in Table 44.4.

The methylxanthines produce only modest bronchodilation. They are chemically related to caffeine and share caffeine's stimulant effect. Methylxanthines are available in forms for PO, parenteral, and rectal administration. Interestingly, theobromine, an ingredient in chocolate, is also a methylxanthine.

Technically, theophylline is the only drug in this class. A second drug, aminophylline, consists of theophylline combined with an inert ingredient that makes it more water soluble. Other than different pharmacokinetics, the two drugs have the same actions and adverse effects.

PROTOTYPE DRUG Theophylline

Classification **Therapeutic:** Bronchodilator
Pharmacologic: Methylxanthine

Therapeutic Effects and Uses: Approved by the FDA in 1940, theophylline is a natural substance found in small amounts in tea. Theophylline relaxes bronchial smooth muscle and may exert some anti-inflammatory action that is beneficial to patients with asthma. It is considered an alternate drug by the NAEPP guidelines to be considered for asthma prophylaxis when more effective drugs fail to bring symptomatic relief. It may be used in combination with a corticosteroid for persistent asthma. Although FDA approved for treating acute bronchospasm, theophylline is not recommended by the NAEPP guidelines because the SABAs are more effective.

Theophylline has several off-label indications. As a respiratory stimulant, theophylline and caffeine may be used to treat sleep apnea in neonates and in adults with chronic heart failure. Given IV, theophylline has been found to reduce neurotoxicity resulting from the drug methotrexate.

Mechanism of Action: Theophylline works by two mechanisms. It relaxes bronchial smooth muscle, which promotes bronchodilation, and it suppresses airway responsiveness to stimuli that promote bronchospasm.

Pharmacokinetics:

Route(s)	PO, parenteral
Absorption	Rapid absorption
Distribution	About 40% protein bound; remainder is distributed well in fluids and less well in body lipids
Primary metabolism	Hepatic (CYP1A2, CYP2E1, CYP3A3)
Primary excretion	Renal
Onset of action	Peak: approximately 60 min (highly variable)
Duration of action	Half-life: 6–10 h (highly variable)

Adverse Effects: Theophylline has a very narrow therapeutic index. Therapeutic levels are 10 to 15 mcg/mL and the toxic level is anything above 20 mcg/mL. Serum theophylline levels should be obtained during therapy. Common adverse effects include nausea and vomiting, headache, irritability, and insomnia. More serious reactions include dysrhythmias, hypotension, and seizures.

Contraindications/Precautions: Theophylline should be used with great caution in patients who have seizure disorders, heart failure, or cardiac dysrhythmias. Theophylline has also been shown to increase the production of gastric acid so use in patients with active peptic ulcer disease is not recommended. Because of the extensive hepatic metabolism, theophylline should be closely monitored in patients with a history of liver disease.

Drug Interactions: Because theophylline is extensively metabolized by CYP450 enzymes, it is subject to numerous drug interactions, including interactions with many common antibiotics (ciprofloxacin, clarithromycin, erythromycin) and antianxiety drugs (diazepam, flurazepam, lorazepam, midazolam). Theophylline also has a number of IV incompatibilities, including emergency medications such as epinephrine, norepinephrine, and isoproterenol. Compatibility of any medication should be checked prior to initiating infusions in the same line. **Herbal/Food:** Foods and beverages containing caffeine will cause additive central nervous system stimulation. St. John's wort may decrease the effectiveness of theophylline.

Pregnancy: Theophylline is not recommended during pregnancy or lactation due to the potential toxicity of the drug and the availability of safer medications for asthma.

Treatment of Overdose: There is no specific antidote to theophylline. Gastric lavage is indicated in the event of an overdose of PO medications. Supportive measures need to be provided for hypotension, shock, dysrhythmias, and other toxic effects. Serum levels should be monitored periodically until they are within normal limits.

Clinician Responsibilities: Key clinical implications for patients receiving theophylline are included in Applied Clinical Judgment: Patients Receiving Pharmacotherapy for Asthma and COPD.

44.11 Monoclonal antibodies are a newer form of biologic therapy for the prevention of asthma symptoms.

A newer approach to treating asthma and COPD is the use of monoclonal antibodies. Monoclonal antibodies are designed to attach to a specific receptor on a target cell or molecule. Most monoclonal antibodies are designed to attack cancer cells. However, several biologics have been designed to attach to inflammatory mediators that reduce allergy symptoms.

Approved in 2003, omalizumab (Xolair) was the first biologic therapy used to treat asthma. Omalizumab attaches to a receptor on immunoglobulin E (IgE). The normal function of IgE is to react to antigens and cause the release of inflammatory chemical mediators from mast cells and basophils. By binding to IgE, omalizumab prevents inflammation and dampens the body's response to allergens that sometimes trigger asthma. This drug is approved for treating allergic rhinitis and moderate to severe, persistent asthma that cannot be controlled effectively with inhaled corticosteroids. A second indication is to treat chronic idiopathic urticaria. Available by the subcutaneous route, injections are scheduled every 2 to 4 weeks. The most common adverse effects include injection-site reaction, upper respiratory tract infections, headache, and pharyngitis. The drug contains a black box warning regarding the potential for anaphylaxis. Animal studies with omalizumab did not show fetal harm. It is not known if this drug is secreted in human milk or if it has any adverse effects on the breastfed neonate.

Approved in 2016, reslizumab (Cinqair) is a monoclonal antibody that binds to interleukin-5 (IL-5). Blocking the activity of IL-5 reduces the inflammatory actions of eosinophils. The drug is reserved for severe, persistent asthma in patients age 18 years and older and who have an eosinophilic phenotype. Eosinophilic asthma is a subtype of asthma in which the sputum contains a high percentage of eosinophils, and it is resistant to standard therapies. Reslizumab is administered by IV injections once every 4 weeks. Oropharyngeal pain is the only common adverse effect. The drug contains a black box warning regarding the potential for anaphylaxis. Animal studies with reslizumab did not show fetal harm. It is not known if this drug is secreted in human milk or if it has any adverse effects on the breastfed neonate.

Other biologics used to treat severe eosinophilic asthma include benralizumab (Fasenra) and mepolizumab (Nucala). Both medications are given by the subcutaneous route, and act by the same mechanism as reslizumab. Dupilumab (Dupixent) is used to treat patients with either eosinophilic or corticosteroid-dependent asthma but it acts by blocking different interleukins: IL-4 and IL-13. Dupilumab is also approved to treat atopic dermatitis (See Chapter 73.)

Pharmacotherapy of Chronic Obstructive Pulmonary Disease

44.12 Chronic obstructive pulmonary disease may be treated with bronchodilators, anti-inflammatory drugs, and mucolytics.

Chronic obstructive pulmonary disease (COPD) is a progressive pulmonary disorder characterized by chronic and recurrent obstruction of airflow. The two most common examples of conditions that cause chronic pulmonary obstruction are **chronic bronchitis**, a condition in which excess mucus is produced in the lower respiratory tract, and **emphysema**, a condition in which there is loss of bronchiolar elasticity and destruction of alveolar walls.

The clinical distinction between chronic bronchitis and emphysema is sometimes unclear because patients may exhibit symptoms of both conditions concurrently. Both conditions are strongly associated with smoking tobacco products (cigarette smoking accounts for 85 to 90% of all cases of nonasthmatic COPD) and, secondarily, breathing air pollutants. In chronic bronchitis, excess mucus is produced in the lower respiratory tract due to the inflammation and irritation from cigarette smoke or pollutants. The airway becomes partially obstructed with mucus, resulting in the classic signs of dyspnea and coughing. An early sign of bronchitis is often a productive cough that occurs on awakening. Gas exchange may be impaired; thus, wheezing and decreased exercise tolerance are additional clinical signs. Microbes thrive in the mucus-rich environment, and pulmonary infections are common.

Because most patients with COPD are lifelong tobacco users, they often have serious comorbid cardiovascular conditions such as heart failure and hypertension. Emphysema is most often the result of years of chronic inflammation and is characterized by loss of elasticity of the bronchioles and damage and loss of alveolar wall structures. The loss of elasticity results in partial collapse of the airways on exhalation, leading to air trapping, and the destruction of alveolar walls leads to decreased perfusion and gas exchange at the alveolus. The patient with emphysema may experience extreme dyspnea from even the slightest physical activity.

Drugs may be used to bring symptomatic relief to patients with COPD, but they do not alter the progression of COPD or cure the disorder. The goals of pharmacotherapy of COPD are to relieve symptoms and avoid complications of the condition. Various classes of drugs are used to treat infections, control cough, and relieve bronchospasm. Most patients receive the same classes of bronchodilators and anti-inflammatory drugs that are prescribed for asthma. A few of the newer drugs and combination drugs are approved only for COPD. These include the following:

- Anoro Ellipta contains umeclidinium and vilanterol (a LABA) and is given by oral inhalation.
- Breo Ellipta is a combination of vilanterol and fluticasone given once daily by oral inhalation.
- Bevespi Aerosphere is a combination of glycopyrrolate (an anticholinergic) and formoterol given by oral inhalation.
- Breztri Aerosphere is an oral inhalation drug containing glycopyrronium, formoterol, and budesonide that is administered twice daily.
- Incruse Ellipta contains umeclidinium (an anticholinergic), which relaxes bronchial smooth muscle to cause bronchodilation. It is administered once daily by oral inhalation.
- Roflumilast (Daliresp) is an oral drug for severe COPD that exhibits anti-inflammatory effects on the airways by inhibiting the enzyme PDE4.
- Stiolto Respimat is a combination of tiotropium and olodaterol given once daily by oral inhalation.

Mucolytics, which are medications given to loosen thick viscous bronchial secretions, and expectorants, which are drugs given to aid in the removal of mucus, are sometimes prescribed (see Chapter 45). Long-term oxygen therapy is prescribed in later stages and it has been shown to decrease mortality in patients with advanced COPD. Antibiotics may be prescribed for patients who experience multiple bouts of pulmonary infections.

Patients with COPD should not receive drugs that have beta-adrenergic antagonist activity because they cause bronchoconstriction. Respiratory depressants such as opioids and barbiturates should also be avoided when possible. An important teaching point for the nurse is to strongly encourage smoking cessation in these patients. Smoking cessation has been shown to slow the progression of COPD and to result in fewer respiratory symptoms; however, it cannot undo damage that has already occurred.

Pharmacotherapy of Cystic Fibrosis

44.13 Newer medications are now available to treat the cause of cystic fibrosis.

Cystic fibrosis (CF) is an autosomal recessive disease caused by a mutation in the cystic fibrosis transmembrane regulator (CFTR) gene. This gene produces a channel protein that helps to maintain a balance of salt and water on epithelial surfaces. Mutations in this gene cause chloride to become trapped inside cells, thus preventing water from hydrating the membrane surface. *CFTR* gene mutations result in highly viscous secretions in exocrine glands in multiple organs, especially the respiratory tract, pancreas, GI tract, and sweat glands. Most patients suffer from chronic lung disease and pancreatic insufficiency. The most frequent cause of death is from end-stage pulmonary disease. About 1900 different mutations of the *CFTR* gene have been identified. The primary pharmacologic goals with CF are to:

- Maintain lung function by use of bronchodilators, mucolytics, antibiotics, and CFTR modifiers.
- Administer nutritional support such as pancreatic enzyme supplements and multivitamin and mineral supplements.

Until recently, pharmacotherapy of CF was entirely symptomatic. In 2012, ivacaftor (Kalydeco) became the first medication to actually treat the underlying cause of the disorder. This drug binds to the defective CFTR protein on the cell surface and holds the channel open so that chloride is able to leave the cell.

Research determined that the majority of the CFTR protein made inside the cell never got transported to the surface to form its channel. Three CFTR modulator medications were subsequently approved for combination therapy that enhance the effectiveness of ivacaftor. These drugs act by changing the shape of the defective CFTR protein so that more reaches the cell surface. These new combinations include:

- Orkambi: contains lumacaftor and ivacaftor
- Symdeko: contains tezacaftor and ivacaftor
- Trikafta: contains elexacaftor, tezacaftor, and ivacaftor

While considered breakthrough medications, there are some disadvantages. These medications are extremely expensive (over $250,000 a year). Furthermore, they are only effective against certain types of *CFTR* mutations.

CONNECTIONS: APPLIED CLINICAL JUDGMENT

Patients Receiving Pharmacotherapy for Asthma and COPD

Key Assessment Data

- History of current condition, including previous history of symptoms and association with seasons, foods, or environmental exposures; baseline vital signs, physical exam findings; history of cardiovascular, cerebrovascular, respiratory disease, diabetes; medication history; pregnancy status. Obtain baseline pulmonary function with pulse oximeter, peak expiratory flowmeter, and arterial blood gases.
- If asthma symptoms are of new onset, particularly in infants and young children, assess for any recent changes in diet, soaps including laundry detergent, laundry softener, cosmetics, lotions, and environmental factors (e.g., pets, travel, or recent carpet cleaning) that may correlate with the onset of symptoms.
- Ongoing assessment during drug therapy should include pulse oximeter, peak expiratory flowmeter, and arterial blood gases and assessment of symptom-related effects on eating, sleep, and activity level.

Desired Therapeutic Outcomes

Improvement is observed and measurable by increased ease of breathing, lessened adventitious breath sounds, improvement in pulmonary function studies, improved signs of peripheral oxygenation and increased activity levels, and maintenance of normal eating and sleep periods.

Minimizing Adverse Effects

- Increasing dyspnea, adventitious breath sounds, diminished oxygenation, or increasing anxiety or confusion may indicate inadequate drug therapy, worsening disease process, or respiratory infection and should be reported immediately.
- Acute asthmatic attacks are managed with quick-acting bronchodilation such as beta$_2$ agonists and the patient must be able to identify the appropriate inhaler to use. Provide written instructions, including drug name and when to use, if both quick-acting and long-acting inhalers are ordered.
- Respiratory difficulty and fatigue associated with hypoxia and the work of breathing may affect appetite, ability to eat during dyspnea, and maintenance of required activities of daily living. Adequate nutrition with calorie-rich, nutrient-dense foods, adequate fluids, frequent rest periods between eating or activity, and a cool room for sleeping, are essential to support optimal health.

Lifespan Considerations

- Older adults may be more sensitive to the drug effects due to existing cardiovascular disease and require more frequent monitoring.
- The older adult male is at higher risk for mechanical obstruction due to an enlarged prostate. The older adult is also at increased risk of constipation due to slowed peristalsis.
- Supervise children under the age of 5 to ensure proper inhaler use.

Diversity Considerations

- Because some drugs such as montelukast and theophylline metabolize through the CYP450 system pathways, monitor ethnically diverse patients to ensure optimal therapeutic effects and to minimize adverse effects

CONNECTIONS: APPLIED CLINICAL JUDGMENT *(continued)*

Patients Receiving Pharmacotherapy for Asthma and COPD

Patient Education

- Immediately report symptoms of deteriorating respiratory status such as increased dyspnea, breathlessness with speech, increased anxiety, or orthopnea.
- Use quick-acting inhalers at the earliest possible appearance of symptoms. Long-acting inhalers or oral therapy may be used to maintain bronchodilation but *do not discard quick-acting inhalers if on long-term maintenance therapy*. They may still be needed for periodic acute attacks.
- Peak expiratory flowmeter or other equipment may be ordered to monitor pulmonary function. Keep a log of the results and bring to each medical appointment.
- Continued regular and consistent administration of all bronchodilation therapy helps to prevent acute attacks. Irregular use may increase the risk or severity of bronchoconstrictive events.
- Use spacers for MDIs as ordered. Rinse the mouth after each use of the inhaler and do not swallow after rinsing. This is especially important if a corticosteroid inhaler is used.
- Supplement drug therapy with nonpharmacologic measures including:
  - Increase fluid intake to liquefy and assist in mobilizing mucus.
  - Eat small, frequent meals of calorie-rich, nutrient-dense foods to prevent fatigue and maintain normal nutrition.
  - Ensure adequate rest periods between eating and activities.
  - Decreased room temperature may assist to ease breathing during sleep.
  - Reduce exposure to allergens where possible.
  - Immediately report any significant change in appetite, inability to maintain normal intake, inadequate sleep periods, or inability to carry out required ADLs.
- Recognize the difference between when a quick-acting or long-acting inhaler is used. Labeling the inhalers may be helpful in identifying each.
- Use proper administration techniques depending on the type of inhaler (e.g., MDI, dry powder), including:
  - Use a spacer if instructed between the MDI and the mouth.
  - Shake the inhaler or load it with a tablet or powder as instructed.
  - If using a bronchodilator and corticosteroid inhalers, use the bronchodilator first, wait 5 minutes, then use the corticosteroid to ensure the drug reaches deeply into the bronchial area.
  - Rinse mouth after using any inhaler.
  - Clean the inhaler at least weekly by running warm water through the plastic mouthpiece after removing the drug canister, shaking out excess water, and allowing to air-dry.
- Carry a wallet identification card or wear medical identification jewelry indicating the presence of asthma or a respiratory condition, any significant allergies or anaphylaxis, and use of inhaler therapy.
- With respect to inhaler technique, it is essential that nurses:
  - Understand how each device works and the techniques required to achieve optimal delivery to the lungs
  - Effectively demonstrate to patients how the devices work
  - Regularly assess technique using inhaler competency and correct bad habits as needed.

Prescribing Considerations

- A stepwise and personalized approach to the selection of the most appropriate inhaler (Figure 44.3) is needed in to maximize disease outcomes with minimal risk for adverse effects.
- Cough suppressants are not recommended for people with COPD as suppressing cough may increase the risk of developing an infection.
- The use of beta-blockers must be carefully weighed against notable risks.

Understanding Chapter 44

Key Concepts Summary

44.1 The physiology of the respiratory system involves two main processes: perfusion and ventilation.

44.2 Asthma is a chronic disease that has both inflammatory and bronchospasm components.

44.3 Inhalation is a common route of administration for pulmonary drugs because it delivers drugs directly to their sites of action.

44.4 The goals of asthma pharmacotherapy are to terminate acute bronchospasms and to reduce the frequency of asthma attacks.

44.5 Beta$_2$-adrenergic agonists are the most effective drugs for relieving acute bronchospasm.

44.6 Inhaled anticholinergics are used for preventing bronchospasm.

44.7 Inhaled corticosteroids are the most effective drugs for the long-term control of asthma.

44.8 Mast cell stabilizers are used for the prophylaxis of asthma and act by preventing the release of histamine.

44.9 The leukotriene modifiers, which are primarily used for asthma prophylaxis, act by reducing the inflammatory component of asthma.

44.10 Methylxanthines were once the mainstay of asthma pharmacotherapy but are now rarely prescribed for the disorder.

44.11 Monoclonal antibodies are a newer form of biologic therapy for the prevention of asthma symptoms.

44.12 Chronic obstructive pulmonary disease may be treated with bronchodilators, anti-inflammatory drugs, and mucolytics.

44.13 Newer medications are now available to treat the cause of cystic fibrosis.

CASE STUDY: Making the Patient Connection

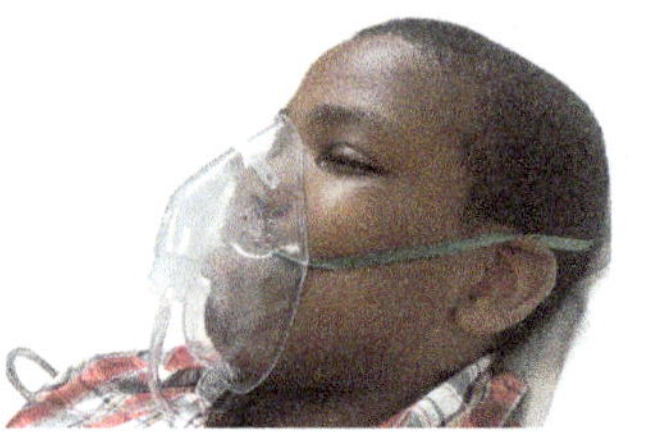

Remember the patient "Nathan Almond" at the beginning of the chapter? Now read the remainder of the case study. Based on the information presented within this chapter, respond to the critical thinking questions that follow.

Nathan is a 12-year-old with a history of asthma, diagnosed 2 years ago. He is an outgoing, active boy and participates in a swim club and a basketball team, but he has had a difficult time adjusting to the limitations of his asthma. He has learned to control acute attacks by using an albuterol (Proventil) MDI, and because his asthma is often triggered by exercise, he has also been using a budesonide (Pulmicort) inhaler and taking montelukast (Singulair).

After competing in his swim meet at the local indoor pool, Nathan began experiencing respiratory distress. He alerted his coach, who retrieved the albuterol inhaler from Nathan's backpack. After two inhalations, Nathan was still in distress and the rescue squad was called.

On admission to the emergency department, Nathan is in obvious distress with pulse oximeter readings of to 91%. He has nasal flaring and bilateral wheezing is heard in his lung fields, pulse rate is 122 beats/min, and he is orthopneic. While treatment is started, the nurse asks him questions that he can nod or shake his head to answer. He shakes his head "no" when asked if he used his budesonide inhaler today and shrugs when asked about his last dose of montelukast.

Critical Thinking Questions

1. Considering his history, medications, and the location where Nathan's asthma attack occurred, what might explain his acute attack?
2. What medications would you anticipate will be prescribed to treat Nathan's acute asthmatic attack and why?
3. What changes might be made to Nathan's medications? What teaching will Nathan and his family need prior to discharge?

Additional Case Study

As the home health nurse, you visit with Mr. Jonas Maxwell weekly to assess his pulmonary status and his adherence to his medication regimen. Jonas has end-stage COPD. He was diagnosed with the disease many years ago and his pulmonary status has deteriorated slowly during the past few years. Despite his healthcare provider's recommendation to change to another medication, Jonas insists that theophylline is the only medication that helps him to breathe. He also uses several MDIs with spacers several times per day.

1. What symptoms would you expect to observe in Jonas if he is experiencing early signs of toxicity?
2. Create a list of things to avoid for an individual who is receiving theophylline therapy.
3. In your own words, how would you describe the function of the spacer used with Jonas's MDI?

Chapter Review

1. A patient with asthma asks which of the prescribed medications should be used in the event of an acute episode of bronchospasm. The nurse will instruct the patient to use:
   1. Albuterol, a beta-agonist bronchodilator, by inhalation.
   2. Beclomethasone, a glucocorticoid anti-inflammatory drug, by inhalation.
   3. Ipratropium, an anticholinergic bronchodilator, by inhalation.
   4. Montelukast, a leukotriene modifier, by mouth.

2. A patient is prescribed a beclomethasone (Qvar) inhaler. Education by the nurse will include:
   1. "Check your heart rate because this drug may cause tachycardia."
   2. "Limit your coffee intake while on this drug."
   3. "Rinse your mouth out well after each use."
   4. "You may feel shaky and nervous after using this drug."

3. The nurse should inform the patient who is prescribed a nebulizer treatment with albuterol (Proventil HFA, VoSpire ER) that a common adverse effect is:
   1. An increased heart rate with palpitations.
   2. A predisposition to infection.
   3. Sedation.
   4. Temporary dyspnea.

4. Vilanterol and fluticasone (Breo Ellipta) has been ordered for a patient with COPD. Because of the combination of drugs, what adverse effects may be expected? (Select all that apply).
   1. Sedation and drowsiness
   2. Tremor and nervousness
   3. Hypotension
   4. Dry mouth and hoarseness
   5. Oropharyngeal candidiasis and increased risk of infections

5. A patient who received a prescription for montelukast (Singulair) returns to his provider's office after 3 days, complaining that "the drug is not working." She reports mild but continued dyspnea and has had to maintain consistent use of her bronchodilator inhaler, albuterol. What does the nurse suspect is the cause of the failure of the montelukast?
   1. The patient is not taking the drug correctly.
   2. The patient is not responding to the drug and will need to be switched to another formulation.
   3. The drug has not had sufficient time of use to have full effects.
   4. The albuterol inhaler is interacting with the montelukast.

6. A 65-year-old patient is prescribed ipratropium (Atrovent) for the treatment of asthma. Which of the following conditions should be reported to the healthcare provider before giving this patient the ipratropium?
   1. A reported allergy to peanuts
   2. A history of intolerance to albuterol
   3. A history of bronchospasms
   4. A reported allergy to chocolate

See Appendix A for answers to critical thinking questions, case study questions and review questions.

References

Asthma and Allergy Foundation of America. (2019). *Asthma facts and figures.* https://www.aafa.org/asthma-facts/

Centers for Disease Control and Prevention. (2016). *Asthma surveillance data.* http://www.cdc.gov/asthma/asthmadata.htm

Har, D., & Lee, M. J. (2019). Systemic reaction rates with omalizumab, subcutaneous immunotherapy, and combination therapy in children with allergic asthma. *Allergy and Asthma Proceedings, 40*, 35–40. https://doi.org/10.2500/aap.2019.40.4173

Maciag, M. C., & Phipatanakul, W. (2019). Preventing the development of asthma: Stopping the allergen march. *Current Opinion in Allergy and Clinical Immunology, 19*, 161–168. https://doi.org/10.1097/ACI.0000000000000501

National Asthma Education and Prevention Program Coordinating Committee. (2020). 2020 focused updates to the asthma management guidelines: A report from the National Asthma Education and Prevention Program Coordinating Committee Expert Panel Working Group. National Heart, Lung, and Blood Institute, National

Institutes of Health. https://www.nhlbi.nih.gov/health-topics/all-publications-and-resources/2020-focused-updates-asthma-management-guidelines

National Center for Health Statistics. (2020). *Asthma.* http://www.cdc.gov/nchs/fastats/asthma.htm

Virchow, J. C. (2019). Allergen immunotherapy (AIT) in asthma. *Seminars in Immunology, 46*, 101334. https:/doi.org/10.1016/j.smim.2019.101334

Selected Bibliography

Barjaktarevic, I. Z., Arredondo, A. F., & Cooper, C. B. (2015). Positioning new pharmacotherapies for COPD. *International Journal of Chronic Obstructive Pulmonary Disease, 10*, 1427–1442. https://doi.org/10.2147/COPD.S83758

Canonica, G. W., Bagnasco, D., Ferrantino, G., Ferrando, M., & Passalacqua, G. (2016). Update on immunotherapy for the treatment of asthma. *Current Opinion in Pulmonary Medicine, 22*, 18–24. https://doi.org/10.1097/MCP.0000000000000227

Carr, T. F., & Kraft, M. (2015). Update in asthma 2014. *American Journal of Respiratory and Critical Care Medicine, 192*(2), 157–163. https://doi.org/10.1164/rccm.201503-0597UP

Centers for Disease Control and Prevention. (2020). *Asthma.* http://www.cdc.gov/nchs/fastats/asthma.htm

Choby, G. W., & Lee, S. (2015). Pharmacotherapy for the treatment of asthma: Current treatment options and future directions. *International Forum of Allergy and Rhinology, 5*(Suppl. 1), S35–S40. https://doi.org/10.1002/alr.21592

Grainge, C., Thomas, P. S., Mak, J. C., Benton, M. J., Lim, T. K., & Ko, F. W. (2016). Year in review 2015: Asthma and chronic obstructive pulmonary disease. *Respirology, 21*, 765–775. https://doi.org/10.1111/resp.12771

Lopes-Pacheco, M. (2020). CFTR modulators: The changing face of cystic fibrosis in the era of precision medicine. *Frontiers in Pharmacology, 10*, 1662. https://doi.org/10.3389/fphar.2019.01662

Morris, M. J. (2019). *Asthma guidelines*. Medscape. http://emedicine.medscape.com/article/296301-guidelines#g1

Sharma, G. D. (2021) *Pediatric asthma*. Medscape. http://emedicine.medscape.com/article/1000997-overview

Shedd, G. C., & Hays, C. N. (2016). The pregnant patient with asthma: Assessment and management. *Journal for Nurse Practitioners, 12*(1), 1–6. https://doi.org/10.1016/j.nurpra.2015.10.019

“I can’t stop coughing, I can’t sleep, and my head hurts. I thought I had a summer cold, but this is just dragging on. It’s affecting my work!”

—*Patient “Nancy Chen”*

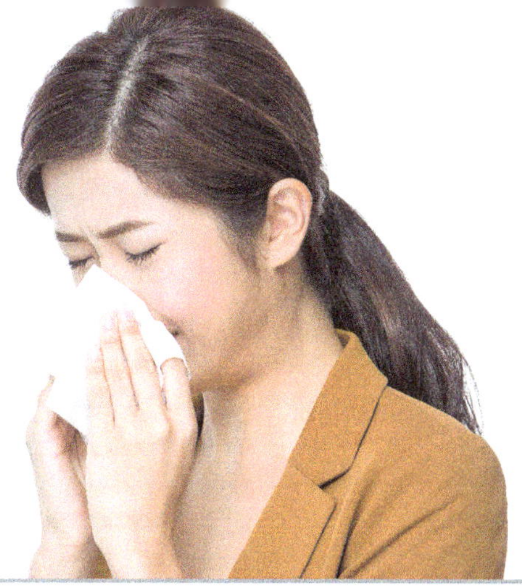

Chapter 45
Pharmacotherapy of Allergic Rhinitis and the Common Cold

Chapter Outline

Learning Outcomes

After reading this chapter, the student should be able to:

1. Identify structures of the upper respiratory tract that serve as body defenses against foreign substances.
2. Describe the common causes and symptoms of allergic rhinitis.
3. Differentiate between H_1 and H_2 histamine receptors.
4. Compare and contrast the first- and second-generation antihistamines.
5. Explain why intranasal corticosteroids are preferred drugs for the treatment of allergic rhinitis.
6. Compare and contrast the oral and intranasal decongestants.
7. Explain why it is usually better to take individual drugs for the common cold rather than a multisymptom combination product.
8. Describe the appropriate use of cough suppressants.
9. Describe the use of drugs prescribed to treat thick bronchial secretions.
10. For each of the classes shown in the chapter outline, identify the prototype and representative drugs and explain the mechanism(s) of drug action, primary indications, contraindications, significant drug interactions, pregnancy data, and important adverse effects.
11. Apply clinical judgment to care for patients receiving pharmacotherapy for allergic rhinitis and the common cold.

Key Terms

Definitions of the terms in bold may be found in the Glossary.

The respiratory system begins at the nose and ends at the respiratory membrane, the dividing line between the alveoli and the pulmonary capillaries. The pharmacotherapy of asthma and chronic obstructive pulmonary disease (COPD), which are conditions of the lower respiratory tract, is discussed in Chapter 44. This chapter examines the drugs used for two conditions that are primarily associated with the upper respiratory tract: allergic rhinitis and the common cold. Because many of these medications are readily available over the counter (OTC), it is essential for the patient to receive effective teaching for their use.

Physiology of the Upper Respiratory Tract

45.1 The upper respiratory tract acts as a defense in preventing systemic infection.

The upper respiratory tract (URT) consists of the nose, nasal cavity, pharynx, and paranasal sinuses. These passageways filter, warm, and humidify air during inhalation. The URT traps particulate matter and many pathogens, preventing them from being carried to the bronchioles and alveoli, where they would have access to the capillaries of the systemic circulation. The mucous membranes of the URT are lined with ciliated epithelium. The cilia projecting from the epithelium are found throughout the nasal passages and help to trap smaller particles. The cilia exert a wavelike motion that sweeps the pathogens and particulate matter upward toward the oropharynx, where they are swallowed when someone coughs or clears the throat. A sneeze clears the nasal passages. The basic structures of the URT are shown in Figure 45.1.

The nasal mucosa is a dynamic structure richly supplied with vascular tissue that is controlled, in part, by the autonomic nervous system. Activation of the sympathetic nervous system constricts the arterioles in the nose, reducing the thickness of the mucosal layer. This serves to widen the airway and allow air to more freely enter the URT. Parasympathetic activation has the opposite effect: The arterioles dilate, and more mucus is produced. This difference is important during therapy with drugs that affect the autonomic nervous system. For example, administration of a sympathomimetic will shrink the nasal mucosa, relieving nasal stuffiness associated with the common cold. These drugs are classified as decongestants. On the other hand, parasympathetic drugs cause increased blood flow to the nose with increased nasal stuffiness and a runny nose as side effects.

The oral mucosa serves an important role in the body's defense against invasion by microbes. Saliva contains immunoglobulins (IgA) and lysozyme, which break

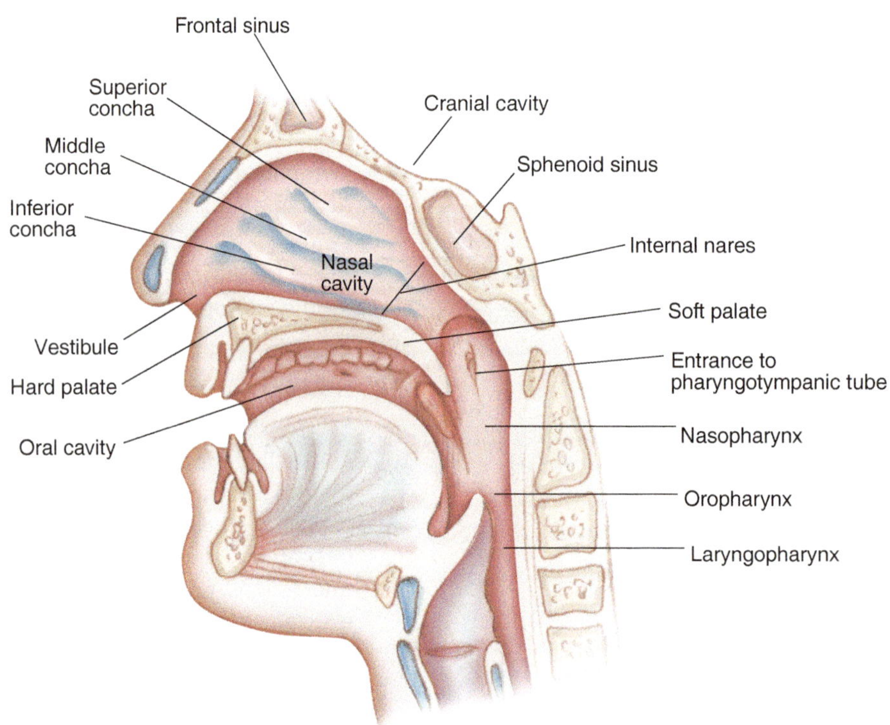

Figure 45.1 The respiratory system.

down bacterial cell walls. Swallowed saliva or nasal mucus exposes microorganisms to the hostile environment of the stomach where they contact high gastric acidity and enzymes that kill them.

The nasal mucosa is also part of the first line of body defense, secreting up to a quart of mucus daily. This fluid is rich in immunoglobulins that are able to neutralize airborne pathogens. The nasal mucosa contains numerous nonspecific body defense cells that can activate complement or engulf microbes. Mast cells, which contain histamine, also line the nasal mucosa, and these play a major role in causing the symptoms of allergic rhinitis.

Pathophysiology of Allergic Rhinitis

45.2 Allergic rhinitis is caused by exposure to an environmental allergen, which leads to symptoms that resemble those of the common cold.

Allergic rhinitis is inflammation of the nasal mucosa due to exposure to allergens. Although not life threatening, allergic rhinitis is a condition that affects millions of people and one that is a common indication for pharmacotherapy.

The symptoms of allergic rhinitis resemble those of the common cold and include tearing, burning, red, swollen, or itching eyes; sneezing; nasal itching or congestion; postnasal drip; cough; and scratchy throat. In addition to the acute symptoms, complications of allergic rhinitis may include loss of taste or smell, sinusitis, hoarseness, and plugged ears. Some people may not obtain restful sleep and awaken very fatigued. Symptoms can be severe enough to cause poor performance in or absence from school or work. Because of the smaller size of their anatomic structures, children are also at increased risk for middle ear infections.

As with other types of allergies, the cause of allergic rhinitis is exposure to an antigen. An antigen, also called an allergen, is anything that is recognized as foreign and provokes a response from the body's defense system. The specific allergen responsible for a patient's allergic rhinitis is often difficult to pinpoint; however, common agents are pollens from weeds, grasses, and trees; mold spores; dust mites; certain foods; and animal dander (skin flakes). Chemical fumes, tobacco smoke, or air pollutants such as ozone are nonallergenic factors that may worsen symptoms. In addition, there is a strong genetic predisposition to allergic rhinitis.

PharmFACT

Allergic rhinitis affects about 19 million adults and over 5 million children in the United States each year. Over 12 million office visits each year have allergic rhinitis as the primary diagnosis. (Centers for Disease Control and Prevention, 2020).

Some patients experience symptoms of allergic rhinitis at specific times of the year when the pollen level is high. These periods are typically in the spring and fall when plants and trees are blooming, thus the name *seasonal* allergic rhinitis. Obviously, the blooming season changes with geographic location and with each species of plant. Patients may need symptom relief for only a few months during the year. When the symptoms are caused by an *outdoor* allergen, the condition is called hay fever. Others are afflicted with allergic rhinitis symptoms throughout the year because they are continuously exposed to *indoor* allergens, such as dust mites, animal dander, or mold. This variation is termed *perennial* allergic rhinitis. These patients may require a treatment plan that includes continuous pharmacotherapy.

It is often not clear whether a patient is experiencing seasonal or perennial allergic rhinitis. Patients with seasonal allergies may also be sensitive to some of the perennial allergens. It is also common for one allergen to sensitize patients to another allergen. For example, during ragweed season, a patient may become hyperresponsive to other allergens such as mold spores or animal dander. The body's response and the symptoms of allergic rhinitis are the same, however, regardless of the specific allergen(s). Allergy testing can help pinpoint the particular allergens responsible for the symptoms and help direct a treatment plan that includes avoiding allergens that cause the symptoms and treating the symptoms.

The fundamental pathophysiology responsible for allergic rhinitis is inflammation of the mucous membranes in the nose, throat, and airways. The nasal mucosa is rich with mast cells and basophils, both of which synthesize and store histamine. The release of histamine and other substances such as leukotrienes occurs after a patient has been exposed to specific allergens. The allergen stimulates the production of high amounts of immunoglobulin E (IgE). The IgE antibodies then bind to the outer surface of mast cells and basophils, thus sensitizing them. Sometime later, when reexposed to an antigen such as pollen, the antigen attaches to the antibody and the antigen–antibody reaction begins. This reaction stimulates a process that begins by mobilizing intracellular calcium and, eventually, the sensitized cells release chemical mediators, including histamine. In certain cases, histamine can be released from mast cells without prior exposure to an antigen (allergen). These nonallergic releases of histamine can occur with cell damage, certain drugs, plasma expanders, or radiographic contrast media.

Patients with allergic rhinitis have greater numbers of mast cells. An immediate (or Type I) hypersensitivity response releases histamine and other chemical mediators such as leukotrienes and prostaglandins from the mast cells and basophils. The body's response to the chemical mediators is to cause vasodilation of arterioles and venules, increase capillary permeability, constrict smooth muscle (bronchioles), increase secretions of glands such as the lacrimals, and act as a neurotransmitter in the central nervous

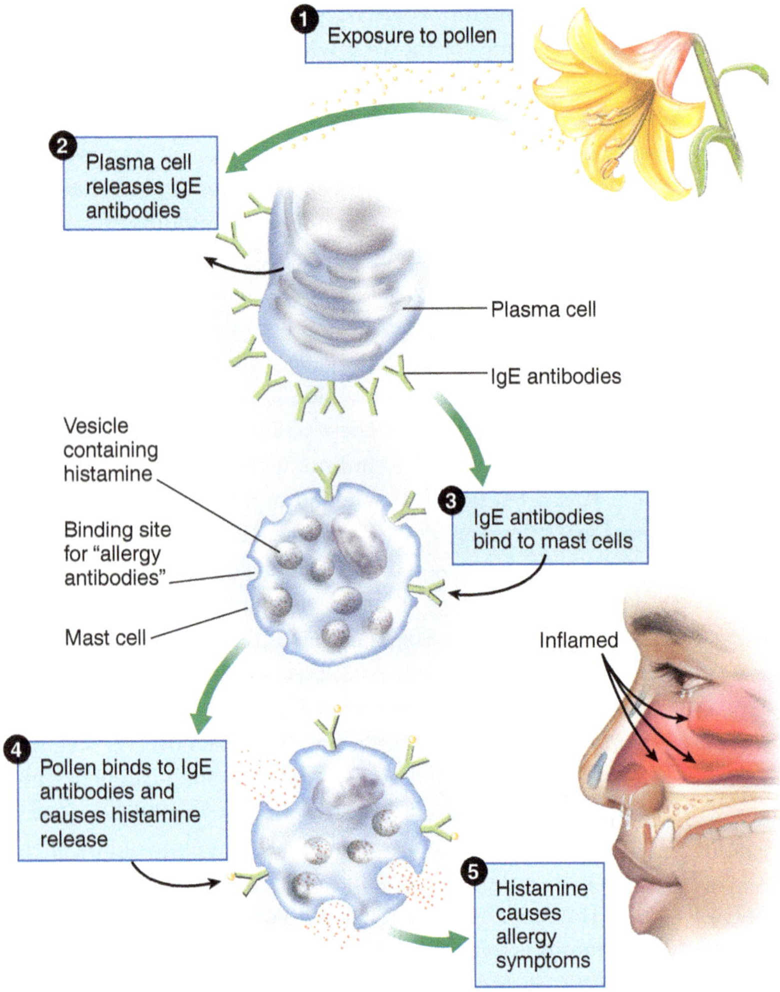

Figure 45.2 Pathophysiology of allergic rhinitis.

system (CNS). These responses, in the case of allergic rhinitis, produce flushing of the skin, sneezing, itching nasal membranes, and watery eyes and may cause drowsiness. A delayed hypersensitivity reaction also occurs 4 to 8 hours after the initial exposure, causing continuous inflammation of the mucosa and adding to the chronic nasal congestion experienced from the allergic response. Because histamine is released during an allergic response, many signs and symptoms of allergy are similar to those of inflammation. The mechanism of allergic rhinitis is illustrated in Figure 45.2.

Pharmacotherapy of Allergic Rhinitis

45.3 Drugs for allergic rhinitis include those that prevent the disorder and those that relieve symptoms.

The therapeutic goals of treating allergic rhinitis are to prevent its occurrence and to relieve symptoms. Drugs that are used to treat allergic rhinitis may thus be grouped into two simple categories: preventers and relievers.

- *Preventers* are used for prophylaxis. These include antihistamines, intranasal corticosteroids, leukotriene modifiers, and mast cell stabilizers.
- *Relievers* are used to provide immediate, though temporary, relief for acute allergy symptoms once they have occurred. Relievers include the oral and intranasal decongestants, which are usually drugs from the sympathomimetic class but may include anticholinergics.

Nurses should help patients identify the sources of the allergy and recommend appropriate actions. These may include removing pets from the home environment or limiting their exposure (such as not allowing pets on furniture); cleaning moldy surfaces; using and routinely cleaning or replacing microfilters on air-conditioning units; and frequent cleaning to remove dust mites from bedding, carpet, or furniture. Although dust mites can never be totally removed from mattresses, regularly decreasing their numbers can help lessen symptoms of allergic rhinitis. It may be interesting to know that dust mites feed primarily on naturally shedding human skin and that it is not the microscopic dust mite itself that a patient inhales and is allergic to, but rather its excrement.

45.4 Antihistamines are widely used to treat allergic rhinitis and other minor allergies.

There are two types of receptors for histamine: H_1 and H_2. Activation of **H_1 receptors** produces the typical symptoms of allergy. Drugs that block H_2 receptors such as ranitidine (Zantac) reduce gastric acid secretion and are used to treat peptic ulcer disease and gastroesophageal reflux disease. This histamine receptor activity is not related to allergic responses and is covered in Chapter 59.

H_1-receptor antagonists, also called *antihistamines*, are drugs that selectively block histamine from reaching its H_1 receptors, thus alleviating allergic symptoms. Because the term *antihistamine* is nonspecific and does not indicate which of the two histamine receptors is affected, *H_1-receptor antagonist* (or *blocker*) is a more accurate name. In clinical practice, as well as in this text, the two terms are used interchangeably. Antihistamines that selectively block H_1 receptors are widely used as OTC remedies for the relief of allergy symptoms, motion sickness, and insomnia. The antihistamines are listed in Table 45.1.

The most frequent therapeutic use of antihistamines is for the treatment of allergies. These medications provide symptomatic relief from the sneezing, runny nose, and

Table 45.1 H_1-Receptor Antagonists for Allergies

Drug	Route and Adult Dose (Maximum Dose Where Indicated)	Adverse Effects
First-Generation Drugs		
brompheniramine (Dimetapp, others)	PO: 4–8 mg q4–6h (max: 40 mg/day)	*Dry mouth, headache, dizziness, urinary retention, thickening of bronchial secretions, nausea and vomiting* Paradoxical excitation (usually in children), sedation, hypersensitivity reactions, hypotension, extrapyramidal symptoms (promethazine), agranulocytosis (brompheniramine, clemastine, promethazine)
chlorpheniramine	PO: 2–4 mg q4–6h (max: 24 mg/day)	
clemastine (Tavist)	PO: 1.34–2.68 mg q12h (max: 8.04 mg/day)	
cyproheptadine	PO: 4–20 mg q6–8h (max: 0.5 mg/kg/day)	
dexchlorpheniramine (Polman)	PO: 2 mg q4–6h (max: 12 mg/day)	
dimenhydrinate (Dramamine)	PO: 50–100 mg q4–6h	
diphenhydramine (Benadryl, others)	PO: 25–50 mg q6–8h (max: 300 mg/day)	
promethazine	PO: 12.5–25 mg q6–24h (max: 100 mg/day)	
Second-Generation Drugs		
azelastine (Astelin, Astepro)	Intranasal: 2 sprays per nostril q12h Ocular: 1 drop in each affected eye bid	*Dry mouth, headache, dizziness, nausea, drowsiness (cetirizine), bitter taste (olopatadine)* Paradoxical excitation, hypersensitivity reactions, hypotension
cetirizine (Zyrtec)	PO: 5–10 mg/day (max: 10 mg/day)	
desloratadine (Clarinex)	PO: 5 mg/day (max: 5 mg/day)	
fexofenadine (Allegra)	PO: 60 mg q12h or 180 mg once daily	
levocetirizine (Xyzal)	PO: 5 mg (1 tablet or 2 teaspoons) once daily	
loratadine (Claritin)	PO: 10 mg/day (max: 10 mg/day)	
olopatadine (Patanase, Pataday)	Intranasal (Patanase): 2 sprays per nostril bid Ocular (Pataday): 1 drop in each affected eye once daily	

Note: *Italics* indicate common adverse effects. Underline indicates serious adverse effects.

itching of the eyes, nose, and throat of allergic rhinitis. Antihistamines are often combined with decongestants and antitussives in OTC cold and sinus medicines. Common OTC antihistamine combinations that are used to treat allergies are listed in Table 45.2.

Antihistamines are most effective when taken prophylactically to *prevent* allergic symptoms. Their effectiveness in reversing allergic symptoms that have already manifested is limited. This is because antihistamines block the effect of histamine at its receptor sites. They do not prevent the release of histamine from mast cells. Their effectiveness may diminish with long-term use.

In addition to producing antihistamine effects, these drugs also easily cross the blood–brain barrier and block cholinergic receptors to cause typical anticholinergic effects. Anticholinergic effects are responsible for certain beneficial effects of antihistamines, such as drying of mucous membranes, which results in less nasal congestion and tearing.

A large number of H_1-receptor antagonists are available as medications. They all have the same basic mechanism of action and are equally effective in treating allergic rhinitis and other mild allergies. Adverse effects are similar but differ in intensity among the various antihistamines. The older, first-generation antihistamines frequently cause significant drowsiness, which can be a limiting adverse effect in some patients. After a few doses tolerance generally develops to sedation. The newer, second-generation antihistamines cause less sedation because they do not cross the blood–brain barrier. Alcohol and other CNS depressants should be used with caution when taking antihistamines

Table 45.2 Selected Over-the-Counter Antihistamine Combinations

Trade Name	Antihistamine	Decongestant	Analgesic
Actifed Cold and Allergy tablets	chlorpheniramine	phenylephrine	—
Benadryl Allergy/Cold	diphenhydramine	phenylephrine	acetaminophen
Chlor-Trimeton Allergy/Decongestant tablets	chlorpheniramine	pseudoephedrine	—
Dimetapp Children's Cold and Allergy	brompheniramine	phenylephrine	—
Sudafed PE Sinus Congestion tablets	diphenhydramine	phenylephrine	—
Triaminic Cold/Allergy	chlorpheniramine	phenylephrine	—
Tylenol Allergy Multi-Symptom Gels	chlorpheniramine	phenylephrine	acetaminophen
Tylenol PM Gelcaps	diphenhydramine	—	acetaminophen

because their sedating effects may be additive, even for the second-generation drugs. Some patients (especially young children) exhibit CNS stimulation, which can cause insomnia, nervousness, and tremors, or even convulsions. Other CNS adverse effects, such as dizziness, confusion, and even fatigue, more commonly affect the older adult.

The second major adverse effect of antihistamines relates to their anticholinergic effects. Excessive drying of mucous membranes can lead to dry mouth, and urinary hesitancy may be troublesome for patients, especially those with prostatic hyperplasia. Diphenhydramine and clemastine exhibit a significant incidence of anticholinergic adverse effects, whereas the second-generation drugs—loratadine, desloratadine, and fexofenadine—produce the least.

Although most antihistamines are given via the oral route (PO), azelastine (Astelin, Astepro) and olopatadine (Patanase) are available by the intranasal route. These drugs are as effective as the PO antihistamines, but because they are applied locally to the nasal mucosa, limited systemic absorption occurs. This may make the intranasal drugs slightly safer than PO antihistamines.

Antihistamines are used as adjuncts to the emergency treatment of anaphylaxis, which is the most severe form of allergic reaction. Although massive histamine release causes bronchoconstriction, edema, hypotension, and other symptoms of anaphylaxis, other inflammatory mediators, including leukotrienes and prostaglandins, contribute to the hypersensitivity response. Because antihistamines do not block these other mediators, antihistamines are effective only as adjunctive therapy in anaphylaxis. They are most effective if given as preventive medications before anaphylaxis for patients who are at high risk of having an allergic response. The major life-threatening symptoms of anaphylaxis are controlled with epinephrine and other vasoconstrictors.

H_1-receptor antagonists are effective in treating a number of other disorders, including the following:

- **Vertigo and motion sickness.** Nausea resulting from vertigo or motion sickness responds well to antihistamines. These drugs act by suppressing the vomiting center in the medulla and depressing the excitability of the neurons of the vestibular apparatus of the inner ear. To be effective, they must be taken prior to the onset of symptoms. Meclizine (Antivert) and dimenhydrinate (Dramamine) are the two most common antihistamines used for this purpose. The pharmacotherapy of nausea is discussed in Chapter 60.
- **Parkinson's disease.** Drugs with significant anticholinergic actions are used to treat mild forms of Parkinson's disease. They are also used to treat the tremor and extrapyramidal adverse effects from conventional antipsychotic drugs. Because diphenhydramine exerts great amounts of anticholinergic action, it is sometimes used to treat these conditions.
- **Insomnia.** Many patients become drowsy after taking first-generation antihistamines. OTC sleep aids usually include antihistamines such as diphenhydramine and doxylamine (Unisom SleepTabs). After a few days, patients will become tolerant to the drowsiness produced by these drugs; thus, they should be used for 2 weeks or less.
- **Urticaria and other skin rashes.** Urticaria or hives is often caused by the release of histamine, and the condition responds well to H_1-receptor blockers. Symptomatic treatment may include any of the first- or second-generation medications, either using PO drugs or topical creams or lotions.

CONNECTIONS: Lifespan Consideration

Antihistamines and Potential Hazards for Older Adults

First-generation antihistamines (FGAs) are found in many OTC combination products. They tend to be more sedating and are often used for this effect in sleep-promoting products. The older adult is also more sensitive to the effects of first-generation antihistamines, and drowsiness, dizziness, and fall risk are possible, as well as cognitive impairment and anticholinergic-related effects such as constipation and dry mouth. For the older adult man, the anticholinergic effects of antihistamines may exacerbate symptoms of an enlarged prostate and worsen urinary symptoms. Particularly concerning is the potential effect on driving and response to hazards. In a study by Hill et al. (2020), antihistamines significantly altered protective maneuvers during driving, such as right-hand turning away from a hazard.

In studying prescribing patterns of FGAs, Cenzar and colleagues (2020) noted that for skin-related conditions, FGAs were prescribed for older adults at the same rate as for younger adults with similar diagnoses, but that primary care providers tended to prescribe FGAs at higher rates than dermatologists. Because a patient may seek care from more than one provider, a medication reconciliation is especially important. It has also been noted that older adults taking FGAs such as diphenhydramine and doxylamine for sleep were not aware of potential safety hazards posed by the drugs (Abraham et al., 2017). When a patient is noted to be taking FGAs on the medication history, assessing driving and transportation needs may be warranted.

Because antihistamines, and particularly FGAs, can pose a significant risk to the older adult, the provider should review all current medications at each encounter, both OTC and prescribed, to assess for any drug interactions and for the use of potentially hazardous medications such as antihistamines. Providing information on the risks, the potential for taking OTC combination products containing similar drugs, and providing a written treatment plan to the patient, in the case that memory issues may be of concern, may decrease both inappropriate use and decrease the risk of adverse effects.

CONNECTION Checkpoint 45.1

Although drugs with anticholinergic action are used to treat Parkinson's disease, they are generally not first-line medications. From what you learned in Chapter 21, name the drug most commonly prescribed for Parkinson's disease and the neurotransmitter it replaces.

PROTOTYPE DRUG Fexofenadine (Allegra)

Classification **Therapeutic:** Drug for allergic rhinitis and minor allergies
Pharmacologic: H_1-receptor antagonist (second generation), antihistamine

Therapeutic Effects and Uses: Approved by the U.S. Food and Drug Administration (FDA) in 1996 for the treatment of seasonal allergic rhinitis, fexofenadine is a second-generation H_1-receptor antagonist with an effectiveness that is equivalent to that of diphenhydramine. Most effective when taken before symptoms develop, fexofenadine reduces the severity of nasal congestion, sneezing, and tearing of the eyes.

The long half-life of fexofenadine—over 14 hours—allows it to be administered once or twice daily. Fexofenadine is available in PO form as regular tablets, orally disintegrating tablets, and as a suspension. In addition to allergic rhinitis, it is also approved to treat chronic idiopathic urticaria. Allegra-D combines fexofenadine with the decongestant pseudoephedrine.

Mechanism of Action: Fexofenadine acts by competing with histamine for binding to histamine (H_1) receptor sites. It does not prevent the release of histamine.

Pharmacokinetics:

Route(s)	PO (capsules, tablets, and suspension)
Absorption	Rapid
Distribution	Does not cross the blood–brain barrier; unknown if secreted in breast milk; 60–70% bound to plasma protein
Primary metabolism	Hepatic
Primary excretion	80% renal, 11% feces
Onset of action	Usually within 1 h
Duration of action	Half-life: 14.4 h; duration: 12–24 h

Adverse Effects: The major advantage of fexofenadine over first-generation antihistamines is that drowsiness is not a major adverse effect. Adverse effects are infrequent and usually minor and include headache, nausea, dyspepsia, and dysmenorrhea. Patients who are taking the drug have an increased incidence of viral infections. Anticholinergic effects such as dry mouth can occur.

Contraindications/Precautions: The only contraindication to fexofenadine is hypersensitivity to this drug. Patients with advanced chronic kidney disease should receive reduced doses.

Drug Interactions: Although considered nonsedating, fexofenadine can still cause drowsiness in certain patients at high doses and if combined with CNS depressants, including alcohol. Concurrent administration with ketoconazole or erythromycin increases the plasma concentrations of fexofenadine. Prolongation of the QT interval has occurred with other antihistamines but is infrequent with this drug. Antacids that contain aluminum or magnesium may interfere with the absorption of fexofenadine. **Herbal/Food:** Absorption may be decreased when taken with grapefruit, orange, or apple juice, thereby reducing the bioavailability of fexofenadine.

Pregnancy: Fexofenadine was not teratogenic in laboratory animals but did reduce the survival rate of offspring. Adverse effects of the drug during pregnancy and lactation are unknown.

Treatment of Overdose: Overdose may cause CNS depression, dry mouth, and dizziness. There is no specific antidote for overdose, and supportive treatment of symptoms is indicated.

Clinician Responsibilities: Key clinical implications for patients receiving fexofenadine are included in Applied Clinical Judgment: Patients Receiving Pharmacotherapy with Antihistamines and for Symptomatic Cough and Cold Relief.

Drugs Similar to Fexofenadine (Allegra)

The second-generation H_1 antagonists include azelastine, cetirizine, desloratadine, loratadine, and olopatadine. Because the first-generation antihistamines are all very similar, the description of diphenhydramine included in this section serves as an example of this group.

Azelastine (Astelin, Astepro): Originally approved in 2000, azelastine is a second-generation H_1 antagonist approved for relief of symptoms caused by seasonal allergic rhinitis. An intranasal formulation (Astepro) was subsequently approved to treat perennial allergic rhinitis and an ophthalmic formulation for allergic conjunctivitis. Dymista is a combination drug that combines azelastine with fluticasone, a corticosteroid. Adverse effects of intranasal azelastine include local effects on the nasal mucosa such as epistaxis (nosebleed), a bitter taste, and postnasal drip. The most common side effects of eyedrop therapy are headache, transient eye stinging, and a bitter taste. The drug can cause drowsiness, especially when combined with CNS depressants or alcohol. Animal studies showed developmental toxicity, embryofetal death, and malformations. Adverse effects on the breastfed neonate are unknown.

Cetirizine (Zyrtec): Approved in 1995, cetirizine is a second-generation antihistamine that is commonly used for treating both seasonal and perennial allergic rhinitis and chronic idiopathic urticaria. In 2017 an ophthalmic form of the drug was approved to treat ocular itching caused by allergic conjunctivitis. It may be used off-label to treat atopic dermatitis and symptoms of allergy-induced asthma. Various PO formulations are available, including tablets to be swallowed, chewable tablets, and syrup. It is well tolerated and approved for children as young as 2 years of age. Adverse effects are uncommon. Cetirizine appears to be somewhat more sedating than other second-generation drugs. Xerostomia and fatigue are additional adverse effects. The drug was moved from prescription to OTC status in 2007. Cetirizine is an active metabolite of hydroxyzine (Vistaril), an older first-generation antihistamine. Animal studies did not show evidence of fetal harm. Because the drug is secreted in milk, caution should be used if breastfeeding.

In 2007, an isomer of cetirizine was approved by the FDA. Levocetirizine (Xyzal) is a PO antihistamine that has the same indications and actions as those of cetirizine but is reported to cause less drowsiness.

Desloratadine (Clarinex): Desloratadine is a nonsedating, second-generation antihistamine that was approved in 2001 for the treatment of both seasonal and perennial allergic rhinitis and chronic idiopathic urticaria. It is the active metabolite of loratadine (Claritin). Desloratadine is administered by the PO route and is approved to treat adults and children ages 6 months and older. Like other second-generation drugs, sedation is minimal and adverse effects are uncommon. Headache, pharyngitis, and xerostomia are the most frequently reported adverse effects. Clarinex-D is an extended-release combination of desloratadine with pseudoephedrine. Desloratadine did not show teratogenicity in laboratory animals. Because the drug is secreted in milk, caution should be used if breastfeeding.

Diphenhydramine (Benadryl, others): Diphenhydramine is a first-generation H_1-receptor antagonist that is commonly used to treat minor symptoms of allergy and the common cold such as sneezing, runny nose, and tearing of the eyes. It exhibits a strong anticholinergic drying action on mucous membranes. OTC diphenhydramine is often combined with an analgesic, decongestant, or expectorant when treating cold symptoms. Diphenhydramine is also used as a topical drug to treat rashes, and intramuscular (IM) and intravenous (IV) forms are available for severe allergic reactions. Elixir and syrup forms are available for administration to young children. Other indications for diphenhydramine include Parkinson's disease, motion sickness, and insomnia. Diphenhydramine can cause significant drowsiness, although this usually diminishes with long-term use. Occasionally diphenhydramine is given to produce drowsiness as a treatment for insomnia. Some patients, especially children, may experience paradoxical excitement. This drug may cause anticholinergic adverse effects such as urinary retention, tachycardia, elevated blood pressure, xerostomia, thickening of bronchial secretions, and blurred vision. Animal studies did not show evidence of teratogenicity or impaired fertility. Beacuse small amounts of this drug enter milk, breastfed neonates should be observed for signs of irritability or drowsiness.

Loratadine (Claritin): Loratadine was the first of the second-generation antihistamines, approved in 1993, to treat seasonal allergic rhinitis and chronic idiopathic urticaria. In 2002, the high safety record of loratadine led to the reclassification of the drug from prescription to OTC. Like other drugs in its class, loratadine causes very little drowsiness, and adverse effects are unusual. It is only available PO and may be administered to children ages 2 and older. Drowsiness and headache may occur at higher doses. Loratadine did not show teratogenicity in laboratory animals. Because the drug is secreted in milk, caution should be used if breastfeeding.

Olopatadine (Patanase, Pataday): Olopatadine is a second-generation H_1 antagonist approved in 1996. The intranasal spray (Patanase) is approved for the treatment of seasonal allergic rhinitis in adults and children 12 years of age and older. Adverse effects of olopatadine include local effects on the nasal mucosa such as epistaxis, a bitter taste, and postnasal drip. Other adverse effects include headache, throat pain, and URT infection. Although uncommon, nasal ulceration and septal perforation are serious adverse effects. In some patients, the drug can cause drowsiness; thus, it should be used with caution when combined with CNS depressants and alcohol. An ophthalmic formulation (Pataday) is approved for the treatment of allergic conjunctivitis. As eyedrops, the drug can cause local effects such as blurred vision, burning or stinging, and dry eyes. Animal studies showed evidence of fetal harm at high doses when given by the PO route. It is not known if this medication enters breast milk when given by the intranasal route.

CONNECTION Checkpoint 45.2

From what you learned in Chapter 44, what is the role of leukotriene antagonists in treating asthma? What drug classes are preferred for this condition?

45.5 Intranasal corticosteroids are preferred drugs for allergic rhinitis because of their effectiveness and safety.

Corticosteroids, also known as glucocorticoids, may be applied directly to the nasal mucosa to prevent symptoms of allergic rhinitis. These drugs are listed in Table 45.3.

Table 45.3 Intranasal Corticosteroids and Miscellaneous Drugs for Allergic Rhinitis

Drug	Route and Adult Dose (Maximum Dose Where Indicated)	Adverse Effects
Intranasal Corticosteroids		
beclomethasone (Qnasl, Qvar Redihaler)	Intranasal: 1 spray bid–qid	*Transient nasal irritation, burning, sneezing, dryness* Hypercorticism (only if large amounts are swallowed), nasal ulceration, oral *Candida* infection, nasal pharyngitis, epistaxis
budesonide (Rhinocort Allergy)	Intranasal: 2 sprays bid	
ciclesonide (Omnaris, Zetonna)	Intranasal: 2 sprays once daily (Zetonna) or bid (Omnaris) (max: 200 mcg/day)	
fluticasone (Flonase)	Intranasal: 1–2 sprays in each nostril once daily	
mometasone (Nasonex)	Intranasal: 2 sprays/day	
triamcinolone (Nasacort Allergy)	Intranasal: 2–4 sprays 4 times daily	
Miscellaneous Drugs		
cromolyn	Intranasal: 1 spray in each nostril tid–qid	*Nasal burning and irritation* Anaphylaxis
ipratropium	Intranasal: 2 sprays per nostril tid–qid	*Transient nasal irritation, burning, sneezing or dryness, cough* Urinary retention, worsening of glaucoma
montelukast (Singulair)	PO: 10 mg/day	*Headache, nausea, diarrhea* No serious adverse effects

Note: *Italics* indicate common adverse effects. Underline indicates serious adverse effects.

Although corticosteroids are very effective at reducing allergy symptoms, their oral and parenteral uses are limited by potentially serious adverse effects. Intranasal formulations of these drugs, however, produce virtually no serious adverse effects. Because of their effectiveness and safety, the intranasal corticosteroids have joined antihistamines as first-line drugs in the therapy of allergic rhinitis; and they are now considered the most effective drug treatment for seasonal and perennial allergic rhinitis. Intranasal corticosteroids are also used for patients undergoing nasal or sinus surgery for their anti-inflammatory action.

When sprayed onto the nasal mucosa, corticosteroids act by multiple mechanisms. They decrease the secretion of inflammatory mediators, reduce tissue edema, and cause a mild vasoconstriction. All corticosteroids are administered with a metered-spray device that delivers a consistent dose of drug per spray. All have equal effectiveness. Unlike sympathomimetics, however, the benefits of inhaled corticosteroids are not immediate. To achieve peak response, 1 to 3 weeks (often longer with perennial rhinitis than seasonal rhinitis) may be required. After the patient's symptoms are controlled, the dose of intranasal corticosteroids is reduced to the lowest amount required to control the symptoms. The intranasal corticosteroids must be taken daily to produce maximum benefit. Rhinocort Aqua, Flonase, and Nasacort AQ are available OTC.

When administered appropriately, the actions of corticosteroids are limited to the nasal passages. The most frequently reported adverse effect is an intense burning sensation in the nose immediately after spraying. Excessive drying of the nasal mucosa may occur, leading to epistaxis.

PROTOTYPE DRUG Fluticasone (Flonase, Veramyst)

Classification **Therapeutic:** Drug for allergic rhinitis, asthma, and COPD
Pharmacologic: Intranasal corticosteroid

Therapeutic Effects and Uses: Approved in 1990, fluticasone is an intranasal corticosteroid that is used for the management of nasal symptoms associated with seasonal and perennial rhinitis. Therapy usually begins with two sprays in each nostril, twice daily, and decreases to one dose per day. Prolonged use of corticosteroids can lead to tolerance to the drug's therapeutic effects.

Veramyst and Dymista are two newer formulations of this drug. Veramyst contains intranasal fluticasone that is approved for the treatment of both seasonal and perennial allergic rhinitis in patients 2 years and older. Veramyst offers the advantage of once-daily dosing along with improvement of both nasal and ocular symptoms associated with allergies. Dymista is a combination drug that contains fluticasone and the antihistamine azelastine. Dymista nasal spray is taken twice daily to treat allergic rhinitis.

Fluticasone is also available in oral inhalation and topical formulations. The oral inhalation product (Flovent) is administered in a metered-dose inhaler (MDI) device for the treatment of asthma and COPD (see Chapter 44). Flovent reduces bronchial inflammation that is characteristic of asthma. In 2013 Breo Ellipta, a combination of fluticasone with vilanterol (a long-acting beta$_2$ agonist), was approved to treat COPD. Topical ointments and creams are applied to the skin for various inflammatory conditions, including atopic dermatitis, eczema, exfoliative dermatitis, psoriasis, and contact dermatitis (see Chapter 73).

Mechanism of Action: Fluticasone acts to decrease local inflammation in the nasal passages through vasoconstrictor and anti-inflammatory mechanisms. It is thought to inhibit mast cells, macrophages, and inflammatory mediators such as prostaglandins, histamine, kinins, and leukotrienes.

Pharmacokinetics:

Route(s)	Intranasal spray, oral inhalation, topical
Absorption	Intranasal: drug is swallowed, with less than 2% absorbed systemically Oral inhalation: 30% reaches systemic circulation Topical: minimal absorption
Distribution	Widely distributed; 91–99% bound to plasma protein
Primary metabolism	Hepatic, extensive first-pass metabolism by CYP3A4
Primary excretion	Feces
Onset of action	12 h to several days
Duration of action	Several days

Adverse Effects: When administered by the intranasal route, adverse effects of fluticasone are uncommon and include headache, cough, nasal ulceration, epistaxis, and local burning. Swallowing large amounts increases the potential for systemic corticosteroid adverse effects (see Chapter 71).

Contraindications/Precautions: The only contraindication to fluticasone is prior hypersensitivity to the drug. Because corticosteroids can mask signs of infection, patients with known bacterial, viral, fungal, or parasitic infections (especially of the respiratory tract) should not receive these drugs until the infection has cleared. Safety has not been established in children under 4 years of age.

Drug Interactions: Concurrent use of fluticasone with an intranasal decongestant increases the risk of nasal irritation or bleeding. Use with ritonavir should be avoided because this drug significantly increases plasma fluticasone levels. **Herbal/Food:** Use with caution with black licorice, which may potentiate the effects of corticosteroids.

Pregnancy: Animal studies showed mixed results depending on the species, route of administration, and dosage. Fluticasone crosses the human placenta but significant adverse effects on the embryo or fetus are unknown. Low amounts of other corticosteroids have been found in milk but adverse effects in breastfed neonates are unknown.

Treatment of Overdose: Overdose with intranasal corticosteroids is unlikely. There is no specific treatment.

Clinician Responsibilities: Key clinical implications for patients receiving fluticasone are included in Applied Clinical Judgment: Patients Receiving Pharmacotherapy with Antihistamines and for Symptomatic Cough and Cold Relief.

Drugs Similar to Fluticasone (Flonase, Veramyst)

All of the intranasal corticosteroids have the same indications, actions, and adverse effects. Due to individual variation, some patients experience more irritation or burning with one drug over another. All are equally effective when administered at their recommended doses. The other intranasal corticosteroids are listed in Table 45.3.

45.6 Cromolyn, ipratropium, and montelukast are alternatives to intranasal corticosteroids in the treatment of allergic rhinitis.

Although most patients with allergic rhinitis are successfully treated with intranasal corticosteroids or antihistamines, several alternatives exist. **Mast cell stabilizers** are drugs that inhibit the release of inflammatory mediators from mast cells. Mast cells contain granules that release histamine and leukotrienes during inflammatory and allergic reactions. Intranasal cromolyn is a mast cell stabilizer approved for the treatment of seasonal or perennial allergic rhinitis. Cromolyn is featured as a prototype in Chapter 44.

Most effective when given prior to allergen exposure, cromolyn has few adverse effects and is now designated as an OTC drug for the treatment of allergy and cold symptoms. It is as effective as antihistamines but less effective than intranasal corticosteroids. This drug is safe and adverse effects are uncommon. A major disadvantage is that cromolyn must be taken four times daily. If a patient is experiencing nasal congestion, a topical decongestant is used prior to administration of cromolyn. When administered by the oral inhalation route, cromolyn is approved for the treatment of asthma.

Ipratropium nasal spray is an anticholinergic drug indicated for the symptomatic relief of rhinorrhea associated with seasonal allergic rhinitis or the common cold. Its actions are limited to decreasing nasal secretions; it does not stop the sneezing, postnasal drip, or itchy throat or eyes characteristic of allergic rhinitis or the common cold. The drug is well tolerated, with epistaxis and nasal dryness experienced by a small percentage of patients. Like other anticholinergics, it should be used with caution in patients with closed-angle glaucoma or with prostatic hyperplasia. The primary use of ipratropium is by the inhalation route as a bronchodilator in the treatment of COPD. It is presented as a prototype drug for this disorder in Chapter 44.

Montelukast (Singulair) is an oral drug that acts by blocking leukotriene receptors. Leukotrienes are associated with inflammation and are responsible for some of the sneezing, nasal itching, and congestion characteristic of allergic rhinitis. Originally approved for the treatment of asthma, allergic rhinitis was subsequently added as an indication. It is approved for both the seasonal and perennial forms of the disease and can be used in children as young as 6 months of age. Like cromolyn, montelukast is not considered as effective as the intranasal corticosteroids. A prototype for this drug is presented in Chapter 44.

Decongestants

45.7 Intranasal and oral sympathomimetics are the most effective drugs for relieving nasal congestion.

Decongestants are drugs that relieve nasal congestion. They are administered by either the PO or intranasal route and are often combined with antihistamines in the pharmacotherapy of allergies or the common cold.

Sympathomimetics (also called adrenergic agonists) with alpha-adrenergic activity are effective at relieving the nasal congestion associated with the common cold and allergic rhinitis when given by either the PO or intranasal route. The intranasal preparations such as oxymetazoline (Afrin) are available OTC as sprays or drops and produce a noticeable response within minutes. The nasal decongestants are listed in Table 45.4.

Intranasal sympathomimetics produce few systemic effects because only minimal amounts of these drugs are absorbed in the circulation. The most serious, limiting adverse effect of the intranasal preparations is **rebound congestion**. In almost all patients, prolonged use causes hypersecretion of mucus and worsening nasal congestion once the drug effects wear off. This leads to a cycle of increased drug use as the condition worsens to obtain the desired effect from these drugs. Because of this rebound congestion, intranasal sympathomimetics should be used for no longer than 3 to 5 days. Patients who develop dependence should be gradually switched to intranasal corticosteroids because they do not cause rebound congestion. The usual technique for switching to intranasal corticosteroids is by stopping the use of the decongestant in one nostril at a time.

When administered PO, sympathomimetics do not produce rebound congestion. Their onset of action by this route, however, is much slower than when administered intranasally, and they are less effective at relieving severe congestion. The possibility of systemic adverse effects is also greater with the PO drugs. Potential adverse effects include HTN and CNS stimulation that may lead to insomnia and anxiety. Pseudoephedrine and phenylephrine are common sympathomimetics found in oral OTC cold and allergy medicines.

The sympathomimetics relieve only nasal congestion and therefore are often combined with antihistamines to control sneezing and tearing. It is interesting to note that some OTC drugs having the same basic name (Neo-Synephrine, Afrin, and Vicks) may contain different sympathomimetics. For example, Neo-Synephrine decongestants with 12-hour duration contain the drug oxymetazoline; Neo-Synephrine preparations that last 4 to 6 hours contain phenylephrine.

Table 45.4 Nasal Decongestants

Drug	Route and Adult Dose (Maximum Dose Where Indicated)	Adverse Effects
naphazoline (Privine)	Intranasal (0.05%): 2 drops or sprays q3–6h	*Intranasal: transient nasal irritation, burning, sneezing, dryness, headache* *Oral: CNS stimulation: nervousness, insomnia, headache, dry mouth* Intranasal: rebound congestion Oral: CNS excitation (in people with coronary artery disease or hypertension [HTN]), tremors, dysrhythmias, tachycardia, difficulty voiding, HTN, and peripheral and visceral vasoconstriction
oxymetazoline (Afrin 12 Hour, Neo-Synephrine 12 Hour, others)	Intranasal (0.05%): 2–3 sprays bid for up to 3 days	
phenylephrine (Afrin 4–6 Hour, Neo-Synephrine 4–6 Hour, others)	Intranasal (0.1%): 1–2 sprays or drops q4h, prn, up to 3 days	
pseudoephedrine (Sudafed)	PO: 30–60 mg q4–6h (max: 240 mg/day) Sustained release: 120 mg q12h	
tetrahydrozoline (Tyzine)	Intranasal: 2–4 drops or sprays q3h	
xylometazoline	Intranasal (0.1%): 1–2 sprays bid (max: 3 doses/day)	

Note: *Italics* indicate common adverse effects. Underline indicates serious adverse effects.

PROTOTYPE DRUG Pseudoephedrine (Sudafed)

Classification **Therapeutic:** Decongestant
Pharmacologic: Sympathomimetic

Therapeutic Effects and Uses: Approved in 1959, pseudoephedrine is available in tablet and elixir formulations. It is often combined with other medications in OTC preparations used to treat allergic rhinitis, sinus congestion, and common cold symptoms. Pseudoephedrine promotes sinus drainage and can open obstructed eustachian tubes in adults and children with chronic otic inflammation. It is also used off-label to prevent otitic barotraumas, pain or damage to the tympanic membrane caused by rapid pressure changes during air travel or diving.

Pseudoephedrine deserves special attention because of its potential for misuse. Pseudoephedrine is the starting chemical for the synthesis of illegal methamphetamine by drug traffickers. Most states require pseudoephedrine products to be kept behind the pharmacy counter, so that pharmacists can monitor sales and distribution. Although still considered OTC, pharmacists are required to keep a log of the names and addresses and check the photo identification of anyone who buys a pseudoephedrine product. At least two states have made pseudoephedrine a prescription drug. Note that these precautions are not being taken because pseudoephedrine itself is a dangerous drug, but instead to limit its availability to illicit makers of methamphetamine. Manufacturers have reformulated their OTC cold medicines to contain phenylephrine rather than pseudoephedrine. Although the two drugs are very similar, it is much more difficult to chemically convert phenylephrine to methamphetamine.

Mechanism of Action: Pseudoephedrine activates alpha$_1$-adrenergic receptors, which causes vasoconstriction in the nasal mucosa, resulting in shrinking of mucosal swelling. It also stimulates beta$_2$-adrenergic receptors of the respiratory tract, which may result in some bronchodilation.

Pharmacokinetics:

Route(s)	PO (tablets, elixir)
Absorption	Well absorbed orally
Distribution	Widely distributed, including in cerebrospinal fluid; crosses the placenta; secreted in breast milk
Primary metabolism	Hepatic
Primary excretion	Renal
Onset of action	30 min; extended release: 60 min
Duration of action	4–8 h; extended release: 12 h

Adverse Effects: Pseudoephedrine is well tolerated at regular dosage levels. Some patients experience CNS stimulation with symptoms of insomnia, restlessness, anxiety, and dizziness. Excitability is especially a concern in infants and young children. At high doses, seizures and psychosis may occur. Other sympathomimetic effects include dysrhythmias, HTN, palpitations, tachycardia, dry mouth, and anorexia. Rebound congestion is not usually a concern with PO decongestants. Serious injury and deaths due to overdose have occurred in children under 2 years of age who received high doses of cough and cold medicines.

Contraindications/Precautions: Pseudoephedrine should not be used by patients with severe HTN, severe coronary artery disease, or hypersensitivity to this drug or by those who take monoamine oxidase inhibitor (MAOI) drugs. Alpha-adrenergic agonists should be used with caution in patients with prostatic enlargement because these drugs increase smooth muscle activity in the prostate gland and may diminish urinary outflow (see Chapter 71). The FDA has issued advisories that nonprescription cough and cold products (including those containing pseudoephedrine) not be used in children under 6 years of age and that they be used with extreme caution in all children.

Drug Interactions: Pseudoephedrine interacts with MAOIs to cause a hypertensive crisis. Use with other sympathomimetic drugs, including caffeine, can lead to additive cardiovascular and CNS stimulation effects. Beta blockers and pseudoephedrine together can result in HTN or severe bradycardia. Concurrent use with tricyclic antidepressants may result in increased cardiovascular toxicity and severe headaches. Pseudoephedrine can antagonize the effects of antihypertensive drugs. Pseudoephedrine should be avoided in patients who are taking nitrates for angina due to the vasoconstriction caused by the stimulation of alpha-adrenergic receptors on systemic blood vessels. Use with digoxin may cause dysrhythmias. **Herbal/Food:** Products containing caffeine can worsen side effects such as nervousness, palpitations and insomnia.

Pregnancy: Human epidemiological studies have not shown evidence of fetal harm, above normal baseline levels. If breastfeeding, the neonate should be monitored for lethargy or irritability and feeding should occur at least 2 hours after taking the medication.

Treatment of Overdose: Overdose may cause coma, seizures, profuse sweating, and dysrhythmias. No specific treatment exists.

Clinician Responsibilities: Key clinical implications for patients receiving pseudoephedrine are included in Applied Clinical Judgment: Patients Receiving Pharmacotherapy with Antihistamines and for Symptomatic Cough and Cold Relief.

Drugs Similar to Pseudoephedrine (Sudafed)

All the sympathomimetic intranasal decongestants have very similar actions and adverse effects. Additional details on this class of drugs are included in Chapter 15.

Drugs for the Common Cold

45.8 The common cold is caused by a virus and is treated with some of the same drugs as those used to treat allergic rhinitis.

The common cold is a viral infection of the upper respiratory tract that produces a characteristic array of annoying symptoms. It is fortunate that the disorder is self-limiting because there is no cure or effective prevention for colds. Therapies used to relieve symptoms include some of the same drug classes used for allergic rhinitis, including antihistamines and decongestants. A few additional drugs, such as those that suppress cough and loosen bronchial secretions, are used for symptomatic cold treatment.

Many OTC preparations are available to treat cold symptoms. These OTC drugs are often made as combinations containing two or more drugs to treat a variety of symptoms. Some common OTC combination products are listed in Table 45.2. The most common ingredients of combination drugs for the common cold are antihistamines and decongestants; caffeine is sometimes added to combat the adverse effect of drowsiness from first-generation antihistamines. The caffeine is omitted from combination drugs if the medication is to be taken at night, for example, NyQuil. Almost all combination drugs contain some form of analgesic, such as acetaminophen, aspirin, or other nonsteroidal anti-inflammatory drug, to help with fever and muscular aches. Many combination products also contain a cough suppressant and an expectorant to help loosen congestion.

The wide variety of combination cold, flu, and sinus products that are available OTC can be confusing for consumers. Multisymptom combination products should be taken only if the patient is experiencing the indicated symptoms. For example, if cough and fever are not present, products that contain cough suppressants, expectorants, or analgesics should not be taken. Consuming combination products without appropriate symptoms can increase the risk of unnecessary adverse effects. It is usually better to take only the drugs needed to treat specific symptoms rather than a combination product.

PharmFACT

Adults average two to four colds per year, while children have six to eight. Colds account for more office visits per year than any other condition (American Lung Association, 2020).

CONNECTIONS: Advanced Practice Application

Ascorbic Acid (Vitamin C) and the Common Cold

Case

Rachel Peterson is a 31-year-old who presents to her primary care nurse practitioner with a 4-day history of fatigue, sore throat, and nasal congestion. She has had no fevers and denies any other symptom. Rachel has heard from her sister that vitamin C may help her but is unsure of the evidence. What information can you provide?

Discussion

Vitamin C is well documented as a prevention and treatment for scurvy. Vitamin C is naturally occurring and found in a variety of foods. Citrus fruits are especially high in vitamin C, as is cranberry. In 1970, Linus Pauling, the only person to win two Nobel prizes, published a book called *Vitamin C and the Common Cold* in which he asserted that the common cold could be almost completely controlled by the adequate intake of ascorbic acid. This book helped the case for vitamin C as a treatment or preventive for the common cold. Since the publication of Pauling's book, many studies have been conducted to test the value of vitamin C in improving the immune system response to viruses that cause the common cold and other disease conditions. Despite being heavily studied, there is scant evidence to support recommending dietary supplementation with vitamin C for more than minimal impact. There is evidence that dietary intake and blood concentrations of vitamin C are associated with reduced risk of cancer, cardiovascular disease, and overall mortality, but these were associated with vitamin C intake from dietary sources, not supplements (Aune et al., 2018).

There are groups of people for whom the Office of Dietary Supplements (2019) at the National Institutes of Health recommend considering the use of vitamin C supplementation. These include those who smoke or are exposed to secondhand smoke, infants fed cow's milk, people who eat a limited variety of foods, or those with conditions that put them at risk for nutritional imbalance, such as malabsorption. Obtaining adequate vitamin C through various foods is the best source and remains the recommendation.

CONNECTIONS: APPLIED CLINICAL JUDGMENT

Patients Receiving Pharmacotherapy with Antihistamines and for Symptomatic Cough and Cold Relief

Key Assessment Data

- History of current condition, including previous history of symptoms and association with seasons, foods, or environmental exposures; baseline vital signs, physical exam findings, presence of fever; history of cardiovascular, cerebrovascular, respiratory disease, diabetes; medication history; pregnancy status. If allergy symptoms are of new onset, particularly for infants and young children, assess for any recent changes in diet, soaps including laundry detergent, laundry softener, cosmetics, lotions, environmental factors (e.g., pets, travel), or recent carpet cleaning.
- Ongoing assessment during drug therapy may include assessment of symptom-related effects on eating, sleep, and activity level.

Desired Therapeutic Outcomes

Improvement is observed and measurable by decreased nasal congestion and drainage, decreased eye watering or itching, decreased nonproductive cough, increased ease of expectorating mucus, clearer nasal passages, and maintenance of normal eating and sleep periods.

Minimizing Adverse Effects

- Increasing dyspnea, adventitious breath sounds, increasing thickness, color, hemoptysis, or increased quantity of sputum may indicate a serious respiratory infection and should be reported immediately.
- Drugs used for symptomatic relief of the common cold are used with extreme caution or are contraindicated in patients with existing respiratory disease, including COPD. A change in the severity of the cough may indicate a worsening disease process or a more serious respiratory infection and should be reported immediately.

Lifespan Considerations

- Older adults may be more sensitive to the drug effects due to existing cardiovascular disease and require more frequent monitoring.
- Children under the age of 6 years should not be given OTC cough and cold preparations routinely unless instructed to do so by the provider. Cough suppressants containing opioids should not be used to treat cough in children under age 18.
- Drowsiness or dizziness from drug effects may occur, increasing the risk of falls, especially in the older adult. Ensure patient safety.

Diversity Considerations

- Because some drugs such as montelukast are metabolized through the CYP450 system pathways, monitor ethnically diverse patients to ensure optimal therapeutic effects and to minimize adverse effects

Patient Education

- Immediately report symptoms of deteriorating respiratory status such as increased dyspnea, breathlessness with speech, increased anxiety, or orthopnea.
- Peak expiratory flowmeter or other equipment may be ordered to monitor pulmonary function. Keep a log of the results and bring to each appointment.
- Any cough accompanied by shortness of breath, increasing congestion, fever, or chest pain should be reported immediately.
- Consider symptoms when reading labels of OTC cold remedies and choose preparations based on current symptoms rather than multi-use remedies.
- Multi-use cold remedies containing acetaminophen must be taken in prescribed doses, should not be taken with other acetaminophen-containing products or if daily alcohol intake exceeds two glasses, and not increased to avoid acetaminophen overdose and potential liver damage.
- Supplement drug therapy with nonpharmacologic measures including:
  - Increase fluid intake to liquefy and assist in mobilizing mucus.
  - Eat small, frequent meals of calorie-rich, nutrient-dense foods to prevent fatigue and maintain normal nutrition.
  - Ensure adequate rest periods between eating and activities.
  - Decreased room temperature may assist to ease breathing during sleep.
  - Reduce exposure to allergens where possible.
  - Immediately report any significant change in appetite, inability to maintain normal intake, inadequate sleep periods, or inability to carry out required ADLs.
  - Report any significant change in the color, consistency, or quantity of expectorated mucus to the healthcare provider.
- Use proper administration techniques, including:
  - *Cough suppressants:* Cough syrups should be swallowed without water and allowed to coat the throat for soothing effects, followed by increased fluid intake 30–60 minutes later. The dose should not be increased beyond the recommended dose to avoid increased risk of adverse effects.
  - *Expectorants:* Syrups should be taken with a full glass of liquid with increased fluid intake throughout the day to assist in thinning mucus for ease of expectoration.
  - *Nasal decongestants:* Nasal passages should be cleared by blowing, followed by the nasal spray. If a second spray is ordered, administer 5 minutes after the first spray. If glucocorticoid or mast cell stabilizer sprays are ordered, the decongestant spray should be used first, followed by the additional drug 5 to 10 minutes later. Spit out any additional drug that drains into the mouth. Discontinue use of decongestant nasal sprays after 3 to 5 days to avoid rebound congestion, unless otherwise ordered by the provider.
- Carry a wallet identification card or wear medical identification jewelry indicating the presence of asthma or a respiratory condition, any significant allergies or anaphylaxis, and use of inhaler therapy.

Prescribing Considerations

- Avoid the use of first-generation antihistamines in children or older adults due to their sedating effects. Dose nonsedating second-generation antihistamines according to body weight rather than age.
- Consider a combination of antihistamines and decongestants for acute rhinitis; however, long-term use of decongestants should be discouraged due to the risk of rebound congestion.
- Antihistamines should be avoided in the first trimester of pregnancy; after that, nonsedating antihistamines are recommended for pregnant and breastfeeding women.
- Prior to prescribing an antihistamine, evaluate elderly patients for comorbidities, concomitant use of medications, differential diagnoses, and assess hepatic and renal function; avoid the use of sedating antihistamines.

Antitussives

45.9 Antitussives are drugs used to suppress the cough reflex.

Cough is a natural reflex mechanism that serves to forcibly remove excess secretions and foreign material from the respiratory system. In diseases such as emphysema and bronchitis, or when liquids have been aspirated into the bronchi, it is not desirable to suppress the normal cough reflex. Dry, hacking, nonproductive coughing, however, can be irritating to the membranes of the throat and trigger inflammation, depriving patients of much-needed rest. It is these types of conditions in which therapy with medications that control cough, known as **antitussives**, is warranted. Although there is clear evidence that antitussives are effective against chronic, nonproductive cough, there is less certainty about their value in treating acute cough due to the common cold (Degeorge, et al.). (2019) Antitussives are classified as opioid or nonopioid and are listed in Table 45.5.

Opioids, the most effective antitussives, act by raising the cough threshold in the CNS. Codeine and hydrocodone are the only opioids prescribed as antitussives. Doses needed to suppress the cough reflex are very low; thus, there is minimal potential for dependence. Most opioid cough mixtures are classified as Schedule III, IV, or V drugs. When used for cough, opioids are always combined with other drugs such as antihistamines, decongestants, and nonopioid antitussives.

In recent years, the use of opioids in controlling cough has declined due to the potential for sedation. significant respiratory depression, overdose, and misuse. The FDA has issued safety warnings that opioids should not be used to treat cough in children under age 18. After reviewing extensive safety data, the FDA determined that the potential risks do not justify any potential benefits for treating cough in children. In children and most adults, cough is managed with nonopioid antitussives that include dextromethorphan and benzonatate. Dextromethorphan is available OTC as a single drug but is usually found as a component of combination, multisymptom cold medications. Benzonatate is a prescription drug. Diphenhydramine (Benadryl) is usually taken for its antihistamine effects, but it also has antitussive action.

Table 45.5 Selected Antitussives and Expectorants

Drug	Route and Adult Dose (Maximum Dose Where Indicated)	Adverse Effects
Antitussives: Opioids		
codeine	PO: 10–20 mg q4–6h prn (max: 120 mg/day)	*Nausea and vomiting, constipation, confusion, dizziness, sedation* Hypotension, seizures, hallucinations, bradycardia, respiratory depression, severe somnolence
hydrocodone combined with homatropine	PO: 5 mL or 1 tablet q4–6h prn (max: 30 mL/day or 6 tablets/day)	
Antitussives: Nonopioids		
benzonatate	PO: 100–200 mg tid (max: 600 mg/day)	*Drowsiness, constipation, GI upset, chest and tongue numbness (if capsules are opened or chewed)* Paradoxical excitation, tremors, euphoria, insomnia
dextromethorphan (Delsym, Robitussin DM, others)	PO: 10–20 mg q4h or 30 mg q6–8h (max: 120 mg/day)	*Drowsiness, headache, GI upset* CNS depression, paradoxical excitation, respiratory depression
Expectorant		
guaifenesin (Mucinex, Robitussin, others)	PO: 200–400 mg q4h (max: 2.4 g/day) PO (extended release): 600–1200 mg q12h (max: 2.4 g/day)	*Drowsiness, headache, GI upset* No serious adverse effects
Mucolytics		
acetylcysteine	Inhalation: 1–10 mL of 20% solution q4–6h or 2–20 mL of 10% solution q4–6h	*Unpleasant odor, nausea, local irritation, stickiness on the face* Severe nausea and vomiting
dornase alfa (Pulmozyme)	Inhalation: 1–2 of 2.5-mg ampules once daily using nebulizer	*Voice alteration, laryngitis, rash* Dyspnea

Note: *Italics* indicate common adverse effects. Underline indicates serious adverse effects.

PROTOTYPE DRUG Dextromethorphan (Delsym, Robitussin DM, Others)

Classification **Therapeutic:** Antitussive
Pharmacologic: Levorphanol derivative

Therapeutic Effects and Uses: Approved in 1954, dextromethorphan is the most frequently used and most effective nonopioid antitussive. Considered as effective as codeine, dextromethorphan carries no risk of dependence. Although used for over 50 years to treat cough, controlled studies examining the effectiveness of dextromethorphan have given mixed results. Its present status is that the FDA considers it a safe and effective cough suppressant when used at recommended doses. It appears to be more effective at reducing nonproductive cough due to chronic throat irritation from tobacco use or emphysema rather than acute cough due to colds.

Reports of dextromethorphan abuse began to appear in the 1990s. Dextromethorphan has been reported to cause a mild stimulant effect at lower doses and altered sensory perceptions and complete dissociative effects (out-of-body–like experiences) at very high doses. The effects typically last 6 to 8 hours. To produce these effects, 10 to 30 times the antitussive dose is used. Additional information on dextromethorphan abuse is presented in Chapter 27.

Mechanism of Action: Dextromethorphan is chemically similar to the opioids and acts directly on the cough center in the medulla to elevate the cough threshold. It has no effect on opioid receptors.

Pharmacokinetics:

Route(s)	PO
Absorption	Readily absorbed orally
Distribution	Unknown; may cross the placenta
Primary metabolism	Hepatic; metabolized by CYP2D6 and CYP3A to active metabolite
Primary excretion	Renal
Onset of action	15–30 min
Duration of action	3–8 h

Adverse Effects: Dextromethorphan has almost no adverse effects at therapeutic doses. Sedation and dizziness have occurred at moderate doses. In abuse situations the drug can cause CNS toxicity with a wide variety of symptoms, including slurred speech, ataxia, hyperexcitability, stupor, respiratory depression, seizures, coma, and toxic psychosis.

Contraindications/Precautions: This medication is extensively metabolized by the liver and should be used cautiously in patients with hepatic impairment. The FDA has issued advisories that nonprescription cough and cold products (including those containing dextromethorphan) not be used in children under 6 years of age and that they be used with extreme caution in all children.

Drug Interactions: Patients who take MAOIs, triptans, or selective serotonin reuptake inhibitors should not take dextromethorphan due to the risk of serotonin syndrome (nausea, changes in blood pressure, and confusion). The drug has an additive CNS depressant effect with alcohol, antihistamines, antidepressants, and opioids. The analgesic effect of opioids can be almost doubled by giving them with dextromethorphan. **Herbal/Food:** Grapefruit juice can raise serum levels of dextromethorphan and cause toxicity.

Pregnancy: Human epidemiological studies show no evidence of fetal harm, above normal baseline levels. This drug enters breast milk but adverse effects on the breastfed neonate are unknown.

Treatment of Overdose: Overdose may result in significant CNS toxicity. Treatment is symptomatic.

Clinician Responsibilities: Key clinical implications for patients receiving dextromethorphan are included in Applied Clinical Judgement: Patients Receiving Pharmacotherapy with Antihistamines and for Symptomatic Cough and Cold Relief.

Drugs Similar to Dextromethorphan (Delsym, Robitussin DM, Others)

The other nonopioid antitussive is benzonatate.

Benzonatate (Tessalon): Approved in 1958, benzonatate is an oral, nonopioid antitussive that acts by a unique mechanism. Chemically related to the local anesthetic tetracaine (Pontocaine), benzonatate suppresses the cough reflex by anesthetizing stretch receptors in the lungs. If chewed, this drug can cause numbing of the mouth and pharynx. Adverse effects are uncommon but may include sedation, nausea, headache, and dizziness. This drug should not be used in children under 10 years of age: Death has been reported from unintentional ingestion in children. Like dextromethorphan, the effectiveness of benzonatate in treating acute cough has not been clearly established. Animal reproduction studies are not available for benzonatate. It is not known if this drug is secreted in milk or if it has adverse effects on the breastfed neonate.

Expectorants and Mucolytics

45.10 Expectorants and mucolytics are used to treat thick bronchial secretions.

Several drugs are available to control excess mucus production. **Expectorants** increase bronchial secretions, and **mucolytics** remove mucus by loosening thick bronchial secretions. These drugs are listed in Table 45.5.

Expectorants reduce the thickness or viscosity of bronchial secretions, thus increasing mucus flow that can then be removed more easily by coughing. The only commonly used OTC expectorant is guaifenesin (Mucinex). Like dextromethorphan, guaifenesin produces few adverse effects and is a common ingredient in many combination multisymptom OTC cold and flu preparations. It is most effective in treating dry, nonproductive cough but may also be of benefit for patients with productive cough. Like the antitussives, the effectiveness of guaifenesin in reducing acute cold symptoms has been questioned. The dosage range used in cold remedies is usually too low to have much positive benefit for patients. Nonprescription cough and cold products (including those containing guaifenesin) should not be used in children under 6 years of age. High doses can induce nausea and vomiting and abdominal pain.

Acetylcysteine is one of the few drugs that directly loosen thick, viscous bronchial secretions. Drugs of this type, known as mucolytics, break down the chemical structure of mucus molecules. The mucus becomes thinner and can be removed more easily by coughing. Acetylcysteine is delivered by the PO and inhalation routes and is not available OTC. It is used in patients who have cystic fibrosis, chronic bronchitis, or other diseases that produce large amounts of thick bronchial secretions. Acetylcysteine is also administered by the IV route (Acetadote) to prevent the development of hepatotoxicity in patients who have received an overdose of acetaminophen. In 2016, a new oral form of the medication (Cetylev) was approved for the same indication. Its use in the pharmacotherapy of acetaminophen toxicity is presented in Chapter 41. Adverse effects include bronchospasm, nausea and vomiting, unpleasant odor, and fever.

A second mucolytic, dornase alfa (Pulmozyme), is an enzyme that was approved in 1993 for the daily management of thick bronchial secretions in patients with cystic fibrosis. Dornase alfa breaks down deoxyribonucleic acid molecules in the mucus, causing it to become less viscous. It is administered by the oral inhalation route. Adverse effects include hoarseness and pharyngitis. This drug is pregnancy category B.

Understanding Chapter 45

Key Concepts Summary

45.1 The upper respiratory tract acts as a defense in preventing systemic infection.

45.2 Allergic rhinitis is caused by exposure to an environmental allergen, which leads to symptoms that resemble those of the common cold.

45.3 Drugs for allergic rhinitis include those that prevent the disorder and those that relieve symptoms.

45.4 Antihistamines are widely used to treat allergic rhinitis and other minor allergies.

45.5 Intranasal corticosteroids are preferred drugs for allergic rhinitis because of their effectiveness and safety.

45.6 Cromolyn, ipratropium, and montelukast are alternatives to intranasal corticosteroids in the treatment of allergic rhinitis.

45.7 Intranasal and oral sympathomimetics are the most effective drugs for relieving nasal congestion.

45.8 The common cold is caused by a virus and is treated with some of the same drugs as those used to treat allergic rhinitis.

45.9 Antitussives are drugs used to suppress the cough reflex.

45.10 Expectorants and mucolytics are used to treat thick bronchial secretions.

CASE STUDY: Making the Patient Connection

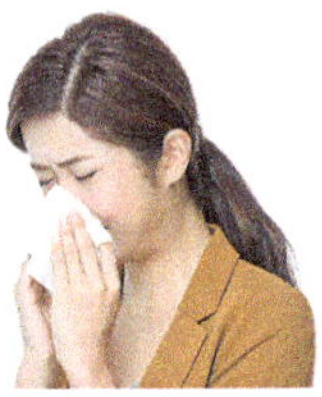

Remember the patient "Nancy Chen" at the beginning of the chapter? Now read the remainder of the case study. Based on the information presented within this chapter, respond to the critical thinking questions that follow.

Nancy Chen is a 32-year-old woman who is in good health except for her current problem. She has come to the urgent care center because of a stuffy nose; red, itchy eyes; and a slightly sore throat. She takes daily calcium supplements but no other medications. She is 1.68 m (5 ft 6 in.) tall and weighs 67 kg (148 lb).

Nancy is a fourth-grade teacher at a local elementary school and is worried about being able to finish her end-of-term activities with the symptoms of a lingering "cold." Her vital signs are as follows: temperature, 37.4°C (99.4°F); pulse, 102 beats/min; respirations, 12 breaths/min; blood pressure, 148/88 mmHg; oxygen saturation, 98%.

After taking her vital signs, Nancy tells the nurse practitioner that her mother-in-law bought her a Neo-Synephrine nasal spray about 10 days ago. It helped, but she tells the nurse that it ran out yesterday and now her nose is even stuffier than before. She had been taking Tylenol but stopped using that, too, because she does not feel like she has a fever and it was not helping much anyway. Nancy says, "I went to the drug store after school and did not stay. I felt so miserable that I could not even figure out what medicine does what and I just wanted to get home. I need some rest so I can take care of my girls, do a good job for my students, and get my report cards done." The nurse practitioner observes that Nancy has a cough, runny nose, and inflamed eyes, which she occasionally rubs during the conversation.

Critical Thinking Questions

1. Considering the history and the initial assessment that the nurse practitioner conducted, what further data would you as the nurse want to gather that are not listed in the scenario?
2. If Nancy has no history of heart disease or HTN and takes no medications to treat those conditions, what do you think might be the cause of her elevated blood pressure and heart rate?
3. Nancy gave her two daughters a golden retriever puppy a few weeks ago. How does this information add to your assessment findings and patient teaching?
4. The nurse practitioner diagnoses Nancy with probable allergic rhinitis and prescribes intranasal fluticasone (Flonase). In addition, the nurse practitioner suggests getting two OTC cough suppressants, one with the main ingredient dextromethorphan and the other one with the main ingredient diphenhydramine. What do you tell Nancy is the reason she is being prescribed each one?

Additional Case Study

A 23-year-old woman arrives at the emergency department with her boyfriend. She is wheezing and short of breath. Her respiratory rate is 23 breaths/min, her heart rate is 104 beats/min, her blood pressure is 88/60 mmHg, and she has hives over most of her body. Her boyfriend says she was eating strawberries and suddenly started having trouble breathing. She has eaten strawberries for years and nothing like this has ever happened before. The healthcare provider prescribes epinephrine for her allergic response.

1. Why did the healthcare provider not prescribe an antihistamine for this allergic response?
2. A second dose of epinephrine is given, and the nurse inserts an IV. With a reduction in her wheezing, the patient's respiratory rate is 18 breaths/min, heart rate is 100 beats/min, and blood pressure is 98/64 mmHg. The healthcare provider prescribes Benadryl, 10 mg IV. Describe why the provider is now prescribing an antihistamine for the patient.

Chapter Review

1. Oxymetazoline (Afrin 12 Hour) has been recommended for a patient with rhinitis. Which points are appropriate to include in the teaching plan? (Select all that apply.)
    1. Take with a full glass of water.
    2. Clear the nose by blowing.
    3. Take the drug at night if drowsiness occurs.
    4. Take for no more than 5 days to prevent rebound congestion.
    5. Effects of the drug may not be noticeable for 2 to 3 weeks.

2. The nurse teaches the patient that which type of OTC cough preparation is not effective on coughs associated with the common cold and allergic rhinitis?
   1. Dextromethorphan
   2. Diphenhydramine
   3. Mucolytics
   4. Pseudoephedrine

3. An older adult man informs the nurse that he is taking diphenhydramine (Benadryl) to reduce seasonal allergy symptoms. The nurse would be most concerned about an increased risk of for this patient.

4. Fexofenadine (Allegra) is prescribed to treat the symptoms of allergic rhinitis for a patient with seasonal allergies. Before teaching the patient about this drug, what condition would the nurse assess for?
   1. A history of osteoporosis
   2. A history of peptic ulcer disease
   3. A history of psoriasis
   4. A history of cardiac disease

5. A patient has been prescribed fluticasone (Flonase) to use with phenylephrine (Neo-Synephrine) nasal inhalers to treat allergic rhinitis. How should the nurse teach the patient to use these drugs?
   1. Fluticasone should be used only if congestion continues after phenylephrine use.
   2. Use fluticasone first, then the phenylephrine after waiting 5 minutes.
   3. Use phenylephrine first, then the fluticasone after waiting 5 minutes.
   4. The drugs may be used in either order.

6. The nurse is teaching the patient about the use of dextromethorphan with guaifenesin (Robitussin DM) syrup for a cough accompanied by thick mucus. Which statement would be part of the patient's teaching?
   1. "Lie supine for 30 minutes after taking the drug."
   2. "Drink minimal fluids to avoid stimulating the cough reflex."
   3. "Take the drug with food for best results."
   4. "Avoid drinking fluids immediately following the syrup and then increase overall fluid intake."

See Appendix A for answers to critical thinking questions, case study questions and review questions.

References

Abraham, O., Schleiden, L., & Albert, S. M. (2017). Over-the-counter medications containing diphenhydramine and doxylamine used by older adults to improve sleep. *International Journal of Clinical Pharmacy, 39*, 808–817. https://doi.org/10.1007/s11096-017-0467-x

American Lung Association. (2020). *Facts about the common cold.* http://www.lung.org/lung-health-and-diseases/lung-disease-lookup/influenza/facts-about-the-common-cold.html

Aune, D., Keum, N., Giovannucci, E., Fadnes, L. T., Boffetta, P., Greenwood, D. C., et al. (2018). Dietary intake and blood concentrations of antioxidants and the risk of cardiovascular disease, total cancer, and all-cause mortality: A systematic review and dose-response meta-analysis or prospective studies. *American Journal of Clinical Nutrition, 108*, 1069–1091. https://doi.org/10.1093/ajcn/nqy097

Centers for Disease Control and Prevention. (2020). *Allergies and hay fever.* https://www.cdc.gov/nchs/fastats/allergies.htm

Cenzar, I., Nkansah-Mahaney, N., Wehner, M., Chren, M. M., Berger, T., Covinsky, K., et al. (2020). A multiyear cross-sectional study of U. S. national prescribing patterns of first-generation sedating antihistamines in older adults with skin diseases. *British Journal of Dermatology, 182*, 763–769. https://doi.org/10.1111/bjd.18042

Degeorge, K.C., Ring, D.J., & Dalrymple, S,N. (2019) Treatment of the common cold. *American Family Physician, 100*, 281-289. https://www.aafp.org/afp/2019/0901/p281.html?wm=3049_b111

Hill, L. L., Andrews, H., Li, G., DiGuiseppi, C. G., Betz, M. E., Strogatz, D., et al. (2020). Medication use and driving patterns in older drivers: Preliminary findings from the LongROAD study. *Injury Epidemiology, 7*, 38. https://doi.org/10.1186/s40621-020-00265-y

Office of Dietary Supplements. (2019). *Vitamin C.* National Institutes of Health. https://ods.od.nih.gov/factsheets/VitaminC-Consumer/

Selected Bibliography

Croke, L. M. (2018). Treatment of seasonal allergic rhinitis: a guideline from the AAAAI/ACAAI joint task force on practice parameters. *American Family Physician, 97*(11), 756–757.

Kawauchi, H., Yanai, K., Wang, D. Y., Itahashi, K., & Okubo, K. (2019). Antihistamines for allergic rhinitis treatment from the viewpoint of nonsedative properties. *International Journal of Molecular Sciences, 20*(1), 213. https://doi.org/10.3390/ijms20010213

Klimek, L., Sperl, A., Becker, S., Mösges, R., & Tomazic, P. V. (2019). Current therapeutical strategies for allergic rhinitis. *Expert Opinion on Pharmacotherapy, 20*(1), 83–89. https://doi.org/10.1080/14656566.2018.1543401

Pauling, L. (1970). *Vitamin C and the common cold.* W. H. Freeman.

Perotin, J. M., Launois, C., Dewolf, M., Dumazet, A., Dury, S., Lebargy, F., et al. (2018). Managing patients with chronic cough: challenges and solutions. *Therapeutics and Clinical Risk Management, 14,* 1041. https://doi.org/10.2147/TCRM.S136036

Smith, J. A., & Badri, H. (2019). Cough: new pharmacology. *Journal of Allergy and Clinical Immunology: In Practice, 7*(6), 1731–1738. https://doi.org/10.1016/j.jaip.2019.04.027

Tomazic, P. V., & Lang-Loidolt, D. (2020). Current and emerging pharmacotherapy for pediatric allergic rhinitis. *Expert Opinion on Pharmacotherapy.* https://doi.org/10.1080/14656566.2020.1808622

Zimlich, R. (2018). FDA restricts opioid-containing cold medicines for children. *Contemporary Pediatrics, 35*(4), 25–26.

Unit 8

Pharmacology of Infectious and Neoplastic Diseases

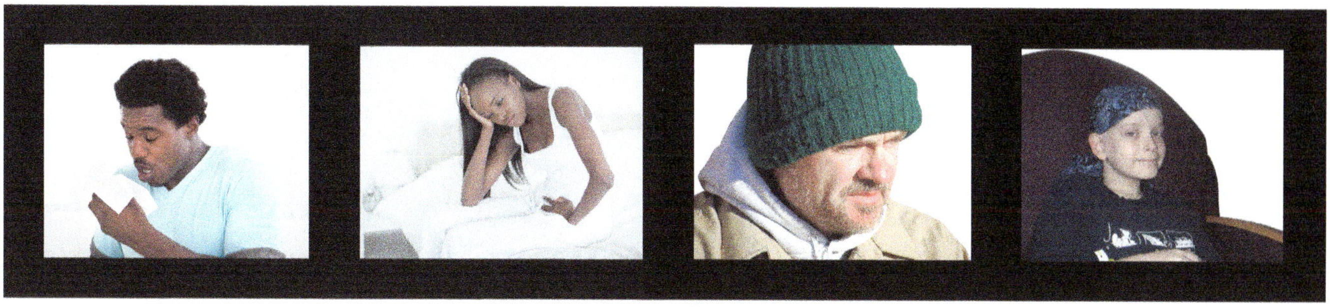

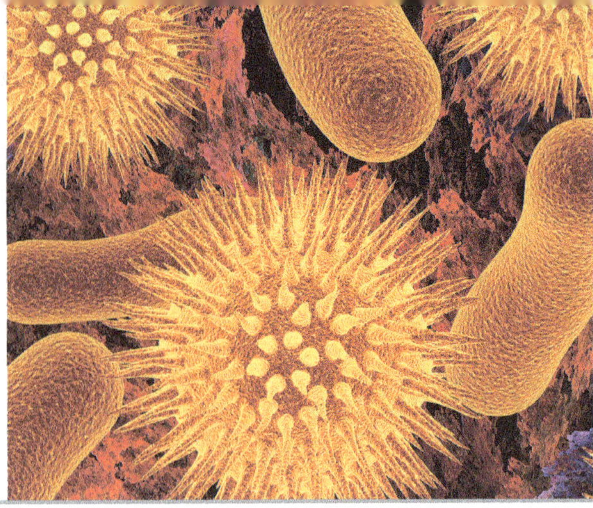

Chapter 46
Basic Principles of Anti-Infective Pharmacotherapy

Chapter Outline

- Pathogenicity and Virulence
- Describing and Classifying Bacteria
- Classification of Anti-Infectives
- Mechanisms of Action of Anti-Infectives
- Acquired Resistance
  - Mechanisms of Resistance
  - Promotion of Resistant Strains
  - Prevention of Resistant Strains
- Indications and Selection of Specific Anti-Infectives
- Host Factors Affecting Anti-Infective Selection
- Superinfections

Learning Outcomes

After reading this chapter, the student should be able to:

1. Explain the mechanisms by which pathogens infect the body.
2. Describe methods for classifying bacteria.
3. Explain the mechanisms by which anti-infective drugs act to kill pathogens or restrict their growth.
4. Describe the clinical significance of bacterial resistance.
5. Identify steps that the nurse can take to limit the development of resistance.
6. Describe the clinical rationale for selecting specific antibiotics.
7. Identify the role of the nurse in preventing, identifying, and treating adverse effects due to antibiotic therapy.
8. Explain how the patient's immune status, local tissue conditions, history of allergic reactions, age, pregnancy status, and genetics influence anti-infective pharmacotherapy.
9. Explain the clinical importance of selecting the correct antibiotic for the individual patient.
10. Describe the development of superinfections.

Key Terms

Definitions of the terms in bold may be found in the Glossary.

The human body has adapted quite well to living in a world teeming with microorganisms. In the air, water, food, and soil, microbes have been essential components of life on the planet for billions of years. In some cases, these microorganisms coexist in intimate contact with human beings. It is estimated that 10^{14} bacterial cells reside inside or on the surface of the body, which is more than the total number of human cells in an average person. Fortunately, of the millions of species of microbes, only a relative few are harmful to human health. The purpose of this chapter is to present the fundamental principles that apply to the pharmacotherapy of infectious diseases.

Pathogenicity and Virulence

46.1 Pathogens cause disease due to their ability to invade tissues or secrete toxins.

The first step in understanding the pharmacotherapy of infectious disease is to review the terminology that is used to describe the organisms. Disease-producing organisms, or **pathogens**, include viruses, bacteria, fungi, unicellular organisms (protozoans), and multicellular animals (e.g., fleas, mites, and worms). Each of these types of pathogens requires a different approach to pharmacotherapy.

Some pathogens are extremely infectious and life-threatening to humans, whereas others simply cause annoying symptoms or none at all. **Pathogenicity**, the ability of an organism to cause disease, depends on an organism's speed of reproduction and its skill in bypassing or overcoming body defenses. Organisms that usually infect only when the body's immune system is suppressed are called *opportunistic* pathogens.

Virulence is a quantitative measure of an organism's pathogenicity. A highly virulent microbe is one that can produce disease when present in very small numbers. Virulent pathogens produce their devastating effects through two primary characteristics: invasiveness and toxicity.

Invasiveness is the ability of a pathogen to grow extremely rapidly and cause direct damage to surrounding tissues by their sheer numbers. Because a week or more may be needed to mount an immune response against the organism, this exponential growth can rapidly overwhelm body defenses and disrupt normal cellular function. Some streptococci, staphylococci, and clostridia secrete hyaluronidase, an enzyme that digests the matrix between human cells, allowing the bacteria to penetrate anatomic barriers more easily. *Staphylococcus aureus* secretes the enzyme coagulase, which causes fibrin to be deposited on its cells, thereby protecting it from phagocytes.

The second characteristic of virulence is the production of toxins. **Exotoxins** are proteins released by bacteria into surrounding tissues that have the ability to inactivate or kill host cells. For example, *Clostridium botulinum*, the organism responsible for botulism, produces one of the most potent toxins known that binds to presynaptic motor neurons to prevent the release of acetylcholine. Cholera toxin from *Vibrio cholerae* causes large amounts of fluid to be secreted into the intestinal lumen. Symptoms of exotoxin-producing bacteria are usually caused by the toxin itself, not the bacteria. For example, patients experience food poisoning by ingesting food containing the toxins produced by the organisms; growth of the bacteria in the body is not required. Most exotoxins are water soluble and can readily enter the blood to cause systemic toxemia.

Endotoxins are harmful nonprotein chemicals that are part of the outer layer of the normal cell wall of gram-negative bacteria. After the bacterial cell dies, endotoxins are liberated into the surrounding tissue and induce macrophages to release large amounts of cytokines, causing generalized inflammation, fever, and chills. Rapid decreases in the number of lymphocytes, leukocytes, and platelets may occur. The initial doses of antibiotic therapy may actually worsen symptoms by lysing bacteria and releasing larger amounts of endotoxins. Even very small amounts of some bacterial endotoxins may disrupt normal cellular activity and, in extreme cases, result in death. Examples of organisms producing endotoxins include *Proteus*, a common cause of urinary tract infections (UTIs), and *Neisseria meningitidis*, the agent that causes meningitis.

Describing and Classifying Bacteria

46.2 Bacteria are described by their staining characteristics, shape, and ability to utilize oxygen.

Because of the enormous number of bacterial species, several descriptive systems have been developed to simplify their study. It is important to learn these classification schemes because drugs that are effective against one organism in a class are likely to be effective against other pathogens in the same class. Common bacterial pathogens and their associated diseases are listed in Table 46.1.

One of the simplest methods of classifying bacteria is to examine them microscopically after a crystal violet Gram stain has been applied to the microbes. Some bacteria contain a thick cell wall composed of peptidoglycan and retain the violet color after staining. These bacteria are called **gram positive** and include *Staphylococcus*, *Streptococcus*, and *Enterococcus*. Bacteria that have thinner cell walls will lose the violet stain and are called **gram negative**. Examples of gram-negative bacteria include *Bacteroides*, *Escherichia*, *Klebsiella*, *Pseudomonas*, and *Salmonella*. The distinction between gram-positive and gram-negative bacteria is a profound one that reflects important biochemical and physiologic differences between the two groups. Many antibiotics are

Table 46.1 Common Bacterial Pathogens

Name of Organism	Disease(s)	Description
Gram-Positive Bacilli		
Bacillus anthracis	Anthrax	Aerobe; appears in cutaneous and respiratory forms
Clostridium	Food poisoning, gas gangrene, tetanus	Anaerobe
Corynebacterium	Diphtheria	Aerobe or anaerobe
Gram-Positive Cocci		
Enterococci	Wounds, UTI, endocarditis, bacteremia	Aerobe; part of host flora of the genitourinary and intestinal tracts; common opportunistic pathogen
Staphylococcus aureus	Pneumonia, food poisoning, impetigo, wounds, bacteremia, endocarditis, toxic shock syndrome, osteomyelitis, UTI	Aerobe; some species are part of host flora on the skin and mucous membranes
Streptococci	Pharyngitis, pneumonia, skin infection, septicemia, endocarditis, otitis media, meningitis in children	Aerobe; some species are part of host flora of the respiratory, genital, and intestinal tracts
Gram-Negative Bacilli		
Bacteroides	Peritonitis, abdominal abscess	Anaerobe; part of host flora of the intestinal, respiratory, and genitourinary tracts
Campylobacter	Gastroenteritis, diarrhea	One of the most common causes of diarrheal illness in the United States
Enterobacter	UTI, blood or lung infections	Aerobe or anaerobe
Escherichia coli	Traveler's diarrhea, UTI, meningitis in children, bacteremia	Part of host flora of the intestinal tract
Haemophilus influenzae	Pneumonia, meningitis in children, bacteremia, otitis media, sinusitis	Some species are part of host flora of the upper respiratory tract
Klebsiella pneumoniae	Pneumonia, UTI	Common opportunistic pathogen; often fatal if not treated aggressively
Proteus mirabilis	UTI, skin infection	Part of host flora of the intestinal tract
Pseudomonas aeruginosa	UTI, skin infection, septicemia	Common opportunistic pathogen
Salmonella enteritides	Food poisoning	Acquired from infected animal products: raw eggs, undercooked meat or chicken
Salmonella typhi	Enteric (typhoid) fever	Acquired from contaminated food or water supplies
Serratia	Hospital-associated infections of wounds and UTI	Aerobic or anaerobic
Shigella	Dysentery	Aerobic or anaerobic; part of host flora of the gastrointestinal (GI) tract
Vibrio cholerae	Cholera	Gram-negative aerobe; acquired from contaminated food or water
Gram-Negative Cocci		
Neisseria gonorrhoeae	Gonorrhea, urethritis, anorectal infection, pelvic inflammatory disease, neonatal eye infection	Gram-negative aerobe; some species are part of host flora of the upper respiratory tract
Neisseria meningitides	Meningitis, particularly in children	Gram-negative aerobe; may result in death within hours of onset of symptoms
Spirilla/Spirochetes		
Borrelia burgdorferi	Lyme disease	Acquired from tick bites
Treponema	Syphilis	Sexually transmitted infection (STI)
Other Organisms		
Chlamydia trachomatis	STIs, eye infection	Gram-negative; most common cause of STIs in the United States
Mycobacterium leprae	Leprosy	Most cases in the United States occur in immigrants from Africa or Asia
Mycobacterium tuberculosis	Tuberculosis	Very high incidence in patients with human immunodeficiency virus (HIV) or acquired immunodeficiency syndrome (AIDS)
Mycoplasma pneumoniae	Pneumonia	Most common cause of pneumonia in patients age 5–35
Rickettsia rickettsii	Rocky mountain spotted fever	Gram-negative; acquired from tick bites

effective against only one of the two groups. For example, gram-negative bacteria are generally susceptible to the tetracycline class but are resistant to the sulfonamides. This generalization, however, quickly breaks down when resistant strains develop.

Bacteria are often described by their basic shape, which can be readily determined microscopically. Those with rod shapes are called *bacilli*, those that are spherical are called *cocci*, and those that are spiral are called *spirilla*. The shape, along with the Gram stain, helps pathologists to identify organisms that are isolated from infectious specimens.

A third factor used to categorize bacteria is their ability to use oxygen. Those that thrive in an oxygen-rich environment are called **aerobic**; those that grow optimally without oxygen are called **anaerobic**. Some organisms have the ability to change their metabolism and survive in either aerobic or anaerobic conditions, depending on their external environment. Antibiotics are often selective for either aerobes or anaerobes.

Classification of Anti-Infectives

46.3 Anti-infective drugs are classified by their susceptible organisms, chemical structures, and mechanisms of action.

Anti-infective is a general term that applies to any medication that is effective against pathogens. In its broadest sense, an anti-infective drug may be used to treat bacterial, fungal, viral, or parasitic infections. To distinguish among the various anti-infectives, these medications are classified as antibacterial, antifungal, antiviral, antiprotozoan, and antihelminthic based on the type of organism they treat.

The most frequent term used to describe an antibacterial drug is *antibiotic*. Technically, **antibiotic** refers to a natural substance produced by a microorganism that can kill other microorganisms. However, many of the newer drugs that are available to treat bacterial infections are now produced synthetically. In clinical practice and in this text, the terms *antibacterial* and *antibiotic* are used interchangeably to refer to any drug that is effective against bacteria.

Classifying drugs only by their susceptible organism, such as an antibacterial, tells us nothing about the properties, actions, or adverse effects of a drug. With over 300 antibacterials available, it is helpful to group these drugs into subclasses that share similar therapeutic properties. Two means of grouping are widely used: chemical classes and pharmacologic classes.

Class names such as aminoglycoside, fluoroquinolone, and sulfonamide refer to the fundamental chemical structure shared by a group of anti-infectives. Anti-infectives that belong to the same chemical class have close structural similarities and usually share similar antibacterial properties and adverse effects. Although chemical names are sometimes long and difficult to pronounce, placing drugs into chemical classes will assist the student in mentally organizing these drugs into distinct therapeutic groups.

Table 46.2 Classification of Anti-Infective Drugs

Mechanism of Action	Chemical Class	Examples
Inhibition of cell wall synthesis	Penicillins Cephalosporins Carbapenems	penicillin G cefotaxime (Claforan) imipenem (Primaxin) isoniazid (INH) vancomycin (Vancocin)
Inhibition of protein synthesis	Aminoglycosides Macrolides Oxazolidinones Tetracyclines	gentamicin erythromycin (E-mycin) linezolid (Zyvox) tetracycline (Achromycin V)
Disruption of plasma membrane	Azoles Polyenes	amphotericin B (Fungizone) fluconazole (Diflucan) nystatin (Mycostatin)
Inhibition of nucleic acid synthesis	Fluoroquinolones	ciprofloxacin (Cipro)
Inhibition of metabolic pathways	Sulfonamides	dapsone (Aczone) trimethoprim-sulfamethoxazole (Bactrim, Septra)

Pharmacologic classes are used to group anti-infectives by their mechanism of action. Like chemical classes, placing an antibiotic into a pharmacologic class allows the nurse to develop a mental framework on which to organize these medications and to predict similar actions and adverse effects. Examples of pharmacologic classes grouped by their mechanisms of action with representative drugs are listed in Table 46.2. It is important for nurses to learn both the chemical class and the pharmacologic class for each antibiotic because this will provide a deeper understanding of each drug's therapeutic action and potential adverse effects.

Mechanisms of Action of Anti-Infectives

46.4 Anti-infective drugs act by selectively targeting a pathogen's metabolism or lifecycle.

Although the immune system provides elaborate defenses against microbial invaders, there are times when the body's defenses become overwhelmed by an infection. Furthermore, there are times when acquiring an infection could be a serious health challenge for a patient, and it is best to prevent it. Whether it is used for treating or preventing disease, the primary goal of anti-infective therapy is to assist the body in eliminating a pathogen. Drugs that accomplish this goal by killing bacteria are called **bactericidal**. Some drugs do not kill pathogens but instead slow their growth, allowing natural body defenses to eliminate the microorganisms. These growth-slowing drugs are called **bacteriostatic**.

Bacterial cells have distinct anatomic and physiologic differences compared to human cells. Bacteria incorporate different chemicals into their membranes and use unique biochemical pathways and enzymes to manage their rapid growth. Even the more complex pathogens such as fungi and protozoans have different cell structures and use certain metabolic pathways not found in human cells. Antibiotics exert selective toxicity by targeting these unique differences between human and bacterial, fungal, and protozoan cells. Through this selective action, these pathogens can be killed, or their growth severely hampered, without any major effects on human cells. Of course, there are limits to this selective toxicity, depending on the specific antibiotic and the dose employed. Adverse effects can be expected from all the anti-infectives. Antibacterials exert their selective toxicity via five major methods: inhibition of cell wall synthesis, inhibition of protein synthesis, disruption of the plasma cell membrane, inhibition of nucleic acid synthesis, and inhibition of metabolic pathways (antimetabolites). This is an oversimplification of antibacterial actions because some of these drugs act by multiple mechanisms and a few act by unknown mechanisms. Furthermore, as new drugs are developed, they often act by new mechanisms and become the only medication in a class. Indeed, although the five major classes encompass the majority of anti-infectives, the "miscellaneous" group of anti-infectives has expanded into a large class (see Chapter 49).

Inhibition of Cell Wall Synthesis

Unlike human cells, bacteria have rigid cell walls that create a high osmotic pressure within the cells. The cell wall primarily consists of **peptidoglycan**, a strong, repeating network of carbohydrate and protein chains found only in bacteria and that contains sugars bound to peptides. Disruption of this wall causes the cell to absorb water and eventually lyse. The presence of a unique cell wall gives several means by which antibiotics may act. Fungi also have a unique cell wall that contains lipids that are not used in human cells.

The penicillins and cephalosporins bind to specific proteins that are essential to building the bacterial cell wall. Vancomycin acts by preventing the formation of peptide chains that are used in the construction of the cell wall. Several drugs that are effective against *Mycobacterium tuberculosis*, including isoniazid, act by inhibiting the incorporation of mycolic acid, an important component of the cell wall of this mycobacterium. Uses of the cell wall inhibitors are presented in Chapter 47.

Inhibition of Protein Synthesis

Both bacterial and human cells conduct protein synthesis, so this may seem an unlikely target for antibiotics. However, proteins are constructed on the surface of ribosomes, and these organelles have different structures in humans and bacteria. This difference in ribosomal structure accounts for the selective toxicity of certain antibiotics for bacterial cells.

The fact that protein synthesis occurs in several steps affords different mechanisms by which antibiotics may act. For example, the tetracyclines interfere with the transfer of ribonucleic acid (RNA), which carries the amino acids to the ribosome. The aminoglycosides change the shape of the ribosome so that protein synthesis is impeded. Drugs that inhibit protein synthesis are discussed in Chapter 48.

Disruption of the Plasma Cell Membrane

A few antibacterial and antifungal medications act by interfering with the pathogen's plasma membrane. For example, when polymyxin B attaches to the phospholipids in bacterial plasma membranes, the permeability of the membrane changes and substances escape from the cell. The antifungal drug amphotericin B shuts down the synthesis of ergosterol, a lipid essential to the integrity of fungal plasma membranes.

Inhibition of Nucleic Acid Synthesis

Although deoxyribonucleic acid (DNA) and RNA synthesis are complex processes that occur in both human and bacterial cells, the molecular structures of the various enzymes required for these processes differ considerably. The largest group of antibiotics that inhibits DNA synthesis is the fluoroquinolones. These drugs affect bacterial DNA gyrase, an enzyme that uncoils DNA during the replication process. The fluoroquinolones are presented in Chapter 49.

Inhibition of Metabolic Pathways (Antimetabolites)

Because they divide rapidly, bacterial cells need a steady supply of nutrients and metabolites. A few drugs structurally resemble these building blocks and "fool" the bacterial cell into using them for growth. The sulfonamide antibiotics resemble para-amino benzoic acid (PABA), a precursor to folic acid. Folic acid, a B vitamin that is essential to human metabolism, is also essential to bacteria. When the bacteria attempt to use the sulfonamides, bacterial protein synthesis is blocked. The sulfonamides are presented in Chapter 50.

Other Mechanisms of Action

Anti-infectives act by a number of other miscellaneous mechanisms. The antifungal drug griseofulvin inhibits the formation of mitotic microtubules. Antiretrovirals such as zidovudine block the synthesis of viral DNA by inhibiting the enzyme reverse transcriptase. Mebendazole kills parasitic worms by preventing their absorption of nutrients.

Pharmacotherapy Illustrated 46.1

Mechanisms of Action of Antimicrobial Drugs

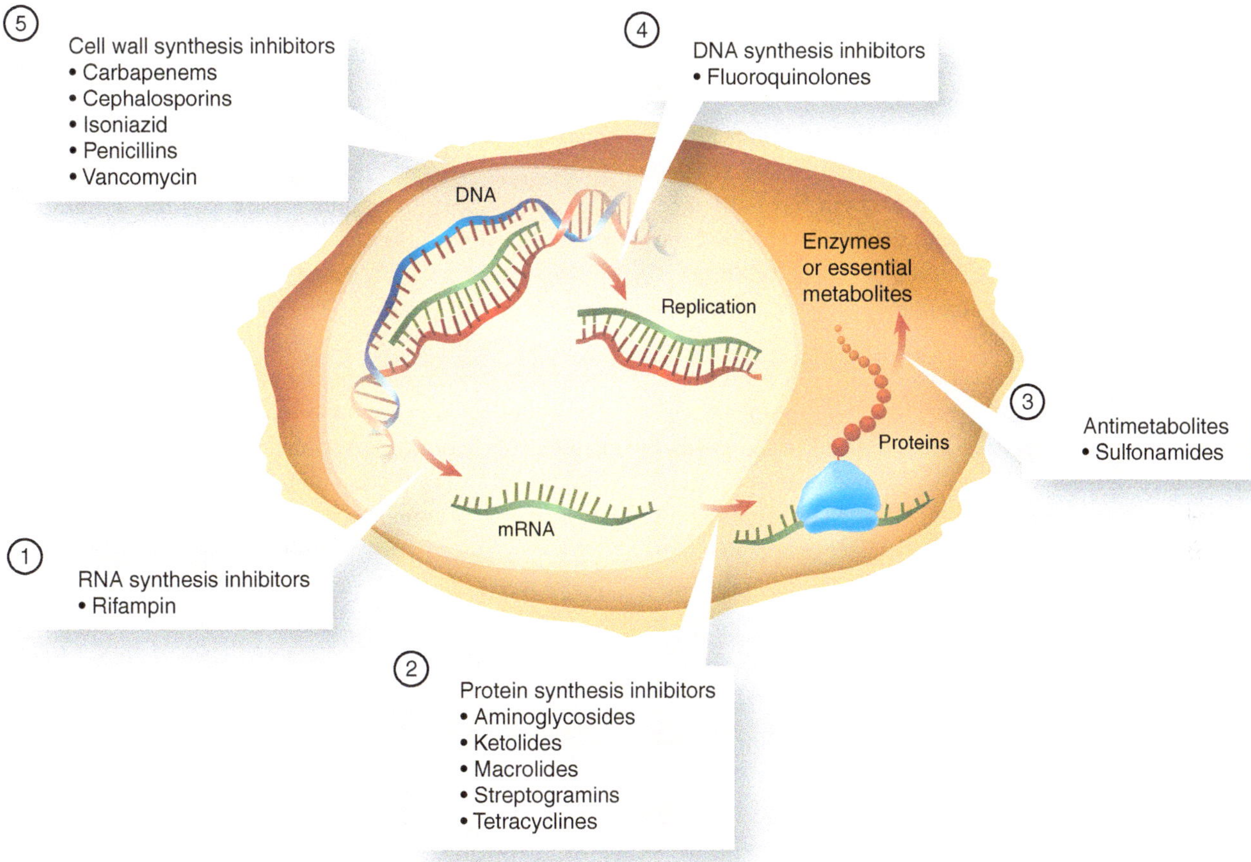

Many other possible mechanisms exist. As the understanding of bacterial physiology increases, it is likely that pharmacologists will develop anti-infectives with entirely new mechanisms of action. The primary mechanisms of action of antibacterial drugs are shown in Pharmacotherapy Illustrated 46.1.

Acquired Resistance

46.5 Acquired resistance is a major clinical problem that is worsened by the inappropriate use of anti-infectives.

In the 1950s, healthcare providers called antibiotics "miracle drugs" and predicted that all infectious disease would one day be eliminated. It did not take long, however, to discover that these miracle drugs were rapidly becoming ineffective. How could a drug that once killed nearly 100% of a species of bacteria soon prove to be ineffective? The answer is acquired resistance.

Acquired resistance is the ability of an organism to become unresponsive over time to the effects of an anti-infective. Resistance can occur in bacteria, fungi, viruses, and protozoans. It is a major clinical problem that is growing in importance.

Mechanisms of Resistance

How can an organism become insensitive to a drug that kills other members of its species? Medicine has discovered a number of mechanisms by which pathogens acquire resistance:

- **Destruction of the drug.** Organisms can produce an enzyme that destroys or deactivates the drug. For example, some bacteria are able to produce beta-lactamase, an enzyme that splits the active portion of the drug molecule. Organisms that produce beta-lactamase are resistant to many of the penicillin and cephalosporin antibiotics.
- **Prevention of drug entry into the pathogen.** Some antibiotics must enter the pathogen to cause their action. Some bacteria have developed enzymes that inactivate the drug as it crosses the cell wall. Others have changed the structure of the channels or pores that the antibiotic

normally uses to enter the cell. Resistance to penicillins and tetracyclines can occur by these methods.

- **Removal by resistance pumps.** Some bacteria have developed a system that rapidly pumps the antibiotic out of the bacterial cell before it can reach intracellular targets such as ribosomes. Resistant bacteria have developed several types of pumps, each of which is used to remove different antibiotics.
- **Alteration of the drug's target site.** Most antibiotics bind to a specific receptor that is located on the cell surface or inside the bacteria. Certain bacteria have changed the shape of these receptors, so they no longer bind the drug. This mechanism of resistance is common for the sulfonamides. For the macrolide antibiotics, mutations have resulted in changes to the structure of the bacterial ribosome, which is the receptor for macrolide binding.
- **Development of alternative metabolic pathways.** Some antibiotics act by depleting the pathogen of an essential substance necessary for growth. Some resistant organisms have survived antibiotic application by synthesizing larger amounts of the essential substance or by finding an alternative means of obtaining it from the environment.

How do bacteria change their physiology to become resistant to antibiotics? The answer lies in the nature of bacterial cell division. Microorganisms have the ability to replicate extremely rapidly. Under ideal conditions *E. coli* can produce a million cells every 20 minutes, or 1×10^{21} cells in only 24 hours. During exponential division, bacteria make frequent errors, or **mutations**, while duplicating their genetic code. These mutations, which occur spontaneously and randomly, occasionally result in a change in physiology that gives a bacterial cell a reproductive advantage over its neighbors. For example, the mutated bacterium may be able to survive in harsher conditions, change the shape of its organelles, or perhaps grow faster than other bacterial cells.

It is possible for such a random mutation to confer drug resistance for a microorganism. Once the mutation produces a resistant strain, the microbes permanently lose sensitivity to that specific drug and often to other drugs in the same pharmacologic and chemical class. Over several decades, these drug-resistant mutants may colonize a large segment of the human population, thus making the medication essentially useless as a first-line antibiotic.

Promotion of Resistant Strains

The widespread and sometimes unwarranted use of antibiotics has promoted the development of drug-resistant bacterial strains. By killing strains of bacteria that are sensitive to the drug, the only bacteria remaining to replicate are those that acquired the mutations that made them insensitive to the effects of the antibiotic. These drug-resistant bacteria are then free to grow, unrestrained by their neighbors that are killed by the antibiotic. Soon the patient develops an infection that is resistant to conventional drug therapy. This concept is shown in Figure 46.1.

After acquiring resistance, the mutated bacterium may pass its resistance gene to other bacteria through **conjugation**, which is the direct transfer of small pieces of circular DNA called plasmids. Through conjugation, it is quite possible for a bacterium that has never been exposed to the antibiotic to become resistant. Furthermore, because conjugation is not species specific, resistance genes may be passed from one species to a totally different species.

It is important to understand that the antibiotic itself does not cause changes in bacterial physiology, nor does the microorganism have a master plan to become resistant or to actively defeat the drug. The mutation occurs randomly—the result of accident and pure chance. The promotion and growth of the resistant strain, however, are not due to chance. The antibiotic kills the surrounding cells that are susceptible to the drug, leaving the mutated bacterium plenty of room to divide and infect. It should also be understood that it is the bacteria that become resistant, not the patient.

Prevention of Resistant Strains

Patients and their healthcare providers play important roles in delaying the emergence of resistance to antibiotics. The Centers for Disease Control and Prevention (CDC) has developed a set of guidelines for preventing antimicrobial resistance in the healthcare setting:

- **Prevent infections when possible.** Nurses must always teach their patients that it is always easier to prevent an infection than to treat one. One important aspect of prevention is getting immunizations to protect against diseases such as influenza, tetanus, polio, measles, and hepatitis B (see Chapter 43). Prevention also includes proper care and hygiene of catheters, which are significant sources of microorganisms and provide portals of entry into the body.
- **Diagnose and treat the infection properly.** Infections should be cultured so that the offending organism can be identified and the correct drug chosen, as discussed in Section 46.7.
- **Use antimicrobials appropriately.** Antibiotics should be prescribed only when there is a clear rationale for their use. The drugs should be taken for the full length of therapy, and the prescription should not be renewed if the infection has been eliminated or prevented. The more often an antibiotic is prescribed in the population, the larger will be the percentage of resistant strains.
- **Prevent transmission.** Nurses can contain infections and stop the spread of the disease in their work settings by using proper infection control procedures. Additionally, nurses should teach their patients the methods of proper hygiene to prevent the transmission of infectious disease in the home and community settings.

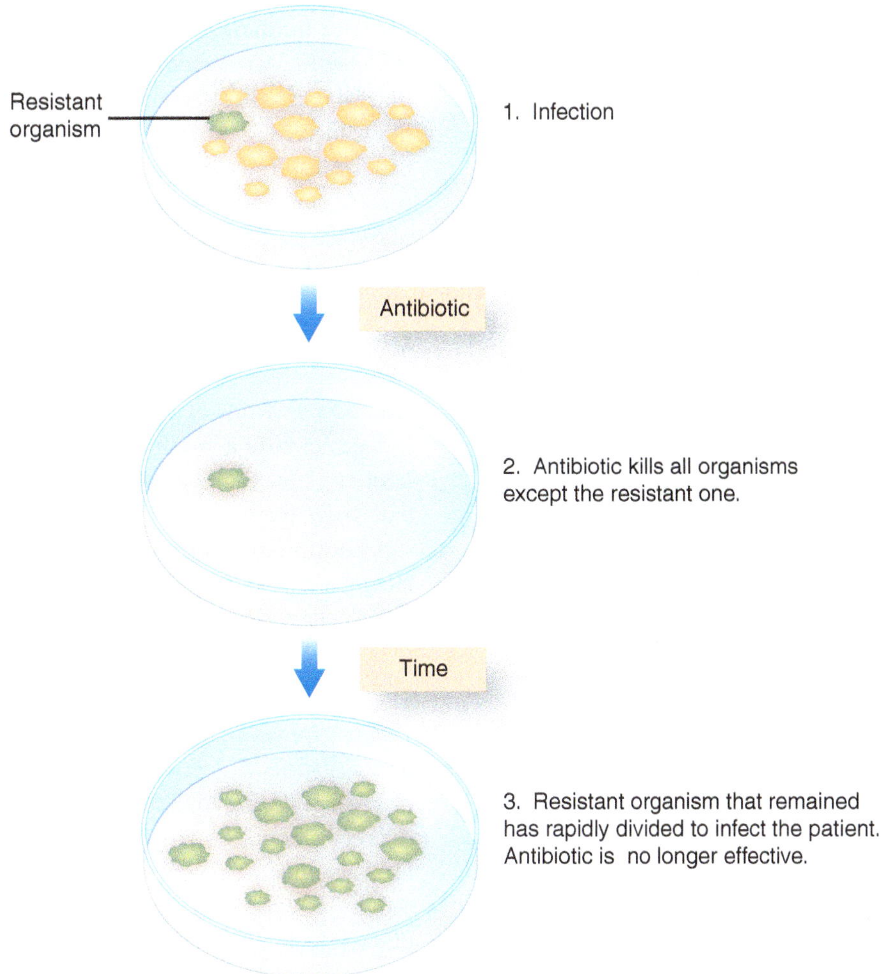

Figure 46.1 Acquired resistance.

46.6 Several resistant strains are major clinical challenges due to the lack of therapeutic options.

Infections that are acquired in a healthcare setting, called **healthcare-associated infections (HAIs)**, are often resistant to common antibiotics. The most common site of HAIs is the urinary tract, followed by surgical wounds, respiratory tract, and the blood (bacteremia). Table 46.3 lists the organisms that are frequently responsible for HAI infections.

The four general sources of HAIs are as follows:

- **Patient flora.** Bacteria normally residing on the skin and in the lung or genitourinary tract
- **Invasive devices.** Urinary catheters, vascular catheters, endotracheal tubes, and endoscopes
- **Medical personnel.** Infected healthcare workers or noninfectious carriers
- **Medical environment.** Contaminated instruments, air, food, or fluids.

Many times, patients are at risk for HAIs caused by resistant organisms. Resistant strains that are especially important to pharmacotherapy include methicillin-resistant

Table 46.3 Common Pathogens Associated with Healthcare-Associated Infections

Pathogen	Infection
Acinetobacter species (spp)	Bacteremia, pneumonia
Clostridioides difficile	Colon
Enterobacter spp	Pneumonia
Enterococcus spp	Urinary tract
Escherichia coli	Bacteremia, pneumonia, urinary tract
Klebsiella pneumoniae	Pneumonia, urinary tract
Pseudomonas aeruginosa	Pneumonia, urinary tract
Staphylococci (coagulase negative)	Bacteremia
Staphylococcus aureus	Bacteremia, pneumonia, surgical wounds

S. aureus, vancomycin-resistant enterococci, carbapenem-resistant Enterobacteriaceae, and *Clostridioides difficile*.

Methicillin-resistant staphylococcus aureus (MRSA): MRSA is a type of bacterium that is resistant to certain antibiotics such as methicillin, amoxicillin, and penicillin. At least 60% of *S. aureus* infections are now resistant to penicillin. The term *methicillin resistant* is still used for these infections despite the fact that methicillin was removed from the market many years ago.

MRSA infections are most frequently acquired in hospitals and long-term care facilities. These hospital-acquired infections (HA-MRSA) occur primarily in patients with weakened immune systems. MRSA infections that occur in nonhospitalized settings are called community-acquired infections. Community-acquired MRSA (CA-MRSA) infections occur in otherwise healthy people and are usually manifested as skin and soft tissue infections, such as pimples and boils. The strains that are responsible for HA-MRSA infections appear to be distinctly different from those that cause CA-MRSA infections; thus, the pharmacotherapy of the two infections differs somewhat.

Therapeutic options for patients with serious MRSA infections are limited. In recent years, MRSA strains have developed resistance to most classes of antimicrobials, including fluoroquinolones, macrolides, aminoglycosides, tetracyclines, and clindamycin. In general, the HA-MRSA strains are resistant to more classes than the CA-MRSA infections. Until recently, vancomycin was the only antibiotic effective for treating serious MRSA infections. Unfortunately, MRSA strains that are also resistant to vancomycin have appeared. Several newer antibiotics, including linezolid (Zyvox), quinupristin-dalfopristin, and daptomycin, are now available to treat multidrug-resistant strains of MRSA.

Vancomycin-resistant enterococci (VRE): Enterococci are normal inhabitants of the human GI tract and the female genital tract. Enterococci are also frequently found in wounds and pressure ulcers in hospitalized patients or nursing home residents. Patients with compromised immune systems are at greatest risk. Because enterococci are hardy organisms, they can survive for prolonged periods on environmental surfaces, and healthcare workers using poor infection control techniques can easily spread them. More than 95% of VRE strains in the United States are *Enterococcus faecium*.

Like MRSA, VRE infections represent a major therapeutic challenge, and treatment options are limited. Strains that are resistant to the most commonly used classes of antibiotics have been isolated. Virtually all are resistant to high levels of ampicillin, which is the conventional treatment for enterococci infections. In the 1990s, vancomycin became the only antibiotic effective against multidrug-resistant VRE strains. Unfortunately, each year finds more VRE strains becoming resistant to vancomycin, and newer antibiotics must be used for these infections.

Carbapenem-resistant enterobacteriaceae (CRE): Enterobacteriaceae colonize the mucosal surfaces and GI tracts of humans and include *E. coli*, *E. aerogenes*, and *K. pneumoniae*. Most members of this family are opportunistic and can cause secondary infections in numerous locations, including the lungs, urinary tract, and blood. Enteric Enterobacteriaceae are responsible for most CRE. CRE secrete carbapenemases, which are a form of beta-lactamase, to inactivate the antibiotics.

CRE have been increasingly observed in hospitals and long-term care facilities, which are the primary transmission sites for these infections. Some CRE are resistant to all drugs in the carbapenem class of antibiotics, which have been considered the drugs of last resort for treating this infection. Indeed, in 2017 a strain was isolated from a patient in the United States that was resistant to all available antimicrobial drugs (pan-resistant) (Chen et al., 2017).

Because most Enterobacteriaceae are resistant to beta-lactam antibiotics and carbapenems, pharmacotherapy may include tigecycline, fosfomycin, aminoglycosides, and polymyxin B. The mortality rate for a CRE infection can be as high as 50%.

***Clostridioides difficile* (*C. difficile*):** Formerly called *Clostridium difficile*, *C. difficile* is the most common microbial cause of HAI, resulting in 500,000 infections. Within a month of diagnosis about 1 in 11 people over age 65 will die of the HAI-acquired *C. diff* infection (CDC, 2020). Those at highest risk for *C. difficile* infection are patients receiving an antibiotic while in a healthcare facility. Infection is attributed to a combination of unnecessary antibiotic use (creatine-resistant strains) and ineffective infection control procedures.

Pharmacotherapy for *C. difficile* includes vancomycin for severe cases and metronidazole and fidaxomicin for moderate or mild infections. In 2016, bezlotoxumab (Zinplava) was approved to prevent relapses, which are very common in patients with *C. difficile* infection. Bezlotoxumab is a monoclonal antibody that binds to *C. difficile* toxin B to prevent its cytotoxic effects. This drug is not an antibiotic but is an adjunct to regular antibiotic therapy for this microbe.

CONNECTION Checkpoint 46.1

From what you learned in Chapter 27, explain the difference between resistance and tolerance.

Indications and Selection of Specific Anti-Infectives

46.7 Selection of the most appropriate antibiotic is essential for effective pharmacotherapy and to limit adverse effects.

It is essential for the healthcare provider to select an antibiotic that will be effective against the specific pathogen that is causing the patient's infection. Selecting an ineffective drug will delay proper treatment, giving the pathogens more time to invade or secrete toxins. For acute infections, treatment delays of just a few hours or days can lead to poorer patient prognosis and even death. Prescribing ineffective antibiotics also promotes the development of resistance and may cause unnecessary adverse effects in the patient.

For the appropriate antibiotic to be chosen, identification of the causative agent is usually necessary. Although gathering data on symptoms is important, many infections produce the same signs early in their course; thus, more exact laboratory means of diagnosis are necessary.

Specimens such as urine, sputum, blood, or pus are examined in the laboratory for the purpose of isolating and identifying specific pathogens. After isolation, the microbe is exposed in the laboratory to different antibiotics to determine the most effective ones. This process of isolating the infectious organism and identifying the most effective antibiotic is called **culture and sensitivity (C&S) testing**. Other laboratory techniques include examination of the blood for specific antibodies, direct antigen detection, and DNA probe hybridization.

Ideally, the pathogen should be identified before anti-infective therapy is begun. However, laboratory testing and identification may take several days and, in the case of viruses, several weeks. Indeed, some pathogens cannot be cultured at all. If the infection is severe, therapy is often begun with a **broad-spectrum antibiotic**, which is one that is effective against a wide variety of different microbial species. After C&S testing is completed, the drug may be changed to a **narrow-spectrum antibiotic**, which is one that is effective against a smaller group of microbes or only the isolated species. In general, narrow-spectrum antibiotics have less effect on **host flora**, thus causing fewer adverse effects. Host flora are microorganisms that normally inhabit the human body.

Anti-infectives should not be prescribed for infections such as the common cold or for disorders for which antibiotics serve no therapeutic advantage. Antibiotics do not affect viral diseases such as the common cold, although many patients with this self-limiting disorder believe that these drugs will speed their recovery. Another example of anti-infective misuse is prescribing antibiotics to patients who have a cough due to chronic bronchitis. It should be understood, however, that healthcare providers may prescribe anti-infectives to prevent a *secondary* infection from developing. For example, an older adult patient with a severe cold may develop a weakened immune response. Thus, the healthcare provider may order an antibiotic not for the viral infection, but to prevent a secondary bacterial infection from developing.

46.8 Depending on the pathogen, anti-infective therapy may be conducted with a single drug or a combination of drugs.

If C&S testing confirms that an infection is caused by only one species of microbe, antibiotic therapy is usually begun with a single drug. In some cases, combining two antibiotics may actually decrease each drug's effectiveness, a phenomenon known as *antagonism*. For example, giving a drug that slows bacterial growth may interfere with an antibiotic that depends on a high bacterial growth rate to produce its bactericidal effect. Use of multiple antibiotics can also promote the emergence of multidrug-resistant strains and produce unnecessary adverse effects.

In well-defined circumstances, combination therapy with multiple antibiotics is warranted. For example, multiple anti-infective drugs are indicated if different species of pathogens are causing the infection. Patients may present with a life-threatening infection of unknown etiology and the healthcare provider may need to prescribe several antibiotics until the specific pathogens can be identified. In some cases, two antibiotics have been shown through clinical research to work synergistically, producing a greater kill rate than would be achieved by either antibiotic given alone. Examples of situations where multidrug therapy is clearly warranted are for the pharmacotherapy of tuberculosis (see Chapter 51) and HIV-AIDS (see Chapter 55).

CONNECTION Checkpoint 46.2

From what you learned in Chapter 5, why would a patient potentially experience fewer adverse effects if given two antibiotics at lower doses, rather than a single antibiotic at a higher dose?

46.9 Anti-infectives may be administered to prevent infections.

In most cases, anti-infectives are given when there is clear evidence of infection. This is because healthcare providers have developed clear rationales for prescribing these drugs to discourage the emergence of resistant strains.

However, anti-infectives are administered to *prevent* infections in certain high-risk patients. In these cases, research has demonstrated that the benefits of infection prophylaxis outweigh the increased risk of adverse effects or the potential for producing resistant strains. Prophylactic anti-infectives are indicated for the following clinical situations:

- Antibiotics for patients with suppressed immune systems, including those with HIV infection, transplant recipients, or profound neutropenia
- Antibiotics for patients with deep puncture wounds such as from dog bites
- Antibiotics for patients with prosthetic heart valves or joint replacements, prior to receiving medical or dental surgery, to prevent bacterial endocarditis
- Antibiotics for patients who are undergoing specific types of surgery, such as cardiovascular, orthopedic, or alimentary canal surgery, where it has been shown that antibiotic use decreases the risk of postoperative infections

- Antimalarial drugs for patients who are traveling to areas of the world where malaria is endemic
- Antitubercular drugs for close personal contacts of patients who have confirmed or suspected active tuberculosis
- Antiretrovirals to prevent the transmission of HIV to newborns when the mother is HIV positive
- Antiretrovirals for postexposure prophylaxis of health-care workers who have a confirmed exposure to HIV-contaminated body fluids.

Prophylactic therapy with anti-infectives is usually conducted using specific protocols that designate the duration of therapy. For example, chloroquine is given 1 week before expected exposure to malaria and continues for 4 weeks following exposure. Zidovudine (AZT) is given to a mother who is HIV positive by week 14 of pregnancy until birth, after which the drug is given to her neonate for 6 weeks. Only in rare cases are anti-infectives given prophylactically for indefinite time periods. Examples include the prevention of infections in patients with suppressed immune systems such as those with HIV infection or those receiving immunosuppressants following an organ transplant.

Host Factors Affecting Anti-Infective Selection

46.10 Patient factors such as host defenses, local tissue conditions, history of allergic reactions, age, pregnancy status, and genetics influence the choice of anti-infective.

The most important factor in selecting an appropriate antibiotic is to be certain that the microbe is sensitive to the bactericidal or bacteriostatic effects of the drug. Once the appropriate drug has been chosen, the nurse must consider a number of host factors that have the potential to significantly influence the success of anti-infective therapy.

Host Defenses

Remember that the primary goal of antibiotic therapy is to kill enough of the pathogen or slow its growth such that natural body defenses can overcome the invading agents. An anti-infective is rarely able to eliminate a pathogen without help from a functioning immune system. Patients with weakened immune defenses often require the administration of prophylactic antibiotics. Should an infection occur in these patients, anti-infective therapy is more aggressive and prolonged. Examples of patients who may require this type of antibiotic therapy include those with AIDS and those with neutropenia caused by immunosuppressive or antineoplastic medications.

Local Tissue Conditions

Anti-infectives must be able to reach the area of infection in sufficient concentrations to be effective; thus, local conditions at the infection site are important to the success of pharmacotherapy. Infections of the central nervous system are particularly difficult to treat because many medications are unable to cross the blood–brain barrier to reach the brain and associated tissues. Injury or inflammation at an infection site can cause tissues to become acidic or anaerobic and have poor circulation. Excessive pus formation or large hematomas can impede drugs from reaching their targets. Pathogens such as mycobacteria, salmonella, toxoplasma, and listeria can reside intracellularly and thus be resistant to antibacterial action.

Factors that hinder the drug from reaching microbes will limit therapeutic success, and adjustments in treatment may be necessary. Increasing the dosage or switching to a different route of drug administration may be indicated. Occasionally, it is necessary to switch to a different antibiotic that is more effective for conditions specific to the infection site.

Allergy History

Although not common, serious hypersensitivity reactions to antibiotics may be fatal. The penicillins are the class of antibacterials that have the highest incidence of allergic reactions: Between 0.7 and 10% of all patients who receive these drugs exhibit some degree of hypersensitivity.

Patient assessment must always include a thorough medication history. A previous acute allergic incident with a drug is highly predictive of future hypersensitivity to the same medication. Because the patient may have been exposed to an antibiotic unknowingly, such as through food products or molds, allergic reactions can occur without any apparent previous exposure. If severe allergy to a drug is established, it is best to avoid all drugs in the same chemical class.

Other Host Factors

Age, pregnancy status, and genetics are additional factors that influence anti-infective pharmacotherapy. Infants and older adults are less able to metabolize and excrete antibiotics; thus, doses are generally decreased. Because of polypharmacy in older patients, this group is more likely to be taking multiple drugs that could interact with antibiotics.

Some antibiotics are readily secreted in breast milk or cross the placenta. For example, tetracyclines taken by the mother can cause teeth discoloration in the newborn, and aminoglycosides can affect hearing. Some anti-infectives are pregnancy category D, such as minocycline, doxycycline, neomycin, and streptomycin. The benefits of antibiotic use in pregnant or lactating women must be carefully weighed against the potential risks to the fetus and neonate.

A genetic absence of certain enzymes can lead to an inability of a patient to metabolize antibiotics to their inactive forms. For example, patients with a deficiency of the enzyme glucose-6-phosphate dehydrogenase should not receive sulfonamides, chloramphenicol, or nalidixic acid due to the possibility of erythrocyte rupture.

CONNECTION Checkpoint 46.3

From what you learned in Chapter 42, what classes of drugs are administered to boost immune function so that the patient is less likely to experience an opportunistic infection?

Superinfections

46.11 Superinfections can occur when an anti-infective antibiotic kills host flora.

Microorganisms that normally inhabit the human body, or host flora, are present on the surface of the skin and in the upper respiratory, genitourinary, and intestinal tracts. Some of these microbes serve useful purposes by producing natural antibacterial substances or by breaking down toxic agents. The various host flora are in competition with each other for physical space and nutrients. This **microbial antagonism** helps protect the host from being overrun by pathogenic organisms.

Antibiotics are unable to distinguish between host flora and pathogenic organisms. When an antibiotic kills the host's normal flora, additional nutrients and space are available for pathogenic microorganisms to grow unchecked. These new, secondary infections caused by antibiotic use are called **superinfections**, or suprainfections. The appearance of a new infection while receiving anti-infective therapy is highly suspicious of a superinfection. Signs and symptoms of superinfection commonly include diarrhea, bladder pain, painful urination, or abnormal vaginal discharges.

Broad-spectrum antibiotics are more likely to cause superinfections because they kill many microbial species, which sometimes include host flora. Organisms that commonly cause superinfections are *Candida albicans* in the vagina, streptococci in the oral cavity, and *C. difficile* in the colon.

Understanding Chapter 46

Key Concepts Summary

46.1 Pathogens cause disease due to their ability to invade tissues or secrete toxins.

46.2 Bacteria are described by their staining characteristics, shape, and ability to utilize oxygen.

46.3 Anti-infective drugs are classified by their susceptible organisms, chemical structures, and mechanisms of action.

46.4 Anti-infective drugs act by selectively targeting a pathogen's metabolism or lifecycle.

46.5 Acquired resistance is a major clinical problem that is worsened by the inappropriate use of anti-infectives.

46.6 Several resistant strains are major clinical challenges due to the lack of therapeutic options.

46.7 Selection of the most appropriate antibiotic is essential for effective pharmacotherapy and to limit adverse effects.

46.8 Depending on the pathogen, anti-infective therapy may be conducted with a single drug or a combination of drugs.

46.9 Anti-infectives may be administered to prevent infections.

46.10 Patient factors such as host defenses, local tissue conditions, history of allergic reactions, age, pregnancy status, and genetics influence the choice of anti-infective.

46.11 Superinfections can occur when an anti-infective antibiotic kills host flora.

References

Centers for Disease Control and Prevention (CDC). (2020). *What is* C. diff? https://www.cdc.gov/cdiff/what-is.html

Chen, L., Todd, R., Kiehlbauch, J., Walters, M., & Kallen A. (2017). Notes from the field: Pan-resistant New Delhi metallo-beta-lactamase-producing *Klebsiella pneumoniae*—Washoe County, Nevada 2016. *Morbidity and Mortality Weekly Report*, *66*, 33. https://doi.org/10.15585/mmwr.mm6601a7

Selected Bibliography

Barlam, T. F., Cosgrove, S. E., Abbo, L. M., MacDougall, C., Schuetz, A. N., Septimus, E. J., et al. (2016). Implementing an antibiotic stewardship program: Guidelines by the Infectious Diseases Society of America and the Society for Healthcare Epidemiology of America. *Clinical Infectious Diseases*, *62*(10), e51–e77. https://doi.org/10.1093/cid/ciw118

Blair, J. M., Webber, M. A., Baylay, A. J., Ogbolu, D. O., & Piddock, L. J. (2015). Molecular mechanisms of antibiotic resistance. *Nature Reviews Microbiology*, *13*, 42–51. https://doi.org/10.1038/nrmicro3380

Cammarota, G., Gallo, A., Ianiro, G., & Montalto, M. (2019). Emerging drugs for the treatment of Clostridium difficile. *Expert Opinion on Emerging Drugs*, *24*(1), 17–28. https://doi.org/10.1080/14728214.2019.1591371

Centers for Disease Control and Prevention. (2020). *About antibiotic/antimicrobial resistance*. https://www.cdc.gov/drugresistance/about.html?CDC_AA_refVal=https%3A%2F%2Fwww.cdc.gov%2Fdrugresistance%2Femerging.html

Chambers, H. F., Eliopoulos, G. M., Gilbert, D. N., Pavia, A., & Saag, M. S. (Eds.). (2018). *The Sanford guide to antimicrobial therapy 2018*. Antimicrobial Therapy, Inc.

Custodio, H. T. (2016). *Hospital-acquired infections*. Medscape. http://emedicine.medscape.com/article/967022-overview#aw2aab6b2b5aa

Davis, C. P. (2019). *MRSA infection*. http://www.emedicinehealth.com/mrsa_infection/article_em.htm

Durante-Mangoni, E., Andini, R., & Zampino, R. (2019). Management of carbapenem-resistant Enterobacteriaceae infections. *Clinical Microbiology and Infection*, *25*(8), 943–950. https://doi.org/10.1097/QCO.0000000000000493

Gupta, A., Cifu, A. S., & Khanna, S. (2018). Diagnosis and treatment of *Clostridium difficile* infection. *Journal of the American Medical Association*, *320*(10), 1031–1032. https://doi.org/10.1001/jama.2018.12194

Trotter, A. J., Aydin, A., Strinden, M. J., & O'Grady, J. (2019). Recent and emerging technologies for the rapid diagnosis of infection and antimicrobial resistance. *Current Opinion in Microbiology*, *51*, 39–45. https://doi.org/10.1016/j.mib.2019.03.001

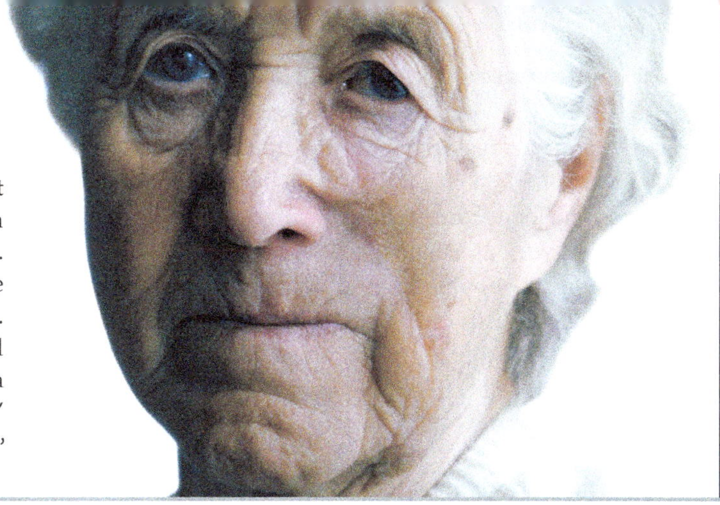

"Last month I underwent surgery for the removal of a skin lesion from my left arm. Unfortunately, I think the wound has become infected. The area is red, swollen, and painful and has a yellowish drainage."

—Patient "Katie Dennison"

Chapter 47
Antibiotics Affecting the Bacterial Cell Wall

Chapter Outline

- Structure of Bacterial Cell Walls
- Penicillins
  - Natural Penicillins
  - **PROTOTYPE** *Penicillin G, p. 821*
  - Broad-Spectrum Penicillins (Aminopenicillins)
  - **PROTOTYPE** *Ampicillin, p. 823*
  - Extended-Spectrum (Antipseudomonal) Penicillins
  - Penicillinase-Resistant (Antistaphylococcal) Penicillins
- Cephalosporins
  - **PROTOTYPE** *Cefazolin (Ancef), p. 826*
- Carbapenems
  - **PROTOTYPE** *Imipenem-Cilastatin (Primaxin), p. 829*
- Miscellaneous Cell Wall Inhibitors
  - **PROTOTYPE** *Vancomycin (Vancocin), p. 830*

Learning Outcomes

After reading this chapter, the student should be able to:

1. Explain the structure of a bacterial cell wall and its importance to pharmacotherapy.
2. Identify the classes of antibiotics that act by affecting the synthesis of the bacterial cell wall.
3. Explain the mechanisms by which antibiotics affect the bacterial cell wall.
4. Compare and contrast the four classes of penicillins.
5. Compare and contrast the five generations of cephalosporins.
6. Identify similarities and differences among drugs in the carbapenem class.
7. For each of the classes shown in the chapter outline, identify the prototype and representative drugs and explain the mechanism(s) of drug action, primary indications, contraindications, significant drug interactions, pregnancy data, and important adverse effects.
8. Apply clinical judgment to care for patients receiving pharmacotherapy with bacterial cell wall inhibitors.

Key Terms

Definitions of the terms in bold may be found in the Glossary.

The discovery and development of the first anti-infective drugs in the mid-1900s was a milestone in the field of medicine. Humans no longer die in massive numbers from infectious organisms such as *Yersinia pestis*, which killed 25% of the known human population in the 14th century due to the bubonic plague. This chapter examines the penicillins, cephalosporins, and other antibiotic drugs that kill bacteria by disrupting their cell walls.

Structure of Bacterial Cell Walls

47.1 Bacterial cell walls consist of layers of carbohydrate and protein chains, which are constructed by enzymes called penicillin-binding proteins.

The cell wall is a structure that sets people apart from the bacterial world. Humans do not have them, but all bacteria do. The osmotic pressure is so high within a bacterial cell that the cell would rupture without the containment of this rigid structure. The cell wall also serves as a barrier to substances that try to enter the cell, including antibiotics. Simply, it protects the bacterial cell from a hostile environment. The cell walls of gram-positive bacteria are very thick, whereas the walls of gram-negative bacteria are thinner. The structure of a bacterial cell wall is illustrated in Figure 47.1.

The primary material in a bacterial cell wall is peptidoglycan, a strong, repeating network of carbohydrate and protein chains that contains sugars bound to peptides. In gram-positive bacteria, peptidoglycan is laid down in repeated layers that are cross-linked to each other to provide greater stability to the wall. The layers may be compared to a fort that is built to provide protection from invaders. A single wall could be easily destroyed, but five or six repeated walls would provide almost impenetrable protection to those inside.

Because of the critical importance of their cell walls, bacteria spend a lot of time and energy building them. At least 30 different bacterial enzymes participate in their construction. Some of these enzymes are targets for penicillins and related antibiotics and are called **penicillin-binding proteins (PBPs)**. Most penicillins affect transpeptidase, which is the final PBP enzyme in the construction of the cell wall that adds the cross-links to the peptidoglycan layers. Without the cross-linking, the cell wall becomes weakened and bulges due to the high osmotic pressure inside the cell. The bacterial cell eventually lyses (ruptures). This process is illustrated in Figure 47.2. Because human cells do not possess cell walls, they do not have PBPs. Therefore, antibiotics that affect the cell wall have selective toxicity toward bacteria.

The PBPs are located on the outside of the plasma membrane of the bacterial cell. This location allows antibiotics to exert their bactericidal effect without actually entering the cell. Although all bacteria have a cell wall, the materials and PBPs used in their construction differ among species. Even slight structural changes to a PBP

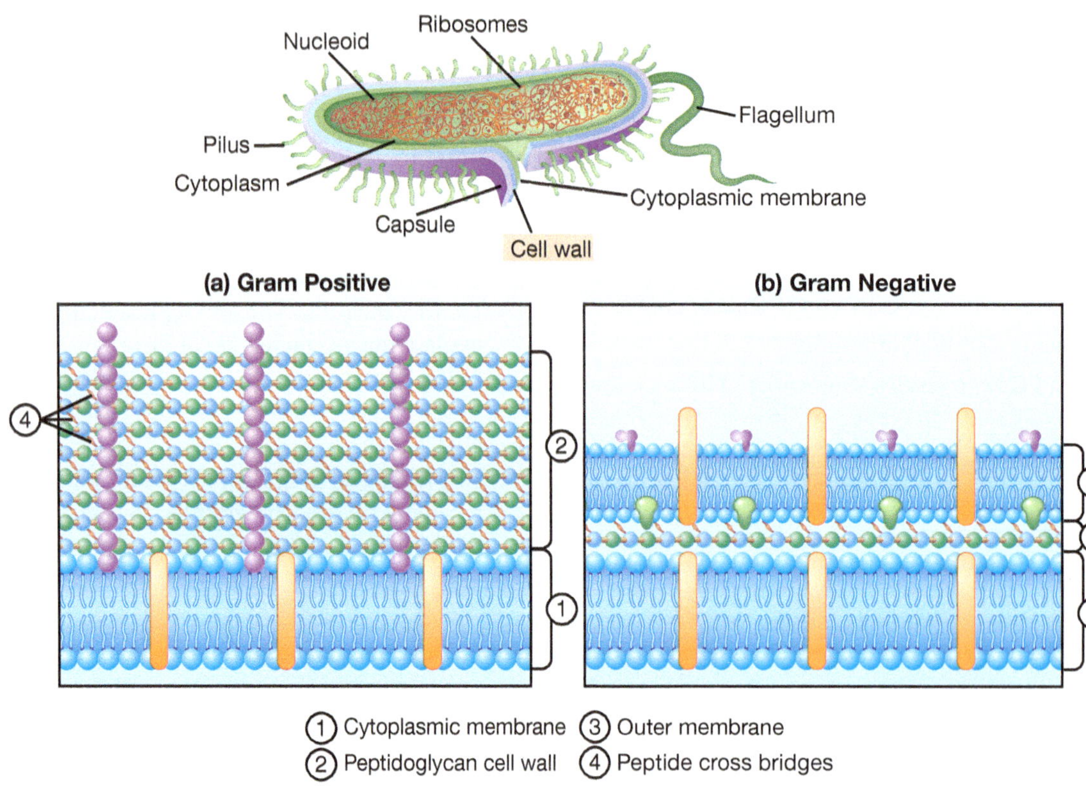

Figure 47.1 The bacterial cell wall: (a) gram-positive bacterium; (b) gram-negative bacterium.

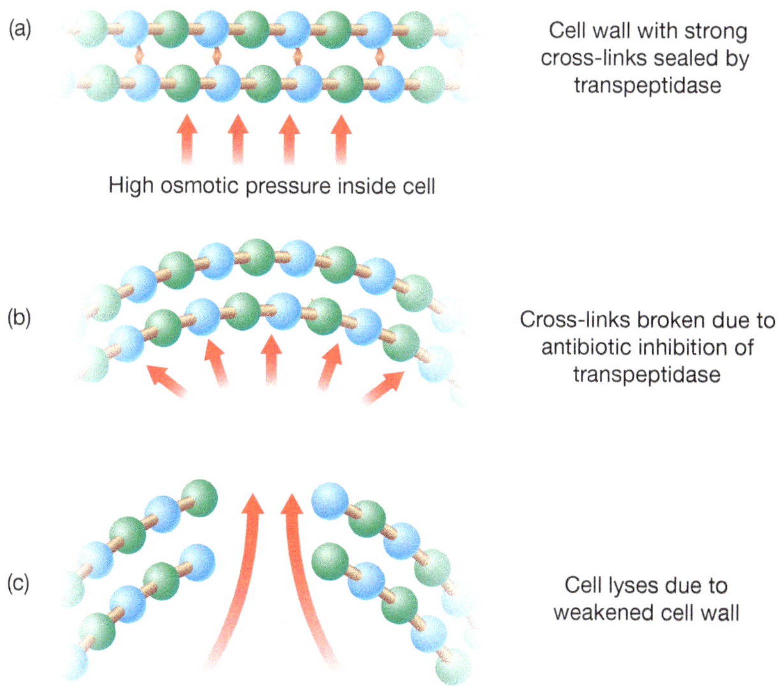

Figure 47.2 Mechanism of penicillin: (a) Bacterial cell wall strengthened by peptide cross-links. (b) Penicillin breaks cross-links. (c) Cell death due to weakened cell walls.

can cause lack of antibiotic binding to the enzyme. This explains why penicillins are not effective against all species of microorganisms. This also provides an explanation as to how an organism develops resistance to the penicillins.

Penicillins

47.2 The penicillins, one of the oldest and safest groups of antibacterials, are primarily active against gram-positive bacteria.

Although not the first anti-infective discovered, penicillin was the first mass-produced antibiotic. Discovered in cultures of the common fungus *Penicillium* in 1929, penicillin was first administered therapeutically in 1941. The medication quickly gathered a reputation as a miracle drug by preventing thousands of deaths from what are now considered minor infections. Penicillins are the most extensively studied of all the antibiotic classes. Doses of the penicillins are listed in Table 47.1.

Penicillins kill bacteria by disrupting their cell walls. The portion of the chemical structure of penicillin that is responsible for its antibacterial activity is called the **beta-lactam ring**. The beta-lactam ring resembles one of the chemical building blocks of peptidoglycan. When the PBP enzyme attempts to add the next "link" in the peptidoglycan chain, it binds to the beta-lactam ring, and construction of the cell wall is terminated. Other antibiotic classes that contain a beta-lactam ring include the cephalosporins, monobactams, and carbapenems, as shown in Figure 47.3. These classes are sometimes grouped together and referred to as beta-lactam antibiotics.

Table 47.1 Penicillins

Drug	Route and Adult Dose (Maximum Dose Where Indicated)	Adverse Effects
Natural Penicillins		
penicillin G benzathine (Bicillin LA)	IM: 1.2 million units as a single dose (max: 2.4 million units/day)	*Rash, pruritus, diarrhea, nausea, fever* Anaphylaxis symptoms including angioedema, circulatory collapse, and cardiac arrest; nephrotoxicity
penicillin G potassium	IM/IV: 2–24 million units divided q4–6h (max: 80 million units/day)	
penicillin G procaine	IM: 600,000–1.2 million units daily (max: 4.8 million units/day)	
penicillin V	PO: 125–250 mg qid (max: 7.2 g/day)	
Broad-Spectrum Penicillins (Aminopenicillins)		
amoxicillin (Amoxil)	PO: 250–500 mg tid (max: 1750 mg/day)	
amoxicillin-clavulanate (Augmentin)	PO: 250- or 500-mg tablet (each with 125 mg clavulanic acid) q8–12h	
ampicillin	PO/IV/IM: 250–500 mg q6h (max: 4 g/day PO or 14 g/day IV/IM)	
ampicillin and sulbactam (Unasyn)	IV/IM: 1.5–3 g q6h	
Extended-Spectrum (Antipseudomonal) Penicillins		
piperacillin	IM/IV: 2–4 g tid–qid (max: 24 g/day)	
piperacillin-tazobactam (Zosyn)	IV: 3.375 g qid over 30 min	
Penicillinase-Resistant (Antistaphylococcal) Penicillins		
dicloxacillin	PO: 125–500 mg qid (max: 4 g/day)	
nafcillin	IV/IM: 500 mg–1 g qid (max: 12 g/day)	
oxacillin	IV: 250–500 mg/kg/day q4–6h (max: 12 g/day)	

Note: *Italics* indicate common adverse effects. Underline indicates serious adverse effects.

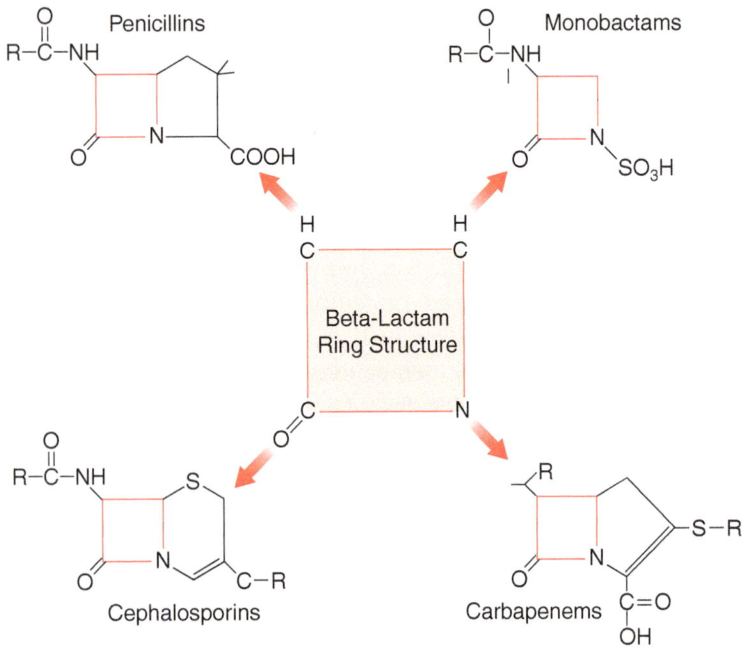

Figure 47.3 Beta-lactam antibiotics: The beta-lactam ring is common to many different classes of antibiotics.

Penicillin lyses the growing bacterial cells that are building cell walls; therefore, it is considered bactericidal. It has much less toxicity, however, on bacterial cells that have already constructed their cell walls. Like all infections, the body's immune defenses are needed to eliminate stable, slow-growing bacterial cells.

Because of their extensive use during the past 80 years, large numbers of resistant bacterial strains have emerged to limit the therapeutic usefulness of the penicillins. There are several mechanisms by which bacteria may become resistant to penicillins. Through mutations, the structures of PBPs have changed such that they no longer bind penicillin.

Another mechanism of resistance is that some bacteria secrete enzymes that split the beta-lactam ring, rendering the antibiotic ineffective. **Beta-lactamase** is the general term used for any of several enzymes produced by bacteria that can split the four-atom beta-lactam ring structure. The action of this enzyme is illustrated in Figure 47.4.

Scientists who first discovered this enzyme named it **penicillinase**, a name that is still frequently used in medicine. Although the terms are sometimes used interchangeably, it should be noted that penicillinase is only one specific type of beta-lactamase—one that splits the ring in penicillin antibiotics. Other forms of beta-lactamase exist that can inactivate cephalosporins, carbapenems, and other antibiotics with this ring structure. In this text, the term *penicillinase* is used when referring to this enzyme's action on penicillins; the term *beta-lactamase* is used when referring to other antibiotics. It should be understood, however, that these are two names for the same enzyme.

To overcome the killing effects of penicillin, some bacteria secrete larger amounts of penicillinase when exposed to antibiotics. In addition, the genes encoding for penicillinase can be transferred to other bacteria through conjugation, thus spreading the development of resistance genes.

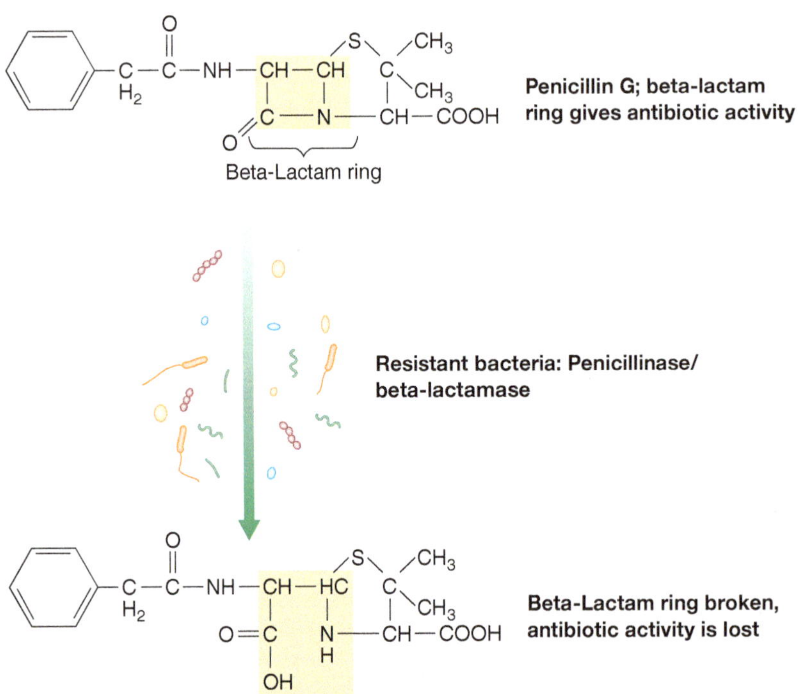

Figure 47.4 Action of penicillinase.

Although each drug in this class has certain unique properties, some generalizations may be made about the penicillins:

- Most are more effective against gram-positive bacteria, although a few have activity against gram-negative bacteria.
- Most have a narrow spectrum of antimicrobial activity.
- They are widely distributed to most body tissues, although only small amounts reach the cerebrospinal fluid (CSF).
- Nearly all are rapidly excreted by the kidneys.
- Most have short half-lives.

Allergic reactions are the most common adverse effects of the penicillins and ones that require careful attention by nurses. The overall incidence of penicillin allergy ranges from 0.7 to 10%. Symptoms range from mild rash and nausea to fever or anaphylaxis. Although the incidence of anaphylaxis is low, from 0.04 to 2%, mortality is high; nurses must take every precaution to identify patients at highest risk. Allergic reactions may occur within minutes after taking the drug, or they may be delayed for several days or weeks.

Prior exposure to penicillin is necessary for an allergic reaction, although this exposure may have occurred inadvertently through exposure to mold or by eating animal products that contain small amounts of penicillin. Allergy to one penicillin increases the risk of allergy to other drugs in this class. There is also a degree of cross hypersensitivity between penicillins and cephalosporins. The nurse should not give penicillin to a patient who has a medical history of serious penicillin allergy. If penicillin must be given due to a patient's condition, and it is unknown if the patient is allergic, skin tests may be used to assess the risk of experiencing a severe allergic reaction. Giving a small amount of penicillin and waiting to see if anaphylaxis develops is not an acceptable method for assessing the probability of allergy. The size of a dose is not related to the severity of the response because even very small amounts can elicit anaphylaxis in susceptible patients. Nurses must always be vigilant in observing for signs of allergy following penicillin administration because there is no infallible method for predicting which patient will experience an allergy to the drug.

Chemical modifications to the original molecule have produced drugs that offer several advantages over the natural penicillins, including the following:

- Penicillinase resistance
- Broader antimicrobial spectrum
- Extended spectrum.

Natural Penicillins

The natural penicillins were the first to be isolated from the fungus *Penicillium*. They are inexpensive and the preferred drugs for susceptible infections.

PROTOTYPE DRUG Penicillin G

Classification **Therapeutic:** Antibacterial
Pharmacologic: Cell wall inhibitor, natural penicillin

Therapeutic Effects and Uses: Approved by the FDA in 1943, penicillin G has a narrow spectrum of activity that includes most gram-positive bacteria. Many gram-negative organisms are resistant to penicillin G. It is a preferred drug for the treatment of infections shown to be susceptible by culture and sensitivity (C&S) testing because it is inexpensive and exhibits few adverse effects. These include susceptible strains of *Staphylococcus*, *Streptococcus*, *Neisseria*, *Actinomyces*, *Bacillus anthracis*, *Clostridium*, *Treponema*, and *Corynebacterium*. Penicillin is given for the prophylaxis of bacterial endocarditis in patients with prosthetic heart valves or congenital heart disease and for those at risk for recurrent bouts of rheumatic fever.

Penicillin G is available as a benzathine, potassium, or a procaine salt; each has slightly different pharmacokinetics. For example, while the intramuscular (IM) administration of penicillin G potassium is rapid, the benzathine and procaine salts are absorbed from an IM site very slowly, over a 24-hour period. However, there is no difference in effectiveness among the three salts because they all dissociate to penicillin G. Penicillin G benzathine CR and penicillin G procaine are administered IM; penicillin G potassium may be administered by either the intravenous (IV) or IM route. Penicillin G potassium was once available by the oral (PO) route, but the drug had low bioavailability due to destruction by gastric acid. Penicillin V and amoxicillin are more stable in acid and are used when oral penicillin therapy is desired.

Mechanism of Action: This drug inhibits bacterial wall synthesis by binding PBPs. Penicillin G is bactericidal and destroyed by penicillinase.

Pharmacokinetics:

Route(s)	IM, IV
Absorption	Rapid absorption (IM)
Distribution	Widely distributed; only small amounts cross the blood–brain barrier; secreted in breast milk; approximately 60% bound to plasma proteins
Primary metabolism	15–30% metabolized, primarily hepatic
Primary excretion	Renal
Onset of action	IM: 15–30 min; IV: immediate
Duration of action	4–6 h; half-life: 20–60 min

Adverse Effects: Penicillin G is well tolerated by most patients and adverse effects are uncommon. Urticaria and delayed skin reactions occasionally occur. The most serious adverse effect is severe hypersensitivity reaction. The anaphylactic response may include cardiovascular collapse; edema of the mouth, tongue, pharynx, and larynx; confusion; seizures; and hallucinations. While most allergic reactions to penicillin occur within minutes after administration, late hypersensitivity reactions may occur several weeks into the regimen.

Contraindications/Precautions: Penicillin G is contraindicated in patients who are allergic to any drug in the penicillin class and is used cautiously in those with hypersensitivity to cephalosporins. In cases where penicillin G is the only effective antibiotic in a patient with a known allergy to the drug, penicillin may be given via a desensitization procedure whereby the dose begins very small and gradually increases. Because 90% of a dose of penicillin G is excreted unchanged by the kidneys through tubular secretion, patients with chronic kidney disease (CKD) must be carefully monitored. Patients with heart failure should not receive the penicillin sodium salt. Hyperkalemia may result with high doses of the penicillin G potassium salt.

Drug Interactions: Penicillin G may decrease the effectiveness of oral contraceptives. Colestipol will decrease the absorption of penicillin. Probenecid decreases the excretion of penicillin G and can lead to antibiotic toxicity. Potassium-sparing diuretics such as spironolactone may cause hyperkalemia when administered with penicillin G potassium. Because penicillins can antagonize the actions of aminoglycoside antibiotics, drugs from these two classes are not administered concurrently. The bacteriostatic action of tetracyclines may inhibit the bactericidal action of penicillin G. **Herbal/Food:** Willow bark and rose hips may decrease the renal clearance of the penicillins.

Pregnancy: Animal reproduction studies and widespread human use of penicillin have not shown significant evidence of adverse effects to the fetus or breastfed neonate. The breastfed infant should be observed for signs of diarrhea, skin rash, and candidiasis.

Treatment of Overdose: No specific therapy is available. Patients are treated symptomatically.

Clinician Responsibilities: Key clinical implications for patients receiving penicillin G are included in Applied Clinical Judgment: Patients Receiving Pharmacotherapy with a Penicillin, Cephalosporin, or Vancomycin Antibiotic.

Drugs Similar to Penicillin G

Other natural penicillins include penicillin G benzathine, penicillin G procaine, and penicillin V. These salts carry the same pregnancy and lactation information as penicillin G.

Penicillin G benzathine (Bicillin LA): Administered only by deep IM injection, penicillin G benzathine is absorbed very slowly, resulting in low peak serum levels with a prolonged duration of action that can last up to 26 days. Neurologic adverse effects have been reported with penicillin G benzathine, including severe agitation, confusion, hallucinations, and seizures. Injections of this drug are painful and injection-site reactions may occur. Permanent neurologic damage occurs if this drug is injected near a nerve. The drug carries a black box warning that it must not be given IV. Bicillin CA consists of a combination of penicillin G benzathine and penicillin G procaine. Both of these salts dissociate to form penicillin G; thus, they share the same actions, indications and adverse effects.

Penicillin G procaine: Approved in 1943, penicillin G procaine is a repository form of penicillin given only by the IM route. Like the benzathine salt, it is absorbed slowly from its injection site and has a prolonged duration of action (15 to 20 hours). It shares the same actions, indications, and adverse effects as penicillin G. The procaine salt is less painful on administration than penicillin G administered by the IM route. Penicillin G procaine can cause neurotoxicity if the drug is unintentionally injected near a nerve. Like the benzathine salt, neurologic adverse effects can occur with penicillin G procaine, including severe agitation, confusion, hallucinations, and seizures. Patients with allergies to the local anesthetic procaine should not receive this drug.

Penicillin V: Penicillin V is nearly identical to penicillin G, except that it is more acid stable, which allows it to be administered PO. However, it should be taken on an empty stomach to maximize absorption. Approved in 1956, it shares the same actions, indications, and adverse effects as penicillin G. Some patients experience nausea and vomiting and diarrhea.

CONNECTION Checkpoint 47.1

From what you learned in Chapter 5, explain how taking a thorough medical history can eliminate some allergic reactions to antibiotics.

Broad-Spectrum Penicillins (Aminopenicillins)

A major limitation of the natural penicillins is their lack of activity against gram-negative organisms. The aminopenicillins, amoxicillin and ampicillin, are effective against gram-positive and certain gram-negative bacilli such as *Haemophilus influenzae, Escherichia coli, Salmonella,* and *Shigella.* This distinction is responsible for them being placed into a separate class called broad-spectrum penicillins.

Aminopenicillins are rapidly inactivated by penicillinase, which limits their therapeutic usefulness, particularly against *Staphylococcus aureus* infections. Despite this limitation, the aminopenicillins are some of the most widely prescribed antibiotics for sinus and upper respiratory and genitourinary tract infections. Their widespread use over many decades has resulted in the emergence of a large number of resistant strains.

Combination drugs have been developed that offer certain advantages over single-drug therapy with aminopenicillins. The fixed-dose combination of Augmentin combines amoxicillin with clavulanate, a beta-lactamase (penicillinase) inhibitor. Another fixed-dose product, Unasyn, contains ampicillin and the beta-lactamase inhibitor sulbactam. By inhibiting penicillinase, these combined drugs allow a greater percentage of the aminopenicillin molecules to reach pathogens and disrupt cell wall synthesis. The beta-lactamase inhibitors are ineffective when used alone and therefore are always used in fixed combination formulations with other drugs.

PROTOTYPE DRUG Ampicillin

Classification **Therapeutic:** Antibacterial
Pharmacologic: Cell wall inhibitor, aminopenicillin

Therapeutic Effects and Uses: Approved in 1963, the actions of ampicillin are similar to those of penicillin G except that ampicillin has a broader spectrum that includes enhanced activity over enterococci, *E. coli*, *Proteus mirabilis*, *Neisseria gonorrhoeae*, *H. influenzae*, *Salmonella*, *Shigella*, and *Bordetella pertussis*. Because a large percentage of resistant strains have developed, ampicillin is no longer a preferred drug for the treatment of gonococcal infections, childhood meningitis, or *Salmonella* or *Shigella* enteritis.

Mechanism of Action: Ampicillin inhibits bacterial wall synthesis by binding PBPs. This drug is bactericidal and inactivated by penicillinase.

Pharmacokinetics:

Route(s)	PO, IM, IV
Absorption	50% absorbed PO
Distribution	Widely distributed; only small amounts cross the blood–brain barrier; secreted in breast milk; plasma protein binding is about 15–20%
Primary metabolism	Largely unmetabolized, 10% hepatic
Primary excretion	Renal
Onset of action	PO: 30–60 min; IM: 15–30 min
Duration of action	Half-life: 1–2 h

Adverse Effects: Ampicillin is a safe drug that rarely produces serious adverse effects. Rash and diarrhea are the most common adverse effects, and diarrhea occurs more frequently with ampicillin than with other aminopenicillins. Pain at the injection site is common. Like all penicillins, anaphylaxis is rare, though potentially fatal. Anaphylactic response may include cardiovascular collapse; edema of the mouth, tongue, pharynx, and larynx; confusion; seizure; and hallucinations. Pseudomembranous colitis (PMC) is an additional rare, though serious, severe adverse effect.

Contraindications/Precautions: Ampicillin is contraindicated in patients who are allergic to any drug in the penicillin class and used cautiously in those with hypersensitivity to cephalosporins. Ampicillin is excreted primarily by the kidneys; therefore, drug therapy must be monitored carefully in patients with CKD.

Drug Interactions: Ampicillin may decrease the effectiveness of oral contraceptives. Probenecid (Probalan) decreases the excretion of ampicillin and can lead to antibiotic toxicity. Penicillins can antagonize the actions of aminoglycoside antibiotics and must be administered at least 2 hours apart. The antibacterial actions of ampicillin are diminished when it is taken concurrently with chloramphenicol, erythromycin, or tetracyclines. **Herbal/Food:** Because food decreases its absorption, ampicillin should be taken on an empty stomach.

Pregnancy: Animal reproduction studies and widespread human use of ampicillin and amoxicillin have not shown significant evidence of adverse effects to the fetus or breastfed neonate. The breastfed infant should be observed for signs of diarrhea, skin rash, and candidiasis.

Treatment of Overdose: No specific therapy is available. Patients are treated symptomatically.

Clinician Responsibilities: Key clinical implications for patients receiving ampicillin are included in Applied Clinical Judgment: Patients Receiving Pharmacotherapy with a Penicillin, Cephalosporin, or Vancomycin Antibiotic.

Drugs Similar to Ampicillin

The only other aminopenicillin is amoxicillin.

Amoxicillin (Amoxil): Approved in 1974, amoxicillin is closely related structurally to ampicillin and has many of the same characteristics. The drug is destroyed by penicillinase-producing organisms. It is more acid stable than ampicillin and offers greater gastrointestinal (GI) absorption with peak serum levels twice as high. It exhibits a lower incidence of diarrhea than ampicillin. Amoxicillin has largely replaced ampicillin, and it is one of the most frequently prescribed antibiotics. Amoxicillin should not be administered to patients with hypersensitivity to any penicillin.

Extended-Spectrum (Antipseudomonal) Penicillins

The only remaining drug in this class, piperacillin, has a broad spectrum of antimicrobial activity similar to that of the aminopenicillins. Its primary advantage is its additional activity against *Pseudomonas aeruginosa*, thus it is called an extended-spectrum or antipseudomonal penicillin. Two other drugs in this class, carbenicillin and ticarcillin, are no longer available in the United States.

P. aeruginosa is an opportunistic pathogen found in air, soil, and water. It can persist on environmental surfaces such as soap residues and hot tubs and can even survive in some antiseptic solutions. *P. aeruginosa* infections may occur anywhere in the body, primarily causing disease in patients whose health is already compromised in some manner. It is responsible for about 10% of all healthcare-associated infections, including serious pneumonia in debilitated patients and a large number of infections in wounds and in patients with extensive burns.

P. aeruginosa has natural resistance to most antibiotics due in part to its ability to rapidly pump out antibiotic molecules that enter its cells. Because *Pseudomonas* infections are often persistent, aggressive combination anti-infective therapy is often indicated. A typical combination includes an aminoglycoside antibiotic with an antipseudomonal penicillin. Because penicillins inactivate aminoglycosides, they must be administered at least 2 hours apart. Other antibiotics such as a cephalosporin or carbapenem may be needed.

Approved in 1981, piperacillin has one of the broadest spectrums of any of the penicillins and is effective against most gram-negative and many gram-positive anaerobic and aerobic microbes. It has been used to treat a variety of serious infections, including those of the skin, blood, sinuses, central nervous system (CNS), respiratory tract, and genitourinary tract. Available by the IM and IV routes, piperacillin is often used in combination with an aminoglycoside antibiotic because together they exert synergistic action on gram-negative microbes. Because penicillinase-producing bacteria are resistant to piperacillin, it is combined with a beta-lactamase inhibitor. Zosyn is a fixed-dose combination with the beta-lactamase inhibitor.

Rash and diarrhea are the most common adverse effects of piperacillin. Electrolytes should be regularly monitored to prevent hypokalemia and hypernatremia. Because this medication can prolong bleeding time, caution must be used when given concurrently with coagulation modifiers. Very high doses may produce confusion and seizures. Localized injection-site reactions include pain, inflammation, phlebitis, and hematomas. Animal studies showed increased numbers of stillbirths with Zosyn, although evidence is insufficient to confirm fetal harm in humans. The breastfed infant should be observed for signs of diarrhea, skin rash, and candidiasis

Penicillinase-Resistant (Antistaphylococcal) Penicillins

This subclass of penicillins includes dicloxacillin, nafcillin, and oxacillin, which are drugs that are effective against penicillinase-producing bacteria. These medications are less effective than penicillin G against non-penicillinase-producing strains and are ineffective against gram-negative bacteria. This narrow spectrum of activity has largely restricted their use to penicillinase-producing strains of *Staphylococcus*. Because they are often the preferred drugs for infections by this organism, they are referred to as antistaphylococcal penicillins. An older drug in this class, cloxacillin (Cloxapen), is no longer marketed in the United States.

The emergence of many methicillin-resistant *S. aureus* (MRSA) strains has severely limited the use of drugs in this class. As discussed in Chapter 46, some MRSA strains are resistant to all penicillins. The first drug developed in the penicillinase-resistant class, called methicillin, was removed from the U.S. market for producing an unacceptable incidence of interstitial nephritis.

Drugs in the penicillinase-resistant class share similar actions and properties with penicillin G. Dicloxacillin is readily absorbed by the PO route, whereas nafcillin and oxacillin are given parenterally. They are rapidly excreted by the kidneys, having a half-life of 30 to 60 minutes. As with all penicillins, hypersensitivity reactions may occur. Some of these drugs are sodium salts, which may cause sodium overload in susceptible patients. PMC has been reported in a small number of patients taking these drugs. Animal reproduction studies and widespread human use of these drugs have not shown evidence of adverse effects to the fetus or breastfed neonate. The breastfed infant should be observed for signs of diarrhea, skin rash, and candidiasis.

Dicloxacillin: Approved in 1968, dicloxacillin is the only penicillinase-resistant penicillin available by the PO route. As with other drugs in this class, its use is primarily limited to the treatment of susceptible staphylococcal infections. It is not effective against MRSA. Nausea and vomiting are commonly reported adverse effects. It should be taken on an empty stomach to enhance absorption. Other adverse effects and contraindications are the same as those of other penicillins. This drug should not be given to a patient with hypersensitivity to any penicillin.

Nafcillin: Approved in 1964, nafcillin is used to treat susceptible infections of the blood, skin, upper and lower respiratory tract, bone and joints, and urinary tract. It is ineffective against MRSA infections. Unlike most penicillins, nafcillin is excreted primarily in the bile; thus, dosage adjustments for patients with hepatic disease are necessary. Because only 10 to 20% of the drug is absorbed when given PO, it is given parenterally. The complete blood count (CBC) must be regularly monitored because nafcillin can cause neutropenia and other blood abnormalities in 10 to 20% of the patients taking it. This drug should not be given to a patient with hypersensitivity to any penicillin.

Oxacillin: Approved in 1962, oxacillin is used to treat a variety of staphylococcal infections of the blood, skin, upper

CONNECTIONS: Using Research in Practice

Environmental Presence of Antibiotics

Recent attention has been focused on the use of antibiotics in the feed of animals raised for consumption, including cattle, pork, and poultry. To maintain a healthy animal, antibiotics may be added to their food source to deter the development of infections. These antibiotics may then be present in the meat itself and may factor into the development of antibiotic resistance in humans.

An overlooked or underappreciated source for antibiotics in the environment is the potential for antibiotics, antibiotic-resistant bacteria (ARBs), or antibiotic-resistant genes (ARGs) to enter the water system through groundwater or sewage treatment facilities. Water runoff from medical facilities, livestock farming and aquaculture, landfills, sewage, and wastewater treatment plants may be a source of antibiotics, ARBs, and ARGs. Zainab and colleagues (2020) found that the antibiotics ciprofloxacin, sulfamethoxazole, erythromycin, and tetracycline were found in groundwater, with sulfonamide and tetracycline ARGs being more prevalent than other antibiotics..

It is difficult to predict the exact risk to humans posed by the presence of antibiotics in groundwater and drinking sources, and the actual risk appears to be very low (Sharma et al., 2019). Judicious use of these drugs and using point-of-care testing to determine the appropriate drug to treat the infection may delay the development of ARBs and ARGs and is a wise strategy to prevent future infections that can't be treated successfully.

and lower respiratory tract, bone and joints, and urinary tract. It is ineffective against MRSA infections. Because oxacillin causes fewer injection-site reactions than nafcillin, it is sometimes the preferred parenteral drug for susceptible strains. Indications and adverse effects are similar to those of other penicillinase-resistant penicillins. This drug should not be given to a patient with hypersensitivity to any penicillin.

Cephalosporins

47.3 The cephalosporins are similar in structure and function to the penicillins and are widely prescribed for gram-negative infections.

Isolated shortly after penicillin, the cephalosporins comprise the largest antibiotic class. Like the penicillins, many cephalosporins contain a beta-lactam ring that is responsible for their antimicrobial activity. In some cephalosporins, the structure of the beta-lactam ring is quite stable and resistant to enzyme destruction. The cephalosporins are bactericidal and inhibit cell wall synthesis by binding to PBPs. Growing bacterial cells are unable to build their cell walls properly, and lysis occurs in the same manner as penicillins. The cephalosporins are listed in Table 47.2.

The primary therapeutic use of the cephalosporins is for gram-negative infections and for patients who are allergic to penicillin or who have penicillin-resistant infections. Over 20 cephalosporins are available, all having similar-sounding names that can challenge even the best memory. Selection of a specific cephalosporin is first based on the sensitivity of the pathogen and, second, on possible adverse effects.

The cephalosporins are classified chronologically by their generations, which are loosely based on differences in their spectrums of microbial activity. It is important to note that the placement of a drug in a particular generation is somewhat arbitrary and has little therapeutic usefulness. Drugs within each generation have different chemical structures, routes of administration, and spectrums of activity. Scientists do not always agree on placement.

CONNECTION Checkpoint 47.2

From what you learned in Chapter 46, what is the primary difference in physiology that distinguishes a gram-positive organism from a gram-negative organism?

Over decades of use, many bacterial strains have developed resistance to the cephalosporins. Like the penicillins, the primary mechanism of resistance is the secretion of beta-lactamase enzymes (sometimes called cephalosporinases). Although third-generation drugs were initially unaffected by beta-lactamase, resistant strains that can inactivate medications in this generation have been identified. None of the cephalosporins has significant activity against MRSA or penicillin-resistant *Streptococcus pneumoniae.*

In general, the cephalosporins are safe drugs with adverse effects similar to those of the penicillins. Allergic reactions are the most common adverse effect. Although sometimes prescribed for patients who are allergic to penicillin, nurses must be aware that 5 to 10% of the patients who are allergic to penicillin will also exhibit hypersensitivity to cephalosporins. Despite this small incidence of cross-allergy, the cephalosporins offer a reasonable alternative for patients who are unable to take penicillin. Cephalosporins are contraindicated, however, for patients who have experienced anaphylaxis following penicillin exposure.

In addition to allergy, rash and GI complaints are common adverse effects of cephalosporins. Nurses should continually assess for the presence of superinfections. Because cephalosporins are secreted in small amounts in breast milk, they should be used with caution in nursing mothers.

Nearly all cephalosporins are eliminated by the kidneys. Earlier-generation cephalosporins exhibited kidney toxicity but this is diminished with the later-generation drugs in this class. Patients with CKD or those who are concurrently receiving nephrotoxic drugs should be monitored

Table 47.2 Cephalosporins

Drug	Route and Adult Dose (Maximum Dose Where Indicated)	Adverse Effects
First Generation		
cefadroxil	PO: 500 mg–1 g once or twice a day (max: 2 g/day)	*Diarrhea, abdominal cramping, nausea, fatigue, rash, pruritus, pain at injection site, oral or vaginal candidiasis* PMC, nephrotoxicity, anaphylaxis
cefazolin (Ancef)	IM/IV: 250 mg–2 g tid (max: 12 g/day)	
cephalexin (Keflex)	PO: 250–500 mg qid (max: 4 g/day)	
Second Generation		
cefaclor	PO: 250–500 mg tid (max: 2 g/day)	
cefotetan (Cefotan)	IV/IM: 1–2 g q12h (max: 6 g/day)	
cefoxitin	IV/IM: 1–2 g q6–8h (max: 12 g/day)	
cefuroxime (Zinacef)	PO (Ceftin): 250–500 mg bid (max: 1 g/day) IM/IV (Zinacef): 750 mg–1.5 g q8h (max: 9 g/day)	
Third Generation		
cefdinir	PO: 300 mg bid (max: 600 mg/day)	
cefixime (Suprax)	PO: 400 mg/day or 200 mg bid (max: 800 mg/day)	
cefotaxime	IM: 1–2 g bid–tid (max: 12 g/day)	
cefpodoxime	PO: 200 mg q12h for 10 days (max: 800 mg/day)	
ceftazidime (Fortaz, Tazicef) ceftazidime-avibactam (Avycaz)	IV/IM: 1–2 mg q8–12h (max: 6 g/day) IV (Avycaz): 2.5 g infused over 2 hr tid (2.0 g ceftazidime, 0.5 g avibactam)	
ceftriaxone	IV/IM: 1–2 g/day in a single or divided dose (max: 4 g/day)	
Fourth and Fifth Generation		
cefepime (Maxipime)	IV/IM: 0.5–1 g q12h for 7–10 days (max: 6 g/day)	
cefiderocol (Fetroja)	IV: 2g tid	
ceftaroline (Teflaro)	IV: 600 mg q12h for 5–14 days	
ceftolozane-tazobactam (Zerbaxa)	IV: 1.5 g q8h	

Note: *Italics* indicate common adverse effects. Underline indicates serious adverse effects.

carefully during therapy with any cephalosporin. Kidney function tests should be evaluated on a regular basis.

Other adverse effects are specific to particular cephalosporins. For example, cefotetan interferes with vitamin K metabolism and increases the risk of bleeding due to hypoprothrombinemia. Nurses must carefully monitor prothrombin time in patients taking these drugs, particularly those who are concurrently taking anticoagulants. Cefotetan produces a disulfiram-like reaction when taken concurrently with alcohol. Cephalosporins cause pain at IM injection sites, and thrombophlebitis can occur when given IV. Over half of the cephalosporins are administered only by the parenteral route.

PROTOTYPE DRUG Cefazolin (Ancef)

Classification **Therapeutic:** Antibacterial
Pharmacologic: Cell wall inhibitor, first-generation cephalosporin

Therapeutic Effects and Uses: Approved in 1973, cefazolin is a beta-lactam antibiotic used for the treatment and prophylaxis of bacterial infections, particularly those that are caused by susceptible gram-positive organisms. Its effectiveness extends to non-penicillinase-producing and penicillinase-producing *S. aureus* and streptococci (except enterococci). Cefazolin is not effective against MRSA. Cefazolin has been used to treat infections of the respiratory tract, urinary tract, skin structures, biliary tract, bones, and joints. It has also been useful in the pharmacotherapy of genital infections, septicemia, and endocarditis. This drug is sometimes used for infection prophylaxis in patients who are undergoing surgical procedures. Cefazolin has a longer half-life than other first-generation cephalosporins, which allows for less frequent dosing. It is one of the most frequently prescribed parenteral antibiotics.

Mechanism of Action: Cefazolin inhibits bacterial wall synthesis by binding to specific PBPs. The drug is bactericidal, exhibits a broad spectrum, and is sensitive to beta-lactamase.

Pharmacokinetics:

Route(s)	IM, IV
Absorption	Well absorbed when given IM
Distribution	Widely distributed; only small amounts cross the blood–brain barrier; crosses the placenta; secreted in breast milk; about 85% bound to plasma protein

Primary metabolism	Not metabolized
Primary excretion	Renal
Onset of action	Immediate
Duration of action	Half-life: 90–135 min

Adverse Effects: Like the penicillins, the cephalosporins are well tolerated by most patients. Rash and diarrhea are the most common adverse effects, and superinfections are likely when the antibiotic is used for prolonged periods. Approximately 1 to 4% of patients will experience some kind of an allergic reaction. Severe hypersensitivity reactions are rare, though potentially fatal. Anaphylactic response may include cardiovascular collapse; edema of the mouth, tongue, pharynx, and larynx; confusion; seizures; and hallucinations. Pain and phlebitis can occur at IM injection sites. However, cefazolin causes less pain than do other cephalosporins. Seizures are a rare, though potentially serious, adverse effect of cephalosporin therapy.

Contraindications/Precautions: Cefazolin is contraindicated in patients who are allergic to any drug in the cephalosporin class and is used cautiously in those with hypersensitivity to penicillins. Because most cefazolin is excreted unchanged by the kidneys, patients with CKD must be carefully monitored.

Drug Interactions: Cefazolin decreases the effectiveness of estrogen-progestin oral contraceptives potentially resulting in contraceptive failure. Concurrent use of cefazolin with nephrotoxic drugs, such as aminoglycosides or vancomycin, increases the risk of nephrotoxicity. Cefazolin may have additive or synergistic antimicrobial action with other antibiotics such as aztreonam, carbapenems, and the penicillins. The anticoagulant effect of warfarin and heparin may be increased if given concurrently with cefazolin. **Herbal/Food:** None known.

Pregnancy: Animal studies showed no evidence of teratogenicity. Because the drug is secreted in human milk, caution should be used if breastfeeding.

Treatment of Overdose: No specific therapy is available. Patients are treated symptomatically.

Clinician Responsibilities (includes all generations of cephalosporins): Key clinical implications for patients receiving cefazolin are included in the Applied Clinical Judgment: Patients Receiving Pharmacotherapy with a Penicillin, Cephalosporin, or Vancomycin Antibiotic.

Drugs Similar to Cefazolin (Ancef)

First generation: First-generation cephalosporins contain a beta-lactam ring; bacteria that produce beta-lactamase are usually resistant to these drugs. They are the most effective cephalosporins against gram-positive bacteria, including staphylococci and streptococci, and are sometimes the preferred drugs for these organisms. First-generation cephalosporins have only moderate activity against gram-negative bacteria. First-generation drugs do not cross the blood–brain barrier to any appreciable extent.

In addition to cefazolin, other first-generation cephalosporins include cefadroxil and cephalexin (Keflex). These drugs are administered parenterally and have the same spectrum of microbial activity. They have the same basic indications (primarily gram-positive bacteria) and are eliminated by the kidneys.

Second generation: Second-generation cephalosporins exhibit a broader spectrum against gram-negative organisms than do the first-generation drugs. They are more potent and less sensitive to beta-lactamase than the first-generation drugs. Like the first-generation cephalosporins, however, they are unable to enter the CSF in sufficient concentration to treat infections of the CNS. In general, the second-generation drugs have largely been replaced by third-generation cephalosporins.

Second-generation cephalosporins include cefaclor, cefotetan (Cefotan), cefoxitin, and cefuroxime (Zinacef). All have the same spectrum of microbial activity and there is little difference among the drugs other than the route of administration (see Table 47.2). The kidneys eliminate all second-generation cephalosporins. Cefoxitin and cefotetan are the most active against *Bacteroides fragilis*.

Third generation: Third-generation cephalosporins exhibit an even broader spectrum against gram-negative bacteria than the second-generation group. They generally have a longer duration of action and are resistant to beta-lactamase. These cephalosporins are sometimes the preferred drugs against infections by *Pseudomonas*, *Klebsiella*, *Neisseria*, *Salmonella*, *Proteus*, and *H. influenzae*. Third-generation drugs are able to enter the CSF to treat CNS infections.

Third-generation cephalosporins are the largest group and include cefdinir, cefixime (Suprax), cefotaxime, cefpodoxime, ceftazidime (Fortaz, Tazicef), and ceftriaxone. The differences among third-generation cephalosporins are minor. Some are available by the PO route, whereas others are given only parenterally (see Table 47.2). Cefixime and ceftriaxone have longer durations that allow for once-daily dosing. Ceftazidime is one of the few third-generation drugs with significant activity against *P. aeruginosa*. Cefotaxime is a preferred drug for certain types of meningitis and for infection prophylaxis in patients who are undergoing surgical procedures.

In 2015, Avycaz, a combination of ceftazidime and avibactam (a beta-lactamase inhibitor), was approved to treat complicated intra-abdominal infections, complicated urinary tract infections (UTIs), and hospital-acquired bacterial pneumonia. Given IV, Avycaz is reserved for infections proven to be susceptible to the drug to reduce the development of resistant strains.

Fourth generation: Cefepime (Maxipime) is the only drug in this generation. It is very similar to third-generation drugs but has a slightly broader spectrum of activity and is more stable against organisms that produce beta-lactamase. It has been used for the treatment of serious infections in hospitalized patients with gram-positive microorganisms such as Enterobacteriaceae and *Pseudomonas*. It is capable of entering the CSF in sufficiently high concentrations to treat CNS infections, but it is not effective against MRSA.

Fifth generation: Fifth-generation cephalosporins are broad-spectrum drugs with extended gram-positive effectiveness. They are designed to be effective against MRSA infections. Ceftaroline (Teflaro), the first drug in this generation, was approved by the FDA in 2010 for acute bacterial skin and skin structure infections and community-acquired bacterial pneumonia. It is effective against a broad spectrum of both gram-positive and gram-negative organisms, including MRSA. Available by the IV route, it is relatively safe, with the most common adverse effects being diarrhea, nausea, and rash. Ceftolozane is a combination drug with tazobactam (Zerbaxa) for the treatment of complicated intra-abdominal infections, hospital-acquired pneumonia, and complicated UTIs.

In 2020, cefiderocol (Fetroja) was approved by the FDA to treat complicated UTIs. While not considered the first of a new generation of cephalosporins, it acts by a novel mechanism that may result in its use in treating infections resistant to many other antibiotics. Cefiderocol was manufactured to contain an attached molecule called a **siderophore** that scavenges soluble iron from the surrounding environment. Why is this important? Bacteria need iron to survive and they produce their own siderophores to gather iron. Once the bacterial siderophore finds iron, it transports it into the bacterial cell. When the cefiderocol siderophore finds iron, the pathogen is "fooled" into transporting the *antibiotic* into the bacterial cell. The cephalosporin then kills the bacteria. The indications for cefiderocol are limited but it is likely this novel approach will be used for the development of other siderophore-containing antibiotics.

Carbapenems

47.4 The carbapenems are resistant to beta-lactamase and are broad-spectrum alternatives to penicillin.

Although the penicillins and cephalosporins comprise the largest groups of drugs affecting the bacterial cell wall, several other antibacterials also act by this mechanism. Doses of these drugs are listed in Table 47.3.

Table 47.3 Carbapenems and Miscellaneous Cell Wall Inhibitors

Drug	Route and Adult Dose (Maximum Dose Where Indicated)	Adverse Effects
Carbapenems		
ertapenem (Invanz)	IV/IM: 1 g/day	*Nausea, diarrhea, headache*
imipenem-cilastatin (Primaxin)	IV: 250–500 mg tid–qid (max: 4 g/day)	Anaphylaxis, superinfections, PMC, confusion, seizures
meropenem (Merrem)	IV: 1–2 g tid (max: 2 g tid)	
Miscellaneous Cell Wall Inhibitors		
aztreonam (Azactam, Cayston)	IM (Azactam): 0.5–2 g bid–qid (max: 8 g/day) Inhalation (Cayston): one vial in nebulizer tid for 28 days	*Nausea and vomiting, rash, thrombophlebitis (Azactam); cough, nasal congestion, wheezing (Cayston)* Anaphylaxis, superinfections, bronchospasm (Cayston)
bacitracin	Topical: Apply thin layer of ointment bid or tid or as solution of 250–1000 units/mL in wet dressing	*Anorexia, nausea and vomiting* Nephrotoxicity, anaphylaxis
dalbavancin (Dalvance)	IV: 1500 mg single dose or 1000 mg followed 1 wk later by 500 mg	*Headache, nausea, diarrhea* Hypersensitivity and infusion-related reactions
fosfomycin (Monurol)	PO: 3 g sachet dissolved in 3–4 oz of water as a single dose	*Nausea, diarrhea, back pain, headache* Anaphylaxis, superinfections
oritavancin (Orbactiv)	IV: 1200 mg single dose given over 3 h	*Headache, nausea and vomiting, diarrhea* Limb and subcutaneous abscesses, hypersensitivity, infusion-related reactions
telavancin (Vibativ)	IV: 10 mg administered over 60 min, once daily for 7–10 days	*Nausea, vomiting and foamy urine* Nephrotoxicity, QT interval prolongation, infusion-related reactions, birth defects
vancomycin (Vancocin)	IV: 500 mg qid; 1 g bid PO: 500 mg–2.0 g in three to four divided doses for 7–10 days	*Nausea and vomiting* Anaphylaxis, superinfections, nephrotoxicity, ototoxicity, red man syndrome

Note: *Italics* indicate common adverse effects. Underline indicates serious adverse effects.

Imipenem (Primaxin), ertapenem (Invanz), and meropenem (Merrem) belong to the carbapenem class of antibiotics. These drugs are bactericidal and have some of the broadest antimicrobial spectrums of any class of antibiotics. They contain a beta-lactam ring and kill bacteria by inhibiting construction of the cell wall. Though similar, the ring in carbapenems has a slightly different structure than other beta-lactam antibiotics that makes it very resistant to destruction by beta-lactamase. These factors allow the carbapenems to provide better activity against serious gram-negative and multidrug-resistant infections than most cephalosporins or penicillins. A disadvantage is that they must be given parenterally. The primary role of the carbapenems is for the treatment of complicated bacterial infections. They are sometimes considered the antibiotics of "last resort" for treating multidrug-resistant infections.

All the carbapenems exhibit a low incidence of adverse effects. Diarrhea, nausea, rashes, and thrombophlebitis at injection sites are the most common adverse effects.

In recent years, bacteria have been isolated that are resistant to the carbapenems. These infections, called carbapenem-resistant Enterobacteriaceae infections, are usually healthcare associated and can be highly lethal (see Chapter 46).

PROTOTYPE DRUG Imipenem-Cilastatin (Primaxin)

Classification **Therapeutic:** Antibacterial
Pharmacologic: Cell wall inhibitor, carbapenem

Therapeutic Effects and Uses: Approved in 1985, imipenem is used for the treatment and prophylaxis of susceptible bacterial infections. Imipenem has a very broad antimicrobial spectrum and is the most widely used carbapenem. Because of its broad spectrum and beta-lactamase resistance, it is effective against most gram-positive and gram-negative microbes, including anaerobic bacteria. It is particularly useful for mixed infections containing both aerobic and anaerobic organisms, including those with *S. aureus*. *P. aeruginosa* and strains of MRSA are also susceptible to imipenem.

Although imipenem contains a beta-lactam ring, it is resistant to the actions of beta-lactamase. This drug, however, is rapidly destroyed by dipeptidase, an enzyme found in the kidney tubules. Concurrent administration of the drug cilastatin, a renal dipeptidase inhibitor, with imipenem prevents the destruction of imipenem and allows for higher serum levels of the antibiotic. Cilastatin possesses no antimicrobial activity of its own. Imipenem is marketed only with cilastatin in a fixed-dose combination (Primaxin).

Primaxin is sometimes combined with antibiotics from other classes, such as the aminoglycosides or cephalosporins, when treating *P. aeruginosa* infections. Primaxin has a short half-life that requires administration every 6 hours.

To enhance the effectiveness of imipenem against resistant organisms, relebactam has been added to imipenem-cilastatin to form the combination drug Recarbrio. Relebactam is a new betalactamase inhibitor with no intrinsic antimicrobial activity. Its function is to prevent imipenem from being destroyed by microbes that secrete beta-lactamase. Recarbrio was approved in 2019 to treat complicated UTIs, complicated intra-abdominal infections, and hospital-acquired pneumonia.

Mechanism of Action: Imipenem inhibits bacterial wall synthesis by binding to specific PBPs. Cilastatin blocks renal dipeptidase, which is the enzyme primarily responsible for the excretion of imipenem. The combination of imipenem-cilastatin is bactericidal.

Pharmacokinetics:

Route(s)	IM, IV
Absorption	Not absorbed PO
Distribution	Widely distributed, including in the CSF; secreted in breast milk; both imipenem and cilastatin cross the placenta
Primary metabolism	Hepatic
Primary excretion	Renal
Onset of action	IM: rapid; IV: immediate
Duration of action	Half-life: 1 h

Adverse Effects: The most frequent adverse effects of imipenem-cilastatin include nausea and vomiting, diarrhea, rash, and pain and phlebitis at the injection site. Rare, though serious, reactions include confusion, seizures, hallucinations, PMC, and anaphylaxis. Anaphylactic response may include cardiovascular collapse and edema of the mouth, tongue, pharynx, and larynx.

Contraindications/Precautions: Imipenem-cilastatin is contraindicated in patients who have experienced a severe allergic reaction to this drug, other carbapenems, cephalosporins, or penicillins. Because the kidneys excrete imipenem-cilastatin, patients with CKD must be carefully monitored and dosages lowered. This drug should be used cautiously in patients with brain lesions, head trauma, or a history of seizures.

Drug Interactions: Certain other antibiotics, including penicillins, cephalosporins, and aztreonam, antagonize the antimicrobial effects of imipenem-cilastatin; therefore, they should not be given concurrently. Concurrent use with cyclosporine, tramadol, theophylline, or ganciclovir may increase the risk of seizures and other CNS effects. Imipenem-cilastatin decreases levels of valproic acid, resulting in seizures. **Herbal/Food:** None known.

Pregnancy: Imipenem-cilastatin is embryotoxic in some laboratory animals, with no evidence of fetal malformations.

Small amounts are secreted in human milk but adverse effects on the breastfed neonate are unknown.

Treatment of Overdose: Overdose may result in ataxia and seizures. Patients are treated symptomatically.

Clinician Responsibilities: Key clinical implications for patients receiving imipenem-cilastatin are included in Applied Clinical Judgment: Patients Receiving Pharmacotherapy with a Penicillin, Cephalosporin, or Vancomycin Antibiotic.

Drugs Similar to Imipenem-Cilastatin (Primaxin)

Other carbapenems include ertapenem and meropenem. Doripenem is no longer available in the United States.

Ertapenem (Invanz): Approved in 2002, ertapenem has a narrower spectrum than the other carbapenems, being active primarily against gram-negative aerobes. Its major advantage is its longer half-life, which allows for once-daily dosing. It is approved for the treatment of serious abdominopelvic and skin infections, community-acquired pneumonia, complicated UTIs, and diabetic foot infections without concomitant osteomyelitis. It is administered by the IV and IM routes. Adverse effects are similar to those of other carbapenems. Ertapenem is contraindicated in patients who have experienced a severe allergic reaction to other carbapenems, cephalosporins, or penicillins. Animal studies did not show evidence of fetal harm. Because this drug is secreted in human milk, caution is urged if breastfeeding.

Meropenem (Merrem): Approved in 1996, meropenem has a similar spectrum of activity to imipenem and is approved for complicated intra-abdominal infections and complicated skin and skin structure infections in adults and bacterial meningitis in children. The drug may be used off-label for other indications. The antimicrobial spectrum of activity of meropenem is similar to that of imipenem. Meropenem may be more active against Enterobacteriaceae, gonococcus, *H. influenzae*, and *P. aeruginosa*. This drug is not destroyed by renal dipeptidase, so it is not administered with cilastatin. Adverse effects are similar to those of imipenem. Meropenem is contraindicated in patients who have experienced a severe allergic reaction to other carbapenems, cephalosporins, or penicillins. It is only available by the IV route. Bolus injections are given IV over 3 to 5 minutes and infusions over 15 to 30 minutes.

In 2017 the FDA approved Vabomere, a combination of meropenem with vaborbactam. Vaborbactam is a new beta-lactamase inhibitor that has no intrinsic antimicrobial activity. Its function is to prevent meropenem from being destroyed by microbes that secrete beta-lactamase. Animal studies with meropenem showed no evidence of fetal harm. Because this drug is secreted in human milk, caution is urged if breastfeeding.

PharmFACT

About 41,000 bloodstream infections occur in hospitalized patients with central lines each year. One in four patients who get a bloodstream infection will die from it (American Nurses Association, n.d.).

Miscellaneous Cell Wall Inhibitors

47.5 Several miscellaneous cell wall inhibitors have activity against resistant microbes.

Several other cell wall inhibitors have important roles in the pharmacotherapy of infections. These drugs comprise a group of mostly unique, distinct antimicrobials.

One of the miscellaneous groups, the lipoglycopeptides, now includes several newer drugs that have similar chemical structures and act by inhibiting peptidoglycan synthesis. The lipoglycopeptides include telavancin (Vibativ), oritavancin (Orbactiv), and dalbavancin (Dalvance). All three drugs are derivatives of vancomycin and contain lipid and carbohydrate chains attached to a peptide.

PROTOTYPE DRUG **Vancomycin (Vancocin)**

Classification **Therapeutic:** Antibacterial
Pharmacologic: Cell wall inhibitor

Therapeutic Effects and Uses: Approved in 1964, vancomycin (Vancocin) is used for the treatment and prophylaxis of susceptible bacterial infections. It is effective against most gram-positive organisms, including *Streptococcus*, *Corynebacterium*, *Clostridium*, *Listeria*, and *Bacillus* species. Vancomycin is usually administered by slow IV infusion for systemic infections because it is not well absorbed from the GI tract. It has been administered off-label by the intrathecal or intraventricular route to treat meningitis. Oral vancomycin is approved for the treatment of antibiotic-induced PMC, which is caused by a toxin produced by *C. difficile*. When given orally, the drug acts locally in the intestine and very little is absorbed into the systemic circulation.

Current protocols restrict the use of vancomycin to severe infections that have become resistant to safer antibiotics. It is anticipated that this restriction will discourage or delay the appearance of resistant strains. Because vancomycin was used infrequently during the first 30 years following its discovery, the incidence of vancomycin-resistant organisms has been less than that of other antibiotics. Vancomycin is the most effective drug for treating MRSA infections. Vancomycin-resistant strains of *S. aureus*, however, have begun to appear in recent years. Vancomycin is often considered a "last resort" antibiotic. Therapeutic options for vancomycin-resistant infections are limited.

Mechanism of Action: Although vancomycin kills bacteria mainly by inhibiting bacterial cell wall synthesis, it also affects the plasma membrane and interferes with ribonucleic acid (RNA) synthesis. The fact that it has multiple mechanisms is probably responsible for the low rate of resistance from the drug. It is bactericidal and only effective against gram-positive organisms such as *S. aureus* and *S. pneumoniae*.

Pharmacokinetics:

Route(s)	IV, PO
Absorption	Poorly absorbed PO
Distribution	Oral form does not usually enter systemic circulation; IV form is widely distributed with small amounts in the CSF; secreted in breast milk; 55% bound to plasma proteins
Primary metabolism	Probably not metabolized
Primary excretion	Renal
Onset of action	IV: immediate
Duration of action	Half-life: 4–8 h

Adverse Effects: Vancomycin may cause a syndrome of flushing, hypotension, tachycardia, and rash on the upper body, a condition called red man syndrome. This syndrome can be minimized by infusing the drug over at least 60 minutes. Other common adverse effects include nausea, rash, fever, and chills. Serious adverse effects include confusion, seizures, and hallucinations. If extravasation occurs, it may lead to tissue necrosis. Ototoxicity is associated with serum concentrations of vancomycin above 60 to 80 mcg/mL. Tinnitus and high-tone hearing loss precede deafness and may progress even after this drug is discontinued. The most susceptible individuals are older adults and those on high doses. Nephrotoxicity can occur in patients with therapeutic concentrations but is more common if trough serum concentrations are kept above 10 mcg/mL. Anaphylactic response may include cardiovascular collapse or edema of the mouth, tongue, pharynx, and larynx.

Contraindications/Precautions: Vancomycin is contraindicated in patients who have experienced previous hypersensitivity to this drug. The nurse must monitor drug therapy carefully in patients with CKD and those with a history of hearing loss.

Drug Interactions: Vancomycin adds to toxicity of aminoglycosides, amphotericin B, cisplatin, cyclosporine, polymyxin B, and other ototoxic and nephrotoxic medications. Vancomycin may increase the risk of lactic acidosis when administered with metformin, especially in patients with CKD. **Herbal/Food:** Unknown.

Pregnancy: Animal studies did not show evidence of fetal harm. Small amounts are secreted in human milk but adverse effects on the breastfed neonate are unknown.

Treatment of Overdose: Because overdose may result in renal impairment, patients are treated supportively to maintain kidney function.

Clinician Responsibilities: Key clinical implications for patients receiving vancomycin are included in Applied Clinical Judgment: Patients Receiving Pharmacotherapy with a Penicillin, Cephalosporin, or Vancomycin Antibiotic.

Drugs Similar to Vancomycin (Vancocin)

Other miscellaneous cell wall inhibitors include aztreonam, bacitracin, dalbavancin, fosfomycin, oritavancin, and telavancin.

Aztreonam (Azactam, Cayston): Approved in 1986, aztreonam has a beta-lactam ring and belongs to a class of antibiotics known as monobactams. Like other cell wall inhibitors, aztreonam binds to specific penicillin-binding proteins to cause a bactericidal effect. Although considered narrow-spectrum antibiotics, monobactams are particularly useful against certain gram-negative aerobes, such as *P. aeruginosa*. Other organisms considered susceptible to aztreonam include *Citrobacter*, *Enterobacter*, *E. coli*, *H. influenzae*, *Neisseria*, *Proteus*, *Providencia rettgeri*, and *Shigella*. Monobactams have little or no activity against gram-positive bacteria or anaerobes. Although they have beta-lactam rings, they do not exhibit cross hypersensitivity with penicillins or cephalosporins. Azactam is administered by the parenteral route and exhibits similar adverse effects as those of other cell wall inhibitors including nausea and vomiting, diarrhea, superinfections such as vaginal candidiasis, and local pain or phlebitis at the injection site. Anaphylaxis and PMC are rare. An inhalation form of the drug, Cayston, was approved in 2010 to improve respiratory symptoms in patients with cystic fibrosis who have *P. aeruginosa* infection. Animal studies did not show evidence of fetal harm. Because this drug is secreted in human milk, caution is urged if breastfeeding.

Bacitracin: Bacitracin is an older antibiotic, approved in 1948, that acts by inhibiting cell wall synthesis. It is combined with polymyxin B in over-the-counter (OTC) first-aid products (Neosporin, Polysporin) and is also available as monotherapy in OTC products such as Bacitracin First Aid. It is effective against a variety of gram-positive and a few gram-negative microbes. Although an IM form is available, bacitracin is almost always used topically due to potential nephrotoxicity (black box warning). In addition to creams and ointments, bacitracin solutions may be used to soak compresses that can be applied to large areas of the skin. Animal studies with topical bacitracin did not show evidence of fetal harm. Adverse effects during lactation are not expected when given by the topical route.

Dalbavancin (Dalvance): Approved in 2014, dalbavancin is a lipoglycopeptide derived from vancomycin that is approved to treat adults with acute bacterial skin and skin structure infections. It is given in one or two IV doses. Susceptible organisms include MRSA and various streptococcus species. The drug is well tolerated, with GI complaints being the most common adverse effects. Animal studies showed embryotoxicity and decreased offspring survival at high doses. It is not known whether this drug is secreted in human milk or if it has adverse effects on the breastfed neonate.

Fosfomycin (Monurol): Approved in 1996, fosfomycin is a cell wall inhibitor that is currently approved for the treatment of uncomplicated UTI and bladder infections in women caused by *E. coli* and *Enterococcus faecalis*. It is given as an oral powder, which is mixed with water and taken PO as a single dose. Adverse effects are minor and include asthenia, nausea and vomiting, diarrhea, headache, and vaginitis. Animal studies at clinically relevant doses showed no evidence of teratogenic effects. It is not known whether this drug is secreted in human milk or if it has adverse effects on the breastfed neonate.

Oritavancin (Orbactiv): Like dalbavancin, oritavancin is a lipoglycopeptide derived from vancomycin that was approved in 2014 to treat adults with acute bacterial skin and skin structure infections. It is given as a single IV infusion. Susceptible organisms include MRSA, various streptococcus species, and *E. faecalis*. Oritavancin may interfere with coagulation blood test results and may cause higher than normal warfarin levels. The use of unfractionated heparin is contraindicated for 5 days after oritavancin administration. Animal studies showed no evidence of fetal harm. It is not known whether this drug is secreted in human milk or if it has adverse effects on the breastfed neonate.

Telavancin (Vibativ): Approved in 2009, telavancin is a synthetic derivative of vancomycin that acts by inhibiting the polymerization and cross-linking of peptidoglycan in bacterial cell walls. It is approved as a once-daily IV infusion for the treatment of complicated skin and skin structure infections caused by gram-negative bacteria, including MRSA. Common adverse effects include taste disturbances, nausea and vomiting, and foamy urine. The use of unfractionated heparin is contraindicated. This drug carries a black box warning regarding its nephrotoxicity and possible risks during pregnancy. Kidney function should be monitored during therapy. Telavancin prolongs the QT interval and it should be used with caution with other medications that cause this effect. Animal studies showed telavancin may cause fetal harm. Women of childbearing potential should have a serum pregnancy test prior to administration and should use effective contraception during therapy and for at least 2 days following the last dose. This drug may impair male fertility.

CONNECTIONS: APPLIED CLINICAL JUDGMENT

Patients Receiving Pharmacotherapy with a Penicillin, Cephalosporin, or Vancomycin Antibiotic

Key Assessment Data

- History of current condition, baseline vital signs, physical exam findings; hepatic, renal, cardiovascular, neurologic, or respiratory disease; pregnancy or breastfeeding. Obtain a drug history and assess signs and symptoms of the current infection, noting location, characteristics, presence or absence of drainage and the character of drainage, duration, and the presence or absence of fever or pain.
- Ongoing assessment during drug therapy should include monitoring appropriate laboratory findings (e.g., CBC, culture and sensitivity, hepatic and renal laboratory values); assess for infections, especially with opportunistic infections such as fungal infections.

Desired Therapeutic Outcomes

Improvement is observed and measurable by fever, pain, or signs and symptoms of infection should begin to diminish after taking the first dose and continue to improve throughout the course of antibiotic therapy.

Minimizing Adverse Effects

- Continued fever may be a sign of worsening infection, adverse drug effects, or antibiotic resistance. Immediately report undiminished fever, changes in level of consciousness (LOC), or febrile seizures.
- Penicillins and cephalosporins may be nephrotoxic. Periodic laboratory testing, and culture and sensitivity tests may be ordered if infections are severe or slow to resolve and to confirm drug therapy is appropriate.
- Anaphylactic reactions are possible, particularly with the first dose of an antibiotic. Residual drug levels, dependent on length of half-life, may cause delayed reactions up to 2 weeks after completing antibacterial therapy.
- Penicillins and cephalosporins may require frequent monitoring to prevent adverse effects. Monitor for nephrotoxicity (e.g., darkened urine, diminished urine output, or weight gain greater than 1 kg [2 lb] in 24 hours).
- Superinfections with opportunistic organisms may occur when normal host flora are diminished or killed by the antibacterial drug. Severe diarrhea may indicate the presence of CDAD (*C. difficile–associated diarrhea*) or PMC, or fungal or yeast infections.
- Penicillins and cephalosporins have an increased risk of neurotoxicity. Monitor for signs and symptoms of neurotoxicity (e.g., dizziness, drowsiness, severe headache, changes in LOC, or seizures).
- Vancomycin hypersensitivity may cause the release of large amounts of histamine. Pretreatment with antihistamines (e.g., diphenhydramine) may be required. IV infusions should be given slowly and monitored closely. Monitor for development of red man syndrome: significantly large area of reddening such as trunk, head, neck, limbs, or gluteal area, especially if associated with decreased blood pressure or tachycardia.
- Penicillins may cause blood dyscrasias with resulting decreases in RBCs, WBCs, or platelets. Monitor for signs and symptoms of blood dyscrasias (e.g., low-grade fever, bleeding, bruising, or significant fatigue).
- Some preparations of penicillin may be based on sodium or potassium salts and may cause hypernatremia and hyperkalemia.

CONNECTIONS: APPLIED CLINICAL JUDGMENT *(continued)*

Patients Receiving Pharmacotherapy with a Penicillin, Cephalosporin, or Vancomycin Antibiotic

Lifespan Considerations

- Age-related physiologic differences may place the young child or older adult at greater risk for nephrotoxicity.
- Older adults may be at increased risk for dizziness related to adverse drug effects, which may increase the risk for falls. Ensure patient safety.
- Some penicillins may significantly reduce the effectiveness of oral contraceptives. Women of childbearing potential taking oral contraceptives should use an alternative form of birth control to prevent pregnancy.

Patient Education

- Report a fever that does not diminish below 37.8°C (100°F) within 3 days, increasing signs and symptoms of infection, or symptoms that remain after taking the entire course of antibacterial therapy. Immediately report febrile seizures, changes in behavior, or changes in LOC r.
- Immediately report any itching, rashes, swelling (particularly of tongue or face), urticaria, flushing, dizziness, syncope, wheezing, throat tightness, or difficulty breathing.
- Increase overall fluid intake. Report any diminished urine output, weight gain of more than 1 kg in a 24-hour period, darkening of urine.
- Report any diarrhea that increases in frequency or amount or contains mucus, blood, or pus. Consult the healthcare provider before taking any antidiarrheal drugs that slow gastric motility because these may cause the retention of harmful bacteria.
- Observe for white patches in the mouth, whitish thick vaginal discharge, itching in the urogenital area, or blistering, itchy rash and report to the healthcare provider.
- Immediately report signs and symptoms of infection such as wounds with redness or drainage, increasing cough, increasing fatigue, white patches on oral mucous membranes, white and itchy vaginal discharge, or itchy blister-like vesicles on the skin.
- Immediately report increasing headache, dizziness, drowsiness, changes in behavior, LOC, or seizures. If dizziness occurs, sit or lie down and do not attempt to stand or walk until the sensation passes.
- Women of childbearing potential on oral contraceptives should consult with their healthcare provider about birth control alternatives if penicillin antibiotics are ordered.
- For known antibacterial allergies, carry a wallet identification card or wear medical identification jewelry indicating allergy.
- Appropriate self-administration of antibiotics includes:
  - Complete the entire course of therapy unless otherwise instructed. Do not share with other family members, and do not stop the medicine when starting to feel better.
  - Avoid or eliminate alcohol. Cephalosporins may cause significant reactions when taken with alcohol, and alcohol increases adverse GI effects of the drug.
  - Take the drug with food or milk but avoid acidic or carbonated beverages to decrease adverse GI effects.
  - Take the medication as evenly spaced throughout each day as feasible.
  - Increase overall fluid intake while taking the antibacterial drug

Prescribing Considerations

- Otitis media (OM): Classify episodes of otitis media as acute OM or OM with effusion; only treat acute OM or if effusions persist for 3 months or more.
- Rhinitis: Antibiotics are not indicated unless it persists without improvement for more than 10 to 14 days.
- Sinusitis: Initial antibiotic treatment of acute sinusitis should use the narrowest-spectrum agent that is effective against the active pathogens.
- Pharyngitis: Antibiotics should not be given to a child with pharyngitis in the absence of diagnosed group A streptococcal infection; penicillin remains the preferred drug for treating group A streptococcal pharyngitis.
- Cough illness and bronchitis: Rarely warrant antibiotic treatment in children; antibiotic treatment for prolonged cough (more than 10 days) in adults may be warranted.

Understanding Chapter 47

Key Concepts Summary

47.1 Bacterial cell walls consist of layers of carbohydrate and protein chains, which are constructed by enzymes called penicillin-binding proteins.

47.2 The penicillins, one of the oldest and safest groups of antibacterials, are primarily active against gram-positive bacteria.

47.3 The cephalosporins are similar in structure and function to the penicillins and are widely prescribed for gram-negative infections.

47.4 The carbapenems are resistant to beta-lactamase and are broad-spectrum alternatives to penicillin.

47.5 Several miscellaneous cell wall inhibitors have activity against resistant microbes.

CASE STUDY: Making the Patient Connection

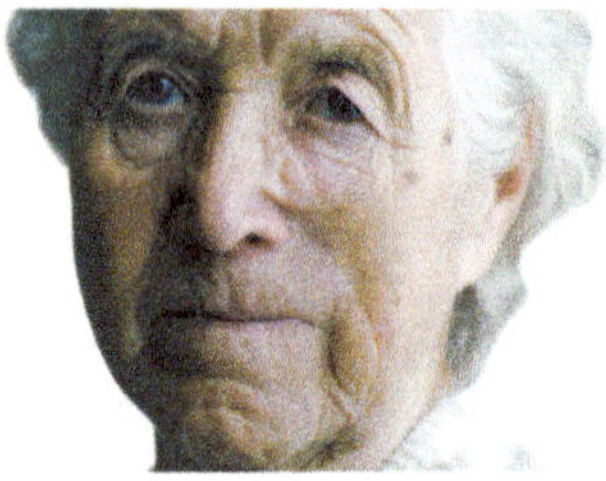

Remember the patient "Katie Dennison" at the beginning of the chapter? Now read the remainder of the case study. Based on the information presented within this chapter, respond to the critical thinking questions that follow.

Katie Dennison is an 83-year-old retired schoolteacher. She was recently seen by her healthcare provider for removal of a noncancerous skin lesion. Now she suspects that the wound on her arm has become infected. She has attempted to report this condition to her healthcare provider. However, due to the holidays she has been unable to reach him. Ms. Dennison presents to a local urgent care center for treatment.

The physical examination and diagnostic tests reveal the following findings: Vital signs are temperature, 38°C (100.9°F); pulse, 110 beats/min; respiratory rate, 20 breaths/min; and blood pressure, 108/68 mmHg. The large dressing on her left arm is saturated with dried yellow-green exudates. Ms. Dennison states that it is painful to move her left arm and that the pain has limited her range of motion in the affected extremity. She is pale and has "paper-thin" fragile skin.

Ms. Dennison reports that she unintentionally got the dressing wet while taking a shower. She did not change the dressing because she was not told to do so by her healthcare provider when the skin lesion was removed. A series of laboratory tests was completed. A sterile dressing was applied to the wound. Ms. Dennison was given an injection of cefazolin (Ancef) and a prescription for antibiotics. She was also instructed to follow up with her healthcare provider within the next 2 to 3 days.

Critical Thinking Questions

1. What factors possibly contributed to the wound infection in this patient?
2. What laboratory tests were probably obtained during this visit to the urgent care center?
3. What information should the nurse provide to the patient concerning the antibiotic?
4. Discuss the mechanism of action for cefazolin.

Additional Case Study

Mrs. Murphy is 80 years old and lives in a retirement community for lower-income older adults. You are the community health nurse visiting with her. As part of your assessment, you ask Mrs. Murphy how she obtains her prescribed medications. The patient explains that most of the time, her neighbor will pick up prescriptions for her. She further explains that in some cases, however, she has "stockpiled" medicines she has been prescribed. When you investigate, you find that the patient has multiple bottles of various types of unused antibiotics. Some of the drugs were prescribed 5 or 6 years ago.

1. Describe how you should respond to this situation.
2. Identify the health teaching needs of this patient regarding stockpiling (saving) antibiotics.

Chapter Review

1. Which instruction should the nurse give a 21-year-old female patient being treated with ampicillin?
    1. Stop taking oral contraceptives because serious adverse effects could occur.
    2. Use oral contraceptives as prescribed because antibiotics do not react with birth control pills.
    3. The antibiotic may decrease the effectiveness of oral contraceptives.
    4. The antibiotic when taken with oral contraceptives causes toxicity.
2. The nurse is caring for a patient who is receiving intravenous vancomycin (Vancocin). Which symptom, if present, may indicate that the patient is experiencing drug-induced ototoxicity?
    1. Erythema of the earlobes and ear canal
    2. Inner ear pruritus after infusion is completed
    3. Tinnitus and dizziness when remaining still
    4. Ocular pain with purulent drainage

3. The patient reports abnormal vaginal discharge after completing a prescription of cefotaxime. For which condition is the patient most likely exhibiting symptoms?

1. Hypersensitivity reaction
2. Superinfection
3. Pseudomembranous colitis
4. Antibiotic toxicity

4. The patient who has been taking cefixime (Suprax) for the past week and a half returns to the provider with reports of "explosive diarrhea, very watery, sometimes with a lot of mucus" up to eight times in the last 2 days. The patient reports significant weakness. For which condition is the patient describing symptoms?

1. Antibiotic-induced peptic ulcer disease
2. Antibiotic-associated malabsorption
3. GI-associated hypersensitivity
4. *Clostridioides difficile*–associated diarrhea

5. The patient who is taking imipenem-cilastatin (Primaxin) reports shortness of breath, mouth and tongue swelling, and generalized itching. For which of the following does the nurse initially assess the patient?

1. Hypersensitivity reaction
2. Blood dyscrasias
3. Beta-lactamase induction
4. Drug toxicity

6. The nurse is teaching a patient who was recently diagnosed with an upper respiratory infection and prescribed ampicillin. The nurse would evaluate the session as being successful if the patient states which of the following?

1. "I should take this medication on an empty stomach with a full glass of water."
2. "I can expect my tongue to become black and furry."
3. "Once I stop coughing, I should stop taking this medication."
4. "If I miss a dose, I should take two doses together to catch up."

See Appendix A for answers to critical thinking questions, case study questions, and review questions.

References

Sharma, B. M., Bečanová, J., Scheringer, M., Sharma A., Bharat, G. K., Whitehead, P.G., et al. (2019). Health and ecological risk assessment of emerging contaminants (pharmaceuticals, personal care products, and artificial sweeteners) in surface and groundwater (drinking water) in the Ganges River Basin, India. *Science of the Total Environment*, *646*, 1459–1467. https://doi.org/10.1016/j.scitotenv.2018.07.235

Zainab, S. M., Junaib, M., Xu, N., & Malik, R. N. (2020). Antibiotics and antibiotic resistant genes (ARGs) in groundwater: A global review on dissemination, sources, interactions, environmental and human health risks. *Water Research*, *187*, 116455. https://doi.org/10.1016/j.watres.2020.116455

Selected Bibliography

Bonomo, R. A. (2019). Cefiderocol: a novel siderophore cephalosporin defeating carbapenem-resistant pathogens. *Clinical Infectious Diseases*, *69*(Suppl. 7), S519–S520. https://doi.org/10.1093/cid/ciz823

Boswihi, S. S., & Udo, E. E. (2018). Methicillin-resistant Staphylococcus aureus: An update on the epidemiology, treatment options and infection control. *Current Medicine Research and Practice*, *8*(1), 18–24. https://doi.org/10.1016/j.cmrp.2018.01.001

Centers for Disease Control and Prevention. (2019). *Healthcare-associated infections: Carbapenem-resistant Enterobacteriaceae in healthcare settings*. http://www.cdc.gov/hai/organisms/cre

Daniels, L. M., & Kufel, W. D. (2018). Clinical review of Clostridium difficile infection: An update on treatment and prevention. *Expert Opinion on Pharmacotherapy*, *19*(16), 1759–1769. https://doi.org/10.1080/14656566.2018.1524872

Durante-Mangoni, E., Andini, R., & Zampino, R. (2019). Management of carbapenem-resistant Enterobacteriaceae infections. *Clinical Microbiology and Infection*, *25*(8), 943–950. https://doi.org/10.1016/j.cmi.2019.04.013

Pachori, P., Gothalwal, R., & Gandhi, P. (2019). Emergence of antibiotic resistance Pseudomonas aeruginosa in intensive care unit; a critical review. *Genes and Diseases*, *6*(2), 109–119. https://doi.org/10.1016/j.gendis.2019.04.001

Shenoy, E. S., Macy, E., Rowe, T., & Blumenthal, K. G. (2019). Evaluation and management of penicillin allergy: A review. *Journal of the American Medical Association*, *321*(2), 188–199. https://doi.org/10.1001/jama.2018.19283

Tumbarello, M., Losito, A. R., & Giamarellou, H. (2018). Optimizing therapy in carbapenem-resistant Enterobacteriaceae infections. *Current Opinion in Infectious Diseases*, *31*(6), 566–577. https://doi.org/10.1097/QCO.0000000000000493

Vardakas, K. Z., Kalimeris, G. D., Triarides, N. A., & Falagas, M. E. (2018). An update on adverse drug reactions related to β-lactam antibiotics. *Expert Opinion on Drug Safety*, *17*(5), 499–508. https://doi.org/10.1080/14740338.2018.1462334

Wiley, K. C., & Villamizar, H. J. (2019). Antibiotic resistance policy and the stewardship role of the nurse. *Policy, Politics, & Nursing Practice*, *20*(1), 8–17. https://doi.org/10.1177/1527154418819251

"Today is the fifth day since I started taking the medication and I'm still having chills and fever. I thought these antibiotics were supposed to get rid of this!"
—*Patient "John Travis"*

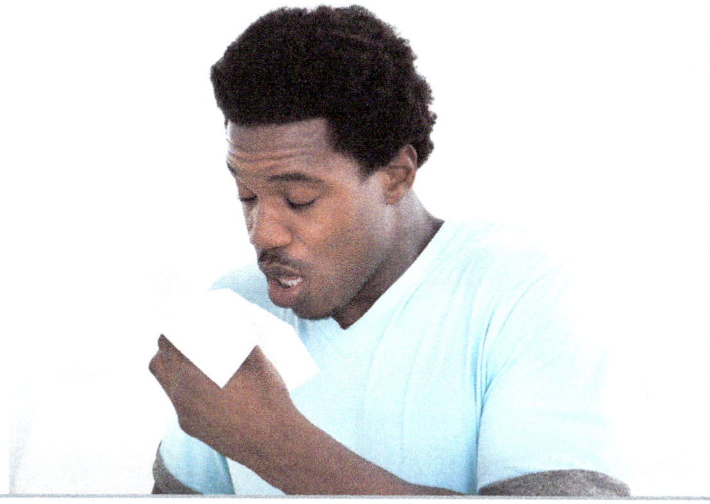

Chapter 48
Antibiotics Affecting Bacterial Protein Synthesis

Chapter Outline

- Mechanisms of Antibiotic Inhibition of Bacterial Protein Synthesis
- Tetracyclines

  PROTOTYPE *Tetracycline (Achromycin V), p. 841*
- Macrolides

  PROTOTYPE *Erythromycin (EryC, Erythrocin, Others), p. 844*
- Aminoglycosides

  PROTOTYPE *Gentamicin, p. 847*
- Miscellaneous Inhibitors of Bacterial Protein Synthesis

Learning Outcomes

After reading this chapter, the student should be able to:

1. Explain the steps in the synthesis of bacterial proteins.
2. Identify the classes of antibiotics that act by inhibiting bacterial protein synthesis.
3. Explain mechanisms by which antibiotics inhibit bacterial protein synthesis.
4. Explain how protein synthesis inhibitors exert selective toxicity toward bacterial, rather than human, cells.
5. Describe means by which bacteria become resistant to protein synthesis inhibitors.
6. For each of the classes shown in the chapter outline, identify the prototype and representative drugs and explain the mechanism(s) of drug action, primary indications, contraindications, significant drug interactions, pregnancy data, and important adverse effects.
7. Apply clinical judgment to care for patients receiving pharmacotherapy with bacterial protein synthesis inhibitors.

Key Terms

Definitions of the terms in bold may be found in the Glossary.

To maintain the extreme metabolic rate required for exponential replication, bacteria must synthesize huge amounts of protein. Antibacterial drugs that inhibit this high rate of protein metabolism can either kill the bacterial cell or slow its replication rate. Tetracyclines, macrolides, and a few miscellaneous drugs are bacteriostatic inhibitors of protein synthesis. The aminoglycosides are bactericidal inhibitors.

Mechanisms of Antibiotic Inhibition of Bacterial Protein Synthesis

48.1 Antibiotics inhibit microbial protein synthesis by binding to the bacterial ribosome.

The importance of protein to a microbe is illustrated by the fact that up to 50% of the dry weight of a bacterial cell consists of protein. Bacterial proteins serve many of the same functions as human proteins. For example, the bacterial enzymes required for all biochemical reactions are proteins. Proteins are studded in the plasma membrane and serve as channels, pores, or transporters, assisting substances as they move into and out of cells. Like human proteins, bacterial proteins are composed of long chains of amino acids.

Several types of proteins, however, are unique to bacteria. Bacterial cells produce protein toxins, which kill other bacteria and can cause serious injury to human cells. The sticky gel-like substance that allows bacterial cells to cling to human epithelial cells on the skin surface, in bronchi, in the gastrointestinal (GI) tract, or in the genitourinary tract consists of proteins combined with carbohydrates. The structure of the bacterial cell wall (see Chapter 47) consists of peptidoglycan layers of protein and carbohydrates that protect the bacterium from its environment. From these examples, it is easy to understand why proteins are critical to bacterial cells.

Knowledge of how proteins are synthesized by bacterial cells is important to understanding how antibiotics act. The basic steps in protein synthesis, or **translation**, are the same in bacteria as they are in humans. Knowledge of translation, which is illustrated in Figure 48.1, is necessary to understand the mechanisms of action of antibiotics that inhibit protein synthesis.

Protein synthesis occurs in the cytoplasm and requires the following three components:

- Messenger ribonucleic acid (mRNA)
- Transfer ribonucleic acid (tRNA)
- Ribosomes, which consist of one large and one small subunit.

The mRNA carries the encoded message for making a protein from the deoxyribonucleic acid (DNA) to the ribosome, which serves as the site for protein construction. The strand of mRNA squeezes between the two ribosomal subunits and begins to move through the subunits. As it does, a tRNA molecule arrives, carrying the specific amino acid that was encoded in the mRNA strand. As the mRNA proceeds through the ribosome, subsequent amino acids are added one at a time to the growing protein chain. This growing chain is known as a polypeptide. Eventually, a "stop signal" is reached on the mRNA strand, which tells

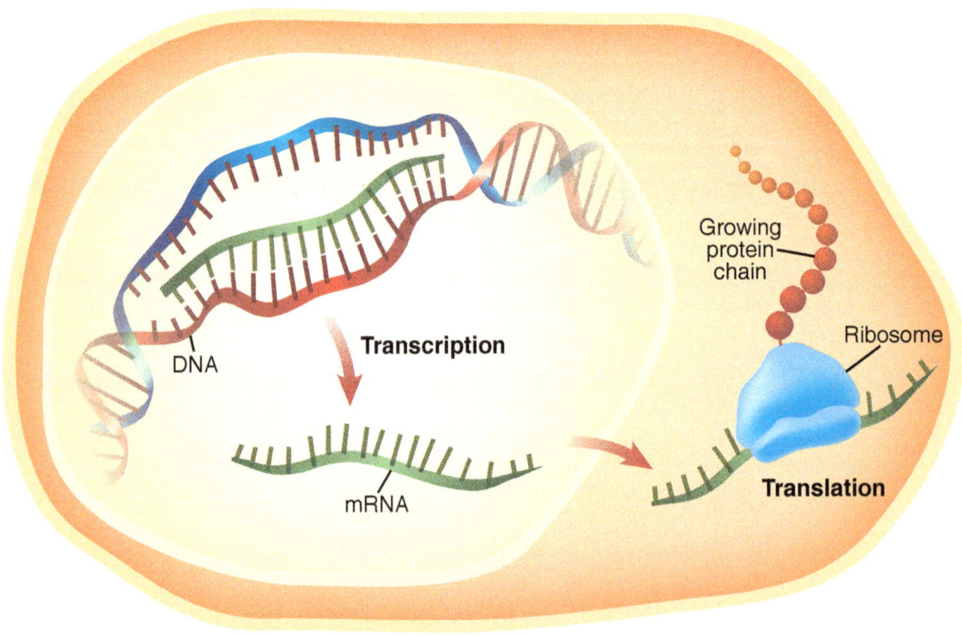

Figure 48.1 Steps in protein synthesis: The DNA is used as a template to make mRNA (transcription). The mRNA is sent to the ribosome to make the protein chain (translation).

the ribosome that the last amino acid has been added and the protein is ready to be released. The protein may be active immediately, or it may be processed to its active form in the Golgi body. The finished protein may be used within the bacterial cell (enzymes) or be exported outside (toxins).

All cells, including bacteria, are able to quickly increase protein synthesis to meet their growth demands or to respond to environmental challenges. For example, a bacterium may receive a message that competitive bacteria are in the vicinity. The gene coding for a toxin or antibiotic may become active, producing large amounts of mRNA and eventually protein toxin, which serves as a defense against the invaders.

If both humans and bacteria conduct continuous protein synthesis, why are antibiotics that inhibit protein synthesis not also toxic to human cells? The answer lies in differences in the structures of the bacterial and human ribosomes. Ribosomes are composed of two subunits, one of which is larger and less dense than the other. In bacteria, these ribosomal components are referred to as 30S and 50S subunits. The letter "S" is a unit of measurement, the **Svedberg unit**, which reflects the ribosome's size or sedimentation rate in a high-speed centrifuge. The entire bacterial ribosome is called a 70S ribosome (Svedberg units are not additive).

All antibiotics that target bacterial protein synthesis do so by affecting the 70S ribosome. Although humans also have ribosomes, their ribosomes are larger and denser than the 70S bacterial ribosome. The 80S human ribosome is mostly unaffected by antibiotics that bind to the bacterial 70S ribosome, thus providing a degree of selective toxicity. Interestingly, human mitochondria do contain a 70S ribosome that is affected by several of these antibiotics, thus explaining some of the adverse effects of these drugs.

About 20 drugs that affect the synthesis of bacterial proteins have been discovered. The different steps at which antibiotics inhibit the production of bacterial proteins are shown in Figure 48.2.

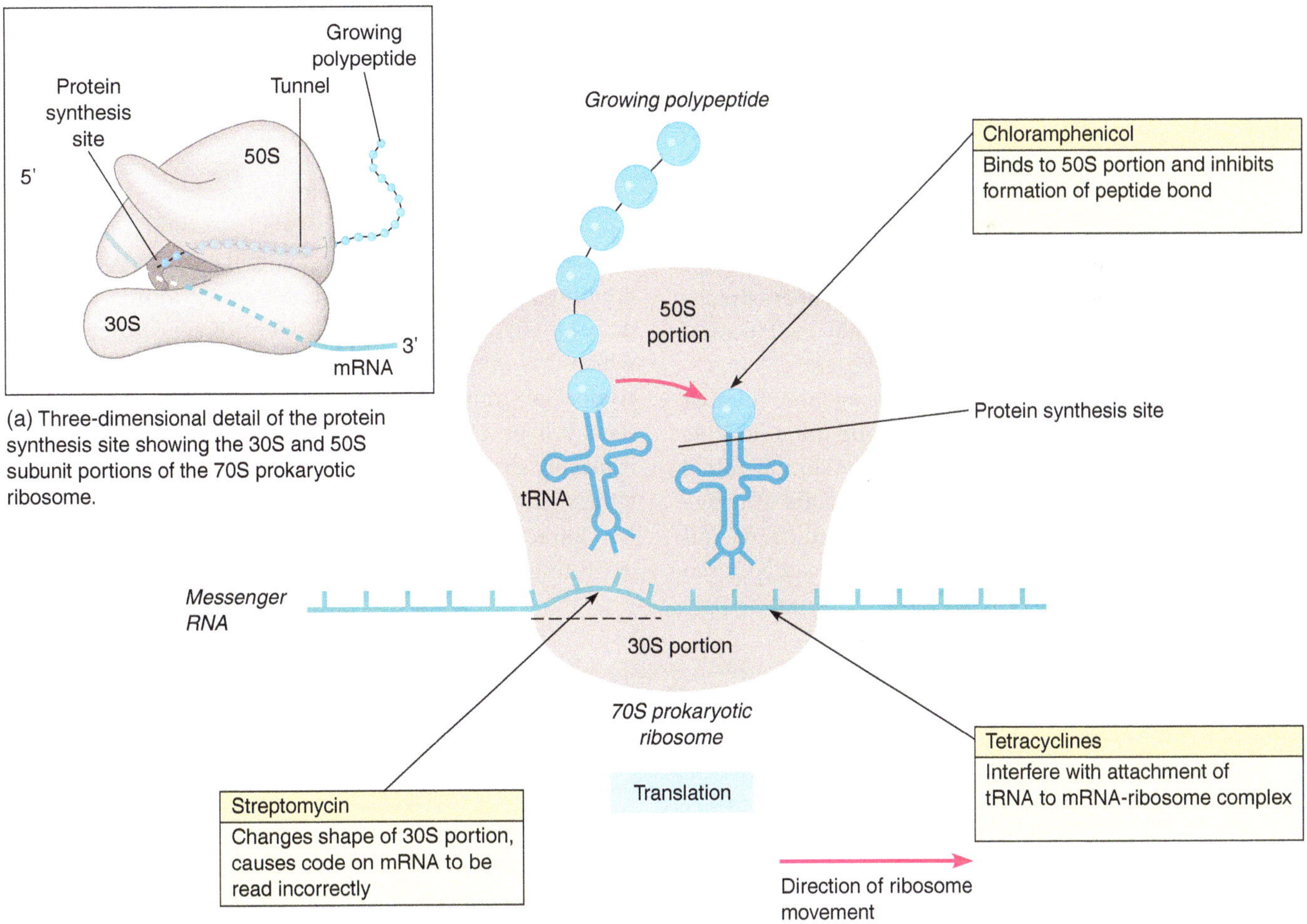

(a) Three-dimensional detail of the protein synthesis site showing the 30S and 50S subunit portions of the 70S prokaryotic ribosome.

(b) In the diagram the black arrows indicate the different points at which chloramphenicol, the tetracyclines, and streptomycin exert their activities.

Figure 48.2 Mechanisms of action of antibiotics inhibiting bacterial protein synthesis.
From Tortora et al. (2010), p. 558. Reprinted by permission of Pearson Education, Inc., Upper Saddle River, NJ.

CONNECTIONS: Using Research in Practice

Traveler's Diarrhea

Traveler's diarrhea (TD) is the most common and predictable travel-related illness (Connor, 2019). TD may or may not have associated symptoms such as fever, nausea and vomiting, or abdominal cramping and, depending on the causative organism, may occur within a few hours to 2 weeks after exposure. It is most often caused by ingesting contaminated food or water or by contact with contaminated surfaces, with poor hygiene in restaurants suspected to be the predominant source. People visiting friends and relatives in other countries may be at higher risk because their stays may be longer, and precautions other travelers take, such as seeing their healthcare provider for prophylactic drugs before travel or avoiding certain local foods, may not be observed (Centers for Disease Control and Prevention [CDC], 2016).

Bacteria are the most common cause of TD; however, viruses, protozoa, and parasites can also be causative agents (Connor, 2019). *Escherichia coli*, *Shigella*, *Campylobacter*, *Salmonella*, and noroviruses are common causes of TD. *Giardia* is the most common protozoal pathogen.

With concern for antibiotic resistance, prophylactic antibiotics may not be recommended for most travelers, because they afford no protection against nonbacterial pathogens. The antibiotic used to treat TD depends on where the patient traveled and the causative bacteria patterns in those areas. Ciprofloxacin and azithromycin are the most commonly prescribed antibiotics for treating TD, although bismuth subsalicylate, commonly found in Pepto-Bismol and Kaopectate, may also be used.

Strategies to decrease risk of contracting TD include practicing frequent hand hygiene with hand sanitizers or antiseptic cloths; avoiding beverages with ice, drinking water that has been boiled, and not using tap water for brushing teeth; and not consuming raw fruits or vegetables that cannot be peeled. Prophylactic antibiotics should be used if diarrhea is severe, and oral rehydration solutions may be needed. Antimotility drugs such as loperamide may also be used but are not recommended for diarrhea containing blood to avoid retaining the causative pathogen.

Tetracyclines

48.2 Tetracyclines have broad antimicrobial activity against many gram-positive and gram-negative bacteria.

The first tetracyclines were extracted from *Streptomyces* in soil samples in 1948. Unfortunately, their widespread use in the 1950s and 1960s resulted in a large number of resistant strains, limiting the current therapeutic usefulness of these drugs.

The tetracyclines are effective against a large number of aerobic and anaerobic gram-negative and gram-positive organisms: They have one of the broadest antimicrobial spectrums of any class of antibiotics. They are effective against some species that are resistant to penicillins and other cell wall inhibitors. Because of widespread bacterial resistance, however, they are the preferred drugs for only a few diseases: Rocky Mountain spotted fever, typhus, cholera, Lyme disease, peptic ulcers caused by *Helicobacter pylori*, and chlamydial infections. In addition, *Treponema pallidum* (syphilis) responds well to tetracycline therapy for patients who are allergic to penicillin. Although traditionally used for gonorrhea, most strains of *Neisseria gonorrhoeae* are now resistant to tetracyclines. Drugs in this class are occasionally used for the treatment of acne vulgaris, for which they are given topically or orally (PO) at low doses. Almost all strains of *Pseudomonas aeruginosa* are resistant to tetracyclines. Once resistance develops to one tetracycline, it usually extends to all drugs in this class. Doses for the tetracyclines are listed in Table 48.1.

Tetracyclines exert a bacteriostatic effect by selectively inhibiting bacterial protein synthesis. As illustrated in

Table 48.1 Tetracyclines

Drug	Route and Adult Dose (Maximum Dose Where Indicated)	Adverse Effects
demeclocycline	PO: 150 mg q6h or 300 mg q12h (max: 2.4 g/day)	*Nausea and vomiting, abdominal cramping, flatulence, diarrhea, mild phototoxicity, rash, dizziness, stinging or burning with topical applications* Anaphylaxis, superinfections, hepatotoxicity, exfoliative dermatitis, permanent teeth discoloration in children
doxycycline (Vibramycin, others)	PO/IV: 100–200 mg bid (max: 200 mg/day)	
eravacycline (Xerava)	IV: 1 mg/kg bid for 4–14 days	
minocycline (Minocin, others)	PO/IV: 100–200 mg bid	
omadacycline (Nuzyra)	IV: 100–300 mg once daily PO: 300–450 mg once daily	
sarecycline (Seysara)	PO: 60–150 mg once daily	
tetracycline (Achromycin V)	PO: 250–500 mg bid–qid (max: 2 g/day)	
tigecycline (Tygacil)	IV: 100 mg, followed by 50 mg q12h	

Note: *Italics* indicate common adverse effects. Underline indicates serious adverse effects.

Figure 48.2, the tetracyclines bind to the 30S bacterial ribosome, thereby preventing the addition of amino acids to the growing polypeptide chain. Resistance to tetracyclines develops when bacteria prevent tetracyclines from concentrating inside their cells, or when their ribosome shape is altered so the antibiotic can no longer bind. In addition to having ribosomes with different structures, human cells lack the active transport system required for tetracyclines to enter their cells. At high doses, however, tetracyclines begin to exert toxicity on human cells.

Most tetracyclines have the same spectrum of antimicrobial activity and similar adverse effects. All except tigecycline and eravacycline may be given PO. Several have topical and parenteral formulations. They are sometimes classified by their duration of action as short acting, intermediate acting, or long acting.

Most PO tetracyclines should be taken on an empty stomach to maximize their absorption. Because gastric distress is relatively common with drugs in this class, patients will often take tetracyclines with food. However, these drugs bind metal ions such as calcium, magnesium, aluminum, and iron, and tetracyclines should not be taken with milk or iron supplements. Food, milk, or other dairy products can reduce drug absorption by 50% or more. Food does not interfere with absorption of the longer-acting drugs doxycycline and minocycline.

Because most tetracyclines are incompletely absorbed, they remain in the GI tract in high concentrations, often killing normal flora in the colon. Tetracycline-induced diarrhea is common and could indicate toxic effects on normal flora or a bowel superinfection. The presence of diarrhea must be monitored carefully due to the possibility of **pseudomembranous colitis (PMC)**. Caused by *C. difficile*, this is a rare, though potentially severe, disorder resulting from therapy with tetracyclines, fluoroquinolones, cephalosporins, and other classes of antibiotics.

When administered parenterally or in high doses, certain tetracyclines can cause hepatotoxicity, especially in patients with preexisting liver disease. Some patients experience photosensitivity during therapy, making their skin especially susceptible to sunburn. Photosensitivity may appear as exaggerated sunburn within minutes to hours of exposure and is often accompanied by a tingling, burning sensation. Because of their broad spectrum, superinfections due to *Candida albicans* are relatively common. Women who are on oral contraceptives may be more susceptible to vaginal candidiasis. Tetracyclines are usually contraindicated in pregnant or lactating women and in children under the age of 8 because these drugs cause yellow-brown teeth discoloration and may slow the overall growth rate in fetuses or children.

CONNECTIONS: Patient Safety

Photosensitivity and Antibiotics

Having fun in the sun may be hazardous to some patients. Photosensitivity is a relatively common adverse reaction to some medications, especially antibiotics. Many pharmacologic therapies have photosensitivity as a possible adverse effect.

Any skin reaction to light is generally defined as photosensitivity. However, this medication-induced adverse effect can present in two categories: phototoxicity and photoallergic reactions. The more common of the two conditions is phototoxicity, which encompasses both sunburn and reactions caused by chemical photosensitizers such as medications. Both reactions are typically manifested by delayed redness and edema followed by hyperpigmentation. Phototoxicity may occur after first exposure to a drug.

Photoallergic reactions are less common. These reactions present as variations of contact dermatitis and are the result of hypersensitivity. In photoallergic reactions, the drug forms an immunogenic complex with cutaneous proteins due to the presence of light energy. Photoallergic reactions tend to become more pronounced with repeat exposures.

What role can nurses play to help patients prevent photosensitivity reactions from occurring?

PROTOTYPE DRUG Tetracycline (Achromycin V)

Classification **Therapeutic:** Antibacterial
Pharmacologic: Bacterial protein synthesis inhibitor, tetracycline

Therapeutic Effects and Uses: Approved by the U.S. Food and Drug Administration (FDA) in 1953, tetracycline is used for the treatment and prophylaxis of susceptible gram-positive and gram-negative bacteria as well as chlamydiae, rickettsiae, mycoplasmas, and certain protozoa. Tetracycline has one of the broadest spectrums of any antibiotic. Its use has increased during the past decade due to its effectiveness against *H. pylori* in the treatment of peptic ulcer disease. Oral and topical preparations are available for treating inflammatory acne vulgaris.

Mechanism of Action: Tetracycline inhibits bacterial protein synthesis by binding to the 30S ribosomal subunit, interfering with the attachment of the tRNA to the mRNA–ribosome complex. The growing amino acid chain is prematurely terminated and protein synthesis is inhibited. Tetracycline is usually considered bacteriostatic, although it can be bactericidal at high concentrations.

Pharmacokinetics:

Route(s)	PO, topical
Absorption	80% is absorbed PO
Distribution	Widely distributed; only small amounts cross the blood–brain barrier; crosses the placenta; secreted in breast milk

Primary metabolism	15–30% metabolized, primarily in the liver
Primary excretion	60% renal, small amounts excreted into bile
Onset of action	1–2 h
Duration of action	Half-life: 6–12 h

Adverse Effects: Being a broad-spectrum antibiotic, tetracycline has a tendency to affect vaginal, oral, and intestinal flora and cause superinfections. Other frequent adverse effects include nausea and vomiting, epigastric burning, diarrhea, discoloration of the teeth, and photosensitivity. Serious adverse reactions include anaphylaxis; fatty degeneration of the liver, producing jaundice; and exfoliative dermatitis. Although not nephrotoxic, tetracycline can worsen kidney impairment in patients with preexisting disease.

Contraindications/Precautions: Tetracycline is contraindicated in patients who are allergic to any drug in the tetracycline class. Tetracycline should not be used during pregnancy. Drug therapy must be monitored carefully in patients with impaired hepatic function or chronic kidney disease (CKD) because this drug is excreted by these routes.

Drug Interactions: Oral supplements, laxatives, or antacids that contain metal ions such as calcium, iron, magnesium, or aluminum reduce the GI absorption and serum levels of oral tetracycline. Tetracycline binds with colestipol and cholestyramine, thereby decreasing the antibiotic's absorption. Tetracyclines decrease the effectiveness of oral contraceptives. **Herbal/Food:** Dairy products interfere with tetracycline absorption. Tetracycline eliminates vitamin K–producing bacteria in the intestines; patients taking warfarin may experience an increased anticoagulant effect.

Pregnancy: Human epidemiological studies have shown an increased risk for spontaneous abortion and adverse effects on fetal skeletal development when given PO. This drug is secreted in human milk and may adversely affect the breastfed neonate. Oral tetracycline should not be used during pregnancy or lactation unless the potential benefits to the mother justify the potential risks to the fetus and neonate. Animal studies have not shown evidence that *topical* tetracycline has adverse effects during pregnancy or lactation.

Treatment of Overdose: No specific therapy is available. Patients are treated symptomatically.

Clinician Responsibilities: Key clinical implications for patients receiving tetracycline are included in Applied Clinical Judgment: Patients Receiving Pharmacotherapy with a Tetracycline, Macrolide, or Aminoglycoside Antibiotic.

Drugs Similar to Tetracycline (Achromycin)

Other tetracyclines include demeclocycline, doxycycline, eravacycline, minocycline, omadacycline, sarecycline, and tigecycline. All drugs in this class have the potential to cause fetal harm and should be used during pregnancy or lactation only if the potential benefits to the mother justifies the potential risks to the fetus or neonate.

Demeclocycline: Approved in 1960, demeclocycline has the same spectrum of antimicrobial action as other tetracyclines. Unrelated to its anti-infective properties, demeclocycline is the only drug in this class used off-label to treat syndrome of inappropriate antidiuretic hormone (SIADH). Because of its blocking action on antidiuretic hormone (ADH), demeclocycline is used to produce diuresis in patients with excess ADH secretion (see Chapter 65). Photosensitivity is more severe with demeclocycline than with other drugs in this class. Demeclocycline undergoes extensive enterohepatic recirculation and is excreted in the bile; thus, doses should be reduced for patients with hepatic impairment.

Doxycycline (Vibramycin, others): Approved in 1967, doxycycline is the safest tetracycline for patients with impaired renal function because it is excreted primarily by nonrenal routes. Normally administered PO, an intravenous (IV) form is available for treating severe infections. It is absorbed well, with or without food, and offers the advantage of once- or twice-daily dosing. Doxycycline is included in the CDC's "Sexually Transmitted Diseases Treatment Guidelines" (2015) for treating chlamydial infections, pelvic inflammatory disease, and penicillin-resistant syphilis. Doxycycline is recommended as an alternative to ciprofloxacin for the prophylactic treatment of *Bacillus anthracis* (anthrax). Adverse effects and contraindications are the same as those of other tetracyclines.

Several other formulations of doxycycline are available. Doryx is an extended-release enteric-coated oral formulation. Oracea is a dual-release capsule, containing immediate- and delayed-release beads for the treatment of inflammatory lesions of the skin associated with rosacea. It is not intended for the treatment or prevention of infections. Atridox is administered as a topical, subgingival controlled-release product for the treatment of chronic periodontitis in adults.

Eravacycline (Xerava): Eravacycline was approved in 2018 for the IV treatment of complicated intra-abdominal infections. To reduce the development of drug-resistant bacteria, eravacycline is reserved for the treatment or prevention of infections known to be susceptible to this antibiotic. The drug is well tolerated, with infusion site reactions and nausea and vomiting being the most common adverse reactions. Other side effects are typical of drugs in this class.

Minocycline (Minocin, others): Approved in 1971, minocycline offers the advantage of once- or twice-daily dosing and may be administered without regard to meals or dairy products. It is the only tetracycline that can cause reversible vestibular toxicity, resulting in dizziness, vertigo, and weakness that can limit therapy. Minocycline is active against some strains of bacteria that are resistant to other drugs in the tetracycline class. Hepatic function laboratory values should be monitored during therapy to assess for hepatotoxicity. Other adverse effects and contraindications are the same as those of other tetracyclines. A microsphere powder formulation, called Arestin, is introduced subgingivally to treat periodontitis. Solodyn, an extended-release tablet, is approved for the treatment of inflammatory lesions associated with moderate to severe acne vulgaris in patients over 12 years of age. Several other formulations are available for the management of rosacea and acne (see Chapter 73).

Omadacycline (Nuzyra): Approved in 2018, omadacycline is indicated for the PO or IV management of bacterial pneumonia and skin and skin structure infections. Because the oral absorption of this drug is greatly diminished by fatty food, the patient should be advised to fast for 4 hours before taking the medication and for 2 hours afterward. No dairy products, antacids, or multivitamins should be consumed for 4 hours after an oral dose. The novel chemical structure of omadacycline confers better activity against strains that show resistance to other drugs in this class. It also causes less nausea and vomiting, which can be dose-limiting adverse effects with some of the tetracyclines.

Sarecycline (Seysara): Sarecycline was approved in 2018 for the management of moderate to severe inflammatory acne in patients ages 9 and above. Given PO, the manufacturer recommends a maximum of 1 year of therapy. Unlike other tetracyclines, sarecycline has a narrow spectrum that causes less disruption of the intestinal and vaginal microbiomes, which may result in fewer adverse effects such as diarrhea and candidiasis.

Tigecycline (Tygacil): Approved in 2005, tigecycline is available only by the IV route, it has more limited indications than other drugs in this class: complicated skin and skin structure infections, complicated intra-abdominal infections, and community-acquired bacterial pneumonia. Tigecycline is effective against certain bacterial strains resistant to other antibiotics, including methicillin-resistant *Staphylococcus aureus* (MRSA) and vancomycin-resistant enterococci (VRE). Nausea and vomiting are the most frequent adverse effects, and these may be severe enough to cause discontinuation of therapy. Life-threatening anaphylaxis and pancreatitis have been reported. Other adverse effects and contraindications are the same as those of other tetracyclines. Hepatic function laboratory values should be monitored during therapy to assess for hepatotoxicity. Tigecycline carries a black box warning that the drug is associated with an increased mortality risk and that its use should be reserved for infections not responsive to other anti-infectives.

PharmFACT

The bubonic plague caused by the bacterium *Yersinia pestis* was responsible for killing approximately 50% of the population during the 5th and 6th centuries AD, and 40% of the population between the 8th and 14th centuries. The plague still occurs sporadically, especially in Africa, but does not cause the same degree of mortality as in past centuries (Dufel, 2015).

Macrolides

48.3 The macrolides are alternatives to penicillin for many gram-positive infections.

Erythromycin (EryC, Erythrocin, others), the first macrolide antibiotic, was isolated from *Streptomyces* organisms in a soil sample in 1952. The name *macrolide* was chosen for this drug class because they all possess an unusually large 14- to 15-atom ring as part of their chemical structure. Doses for the macrolides are listed in Table 48.2.

Macrolides are considered alternative drugs for patients who are allergic to penicillin. They are widely prescribed, although they are the preferred drugs for relatively few diseases. Most effective against gram-positive bacteria, common indications for macrolides include the treatment of whooping cough, diphtheria, Legionnaire's disease, and infections by streptococci, *Haemophilus influenzae*, *Mycoplasma pneumoniae*, and chlamydia. Clarithromycin is one of several antibiotics used to treat peptic ulcer disease due to its activity against *H. pylori* (see Chapter 59). The macrolides are first-line drugs for the prophylaxis of recurring rheumatic fever in patients who are allergic to penicillins. Fidaxomicin (Dificid) is approved for treatment of *C. difficile*–associated diarrhea (CDAD).

The macrolides inhibit bacterial protein synthesis by binding to the 50S ribosomal subunit, thus preventing movement of the ribosome along the mRNA. Macrolides do not bind to human ribosomes, thus offering a degree of selective toxicity. These drugs are usually bacteriostatic, though they may be bactericidal depending on the dose and the target organism.

The newer macrolides have a longer half-life and generally cause less GI irritation than erythromycin, which is the original drug from which macrolides were synthesized. Azithromycin (Zithromax) has an extended half-life such that it can be administered for only 5 days rather than the 10-day therapy required for most antibiotics. A single dose of azithromycin is effective against *N. gonorrhoeae*. The brief duration of therapy increases patient adherence.

Like most of the older antibiotics, macrolide-resistant strains are becoming more common. Many microbes develop resistance to macrolides by pumping them out of the cell before the antibiotic has a chance to reach an

Table 48.2 Macrolides

Drug	Route and Adult Dose (Maximum Dose Where Indicated)	Adverse Effects
azithromycin (Zithromax)	PO (Zithromax): 500 mg for 1 dose, then 250 mg/day for 4 days PO (Zmax): 2 g single dose	*Nausea and vomiting, diarrhea, abdominal cramping, dry skin or burning (topical route)* <u>Anaphylaxis, ototoxicity, PMC, hepatotoxicity, superinfections, dysrhythmias</u>
clarithromycin	PO (regular release): 250–500 mg bid PO (extended release): 1000 mg once daily	
erythromycin (EryC, Erythrocin, others)	PO: 250–500 mg bid or 333 mg tid	
fidaxomicin (Dificid)	PO: 200 mg bid for 10 days	*Nausea and vomiting, abdominal pain* <u>GI bleeding, anemia, neutropenia, anaphylaxis</u>

Note: *Italics* indicate common adverse effects. <u>Underline</u> indicates serious adverse effects.

effective concentration. In some cases, bacteria have modified the shape of their 50S ribosomal subunit so that it no longer binds the drug.

The macrolides are well tolerated and considered to be one of the safest antibiotic classes. The most common adverse effects are GI related and include nausea and vomiting, abdominal cramping, and diarrhea. These GI symptoms occur whether the drug is administered PO or IV. Taking the drug with food can significantly inhibit absorption; thus, these drugs should be taken on an empty stomach.

Many macrolides have an enteric coating, which serves two purposes. First, the coating allows the drug to dissolve in the small intestine rather than the stomach, causing less gastric irritation. Second, the macrolides are inactivated in gastric acid, and the enteric coating allows it to avoid destruction and reach the small intestine where they are readily absorbed in the alkaline environment.

Macrolides are metabolized and concentrated in the liver and excreted into bile. Because macrolides decrease the hepatic metabolism of other drugs, a number of drug–drug interactions are possible. When macrolides prevent the conversion of drugs to their less active form, the serum levels of these other drugs will increase and cause potential toxicity. For example, warfarin (Coumadin) is extensively metabolized to its inactive form in the liver. If given concurrently with erythromycin, the destruction of warfarin is diminished and greater amounts of "active" warfarin remain in the blood for longer periods. Because warfarin increases bleeding time, this could result in prolonged bleeding in a patient. In general, doses of drugs that are metabolized in the liver should be reduced, or at least carefully monitored, if they are given concurrently with macrolides.

CONNECTION Checkpoint 48.1

From what you learned in Chapter 38, what type of laboratory monitoring should be done for a patient who is taking warfarin concurrently with a macrolide?

PROTOTYPE DRUG Erythromycin (EryC, Erythrocin, Others)

Classification **Therapeutic:** Antibacterial
Pharmacologic: Bacterial protein synthesis inhibitor, macrolide

Therapeutic Effects and Uses: Erythromycin (called erythromycin base) is indicated for the treatment and prophylaxis of susceptible bacterial infections. The main application for erythromycin is for patients who are allergic to penicillins or who may have a penicillin-resistant infection. It has a spectrum similar to that of the penicillins and is effective against most gram-positive bacteria, including susceptible strains of *Staphylococcus* and *Streptococcus*. Susceptible gram-negative strains include *N. gonorrhoeae* and *H. influenzae*. It is a first-line drug for infections from *Bordetella pertussis* (whooping cough), *Legionella pneumophila* (Legionnaire's disease), *M. pneumoniae*, and *Corynebacterium diphtheriae*.

All oral forms of erythromycin are considered to have equal effectiveness. Topical and ophthalmic formulations are also available. Erythromycin is available in a number of salts:

- Erythromycin stearate and erythromycin ethylsuccinate (EryPed) are acid stable and more readily absorbed in the stomach than erythromycin base. These forms are converted to the base form in the liver before they become bacteriostatic. The stearate salt should be taken on an empty stomach, whereas the ethylsuccinate salt may be taken without regard to food.
- Erythromycin lactobionate is given IV when the patient is unable to take oral medications, or when the infection is severe enough to warrant a faster onset of action.

Mechanism of Action: Erythromycin inhibits bacterial protein synthesis by binding to the 50S ribosomal subunit. Erythromycin is considered bacteriostatic but may be bactericidal in high doses.

Pharmacokinetics:

Route(s)	PO, topical, IV
Absorption	Readily absorbed PO; enteric coated
Distribution	Widely distributed; only small amounts cross the blood–brain barrier; secreted in breast milk
Primary metabolism	Hepatic metabolism (CYP3A); concentrates in the liver and bile
Primary excretion	Bile
Onset of action	1 h
Duration of action	Half-life: 1.5–2 h

Adverse Effects: The most common adverse effects from erythromycin are nausea and vomiting and abdominal cramping, although these are rarely serious enough to cause discontinuation of therapy. Concurrent administration with food reduces these adverse effects. When given by the IV route, phlebitis and intense pain at the injection site are common. Anaphylaxis is possible. Hearing loss, vertigo, and dizziness may be experienced when using high doses, particularly in older adults and in those with impaired hepatic or renal excretion. High doses of IV erythromycin may be cardiotoxic and pose a risk for torsades de pointes, which is a type of dysrhythmia that is potentially fatal. Like nearly all other antibiotics, PMC is possible with the use of erythromycin.

Contraindications/Precautions: Erythromycin is contraindicated in patients with hypersensitivity to drugs in the macrolide class and for those who are taking terfenadine, astemizole, or cisapride. Drug therapy must be monitored carefully in patients with impaired hepatic or biliary function, due to the possibility of **cholestatic hepatitis**, a type of liver inflammation caused by obstruction of the bile ducts. Because macrolides have been shown to prolong the QT interval, erythromycin should be used with caution in patients with known prolongation of the QTc interval, a history of torsades de pointes, bradydysrhythmias, or uncompensated heart failure.

Drug Interactions: Erythromycin inhibits hepatic CYP450 metabolic enzymes and can interact with many drugs. When used concurrently with erythromycin, the serum levels and toxicities of alfentanil, carbamazepine, cyclosporine, fentanyl, estradiol, and methadone may increase. Because erythromycin may increase the effects of digoxin or warfarin, leading to abnormal bleeding, the doses of these anticoagulants may need to be lowered. Erythromycin should not be taken with clarithromycin because both drugs increase the QTc interval. The concurrent use of erythromycin with lovastatin or simvastatin is contraindicated because it increases the risk of myopathy and rhabdomyolysis. Because fluconazole also inhibits CYP3A4, especially at high dosages, its concurrent use with erythromycin is contraindicated. **Herbal/Food:** Grapefruit juice may increase the bioavailability of erythromycin.

Pregnancy: Erythromycin did not show evidence of significant fetal harm in laboratory animals. Human observational studies suggest there may be a risk for cardiovascular, GI, and urinary malformations when taken during the first trimester. This drug is secreted in human milk and breastfed neonates should be observed for irritability, diarrhea, and candidiasis.

Treatment of Overdose: No specific therapy is available. Patients are treated symptomatically.

Clinician Responsibilities: Key clinical implications for patients receiving erythromycin are included in Applied Clinical Judgment: Patients Receiving Pharmacotherapy with a Tetracycline, Macrolide, or Aminoglycoside Antibiotic.

Drugs Similar to Erythromycin (EryC, Erythrocin, Others)

Other macrolides include azithromycin, clarithromycin, and fidaxomicin. The macrolide dirithromycin (Dynabac) is no longer available in the United States.

Azithromycin (Zithromax): Approved in 1991, azithromycin has a long duration of action that allows for less frequent dosing. A "Tri-pak" consists of three 500-mg tablets (taken over 3 days) and a "Z-pak" contains six 250-mg tablets (taken over 5 days). For acute otitis media in children, a single dose has been found to be as effective as 3- or 5-day regimens. An IV form for infusions is available for the treatment of pelvic inflammatory disease and community-acquired pneumonia. An ophthalmic solution (AzaSite) is available for treating bacterial conjunctivitis. Azithromycin demonstrates greater activity over gram-negative organisms than erythromycin.

Azithromycin causes less nausea than erythromycin and may be taken with or without food. The extended-release oral suspension should be administered on an empty stomach. Serious and sometimes fatal hepatotoxicity has been reported and liver function tests should be monitored during therapy. The most common adverse effects are diarrhea, nausea, and abdominal pain. Azithromycin has been shown to prolong the QTc interval, which can increase the risk of cardiac dysrhythmia, especially when used in patients with known prolongation of the QTc interval, a history of torsades de pointes, bradydysrhythmias, or uncompensated heart failure. Patients with a known hypersensitivity to any macrolide should not receive azithromycin. Studies in laboratory animals showed no evidence of significant fetal harm. This drug is secreted in human breast milk and breastfed neonates should be observed for irritability, diarrhea and candidiasis.

Clarithromycin: Approved in 1991, clarithromycin is similar to erythromycin but causes significantly less nausea, and the regular-release tablets may be taken with or without food. The drug is commonly prescribed for infections of the respiratory tract, sexually transmitted infections, *H. pylori*–associated peptic ulcer disease, and otitis media. An extended-release (XL) formulation is used to treat sinusitis, chronic bronchitis, and community-acquired pneumonia. The XL form should be administered with food because this increases its absorption. The most frequent adverse effects with clarithromycin are diarrhea, nausea, abnormal taste, dyspepsia, abdominal discomfort, and headache. Like erythromycin, clarithromycin is metabolized by CYP450 enzymes and a significant number of drug–drug interactions may occur. Patients with a known hypersensitivity to any macrolide should not receive clarithromycin. Animal studies showed fetal harm and human epidemiological studies suggest evidence for increased spontaneous abortions when taken during the first trimester. This drug is secreted in human milk and breastfed neonates should be observed for irritability, diarrhea, and candidiasis. Clarithromycin should not be used during pregnancy unless the potential benefits to the mother justify the potential risks to the fetus or neonate.

Fidaxomicin (Dificid): Fidaxomicin was approved in 2011 specifically for infections proven or strongly suspected to be caused by *C. difficile*. The drug should be prescribed only for this indication because other uses could encourage the development of resistant strains. Taken as an oral tablet, the drug is not significantly absorbed and remains in the digestive tract where it produces its effects on *C. difficile*. Fidaxomicin appears to have equal efficacy to vancomycin, the primary antibiotic used to treat CDAD. Relapses are less frequent than with vancomycin. The drug is well tolerated, with the most frequent adverse effects being nausea and vomiting, abdominal pain, and GI bleeding. Animal studies did not show evidence of embryofetal toxicity. It is not known if this drug is secreted in milk or has any adverse effects on the breastfed neonate.

Aminoglycosides

48.4 The aminoglycosides are effective against aerobic gram-negative organisms but have the potential to cause ototoxicity and nephrotoxicity.

The first aminoglycoside, streptomycin, was named after *Streptomyces griseus*, the soil organism from which it was isolated in 1943. Once widely used, streptomycin is now reserved for the treatment of tuberculosis (TB) due to the development of safer alternatives and the appearance of a large number of resistant strains. Other aminoglycosides have since been isolated, and several have been produced semisynthetically. All have a common chemical structure of two or more amino sugars with a glycosidic, or sugar, link. The differences in spelling of some of these drugs, *-mycin* and *-micin*, reflects the different organisms from which the drugs were originally isolated. Doses for the aminoglycosides are listed in Table 48.3.

Aminoglycosides bind irreversibly to the 30S ribosomal subunit of bacteria, changing its shape and preventing the initiation stage of protein synthesis. Some drugs in this class also affect the 50S subunit. In addition, these antibiotics cause mRNA to be read incorrectly, resulting in abnormal proteins that are subsequently inserted into the bacterial plasma membrane, causing it to leak. Whereas most antibiotics that affect protein synthesis are bacteriostatic, aminoglycosides are bactericidal.

Although they have the ability to kill many different bacterial species, the aminoglycosides are considered narrow-spectrum drugs because they are normally reserved for serious systemic infections caused by aerobic gram-negative organisms, such as *Pseudomonas* and members of the Enterobacteriaceae family, which includes *E. coli*, *Serratia*, *Proteus*, and *Klebsiella*. Aminoglycosides are ineffective against most gram-positive bacteria. Because oxygen is required for aminoglycoside antibiotics to be transported inside bacterial cells, this class of drugs is ineffective against anaerobes.

Table 48.3 Aminoglycosides

Drug	Route and Adult Dose (Maximum Dose Where Indicated)	Adverse Effects
amikacin (Arikayce)	IV/IM: 5–7.5 mg/kg as a loading dose, then 7.5 mg/kg bid Inhalation (Arikayce): 590 mg (one vial) daily	*Pain or inflammation at the injection site, rash, fever, nausea, diarrhea, dizziness, tinnitus* Anaphylaxis, nephrotoxicity, irreversible ototoxicity, superinfections
gentamicin	IV/IM: 1.5–2 mg/kg as a loading dose, then 1–2 mg/kg bid–tid	
neomycin	PO: 4–12 g/day in divided doses	
paromomycin	PO: 7.5–12.5 mg/kg tid	
plazomicin (Zemdri)	IV: 15–20 mg given over 30 minutes once daily	
streptomycin	IM: 15 mg/kg up to 1 g as a single dose	
tobramycin (Tobrex)	IV/IM: 1 mg/kg tid (max: 5 mg/kg/day)	

Note: *Italics* indicate common adverse effects. Underline indicates serious adverse effects.

Most aminoglycosides are polar compounds that are poorly absorbed from the GI tract. Less than 1% of an oral dose is absorbed; therefore, they must be administered parenterally to treat systemic infections. Because aminoglycosides travel through the alimentary canal unchanged, they are occasionally given PO to sterilize the bowel prior to intestinal surgery. Neomycin is available for topical infections of the skin, eyes, and ears. Paromomycin is given PO for the treatment of parasitic infections.

Due to their polar nature, aminoglycosides are unable to enter most human cells. Although distributed to most body fluids, not enough of the drugs enter the cerebrospinal fluid (CSF) for them to treat central nervous system infections. Aminoglycosides can, however, cross the placenta. If taken late in pregnancy, streptomycin can cause hearing loss in the child. In addition, aminoglycosides concentrate in renal tissue, which leads to potential nephrotoxicity.

Resistance develops quickly when aminoglycosides are administered as monotherapy. Resistance occurs when a species acquires an ability to degrade the antibiotic. Once degraded by the bacterial enzymes, these drugs are unable to bind with the bacterial ribosome. Some resistance also occurs when mutations change the shape of the bacterial ribosome so that it no longer binds the aminoglycoside. The emergence of aminoglycoside-resistant strains of *Enterococcus faecalis* and *Enterococcus faecium* has become a serious clinical problem because there are few therapeutic alternatives to treat these infections. Once resistance develops to an aminoglycoside, the mutant strain of infection is usually resistant to the other drugs in this class. An exception is amikacin, which appears to act against gentamicin-resistant strains.

Several techniques have been used to increase the effectiveness of the aminoglycosides. Administering these drugs in one large dose per day rather than smaller divided doses results in a greater bactericidal effect and fewer resistant microbes. A second technique is to administer aminoglycosides and penicillins concurrently (though not mixed in the same IV solution). The penicillin weakens the cell wall, allowing a greater amount of aminoglycoside to enter and reach its ribosomal targets.

Aminoglycosides are excreted almost exclusively by the kidneys. Because certain tissues bind the drugs very tightly, renal excretion may be prolonged up to 20 days after discontinuation of the drug. Although serum drug levels may fall below what is considered a minimally effective concentration, some antimicrobial activity continues during this time. This is known as a **postantibiotic effect**.

The clinical applications of the aminoglycosides are limited by their potential to cause serious adverse effects. The degree and types of toxicity are similar for all drugs in this class. For example, all aminoglycosides can impair both hearing and balance. Damage to sensory cells in the cochlea causes hearing loss. Balance is affected by damage to sensory cells in the vestibular apparatus of the inner ear. As many as 25% of patients who are taking aminoglycoside antibiotics may experience some ototoxicity. This effect is more prominent when the medications are used for longer than 10 days, or when the patient has preexisting kidney impairment, causing high serum drug levels. The damage to sensory cells is cumulative; repeated doses of the drug can damage increasing numbers of cells. Because many older adults have some degree of preexisting hearing impairment, permanent deafness may occur in this group. Signs of impending inner ear damage include high-pitched tinnitus, headache, nausea and vomiting, and vertigo. Signs of ototoxicity may continue for several weeks after the drugs are discontinued. If hearing and balance functions are not carefully monitored during therapy and proper interventions are not implemented, the ototoxicity may become irreversible.

One of the most serious adverse effects of aminoglycosides is nephrotoxicity. Aminoglycosides directly injure renal tubule cells, and this nephrotoxicity may be severe, affecting up to 26% of patients receiving these antibiotics. As expected, patients who are receiving higher doses for longer periods are most affected. Those with CKD or who are receiving concurrent therapy with other nephrotoxic drugs must be monitored carefully: Regular evaluation of urinalysis, blood urea nitrogen (BUN), and serum creatinine results is essential. Serum drug concentrations should be obtained regularly and doses adjusted accordingly to prevent permanent damage. If recognized early, renal damage caused by aminoglycosides is reversible. Impaired kidney function may cause drug serum levels to rise, thus increasing the risk or worsening of ototoxicity.

A less common though serious adverse effect of aminoglycosides is neuromuscular blockade. Aminoglycosides inhibit the release of acetylcholine at synapses. Giving other drugs that affect acetylcholine release, such as anesthetics or neuromuscular blockers (see Chapter 26), can result in profound apnea and prolonged muscle paralysis. Because they have fewer acetylcholine receptors, patients with myasthenia gravis are especially at risk. To avoid the problem, aminoglycosides may be discontinued prior to surgery. IV calcium salts have been found to reverse aminoglycoside-induced neuromuscular blockade.

CONNECTION Checkpoint 48.2

From what you learned in Chapter 14, name the prototype drugs classified as neuromuscular blockers. Is muscle paralysis occurring at a nicotinic or muscarinic synapse?

PROTOTYPE DRUG Gentamicin

Classification **Therapeutic:** Antibacterial
Pharmacologic: Bacterial protein synthesis inhibitor, aminoglycoside

Therapeutic Effects and Uses: Approved in 1966, gentamicin is used for the treatment and prophylaxis of susceptible bacterial infections. It is prescribed primarily for serious infections caused by aerobic, gram-negative bacilli. Activity includes *Enterobacter*, *E. coli*, *Klebsiella*, *Citrobacter*, *Pseudomonas*, and *Serratia*. Gentamicin is effective against a few gram-positive bacteria, including some strains of MRSA. It has no activity against anaerobes. This drug is not absorbed by the PO route. A topical formulation (Genoptic) is available for infections of the external eye. Ointments and creams are available for minor skin infections.

Therapy with parenteral gentamicin is generally limited to those cases in which a less toxic alternative is not available. Resistance to gentamicin is increasing, and some patients show cross-resistance to other aminoglycosides such as tobramycin. Gentamicin is sometimes given concurrently with a beta-lactam antibiotic such as a penicillin or cephalosporin to improve bacterial kill and to delay resistance.

Mechanism of Action: Gentamicin inhibits bacterial protein synthesis by binding to the 30S ribosomal subunit. Gentamicin is bactericidal in that it causes premature termination of the growing polypeptide chain.

Pharmacokinetics:

Route(s)	Intramuscular (IM), IV, topical (ophthalmic)
Absorption	Not absorbed PO; readily absorbed IM
Distribution	Distributed to most body tissues and fluids, except the CSF; concentrates in the kidney and inner ear; crosses the placenta; small amounts secreted in breast milk
Primary metabolism	Not metabolized
Primary excretion	Renal
Onset of action	Rapid
Duration of action	Half-life: 3–4 h

Adverse Effects: Resistance to gentamicin is increasing and some cross-resistance among aminoglycosides has been reported. Rash, nausea and vomiting, and fatigue are the most common adverse effects. **Black Box Warnings:** Adverse effects from parenteral gentamicin may be severe and include the following:

- Neurotoxicity may manifest as ototoxicity and produce a loss of hearing or balance, which may become permanent with continued use. Tinnitus, vertigo, and persistent headaches are early signs of ototoxicity. The risk of neurologic effects is higher in patients with CKD. Other signs of neurotoxicity include paresthesias, muscle twitching, and seizures. Concurrent use with other neurotoxic drugs should be avoided.
- Neuromuscular blockade and respiratory paralysis are possible, and the drug may cause severe neuromuscular weakness that lasts for several days.
- Nephrotoxicity is possible. Signs of reduced kidney function include oliguria, proteinuria, and elevated BUN and creatinine levels. Nephrotoxicity is of particular concern to patients with preexisting kidney disease and may limit pharmacotherapy. Concurrent use with other nephrotoxic drugs should be avoided.

Contraindications/Precautions: Gentamicin is contraindicated in patients who are hypersensitive to aminoglycosides. Drug therapy must be monitored carefully in patients with CKD or in those with preexisting hearing loss. Gentamicin should not be used in pregnant or breastfeeding patients.

Drug Interactions: Concurrent use with other nephrotoxic drugs such as acyclovir, amphotericin B, capreomycin, cisplatin, cyclosporine, salicylates, polymyxin B, or vancomycin increases the risk of nephrotoxicity. Other drugs affecting the eighth cranial nerve such as ethacrynic acid and furosemide will increase the risk of ototoxicity if given concurrently with gentamicin. Penicillins can inactivate aminoglycosides if they are mixed together in the same solution. Antiemetics such as dimenhydrinate, meclizine, promethazine, and scopolamine may block the nausea characteristic of vestibular toxicity or motion sickness, thus masking the signs of aminoglycoside-induced ototoxicity. **Herbal/Food:** No significant interactions are known.

Pregnancy: Parenteral use of gentamicin may cause fetal harm in humans, including potential ototoxicity and nephrotoxicity. Because small amounts of this drug are secreted in human milk, caution should be used when breastfeeding. Gentamicin should not be used during pregnancy unless the potential benefits to the mother justify the potential risks to the fetus or neonate.

Treatment of Overdose: Overdose can result in serious kidney damage and ototoxicity. No specific therapy is available. Patients are treated symptomatically.

Clinician Responsibilities: Key clinical implications for patients receiving gentamicin are included in Applied Clinical Judgment: Patients Receiving Pharmacotherapy with a Tetracycline, Macrolide, or Aminoglycoside Antibiotic.

Drugs Similar to Gentamicin

Other aminoglycosides include amikacin, neomycin, paromomycin, plazomicin, streptomycin, and tobramycin. Kanamycin is no longer available in the United States. All aminoglycosides have similar spectrums of activity and adverse effects. Systemic forms carry similar black box warnings and pregnancy recommendations as gentamicin.

Amikacin: Approved in 1976, amikacin has the broadest spectrum in this class and is sometimes effective against organisms that have developed resistance to other aminoglycosides. Amikacin has been used to treat multidrug-resistant TB. It is administered by the IV and IM routes. Indications, contraindications, and adverse effects (including the black box warning) are nearly the same as those for gentamicin. In 2018, amikacin liposomal (Arikayce) was approved to treat Mycobacterium avium complex lung disease. Given by nebulizer, Arikayce carries an additional black box warning that the drug may cause pneumonitis, bronchospasm, worsening of underlying lung disease, and hemoptysis.

Neomycin: Approved in 1952, neomycin is widely used for topical infections as an over-the-counter (OTC) ointment combined with polymyxin B and bacitracin (Neosporin). It is also combined in OTC creams with hydrocortisone for minor skin irritations and insect bites. Not available in parenteral form due to its toxicity, neomycin may be used orally to sterilize the bowel. Oral neomycin can cause headache, lethargy, and nausea and vomiting.

Paromomycin: Approved in 1959, paromomycin is most active against gram-negative aerobic bacteria (with the exception of *Pseudomonas*). When administered PO, the drug is not absorbed and 100% is recovered in the feces. The primary use of this drug is for sterilizing the bowel and treating intestinal parasitic infections caused by protozoans and tapeworms. Because this drug is not absorbed systemically, it does not carry the same pregnancy warnings and black box warnings as other aminoglycosides.

Plazomicin (Zemdri): Plazomicin is an aminoglycoside approved in 2018 to treat complicated urinary tract infections that are often resistant to other antibiotics. Plazomicin has a novel chemical structure that increases its effectiveness against resistant microbes. It is administered by IV infusion over 4 to 7 days. The most common adverse reactions are reduced kidney function, hypertension (HTN), headache, and nausea and vomiting.

Streptomycin: The use of streptomycin, the first aminoglycoside approved in 1945, has been greatly reduced since 1993. It is rarely used due to a large number of resistant strains and its high risk for ototoxicity. It is most often used in combination with other drugs in the pharmacotherapy of multidrug-resistant TB.

Tobramycin (Tobrex): Approved in 1975, tobramycin has a spectrum of activity similar to that of gentamicin, but it is more effective against *P. aeruginosa* than gentamicin. Most often administered parenterally, tobramycin is also available as an ophthalmic solution (Aktob, Tobrex) and in nebulizer form (TOBI) for patients with cystic fibrosis who have *Pseudomonas* infections. Tobradex is an ophthalmic suspension combing tobramycin with dexamethasone for treating inflammatory bacterial infection of the external eye. Adverse effects of parenteral formulations (including the black box warning) and contraindications are similar to those of gentamicin.

PharmFACT

This chapter discusses antibiotics selective for bacterial protein synthesis. However, bacteria can fight back. *C. diphtheriae* produces a toxin that targets *human* protein synthesis and is so potent that a single molecule can kill a human cell (Madigan et al., 2018).

Miscellaneous Inhibitors of Bacterial Protein Synthesis

48.5 Several inhibitors of protein synthesis are effective against resistant infections but may have significant adverse effects that limit their use.

Several bacterial protein synthesis inhibitors do not belong to the tetracycline, macrolide, or aminoglycoside classes. These miscellaneous drugs, listed in Table 48.4, have varying spectrums of activity and adverse effect profiles and are considered individually.

Chloramphenicol: Chloramphenicol is an older, broad-spectrum antibiotic that was approved in 1960. It binds to the 50S subunit of the bacterial ribosome and may be bacteriostatic or bactericidal, depending on species and dose. Administered IV for serious infections, chloramphenicol is effective in treating salmonellae, rickettsiae, streptococci, typhoid fever, and meningitis caused by *H. influenzae*. This drug was widely used before it was found to be associated with bone marrow suppression and a small, though fatal, incidence of aplastic anemia. Chloramphenicol carries a black box warning that serious and fatal blood dyscrasias have been reported with the drug. Peak and trough serum levels should be monitored regularly during therapy to avoid serious adverse effects. Chloramphenicol is now reserved for meningitis and other infections in which the benefits of the drug may justify the risks of serious drug toxicity.

Another serious toxicity from chloramphenicol is **gray baby syndrome**. Most often seen in preterm or newborn infants, this syndrome occurs when the baby's liver is unable to metabolize or excrete this drug. Symptoms include failure to feed, abdominal distention, cyanosis, and cardiovascular collapse. The syndrome is rapidly fatal and can cause death in just a few hours. If done early, discontinuing chloramphenicol therapy can reverse the syndrome. This drug should only be taken during pregnancy if the potential benefits to the mother justify the risks to the fetus or neonate.

Clindamycin (Cleocin, others): Approved in 1970, clindamycin acts on the 50S bacterial ribosomal subunit in

Table 48.4 Miscellaneous Inhibitors of Bacterial Protein Synthesis

Drug	Route and Adult Dose (Maximum Dose Where Indicated)	Adverse Effects
chloramphenicol	IV: 50 mg/kg/day divided q6h	*Nausea, and vomiting, diarrhea* Anaphylaxis, superinfections, pancytopenia, bone marrow depression, aplastic anemia
clindamycin (Cleocin, others)	PO: 150–450 mg qid IV: 600–1200 mg/day in divided doses	*Nausea and vomiting, diarrhea, rash, burning, pruritus (topical forms)* Anaphylaxis, superinfections, cardiac arrest, PMC, blood dyscrasias
lefamulin (Xenleta)	PO: 600 mg bid IV: 150 mg given over 60 min bid	*Diarrhea, nausea, injection site reactions, elevated hepatic enzymes* Embryo-fetal toxicity, QTc prolongation
lincomycin (Lincocin)	IM: 600 mg q12–24h (max: 8 g/day)	*Nausea, vomiting, diarrhea* Anaphylaxis, superinfections, cardiac arrest, PMC, blood dyscrasias
linezolid (Zyvox)	IV: 600 mg q12h (max: 1200 mg/day)	*Nausea and diarrhea, headache* Anaphylaxis, superinfections, PMC, blood dyscrasias
quinupristin-dalfopristin (Synercid)	IV: 7.5 mg/kg infused over 60 min q8h	*Pain and inflammation at the injection site, myalgia, arthralgia, diarrhea* Superinfections, PMC
tedizolid (Sivextro)	PO/IV: 200 mg once daily	*Nausea and vomiting, headache, diarrhea, dizziness* Anemia, hypersensitivity, CDAD

Note: *Italics* indicate common adverse effects. Underline indicates serious adverse effects.

a manner similar to that of the macrolides. It is usually bacteriostatic. A first-line drug for abdominal infections caused by *Bacteroides fragilis*, it is also effective against *Fusobacterium*, *Actinomyces*, and *Clostridium*.

Three salts of clindamycin are available: clindamycin hydrochloride (PO), clindamycin palmitate (PO), and clindamycin phosphate (parenteral or topical). The topical form of clindamycin is available as a gel, lotion, or foam for the treatment of acne vulgaris. A single-dose suppository vaginal cream (Clindesse) is approved for bacterial vaginosis.

Once widely prescribed as a penicillin alternative, the use of clindamycin is now limited due to the development of resistant strains, a high incidence of diarrhea, and a potential risk of drug-induced PMC caused by *C. difficile*, which can be fatal (black box warning). It is generally used only when safer alternatives are not effective. Patients must be instructed to immediately report incidences of diarrhea during therapy. If PMC is suspected, clindamycin is discontinued and the patient is placed on a drug that is effective against *C. difficile* such as vancomycin. When given either IV or PO during the first trimester of pregnancy, clindamycin was associated with an increased incidence of congenital malformations. Because this drug is secreted in human milk and has the potential to cause adverse effects on the neonate, breastfeeding is not recommended. No pregnancy or lactation information is available on the topical forms of the drug.

Lefamulin (Xenleta): Approved in 2019, lefamulin is indicated for the treatment of community-acquired bacterial pneumonia. Lefamulin may be given by the oral or IV route, with diarrhea, nausea, injection site reactions, and elevated hepatic enzymes being the most common adverse effects. Caution should be used if given concurrently with other medications that prolong the QTc interval. Animal studies showed that lefamulin may be embryofetal toxic. Because this drug is secreted in milk, breastfeeding is not recommended. Females with childbearing potential should have a pregnancy test prior to starting therapy and use effective contraception during therapy and for 2 days after discontinuing the drug.

Lincomycin (Lincocin): Approved in 1964, lincomycin is chemically similar to clindamycin. Lincomycin may be used for patients who cannot take penicillins or cephalosporins, but it offers no therapeutic advantages over clindamycin. The drug is rarely prescribed due to a relatively high incidence of serious adverse effects, especially PMC (black box warning). It is available by parenteral routes. Animal studies showed no evidence of fetal harm. Because lincomycin is secreted in human milk, breastfeeding is not recommended.

Linezolid (Zyvox): Approved in 2000, linezolid is in a class of antibiotics called oxazolidinones that act by binding to the bacterial 50S ribosome at the 23S portion. Oxazolidinones are unique among antibiotics in that they prevent the first event in protein synthesis, which is the formation of an initiation complex. Linezolid is believed to be bactericidal. Linezolid is important because it is effective against infections that have become resistant to most other antibiotics, including MRSA and VRE. It is less effective against gram-negative organisms. Oral and IV formulations are available.

Adverse effects are usually minor and related to GI distress. Because this drug can cause transient dose-related myelosuppression, laboratory blood counts should be frequently monitored during therapy. Linezolid is a nonselective inhibitor of monoamine oxidase (MAO) and may cause HTN in some patients. Risk for HTN and palpitations is increased if the patient is taking sympathomimetics concurrently with linezolid; thus, these medications should be avoided. Patients with diabetes should be cautioned about possible hypoglycemic events while taking linezolid. Animal studies showed that linezolid is embryofetal toxic at high doses. Because this drug is secreted in milk, caution should be used if breastfeeding and the infant should be monitored for diarrhea and vomiting.

Quinupristin-dalfopristin (Synercid): Approved in 1999, quinupristin-dalfopristin is a fixed-dose bactericidal combination used for therapy of life-threatening *E. faecium* infections that are vancomycin resistant and for complicated infections caused by MRSA or *Streptococcus pyogenes*. It belongs to a class of antibiotics called *streptogramins* that act by binding the 50S bacterial ribosome in a manner similar to that of the macrolides. The combination of the two antibiotics is truly synergistic: The combination has 16 times more antimicrobial activity compared to either drug used alone. Synercid is bactericidal and only available by the IV route.

Joint and muscle pain, diarrhea, rash, and pain at the infusion site are common adverse effects. Venous irritation may be severe. Synercid inhibits hepatic drug metabolism enzymes, resulting in numerous drug–drug interactions. The nurse should use caution when administering drugs concurrently with Synercid because those that rely on hepatic metabolism for detoxification may build to toxic levels in the blood. In addition, some cases of PMC have been reported. Quinupristin-dalfopristin carries a black box warning that it should be reserved for serious or life-threatening vancomycin-resistant *E. faecium* infections. Despite its potential for adverse effects, quinupristin-dalfopristin serves an important role in treating multidrug-resistant gram-positive pathogens, which have become a major clinical challenge. Animal studies did not show evidence of fetal harm. This drug is secreted in milk but adverse effects on the breastfed neonate are unknown.

Tedizolid (Sivextro): Like linezolid, tedizolid is a member of the oxazolidinone class that binds to and inhibits the 50S bacterial ribosome. Tedizolid was approved in 2014 for the treatment of skin and skin structure infections, including MRSA strains, *Streptococcus* strains, and *E. faecalis*. Available IV or PO, the drug is well tolerated, with nausea and vomiting and GI complaints being the most common side effects. Animal studies showed tedizolid to be fetotoxic. This drug is secreted in milk but adverse effects on the breastfed neonate are unknown.

CONNECTIONS: APPLIED CLINICAL JUDGMENT

Patients Receiving Pharmacotherapy with a Tetracycline, Macrolide, or Aminoglycoside Antibiotic

Key Assessment Data

- History of current condition, baseline vital signs, physical exam findings; hepatic, renal, cardiovascular, neurologic, or respiratory disease; pregnancy or breastfeeding. Obtain a drug history and assess signs and symptoms of the current infection, noting location, characteristics, presence or absence and the character of drainage, duration, and the presence or absence of fever or pain.
- Ongoing assessment during drug therapy should include monitoring appropriate laboratory findings (e.g., CBC, culture and sensitivity, hepatic and renal laboratory values); assess for infections, especially with opportunistic infections such as fungal infections.

Desired Therapeutic Outcomes

Improvement is observed and measurable by reduction in fever, pain, or signs and symptoms of infection, which should begin to diminish after taking the first dose and continue to improve throughout the course of antibiotic therapy.

Minimizing Adverse Effects

- Continued fever may be a sign of worsening infection, adverse drug effects, or antibiotic resistance. Immediately report undiminished fever, changes in level of consciousness (LOC).
- Anaphylactic reactions are possible, particularly with the first dose of an antibiotic. Residual drug levels, dependent on length of half-life, may cause delayed reactions up to 2 weeks after completing therapy.
- Superinfections with opportunistic organisms may occur when normal host flora are diminished or killed by the antibacterial drug. Severe diarrhea may indicate the presence of CDAD (*C. difficile*–associated diarrhea) PMC, or fungal or yeast infections.
- Esophagitis or esophageal ulceration may occur secondary to tetracycline use. Monitor for significant throat irritation.
- Erythromycin and some related drugs may prolong the QTc interval and increase the risk for potentially fatal dysrhythmias. Monitor electrolytes, pulse, and ECG, if indicated.
- Erythromycin and aminoglycosides have an increased risk of ototoxicity. Monitor for signs and symptoms (e.g., dizziness, vertigo, tinnitus, or diminished hearing).
- Tetracyclines may cause significant dermatologic effects including Stevens–Johnson syndrome. Monitor for dermatologic effects including red or purplish skin rash, blisters, or sunburn.

(continued)

CONNECTIONS: APPLIED CLINICAL JUDGMENT *(continued)*

Patients Receiving Pharmacotherapy with a Tetracycline, Macrolide, or Aminoglycoside Antibiotic

Lifespan Considerations

- Age-related physiologic differences may place the young child or older adult at greater risk for nephrotoxicity.
- Older adults may be at increased risk for dizziness related to adverse drug effects, which may increase the risk of falls. Ensure patient safety.
- Tetracyclines affect fetal bone growth and teeth development, causing permanent yellowish-brown staining of teeth. Tetracycline use in children under age 8 or 9 should be avoided.
- Erythromycin antibiotics may significantly reduce the effectiveness of oral contraceptives, and a secondary method to prevent conception should be used.

Diversity Considerations

- Because erythromycin metabolizes through the CYP450 system pathways, monitor ethnically diverse patients to ensure optimal therapeutic effects and to minimize adverse effects. Erythromycin also inhibits CYP450 enzymes and is known to increase the effects of some drugs such as anticoagulants and digoxin and decrease others. Grapefruit juice taken concurrently with erythromycin may increase drug levels.

Patient Education

- Report a fever that does not diminish below 37.8°C (100°F) within 3 days, increasing signs and symptoms of infection, or symptoms that remain after taking the entire course of antibacterial therapy. Immediately report febrile seizures, changes in behavior, or changes in LOC to the healthcare provider.
- Immediately report any itching, rashes, swelling (particularly of tongue or face), urticaria, flushing, dizziness, syncope, wheezing, throat tightness, or difficulty breathing.
- Increase overall fluid intake. Report any diminished urine output, weight gain of more than 1 kg (2 lb) in a 24-hour period, darkening of urine.
- Report any diarrhea that increases in frequency or amount or contains mucus, blood, or pus. Consult the healthcare provider before taking any antidiarrheal drugs that slow gastric motility because these may cause the retention of harmful bacteria.
- Observe and report white patches in the mouth, whitish thick vaginal discharge, itching in the urogenital area, or blistering itchy rash and report to the healthcare provider.
- Immediately report increasing headache, dizziness, drowsiness, changes in behavior, LOC, or seizures. If dizziness occurs, sit or lie down and not attempt to stand or walk until the sensation passes.
- Women who are pregnant, or attempting pregnancy, should not take tetracycline antibiotics due to adverse effects to the developing fetus.
- Women of childbearing age taking oral contraceptives should consult their healthcare provider about birth control alternatives if erythromycin antibiotics are used.
- For known antibacterial allergies, carry a wallet identification card or wear medical identification jewelry indicating allergy.
- Appropriate self-administration of antibiotics includes:
  - Complete the entire course of therapy unless otherwise instructed. Do not share with other family members, and do not stop the medicine when starting to feel better.
  - Patients taking erythromycin or aminoglycoside antibiotics should immediately report dizziness, vertigo, tinnitus, or diminished hearing to the healthcare provider.
  - Do not take tetracycline with milk products, iron-containing preparations such as multivitamins, or with antacids. Take the tetracycline 1 hour before or 2 hours after consuming these products.
  - If tetracycline antibiotics are ordered, wear sunscreen and protective clothing for sun exposure and avoid tanning beds. Immediately report any severe sunburn or rashes.
  - Take the medication as evenly spaced throughout each day as feasible.
  - Increase overall fluid intake while taking the antibacterial drug

Prescribing Considerations

- Tetracyclines and aminoglycosides may be nephrotoxic; macrolides may be hepatotoxic. Periodic culture and sensitivity (C&S) tests may be ordered if infections are severe or are slow to resolve to confirm appropriate therapy. Peak and trough drug levels will be monitored for aminoglycosides to prevent severe adverse effects.
- Aminoglycosides have an increased risk of neurotoxicity. Reduce dosage or change medications at first signs of nephrotoxicity.

Understanding Chapter 48

Key Concepts Summary

48.1 Antibiotics inhibit microbial protein synthesis by binding to the bacterial ribosome.

48.2 Tetracyclines have broad antimicrobial activity against many gram-positive and gram-negative bacteria.

48.3 The macrolides are alternatives to penicillin for many gram-positive infections.

48.4 The aminoglycosides are effective against aerobic gram-negative organisms but have the potential to cause ototoxicity and nephrotoxicity.

48.5 Several inhibitors of protein synthesis are effective against resistant infections but may have significant adverse effects that limit their use.

CASE STUDY: Making the Patient Connection

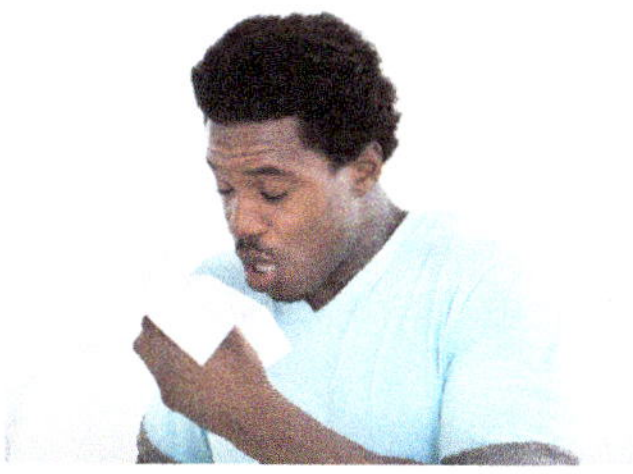

Remember the patient "John Travis" at the beginning of the chapter? Now read the remainder of the case study. Based on the information presented within this chapter, respond to the critical thinking questions that follow.

John Travis, a 31-year-old high school teacher, has had an upper respiratory infection for the past 2 weeks. Although he has seen his healthcare provider, he does not seem to be improving. He is convinced that if he takes the antibiotic just 1 more day, he will surely improve. However, after 5 days of drug therapy, John continues to experience chills, fever, and a productive cough. His wife insisted that he return to the clinic for further evaluation and treatment.

At the clinic the patient's physical examination and diagnostic tests reveal the following findings: temperature, 39.2°C (102.6°F); pulse rate, 112 beats/min; respiratory rate, 30 breaths/min; and blood pressure, 134/88 mmHg. John is visibly short of breath and is experiencing intermittent coughing episodes. On auscultation of his lung fields, bilateral crackles and wheezes are discovered. His white blood cell (WBC) count is 14,400 mm^3. A chest x-ray is taken to confirm a diagnosis of pneumonia and reveals right lower lobe infiltrates (white areas in the lung that indicate infection).

The patient is diagnosed with bacterial pneumonia. John is hospitalized and prescribed IV antibiotic therapy. On the second hospital day you are assigned to care for John. He and his wife have multiple questions about the drug therapy prescribed.

Critical Thinking Questions

1. Why did the first antibiotic prescribed not cure the infection?
2. The patient has been told that a sputum specimen is needed for a "C and S" and asks what that is. What will the nurse teach him about this test and why it is needed?
3. John has been told that laboratory personnel will be collecting blood for a peak and trough level this afternoon and in the morning. How would the nurse explain this laboratory test to the patient?
4. What symptoms would indicate that the patient's condition is worsening? What additional testing is warranted?

Additional Case Study

Mr. Klein is an 85-year-old man seen in the outpatient clinic for an acute infection. He has informed the healthcare provider that he is allergic to a variety of antibiotics and is subsequently prescribed erythromycin estolate. The patient is a recovering alcoholic who has been abstinent for 10 years.

1. What is the significance of Mr. Klein's history of alcoholism?
2. What possible adverse effect should the nurse instruct the patient to watch for?
3. What laboratory diagnostic studies may be indicated for this patient?

Chapter Review

1. While teaching the patient about taking oral tetracycline, which of the following does the nurse advise the patient to do?
   1. Consume calcium-rich products to decrease the duration of the antibacterial effect.
   2. Use a soft-bristle toothbrush and floss teeth gently to remove staining on teeth.
   3. Report any ringing in the ears or dizziness.
   4. Avoid direct exposure to sunlight and apply sunblock when outdoors.
2. The nurse determines that the patient understands the use of azithromycin (Zithromax) when the patient makes which statement?
   1. "It only needs to be taken once daily because it lasts longer."
   2. "It causes more nausea than most other antibiotics in this classification."
   3. "It must be taken on an empty stomach."
   4. "It is ineffective if taken with calcium-rich foods."

3. The patient is receiving amikacin for a bacterial infection. Which adverse effects does the nurse include in the plan of care to monitor the patient's status?
   1. Weight gain
   2. Visual disturbances
   3. Mental depression
   4. Urinary frequency

4. The healthcare provider orders gentamicin for a patient with a postoperative wound infection. Which laboratory result should prompt the nurse to consult with the prescriber about possible nephrotoxicity of this drug?
   1. Elevated serum creatinine level
   2. Decreased BUN level
   3. Increased white blood cell count
   4. Elevated serum iron level

5. The patient has received a prescription for tetracycline for treatment of acne. The nurse will teach the patient to avoid taking the tetracycline concurrently with ________.

6. The patient is receiving gentamicin IV for a serious infection. While the patient is receiving this drug, what assessment data will the nurse gather to monitor for adverse effects? (Select all that apply.)
   1. Serum creatinine
   2. Signs of muscle weakness
   3. Liver function studies
   4. Urine output
   5. Hearing and balance assessments

See Appendix A for answers to critical thinking questions, case study questions, and review questions.

References

Centers for Disease Control and Prevention (CDC). (2016). *Visiting friends or relatives in a foreign country*. https://wwwnc.cdc.gov/travel/page/vfr

Centers for Disease Control and Prevention (CDC). (2019). *Sexually transmitted diseases treatment guidelines*. https://www.cdc.gov/std/tg2015

Connor, B. A. (2019). *Travelers' diarrhea*. Centers for Disease Control and Prevention. https://wwwnc.cdc.gov/travel/yellowbook/2020/preparing-international-travelers/travelers-diarrhea

Dufel, S. E. (2015). *CBRNE—plague*. Medscape. http://emedicine.medscape.com/article/829233-overview

Madigan, M. T., Bender, K. S., Buckley, D. H., Sattley, W. M., & Stahl, D. A. (2018). *Brock biology of microorganisms* (15th ed.). Pearson.

Selected Bibliography

Aberra, F. N. (2019). Clostridioides difficile *colitis*. Medscape. http://emedicine.medscape.com/article/186458-overview

Germovsek, E., Barker, C. I., & Sharland, M. (2017). What do I need to know about aminoglycoside antibiotics? *Archives of Disease in Childhood-Education & Practice, 102*, 89–93. https://doi.org/10.1136/archdischild-2015-309069

Golkar, T., Zieliński, M., & Berghuis, A. M. (2018). Look and outlook on enzyme-mediated macrolide resistance. *Frontiers in Microbiology, 9*, 1942. https://doi.org/10.3389/fmicb.2018.01942

Hashempour-Baltork, F., Hosseini, H., Shojaee-Aliabadi, S., Torbati, M., Alizadeh, A. M., & Alizadeh, M. (2019). Drug resistance and the prevention strategies in food borne bacteria: An update review. *Advanced Pharmaceutical Bulletin, 9*(3), 335. https://doi.org/10.15171/apb.2019.041

Markley, J. L., & Wencewicz, T. A. (2018). Tetracycline-inactivating enzymes. *Frontiers in Microbiology, 9*, 1058. https://doi.org/10.3389/fmicb.2018.01058

Restrepo, M. I., Sole-Violan, J., & Martin-Loeches, I. (2016). Macrolide therapy of pneumonia: Is it necessary, and how does it help? *Current Opinion in Infectious Diseases, 29*, 212–217. https://doi.org/10.1097/QCO.0000000000000250

Shankar, C., Nabarro, L. E., Anandan, S., & Veeraraghavan, B. (2017). Minocycline and tigecycline: What is their role in the treatment of carbapenem-resistant gram-negative organisms? *Microbial Drug Resistance, 23*, 437–446. https://doi.org/10.1089/mdr.2016.0043

Thung, I., Aramin, H., Vavinskaya, V., Gupta, S., Park, J. Y., Crowe, S. E., & Valasek, M. A. (2016). Review article: The global emergence of *Helicobacter pylori* antibiotic resistance. *Alimentary Pharmacology & Therapeutics, 43*, 514–533. https://doi.org/10.1111/apt.13497

Tortora, G., Funke, B., & Case, C. (2021). *Microbiology: An introduction* (13th ed.). Pearson.

"Every morning for the last month I have had terrible headaches with pain directly on my forehead. Then my upper jaw and cheeks became tender to touch and my teeth ached."
—*Patient "Mike Springs"*

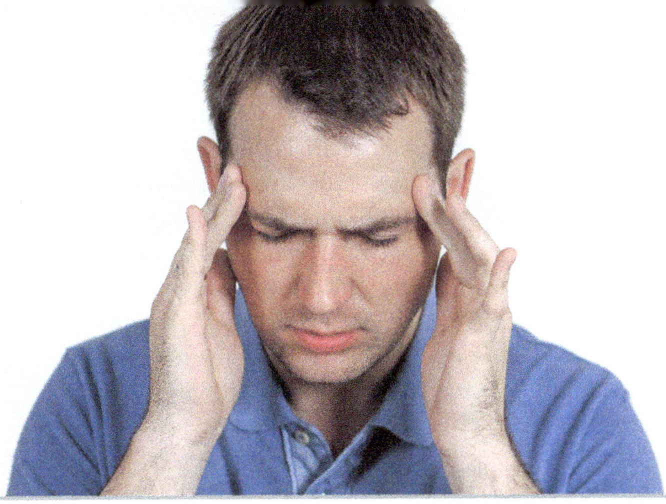

Chapter 49
Fluoroquinolones and Miscellaneous Antibacterials

Chapter Outline

- Bacterial DNA Replication
- Inhibition of DNA Replication
- Fluoroquinolones
  PROTOTYPE *Ciprofloxacin (Cipro), p. 859*
- Miscellaneous Antibacterials

Learning Outcomes

After reading this chapter, the student should be able to:

1. Explain the steps in bacterial DNA replication.
2. Identify the classes of drugs that act by affecting bacterial DNA replication.
3. Explain mechanisms by which fluoroquinolones inhibit bacterial DNA replication.
4. Describe means by which bacteria become resistant to fluoroquinolones.
5. For each of the classes shown in the chapter outline, identify the prototype and representative drugs and explain the mechanism(s) of drug action, primary indications, contraindications, significant drug interactions, pregnancy data, and important adverse effects.
6. Explain the nurse's role in the safe administration of fluoroquinolones.
7. Apply clinical judgment to care for patients receiving pharmacotherapy with fluoroquinolones and miscellaneous antibacterials.

Key Terms

Definitions of the terms in bold may be found in the Glossary.

With resistance to other antibacterials developing rapidly, drugs in the fluoroquinolone class have become increasingly important in the pharmacotherapy of infectious diseases. Fluoroquinolones are bactericidal and are effective against many gram-positive and gram-negative microbes. They affect bacterial deoxyribonucleic acid (DNA) synthesis and are particularly useful in the management of respiratory, genitourinary, and gastrointestinal (GI) infections.

Bacterial DNA Replication

49.1 Bacterial DNA replication requires several different enzymes to uncoil, unwind, and duplicate the DNA.

Under optimal conditions, many pathogenic bacteria can divide every 1 to 3 hours. Under highly favorable conditions, *Escherichia coli* divides every 20 minutes, producing a billion cells in only 10 hours. The most critical step in bacterial reproduction is duplicating the DNA so that each daughter cell contains the same genetic material. Thus, bacteria are in the process of continuously replicating their DNA as well as constructing cell walls and synthesizing proteins.

Like human DNA, bacterial DNA uses the four bases—adenine, guanine, cytosine, and thymidine—and is arranged in a double-helical formation. Most bacteria, however, contain a single circular chromosome, as illustrated in Figure 49.1. The helix is then twisted and coiled. This highly twisted arrangement is called a **supercoil**. The supercoiled arrangement is necessary for all the DNA to fit into the small bacterial cell. However, this supercoil must be relaxed and the two helices unwound immediately prior to replicating its DNA, so that duplication enzymes can reach the bases.

A large number of enzymes are needed for DNA replication, and some of these enzymes are targets for antibiotics. This is a complex process but may be simplified in four steps. The enzymes involved in this four-step process afford different sites at which drugs may act.

1. *Unwind:* The enzyme **DNA helicase** speeds down the DNA, unwinding the two strands.
2. *Relax:* Working just ahead of helicase, **DNA gyrase** (also called **topoisomerase II**) relaxes the supercoils.
3. *Replicate:* The enzyme **DNA polymerase** adds the precursor bases to replicate the original DNA and form new DNA strands.
4. *Migrate:* The two newly formed strands are interlocked until the enzyme **topoisomerase IV** frees them to migrate to opposite sides of the cell, where they are segregated into the two daughter cells.

Inhibition of DNA Replication

49.2 Drugs have been discovered that inhibit different steps in bacterial DNA replication.

Blocking the DNA replication of a pathogen is a common mechanism used by drugs across several different therapeutic classes. Drugs can block bacterial DNA replication in three basic ways:

- They can inhibit the synthesis or availability of precursor bases or nucleotides.
- They can bind to bacterial DNA, preventing the relaxation and uncoiling processes required for replication.
- They can bind to enzymes of DNA replication, halting the formation of new DNA strands.

A number of drugs employed in cancer chemotherapy act by mimicking precursor molecules or by interacting with DNA. Cytarabine and fluorouracil resemble nucleotides and are mistakenly incorporated into newly formed DNA strands. Daunorubicin (Cerubidine) and bleomycin are highly toxic antibiotics that interact with DNA to physically block replication. Although classified as antibiotics, these drugs are too toxic to be used for infections but have

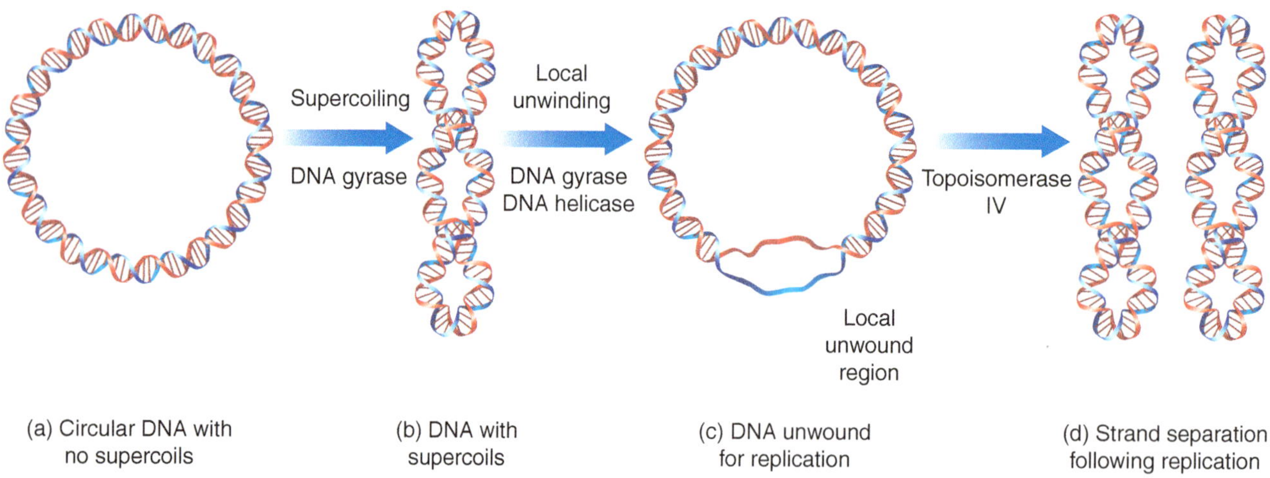

Figure 49.1 The unwinding and replication of bacterial DNA.

therapeutic indications in the chemotherapy of specific types of cancer.

Several drugs act by inhibiting enzymes involved in DNA replication. Acyclovir (Zovirax) inhibits the DNA polymerase of herpesvirus and is a leading drug for treating this infection (see Chapter 54). Irinotecan (Camptosar) and etoposide (VePesid) are antineoplastic drugs that act by inhibiting topoisomerase I, an enzyme that helps repair DNA damage. By binding in a complex with topoisomerase and DNA, these antineoplastics cause strand breaks that accumulate and permanently damage the DNA.

The fluoroquinolone antibiotics act on two enzymes in the DNA replication process. First, they bind to DNA gyrase, inhibiting its ability to relax the supercoiling of the bacterial DNA. When the replication enzymes reach an area still in a supercoiled state, replication terminates. A second mechanism is binding to topoisomerase IV. When this occurs, the two daughter DNA strands cannot migrate to opposite sides of the cell, and division cannot be completed. It is thought that fluoroquinolones inhibit DNA gyrase in gram-negative organisms and inhibit topoisomerase IV in gram-positive organisms. However, this is likely an oversimplification of their exact mechanism. These drugs have no effect on human enzymes involved in DNA replication because of significant differences in the chemical structures of the human and bacterial enzymes. These differences account for their selective toxicity on bacteria and their favorable safety profile.

Fluoroquinolones

49.3 Fluoroquinolones are antibiotics whose therapeutic applications have expanded in recent years to treat many gram-positive and gram-negative infections.

The first drug in this class, nalidixic acid (NegGram), was approved by the U.S. Food and Drug Administration (FDA) in 1962. Classified as a quinolone, the use of nalidixic acid was restricted to treating urinary tract infections (UTIs). Although no longer available, nalidixic acid is important because it served as a building block for the synthesis of other drugs in this class.

In the late 1980s, the development of quinolones with a fluorine side chain resulted in drugs with wider spectrums of activity and longer durations of action. The fluoroquinolones, listed in Table 49.1, have become an increasingly important class of antibiotics in the past two decades. Fluoroquinolones are bactericidal and affect bacterial DNA synthesis by inhibiting both DNA gyrase and topoisomerase IV.

The generations of fluoroquinolones are based on their antibacterial spectrums. All fluoroquinolones have activity against gram-negative pathogens, with the newer generations being significantly more effective against gram-positive bacteria. The distinctions among the generations are listed in Table 49.2. Some of the newer fluoroquinolones were developed and approved primarily for the treatment of respiratory infections.

Table 49.1 Fluoroquinolones

Drug	Route and Adult Dose (Maximum Dose Where Indicated)	Adverse Effects
First Generation (no longer available)		
Second Generation		
ciprofloxacin (Cipro)	PO (regular release): 250–750 mg bid (max: 1500 mg/day) PO (extended release): 500–1000 mg once daily Drops (ophthalmic solution): 1–2 drops q2h while awake for 2 days, then q4h for the next 5 days	*Nausea, headache, diarrhea, rash, insomnia, pain and inflammation at injection site, local burning, stinging, corneal irritation (ophthalmic)* Anaphylaxis, tendon rupture, superinfections, photosensitivity, pseudomembranous colitis (PMC), seizure, peripheral neuropathy, hepatotoxicity, exacerbation of myasthenia gravis, toxic psychosis
ofloxacin	PO/IV: 200–400 mg bid (max: 800 mg/day) Drops (ophthalmic solution): 1–2 drops q2–4h in affected eye Drops (otic solution): 5–10 drops in affected ear daily	
Third Generation		
gatifloxacin (Zymar, Zymaxid)	Drops (ophthalmic solution): 1 drop in each affected eye q2–4h	
levofloxacin	PO/IV: 250–750 mg/day (max: 750 mg/day)	
Fourth Generation		
besifloxacin (Besivance)	Drops (ophthalmic solution): 1 drop in each affected eye q8h	
delafloxacin (Baxdela)	PO: 450 mg bid IV: 300 mg bid given over 60 minutes	
finafloxacin (Xtoro)	Drops (otic solution): 4 drops in affected ear bid	
gemifloxacin (Factive)	PO: 320 mg/day (max: 320 mg/day)	
moxifloxacin (Moxeza, Vigamox)	PO/IV: 400 mg/day once daily (max: 400 mg/day) Drops (ophthamic solution): 1 drop in affected eye tid (Vigamox) or bid (Moxeza)	

Note: *Italics* indicate common adverse effects. Underline indicates serious adverse effects.

Table 49.2 Generations of Fluoroquinolones

Generation	Example	Route of Administration	Spectrum of Activity	Indications
First generation	nalidixic acid	Oral	Enterobacteriaceae	No longer available
Second generation	ciprofloxacin	Oral and IV	Enterobacteriaceae, atypical pathogens, *Pseudomonas aeruginosa*	Complicated UTI, gastroenteritis with severe diarrhea, sexually transmitted infections (STIs)
Third generation	levofloxacin	Oral and IV	Enterobacteriaceae, atypical pathogens, some streptococci	Complicated UTI, gastroenteritis with severe diarrhea, STIs, community-acquired pneumonia
Fourth generation	moxifloxacin	Oral	Enterobacteriaceae, atypical pathogens, some streptococci, methicillin-resistant *S. aureus* (MRSA), anaerobes	Bacterial conjunctivitis (ophthalmic drops), acute bacterial sinusitis, exacerbations of chronic bronchitis, community-acquired pneumonia, skin and skin structure infections

Clinical applications of fluoroquinolones include infections of the respiratory, GI, and genitourinary tracts and some skin and soft tissue infections. Their effectiveness against gram-negative organisms makes them preferred drugs in the treatment of uncomplicated UTIs (see Chapter 50). Moxifloxacin is effective against anaerobes, a group of bacteria that are often difficult to treat. Ciprofloxacin (Cipro) is the fluoroquinolone usually selected for infections by *Pseudomonas aeruginosa*. Recent studies have suggested that some fluoroquinolones may be effective against *Mycobacterium tuberculosis*, although the FDA has not approved these drugs for this indication.

Along with doxycycline, streptomycin, and penicillin, several fluoroquinolones are indicated for pathogens that could potentially be of benefit following a bioterrorism incident. Ciprofloxacin (Cipro) is a preferred drug for postexposure prophylaxis to *Bacillus anthracis*, the causative agent of anthrax. Ciprofloxacin is also indicated for postexposure prophylaxis to other potential biologic warfare pathogens such as *Yersinia pestis* (plague), *Francisella tularensis* (tularemia), and *Brucella melitensis* (brucellosis). Details on the pharmacotherapy of bioterrorism agents are presented in Chapter 75.

Several fluoroquinolones are well absorbed orally and may be administered either once or twice a day, making them ideal for outpatient therapy. The serum levels of these drugs after oral (PO) administration are nearly equivalent to the levels achieved during IV administration. This allows for a rapid, smooth transition from IV therapy to oral therapy, potentially decreasing the length of the hospital stay. Like aminoglycosides, fluoroquinolones exhibit a postantibiotic effect. Their bactericidal actions continue after serum levels fall to below minimum inhibitory concentrations. Once available by the PO route, gatifloxacin is now formulated as an ophthalmic solution.

In the 1990s, fluoroquinolones came into widespread use because they were well tolerated, and few serious adverse effects were reported. Over time, several uncommon, although very serious, adverse effects were discovered. Since that time, almost half the fluoroquinolones approved by the FDA have been discontinued in the United States due to safety concerns. As part of the black box warning for all oral and IV fluoroquinolones, the risk for serious adverse effects generally outweighs the benefits for patients with acute bacterial sinusitis, acute exacerbation of chronic bronchitis, and uncomplicated UTIs. Fluoroquinolones should only be used for these indications when there are no alternative treatment options.

Cartilage toxicity: Animal studies have suggested that fluoroquinolones can affect the extracellular matrix of cartilage during development, and tendon toxicity has been reported in children using these drugs. Although these abnormalities ceased upon termination of antibiotic therapy, fluoroquinolones are not approved for patients under age 18, and their use in children is restricted to instances where the benefits of pharmacotherapy clearly outweigh the potential risks.

Although rare, tendon abnormalities have also been reported in adults. Tendinitis and rupture of the shoulder, hand, and Achilles tendons have occurred several months after discontinuation of therapy. The FDA requires safety labeling that states patients older than 65 years are at increased risk for severe tendon disorders and that this risk is further increased by concurrent use of corticosteroids. Musculoskeletal complaints should be carefully monitored during therapy with fluoroquinolones, and patients should be advised to report unexplained joint or tendon pain.

GI toxicity: GI symptoms such as nausea and vomiting and diarrhea occur in as many as 20% of patients taking fluoroquinolones. Although food does not affect their absorption, certain multivitamins or mineral supplements containing calcium, zinc, iron, aluminum, and magnesium can delay absorption of the antibiotic by as much as 90%. Substances containing these minerals should not be administered at the same time as fluoroquinolones.

The FDA has issued required safety labeling for certain antimicrobials to warn of the risk for *Clostridioides difficile*–associated diarrhea (CDAD). This safety labeling applies to most fluoroquinolones as well as drugs from many other antibiotic classes.

Hypersensitivity reactions: Certainly not unique to fluoroquinolones, hypersensitivity may occur to any antibiotic.

Although the FDA has always required label warnings on quinolones for the risk of hypersensitivity reactions that occur after the first dose, new labels warn of the rare risk for serious, and sometimes fatal, events after multiple doses.

Cardiotoxicity: Some of the most serious adverse effects of drugs in this class are dysrhythmias (moxifloxacin). Several of the drugs in this class were removed from the market due to the potential for fatal dysrhythmias. Nearly all fluoroquinolones prolong the QTc interval.

Nervous system toxicity: Central nervous system (CNS) effects such as dizziness, headache, and sleep disturbances affect 1 to 8% of patients. Seizures, hallucinations, high intracranial pressure, confusion, and toxic psychoses have been reported in patients taking fluoroquinolones. These drugs should be used with caution in patients with preexisting seizure disorders. In 2013, the FDA issued a safety warning that serious nerve damage (peripheral neuropathy) caused by oral or parenteral fluoroquinolones may be permanent.

Phototoxicity: Moderate to severe phototoxicity may occur in patients exposed to direct or indirect sunlight or to sunlamps during or following treatment with fluoroquinolones. Recovery may take several weeks.

Hepatotoxicity: Some of the fluoroquinolones elevate hepatic enzymes, which usually return to normal 1 to 2 months after completion of therapy. Liver damage, including fatal hepatic failure, is a potential risk.

Resistance: Like other antibiotics, the incidence of resistant bacterial species has been increasing and can occur by multiple mechanisms. Mutations to DNA gyrase can alter its ability to bind fluoroquinolones, thus rendering the drug less effective. Some bacteria have developed resistance pumps that remove fluoroquinolones from inside their cells, whereas others have developed a cell wall structure that is less permeable to the drugs. Because of the large number of resistant strains, the Centers for Disease Control and Prevention no longer recommends fluoroquinolones for the treatment of gonorrhea. Resistance to one fluoroquinolone sometimes confers resistance to all drugs in this class; therefore, resistance is becoming a limiting factor in the clinical utility of these drugs.

PROTOTYPE DRUG Ciprofloxacin (Cipro)

Classification **Therapeutic:** Antibacterial
Pharmacologic: Bacterial DNA replication inhibitor, fluoroquinolone

Therapeutic Effects and Uses: Ciprofloxacin is a second-generation fluoroquinolone approved in 1987 that is the most widely used drug in this class. It is prescribed for UTI, sinusitis, pneumonia, skin infections, bone and joint infections, infectious diarrhea, and certain eye infections. It is a broad-spectrum antibiotic that is most effective against gram-negative organisms. It is active against *Enterobacter*, *Citrobacter*, *E. coli*, *Haemophilus*, *Klebsiella*, *Proteus*, *Staphylococcus*, *Shigella*, *Salmonella*, *Neisseria*, and *Serratia* species. It is poorly effective against *Streptococcus pneumoniae* and is inactive against most anaerobic bacteria. Ciprofloxacin is a preferred drug for postexposure prophylaxis of inhalational *B. anthracis* spores. It is generally not a first-line drug for children when given PO of IV due to an increased risk for arthropathy.

Ciprofloxacin is available by the oral, IV, ophthalmic, and otic routes. As an ophthalmic solution (Ciloxan), it is used to treat corneal ulcers and conjunctivitis due to *Staphylococcus*, *Haemophilus*, and *Pseudomonas*. An otic suspension (Ciprodex) is a combination of ciprofloxacin and dexamethasone to treat acute otitis media and acute otitis externa in children ages 6 months and older. Cipro HC otic combines ciprofloxacin with hydrocortisone to treat adults and children with acute otitis media. Ciprofloxacin extended release is a once-daily formulation. It is approved for 3-day therapy of acute uncomplicated UTI or 7 days for complicated UTI.

Mechanism of Action: By inhibiting bacterial DNA gyrase and topoisomerase, ciprofloxacin affects bacterial replication and DNA repair. Ciprofloxacin is usually considered bactericidal and exhibits a prolonged postantibiotic effect.

Pharmacokinetics:

Route(s)	PO, IV, ophthalmic and otic drops
Absorption	60–80% absorbed
Distribution	Widely distributed to all body fluids; crosses the placenta; secreted in breast milk; small amounts in cerebrospinal fluid; 20–40% bound to plasma proteins
Primary metabolism	Mostly unchanged; small amounts of hepatic metabolism
Primary excretion	Primarily renal; 15% by biliary route
Onset of action	Rapid
Duration of action	12 h

Adverse Effects: Ciprofloxacin is well tolerated by most patients, and serious adverse effects are uncommon. GI adverse effects, such as nausea and vomiting and diarrhea, may occur in patients taking high doses. Ciprofloxacin may be administered with food to diminish adverse GI effects. The patient should not, however, take this drug with antacids or mineral supplements because drug absorption will be diminished. Some patients report phototoxicity, headache, and dizziness. Like most antibiotics, ciprofloxacin can cause serious PMC. Although rare, seizures and toxic psychosis have been reported in patients receiving fluoroquinolones. Geriatric patients are at increased risk to developing severe tendon rupture. **Black Box Warning:** Tendinitis and tendon rupture may occur in patients of all ages. Risk is especially high in patients over age 60; in kidney, heart, and lung transplant recipients; and in those receiving concurrent corticosteroid therapy. Fluoroquinolones may cause extreme muscle weakness in patients with myasthenia gravis. Ciprofloxacin should not be used for the following conditions, unless no alternatives exist: acute exacerbation of chronic bronchitis, acute uncomplicated cystitis, and acute sinusitis.

Contraindications/Precautions: Ciprofloxacin is contraindicated in patients who are hypersensitive to fluoroquinolones and in pregnant patients. Drug therapy must be monitored carefully in patients with suspected CNS disorders because this drug can be neurotoxic at high doses and can cause seizures when given by rapid IV infusion. Although prescribed for patients with UTIs, the drug should be used with caution in patients with serious chronic kidney disease because this drug is excreted by this route and may accumulate to toxic levels. Fluoroquinolones should be used with caution in patients with myasthenia gravis because they may greatly exacerbate muscle weakness.

Drug Interactions: Concurrent administration with warfarin may increase anticoagulant effects and result in bleeding due to the decreased metabolism of warfarin. Antacids and vitamin supplements containing calcium or aluminum, iron or zinc sulfate, and sucralfate decrease the absorption of ciprofloxacin, thus causing decreased effectiveness of the antibiotic. Ciprofloxacin slows the hepatic metabolism of xanthines, including caffeine, theophylline, and theobromine. **Herbal/Food:** Patients ingesting large quantities of caffeinated products may experience excessive nervousness, anxiety, or tachycardia. Calcium-fortified juices may interfere with absorption of the antibiotic.

Pregnancy: Animal studies showed fetal toxicity in some species but not in others. Results of human epidemiological studies also varied: some showed an increase in spontaneous abortions and congenital malformations, whereas others showed no fetal toxicity. Because ciprofloxacin is secreted in human milk, caution should be used if breastfeeding.

Treatment of Overdose: No specific therapy is available; patients are treated symptomatically.

Clinician Responsibilities: Key clinical implications for patients receiving ciprofloxacin are included in Applied Clinical Judgment: Patients Receiving Pharmacotherapy with Fluoroquinolones.

Drugs Similar to Ciprofloxacin (Cipro)

Other fluoroquinolones include besifloxacin, delafloxacin, finafloxacin, gatifloxacin, gemifloxacin, levofloxacin, moxifloxacin, and ofloxacin. When administered for systemic indications, these drugs have actions and adverse effects that are very similar to those of ciprofloxacin. A black box warning regarding possible tendon rupture is included for all oral and parenteral drugs in this class. Included below is ozenoxacin, which is a quinolone with the same mechanism of action as the fluoroquinolones.

Besifloxacin (Besivance): Approved in 2009, besifloxacin is available as a 0.6% ophthalmic suspension for the treatment of bacterial conjunctivitis. The most frequently reported adverse reaction is conjunctival redness. Prolonged use may lead to overgrowth of resistant microbes. Patients should be advised to discontinue use of contact lenses during therapy. Very little is absorbed systemically.

Delafloxacin (Baxdela): Delafloxacin was approved in 2017 to treat skin and skin structure infections. It is effective against a large number of gram-positive and gram-negative bacteria and has the highest activity of any fluoroquinolone against MRSA. The most frequent adverse effects include nausea and vomiting, diarrhea, and headache. Delafloxacin carries black box warnings similar to the other systemic drugs in this class. Animal studies showed no evidence of fetal toxicity. This drug is secreted in animal milk, but adverse effects on the breastfed neonate are unknown.

Finafloxacin (Xtoro): Finafloxacin was approved in 2014 for the treatment of acute otitis externa caused by *P. aeruginosa* or *Staphylococcus aureus*. It is used for 7 days and rarely causes any adverse effects. Prolonged use may lead to an overgrowth of nonsusceptible organisms. Very little is absorbed systemically.

Gatifloxacin (Zymar, Zymaxid): Once available by the oral and parenteral routes, gatifloxacin is now approved only as an ophthalmic solution for the treatment of bacterial conjunctivitis. The most frequently reported adverse reactions after ophthalmic administration include increased worsening of conjunctivitis, eye irritation, dysgeusia, and eye pain. Patients should be advised to discontinue use of contact lenses during therapy. Prolonged use may lead to overgrowth of resistant microbes. Very little is absorbed systemically.

Gemifloxacin (Factive): Gemifloxacin was approved in 2003 for acute bacterial exacerbations of chronic bronchitis and community-acquired pneumonia. It is more effective against gram-positive bacteria, most importantly *S. pneumoniae* and *S. aureus*, than many other drugs in this class. To reduce the development of drug-resistant strains, the manufacturer recommends that gemifloxacin be used to treat only infections proven susceptible to the drug. Available PO, the drug undergoes minimal metabolism by the liver and is excreted almost equally by the kidneys and in the feces. Diarrhea, rash, and nausea are the most common adverse effects. It is contraindicated in patients with certain dysrhythmias, due to its effects on cardiac conduction. Other contraindications and adverse effects (including the black box warning) are similar to those of ciprofloxacin. Animal studies showed fetal malformations and growth retardation. This drug is secreted in animal milk, but adverse effects on the breastfed neonate are unknown. Gemifloxacin is not recommended during pregnancy or lactation unless the potential benefits to the mother justify the potential risks to the fetus or neonate.

Levofloxacin: Approved in 1996, levofloxacin is prescribed for UTI, acute pyelonephritis, chronic bacterial prostatitis, hospital-acquired and community-acquired pneumonia, acute bacterial sinusitis, acute bacterial exacerbation of chronic bronchitis, skin infections, and bacterial conjunctivitis. It is available for PO, IV, and ophthalmic administration. Levofloxacin has a long half-life that allows for once-daily dosing. The most common adverse effects are nausea, headache, diarrhea, insomnia, constipation, and dizziness. Adverse effects of ophthalmic levofloxacin include transient blurred vision, foreign body sensation, headache, burning, pharyngitis, and photophobia. Caution should be used for patients with certain dysrhythmias due to its effects on cardiac conduction. Although rare, hematologic toxicity, including agranulocytosis and thrombocytopenia, hepatotoxicity, and nephrotoxicity, may occur after multiple doses. Other contraindications and adverse effects for the oral and IV forms (including the black box warning) are the same as those of ciprofloxacin. Animal studies showed increased fetal mortality at high doses. Results of some human epidemiological studies with systemic fluoroquinolones showed an increase in spontaneous abortions and congenital malformations. Because levofloxacin is secreted in human milk and could cause adverse effects in the neonate, breastfeeding is not recommended.

Moxifloxacin (Moxeza, Vigamox): Approved in 1999, moxifloxacin is prescribed for skin infections, intra-abdominal infections, community-acquired pneumonia, acute sinusitis, and acute bacterial exacerbation of chronic bronchitis. It is available by the oral and IV routes and as an ophthalmic preparation (Moxeza, Vigamox) for bacterial conjunctivitis. The most common adverse effects are dizziness, diarrhea, and nausea and vomiting. For the ophthalmic drops, eye irritation, pyrexia, and conjunctivitis are the common adverse effects. Like gemifloxacin, it is contraindicated in patients with certain dysrhythmias due to its effects on cardiac conduction. Other contraindications and adverse effects for the oral and IV forms (including the black box warning) are the same as those of ciprofloxacin. Animal studies showed evidence of fetotoxicity. This drug is secreted in animal milk but its effects on the breastfed neonate are unknown. Moxifloxacin is not recommended during pregnancy or lactation unless the potential benefits to the mother justify the potential risks to the fetus or neonate.

CONNECTIONS: Patient Safety

Levofloxacin

Yesterday, Mrs. Rackey received the first dose of IV levofloxacin. While receiving the medication, she reported itching and a slight swelling of the tongue and lips (angioedema). However, later that day she had no discomfort or presence of the previous symptoms. She will receive the second dose of the medication again this morning. What should the nurse do?

Ofloxacin: Approved in 1990, ofloxacin is indicated for acute bacterial exacerbations of chronic bronchitis, community-acquired pneumonia, chlamydial infections of the reproductive tract, acute pelvic inflammatory disease, cystitis, complicated UTI, prostatitis, superficial ocular infections (ophthalmic solution), and otitis media (otic solution). The most common adverse effects are nausea, headache, insomnia, dizziness, and rash. The otic preparation can cause otic pruritus. Other contraindications and adverse effects for the oral and IV forms (including the black box warning) are the same as those of ciprofloxacin. It is available for the PO, IV, ophthalmic, and otic routes. Results of some human epidemiological studies with systemic fluoroquinolones showed an increase in spontaneous abortions and congenital malformations. Because ofloxacin is secreted in human milk and could cause adverse effects in the neonate, breastfeeding is not recommended.

Ozenoxacin (Xepi): Ozenoxacin was approved in 2017 for the topical treatment of impetigo caused *by S. aureus or S. pyogenes*. This medication is a quinolone (lacking a fluorine atom), but it acts by the same mechanism as the fluoroquinolones. The cream is applied to the affected area twice a day for 5 days. Ozenoxacin is not absorbed systemically.

Miscellaneous Antibacterials

49.4 A number of miscellaneous antibacterials have specific clinical indications.

Several drugs act by miscellaneous mechanisms or are the only drugs in their class. Doses for the miscellaneous drugs are listed in Table 49.3.

Daptomycin (Cubicin): Approved in 2003, daptomycin belongs to a class of antibiotics known as the cyclic lipopeptides. The spectrum of activity of daptomycin includes a wide variety of gram-positive pathogens. It is indicated for the treatment of complicated skin and skin structure infections caused by organisms such as *S. aureus*,

Table 49.3 Miscellaneous Antibacterials

Drug	Route and Adult Dose (Maximum Dose Where Indicated)	Adverse Effects
daptomycin (Cubicin)	IV: 4–6 mg/kg once q24h for 7–14 days	*Insomnia, diarrhea, headache, abnormal liver function tests, elevated CPK, edema* Anaphylaxis, superinfections, renal failure, myopathy, jaundice, PMC
metronidazole (Flagyl)	Anaerobic infections: PO: 7.5 mg/kg q6h (max: 4 g/day) IV 7.5–15 mg/kg q6h (max: 4 g/day)	*Dizziness, headache, anorexia, abdominal pain, metallic taste and nausea,* Candida *infections* Seizures, peripheral neuropathy, leukopenia
polymyxin B	IV: 15,000–25,000 units/kg/day divided q12h IM: 25,000–30,000 units/kg/day divided q4–6h	*Urticaria* Nephrotoxicity, neurotoxicity (confusion, blurred vision, paresthesias, paralysis), superinfections
rifampin (Rifadin, Rimactane)	PO/IV: 600 mg/day	*Nausea and vomiting, heartburn, anorexia, diarrhea, orange discoloration of the urine, sweat, and tears* PMC, renal failure, hepatotoxicity, blood dyscrasias, possible fetotoxicity
secnidazole (Solosec)	PO: 2 g packet taken once	*Vulvovaginal candidiasis and pruritus, headache, nausea and vomiting, dyspepsia* History of hypersensitivity

Note: *Italics* indicate common adverse effects. Underline indicates serious adverse effects.

including MRSA, *Streptococcus pyogenes*, and *Enterococcus faecalis* (vancomycin-susceptible strains only). Daptomycin is bactericidal and its mechanism of action is clearly distinct from that of any other antibiotic. When binding to bacterial membranes, daptomycin causes a rapid depolarization of membrane potential, leading to inhibition of protein, DNA, and ribonucleic acid (RNA) synthesis. It is given only by IV infusion. The most serious adverse effects are abnormal liver function tests, elevated creatine phosphokinase (CPK), dyspnea, and pneumonia. Myopathy has been recorded in a small percentage of patients taking daptomycin; therefore, the nurse should carefully monitor for muscle pain or weakness. The drug should be withheld if the CPK becomes elevated above 1000 units/L. Animal studies showed no evidence of fetal harm. Daptomycin is secreted in human milk but adverse effects on the breastfed neonate are unknown.

Metronidazole (Flagyl): Approved in 1963, metronidazole is effective against a large number of anaerobes. It acts by interfering with the DNA and RNA synthesis of pathogens. Metronidazole is one of only a few drugs that have dual activity against both bacteria and multicellular parasites. It is a preferred drug for trichomoniasis, giardiasis, and amebiasis. Unlike most antibiotics, resistance to metronidazole is uncommon. When given orally, adverse effects are generally minor and include nausea, dry mouth, and headache. High doses can produce neurotoxicity.

As an antibacterial, metronidazole has two indications: serious infections due to anaerobic bacteria and peptic ulcer disease. Few antibacterials are effective against anaerobes because the organisms reside in sites that have tissue destruction and a poor blood supply. Anaerobic bacteria are common causes of abscesses, gangrene, diabetic skin ulcers, and deep wound infections. Serious intra-abdominal infections or septicemia due to *Bacteroides* and streptococci often respond well to IV infusions of the drug. It is a preferred drug for managing CDAD. Metronidazole has found a relatively new use in the treatment of *Helicobacter pylori* infections of the stomach associated with peptic ulcer disease. The drug carries a black box warning that it causes cancer in laboratory animals. Metronidazole is featured as a prototype drug in Chapter 53. Animal studies showed no evidence of fetal harm. Metronidazole is secreted in human milk. Due to potential tumor production in animal studies, breastfeeding is not recommended.

Polymyxin B: Approved in 1951, polymyxin B is an older, bactericidal drug that acts by disrupting the bacterial cell membrane. The drug is able to penetrate the phospholipid layer, make the membrane leaky, and cause the death of the bacterium. Although parenteral formulations are available, polymyxin B is rarely prescribed by these routes due to potential nephrotoxicity and neurotoxicity (black box warnings). Its primary application is in the treatment of topical infections of the skin, mucous membranes, or eye caused by gram-negative organisms. It is not effective against gram-positive microbes. It is combined with bacitracin and neomycin in common OTC first-aid products such as Neosporin Ointment, Bactine

Antibiotic, and Polysporin. Topical application, including to denuded skin, results in negligible systemic absorption. Polymyxin B is combined with neomycin and hydrocortisone in prescription otic preparations. Data on the safety of polymyxin B during pregnancy and lactation are not available.

Rifampin (Rifadin, Rimactane): Approved in 1958, rifampin is administered PO or IV and is usually associated with the pharmacotherapy of tuberculosis. The drug, however, is effective against a wide range of both gram-positive and gram-negative organisms. As an antibacterial, it is used for prophylaxis in contacts of patients with *Haemophilus influenzae* type B and for the prophylaxis of asymptomatic carriers of meningococcal disease. Occasionally, it is used for Legionnaire's disease or when therapy with other antibiotics is unsuccessful. The reason its applications are limited is because of the rapid development of resistance, which can appear after only a few days of therapy. A flu-like syndrome develops in about half the patients receiving the drug. Rifampin acts by inhibiting bacterial RNA polymerase, the enzyme that makes bacterial RNA. The use of rifampin in the pharmacotherapy of tuberculosis is presented in Chapter 51. Animal studies showed that rifampin is embryotoxic and teratogenic. Rifampin is not recommended during pregnancy or lactation unless the potential benefits to the mother justify the potential risks to the fetus or neonate.

Secnidazole (Solosec): Secnidazole was approved in 2017 for one indication: bacterial vaginosis, the most common gynecologic infection in women of childbearing age. This drug is classified as a nitroimidazole, the same class as metronidazole and tinidazole (an antiparasitic drug). Secnidazole is taken as a single dose of oral granules, sprinkled on applesauce, yogurt, or pudding. It is as effective as metronidazole, which has been the standard treatment for bacterial vaginosis for many years. About 10% of patients will acquire vulvovaginal candidiasis. Animal studies showed no evidence of fetal harm. Because secnidazole is secreted in human milk, it is recommended that breastfeeding be suspended for 96 hours after a dose.

CONNECTIONS: APPLIED CLINICAL JUDGMENT

Patients Receiving Pharmacotherapy with Fluoroquinolones

Key Assessment Data

- History of current condition, baseline vital signs, physical exam findings; hepatic, renal, cardiovascular, neurologic, or respiratory disease; pregnancy or breastfeeding. Obtain a drug history and assess signs and symptoms of the current infection, noting location, characteristics, presence or absence and the character of drainage, duration, and the presence or absence of fever or pain.
- Ongoing assessment during drug therapy should include monitoring appropriate laboratory findings (e.g., complete blood count, culture and sensitivity (C&S), hepatic and renal laboratory values); assess for infections, especially with opportunistic infections such as fungal infections.

Desired Therapeutic Outcomes

Improvement is observed and measurable by reduction in fever, pain, or signs and symptoms of infection, which should begin to diminish after taking the first dose and continue to improve throughout the course of antibiotic therapy.

Minimizing Adverse Effects

- Continued fever may be a sign of worsening infection, adverse drug effects, or antibiotic resistance. Immediately report undiminished fever or changes in level of consciousness (LOC).
- Fluoroquinolones may be nephrotoxic. Periodic C&S tests may be ordered if infections are severe or are slow to resolve to confirm appropriate therapy. Monitor for nephrotoxicity (e.g., darkened urine, diminished urine output, or weight gain greater than 1 kg [2 lb] in 24 hours).
- Anaphylactic reactions are possible, particularly with the first dose. Residual drug levels, dependent on length of half-life, may cause delayed reactions up to 2 weeks after completing therapy.
- Superinfections with opportunistic organisms may occur when normal host flora are diminished or killed by the antibacterial drug. Severe diarrhea may indicate the presence of CDAD, PMC, or fungal or yeast infections.
- Fluoroquinolones have an increased risk of neurotoxicity. Previous seizure disorders or head injuries may increase this risk. Persistent or increasing headaches should be immediately reported. Peripheral neuropathies may be permanent.
- Fluoroquinolones have been associated with tendinitis and tendon rupture, especially of the Achilles tendon. Monitor for joint, tendon, leg, or heel pain or difficulty with movement or walking in patients.
- Fluoroquinolones decrease the metabolism of warfarin and may increase anticoagulation effects and risk of bleeding. Monitor for anticoagulation effects if the patient is on warfarin.
- Fluoroquinolones may cause significant dermatologic effects including Stevens–Johnson syndrome. Monitor for dermatologic effects including red or purplish skin rash, blisters, or sunburn.

Lifespan Considerations

- Age-related physiologic differences may place the young child or older adult at greater risk for nephrotoxicity.
- Older adults may be at increased risk for dizziness related to adverse drug effects, which may increase the risk of falls. Ensure patient safety.
- The older adult is at greater risk for tendinitis and tendon rupture.

(continued)

CONNECTIONS: APPLIED CLINICAL JUDGMENT *(continued)*

Patients Receiving Pharmacotherapy with Fluoroquinolones

Patient Education

- Report a fever that does not diminish below 37.8°C (100°F) within 3 days, increasing signs and symptoms of infection, or symptoms that remain after taking the entire course of antibacterial therapy. Immediately report febrile seizures, changes in behavior, or changes in LOC.
- Immediately report any itching, rashes, swelling (particularly of tongue or face), urticaria, flushing, dizziness, syncope, wheezing, throat tightness, or difficulty breathing.
- Increase overall fluid intake. Report any diminished urine output, weight gain of more than 1 kg (2 lb) in a 24-hour period, and darkening of urine.
- Report any diarrhea that increases in frequency or amount or contains mucus, blood, or pus. consult the healthcare provider before taking any antidiarrheal drugs that slow gastric motility because these may cause the retention of harmful bacteria.
- Report signs and symptoms of infection such as wounds with redness or drainage, increasing cough, increasing fatigue, white patches on oral mucous membranes, white and itchy vaginal discharge, or itchy blister-like vesicles on the skin.
- Immediately report increasing headache, dizziness, drowsiness, changes in behavior, LOC, or seizures. If dizziness occurs, sit or lie down and do not attempt to stand or walk until the sensation passes.
- Immediately report any significant or increasing joint, tendon, heel, lower leg, or calf pain or difficulty moving or walking.
- Wear sunscreen and protective clothing for sun exposure and avoid tanning beds. Immediately report any severe sunburn or rashes.
- For known antibacterial allergies, carry a wallet identification card or wear medical identification jewelry indicating allergy.
- Appropriate self-administration of antibiotics includes:
  - Complete the entire course of therapy unless otherwise instructed. Do not share with other family members, and do not stop the medicine when starting to feel better.
  - Take the drug with food but avoid taking the drug concurrently with dairy products or calcium-fortified juices, which may decrease absorption. Take the fluoroquinolone 1 hour before or 2 hours after consuming these products.
  - Do not take antacids or preparations containing iron or zinc at the same time as the fluoroquinolone dose.
  - Take the medication as evenly spaced throughout each day as feasible.
  - Increase overall fluid intake while taking the antibacterial drug

Prescribing Considerations

- Avoid prescribing these medications for patients with a history of prolonged QTc syndrome.
- Evaluate liver function before initiating fluoroquinolone therapy and avoid prescribing these antibiotics for patients at increased risk for hepatotoxicity.
- Monitor older adults, particularly if they have atherosclerosis or epilepsy.

Understanding Chapter 49

Key Concepts Summary

49.1 Bacterial DNA replication requires several different enzymes to uncoil, unwind, and duplicate the DNA.

49.2 Drugs have been discovered that inhibit different steps in bacterial DNA replication.

49.3 Fluoroquinolones are antibiotics whose therapeutic applications have expanded in recent years to treat many gram-positive and gram-negative infections.

49.4 A number of miscellaneous antibacterials have specific clinical indications.

CASE STUDY: Making the Patient Connection

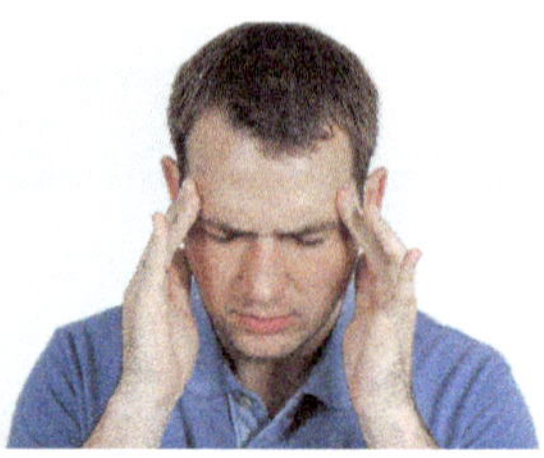

Remember the patient "Mike Springs" at the beginning of the chapter? Now read the remainder of the case study. Based on the information presented within this chapter, respond to the critical thinking questions that follow.

Mike Springs presents to the local health clinic. He is a 38-year-old man who has no history of chronic illness. His vital signs are normal with the exception of a slight increase in body temperature, 37.3°C (99.2°F). He denies shortness of breath. However, his nasal passages are congested, causing him to "mouth breathe." Until this most recent illness, Mike had started efforts toward a healthier lifestyle and weight reduction. He is now jogging for exercise and taking vitamin tablets. He is diagnosed with acute sinusitis, and the healthcare provider orders ciprofloxacin PO 500 mg twice daily for 10 days. Additional medications prescribed include a nasal decongestant and a mild analgesic.

As Mike is leaving the health clinic, he comments that he is responsible for multiple corporate offices and will soon be traveling. He is worried about remembering to take the medication and admits to a history of nonadherence to therapy regimens because of his forgetfulness.

Critical Thinking Questions

1. Prepare a patient teaching handout for Mike that provides him with information about the antibiotics he is being prescribed.
2. Mike asks you, the nurse, if he should continue jogging and taking vitamins. What would you advise?
3. What tips can you provide someone who forgets to take scheduled medications?

Additional Case Study

Carolyn Ijams is doing her spring cleaning. As she is arranging the contents of her medicine cabinet, she notices a bottle of ciprofloxacin ophthalmic drops that is about half-used. She wonders whether she should keep it and asks you, the nurse who lives next door, what she should do.

1. Should Carolyn keep the ciprofloxacin drops? What would you want to know before making a recommendation?
2. What would you teach Carolyn about the use of ophthalmic drops such as ciprofloxacin?

Chapter Review

1. The patient is prescribed ciprofloxacin (Cipro) and is instructed to take each dose of medication as evenly spaced apart during the day as possible. The nurse recognizes that this instruction is essential because:
    1. The medication can cause sleep pattern disturbances.
    2. Pathogenic bacteria have extremely rapid growth and reproduction rates.
    3. Superinfections may develop if a dose of the medication is missed.
    4. Allergic reactions are more likely to occur if a dose is missed.
2. The patient is prescribed ofloxacin (Floxin) for treatment of acute bronchitis. The patient tells the nurse that he experienced an allergic reaction when he took ciprofloxacin previously. As reported by the patient, which of the following would be most indicative of an allergic reaction to this drug group? (Select all that apply.)
    1. Headache
    2. Nausea and vomiting
    3. Itching without visible rash
    4. Swelling of lips or tongue
    5. Nervousness or anxiety
3. The nurse is instructing a patient on a new prescription for ciprofloxacin (Cipro) and will include which instructions? (Select all that apply.)
    1. Increase fluid intake to 2 to 3 liters per day.
    2. Avoid consuming dairy products or antacids when you take the antibiotic.
    3. Limit vitamin C intake in both dietary and oral vitamin forms.
    4. Take the pill with an antihistamine to avoid adverse effects.
    5. Coffee or tea without milk, cream, or coffee-lightener is the preferred beverage for taking the antibiotic dose.
4. A patient has been receiving levofloxacin IV for septicemia for 2 weeks and will be given the drug orally at home. Which discharge instruction would be most appropriate for the nurse to give this patient?
    1. Report any unusual joint or tendon pain or difficulty with movement or walking.
    2. Take a daily multivitamin supplement with the levofloxacin.
    3. Exposure to direct sunlight will help increase absorption of vitamin D, which is impaired by this medication.
    4. Limit fluid intake to less than 1500 mL per day.
5. A patient has been given a prescription for ciprofloxacin. The nurse checks the patient's history because this drug should be used cautiously, or is contraindicated, in patients with what condition?
    1. A history of anxiety disorder and nervousness
    2. Patients over the age of 65
    3. A history of penicillin allergy
    4. Patients with myasthenia gravis

6. Which is the most important goal of nursing care for a patient receiving polymyxin B ointment on a laceration?

1. Promote wound healing.
2. Sterilize the skin and mucous membranes.
3. Prevent allergic reaction.
4. Maximize pain relief.

See Appendix A for answers to critical thinking questions, case study questions, and review questions.

Selected Bibliography

Alves, C., Mendes, D., & Marques, F. B. (2019). Fluoroquinolones and the risk of tendon injury: a systematic review and meta-analysis. *European Journal of Clinical Pharmacology*, *75*(10), 1431–1443. https://doi.org/10.1007/s00228-019-02713-1

Aschenbrenner, D. S. (2019). New warning for fluoroquinolone antibiotics. *American Journal of Nursing*, *119*(4), 20. https://doi.org/10.1097/01.NAJ.0000554544.80148.ee

Coudray, M. S., & Madhivanan, P. (2020). Bacterial vaginosis—A brief synopsis of the literature. *European Journal of Obstetrics and Gynecology and Reproductive Biology*, *245*, 143–148. https://doi.org/10.1016/j.ejogrb.2019.12.035

Gorelik, E., Masarwa, R., Perlman, A., Rotshild, V., Abbasi, M., Muszkat, M., & Matok, I. (2019). Fluoroquinolones and cardiovascular risk: a systematic review, meta-analysis and network meta-analysis. *Drug Safety*, *42*(4), 529–538. https://doi.org/10.1007/s40264-018-0751-2

Jackson, M. A., Schutze, G. E., & Committee on Infectious Diseases. (2016). The use of systemic and topical fluoroquinolones. *Pediatrics*, *138*, e20162706. https://doi.org/10.1542/peds.2016-2706

Madigan, M. T., Bender, K. S., Buckley, D. H., Sattley, W. M., & Stahl, D. A. (2018). *Brock biology of microorganisms* (15th ed.). Pearson.

Martin, L. T., Vincent, S., Gillian, S., Moore, K., Ratermann, D., & Droege, C. A. (2019). Pharmacologic approach to management of *Clostridium difficile* infection. *Critical Care Nursing Quarterly*, *42*(1), 2–11. https://doi.org/10.1097/CNQ.0000000000000232

Meesters, K., Raes, A. M., & Walle, J. G. V. (2019). What do I need to know about fluoroquinolones for children? *Archives of Disease in Childhood-Education and Practice*, *104*(5), 254–258. http://dx.doi.org/10.1136/archdischild-2017-313513

Yang, Y., Feye, K. M., Shi, Z., Pavlidis, H. O., Kogut, M., Ashworth, A. J., & Ricke, S. C. (2019). A historical review on antibiotic resistance of foodborne Campylobacter. *Frontiers in Microbiology*, *10*, 1509. https://doi.org/10.3389/fmicb.2019.01509

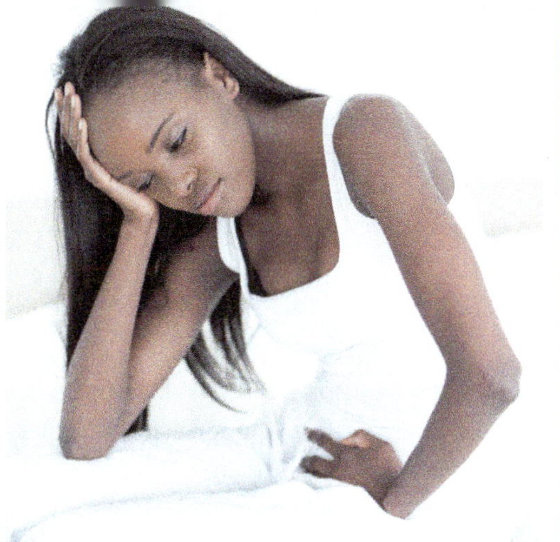

"It seems that I have been sick all winter. Yesterday, when I began having a fever, I took some antibiotic tablets that a doctor prescribed when I was sick last month. I'm sure glad I didn't take all of the prescription and had some of the pills left to take."
—*Patient "Amoya Deboissiere"*

Chapter 50
Sulfonamides and the Pharmacotherapy of Urinary Tract Infections

Chapter Outline

Learning Outcomes

After reading this chapter, the student should be able to:

1. Classify types of urinary tract infections based on their anatomic location.
2. Explain the epidemiology and pathogenesis of urinary tract infections.
3. Compare and contrast the pharmacotherapy of complicated versus uncomplicated urinary tract infections.
4. Identify the classes of antibiotics used to treat urinary tract infections.
5. Describe modifications in the pharmacotherapy of urinary tract infections for infants and children, pregnant women, older adults, and those with recurring infections.
6. Explain why folic acid inhibitors exert selective toxicity toward bacterial cells.
7. For each of the classes shown in the chapter outline, identify the prototype and representative drugs and explain the mechanism(s) of drug action, primary indications, contraindications, significant drug interactions, pregnancy data, and important adverse effects.
8. Apply clinical judgment to care for patients receiving pharmacotherapy for urinary tract infections.

Key Terms

Definitions of the terms in bold may be found in the Glossary.

Urinary tract infections (UTIs) account for an estimated 7 million office visits and 100,000 hospitalizations per year, making them the most common type of bacterial infection. Although antimicrobial therapy of these infections is often straightforward, UTI is becoming a major clinical challenge in this era of increasing antibiotic resistance. This chapter examines the types of patients most likely to acquire UTIs and the anti-infective therapy that is most effective against them.

Pathophysiology of Urinary Tract Infections

50.1 Infections can occur in any portion of the urinary tract.

The urinary tract consists of the kidneys, ureters, urinary bladder, and urethra. The male and female urinary tracts are identical, with the exception of the urethra, which is shorter in the female and located closer to the anus. This anatomic difference results in the periurethral region of the female being populated by bacteria that are normally restricted to the gastrointestinal (GI) tract and could cause UTIs. In addition to the male having a longer urethra, the scrotum provides a physical barrier between the urethra and the anus. These anatomic differences result in a higher risk of UTI in females.

The continuous, peristaltic flow of urine from the kidneys, down the ureters, into the bladder, and voiding through the urethra provide formidable barriers to harmful microorganisms, or **uropathogens**, attempting to invade the urinary system. Although it is indeed difficult for uropathogens to go against the flow of urine and reach beyond the proximal portion of the urethra, this is the means by which the large majority of UTIs are acquired. Infections that travel from the urethra to the bladder or kidney are known as retrograde or ascending infections. The most successful uropathogens are those that secrete sticky adhesion proteins or that have structures called fimbriae that allow them to adhere to the epithelial lining of the urinary tract. Occasionally, pathogens traveling through the blood can infect the kidney. This mode of infection is called the hematogenous route and is responsible for about 5% of all UTIs.

Any portion of the urinary tract may be infected by uropathogens. Infection of the urethra, or **urethritis**, presents as discomfort during voiding and occurs in both men and women. It is usually distinguished from a bladder infection, or **cystitis**, because it causes less voiding urgency than cystitis and has a more gradual onset of symptoms. Urethritis is often a sign of a sexually transmitted infection.

A cluster of complaints known as **irritative voiding symptoms** accompanies cystitis. Occurring in both men and women, symptoms include dysuria and increased voiding urgency and frequency. Despite the increased urgency and frequency, only small volumes of urine are voided during each attempt. During and immediately following voiding, burning or aching may occur. The patient may have suprapubic tenderness upon palpation. Urinalysis usually identifies the presence of an offending uropathogen, or **bacteriuria**, as well as other signs of infection such as pyuria, hematuria, and changes in urine pH, nitrites, or proteins.

In women, symptoms of cystitis are frequently reported following intercourse with a new sexual partner. In men, cystitis is likely to occur following anal intercourse. Cystitis in men may be accompanied by acute **prostatitis**. Normally recognized by palpating the prostate, which will be tender during manual examination, prostatitis may include fever and has the potential to cause urinary obstruction as the prostate swells.

Bacteria that ascend the ureter and reach the kidney can cause **pyelonephritis**, an inflammation of the kidney, pelvis, and other renal cells. Irritative voiding symptoms occur, along with other signs similar to cystitis. More severe symptoms are manifested as nausea and vomiting, fever, chills, and acute costovertebral angle and flank tenderness. Because acute pyelonephritis may lead to shock, aggressive anti-infective therapy may be required.

Pharmacotherapy of Urinary Tract Infections

50.2 Choice of pharmacotherapy for acute urinary tract infection depends on the severity of the infection and the presence of coexisting conditions.

In addition to describing UTIs by their location, these infections are also classified as complicated or uncomplicated. The classification is an important clinical distinction because the pharmacotherapy for complicated UTI and uncomplicated UTI is quite different.

Acute Uncomplicated Cystitis

Acute uncomplicated cystitis (AUC) occurs in patients who have no serious or chronic health disorders that might impact the spread of the uropathogen or the treatment of the UTI. These infections occur mostly in women of reproductive age, with the highest incidence occurring from 18 to 24 years of age. Adult men rarely have AUC. Common risk factors for AUC include the following:

- Frequent sexual activity
- Use of spermicides for contraception
- Incontinence
- Estrogen deficiency.

In many cases, a diagnosis of AUC is made by the healthcare provider based on symptoms and history alone, without laboratory testing. Women who have experienced a prior AUC are often able to self-diagnose. Rapid dipstick tests are available to examine for the presence of infection. *Escherichia coli* is the most common causative agent for AUC, being responsible for 80 to 90% of UTIs. *Staphylococcus saprophyticus* is isolated in about 10 to 15% of the cases. The most frequent uropathogens are listed in Table 50.1. Follow-up of AUC is usually by routine office visit; no additional testing is required if the symptoms promptly resolve.

The selection of an initial antibiotic and duration of therapy for AUC vary among healthcare providers. The choice may be customized to an institution or community, based on local antibiotic resistance patterns and practitioner experience. Single-dose or short-course therapy is preferred for patient convenience and to maximize adherence.

Asymptomatic bacteriuria is frequently discovered on a routine urinalysis: Estimates range from 1 to 2% of young adult women to as high as 60% of women over age 60. In general, asymptomatic bacteriuria is not treated with medications because very few of these patients will progress to symptomatic UTI. Widespread therapy would be costly and promote resistant strains in the community. Certain populations of patients, however, are treated when asymptomatic bacteriuria is discovered. These include pregnant women, those undergoing urologic procedures, and patients who are immunosuppressed or in otherwise poor health.

Three drug regimens are considered first-line therapy for AUC. The traditional choice is trimethoprim-sulfamethoxazole (TMP-SMZ), a fixed-dose combination drug that is featured as a prototype in Section 50.4. Given as a 3-day regimen, TMP-SMZ is effective at eliminating most of the common species of uropathogens. The occurrence of many resistant strains, however, has limited its use as a first-line drug.

In communities where TMP-SMZ resistance is high (over 20%), a urinary antiseptic such as nitrofurantoin taken for 5 to 7 days is effective. Nitrofurantoin is featured as a prototype in Section 50.5. If adherence is an issue, a single dose of fosfomycin (Monurol) has proven effective for many patients. Fosfomycin blocks cell wall synthesis, and its only indication is UTI.

Fluoroquinolones are highly effective at treating UTI, however, they are considered second-line antibiotics for AUC due to the existence of resistant strains. They are still considered first-line drugs for *complicated* UTIs. Indeed, practitioners are concerned that if fluoroquinolones are used too frequently for AUC, it will increase the number of resistant strains so the drugs will no longer be effective against more serious infections. Fluoroquinolones useful in treating AUC include ciprofloxacin (Cipro XR), ofloxacin, and levofloxacin. Additional details about the fluoroquinolones are presented in Chapter 49.

Beta-lactam antibiotics are alternate therapies for AUC that are employed when other therapies are ineffective or contraindicated. These drugs are usually given for 7 to 10 days. Choices include amoxicillin-clavulanate, cefaclor, cefdinir, cefpodoxime, and cefuroxime.

CONNECTION Checkpoint 50.1

From what you learned in Chapter 49, what black box warning accompanies the oral and parenteral fluoroquinolones?

Table 50.1 Most Common Uropathogens

Uncomplicated UTI	Complicated UTI
E. coli	*E. coli*
S. saprophyticus	Enterobacteriaceae
Klebsiella	*Klebsiella*
Proteus mirabilis	Group B streptococci
Enterobacter	*Enterococcus*
	Pseudomonas
	Proteus mirabilis

Complicated Urinary Tract Infection

Complicated urinary tract infections (C-UTIs) are defined as infections that occur in a patient who has an underlying condition that increases the risk of treatment failure. C-UTIs may require aggressive pharmacotherapy, often involving more toxic drugs, higher doses, or prolonged therapy. Coexisting conditions that may influence pharmacotherapy include the following:

- Structural or functional abnormalities in the genitourinary tract such as neurogenic bladder, benign prostatic hyperplasia (BPH), kidney tumor, or urinary stones
- Indwelling urinary catheters
- Older patients with generally ill health
- Recurring urinary infections
- Identification of resistant uropathogens
- Patients with poor toileting or periurethral hygiene
- All UTIs in men.

Although nearly all uncomplicated UTIs are caused by *E. coli* and *S. saprophyticus*, C-UTIs are caused by a wider variety of uropathogens (see Table 50.1). Hospital-acquired C-UTIs are sometimes caused by organisms such as *Klebsiella*, *Enterobacter*, *Proteus*, and *Pseudomonas*. When treating C-UTIs, a urine sample should be obtained to identify the specific microbe and the most effective antibiotic based on culture and sensitivity (C&S) testing. Therapy is often begun with a broad-spectrum anti-infective, then adjusted based on C&S results. Patients who have mild or moderate C-UTIs can be treated with the same medications used for AUC: TMP-SMZ, nitrofurantoin, or a fluoroquinolone. A newer treatment approved in 2017 is Vabomere, a combination that contains meropenem and vaborbactam, a beta-lactamase inhibitor. Therapy for C-UTI is continued for 10 to 14 days to be certain that all uropathogens have been eliminated. Severe disease requires hospitalization with parenteral administration of fluoroquinolones, aminoglycosides, cephalosporins, or ampicillin, depending on the sensitivity of the microbe. Follow-up urine cultures are performed several weeks after completion of therapy to ensure that the uropathogen has been eliminated.

PharmFACT

Although men have a much lower overall incidence of UTI than women, the presence of prostatic hyperplasia or catheterization in men over age 50 dramatically increases the risk of UTI (Brusch, 2020).

Modified Pharmacotherapy for Specific Populations

50.3 Infants, children, pregnant women, older adults, and those with recurring urinary tract infections require modifications to standard pharmacotherapy.

Certain populations require special consideration when selecting and initiating a course of pharmacotherapy to treat UTI. These include infants, children, pregnant women, older adults, and those with recurring infections.

Infants and Children

Although UTIs occur most frequently in sexually active adult women, they are also relatively common in infants and children. More than 2% of boys have a UTI before 12 months of age, a higher percentage than girls of the same age. As many as 3% of all and 1% of boys experience a UTI during their school-age years. A concern with pediatric patients is that repeated UTIs may cause scarring of the kidneys, resulting in hypertension (HTN) later in life. With this possibility in mind, healthcare providers have a goal of preventing recurring infections in children.

As in adults, *E. coli* causes most pediatric UTIs. Therapeutic options, however, are more limited in children. TMP-SMZ and nitrofurantoin are effective in children. However, fluoroquinolones are contraindicated in children under age 18 because they have been found to affect cartilage development. The safety and efficacy of fosfomycin has not been established in children younger than 12 years old. Recurring UTIs in infants and children may require prolonged, prophylactic antibiotic therapy.

Pregnancy

During pregnancy, the enlarging uterus creates pressure on the urinary bladder, which increases the size of the ureters and promotes urinary stasis and reflux. UTIs in pregnant women are a risk factor for prematurity and newborn low birth weight. In addition, pyelonephritis is one of the most frequent reasons for hospitalization during pregnancy.

Urinary screening is routinely performed by the 16th week of pregnancy. Discovery of high levels of bacteria in the urine is an indication for antimicrobial therapy, even if the patient is asymptomatic at the time of testing. A follow-up culture is performed 1 to 2 weeks after therapy is completed. Continued asymptomatic bacteriuria is predictive of the development of symptomatic UTI later in pregnancy. Therapy for asymptomatic bacteriuria is continued until cultures are negative or until delivery.

During pregnancy, C&S testing may be conducted to identify the most effective antibiotic. First-line, broad-spectrum medications include nitrofurantoin, amoxicillin-clavulanate, cephalexin, and fosfomycin. Ampicillin is also considered a first-line drug if the organism is shown to be susceptible to this antibiotic. All the first-line drugs are given for 5 to 7 days except fosfomycin, which is a single dose. Fluoroquinolones are contraindicated during pregnancy due to possible growth inhibition in the fetus, and TMP-SMZ is contraindicated during the first trimester. Asymptomatic patients are sometimes given a shorter treatment of 1 to 3 days.

CONNECTION Checkpoint 50.2

From what you learned in Chapter 47, if a pregnant patient has a history of allergy to ampicillin, should the nurse administer a cephalosporin such as ceftriaxone for UTI?

Older Adults

UTIs are common in the geriatric population, especially for those in long-term care (LTC) facilities. Factors that predispose older adults to UTI are BPH, increased postvoid residual urine, and urinary incontinence. Residents of LTC facilities may have chronic diseases that require the use of indwelling catheters or IV lines. The large percentage of patients receiving antibiotics in these facilities promotes the emergence of multidrug-resistant strains, which can be difficult to eliminate in the LTC setting.

Pharmacotherapy in the geriatric population is conducted in the same manner as for younger adults, if the patient is otherwise healthy. Asymptomatic bacteriuria is generally not treated unless the patient has an underlying comorbid condition. Asymptomatic bacteriuria is present in 30 to 50% of older adults, and such widespread therapy would promote the emergence of resistant strains.

Older adults in generally poor health and those with certain coexisting conditions receive more aggressive pharmacotherapy. These patients may exhibit atypical symptoms, such as altered mental status, sudden incontinence, or nausea and vomiting. If immunosuppressed, an antibiotic may be prescribed for prophylaxis against pneumonia, UTIs, and skin and soft tissue infections, which are the three most common infections in LTC facilities. Because of the prevalence of resistant strains, patients in an LTC setting with symptomatic UTI should undergo C&S testing to determine the most effective course of therapy. Pharmacotherapy may be prolonged and continue until urine cultures are negative.

By providing a direct route of entry to the bladder for uropathogens, catheter-associated UTI is one of the common hospital-acquired infections. Because the risk of infection increases over time, the catheter should be removed as soon as feasible. Patients with catheters should be carefully monitored for signs of UTI. Periodic urinalysis testing should be conducted to check for bacteriuria. A positive urine culture, with or without urinary tract symptoms, is an indication for removal of the catheter (if feasible) and initiation of pharmacotherapy.

Patients with Recurring Urinary Tract Infections

One in five patients with a UTI will experience a subsequent UTI within 6 months. Recurring UTIs are classified as either relapses or reinfections. A *relapse* occurs when the patient experiences a second UTI within 2 weeks after completing pharmacotherapy for the original infection. Normally, a relapse is caused by failure of the initial treatment to totally eliminate the uropathogen. A *reinfection* occurs when the patient recovers from the original infection but acquires another infection weeks or months later. Reinfections may be caused by the original microbe or by a different uropathogen.

Recurrent UTIs require extended antimicrobial therapy, either with the original antibiotic or with a different medication. It is necessary to identify the pathogen in order to examine for resistant strains.

Women who experience two or more UTIs within 6 months, or three or more UTIs over the course of a year, may be candidates for prophylactic therapy. Choices for prophylaxis include administration of antibiotics at low doses either on a daily or three-times-per-week schedule. Another option is to allow the woman to initiate therapy herself. With this type of treatment, the patient is provided with a single-dose or 3-day course of therapy, which is initiated by the woman after each act of coitus, or when symptoms first develop. Patients should be advised to see their healthcare provider if symptoms worsen, or if they do not resolve during prophylactic therapy because this may be a sign of a more serious infection.

Sulfonamides

50.4 Sulfonamides are the traditional preferred drugs for urinary tract infections, but resistance limits their usefulness.

The discovery of the sulfonamides, also called sulfa drugs, in the 1930s heralded a new era in the treatment of infectious disease. Effective against both gram-positive and gram-negative bacteria, the sulfonamides significantly reduced mortality from susceptible microbes and earned its discoverer a Nobel Prize in medicine in 1938. Doses for the sulfonamides are listed in Table 50.2.

Sulfonamides are active against a broad spectrum of microorganisms including some staphylococci, many streptococci (except *Enterococcus faecalis*), *Haemophilus influenzae*, *Nocardia*, most Enterobacteriaceae, *Neisseria*, and *Chlamydia*. Sulfonamides have also been used to treat mycobacterial infections and some protozoans such as *Toxoplasma gondii*. Drugs in this class are also given for treatment and prophylaxis of *Pneumocystis jiroveci* pneumonia and *Shigella* infections of the small bowel. The nurse should keep in mind that although these drugs are approved by the U.S. Food and Drug Administration (FDA) to treat many different species of bacteria, the sensitivity of specific strains to sulfonamides in a particular community setting must be confirmed.

Sulfonamides suppress bacterial growth by inhibiting the synthesis of folic acid, or folate. In human physiology, folic acid is a water-soluble vitamin that serves a critical role as a coenzyme in the synthesis of ribonucleic acid (RNA) and deoxyribonucleic acid (DNA). But if folic acid is essential to both humans and bacteria, why are the sulfonamides not acutely toxic to humans? The answer lies in differences in the metabolic pathways in humans and bacteria.

Humans must obtain "premade" folic acid by eating foods rich in this vitamin. Humans are unable to synthesize this essential nutrient "from scratch." Bacteria, on the other hand, make their own folic acid using simpler precursor molecules. The basic steps in this pathway are shown in Figure 50.1. Sulfonamides inhibit the enzyme in step 1; the drug trimethoprim inhibits the enzyme in step 3. Note how closely the sulfonamides resemble the precursor molecule, **para-aminobenzoic acid (PABA)**, in Figure 50.2. It is easy to see how an enzyme could confuse the two similar

Table 50.2 Sulfonamides and Other Drugs Used for Urinary Tract Infections

Drug	Adult Dose (Maximum Dose Where Indicated)	Adverse Effects
Sulfonamides		
silver sulfadiazine (Silvadene, Thermazene)	Topical: Apply 1% cream 1–2 times per day to burn wounds to a thickness of 1.5 mm	*Nausea and vomiting, anorexia, rash, crystalluria, burning or stinging with topical and ophthalmic solutions* Anaphylaxis, Stevens–Johnson syndrome (SJS), blood dyscrasias, fulminant hepatic necrosis, hyperkalemia
sulfacetamide (Klaron)	Ophthalmic: 1–3 drops or ½ in ointment in affected eye q2–4 h Topical (Klaron): Apply thin film to area bid	
sulfadiazine	PO: Loading dose: 2–4 g Maintenance dose: 2–4 g/day in four to six divided doses	
sulfasalazine (Azulfidine)	PO: 1–2 g/day in 4 divided doses	
trimethoprim (Primsol)	PO: 100–200 mg daily	
trimethoprim-sulfamethoxazole (TMP-SMZ) (Bactrim, Septra)	PO: 160 mg TMP/800 mg SMZ bid IV: 8–10 mg/kg/day TMP, q6–12h infused over 60–90 min	
Urinary Antiseptics and Miscellaneous Drugs		
fosfomycin (Monurol)	PO: 3-g sachet dissolved in 3–4 oz of water as a single dose	*Nausea, diarrhea, back pain, headache* Anaphylaxis, superinfections
meropenem and vaborbactam (Vabomere)	IV: 2 g meropenem and 2 g vaborbactam tid	*Headache, phlebitis, infusion site reactions, diarrhea* Anaphylaxis, seizures
methenamine hippurate (Hiprex) or mandelate (Mandelamine)	PO: 1 g bid (hippurate) or 1 g qid (mandelate)	*Nausea and vomiting, diarrhea, increased urinary urgency* Anaphylaxis, crystalluria
nitrofurantoin (Furadantin) and nitrofurantoin macrocrystals (Macrobid, Macrodantin)	PO: 50–100 mg qid (max: 7 mg/kg/day)	*Nausea and vomiting, anorexia, dark urine, rash* Anaphylaxis, superinfections, hepatic necrosis, interstitial pneumonitis, SJS, hemolytic anemia

Note: *Italics* indicate common adverse effects. Underline indicates serious adverse effects.

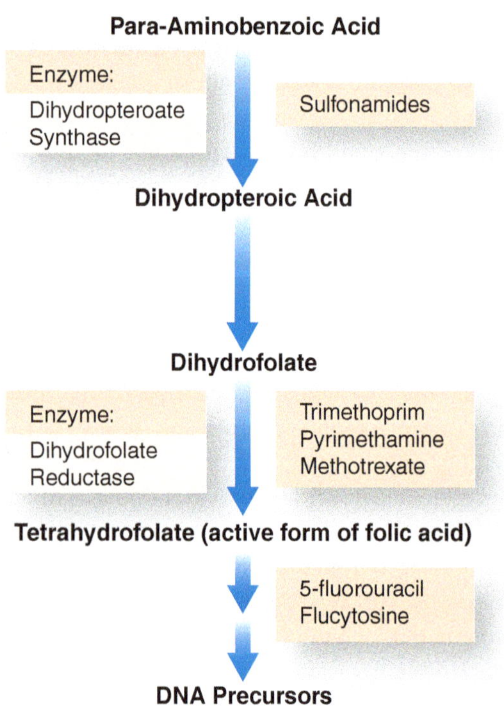

Figure 50.1 Drug inhibition of folic acid metabolism. Drugs inhibit multiple steps in the metabolic pathway leading to folic acid.

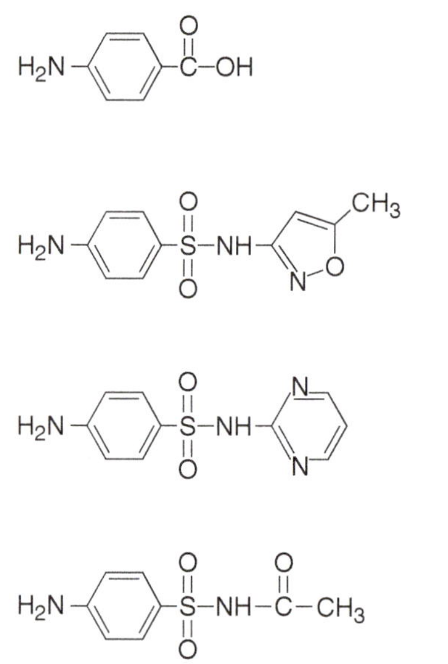

Figure 50.2 Chemical similarities between para-aminobenzoic acid and sulfonamides.

molecules. Once the enzyme binds to the sulfonamide, however, folic acid synthesis stops, and bacterial growth slows. This explains why these drugs are bacteriostatic; they slow bacterial growth rather than kill the cells.

The widespread use of sulfonamides for over 60 years resulted in a substantial number of resistant strains. The mechanism of acquired resistance to sulfonamides is most often a mutation in the enzyme performing step 1 of folic acid synthesis. Mutant enzymes can still bind to PABA but can no longer bind to sulfonamides. Resistance to one sulfonamide may confer resistance to all members of this class.

In addition to resistance, several other factors have led to a significant decline in the use of sulfonamides. The development of the penicillins, cephalosporins, fluoroquinolones, and macrolides gave practitioners larger choices of antibiotics, some of which exhibited an improved safety profile over the sulfonamides. Approval of the combination antibiotic TMP-SMZ marked a resurgence in the use of sulfonamides in treating UTIs. Decades of widespread use, however, have now resulted in a large number of strains resistant to TMP-SMZ. In communities with high resistance rates, TMP-SMZ is no longer a first-line drug, unless C&S testing determines it to be the most effective drug for the specific uropathogen.

Sulfonamides are classified by their absorption and excretion characteristics. These subclasses include:

- Oral (PO) drugs that are readily absorbed
- PO drugs that are incompletely absorbed
- Topical drugs.

Medications that are readily absorbed after a PO dose include TMP-SMZ and sulfadiazine. These sulfonamides are distributed to most tissues in the body, and the amount of plasma protein binding may be significant. Once hepatic enzymes convert these drugs to inactive metabolites, the drugs are excreted rapidly by the kidney.

One sulfonamide comprises the second subclass. Sulfasalazine (Azulfidine) remains mostly unabsorbed in the alimentary canal (only 10 to 15% is absorbed), where it is used to treat mild to moderate ulcerative colitis. It is also approved as a disease-modifying antirheumatic drug.

The third subclass includes topical sulfonamides. Silver sulfadiazine (Silvadene, Thermazene) is used for the prophylaxis and treatment of topical infections resulting from wounds or burns. Mafenide (Sulfamylon) is applied topically over burn wounds. Topical sulfonamides may be absorbed across denuded skin, resulting in significant plasma drug levels. Sulfacetamide is a topical sulfonamide used to treat either conjunctivitis or acne. Blephamide is a combination drug with sulfacetamide and prednisolone indicated for ocular infections that have inflammation as a significant component.

CONNECTIONS: Patient Safety

Trimethoprim-Sulfamethoxazole (Bactrim, Septra)

The nurse is preparing to administer TMP-SMZ to a patient with a UTI. Before giving the medication, the nurse reviews the patient's chart. The nurse notices that the patient is afebrile with a normal pulse, blood pressure, and respiratory rate. The most recent culture indicates a decline in the number of bacteria present in the urine. Other information found in the medical record indicates that the patient routinely takes medication for HTN and arthritis. The patient has also reported allergies to chocolate and thiazide diuretics. Should the nurse give the medication as prescribed?

In general, the sulfonamides are safe drugs; however, some adverse effects may be serious. Of most concern are adverse effects on the urinary tract, hypersensitivity reactions, and blood abnormalities. Nausea and vomiting and anorexia may also occur.

Drugs in this class must be used with caution in patients with chronic kidney disease (CKD). Sulfonamides have a low solubility, which may cause **crystalluria**, crystals that form in the urine and potentially obstruct the kidneys or ureters. The risk is higher in dehydrated patients and when urine pH is abnormally low. To decrease the possibility of crystalluria, fluids in amounts up to 3000 mL/day should be encouraged to achieve a urinary output of 1500 mL in 24 hours.

Although not common, sulfonamides can cause potentially fatal blood abnormalities such as aplastic anemia, acute hemolytic anemia, and agranulocytosis. Baseline and periodic blood laboratory values should be assessed to prevent the development of anemia or other hematologic disorders. Patients with preexisting myelosuppression should be monitored carefully during therapy because this increases the risks associated with drug-induced bone marrow depression.

Hypersensitivity to sulfa drugs is well documented. These drugs cause a number of dermal reactions ranging from urticaria to photosensitivity and exfoliative dermatitis. Patients may develop fever and malaise. Cross sensitivity exists with diuretics, such as acetazolamide and the thiazides, and with sulfonylurea antidiabetic drugs. These medications should be avoided in patients with a history of hypersensitivity to sulfonamides because this can induce SJS. At the first signs of rash, patients should be instructed to stop taking the drug and contact their healthcare provider.

Most sulfonamides readily cross the placenta and have the potential to interfere with folate metabolism in the fetus or neonate. They are contraindicated for infants less than 2 months of age and for pregnant patients near term because sulfonamides displace bilirubin from plasma proteins. The displaced, free bilirubin is toxic to the brain and causes kernicterus, a serious type of jaundice.

PROTOTYPE DRUG Trimethoprim-Sulfamethoxazole (Bactrim, Septra)

Classification **Therapeutic:** Antibacterial
Pharmacologic: Folic acid inhibitor, sulfonamide

Therapeutic Effects and Uses: Approved in 1973, TMP-SMZ is a folic acid inhibitor containing a fixed-dose combination of trimethoprim (TMP) and sulfamethoxazole (SMZ), a sulfonamide. The drug is commonly used for UTI prophylaxis and in the pharmacotherapy of complicated and uncomplicated UTI, depending on the sensitivity of the specific uropathogen. It is also approved for the treatment and prophylaxis of *P. jiroveci* pneumonia, *Shigella* infections of the small bowel, traveler's diarrhea due to *E. coli*, and for acute exacerbations of chronic bronchitis due to *Streptococcus pneumoniae* or *H. influenzae*. The drug is used off-label for many other indications, depending on the sensitivity of the microbe. PO and IV formulations are available.

Mechanism of Action: Both SMZ and TMP are inhibitors of the bacterial metabolism of folic acid. Each drug inhibits a separate enzyme in the metabolic pathway, creating a synergistic combination: A greater bacterial kill is achieved by the fixed combination than would be achieved with either drug used separately. Because humans obtain folate in their diets, these medications are selective toward bacterial folate metabolism.

Pharmacokinetics:

Route(s)	PO, IV
Absorption	Readily absorbed
Distribution	Widely distributed to all body fluids, including cerebrospinal fluid; crosses the placenta; secreted in breast milk; protein binding is 70% (SMZ) and 44% (TMP)
Primary metabolism	Hepatic
Primary excretion	Renal
Onset of action	PO: 1–4 h
Duration of action	Half-life: 8–10 h (TMP) and 10–13 h (SMZ)

Adverse Effects: Nausea and vomiting are the most common adverse effects of TMP-SMZ therapy. These normally diminish with time but may require treatment or cause discontinuation of therapy. Hypersensitivity is relatively common and usually manifests as skin rash, pruritus, and fever. Severe hypersensitivity reactions such as anaphylaxis, SJS, epidermal necrolysis, agranulocytosis, aplastic anemia, and allergic myocarditis have been reported. The drug should be discontinued at the first appearance of a skin rash. To prevent crystalluria and potential damage to tubular cells, it is important to maintain dilute urine during therapy to reduce the concentration of the drugs as they travel through the renal tubule. Due to the potential for photosensitivity, the patient should avoid direct sunlight during therapy.

Contraindications/Precautions: An allergy history should be taken prior to administration because TMP-SMZ is contraindicated in patients with hypersensitivity to sulfites, sulfonamides, or chemically related drugs such as thiazide diuretics. TMP-SMZ is contraindicated in patients with folate deficiency anemia since a folic acid inhibitor would worsen this condition. This medication is contraindicated in patients with severe CKD because this is the primary route of drug excretion and the drug may accumulate to toxic levels in these patients. It should be used with caution in patients with hepatic impairment because the liver metabolizes TMP-SMZ. Trimethoprim decreases potassium excretion and is contraindicated in patients with hyperkalemia. Caution must be used when treating patients infected with human immunodeficiency virus (HIV) because these patients have a greater incidence of serious adverse effects than others.

Drug Interactions: TMP and SMZ may enhance the effects of oral anticoagulants. Since methotrexate also interferes with folate metabolism, concurrent use with TMP-SMZ increases the risk of toxicity. TMP-SMZ exerts a potassium-sparing effect on the nephron and should be used with caution with diuretics such as spironolactone (Aldactone) to prevent hyperkalemia. TMP-SMZ may increase the hypoglycemic response to sulfonylureas due to displacement from protein-binding sites or inhibition of metabolism. **Herbal/Food:** Potassium supplements should not be taken during therapy, unless directed by the healthcare provider.

Pregnancy: Some human epidemiological data suggest there may be an association between use of TMP-SMV in the first trimester and congenital malformations and increased spontaneous abortions. Because metabolites of this drug are secreted in human milk, caution should be used if breastfeeding. TMP-SMV should not be used during pregnancy or lactation unless the potential benefits to the mother justify the potential risks to the fetus or neonate.

Treatment of Overdose: Acidification of the urine will increase the renal elimination of trimethoprim. If signs of bone marrow depression occur during high-dose therapy, 5 to 15 mg of leucovorin should be given daily.

Clinician Responsibilities: Key clinical implications for patients receiving TMP-SMZ are included in Applied Clinical Judgment: Patients Receiving Pharmacotherapy for Urinary Tract Infection.

Drugs Similar to Trimethoprim-Sulfamethoxazole (Bactrim, Septra)

Other orally absorbed sulfonamides include sulfacetamide, sulfadiazine, sulfasalazine, and trimethoprim. Sulfisoxazole and sulfadoxine-pyrimethamine (Fansidar) have been withdrawn from the US market.

Sulfacetamide: Sulfacetamide is a topical sulfonamide used to treat either conjunctivitis or acne. For conjunctivitis or other external eye infection a solution or ointment is applied. Blephamide is a combination drug with sulfacetamide and prednisolone indicated for ocular infections that have inflammation as a significant component. Sulfacetamide (Klaron) is applied as a cream for acne vulgaris or seborrheic dermatitis. It is not known if topical sulfonamides cause fetal harm or have adverse effects on the breastfed neonate.

Sulfadiazine: Approved in 1941, sulfadiazine is a short-acting, oral sulfonamide that is given every 4 to 6 hours. It has a broad spectrum and is used for diverse infections, including UTI, nocardiosis, meningococcal meningitis, cerebral toxoplasmosis (in combination with pyrimethamine), and resistant malaria. Sulfadiazine is usually prescribed only when safer anti-infectives have failed to produce a therapeutic effect and C&S testing has determined the organism to be sensitive to the drug. Like other sulfonamides, hypersensitivity may be a limitation to therapy. Sulfadiazine is poorly soluble in urine and causes more crystalluria than other sulfonamides. Adequate fluid intake and frequent urinary testing are essential to avoid nephrotoxicity. Sulfadiazine carries a black box warning that it should be discontinued at the first sign of a skin rash due to the possibility for SJS. Animal studies and some human epidemiological data suggest this drug may cause fetal harm. Because sulfonamides are secreted in human milk, caution should be used if breastfeeding.

Silver sulfadiazine (Silvadene, Thermazene) is a topical cream indicated as an adjunct for the prevention and treatment of wound sepsis in patients with second- and third-degree burns. Adverse effects are rare when the cream is applied over small areas. However, when the drug is applied over large, denuded areas, some of the topical medication is absorbed and systemic adverse effects may occur.

Sulfasalazine (Azulfidine): Sulfasalazine is a prodrug that is converted by bacteria in the colon to two active metabolites: sulfapyridine and 5-aminosalicylic acid (5-ASA). These metabolites have significant anti-inflammatory properties. Most of the drug and metabolites remain in the intestine, where they reduce inflammation due to ulcerative colitis. A portion is absorbed and can bring relief to patients with rheumatoid arthritis. This drug is a prototype in Chapter 60. Human epidemiological studies have not found evidence of adverse pregnancy outcomes above baseline levels. Because metabolites of this drug are secreted in human milk, caution should be used if breastfeeding and the neonate should be observed for diarrhea and bloody stools.

Trimethoprim (Primsol): In addition to being part of the TMP-SMZ combination, trimethoprim is also available as monotherapy for treating uncomplicated UTI and acute otitis media in children due to *S. pneumoniae* or *H. influenzae*. It has been used off-label for the treatment of traveler's diarrhea and for *Pneumocystis* pneumonia, in combination with either sulfamethoxazole or dapsone. Rash and pruritus are common adverse effects, and these may appear 1 to 2 weeks after therapy has begun. Some patients experience nausea and vomiting and diarrhea. Polytrim is a combination of trimethoprim with polymyxin B in an ophthalmic solution for ocular infections.

CONNECTIONS: Complementary and Alternative Therapies

Cranberry

Description

Cranberry shrubs grow in diverse climates ranging from bogs to forests. The ripe berry is used for its potential medicinal effects.

History and Claims

Native Americans used the berries to treat wounds and to cure anorexia and other digestive complaints. In the early 1900s, it was noted that the acidity of urine increases after eating cranberries, thus began the belief that cranberry juice is a natural cure for UTIs.

Standardization

The herb is taken as juice or dried extract. Doses generally range from 120 to 4000 mL of juice or 400 to 500 mg of the extract daily.

Evidence

Cranberry contains a significant amount of vitamin C and other antioxidants that can promote health. Recently, specific chemicals found in cranberry juice (e.g., proanthocyanidins) have demonstrated the ability to prevent the bacteria from sticking to the walls of the bladder (González de Llano et al., 2019). This makes it more difficult for the bacteria to colonize and reproduce and may help reduce symptoms related to the inflammatory response caused by the bacteria (Mantzorou & Giaginis, 2018). In addition to cranberries and cranberry juice products, cranberry tablets are also available, although the consumer is encouraged to read product labels to ensure the tablets are not merely cranberry-flavored. While antibiotics are required to successfully treat UTIs, and cranberry alone cannot provide an effective treatment, cranberry products may have a role in preventing such infections (Wawrysiuk et al., 2019). In 2020, the FDA began to allow limited health claims on certain cranberry products to include wording on the potential of the product to reduce the risk of UTIs (FDA, 2020).

Cranberry should be used cautiously by people who take anticoagulants such as warfarin because of the potential for interactions (National Center for Complementary and Integrative Health, 2020). It has also been noted that patients who are susceptible to developing kidney stones may be at higher risk for stone formation from cranberry tablets, with or without vitamin C added, as they increase urinary oxalate excretion (Redmond et al., 2019). GI intolerance and weight gain from extra caloric intake from the juice seem to be the dominant reasons for discontinuing the cranberry product.

Urinary Antiseptics

50.5 Urinary antiseptics are anti-infective drugs used exclusively for urinary tract infections.

As has been noted throughout this text, most medications are totally or partially excreted by the kidneys. The majority of drugs and their metabolites travel through the urinary system, producing little or no effect on the renal tubular cells or the other parts of the kidney. For the small class of drugs known as the urinary antiseptics, however, the urinary system is their target tissue. Being able to reach the urinary tract in high concentrations is essential to their therapeutic success.

Urinary antiseptics are given by the PO route for their antibacterial action in the urinary tract. While they do not reach high enough levels in the blood to be effective for systemic infections, the kidney concentrates the drugs; thus, their actions are specific to the urinary system. Urinary antiseptics reach therapeutic levels in the kidney tubules, and their anti-infective action continues as they travel to the urinary bladder.

The advantage of the urinary antiseptics is that they are able to treat local infections in the urinary tract without reaching high levels in the blood that might produce systemic toxicity. Although not considered first-line drugs for UTI, they serve important roles as secondary medications, especially in patients who present with infections resistant to TMP-SMZ or the fluoroquinolones.

PROTOTYPE DRUG **Nitrofurantoin (Furadantin) and Nitrofurantoin Macrocrystals (Macrobid, Macrodantin)**

Classification **Therapeutic:** Antibacterial
Pharmacologic: Urinary tract antiseptic

Therapeutic Effects and Uses: Nitrofurantoin is an older drug that is indicated for the treatment of AUC, most commonly for the prophylaxis of recurrent infections. Nitrofurantoin is active against *E. coli*, *S. saprophyticus*, and many other strains of gram-positive and gram-negative aerobes. It is not effective against the *Pseudomonas*, *Proteus*, or *Serratia* species. It is not indicated for the treatment of pyelonephritis.

Nitrofurantoin is available in three formulations: a microcrystalline form (Furadantin), a regular-release macrocrystalline form (Macrodantin), and a sustained-release macrocrystalline form (Macrobid). The macrocrystalline form is more slowly absorbed than the microcrystalline form and produces fewer GI-related adverse effects.

Despite being approved by the FDA in 1953, development of resistance has not been a significant problem. The broad-based mechanism of action may explain the relative lack of acquired bacterial resistance to nitrofurantoin. Multiple mutations at diverse locations of the bacterial chromosome would be necessary for a bacterium to acquire such resistance. Cross resistance with other antibiotics is very rare.

Mechanism of Action: Nitrofurantoin acts by several unique mechanisms. When bacteria break down nitrofurantoin, the drug is converted to highly reactive intermediates. These intermediates attack bacterial ribosomal proteins. The drug inhibits bacterial protein synthesis, aerobic energy metabolism, DNA synthesis, RNA synthesis, and formation of the cell wall. Nitrofurantoin is bactericidal in the urine at therapeutic doses.

Pharmacokinetics:

Route(s)	PO
Absorption	Readily absorbed
Distribution	Widely distributed to body fluids; crosses the placenta; secreted in breast milk; 60% bound to plasma proteins
Primary metabolism	Hepatic
Primary excretion	Renal
Onset of action	30 min
Duration of action	Half-life: 20 min

Adverse Effects: Nitrofurantoin has the potential to produce many adverse effects. The most frequent include hypersensitivity reactions, anorexia, headache, rash, and nausea and vomiting. Pulmonary toxicity is a serious adverse effect and may include interstitial pneumonitis, persistent cough, and pulmonary fibrosis. Chronic pulmonary toxicity may not appear until months or years after therapy has been completed. Hepatotoxicity is rare, though potentially fatal, and may include cholestatic jaundice, hepatic necrosis, or hepatitis.

Contraindications/Precautions: Because nitrofurantoin is excreted by the kidneys, significant renal impairment (creatinine clearance under 60 mL/min or significant elevated serum creatinine) is a contraindication. Successful treatment depends on achieving high amounts of drug in the urine, which will not occur in patients with oliguria or anuria. Because of the possibility of hemolytic anemia due to immature erythrocyte enzyme systems, the drug is contraindicated in pregnant patients or in neonates less than 1 month of age.

This drug should be used with caution in patients with preexisting pulmonary disease, and pulmonary function should be closely monitored throughout therapy. Although rare, reports have cited diffuse interstitial pneumonitis or pulmonary fibrosis as causes of death in patients receiving nitrofurantoin.

Nitrofurantoin should be used with caution in patients with preexisting hepatic disease. The drug should be discontinued immediately if changes are noted in liver function tests.

Drug Interactions: Nitrofurantoin should not be given with antacids containing magnesium because absorption will be decreased. Concurrent administration with fluoroquinolones may result in antagonism and a decreased drug effect. **Herbal/Food:** Unknown.

Pregnancy: Animal studies have not shown evidence of fetal harm. Use of this drug is contraindicated at term and when labor onset is imminent due to the potential inducement of hemolytic anemia in the newborn. Breastfeeding of neonates younger than 1 month is not recommended.

Treatment of Overdose: Adequate fluid intake should be provided to ensure renal excretion of the drug. In extreme cases, dialysis may be of value in removing nitrofurantoin.

Clinician Responsibilities: Key clinical implications for patients receiving nitrofurantoin are included in Applied Clinical Judgment: Patients Receiving Pharmacotherapy for Urinary Tract Infection.

Drugs Similar to Nitrofurantoin (Furadantin) and Nitrofurantoin Macrocrystals (Macrobid, Macrodantin)

Other urinary antiseptics include fosfomycin and methenamine.

Fosfomycin (Monurol): Approved in 1996, fosfomycin is used for the treatment of uncomplicated UTI caused by susceptible strains of *E. coli* and *E. faecalis*. Technically classified as a cell wall inhibitor (see Chapter 47), it reaches high concentrations in the urine and bladder. Thus, it is sometimes called a bladder antiseptic. It is administered as a single PO dose. The most frequent adverse effects are diarrhea, headache, vaginitis, nausea, rhinitis, and pain. Animal studies using clinically relevant doses showed no evidence of teratogenic effects. It is not known whether this drug is secreted in human milk or if it has adverse effects on the breastfed neonate.

Methenamine (Hiprex, Urex): Methenamine is an older drug approved in 1939 that is available as hippurate (Hiprex) or mandelate (Urex) salts. In the very acidic environment of urine, methenamine hippurate is metabolized to formaldehyde, a breakdown product toxic to microorganisms. The hippurate salt becomes an acid in the urine, thus providing an even greater environment (lower pH) for the generation of formaldehyde. At therapeutic doses, methenamine is a safe drug, although higher doses can result in dysuria, nausea and vomiting, and hematuria.

The only clinical application of methenamine is for prophylactic treatment of recurrent UTI, especially those with neurogenic bladder. Preventive therapy with methenamine is instituted after eradication of the infection by other appropriate anti-infectives. It is effective against most bacteria typically responsible for UTI. Urease-positive bacteria such as *Proteus* are resistant because they produce ammonia in the urine, which prevents the formation of formaldehyde. Concurrent therapy of methenamine with sulfamethoxazole is contraindicated because the combination promotes crystalluria. Animal and human studies have not shown evidence of fetal harm. Although methenamine is secreted in human milk, adverse effects on the breastfed neonate are unknown.

CONNECTIONS: APPLIED CLINICAL JUDGMENT

Patients Receiving Pharmacotherapy for Urinary Tract Infection

Key Assessment Data

- History of current condition, baseline vital signs, physical exam findings; hepatic or renal disease, diabetes, AIDS, folic acid–deficiency anemia; pregnancy or breastfeeding. Obtain a drug history and assess signs and symptoms of the current infection, noting location, characteristics, presence or absence and duration of hematuria or pyuria and the presence or absence of fever or pain.
- Ongoing assessment during drug therapy should include monitoring appropriate laboratory findings (e.g., complete blood count, C&S, hepatic and renal laboratory values); assess for infections, especially with opportunistic infections such as fungal infections.

Desired Therapeutic Outcomes

Improvement is observed and measurable by reduction in fever, pain, or signs and symptoms of infection should begin to diminish after taking the first dose and continue to improve throughout the course of antibiotic therapy.

Minimizing Adverse Effects

- Continued fever may be a sign of worsening infection, adverse drug effects, or antibiotic resistance. Immediately report undiminished fever, changes in level of consciousness (LOC).
- Anaphylactic reactions are possible, particularly with the first dose of an antibiotic. Residual drug levels, dependent on length of half-life, may cause delayed reactions up to 2 weeks after completing therapy.
- Superinfections with opportunistic organisms may occur when normal host flora are diminished or killed by the antibacterial drug. Severe diarrhea may indicate the presence of *C. difficile*–associated diarrhea, pseudomembranous colitis, or fungal or yeast infections.
- Sulfonamides may cause significant dermatologic effects including SJS. Monitor for dermatologic effects including red or purplish skin rash, blisters, or sunburn.
- Large areas of treatment with topical sulfonamides for burns or infected wounds may result in excessive absorption of the drug, resulting in systemic effects. Stinging or burning may occur on application of the cream but does not indicate a systemic effect.
- Sulfonamides exert a potassium sparing effect on the kidney and may cause hyperkalemia in patients taking potassium sparing diuretics or angiotensin-converting enzyme (ACE) inhibitors. The drugs also increase the hypoglycemic effect of sulfonylureas used orally for diabetes.

(continued)

CONNECTIONS: APPLIED CLINICAL JUDGMENT *(continued)*

Patients Receiving Pharmacotherapy for Urinary Tract Infection

Lifespan Considerations
- Age-related physiologic differences may place the young child or older adult at greater risk for nephrotoxicity.

Patient Education
- Report a fever that does not diminish below 37.8°C (100°F) within 3 days, increasing signs and symptoms of infection, or symptoms that remain after taking the entire course of antibacterial therapy. Immediately report febrile seizures, changes in behavior, or changes in LOC.
- Immediately report any itching, rashes, swelling (particularly of tongue or face), urticaria, flushing, dizziness, syncope, wheezing, throat tightness, or difficulty breathing.
- Increase overall fluid intake. Report any diminished urine output, weight gain of more than 1 kg (2 lb) in a 24-hour period, and darkening of urine.
- Report any diarrhea that increases in frequency or amount or contains mucus, blood, or pus. Consult the healthcare provider before taking any antidiarrheal drugs that slow gastric motility because these may cause the retention of harmful bacteria.
- Observe and report any white patches in the mouth, whitish thick vaginal discharge, itching in the urogenital area, or blistering itchy rash.
- Wear sunscreen and protective clothing for sun exposure and avoid tanning beds. Immediately report any severe sunburn or rashes.
- Patients with diabetes who rely on PO medication with sulfonylureas (e.g., glyburide) should monitor their blood glucose more frequently and be aware of subtle signs of possible hypoglycemia (e.g., nervousness, irritability). Any consistent changes in their blood glucose levels while on a sulfonamide antibiotic should be reported.
- For known antibacterial allergies, carry a wallet identification card or wear medical identification jewelry indicating allergy.
- Appropriate self-administration of antibiotics includes:
  - Complete the entire course of therapy unless otherwise instructed. Do not share with other family members, and do not stop the medicine when starting to feel better.
  - Take the medication as evenly spaced throughout each day as feasible.
  - Patients also taking potassium-sparing diuretics (e.g., spironolactone) or ACE inhibitors (e.g., lisinopril) should avoid foods high in potassium and avoid the use of salt substitutes, which often contain potassium salts.
  - If antibiotic cream is ordered, apply a thin layer to the affected area and cover with a dry dressing.
  - Increase overall fluid intake while taking the antibacterial drug

Prescribing Considerations
- Sulfonamides may be nephrotoxic. Periodic C&S tests should be ordered if infections are severe or are slow to resolve to confirm appropriate therapy. Reduce dosage or change medications at first signs of nephrotoxicity.
- Sulfonamides may increase the effects of warfarin, resulting in an increased risk of bleeding. Reduce dosage or change medications at first signs of significant changes in coagulation or bleeding studies.
- Persistent UTI that includes hematuria or vaginal discharge with pruritus are indications for referral to appropriate specialties to rule out possible malignancy or sexually-transmitted infection.

Understanding Chapter 50

Key Concepts Summary

50.1 Infections can occur in any portion of the urinary tract.

50.2 Choice of pharmacotherapy for acute urinary tract infection depends on the severity of the infection and the presence of coexisting conditions.

50.3 Infants, children, pregnant women, older adults, and those with recurring urinary tract infections require modifications to standard pharmacotherapy.

50.4 Sulfonamides are the traditional preferred drugs for urinary tract infections, but resistance limits their usefulness.

50.5 Urinary antiseptics are anti-infective drugs used exclusively for urinary tract infections.

CASE STUDY: Making the Patient Connection

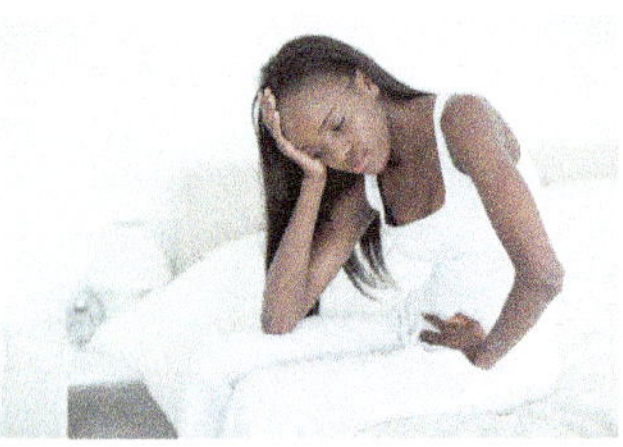

Remember the patient "Amoya Deboissiere" at the beginning of the chapter? Now read the remainder of the case study. Based on the information presented within this chapter, respond to the critical thinking questions that follow.

Amoya Deboissiere is a 32-year-old woman who has experienced frequent UTIs. Amoya is married with two children and works as a branch manager in a local bank.

In the clinic, Amoya's physical examination reveals the following findings: temperature, 38.4°C (101.2°F); pulse, 106 beats/min; respiratory rate, 18 breaths/min; and blood pressure 112/74 mmHg. She reports having a fever, chills, dysuria, urinary frequency, urinary urgency, and suprapubic pain. Amoya also reports seeing a small amount of blood in the urine and the sensation of incomplete bladder emptying. She states that recently her urine has become cloudy and smells bad.

As you continue your interview with the patient, she states, "I can't believe I have another UTI. I had one just last month." The urinalysis reveals microscopic bacteriuria (greater than 10^5/mL). A urine culture is also collected during this visit, and the results will be reported within 48 hours. The patient's preliminary diagnosis is recurrent UTI, and she receives a prescription for TMP-SMZ (Bactrim, Septra).

Critical Thinking Questions

1. How should you respond to the patient's statements about the recurrent infections?
2. What health teaching regarding antibiotic therapy should you stress to this patient?
3. What information should you give patients about saving medications?

Additional Case Study

Dorothy Janes is an 80-year-old woman admitted to your unit for HTN and a history of stroke with residual right-sided weakness. She is alert and oriented to person, time, and place but requires assistance with ambulation due to a history of falls. Her healthcare provider ordered Dorothy to be restricted to bedrest with bathroom privileges with assistance. When the patient's daughter comes to visit, she tells you that sometimes her mother has urinary incontinence due to her inability to walk to the bathroom by herself when the urge to urinate occurs. She wants to know if her mother can have a urinary catheter inserted to prevent accidents.

1. How would you respond to the daughter's request for her mother to have a urinary catheter inserted?
2. Brainstorm nursing actions that you could implement to avoid urinary incontinence for this patient.

Chapter Review

1. An older patient is prescribed sulfasalazine (Azulfidine). Knowing that one of the major adverse effects of this drug is crystalluria, what should the nurse instruct the patient to do?
   1. Limit intake of foods high in calcium such as milk, cheese, and yogurt.
   2. Avoid changing positions (lying down, sitting, or standing) rapidly.
   3. Increase fluid intake to 2 to 3 L per day.
   4. Avoid consuming alcoholic beverages while taking this medication.

2. The nurse understands that which of the following is the main purpose of nitrofurantoin (Furadantin)?
   1. Prevent recurrent urinary tract infections.
   2. Relieve the pain associated with urinary tract infections.
   3. Promote effective urinary elimination and prevent stasis.
   4. Reduce pathogenic microorganisms specific to pyelonephritis.

3. The nurse is collecting health data from a patient with diabetes who has a urinary tract infection before starting an order for trimethoprim-sulfamethoxazole (Bactrim, Septra). Which questions asked by the nurse would be most important? (Select all that apply.)
   1. "Have you ever had migraine headaches?"
   2. "Are you allergic to any sulfa drugs?"
   3. "Do you empty your bladder before and after sexual intercourse?"
   4. "When was your last menstrual period?"
   5. "What drugs do you use to manage your diabetes?"

4. The nurse is providing the patient with discharge instructions concerning silver sulfadiazine (Silvadene) cream, which has been ordered to treat a significant skin infection. Which statement by the patient indicates to the nurse that the teaching session was effective?
   1. "I should use this cream on noninfected surfaces surrounding the infection to prevent additional infection."
   2. "If I experience stinging or burning, I should stop the drug and report that to my doctor immediately as a drug allergy."
   3. "If I experience any nausea that continues for more than 24 hours, I will contact my doctor."
   4. "I must avoid foods high in potassium."

5. The patient is to receive nitrofurantoin (Furadantin) for a urinary tract infection. A nurse should question the order for the patient with which condition?
   1. Pulmonary disease
   2. Diabetes
   3. Rheumatoid arthritis
   4. Angina and HTN

6. A patient taking trimethoprim-sulfamethoxazole develops a reddish-purplish papular rash surrounded by areas of erythema. The rash should be evaluated by the provider because it may indicate which skin condition?
   1. A fungal superinfection
   2. Viral skin eruptions
   3. Dermatologic toxicity including SJS
   4. Nonadherence with drug therapy

See Appendix A for answers to critical thinking questions, case study questions, and review questions.

References

Brusch, J. L. (2020). *Urinary tract infection in males.* Medscape. http://emedicine.medscape.com/article/231574-overview

Foxman, B., Cronenwett, A. E., Spino, C., Berger, M. B., & Morgan, D. M. (2015). Cranberry juice capsules and urinary tract infection after surgery: Results of a randomized trial. *American Journal of Obstetrics and Gynecology, 213*(2), 194.e1–194.e8. https://doi.org/10.1016/j.ajog.2015.04.003

González de Llano, D., Khoo, C., Moreno-Arribas, M. V., & Bartolomé, B. (2019). Some new findings regarding the antiadhesive activity of cranberry phenolic compounds and their microbial-derived metabolites against uropathogenic bacteria. *Journal of Agricultural and Food Chemistry, 67*, 2166–2174. https://doi.org/10.1021/acs.jafc.8b05625

Mantzorou, M., & Giaginis, C. (2018). Cranberry consumption against urinary tract infections: Clinical state-of-the-art and future perspectives. *Current Pharmaceutical Biotechnology, 19*, 1049–1063. https://doi.org/10.2174/1389201020666181206104129

National Center for Complementary and Integrative Health. (2020). *Cranberry.* https://nccih.nih.gov/health/cranberry

Redmond, E. J., Murphy, C. F., Leonard, J., Faulds, K., Abdelfadil, S., Crowley, V. E., et al. (2019). The influence of dietary supplementation with cranberry tablets on the urinary risk for nephrolithiasis. *World Journal of Urology, 37*, 561–566. https://doi.org/10.1007/s00345-018-2344-1

U.S. Food and Drug Administration. (2020). *FDA allows qualified health claim for certain cranberry products and urinary tract infections.* https://www.fda.gov/food/cfsan-constituent-updates/fda-announces-qualified-health-claim-certain-cranberry-products-and-urinary-tract-infections

Wawrysiuk, S., Naber, K., Rechberger, T., & Miotia, P. (2019). Prevention and treatment of uncomplicated lower urinary tract infections in the era of increasing antimicrobial resistance – non-antibiotic approaches: A systematic review. *Archives of Gynecology and Obstetrics, 300*, 821–828. https://doi.org/10.1007/s00404-019-05256-z

Selected Bibliography

Angelescu, K., Nussbaumer-Streit, B., Sieben, W., Scheibler, F., & Gartlehner, G. (2016). Benefits and harms of screening for and treatment of asymptomatic bacteriuria in pregnancy: A systematic review. *BMC Pregnancy and Childbirth, 16*, 336. https://doi.org/10.1186/s12884-016-1128-0

Brusch, J. L. (2020). *Urinary tract infection (UTI) and cystitis (bladder infection) in females.* Medscape. http://emedicine.medscape.com/article/233101-overview

Girard, R., Gaujard, S., Pergay, V., Pornon, P., Gaujard, G. M., Vieux, C., et al. (2015). Controlling urinary tract infections associated with intermittent bladder catheterization in geriatric hospitals. *Journal of Hospital Infection, 90*, 240–247. https://doi.org/10.1016/j.jhin.2015.02.008

Heppner, P. E., Schnepper, L., Langer, K., Fritzlar, S., & Deppa, B. (2020). Evidence of antimicrobial stewardship in the treatment of uncomplicated urinary tract infection. *Journal for Nurse Practitioners, 16*(9), E153–E157. https://doi.org/10.1016/j.nurpra.2020.06.003

Herzig, C., Dick, A., Castle, N., & Stone, P. (2016). Policies and practices to reduce urinary tract infections in nursing homes. *American Journal of Infection Control, 44*(6, Suppl.), S20. https://doi.org/10.1016/j.ajic.2016.04.169

Khan, A., Jhaveri, R., Seed, P. C., & Arshad, M. (2019). Update on associated risk factors, diagnosis, and management of recurrent urinary tract infections in children. *Journal of the Pediatric Infectious Diseases Society*, *8*(2), 152–159. https://doi.org/10.1093/jpids/piy065

Matulay, J. T., Mlynarczyk, C. M., & Cooper, K. L. (2016). Urinary tract infections in women: Pathogenesis, diagnosis, and management. *Current Bladder Dysfunction Reports*, *11*, 53–60. https://doi.org/10.1007/s11884-016-0351-x

Owens, D. K., Davidson, K. W., Krist, A. H., Barry, M. J., Cabana, M., Caughey, A. B., et al. (2019). Screening for asymptomatic bacteriuria in adults: US Preventive Services Task Force recommendation statement. *Journal of the American Medical Association*, *322*(12), 1188–1194. https://doi.org/10.1001/jama.2019.13069

Platte, R.O. (2019). *Urinary tract infections in pregnancy treatment and management.* Medscape. https://emedicine.medscape.com/article/452604-treatment

Tullus, K., & Shaikh, N. (2020). Urinary tract infections in children. *The Lancet*, *395*(10237), 1659–1668. https://doi.org/10.1016/S0140-6736(20)30676-0

Wagenlehner, F. M., Johansen, T. E. B., Cai, T., Koves, B., Kranz, J., Pilatz, A., & Tandogdu, Z. (2020). Epidemiology, definition and treatment of complicated urinary tract infections. *Nature Reviews Urology*, *17*, 586–600. https://doi.org/10.1038/s41585-020-0362-4

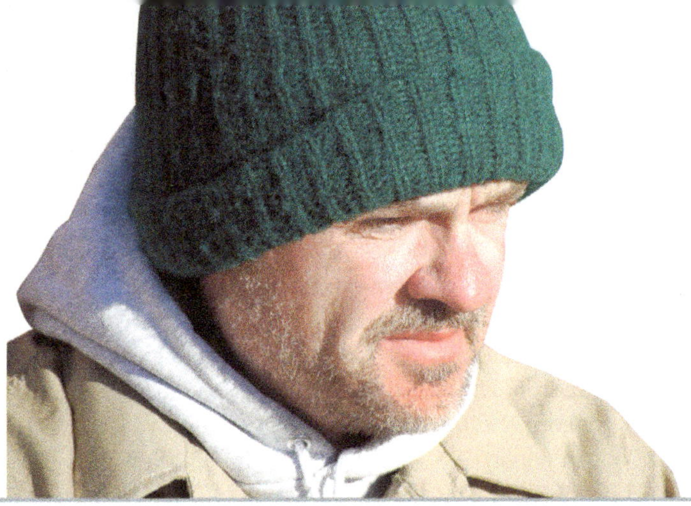

"A few years ago, I lost my job and was unable to pay my rent. Since then, you could say that I'm homeless. I try to spend my nights at the shelter, but it is sometimes too crowded and so I sleep on the street. About a month ago, I started feeling sick with a cough and fever. I'm exhausted and I have no energy."
—*Patient "Sam Myers"*

Chapter 51
Pharmacotherapy of Mycobacterial Infections

Chapter Outline

Learning Outcomes

After reading this chapter, the student should be able to:

1. Compare and contrast the types of infections caused by mycobacteria.
2. Explain the pathogenesis of tuberculosis.
3. Describe how the pharmacotherapy of tuberculosis differs from that of bacterial infections.
4. Identify the most common drug regimens for treating tuberculosis.
5. Describe the pathogenesis and treatment of leprosy.
6. Describe the pathogenesis and treatment of infections caused by *Mycobacterium avium* complex.
7. Explain significant patient variables that must be considered for effective pharmacotherapy with antimycobacterial drugs.
8. For each of the classes shown in the chapter outline, identify the prototype and representative drugs and explain the mechanism(s) of drug action, primary indications, contraindications, significant drug interactions, pregnancy data, and important adverse effects.
9. Apply clinical judgment to care for patients receiving pharmacotherapy for mycobacterial infections.

Key Terms

Definitions of the terms in bold may be found in the Glossary.

Mycobacterial infections have been responsible for considerable human suffering and death throughout history. Mycobacterial disease was once called *consumption* because of its ability to cause the body to waste away if left untreated. Although these infections usually respond to modern anti-infectives, therapy is prolonged, and resistant organisms have emerged as major clinical challenges. Despite the effective treatments available for the disease, tuberculosis (TB) still claims about 1.8 million lives each year worldwide. This chapter examines the pharmacotherapy of the three primary infections caused by mycobacteria.

PharmFACT

More than 9200 new cases of tuberculosis are reported each year in the United States. The incidence has decreased every year since 1992 (Centers for Disease Control and Prevention [CDC], 2018).

Types of Mycobacterial Infections

51.1 Several species of mycobacteria are important human pathogens.

The genus *Mycobacterium* consists of over 150 species of aerobic organisms that have in common a unique and complex lipid, **mycolic acid**, which covers their cell surfaces. This waxy coating, comprising up to 40% of the cell's weight, protects the mycobacterium, making it resistant to many disinfectants, including chlorinated water. About 10 are potential human pathogens.

The most common human mycobacterial pathogen is *Mycobacterium tuberculosis. M. tuberculosis* was identified as being the cause of TB by Robert Koch, a pioneering microbiologist, in 1882.

Nontuberculosis diseases caused by mycobacteria are known as **atypical mycobacterial infections (AMIs)**. These are considered opportunistic infections because they most often appear in people with compromised immune defenses. As the infections from the human immunodeficiency virus (HIV) appeared during the 1980s and 1990s, the once-rare AMIs began to rise in frequency. In addition to HIV infection, AMIs sometimes occur in patients who are undergoing antineoplastic or immunosuppressive therapy.

Mycobacterium leprae is an AMI that was identified as the causative agent of leprosy by G. A. Hansen in 1873. Leprosy is still sometimes called Hansen's disease, after its discoverer. The pharmacotherapy of leprosy is presented in Section 51.6.

Unlike *M. tuberculosis* and *M. leprae*, which have been described since antiquity, the characterization of ***Mycobacterium avium* complex (MAC)** infection is relatively recent. MAC usually arises as a secondary infection due to the immunosuppression caused by HIV. MAC consists of two predominant species, *M. avium* and *Mycobacterium intracellulare*. The pharmacotherapy of MAC is discussed in Section 51.7.

Several other mycobacteria species can cause AMIs in humans, but their incidence is rare. *Mycobacterium kansasii* is the second most common cause of AMI in patients with HIV. *Mycobacterium bovis* is usually acquired from the ingestion of raw, unpasteurized milk. Infections by *M. kansasii* or *M. bovis* cause respiratory symptoms that are almost identical to those of TB.

Mycobacterium scrofulaceum usually affects children 1 to 3 years of age. The target for this pathogen is the lymph nodes, and infants have mild symptoms, such as low-grade fever. Infections by *Mycobacterium chelonae* and *Mycobacterium abscessus* can cause a variety of clinical syndromes including respiratory disease, local skin disease, osteomyelitis, joint infections, and ocular disease. Surgical-site infections due to *M. chelonae* are well documented.

Pathogenesis and Diagnosis of Tuberculosis

51.2 Tuberculosis is a respiratory infection that exhibits both active and latent stages.

Tuberculosis (TB) is a highly contagious infection caused by the organism *M. tuberculosis*. Although TB has been a major killer throughout human history, its incidence declined in the United States during most of the 20th century. With the appearance of HIV, however, the incidence of TB greatly increased. Immigration from areas of the world where TB is endemic also contributes to increases in this disease in the United States.

Patients acquire *M. tuberculosis* by inhaling infected droplets through sneezing, coughing, and even talking. The organism can remain alive in these droplets for several hours outside the body. Unlike most species of mycobacteria, however, *M. tuberculosis* is not an environmental pathogen. It must reside in a living host to survive and reproduce. Left untreated, it is estimated that each individual infected with active TB will spread the disease by close contact to 10 to 15 other people over the course of a year (World Health Organization [WHO], 2020c).

TB infections may be classified as primary or postprimary. A *primary* TB infection occurs when the patient inhales mycobacteria from an individual with an active TB infection. The slow-growing mycobacteria activate cells of the immune response, which isolate the microorganisms by creating a wall of macrophages around them. In an attempt to neutralize the mycobacteria, the macrophages ingest them. The pathogens, however, can grow *inside* the macrophages, despite the presence of an ongoing immune response. An acute respiratory infection develops, with symptoms presenting as pneumonia. In those with healthy immune systems, the primary infection lasts a few weeks and then subsides.

Although the macrophages are eventually successful in isolating the pathogen, granulomatous lesions called **tubercles** are formed in the lung. Tissue within the tubercles undergoes necrosis, causing cavities within the lung, which can be identified on chest radiographs. The mycobacteria often become dormant, lying inside the tubercles for an extended time. Indeed, people can retain latent, inactive mycobacteria in tubercles for an entire lifetime.

If the immune system becomes suppressed later in life, the dormant mycobacteria may enter a *postprimary* or *reactivation* stage. Once reactivated, *M. tuberculosis* can be disseminated throughout the body via the blood or lymphatic system. Lymph nodes and organs of the genitourinary system are the most common nonrespiratory sites, although infections of the bone marrow and liver are possible. Reactivation frequently occurs in patients with HIV infection, those with poor nutritional status, and those who have terminal or debilitating diseases. The pathogenesis of TB is illustrated in Pharmacotherapy Illustrated 51.1.

PharmFACT

People with HIV are 19 times more likely to develop active TB than those not infected by HIV (WHO, 2020c).

Many patients remain asymptomatic following a primary TB infection. Indeed, only about 30% of those experiencing a primary TB infection will develop a latent infection and only 5 to 10% of these patients will progress to the reactivation stage (Bibbins-Domingo et al., 2016). In others, the disease progresses so gradually that the individual may not seek medical intervention until it becomes advanced. Symptoms of reactivation are nonspecific and include anorexia, weight loss, night sweats, fatigue, and low-grade fever. Cough becomes progressively worse, producing infectious sputum.

TB is diagnosed by several different means. Each of the following tests has advantages and drawbacks:

- **Tuberculin skin test (purified protein derivative [PPD]).** A positive PPD indicates the presence of memory T cells to *M. tuberculosis* but cannot determine whether the disease is active or latent. Once a positive PPD occurs, the test will always be positive

Pharmacotherapy Illustrated **51.1**

The Pathogenesis of Tuberculosis

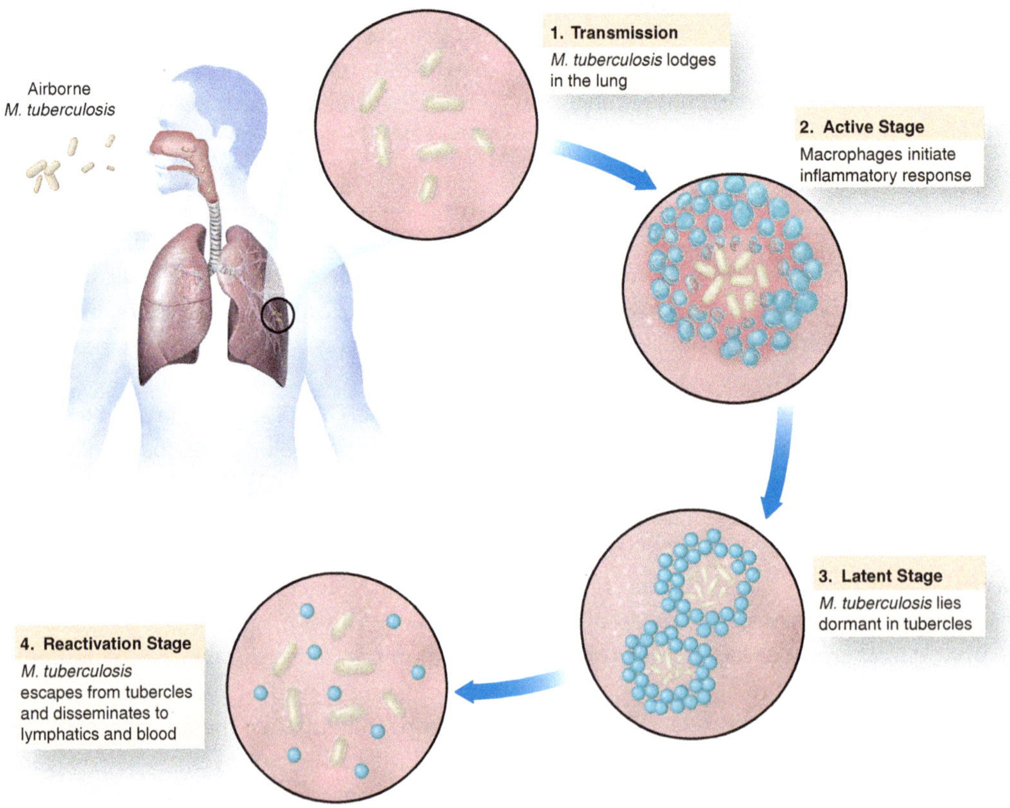

due to the presence of these memory T cells, and the patient should never have subsequent PPDs because skin damage may result. Although inexpensive, the PPD test requires that the patient return to have the results examined.

- **Sputum culture.** Sputum is obtained to culture and identify *M. tuberculosis*. Unfortunately, samples may be negative even when the patient has confirmed TB. Because *M. tuberculosis* grows very slowly on cultured media, results may take 2 to 8 weeks to produce results.
- **Chest radiography.** Both active and chronic TB infections produce changes in the lung that can be identified on chest radiographs. X-ray evidence is not always specific to TB, however, and other diagnostic evidence is needed to confirm the disease. Annual chest x-rays are often used to exclude active TB in patients who exhibit positive PPDs.
- **Nucleic acid amplification tests.** Diagnostic laboratory tests such as the Amplified *Mycobacterium Tuberculosis* Direct Test can identify the presence of *M. tuberculosis* RNA in a sputum specimen in 2 to 4 hours. Because these tests are rapid, they allow for earlier treatment of infected patients.
- **Interferon gamma release assay (IGRA).** The IGRA measures the response of the immune system to a sample of the patient's blood. Large amounts of interferon released by the immune cells during the IGRA test suggest a TB infection. Test results are ready in about 24 hours.

CONNECTION Checkpoint 51.1

From what you learned in Chapter 42, identify immunosuppressant drugs that may cause TB to enter the reactivation stage in a patient who is receiving pharmacotherapy with these drugs.

Pharmacotherapy of Tuberculosis

51.3 The pharmacotherapy of tuberculosis requires special dosing regimens and schedules.

The primary goal of TB pharmacotherapy is to eliminate all tubercle mycobacteria, while avoiding the emergence of resistant strains. This involves an initial or induction phase of therapy during which the actively dividing microbes are killed, and a continuation phase in which the remaining dormant mycobacteria are eliminated. Special pharmacotherapeutic strategies are required to successfully eradicate this persistent pathogen.

The pharmacotherapy of TB differs from that of other bacterial infections because the thick mycolic acid layer surrounding the mycobacterium is resistant to penetration by anti-infectives. For the drugs to reach the mycobacteria isolated in tubercles and inside macrophages, pharmacotherapy must continue for 6 to 12 months. Although the patient is not infectious this entire time and, indeed, may have no symptoms, it is critical that therapy be continued for the entire period. Patients who develop multidrug-resistant infections may require therapy for as long as 2 years.

A second difference in the therapy of TB is that a minimum of two—and sometimes as many as seven—antimycobacterial drugs may be necessary. During the long treatment period, different combinations of drugs are used. Combination drug therapy is necessary because mycobacteria grow slowly and often develop resistance during the course of treatment. The incidence of multidrug-resistant TB is increasing. In some communities, as many as 10% of patients have infections resistant to at least one antituberculosis medication. The use of multiple drugs that kill mycobacteria by different mechanisms lowers the potential for resistance and increases pharmacotherapeutic success. Figure 51.1 illustrates the use of combination therapy during tuberculosis therapy. Doses for the antimycobacterial drugs are listed in Table 51.1.

A third difference in therapy is that antimycobacterial drugs are used extensively for *preventing* the disease, in addition to treating active infections. Because of the acute infectious nature of TB, prophylactic therapy is indicated for close contacts or family members of recently diagnosed patients. Therapy of infected patients and all close contacts begins immediately after a positive diagnosis has been established. Patients with compromised immune function, such as those with HIV infection or those who are receiving

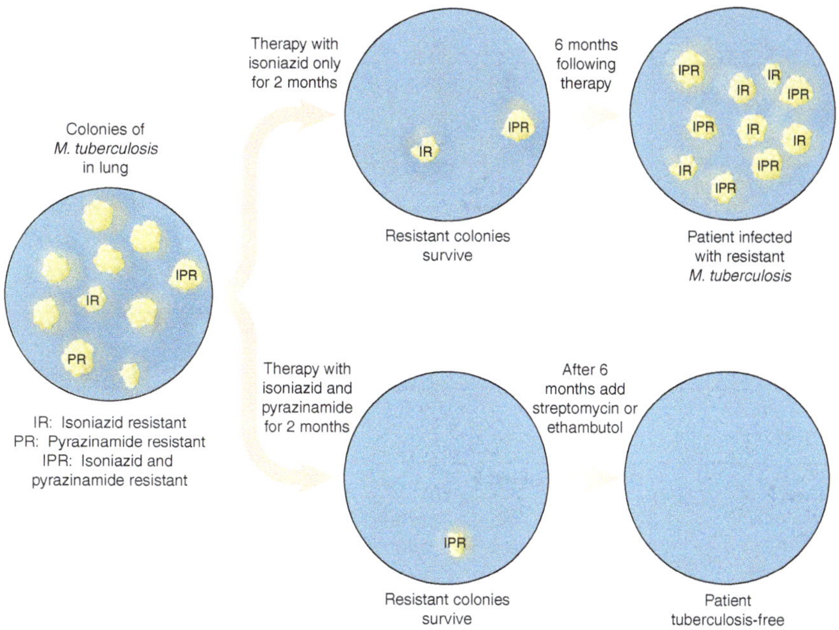

Figure 51.1 Use of combination therapy during tuberculosis therapy to avoid resistance.

Table 51.1 Antimycobacterial Drugs

Drug	Route and Adult Dose (Maximum Dose Where Indicated)	Adverse Effects
First-Line Drugs		
ethambutol (Myambutol)	PO: 15–25 mg/kg/day (max: 1600 mg for daily therapy)	*Nausea and vomiting, headache, dizziness* Anaphylaxis, optic neuritis (decreased acuity, color blindness, or visual defects)
isoniazid (INH)	Latent TB: PO: 300 mg/day or 900 mg twice weekly for 6–9 months Active TB: PO: Daily therapy: 5 mg/kg/day or 300 mg/day; if given by DOT: 15 mg/kg or 900 mg twice weekly	*Nausea, vomiting, diarrhea, epigastric pain* Anaphylaxis, peripheral neuropathy, optic neuritis, hepatotoxicity, blood dyscrasias
pyrazinamide (PZA)	PO: 5–15 mg/kg tid–qid (max: 2 g/day)	*Nongouty polyarthralgia, increase in serum uric acid, rash* Anaphylaxis, hepatotoxicity, fatal hemoptysis, hemolytic anemia
rifabutin (Mycobutin)	TB prophylaxis: PO: 300 mg once daily (max: 600 mg/day) Active TB: 1st phase PO: 5 mg/kg/day 2nd phase PO: 5 mg/kg/day or twice weekly (max: 300 mg/day)	*Nausea and vomiting; epigastric pain; anorexia; diarrhea; orange discoloration of the urine, sweat, and tears; pyuria; hematuria; urinary tract infection; proteinuria; hypoglycemia* Pseudomembranous colitis (PMC), acute renal failure, hepatotoxicity, hyperuricemia, lymphopenia, neutropenia, anemia
rifampin (Rifadin, Rimactane)	Latent TB: PO: 600 mg/day or 900 mg twice weekly for 4 months Active TB: PO: 10 mg/kg/day or 600 mg/day IV and PO are same dose, but IV needs to be given over 30 min to 3 h and the final concentration should not exceed 6 mg/mL	
rifapentine (Priftin)	PO: 600 mg (four 150-mg tablets) given twice a week for 2 months with an interval of no less than 72 h between doses, then once a week for 4 months	
Second-Line Drugs		
amikacin	Intramuscular (IM): 10–15 mg/kg daily for 2 wk in a large muscle	Pain or inflammation at injection site, rash, fever, nausea, diarrhea, dizziness, tinnitus Anaphylaxis, nephrotoxicity, PMC, ototoxicity
aminosalicylic acid (Paser)	PO: 150 mg/kg/day in three to four equally divided doses (max: 8 g/day)	*GI intolerance, anorexia, diarrhea, fever, leukopenia* Hypersensitivity, inhibition of vitamin B_{12} absorption, hepatotoxicity
bedaquiline (Sirturo)	PO: 400 mg once daily for 2 wk then 200 mg 3 times/wk for 22 wk	*Nausea, arthralgia, headache* QT prolongation, increased risk of death, hepatotoxicity
capreomycin (Capastat)	IM: 1 g/day (max: 20 mg/kg/day) for 60–120 days, then 1 g 2–3 times/wk	*Rash, pain and inflammation at injection site, tinnitus* Blood dyscrasias, nephrotoxicity, ototoxicity, increase in urination, thirst
ciprofloxacin (Cipro)	PO: 250–750 mg bid	*Nausea and vomiting, diarrhea, rash, restlessness, pain and inflammation at injection site, local burning, stinging and corneal irritation (ophthalmic)* Anaphylaxis, tendon rupture, superinfections, photosensitivity, PMC, seizure, peripheral neuropathy, hepatotoxicity
cycloserine (Seromycin)	PO: 250–500 mg every 12 h for 2 wk (max: 1 g/day)	*Drowsiness, headache, lethargy* Convulsions, psychosis, confusion
ethionamide (Trecator)	PO: 750 mg/day (max: 1 g given in 3–4 divided doses)	*Nausea and vomiting, epigastric pain, diarrhea* Convulsions, hallucinations, mental depression, hepatotoxicity
ofloxacin	PO: 200–400 mg bid	(See ciprofloxacin.)
streptomycin	IM: 15–30 mg/kg (max: 1–2 g/day) DOT: twice-weekly IM: 25–30 mg/kg (max: 1.5 g) DOT: 3 times/wk IM: 25–30 mg/kg	*Nausea and vomiting, pain at injection site, drowsiness, headache* Anaphylaxis, ototoxicity, profound central nervous system depression in infants, respiratory depression, exfoliative dermatitis, nephrotoxicity, teratogenicity

Note: *Italics* indicate common adverse effects. Underline indicates serious adverse effects.

immunosuppressant drugs, may also receive preventive treatment with antimycobacterials. A short-term therapy of 2 months, consisting of combination therapy with isoniazid (INH) and pyrazinamide, is approved for TB prophylaxis in patients who are HIV positive.

A major concern with TB pharmacotherapy is ensuring that patients fully adhere to the prescribed regimen. Nonadherence to pharmacotherapy is the most common cause of treatment failure in patients with TB. In high-risk patients, directly observed therapy is necessary, which requires that a healthcare provider directly observe the patient swallowing the medication, whether in the hospital, office, or home care setting. Nurses serve essential roles in providing education about this disorder to their patients and stressing the importance of adherence.

First-Line Antituberculosis Drugs

51.4 First-line or primary antituberculosis drugs are the most efficacious and safest drugs for treating *M. tuberculosis* infections.

Medications for TB are placed into two categories. The safer and more effective medications are called *first-line drugs*. A second group of medications, which exhibit greater toxicity, is less effective and prescribed when resistance develops to the first-line drugs. The *second-line drugs* are discussed in Section 51.5.

The pharmacotherapy regimen for TB depends on drug sensitivity, disease stage, and the patient's immune status. Ideally, results of culture and sensitivity (C&S) testing should be obtained prior to treatment because of the possibility of drug-resistant strains. Definitive C&S results may take several weeks, however, and treatment must begin immediately. Therefore, the initial selection of pharmacotherapy is based on the experience of the prescriber and later adjusted when laboratory results become available.

Standard Regimen

The standard regimen applies to patients who have a positive diagnosis of TB, or who have symptomology strongly suspicious of a TB infection. This therapy is recommended by the American Thoracic Society, the CDC, and the Infectious Diseases Society of America (Nahid et al., 2016). The preferred regimen for patients with confirmed TB caused by drug-susceptible organisms includes the following:

- *Intensive phase.* Two months of daily therapy with isoniazid (INH), rifampin (Rifadin, Rimactane), pyrazinamide (PZA), and ethambutol (Myambutol). If C&S results show that the strain is sensitive to isoniazid and rifampin, ethambutol is dropped from the regimen.
- *Continuation phase.* Four months of therapy with isoniazid and rifampin, two to three times per week.

The above regimen cures more than 95% of these patients. The preferred administration schedule is to take the medications once daily, for 7 days/week. Because of the importance of taking the medication daily, many clinics actually observe the patient taking the drug, a practice called direct-observed therapy (DOT). If adherence is a problem, giving the medication 5 days/week using DOT is acceptable.

Patients Who Are HIV Positive

Routine HIV testing should be done on all new patients with confirmed TB. Coinfection with both TB and HIV can have mortal consequences: Worldwide, about 33% of patients with HIV die of TB infection (WHO, 2019). Patients who are HIV positive often respond to the standard 6-month regimen. Because nonadherence has been frequently reported, DOT is recommended for patients who are HIV positive. In addition, patients taking numerous antiretroviral drugs are at greater risk for drug–drug interactions and must be monitored carefully. For example, rifampin and rifabutin are considered essential to TB elimination in this population, yet they can increase the metabolism of some antiretrovirals and decrease their effectiveness against HIV. Certain drug combinations, such as rifampin with single protease inhibitors, should be avoided to the extent possible or dosages adjusted accordingly. Nurses treating patients with HIV infection who also have TB should regularly consult recent pharmacology sources to identify the many drug–drug interactions because serious adverse effects can compromise the success of pharmacotherapy.

Pregnant and Breastfeeding Patients

Pregnant women with TB are at risk because medication choices are fewer. Indeed, all four primary drugs cross the placenta and no adequate and well-controlled studies have been conducted on their safety during pregnancy. The safety of pyrazinamide during pregnancy has not been established, although it is used extensively in other countries. Although ethambutol has been used successfully without adverse fetal effects, high doses in laboratory animals produced a low incidence of birth defects; therefore, it is used in pregnancy only if C&S testing shows it to be effective. Streptomycin is contraindicated during pregnancy because it can cause hearing impairment in the newborn. As with all pharmacotherapy during pregnancy, the healthcare provider must weigh the potential benefits of therapy for the mother with the potential risks to the fetus.

Fortunately, only small amounts of the first-line medications enter breast milk and they have not been shown to have adverse effects on the breastfed neonate. Pregnant patients should receive isoniazid therapy supplemented with pyridoxine (vitamin B_6), which has been shown to prevent peripheral neuropathy.

Patients with Latent Tuberculosis

Treatment of latent TB reduces the risk that the infection will progress to its reactivation stage, thereby helping to prevent transmission of the disease. Although it would seem prudent to treat everyone suspected of having latent TB, pharmacotherapy is expensive and carries the risk of adverse drug reactions. Furthermore, not everyone with latent TB will progress to active disease. Patients with a possible latent TB infection are screened and treated only if they fall into a high-risk category. High-risk categories include patients who are HIV positive, those receiving immunosuppressive drugs, employees and residents of nursing homes, those living in residential facilities for patients with HIV infection, those living in prisons, people born in countries where TB is endemic, and those who have been in close contact with patients with active TB. Pharmacotherapy of latent TB normally includes one of the following regimens (Sterling et al., 2020):

- Three months of once-weekly therapy with isoniazid and rifapentine.
- Three months of daily isoniazid and rifampin.
- Four months of daily therapy with rifampin.
- Six or 9 months of daily isoniazid; considered an alternate therapy due to a higher risk of toxicity and lower adherence rates.

PROTOTYPE DRUG Isoniazid (INH)

Classification **Therapeutic:** Antituberculosis drug, antimycobacterial
Pharmacologic: Mycolic acid inhibitor

Therapeutic Effects and Uses: Approved by the U.S. Food and Drug Administration (FDA) in 1952, isoniazid remains a first-line drug for the treatment of *M. tuberculosis* infections because decades of experience have shown it to have a superior safety profile and to be the most effective, single drug for the disease. Isoniazid is used exclusively for the treatment and prophylaxis of mycobacterial infections. Isoniazid may be used alone for chemoprophylaxis or in combination with other antituberculosis drugs for treating active disease. When used for prophylaxis, therapy may continue for as long as a year. While resistance to isoniazid can develop during therapy, the incidence is only about 10%. Treatment of active disease requires multidrug therapy.

The main route of metabolism of isoniazid is through enzymatic acetylation in the liver. **Acetylation** is a general biochemical process that adds a two-carbon chain to a drug molecule, which usually renders the medication less effective or allows it to be excreted more easily. Not all people are able to acetylate isoniazid at the same rate because of genetic differences in the activity of acetyltransferase, the hepatic enzyme that performs this action. Those of Japanese and Inuit descent often have increased enzyme activity and are known as *fast acetylators*. Those with decreased activity—*slow acetylators*—are most commonly of Scandinavian, North African Caucasian, or Jewish descent. The half-life of isoniazid ranges from 70 minutes in fast acetylators to 2 to 5 hours in slow acetylators. Fortunately, isoniazid is safe across a wide range of doses, and these variations do not generally result in toxicity. For optimal therapy, however, doses should be lowered in slow acetylators to avoid adverse effects and increased in fast acetylators to keep plasma levels consistently in the therapeutic range. Dosage reductions should also occur in any patient with significant hepatic impairment because of diminished acetylation. The acetylation of isoniazid is illustrated in Figure 51.2.

Mechanism of Action: Isoniazid acts by inhibiting the synthesis of mycolic acid, an essential cell wall component of mycobacteria. Because mycolic acids are unique to mycobacteria, isoniazid has no activity for other microbial species. It is bactericidal for rapidly dividing organisms but bacteriostatic for dormant mycobacteria.

Pharmacokinetics:

Route(s)	Oral (PO) and IM (only if PO is unavailable)
Absorption	Readily absorbed
Distribution	Widely distributed (can even enter the necrotic lung tubercles that are characteristic of TB); crosses the placenta and enters the central nervous system; secreted in breast milk; about 15% bound to plasma protein
Primary metabolism	Metabolized by acetylation in the liver
Primary excretion	Renal (75%)
Onset of action	Rapid
Duration of action	Half-life: 1–4 h

Adverse Effects: Isoniazid exhibits few serious adverse effects. Common adverse effects include rash and fever. Neurotoxicity is a concern during therapy, and patients may exhibit paresthesia of the feet and hands, convulsions, optic neuritis, dizziness, coma, memory loss, and various psychoses. A major factor responsible for the neurotoxicity of isoniazid is the ability of the drug to cause a deficiency of activated pyridoxine (vitamin B_6), which is required for synthesis of the neurotransmitter gamma-aminobutyric acid (GABA). Many practitioners routinely prescribe pyridoxine during isoniazid therapy to prevent the development of peripheral neuropathy. Pyridoxine is considered the antidote for reversing acute nervous system effects of isoniazid overdose. Blood dyscrasias such as

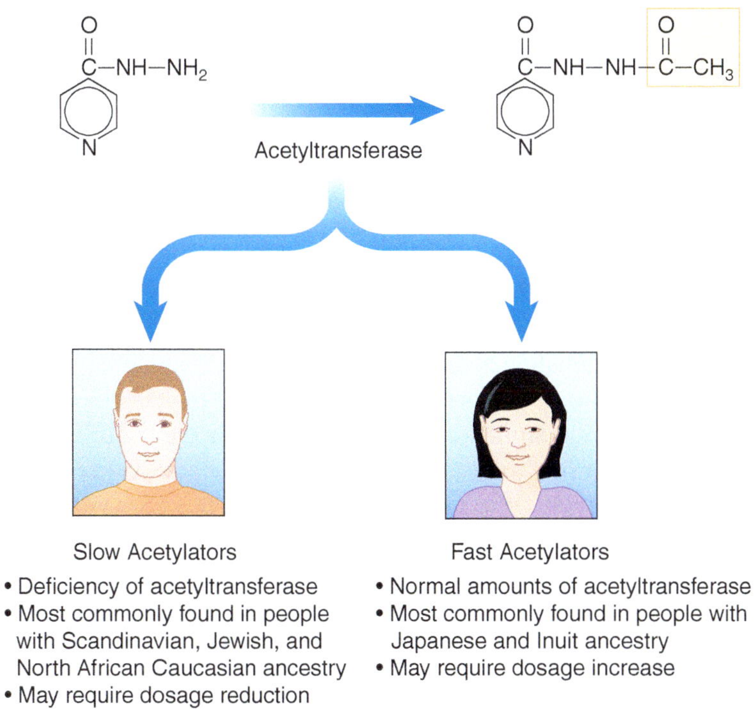

Figure 51.2 Variation in the acetylation of isoniazid.

agranulocytosis and aplastic anemia may occur, although they are uncommon. **Black Box Warning:** Although rare, hepatotoxicity is a potentially fatal adverse effect; thus, the patient should be monitored carefully for jaundice, fatigue, elevated hepatic enzymes, or loss of appetite. Liver enzyme tests are usually performed monthly during therapy to identify early hepatotoxicity. Hepatotoxicity usually appears in the first 1 to 3 months of therapy but may occur at any time during treatment. Older adults and those with daily alcohol consumption are at greater risk of developing hepatotoxicity.

Contraindications/Precautions: Isoniazid has no absolute contraindications other than previous allergy to the drug. Pharmacotherapy must be monitored carefully in patients with a history of chronic hepatic disease because the liver metabolizes the drug and fatal hepatitis has been reported. Serum aspartate aminotransferase (AST) levels should be monitored regularly during therapy in high-risk patients. If AST levels rise to three times baseline levels, liver damage is likely, and isoniazid should be discontinued. Patients with significant chronic kidney disease (CKD) usually require lower doses because the kidneys excrete the drug. Patients with seizure disorders should be carefully monitored because isoniazid can increase the incidence of seizures. Patients with a history of seizures often receive pyridoxine supplementation to prevent seizures during isoniazid therapy.

Drug Interactions: Isoniazid is a potent inhibitor of hepatic metabolic enzymes (CYP2C19 and CYP3A4) and is associated with numerous drug–drug interactions. Before adding a new drug to the regimen, the nurse should consult a drug guide for potential interactions. Aluminum-containing antacids should not be administered concurrently because they can decrease the absorption of isoniazid. Azole antifungals should not be used concurrently with isoniazid because this results in decreased levels of antifungals. Alcohol use should be avoided because it can increase the risk of hepatotoxicity. Isoniazid inhibits the metabolic breakdown of phenytoin, which may cause the anticonvulsant to build to toxic levels, an effect that occurs more often in slow acetylators. Isoniazid can increase serum levels of carbamazepine and cause toxicity. **Herbal/Food:** Food decreases the absorption of isoniazid.

Pregnancy: Extensive human use has not shown isoniazid to cause malformations or harmful fetal effects above baseline levels. Small amounts of the drug are secreted in human milk, although it has not been shown to adversely affect the breast-fed neonate.

Treatment of Overdose: Isoniazid overdose may be fatal, and treatment is mostly symptomatic. Pyridoxine may be infused in a dose equal to that of the isoniazid overdose to prevent seizures and to correct metabolic acidosis. The dose may be repeated several times until the patient regains consciousness.

Clinician Responsibilities: Key clinical implications for patients receiving isoniazid are included in Applied Clinical Judgment: Patients Receiving Pharmacotherapy for Tuberculosis.

Drugs Similar to Isoniazid (INH)

Other first-line antituberculosis drugs include ethambutol, pyrazinamide, rifabutin, rifampin, and rifapentine.

Ethambutol (Myambutol): Approved in 1967, ethambutol is included in multidrug regimens for TB because it is sometimes active against organisms that are resistant to other first-line drugs. It is also effective against atypical mycobacteria such as *M. kansasii*. The mechanism of action of ethambutol is believed to be due to the inhibition of cell wall synthesis and RNA synthesis. It is always given with other antimycobacterials because resistance develops rapidly if the drug is given as monotherapy. It is rapidly absorbed, distributed to most tissues, and excreted by both renal and fecal routes. Ethambutol has a short half-life of 1 to 4 hours; therefore, it should be taken daily.

Ethambutol has a unique adverse effect of optic neuritis that affects visual acuity and the ability to distinguish red from green. This effect is dose related, may be unilateral or bilateral, and is usually reversible when therapy is discontinued. A baseline ophthalmic examination should be conducted prior to therapy. Ethambutol may decrease the excretion of uric acid, causing hyperuricemia; patients with a history of gout should be closely monitored. This drug has few other significant adverse effects. Extensive human use has not shown ethambutol to cause malformations or harmful fetal effects above baseline levels. Small amounts of the drug are secreted in human milk, although it has not been shown to adversely affect the breastfed neonate.

Pyrazinamide (PZA): Pyrazinamide is an older drug approved in 1955 that may be used for the initial therapy of active or advanced TB in combination with other antimycobacterials. It is usually taken in combination with rifampin, ethambutol, and INH. If used alone, resistance develops rapidly. Like isoniazid, it acts by inhibiting the synthesis of mycolic acid in *M. tuberculosis*. Given PO, it is distributed to all body fluids and is excreted by the kidneys.

Pyrazinamide causes some degree of dose-related hepatotoxicity in as many as 15% of patients. Caution should be observed when giving pyrazinamide to patients with preexisting hepatic disease, and frequent laboratory monitoring of liver enzymes must be performed. Frequent use of ethanol increases the risk of hepatotoxicity. Hyperuricemia may occur because the drug slows the excretion of uric acid. Uric acid levels should be monitored, and the nurse should assess for signs of gout or arthralgia, which can occur in up to 40% of the patients taking this drug. Animal studies have shown fetotoxicity. The drug is recommended during pregnancy only if the potential benefits to the mother justify the potential risks to the fetus or neonate.

Rifampin (Rifadin, Rimactane): Rifampin is used widely in combination with other drugs in the first-line treatment of TB: It is rarely given as monotherapy for the short-course therapy of latent *M. tuberculosis* infections. Rifampin exerts its bactericidal effects by inhibiting RNA synthesis. In addition to treating TB, rifampin is a broad-spectrum antibiotic approved for the short-term treatment of meningococci from the nasopharynx of asymptomatic carriers of *Neisseria meningitidis*. When given to meningococcal carriers, the length of therapy is only 2 days. Off-label uses include chemoprophylaxis of contacts of patients with *Haemophilus influenzae* type B and the treatment of Legionnaire's disease. It is also used to treat leprosy, in combination with dapsone. The drug should be used only when the infectious microbe has been demonstrated to be susceptible to the effects of the medication. In 2019 Talicia was approved, which is a combination of rifampin, amoxicillin, and omeprazole. This medication is used to treat infection by *Helicobacter pylori*.

Rifampin is administered by either the PO or intravenous (IV) routes. Hypersensitivity reactions cause flulike symptoms in as many as 50% of the patients taking rifampin. Rash and urticaria are relatively common. Rifampin can be hepatotoxic, and caution must be used when administering the drug to patients with preexisting liver disease or who are taking other hepatotoxic antituberculosis drugs such as isoniazid and pyrazinamide. Rifampin is a potent inducer of cytochrome P450 (CYP450) enzymes. Thus, it has the potential to increase the metabolism of other drugs metabolized by the liver, such as some antiretrovirals for HIV infection, warfarin, and oral contraceptives. Because resistance develops rapidly, rifampin is almost always given in combination with other drugs. Animal studies showed evidence of congenital malformations and embryotoxicity. If given to women in the last trimester, it may cause postnatal hemorrhage in the mother and neonate. Animal studies showed evidence of tumors in breastfed offspring. Rifampin is recommended during pregnancy only if the potential benefits to the mother justify the potential risks to the fetus or neonate.

Rifabutin (Mycobutin) and Rifapentine (Priftin): These two PO drugs are closely related to rifampin, act by the same mechanism, and cause the same adverse effects, including induction of CYP450 enzymes and potential hepatotoxicity.

CONNECTIONS: Community-Oriented Practice

Lessons Learned from COVID-19 May Aid in TB Control

The response to the pandemic caused by SARS-CoV-2 (COVID-19) overwhelmed the public health communities and shifted attention and resources away from other diseases still very much present and spreading, such as TB. As a leading cause of death, TB remains in the top 10 causes worldwide (WHO, 2020a). Tuberculosis has not disappeared as the COVID-19 pandemic continues and South-East Asia and Africa account for almost 70% of cases worldwide (WHO, 2020b). As testing, tracing, and drug therapies are diverted to COVID-19 and away from TB control, the potential for the spread of the disease, as well as drug-resistant organisms, rises.

But even as the focus of attention moves away from TB and other global diseases to mitigation and management of COVID-19, lessons learned from the response to the pandemic may help to change the way TB is managed and controlled. Social distancing to prevent the spread of TB, contact-tracing measures to determine others in the community who may also need treatment, and the use of modeling to predict disease severity or successful treatment options may be more fully implemented as strategies for TB control. The hope is that communities, public health professionals, and governments can work together and learn from the efforts used for COVID-19 to improve control of other worldwide diseases (Togun et al., 2020).

There is a high level of cross resistance among rifampin, rifabutin, and rifapentine, which, collectively, are called **rifamycin derivatives**. They are always used in combination with other antituberculosis medications.

Approved in 1998, rifapentine is used only for the pharmacotherapy of TB and has a longer half-life than rifampin, thus offering the advantage of twice-a-week dosing. Rifabutin was approved in 1992 for the prophylaxis of MAC in patients infected with HIV. It offers little advantage over rifampin, other than it is thought to have less effect on hepatic enzymes. Animal studies with rifabutin and rifapentine showed embryotoxicity and major skeletal malformations. Breastfeeding should be conducted with caution.

Combination drugs: Rifamate is a combination medication that contain isoniazid and rifampin. Rifater is a tablet containing isoniazid, rifampin, and pyrazinamide. Combining multiple drugs into a single capsule or pill increases their ease of use and promotes patient adherence to therapy.

Second-Line Antituberculosis Drugs

51.5 Second-line antituberculosis drugs are used when resistance develops to the first-line drugs.

If a patient develops multidrug-resistant strains of *M. tuberculosis* during the course of therapy, second-line antibiotics are added to the regimen. These medications are either more toxic or less effective than the first-line drugs. Some of them are occasionally included as part of the initial course of therapy if C&S testing demonstrates their effectiveness. As a general rule, a single antituberculosis drug should never be added to a regimen that has failed to control the mycobacterial infection. At least two, and preferably three, new medications to which the organism is likely to be susceptible should be added.

Aminoglycosides: Amikacin and streptomycin are aminoglycosides used as both antibacterials and antituberculosis drugs. Like other second-line drugs, they are used for multidrug-resistant TB and always in combination with other antimycobacterials. They are administered parenterally because they are not absorbed when given by the PO route.

Approved in 1945, streptomycin has the distinction of being the first clinically effective drug used to treat TB. It was soon noticed, however, that resistance developed quickly when streptomycin was used as monotherapy. Streptomycin is now a second-line TB drug primarily because of the emergence of numerous streptomycin-resistant strains of *M. tuberculosis* and the need to administer the drug by the IM route. Other indications for streptomycin include tularemia, plague, brucellosis, and subacute bacterial endocarditis.

Streptomycin has a black box warning that renal function tests must be regularly assessed because the drug can accumulate to toxic levels in patients with CKD. Additionally, the warning states that concurrent use with nephrotoxic or neurotoxic drugs should be avoided. IM injection of the drug is painful and can produce sterile abscesses at the site of injection. Also of serious concern is ototoxicity, which can cause tinnitus, deafness, and vertigo.

Amikacin is an aminoglycoside antibiotic. Like other aminoglycosides, amikacin is nephrotoxic, and kidney function must be monitored regularly during therapy. It is also ototoxic and can cause deafness and balance abnormalities. In 2018, amikacin liposomal (Arikayce) was approved to treat Mycobacterium avium complex lung disease. The risk of ototoxicity is greater in patients with impaired renal function.

Aminosalicylic acid (Paser): Aminosalicylic acid (or para-aminosalicylic acid) was widely used to treat TB until more effective and safer drugs were discovered. It is structurally similar to para-aminobenzoic acid and is thought to have a similar mechanism of action as the sulfonamides. Aminosalicylic acid is given PO, but it has a half-life of only 1 hour. The drug is available as delayed-release granules that are taken several times a day.

The use of aminosalicylic acid is limited to the treatment of multidrug-resistant strains of *M. tuberculosis*. Higher doses can inhibit the acetylation of isoniazid, especially in patients who are rapid acetylators. Concurrent therapy of aminosalicylic acid with isoniazid, however, does not affect the serum level, half-life, or excretion of isoniazid.

Aminosalicylic acid has many adverse effects, the most common of which are gastrointestinal (GI) related and include nausea and vomiting, diarrhea, and abdominal pain. Taking the drug with food can diminish these types of adverse effects. Hypersensitivity is observed in up to 15% of patients and may begin with a rapid onset of high fever, lethargy, and joint pain. Aminosalicylic acid reduces the absorption of vitamin B_{12} by as much as 50%; thus, vitamin B_{12} supplements are indicated during long-term therapy. Animal studies showed this drug to be embryotoxic and cause fetal malformations. Breastfeeding is not recommended.

CONNECTION Checkpoint 51.2

From what you learned in Chapter 50, the synthesis of what essential vitamin is inhibited by the sulfonamides? What is the primary indication for sulfonamide pharmacotherapy?

Bedaquiline (Sirturo): Bedaquiline was approved in 2013 for the treatment of multidrug-resistant TB. Bedaquiline is always used in combination with at least three other antituberculosis drugs. It should not be used to treat TB strains that are sensitive to first-line drugs, for latent TB, or for nontuberculous mycobacterial infections. It is generally well tolerated, with nausea, headache, and joint pain being the most common side effects. However, the drug carries a black box warning because patients receiving the drug appear to have an increased risk of mortality. In addition, bedaquiline prolongs the QTc interval, which is associated with dysrhythmias in some patients. Animal studies did not show evidence of fetal harm. It is not known if this drug is secreted in human milk or if it has adverse effects on the breastfed neonate.

Capreomycin (Capastat): Approved in 1971, the only indication for capreomycin is the pharmacotherapy of multidrug-resistant strains of *M. tuberculosis*. Capreomycin is always given with other antimycobacterials because resistance quickly develops if it is administered as monotherapy. It is given only by IM injection. Because it is usually administered daily for the first 120 days of therapy, care must be taken to inject the drug deep into a large muscle mass and to rotate injection sites.

Capreomycin has a black box warning that the drug exhibits both neurotoxicity and nephrotoxicity. The drug is ototoxic, causing tinnitus and high-frequency hearing loss in up to 9% of patients. Auditory and vestibular function should be assessed prior to starting therapy and retested at least every other month during therapy. Nephrotoxicity is more common with capreomycin than with streptomycin. Older adults are generally more susceptible to the nephrotoxic effects of capreomycin, and the maximal daily dosage should be reduced. Other nephrotoxic drugs such as aminoglycosides should be avoided during capreomycin pharmacotherapy. Renal function tests should be monitored regularly and the drug discontinued if blood urea nitrogen levels exceed 30 mg/dL. Because of these adverse effects, capreomycin is sometimes referred to as a last-line drug for TB. Capreomycin is teratogenic in laboratory animals. It is not known if this drug is secreted in human milk or if it has adverse effects on the breastfed neonate.

Cycloserine (Seromycin): Approved over 50 years ago, cycloserine is a PO drug used in the pharmacotherapy of multidrug-resistant strains of *M. tuberculosis*. The drug, which resembles the common amino acid D-alanine, acts by blocking mycobacterial cell wall synthesis. In addition to being an antimycobacterial, cycloserine is also effective against certain gram-negative and gram-positive bacteria and may be used to treat urinary tract infections that are unresponsive to safer antibiotics. It is taken PO, usually twice daily.

Cycloserine use is limited because the difference between a toxic dose and an effective dose is small. Of most concern is neurotoxicity, which can manifest as different symptoms, including headache, lethargy, convulsions, psychotic states with suicidal ideation, depression, confusion, tremor, and paranoid reactions. Concurrent administration of isoniazid and ethionamide can increase the risk of neurotoxicity. The drug is contraindicated in patients with preexisting psychoses or epilepsy because it may worsen these disorders. Because of its toxicity, serum levels of cycloserine are measured frequently during therapy, with normal levels ranging from 25 to 35 mcg/mL. Patients with serious CKD should not receive this drug because the primary route of excretion of this drug is via the kidneys. Animal studies did not show evidence of fetal harm. It is not known if this drug is secreted in human milk or if it has adverse effects on the breastfed neonate.

Ethionamide (Trecator): Approved in 1962, ethionamide is a PO drug used as a second-line drug in the pharmacotherapy of multidrug-resistant TB or when patients are unable to tolerate first-line drugs. Ethionamide is always used in combination with other antituberculosis drugs because resistance develops rapidly if given alone. It is thought to act by inhibiting mycobacterial protein synthesis. The drug only has a 3-hour half-life and therefore must be administered several times daily.

The most common and limiting adverse effects of ethionamide are GI related and include nausea and vomiting, diarrhea, abdominal pain, excessive salivation, metallic taste, anorexia, and weight loss. GI effects may be diminished by decreasing dosage, by taking the drug with food, or by the concurrent administration of an antiemetic. Concomitant administration of pyridoxine is recommended to decrease the incidence of peripheral neuropathy. Depression and drowsiness are common, and seizures have been reported with ethionamide. Hepatic function should be monitored regularly because hepatitis occurs in about 5% of patients taking the drug. Alcohol use should be discouraged during ethionamide therapy because of additive harmful effects on the liver. Ethionamide is teratogenic in laboratory animals. It is not known if this drug is secreted in human milk or if it has adverse effects on the breastfed neonate.

Fluoroquinolones: Ciprofloxacin (Cipro) and ofloxacin have undergone considerable testing for use as antituberculosis drugs. Many multidrug-resistant strains of *M. tuberculosis* are sensitive to the actions of the fluoroquinolones. Because this class of antibiotics is used widely in the pharmacotherapy of bacterial infections, there is concern in the medical community that use of these drugs for TB could produce resistant strains of other pathogens in addition to *M. tuberculosis*. Although they are sometimes given for multidrug-resistant TB, they have not been approved by the FDA for this indication. They are the safest of the second-line drugs available for this infection.

Pretomanid: Approved in 2019, pretomanid is indicated to treat highly drug-resistant TB. It is not indicated for latent TB or TB sensitive to other medications. It must be given as a three-drug regimen called BPaL, consisting of bedaquiline, pretomanid, and linezolid. All three of these drugs are given PO, and therapy is for 26 weeks. Adverse effects with BPaL include myelosuppression, hepatotoxicity, QTc prolongation, and peripheral and optic neuropathy. Pretomanid should only be administered during pregnancy and lactation if the potential benefits to the mother justify the potential risks to the fetus or neonate.

CONNECTIONS: APPLIED CLINICAL JUDGMENT

Patients Receiving Pharmacotherapy for Tuberculosis

Key Assessment Data

- History of current condition, baseline vital signs, physical exam findings; hepatic, renal, cardiovascular, neurologic, or respiratory disease; HIV; alcohol use; pregnancy or breastfeeding. Obtain a drug history and assess signs and symptoms of the current infection, noting symptoms, duration, or any recent changes.
- Ongoing assessment during drug therapy should include monitoring appropriate laboratory findings (e.g., complete blood count, C&S, hepatic and renal laboratory values).

Desired Therapeutic Outcomes

Improvement is observed and measurable by diminished fever, cough, sputum, and other signs and symptoms of infection.

Minimizing Adverse Effects

- Increasing signs of infection may signify drug resistance or nonadherence to the drug regimen. Immediately report undiminished fever, increases in sputum production, hemoptysis, or increase in adventitious breath sounds.
- Antituberculosis drugs are hepatic, renal, or ototoxic and require frequent monitoring to prevent adverse effects. Increasing fluid intake will help prevent drug accumulation in the kidneys.
- Isoniazid may increase glucose levels. Patients with diabetes may require a change in their antidiabetic drug routine.
- Ethambutol and pyrazinamide decrease the renal excretion of uric acid, and hyperuricemia may result. Monitor for signs and symptoms of gout and increase overall fluid intake.
- Isoniazid may interact with foods high in tyramine and cause palpitations, flushing, and hypertension. Monitor BP more frequently and provide dietary instruction.
- Rifampin may turn body fluids (tears, sweat, saliva, urine) reddish orange. The effect is harmless but may stain soft, hydrophilic contact lenses or clothing.

Lifespan Considerations

- Age-related physiologic changes may affect the drug's metabolism or excretion in older adults. Periodic C&S tests may be ordered if infections are severe or are slow to resolve to confirm appropriate therapy. Levels of drugs with known severe adverse effects will be monitored.
- Older adults may be at increased risk for dizziness related to adverse drug effects, which may increase the risk for falls. Ensure patient safety.

Diversity Considerations

- Isoniazid metabolizes through the CYP450 system pathway and requires more frequent monitoring in ethnically diverse patients to ensure optimal therapeutic effects and to minimize adverse effects.

Patient Education

- Report a fever that does not diminish below 37.8°C (100°F), continued symptoms of disease (e.g., night sweats, fatigue), or increased sputum production.
- Immediately report any itching, rashes, swelling (particularly of tongue or face), urticaria, flushing, dizziness, syncope, wheezing, throat tightness, or difficulty breathing.
- Increase overall fluid intake. Report any diminished urine output, weight gain of more than 1 kg (2 lb) in a 24-hour period, and darkening of urine.
- Report any nausea or vomiting; yellowing of the skin or sclera; abdominal pain; light or clay-colored stools; diminished urine output; darkening of urine; ringing, humming, or buzzing in the ears; dizziness; or vertigo.
- Immediately report numbness or tingling in peripheral extremities, blurred vision, changes in visual color sense, or changes in visual acuity.
- Patients with diabetes should test their glucose levels more frequently, reporting any consistent elevations.
- Report signs and symptoms of gout such as inflammation and pain around joints, redness, or swelling, particularly of toes or fingers. Increase fluid intake, avoid foods high in purine, eliminate alcohol consumption, and avoid increased vitamin C intake or supplementation.
- If isoniazid is taken, avoid foods containing tyramine, such as aged cheese, smoked and pickled fish, beer, red wine, bananas, and chocolate, and immediately report any severe headache.
- Appropriate self-administration of antituberculosis drugs includes:
  - Complete the entire course of therapy unless otherwise instructed. The duration of the required therapy may be quite lengthy, but it is necessary to prevent active infection. Do not stop taking the medicine when starting to feel better.
  - Do not share the medicine with other family members. If there is reason to believe they need medication, they should be assessed by a healthcare provider.
  - Eliminate alcohol while on these medications. Antituberculosis drugs cause significant reactions when taken with alcohol.
  - Take the drug with food or milk but avoid acidic beverages. If instructed to take the drug on an empty stomach, take with a full glass of water.
  - Take the medication as evenly spaced throughout each day as feasible.

Prescribing Considerations

- Neurotoxicity and peripheral and optic neuritis are adverse effects of antituberculosis drugs. Prescribe vitamin B_6 to decrease the risk of peripheral neuropathy, especially that associated with isoniazid use. Monitor visual acuity and color vision sense in patients taking ethambutol.
- Alteration in dosing of anti-TB drugs is commonly necessary in patients with CKD or end-stage renal disease (ESRD) requiring hemodialysis. The dosage of anti-TB drugs should not be decreased because the peak serum concentrations may be low and smaller doses may decrease drug efficacy. Instead, the dosing interval of anti-TB drugs should be increased.
- The treatment of TB disease in patients with advanced liver disease requires expert consultation.

Drugs for Leprosy

51.6 Leprosy is caused by a mycobacterium and is treated by a multidrug regimen.

Leprosy is a chronic infection caused by *M. leprae*. Leprosy has been known for thousands of years, but the term *leper* has been used by different cultures to designate someone sinful or unclean, not necessarily someone with the disease we now call leprosy.

Although rare in the United States, it is estimated that 6 million people worldwide have leprosy. Patients with leprosy present with large, macular skin lesions. The organism invades peripheral nervous tissue, resulting in loss of sensation or paresthesia. If left untreated, the infection causes extreme disfigurement and bone resorption, resulting in loss of digits.

Leprosy may be infectious or noninfectious, depending on the stage of the disease and the progress of pharmacotherapy. Although the mode of transmission is not clear, *M. leprae* is likely spread by the respiratory route. The disease may have a very long incubation period extending from several months to years.

PharmFACT

Fewer than 200 cases of leprosy are reported in the United States each year. Most cases are diagnosed in immigrants from countries where leprosy is endemic; however, some patients acquire the disease from armadillos, which are a reservoir for the disease (Smith, 2020).

There are two types of leprosy, and pharmacotherapy differs for each. *Lepromatous* leprosy occurs in patients with defective cell-mediated immunity and is characterized by a slow, progressive development of nodular skin lesions and nerve involvement. Because the patient has an impaired immune system, the mycobacteria may disseminate throughout the body and cause death. *Tuberculoid* leprosy is less progressive and may have long periods of remission followed by reactivation with more severe nerve involvement. These patients have an intact cell-mediated immune response; thus, the disease is more benign and less often fatal.

Like tuberculosis, leprosy is treated with prolonged combination pharmacotherapy because monotherapy causes rapid development of resistant strains. Although improvement in skin lesions may occur within a few months, therapy must continue during the entire treatment period to eliminate all the mycobacteria. Follow-up may continue for 3 years or longer after the completion of pharmacotherapy. A typical regimen includes the following:

- **Lepromatous leprosy.** Initial three-drug regimen that includes dapsone and rifampin given for 2 to 5 years.
- **Tuberculoid leprosy.** Initial two-drug regimen with dapsone and rifampin for 6 to 12 months, followed by dapsone alone for 2 to 3 years.

Other drugs may be substituted when the patient cannot tolerate the standard regimen. Ofloxacin, clarithromycin, and minocycline are antibacterials that have activity against *M. leprae* and may be used during the long course of leprosy pharmacotherapy.

During the first year of pharmacotherapy, skin lesions may actually worsen because of activation of the cell-mediated immune response. Skin edema may occur, and new lesions may appear on normal skin. Most of these reactions occur because immune cells are attacking antigens released by the mycobacteria. If this occurs, corticosteroids such as prednisone are added to the regimen to reduce the severe inflammation.

PROTOTYPE DRUG Dapsone

Classification **Therapeutic:** Antileprosy drug, antimycobacterial, antiacne drug
Pharmacologic: Folic acid inhibitor

Therapeutic Effects and Uses: Approved in 1955, dapsone is a first-line drug for the treatment of *M. leprae* infections, usually in combination with other antileprosy drugs. It has several off-label uses that include the chemoprophylaxis of malaria in combination with pyrimethamine. In combination with trimethoprim, dapsone is used for the prophylaxis and treatment of *Pneumocystis jiroveci* pneumonia in patients with HIV infection. It may take 3 to 6 months of dapsone therapy before symptoms begin to improve. Pharmacotherapy for the prophylaxis of toxoplasmosis combines dapsone, pyrimethamine, and leucovorin. Dapsone 5% gel (Aczone) is approved as topical therapy for acne vulgaris.

Dapsone is the primary therapy for dermatitis herpetiformis and for autoimmune disease characterized by severe blistering skin lesions. Although its name implies herpes simplex virus as a causative agent, the etiology of the disorder is sensitivity to gluten in the diet. Gluten is a protein found in wheat products.

Mechanism of Action: The mechanism of action of dapsone is incompletely understood but is thought to be the same as that of the sulfonamides: inhibition of folic acid metabolism.

Pharmacokinetics:

Route(s)	PO
Absorption	Readily absorbed
Distribution	Widely distributed; crosses the placenta; secreted in breast milk; up to 90% protein bound
Primary metabolism	Hepatic, through acetylation by CYP2E1 and CYP3A4
Primary excretion	Renal, with small amounts in the feces
Onset of action	4–8 h
Duration of action	Half-life: 20–30 h

Adverse Effects: The most frequent adverse effects of oral dapsone relate to the hematologic system: dose-related hemolysis and methemoglobinemia with cyanosis. Aplastic anemia and agranulocytosis are rare, though potentially severe, adverse effects. Toxic hepatitis has been reported. The drug concentrates in the skin, causing dermatologic reactions that include photosensitivity and toxic epidermal necrolysis. When administered topically, the most frequent side effects are erythema and skin dryness.

Contraindications/Precautions: Contraindications include hypersensitivity to dapsone or related drugs, such as sulfonamides. Because of its adverse effects on the hematologic system, caution should be used in treating patients with preexisting blood disorders. Frequent blood assessments are conducted during therapy to avoid serious adverse effects. Frequent liver enzyme testing should be conducted to monitor for hepatotoxicity, especially in patients with preexisting liver impairment.

Drug Interactions: Some patients receiving pyrimethamine and dapsone concurrently developed agranulocytosis during the second and third month of therapy; therefore, concurrent administration of these drugs must be carefully monitored. Increased dapsone levels have been reported in patients receiving trimethoprim, and patients receiving this combination may be at increased risk for dapsone toxicity. Rifampin may significantly reduce serum levels of dapsone. The H_2-receptor blockers such as ranitidine will decrease gastric pH and lower the effectiveness of dapsone. **Herbal/Food:** Dapsone levels may be decreased by St. John's wort.

Pregnancy: Significant human experience with dapsone has not shown fetal abnormalities, although these were not well-controlled studies. Because dapsone enters human milk and can cause hemolytic reactions in the neonate, breastfeeding is not recommended.

Treatment of Overdose: Acute overdose may result in cyanosis, which is treated by the slow IV administration of 1–2 mg/kg of methylene blue.

Drugs Similar to Dapsone

Dapsone and rifampin are the primary drugs for leprosy. Rifampin is also used for TB and is discussed in Section 51.4. Clofazimine was used to treat leprosy and MAC infections for several decades but it is no longer available in the United States.

Drugs for *Mycobacterium avium* Complex Infections

51.7 *Mycobacterium avium* complex infections are common in patients with impaired immune function.

MAC is the most common cause of lung disease due to atypical mycobacterial infections. Although rare in healthy people, MAC is a frequent cause of infection among those with impaired immune systems and is an expected complication in many patients with HIV infection. It is also found in higher incidence in patients with chronic obstructive pulmonary disease. The infection is caused by *M. avium*, *M. intracellulare*, or a combination of atypical mycobacteria.

Unlike TB, MAC infections are not believed to be contagious or spread by human-to-human contact. The mode of transmission is not understood, although the organisms are widely distributed in soil and water and these may be the primary sources of infection. Once inside the body, MAC resides in the lungs like *M. tuberculosis*, and the initial respiratory symptoms are identical. The pathogen may travel through the lymphatics and bloodstream to infect any organ. The frequency of disseminated MAC disease has been markedly reduced because of successes in the pharmacotherapy of HIV infection.

Treatment of MAC should include at least two drugs (and often three or four) because monotherapy has been shown to promote the emergence of resistant strains. Treatment is continued for at least 1 year, and relapse rates for treating pulmonary MAC are high. Primary drugs for this infection include the following:

- **Macrolide antibiotics.** Clarithromycin and azithromycin are relatively safe and effective against MAC and are included in most regimens. High doses of clarithromycin (1000 mg bid) are associated with increased mortality rates.
- **Ethambutol (Myambutol).** Usually used for TB, this drug may be combined with clarithromycin in the pharmacotherapy of MAC.
- **Rifabutin (Mycobutin).** If a third drug is needed, rifabutin is often effective. Rifabutin, however, can cause many drug interactions, and high doses (600 mg/day) are associated with greater risk of serious uveitis with eye pain. Rifabutin is approved only for the prophylaxis of MAC in patients with HIV infection, although it is also used off-label to treat active infections.
- **Aminoglycosides.** Streptomycin and amikacin are indicated for severe MAC lung disease, especially in patients with HIV infection.

Understanding Chapter 51

Key Concepts Summary

51.1 Several species of mycobacteria are important human pathogens.

51.2 Tuberculosis is a respiratory infection that exhibits both active and latent stages.

51.3 The pharmacotherapy of tuberculosis requires special dosing regimens and schedules.

51.4 First-line or primary antituberculosis drugs are the most efficacious and safest drugs for treating *M. tuberculosis* infections.

51.5 Second-line antituberculosis drugs are used when resistance develops to the first-line drugs.

51.6 Leprosy is caused by a mycobacterium and is treated by a multidrug regimen.

51.7 *Mycobacterium avium* complex infections are common in patients with impaired immune function.

CASE STUDY: Making the Patient Connection

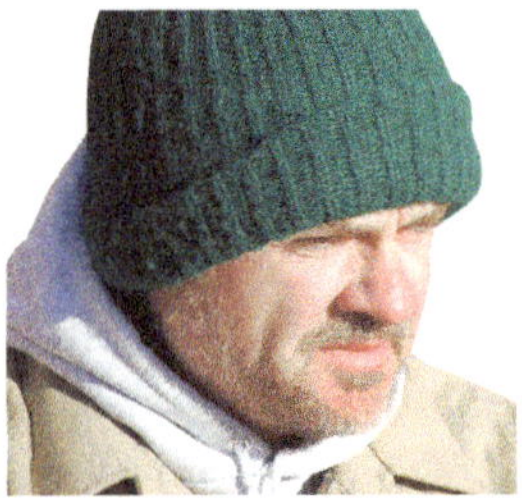

Remember the patient "Sam Myers" at the beginning of the chapter? Now read the remainder of the case study. Based on the information presented within this chapter, respond to the critical thinking questions that follow.

Sam Myers is a 58-year-old man who is homeless and spends some nights in shelters and some nights on the street. For the past 6 weeks, he has experienced anorexia, weight loss, and low-grade fever. He comes to the local church health center and presents with a productive cough that has progressively worsened.

A history and physical examination are completed with an evaluation for TB. The physical examination reveals the following findings: The patient's height is 1.9 m (6′1″) and his weight is 56.2 kg (124 lb). He is emaciated and obviously malnourished. His vital signs are blood pressure, 112/82 mmHg; heart rate, 102 beats/min; respiratory rate, 26 breaths/min; and body temperature, 38.2°C (100.9°F). On auscultation, crackles are heard in the upper lung fields. The patient is experiencing moderate dyspnea. Sam's chest x-ray reveals multiple calcifications and two cavitary masses in the apical posterior segments of the upper lobes of the lungs with lymphadenopathy also present. Sam admits to drinking alcohol and smoking at least one pack of cigarettes every day. He is admitted to a local acute care hospital for treatment of pulmonary TB.

Critical Thinking Questions

1. Describe the mechanism of transmission for *M. tuberculosis*.
2. Discuss how Sam's living conditions predispose him to pulmonary TB.
3. Why is Sam at high risk for hepatic-related adverse drug effects?

Additional Case Study

Georgia Sully has been diagnosed with an active TB infection after several months of increasing fevers, night sweats, productive cough, and weight loss. She is prescribed isoniazid (INH), ethambutol (Myambutol), rifampin (Rifadin), and pyrazinamide (PZA) for 6 months. She is also given instructions to take a daily dose of pyridoxine (vitamin B_6). She lives in a state that requires DOT for all patients receiving treatment for active TB.

1. Georgia is worried and questions the nurse about why she is receiving four different drugs for her tuberculosis. How would you respond?
2. Discuss why Georgia is receiving vitamin B_6 supplements.
3. Georgia asks what "directly observed therapy" is and why she needs it. What would you explain about DOT?

Chapter Review

1. A patient who is receiving isoniazid (INH) reports tingling and numbness of the fingers and toes. The nurse knows that these symptoms are most likely due to the drug's ability to:
    1. Increase the sensitivity of nerve endings.
    2. Decrease the activity of pyridoxine (vitamin B_6).
    3. Accelerate the excretion of neurotransmitters.
    4. Enhance skin receptors for ascorbic acid (vitamin C).

2. Ethambutol (Myambutol) has been included as part of a multidrug regimen to treat a patient with active tuberculosis. Prior to starting this drug, which screening tests should the patient have? (Select all that apply.)
    1. Coagulation studies
    2. Sputum cultures
    3. Uric acid level
    4. Hepatic function tests
    5. Vision acuity and vision color sense screening

3. A patient is identified as a possible slow acetylator and will be closely followed after beginning isoniazid therapy for latent tuberculosis. To ensure that this patient does not experience adverse effects related to the acetylation process, both ______________ and ______________ will be monitored frequently.

4. A patient with HIV infection who also has a *Mycobacterium avium* complex infection is started on clarithromycin and ethambutol (Myambutol). What appropriate teaching should the nurse give this patient?
    1. You will remain contagious until drug treatment is completed.
    2. These drugs will be required only for a short period of time, approximately 2 to 3 weeks.
    3. Drug therapy will be stopped if CD4 counts drop below 50 cells/mL.
    4. It will be necessary to continue these drugs for a prolonged period of time to adequately treat the infection.

5. The patient is diagnosed with *Mycobacterium leprae* (leprosy) and is being treated with dapsone. Which nursing assessment findings would indicate that the patient is experiencing adverse effects from this therapy?
    1. Discoloration of skin, cornea, and conjunctiva
    2. Chronic constipation, chills, and dehydration
    3. Hypoglycemia, impaired memory, and impotence
    4. Memory loss, nervousness, and pruritus

6. Patients with diabetes who take isoniazid (INH) may require more frequent monitoring of blood glucose levels. What effect does isoniazid have on glucose levels?
    1. It may decrease glucose levels.
    2. It has no known effects on glucose levels.
    3. It may increase glucose levels.
    4. It causes rapid rises and falls of glucose levels.

See Appendix A for answers to critical thinking questions, case study questions and review questions.

References

Centers for Disease Control and Prevention (CDC). (2019). *Trends in tuberculosis, 2018.* https://www.cdc.gov/tb/publications/factsheets/statistics/tbtrends.htm

Nahid, P., Dorman, S. E., Alipanah, N., Barry, P. M., Brozek, J. L., Cattamanchi, A., et al. (2016). Official American Thoracic Society/Centers for Disease Control and Prevention/Infectious Diseases Society of America clinical practice guidelines: Treatment of drug-susceptible tuberculosis. *Clinical Infectious Diseases, 63*(7), e147–e195. https://doi.org/10.1093/cid/ciw376

Smith, D. S. (2020). *Leprosy*. Medscape. http://emedicine.medscape.com/article/220455-overview

Sterling, T. R., Njie, G., Zenner, D., Cohn, D. L., Reves, R., Ahmed, A., et al. (2020). Guidelines for the treatment of latent tuberculosis infection: Recommendations from the National Tuberculosis Controllers Association and CDC, 2020. *MMWR Recommendations and Reports, 69*(No. RR-1), 1–11. http://dx.doi.org/10.15585/mmwr.rr6901a1external icon

Togun, T., Kampmann, B., Stoker, N. G., & Lipman, M. (2020). Anticipating the impact of the COVID-19 pandemic on TB patients and TB control programmes. *Annals of Clinical Microbiology and Antimicrobials, 19*, 21. https://doi.org/10.1186/s12941-020-00363-1

World Health Organization (WHO). (2019). *HIV-associated tuberculosis*. https://www.who.int/tb/areas-of-work/tb-hiv/tbhiv_factsheet.pdf?ua=1

World Health Organization (WHO). (2020a). *Causes of death*. https://www.who.int/data/gho/data/themes/topics/causes-of-death

World Health Organization (WHO). (2020b). *Global tuberculosis report 2020*. https://www.who.int/tb/publications/global_report/en/

World Health Organization (WHO). (2020c). *Tuberculosis key facts*. https://www.who.int/news-room/fact-sheets/detail/tuberculosis

Selected Bibliography

Centers for Disease Control and Prevention (CDC). (2018). *Tuberculosis (TB)*. https://www.cdc.gov/tb/default.htm

Centers for Disease Control and Prevention (CDC). (2020). *Latent tuberculosis infection: A guide for primary health providers*. https://www.cdc.gov/tb/publications/ltbi/ltbiresources.htm

Foster-Chang, S., & Balmer, J. (2020). Updated tuberculosis screening guidelines for health care personnel. *Workplace Health & Safety*, *68*(7). https://doi.org/10.1177/2165079920913892

Koirala, J. (2019). *Mycobacterium avium complex (MAC)*. Medscape. http://emedicine.medscape.com/article/222664-overview

Pettit, A. C., Shepherd, B. E., & Sterling, T. R. (2018). Treatment of drug-susceptible tuberculosis among people living with human immunodeficiency virus infection: an update. *Current Opinion in HIV and AIDS*, *13*(6), 469. https://doi.org/10.1097/COH.0000000000000506

Rokadiya, S., Millar, F. R., & Tiberi, S. (2018). Non-tuberculous mycobacterial pulmonary disease: a clinical update. *British Journal of Hospital Medicine*, *79*(8), C118–C122. https://doi.org/10.1016/j.jiac.2019.11.004

Singh, R., Dwivedi, S. P., Gaharwar, U. S., Meena, R., Rajamani, P., & Prasad, T. (2020). Recent updates on drug resistance in Mycobacterium tuberculosis. *Journal of Applied Microbiology*, *128*(6), 1547–1567. https://doi.org/10.1111/jam.14478

World Health Organization (WHO). (2019). *Global tuberculosis report 2019*. https://www.who.int/tb/publications/factsheet_global.pdf?ua=1

"Since I started chemotherapy, these white patches have appeared on my tongue and sometimes my throat burns when I swallow. So I decided to come to the clinic to find out what's going on with me."
—*Patient "Sarah Williams"*

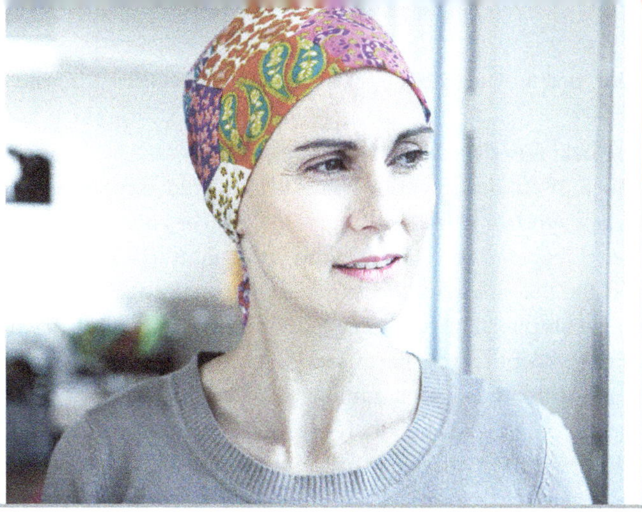

Chapter 52
Pharmacotherapy of Fungal Infections

Chapter Outline

Learning Outcomes

After reading this chapter, the student should be able to:

1. Compare and contrast the pharmacotherapy of fungal and bacterial infections.
2. Classify mycoses based on the location of the infection and the causative organism.
3. Compare and contrast the pharmacotherapy of systemic and superficial fungal infections.
4. Identify the types of patients at greatest risk of acquiring serious fungal infections.
5. Describe the nurse's role in the pharmacologic management of fungal infections.
6. For each of the classes shown in the chapter outline, identify the prototype and representative drugs and explain the mechanism(s) of drug action, primary indications, contraindications, significant drug interactions, pregnancy data, and important adverse effects.
7. Apply clinical judgment to care for patients receiving pharmacotherapy for fungal infections.

Key Terms

Definitions of the terms in bold may be found in the Glossary.

The past few decades have seen a dramatic rise in the incidence of fungal infections due to acquired immunodeficiency syndrome (AIDS), aggressive cancer chemotherapy, the widespread use of indwelling intravenous (IV) catheters, and the use of broad-spectrum antibiotics. Fungi are much more complex than bacteria and require a different approach to pharmacotherapy. Because of these structural and functional differences, most antibacterial drugs are ineffective against fungi. Although there are fewer drugs to treat fungal infections, the available medications are usually effective.

Characteristics of Fungi and Fungal Infections

52.1 Serious fungal infections are uncommon in people with healthy immune defenses.

Fungi are single-celled or multicellular organisms that serve essential roles on the planet as decomposers of dead plants and animals, returning their elements to the soil for recycling. Fungi include mushrooms, yeasts, and molds. Although 100,000 to 200,000 species of fungi exist in soil, air, and water, only about 50 species are associated with disease in humans. A few species of fungi survive as part of the normal host flora on the skin, mouth, and urogenital tract.

Unlike bacteria, which produce toxins or grow rapidly to overwhelm hosts' defenses, some fungi grow slowly and infections may progress for many months before symptoms develop. With a few exceptions (such as athlete's foot), fungal infections are not easily transmitted through casual contact. In addition to causing infections, fungal antigens may trigger hypersensitivity responses in susceptible patients, resulting in allergies to mold or mildew. A few fungi, such as *Aspergillus flavus*, secrete toxins that can cause illness in humans through ingestion of contaminated grains or other foods.

The human body is remarkably resistant to infection by these organisms and patients with healthy immune defenses experience few serious fungal diseases. However, patients with a suppressed immune system (immunocompromised), especially those infected with human immunodeficiency virus (HIV), may experience frequent fungal infections and require aggressive pharmacotherapy. A systemic fungal infection in an immunocompromised patient may be rapidly fatal.

The species of pathogenic fungi that attack hosts with healthy immune defenses are often distinct from those that infect immunocompromised patients. Patients with intact immune defenses are afflicted with community-acquired infections such as sporotrichosis, blastomycosis, histoplasmosis, and coccidioidomycosis. Opportunistic fungal infections acquired in a hospital setting are more likely to be candidiasis, aspergillosis, cryptococcosis, and mucormycosis. Thus, assessing the immune status of a patient may help in diagnosing the specific infection and in determining the course of pharmacotherapy. Table 52.1 lists the species of fungi that most commonly cause disease in humans.

Table 52.1 Fungal Pathogens

Name of Fungus	Description
Systemic	
Aspergillus fumigatus and other species	Aspergillosis: Opportunistic; most commonly affects the lungs but can spread to other organs
Blastomyces dermatitides	Blastomycosis: Begins in the lungs and spreads to other organs
Candida albicans and other species	Candidiasis: Most common opportunistic fungal infection; may affect nearly any organ
Coccidioides immitis	Coccidioidomycosis: Begins in the lungs and spreads to other organs
Cryptococcus neoformans	Cryptococcosis: Opportunistic; begins in the lungs but is the most common cause of meningitis in patients with AIDS
Histoplasma capsulatum	Histoplasmosis: Begins in the lungs and spreads to other organs
Mucorales species	Mucormycosis: Opportunistic; affects blood vessels, causes sinus infections, stomach ulcers, and other disorders
Pneumocystis jirovecii	*Pneumocystis* pneumonia: Opportunistic; primarily pneumonia of the lung but can spread to other organs
Superficial	
Candida albicans and other species	Candidiasis: Affects the skin, nails, oral cavity (thrush), vagina
Epidermophyton floccosum	Athlete's foot (tinea pedis), jock itch (tinea cruris), and other skin infections
Microsporum species	Ringworm of the scalp (tinea capitis)
Trichophyton species	Affects the scalp, skin, and nails
Subcutaneous and Cutaneous	
Sporothrix schenckii	Sporotrichosis: Primarily affects the skin and superficial lymph nodes
Mixed species	Chromoblastomycosis: Chronic skin mycosis found in tropical and subtropical climates

PharmFACT

Certain medications can weaken the immune system and increase the risk of a fungal infection. Patients taking antineoplastics, corticosteroids, and tumor necrosis factor (TNF) inhibitors such as adalimumab (Humira) should be monitored for mycoses during therapy (Centers for Disease Control and Prevention [CDC], 2020).

52.2 Mycoses are classified as superficial, subcutaneous, or systemic.

Fungal infections are called **mycoses** (singular, *mycosis*). A simple and useful method of classifying fungal infections is to consider them as superficial, subcutaneous, or systemic.

Superficial mycoses affect the scalp, skin, nails, and mucous membranes such as the oral cavity and vagina. Only the surface layers of these regions are affected. Mycoses of this type are often treated with topical drugs because these medications can penetrate into the keratin layer of the skin while producing few systemic adverse effects.

Subcutaneous and cutaneous mycoses are infections that affect deeper skin layers, including the dermis and subcutaneous layers. Often, the organisms that cause subcutaneous and cutaneous infections are different from those that cause superficial infections, as listed in Table 52.1. Because these fungal species often reside in soil, gardeners or people working in occupations involving exposure to soil can acquire these infections through cuts or abrasions on their skin. In addition, these infections occur in greater incidence in regions where the population travels barefoot. Topical antifungal preparations may not penetrate deep enough to reach the pathogen, thus oral (PO) antifungal therapy may be indicated. Some textbooks consider subcutaneous mycoses as subtypes of superficial mycoses.

Systemic mycoses are those that affect internal organs, typically the lungs, brain, and digestive organs. These infections often originate in the lungs, through inhalation of fungal spores. Although less common than superficial or subcutaneous mycoses, systemic fungal infections affect multiple body systems and may be fatal to patients with severely suppressed immune systems. Invasive systemic mycoses require aggressive PO or parenteral medications that produce more adverse effects than the topical drugs.

Historically, antifungal drugs used for superficial infections were clearly distinct from those prescribed for systemic infections. In recent years, this distinction has blurred. Some of the newer antifungals may be used for superficial, subcutaneous, or systemic infections. Furthermore, some superficial infections may be treated with parenteral, oral, or topical drugs. This therapeutic division, however, is still useful because it separates the pharmacotherapy of relatively benign infections (superficial) from those that may be life-threatening (systemic).

52.3 Antifungal drugs act by disrupting the fungal cell membrane or wall, affecting fungal enzymes, or disrupting replication.

Biologically, fungi are classified as eukaryotes: Their cellular organelles and metabolic pathways are more similar to those of humans than those of bacteria. Antibiotics that are efficacious against bacteria are ineffective in treating mycoses due to these differences in physiology; thus, an entirely different set of drugs is needed to eliminate fungal pathogens.

Like antibacterials, the antifungal drugs may either slow the growth of the organisms (fungistatic) or kill them (fungicidal). The five mechanisms of action of the antifungal drugs are illustrated in Pharmacotherapy Illustrated 52.1.

Pharmacotherapy Illustrated 52.1

Mechanisms of Action of Antifungal Drugs

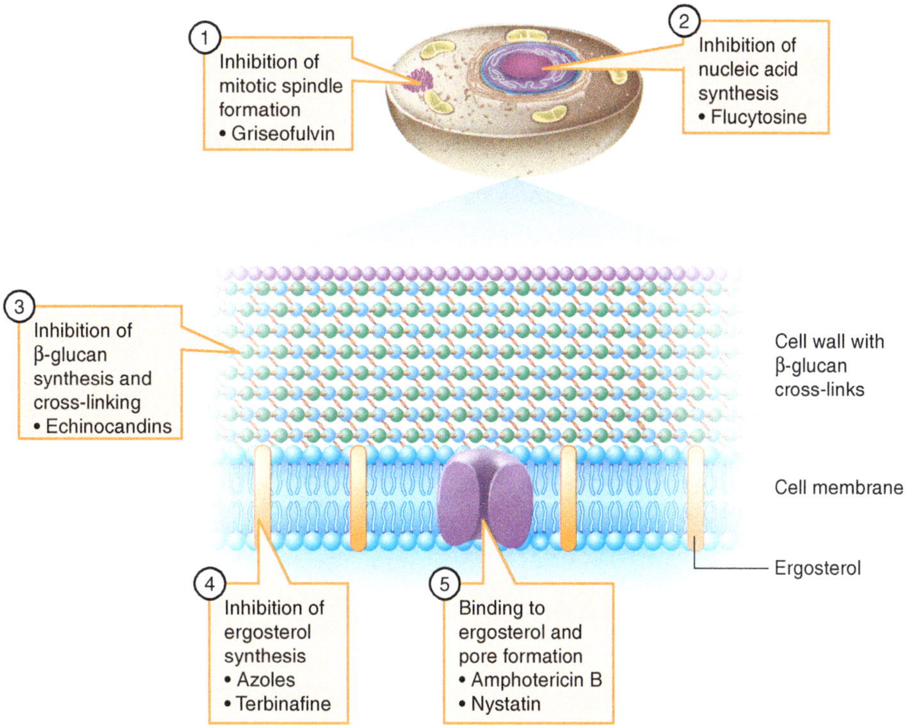

One important difference between fungal cells and human cells is the specific steroid used in constructing plasma membranes. While cholesterol is essential for animal cell membranes, **ergosterol** is present in fungi. The largest class of antifungals, the azoles, inhibits ergosterol biosynthesis, causing the fungal plasma membrane to become porous or leaky. Amphotericin B, terbinafine (Lamisil), and nystatin also act by this mechanism.

Caspofungin (Cancidas) disrupts fungal cell walls by inhibiting the synthesis of **β-glucan**, an essential component that shapes and strengthens the cell wall. Without sufficient β-glucan, the wall weakens and becomes porous, causing the death of the cell. Chitin is another material in the cell wall of fungi. The polyoxins are fungicides that interfere with chitin synthesis and are widely used in agriculture.

Some antifungals act by mechanisms that take advantage of enzymatic differences between fungi and humans. In fungi, flucytosine (Ancobon) is converted to the potent antimetabolite fluorouracil, which inhibits both deoxyribonucleic acid (DNA) and ribonucleic acid (RNA) synthesis. Humans do not have the enzyme necessary for this conversion. Fluorouracil itself is a common antineoplastic medication (see Chapter 57).

A final mechanism is used by the drug griseofulvin (Gris-PEG). This drug is incorporated into newly formed keratin where it protects against fungal invasion. Once it has entered the fungal cell, it disrupts the mitotic spindle, preventing replication.

CONNECTION Checkpoint 52.1

From what you learned in Chapter 47, what major classes of antibacterials act by disrupting cell walls? Why are these drugs not effective against fungi?

Drugs for Systemic Fungal Infections

52.4 Systemic or invasive fungal disease may require intensive pharmacotherapy for extended periods.

Because human body defenses provide a formidable barrier to fungi, systemic mycoses are rarely encountered in individuals with healthy immune systems. The AIDS epidemic, however, resulted in the frequent clinical occurrence of previously rare mycoses, such as cryptococcosis and coccidioidomycosis. The opportunistic disease in patients with AIDS spurred the development of several new drugs for systemic fungal infections. In addition to occurring in patients with HIV infection, others who may experience systemic mycoses include those receiving prolonged therapy with

CONNECTIONS: Advanced Practice Application

Asthma and Exposure to Fungal Pathogens

Case

Tyler, a 9-year-old boy, presents to our pediatric pulmonology clinic with severe persistent asthma and atopic dermatitis that he has had since he was 2 years old. He has been hospitalized 3 times for his asthma in the past 18 months. He lives in an older apartment in a major metropolitan city and his mother believes that the mold in the windows may be making Tyler worse. Results of pulmonary-function tests (PFTs) confirm the asthma diagnosis (he improved after bronchodilator therapy). He has been treated for asthma by his pediatrician in a stepwise fashion, eventually requiring high-dose inhaled corticosteroids, long-acting β agonists, leukotriene receptor antagonists, and antihistamines. Despite these medications, Tyler continues to exhibit daily symptoms that require frequent bursts of high-dose systemic steroids. Because his skin testing was positive for *Aspergillus*, he was started on 100 mg of itraconazole by mouth twice a day. Within 6 weeks, Tyler reported complete resolution of symptoms, and after 6 months on itraconazole, his systemic steroids were weaned and he was maintained on inhaled corticosteroids, long-acting β agonists, and leukotriene receptor antagonists. Throughout the 6-month treatment period, he experienced only one exacerbation. The family will be relocating to a new apartment at the end of their lease in 1 month. Why did the itraconazole help control Tyler's asthma?

Discussion

Asthma is a serious public health problem affecting people of all ages. When uncontrolled, asthma can lead to severe limitation on activities of daily life and may even be fatal. Uncontrolled asthma generally affects only a small percentage of the total asthma population. It is difficult to treat, prone to recurrent exacerbations, and contributes disproportionately to the overall costs of asthma. Exposure to environmental fungal spores has been associated with worsening asthma severity, including worsening lung function, increased hospital admissions, and asthma-related deaths (Jara, 2017; Tham, 2017).

Preventing exposure to fungal pathogens is the ideal clinical strategy (CDC, 2019):

- Keep humidity levels as low as you can.
- Use exhaust fans that vent outside your home in the kitchen and bathroom.
- Clean and dry out your home thoroughly and quickly after flooding.
- Add mold inhibitors to paints before applying.
- Clean bathrooms with mold-killing products.
- Remove or replace carpets and upholstery that have been soaked and cannot be dried promptly.

corticosteroids, having extensive burns, receiving antineoplastic drugs, having indwelling vascular catheters, or receiving organ transplants. Prophylactic antifungal therapy is sometimes indicated for these high-risk patients.

Pharmacotherapy of systemic mycoses is often continued for many months to ensure that the fungus is eliminated. Unlike the superficial antifungal medications, systemic drugs have the potential to cause serious adverse effects and therapy must be carefully monitored. The systemic antifungal drugs are listed in Table 52.2.

Pharmacologic options for serious systemic mycoses are limited. Amphotericin B has been the traditional preferred drug for systemic fungal infections since the 1960s. Azole drugs such as itraconazole, however, are considerably safer and have become preferred drugs for less severe infections. Although rarely used as a monotherapy, flucytosine (Ancobon) is sometimes used in combination with amphotericin B in the pharmacotherapy of severe *Candida* infections. Voriconazole (Vfend) is the preferred drug for treating invasive aspergillosis, a rare though particularly lethal mycosis with a high mortality rate. In 2015, isavuconazonium (Cresemba) was approved by the U.S. Food and Drug Administration (FDA) as an alternative option for treating invasive aspergillosis.

PROTOTYPE DRUG Amphotericin B Deoxycholate

Classification **Therapeutic:** Antifungal (systemic type)
Pharmacologic: Polyene

Therapeutic Effects and Uses: Approved in 1957, amphotericin B has a broad spectrum of activity that includes most fungi that are pathogenic to humans. It has been the traditional preferred drug for treating severe systemic mycoses and may also be indicated as prophylactic antifungal therapy for patients with severe immunosuppression. Because it is not absorbed from the gastrointestinal (GI) tract, it is normally given by IV infusion. Fungal resistance to amphotericin B is not a major clinical problem.

Table 52.2 Drugs for Systemic Mycoses

Drug	Route and Adult Dose (Maximum Dose Where Indicated)	Adverse Effects
amphotericin B (Abelcet, AmBisome)	IV: 0.3–1.5 mg/kg/day, infused over 2–4 h (max: 1.5 mg/kg/day) IV (Abelcet): 5 mg/kg/day IV (Ambisome): 3–5 mg/kg/day	*Hypokalemia, hypomagnesemia, rash, fever and chills, nausea and vomiting, anorexia, headache* Nephrotoxicity, liver failure, anaphylaxis, cardiac arrest, thrombocytopenia, leukopenia, agranulocytosis, anemia
anidulafungin (Eraxis)	Candidemia: IV: 200 mg on day 1, then 100 mg/day for 14 days Esophageal candidiasis: IV: 100 mg on day 1, then 50 mg/day for 7–14 days	*Diarrhea, nausea and vomiting, mild allergic reactions, hypokalemia* Neutropenia, dysrhythmias, hepatic impairment, anaphylaxis
caspofungin (Cancidas)	IV: 70 mg on day 1, then 50 mg/day infused over 1 h for 14 days	*Fever, chills, diarrhea, increased serum alkaline phosphatase, hypokalemia* Anaphylaxis, hepatic impairment
flucytosine (Ancobon)	PO: 25 mg/kg every 6 h to reach a peak concentration of 50–100 mcg/mL	*Nausea and vomiting, headache* Blood dyscrasias, cardiac toxicity, renal failure, psychosis
micafungin (Mycamine)	IV: 150 mg/day over 1 h for active *Candida* infection; 50 mg/day over 1 h for *Candida* prophylaxis	*Headache, fever, nausea and vomiting, diarrhea, rash* Thrombocytopenia, hemolytic anemia, anaphylaxis, hepatic and renal failure
Azoles		
fluconazole (Diflucan)	PO/IV: 200–400 mg on day 1, then 100–200 mg/day for 2–4 wk PO (for vaginal candidiasis): 150 mg single dose	*Fever, chills, rash, dizziness, drowsiness, nausea and vomiting, diarrhea* Hepatotoxicity, anaphylaxis, blood dyscrasias, visual disturbances (voriconazole), dysrhythmias (posaconazole, voriconazole)
isavuconazonium (Cresemba)	PO/IV: 372 mg/day	
itraconazole (Sporanox, Tolsura)	PO (Sporanox): 200 mg/day (max: 400 mg/day) PO (Tolsura): 130 mg/day (max: 260 mg/day)	
ketoconazole (Nizoral)	PO: 200–400 mg/day	
posaconazole (Noxafil)	PO (delayed-release tablet): 100–300 mg/day (max: 400 mg/day) IV: 300 mg 1–2 times/day	
voriconazole (Vfend)	IV: 6 mg/kg on day 1, then 4 mg/kg q12h PO (maintenance dose): 200 mg q12h	

Note: *Italics* indicate common adverse effects. Underline indicates serious adverse effects.

To reduce the toxicity of amphotericin B, the original molecule has been formulated with two different types of lipid "delivery vehicles":

- **Liposomal amphotericin B (AmBisome).** Consists of closed spherical vesicles. Amphotericin B is integrated into the membrane, as illustrated in Figure 52.1.
- **Amphotericin B lipid complex (Abelcet).** Contains amphotericin B complexed with two phospholipids in a 1:1 ratio.

The principal advantage of the lipid formulations is reduced nephrotoxicity and less infusion-related fever and chills. The reduced toxicity is believed to be due to the decreased plasma levels of the drug. Macrophages ingest the lipid formulations and deliver the medication to its fungal targets before it can accumulate to high serum levels that cause toxicity. Because of their expense, however, the lipid preparations are not considered first-line drugs and are generally used only after therapy with other antifungals has failed.

Mechanism of Action: Amphotericin B acts by binding to ergosterol in fungal cell membranes, causing them to become permeable.

Pharmacokinetics:

Route(s)	IV, topical
Absorption	Not absorbed topically
Distribution	Widely distributed; very little enters the cerebrospinal fluid (CSF) or amniotic fluid; about 90% bound to plasma protein
Primary metabolism	Hepatic
Primary excretion	Renal
Onset of action	IV: immediate
Duration of action	Half-life: 24–48 h; drug may persist several weeks after therapy is discontinued

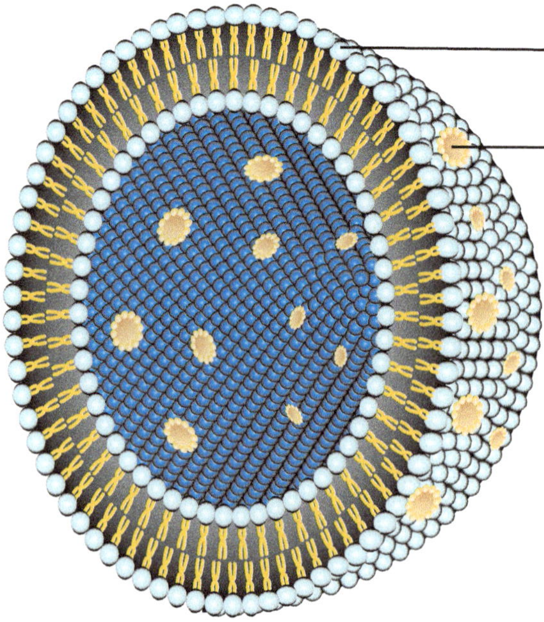

Figure 52.1 Liposomal amphotericin B: Drug molecules are embedded in the phospholipid bilayer.

Adverse Effects: Amphotericin B can produce frequent and sometimes serious adverse effects. At the onset of therapy, as many as 50% of patients experience acute, infusion-related fever and chills, vomiting, anorexia, and headache. These symptoms usually subside as treatment continues. Phlebitis is also common during IV therapy, and alternate-day dosing is sometimes needed to reduce this adverse effect. Amphotericin B can cause ototoxicity, potentially affecting both branches, cochlear and vestibular, of cranial nerve VIII.

The most serious toxic effects of amphotericin B are on the kidney. Some degree of nephrotoxicity is observed in 80% of patients taking amphotericin B; thus, laboratory tests of kidney function are regularly performed throughout the treatment period. Electrolyte imbalance, especially hypokalemia and hypomagnesemia, may develop as a result of renal damage and place the patient at greater risk of developing life-threatening dysrhythmias and cardiac arrest. Concurrent therapy with other medications that reduce liver or renal function, such as aminoglycosides, is not recommended.

Amphotericin B is occasionally hepatotoxic. Anaphylaxis is possible, and cardiac arrest has been reported. Blood abnormalities, including thrombocytopenia, leukopenia, agranulocytosis, and anemia, are potentially serious adverse effects. **Black Box Warning:** The nonliposomal form of this drug should only be used for patients with a progressive and potentially life-threatening fungal infection. Caution should be exercised to prevent overdosage.

Contraindications/Precautions: Amphotericin B should be infused slowly, over 2 to 6 hours, because hypotension, hypokalemia, and shock may result if the medication is administered too rapidly. The drug should be withheld if blood urea nitrogen exceeds 40 mg/dL or if serum creatinine rises above 3 mg/dL.

Drug Interactions: Drug interactions with amphotericin B focus on worsening two of its potentially serious adverse effects: nephrotoxicity and hypokalemia. For example, concurrent therapy with aminoglycosides, cyclosporine, acyclovir, carboplatin, and tacrolimus is not recommended. Corticosteroids, skeletal muscle relaxants, and thiazole may potentiate hypokalemia caused by amphotericin B. Drug-induced hypokalemia will also increase the risk of digoxin toxicity. Because animal studies have indicated an antagonistic effect between amphotericin B and certain azoles (imidazoles), concurrent therapy with this class of antifungals is usually avoided. **Herbal/Food:** Unknown.

Pregnancy: Human experience with this drug during pregnancy is limited, but the data have not shown evidence of fetal harm. It is not known if this drug is secreted in human milk or if it has any adverse effects on the breastfed neonate.

Treatment of Overdose: Overdose may result in cardiorespiratory arrest. No specific therapy is available. Patients are treated symptomatically.

Clinician Responsibilities: Key clinical implications for patients receiving amphotericin B are included in Applied Clinical Judgment: Patients Receiving Pharmacotherapy with Antifungals.

Drugs Similar to Amphotericin B Deoxycholate

Other systemic antifungals include the β-glucan synthesis inhibitors, flucytosine, and certain azole drugs (see Section 52.5).

β-Glucan synthesis inhibitors: Caspofungin (Cancidas), micafungin (Mycamine), and anidulafungin (Eraxis) belong to a class of antifungals called echinocandins or β-glucan synthesis inhibitors. Given only by slow IV infusion, the echinocandins are better tolerated than amphotericin B and do not exhibit significant nephrotoxicity or hepatotoxicity.

Caspofungin was approved in 2001 and is particularly effective against invasive *Candida* and *Aspergillus* species. It is effective against some fungal species that have developed resistance to amphotericin B and the azoles. Adverse effects with caspofungin include fever, rash, and infusion-related reactions such as phlebitis, diarrhea, headache, and nausea. Caution should be used when administering caspofungin to patients with hepatic impairment.

Micafungin, approved in 2005, is used to treat acute disseminated candidiasis, esophageal candidiasis, and *Candida* infections in patients undergoing bone marrow transplants. Micafungin causes transient increases in hepatic enzymes, headache, and nausea and vomiting. Rare, serious cases of renal and hepatic impairment and hematologic toxicity have occurred with micafungin.

Anidulafungin was approved in 2006 for candidemia and other systemic *Candida* infections as esophageal candidiasis and intra-abdominal abscess. The drug is generally well tolerated with adverse reactions occurring in 2% or less of patients. These adverse effects are generally not severe and include fever, diarrhea, hypokalemia, and increases in liver function test values.

Animal studies showed evidence of fetal harm with β-glucan synthesis inhibitors. It is not known if these drugs are secreted in human milk or if it they have any adverse effects on the breastfed neonate.

Flucytosine (Ancobon): Unlike amphotericin B and the β-glucan synthesis inhibitors, which must be given parenterally, flucytosine is well absorbed from the GI tract. Approved in 1990, flucytosine is structurally similar to cytosine, a nucleotide used in DNA synthesis. When the fungus attempts to use flucytosine to construct its DNA, cell division is inhibited. It is approved to treat septicemia and pulmonary and urinary tract infections due to *Candida* and *Cryptococcus* species. Unfortunately, resistance to flucytosine can be a major clinical problem. The drug is sometimes used in combination with amphotericin B to reduce the potential for treatment failure due to resistance. Combination therapy also permits the use of lower doses of amphotericin B, thus reducing the risk of nephrotoxicity.

Although adverse GI effects are common with flucytosine, they are usually not severe. The drug carries a black box warning that extreme caution should be used in patients with chronic kidney disease (CKD). The warning urges close monitoring of hematologic, renal, and hepatic status during therapy. Flucytosine can cause bone marrow toxicity, leukopenia, agranulocytosis, and thrombocytopenia. Serum concentrations of flucytosine should be less than 100 g/mL to avoid bone marrow suppression. Flucytosine may cause hepatitis and elevate serum levels of hepatic enzymes. Animal studies showed that flucytosine causes embryotoxicity and teratogenicity. Because this medication is secreted in human milk and may cause potential adverse effects in the neonate, breastfeeding is not recommended.

Drugs for Both Systemic and Superficial Fungal Infections

52.5 Azoles are the preferred drugs for many mycoses due to their efficacy and favorable safety profile.

The **azole** class is the largest and most versatile group of antifungals. These drugs have broad spectrums and are used to treat nearly any systemic, subcutaneous, or superficial fungal infection. They have replaced many of the older antifungals because they can be administered PO and have a superior safety profile.

The azoles are sometimes grouped by chemical or therapeutic classes. The azoles form two distinct chemical classes, as follows:

- *Imidazoles:* Butoconazole, clotrimazole, econazole, ketoconazole, miconazole, oxiconazole, sulconazole, and ticonazole
- *Triazoles:* Fluconazole, isavuconazonium, itraconazole, posaconazole, terconazole, and voriconazole.

The triazoles are more slowly metabolized and elicit fewer adverse effects than the imidazoles. In clinical practice, imidazoles and triazoles exhibit the same spectrum of activity and act by the same mechanism.

A second method of classifying azoles is by their therapeutic utility as either systemic or topical drugs. Isavuconazonium (Cresemba) is only used systemically. Fluconazole (Diflucan), itraconazole (Sporanox), ketoconazole (Nizoral), posaconazole (Noxafil), and voriconazole (Vfend) are used for both systemic and topical infections. The remainder of the azoles are prescribed for superficial infections (see Section 52.6).

Azoles interfere with the biosynthesis of ergosterol, which is essential for the construction of fungal cell membranes. By depleting the fungal cells of ergosterol, fungal growth is impaired.

The systemic azoles have a spectrum of activity similar to that of amphotericin B, are less toxic, and have the major advantage that they can be administered PO. Because of these characteristics, some of the azoles have replaced amphotericin B in the pharmacotherapy of less serious systemic fungal infections.

The most common adverse effects of the systemic azoles are nausea and vomiting, which occur in 10 to 20% of patients. Giving the drugs with food or in divided doses may relieve minor GI distress. Severe nausea may require dose reduction or the concurrent administration of an antiemetic. Asymptomatic elevations of serum aminotransferase levels are common during therapy. Anaphylaxis and rash have been reported. Fatal drug-induced hepatitis has occurred with ketoconazole, though the incidence is rare and has not been reported with the other systemic azoles. Because of this, itraconazole has largely replaced ketoconazole in the therapy of systemic mycoses. With all the systemic azoles, liver function tests should be obtained before therapy begins and throughout the course of treatment. Azoles may affect glycemic control, so blood glucose should be monitored regularly in patients with diabetes and those with metabolic syndrome.

Various reproductive abnormalities have been reported with systemic azoles, including menstrual irregularities, gynecomastia in men, and drops in plasma testosterone levels. Decreased libido and temporary sterility in men are other potential adverse effects.

PROTOTYPE DRUG Fluconazole (Diflucan)

Classification **Therapeutic:** Antifungal
Pharmacologic: Inhibitor of fungal cell membrane synthesis, triazole (azole)

Therapeutic Effects and Uses: Approved in 1990, fluconazole is available as tablets, oral suspension, and IV injection. It is particularly effective against *Candida albicans* and is used to treat oropharyngeal candidiasis, esophageal candidiasis, vulvovaginal candidiasis, and various systemic infections by this species. It is also effective against cryptococcal meningitis and may be used for mycoses that are resistant to other antifungals. Fluconazole is less effective against non-*albicans Candida* species, which account for a significant percentage of opportunistic fungal infections. The drug is approved for prophylaxis of fungal infections in patients with HIV infection, those undergoing bone marrow transplants, and those receiving antineoplastic drugs.

Fluconazole offers several advantages over other systemic antifungals. It is rapidly and completely absorbed when given PO and is also available by the IV route. Compared to itraconazole and ketoconazole, it more easily penetrates body membranes to reach infections in the central nervous system (CNS), bone, eye, urinary tract, and respiratory tract.

Mechanism of Action: Like other azoles, fluconazole acts by interfering with the synthesis of ergosterol.

Pharmacokinetics:

Route(s)	IV, PO
Absorption	Readily absorbed PO
Distribution	Widely distributed, including the CSF; secreted in breast milk; 12% bound to plasma protein
Primary metabolism	Hepatic
Primary excretion	Renal
Onset of action	Peak effect: 1–2 h
Duration of action	Half-life: 20–50 h

Adverse Effects: Fluconazole causes few serious adverse effects. Nausea and vomiting and diarrhea are reported at high doses. Because the kidneys excrete most of the drug, it should be used cautiously in patients with CKD. Hepatotoxicity with fluconazole is less common than with ketoconazole. Stevens–Johnson syndrome (SJS) has been reported in patients with immunosuppression.

Contraindications/Precautions: The only contraindication to fluconazole is hypersensitivity to the drug or another azole. Fluconazole should be used with caution in patients with hepatic impairment because the drug is metabolized in the liver: Hepatic injury has occurred with this drug. When given by the IV route, fluconazole is usually prepared without added medications because it is incompatible with a number of drugs. Patients with hypokalemia should be treated with caution because fluconazole may worsen this electrolyte imbalance.

Drug Interactions: Fluconazole is a strong inhibitor of CYP2C9, CYP2C19, and CYP3A4; therefore, it has the potential to interact with several drugs. Use with warfarin (Coumadin) may increase prothrombin time and cause increased risk for bleeding. Hypoglycemia may result if fluconazole is administered concurrently with certain oral hypoglycemics, including glyburide. Fluconazole levels may be decreased with concurrent rifampin or cimetidine use. The effects of fentanyl, benzodiazepines, tricyclic antidepressants, or methadone may be prolonged with concurrent administration of fluconazole. This drug increases the serum level of phenytoin; careful monitoring of phenytoin concentrations is recommended to avoid CNS toxicity. Rifampin increases the metabolism of fluconazole; thus, the dose of fluconazole may need to be increased to maintain therapeutic plasma levels. Concurrent use of fluconazole and erythromycin is contraindicated because the combination can increase the level and effect of erythromycin and increase the QT interval. **Herbal/Food:** Unknown.

Pregnancy: High-dose therapy with this drug during the first trimester is teratogenic in humans. Taking a single oral dose for vulvovaginal candidiasis has been associated with a higher risk for spontaneous abortion. This drug is secreted in human milk but adverse effects on the breastfed neonate are unknown. Fluconazole should not be used during pregnancy or lactation unless the potential benefits for the mother justify the potential risks to the fetus or neonate.

Treatment of Overdose: No specific therapy is available; patients are treated symptomatically. Dialysis can be used to lower serum drug level.

Clinician Responsibilities: Key clinical implications for patients receiving fluconazole are included in Applied Clinical Judgment: Patients Receiving Pharmacotherapy with Antifungals.

Drugs Similar to Fluconazole (Diflucan)

Other systemic azoles include isavuconazonium, itraconazole, ketoconazole, posaconazole, and voriconazole. All of the systemic azoles have shown evidence of embryotoxicity and fetotoxicity in laboratory animals. Most are secreted in the milk of animals, although it is not known if these drugs cause adverse effects on the breastfed neonate. When given systemically, these medications should not be used during pregnancy and lactation unless the potential benefits to the mother justify the potential risks to the fetus or neonate. It should be noted, however, that these medications are sometimes used to treat serious, life-threatening infections

Isavuconazonium (Cresemba): Isavuconazonium is a prodrug that is rapidly converted to its active form, isavuconazole, by enzymes in the blood. Given either PO or IV, it was approved in 2015 to treat invasive aspergillosis and mucormycosis infections. Because isavuconazole is a substrate for CYP450 enzymes 3A4 and 3A5, the drug should not be administered concurrently with CYP3A4 inhibitors such as ketoconazole or carbamazepine. Frequent adverse effects include nausea and vomiting, diarrhea, headache, and elevated hepatic laboratory test results. Serious hepatotoxicity has been reported. Women of childbearing potential should use effective contraception during therapy and for 28 days following the last dose.

Itraconazole (Sporanox, Tolsura): Approved in 1992, itraconazole is available as capsules, PO solution, and IV injection. Its spectrum is similar to that of other azoles, except it may have greater activity against *Aspergillus*. It is metabolized in the liver to hydroxyitraconazole, which also has antifungal activity. Because the drug may take 2 or more weeks to reach therapeutic levels, a loading dose is infused when treating invasive mycoses. The PO capsules should be taken with food to enhance absorption; however, the PO solution should be taken on an empty stomach. Both PO formulations require an acidic stomach environment for absorption and thus should not be taken concurrently with drugs or foods that decrease stomach acidity. Onmel is an oral formulation approved for 12 consecutive weeks of therapy for fungal infections of the toenail.

The most common adverse effects of itraconazole are GI related, especially nausea, which occurs in about 10% of patients. Hepatotoxicity is a rare, though potentially serious, adverse effect, which warrants periodic monitoring of liver laboratory tests. Itraconazole carries a black box warning that the drug should be discontinued if any signs of cardiotoxicity or heart failure arise during therapy. The warning also states that care should be taken when administering itraconazole with other medications, since numerous drug–drug interactions have been reported. Concurrent administration of itraconazole with benzodiazepines or statins is contraindicated. Itraconazole is contraindicated during pregnancy for the treatment of onychomycosis. Women of childbearing potential should use effective contraception during therapy and for 60 days following the last dose.

Ketoconazole (Nizoral): Approved in 1981, ketoconazole is available as tablets for systemic mycoses and as a topical preparation for superficial mycoses. The topical drugs are used to treat dandruff and various tinea infections (see Section 52.6). PO ketoconazole requires an acidic stomach environment for absorption and thus should not be taken concurrently with drugs or foods that decrease stomach acidity. As a systemic drug, it is reserved for invasive mycoses because it is the most hepatotoxic of the azoles. The most common adverse effects are nausea and vomiting, which can affect over 50% of patients taking high doses of the drug.

Ketoconazole carries several black box warnings. In 2013 and in 2016, the FDA issued a safety alert that the oral form of the drug should not be used to treat skin and nail mycoses because ketoconazole has been associated with serious hepatotoxicity that can result in death or the need for liver transplantation. Hepatic function must be monitored regularly during therapy and it should not be used in patients with acute or chronic liver disease. Ketoconazole reduces the amount of corticosteroids secreted by the adrenal glands, which can cause symptoms of adrenal insufficiency. Ketoconazole may interact with other medications to cause serious drug–drug interactions; all drugs taken while undergoing ketoconazole treatment must be monitored for potential interactions. Ketoconazole tablets are only indicated for serious infections, and only when safer antifungals have been proven ineffective. These safety warnings do not apply to the topical forms of the drug.

Posaconazole (Noxafil): Posaconazole is a newer azole, approved in 2013, that has one of the broadest spectrums of activity of any azole. As delayed-release tablets, the drug is approved for prophylaxis of invasive *Aspergillus* and *Candida* infections, which can be life-threatening in patients with severely compromised immune systems. An oral suspension is approved for the treatment of oropharyngeal candidiasis. It is also given by the IV route for invasive infections. Caution must be used when treating patients taking calcineurin inhibitors such as tacrolimus or cyclosporine because posaconazole can increase the serum concentrations of these drugs and cause calcineurin toxicity. Posaconazole should also be used with caution in patients with dysrhythmias because the drug can prolong the QT interval. Its use is contraindicated in patients taking sirolimus, statins, and ergot alkaloids. Common adverse effects include fever, diarrhea, and nausea.

Voriconazole (Vfend): Approved in 2002, voriconazole is a second-generation triazole synthesized from fluconazole that is approved to treat invasive *Aspergillus* infections and serious *Candida* infections. It is believed to be safer and more effective than amphotericin B for these indications. It is available by PO and slow IV infusion. Extreme caution should be used when administering voriconazole to patients with severe renal or hepatic impairment because this can result in toxic accumulation of the drug. The most frequent adverse events affect vision: enhanced brightness, changes in color vision, and blurred vision. Headache, nausea and vomiting, and rash are also common adverse effects. Although visual impairment occurs in 35 to 45% of patients, it is reversible following discontinuation of therapy. Dermatologic toxicity includes photosensitivity and the potential for SJS. Because it participates in many drug interactions, the nurse should seek information from a current drug guide when administering voriconazole concurrently with other medications. Women of childbearing potential should use effective contraception during therapy and for 60 days following the last dose.

CONNECTION Checkpoint 52.2

Antifungal medications are sometimes administered to patients taking calcineurin inhibitors such as tacrolimus. From what you learned in Chapter 42, what is the primary indication for the calcineurin inhibitors?

Drugs for Superficial Fungal Infections

52.6 Drugs for superficial mycoses are safe and effective at eliminating fungi on the skin, nails, or mucous membranes.

Superficial fungal infections of the hair, scalp, nails, and the mucous membranes of the mouth and vagina are rarely medical emergencies. Infections of the nails may be ongoing for months or even years before a patient seeks treatment. Unlike systemic fungal infections, superficial infections may occur in any patient, not just those who have suppressed immune systems. Drugs used to treat superficial mycoses are listed in Table 52.3.

Superficial antifungal drugs are much safer than their systemic counterparts because penetration into the deeper layers of the skin is limited, and only small amounts are absorbed into the circulation. Many are available as over-the-counter (OTC) creams, gels, and ointments. If the infection has spread into the deeper skin layers, PO antifungal drugs are indicated. Extensive superficial or subcutaneous mycoses are sometimes treated with both PO and topical antifungal drugs to ensure that the infection is eliminated from deeper skin layers.

Dermatophytosis: Fungal infection of the skin and hair is called **dermatophytosis**. These infections are named by their Latin terms, beginning with *tinea*. For example, tinea capitis is an infection of the scalp, and tinea pedis is an infection of the feet.

Fungi that cause dermatophytosis grow in the keratin layer of the skin. Because fungi multiply more rapidly in warm, moist areas, dermatophytosis occurs more frequently during the summer months and in warmer climates. It tends to favor skin creases that stay moist due to sweat or following bathing. Because relapse rates following pharmacotherapy are high, the patient should be taught proper personal hygiene measures to help eliminate the pathogen. These include frequent bathing with thorough drying of the infected area, the use of separate towels for the groin area, and wearing loose clothing.

Tinea corporis is an infection in which the fungus invades relatively hairless skin. The fungus typically appears as a ring pattern, thus resulting in the name *ringworm*. Transmission may occur through direct contact with infected animals (especially cats and dogs), infected humans, or contaminated furniture or clothing. The most common pathogens are *Trichophyton* and *Microsporum* species. Topical therapies are usually successful in controlling tinea corporis. In cases of inflammatory lesions, oral therapy with griseofulvin (Gris-PEG), terbinafine (Lamisil), itraconazole (Sporanox), or fluconazole (Diflucan) is recommended.

Tinea cruris, commonly called *jock itch*, is a form of tinea corporis that occurs in the groin, perineum, and perianal

Table 52.3 Selected Drugs for Superficial Mycoses

Drug	Route and Adult Dose (Maximum Dose Where Indicated)	Adverse Effects
butenafine (Mentax)	Topical: Apply daily for 2–4 wk for tineas	*Drying of skin, stinging sensation at application site, pruritus, urticaria, contact dermatitis* Granulocytopenia (griseofulvin), cholestatic hepatitis (oral terbinafine), neutropenia (oral terbinafine)
ciclopirox cream, gel, shampoo (Loprox), or nail lacquer (Penlac)	Topical: Apply cream bid for 4 wk for tineas Topical: Apply lacquer to nail for 48 wk for onychomycosis	
griseofulvin (Gris-PEG)	PO: 330–375 mg ultramicrosize daily for tineas and onychomycosis	
naftifine (Naftin)	Topical: Apply cream daily or gel bid for 4 wk for tineas	
nystatin topical powder (Nystop); oral suspension, capsule; cream or ointment	Suspension PO: 400,000–600,000 units 4 times/day Topical: Apply bid–tid to the affected area Capsule: PO: 500,000 to 1 million units q6h Vaginal tablets: Insert 1 tablet daily for 2 wk	
tavaborole (Kerydin)	Topical: Apply 5% solution once daily for 48 wk	
terbinafine (Lamisil)	Topical: Apply once daily or bid for 7 wk for tineas PO: 250 mg/day for 6–12 wk for onychomycosis	
undecylenic acid (Fungi-Nail, Gordochom, others)	Topical: Apply once daily or bid for tineas for up to 4 wk	
Azoles		
butoconazole (Gynazole)	Intravaginal: 1 applicator as a single dose	*Drying of the skin, stinging sensation at application site, pruritus, urticaria, contact dermatitis* Topical drugs exhibit few serious adverse effects except hypersensitivity
clotrimazole topical cream; intravaginal; troche	Topical: Apply 1% cream bid for 4 wk Intravaginal: 1 applicator for 7 days; one 100-mg tablet vaginally for 7 days or one 500-mg tablet once Troche: Dissolve one in the mouth over 15–30 min	
econazole (Ecoza, Spectazole)	Topical: Apply 1% cream bid for 4 wk for tineas or cutaneous candidiasis	
efinaconazole (Jublia)	Topical: Apply 10% solution to affected nails once daily for 48 wk	
fluconazole (Diflucan)	PO: 150 mg once, for vulvovaginal candidiasis (VVC)	
itraconazole (Sporanox)	PO: 200 mg daily for 1–2 wk for OPC PO: 200 mg daily for 3 days for VVC PO: 200 mg daily for 3 months for onychomycosis	
ketoconazole (Nizoral)	Topical: Apply 2% cream or shampoo 1–2 times/day to affected area for tineas	
luliconazole (Luzu)	Topical: Apply 1% cream once daily for 2 wk for tineas	
miconazole (Monistat-3, Oravig, Vusion)	Topical: Apply 2% cream bid for 2–4 wk Intravaginal (Monistat-3): Insert 1 suppository daily for 3 days for VVC Buccal (Oravig): Apply 1 tablet to the gum region daily for 2 wk for oral candidiasis	
oxiconazole (Oxistat)	Topical: Apply 1% cream daily for 2 months for tineas and cutaneous candidiasis	
sulconazole (Exelderm)	Topical: Apply 1% cream once daily or bid for 2–6 wk for tineas	
terconazole (Terazol)	Intravaginal: 1 applicator for 3–7 days for VVC	
tioconazole (Vagistat-1)	Intravaginal: 1 applicator as a single dose	

Note: *Italics* indicate common adverse effects. Underline indicates serious adverse effects.

region. Topical powders and creams are usually sufficient to cure tinea cruris. PO antifungal drugs such as griseofulvin, terbinafine, itraconazole, or fluconazole may be necessary for severe cases.

Tinea pedis, commonly called *athlete's foot*, is a type of tinea corporis occurring on the feet, principally between the toes and on the sole. It is associated with the wearing of shoes and contact with infected bath or pool floors. Tinea pedis is the most common dermatomycosis, affecting about 70% of adults at some time during their life. Topical antifungals are effective for noninflammatory tinea pedis. PO therapy is sometimes used to treat more severe infections and areas such as the soles. Typical therapy includes terbinafine (Lamisil) or itraconazole (Sporanox) for 2 to 4 weeks.

Tinea capitis involves the hair of the head, eyebrows, or eyelashes and primarily affects children between 4 and 14 years of age. *Trichophyton* is responsible for more than 90% of cases. In contrast with other dermatophytosis, tinea capitis is routinely treated with PO drugs. Typical regimens include the following:

- Griseofulvin: 10 mg/kg/day for 8 to 10 weeks
- Itraconazole: 5 mg/kg/day for 1 to 4 weeks
- Terbinafine: 62.5 to 250 mg/day for 4 weeks.

Onychomycosis: **Onychomycosis**, or *tinea unguium*, is the invasion of the nail plate by a fungus. It is a common infection, affecting 2 to 3% of Americans. Rates among men are twice that of women, and infections increase with age. The higher incidence in older patients is believed to be due to reduced peripheral circulation, general inactivity, increased nail trauma, and difficulty (or inability) in maintaining proper nail hygiene. One in four patients with diabetes will acquire onychomycosis, likely due to reduced circulation to the area.

The most common fungal pathogens responsible for onychomycosis are *Trichophyton* and *Epidermophyton* species. Although any part of the nail may be affected, most commonly the infection begins with invasion of the hyponychium, the place where the nail separates from the nail bed. Toenails are more often affected than fingernails. The nail becomes markedly disfigured and distorted.

Although certainly not a life-threatening infection, onychomycosis is one of the most difficult superficial fungal infections to treat. Nails grow slowly and the nail plate is hard, preventing antifungal drugs from penetrating. The traditional medication for onychomycosis has been griseofulvin, but this drug has a narrow spectrum of activity and has been largely replaced by newer therapies. The preferred therapies include terbinafine (Lamisil) and itraconazole (Sporanox). Both of these drugs are absorbed into the nail matrix and remain active for several months. These oral therapies have shorter treatment regimens and higher cure rates than the topical drugs. Terbinafine is administered once daily for 6 to 12 weeks. Itraconazole is taken twice daily for 1 week for fingernails or 12 weeks for toenails.

Topical drugs may be indicated if less than half the nail plate is infected or if the patient is unable to tolerate the oral therapies. Topical and oral medications may be administered concurrently for persistent infections. The preferred topical medications include efinaconazole (Jublia), ciclopirox nail lacquer (Penlac), and tavaborole (Kerydin). These three topical drugs are applied daily for 48 weeks.

PharmFACT

The overall incidence of onychomycosis is highly age dependent. The incidence is 90% in older adults and less than 3% in those under age 18 (Tosti, 2018).

Superficial candidiasis: Although at least 10 species of *Candida* cause disease in humans, *C. albicans* is responsible for nearly 100% of cases of oropharyngeal fungal infections and at least 90% of cases of vulvovaginal candidiasis. A small yeast, *Candida* is often found as part of normal host flora on body surfaces. *Candida* species are the most common pathogens causing fungal disease in patients with compromised immune defenses.

Oropharyngeal candidiasis (OPC) is an oral mycosis, sometimes called *thrush*. About 50% of people carry *Candida* in the mouth as part of their host flora. Infection occurs when the patient's immune defenses are weakened; thus, the highest incidence of OPC is seen in patients with HIV infection, diabetes, or cancer and in hospitalized patients. Patients taking inhaled corticosteroids are also at greater risk because these drugs cause a local immunosuppression in the oral cavity. Although not life-threatening, OPC may predispose a patient to esophageal candidiasis, which is a serious, invasive mycosis.

Several options are available for the pharmacotherapy of OPC. Topical therapy is generally preferred and is often successful for milder, uncomplicated infections. Troches and PO suspensions are the most common formulations for topical therapy. Symptoms generally subside in 2 to 3 days, but the nurse should encourage the patient to complete the full 1- to 2-week course of therapy. Preferred treatments for mild OPC include miconazole buccal tablet (Oravig), nystatin PO suspension, or clotrimazole troche. Moderate to severe OPC is generally treated with oral fluconazole (Diflucan). Alternatives include suspensions of itraconazole (Sporanox) or posaconazole.

Candida species are part of the normal vaginal flora in about 50% of healthy women. Because vulvovaginal candidiasis (VVC) occurs in both healthy and immunosuppressed women, it is not considered an opportunistic infection. The biggest risk factors for VVC are sexual activity, pregnancy, diabetes mellitus, the use of oral contraceptives with high

CONNECTIONS: Lifespan Considerations

Oropharyngeal Candidiasis in Infants

Oropharyngeal candidiasis (OPC or thrush) is commonly seen in infants. It is often difficult to distinguish from milk and appears as white patches on the tongue, palate, and inner aspects of the cheeks. Frequently, the infant with thrush may refuse to suck or feed because of mouth irritation. Transmission of this fungal infection may occur during a vaginal birth when the infant comes in contact with the mother's normal flora, or during feedings, including breastfeeding. In most cases, thrush is self-limiting and resolves spontaneously. However, it may take as long as 2 months to resolve, during which time it may spread to the larynx, trachea, bronchi, lungs, and GI tract.

The condition is treated with good hygiene, application of a fungicide, and correction of any underlying causes. Because the mother is often the source of the infection, she should also be treated to prevent reinfections. Fluconazole (Diflucan) and nystatin are commonly used, including for topical treatment of the nipple area of the mother if the thrush continues.

Antifungal medications should be administered to the infant after feedings. When possible, sips of water may be useful to rinse away milk sugars and proteins after the feeding. Using an applicator or syringe, the medication should be distributed over the entire surface of the oral mucosa and tongue. After swabbing the area, the remainder of the dose is then deposited in the infant's mouth to be swallowed to treat any more extensive infection.

estrogen content, and broad-spectrum antibiotics. *Candida* may be transmitted to male sexual partners. Its highest incidence occurs between the ages of 30 and 40. *C. albicans* is by far the most common species, although *Candida glabrata* is an emerging pathogen for VVC.

Several effective topical drugs for VVC are available without a prescription. The various topical regimens have equal effectiveness in treating VVC, with response rates of 80 to 90%. Many women prefer PO therapies because of their convenience. Oral therapy has the same efficacy as topical treatment.

Regimens for VVC are classified by their duration of therapy. The most popular therapies are 1-day PO regimens, due to their ease of use. Although 1-day treatments are effective for most women with VVC, this brief therapy has limitations. Because 1-day treatments may take up to 48 hours to produce relief, faster-acting topical drugs may be more beneficial for patients with severe symptoms. In addition, patients with complicated, persistent, or severe infections require 10 to 14 days of therapy for successful elimination of the pathogen, regardless of the route of administration. Typical therapies for VVC include the following:

- Single topical application: ticonazole 6.5% ointment; butoconazole 2% cream (sustained release formulation); miconazole 2% cream
- Single PO dose: fluconazole, one 150-mg tablet; itraconazole, 200 mg bid for 1 day; clotrimazole, one 500-mg tablet for 1 day
- Multiday regimens: clotrimazole, 1% cream or 100-mg tablets for 1 to 7 days; miconazole, 2% cream or 100- to 200-mg suppositories for 1 to 7 days; or nystatin, 100,000-unit vaginal tablet daily for 7 to 14 days

Because recurrent VVC may occur in 5% of patients treated for this infection, cultures may be necessary to identify the specific pathogen. Treatment begins with a 14-day induction phase that uses the same drugs as for nonrecurring infections. A maintenance phase follows, typically with azole antifungals taken once weekly (fluconazole) or once monthly (itraconazole) for 6 months.

PharmFACT

Three of every four women will experience vulvovaginal candidiasis at least once during their lifetime (Hidalgo, 2020).

CONNECTION Checkpoint 52.3

From what you learned in Chapter 46, why might broad-spectrum antibacterial therapy cause a *Candida* infection of the vagina?

PROTOTYPE DRUG **Nystatin (Nystop)**

Classification **Therapeutic:** Antifungal, superficial type
Pharmacologic: Polyene

Therapeutic Effects and Uses: Approved in 1954, nystatin belongs to the same chemical class as amphotericin B, the polyenes. Although it acts by the same mechanism as the polyenes, nystatin has very different indications and is available in a wider variety of formulations, including cream, ointment, powder, tablets, capsules, and oral suspension. Too toxic for parenteral administration, it is usually used topically to treat *Candida* infections of the vagina, skin, and mouth because it is not absorbed in these areas. Although available as vaginal tablets, the azoles have largely replaced nystatin due to their higher efficacy. PO suspensions are available to treat OPC, using a swish-and-swallow technique. It is available as tablets to treat candidiasis of the intestine, since it travels through the GI tract without being absorbed. It is not effective for treating onychomycosis. Mykacet is a topical cream containing nystatin and triamcinolone.

Mechanism of Action: Nystatin binds to sterols in the fungal cell membrane, allowing leakage of intracellular contents across the weakened membrane.

Pharmacokinetics:

Route(s)	PO suspension, capsules, troches, topical creams, and vaginal tablets; PO tablets for intestinal infections
Absorption	Poorly absorbed
Distribution	Not distributed
Primary metabolism	Not metabolized
Primary excretion	Excreted unchanged in the feces
Onset of action	Rapid
Duration of action	Half-life: 6–12 h

Adverse Effects: When given topically, nystatin produces few adverse effects other than minor skin irritation and burning at the site of application. There is a high incidence of contact dermatitis, related to the preservatives found in some of the formulations. When given PO, it may cause diarrhea, and nausea and vomiting.

Contraindications/Precautions: The only contraindication to nystatin therapy is hypersensitivity to the drug.

Drug Interactions: Unknown.

Pregnancy: Animal reproduction studies have not been conducted on this drug, and it is not known if it has any adverse effects on lactation.

Treatment of Overdose: No specific therapy is available; patients are treated symptomatically.

Clinician Responsibilities: Key clinical implications for patients receiving nystatin are included in Applied Clinical Judgment: Patients Receiving Pharmacotherapy with Antifungals.

Drugs Similar to Nystatin (Nystop)

Other superficial antifungals include griseofulvin, terbinafine, topical azoles, and several miscellaneous drugs. In general, topical antifungals are safe to use during pregnancy and lactation because very little is absorbed systemically. However, this is not always the case and women should always check with their practitioner prior to taking any antifungal medication during pregnancy.

Griseofulvin (Gris-PEG): Approved in 1959, griseofulvin is an inexpensive antifungal that is indicated for the PO therapy of mycoses of the hair, skin, and nails that have not responded to conventional topical preparations. It is not given topically because the drug is unable to penetrate into the deeper skin layers when given by this route. In an attempt to reduce adverse GI effects and increase its bioavailability, griseofulvin is available as ultramicrosize particles (Gris-PEG) that are almost 100% absorbed.

The length of treatment for tinea pedis is 4 to 8 weeks and for tinea unguium, 3 to 6 months. Griseofulvin is deposited in keratin, where it accumulates and inhibits mitosis of the fungal cells. It exhibits few adverse effects, other than headache. Although rare, hepatitis and neutropenia have been reported with prolonged therapy. Griseofulvin has a higher incidence of long-term adverse effects and has a greater relapse rate than some other superficial antifungal drugs. Animal studies showed that griseofulvin causes embryotoxicity and teratogenicity. Because this medication is secreted in animal milk and may cause potential adverse effects in the neonate, breastfeeding is not recommended. Women with childbearing potential are advised to use contraception during therapy and for 30 days following the last dose.

Terbinafine (Lamisil): Approved in 1993, terbinafine may be administered by the PO or topical route. Terbinafine belongs to a chemical class called allylamines that act by inhibiting ergosterol biosynthesis. The PO form of the drug is available by prescription to treat onychomycosis. The drug rapidly accumulates in nails, although therapy of persistent onychomycosis may require 6 to 12 weeks. The cure rate for onychomycosis is 50 to 70%, which is higher than that for griseofulvin. Oral preparations are well tolerated, with nausea and vomiting, abdominal pain, and diarrhea being the most common adverse effects. Rare, though serious, adverse effects include SJS, blood dyscrasias, and hepatic failure.

Nonprescription formulations such as Lamisil AT include topical creams and sprays for treating tinea corporis, tinea pedis, and tinea cruris. Adverse effects are rare with topical terbinafine; irritation or urticaria occurs in less than 1% of patients. The drug is not absorbed when administered topically. Animal studies did not show evidence of fetal harm.

Topical azoles: Eleven azoles are used to treat superficial mycoses. Itraconazole, voriconazole, posaconazole, and fluconazole may be used PO to treat superficial mycoses, whereas the others are for topical use only. Among the topical drugs, all have equal effectiveness and similar adverse effects. Miconazole and clotrimazole are preferred drugs available OTC for vulvovaginal *Candida* infections, although a number of other azoles are available that are equally effective. Transient burning and irritation at the application sites are the most common adverse effects of the topical azoles.

Miscellaneous topical antifungals: Several drugs are less commonly used for superficial fungal infections. These medications are applied topically, for tineas, or intravaginally, for VVC. The doses and indications for these drugs are shown in Table 52.3.

CONNECTIONS: APPLIED CLINICAL JUDGMENT

Patients Receiving Pharmacotherapy with Antifungals

Key Assessment Data

- History of current condition, baseline vital signs, physical exam findings; hepatic, renal, cardiovascular, neurologic, respiratory disease; pregnancy or breastfeeding. Obtain a drug history and assess signs and symptoms of the current infection, noting symptoms, duration, or any recent changes.
- Ongoing assessment during drug therapy should include monitoring appropriate laboratory findings (e.g., complete blood count, hepatic and renal laboratory values).

Desired Therapeutic Outcomes

Improvement is observed and measurable by diminished fever, other signs and symptoms of infection, surface lesions are improving or cleared.

Minimizing Adverse Effects

- Hypotension, tachycardia, dysrhythmias, cardiac collapse, and cardiac arrest are possible adverse effects of antifungal drugs given IV. Frequent monitoring may be needed when drug is given IV.
- IV antifungal medication is irritating to the vein and the IV site should be monitored frequently.
- Azole antifungals may increase glucose levels. Patients with diabetes may require a change in their antidiabetic drug routine.
- Antifungals given systemically may cause ototoxicity and require frequent monitoring to prevent hearing loss.

Lifespan Considerations

- Age-related physiologic changes may affect the drug's metabolism or excretion in older adults.
- Older adults may be at increased risk for dizziness related to adverse drug effects, which may increase the risk for falls. Ensure patient safety.

Diversity Considerations

- Fluconazole given systemically metabolizes through the CYP450 system pathway and requires more frequent monitoring in ethnically diverse patients to ensure optimal therapeutic effects and to minimize adverse effects.

Patient Education

- Oral antifungals may require several months of treatment. Complete the entire course of therapy and return to the provider if symptoms have not resolved.
- Rise from lying to sitting or standing slowly to avoid dizziness or falls if hypotension is noted. If dizziness occurs, sit or lie down and do not attempt to stand or walk until the sensation passes.
- Promptly report any chills, nausea, tremors, palpitations, or headache. Immediately report any itching, rashes, swelling (particularly of tongue or face), urticaria, flushing, dizziness, syncope, wheezing, throat tightness, or difficulty breathing.
- Increase overall fluid intake. Report weight gain of more than 1 kg (2 lb) in a 24-hour period.
- Report any nausea and vomiting; yellowing of the skin or sclera; abdominal pain; light or clay-colored stools; diminished urine output; darkening of urine; ringing, humming, or buzzing in the ears; dizziness; or vertigo.
- Patients with diabetes should test their glucose levels more frequently, reporting any consistent elevations to the healthcare provider.
- Appropriate self-administration of antifungal drugs includes:
  - Complete the entire course of therapy unless otherwise instructed. The duration of the required therapy may be quite lengthy. Do not stop taking the medicine when starting to feel better.
  - Eliminate alcohol while on these medications.
  - Take the drug with food or milk but avoid acidic or carbonated beverages.
  - Dissolve oral antifungal lozenges (troches) in the mouth, or rinse with liquids after meals and at bedtime. If dentures are worn, remove them before using the drug and leave them out overnight. Swish the liquid drug around the mouth and hold in the mouth at least 2 minutes before expectorating. Do not swallow unless instructed to do so by the provider and do not rinse the mouth with water afterward.
  - Apply a thin, even layer of topical antifungals to the affected area. Do not use occlusive dressings.

Prescribing Considerations

- Some antifungals may be hepatotoxic and nephrotoxic. Antifungals, particularly when given IV, may cause electrolyte imbalances, especially hypokalemia and hypomagnesemia, and electrolyte replacement may be needed. Adequate hydration is necessary to prevent adverse renal effects, and monitor electrolytes while on IV therapy.
- Anaphylactic reactions are possible and most common with the first dose given by IV infusion. A test dose of a small amount given slowly may be given before the main infusion. Premedication, including antipyretics, antihistamines, corticosteroids, and antiemetics, may be required to prevent reactions.
- Itraconazole is noted to have a negative inotropic effect and should not be administered in patients with congestive heart failure.

Understanding Chapter 52

Key Concepts Summary

52.1 Serious fungal infections are uncommon in people with healthy immune defenses.

52.2 Mycoses are classified as superficial, subcutaneous, or systemic.

52.3 Antifungal drugs act by disrupting the fungal cell membrane or wall, affecting fungal enzymes, or disrupting replication.

52.4 Systemic or invasive fungal disease may require intensive pharmacotherapy for extended periods.

52.5 Azoles are the preferred drugs for many mycoses due to their efficacy and favorable safety profile.

52.6 Drugs for superficial mycoses are safe and effective at eliminating fungi on the skin, nails, or mucous membranes.

CASE STUDY: Making the Patient Connection

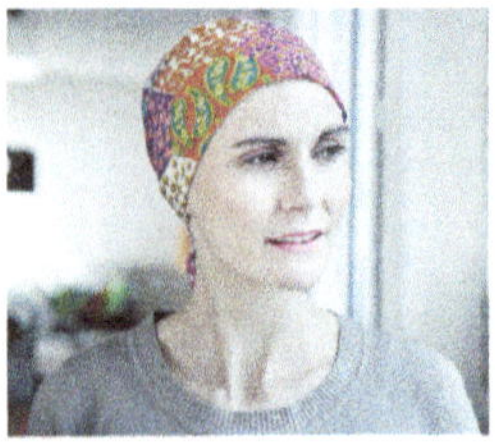

Remember the patient "Sarah Williams" at the beginning of the chapter? Now read the remainder of the case study. Based on the information presented within this chapter, respond to the critical thinking questions that follow.

Sarah Williams is a 54-year-old woman with lung cancer who recently finished her second round of chemotherapy. She comes to her appointment at the oncology clinic with concerns about white patches on her tongue and mouth. She states that her mouth is not sore, but her throat burns when she swallows. This has made it very difficult for her to eat and drink.

A history and physical examination are completed. She is 5′3′′ tall and weighs 52.7 kg (116 lb). The healthcare provider evaluates Sarah for oropharyngeal candidiasis. Sarah was diagnosed with lung cancer several months prior and is taking chemotherapy and corticosteroids. Upon initial assessment, her vital signs are normal, and she has no complaints except her expressed concerns about her mouth and throat. She has worn dentures for about 5 years.

Critical Thinking Questions

1. What are the signs and symptoms that you, as the nurse, look for to determine if Sarah is experiencing oropharyngeal candidiasis?
2. Why do you think that Sarah is at risk for this type of infection?
3. What treatment do you anticipate that Sarah will receive? What patient teaching will she need regarding this treatment?

Additional Case Study

Sean Seales is a 23-year-old patient with Hodgkin's lymphoma who is undergoing chemotherapy. He has experienced chills and fever with increasing fatigue for the past several days. Sean was assessed by his oncologist and was hospitalized for possible early sepsis. He is neutropenic and will be started on IV antibiotics and fluconazole (Diflucan) IV.

1. Why was Sean started on both IV antibiotics and antifungal medication?
2. What possible adverse effects might Sean experience from the fluconazole (Diflucan)? As his nurse, what will you monitor?

Chapter Review

1. A patient is admitted to the intensive care unit for systemic fungal infections. Amphotericin B has been ordered and the nurse will administer this drug slowly IV. When administered too rapidly, amphotericin B may cause what significant adverse effects? (Select all that apply.)

1. Laryngeal spasms
2. Hypotension
3. Hypokalemia
4. Shock
5. Hypoglycemia

2. A patient with AIDS has been given a prescription for oral fluconazole (Diflucan) to prevent *Candida* infection. Considering the patient's primary diagnosis and the order for fluconazole, what essential teaching will the nurse provide?

1. Keep a food diary and request antinausea medication if eating becomes problematic.
2. Maintain regular low-impact exercise daily to avoid loss of muscle mass.
3. Wear a high-filtration mask if going out in public.
4. Avoid all fat-based soaps and allow the body to air-dry after bathing.

3. Nystatin suspension has been ordered for treatment of thrush (oropharyngeal *Candida*) in a 6-week-old infant. What instructions should the caregiver receive? (Select all that apply.)

1. Give the infant a small amount of water after feedings and before the drug to rinse the mouth.
2. Using an applicator or syringe, distribute the solution around the mouth and tongue, allowing the infant to swallow the remainder.
3. Chill the suspension in the refrigerator before giving for better taste.
4. Give the suspension before feeding the infant to prevent adverse GI effects.
5. Add the suspension to a bottle of formula for easier administration.

4. The nurse is caring for a patient with onychomycosis who is receiving oral terbinafine (Lamisil) for treatment. The patient questions the need for 3 months' worth of pills. What is the nurse's best response?
   1. "The healthcare provider will evaluate the nails monthly and stop treatment earlier if warranted."
   2. "It is cheaper to buy more pills at one time than on a monthly schedule."
   3. "The extensive prescription avoids the need for shorter term, potentially toxic doses."
   4. "Nails grow slowly and the nail beds must receive adequate length of treatment to eliminate the infection."
5. The nurse knows that pretreatment with corticosteroids, antihistamines, and antipyretics prior to the administration of amphotericin B is given for what effect?
   1. To enhance the effectiveness of amphotericin B
   2. To eliminate toxic by-products of amphotericin B
   3. To reduce the severity of adverse effects associated with amphotericin B
   4. To increase the half-life of amphotericin B
6. A patient with diabetes treated with oral antidiabetic medications is receiving oral fluconazole (Diflucan) for treatment of long-standing tinea cruris (jock itch). The nurse will instruct the patient to monitor blood sugar more frequently while on this drug because of what potential drug effects?
   1. Fluconazole antagonizes the effects of antidiabetic drugs.
   2. Fluconazole may increase blood sugar levels.
   3. Fluconazole may decrease blood sugar levels.
   4. Fluconazole may enhance the effects of antidiabetic drugs.

See Appendix A for answers to critical thinking questions, case study questions, and review questions.

References

Centers for Disease Control and Prevention (CDC). (2019). *Aspergillosis risk & prevention*. https://www.cdc.gov/fungal/diseases/aspergillosis/risk-prevention.html

Centers for Disease Control and Prevention (CDC). (2020). *Medications that weaken your immune system and fungal infections*. https://www.cdc.gov/fungal/infections/immune-system.html

Hidalgo, J. A. (2020). *Candidiasis*. Medscape. http://emedicine.medscape.com/article/213853-overview

Jara, P. (2017). Relation of indoor and outdoor airborne fungal spore levels in the Kansas City metropolitan area. *Allergy and Asthma Proceedings*, *38*(2), 130–135. https://doi.org/10.2500/aap.2017.38.4030

Tham, K. (2017). The role of outdoor fungi on asthma hospital admissions in children and adolescents: A 5-year time stratified case-crossover analysis. *Environmental Research*, *154*, 42–49. https://doi.org/10.1016/j.envres.2016.12.016

Tosti, A. (2020). *Onychomycosis*. Medscape. http://emedicine.medscape.com/article/1105828-overview

Selected Bibliography

Berman, J., & Krysan, D. J. (2020). Drug resistance and tolerance in fungi. *Nature Reviews Microbiology*, *18*, 319–331. https://doi.org/10.1038/s41579-019-0322-2

Flowers, R. H. (2020). *Cutaneous candidiasis*. Medscape. https://emedicine.medscape.com/article/1090632-overview

Gupta, A. K., Stec, N., Summerbell, R. C., Shear, N. H., Piguet, V., Tosti, A., & Maria Piraccini, B. (2020). Onychomycosis: A review. *Journal of the European Academy of Dermatology and Venereology*, *34*(9), 1972–1990. https://doi.org/10.1111/jdv.16394

Jenks, J. D., & Hoenigl, M. (2018). Treatment of aspergillosis. *Journal of Fungi*, *4*(3), 98. https://doi.org/10.3390/jof4030098

Nicola, A. M., Albuquerque, P., Paes, H. C., Fernandes, L., Costa, F. F., Kioshima, E. S., et al. (2019). Antifungal drugs: New insights in research and development. *Pharmacology & Therapeutics*, *195*, 21–38.

Pappas, P. G., Lionakis, M. S., Arendrup, M. C., Ostrosky-Zeichner, L., & Kullberg, B. J. (2018). Invasive candidiasis. *Nature Reviews Disease Primers*, *4*, 18026. https://doi.org/10.1038/nrdp.2018.26

Robbins, N., Wright, G. D., & Cowen, L. E. (2017). Antifungal drugs: The current armamentarium and development of new agents. In J. Heitman, B. J. Howlett, P. W. Crous, E. H. Stukenbrock, T. Y. James, & N. A. R. Gow (Eds.), *The fungal kingdom* (pp. 903–922). ASM Press.

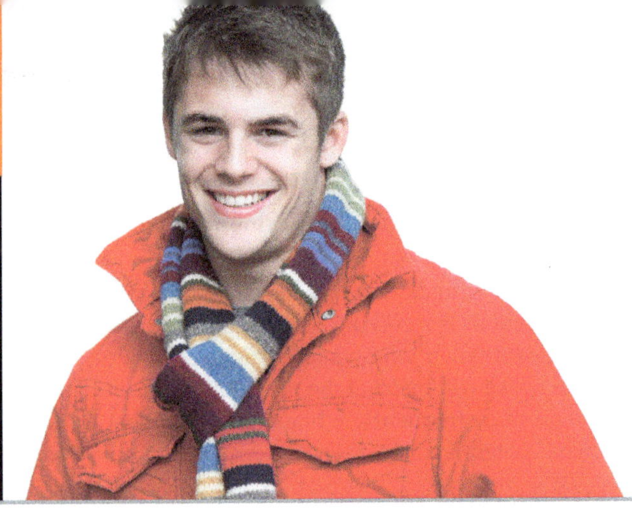

"Sure, I've thought about the possibility I may catch something on this trip to Brazil. But it's the chance of a lifetime!"

—Patient "Trevor Skales"

Chapter 53
Pharmacotherapy of Protozoan and Helminthic Infections

Chapter Outline

Learning Outcomes

After reading this chapter, the student should be able to:

1. Identify features of protozoa and helminths that distinguish them from bacteria.
2. Identify protozoan and helminthic infections that may benefit from pharmacotherapy.
3. Explain why an understanding of *Plasmodium*'s lifecycle is important to the successful pharmacotherapy of malaria.
4. Explain the etiology, pathogenesis, and pharmacotherapy of amebiasis, giardiasis, cryptosporidiosis, toxoplasmosis, trichomoniasis, trypanosomiasis, and leishmaniasis.
5. Explain the etiology, pathogenesis, and pharmacotherapy of ascariasis, enterobiasis, hookworm, and tapeworm infections.
6. Describe the nurse's role in the pharmacologic management of protozoan and helminthic infections.
7. For each of the classes shown in the chapter outline, identify the prototype and representative drugs and explain the mechanism(s) of drug action, primary indications, contraindications, significant drug interactions, pregnancy data, and important adverse effects.
8. Apply clinical judgment to care for patients receiving pharmacotherapy for protozoan and helminthic infections.

Key Terms

Definitions of the terms in bold may be found in the Glossary.

Protozoa and parasitic worms, or helminths, are more complex than bacteria and cause significant morbidity and mortality worldwide. Pharmacotherapy is complicated by the lifecycles of the organisms, during which they may change form and travel to infect distant organs. Some may remain infectious in contaminated soil or water for months or years. With few exceptions, the anti-infective drugs used to treat these disorders are different from those for bacterial or fungal infections.

Classification and Pathogenesis of Protozoan Infections

53.1 Protozoa are diverse, single-celled organisms that can cause widespread disease.

A **protozoan** is a single-celled organism that inhabits water, soil, and animal hosts. Although only a few of the more than 20,000 species are pathogenic in humans, they cause significant morbidity and mortality in Africa, South America, Central America, and Asia. These parasites thrive in conditions where sanitation and personal hygiene are poor and population density is high. The nurse needs to be familiar with these infections because travelers may acquire protozoan diseases overseas and bring them back to the United States and Canada. In addition, some of the protozoan infections frequently occur in patients with immunosuppression, such as those in the advanced stages of acquired immunodeficiency syndrome (AIDS) or those receiving chemotherapy or immunosuppressants. Selected protozoan infections important to human health are listed in Table 53.1.

Protozoa are an extremely diverse group of organisms, with each class having very different physiologies and survival strategies. Drugs that are effective against one species of protozoan are often not effective against others.

Some pathogenic protozoa have complex lifecycles. The active, growing stage during which the organism feeds, often at the expense of its host, is the **trophozoite** stage. When faced with adverse conditions, some protozoa can form protective capsules called **cysts** that allow the organism to survive in harsh environments in a dormant state for prolonged time periods. Both trophozoite and cyst forms may reside within the human body simultaneously; however, some protozoa enter the cyst stage after they exit the human body through coughing, sneezing, or fecal excretion. Protozoa remain in the cyst form until the organism is able to reinfect another host. When cysts occur inside the host, the parasite is often resistant to drug therapy.

Several of the major protozoan infections are spread by **vectors**, organisms that harbor the pathogen and carry it from one host to another. Some vectors, such as house flies, simply pick up pathogens on their feet and transport them to human food or water. In other cases, the protozoan lives and multiplies inside the insect, which serves as an

Table 53.1 Selected Protozoan Infections

Name of Disease and Protozoan Species	Description	Source of Infection
Amebiasis *Entamoeba histolytica*	Primarily infects the large intestine, causing severe diarrhea; commonly travels to the liver to form liver abscesses; rarely travels to other organs such as the brain, lungs, or kidney	Fecal-contaminated water
Cryptosporidiosis *Cryptosporidium parvum*	Infects the intestines, causing diarrhea; often seen in immunocompromised patients	Fecal-contaminated water; humans and other animals
Giardiasis *Giardia lamblia*	Infects the intestines, causing malabsorption, fatigue, and abdominal pain	Fecal-contaminated water
Leishmaniasis *Leishmania* (various species)	Affects many body systems including the skin, liver, spleen, or blood depending on the species	Bite of sand fly
Malaria *Plasmodium* (various species)	Infects red blood cells (RBCs) to cause fever, chills, and fatigue; some *Plasmodia* invade the liver and other tissues	Bite of female *Anopheles* mosquito
Toxoplasmosis *Toxoplasma gondii*	Can invade any organ; causes a fatal encephalitis in immunocompromised patients	Congenital transmission; cat feces
Trichomoniasis *Trichomonas vaginalis*	Common sexually transmitted infection (STI) that causes vaginitis in women and urethritis in men	Transmission through sexual contact with infected fluids
Trypanosomiasis *Trypanosoma brucei* (African) *Trypanosoma cruzi* (American)	The American form (Chagas' disease) invades cardiac tissue and autonomic ganglia; the African form (sleeping sickness) causes fatigue and central nervous system (CNS) depression	Bite of the kissing bug (American) or the tsetse fly (African)

intermediate host. The protozoan *Plasmodium*, for example, reproduces in the gut of a mosquito and is transmitted to humans during a mosquito bite, causing malaria. The discovery that mites, ticks, or insects could spread infections was a major advance in medicine because researchers then realized that disease outbreaks could be prevented or controlled by eliminating the vectors.

53.2 The female *Anopheles* mosquito is the carrier of several species of *Plasmodium*, the parasite responsible for malaria.

Although rare in the United States and Canada, about 218 million cases of malaria occur annually worldwide. Although malaria was declared eliminated in the United States in the early 1950s, approximately 1500 to 2000 cases are diagnosed each year. Almost all cases occur in infected immigrants or travelers who bring the disease into the United States from regions where the disease is endemic.

PharmFACT

In 2018 the estimated number of malaria deaths worldwide was 405,000. Children under age 5 accounted for 67% of these deaths (World Health Organization, 2020).

Malaria is caused by five species of the protozoan *Plasmodium*. Each species has a characteristic geographical distribution and pattern of infection, although several species may coexist in the same location. *Plasmodium vivax*, the most common malarial species, occurs predominantly in India, Pakistan, and Central America. *Plasmodium falciparum* occurs with greater incidence in Africa, South America, Haiti, and the Dominican Republic. Although less common, *P. falciparum* causes the most severe symptoms, including a significant number of deaths in endemic areas, and is often more resistant to antimalarial drugs than the other *Plasmodium* species. The other three species, *Plasmodium malariae, Plasmodium knowlesi*, and *Plasmodium ovale*, are less common, and current medical sources should be consulted for information on these species.

The carrier of *Plasmodium* is a mosquito. *Plasmodium* resides in the gut of the female *Anopheles* mosquito where it matures to its infective form, called a **sporozoite**. When the mosquito bites a human, some of the sporozoites, contained in mosquito saliva, are injected.

Once inside the human host, the blood carries the sporozoites to the liver, where they multiply and transform into millions of progeny called **merozoites**. There is an incubation period of 1 to 6 weeks following the mosquito bite, during which the patient experiences no ill effects.

After the incubation period, merozoites are released into the blood, where they enter RBCs and multiply. The infected erythrocytes eventually rupture, releasing more merozoites and causing acute symptoms. This is the **erythrocytic stage** of the infection. The bite of another *Anopheles* mosquito can pick up the merozoites from infected human blood, and the cycle begins anew. *P. vivax* can remain in body tissues for extended periods and cause relapses months, or even years, after the initial infection. Unlike the human host, which can experience severe illness, the mosquito is unaffected by the presence of *Plasmodium*. The lifecycle of *Plasmodium* is shown in Figure 53.1.

Symptoms of *P. vivax* malaria occur in a predictable, cyclic manner every 48 hours. This is because the merozoites grow and rupture erythrocytes on a regular time schedule. The uncomplicated or classic malaria attack lasts 6 to 10 hours and occurs in the following stages:

- *Cold stage:* Intense chills and shivering
- *Hot stage:* Fever, headache, vomiting; possible seizures in young children
- *Sweating stage:* Profuse diaphoresis, followed by return to normal body temperature and fatigue.

Complicated malaria may involve multiple organ failures and can be fatal. Nervous system involvement, called cerebral malaria, leads to abnormal behaviors, impairment of consciousness, seizures, or coma. Loss of large numbers of erythrocytes can cause severe anemia. Pulmonary edema and renal failure can occur. Complicated symptoms are nearly always indicative of infection by *P. falciparum*; the other three species rarely cause severe manifestations or death.

Drugs for Malaria

53.3 The three goals of malaria pharmacotherapy are chemoprophylaxis, treatment of acute attacks, and prevention of relapses.

Pharmacotherapy of malaria attempts to interrupt the complex lifecycle of *Plasmodium*. Treatment becomes increasingly challenging as the parasite enters different phases of its lifecycle. The goals of antimalarial therapy depend on the stage of the infection. These goals include chemoprophylaxis, treatment of acute attacks, and prevention of relapse. Drugs for malaria are listed in Table 53.2.

Chemoprophylaxis: A rule of thumb to remember about malaria (and many other infectious diseases) is that it is much easier to prevent than to treat. The Centers for Disease Control and Prevention (CDC) recommends that travelers to infested areas receive prophylactic antimalarial drugs prior to travel, during their visit, and for at least 1 week after leaving. The recommended drug depends on the specific country being visited (CDC, 2019). For many decades, chloroquine (Aralen) was the preferred drug for prophylaxis, but most regions now have a high incidence of chloroquine-resistant strains of *Plasmodium*. Chloroquine for chemoprophylaxis has been largely replaced by other effective antimalarials, including

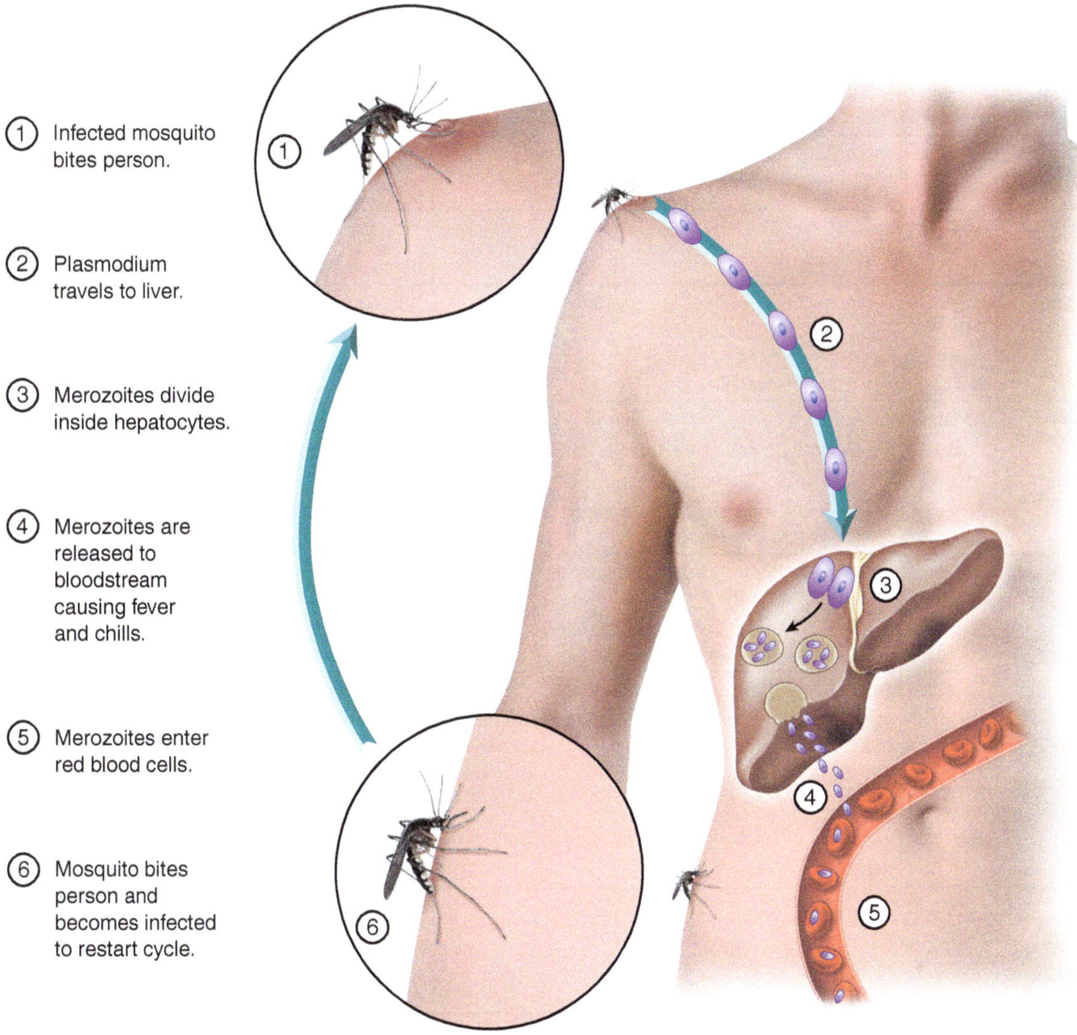

Figure 53.1 Lifecycle of *Plasmodium*.

atovaquone-proguanil (Malarone), doxycycline, primaquine, tafenoquine (Arakoda), and mefloquine.

Treatment of acute attacks: Once a *Plasmodium* infection has been diagnosed, pharmacotherapy of malaria is most successful when it is begun immediately. Classic malaria symptoms in a patient with a history of recent travel to an endemic region are sufficient evidence to begin antimalarial therapy, without waiting for laboratory confirmation.

Medications are used to interrupt the erythrocytic stage and eliminate the merozoites from RBCs. Elimination will break the lifecycle of the protozoan and stop the acute symptoms. Chloroquine is a preferred antimalarial for treating the acute stage of the disease, if the infection was acquired in a region without chloroquine resistance. Options available for treating chloroquine-resistant infections include artesunate, mefloquine, artemether-lumefantrine, atovaquone-proguanil, and quinine sulfate (with an antibiotic such as tetracycline, doxycycline, or clindamycin).

Patients with severe or complicated malaria are treated aggressively with high doses of antimalarials. IV artesunate is the preferred drug, although it may not be available at all hospitals. While waiting for artesunate to arrive, the patient should receive artemether-lumefantrine.

Prevention of relapse: In some types of malaria, the liver can harbor a dormant stage called the **hypnozoite**, for several years after the initial infection. The hypnozoites are unresponsive to treatment with most antimalarials, and the patient will almost always experience subsequent attacks. Complete removal of all forms of *Plasmodium* from the body (including the hypnozoites) is called a **radical cure**. Treatment for the radical cure begins before or immediately after pharmacotherapy for the acute attack has been completed.

Two drugs are approved for radical cure. The traditional drug is primaquine; however, this drug must be taken for 14 days, which results in low adherence. In 2018 tafenoquine (Krintafel) was approved for radical cure. Although it belongs to the same chemical class as primaquine, it requires only a single dose, which is a major breakthrough in malaria pharmacotherapy.

Table 53.2 Drugs for Malaria

Drug	Route and Adult Dose (Maximum Dose Where Indicated)	Adverse Effects
artemether-lumefantrine (Coartem)	For acute infections: PO: 4 tablets as an initial dose followed by 4 tablets 8 h later, then 4 tablets bid for the following 3 days	*Headache, anorexia, dizziness, asthenia, arthralgia, myalgia* QT prolongation, hypersensitivity reactions
artesunate	IV: 2.4 mg at 0, 12, and 24 h then once per day	*Increased transaminase, hyperbilirubinemia, leukocytosis* Acute renal failure, hemolytic anemia
atovaquone-proguanil (Malarone)	For acute infections: PO: 4 tablets as a single daily dose for 3 days For prophylaxis: PO: 1 tablet/day starting 1–2 days before travel and continuing 7 days following return	*Nausea, vomiting, abdominal pain, diarrhea, headache, myalgia* Neutropenia, hypotension
chloroquine (Aralen)	For acute infections: PO: 600-mg initial dose, then 300 mg at 6, 24, and 48 h IM: 200 mg q6h prn (max: 800 mg/24 h) For prophylaxis: PO: 300 mg starting 2 wk before travel and continuing 7–14 days following return	*Nausea and vomiting; diarrhea; visual changes including blurred vision, photophobia, difficulty focusing* Hemolytic anemia in patients with G6PD deficiency; irreversible retinal damage
hydroxychloroquine (Plaquenil)	For acute infections: PO: 620-mg initial dose, then 310 mg at 6, 18, and 28 h For prophylaxis: PO: 310 mg starting 2 wk before travel and continuing 4–6 wk following return	
mefloquine	For acute infections: PO: 1250 mg as a single dose For prophylaxis: PO: 250 mg once a week for 4 wk before travel; continuing 250 mg every other week during travel and 2 doses following return	*Nausea and vomiting, diarrhea, myalgia, dizziness, anorexia, abdominal pain* Atrioventricular block, bradycardia, tachycardia, psychosis
primaquine	For acute infection: PO: 15 mg/day for 2 wk For prophylaxis: PO: 15 mg/day following return for 14 days	*Nausea and vomiting, diarrhea, myalgia, headache, anorexia, abdominal pain* Hemolytic anemia in patients with G6PD deficiency
quinine (Qualaquin)	For acute infections: PO: 650 mg tid for 7 days	*Nausea and vomiting, diarrhea* Cinchonism (tinnitus, ototoxicity, vertigo, fever, visual impairment), hypothermia, coma, cardiovascular collapse, agranulocytosis
tafenoquine (Arakoda, Krintafel)	PO (Arakoda): 200 mg given 3 days before travel, 1 week during travel, and 1 week after travel PO (Krintafel): 300 mg once	*Nausea and vomiting, headache, dizziness, motion sickness* Hemolytic anemia in patients with G6PD deficiency, psychiatric symptoms

Note: *Italics* indicate common adverse effects. Underline indicates serious adverse effects.

CONNECTION Checkpoint 53.1

From what you learned in Chapter 48, what adverse effects of tetracyclines, such as doxycycline, cause these drugs to be used with caution during pregnancy?

PROTOTYPE DRUG Chloroquine (Aralen)

Classification **Therapeutic:** Antimalarial drug
Pharmacologic: Heme complexing drug

Therapeutic Effects and Uses: Developed in response to the high incidence of malaria among American soldiers in the Pacific islands during World War II, chloroquine has been the traditional prototype medication for malarial prophylaxis and treatment for over 70 years. Chloroquine is very effective in treating acute symptoms of the erythrocytic stage but has no activity against dormant *P. vivax* or *P. ovale*. It can reduce the high fever of patients in the acute stage in less than 48 hours. It is also effective for the chemoprophylaxis of malaria caused by *P. malariae* and sensitive strains of *P. falciparum*, when taken 2 weeks before entering an endemic area and continuing 4 to 6 weeks after leaving. Chloroquine is used only for patients who acquired malaria in a region without chloroquine resistance.

Mechanism of Action: Chloroquine concentrates in the food vacuoles of *Plasmodia* residing in human RBCs. Once in the vacuole, the drug likely prevents the destruction of heme and other proteins, which then build to toxic levels within the parasite. The anti-inflammatory effects of chloroquine occur because the drug inhibits the actions of histamine and serotonin as well as prostaglandin synthesis.

Pharmacokinetics:

Route(s)	Oral (PO), intramuscular (IM)
Absorption	Rapid and completely absorbed
Distribution	Widely distributed; crosses the placenta; secreted in breast milk
Primary metabolism	Hepatic; two active metabolites

Primary excretion	Renal
Onset of action	Peak effect: 1–2 h
Duration of action	Half-life: 70–120 h

Adverse Effects: Chloroquine exhibits few serious adverse effects at low to moderate doses. Nausea and diarrhea may occur. At higher doses, CNS and cardiovascular toxicity may be observed. Symptoms include confusion, delirium, convulsions, reduced reflexes, hypotension, and dysrhythmias. Blood dyscrasias are possible. Chloroquine can cause retinal toxicity, including blurred vision, photophobia, and difficulty focusing.

Contraindications/Precautions: Patients with preexisting retinal field changes should not receive chloroquine because the drug concentrates in this tissue and high doses can cause irreversible retinal damage. Because this drug can affect heme metabolism, it is contraindicated in patients with porphyria. Patients with known glucose-6-phosphate dehydrogenase (G6PD) deficiency should be treated cautiously, if at all, because chloroquine may cause hemolysis in these patients. Because chloroquine is metabolized in the liver, patients with chronic alcoholism or hepatic impairment should be monitored regularly. It is also contraindicated in patients with chronic kidney disease (CKD) and in those with hypersensitivity to the drug. Patients with preexisting hematologic disease should be treated with caution because chloroquine may cause blood dyscrasias.

Drug Interactions: Antacids and laxatives containing aluminum and magnesium can decrease absorption and must not be given within 4 hours of oral chloroquine administration. Because chloroquine is associated with an increased risk for QT prolongation and torsades de pointes, it should not be administered concurrently with other drugs known to prolong the QT interval, such as many antidysrhythmics, phenothiazines, and beta-adrenergic agonists. **Herbal/Food:** Unknown.

Pregnancy: This drug showed embryofetal toxicity in laboratory animals. Chloroquine is secreted in human milk and small amounts may remain in milk for up to a month following the last dose. Travel to malaria endemic regions is not recommended during pregnancy, however, the small doses used for prophylactic therapy are generally considered safe.

Treatment of Overdose: Chloroquine overdose may be fatal. Symptomatic treatment includes anticonvulsants and vasopressors for shock. Ammonium chloride may be used to acidify the urine to hasten excretion of chloroquine.

Clinician Responsibilities: Key clinical implications for patients receiving chloroquine are included in Applied Clinical Judgment: Patients Receiving Pharmacotherapy for Protozoan and Helminthic Infections.

Drugs Similar to Chloroquine (Aralen)

Other antimalarials include artemether-lumefantrine, artesunate, atovaquone-proguanil, hydroxychloroquine, mefloquine, primaquine, quinine, and tafenoquine.

Artemether-lumefantrine (Coartem): In 2009, the U.S. Food and Drug Administration (FDA) approved the use of a fixed-dose combination of artemether and lumefantrine to treat acute, uncomplicated malaria. Artemether is prepared from substances obtained from the Chinese herb *Artemisia annua*, which has been known to have antimalarial properties for over a thousand years. Lumefantrine extends the half-life of the combination drug. Coartem is very effective and is the preferred option for treating chloroquine-resistant infections. This drug is approved for treatment, not prevention, of malaria. Side effects are generally mild. Because artemether-lumefantrine prolongs the QT interval, it should be used with caution in patients with cardiac impairment. Extensive human data have not shown evidence for an increase in adverse pregnancy outcomes or teratogenicity above the baseline rate. It is not known if this drug is secreted in human milk and adverse effects on the breastfed neonate are unknown.

Artesunate: Artesunate was approved in 2020 by IV bolus for the initial treatment of severe malaria. Therapy with artesunate is followed by a complete course of an appropriate oral antimalarial treatment. It is not active against the hypnozoite stage of *Plasmodium*. Cases of serious hemolytic anemia have been reported up to 4 weeks after treatment. Artesunate showed embryofetal toxicity in laboratory animals. This drug is secreted in human milk, although adverse effects on the breastfed neonate are unknown.

Atovaquone-proguanil (Malarone): The fixed-dose combination drug Malarone was approved in 2000 for the prevention and treatment of malaria. Malarone may be given for prophylaxis or to lessen the severity of acute symptoms. For acute attacks, a 3-day regimen is usually sufficient. For prevention, the drug is begun 1 to 2 days before entering an endemic region and continued for 7 days after returning. The drug combination rarely produces serious adverse effects; rash and gastrointestinal (GI) upset are the two most common complaints. Atovaquone (Mepron) is approved as monotherapy to treat *Pneumocystis jiroveci* pneumonia in patients who are intolerant to trimethoprim-sulfamethoxazole (TMP-SMZ). Animal studies did not show evidence of embryofetal harm or teratogenicity. Proguanil is secreted in human milk, although adverse effects on the breastfed neonate are unknown.

Hydroxychloroquine (Plaquenil): As its name implies, hydroxychloroquine is closely related to chloroquine and has essentially the same actions. Approved in 1955, it is indicated for the prevention and treatment of malaria. Like chloroquine, retinal toxicity is a concern. Hydroxychloroquine is also prescribed to treat patients with cutaneous and systemic forms of systemic lupus erythematosus and for rheumatoid arthritis. It is administered by the oral (PO) route. In 2020, hydroxychloroquine was used to treat infection from the COVID-19 virus. Use of the drug did not demonstrate any improvement in clinical outcomes and the FDA withdrew emergency approval for this indication. Human data have not shown evidence for an increase in adverse pregnancy outcomes or teratogenicity above the baseline rate. This drug is secreted in human milk, although adverse effects on the breastfed neonate are unknown.

Mefloquine: Approved in 1989, mefloquine was developed during the Vietnam War to protect American soldiers from multidrug-resistant *P. falciparum* malaria. It is approved for both treatment and prophylaxis. Prophylactic dosing begins 1 week before entering an endemic area and continues for 4 weeks after leaving. Because of the rapid emergence of resistant strains, it is reserved for multidrug-resistant strains of *Plasmodium*. Nausea and vomiting are the most common adverse effects. The primary limitation of mefloquine is nervous system toxicity, including dizziness, nightmares, aggression, and psychoses, which can appear at high doses. Patients with preexisting psychiatric disorders should not take mefloquine. Extensive human experience has not shown evidence for an increase in adverse pregnancy outcomes or teratogenicity above the baseline rate. This drug is secreted in human milk, although adverse effects on the breastfed neonate are unknown.

Primaquine: Approved in 1951, primaquine is a preferred drug for preventing relapses caused by dormant *P. vivax* in the liver. Because it has no activity against the blood forms of *Plasmodium*, it must always be used in combination with other antimalarials. Standard therapy is for 14 days, although 5-day regimens have proved successful. The drug is well tolerated, even at high doses. The most serious adverse effect is hemolytic anemia in patients who are deficient in G6PD. Unlike some of the other drugs in this class, resistance is not a major clinical problem with primaquine. It is also used to treat *P. jiroveci* pneumonia in combination with clindamycin. All patients should be screened for G6PD deficiency prior to therapy. Studies showed an increase in abortions when given to pregnant laboratory animals, but no fetotoxicity or teratogenicity. This drug is contraindicated for breastfeeding if the infant is found to have G6PD deficiency or if the neonate's status is unknown.

Quinine (Qualaquin): First described in the 1600s, quinine is the oldest drug used to treat malaria, and it is still obtained from the bark of the South American cinchona tree. Although safer alternatives have since been discovered, quinine is still used for chloroquine-resistant *Plasmodia*, in combination with other antimalarials. It is approved only for the treatment (not prophylaxis) of uncomplicated malaria caused by *P. falciparum*. Cinchonism, a syndrome characterized by tinnitus, deafness, headache, vision abnormalities, and diarrhea, can occur at therapeutic doses. A major limiting factor is cardiotoxicity, which produces quinidine-like dysrhythmias at high doses. In 2017 an IV form of this drug, quinidine gluconate, was withdrawn from the U.S. market. Extensive human data have not shown evidence for an increase in adverse pregnancy outcomes or teratogenicity above the baseline rate. Small amounts of this drug are secreted in human milk, although adverse effects on the breastfed neonate are unknown.

Tafenoquine (Arakoda, Krintafel): Tafenoquine was approved in 2018 for two indications: prophylaxis of malaria (Arakoda) and for the prevention of malaria relapses (Krintafel). Arakoda is given prior to, during, and after travel to a region where malaria is endemic. Krintafel is given on the first or second day of treatment for acute malarial symptoms. Like primaquine, the drug is well tolerated, with the most serious adverse effect being hemolytic anemia in patients who are deficient in G6PD. All patients should be screened for G6PD deficiency prior to therapy. Animal studies showed an increase in abortions, but no fetotoxicity or teratogenicity. This drug is contraindicated for breastfeeding if the infant is found to have G6PD deficiency or if the neonate's status is unknown.

Drugs for Nonmalarial Protozoan Infections

53.4 Amebiasis, giardiasis, and cryptosporidiosis are caused by intestinal parasites and are usually acquired through contaminated water or food.

Although infection by *Plasmodium* is the most significant protozoan disease worldwide, infections caused by other protozoa affect significant numbers of people in endemic areas. Each of the organisms has unique differences in its distribution pattern and physiology.

Many areas of the world do not enjoy the high level of sanitation found in the United States and Canada. In developing countries, drinking water may not be disinfected before consumption and may be contaminated with pathogens from animal waste. In regions with poor sanitation, infectious diseases are endemic and contribute significantly to mortality, especially in children, who are often more susceptible to the pathogens. Amebiasis, giardiasis, and cryptosporidiosis are protozoan infections of the intestines, spread primarily by poor sanitation.

PharmFACT

It is estimated that 50 million cases of amebiasis occur each year worldwide, resulting in 100,000 deaths annually. Worldwide, it is the second leading cause of death due to parasitic diseases (Dhawan, 2019).

Amebiasis: Although not endemic to the United States, as much as 10% of the world's population is infected with this protozoan disease. The infection may be carried to the United States by travelers from regions where the disease is endemic, such as Mexico, India, western and southern Africa, and portions of Central and South America. The parasite is spread by ingesting fecally contaminated food or drinking water

Amebiasis begins when an individual ingests cysts of *Entamoeba histolytica*. The trophozoite form of the protozoan invades the colon mucosa, causing ulcerations and considerable abdominal pain, cramping, and bloody diarrhea. Cysts are expelled in the feces. Diagnosis of amebiasis is generally through identification of the trophozoites in the stool; however, serum and stool antigen detection tests specific for *E. histolytica* are available. The lifecycle of *E. histolytica* is illustrated in Figure 53.2.

Although rare, the trophozoite may gain access to the general circulation through colon ulcers and travel to other organs, particularly the liver, where it produces hepatic abscesses. Liver involvement causes high fever and right upper quadrant pain. Other possible sites of infection include the brain, genitalia, and lung.

Regimens for amebiasis include combination therapy with two to three drugs to eliminate the parasites from their many potential sites. The most commonly prescribed medication for both intestinal and hepatic amebiasis is metronidazole, due to its safety and efficacy. In cases of acute disease, IV metronidazole may be administered concurrently with an opioid to control severe diarrhea. Tinidazole (Tindamax) is an option for patients unable to take metronidazole.

If the infection is limited to the intestine, paromomycin is a preferred drug because it is able to reach high concentrations in the intestinal lumen without producing significant systemic toxicity. This drug is also prescribed to eliminate the protozoan in patients who are asymptomatic carriers of the infection.

Pharmacotherapy for amebiasis is continued until multiple negative stool specimens are obtained. Drugs for amebiasis and other nonmalarial protozoan infections are listed in Table 53.3.

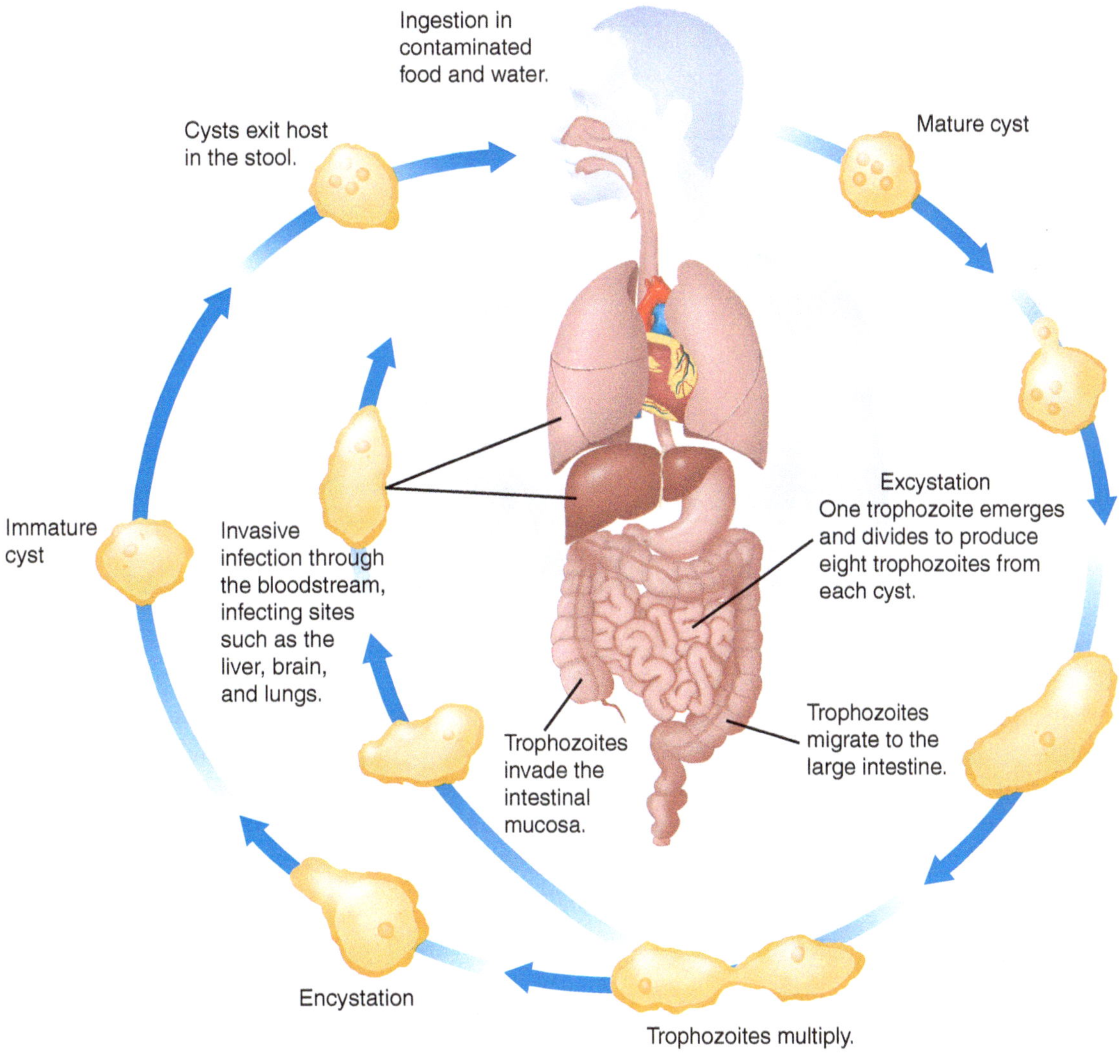

Figure 53.2 Lifecycle of *Entamoeba histolytica*.

Table 53.3 Drugs for Nonmalarial Protozoan Infections

Drug	Infection	Route and Adult Dose (Maximum Dose Where Indicated)	Adverse Effects
eflornithine*	African trypanosomiasis	IV: 100 mg/kg injected over at least 45 min q6h for 14 days	*Nausea and vomiting, diarrhea* Blood dyscrasias, seizures, ototoxicity
melarsoprol* (Arsobal)	African trypanosomiasis	IV: 2–3.6 mg/kg for 3 days, then repeated on day 7 and days 10–21	*Fever, albuminuria, transient arthralgias, dermatitis* Encephalopathy, increased mental excitement, twitching, confusion, tremor, seizures
metronidazole (Flagyl)	Amebiasis, trichomoniasis, giardiasis, Gardnerella vaginitis	For giardiasis: PO: 500 mg bid for 7 days For amebiasis: PO: 500–750 mg tid for 5–10 days	*Dizziness, headache, anorexia, abdominal pain, metallic taste, nausea* Seizures, peripheral neuropathy
miltefosine (Impavido)	Leishmaniasis	PO: 100–150 mg daily for 28 days	*Skin rash, elevated transaminases and creatinine levels, reduced sperm counts* Stevens–Johnson syndrome, melena, thrombocytopenia, embryofetal toxicity
nifurtimox (Lampit)	American trypanosomiasis	PO: 8–10 mg/kg 3–4 times/day for 30–60 days	*Rash, dizziness, headache, nausea and vomiting* Seizures, paresthesia with myalgia, pneumonia, embryofetal toxicity
nitazoxanide (Alinia)	Diarrhea caused by cryptosporidiosis or giardiasis in children	PO: 100–200 mg q12h for 3 days	*Abdominal pain, diarrhea, nausea and vomiting, headache* No serious adverse effects
paromomycin	Intestinal amebiasis	PO: 25–35 mg/kg divided in 3 doses for 5–10 days	*Nausea and vomiting, headache, diarrhea, abdominal cramps* Ototoxicity, nephrotoxicity
pentamidine (NebuPent, Pentam)	*Pneumocystis* pneumonia, trypanosomiasis, leishmaniasis	IM/IV: 4 mg/kg/day for 14–21 days Inhaled: 300 mg per nebulizer every 3–4 wk	*Cough, bronchospasm* Hypoglycemia, severe hypotension, kidney failure, pneumothorax
pyrimethamine (Daraprim)	Toxoplasmosis	PO: 50–75 mg for 1–3 wk, then 25–37.5 mg for 4–5 wk	*Nausea and vomiting, diarrhea, rash* Folic acid deficiency, blood dyscrasias
sodium stibogluconate (Pentostam)*	Leishmaniasis	IV or IM: 20 mg/kg/day for 20 days	*Nausea and vomiting, diarrhea, anorexia, cough, substernal pain* ECG changes, pneumonia, blood dyscrasias
suramin* (Germanin)	African trypanosomiasis	IV: 1 g on days 1, 3, 7, 14, and 21	*Nausea and vomiting, malaise, fatigue, fever, diarrhea, rash* Loss of consciousness, seizures, nephrotoxicity, adrenal insufficiency, blood dyscrasias, hepatotoxicity, severe hypersensitivity reactions
tinidazole (Tindamax)	Amebiasis, giardiasis, trichomoniasis, bacterial vaginosis	For amebiasis: PO: 2 g/day for 3 days For giardiasis or trichomoniasis: PO: 2 g as single dose For vaginosis: PO: 2 g/day for 3 days	*Anorexia, constipation, dyspepsia, dizziness, bitter or metallic taste, nausea and vomiting* Seizures, peripheral neuropathy, angioedema

Note: *Italics* indicate common adverse effects. Underline indicates serious adverse effects.

* Denotes a drug that is only available through the CDC.

Giardiasis: Giardiasis is an infection caused by the protozoan *Giardia lamblia* that has much in common with amebiasis. They are both endemic to regions with poor sanitation, where the water supply is contaminated with human feces. Both affect the intestine, causing acute cramping pain, severe diarrhea, fatigue, and marked weight loss. Both have a trophozoite and cyst stage, with no intermediate host or vector. Identification of *Giardia* trophozoites or cysts in the stool can help distinguish between the two diseases. Another potential cause of giardiasis in the United States is the unsanitary handling of soiled diapers in daycare centers. It is interesting to note that *Giardia* was the very first protozoan discovered, originally identified by the inventor of the microscope, Antonie van Leeuwenhoek, in the 1600s.

More common than amebiasis, giardiasis is the most common intestinal parasite responsible for diarrhea symptoms throughout the world. When contaminated food or water is ingested, the acidic environment of the stomach causes the parasite to transform from the cyst to the trophozoite stage. The incubation period is 1 to 3 weeks, and symptoms last 2 to 6 weeks.

Infections of *G. lamblia* remain localized to the intestine and are often self-limiting. A chronic form of giardiasis, however, can last for months and lead to malabsorption, steatorrhea, weakness, and chronic diarrhea. Although giardiasis is not fatal, it can weaken patients and make them susceptible to infection by opportunistic pathogens. Family members of infected patients, food handlers, and daycare workers who are asymptomatic carriers should receive treatment.

Pharmacotherapy of giardiasis includes metronidazole (Flagyl), tinidazole (Tindamax), and nitazoxanide (Alinia). Diarrhea generally stops within 48 hours after pharmacotherapy is initiated and a typical regimen continues for 3 to 5 days. Follow-up stool specimens are analyzed to confirm that the pharmacotherapy has been successful. For persistent cases, therapy may last 3 to 4 weeks.

PharmFACT

Someone infected with giardiasis may shed as many as 10 billion *Giardia* cysts each day for several months. It is believed that swallowing as few as 10 cysts might cause someone to develop symptoms of giardiasis (CDC, 2019).

Cryptosporidiosis: Cryptosporidiosis is an infection caused by the protozoan *Cryptosporidium parvum* that causes severe diarrhea. Like *E. histolytica* and *G. lamblia*, *C. parvum* is primarily an intestinal parasite, acquired through the consumption of fecally contaminated food or water. It has also been isolated from recreational water and has even been found in municipal water supplies. Cysts of *C. parvum* survive harsh conditions, including chlorination of water. Although only about 3000 cases of cryptosporidiosis are reported in the United States each year, it is responsible for a significant proportion of infectious diarrhea worldwide.

In patients with healthy immune systems, the disease is self-limiting and no antiprotozoan drugs are necessary to remove the parasite. Pharmacotherapy of cryptosporidiosis is targeted at stopping the severe diarrhea through the symptomatic use of antidiarrheal drugs. In addition to opioids, nitazoxanide is approved to treat diarrhea from this parasite.

In immunosuppressed patients, cryptosporidiosis has a high mortality rate. In addition, the disease can spread to other tissues, especially the gallbladder and biliary tree. Antiprotozoan drug therapy is necessary for these patients, with paromomycin being a preferred medication. Other drugs that may be of benefit include azithromycin and nitazoxanide. Combination therapy with these drugs may continue for 14 to 28 days, depending on patient response.

PROTOTYPE DRUG Metronidazole (Flagyl)

Classification **Therapeutic:** Anti-infective, antiprotozoan
Pharmacologic: Nitroimidazole drug

Therapeutic Effects and Uses: Approved in 1963, metronidazole is the prototype medication for amebiasis, being effective against both the intestinal and hepatic phases of the disease. Resistant forms of *E. histolytica* have not yet emerged as a clinical problem with metronidazole. Metronidazole is also a preferred drug for giardiasis (off-label) and trichomoniasis.

In addition to its classification as an antiprotozoan drug, metronidazole has strong activity against anaerobic bacteria and may be given PO or IV to treat a number of serious respiratory, bone, skin, and CNS infections. A vaginal gel (Nuvessa) is available as a single dose to treat bacterial vaginosis.

Topical forms of metronidazole (MetroGel, MetroLotion, Noritate) are used to treat rosacea, a chronic, inflammatory condition characterized by skin reddening and hyperplasia of the sebaceous glands, particularly around the nose and face. MetroGel-vaginal is approved to treat susceptible vaginal infections. Pylera (metronidazole, bismuth, and tetracycline) is approved to eradicate *Helicobacter pylori*, an infection associated with peptic ulcer disease.

Off-label uses of metronidazole include the pharmacotherapy of pseudomembranous colitis, Crohn's disease, and colitis. When used for intestinal pathogens, metronidazole therapy is sometimes followed by administration of iodoquinol to more effectively eliminate residual parasites harbored in the colon.

Mechanism of Action: Metronidazole enters pathogens and binds to deoxyribonucleic acid (DNA), ribonucleic acid (RNA), and intracellular proteins. Cell death is likely the result of an absence of DNA repair and abnormalities in RNA synthesis.

Pharmacokinetics:

Route(s)	PO, IV, topical
Absorption	Well-absorbed PO (80%)
Distribution	Widely distributed, including cerebrospinal fluid (CSF) and abscesses; crosses the placenta; secreted in breast milk
Primary metabolism	Hepatic: 30–60%
Primary excretion	Renal: 77%; feces: 6–15%
Onset of action	PO/IV: rapid; topical: 3 weeks
Duration of action	PO/IV: 6–8 h; topical: 12 h

Adverse Effects: Although adverse effects occur frequently during metronidazole therapy, most are not serious enough to cause discontinuation of the drug. The most common adverse effects are anorexia, nausea and vomiting, diarrhea, abdominal pain, dizziness, and headache. Dryness of the mouth and an unpleasant metallic taste may be experienced. Seizures and peripheral neuropathy have been reported. Patients receiving the drug by the IV route should be monitored for injection-site reactions. Use of the vaginal gel may lead to vaginal candidiasis in more than 10% of patients. **Black Box Warning:** Metronidazole (oral and parenteral) is carcinogenic in laboratory animals and should be used only for approved indications.

Contraindications/Precautions: Although rare, metronidazole can cause bone marrow suppression. Thus, it is contraindicated for patients with blood dyscrasias. Complete blood counts (CBCs) should be monitored during therapy to rule out any developing leukopenia. Metronidazole crosses the blood–brain barrier and is contraindicated in patients with active CNS pathology. The drug should be discontinued if signs of CNS toxicity appear. Liver function tests should be carefully monitored in patients with alcoholism or hepatic impairment because metronidazole is extensively metabolized in the liver. Doses of metronidazole should be lowered in these patients. The injectable form contains significant amounts of sodium, which can lead to edema in patients with heart failure.

Drug Interactions: Concurrent administration with PO anticoagulants can potentiate hypoprothrombinemia; thus, warfarin doses may require adjustment. Alcohol use may elicit a disulfiram-like reaction. Concurrent use with disulfiram can induce acute psychosis. This includes medications such as cough remedies that contain alcohol. Because metronidazole may elevate lithium levels, doses of lithium may need to be decreased to avoid toxicity. **Herbal/Food:** The extended release form of the drug should be taken on an empty stomach.

Pregnancy: Animal studies showed no evidence of fetal harm. Human data suggests there may be some fetal risk when given during the first trimester. This drug is secreted in human milk. Systemic metronidazole should only be given during pregnancy if the potential benefits to the mother justify the potential risks to the fetus or neonate.

Treatment of Overdose: No specific therapy for overdose is available. Patients are treated symptomatically.

Clinician Responsibilities: Key clinical implications for patients receiving metronidazole are included in Applied Clinical Judgment: Patients Receiving Pharmacotherapy for Protozoan and Helminthic Infections.

Drugs Similar to Metronidazole (Flagyl)

Other selected antiprotozoan drugs for amebiasis, giardiasis, or cryptosporidiosis include nitazoxanide, paromomycin, and tinidazole. Iodoquinol was used to treat amebiasis for many years but is no longer available in the United States.

Nitazoxanide (Alinia): Approved in 1996, nitazoxanide is approved for the treatment of infectious diarrhea caused by cryptosporidiosis and giardiasis in adults and children. For children, it is formulated as a PO suspension. Off-label uses include diarrhea caused by other agents such as *E. histolytica* and *Clostridioides difficile*. A typical regimen is 500 mg bid for 3 days. The drug is well tolerated, with abdominal pain and GI distress being the most common adverse effects. Animal studies did not show evidence of fetotoxicity. It is not known if this drug is secreted in milk or if it has adverse effects on the breastfed neonate.

Paromomycin: Approved in 1959, paromomycin is a broad-spectrum aminoglycoside antibiotic with antiprotozoan activity. The drug has activity against most gram-negative bacteria (except *Pseudomonas aeruginosa*), many gram-positive bacteria, some protozoa, and many parasitic worms. Because it is poorly absorbed from the GI tract, PO dosing is used to kill intestinal bacteria, protozoa, and helminths. It is approved for the treatment of intestinal *E. histolytica* infections, with a typical regimen consisting of 10 to 14 days of therapy. The drug has an orphan drug designation for treating multidrug-resistant tuberculosis and *Mycobacterium avium* complex infections. The most common adverse effects are GI related: nausea and vomiting, cramping, and diarrhea. Like other aminoglycosides, the drug may exhibit ototoxicity and nephrotoxicity. Paromomycin is not absorbed, therefore no adverse effects during pregnancy or lactation would be expected.

Tinidazole (Tindamax): Approved in 2004, tinidazole is in the same chemical class as metronidazole but has a longer half-life that allows for less frequent dosing intervals. Like metronidazole, tinidazole exhibits both antibacterial and antiprotozoan activity. It is highly active against *E. histolytica*, *T. vaginalis*, *G. lamblia*, and certain anaerobic bacteria. Typical regimens include single PO doses for giardiasis and trichomoniasis and 3-day therapy for amebiasis. In 2007, Tindamax was approved to treat bacterial vaginosis, the most common vaginal infection in the United States. Tinidazole interacts with anticoagulants to increase the risk of bleeding. When taken concurrently with alcohol, a disulfiram-like reaction occurs. Adverse effects are mild and include a bitter or metallic taste and GI distress. Tinidazole carries a black box warning that the drug is carcinogenic in laboratory animals and should be used only for approved indications. Tinidazole is contraindicated during the first trimester of pregnancy and should be used with caution in the second and third trimesters. Because tinidazole is secreted in human milk, breastfeeding is not recommended during therapy and for 72 hours after the last dose.

53.5 Other protozoan infections that can cause significant disease include toxoplasmosis, trichomoniasis, trypanosomiasis, and leishmaniasis.

Protozoa can invade nearly any tissue in the body. As discussed earlier in this chapter, *Plasmodia* prefer erythrocytes, *Giardia* the colon, and *Entamoeba* travel to the liver. This section presents less common protozoa that invade additional sites. These infections include toxoplasmosis, trichomoniasis, trypanosomiasis, and leishmaniasis.

Toxoplasmosis: Toxoplasmosis is an infection caused by the protozoan *Toxoplasma gondii*. The domestic cat is an intermediate host to the parasite and serves as a primary means of transmission to humans. The only method of direct human-to-human transmission is from an infected mother to her fetus.

The cycle of *Toxoplasma* infection begins when a cat ingests cysts of *T. gondii*, either through fecally contaminated food or in the flesh of their prey. Once inside the cat, the cysts become trophozoites and invade the small intestine. The cysts are excreted and become infectious after they leave the cat's body. *Toxoplasma* cysts can remain infectious in the environment for up to a year.

Toxoplasmosis can occur if humans are exposed to contaminated cat feces, or if they eat raw or undercooked meat containing the cysts. In healthy people, toxoplasmosis is usually asymptomatic or presents with flulike symptoms that rarely require treatment. Those who are pregnant or immunosuppressed, however, require pharmacotherapy because the disease can cause significant morbidity in these populations.

Once *T. gondii* enters the body, it can invade nearly any organ. The most frequent sign is nonspecific lymphadenopathy. In immunosuppressed patients the brain is sometimes affected, resulting in a variety of CNS symptoms from headache to seizures. The cysts can form necrotic regions in the brain, resulting in focal neurologic abnormalities and changes in mental status. Fatal encephalitis from *Toxoplasma* infection was common in the early years of the AIDS epidemic. Lung infections were also frequent in these patients.

A pregnant patient acquiring *Toxoplasma* during the first two trimesters of pregnancy is at high risk of transmitting the infection to her fetus. The protozoan may cause stillbirth or abortion. Babies may present with ocular toxoplasmosis, a form of the infection that occurs when the cysts are deposited near the retina. Approximately 85% of the newborns who appear normal will develop brain or eye infections from *T. gondii*, sometimes years after birth.

The most effective regimen for acute toxoplasmosis is pyrimethamine (Daraprim) for 4 to 5 weeks. Clarithromycin, azithromycin, or a sulfonamide may be added to the regimen in combination with pyrimethamine or as alternatives. Leucovorin is a form of folic acid that is added to the regimen to reduce the potential for pyrimethamine-induced bone marrow suppression. Because relapse rates for toxoplasmosis in patients with AIDS approach 100%, lifelong prophylaxis may be necessary.

Trichomoniasis: Trichomoniasis is a parasitic infection caused by the protozoan *T. vaginalis*. It is a common STI, affecting approximately 15% of women visiting clinics in the United States (2.5 to 3 million women).

Because *T. vaginalis* can survive on moist surfaces for several hours, the infection may also be spread by nonsexual means, although this mode of transmission is believed to be uncommon. In addition, there is a small risk of transmission of the infection from mother to baby during childbirth. Thus, trichomoniasis in pregnant patients is usually treated.

Trichomoniasis most commonly presents with malodorous vaginal discharge, accompanied by vulvar pruritus. Intense scratching may cause erythema and secondary infections in surrounding areas. Dysuria and discomfort during intercourse are common. Fifty percent of *Trichomonas* infections are asymptomatic or subclinical. Most infections in men are asymptomatic, or small amounts of urethral discharge may be noted. Because of the nonspecific nature of the symptoms, diagnosis may be difficult. Culturing of the vaginal discharge is conducted in patients who do not respond to standard therapy, and a specific monoclonal antibody test is available.

With pharmacotherapy, cure rates for trichomoniasis are high. A single PO dose of metronidazole has been demonstrated to be as effective as prolonged therapy and more effective than topical drugs. However, the higher amount administered as a single dose causes a greater incidence of adverse effects, particularly GI upset. For these patients, 7 days of metronidazole therapy at a lower daily dose is equally effective and produces less GI upset. Therapy should also include the patient's sexual partners, even if they are asymptomatic, to break the cycle of reinfection.

Trypanosomiasis: Trypanosomiasis is actually two distinct parasitic infections: American and African trypanosomiasis. The two infections are caused by different organisms and have different vectors, clinical manifestations, and treatments.

American trypanosomiasis, or Chagas' disease, is caused by *Trypanosoma cruzi*, a parasite found throughout central and northern South America, Central America, and Mexico. The disease is a growing health concern in the United States. The vector for Chagas' disease is the "kissing" bug that ingests *T. cruzi* when it feeds on an infected human. The protozoan reproduces in the bug and is transmitted when the vector defecates on the host's skin at the same time that it feeds. *T. cruzi* usually enters the human host by being rubbed into the vector's bite, an open cut, or the mucous membranes of the eye, nose, or mouth. Other carriers are suspected for *T. cruzi*, including dogs, cats, and rodents. It is estimated that 50,000 people die each year from the infection.

Acute Chagas' disease occurs more commonly in children and presents as a granuloma at the entry site, lymphadenopathy, and hepatomegaly. The acute form is not common and is often self-limiting. If pharmacotherapy is initiated, the preferred drugs are benzimidazole and nifurtimox, which are available only from the CDC.

Pharmacotherapy for the acute phase is prolonged, at 60 to 100 days.

The chronic stage of Chagas' disease may appear decades after the initial infection. Signs and symptoms include cardiomyopathy and degeneration of autonomic ganglia that can result in megacolon, megaesophagus, and uncoordinated peristalsis. Unfortunately, medications will not cure the chronic phase, which is treated symptomatically.

African trypanosomiasis, commonly known as sleeping sickness, is caused by two subspecies of the protozoan *Trypanosoma brucei*. The infection is transmitted to humans by the bite of a tsetse fly carrying *T. brucei*. African trypanosomiasis is restricted to sub-Saharan Africa, and its incidence ranges from 20,000 to 300,000 new infections annually, with about 50,000 deaths a year due to the infection.

Symptoms of *T. brucei* infection include a chancre at the site of the insect bite, extreme malaise (thus the name "sleeping sickness"), intermittent fever, muscle aches, weight loss, and body rash. The parasitic invasion may reach the CNS, causing personality changes, confusion, encephalitis, coma, and possibly death. The infection also affects the liver, heart, and other organs.

Early stages of *T. brucei* infection may be treated with suramin (Germanin) or pentamidine (Pentam). The standard drug for treating the late CNS manifestations is melarsoprol (Arsobal), a medication that has several toxic adverse effects. Eflornithine, the first new drug for *T. brucei* in over 50 years, also causes serious adverse effects. In 2020 the FDA approved nifurtimox (Lampit) for the treatment of Chagas' disease in children ages birth to 18 years.

Leishmaniasis: Most prevalent in Afghanistan, Bangladesh, Bolivia, Brazil, India, Iran, Peru, Saudi Arabia, Sudan, and Syria, leishmaniasis is an infection caused by about 20 different species of the protozoan *Leishmania*. Worldwide, 350 million people are believed to be afflicted with the disease. Carriers for *Leishmania* include dogs, foxes, squirrels, and rodents. The disease is transmitted to humans by the bite of the sand fly. Two primary forms of leishmaniasis have been identified, based on clinical signs and symptoms:

- *Visceral leishmaniasis.* Begins as a skin lesion but progresses to infect the spleen, liver, bone marrow, and lymph nodes. Visceral leishmaniasis is transmitted by contaminated blood or needlesticks and may occur in patients with advanced AIDS. It is usually fatal if untreated. This type most commonly occurs in Bangladesh, India, and Nepal.
- *Cutaneous leishmaniasis.* Characterized by skin lesions that spontaneously heal in 2 to 10 months. May progress to ulcers of the mucous membranes of the nose, pharynx, or oral cavity. Occurs mostly in Middle East countries such as Afghanistan, Iran, and Saudi Arabia but is also found in southern Texas, Central America, and South America.

CONNECTIONS: Community-Oriented Practice

Naegleria fowleri ("Brain-Eating Amoeba") Infections

The amoeba *Naegleria fowleri* causes primary amebic meningoencephalitis and is almost always fatal. Infection occurs when water from freshwater lakes, rivers, or hot springs enters through the nose and into the brain. It causes symptoms within 2 to 15 days after exposure and signs and symptoms include nausea and vomiting, fever, sudden severe headache, nasal congestion or discharge, and changes in taste or smell, progressing to symptoms of meningitis and encephalitis such as seizures, confusion, stiff neck, and sensitivity to light (Mayo Clinic, 2020). While many people are exposed every year through swimming or water sports in freshwater bodies of water, it is not known why some people develop the infection and others do not. *N. fowleri* has also been found in treated drinking water systems (Cope et al., 2019). It has been noted that children, those who participate in water activities during summer months, and people who use nasal irrigators have a higher risk of developing the disease. Diagnosis is based on a lumbar puncture and analysis of CSF. Treatment of the disease includes the use of amphotericin B, given IV or intrathecally, which kills the amoebas; other antifungal drugs; and antibiotics. The infection must be detected earlier as the disease is usually fatal, even with treatment.

Because protozoal diseases such as *N. fowleri* are usually associated with conditions where sanitation may be lacking, many people may not realize that common activities such as swimming in lakes or using nasal irrigators may introduce the infection. For outdoor recreational activities, even in public swimming pools, holding the nose shut or nose clips used for jumping or diving into the water, avoiding swimming or diving in freshwater bodies of water, and using cooled, boiled water or distilled water when using nasal irrigators is recommended.

The CDC recommends sodium stibogluconate (Pentostam) as the standard treatment for visceral leishmaniasis. This drug is available only through the CDC. Stibogluconate must be administered by the IV or IM routes for 4 to 6 weeks, which makes the treatment of visceral leishmaniasis procedurally difficult in underdeveloped countries where the disease is most prevalent. In addition, resistance is common. Relapse may occur as long as 10 years after the initial exposure. Alternative pharmacotherapy (off-label) for visceral leishmaniasis includes amphotericin B, pentamidine (Pentam), and IM paromomycin.

Cutaneous leishmaniasis generally heals spontaneously in 5 to 12 months in immunocompetent patients and does not require pharmacotherapy. For severe cases, pharmacotherapy includes many of the same drugs used for the visceral form. In 2014, miltefosine (Impavido) became the first FDA-approved drug to treat cutaneous leishmaniasis.

PROTOTYPE DRUG **Pyrimethamine (Daraprim)**

Classification **Therapeutic:** Antiprotozoan
Pharmacologic: Folic acid antagonist

Therapeutic Effects and Uses: Available for over 30 years, pyrimethamine is a preferred PO drug for treating toxoplasmosis. Acute toxoplasmosis is treated for 2 to 4 weeks, whereas chronic stages that exhibit organ involvement may require months of therapy.

Pyrimethamine is primarily effective against the acute phase of *T. gondii* infection and is less effective once the protozoan has entered the cystic phase of its lifecycle. To boost its efficacy, pyrimethamine is sometimes combined with other anti-infectives such as a sulfonamide, clarithromycin, clindamycin, or azithromycin.

Fansidar, a fixed-dose combination drug containing pyrimethamine and sulfadoxine, has been discontinued in the United States due to the large number of malarial strains that are resistant to it.

Mechanism of Action: Pyrimethamine inhibits the synthesis of folic acid in protozoa, thus inhibiting cell division.

Pharmacokinetics:

Route(s)	PO
Absorption	Pyrimethamine is well absorbed
Distribution	Widely distributed; crosses the placenta; secreted in breast milk; over 80% bound to plasma protein
Primary metabolism	Hepatic
Primary excretion	Kidneys
Onset of action	1 h
Duration of action	Half-life: 100 h

Adverse Effects: Common adverse effects of pyrimethamine include nausea and vomiting, anorexia, abdominal cramping, and rash. Serious adverse effects such as folic acid deficiency, megaloblastic anemia, pancytopenia, thrombocytopenia, and leukopenia may occur.

Contraindications/Precautions: Because pyrimethamine is a folic acid inhibitor, it is contraindicated in patients with preexisting megaloblastic anemia caused by folate deficiency. To prevent the development of anemia during therapy, leucovorin is administered concurrently. Pyrimethamine can stimulate the CNS and cause seizures. Therefore, it is used with caution in patients with seizure disorders. It should be used with caution in patients with significant CKD or hepatic impairment and in those with G6PD deficiency.

Drug Interactions: Few significant drug interactions occur with pyrimethamine. Other folic acid antagonists such as TMP-SMZ should not be used concurrently because this will increase the possibility of severe folic acid depletion in the patient. Folic acid supplements should not be given because they will reduce the effectiveness of pyrimethamine. The drug increases the half-life of phenytoin and may cause phenytoin toxicity. **Herbal/Food:** Unknown.

Pregnancy: This drug is teratogenic in laboratory animals. Because pyrimethamine is secreted in human milk, breastfeeding is not recommended.

Treatment of Overdose: Overdose can cause seizures and serious blood dyscrasias. Parenteral diazepam may be used to control seizures and leucovorin may be administered to prevent folic acid deficiency.

Clinician Responsibilities: Key clinical implications for patients receiving pyrimethamine are included in Applied Clinical Judgment: Patients Receiving Pharmacotherapy for Protozoan and Helminthic Infections.

Drugs Similar to Pyrimethamine (Daraprim)

Other selected antiprotozoan drugs for toxoplasmosis, trichomoniasis, trypanosomiasis, or leishmaniasis include eflornithine, melarsoprol, nifurtimox, sodium stibogluconate, and suramin. All these drugs are available from the CDC, with the exception of nifurtimox.

Eflornithine (Ornidyl): Eflornithine is prescribed for African trypanosomiasis, especially late-occurring CNS disease. It is less toxic than melarsoprol, but it is more expensive and is thus considered for therapy when melarsoprol fails to provide relief. Given by the IV route, therapy is continued for 7 to 14 days. Close medical supervision is required to monitor for the many serious adverse reactions, such as anemia, diarrhea, seizures, and vomiting. Unrelated to its antiprotozoan action, eflornithine cream (Vaniqa) was approved by the FDA in 2000 as the first topical prescription treatment for women with unwanted facial hair. Adverse effects from the topical formulation are mild and transient.

Melarsoprol (Arsobal): Melarsoprol was approved in 1949 for the late CNS stages of African trypanosomiasis. It is one of only a few antiprotozoan drugs that can cross the blood–brain barrier to reach the parasite in the CNS. Melarsoprol contains arsenic, an element acutely toxic to life-forms. The most common regimen is a series of three IV injections administered with a rest period of 8 to 10 days between each series. Melarsoprol is a toxic drug and severe adverse effects are possible, including fatal encephalopathy, convulsions, coma, thrombophlebitis, and necrosis at the injection site, if the drug is extravasated. Significant drug resistance has developed to melarsoprol.

Nifurtimox (Lampit): Nifurtimox received accelerated approval from the FDA in 2020 for the treatment of American trypanosomiasis in pediatric patients age birth to 18. It is given PO for 30 to 60 days. Adverse effects include nausea and vomiting, anorexia, and neurologic disturbances. Only 50 to 70% of patients will respond favorably to nifurtimox therapy, indicating a need for additional drugs for this infection. This drug may cause fetal harm and is not recommended during pregnancy or lactation. Females with reproductive potential should submit a negative pregnancy test prior to initiating treatment.

Sodium stibogluconate (Pentostam): Sodium stibogluconate is the traditional drug for treating leishmaniasis; however, decades of use have led to near-total resistance in certain strains of *Leishmania*. The drug must be given parenterally for 2 to 3 weeks. The most common adverse effects are pain at the injection site, pancreatitis, muscle and joint pain, and decreases in white blood cell (WBC) and RBC counts. Treatment failures and relapses are common, indicating a need for more effective drugs for this infection.

Suramin (Germanin): Discovered in 1921, suramin is one of the oldest drugs for African trypanosomiasis. It is used exclusively for pharmacotherapy of the initial phase of the infection, since it is unable to cross the blood–brain barrier to treat the CNS symptoms characteristic of late disease. The usual regimen is one IV injection per week for 5 weeks. Renal toxicity, nausea, and malaise are common during infusions.

CONNECTION Checkpoint 53.2

Sulfonamides have been used as common antibiotics for many decades. From what you learned in Chapter 50, what are the primary indications for sulfonamide pharmacotherapy?

Classification and Pathogenesis of Helminthic Infections

53.6 Helminthic infections cause significant intestinal disease, particularly in areas with poor sanitation.

Helminths consist of various species of parasitic worms. Unlike the single-celled protozoa, helminths have many cells, and thus their anatomy, physiology, and lifecycles are more complex. Diseases caused by these pathogens affect more than 2 billion people worldwide and are quite common in areas of the world lacking high standards of sanitation. Helminth infections in the United States and Canada are neither common nor fatal, although drug therapy may be indicated.

Like protozoa, helminths have different stages in their lifecycles, which include both immature and mature forms. Typically, the immature forms enter the body through the skin or the digestive tract. Most attach to the intestinal tract, although some form cysts in skeletal muscle or in organs such as the liver. Helminths are classified as roundworms (nematodes), flukes (trematodes), or tapeworms (cestodes).

Ascariasis: Ascariasis, caused by the roundworm *Ascaris lumbricoides*, is the most common helminth disease worldwide, affecting more than 1.4 billion people. This parasite is endemic to Latin America and Asia and afflicts 4 million Americans, generally in the warm climates of the Southeast. This infection occurs most commonly in children between the ages of 3 and 8 years, because this group is most likely to be exposed to contaminated soil without proper hand hygiene. Although fatalities are rare in the United States, severe infections can lead to complete intestinal obstruction if left untreated. Worldwide, it is estimated that ascariasis causes approximately 60,000 deaths annually, mostly in children.

Transmission of *A. lumbricoides* occurs when an individual unintentionally ingests eggs from the parasite. Once in the stomach, immature worms hatch from the eggs, and larvae attach to the intestinal wall. The larvae can travel through veins and lymphatics and be carried to the lungs, where they burrow through alveolar walls and migrate up the bronchi. Once reaching the throat, the larvae are swallowed and the cycle begins again.

A. lumbricoides develops into adult worms in the intestines. The female adult worm, which can grow to over 40 cm (16 in.) in length, lays as many as 240,000 eggs daily, which enter the feces. Under unsanitary conditions, *Ascaris* eggs reach soil where they may remain infective for years. The lifecycle of *Ascaris* is shown in Figure 53.3.

Ascariasis presents with both pulmonary and intestinal symptoms. As the larvae reach the lungs, the patient experiences cough, dyspnea, and low-grade fever. The intestinal phase is asymptomatic until large masses of worms are present. Vague upper abdominal pain, distention, and occasional vomiting may be present. Diagnosis is through identification of *Ascaris* eggs or worms in the feces. Occasionally, a worm is observed passing through the anus, mouth, or nose.

Pharmacotherapy for ascariasis is generally successful in eliminating the helminth from the body, without causing significant adverse effects. Oral mebendazole (Emverm) for 3 days is the standard treatment, with albendazole (Albenza) and ivermectin as alternative medications. Stools are rechecked 2 weeks after therapy is completed to confirm elimination of the roundworms. When possible, pregnant patients are treated after the first trimester to minimize risks to the fetus.

Enterobiasis: Infection by the pinworm *Enterobius vermicularis* is the most common helminth infection in the United States, afflicting as many as 40 million people, mostly children. The disease causes intense perineal itching due to the presence of deposited *Enterobius* eggs or migrating female worms. The itching is worse at night and may cause restlessness, enuresis, and insomnia. Diagnosis is by identification of eggs on the perianal skin or worms in the stool.

Transmission of *Enterobius* is by diapers, toys, hands, or food contaminated with the eggs. After ingestion, eggs hatch in the duodenum within 6 hours and worms mature in 2 weeks. Only 1 cm in size, adult worms infest the terminal ileum and colon. The female worm is either expelled during defecation or migrates to the perineum where 11,000 eggs per day

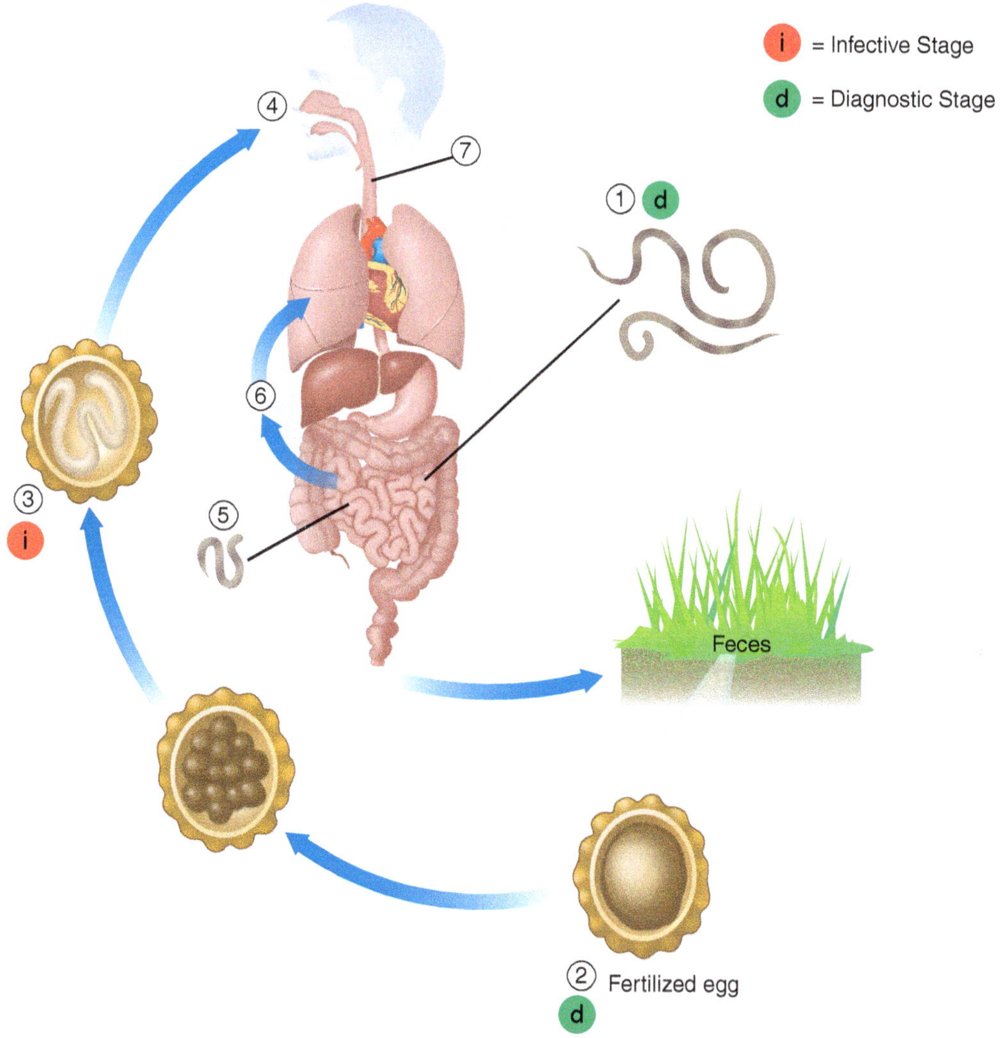

Figure 53.3 Lifecycle of *Ascaris*: Adult worms (1) live in the lumen of the small intestine. A female may produce as many as 240,000 eggs per day, which are passed with the feces (2). Fertile eggs become infective after 18 days to several weeks (3), depending on the environmental conditions (optimal: moist, warm, shaded soil). After infective eggs are swallowed (4), the larvae hatch (5), invade the intestinal mucosa, and are carried via circulation to the lungs (6). The larvae mature further in the lungs (10 to 14 days), ascend the bronchial tree to the throat, and are swallowed (7). Upon reaching the small intestine, they develop into adult worms.

may be released. After leaving the body, *Enterobius* eggs can remain infectious in the environment for up to 3 weeks. If proper hygiene is not observed, eggs deposited under the fingernails during scratching may be placed in the mouth, renewing the infectious cycle. Like ascariasis, enterobiasis is more common in children, due to the inattention to hand hygiene. Enterobiasis, however, does not cause mortality.

Pharmacotherapy of enterobiasis includes mebendazole (Emverm) or albendazole (Albenza). A single dose is usually sufficient to eradicate the pinworms, although the dose may be repeated in 2 weeks to maximize therapeutic success. Antipruritic ointments are available for topical application to the perianal region for symptomatic relief of pruritus. Asymptomatic infestation of other household members is frequent; therefore, it is prudent for all close contacts to receive antihelminthic treatment.

Hookworms: Two human hookworms, *Ancylostoma duodenale* and *Necator americanus*, infect 900 million people each year worldwide, usually in warm subtropical and tropical regions. Only about 1 cm in length, the adult hookworms live in the small intestine of the host. The female produces about 10,000 to 25,000 eggs per day, which are passed in the feces. Five days after exiting the body, hookworm eggs hatch and develop into an infective stage. The parasite is transmitted when an infective larva penetrates the skin, often that of a child walking barefoot through contaminated soil. Diagnosis of infestation is confirmed by identification of hookworm eggs in the feces.

The initial symptom of hookworm infection is an itchy rash called "ground itch" at the site of skin penetration. As larvae migrate through the host's blood, they travel to the lung and up to the throat, where they are swallowed and eventually end up in the small intestine. Pulmonary symptoms include cough, blood-tinged sputum, and low-grade fever. Later symptoms include vague abdominal pain, anorexia, and diarrhea.

The mouthparts of hookworms are modified cutting plates that cause hemorrhage when the worms attach to the intestinal mucosa to suck blood from the host. Children are particularly affected by the loss of blood. Although not directly fatal, hookworm infections can weaken the body by causing anemia and may cause death from infection by opportunistic pathogens.

The larvae of dog and cat hookworms can also infect humans, although they will not mature into adult worms in the human host. Transmitted to humans through contaminated soil or cat litter, these larvae remain in the skin where they migrate for many weeks and cause intense itching. This results in a condition known as *cutaneous larva migrans* or "creeping eruption."

Mebendazole (Emverm) and albendazole (Albenza) are preferred drugs for hookworm infections. Albendazole is given as a single dose; mebendazole therapy is generally for 3 days. Iron supplements and antianemic drugs may be necessary for patients who have lost an extensive amount of blood.

Tapeworms: Taeniasis is a parasitic infection caused by several species of tapeworms. Tapeworms are acquired when consuming raw or undercooked beef, pork, or fish. Some of the tapeworms reach enormous lengths; the beef tapeworm, *Taenia saginata*, grows to 25 meters (82 feet) and the pork tapeworm, *Taenia solum*, is 7 meters (23 feet).

Tapeworm infections may be asymptomatic or produce nonspecific symptoms such as nausea, diarrhea, hunger, fatigue, or abdominal pain. Larval cysts of *T. solium* can infect the brain, resulting in a disease called cysticercosis, which is a major cause of adult-onset seizures in low-income countries. Diagnosis of tapeworm infections is through identification of perianal eggs or by finding tapeworm eggs in a stool specimen.

The treatment of choice for most tapeworm infections is a single dose of praziquantel (Biltricide). For some infections, a laxative is given 2 hours after treatment to remove all parts of the worm and its eggs.

Other helminthic infections: Several other helminths cause significant disease worldwide in areas where sanitation is inadequate and food-handling techniques are poor. Drugs used to treat these infections are either the same as those described previously or are only available in other countries. Nurses traveling to these regions should consult medical sources for the most up-to-date pharmacotherapeutic information.

Drugs for Helminthic Infections

53.7 Antihelminthic drugs are usually successful in rapidly eliminating parasites and have few serious adverse effects.

Drugs used to treat worm infections are called *antihelminthics*. Pharmacotherapy is not indicated for all helminthic infections because some are self-limiting and the adult parasites die without reinfecting the host. When the infestation is severe or if complications occur, however, drug therapy is initiated. Complications caused by extensive infestations may include physical obstruction in the intestine, malabsorption, extensive loss of blood, increased risk for opportunistic bacterial infections, and severe fatigue. Pharmacotherapy is targeted at killing the parasites locally in the intestine and systemically in the tissues and organs they have invaded. Some antihelminthics have a broad spectrum and are effective against multiple species of worms, whereas others are indicated for a single species. Resistance is not a clinical problem with antihelminthics. Drugs for helminthic infections are listed in Table 53.4.

Because helminthic infections are often the result of poor sanitation or unhealthy hygiene habits, assessment of the patient's living conditions should be conducted. Often, all family members and close contacts of the patient should be treated in order to prevent reinfestation. Family teaching

Table 53.4 Drugs for Helminthic Infections

Drug	Route and Adult Dose (Maximum Dose Where Indicated)	Adverse Effects
albendazole (Albenza)	PO: 400 mg bid with meals (max: 800 mg/day)	*Abnormal liver function tests, abdominal pain, nausea and vomiting* Agranulocytosis, leukopenia
ivermectin (Sklice, Soolantra, Stromectol)	PO: 150–200 mcg/kg as a single dose	*Fever, pruritus, dizziness, arthralgia, lymphadenopathy* Acute allergic or inflammatory response
mebendazole (Emverm)	PO: 100 mg as a single dose or 100 mg bid for 3 days	*Abdominal pain, diarrhea, rash* Angioedema, convulsions, agranulocytosis, neutropenia
praziquantel (Biltricide)	PO: 5 mg/kg as a single dose or 25 mg/kg tid	*Headache, dizziness, malaise, fever, abdominal pain* Cerebrospinal reaction syndrome

Note: *Italics* indicate common adverse effects. Underline indicates serious adverse effects.

about ways to prevent reinfestation is essential to break the lifecycle of the parasite.

PROTOTYPE DRUG **Mebendazole (Emverm)**

Classification **Therapeutic:** Antihelminthic
Pharmacologic: Microtubule inhibitor

Therapeutic Effects and Uses: Mebendazole and albendazole belong to the same chemical family, known as the benzimidazoles. Although the two benzimidazoles have similar properties and spectrums of action, mebendazole is the most widely prescribed in the United States.

Approved in 1974, mebendazole is used in the treatment of a wide range of helminthic infections, including those caused by roundworm (ascariasis), pinworm (enterobiasis), and hookworm species. As a broad-spectrum drug it is particularly valuable in mixed helminthic infections, which are common in areas with poor sanitation. It is effective against both the adult and larval stages of these parasites. For pinworm infections, a single dose is taken, followed by a second dose in 2 weeks. Other helminthic infections require 3 consecutive days of therapy. It may be prescribed off-label for tapeworm infections.

Mebendazole is poorly absorbed after PO administration, which allows it to maintain high concentrations in the intestine without causing systemic adverse effects.

Mechanism of Action: Mebendazole kills helminths by several biochemical mechanisms, including inhibition of glucose transport and uncoupling of energy metabolism in the parasite's mitochondria. The drug binds to β-tubulin and is thought to disrupt the microtubular network in parasitic cells.

Pharmacokinetics:

Route(s)	PO
Absorption	Poorly absorbed
Distribution	Very little reaches the systemic circulation; 95% bound to plasma proteins
Primary metabolism	Hepatic
Primary excretion	Feces
Onset of action	Rapid
Duration of action	Half-life: 3–9 h

Adverse Effects: Because so little of the drug is absorbed, mebendazole does not cause serious systemic adverse effects. As the worms die, some abdominal pain, distention, and diarrhea may be experienced. Rare cases of seizures, agranulocytosis, neutropenia, and angioedema have been reported.

Contraindications/Precautions: Other than hypersensitivity, there are no contraindications for mebendazole. Because it is metabolized by the liver, patients with serious hepatic impairment should be monitored carefully. The drug is a potent teratogen in laboratory animals and should be avoided during pregnancy, especially the first trimester. Use in children under 2 years of age is not advised.

Drug Interactions: Carbamazepine and phenytoin can increase the metabolism of mebendazole, although dosage adjustment is not required because so little mebendazole is absorbed.

Pregnancy: Animal studies showed embryofetal toxicity. Human experience has not shown evidence of fetal harm. Small amounts of this drug are secreted in human milk, although adverse effects on the breastfed neonate are unknown.

Treatment of Overdose: No specific therapy is available; patients are treated symptomatically.

Clinician Responsibilities: Key clinical implications for patients receiving mebendazole are included in Applied Clinical Judgment: Patients Receiving Pharmacotherapy for Protozoan and Helminthic Infections.

Drugs Similar to Mebendazole (Emverm)

Other selected drugs for helminthic infections include albendazole, ivermectin, and praziquantel. Bithionol (Bitin) is an antihelminthic available from the CDC for treating *Fasciola hepatica* (a liver fluke). Also available through the CDC, diethylcarbamazine (Hetrazan) is only used to treat helminthic infections known as lymphatic filariasis, which are caused by various species of threadlike worms found in tropical climates. Pyrantel has been discontinued in the United States,

Albendazole (Albenza): Approved in 1996, albendazole belongs to the same chemical class as mebendazole. It is incompletely absorbed when given PO, although enough of the drug is distributed to kill parasitic cysts in some tissues. It is a first-line drug for larval forms of the beef tapeworm *T. solium* and for hydatid cysts in the liver that form following infection by the dog tapeworm *Echinococcus granulosus*. It is often prescribed off-label for other helminthic infections. Albendazole is well tolerated and exhibits few adverse effects. The most common adverse effect is a transient increase in serum aminotransferase activity caused by its effects on liver function. Albendazole is embryotoxic and teratogenic in laboratory animals. Effective contraception is advised during therapy and at least 3 days after the last dose. This drug is secreted in human milk, although adverse effects on the breastfed neonate are unknown.

Ivermectin (Stromectol): Approved in 1996, ivermectin has become a mainstay in the pharmacotherapy of several helminthic infections due to its superior safety profile and single-dose efficacy. It is a preferred drug for treating onchocerciasis or "river blindness," an especially debilitating filarial infection in Africa, Latin America, and the Middle East. Annual doses have caused a significant reduction of this disease in endemic areas. It is used (off-label) for the therapy of *cutaneous larva migrans*, or "creeping eruption." Because of its wide spectrum of action, it is of great importance in treating mixed helminthic infections. Two topical formulations include Sklice for lice infestation and Soolantra for the inflammatory lesions of rosacea. Adverse effects are minor and include fever, rash, and pruritus resulting from allergic and inflammatory reactions to the death of the parasites. In animal studies, oral ivermectin caused fetal harm. Because small amounts are secreted in human milk, breastfeeding is not recommended. Topical solutions have not been examined for adverse effects on pregnancy.

Praziquantel (Biltricide): Approved in 1982, praziquantel is a broad-spectrum antihelminthic for schistosomiasis, a helminthic infection caused by blood flukes that affects 200 million people worldwide. People acquire the parasite by bathing or swimming in fecally contaminated water. Although not found in the United States, the parasite is endemic to tropical regions across the globe, causing chronic ill health. Praziquantel is also approved for Chinese liver fluke infections and is prescribed worldwide for other helminthic infections. It is a safe medication, with dizziness, headache, and abdominal pain being the most common adverse effects. Human studies showed no evidence of fetal harm above baseline level. Because this drug is secreted in human milk, breastfeeding should be done with caution.

CONNECTIONS: APPLIED CLINICAL JUDGMENT

Patients Receiving Pharmacotherapy for Protozoan and Helminthic Infections

Key Assessment Data

- History of current condition, baseline vital signs, physical exam findings; hepatic, renal, cardiovascular, neurologic, hematologic, or respiratory disease; pregnancy or breastfeeding. Obtain a drug history and assess signs and symptoms of the current infection, noting location, characteristics, presence or absence and the character of drainage, duration, and the presence or absence of fever or pain.
- Obtain a travel history, noting dates of travel and when current symptoms started in relation to travel (i.e., before, during, or after travel). Assess signs and symptoms of current infection and assess family members or others living in the home.

Desired Therapeutic Outcomes

Improvement is observed and measurable by reduction in diarrhea, chills, fever, muscle pain which should begin after taking the first dose and continue to improve throughout the course of antibiotic therapy.

Minimizing Adverse Effects

- Continued fever may be a sign of worsening infection, adverse drug effects, or antibiotic resistance. Immediately report undiminished fever, changes in level of consciousness (LOC), or febrile seizures.
- Anaphylactic reactions are possible, particularly with the first dose of the drug. As parasites die, increasing diarrhea, abdominal pain, or chills may occur.
- Periodic vision and retinal screening is required with chloroquine therapy because the drug can cause irreversible damage to the retina.
- Some antimalarials may cause dysrhythmias and hypotension. Periodic ECG monitoring may be required.
- Alcohol use, especially in patients on metronidazole, may cause a disulfiram-like reaction with excessive nausea and vomiting and possible hypotension.
- Bone marrow suppression is an adverse effect and may cause blood dyscrasias with resulting decreases in RBCs, WBCs, or platelets. Periodic monitoring of CBC may be required.
- Sexually transmitted infections may be reintroduced by an untreated sexual partner. Assess the patient's sexual partners for infection and treat current partners to avoid reinfection.
- Families with young children should practice scrupulous hand hygiene and proper disposal of diapers and notify daycare or childcare providers of the infection. Assess family pets that may carry infection and also require treatment.

Lifespan Considerations

- Age-related physiologic differences may place the older adult at greater risk for hepatotoxicity or nephrotoxicity.

Patient Education

- Report a fever that does not diminish below 37.8°C (100°F) within 3 days, increasing signs and symptoms of infection, or symptoms that remain after taking the entire course of drug therapy.
- Immediately report any itching, rashes, swelling (particularly of tongue or face), urticaria, flushing, dizziness, syncope, wheezing, throat tightness, or difficulty breathing.
- Increase overall fluid intake. Report any diminished urine output, weight gain of more than 1 kg (2 lb) in a 24-hour period. Avoid or eliminate alcohol use.
- Immediately report any severe nausea and vomiting, yellowing of the skin or sclera, abdominal pain, light- or clay-colored stools, diminished urine output, or darkening of urine.
- Report any low-grade fevers, sore throat, rashes, bruising or increased bleeding, or unusual fatigue or shortness of breath, especially after taking drug therapy for a prolonged period.
- Immediately contact the provider if blurring, difficulty focusing, or photophobia is severe, continues, or worsens.
- Immediately report increasing headache, dizziness, drowsiness, changes in behavior, LOC, or seizures. If dizziness occurs, sit or lie down and do not attempt to stand or walk until the sensation passes.
- Veterinary assessment of family pets, even if asymptomatic, may be required to avoid reinfection.
- Appropriate self-administration includes:
  - Complete the entire course of therapy unless otherwise instructed. Do not share with other family members, and do not stop the medicine when starting to feel better.
  - Take the drug with food but avoid alcohol or acidic beverages. If the drug is to be taken on an empty stomach, take with a full glass of water.
  - Increase overall fluid intake while taking the drug.

CONNECTIONS: APPLIED CLINICAL JUDGMENT *(continued)*

Patients Receiving Pharmacotherapy for Protozoan and Helminthic Infections

Prescribing Considerations

- Ongoing assessment during drug therapy should include monitoring appropriate laboratory findings (e.g., CBC, fecal ova and parasites, hepatic and renal laboratory values).
- Periodic culture and sensitivity or fecal ova and parasite tests may be needed if infections are severe or are slow to resolve to confirm appropriate therapy.

Understanding Chapter 53

Key Concepts Summary

53.1 Protozoa are diverse, single-celled organisms that can cause widespread disease.

53.2 The female *Anopheles* mosquito is the carrier of several species of *Plasmodium*, the parasite responsible for malaria.

53.3 The three goals of malaria pharmacotherapy are chemoprophylaxis, treatment of acute attacks, and prevention of relapses.

53.4 Amebiasis, giardiasis, and cryptosporidiosis are caused by intestinal parasites and are usually acquired through contaminated water or food.

53.5 Other protozoan infections that can cause significant disease include toxoplasmosis, trichomoniasis, trypanosomiasis, and leishmaniasis.

53.6 Helminthic infections cause significant intestinal disease, particularly in areas with poor sanitation.

53.7 Antihelminthic drugs are usually successful in rapidly eliminating parasites and have few serious adverse effects.

CASE STUDY: Making the Patient Connection

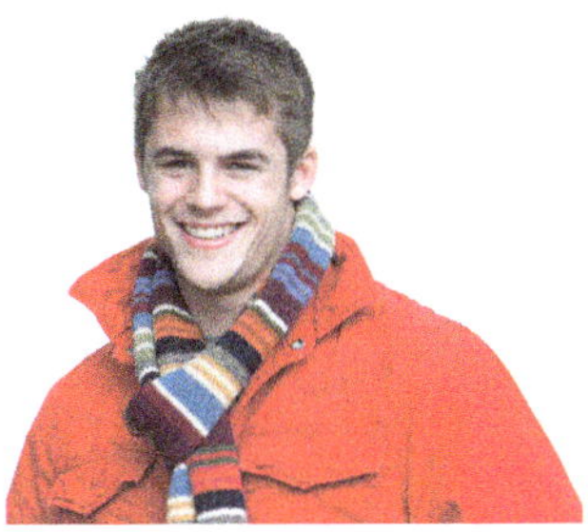

Remember the patient "Trevor Skales" at the beginning of the chapter? Now read the remainder of the case study. Based on the information presented within this chapter, respond to the critical thinking questions that follow.

Trevor Skales is a 23-year-old man with an upcoming month-long eco tour vacation planned to a rain forest in South America. He has been planning and researching this trip since he graduated from college and will be leaving in 3 weeks with two college friends. He knows about the possible endemic diseases in the area including tuberculosis, dengue fever, leishmaniasis, leprosy, and malaria. He discusses the trip with his healthcare provider who determines that malaria carries the biggest threat for transmission during Trevor's vacation.

Trevor has had a complete physical examination and is up to date on all required vaccinations. His provider has also screened for the possibility of a G6PD deficiency, and he has had a thorough eye examination. The provider has ordered chloroquine (Aralen) for Trevor. He is to begin taking it 2 weeks before his trip, every week throughout his trip, and for 1 month after returning home.

Critical Thinking Questions

1. Why was chloroquine ordered for Trevor before he has started his trip?
2. Why are special screening for G6PD deficiency and an eye examination important?
3. Trevor asks why he needs to continue to take the chloroquine after he returns home. As his nurse, what would you teach him about the drug dosing schedule and about symptoms to watch for?
4. What adverse effects are associated with chloroquine therapy?

Additional Case Study

Mary Porter is a 19-year-old woman who visits the local clinic with malodorous vaginal discharge, accompanied by vulvar pruritus. She also reports dysuria and discomfort during sexual intercourse. Mary is diagnosed with trichomoniasis and started on metronidazole (Flagyl).

1. Why are female patients more likely to contract trichomoniasis?
2. What health teaching would you provide to the patient who is being treated for trichomoniasis?
3. Develop a list of adverse effects this patient may experience while taking metronidazole.

Chapter Review

1. The patient is taking atovaquone-proguanil (Malarone) prophylactically before traveling to a developing country and asks the nurse how long the drug will need to be taken after returning from the trip. Which response from the nurse would be correct?

1. Recommended for 7 days after returning from the malaria-infested location.
2. Not necessary after leaving the location.
3. Suggested for 3 days after returning from the trip.
4. Optional unless the patient reports symptoms of malaria.

2. A patient has been started on hydroxychloroquine (Plaquenil) for prevention of malaria on an overseas trip. In addition to the prevention and treatment of malaria, hydroxychloroquine is also indicated for what other conditions? (Select all that apply.)

1. Systemic lupus erythematosus
2. Roundworm infections
3. Urinary tract infections
4. Rheumatoid arthritis
5. Leishmaniasis infections

3. A patient is being treated with metronidazole (Flagyl) for *Giardia lamblia* infection. When instructing the patient about this drug, the nurse should caution about the possibility of which adverse reaction?

1. Flatus and intestinal bloating
2. Halitosis
3. Unpleasant metallic taste
4. Alopecia

4. The patient is diagnosed with toxoplasmosis and will be treated with pyrimethamine (Daraprim). Because of significant adverse effects, what teaching should the nurse give this patient?

1. Increase intake of fiber-rich foods to prevent constipation.
2. Report unusual bruising, fatigue, sores that do not heal, or low-grade fever.
3. Increase fluid intake to 3 L per day.
4. Schedule eye examinations every 6 months for 2 years after taking this drug.

5. A 6-year-old boy is diagnosed with an *Enterobius vermicularis* (pinworm) infection and has been prescribed mebendazole (Emverm). What appropriate instructions should the nurse give the boy's caregiver?

1. The drug will be continued for 2 weeks and then a stool sample will be retested.
2. Because the infection is not easily transmitted, it is not necessary to test or treat family members.
3. Eliminate all citrus and dairy products while this medication is taken.
4. Wash all bedding and undergarments thoroughly after the medication is given.

6. A nurse is monitoring a patient receiving metronidazole (Flagyl) for potential adverse effects. Which symptom, if present, would cause the nurse to discontinue the medication and notify the prescriber?

1. Ataxia and confusion
2. Nausea and diarrhea
3. Anorexia and thirst
4. Weight gain and irritability

See Appendix A for answers to critical thinking questions, case study questions and review questions.

References

Centers for Disease Control and Prevention (CDC). (2019). *Malaria information and prophylaxis by country*. https://www.cdc.gov/malaria/travelers/country_table/a.html

Cope, J. R., Kahler, A. M., Causey, J., Williams, J. G., Kihlken, J., Benjamin, C., et al. (2019). Response and remediation actions following the detection of Naegleria fowleri in two treated drinking water distribution systems, Louisiana 2013–2014. *Journal of Water and Health*, *17*, 777–787. https://doi.org/10.2166/wh.2019.239

Dhawan, V. K. (2019). *Amebiasis*. Medscape. https://emedicine.medscape.com/article/212029-overview

Mayo Clinic (2020). *Naegleri infection*. https://www.mayoclinic.org/diseases-conditions/naegleria-infection/symptoms-causes/syc-20375470

World Health Organization. (2020). *Malaria: Key facts*. https://www.who.int/news-room/fact-sheets/detail/malaria

Selected Bibliography

Antczak, M., Dzitko, K., & Długońska, H. (2016). Human toxoplasmosis—searching for novel chemotherapeutics. *Biomedicine & Pharmacotherapy*, *82*, 677–684. doi.10.1016/j.biopha.2016.05.041

Centers for Disease Control and Prevention (CDC). (2018). *Parasites—neglected parasitic infections (NPIs)*. http://www.cdc.gov/parasites/npi/index.html

Centers for Disease Control and Prevention (CDC). (2020). *Malaria treatment: Guidelines for clinicians*. https://www.cdc.gov/malaria/diagnosis_treatment/clinicians1.html

Chakravarty, J., & Sundar, S. (2019). Current and emerging medications for the treatment of leishmaniasis. *Expert Opinion on Pharmacotherapy*, *20*(10), 1251–1265. https://doi.org/10.1080/14656566.2019.1609940

Defendi, G. L. (2016). *Trypanosomiasis*. Medscape. http://emedicine.medscape.com/article/ 1000389-overview

Dora-Laskey, A. (2019). *Ascaris lumbricoides*. Medscape. http://emedicine.medscape.com/article/788398-overview

Herchline, T.E. (2020). *Malaria medication*. Medscape. https://emedicine.medscape.com/article/221134-medication#showall

Holla, S. N., Kishore, M. K. K., & Amberkar, M. B. (2016). Pharmacotherapy of opportunistic infections in HIV patients: A review. *Journal of Applied Pharmaceutical Science*, *6*, 227–236. https://doi.org/10.7324/JAPS.2016.60934

John, C. C. (2020). Treatment of severe malaria in the United States. *Annals of Internal Medicine*, *172*(3), 224–225. https://doi.org/10.7326/L19-0674

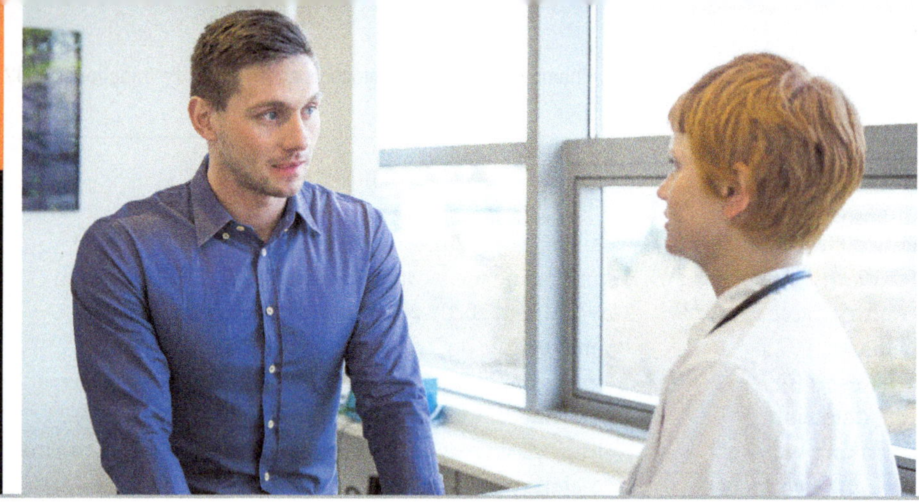

"The cold sores are painful and embarrassing. Is there any medication I can take to prevent them from returning?"
—*Patient "Richard Palmer"*

Chapter 54
Pharmacotherapy of Non-HIV Viral Infections

Chapter Outline

Learning Outcomes

After reading this chapter, the student should be able to:

1. Describe the major structural components of viruses.
2. Identify viral infections that benefit from pharmacotherapy.
3. Explain the five principal stages in the pathogenesis of a viral infection.
4. Explain general principles related to the pharmacotherapy of viral infections.
5. Describe the nurse's role in the pharmacologic management of patients receiving medications for herpesviruses, influenza viruses, hepatitis viruses, and coronavirus-19.
6. For each of the classes shown in the chapter outline, identify the prototype and representative drugs and explain the mechanism(s) of drug action, primary indications, contraindications, significant drug interactions, pregnancy data, and important adverse effects.
7. Apply clinical judgment to care for patients receiving pharmacotherapy for viral infections.

Key Terms

Definitions of the terms in bold may be found in the Glossary.

Viruses are tiny infectious agents capable of causing disease in humans and other organisms. Because they possess only a few simple molecules, viruses use host enzymes and cellular mechanisms to replicate. Although the number of antiviral drugs has increased dramatically in recent years due to research into acquired immunodeficiency syndrome (AIDS), antiviral drugs remain the least effective of all the anti-infective classes. This chapter examines the pharmacotherapy of non–human immunodeficiency virus (HIV) viral infections, including herpesviruses, influenza viruses, and hepatitis viruses. Drugs for HIV infection are presented in Chapter 55.

Characteristics of Viruses

54.1 Viruses are infectious agents with simple structures.

Viruses are nonliving agents that do not contain any of the cellular organelles necessary for self-survival that are present in living organisms. Viruses infect bacteria, plants, and animals by entering a host cell and then using the enzymes inside that cell to replicate. Thus, viruses are **intracellular parasites**: They must be inside a host cell to cause infection. A mature infective virus particle is called a **virion**. Figure 54.1 shows the basic structure of a virus.

The structure of viruses is quite primitive, compared to even the simplest bacterial cell. The virus is surrounded by a protein coat or **capsid**, which helps to protect it from the surrounding environment. The structural proteins or glycoproteins that comprise the capsid are arranged in distinct, repeating subunits. These proteins help the virus attach to the cell membrane of its host.

All viruses contain genes, which carry the genetic information needed for viral replication, either in the form of ribonucleic acid (RNA) or deoxyribonucleic acid (DNA). Most possess only a few dozen genes.

Some viruses have an envelope surrounding the capsid and genetic material. The viral envelope consists of phospholipids, glycoprotein, and protein "spikes." The phospholipids are actually derived from the host cell membrane as the virus buds off the host cell. The protein spikes are entirely viral in nature. Recognized as foreign by the host's immune system, viral proteins trigger body defenses that attempt to remove the invader.

Although the host cell supplies most of the metabolic machinery needed by the virus, virions contain a few enzymes that serve key roles in the infection process. These enzymes are virus specific and assist the pathogen in entering the host cell, duplicating its genetic material, inserting its genes into the host's chromosome, or assembling newly formed virions. These unique viral enzymes serve as important targets for antiviral drug action.

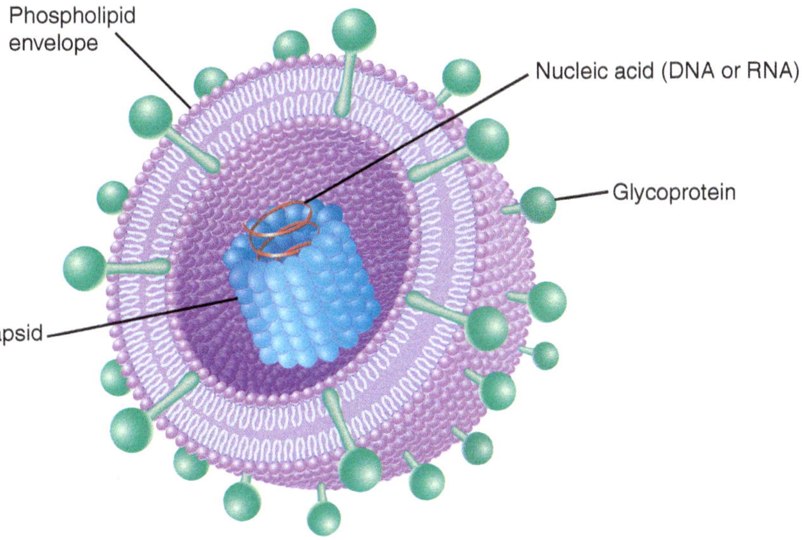

Figure 54.1 General structure of a virus.

54.2 The replication cycle of a virus occurs in five stages.

Despite their simple structures, viruses are diverse, each having a distinct spectrum of infection. Although some viruses are lethal, others can coexist with their host and produce no detectable symptoms. Only a handful of viruses cause significant disease in humans. Selected human pathogenic viruses are listed in Table 54.1. Not all viral infections warrant pharmacotherapy. Viruses that may be treated with antiviral medications include herpes simplex, cytomegalovirus, Epstein-Barr, varicella zoster, respiratory syncytial virus, and hepatitis.

Despite their diversity, certain stages are common to most viral infections, as shown in Figure 54.2. The first stage is attachment of the virus to its host cell. In this stage, the proteins on the surface of the virion fuse with protein receptors on the host cell. This attachment is very specific; the "attachment receptor" may be found only in a single species of plant, bacteria, or animal, or even on a single type of cell within an organism. This specificity is why most viruses infect only one species, although a few viruses can mutate and cross species, as is likely the case for HIV.

The second stage of viral infection is penetration of the viral genes and enzymes into the host cell. For some viruses, the entire virion enters the cell, whereas others simply "inject" their genes and enzymes into the host cell.

The third stage is synthesis of viral nucleic acid and proteins by the host cell. Immediately after penetration, a few viral

Table 54.1 Selected Human Viral Diseases

	Virus	Description
DNA viruses	Adenoviruses 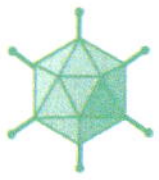	More than 40 species that primarily infect the human upper respiratory tract but can also cause conjunctivitis, gastrointestinal (GI) infections, hemorrhagic cystitis, and serious infections in neonates
	Hepadnaviruses 	Family of viruses that causes hepatitis B by invading hepatocytes; primarily transmitted by injection of infected blood or by use of contaminated needles
	Herpesviruses 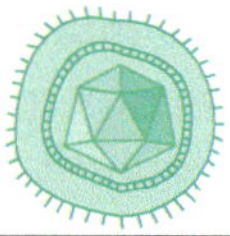	Family of viruses that causes cold sores, genital herpes, infectious mononucleosis, chickenpox, and shingles
	Papovaviruses 	Family of viruses that can cause tumors or warts
	Poxvirus 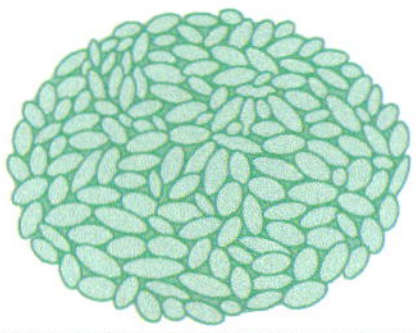	Responsible for smallpox, monkeypox, and molluscum contagiosum (a sexually transmitted infection)
RNA viruses	Arenaviruses 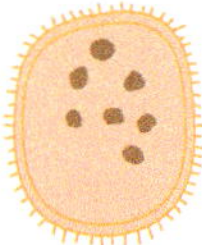	Family of 15 viruses, one of which causes Lassa fever, a severe form of epidemic hemorrhagic fever that is highly fatal
	Coronaviruses 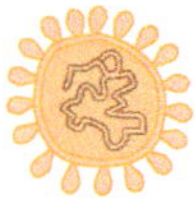	Family of viruses, some of which cause upper respiratory tract infections that can range from mild to lethal
	Myxoviruses and paramyxoviruses 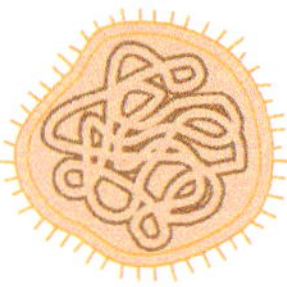	Family of viruses that includes the influenza virus, respiratory syncytial virus, measles virus, and mumps virus
	Orthomyxoviruses 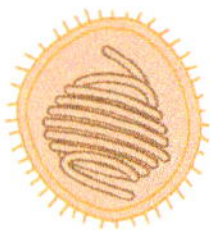	Responsible for human influenza and avian (bird) flu
	Picornaviruses 	Large family of viruses that can cause hepatitis A, polio, common cold, meningitis, and myocarditis
	Reoviruses 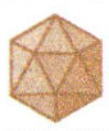	Large family of viruses that can cause upper respiratory symptoms and gastroenteritis in infants
	Retroviruses 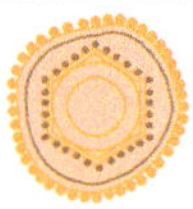	Virus family that includes HIV, the virus responsible for AIDS

proteins are constructed, which assist in duplication of the viral DNA or RNA. Following duplication of the viral genetic material, two possible events may occur. The virus may immediately begin replicating itself by making viral capsid proteins and viral enzymes and then assembling more virions. In some cases, however, the viral DNA enters the nucleus of the host cell, where it inserts into the chromosome and remains for a period of time ranging from weeks to years before it proceeds to the replication stage. Once the viral DNA integrates into the host chromosome, it is called a **provirus**.

Assembly is the fourth stage of viral infection. All the viral components, structural proteins, enzymes, and nucleic acids are packaged and made ready for leaving the cell.

The final stage is the release of virions from the host cell. The number of virions may be so large that the cell bursts, releasing all the infectious particles at one time, killing the cell. In other cases, the virions bud off the host's plasma membrane in a slower, continuous process that does not result in death of the host cell.

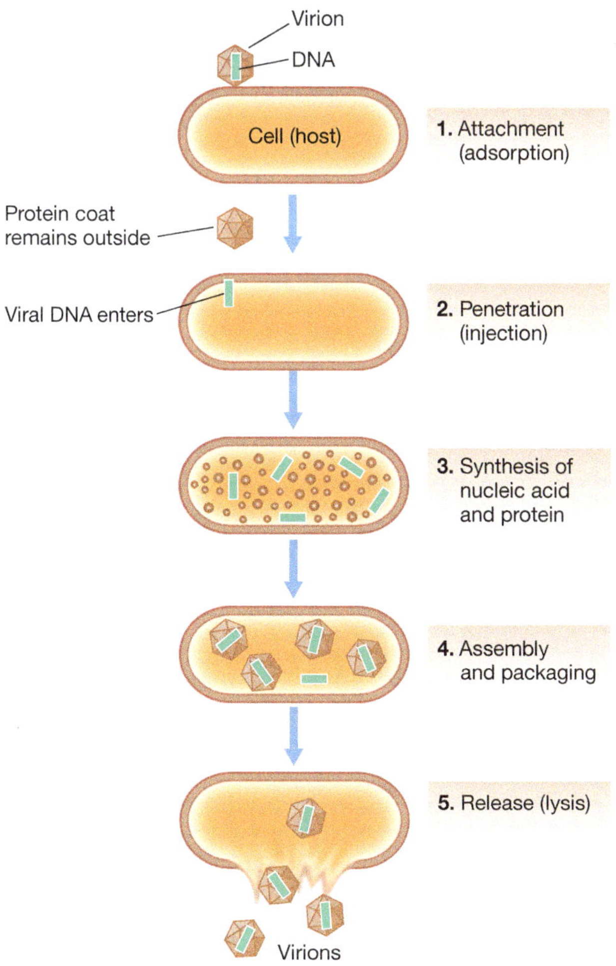

Figure 54.2 The five stages of viral infection.

From Madigan and Martinko (2006). Reprinted and electronically reproduced by permission of Pearson Education, Inc., Upper Saddle River, NJ.

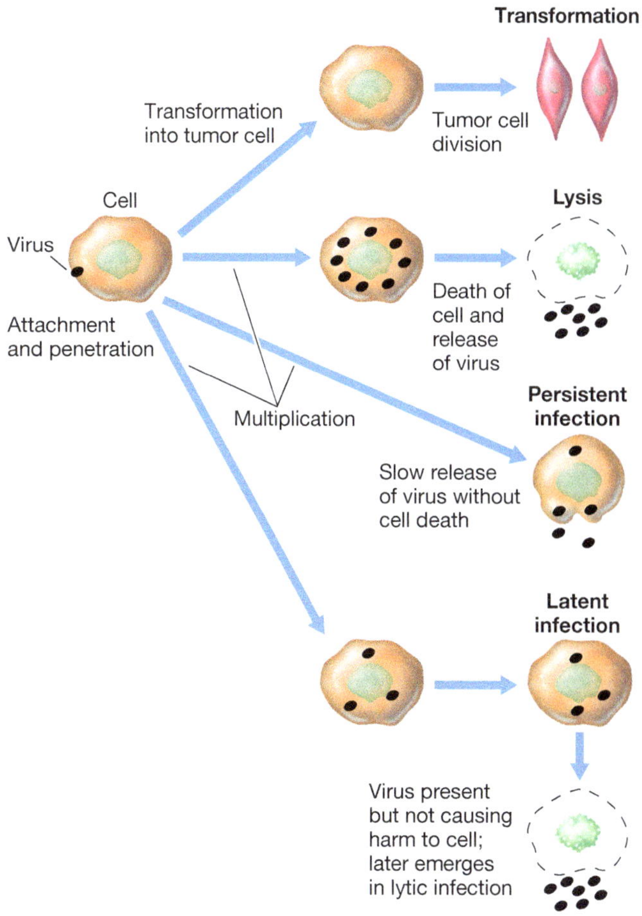

Figure 54.3 Effects of viruses on their host cells.

From Madigan and Martinko (2006). Reprinted and electronically reproduced by permission of Pearson Education, Inc., Upper Saddle River, NJ.

Pharmacotherapy of Non-HIV Viral Infections

54.3 Antiviral drugs target a specific viral structure or stage of its replication cycle.

Viruses can produce significant effects on their host cells, as illustrated in Figure 54.3. Some viral infections, such as the common cold, cause acute symptoms but they are self-limiting. While symptoms may be annoying, they resolve in 7 to 10 days and the virus causes no permanent effects if the patient is otherwise healthy. For these viral infections, medication is not warranted due to the expense and the possibility of producing adverse drug effects.

Some viral infections are not self-limiting, and drug therapy can be used to prevent the infection or alleviate symptoms. For example, HIV is uniformly fatal if left untreated. Certain hepatitis viruses can result in permanent liver damage and increase a patient's risk of hepatocellular carcinoma. Although not life-threatening in most patients, herpesviruses can cause significant pain and, in the case of ocular herpes, permanent disability. Some viruses may even transform normal cells into tumor cells.

Antiviral therapy is targeted to a specific structure of the virus or an aspect of its replication cycle. For example, antiviral drugs are available that inhibit specific viral enzymes or change the shape of proteins that can prevent attachment to the host cell.

Another approach to treating viral infections is to boost the immune system's response to viral antigens. Prevention of some viral infections can be accomplished through vaccines, which prepare body defenses in advance of the infection (see Chapter 43). Treatment of acute disease may utilize immunomodulators such as interferons (IFNs) that enhance aspects of the immune response. These are of particular value in treating hepatitis (see Section 54.6).

Antiviral pharmacotherapy can be extremely challenging due to the rapid mutation rates of viruses, which can quickly render medications ineffective. Also complicating therapy is the intracellular nature of the virus, which makes it difficult for drugs to find their targets without giving excessively high doses that injure normal cells. Antiviral drugs have narrow spectrums of activity, usually limited

CONNECTIONS: Patient Safety

Adverse Reaction to Vaccination

A 62-year-old woman receives a shingles vaccine (Zostavax). Two weeks later, a severe blistering rash develops along the patient's anterior chest wall. The patient also reports having a headache and flulike symptoms, but no fever. On examination, the lesions are confirmed to be herpes zoster and drug therapy with acyclovir (Zovirax) is initiated.

What is a potential cause for the occurrence of herpes zoster after receiving the shingles vaccine? What could the healthcare provider have done differently to prevent such an occurrence?

to one specific virus. For most of the viral pathogens, pharmacologic cures are not possible; thus, antivirals remain the least effective of all the anti-infective classes.

Drugs for Herpesviruses

54.4 Pharmacotherapy can lessen the severity of acute herpes simplex infections and prolong latency.

Herpes simplex viruses (HSVs) are a family of DNA viruses that cause blister-like lesions on the skin, genitals, and mucous membranes. Herpesviruses are usually acquired through direct physical contact with an infected individual, but they can also be transmitted from infected mothers to their newborns, sometimes resulting in severe central nervous system (CNS) disease. Neonatal herpes infection is estimated to have a mortality rate of 50%. The herpesvirus family includes the following:

- **HSV type 1 (HSV-1).** Primarily infections of the eye and mouth and lip "cold sores," although it may also cause genital infections
- **HSV type 2 (HSV-2).** Primarily genital infections
- **Cytomegalovirus (CMV).** Affects multiple body systems in immunosuppressed patients
- **Varicella-zoster virus (VZV).** Shingles (zoster) and chickenpox (varicella)
- **Epstein-Barr virus (EBV).** Infectious mononucleosis and a form of cancer known as Burkitt's lymphoma
- **Herpesvirus type 6.** Roseola in children and hepatitis or encephalitis in immunosuppressed patients.

Humans are believed to be the only reservoir for HSV. Following its initial entrance into the human host, HSV may remain in a latent, asymptomatic, nonreplicating state in sensory or autonomic nerve root ganglia for many years. Infection is lifelong. Immunosuppression, physical challenge, or emotional stress can promote active replication of the virus and the reappearance of the characteristic lesions. Complications include secondary infections of nongenital tissues.

The pharmacologic goals for the management of herpes infections are twofold: to relieve acute symptoms and to prevent recurrences. Note that the antiviral drugs used to treat herpesvirus do not cure the patient; the virus remains inside infected neurons for the remainder of the patient's life.

Treatment of acute herpesvirus infection: Pharmacotherapy of initial acute HSV-1 and HSV-2 infections includes 7 to 10 days of oral antiviral therapy. Commonly prescribed antivirals for HSV and VZV include acyclovir (Zovirax), famciclovir, and valacyclovir (Valtrex). Topical forms of several antivirals are available for local application to herpes lesions, although they are not as effective as the oral medications. In immunocompromised patients, intravenous (IV) medications may be indicated; however, these drugs have a higher risk of serious adverse effects. Antiviral drugs for HSV infections are listed in Table 54.2.

PharmFACT

In the United States about one out of six people age 14 to 49 are infected with genital herpes. This rate has remained stable during the past decade (Centers for Disease Control and Prevention [CDC], 2017a).

Because of the severity of neonatal herpes infections, pregnant women with the infection are sometimes treated with antivirals. The most extensive clinical experience during pregnancy has been with acyclovir, which has not been associated with teratogenic effects. The safety and effectiveness of these drugs during pregnancy, however, have not been clearly established. The greatest risk for transmission of HSV occurs when the mother acquires the infection late in the pregnancy.

Herpes of the eye is the most common infectious cause of corneal blindness in the United States. Ocular herpes causes a painful, inflamed lesion on the eyelid or surface of the eye. Prompt treatment with antiviral drugs can stop the herpesvirus from multiplying and destroying epithelial cells. Like genital herpes, once patients acquire ocular herpes, they often experience recurrences, which may occur years after the initial symptoms.

Pharmacotherapy of ocular herpes is through the local application of drops or ointment. The goal of therapy is to prevent permanent visual disability by limiting corneal involvement of the infection. Trifluridine (Viroptic) and ganciclovir (Zirgan) are available in ophthalmic formulations. Eyedrops containing steroids may be used concurrently with the antiviral to reduce inflammation. Oral acyclovir is used in situations where topical drops or ointments are contraindicated. Uncomplicated ocular herpes resolves after 1 to 2 weeks of pharmacotherapy.

Prophylaxis of herpesvirus infection: Due to the expense and potential adverse effects, antiviral drugs are

Table 54.2 Drugs for Herpesvirus Infections

Drug	Route and Adult Dose (Maximum Dose Where Indicated)	Adverse Effects
Systemic Drugs		
acyclovir (Zovirax)	Initial episode: PO: 200 mg q4h for 10 days or 400 tid for 5–10 days Mild HSV labialis (cold sore or fever blister) or mild genital or perirectal HSV: PO: 400 tid for 7 days Severe genital or perirectal HSV: IV: 5–10 mg/kg q8h for 7–14 days	*Nausea and vomiting, diarrhea, headache, pain, inflammation at injection sites (parenteral drugs)* Thrombocytopenic purpura or hemolytic uremic syndrome, nephrotoxicity, seizures (foscarnet), electrolyte imbalances (foscarnet), hematologic toxicity or bone marrow suppression (ganciclovir, valganciclovir), neutropenia (cidofovir)
cidofovir	IV: 5 mg/kg once weekly for 2 wk	
famciclovir	PO: 500 mg tid for 7 days (max: 1500 mg/day)	
foscarnet (Foscavir)	IV: 40–60 mg/kg infused over 1–2 h tid (max: 180 mg/kg/day)	
ganciclovir (Cytovene, Zirgan)	IV: 5 mg/kg infused over 1 h bid (max: 6 mg/kg/dose) PO: 1000 mg tid (max: 3000 mg/day) Topical (Zirgan): 1 drop in the affected eye 3–5 times/day	
valacyclovir (Valtrex)	PO: 1 g tid (max: 3 g/day)	
valganciclovir (Valcyte)	PO: 900 mg once daily (max: 900 mg/day; 1800 mg/day during CMV retinitis induction therapy)	
Topical Drugs		
docosanol (Abreva)	Topical: 10% cream applied to cold sore up to 5 times/day for 10 days	*Burning, irritation, or stinging at site of application, headache* Photophobia, keratopathy, edema of eyelids (ocular drugs)
penciclovir (Denavir)	Topical: Apply q2h while awake for 4 days	
trifluridine (Viroptic)	Topical: 1 drop in each eye q2h during waking hours (max: 9 drops/day)	

Note: *Italics* indicate common adverse effects. Underline indicates serious adverse effects.

not routinely prescribed for prophylaxis. However, patients who experience particularly severe or frequent recurrences (more than six episodes per year) may receive low doses of prophylactic antivirals. Chronic suppressive therapy may also benefit immunocompromised patients, such as those undergoing antineoplastic therapy or those with AIDS.

CONNECTION Checkpoint 54.1

From what you learned in Chapter 3 about the pharmacokinetics of topical drugs, why are topical medications not as effective as oral drugs in the case of herpes infections?

PROTOTYPE DRUG Acyclovir (Zovirax)

Classification **Therapeutic:** Antiviral for herpesviruses
Pharmacologic: Nucleoside (deoxyguanosine) analog

Therapeutic Effects and Uses: Approved by the U.S. Food and Drug Administration (FDA) in 1982 as one of the first antiviral medications, the activity of acyclovir is limited to the herpesviruses, for which it is a preferred drug. It is most effective against HSV-1 and HSV-2 and effective only at high doses against CMV and VZV. Acyclovir has no activity against HIV.

Acyclovir decreases the duration and severity of acute herpes symptoms. When given for prophylaxis, it decreases the frequency of herpes recurrences, but it does not completely eradicate the virus from the body. It is available in topical form for placing directly on active lesions, in oral (PO) form for prophylaxis, and in an IV form for severe conditions such as herpes simplex encephalitis. Because of its 2.5- to 5-hour half-life, acyclovir is sometimes administered PO up to five times a day. PO formulations include capsule, tablet, and oral suspension. A 5% ointment is available for application to cold sores.

Mechanism of Action: Acyclovir is a nucleoside analog that inhibits viral replication by affecting two viral enzymes. First, it enters the host cell where it is activated by a viral enzyme known as thymidine kinase. The activated drug molecule resembles dGTP, one of the building blocks for DNA. As the virus begins to construct its DNA, it uses acyclovir, rather than dGTP. Once the acyclovir is inserted into the growing DNA chain, viral DNA synthesis is terminated, thus stopping the replication cycle of the virus. Simply stated, acyclovir acts by preventing viral DNA synthesis.

Pharmacokinetics:

Route(s)	PO, IV, topical
Absorption	15–30% is absorbed PO, minimal topical absorption
Distribution	Widely distributed, including cerebrospinal fluid (CSF); crosses the placenta; secreted in breast milk; 9–33% bound to plasma protein
Primary metabolism	Not metabolized

Primary excretion	Renal excretion, unchanged
Onset of action	Peak effect: 1.5–2 h
Duration of action	4–8 h

Adverse Effects: Acyclovir has few adverse effects when it is administered topically or PO. Nausea and vomiting, fatigue, and elevated hepatic enzymes have been reported. Minor skin irritation, rash, and localized pruritus may occur with the dermatologic formulations.

When given by the IV route, acyclovir is associated with nephrotoxicity, and frequent laboratory tests should be performed to monitor renal function. Ensuring that the infusion is administered slowly and that the patient is properly hydrated can lessen the potential for IV toxicity. Neurotoxicity has also been reported at high doses when acyclovir is given IV, including dizziness, confusion, delirium, and coma.

Contraindications/Precautions: Acyclovir should be used with caution in patients with chronic kidney disease (CKD) because the antiviral is excreted entirely by the kidneys. Doses should be lowered in these patients and proper hydration should be implemented to prevent crystalluria.

Drug Interactions: Acyclovir interacts with only a few drugs. Probenecid decreases acyclovir elimination and can lead to toxic levels of the antiviral. Zidovudine may increase drowsiness and lethargy. Systemic acyclovir may result in additive nephrotoxicity if used with other drugs affecting renal function such as aminoglycosides. **Herbal/Food:** Unknown.

Pregnancy: Animal studies showed no evidence of fetal harm. Human experience found no evidence of fetal harm above baseline levels. Although the drug is secreted in human milk, significant adverse effects have not been reported in breastfed neonates.

Treatment of Overdose: Overdose may result in coma, seizures, and renal failure. No specific therapy is available; hemodialysis may be initiated.

Clinician Responsibilities: Key clinical implications for patients receiving acyclovir are included in Applied Clinical Judgment: Patients Receiving Pharmacotherapy with Antivirals for Non-HIV Viral Infections.

Drugs Similar to Acyclovir (Zovirax)

Other antivirals effective for treating herpesvirus infections include cidofovir, docosanol, famciclovir, foscarnet, ganciclovir, penciclovir, trifluridine, valacyclovir, and valganciclovir.

Cidofovir: Once activated, cidofovir resembles a natural nucleoside (dCTP) and is incorporated into the viral DNA chain, causing premature termination. Approved in 1996, its use is restricted to the prevention or treatment of CMV retinitis in patients with AIDS, although it has been used off-label to treat HSV, Epstein-Barr, and other viruses. Cidofovir is available only by the IV route. It has an extended intracellular half-life that permits once-weekly dosing, versus foscarnet or ganciclovir, which must be infused daily. Common adverse effects include rash, headache, alopecia, chills, anorexia, and anemia. Cidofovir carries a black box warning that the primary dose-limiting adverse effect is nephrotoxicity, which occurs in a significant percentage of patients receiving the drug. Other drugs that cause nephrotoxicity should be avoided during therapy and serum creatinine and urine protein should be monitored within 48 hours of each dose. The black box warning also states that the patient should be monitored for neutropenia during therapy. Cidofovir causes embryofetal toxicity in laboratory animals. It is not known if this drug is secreted in human milk or if it causes adverse effects in the breastfed neonate. Women of childbearing potential should use effective contraception during therapy and for 30 days following the last dose. Men taking this drug have a risk for male-mediated teratogenicity and possible infertility; therefore, barrier contraception should be used during and for 3 months following the last dose.

Docosanol (Abreva): Approved in 2000, docosanol is a nonprescription drug for cold sores and fever blisters. Available as a 10% cream, the drug shortens the healing time and duration of symptoms of the lesions. It acts by blocking the fusion of HSV with its target cells, which is a very different mechanism than other drugs in this class. Docosanol is not absorbed from the skin; thus, no significant systemic adverse effects occur. Animal studies during pregnancy or lactation are not available for this drug.

Famciclovir: Famciclovir inhibits viral DNA synthesis in a manner similar to acyclovir, although it has a longer half-life that permits less frequent dosing. Approved in 1994, it is a prodrug, being activated to penciclovir after GI absorption. When used PO for treating acute genital herpes, it reduces the severity of symptoms and shortens the healing time of the lesions. It is also used for prophylaxis of genital herpes and for treatment of acute herpes zoster (shingles). In herpes zoster management, famciclovir shortens healing time from 7 to 5 days and reduces pain. It is well tolerated, with headache, nausea and vomiting, and diarrhea being the most common adverse effects. Animal studies showed no evidence of fetal harm. It is not known if this drug is secreted in human milk or if it causes adverse effects in the breastfed neonate.

Foscarnet (Foscavir): Approved in 1991, foscarnet is an IV medication that is effective against CMV and herpesviruses. It is indicated for CMV retinitis, acyclovir-resistant infections, and HSV infections in patients with AIDS. Off-label uses include nonocular CMV infections and VZV infections in patients with AIDS. Foscarnet exhibits greater toxicity than ganciclovir and has a short half-life that requires daily infusions throughout the therapy period. Headache, nausea and vomiting, and diarrhea are common during therapy. Foscarnet carries a black box warning that nephrotoxicity is a dose-limiting adverse effect that occurs in about 30% of the patients receiving the drug. Serum creatinine must be monitored carefully during therapy. Foscarnet is highly ionized in body fluids and may interfere with mineral and electrolyte metabolism, including serum calcium, phosphate, potassium, and magnesium levels. Electrolyte abnormalities with foscarnet use have been associated with seizures and cardiac abnormalities; thus, regular monitoring of serum electrolytes is essential. Animal studies showed a small risk for skeletal anomalies. This drug is secreted in animal milk, although adverse effects on the breastfed neonate are unknown.

Ganciclovir (Cytovene, Zirgan): Approved in 1989, ganciclovir is structurally similar to acyclovir and has the same mechanism of action. It is indicated for acute treatment of CMV retinitis and for prophylaxis of CMV infection in immunosuppressed patients. Initial therapy is conducted by IV infusion, followed by PO doses for continued therapy. Ganciclovir has a short half-life and must be administered daily by slow IV infusion during the treatment period. Diarrhea, nausea and vomiting, anorexia, abnormal dreams, anxiety, and confusion are frequent adverse effects. A black box warning for ganciclovir states that the principal dose-limiting adverse effect is bone marrow suppression, which can manifest as anemia, neutropenia, thrombocytopenia, or pancytopenia. Complete blood counts (CBCs) and platelet counts must be carefully monitored to assess for leukopenia and thrombocytopenia because these adverse effects occur in up to 40% of patients taking ganciclovir. Ganciclovir is a known teratogen in laboratory animals. Because of the potential for serious adverse effects in the neonate, breastfeeding is not recommended. Women with childbearing potential should use effective contraception during treatment and for 30 days after the last dose. Similarly, men should use barrier contraception for at least 30 days following treatment with ganciclovir.

Penciclovir (Denavir): Approved in 1996, penciclovir is the active metabolite of famciclovir and acts by the same mechanism. Unlike famciclovir, which is taken PO, penciclovir is available by prescription only as a 1% cream to apply to recurrent cold sores on the lips or face. To be effective, it should be applied to lesions every 2 hours while awake. It should not be applied to lesions on mucous membranes of the nose or mouth. Penciclovir is not absorbed from the skin; thus, it should not affect pregnancy or lactation.

Trifluridine (Viroptic): Approved in 1980, trifluridine is a 1% ophthalmic solution indicated for primary keratoconjunctivitis and recurrent epithelial keratitis due to HSV types 1 and 2. The drug has no systemic adverse effects and causes only minor eye irritation. Lonsurf is a PO combination of trifluridine and tipiracil indicated for metastatic colorectal cancer. Animal testing showed no evidence of fetal harm when administered by the ophthalmic route.

Valacyclovir (Valtrex): Approved in 1995, valacyclovir is a prodrug that is rapidly transformed into acyclovir after oral absorption. It offers the advantage of greater absorption and higher plasma levels than acyclovir. It has the same mechanism of action, indications, adverse effects, and pregnancy data as acyclovir. It was originally approved to treat herpes zoster (shingles), but its indications have since been expanded to include initial and recurrent episodes and prophylaxis of herpes genitalis and herpes labialis.

Valganciclovir (Valcyte): Approved in 2001, valganciclovir is a prodrug that is rapidly converted to ganciclovir after absorption. Given PO, it has the same mechanism of action, indications (CMV), adverse effects, and pregnancy data as ganciclovir. Patients must be monitored carefully for neutropenia and anemia during therapy. Patients may exhibit cross resistance between the two drugs. The black box warnings given for ganciclovir also apply for valganciclovir.

Drugs for Influenza Viruses

54.5 Pharmacotherapy of influenza viruses includes drugs to prevent infection as well as drugs to treat active infections.

Influenza, or *flu*, is a viral infection characterized by acute symptoms that include sore throat, sneezing, coughing, fever, and chills. The infectious virions are easily transmitted via airborne droplets or by hand-to-hand contact. In immunosuppressed patients, an influenza infection may be fatal, and flu outbreaks in long-term care facilities can be devastating. In 1919, a worldwide outbreak of influenza killed about 20 million people.

The influenza viruses contain single-stranded RNA genetic material and have an envelope that contains two types of protein spikes important for pharmacotherapy. One spike contains **hemagglutinin**, an enzyme that facilitates the attachment of the virus to host cells. The other protein spike is composed of an enzyme called **neuraminidase**, which assists the virus in exiting the host cell. Continual mutations to the chemical structures of these spikes create new influenza strains that are able to evade the immune system. New strains are named by the hemagglutinin (H) and neuraminidase (N) proteins. For example, the Spanish flu subtype is H1N1, whereas the avian (bird) flu subtype is H5N1. The best approach to influenza infection is prevention through annual vaccination. Detailed information about influenza vaccination is presented in Chapter 43.

CONNECTION Checkpoint 54.2

From what you learned in Chapter 43, explain the difference between a live and an attenuated vaccine.

Only a few antiviral drugs are available to treat influenza. Although these antiviral medications may be useful in preventing influenza or decreasing the severity of influenza symptoms, they should not be considered substitutes for vaccination. The drug amantadine (Symmetrel) has been available to prevent and treat influenza A since 1966. Due to a high level of viral resistance to amantadine and rimantadine, the CDC (2017b) no longer recommends that they be used routinely for prophylaxis or treatment of influenza type A. Because of their expense and the possibility of adverse effects, these drugs are prescribed only for patients who are at risk for the severe complications of influenza. Antivirals for influenza are listed in Table 54.3.

The neuraminidase inhibitors are used to treat active influenza infections. Neuraminidase is a viral enzyme that allows newly formed, mature virions to bud from infected cells and disperse throughout the respiratory system. Neuraminidase also promotes the penetration of the virus into respiratory epithelial cells and prevents viral inactivation by respiratory mucus. When viral neuraminidase is inhibited, the virions will cling to the surface of the host cell and be noninfectious.

Given within 48 hours of the onset of symptoms, the neuraminidase inhibitors, oseltamivir (Tamiflu), peramivir (Rapivab), and zanamivir (Relenza), will shorten the normal 7-day duration of influenza symptoms to 5 days. Oseltamivir is given PO, peramivir is by IV infusion, and zanamivir is inhaled. Oseltamivir is the only antiviral approved to treat both A and B influenza viruses in patients 12 months of age and older. Cross resistance has been reported between the three drugs in this class. Because these drugs are expensive and produce only modest results, prevention through vaccination remains the best alternative.

A second mechanism of action for managing influenza was approved in 2018. Baloxavir (Xofluza) inhibits polymerase acidic endonuclease, a viral enzyme required for influenza replication.

It is important to remember that these antivirals are not effective against the common cold virus. About 200 different viruses, including rhinoviruses, cause symptoms characteristic of the common cold. Despite considerable attempts to develop a vaccine to prevent this annoying infection, success has not yet been achieved. Some drugs, however, may relieve symptoms of the common cold, and these were presented in Chapter 45.

PROTOTYPE DRUG Amantadine (Symmetrel)

Classification **Therapeutic:** Antiviral for influenza
Pharmacologic: Viral replication inhibitor

Therapeutic Effects and Uses: Amantadine has both therapeutic and prophylactic applications for influenza infections. When given during an active infection, amantadine significantly reduces the duration of influenza symptoms. Amantadine is sometimes used immediately following influenza vaccination to give the patient protection during the 2 weeks it takes for protective antibodies to the vaccine to develop.

Amantadine is occasionally prescribed for patients at high risk for influenza exposure. This includes immunocompromised patients, long-term care residents, healthcare workers, and close personal contacts of high-risk patients. Furthermore, the CDC has recommended that the

Table 54.3 Drugs for Influenza Infections

Drug	Route and Adult Dose (Maximum Dose Where Indicated)	Adverse Effects
Influenza Prophylaxis		
amantadine (Symmetrel)	PO: 100 mg q12h continued for at least 10 days after exposure (max: 400 mg/day)	*Nausea, dizziness, nervousness, difficulty concentrating, insomnia*
rimantadine (Flumadine)	PO: 100 mg bid (max: 200 mg/day)	Leukopenia, hallucinations, orthostatic hypotension, seizures
Influenza Treatment		
baloxavir (Xofluza)	PO: 40–80 mg single dose	*Diarrhea, bronchitis, nasopharyngitis* No serious adverse effects
oseltamivir (Tamiflu)	Treatment: PO: 75 mg q12h for 5 days Prophylaxis: PO: 75 mg once daily for at least 7 days following close contact, or up to 6 wk during a community outbreak	*Nausea and vomiting, diarrhea, dizziness* Bronchitis, bronchospasm, serious skin hypersensitivity reactions, neuropsychiatric events and abnormal behavior (peramivir), Stevens–Johnson syndrome (peramivir)
peramivir (Rapivab)	IV: 600 mg once	
zanamivir (Relenza)	Treatment: Two 5-mg inhalations bid for 5 days Prophylaxis: One 5-mg inhalation q24h	

Note: *Italics* indicate common adverse effects. Underline indicates serious adverse effects.

distribution of the drug be further restricted due to the large number of influenza strains becoming resistant to amantadine. This drug should not be used as a substitute for influenza virus vaccination.

Quite by accident, amantadine was found to have anticholinergic effects that can benefit patients with Parkinson's disease. Although approved for this disorder, the effectiveness of amantadine in relieving symptoms of Parkinson's disease is modest and it is not a first-line drug for this disorder (see Chapter 21).

Mechanism of Action: The precise mechanism of action of amantadine is not known. It is thought to inhibit viral replication by preventing uncoating, although it may also affect assembly of new virions. The antiparkinsonism effects are likely due to the drug's ability to release dopamine and norepinephrine from neuronal storage sites and possibly prevent their reuptake.

Pharmacokinetics:

Route(s)	PO
Absorption	Completely absorbed
Distribution	Widely distributed, including CSF; crosses the placenta; secreted in breast milk
Primary metabolism	Not metabolized
Primary excretion	Renal
Onset of action	48 h
Duration of action	Half-life: 20–50 h

Adverse Effects: Up to 33% of patients experience CNS effects that may include insomnia, dizziness, lightheadedness, nervousness, loss of concentration, and mental confusion. These symptoms quickly resolve when treatment is stopped. Amantadine can worsen mental problems in patients with a history of psychiatric disorders or substance abuse and cause or increase suicidal ideation. In patients with CKD, the drug can build to toxic levels, resulting in symptoms such as visual or auditory hallucinations, seizures, coma, or dysrhythmias. Dosage adjustment in these patients is necessary to avoid toxicity. Older adults exhibit a higher incidence of adverse effects and often require reduced dosages.

Contraindications/Precautions: Amantadine should be used cautiously in patients with CNS disease, suicidal ideation, or psychiatric disorders, including seizures or psychoses, because the antiviral may worsen these conditions. Because the drug is excreted almost entirely by the kidneys, patients with CKD must be monitored regularly. Although rare, amantadine has caused peripheral edema and heart failure and therefore should be used with caution in patients with preexisting cardiac disease. The drug should not be abruptly withdrawn in patients with Parkinson's disease because symptoms of parkinsonism may dramatically worsen.

Drug Interactions: Patients should avoid alcohol use while taking amantadine because the combination can lead to increased CNS toxicity, including dizziness, confusion, and orthostatic hypotension. Anticholinergic drugs will exhibit additive effects with amantadine. Dopamine antagonists will reduce the antiparkinson effects of amantadine. Coadministration with trimethoprim-sulfamethoxazole may impair renal clearance of amantadine, resulting in higher plasma concentrations of the antiviral. **Herbal/Food:** Unknown.

Pregnancy: Amantadine is embryotoxic and teratogenic in laboratory animals. Because this drug is secreted in human milk, breastfeeding is not recommended. Women of childbearing potential should use effective contraception during treatment and for 5 days after the last dose.

Treatment of Overdose: Overdose of amantadine can result in serious CNS toxicity and death. Physostigmine may be administered by the IV route to control some of the CNS symptoms, and anticonvulsants may be necessary. Administration of acidic drugs enhances the renal excretion of the drug. Antidysrhythmics and antihypertensives may be administered to manage cardiovascular toxicity.

Clinician Responsibilities: Key clinical implications for patients receiving amantadine are included in Applied Clinical Judgment: Patients Receiving Pharmacotherapy with Antivirals for Non-HIV Viral Infections.

Drugs Similar to Amantadine (Symmetrel)

Other drugs for treating influenza include baloxavir, oseltamivir, peramivir, rimantadine, and zanamivir.

Baloxavir (Xofluza): Approved in 2018 for patients age 12 and older, baloxavir acts by blocking a key influenza enzyme needed for viral replication. Like other influenza treatments, it must be taken within 48 hours of the first appearance of symptoms. The drug is well tolerated, with diarrhea and bronchitis being the most common adverse effects. It has equal efficacy to drugs in the neuraminidase inhibitor class and has an advantage of being administered only once by the PO route. Animal studies showed no fetal toxicity. This drug is secreted in animal milk, although adverse effects on the breastfed neonate are unknown.

Oseltamivir (Tamiflu): Oseltamivir is a neuraminidase inhibitor available as a PO suspension or capsule that is indicated for the treatment of influenza A or B in patients over 12 months of age. It is also approved for influenza chemoprophylaxis in patients age 12 months and older. Approved in 1999, the drug must be started within 48 hours of the onset of flu symptoms to be effective. Symptoms in patients infected with influenza resolve about 1.3 days (30%) faster if oseltamivir is administered. The drug is well tolerated, with nausea and vomiting and diarrhea being the most common adverse effects. Oseltamivir should not be administered until 2 weeks after administration of the live attenuated influenza vaccine. Animal studies showed no fetal toxicity. Small amounts of this drug are secreted in human milk, although adverse effects on the breastfed neonate are unknown.

Peramivir (Rapivab): Approved in 2014, peramivir is a neuraminidase inhibitor given by a single IV infusion for the treatment of influenza in patients age 18 and older. Like other drugs in this class, peramivir must be administered within 48 hours of the onset of flu symptoms to be effective. Although the most common side effect is diarrhea, some patients have experienced neuropsychiatric events such as hallucinations, delirium, and abnormal behavior. Serious hypersensitivity skin reactions have occurred with peramivir. Animal studies did not show fetal harm when given by bolus injection. This drug is secreted in animal milk, although adverse effects on the breastfed neonate are unknown.

Rimantadine (Flumadine): Approved in 1993, rimantadine is chemically similar to amantadine and acts by a similar mechanism. It is approved for the treatment of influenza A infections in adults and for prophylaxis in children. Formulations include tablets as well as syrup for pediatric use. Like amantadine, it is not effective against influenza B. Rimantadine is less toxic than amantadine, with GI complaints such as nausea and vomiting and abdominal pain being most commonly reported. Older adults experience more adverse effects to rimantadine; thus, doses in this population should be reduced. Like amantadine, the CDC has recommended that prophylactic use of rimantadine be restricted due to the appearance of resistant viral strains. At high doses rimantadine showed embryofetal toxicity in animal studies. This drug is secreted in animal milk, although adverse effects on the breastfed neonate are unknown.

Zanamivir (Relenza): Zanamivir is a neuraminidase inhibitor available as an inhaled, powdered formulation. It was initially approved in 1999 for the treatment of active influenza infections in patients age 7 and older and subsequently approved for influenza prophylaxis. Like oseltamivir, the drug must be started within 48 hours of the onset of flu symptoms to be effective. Symptoms in patients infected with influenza resolve 1 to 2 days faster if zanamivir is administered. Zanamivir is well tolerated and devoid of significant adverse effects in most patients. Those with preexisting respiratory disease should use zanamivir with caution because the drug may initiate bronchospasm in these patients and the use of a bronchodilator may be indicated. Zanamivir should not be administered until 2 weeks after administration of the live attenuated influenza vaccine. Animal studies showed no fetal toxicity. This drug is secreted in animal milk, however, adverse effects on the breastfed neonate are not expected since this medication is poorly absorbed by the oral route.

Drugs for Hepatitis Viruses

Hepatitis, or inflammation of the liver, may be caused by drugs, alcohol, autoimmune disorders, metabolic diseases, or infections. Viral hepatitis is a common infection caused by several different viruses. Although each virus has its own unique clinical features, they all invade hepatocytes, producing the same symptoms.

Hepatitis may be classified as acute or chronic. Symptoms of acute hepatitis include fever, chills, fatigue, anorexia, nausea and vomiting. Chronic hepatitis may result in prolonged fatigue, jaundice, liver cirrhosis, and, ultimately, hepatic failure. Neonates and immunocompromised patients are at higher risk for developing chronic hepatitis. Some patients infected with hepatitis viruses, especially children, are asymptomatic.

The three primary types of viral hepatitis are hepatitis A (HAV), hepatitis B (HBV), and hepatitis C (HCV). These types are summarized in Table 54.4.

54.6 Hepatitis A is managed through vaccines, supporting measures, and postexposure immunoglobulins.

Hepatitis A, an RNA virus, is spread by the oral–fecal route and causes epidemics in regions of the world having poor sanitation. Outbreaks in the United States, however, are most often sporadic events caused by contaminated food.

HAV has an incubation period of 2 to 4 weeks. During this period, and for 1 to 10 days after symptoms appear, the virus is excreted in the stool and the patient is infectious. Clinical presentation includes an abrupt onset of nausea, anorexia, fatigue, and right upper quadrant pain. Hyperbilirubinemia and very high serum transaminase values are usually observed. Diagnosis is confirmed by the presence of anti-HAV antibodies.

HAV is the most common cause of acute hepatitis in the United States. Although some patients require some hospitalization for symptoms related to the infection, most recover without treatment and develop lifelong immunity to HAV. Fatalities due to chronic disease are rare, with only a small number of patients developing liver failure. Thus, HAV is considered an acute disease, having no significant chronic form. This makes HAV very different from hepatitis B or C.

Like all forms of hepatitis, the best approach for HAV is prevention. HAV vaccine (Havrix, VAQTA) has been available since 1995. When a booster is given 6 to 12 months after the initial dose, close to 100% immunity is obtained. The availability of the HAV vaccine has led to a dramatic drop in the rate of this infection in the United States. Details on immunization for HAV are presented in Chapter 43.

No antiviral drugs are necessary to treat acute HAV infection because symptoms resolve in about 2 to 3 months.

Table 54.4 Summary of Viral Hepatitis Types

Type	Transmission	People at Risk	Prevention	Treatment
Hepatitis A	Primarily through food or water contaminated by feces from an infected individual; rarely, it spreads through contact with infected blood	International travelers; people living in areas where hepatitis A outbreaks are common; people who live with or have sex with an infected individual; and, during outbreaks, daycare children and employees, men who have sex with men, and injection drug users	Hepatitis A vaccine; also, avoiding tap water when traveling internationally and practicing good hygiene and sanitation	Hepatitis A usually resolves on its own over several weeks
Hepatitis B	Through contact with infected blood, through sex with an infected individual, and from mother to child during childbirth	People who have sex with an infected individual, injection drug users, children of immigrants from disease-endemic areas, infants born to infected mothers, people who live with an infected individual, healthcare workers, hemodialysis patients, people who received a transfusion of blood or blood products before July 1992 or clotting factors made before 1987, and international travelers	Hepatitis B vaccine	Chronic hepatitis B: drug treatment with PegIFN alfa 2a, tenofovir disoproxil, tenofovir alafenamide or entecavir Acute hepatitis B usually resolves on its own; severe cases can be treated with lamivudine
Hepatitis C	Primarily through contact with infected blood; less commonly, through sexual contact and childbirth	Injection drug users, people who have sex with an infected individual, people who have multiple sex partners, healthcare workers, infants born to infected women, hemodialysis patients, and people who received a transfusion of blood or blood products before July 1992 or clotting factors made before 1987	There is no vaccine for hepatitis C; the only way to prevent the disease is to reduce the risk of exposure to the virus. This means avoiding behaviors like sharing drug needles or sharing personal items like toothbrushes, razors, and nail clippers with an infected individual	Chronic hepatitis C: Drug treatment with pegIFN alone or combination treatment with pegIFN and the drug ribavirin Acute hepatitis C: Treatment is recommended if it does not resolve within 2–3 months

For someone who has been recently exposed to HAV, hepatitis A immunoglobulin (HAIg), a concentrated solution of antibodies, may provide some degree of passive immunity. HAV immunoglobulin is administered as prophylaxis for people traveling to endemic areas and to close personal contacts of infected patients to prevent transmission of the virus. A single IM dose of HAIg can provide prophylaxis for about 3 months. If taken within 2 weeks of exposure to the virus, the immunoglobulins are 85% effective at preventing HAV infection. Serious adverse effects to HAV immunoglobulins are rare.

CONNECTION Checkpoint 54.3

From what you learned in Chapter 43, what is an immunoglobulin? Name some other disease or conditions treated with immunoglobulins.

54.7 Hepatitis B is managed through vaccines, antiviral drugs, and postexposure immunoglobulins

Hepatitis B is caused by a DNA virus. Although transmission in the United States is primarily through exposure to contaminated blood and body fluids, in endemic regions of the world the infection is widely transmitted by the perinatal route and from child to child.

The incubation period in adults is 1 to 6 months, whereas in children the asymptomatic period may last decades. Symptoms of acute HBV infection are indistinguishable from those of other hepatitis viruses and include anorexia, nausea and vomiting, fatigue, jaundice, and abdominal pain. Ninety-five percent of acute HBV infections in adults resolve with complete recovery and do not progress to chronic disease. Lifelong immunity to HBV is usually acquired following resolution of the infection. Treatment of acute HBV infection is symptomatic.

Chronic HBV infection may be asymptomatic, and it may take 10 years or longer before the chronic stage develops. HBV has a much greater incidence of chronic hepatitis and a greater mortality rate than does HAV. Although adults rarely progress from acute to chronic hepatitis, infants who acquire the infection have a 90% probability of progressing to chronic hepatitis later in life. If untreated, chronic HBV infection often progresses to hepatic cirrhosis and a small percentage will develop hepatocellular carcinoma.

Diagnosis of HBV infection is by the presence of several serologic markers, some of which are also used to guide pharmacotherapy.

- Hepatitis B surface antigen (HBsAg) is a protein on the surface of the virus. A seropositive test for HBsAg means the person is infected with HBV.

- Hepatitis Be antigen (HBeAg) is a protein found just under the viral capsid. A seropositive test for HBeAg means that the virus is actively replicating and the person is infectious. As treatment progresses, a falling level (or disappearance) of HBeAg suggests that pharmacotherapy has been successful.
- HBV DNA is a test that quantitates the amount of HBV infection. Elevated HBV DNA levels suggest that the virus is actively replicating. As treatment progresses, a falling level of HBV DNA suggests that pharmacotherapy has been successful.

Like HAV, the best therapy for HBV infection is prevention through immunization. HBV vaccine (Engerix-B, Recombivax HB) consists of preparations of HBsAg, rather than inactivated virus. Combination vaccines that contain HBV vaccine include Comvax (hepatitis B–*Haemophilus influenzae* type b conjugate vaccine), Pediarix (hepatitis B; diphtheria, tetanus, acellular pertussis [DTaP]; and inactivated poliovirus vaccine), and Twinrix (HAV and HBV vaccine). Additional details on HBV and a prototype feature for hepatitis B vaccine are presented in Chapter 43.

For someone who has been recently exposed to HBV, prophylactic therapy with hepatitis B immunoglobulins (HBIg) may be initiated. Indications for HBIg therapy include probable exposure to HBV through the perinatal, sexual, or parenteral routes, or known exposure of an infant to a caregiver with HBV. To be effective, HBIg should be administered within 24 hours after parenteral exposure to HBV, within 2 weeks of sexual contact, or to newborns of HBV-positive mothers 12 hours postpartum.

The treatment goal for chronic HBV infection is to achieve sustained suppression of HBV DNA to prevent the development of cirrhosis or carcinoma. Pharmacotherapy is conducted with the drugs listed in Table 54.5. The two basic strategies to eliminate HBV are to stop viral replication (i.e., suppress viral load) with antivirals or to boost body defenses with immunomodulators. The following antiviral drugs have demonstrated the greatest effectiveness at reducing HBV DNA levels and are thus considered first-line drugs for chronic HBV infection: PegIFN alfa 2a (Pegasys), tenofovir disoproxil (Viread), tenofovir alafenamide (Vemlidy), and entecavir (Baraclude).

The remaining medications for HBV infection are considered second-line drugs because they exhibit lower effectiveness, increased adverse effects, or greater resistance than the first-line drugs. Adefovir dipivoxil (Hepsera) and lamivudine (Epivir) may be useful when resistance to the first-line drugs develops or when used in combination with

Table 54.5 Drugs for Viral Hepatitis

Drug	Route and Adult Dose (Maximum Dose Where Indicated)	Adverse Effects
Antivirals for Hepatitis B Infection		
adefovir dipivoxil (Hepsera)	PO: 10 mg once daily	*Headache, nausea, dizziness, fatigue, diarrhea* Lactic acidosis (adefovir, tenofovir), loss of bone mineral density (tenofovir), pancreatitis (lamivudine), hepatomegaly with steatorrhea (lamivudine, entecavir, tenofovir), nephrotoxicity (adefovir), hematuria (adefovir)
entecavir (Baraclude)	PO: 0.5–1 mg once daily	
lamivudine (Epivir)	PO: 150 mg bid	
tenofovir alafenamide (Vemlidy)	PO: 25 mg once daily with food	
tenofovir disoproxil (Viread)	PO: 300 mg once daily	
Antivirals for Hepatitis C Infection		
elbasvir plus grazoprevir (Zepatier)	PO: 1 tablet daily (50 mg elbasvir, 100 mg grazoprevir)	*Asthenia, fatigue, headache, nausea* HBV reactivation, anemia (Epclusa, Zepatier), fulminant hepatitis, cardiac arrest (ribavirin), hemolytic anemia (ribavirin), apnea (ribavirin), hepatic decompensation (ombitasvir-paritaprevir-ritonavir)
glecaprevir plus pibrentasvir (Mavyret)	PO: 3 tablets once daily (300 mg glecaprevir, 120 mg pibrentasvir)	
ledipasvir plus sofosbuvir (Harvoni)	PO: 1 tablet daily (90 mg ledipasvir, 400 mg sofosbuvir)	
ombitasvir plus paritaprevir, ritonavir, and dasabuvir (Viekira Pak)	PO: 2 tablets ombitasvir (12.5 mg) paritaprevir (75 mg) ritonavir (50 mg) and one tablet dasabuvir (250 mg)	
ribavirin (Rebetol, Virazole)	PO: 800–1200 mg in 2 divided doses	
sofosbuvir (Sovaldi)	PO: 400 mg once daily	
sofosbuvir plus velpatasvir (Epclusa):	PO: 1 tablet daily (400 mg sofosbuvir, 100 mg velpatasvir)	
sofosbuvir plus velpatasvir and voxilaprevir (Vosevi)	PO: 1 tablet daily (400 mg sofosbuvir, 100 mg velpatasvir, 100 mg voxilaprevir)	
Interferons		
IFN alfa-2b (Intron A)	IM/subcutaneous: 2 million units/m^2 3 times/wk	*Flulike symptoms, myalgia, fatigue, headache, anorexia, diarrhea* Myelosuppression, thrombocytopenia, suicide ideation, anaphylaxis, hepatotoxicity
pegIFN alfa-2a (Pegasys)	Subcutaneous: 180 mcg once weekly for 48 wk	

Note: *Italics* indicate common adverse effects. Underline indicates serious adverse effects.

those drugs. Clinical guidelines for the treatment of chronic HBV infection continue to evolve as data from long-term research becomes available.

Interferons (IFNs) are immunomodulatory proteins secreted by macrophages, B lymphocytes, and other body defense cells in response to viral infection. Actions of IFNs include suppression of cell division, inhibition of viral replication, and enhancement of macrophage and T-lymphocyte activity. Only the alpha family of IFNs is used in hepatitis therapy, and each IFN has slightly different applications and indications. Information on IFNs used for other indications may be found in Chapter 42.

PROTOTYPE DRUG Tenofovir (Vemlidy, Viread)

Classification **Therapeutic:** Antiviral
Pharmacologic: Reverse transcriptase inhibitor

Therapeutic Effects and Uses: Originally approved for the treatment of HIV in 2001, tenofovir diproxil (Viread) was approved in 2008 to treat chronic HBV in adults and in children 12 years and older. Tenofovir diproxil is given PO, usually in combination with other drugs. When used to treat HIV infection, tenofovir is always combined with at least two other drugs to delay the development of HIV resistance (see Chapter 55). Tenofovir is a preferred drug for treating combined HIV–HBV infections due to its dual effectiveness.

Tenofovir alafenamide (Vemlidy) is a newer formulation that has equivalent effectiveness to tenofovir diproxil. Compared to the original formulation, tenofovir alafenamide exhibits lower nephrotoxicity, has less effect on bone mineral density, and uses one-tenth the dose. Tenofovir alafenamide is not approved for HIV infection. Tenofovir alafenamide is expected to replace tenofovir disoproxil in many fixed-dose combinations.

Both salts of tenofovir are first-line therapies for treating chronic HBV infection. A major advantage of tenofovir over other drugs for chronic HBV infection is that resistance is relatively low during long-term therapy.

Mechanism of Action: Resembling a natural nucleoside, tenofovir inhibits viral DNA synthesis by inhibiting the reverse transcriptase enzyme.

Pharmacokinetics:

Route(s)	PO (diproxil salt)
Absorption	25% absorbed; taking the drug with high-fat meals increases absorption to 40%
Distribution	Distribution to milk and CSF is unknown; minimal protein binding
Primary metabolism	Not metabolized by hepatic CYP450 enzymes
Primary excretion	Renal
Onset of action	Unknown; peak plasma levels reached in 1 h
Duration of action	12 h

Adverse Effects: The most frequent adverse effects include abdominal pain, nausea and vomiting, pruritus, and dizziness. Because tenofovir diproxil may cause or worsen kidney disease, renal function should be monitored prior to initiating therapy and periodically during treatment. Decreases in bone mineral density have been recorded with tenofovir diproxil, which may cause fractures in patients with osteoporosis. **Black Box Warning:** Tenofovir can cause a type of liver abnormality called lactic acidosis and severe hepatomegaly with steatosis. Although rare, this type of hepatotoxicity has resulted in several deaths. Also part of the warning, tenofovir may cause acute exacerbations of hepatitis B in patients who are coinfected with HBV and HIV and who discontinue this drug abruptly.

Contraindications/Precautions: There are no contraindications to the use of tenofovir. However, patients with CKD should receive a lower dose and be monitored frequently for changes in urinary laboratory values. Hepatic enzyme values should be monitored regularly during therapy. If any signs of lactic acidosis or hepatotoxicity are noted, the drug should be immediately discontinued.

Drug Interactions: Tenofovir should not be used concurrently with Atripla, Complera, Stribild, or Truvada; these are combination drugs for HIV that contain tenofovir as one of their components. **Herbal/Food:** May be taken with or without food, although food increases the rate of drug absorption.

Pregnancy: Animal studies showed no evidence of fetal harm. It is not known if this drug is secreted in milk or if it causes adverse effects on the breastfed neonate.

Treatment of Overdose: There is no antidote for tenofovir overdose. Patients are treated symptomatically.

Clinician Responsibilities: Key clinical implications for patients receiving tenofovir are included in Applied Clinical Judgment: Patients Receiving Pharmacotherapy with Antivirals for Non-HIV Viral Infections.

Drugs Similar to Tenofovir (Vemlidy, Viread)

Other antivirals for chronic HBV infection include adefovir dipivoxil, entecavir, and lamivudine. Daclatasvir (as monotherapy), simeprevir, and telbivudine have been discontinued. Although structurally different, the IFNs are discussed with this group because they are used to treat chronic hepatitis.

Adefovir dipivoxil (Hepsera): Approved in 2002, adefovir structurally resembles a natural nucleotide and inhibits viral DNA synthesis of HBV. It is active against several species of viruses, although it is approved only for the oral therapy of chronic HBV infection that shows evidence of active viral replication. Adefovir is an antiviral alternative for patients who have developed resistance to first-line antivirals. Other than headache and abdominal pain, the drug is well tolerated. Resistance has not been a clinical problem. This drug has a black box warning that in patients with preexisting CKD, urinary laboratory values should be monitored regularly. Severe exacerbation of hepatitis has been reported in patients who have discontinued therapy with adefovir and some other antivirals. Lactic acidosis and hepatomegaly with steatosis have resulted in several deaths in patients taking adefovir. Animal studies showed no evidence of fetal harm. It is not known if this drug is secreted in milk or if it causes adverse effects on the breastfed neonate.

Entecavir (Baraclude): Entecavir was approved in 2005 for the treatment of chronic HBV that exhibits evidence of active viral replication. Indications for entecavir were expanded in 2010 to include its use as a pretreatment for chronic HBV in patients with decompensated liver disease. Like lamivudine, entecavir is a reverse transcriptase inhibitor that blocks viral DNA synthesis. Given PO, the drug is well tolerated and the most common adverse effects include nausea, headache, fatigue, and dizziness. A major advantage of this drug is that viral resistance is very low. Because of its effectiveness and relatively high safety profile, entecavir has become a first-line drug in the pharmacotherapy of HBV infection. A black box warning indicates that fatal lactic acidosis and severe hepatomegaly with steatosis have been reported. Exacerbation of hepatitis may occur following discontinuation of therapy with antivirals. Entecavir is not recommended for patients coinfected with HIV who are not receiving pharmacotherapy for HIV. Animal studies showed no evidence of fetal harm. This drug is secreted in animal milk, although adverse effects on the breastfed neonate are unknown.

Lamivudine (Epivir): Originally approved for HIV infection in combination with other antiviral drugs in 1995, lamivudine was later approved for chronic HBV infections that have evidence of viral replication and active liver inflammation. Lamivudine is given PO, often in combination with other drugs. Compared to tenofovir, patients on lamivudine are more likely to develop resistant strains during long-term therapy. The dose recommended for treating HBV (100 mg/day) is much less than that recommended for treating HIV (300 mg/day). Its use in treating HIV is discussed in Chapter 55.

Most patients tolerate lamivudine well, with the most frequent side effects being nausea and vomiting, abdominal pain, and diarrhea. Ear, nose, and throat infections and fatigue may occur in as many as 25% of patients taking the drug. Lamivudine carries the same black box warning as tenofovir. Both can cause lactic acidosis and severe hepatomegaly with steatosis. In addition, both of these drugs cause severe exacerbations of hepatitis B in patients who are coinfected with HBV and HIV and who discontinue this drug abruptly. Hepatic enzyme values should be monitored regularly during therapy. If any signs of lactic acidosis or hepatotoxicity are noted, the drug should be immediately discontinued. Animal studies showed no evidence of fetal harm. This drug is secreted in animal milk but adverse effects on the breastfed neonate are unknown.

Interferons: Several IFNs are commercially available as drugs through recombinant DNA technology. All IFNs carry a black box warning that the drug may cause or worsen serious neuropsychiatric, autoimmune, ischemic, and infectious disorders. Additional information on these drugs is presented in Chapter 42.

- **IFN alfa-2b (Intron A).** This drug is approved for chronic HBV infection. After 4 months of pharmacotherapy, approximately one-third of patients will experience long-term loss of HBV DNA and HBsAg. In the second or third month of therapy, patients may experience an exacerbation of symptoms, probably due to removal of infected hepatocytes by the immune system. Patients most likely to respond to IFN therapy include those with a low viral load (HBV less than 20 copies/mL) and ALT greater than 100. Although the majority of patients respond to IFN monotherapy with normalization of transaminases and a reduction in liver degeneration, relapse rates are high. IFN alfa-2b is also approved to treat chronic HCV infection. Combination therapy with ribavirin increases the therapeutic success rate. Interferon alfa-2b is also used to treat hairy cell leukemia, follicular lymphoma, malignant melanoma, condylomata acuminata, and Kaposi's sarcoma. A prototype feature for this drug is presented in Chapter 42.
- **PegIFN alfa-2a (Pegasys) and pegIFN alfa-2b (PegIntron).** These drugs are pegylated formulations of IFNs that produce a more sustained serum drug level over a longer period of time than the nonpegylated formulations. Pegylation permits the IFN to maintain a consistently high serum level and to be administered less frequently. The peg molecule is inert and does not influence antiviral activity. Pegasys and PegIntron are believed to be equivalent in terms of efficacy.

Approved indications for pegIFN alfa-2a include chronic HBV and HCV infections that show evidence that the virus is replicating. PegIFN alfa-2b is indicated for the treatment of chronic hepatitis C in patients 3 years or older with compensated liver disease. PegIFN alfa-2b is usually given in combination with ribavirin over a period of 24 to 48 weeks. Actions and adverse effects are the same as those for IFN alfa-2b.

54.8 Hepatitis C is managed through combinations of antiviral drugs.

Transmitted primarily through exposure to infected blood or body fluids, *hepatitis C* is more common than HBV. About 40 to 50% of all patients with HIV infection are coinfected with HCV. Perinatal transmission rates are very low.

The incubation period for HCV is about 50 days. Like other hepatitis infections, HCV symptoms include nausea, vomiting, anorexia, and jaundice. Although acute symptoms occasionally accompany an HCV infection, the majority of patients are asymptomatic. About 70% of patients infected with HCV proceed to chronic hepatitis C, and up to 20% may progress to cirrhosis. HCV is the most common cause of chronic hepatitis and is the leading indication for liver transplants.

Unlike HAV and HBV, no vaccine is available for hepatitis C. In addition, postexposure prophylaxis of HCV with immunoglobulins is not recommended because its effectiveness has not been demonstrated. At least six different viral genotypes (and more than 50 subtypes) have been identified for HCV. HCV genotype 1 accounts for 75% of the infections in the United States. Genotyping is common for chronic HCV infection because it helps guide the appropriate treatment.

Current pharmacotherapy for chronic HCV infection includes combination therapy with two or three antiviral drugs concurrently. Combination therapy has been found to produce a more sustained viral suppression than monotherapy. Indeed, 12 or more weeks of pharmacotherapy can produce a complete cure for HCV infection. Ribavirin may be added to the regimen, in patients experiencing relapses following a previous treatment. Clinical visits are performed monthly during therapy to monitor for adherence and for side effects.

- *elbasvir plus grazoprevir (Zepatier)*: Approved in 2016, most patients receive 12 weeks of therapy. The addition of ribavirin is recommended for some patients.
- *glecaprevir plus pibrentasvir (Mavyret)*: Approved in 2017, patients receive 8 to 16 weeks of therapy. Mavyret is a pangenotypic medication that is effective against genotypes 1–6 HCV.
- *ledipasvir plus sofosbuvir (Harvoni)*: Approved in 2014, this is a 12- to 24-week regimen.
- *ombitasvir plus paritaprevir, ritonavir, and dasabuvir (Viekira Pak)*: Approved in 2014 for genotype 1 chronic hepatitis C, this combination regimen is 12 to 24 weeks. It is available with or without ribavirin. The addition of ribavirin is recommended for some patients, based on prior treatment history.
- *sofosbuvir plus velpatasvir (Epclusa)*: Approved in 2016, this is a 12-week regimen. The addition of ribavirin is recommended for some patients. Epclusa is a pangenotypic medication that is effective against genotypes 1–6 HCV.
- *sofosbuvir plus velpatasvir and voxilaprevir (Vosevi)*: Approved in 2017, this is a 12-week regimen. Vosevi is a pangenotypic medication that is effective against genotypes 1–6 HCV.

Ribavirin (Rebetol, Virazole): Ribavirin resembles a natural nucleoside and inhibits the viral synthesis of both DNA and RNA. Unlike many antivirals, it has a broad spectrum of activity against both RNA and DNA viruses. Ribavirin is given PO when treating HCV, always in combination with alfa IFNs. The inhalation form (Virazole) is approved to treat severe infections from the respiratory syncytial virus. Off-label uses include treatment of influenza, herpes, and other viruses. The drug can affect the heart and should be used with caution in patients with preexisting cardiac disease. A black box warning states that hemolytic anemia is a serious adverse effect, and patients must be assessed regularly for changes in laboratory blood values. Ribavirin has produced embryotoxicity and fetal defects in every animal studied. Indeed, pregnant healthcare workers should not care for patients receiving aerosolized ribavirin due to the risk of incidental exposure. Female patients and female partners of male patients should use two forms of contraception during therapy and for 6 months after therapy is stopped. Breastfeeding is contraindicated during therapy due to the potential for serious adverse effects in the neonate.

Sofosbuvir (Sovaldi): Sofosbuvir is a first-line drug for chronic HCV due to its effectiveness against several genotypes, its once-daily dosing regimen, and its minimal adverse effects. Sofosbuvir is an inhibitor of viral RNA polymerase, the enzyme required for the virus to make RNA. Approved in 2013 for the treatment of chronic HCV infection, it is always used in combination therapies, often with ribavirin or peginterferon. Fatigue and headaches are the most common side effects when used in combination with ribavirin. Several PO fixed-dose combinations are also approved for chronic hepatitis C infection: sofosbuvir with velpatasvir (Epclusa) and sofosbuvir with velpatasvir and voxilaprevir (Vosevi). Sofosbuvir is contraindicated during pregnancy when used in combination with ribavirin.

Drugs for Coronavirus-19 Infections

54.9 Therapies are emerging for the prevention and treatment of coronavirus-19 infections.

In 2020 a novel coronavirus, COVID-19, caused millions of infections and deaths across the world. This infection had not been previously reported, and no prevention or treatment existed at the time of its appearance. Rapidly spreading by airborne droplets, the primary transmission is through the respiratory system. Symptoms occur 2 to 14 days after exposure and range from mild flulike symptoms to life-threatening respiratory failure.

At the time of publishing this text, physicians and scientists were searching for effective treatments, other than supportive measures. The following therapies are available, some through emergency-use authorizations.

- *remdesivir (Veklury)*: An antiviral drug given by the intravenous route for patients requiring hospitalization.
- *baricitinib (Olumiant)*: An inhibitor of the enzyme Janus kinase (JAK) used in combination with remdesivir to shortens the time of recovery in hospitalized patients.

- *Convalescent plasma:* Plasma collected from people who have recovered from COVID-19 infection, which contains antibodies to the virus. Evidence for the effectiveness of this treatment is inconclusive.
- *bamlanivimab and etesevimab:* Two monoclonal antibodies administered together for nonhospitalized patients with mild to moderate symptoms who are at high risk to progressing to severe COVID-19 disease.
- *casirivimab and imdevimab:* Two monoclonal antibodies administered together by IV infusion for nonhospitalized patients with mild to moderate symptoms who are at high risk to progressing to severe COVID-19 disease.

Vaccines for COVID-19 began to be distributed in late 2020 and were introduced on a wide scale in 2021. The student should check frequently for current updates regarding prevention and treatment of COVID-19.

CONNECTIONS: APPLIED CLINICAL JUDGMENT

Patients Receiving Pharmacotherapy with Antivirals for Non-HIV Viral Infections

Key Assessment Data

- History of current condition, baseline vital signs, physical exam findings; immunizations; respiratory, neurologic, hepatic, or renal disease; pregnancy or breastfeeding. Obtain a drug history, including OTC and alcohol use.
- Ongoing assessment during drug therapy should include monitoring appropriate laboratory findings (e.g., CBC, hepatic and renal laboratory values) and bone mineral density.

Desired Therapeutic Outcomes

Improvement is observed and measurable by diminishing signs of original infection, maintenance of normal appetite and fluid intake, and increasing energy level.

Minimizing Adverse Effects

- Antiviral drugs may cause hepatotoxicity or nephrotoxicity. Loss of bone mineral density may also occur with some drugs.
- Hemolytic anemia is a serious adverse effect of ribavirin and frequent CBCs or red blood cell counts should be monitored.
- Acyclovir and other antiviral drugs may be nephrotoxic and adequate hydration is essential to prevent adverse renal effects, especially if the drug is given IV.
- Lactic acidosis is a possible life-threatening adverse effect of tenofovir, lamivudine, and similar drugs. Monitor for abdominal pain, anxiety, fatigue, palpitations, lethargy, rapid breathing and heart rate, weakness, chest pain or tightness, fever, or shortness of breath.
- Acyclovir, especially when given IV, may be neurotoxic. Assess for changes in level of consciousness, disorientation, confusion, or tremors.
- Bone marrow suppression may occur and may cause blood dyscrasias with resulting decreases in red blood cells, white blood cells, or platelets.
- Adverse GI effects are common, and the patient may also have disease-related effects. Maintaining adequate nutrition and fluids is essential to healing. Lamivudine is known to cause or worsen pancreatitis, particularly in children with a history of pancreatitis.
- Increasing fever, especially when accompanied by worsening symptoms, may be a sign of worsening infection or adverse drug effects.

Lifespan Considerations

- Older adults may be at increased risk for hypotension, and dizziness may increase the risk for falls.
- Age-related physiologic changes increase the risk of adverse renal and hepatic effects in the older adult.
- Embryotoxicity and fetal defects occur with ribavirin. Female patients and female partners of male patients should use two forms of contraception during therapy and for 6 months after therapy is stopped. Breastfeeding is contraindicated during therapy due to the potential for serious adverse effects in the neonate. Pregnant healthcare workers should not care for patients receiving aerosolized ribavirin due to the risk of incidental exposure.

Patient Education

- Report a fever that does not diminish below 37.8°C (100°F) or per provider's instructions, an inability to maintain hydration or nutrition, or dizziness to the healthcare provider.
- Rise from lying to sitting or standing slowly to avoid dizziness or falls. If dizziness occurs, sit or lie down and do not attempt to stand or walk until the sensation passes. Report increasing lethargy, disorientation, confusion, changes in behavior or mood, slurred speech, tremors, or ataxia. Report any changes in behavior, confusion, delusion, or expressed thoughts of suicide.
- Immediately report any nausea, vomiting, yellowing of the skin or sclera, abdominal pain, light- or clay-colored stools, diminished urine output, or darkening of urine.
- Increase fluid intake to 2 to 3 L/day. Avoid or eliminate alcohol.
- Report any low-grade fevers, sore throat, rashes, bruising or increased bleeding, unusual fatigue, or shortness of breath, especially if on drug therapy for a prolonged period.
- Drug routines for HCV will require 12 to 24 weeks of administration. The drug should be taken as ordered and not stopped unless directed by the healthcare provider.
- For HBV, prevention through the use of vaccination is the preferred strategy and many school districts require the vaccination before the child starts school. HAV is also a vaccine-preventable disease and the vaccine may be required as well.
- Report symptoms of lactic acidosis such as abdominal pain, anxiety, fatigue, palpitations, lethargy, rapid breathing and heart rate, weakness, chest pain or tightness, fever, or shortness of breath.
- Avoid acidic foods and beverages, carbonated drinks, or excessively hot or cold foods and beverages that may cause mouth irritation. Eat small, frequent meals, which may be better tolerated than fewer, larger meals.
- Genital HSV infections may be transmitted even in the asymptomatic period. Practice abstinence or always use barrier protection during sexual activity even if genital lesions are not present. Consult with the healthcare provider about suppressive therapy.
- Take the medication as follows:
  - Complete the entire course of therapy unless otherwise instructed. This is especially important in the treatment of HCV to achieve a cure. Suppressive therapy with other antivirals may be used to maintain a symptom-free period. Do not stop the medicine when starting to feel better.
  - Do not share the medicine with other family members. If there is reason to believe they need medication, they should be assessed by a healthcare provider.
  - Take the medication as evenly spaced throughout each day as feasible.
  - Increase overall fluid intake while taking these drugs.
  - If using ointments or creams, wash hands well before applying and again after application. If family or caregivers administer the medicine, gloves should be worn.

CONNECTIONS: APPLIED CLINICAL JUDGMENT *(continued)*

Patients Receiving Pharmacotherapy with Antivirals for Non-HIV Viral Infections

Prescribing Considerations

- Appearance of CNS or psychiatric symptoms such as suicidal thoughts have been known to occur with amantadine or interferon and may require dosage reduction or substitution.
- Patients being treated for HBV or HCV should receive frequent kidney and liver testing. Signs of worsening kidney or liver failure require dosage reduction or substitution.

Understanding Chapter 54

Key Concepts Summary

54.1 Viruses are infectious agents with simple structures.

54.2 The replication cycle of a virus occurs in five stages.

54.3 Antiviral drugs target a specific viral structure or stage of its replication cycle.

54.4 Pharmacotherapy can lessen the severity of acute herpes simplex infections and prolong latency.

54.5 Pharmacotherapy of influenza viruses includes drugs to prevent infection as well as drugs to treat active infections.

54.6 Hepatitis A is managed through vaccines, supporting measures, and postexposure immunoglobulins.

54.7 Hepatitis B is managed through vaccines, antiviral drugs, and postexposure immunoglobulins.

54.8 Hepatitis C is managed through combinations of antiviral drugs.

54.9 Therapies are emerging for the prevention and treatment of coronavir-19 infections.

CASE STUDY: Making the Patient Connection

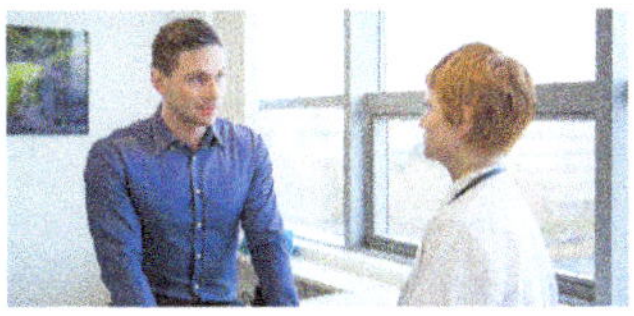

Remember the patient "Richard Palmer" at the beginning of the chapter? Now read the remainder of the case study. Based on the information presented within this chapter, respond to the critical thinking questions that follow.

Richard Palmer, a 19-year-old university student, has come to the health clinic. He states that he gets cold sores at least six to eight times per year. He informs the nurse that the cold sores usually start with lip pain or tingling, often followed by small, painful, fluid-filled blisters on a raised, red, painful area of his lip. The blisters usually last 2 to 3 days, then form yellowish crusts that slough off to reveal pinkish skin.

With his final exams coming up, Richard admits to feeling stressed. He also works part time serving at a local restaurant to help meet the expenses of college. Like other college students his age, Richard eats on the run and seldom sleeps more than 4 to 5 hours per night. His weekends are even more hectic with the job, school, and social activities. Richard requests something to help rid him of the existing cold sore immediately.

Critical Thinking Questions

1. How would you explain the mode of transmission and onset of symptoms for herpes simplex viruses to Richard?
2. How would you respond when Richard asks, "Is there any medication that I can take to prevent the cold sores from returning?"
3. Topical acyclovir is prescribed for this patient. What patient education would you provide?

Additional Case Study

Jeanie Schinkle is a 43-year-old factory worker who has just started a new job. Today, she presents to employee health services with a fever (T 38.3°C [101.1°F]), headache, myalgia, and cough that developed less than 24 hours ago.

As she is talking to the nurse, she expresses concern that she will lose her job if she is absent from work. "If only I had taken the flu shot, maybe I would not have gotten sick," says Jeanie.

1. Is Jeanie a possible candidate for oseltamivir (Tamiflu)? Why or why not?
2. What health teaching should the nurse provide Jeanie about the flu?

Chapter Review

1. Acyclovir (Zovirax) has been ordered intravenously for a patient with a herpes zoster infection to the upper torso and face. Which nursing intervention will help prevent a common adverse effect?

1. Administer the drug slowly IV over an hour and encourage fluid intake throughout the day.
2. Keep skin areas dry to prevent fungal overgrowth.
3. Administer antihistamines 1 hour before giving the infusion to prevent itching.
4. Assess visual acuity periodically and provide for eye comfort such as lubricating eye drops.

2. The patient is receiving elbasvir-grazoprevir (Zepatier) for hepatitis C virus. Which statement by the nurse is correct?

1. "Neither the topical nor the intravenous form of Zepatier will prevent the spread of hepatitis C virus."
2. "The patient will receive a 12- to 16-month course of therapy with Zepatier."
3. "Zepatier may be used in combination with ribavirin."
4. "The most common adverse effects of Zepatier are fatigue, rash, and dizziness."

3. Which assessment data would be most important for the nurse to monitor frequently in the patient receiving amantadine (Symmetrel)? (Select all that apply.)

1. White blood cell and platelet counts
2. Serum creatinine and urine output
3. Mental status and level of consciousness
4. Sodium and potassium levels
5. Lung sounds and signs of peripheral edema

4. The patient has received a prescription for zanamivir (Relenza) for flu symptoms but tells the nurse, "I think I can hold off on starting this; I don't feel that bad yet." What would be the nurse's best response?

1. "That should be fine, and the drug has a stable shelf-life so it can be saved for later infections."
2. "It can be saved for later, but you will also require an additional antibiotic to treat the symptoms at that point."
3. "It can be started within 2 weeks after the onset of symptoms."
4. "To be effective, it must be started within 48 hours after the onset of symptoms."

5. A patient with chronic HBV has been prescribed tenofovir disoproxil (Viread). The nurse will teach the patient to immediately report symptoms of what adverse and potentially life-threatening drug effect?

1. Systemic yeast infection
2. Lactic acidosis
3. Heart failure
4. Ventricular dysrhythmias

6. The patient is receiving ribavirin for treatment of chronic HBV. Which manifestation, if present in the patient, would the nurse conclude is an adverse effect of this medication?

1. Neurologic symptoms such as headaches and dizziness
2. Respiratory symptoms such as dyspnea and congestion
3. Skin disruptions such as acne and ulcerations
4. Hematologic symptoms such as excessive fatigue or dizziness

See Appendix A for answers to critical thinking questions, case study questions and review questions.

References

Centers for Disease Control and Prevention (CDC). (2017a). *Genital herpes—CDC fact sheet*. http://www.cdc.gov/std/herpes/stdfact-herpes.htm

Centers for Disease Control and Prevention (CDC). (2017b). *Influenza antiviral medications: Summary for clinicians*. https://www.cdc.gov/flu/professionals/antivirals/summary-clinicians.htm

Centers for Disease Control and Prevention (CDC). (2019). *Surveillance or viral hepatitis – United States, 2017*. https://www.cdc.gov/hepatitis/statistics/2017surveillance/index.htm#hepatitisB

Selected Bibliography

American Association for the Study of Liver Diseases. (2020). *Welcome to HCV guidelines*. https://www.hcvguidelines.org

Ayoyade, F. O. (2018). *Herpes simplex*. Medscape. http://emedicine.medscape.com/article/218580-overview

Centers for Disease Control and Prevention (CDC). (2020). *Genital herpes*. https://www.cdc.gov/std/herpes/default.htm

Ghany, M. G., Strader, D. B., Thomas, D. L., & Seeff, L. B. (2009). Diagnosis, management, and treatment of hepatitis C: An update. *Hepatology, 49*(4), 1335–1374. https://doi.org/10.1002/hep.22759

Lachiewicz, A. M., & Srinivas, M. L. (2019). Varicella-zoster virus post-exposure management and prophylaxis: A review. *Preventive Medicine Reports, 16*, 101016. https://doi.org/10.1016/j.pmedr.2019.101016

Li, H., Yan, L., Shi, Y., Lv, D., Shang, J., Bai, L., & Tang, H. (2020). Hepatitis B virus infection: Overview. In H. Tang (Ed.), *Hepatitis B virus infection: Molecular virology to antiviral drugs* (pp. 1–16). Springer.

Madigan, M., & Martinko, J. (Eds.). (2006). *Brock biology of microorganisms* (11th ed.). Pearson.

Ning, Q., Wu, D., Wang, G. Q., Ren, H., Gao, Z. L., Hu, P., et al. (2019). Roadmap to functional cure of chronic hepatitis B: An expert consensus. *Journal of Viral Hepatitis, 26*(10), 1146–1155. https://doi.org/10.1111/jvh.13126

Nguyen, H. H. (2020). *Influenza*. Medscape. http://emedicine.medscape.com/article/219557-overview

Pyrsopoulos, N. T. (2018). *Hepatitis B*. Medscape. http://emedicine.medscape.com/article/ 177632-overview

Samies, N. L., & James, S. H. (2020). Prevention and treatment of neonatal herpes simplex virus infection. *Antiviral Research, 176*, 104721. https://doi.org/10.1016/j.antiviral.2020.104721

Samji, N, S. (2017). *Viral hepatitis*. Medscape. http://emedicine.medscape.com/article/775507-overview

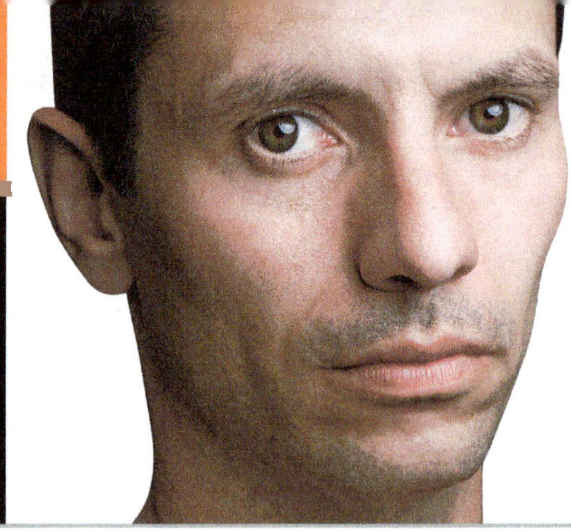

"Yeah, I admit it. I'm scared and practically out of my mind with worry. I've known several people who have died because of AIDS. What if this happens to me?"
—*Patient "Ryan Orre"*

Chapter 55
Pharmacotherapy of HIV Infection and AIDS

Chapter Outline

- Pathogenesis of HIV Infection
- General Principles of HIV Pharmacotherapy
- Classification of Antiretroviral Drugs
- Antiretroviral Drugs
  - Nucleoside and Nucleotide Reverse Transcriptase Inhibitors
  - **PROTOTYPE** *Zidovudine (AZT, Retrovir), p. 965*
  - Nonnucleoside Reverse Transcriptase Inhibitors
  - **PROTOTYPE** *Efavirenz (Sustiva), p. 967*
  - Protease Inhibitors
  - **PROTOTYPE** *Lopinavir with Ritonavir (Kaletra), p. 969*
  - Entry Inhibitors, Integrase Inhibitors, and Attachment Inhibitors
- Prophylaxis of HIV Infections
  - Occupational Exposure Prophylaxis
  - Nonoccupational Exposure Prophylaxis
  - Preexposure Prophylaxis
  - Perinatal Transmission Prophylaxis
- Pharmacotherapy of Opportunistic Infections Associated with HIV and AIDS

Learning Outcomes

After reading this chapter, the student should be able to:

1. Describe the primary steps in the pathogenesis of HIV infection.
2. Explain the therapeutic goals for HIV pharmacotherapy.
3. Identify reasons for virologic failure during HIV pharmacotherapy.
4. Describe the advantages of antiretroviral therapy in the pharmacotherapy of HIV infection.
5. Compare and contrast the classes of antiretroviral medications.
6. Explain the protocol and rationale for prophylaxis following possible occupational and nonoccupational exposure to HIV.
7. Explain recent advances in the preexposure prophylaxis of HIV infection.
8. Describe the antiretroviral protocols used for reducing the risk of perinatal transmission and for treating neonates with HIV infection.
9. Identify opportunistic infections commonly acquired by patients with HIV infections and the drugs used to treat them.
10. Describe the nurse's role in the pharmacologic management of patients receiving antiretroviral medications.
11. For each of the classes shown in the chapter outline, identify the prototype and representative drugs and explain the mechanism(s) of drug action, primary indications, contraindications, significant drug interactions, pregnancy data, and important adverse effects.
12. Apply clinical judgment to care for patients receiving pharmacotherapy for HIV infection or AIDS.

Key Terms

Definitions of the terms in bold may be found in the Glossary.

Recognized by the medical community as a distinct disease in 1981, the first documented case of **acquired immunodeficiency syndrome (AIDS)** has since been traced back to 1959. The syndrome is characterized by profound immunosuppression, leading to opportunistic infections (OIs) and malignancies not commonly experienced by people with intact immune defenses. The **human immunodeficiency virus (HIV)** was quickly identified as the causative agent for AIDS. HIV infection has resulted in a tragic, worldwide epidemic, causing the deaths of millions of people. The infection continues to be a major public health challenge.

PharmFACT

About 1.17 million Americans are living with HIV; 13% do not know they are infected (Centers for Disease Control and Prevention [CDC], 2020b).

Pathogenesis of HIV Infection

55.1 HIV causes a profound loss of immune function.

The two primary types of HIV are HIV-1 and HIV-2. Because more than 99% of the global AIDS cases are caused by HIV-1, the discussion in this text applies only to HIV-1. HIV uses the same stages of viral infection described in Chapter 54. There are, however, additional details that are important to understanding the pharmacotherapy of HIV infection.

Transmission: HIV infection occurs by exposure to contaminated body fluids, most commonly blood or semen because these fluids have the highest concentration of the virus. Transmission may occur through sexual activity or through contact of infected fluids with broken skin, mucous membranes, or needlesticks. Newborns of a mother infected with HIV may acquire the virus during birth or breastfeeding. Although in the United States the majority of patients with HIV infection are men who have sex with other men, heterosexual transmission is significant and is the predominant means of acquiring the infection in developing countries.

PharmFACT

About 38,000 new cases of AIDS are diagnosed each year in the United States. Approximately 69% of these involve male-to-male sexual contact. However, about one in every four people who acquire this disease is a woman who acquired the infection through heterosexual contact (CDC, 2020).

Replication cycle: Like other viruses, HIV must infect a host cell to duplicate its genetic material and assemble more virus particles (virions). Knowledge of the replication cycle of HIV, which is shown in Pharmacotherapy Illustrated 55.1, is critical to understanding the pharmacotherapy of HIV infection.

The first stage of HIV pathogenesis is the attachment of the virus to its preferred target: the **CD4 receptor** on the surface of T4 lymphocytes. (Note that the terms *CD4 cells*, *T4 cells*, and *T4 lymphocytes* are used interchangeably in this text.) During this initial stage, structural proteins on the surface of HIV fuse with the CD4 receptor. Because these receptors are also present on monocytes, macrophages, and dendritic cells, multiple cell types become infected. In addition to the CD4 receptor, coreceptors known as CCR5 and CXCR4 have been discovered that assist HIV in binding to the T4 lymphocyte.

The second stage of pathogenesis is the penetration of HIV into the T4 lymphocyte. The virus uncoats and the single-stranded ribonucleic acid (RNA) genetic material enters the host cell. HIV converts its RNA strands to double-stranded deoxyribonucleic acid (DNA), using the viral enzyme **reverse transcriptase**. Only a few viruses are able to construct DNA from RNA; no bacteria, plants, or animals are able to perform this unique metabolic function. All living organisms make RNA from DNA. Because of their "backward" or reverse DNA synthesis, these viruses are called *retroviruses* and drugs used to treat HIV infections are called **antiretrovirals**. Although unique to HIV, reverse transcriptase is an inefficient enzyme that makes many errors when converting the viral RNA to double-stranded DNA. The enzyme has no "proofreading" ability, which allows errors in the viral genetic code to accumulate. This produces a high mutation rate, making it difficult to develop effective vaccines.

The viral DNA eventually enters the nucleus of the T4 lymphocyte where it becomes incorporated into the host's chromosomes. This action is performed by HIV **integrase**, another enzyme unique to HIV. Once incorporated into human chromosomes, the HIV is called a provirus, and it remains for the lifetime of the cell. It is impossible to recognize the HIV provirus or remove it once it has entered the cell. Indeed, despite the fact that the T4 lymphocyte is infected with a deadly virus, the host's immune system is unable to effectively remove the defective cells.

This *latent phase* of the infection may last only a few weeks or it may continue for decades. During this phase, patients are asymptomatic and do not realize they are infected. It was once thought that the virus was truly

Pharmacotherapy Illustrated 55.1

Replication of HIV

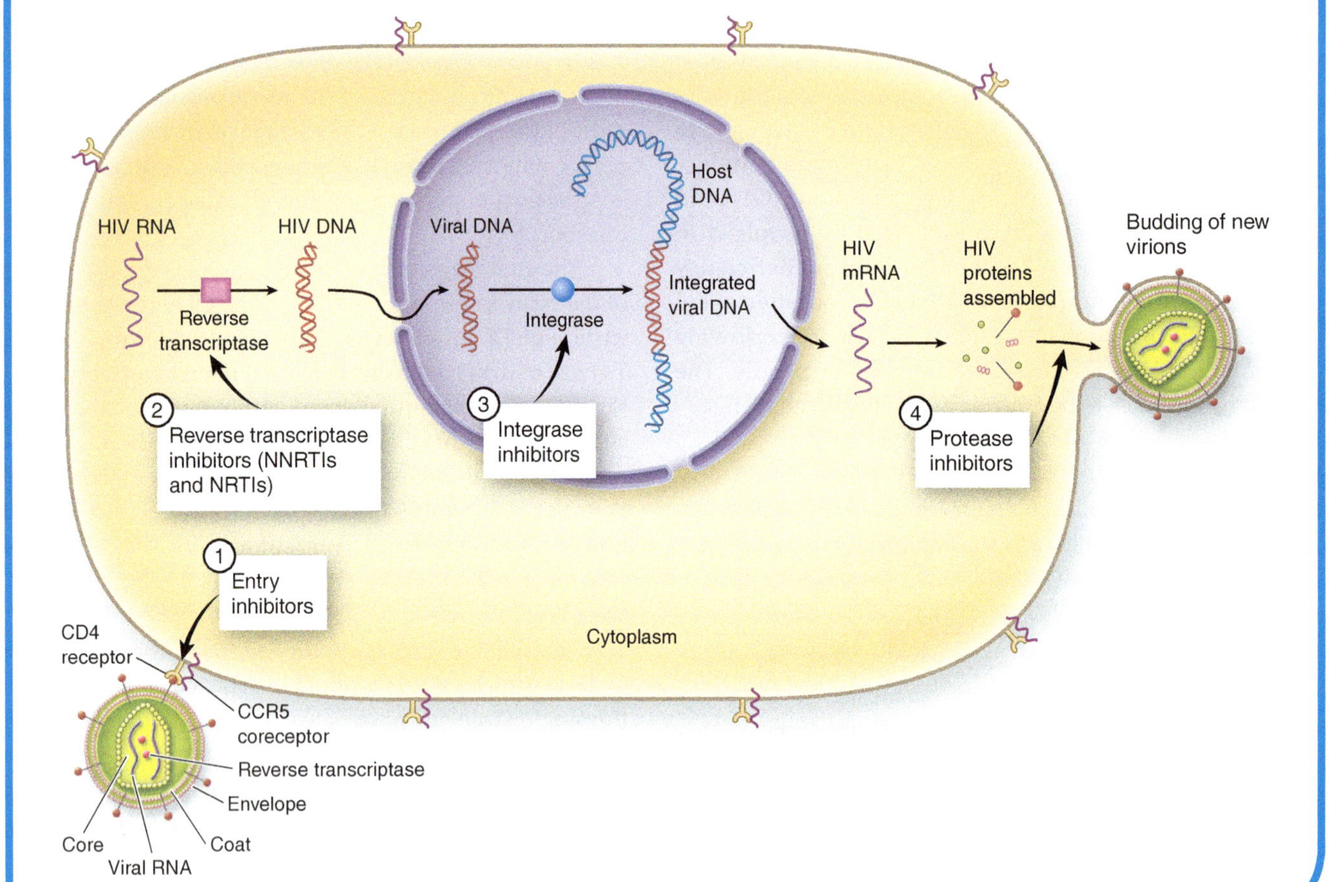

"silent" during the latent phase, but continuous HIV replication and immune system damage are occurring.

At some point, the latent provirus becomes activated and produces large amounts of viral messenger RNA, with the first strands producing viral proteins that amplify the replication process. All structural components of HIV are subsequently synthesized, and the cell is ready to assemble more virions.

The individual structural components of HIV migrate to the plasma membrane of the host cell, where they are packaged and eventually bud from the host cell. The new virions, however, are not yet infectious. As a final step, the viral enzyme **protease** cleaves some of the larger proteins to smaller, functional forms. Once budding occurs, the immune system recognizes that the cell is infected and kills the T4 lymphocyte. Unfortunately, it is too late; it is estimated that a patient infected with HIV may produce as many as 10 billion new virions every day, and the immune system becomes overwhelmed by the infection.

Symptoms: The immune system recognizes invasion by the virus and mounts an immediate defense, resulting in an acute inflammatory response that rids the body of many of the infectious virions. It is estimated that a billion HIV virions are destroyed each day during this early stage. Patients experience sore throat, fever, rash, malaise, and weight loss that may last several weeks. However, because patients often mistake these vague symptoms for the common cold or flu, they do not realize that HIV infection has occurred and rarely seek medical intervention. Symptoms during this initial phase, which lasts 2 to 4 weeks, are known as the **acute retroviral syndrome**. Although body defenses may suppress the viral invasion, tragically they are unable to eliminate the virus.

Progression to AIDS is characterized by gradual destruction of the immune system, as measured by the steady decline in the number of CD4 lymphocytes. Unfortunately, the CD4 lymphocyte is the primary cell coordinating the immune response for both the humoral and cell-mediated branches of the immune system. When the CD4 cell count falls below a critical level, the patient begins to experience opportunistic bacterial, fungal, and viral diseases and certain malignancies. Left untreated, the patient eventually is unable to mount any immune defense, and death occurs.

CONNECTION Checkpoint 55.1

Patients who are receiving immunosuppressant drugs have low white blood cell counts and, like patients with AIDS, are at risk for contracting OIs. From what you learned in Chapter 42, what are the major indications for immunosuppressant therapy?

General Principles of HIV Pharmacotherapy

55.2 Treatment of HIV infection is challenging due to the latent nature of the virus and the development of resistant strains.

The widespread appearance of HIV infection in 1981 created enormous challenges for public health and an unprecedented need for the development of new antiretroviral drugs. HIV infection is unlike any other viral disease because it is sexually transmitted, uniformly fatal if untreated, and demands a continuous supply of new drugs for patient survival. Although the infection can be managed as a chronic disease, stopping antiretroviral therapy always results in a rapid rebound in HIV replication.

While pharmacotherapy for HIV infection has not produced a total cure, it has resulted in significant therapeutic successes. With antiretroviral therapy, patients with HIV infection may live symptom free with their disease for decades. In many cases, the sexual transmission of the virus can be prevented by medications that keep the viral load low. Transmission of the virus from a mother infected with HIV to her newborn has been reduced dramatically due to intensive drug therapy of the mother prior to delivery and of the baby immediately following birth. Along with better patient education and prevention, successes in pharmacotherapy have produced a steady decline in the annual death rate due to AIDS in the United States from a high of almost 41,000 in 1985 to around 16,000 now.

Goals for the pharmacotherapy of HIV infection include the following:

- Reduce HIV-related morbidity and prolong survival.
- Improve the quality of life.
- Restore and preserve natural functions of the immune system.
- Suppress plasma HIV viral load to the maximum extent possible.
- Prevent HIV transmission.

Initiation of antiretroviral therapy: Current guidelines recommend that antiretroviral therapy be initiated immediately after diagnosis because early treatment can delay the onset of symptoms and the progression to AIDS. Serious, life-threatening OIs can be prevented with early treatment. Most importantly, early treatment reduces the risk of transmission to sexual partners and helps to lower the risk for perinatal transmission of the virus. The CDC recommends HIV testing for persons age 15 to 65 years old and for all pregnant individuals.

Patients experiencing their first treatment for HIV infection are called antiretroviral *naive*. Medication choices for antiretroviral-naive patients are often different from that for antiretroviral-experienced patients because drug-resistant strains of HIV develop during therapy.

Monitoring the progress of antiretroviral therapy: The two laboratory tests used to guide pharmacotherapy are CD4 cell count and measurement of HIV RNA in the plasma (CDC, 2014). Figure 55.1 illustrates the progression of these two values during an untreated HIV infection.

The number of CD4 lymphocytes estimates the degree of immune system damage caused by the virus. It also

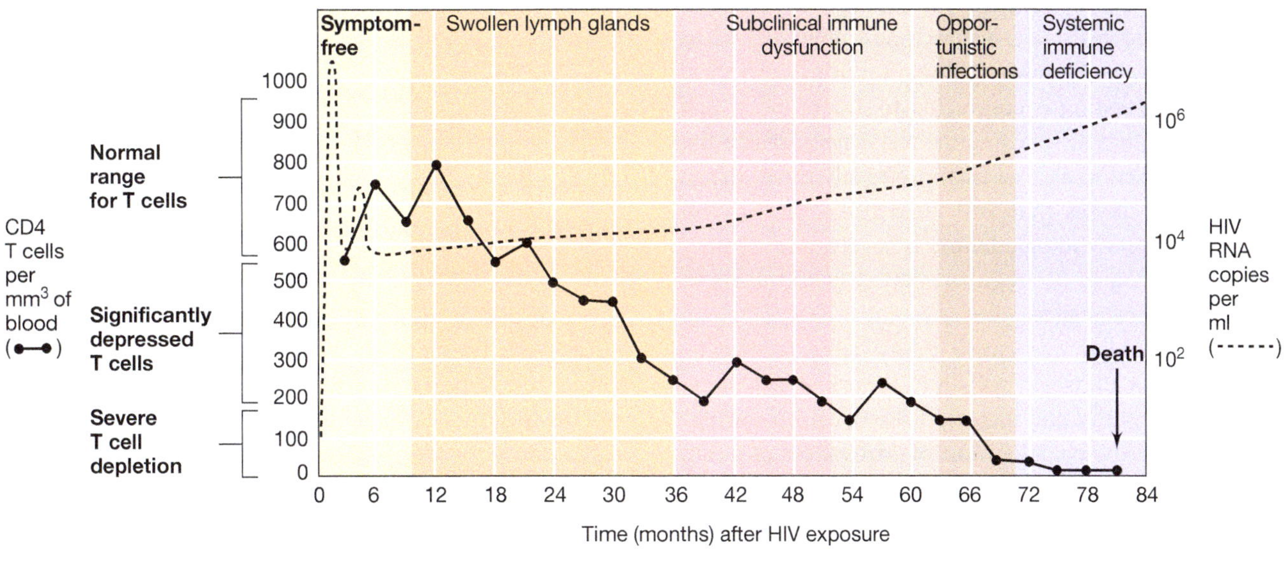

Figure 55.1 Decline of CD4 lymphocyte and progression of untreated HIV infection.
From Madigan et al. (2018). Reprinted by permission of Pearson Education, Inc., Upper Saddle River, NJ.

guides the healthcare provider in determining the need to initiate prophylaxis for OIs. Normal CD4 lymphocyte values range from 500 to 1600 cells/m^3. Patients with HIV infection whose CD4 counts fall below 200 cells/m^3 are at high risk for OIs. Once treatment succeeds in raising the CD4 cell count above the level for OI risk, this laboratory test is conducted every 6 to 12 months.

The **viral load** is determined by measuring the amount of HIV RNA in the blood, which provides an estimate of how rapidly the virus is replicating in the body. Plasma viral load is considered the most reliable indicator of response to drug treatment. The goal of antiretroviral therapy is to reduce plasma HIV RNA to undetectable levels or less than 200 copies/mL. Maintaining the viral load at an undetectable level prevents the sexual transmission of the virus to sexual partners. This is referred to as **treatment as prevention**. Once a patient is stabilized on a suppressive regimen, the viral load is assessed every 3 to 6 months.

Treatment as prevention only applies to sexual transmission of HIV. It does not prevent the transmission of the virus from blood exposure such as sharing needles. It also does not apply to perinatal or breastfeeding transmission.

Reasons for virologic failure: Because antiretroviral therapy does not totally eliminate the virus from the body, patients may experience relapses during therapy. **Virologic failure** is defined as a persistent HIV RNA level above 200 copies/mL while receiving HIV pharmacotherapy. Factors responsible for virologic failures include emergence of resistant HIV strains, adverse effects of the medications, lack of adherence to drug therapy, and drug interactions (including interactions with food, supplements, and other medications). Determining the reason for the failure can be challenging for the healthcare provider.

Drug resistance has become a serious challenge in treating HIV infection. When standard therapies fail, viral resistance should always be considered as a potential cause. Baseline HIV drug resistance testing is recommended when patients enter care. Should virologic failure occur, viral genotypic drug testing is conducted to determine which mutated viral genes are causing the resistance. Ideally, the patient is switched to at least two (preferably three) drugs from chemical classes that will yield full antiretroviral activity. Unless the virologic failure is severe, adding only a single new drug to the regimen may lead to the rapid development of resistance.

Antiretroviral drugs cause many adverse effects, including nausea, diarrhea, rash, lipid abnormalities, hepatotoxicity, neuropathy, and increased risk of cardiovascular events. Patients always take multiple drugs, which often interact with other medications to cause additional adverse effects. Identifying the specific drug interaction causing a toxic effect is challenging. Serious adverse effects often require an immediate change in pharmacotherapy. Other times, a simple adjustment, such as changing the amount per dose or spacing doses further apart, may prevent or eliminate the adverse effect or drug interaction. Adding antinausea or antidiarrheal drugs to the regimen can diminish some of the more common adverse effects.

To be successful, antiretroviral therapy requires strict patient adherence to a complex regimen. Unfortunately, many factors have the potential to affect adherence. Some antiretroviral drugs have inconvenient schedules and must be taken three to four times per day or be given parenterally. Some are very expensive or simply not available to patients in developing countries. Others make the patients feel quite ill; patients may actually feel much better (at least temporarily) when they are not taking the drugs. Given these complicating factors, and the prospect of a lifetime of drug therapy, it is easy to understand why adherence to the medication regimen is difficult, even for a motivated patient.

Sexual lifestyle adjustments: Patients with HIV infection may face serious mental health challenges because of their illness. Most patients are young and sexually active. Knowing that they may die prematurely of the infection and that they could kill others through unsafe sexual practices is difficult to accept. Many patients benefit from psychotherapy, and all benefit from compassionate, nonjudgmental nursing care. Teaching patients with HIV infection or AIDS how to care for themselves and how to protect others from their disease is a major task of the nurse.

When first starting pharmacotherapy, the patient should abstain from sexual activity or use other forms of barrier prevention for at least 6 months and until the viral load is less than 200 copies/mL (or undetectable). Some practitioners recommend that the patient demonstrate *sustained suppression* of HIV RNA before resuming sexual activity. If HIV-RNA rises above 200 copies/mL the patient should implement abstinence or other protective measures. If a patient is intending to use treatment as prevention, they must understand that strict adherence to the therapeutic regimen is required.

Classification of Antiretroviral Drugs

55.3 Seven classes of antiretroviral drugs are available to treat HIV infection.

Antiretroviral drugs target specific phases of the HIV replication cycle. The standard pharmacotherapy for HIV infection includes aggressive treatment with multiple drugs concurrently, a regimen called **antiretroviral therapy (ART)**, formerly called highly active antiretroviral therapy. The goal of ART is to drastically reduce the replication of HIV, so that plasma HIV RNA is reduced to its lowest possible level. The concurrent use of medications from several classes reduces the probability that HIV will become resistant to treatment.

Should a patient reach a stage where HIV RNA levels are low or undetectable, it is important for the nurse to stress to the patient that the disease has not been cured and that ART must be continued for the remainder of the lifetime of the patient.

Antiretroviral drugs, listed in Table 55.1, are classified into the following groups, based on their mechanism of action:

- Nucleoside and nucleotide reverse transcriptase inhibitors (NRTIs and NtRTIs)
- Nonnucleoside reverse transcriptase inhibitors (NNRTIs)

Table 55.1 Antiretroviral Drugs for HIV Infection

Drug	Route and Adult Dose (Maximum Dose Where Indicated)	Adverse Effects
Nucleoside and Nucleotide Reverse Transcriptase Inhibitors (NRTIs, NtRTIs)		
abacavir (Ziagen)	PO: 300 mg bid (max: 600 mg/day)	*Fatigue, generalized weakness, myalgia, nausea, vomiting, headache, abdominal pain, anorexia, rash, sleep disorders* Bone marrow suppression, neutropenia, anemia, granulocytopenia, lactic acidosis–hepatic steatosis, neurotoxicity, peripheral neuropathy (stavudine), pancreatitis (didanosine, lamivudine), hepatotoxicity (stavudine), multi-organ hypersensitivity syndrome (abacavir), immune reconstitution syndrome (abacavir)
didanosine	PO: 200–400 mg once daily on an empty stomach	
emtricitabine (Emtriva)	PO: 200 mg once daily (max: 200 mg/day)	
lamivudine (Epivir)	PO: 150 mg bid (max: 300 mg/day)	
stavudine (Zerit)	PO: 40 mg bid (max: 80 mg/day)	
tenofovir disoproxil (Viread)	PO: 300 mg once daily	
zidovudine (AZT, Retrovir)	PO: 200 mg q4h (1200 mg/day); after 1 month may reduce to 100 mg q4h (600 mg/day) IV: 1–2 mg/kg q4h (1200 mg/day)	
Nonnucleoside Reverse Transcriptase Inhibitors (NNRTIs)		
doravirine (Pifeltro)	PO: 100 mg once daily	*Rash, fever, nausea, diarrhea, headache, stomatitis* Paresthesia, hepatotoxicity, Stevens–Johnson syndrome (SJS), central nervous system (CNS) toxicity (efavirenz), severe depression (rilpivirine)
efavirenz (Sustiva)	PO: 600 mg/day (max: 600 mg/day)	
etravirine (Intelence)	PO: 200 mg bid following a meal (max: 400 mg/day)	
nevirapine (Viramune XR)	PO: 200 mg/day for 14 days, then increase to bid	
rilpivirine (Edurant)	PO: 25 mg once daily	
Protease Inhibitors (PIs)		
atazanavir (Reyataz)	PO: 300 mg plus 100 mg ritonavir daily with food	*Nausea and vomiting, diarrhea, abdominal pain, headache, dyslipidemia* Anemia, leukopenia, deep venous thrombosis, pancreatitis, lymphadenopathy, hemorrhagic colitis, cardiac arrest (atazanavir), immune reconstitution syndrome (saquinavir), QT and PR interval prolongation (saquinavir)
darunavir (Prezista)	PO: 600 mg taken with 100 mg ritonavir bid with food	
fosamprenavir (Lexiva)	PO: 700–1400 mg bid in combination with 100 mg ritonavir bid (max: 2800 mg/day)	
lopinavir with ritonavir (Kaletra)	PO: 800 lopinavir and 200 mg ritonavir given once or twice daily	
nelfinavir (Viracept)	PO: 750 mg tid with a meal	
ritonavir (Norvir)	PO: 600 mg bid (max: 1200 mg/day)	
saquinavir (Invirase)	PO: 1000 mg bid (max: 2000 mg/day)	
tipranavir (Aptivus)	PO: 500 mg taken with 200 mg ritonavir bid with food (max: 2000 mg/day)	
Entry Inhibitors and Attachment Inhibitors		
enfuvirtide (Fuzeon)	Subcutaneous: 90 mg bid	*Local injection-site reactions, nausea, diarrhea, fatigue* Hypersensitivity, neutropenia, thrombocytopenia, nephrotoxicity, pneumonia
fostemsavir (Rukobia)	PO: 600 mg bid	*Nausea* QT prolongation, transaminase elevation, immune reconstitution syndrome
ibalizumab (Trogarzo)	IV: loading dose 2,000 mg followed by maintenance dose 800 mg q 2 weeks	*Nausea, dizziness, diarrhea, rash* Immune reconstitution syndrome
maraviroc (Selzentry)	PO: 150–600 mg bid (max: 1200 mg/day)	*Respiratory tract infections, cough, pyrexia, rash, dizziness* Hepatotoxicity, myocardial infarction, severe hypersensitivity reactions
Integrase Inhibitors		
bictegravir	PO: only available in combination therapy	—
cabotegravir (Vocabria)	PO (loading dose): 30 mg once IM (with rilpivirine): 400–600 mg monthly	*Headache, nausea, abnormal dreams, anxiety, insomnia* Hepatotoxicity, depression, hypersensitivity
dolutegravir (Tivicay)	PO: 50 mg once daily	*Insomnia, headache* Severe hypersensitivity reactions, hepatotoxicity, embryofetal toxicity, immune reconstitution syndrome
elvitegravir	PO: only available in combination therapy	—
raltegravir (Isentress)	PO: 400–600 mg bid (max: 1200 mg/day)	*Headache, diarrhea, nausea, fatigue, insomnia* Severe skin and hypersensitivity reactions, myopathy, rhabdomyolysis, immune reconstitution syndrome

Note: *Italics* indicate common adverse effects. Underline indicates serious adverse effects.

- Protease inhibitors (PIs)
- Entry inhibitors (includes fusion inhibitors and CCR5 antagonists)
- Attachment inhibitors
- Integrase inhibitors.

Throughout the AIDS epidemic, pharmacotherapeutic regimens for treating the infection have continuously evolved based on ongoing research. Recommendations vary based on comorbid conditions such as hepatitis, tuberculosis, liver disease, or kidney disease. In current clinical practice, the following regimens have been shown to be the most successful choices for the *initial* therapy of HIV infection (Panel on Antiretroviral Guidelines for Adults and Adolescents, 2019):

- Bictegravir/tenofovir alafenamide/emtricitabine
- Dolutegravir/abacavir/lamivudine (only for individuals who are HLA-B*5701 negative)
- Dolutegravir plus (emtricitabine or lamivudine) plus tenofovir alafenamide or tenofovir disoproxil
- Dolutegravir/lamivudine (except for individuals with HIV RNA >500,000 copies/mL)
- Raltegravir plus emtricitabine or lamivudine plus tenofovir alafenamide or tenofovir disoproxil.

Although the preceding drug combinations are preferred, divergence to other regimens is necessary, depending on comorbid conditions and as resistant strains develop. The pharmacotherapy of HIV infection is evolving, and healthcare providers are still learning which drug combinations are most effective. The nurse should always review the latest medical literature before treating patients with HIV infection.

To improve adherence and to make the regimen more convenient for patients, the pharmaceutical companies have created many fixed-dose regimens combined into a single tablet or capsule. Some of these combinations are shown in Table 55.2.

Pharmacokinetic variables become very important when treating patients with HIV and can, in fact, contribute in a major way to the success or failure of ART. The bioavailability of some antiretrovirals is greatly affected by food in the stomach. The absorption of certain antiretrovirals (e.g., efavirenz) is decreased in the presence of food. Some (e.g., lopinavir) have a significantly increased absorption with high-fat meals and many others (e.g., dolutegravir) are not affected by the presence of food.

In addition to changes in absorption, most antiretrovirals are metabolized by the liver. Several can significantly increase or decrease the hepatic metabolism of other drugs, resulting in potential drug–drug interactions. These effects differ, even within the same drug class. For example, nevirapine induces the hepatic CYP450 enzyme system, thus decreasing the levels of other drugs. Predicting and avoiding complex drug interactions in patients with HIV requires truly skilled and dedicated nurses and other healthcare providers who are current on the most recent medical literature.

Two drugs, ritonavir and cobicistat, are given concurrently with antiretrovirals primarily for the purpose of inhibiting liver enzymes that would inactivate the antiretroviral. Ritonavir and cobicistat raise the serum concentration of other antiretrovirals. These drugs are called **pharmacokinetic enhancers** or boosters. For example, giving cobicistat with atazanavir enhances the actions of

Table 55.2 Combination Drugs for HIV Infection

Trade Name	NRTIs and NtRTIs	NNRTIs	PIs	Integrase Inhibitors	Pharmacokinetic Booster
Atripla	emtricitabine, tenofovir disoproxil	efavirenz	—	—	—
Biktarvy	emtricitabine, tenofovir alafenamide	—	—	bictegravir	—
Carbenuva	—	rilpivirene	—	cabotegravir	—
Combivir	zidovudine, lamivudine	—	—	—	—
Complera	emtricitabine, tenofovir disoproxil	rilpivirine	—	—	—
Delstrigo	lamivudine, tenofovir disoproxil	doravirine	—	—	—
Descovy	emtricitabine, tenofovir alafenamide	—	—	—	—
Epzicom	abacavir, lamivudine	—	—	—	—
Evotaz	—	—	atazanavir	—	cobicistat
Genvoya	emtricitabine, tenofovir alafenamide	—	—	elvitegravir	cobicistat
Juluca	—	rilpivirine	—	dolutegravir	—
Kaletra	—	—	lopinavir	—	ritonavir
Odefsey	emtricitabine, tenofovir alafenamide	rilpivirine	—	—	—
Prezcobix	—	—	darunavir	—	cobicistat
Stribild	emtricitabine, tenofovir disoproxil	—	—	elvitegravir	cobicistat
Triumeq	abacavir, lamivudine	—	—	dolutegravir	—
Trizivir	abacavir, zidovudine, lamivudine	—	—	—	—
Truvada	emtricitabine, tenofovir disoproxil	—	—	—	—

atazanavir. It also allows for lower doses of atazanavir, which lowers the potential for adverse drug effects. Cobicistat itself has no antiretroviral activity. The other booster, ritonavir, does have some antiretroviral activity of its own.

Antiretroviral Drugs

55.4 Reverse transcriptase inhibitors block the synthesis of viral DNA.

Following entry into a T4 lymphocyte, the single-stranded viral RNA is used as a template to synthesize double-stranded proviral DNA. HIV virions come "prepackaged" with reverse transcriptase, the enzyme necessary to perform this critical step. Because reverse transcriptase is a viral enzyme not found in human cells, researchers have been able to design drugs with the ability to selectively inhibit viral replication.

The synthesizing of proviral DNA requires biochemical building blocks known as nucleosides and nucleotides. Nucleosides and nucleotides form the backbone of the DNA molecule and are composed of the four bases, adenine, guanine, thymine, and cytosine. These same nucleosides and nucleotides are used to make human DNA.

Drugs in the nucleoside and nucleotide reverse transcriptase inhibitor classes (NRTIs and NtRTIs) chemically resemble the natural building blocks of DNA. In essence, reverse transcriptase is "tricked" into inserting these drugs into the proviral DNA strand. When the "fake" nucleosides and nucleotides are used to build DNA, however, the proviral DNA chain is prematurely terminated. Hence, the viral DNA chain is unable to insert into the host chromosome. Reverse transcriptase inhibitors have less effect on the progression of the infection if the proviral DNA has already been integrated into the host chromosome.

Of the 30 medications available for HIV infection, tenofovir and emtricitabine are effective drugs for reducing viral load and are included in many treatment regimens for the initial therapy. With the exception of zidovudine, which may be used as monotherapy to prevent the perinatal transmission of HIV, the NRTIs and NtRTIs are always used in multidrug combinations with drugs from other classes.

The NRTIs are prodrugs. They must first be metabolized to their active, triphosphate form inside their target cells before they become effective. Unlike many other antiretrovirals, the NRTIs do not interact extensively with other drugs undergoing hepatic metabolism. The NtRTIs are nucleotide inhibitors that are already in their active, triphosphate forms; thus, no metabolic activation is necessary. Tenofovir is the only NtRTI approved for HIV therapy, although a second drug in this class, adefovir, is available for treating hepatitis B virus (HBV) infection.

As a class, the NRTIs are well tolerated, although nausea, vomiting, diarrhea, headache, and fatigue are common during the first few weeks of therapy. Some of the serious adverse effects of NRTIs are caused by **mitochondrial toxicity**. NRTIs inhibit the enzyme mitochondrial polymerase, which is responsible for the replication of DNA in mitochondria. This small, obscure DNA molecule encodes subunits for mitochondrial enzymes in the respiratory chain, which generates ATP. All the NRTIs have been associated with a low incidence of an unusual form of mitochondrial toxicity known as lactic acidosis–hepatic steatosis. This syndrome, which occurs more commonly in those with preexisting hepatic impairment, includes lipid deposits in the liver, elevated transaminase values, and possible hepatic failure. Symptoms are often vague and include nausea, right upper quadrant pain, and myalgia. Liver function tests should be monitored regularly because fatalities have resulted from this adverse effect.

Another manifestation of mitochondrial toxicity from NRTIs is **lipodystrophy**, a disorder in which fat is redistributed in specific areas of the body. Areas such as the face, arms, and legs tend to lose fat, while the abdomen, breasts, and base of the neck (buffalo hump) develop excess fat. The fat redistribution may be associated with hyperlipidemia and hyperglycemia. Tesamorelin (Egrifta), a drug similar to growth hormone, may be prescribed to reduce the excess abdominal fat in patients with lipodystrophy who are infected with HIV.

PROTOTYPE DRUG **Zidovudine (AZT, Retrovir)**

Classification **Therapeutic:** Antiretroviral
Pharmacologic: Nucleoside reverse transcriptase inhibitor

Therapeutic Effects and Uses: Zidovudine was first discovered in the 1960s and its antiviral activity was demonstrated prior to the AIDS epidemic. It was approved in 1987 for the treatment of HIV infection in combination with other antiretrovirals, as well as for prevention of the transmission of HIV from mother to fetus or neonate.

Because of its widespread use since the beginning of the AIDS epidemic, HIV strains resistant to zidovudine are common. There is a high degree of cross resistance between zidovudine and other NRTIs. Current treatment guidelines for patients newly diagnosed with HIV infection do not include zidovudine as a first-line drug due to the potential for resistance. Zidovudine is administered to pregnant, HIV-infected women just prior to delivery to reduce the risk for perinatal transmission of the virus (see Section 55.10).

Mechanism of Action: Structurally, zidovudine resembles thymidine, one of four nucleoside building blocks of DNA. As the reverse transcriptase enzyme begins to synthesize viral DNA, it mistakenly uses zidovudine instead of thymidine, thus terminating the growing chain and creating a defective proviral DNA strand.

Pharmacokinetics:

Route(s)	Intravenous (IV), oral (PO)
Absorption	Readily absorbed
Distribution	Widely distributed, including cerebrospinal fluid (CSF); secreted in breast milk
Primary metabolism	Hepatic
Primary excretion	Renal
Onset of action	Peak effect: 1–2 h
Duration of action	Half-life: 1 h

Adverse Effects: Many patients experience headache, anorexia, nausea, and diarrhea. Patients may report fatigue, myalgia, and generalized weakness. It is often difficult to determine if adverse effects are due to zidovudine, other drugs the patient is taking concurrently, or the progression of the HIV infection. **Black Box Warnings:** Rare cases of fatal lactic acidosis with severe hepatomegaly and steatosis have been reported with zidovudine and other drugs in this class. Bone marrow suppression may result in neutropenia or severe anemia. Myopathy may occur with long-term use.

Contraindications/Precautions: Because zidovudine can suppress bone marrow function after 4 to 6 weeks of therapy, it should be used with caution in patients with preexisting anemia or neutropenia. Blood counts and other laboratory blood tests should be monitored frequently during therapy to prevent hematologic toxicity. Patients with significant chronic kidney disease (CKD) or hepatic impairment require a reduction in dosage because zidovudine may accumulate to toxic levels in these patients. Discontinuation of therapy should always be conducted under the guidance of a healthcare provider.

Drug Interactions: Zidovudine interacts with many drugs. Concurrent administration with other drugs that depress bone marrow function—such as ganciclovir, interferon-alfa, dapsone, flucytosine, or vincristine—should be avoided due to cumulative immunosuppression. Ribavirin and doxorubicin compete for intracellular activation sites and will diminish the effects of zidovudine. Probenecid, fluconazole, atovaquone, valproic acid, amphotericin B, and aspirin increase the blood levels of zidovudine and may increase the adverse effects of the antiretroviral. Other antiretroviral drugs may contribute to the lactic acidosis and hepatomegaly caused by zidovudine. **Herbal/Food:** Zidovudine should be used with caution with herbal supplements such as St. John's wort, which may cause a decrease in antiretroviral activity.

Pregnancy: Human data has not shown evidence of pregnancy-related adverse events above baseline levels. Breastfeeding is not recommended due to the possibility of transmitting HIV to the nursing infant.

Treatment of Overdose: No specific therapy is available; patients are treated symptomatically.

Clinician Responsibilities: Key clinical implications for patients receiving zidovudine are included in Applied Clinical Judgment: Patients Receiving Pharmacotherapy with Antiretrovirals.

Drugs Similar to Zidovudine (AZT, Retrovir)

Other NRTIs and NtRTIs include abacavir, didanosine, emtricitabine, lamivudine, stavudine, and tenofovir disoproxil. All of the NRTIs and NtRTIs are used in combination with other antiretrovirals. Fixed-dose combinations with NRTIs and NtRTIs are shown in Table 55.2.

All drugs in this class carry a black box warning for lactic acidosis–hepatic steatosis. Some carry additional warnings. Breastfeeding is not recommended due to the possibility of transmitting HIV to the nursing infant.

Abacavir (Ziagen): Abacavir chemically resembles the natural nucleoside guanosine and is indicated for the treatment of HIV infection as part of a multidrug regimen. Approved in 1998, it is given PO once or twice daily and is widely distributed throughout the body, including CSF.

The most common adverse effects are gastrointestinal (GI) and include nausea and vomiting, anorexia, and diarrhea. Alcohol use during abacavir therapy should be avoided because blood levels of the antiretroviral can increase as much as 40%. Abacavir carries a black box warning regarding the potential for multi-organ hypersensitivity reactions. This unique hypersensitivity syndrome occurs in 4 to 6% of patients taking the drug. Symptoms, which include fever, rash, dyspnea, cough, or GI distress, occur within the first 6 weeks of treatment. It is essential that the medication be immediately discontinued should allergy be suspected because deaths have occurred from this syndrome. Animal studies showed fetal malformations and developmental toxicity.

Didanosine: Approved in 1991, didanosine chemically resembles the naturally occurring nucleoside inosine and is indicated for the treatment of HIV infection as part of a multidrug regimen. Given orally once daily, it should be administered on an empty stomach to enhance absorption. Didanosine is not a preferred drug for treating HIV.

Diarrhea and peripheral neuropathy involving numbness and tingling in the hands and feet are common adverse effects occurring in over 20% of patients taking the drug. This drug has black box warnings that include pancreatitis, which may occur in up to 10% of patients. Patients should be carefully monitored for signs and symptoms that may suggest pancreatitis, such as nausea and vomiting, elevated serum amylase, and increased serum triglycerides, because deaths have occurred due to this disorder. Animal studies did not show evidence of fetal harm.

Emtricitabine (Emtriva): Approved in 2003, emtricitabine is a cytosine analog, also known as FTC, which is approved for the treatment of HIV infection as part of a multidrug regimen. Although chemically similar to lamivudine, it has the advantages of once-daily dosing and fewer adverse effects. The most frequently reported adverse effects are nausea, headache, dizziness, depression, rhinitis, skin rash, and skin discoloration on the palms and soles. Of the NRTIs, emtricitabine is believed to have the least mitochondrial toxicity. Emtricitabine carries a black box warning that it should not be administered to patients coinfected with HBV because severe exacerbations of HBV symptoms may occur after discontinuation of emtricitabine. Emtricitabine is a first-line drug for initial HIV therapy. Animal studies did not show evidence of fetal harm.

Lamivudine (Epivir): Also known as 3TC, lamivudine is a chemical analog of cytosine, a naturally occurring nucleoside. Approved in 1995, lamivudine is rapidly absorbed PO and better tolerated than most NRTIs. Minor adverse effects include transient insomnia and headache. Because serious adverse effects from lamivudine are uncommon, it has been a widely used component of ART regimens. This drug is also approved for treatment of HBV (Epivir HBV) (see Chapter 54). The dose recommended for treating HBV (100 mg/day) is much less than that recommended for treating HIV (300 mg/day). Its primary disadvantage is rapid emergence of resistance. A black box warning states that severe exacerbations of HBV illness may occur when the drug is withdrawn from patients infected with HIV. Human data have not shown evidence of pregnancy-related adverse events above baseline levels.

Stavudine (Zerit): Approved in 1994, stavudine is a chemical analog of thymidine, a naturally occurring nucleoside that is approved for the treatment of HIV infection as part of a multidrug regimen. Given orally, the use of stavudine has declined because the drug exhibits greater mitochondrial toxicity than others in this class. Of special concern is a high degree of lipodystrophy, evidenced by excessive loss of fat tissue, which persists long after the drug is discontinued. Headache and peripheral neuropathy occur in 50% or more of patients taking the drug. A black box warning includes serious pancreatitis that may occur if this drug is given concurrently with didanosine. Animal studies did not show evidence of fetal harm when given at clinically relevant doses.

Tenofovir diproxil (Viread) and tenofovir alefenamide (Vemlidy): Approved in 2001, tenofovir diproxil is an NtRTI that is indicated in combination with other antiretrovirals for the treatment of HIV infection in adults and children 2 years of age and older. Tenofovir is administered PO on an empty stomach to increase absorption. Tenofovir is a preferred drug for the initial treatment of HIV infection and chronic HBV infection, for which it is a prototype drug in Chapter 54.

The most frequently reported adverse effects of tenofovir are nausea and vomiting, depression, and diarrhea. Because tenofovir has less effect on mitochondrial enzymes than other drugs in this class, it is better tolerated. Tenofovir disoproxil can lower bone mineral density, placing the patient at risk for osteopenia or bone fractures. Due to nephrotoxicity, the use of tenofovir disoproxil in patients with CKD should be carefully monitored, and it should be used cautiously in patients receiving other nephrotoxic drugs. A black box warning states that severe exacerbations of HBV illness may occur when tenofovir is withdrawn from patients with HIV infection. Animal studies did not show evidence of fetal harm.

In 2016, a new salt of tenofovir became available. Tenofovir alafenamide, has equivalent effectiveness but exhibits fewer adverse effects on the kidney and on bone mineral density. Tenofovir alafenamide is available as monotherapy (Vemlidy) for the treatment of chronic hepatitis B infection. To treat HIV infection, the drug is available in several fixed-dose combinations (see Table 55.2).

55.5 The nonnucleoside reverse transcriptase inhibitors block viral DNA replication by binding to reverse transcriptase.

The nonnucleoside reverse transcriptase inhibitors (NNRTIs) act by a mechanism distinct from the NRTIs. Drugs in this class bind in proximity to the active site of reverse transcriptase, causing a change in shape of the enzyme molecule. Because of this structural change, reverse transcriptase is unable to add nucleotides to the proviral DNA chain, resulting in a direct inhibition of enzyme function.

Because resistance develops rapidly to NNRTIs, they are always used in combination with other antiretrovirals. Resistance to one NNRTI often confers resistance to all drugs in this class.

The NNRTIs are generally well tolerated and exhibit few serious adverse effects. The adverse effects are different than those of the NRTIs. Rash is common with NNRTIs and rare cases of SJS have been reported. They all affect hepatic metabolism, increasing the risk of drug–drug interactions. Liver function should be regularly assessed, especially in patients with preexisting liver disease.

PROTOTYPE DRUG **Efavirenz (Sustiva)**

Classification **Therapeutic:** Antiretroviral
Pharmacologic: Nonnucleoside reverse transcriptase inhibitor

Therapeutic Effects and Uses: Approved in 1998, efavirenz is given PO in combination with other antiretrovirals in the treatment of HIV infection. Efavirenz has the advantage of once-daily dosing and penetration into CSF.

Indications for efavirenz have been extended to include pediatric patients who are 3 months and older and weigh at least 3.5 kg (7.7 lb).

Resistance to NNRTIs can develop rapidly and cross resistance among drugs in this class can occur. High-fat meals increase the absorption by over 20%, which may result in toxicity. Because of this, efavirenz should be taken on an empty stomach.

Mechanism of Action: Efavirenz binds directly to reverse transcriptase, disrupting the shape of the enzyme's active site. This inhibition prevents viral DNA from being synthesized from HIV RNA.

Pharmacokinetics:

Route(s)	PO
Absorption	Readily absorbed
Distribution	Widely distributed, including CSF; unknown if secreted in breast milk; 99% bound to plasma protein
Primary metabolism	Hepatic (CYP3A4 and CYP2B6)
Primary excretion	Renal
Onset of action	Peak effect: 3–5 h
Duration of action	Half-life: 52–76 h

Adverse Effects: CNS adverse effects are observed in at least 50% of patients when first initiating therapy, including sleep disorders, nightmares, dizziness, reduced ability to concentrate, and delusions. CNS adverse effects usually diminish after 3 to 4 weeks of therapy. Like other drugs in this class, rash is common and must be monitored carefully.

Contraindications/Precautions: Liver function should be monitored during therapy due to the risk for hepatotoxicity. Efavirenz should be used cautiously in patients with a history of seizures.

Drug Interactions: Efavirenz induces CYP3A4 and can interact with drugs that are substrates for, or antagonists of, this isozyme. Patients who are receiving antiepileptic medications metabolized by the liver, such as carbamazepine, phenytoin, and phenobarbital, may require periodic monitoring of plasma levels because efavirenz may increase the incidence of seizures. Efavirenz can decrease serum levels of the following: statins, methadone, sertraline, and calcium channel blockers. CNS adverse effects of efavirenz are worsened if the patient takes psychotropic drugs or consumes alcohol. Levels of warfarin may either increase or decrease. **Herbal/Food:** Efavirenz should be used with caution with herbal supplements, such as St. John's wort, which may cause a decrease in antiretroviral activity.

Pregnancy: Human data suggests that this drug can cause neural tube defects when taken during pregnancy. Patients of childbearing potential should be advised to use reliable methods of birth control during therapy and for 12 weeks after the drug is discontinued.

Treatment of Overdose: No specific therapy is available; patients are treated symptomatically.

Clinician Responsibilities: Key clinical implications for patients receiving efavirenz are included in Applied Clinical Judgment: Patients Receiving Pharmacotherapy with Antiretrovirals.

Drugs Similar to Efavirenz (Sustiva)

Other NNRTIs include doravirine, etravirine, nevirapine, and rilpivirine. Delavirdine (Rescriptor) was discontinued in 2018.

Doravirine (Pifeltro): Approved in 2018, doravirine is indicated for HIV infection in treatment-naive patients. Given PO, the drug is usually well tolerated with nausea, dizziness, fatigue, and diarrhea being the most frequent adverse effects. Being new, it has the advantage of being effective against HIV strains resistant to other NNRTIs. Animal studies showed no evidence of fetal harm.

Etravirine (Intelence): Approved in 2008, etravirine is used in combination with other antiretroviral drugs in the pharmacotherapy of HIV infection. It is approved only for treatment-experienced adults. Because the fasting state can increase absorption of the drug significantly and cause potential toxicity, it should always be taken with food. It is excreted primarily in the feces; therefore, no dose adjustment is necessary in patients with CKD. Because etravirine can decrease hepatic metabolism, many drug–drug interactions are possible, including those listed for efavirenz. The drug does not exhibit the hepatotoxicity of nevirapine or the CNS toxicity of efavirenz. The drug is generally well tolerated, with the most frequently reported adverse effect being rash. Animal studies showed no evidence of fetal harm.

Nevirapine (Viramune XR): Nevirapine was approved in 1996 for the treatment of HIV infection in combination with other antiretroviral drugs. By inducing CYP450 enzymes, nevirapine increases its own breakdown; thus, dosage may need to be increased after several weeks of therapy to maintain its effectiveness. In addition, because the metabolism of protease inhibitors is decreased, dosage adjustments in these antiretrovirals may be necessary. Unlike some other antiretrovirals that negatively impact lipid metabolism, nevirapine may improve the lipid profile by increasing high-density lipoprotein cholesterol levels. Common adverse effects include nausea, diarrhea, fever, fatigue, and rash, which is occasionally severe enough to require discontinuation of therapy. A black box warning states that during the first 18 weeks of therapy, the patient should be carefully monitored for hepatic function due to potentially life-threatening hepatotoxicity. Patients with a history of liver disease are at greater risk for nevirapine-induced hepatotoxicity. In addition, severe dermal reactions, including SJS, have been reported. Serum transaminase levels should be checked for all patients developing a rash in the first 18 weeks. Animal studies showed no evidence of fetal harm.

Rilpivirine (Edurant): Rilpivirine was approved in 2011 for the treatment of HIV infection in treatment-naive patients with HIV RNA levels of less than 100,000 copies/mL at the start of therapy. It is a PO drug that offers the convenience of once-daily dosing. The most common adverse effects are depression, insomnia, headache, and rash. Patients should be monitored for severe depression and possible suicide ideation during therapy. Liver function should be monitored during therapy due to the risk for hepatotoxicity. Because rilpivirine can decrease hepatic CYP metabolism, many drug–drug interactions are possible. Animal studies showed no evidence of fetal harm.

55.6 Protease inhibitors prevent HIV protease from completing the final step in HIV maturation.

Near the end of its replication cycle, HIV has synthesized all the necessary components to create new virions. As the newly formed virions bud from the host cell and are released into the surrounding extracellular fluid, one final step remains before the HIV matures and becomes infectious: A long polypeptide chain must be cleaved to produce the final HIV proteins. The enzyme performing this step is HIV protease.

Drugs in the protease inhibitor class attach to the active site of HIV protease, thus preventing the final synthesis of HIV proteins. Without this final step in HIV maturation, the virions are noninfectious. When combined with other antiretroviral drug classes in an ART regimen, the PIs are capable of significantly lowering plasma HIV RNA levels.

Although widely used in antiretroviral combinations, the PIs have been replaced by integrase inhibitors in the initial recommendations for HIV treatment. PIs have the potential to cause more drug–drug interactions than other antiretrovirals and widespread resistance (and cross resistance) has developed that have reduced their effectiveness. In general, they are well tolerated, with GI complaints being the most common adverse effects. Lipodystrophies are common, including elevated cholesterol and triglyceride levels and abdominal obesity. Some of the PIs are associated with hyperglycemia and can cause diabetes or worsen existing diabetes. Blood glucose levels should be monitored regularly in patients taking PIs.

The available PIs are very similar but there are some noticeable differences in pharmacokinetic properties and adverse effect profiles. Cross resistance among the PIs may occur.

PIs most often include low doses of ritonavir or cobicistat, which are classified as pharmacokinetic boosters or enhancers. The addition of small amounts of these boosters allows longer dosing intervals and increases the plasma concentration of the PI.

PROTOTYPE DRUG Lopinavir with Ritonavir (Kaletra)

Classification **Therapeutic:** Antiretroviral
Pharmacologic: Protease inhibitor

Therapeutic Effects and Uses: Approved in 2000, Kaletra is a combination drug containing the protease inhibitors lopinavir and ritonavir. Lopinavir is the active component of the combination. Ritonavir inhibits the hepatic breakdown of lopinavir, thus permitting serum levels of lopinavir to increase by more than 100-fold. Kaletra tablets may be taken with or without food, but the oral solution form must be taken with a meal to enhance absorption. It has an extended half-life that allows for once- or twice-daily dosing.

Mechanism of Action: By effectively inhibiting HIV protease, the final step in the assembly of an infectious HIV virion is prevented.

Pharmacokinetics:

Route(s)	PO
Absorption	Readily absorbed (but quickly destroyed through hepatic first-pass metabolism)
Distribution	Widely distributed; 98% bound to plasma proteins
Primary metabolism	Hepatic (lopinavir is metabolized by CYP3A; ritonavir inhibits CYP3A)
Primary excretion	Renal (10%); feces (83%)
Onset of action	Peak effect: 3–4 h
Duration of action	Half-life: 5–6 h

Adverse Effects: Kaletra is well tolerated, with the most frequently reported problem being diarrhea. Headache and GI-related effects are common, including nausea and vomiting, dyspepsia, and abdominal pain. Kaletra may cause or worsen symptoms of diabetes mellitus, and hyperglycemia has been reported. Lipodystrophy syndrome occurs in many patients receiving long-term therapy with PIs and large increases in total cholesterol and triglycerides may occur during therapy. This syndrome is associated with hyperglycemia and fat redistribution. Kaletra should be used with caution in patients with cardiac disease because the drug can prolong the PR interval and cause third-degree heart block. Pancreatitis is a rare, though potentially fatal, adverse event.

Contraindications/Precautions: Because of its extensive hepatic metabolism, patients with liver impairment, especially those with preexisting viral hepatitis, should be carefully monitored. Hepatic enzyme levels should be regularly evaluated in these patients to prevent hepatic failure. Patients with diabetes should be monitored regularly because Kaletra may exacerbate this condition.

Drug Interactions: Lopinavir is extensively metabolized by hepatic CYP3A, and drugs that undergo hepatic metabolism may interact with Kaletra. Drugs that increase hepatic CYP450 enzymes will reduce the effectiveness of the antiretroviral. These include nevirapine, efavirenz, barbiturates, rifampin, rifabutin, phenytoin, and carbamazepine. Conversely, drugs that inhibit the CYP450 enzymes will increase levels of lopinavir, including alfuzosin, ketoconazole, delavirdine, and ritonavir. Statins should not be administered with Kaletra due to an increased risk for myopathy. Concurrent use of rifampin may lower the effectiveness of Kaletra. Potentially life-threatening dysrhythmias may occur if Kaletra is used concurrently with other medications that prolong the QT interval. Kaletra may increase adverse effects associated with selective serotonin reuptake inhibitors (SSRIs), tricyclic antidepressants, and phenothiazines. **Herbal/Food:** St. John's wort should be used with caution because it may decrease antiretroviral activity.

Pregnancy: Kaletra is embryotoxic and fetotoxic in laboratory animals. Human data has not shown evidence of fetal harm above baseline levels.

Treatment of Overdose: No specific therapy is available; patients are treated symptomatically.

Clinician Responsibilities: Key clinical implications for patients receiving lopinavir with ritonavir are included in Applied Clinical Judgment for Patients Receiving Pharmacotherapy with Antiretrovirals.

Drugs Similar to Lopinavir with Ritonavir (Kaletra)

Other PIs include atazanavir, darunavir, fosamprenavir, nelfinavir, ritonavir, saquinavir, and tipranavir. Amprenavir (Agenerase) and indinavir (Crixivan) have been discontinued in the United States.

Atazanavir (Reyataz): Approved in 2003, atazanavir offers the advantages of once- or twice-daily dosing and fewer adverse effects on lipid levels than other PIs. Headache, insomnia, dizziness, myalgia, depression, fever, and nausea are common adverse effects. Atazanavir increases bilirubin levels, and cholelithiasis is possible. Liver function should be regularly monitored during therapy. Atazanavir has been shown to prolong the PR interval of the electrocardiogram and produce first-degree atrioventricular block and other conduction abnormalities. The drug should be discontinued if rash occurs due to the risk for SJS. Atazanavir may cause hyperglycemia and worsen the symptoms of diabetes. Other adverse effects, contraindications, and drug interactions are similar to those of lopinavir. Animal studies and human data have not shown evidence of fetal harm.

Darunavir (Prezista): Approved in 2006, the PI darunavir is indicated for the treatment of HIV infection in adults and in children ages 3 years and older. Darunavir must be concurrently administered with ritonavir. Although cross resistance has been reported, darunavir retains some activity against viral strains resistant to other PIs. Because both darunavir and ritonavir decrease hepatic metabolism, numerous drug–drug interactions are possible. Darunavir should be administered with food to increase its absorption. Diarrhea, nausea and vomiting, rash, and headache are the most common adverse effects. Because drug-induced hepatitis has been reported with this drug, hepatic enzymes should be monitored regularly. Severe rashes are possible, and these call for discontinuation of therapy. Other adverse effects, contraindications, and drug interactions are similar to those of lopinavir. Animal studies showed no evidence of fetal harm.

Fosamprenavir (Lexiva): Approved in 2003, fosamprenavir is administered with low doses of ritonavir as a booster. Both tablet and oral solution formulations are available and fosamprenavir may be taken with or without food. Like other PIs, fosamprenavir affects the hepatic metabolism of many drugs, making interactions likely. The drug can cause hyperglycemia and thus should be used cautiously in patients with diabetes. Other adverse effects, contraindications, and drug interactions are similar to those of lopinavir. In laboratory animals, fosamprenavir increased abortions, caused skeletal malformations and decreased offspring survival.

Nelfinavir (Viracept): Approved in 1997, nelfinavir was one of the most frequently used PIs for many years. Its use has declined because newer PIs offer a lower pill burden and fewer adverse effects. Nelfinavir is given PO, usually with meals, in order to increase drug absorption. Unlike some other antiretrovirals, nelfinavir is 98% bound to plasma proteins and excreted almost entirely in the feces. Because large amounts of the drug and its metabolites reach the colon, frequent diarrhea is possible and antidiarrheal medications may be indicated. Patients taking oral contraceptives should be advised to use a second method of birth control because nelfinavir decreases plasma levels of ethinyl estradiol. Patients with diabetes should be monitored carefully due to the hyperglycemic effect of the antiretroviral. Animal studies showed no evidence of fetal harm.

Ritonavir (Norvir): Approved in 1995, ritonavir is well absorbed orally and is available in both capsule and solution formulations. The use of ritonavir is limited to enhancing the function of other PIs. The drug undergoes extensive hepatic metabolism and is excreted primarily in the feces. Like other PIs, ritonavir inhibits CYP450 hepatic metabolizing enzymes, which reduces the elimination of many drugs. When acting by this mechanism, ritonavir acts as a pharmacokinetic enhancer or booster. This is used to advantage in dual PI regimens. Giving low doses of ritonavir to boost serum levels of other PIs permits lower doses of the second PI. Ritonavir increases several other drug-metabolizing enzymes in the liver; therefore, drug–drug interactions are common.

Most of the adverse effects of ritonavir are GI related and may limit therapy. Peripheral and perioral paresthesias are possible. Because ritonavir induces enzymes that increase its own metabolism, its effectiveness will diminish unless doses are increased. Animal studies and human data have not shown evidence of fetal harm.

Saquinavir (Invirase): Saquinavir was the original protease inhibitor approved by the FDA in 1995. Boosting with ritonavir increases the serum levels of saquinavir, making the drug more effective. Resistance to saquinavir develops with continued use and may induce cross resistance with other PIs. Saquinavir is well tolerated, with the most frequently reported problems being GI related, such as nausea, vomiting, dyspepsia, and diarrhea. Other adverse effects are similar to those of lopinavir. Because of its extensive hepatic metabolism, patients with liver impairment should be carefully monitored. Animal studies have not shown evidence of fetal harm.

Tipranavir (Aptivus): Approved in 2005, tipranavir is indicated for the management of HIV infection in treatment-experienced patients and those with strains of HIV that are resistant to more than one PI. To boost antiretroviral activity, it is administered with ritonavir. Tipranavir capsules and solution can be taken without regard to food but the tablets should be taken with a high-fat meal to enhance absorption. The most common adverse effects are diarrhea, nausea, vomiting, pyrexia, fatigue, headache, and abdominal pain. Tipranavir contains sulfur and should be used with caution in patients with allergies to sulfa drugs. The drug has been associated with the development or worsening of diabetes, elevations in cholesterol and triglycerides, and lipodystrophies. Tipranavir inhibits platelet aggregation and should be used with caution in patients who may be at risk of increased bleeding from trauma, surgery, or other medical conditions or who are receiving anticoagulants or antiplatelet drugs. The drug should be discontinued if a severe skin rash occurs. Black box warnings state that tipranavir has been associated with intracranial hemorrhage. Caution should be used when prescribing it to patients with elevated transaminases or pre-existing hepatic impairment. The black box warning also notes that patients coinfected with hepatitis B or hepatitis C have a higher risk for hepatotoxicity. Tipranavir showed teratogenicity in laboratory animals.

55.7 Integrase inhibitors, entry inhibitors, and attachment inhibitors are newer strategies for managing HIV infections.

Because HIV develops resistance to many antiretrovirals, scientists have been looking intensively for unique mechanisms of drug action. In recent years, several new mechanisms have been discovered. The role of these drugs in treating HIV infection is evolving.

Integrase inhibitors: In 2007, the FDA approved the first drug in a class of antiretrovirals called integrase inhibitors or integrase strand transfer inhibitors. The HIV integrase enzyme transfers the proviral DNA to the human chromosome where it is inserted. Their high level of effectiveness and tolerability have resulted in the integrase inhibitors becoming first-line antiretrovirals for the therapy of HIV infection.

Raltegravir (Isentress), the first integrase inhibitor, is indicated for combination therapy with other antiretroviral drugs for the treatment of HIV infection in adult and pediatric patients. It may be administered with or without food. Insomnia, fatigue, headache, and GI-related symptoms such as diarrhea and nausea are the most frequently reported adverse effects. Caution should be used when administering this drug to patients with myopathy or rhabdomyolysis because raltegravir may worsen these conditions. Animal studies with raltegravir did not show evidence of fetal harm.

Other integrase inhibitors include dolutegravir (approved in 2013), bictegravir (approved in 2018), and elvitegravir (approved in 2012). Dolutegravir (Tivicay) is a first-line drug for treatment-naive and treatment-experienced adults and children at least 4 weeks of age. It has a higher genetic barrier to resistance than the other integrase inhibitors. The drug may cause serious hepatotoxicity, especially in patients with underlying hepatitis B or C. Dolutegravir did not show evidence of fetal harm in laboratory animals.

Bictegravir (Biktarvy) and elvitegravir (Genvoya, Stribild) are only available in fixed-dose combination tablets with other antivirals.

In 2021 the FDA approved Carbenuva, an extended-release combination of the integrase inhibitor cabotegravir and rilpivirine. This combination therapy is the first complete injectable regimen for HIV infection that is administered once monthly. Given to patients who have viral suppression, Carbenuva removes the daily burden of taking multiple pills.

Entry inhibitors: For HIV to begin its infectious cycle, the very first steps are to attach to the CD4 lymphocyte, fuse with its membrane, and "inject" the viral RNA into the human cell. Entry inhibitors block the entry of the viral nucleic acid into the T4 lymphocyte. The two drugs in this class block the entry by different mechanisms.

Approved in 2003, enfuvirtide (Fuzeon) blocks the fusion of the viral membrane with the bilipid layer of the CD4 plasma membrane. Because this mechanism is very different from other antiretrovirals, patients resistant to other drug classes may be sensitive to the effects of enfuvirtide. The use of enfuvirtide is limited because it must be given by subcutaneous injection twice daily. Its current use is for treating HIV infections in treatment-experienced patients with strains resistant to other antiretrovirals. Almost every patient taking enfuvirtide will experience an injection-site reaction, usually during the first week of therapy. These reactions may involve severe pain, pruritus, erythema, cysts, abscesses, and cellulitis. Nausea, diarrhea, and fatigue are other common adverse effects. Patients should be carefully monitored for lung infections because an increased incidence of pneumonia has been reported in patients taking enfuvirtide. No significant drug interactions have been found with enfuvirtide. Dolutegravir did not show evidence of fetal harm in laboratory animals.

The second entry inhibitor, maraviroc (Selzentry), was developed in 2007 after scientists discovered that HIV needs coreceptors (in addition to the CD4 receptor) to enter human cells. Found on the surface of T-lymphocytes, CCR5 is one of the coreceptors that is required for HIV entry. Maraviroc is the first of a class of HIV drugs called CCR5 coreceptor antagonists. This drug selectively blocks CCR5, preventing HIV from entering. Before treatment is initiated, the patient must receive a tropism assay (CCR5-tropic HIV-1), which is used to determine if maraviroc will be effective. Some strains of HIV can enter through receptors other than CCR5; maraviroc will not be effective against these strains. The drug is well tolerated, with the most frequently reported adverse effects being upper respiratory tract infections, cough, pyrexia, rash, and dizziness. Caution should be used when administering this drug to patients with preexisting cardiac disease because the drug may increase the risk for myocardial ischemia or infarction. Maraviroc carries a black box warning regarding the possibility of hepatotoxicity, which may be preceded by signs of severe rash or a systemic allergic reaction. Maraviroc did not show evidence of fetal harm in laboratory animals.

Attachment inhibitors: One of the newer therapies to treat HIV treatment-experienced patients is through the use of HIV attachment inhibitors. Two drugs have been approved in this class, although they act by very different mechanisms. Fostemsavir prevents the viral connection *before* it occurs whereas ibalizumab prevents the entry of the virus *after* it has attached. Ibalizumab is sometimes called a postattachment inhibitor.

Approved in 2020, fostemsavir (Rokubia) binds directly to the gp120 protein on the viral envelope. This protein is required for attachment to the CD4 lymphocyte. It is given PO and is only indicated for treatment-experienced patients with multidrug-resistant HIV.

Approved in 2018, ibalizumab (Trogarzo) is a monoclonal antibody that binds to a region of the CD4 receptor *after* the virus attaches. This drug changes the shape of the receptor so that HIV cannot enter the human cell. It is given every 2 weeks by IV infusion. Like fostemsavir, ibalizumab is only indicated for treatment-experienced patients with multidrug-resistant HIV.

CONNECTIONS: APPLIED CLINICAL JUDGMENT

Patients Receiving Pharmacotherapy with Antiretrovirals

Key Assessment Data

- History of current condition, baseline vital signs, physical exam findings; immunizations; respiratory, neurologic, hepatic, or renal disease; pregnancy or breastfeeding. Obtain a drug history, including over-the-counter medications and alcohol use.
- Ongoing assessment during drug therapy should include monitoring appropriate laboratory findings: complete blood count, CD4 count, HIV viral load (HIV RNA), culture and sensitivity for any concurrent infections, hepatic and renal function studies, lipid levels, serum amylase, and glucose.

Desired Therapeutic Outcomes

Improvement is observed and measurable by CD4 counts and HIV RNA within acceptable limits, ability to attend to normal activities of daily living, and absence of signs and symptoms of concurrent infections.

Minimizing Adverse Effects

- Because drug resistance can develop over time, CD4, HIV RNA, and the treatment regimen will be assessed periodically to ensure treatment continues to be effective.
- Drugs used for the treatment of HIV may be hepatotoxic and nephrotoxic.
- Monitor for hypersensitivity and allergic reactions, especially with the first dose of any antiretroviral or protease inhibitor. Continue to monitor the patient as needed based on drug used or patient condition. Anaphylactic reactions are possible, and reactions may not always be predictable.
- Lactic acidosis is a possible life-threatening adverse effect of NRTIs and NtRTIs. Monitor for abdominal pain, anxiety, fatigue, palpitations, lethargy, rapid breathing and heart rate, weakness, chest pain or tightness, fever, or shortness of breath.
- Bone marrow suppression may occur and may cause blood dyscrasias with resulting decreases in red blood cells, white blood cells, or platelets.
- HIV drugs may cause significant dermatologic effects including stomatitis and SJS, a potentially fatal condition. Monitor for dermatologic effects such as red or purplish skin rash, blisters, or peeling skin, including oral mucous membranes. Assess oral mucous membranes for signs of stomatitis because drug effects or immunosuppression may result in overgrowth of oral flora.
- Some HIV drugs cause peripheral neuropathy and have neurologic adverse effects. Frequent monitoring is needed to prevent or minimize adverse effects.
- GI effects are common adverse effects of most antiretrovirals and PIs. Some antiretroviral drugs may cause pancreatitis. Serum amylase and lipid levels should be monitored periodically.
- Many antiretroviral drugs may cause hyperglycemia. Patients with diabetes may require a change in their antidiabetic drug regimen. Lipodystrophy syndrome occurs in many patients receiving long-term therapy with many antiretroviral drugs, and large increases in total cholesterol and triglycerides may occur during therapy.
- Some antiretroviral drugs may significantly reduce the effectiveness of oral contraceptives. Women of childbearing age should use an alternative form of birth control to prevent pregnancy.

CONNECTIONS: APPLIED CLINICAL JUDGMENT *(continued)*

Patients Receiving Pharmacotherapy with Antiretrovirals

Lifespan Considerations

- Older adults may be at increased risk for hypotension, and dizziness may increase the risk of falls.
- Age-related physiologic changes increase the risk of adverse renal and hepatic effects in the older adult.

Diversity Considerations

- Because many drugs for HIV metabolize through the CYP450 system pathways, frequent monitoring in ethnically diverse patients is needed to ensure optimal therapeutic effects and to minimize adverse effects.

Patient Education

- The treatment plan will be reviewed periodically, and the drugs used may change if drug resistance is suspected.
- Report a fever that does not diminish below 37.8°C (100°F) or per provider's instructions, an inability to maintain hydration or nutrition, or dizziness to the healthcare provider.
- Rise from lying to sitting or standing slowly to avoid dizziness or falls. If dizziness occurs, sit or lie down and do not attempt to stand or walk until the sensation passes. Report increasing lethargy, disorientation, confusion, changes in behavior or mood, slurred speech, tremors, or ataxia. Report any changes in behavior, confusion, delusion, or expressed thoughts of suicide.
- Immediately report any nausea and vomiting, yellowing of the skin or sclera, abdominal pain, light- or clay-colored stools, diminished urine output, or darkening of urine.
- Increase fluid intake to 2 to 3 L/day. Eliminate alcohol.
- Report any low-grade fevers, sore throat, rashes, bruising or increased bleeding, unusual fatigue, or shortness of breath, especially if on drug therapy for a prolonged period.
- Report symptoms of lactic acidosis such as abdominal pain, anxiety, fatigue, palpitations, lethargy, rapid breathing and heart rate, weakness, chest pain or tightness, fever, or shortness of breath.
- Avoid acidic foods and beverages, carbonated drinks, or excessively hot or cold foods and beverages that may cause mouth irritation. Eat small, frequent meals, which may be better tolerated than fewer, larger meals.
- Patients with diabetes should test blood glucose level more frequently, reporting any consistent elevations.
- Take the medication as follows:
  - Complete the entire course of therapy unless otherwise instructed. Suppressive therapy may be used to maintain a symptom-free period. Do not stop the medicine when starting to feel better.
  - Do not share medicine with other family members. If there is reason to believe they need medication, they should be assessed by a healthcare provider.
  - Take the medication as evenly spaced throughout each day as feasible.
  - Increase overall fluid intake while taking these drugs and eliminate alcohol, which can cause significant reactions when taken with alcohol.

Prescribing Considerations

- Be aware of potential interactions between specific antiretroviral medications and hormonal contraceptives that could lower contraceptive efficacy.
- Treatment should be started based on a person's informed decision to initiate ART; ART initiation is rarely urgent, however it may need to be expedited in certain circumstances, such as serious ill health and for pregnant women in labor.

Prophylaxis of HIV Infections

55.8 Postexposure prophylaxis of HIV infection is designed to prevent transmission in specific occupational and nonoccupational settings.

Since the start of the AIDS epidemic, nurses and other healthcare workers caring for patients with HIV infection or AIDS have been concerned about acquiring the disease from their patients. Fortunately, if proper precautions are observed, the disease is rarely transmitted from patient to healthcare worker. Accidents have occurred, however, in which the healthcare provider has acquired the infection by exposure to the blood or body fluids of patients infected with HIV. Estimates of the risk for transmission to the heathcare provider following occupational HIV exposure is 0.3% for percutaneous exposure and 0.09% for mucous membrane exposure.

Occupational Postexposure Prophylaxis

For prevention to be most successful, postexposure prophylaxis (PEP) should be started within 72 hours after exposure to a source individual who is known or suspected to be HIV positive. Although the exact interval remains undefined, longer periods allow the infection to progress to stages where prophylaxis would not be successful. The healthcare worker should obtain a baseline HIV viral load as soon as possible after exposure.

If the HIV status of the source individual is unknown, PEP is decided case by case, based on the type of exposure (percutaneous or mucous membrane) and the likelihood the blood contained HIV. With the advent of rapid HIV diagnosis, results from the source patient may become available as quickly as 30 minutes. If locating or testing the source patient is delayed, PEP should begin immediately. If confirmed that the exposure contained HIV-infected blood, a 4-week course of ART is recommended.

A three-drug antiviral regimen is recommended. The first-line therapy for PEP consists of a dual NRTI backbone (tenofovir disoproxil/emtricitabine [Truvada]) plus an integrase strand inhibitor (raltegravir [Isentress]). Consensus on the optimal regimen for occupational PEP is still evolving, and many alternative regimens are possible.

Nonoccupational Postexposure Prophylaxis

Guidelines have been established for antiviral PEP of HIV following sexual, injection drug use, or other nonoccupational exposure to HIV (CDC, 2016b). These guidelines are largely based on animal studies and analysis of the existing data for occupational exposure. Because nonoccupational postexposure prophylaxis (nPEP) is expensive and may result in adverse drug effects, it is recommended only when meeting specific criteria.

- Prior to starting nPEP, the HIV status of the potentially exposed person should be determined (using a rapid HIV diagnostic test) because the person may have already acquired HIV and not be aware of it.
- The exposure must have occurred no later than 72 hours before antiretroviral therapy is initiated.
- The nature of the nonoccupational exposure must present a substantial risk for HIV acquisition.
- The source of the blood or body fluids must be known to be HIV positive. If possible, given the short time frame, the source person should be requested to consent to rapid HIV testing.

Individuals offered nPEP receive a 28-day, three-drug antiviral regimen. The preferred regimen for nPEP consists of tenofovir disoproxil or tenofovir alafenamide with emtricitabine plus an integrase strand inhibitor (raltegravir). Many alternative regimens are possible.

Preexposure Prophylaxis

55.9 Preexposure prophylaxis is effective in preventing HIV transmission in certain groups.

Significant research has been conducted to determine if HIV infection can be *prevented* by medications. The goal of preventing HIV infection is an important one to consider because prevention is always preferable to treatment. This type of therapy is called preexposure prophylaxis (PrEP).

Preexposure prophylaxis may be beneficial for someone who is HIV negative who has a sexual partner who is HIV positive or if someone has multiple sexual partners whose HIV status is unknown. The PrEP drugs are 99% effective in reducing HIV transmission from a sexual partner. However, they are only 74% effective in reducing transmission among people who inject drugs. The medications must be taken continuously on a daily basis. The cost of PrEP medication is approximately $2,000 per month which can present a major barrier for many patients.

There are two drugs currently approved for PrEP. Approved in 2004, Truvada is a combination of emtricitabine and tenofovir diproxil. Truvada is indicated to reduce the risk of sexually transmitted HIV infection. In 2016, it was approved to treat HIV infection, in combination with other antiretrovirals.

Approved in 2015, Descovy is a combination of emtricitabine and tenofovir alafenamide. Like Truvada, Descovy is approved to treat HIV infection, when combined with other antiretrovirals. However, Descovy for PrEP is only approved to prevent HIV transmission in gay and bisexual cis men and transgender women. In simple terms, this means that Descovy is not indicated to prevent HIV transmission during penile-vaginal sex.

Perinatal Transmission Prophylaxis

55.10 The risk of perinatal transmission of HIV can be markedly reduced by optimizing antiretroviral therapy during pregnancy.

When pregnancy occurs, the therapeutic outcomes focus on aggressively lowering the viral load in the mother while preventing the transmission of HIV to the unborn child. Lowering the maternal viral load to less than 50 copies/mL reduces the risk of HIV transmission to the baby to less than 1%.

If the woman is currently on fully suppressive ART when becoming pregnant, the current regimen is usually continued. Doses may need adjusting due to potential pharmacokinetic changes that occur during pregnancy. If not already on ART, current guidelines recommend that therapy begin as early in pregnancy as possible. Preferred protocols for the pregnant individual include one of two regimens: an integrase inhibitor regimen or a protease inhibitor regimen. Both of these regimens include a preferred dual NRTI backbone.

- *Integrase strand inhibitor regimen*
  - Choice 1: dolutegravir/abacavir/lamivudine or dolutegravir plus a NRTI backbone.
  - Choice 2: raltegravir plus a NRTI backbone

- *Protease inhibitor regimen*
  - Choice 1: atazanavir/ritonavir plus a NRTI backbone
  - Choice 2: darunavir/ritonavir plus a NRTI backbone.

- *Dual NRTI backbone*
  - Choice 1) abacavir/lamivudine
  - *Choice 2:* tenofovir diproxil/lamivudine or tenofovir disoproxil/emtricitabine.

Women on antepartum ART should continue to receive the regimen during labor and delivery. If the patient's HIV RNA level is greater than 1000 copies/mL, an infusion of zidovudine is begun about 3 hours before scheduled cesarean delivery. Zidovudine readily crosses the placenta and is effective at reducing the risk for perinatal transmission.

Women with unknown HIV status should undergo rapid HIV testing during labor. If confirmed to be HIV positive, an immediate infusion of intrapartum zidovudine is begun.

Antiretroviral therapy of neonates born to mothers infected with HIV should begin within 6 hours after delivery (Panel on Treatment of HIV-Infected Pregnant Women and Prevention of Perinatal Transmission, 2016). Current recommendations include the following:

- If the mother had been receiving antiretroviral therapy and viral load was suppressed (less than 50 copies/mL) prior to delivery, the infant receives 4 weeks of prophylactic zidovudine.
- If the mother had not been receiving antiretroviral therapy prior to delivery, the infant receives 6 weeks of *presumptive* antiretroviral therapy with zidovudine/lamivudine, plus either nevirapine *or* raltegravir.
- Infant treatment is discontinued immediately if the supplemental testing confirms the mother to be HIV negative.

The CDC advises that mothers with HIV infection not breastfeed their infants because this is a possible route of HIV transmission, and many antiretrovirals are secreted in breast milk (Panel on Treatment of HIV-Infected Pregnant Women and Prevention of Perinatal Transmission, 2016).

Definitive diagnosis on infants with perinatal HIV exposure who are less than 18 months of age requires HIV RNA or HIV DNA nucleic acid testing. Diagnostic testing at birth, 1 to 2 months, and 4 to 6 months is recommended. Some practitioners continue testing at 12 months and 18 months. If diagnostic testing reveals that the infant is not infected before the 6-week prophylactic treatment period is completed, zidovudine therapy is discontinued. On the other hand, if HIV diagnosis is confirmed during this period, the infant is switched to three-drug ART.

Providers caring for patients who have had an exposure can call the PEPline (1-888-448-4911) for advice on its management. It is important that providers prescribing PEP discuss with their patients the risks, benefits, and possible side effects of PEP and follow patients closely to make sure they take their regimen correctly.

Pharmacotherapy of Opportunistic Infections Associated with HIV and AIDS

55.11 Loss of immune function due to HIV often results in opportunistic infections that require anti-infective therapy.

In the early 1980s, all patients with AIDS acquired serious OIs from pathogenic bacteria, viruses, fungi, and protozoans. Profound loss of immune function allowed dormant pathogens to flourish and also lowered the defense barriers for infection by newly acquired organisms. Often, the presentation of an acute OI was the reason the patient first sought medical attention for HIV disease. For example, in the early years of the epidemic, 70 to 80% of all patients with AIDS developed *Pneumocystis* pneumonia, which carried a mortality rate of up to 40% in these patients. Since the advent of ART, *Pneumocystis* pneumonia is now rare.

OIs still occur in patients with HIV infection and AIDS; however, they are less common and mortality is diminished. This is because ART increases the numbers of CD4 lymphocytes, allowing patients with HIV infection to maintain a higher level of immunologic defense. In addition, the

CONNECTIONS: Advanced Practice Application

HIV and Occupational Exposure

Case

Katrina King, MPH, RN was working at a community event testing for HIV when a coworker was having trouble getting blood from a client. Katrina offered to help and was successful on the first attempt using a butterfly needle. She then removed the needle and while putting pressure on the patient's arm to stop the bleeding, she reached behind her to place the used needle in the sharps box and was stuck in the hand by another needle in the box. She immediately rinsed the area and reports to you, one of the occupational health nurse practitioners for the health system Katrina works for. What can you share with her about her risk of transmission?

Discussion

While it is true that healthcare workers are at risk of acquiring HIV infection from their patients, this risk is exceedingly small. Only 58 cases of confirmed occupational HIV transmission to healthcare personnel have been reported in the United States and based on the most recent data available, only one confirmed case has been reported since 1999 (CDC, 2019b).

The CDC (2019b) recommendations for the prevention of transmission of HIV in the workplace are that healthcare workers follow universal precautions to avoid contact with potentially infectious blood and if a healthcare worker experiences significant percutaneous or mucous membrane exposure to blood from any patient, they should undergo serological screening for potential bloodborne agents, including HIV, and be monitored with standardized follow-up. This may include postexposure prophylaxis. (See Section 55.8.)

Table 55.3 Pharmacotherapy of Selected Opportunistic Infections in Patients with HIV and AIDS

Disease	Preferred Drug(s) for Prevention	Comments
Bacterial enteric infections	PO: fluoroquinolone (ciprofloxacin preferred) or ceftriaxone	Most common pathogens are *Salmonella*, *Campylobacter*, and *Shigella*
Bacterial respiratory infections	Pneumococcal vaccine (PCV or PPV); inactivated influenza vaccine	Most common pathogens are *S. pneumoniae* and *H. influenzae*
Candidiasis (mucocutaneous)	PO: fluconazole	Topical azoles may be used for vulvovaginal or oropharyngeal disease
Cryptococcosis	No prevention recommended; treatment is with amphotericin B with flucytosine for 2 wk, followed by fluconazole for 8 wk	Lifelong prophylaxis with fluconazole is indicated in certain patients
Cryptosporidiosis	Antiretroviral regimen should be optimized	HIV-infected patients should drink only purified water free from possible bacteria
Herpes simplex	PO: famciclovir or acyclovir for 7–14 days	IV therapy is indicated in severe infections
Histoplasmosis (disseminated)	PO: itraconazole daily	Lifelong prophylaxis with itraconazole is indicated in certain patients
Pneumocystis pneumonia (PCP)	PO: trimethoprim-sulfamethoxazole (TMP-SMZ) for 21 days	Lifelong prophylaxis is indicated in certain patients; pentamidine IV may be used for severe cases
Syphilis	IM: benzathine penicillin	If allergic to penicillin, penicillin desensitization is attempted or doxycycline is substituted
Toxoplasma gondii encephalitis	PO: TMP-SMZ	Pyrimethamine and clindamycin are alternative drugs

anti-infective pharmacotherapy of OIs has evolved due to a better understanding of these diseases. Patients with CD4 counts below 200 cells/mcL may be placed on prophylactic antibiotics because the risk of an OI in these patients is very high. Most other patients with HIV infection are monitored carefully for signs of infectious disease and treated as symptoms indicate.

Drugs used for treating OIs have been presented in previous anti-infective chapters. The CDC publishes detailed, updated recommendations for prevention and treatment of OIs in patients with HIV infection (CDC, 2020a). A list of preferred drugs for selected OIs is given in Table 55.3.

Understanding Chapter 55

Key Concepts Summary

55.1 HIV causes a profound loss of immune function.

55.2 Treatment of HIV infection is challenging due to the latent nature of the virus and the development of resistant strains.

55.3 Five classes of antiretroviral drugs are available to treat HIV infection.

55.4 Reverse transcriptase inhibitors block the synthesis of viral DNA.

55.5 The nonnucleoside reverse transcriptase inhibitors block viral DNA replication by binding to reverse transcriptase.

55.6 Protease inhibitors prevent HIV protease from completing the final step in HIV maturation.

55.7 Integrase inhibitors, entry inhibitors, and attachment inhibitors are newer strategies for managing HIV infections.

55.8 Postexposure prophylaxis of HIV infection is designed to prevent transmission in specific occupational and nonoccupational settings.

55.9 Preexposure prophylaxis is effective in preventing HIV transmission in certain groups.

55.10 The risk of perinatal transmission of HIV can be markedly reduced by optimizing antiretroviral therapy during pregnancy.

55.11 Loss of immune function due to HIV often results in opportunistic infections that require anti-infective therapy.

CASE STUDY: Making the Patient Connection

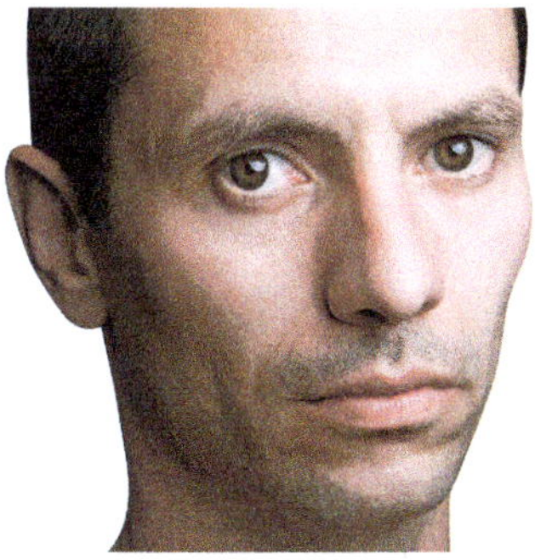

Remember the patient "Ryan Orre" at the beginning of the chapter? Now read the remainder of the case study. Based on the information presented within this chapter, respond to the critical thinking questions that follow.

Ryan Orre is a 37-year-old single man who has come to his healthcare provider because of the recent onset of a chronic sore throat and flulike symptoms, including swollen lymph nodes in the neck and armpits, tiredness, fever, and night sweats. During this office visit, Ryan appears extremely anxious and troubled.

When questioned about his apparent nervousness, Ryan states, "You don't understand; I'm gay. But I've always been very careful and practice safe sex. What if I have AIDS? What will I do? I don't want to die." The healthcare provider acknowledges Ryan's fears and spends additional time allowing Ryan to express his concerns. The process of diagnosing HIV infection is discussed with the patient and initiated.

Ryan's medical history reveals that he is allergic to penicillin, which results in rash and pruritus. Although Ryan does not currently take any prescribed medications, he recently started multivitamin and nutritional supplements due to a recent loss of weight. The patient denies any current recreational drug use but admits that he occasionally used IV drugs during his college years. He has not used them in the past 8 years. No past history of medical or psychiatric illness exists. He has never had surgery.

Ryan does not use tobacco products. He reports drinking alcoholic beverages several times weekly but never to excess. Ryan explains that he has had several male sexual partners over the past 10 years but feels that he has been consistent in his use of condoms. He currently lives alone and works as a sales representative with a local computer firm. A series of laboratory diagnostic tests found the following abnormal results: plasma HIV RNA >10,000 copies/mL and CD4 count of 550/mm^3. Ryan is hospitalized with the preliminary diagnosis of sepsis and to rule out HIV. A test for HIV viral load is ordered.

Critical Thinking Questions

1. You are the nurse caring for Ryan in the hospital. On the first evening, he asks if you think his provider will be prescribing antiretroviral therapy. Given this situation, how would you explain the factors that determine when antiretroviral therapy should be initiated?
2. Ryan's CD4 count is still within low-normal range, but his HIV viral load (plasma HIV RNA) comes back significantly increased, indicating HIV infection. After talking with the provider, Ryan asks you to explain again the difference between HIV infection and AIDS. How would you explain this?
3. Ryan's provider has decided to start him on antiretroviral therapy and Ryan will begin taking efavirenz (Sustiva), tenofovir disoproxil (Viread), and emtricitabine (Emtriva). What will be the best method of teaching Ryan about these drugs? What other factors should be considered when talking with Ryan?

Additional Case Study

Alexa Trihan is referred to an HIV clinic after she is diagnosed at the free clinic she goes to for medical care as having HIV infection, most likely acquired by IV drug use. She is prescribed antiretroviral therapy using an ART regimen. Although the healthcare provider has explained the therapy, Alexa's anxiety results in her inability to comprehend the entire explanation provided. Alexa begins asking you, her nurse, questions about ART.

1. Using simple language, how would you, as Alexa's nurse, explain HIV and ART?
2. Explain the concept of treatment as prevention to Alexa.
3. Alexa tells you that she may be pregnant. How will this potentially affect her treatment?

Chapter Review

1. A 29-year-old has been diagnosed with HIV infection and will begin dolutegravir (Tivicay) for treatment as prevention purposes. Teaching for this patient should include what important information?

1. It has no serious adverse effects, but drug levels will be monitored.
2. It may be stopped once the viral load (HIV RNA) is below 200 copies/mL.
3. The medication schedule can be adjusted daily depending on my activities.
4. Sexual abstinence or barrier methods should be used until the viral load is maintained at less than 200 copies/mL.

2. A patient has been taking lopinavir with ritonavir (Kaletra) for the past 8 years and has noticed a redistribution of body fat in the arms, legs, and abdomen (lipodystrophy). In addition to this effect, the nurse knows that this drug may be associated with which additional adverse effects? (Select all that apply.)

1. CKD
2. Hyperglycemia
3. Pancreatitis
4. Bone marrow suppression
5. Hepatic failure

3. Emtricitabine (Emtriva) is included as part of an ART regimen for a patient newly diagnosed with HIV. While lower in toxicity than other NRTIs, a potentially fatal adverse effect known to occur is:

1. Ventricular cardiac dysrhythmias.
2. Pulmonary fibrosis.
3. Necrotic bowel syndrome.
4. Lactic acidosis.

4. Protease inhibitor–based regimens have been shown to be a successful choice for the initial therapy of HIV infection. Which adverse effects are common with this regimen?

1. Fatigue, generalized weakness, myalgia
2. Headache, diarrhea, nausea, fatigue, insomnia
3. Nausea and vomiting, diarrhea, abdominal pain, headache
4. Respiratory tract infections, cough, pyrexia, rash, dizziness

5. The nurse is planning a teaching session with a patient who will be receiving ART. Which of the following should be included in the teaching plan? (Select all that apply.)

1. Avoid crowds and other people with colds, flu, and other infections.
2. Notify the healthcare provider at the first sign of any rash.
3. The medications will reduce transmission of the disease.
4. The drugs will be stopped periodically to give the immune system a chance to respond.
5. Herbal supplements will not interfere with this therapy.

6. The strategies for managing and treating HIV infection during pregnancy have changed as more is learned about the disease. As the nurse teaching a group of new graduate nursing employees, which of the following information would you provide? (Select all that apply.)

1. Due to toxicities, HIV therapy will be initiated after delivery and only after confirming the infant's viral load.
2. Mothers with HIV infection are started on HIV as early as possible in pregnancy.
3. Infants born to mothers with HIV infection will start on HIV therapy as soon as possible after delivery.
4. Treatment of an infant born to a mother who was not on antiretroviral therapy during pregnancy will be continued for 6 months.
5. Due to toxicities, newborns should be breastfed only so that any drug therapy the mother is receiving will be passed to the infant through the breast milk.

See Appendix A for answers to critical thinking questions, case study questions, and review questions.

References

Centers for Disease Control and Prevention (CDC). (2014). *Guidelines for the use of antiretroviral agents in adults and adolescents living with HIV: Laboratory testing.* https://clinicalinfo.hiv.gov/en/guidelines/adult-and-adolescent-arv/plasma-hiv-1-rna-viral-load-and-cd4-count-monitoring

Centers for Disease Control and Prevention (CDC). (2016b). *Updated guidelines for antiretroviral postexposure prophylaxis after sexual, injected drug use of other nonoccupational exposure to HIV—United States, 2016.* https://stacks.cdc.gov/view/cdc/38856

Centers for Disease Control and Prevention (CDC). (2019a). *Guidelines for the use of antiretroviral agents in adults and adolescents living with HIV: Antiretroviral therapy to prevent sexual transmission of HIV.* https://clinicalinfo.hiv.gov/en/guidelines/adult-and-adolescent-arv/antiretroviral-therapy-prevent-sexual-transmission-hiv

Centers for Disease Control and Prevention (CDC). (2019b). *HIV and occupational exposure.* https://www.cdc.gov/hiv/workplace/healthcareworkers.html

Centers for Disease Control and Prevention (CDC). (2020a). *Guidelines for the prevention and treatment of opportunistic infections in HIV-infected adults and adolescents.* https://clinicalinfo.hiv.gov/en/guidelines/adult-and-adolescent-opportunistic-infection/whats-new-guidelines

Centers for Disease Control and Prevention (CDC). (2020b). *HIV in the United States: At a glance.* https://www.cdc.gov/hiv/statistics/overview/ataglance.html

Madigan, M. T., Bender, K. S., Buckley, D. H., Stately, W. M., & Stahl, D. A. (Eds.). (2018). *Brock biology of microorganisms* (15th ed.). Pearson Education.

Panel on Antiretroviral Guidelines for Adults and Adolescents. (2019). *Guidelines for the use of antiretroviral agents in HIV-1-infected adults and adolescents.* Centers for Disease Control and Prevention. https://clinicalinfo.hiv.gov/en/guidelines/adult-and-adolescent-arv/what-start-initial-combination-regimens-antiretroviral-naive?view=brief

Panel on Treatment of HIV-Infected Pregnant Women and Prevention of Perinatal Transmission. (2016). *Recommendations for use of antiretroviral drugs in pregnant HIV-1-infected women for maternal health and interventions to reduce perinatal HIV transmission in the United States.* Centers for Disease Control and Prevention. https://aidsinfo.nih.gov/guidelines/html/3/perinatal-guidelines/187/infant-antiretroviral-prophylaxis

Selected Bibliography

Castor, D., Meyers, K., & Allen, S. (2020). The only way is up: priorities for implementing long-acting antiretrovirals for HIV prevention and treatment. *Current Opinion in HIV and AIDS, 15*(1), 73. https://doi.org/10.1097/COH.0000000000000601

Centers for Disease Control and Prevention (CDC). (2016). *Updated guidelines for antiretroviral postexposure prophylaxis after sexual, injection drug use, or other nonoccupational exposure to HIV—United States, 2016.* http://www.cdc.gov/hiv/pdf/programresources/cdc-hiv-npep-guidelines.pdf

LeMessurier, J., Traversy, G., Varsaneux, O., Weekes, M., Avey, M. T., Niragira, O., et al. (2018). Risk of sexual transmission of human immunodeficiency virus with antiretroviral therapy, suppressed viral load and condom use: A systematic review. *Canadian Medical Association Journal, 190*(46), E1350–E1360. https://doi.org/https://doi.org/10.1503/cmaj.180311

O'Byrne, P., MacPherson, P., Orser, L., Jacob, J. D., & Holmes, D. (2019). PrEP-RN: Clinical considerations and protocols for nurse-led PrEP. *Journal of the Association of Nurses in AIDS Care, 30*(3), 301. https://doi.org/10.1097/JNC.0000000000000075

Max, B. (2020). Update of HIV integrase inhibitors for the treatment of HIV-1 infection. *Future Virology, 14*(10). https://www.futuremedicine.com/doi/10.2217/fvl-2019-0077

Panel on Antiretroviral Therapy and Medical Management of HIV-Infected Children. (2016). *Guidelines for the use of antiretroviral agents in pediatric HIV infection.* Centers for Disease Control and Prevention. https://aidsinfo.nih.gov/contentfiles/lvguidelines/pediatricguidelines.pdf

Phanuphak, N., & Gulick, R. M. (2020). HIV treatment and prevention 2019: Current standards of care. *Current Opinion in HIV and AIDS, 15*(1), 4–12. https://doi.org/10.1097/COH.0000000000000588

Rathburn, R. C. (2020). *Antiretroviral therapy for HIV infection.* Medscape. http://emedicine.medscape.com/article/1533218-overview

Saag, M. S., Benson, C. A., Gandhi, R. T., Hoy, J. F., Landovitz, R. J., Mugavero, M. J., et al. (2018). Antiretroviral drugs for treatment and prevention of

HIV infection in adults: 2018 recommendations of the International Antiviral Society–USA Panel. *Journal of the American Medical Association, 320*(4), 379–396. https://doi.org/10.1001/jama.2018.8431

Weber, D. J., & Rutala, W. A. (2016). Occupational health update: Focus on preventing the acquisition of infections with pre-exposure prophylaxis and postexposure prophylaxis. *Infectious Disease Clinics of North America, 30*, 729–757. https://doi.org/10.1016/j.idc.2016.04.008

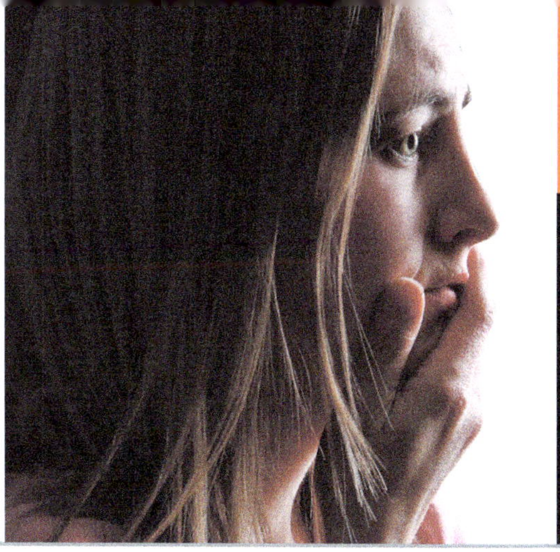

"When the doctor first told me that I had cancer, I was scared. Now after hearing all of the things that the chemotherapy can do to my body, I'm petrified."
—Patient "Cheryl Ogen"

Chapter 56
Basic Principles of Antineoplastic Therapy

Chapter Outline

- Characteristics of Cancer
- Etiology of Cancer
- Detection and Prevention of Cancer
- Goals of Chemotherapy
- Staging and Grading of Cancer
- The Cell Cycle and Growth Fraction
- Cell Kill Hypothesis
- Improving the Success of Chemotherapy
  - Combination Chemotherapy
  - Dosing Schedules
  - Route of Administration
- Toxicity of Antineoplastic Drugs
  - Hematologic System
  - Gastrointestinal Tract
  - Cardiopulmonary System
  - Urinary System
  - Reproductive System
  - Nervous System
  - Skin and Soft Tissue
  - Other Adverse Effects

Learning Outcomes

After reading this chapter, the student should be able to:

1. Compare and contrast the differences between normal cells and cancer cells.
2. Identify etiologic factors associated with an increased incidence of cancer.
3. Construct a table categorizing the major primary and secondary means of cancer prevention.
4. Compare and contrast the following goals of chemotherapy: cure, control, palliation, prophylaxis, adjuvant therapy, and neoadjuvant therapy.
5. Explain the purposes of staging and grading cancers.
6. Explain the significance of growth fraction and the cell cycle to the success of chemotherapy.
7. Assess the ability of antineoplastic drugs to achieve a total cancer cure based on the cell kill hypothesis.
8. Explain how special protocols increase the effectiveness of chemotherapy.
9. Discuss the types of toxicity and adverse effects of chemotherapeutic drugs on the various organ systems.

Key Terms

Definitions of the terms in bold may be found in the Glossary.

Cancer is one of the most feared diseases in society for a number of valid reasons. In the United States, cancer accounts for one out of every four deaths. It is often silent, producing no symptoms until it reaches an advanced stage. It sometimes requires painful and disfiguring treatments such as surgery or radiation. Cancer may strike at an early age, even during infancy, to deprive patients of a normal lifespan. Perhaps worst of all, the medical treatment of cancer often cannot offer a cure, and progression to death is sometimes slow and psychologically difficult for patients and their loved ones.

Despite its feared status, many successes have been made in the diagnosis and treatment of cancer. Modern treatment methods result in a cure for nearly two of every three people and the 5-year survival rate has steadily increased for most types of cancer. This chapter examines the basic principles of cancer therapy. Chapter 57 examines the medications used to treat cancer.

PharmFACT

The American Cancer Society (Siegel et al., 2020) estimates that 1,806,590 new cancer cases occur each year in the United States (not including basal cell or squamous cell skin cancer). More than 606,520 deaths occur annually (about 1600 people per day).

Table 56.1 Classification and Naming of Tumors

Name	Description	Examples
Benign tumor	Slow growing; does not metastasize and rarely requires drug treatment	Adenoma, papilloma, lipoma, osteoma, meningioma
Carcinoma	Cancer of epithelial tissue; most common type of malignant neoplasm; grows rapidly and metastasizes	Malignant melanoma, renal cell carcinoma, adenocarcinoma, hepatocellular carcinoma
Glioma	Cancer of glial (interstitial) cells in the central nervous system	Telangiectatic glioma, brainstem glioma, posterior pituitary gland, or retina
Leukemia	Cancer of the blood-forming cells in bone marrow; may be acute or chronic	Myelocytic leukemia, lymphocytic leukemia
Lymphoma	Cancer of lymphoid tissue	Hodgkin's disease, lymphoblastic lymphoma
Sarcoma	Cancer of connective tissue; grows extremely rapidly and metastasizes early in the progression of the disease	Osteogenic sarcoma, fibrosarcoma, Kaposi's sarcoma, angiosarcoma

Characteristics of Cancer

56.1 Cancer is characterized by rapid, uncontrolled growth of cells that eventually invade normal tissues and metastasize.

A **tumor** is a swelling, an abnormal enlargement, or a mass. The word **neoplasm** is often used interchangeably with *tumor*. Tumors may be benign or malignant. Whereas benign tumors are usually slow growing, remain localized, and rarely cause death, malignant tumors grow rapidly, are invasive, and will kill the host if left untreated. Malignant tumors are classified as carcinomas or sarcomas. Examples of various types of benign and malignant tumors are listed in Table 56.1.

Cancer or carcinoma is a disease characterized by abnormal, uncontrolled cell division. Cell division is a normal process that occurs extensively in most body tissues from conception to late childhood. At some point in time, whether it occurs during fetal life, childhood, or adulthood, the degree of cell division in every tissue must be controlled.

Each cell in the body has the ability to regulate its growth (proliferation) by turning specific genes on and off. For example, growth-promoting genes can be turned on when it is necessary to replace wornout cells, as in the case of blood stem cells, skin epithelial cells, and the lining of the digestive tract. Growth suppressor genes are responsible for slowing the duplication rate and can completely shut down replication, as in the case of muscle cells and most neuron cells. If the suppressor genes become damaged or mutated and do not slow down or stop cell growth, the cells will undergo abnormal proliferation. Because of the critical importance of cell growth to life, it is likely that each cell has multiple genes that regulate division, all of which are responsive to various chemical signals or messages originating from both inside and outside the cell.

Cancer is thought to result from damage to the genes controlling cell growth. Once damaged, cells may become unresponsive to the chemical signals that normally check growth. The cancer cells lose their normal functions, dividing rapidly and invading surrounding tissues. Unlike most normal cells, cancerous cells are able to move to other places in the body. The abnormal cells often travel to distant sites where they populate new tumors, a process called **metastasis**. Figure 56.1 illustrates some characteristics of cancer cells.

Each time a cell divides, it loses a small amount of deoxyribonucleic acid (DNA) at the end of each chromosome. These regions of "extra" repetitive DNA, called **telomeres**, serve to protect the vital sequences of DNA from being destroyed. Average reproducing cells are able to undergo mitosis 50 to 60 times before the cell loses the protective telomeres. Certain human stem cells contain the enzyme **telomerase**, which can lengthen the DNA chains and allow continued replication. Interestingly, this enzyme is not produced in mature cells, which dooms the cells to eventual death. As aging progresses, the telomeres become shorter and shorter and organ degeneration occurs.

Cancer cells are different from normal cells in that they do not die as quickly and can divide and form new cancer

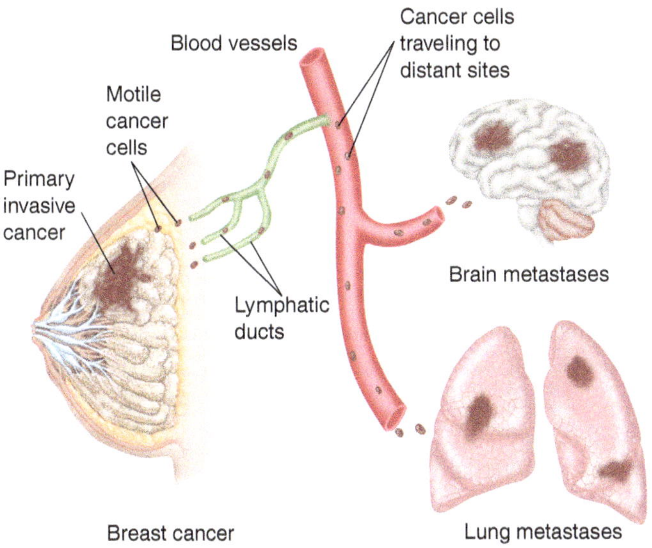

Figure 56.1 Invasion and metastasis by cancer cells.

cells indefinitely. One explanation for this difference is that most cancer cells produce large amounts of telomerase, which continues to add pieces to the telomeres so that the cell can continue to divide. It is believed that the cancer cell begins to produce telomerase soon after it has mutated and that this may be an important factor in the progression to cancer.

To divide rapidly (and indefinitely), cancer cells need an adequate supply of nutrients. Solid tumors need to create a new capillary network to "feed" themselves. The process of **angiogenesis**, which is the formation of new blood vessels, is controlled by a cascade of events. Some factors that are secreted by cells promote angiogenesis, whereas others inhibit it. Cancer cells have the ability to control angiogenesis by causing normal cells to secrete large amounts of vascular endothelial growth factors (VEGFs), which promote the formation of new capillaries. Thus, solid tumors establish their own blood supply, which not only brings in nutrients but also provides an "escape route" during metastasis. Several antineoplastic drugs are used to block VEGF, which "starves" the growing tumor. Examples include bevacizumab (Avastin), aflibercept (Eylea), and pazopanib (Votrient).

Etiology of Cancer

56.2 The etiology of cancer may be chemical, physical, or biologic.

Numerous factors cause cancer or are associated with a higher risk for acquiring the disease. Agents that cause cancer are called **carcinogens**.

Many chemical carcinogens have been identified. For example, chemicals in tobacco smoke are responsible for about one-third of all cancers in the United States. Alcohol ingestion has also been linked to certain cancers, including esophageal, oral, breast, and liver cancers. Chemicals such as asbestos and benzene have been associated with a higher incidence of cancer in the workplace. In some cases, the site of the cancer may be distant from the entry location, as is the case with bladder cancer, which is caused by the inhalation of certain industrial chemicals.

A number of physical factors are also associated with cancer. For example, exposure to large amounts of x-rays is associated with a higher risk of leukemia. Ultraviolet (UV) light from the sun is a common cause of skin cancer.

Viruses and bacteria are estimated to cause 15 to 20% of all human cancers. The common bacterium *Helicobacter pylori* is associated with a higher incidence of gastric cancer. Examples of viruses include hepatitis B and C, Epstein-Barr, human papillomavirus (HPV), and human T-lymphotrophic viruses. If patients remain free from infection with these viruses, their chances of developing certain types of cancer diminish greatly. For example, a vaccine against HPV is available to prevent infection from the two major types of HPV that cause cervical cancer and genital warts. On the other hand, factors that depress immune function, such as the human immunodeficiency virus or immunosuppressant drugs given after transplant surgery, may promote the growth of cancer cells.

Some cancers have a strong genetic component. The fact that twins or close relatives may acquire the same type of cancer suggests that certain genes may confer a predisposition to the condition. These abnormal genes interact with chemical, physical, and biologic agents to promote the formation of cancer. Gender can also be considered a risk factor for certain types of cancer. For instance, breast cancer is more commonly associated with women, whereas bladder cancer is more frequent in men.

Although the development of cancer has a genetic component, it is also greatly influenced by factors in the environment. Maintaining or adopting healthy lifestyle habits may reduce the risk of acquiring cancer. Following proper nutrition, avoiding chemical and physical risks (especially tobacco), and maintaining a regular schedule of health checkups can help prevent cancer from developing into a fatal disease.

Detection and Prevention of Cancer

56.3 The keys to successful cancer treatment are prevention and early detection.

If allowed to grow unchecked and untreated, cancer is eventually fatal in nearly 100% of those who acquire it. The keys to successful cancer treatment are prevention and early detection. Prevention of cancer falls into two categories: primary prevention and secondary prevention.

Primary prevention of cancer includes interventions that keep cancer from ever developing. Interventions for primary prevention are targeted at avoiding known carcinogens and promoting a healthy lifestyle. Examples of primary prevention include the following:

- Health counseling and education delivered by the nurse and nurse practitioner
- Elimination of tobacco use to prevent lung, oral, and other cancers
- Receiving the HPV vaccination to prevent cervical cancer and other cancers
- Maintaining a healthy diet low in saturated fat and processed meats and high in fresh vegetables and fruits
- Maintaining weight within recommended levels
- Decreasing excess stress
- Avoiding chronic or prolonged exposure to direct sunlight or wearing protective clothing or sunscreen. Avoiding use of UV-emitting indoor tanning devices.
- Limiting alcohol consumption to prevent cancers of the liver, colon, rectum, and other regions.

Secondary prevention includes interventions leading to the discovery and control of cancerous or precancerous lesions while they are small and localized. Examples of secondary prevention include the following:

- Receiving a Papanicolaou (Pap) as recommended by the healthcare provider
- Receiving a screening colonoscopy, according to the schedule recommended by the healthcare provider
- Receiving mammograms, according to the schedule recommended by the healthcare provider
- Receiving prostate screening, as recommended by the healthcare provider
- Performing or receiving regular skin examinations to check for abnormal lesions.

CONNECTION Checkpoint 56.1

From what you learned in Chapter 43, describe the recommended immunization schedule for receiving the HPV vaccine.

Goals of Chemotherapy

56.4 The three primary goals of chemotherapy are cure, control, and palliation.

Pharmacotherapy of cancer is sometimes simply referred to as **chemotherapy**. Transported through the blood, drugs have the potential to reach cancer cells in virtually any location. Certain chemotherapeutic drugs are specifically designed to be able to cross the blood–brain barrier to reach brain tumors. Others are instilled directly into body cavities such as the urinary bladder to bring the highest dose possible to the cancer cells without producing systemic adverse effects. Chemotherapy has three general goals: cure, control, and palliation.

When diagnosed with cancer, the primary goal desired by most patients is to achieve a complete cure; that is, permanent removal of all cancer cells from the body. The possibility for cure is much greater if a cancer is identified and treated when the tumor is small and localized to a well-defined region. The 5-year survival rates for nearly all types of cancers have increased in the past two decades due to improved detection and more effective therapies. Examples in which chemotherapy has been used successfully as curative treatment include Hodgkin's lymphoma, certain leukemias, and choriocarcinoma.

PharmFACT

The highest 5-year survival rates are for cancers of the prostate, melanoma, and female breast cancer. The lowest survival rates are for pancreatic, liver, and lung cancers (Siegel et al., 2020).

When cancer has progressed and cure is not possible, a second goal of chemotherapy is to control or manage the disease. Although the cancer is not eliminated, preventing the growth and spread of the tumor may extend a patient's life. Essentially, the cancer is managed as a chronic disease, such as hypertension or diabetes.

In its advanced stages, cure or control of the cancer may not be achievable. For these patients, chemotherapy is used as **palliation**. Chemotherapy drugs are administered to reduce the size of the tumor, easing the severity of pain and other tumor symptoms and thus improving the quality of life. Examples of advanced cancers for which palliation is frequently used include osteosarcoma, pancreatic cancer, and Kaposi's sarcoma.

Chemotherapy may be used alone or in combination with other treatment modalities such as surgery or radiation therapy. Surgery is especially useful for removing solid tumors that are localized. Surgery lowers the number of cancer cells in the body so that radiation therapy and pharmacotherapy can be more successful. The process of removing only a portion of a tumor is referred to as *debulking*. Surgery is not an option for tumors of blood cells or when it would not be expected to extend a patient's lifespan or improve the quality of life.

Approximately 50% of patients with cancer receive radiation therapy as part of their treatment. Radiation therapy is most successful and produces the fewest adverse effects for cancers that are localized when high doses of ionizing radiation can be aimed directly at the tumor and be confined to a small area. Radiation treatments are frequently prescribed postoperatively to kill cancer cells that may remain following an operation. Radiation is sometimes given as palliation for inoperable cancers to shrink the size of a tumor that may be pressing on vital organs and to relieve pain, difficulty breathing, or difficulty swallowing.

Adjuvant chemotherapy is the administration of antineoplastic drugs after surgery or radiation therapy. The purpose of adjuvant chemotherapy is to rid the body of any cancerous cells that were not removed during the surgery or to treat any micrometastases that may be developing.

Neoadjuvant chemotherapy is the administration of antineoplastic drugs before surgery or radiation therapy with the goal of shrinking a large tumor to a more manageable size. This may also be done if the tumor has invaded vital tissue around it, such as may happen with brain tumors. Shrinking the tumor preoperatively results in less surgical invasion when removing the tumor.

In a few cases, drugs are given as chemoprophylaxis with the goal of preventing cancer from occurring in patients at high risk for developing tumors. For example, patients with a close family history of breast cancer who have had a primary breast cancer removed may receive tamoxifen, even if there is no evidence of metastases. Tamoxifen has been shown to prevent the recurrence of breast cancer in these patients. Chemoprophylaxis of cancer is uncommon because most of these drugs have potentially serious adverse effects.

CONNECTION Checkpoint 56.2

Corticosteroids are administered to most patients who are receiving tissue or organ transplants. From what you learned in Chapter 42, what is the rationale for administering corticosteroids to these patients?

Table 56.2 Staging of Cancer*

T Category: Describes the Primary Tumor	
TX	Primary tumor cannot be assessed
T0	No evidence of primary tumor
T_{is}	Tumor is confined to the primary area
T1–T4	Tumor has invaded areas surrounding the primary tumor (number based on extent and size of the tumor)
N Category: Describes Whether or Not the Cancer Has Spread to Lymph Nodes	
NX	Nearby lymph nodes cannot be assessed
N0	Regional lymph nodes do not contain cancer
N1–N3	Primary tumor has spread to regional lymph nodes
M Category: Describes Whether or Not Distant Metastases Are Present	
MX	Distant metastases cannot be assessed
M0	No distant metastases were found
M1	Distant metastases are present

*The exact staging of a tumor varies somewhat with each specific type of cancer. Most have multiple subcategories to better define the tumor.

Staging and Grading of Cancer

56.5 Cancers are described by their stage and grade.

Staging and grading must be done to determine the extent to which a cancer has invaded the body. These processes are performed on the initial diagnosis of cancer to determine the optimum course of therapy and predict patient outcomes.

Staging is the process of determining where the cancer is located and the extent of its invasion. Staging helps the healthcare provider to more accurately communicate the prognosis of the disease with the patient and helps to determine the best course of treatment.

During the staging of solid tumors, diagnostic testing determines the size of the tumor, whether the tumor has invaded surrounding tissue, the involvement of lymph nodes, and the presence or absence of metastasis (Table 56.2). The patient's disease is assigned numerical values for the tumor (T), node (N), and metastasis (M). Once these are determined, an overall stage is assigned: I, II, III, or IV. Stage I is assigned to cancers that are the least invasive and have the best prognosis. Stage IV is given for cancers that are the most aggressive and have the poorest prognosis.

Restaging may be done after surgical removal of the cancer or following additional testing. The new stage classification is added to the original stage, but it does not replace it. The new stage, however, will help guide treatment options and determine survival predictions.

Grading is a process that examines potential cancer cells under a microscope and compares their appearance to normal parent cells. Normal cells are highly differentiated: They have developed, become fully mature, look like the parent cell, and carry on the functions of the parent cell. For example, it is very easy to distinguish a liver cell from a muscle cell or a nerve cell microscopically. When a normal cell becomes cancerous, however, it gradually changes and becomes less differentiated in both structure and function. Once fully undifferentiated, the cancer cell will look very different from the parent cell from which it came and will not carry on the functions of the parent cell.

In the grading process, if the biopsy cells appear differentiated and very similar to the parent cells, the tumor is classified as a Grade 1 (G1) and has the best prognosis. G4 cells are grossly abnormal and clearly different from normal cells. Patients with these malignant and aggressive cells have the worst prognosis. The different grades are described in Table 56.3.

Grading has certain limitations. For instance, solid tumors often contain many different types of cells that vary in appearance, from near normal to grossly abnormal. One part of the tumor may have cells consistent with G2, whereas other parts of the same tumor may have cells consistent with G4. Unlike staging, grading may change over time as the tumor evolves.

Table 56.3 Grading of Cancer Cells

Grade	Description
GX	Grade cannot be determined
G0	Carcinoma in situ: the cancer is localized and has not spread.
G1	Well differentiated: The cancer cells look like normal cells and are replicating slowly
G2	Moderately differentiated: The cancer cells look somewhat like normal cells and are replicating moderately fast
G3	Poorly differentiated: The cancer cells look clearly different from normal cells and are replicating rapidly
G4	Undifferentiated: The cancer cells do not look anything like normal cells and are replicating aggressively

The Cell Cycle and Growth Fraction

56.6 Many antineoplastic drugs are more effective when given at specific stages of the cell cycle and in tumors with a high growth fraction.

Both normal and cancerous cells go through a sequence of events known as the cell cycle, which is illustrated in Figure 56.2. Knowledge of the cell cycle is important to understanding the effectiveness of anticancer drugs.

In simplest terms, a cell is either performing its daily functions or it is undergoing cell division. Certain cellular activities occur in between these two basic functions of the cell that allow its lifecycle to be divided into five stages or phases:

Stage G_0. Although sometimes called the resting phase, G_0 is the phase during which cells conduct their everyday activities such as metabolism, impulse conduction, contraction, or secretion. A cell may enter its G_0 phase at any point in the cycle and remain there for extended periods, depending on the specific tissue and surrounding cellular signals. Cells spend most of their lifetime in the G_0 phase.

Stage G_1 (gap 1). If a cell receives a signal to divide, it leaves the G_0 phase and enters the G_1 phase, during which it synthesizes the ribonucleic acid, proteins, and other components needed to duplicate its DNA.

Stage S (synthesis). During the S phase the cell duplicates its DNA.

Stage G_2 (gap 2). During the G_2 or premitotic phase, the cell makes additional proteins and the spindle apparatus that are necessary for cell division or mitosis.

Stage M (mitosis). The cell undergoes mitosis, which includes prophase, metaphase, anaphase, and telophase. Following mitosis in the M phase, the cell has split into two identical cells that will either start the process over at the G_1 phase or enter the G_0 phase, depending on the needs of the body. This is the briefest stage of the cell cycle.

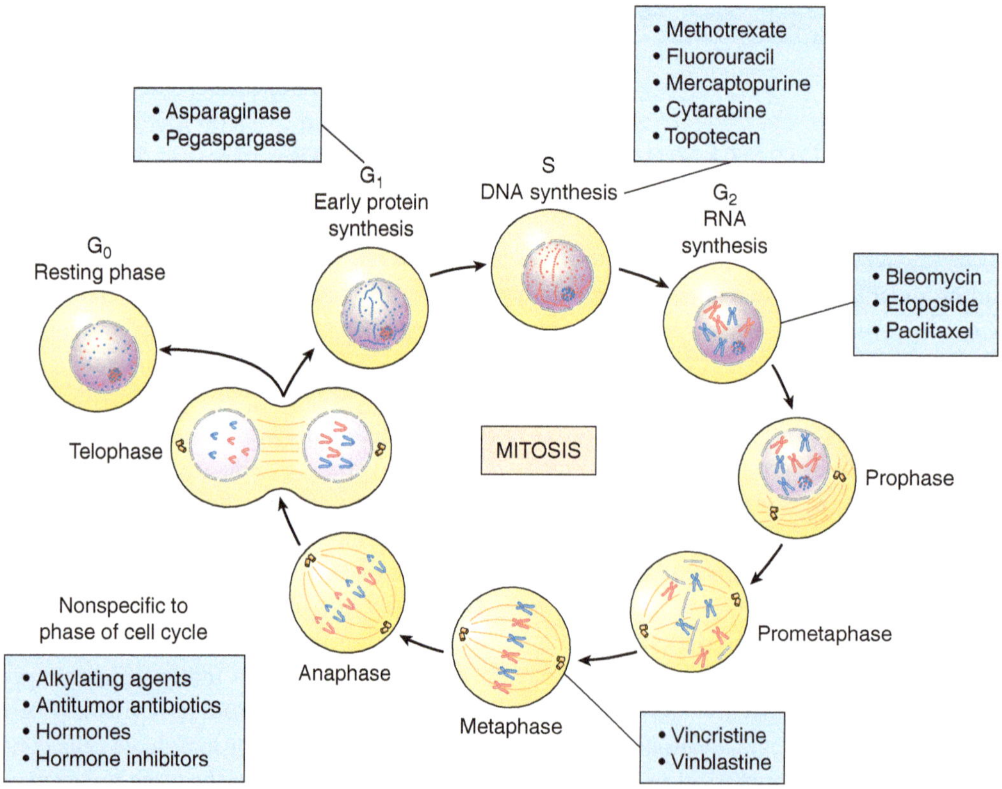

Figure 56.2 Antineoplastic drugs and the cell cycle.

The actions of some antineoplastics are specific to certain phases of the cell cycle, whereas others are mostly independent of the cell cycle. Cell-cycle-specific drugs kill the most cancer cells when they are administered in divided but frequent doses. Cell-cycle-specific drugs are most effective in treating hematologic malignancies and other cancers that have a relatively large proportion of cells proliferating at any given point in time. Examples include mitotic inhibitors such as vincristine (Oncovin), which affect cells in the M phase, and antimetabolites such as fluorouracil (Adrucil), which are most effective against cells during the S phase. In general, cell-cycle-specific drugs are not effective against tumors that have a large percentage of resting cells.

Cell-cycle-nonspecific drugs can kill cancer cells in any stage of the cell cycle, including the G_0 resting phase. Often, these drugs are incorporated into resting cancer cells and have no effects until the cells attempt to divide. These drugs act relatively slowly and are given intermittently to give normal cells an opportunity to recover. The effects of alkylating agents such as cyclophosphamide (Cytoxan), antitumor antibiotics, and hormonal therapies are generally independent of the phases of the cell cycle.

The **growth fraction** is a measure of the number of cells undergoing mitosis in a tissue. It is a ratio of the number of replicating cells to the number of resting cells. Antineoplastic drugs are more toxic to tissues and tumors with high growth fractions. For example, certain leukemias and lymphomas have a high growth fraction and therefore have a greater antineoplastic success rate. Solid tumors such as breast and lung cancer generally have a low growth fraction; therefore, they are less sensitive to antineoplastic drugs. Because certain normal tissues, such as hair follicles, bone marrow, and the gastrointestinal (GI) epithelium, also have high growth fractions, they are sensitive to the effects of the antineoplastics.

With large solid tumors, a high percentage of the cells have entered the G_0 phase, causing the tumor to have a lower growth fraction. Chemotherapeutic drugs are not as effective against cells that are in the G_0 phase. To improve the success of chemotherapeutic drugs, the tumor may be debulked. When a tumor is debulked, a portion is removed surgically, causing the remaining cells to move into the active phases of mitosis. Once the cells enter into mitosis, the chemotherapeutic drugs can more effectively kill the cancer cells.

Cell Kill Hypothesis

56.7 The goal of chemotherapy is to kill as many cancer cells as possible while sparing normal cells.

Measurement of the success of chemotherapy is dependent on the therapeutic goal. If the desirable outcome is a total cure, then success is measured by how long the patient remains cancer free following treatment. If the goal is palliation, success is measured by the degree to which the patient's quality of life is improved. Because chemotherapy is often prolonged and physically challenging, it is crucial that the patient understand the goals of treatment and how they will be measured. In cases of palliation, the patient must weigh whether the adverse effects associated with treatment are worth the anticipated increase in the quality of life.

Patients who are undergoing chemotherapy usually receive several rounds of treatment spaced over a designated time, usually several weeks or months. This is because each round of chemotherapy kills a set percentage of cancer cells, usually those that are rapidly dividing at the time of treatment. Subsequent rounds kill additional cells. Another reason is that chemotherapy always damages normal cells and can cause serious adverse effects. Patients need time to recover between treatments. For example, neutrophils are especially sensitive to chemotherapy and a patient's absolute neutrophil count (ANC) will usually plummet after a therapy session. Intervals between treatments allow the body to make more neutrophils so that body defenses are able to fight infections.

The **cell kill hypothesis** is a theoretical model that predicts the ability of antineoplastic drugs to eliminate cancer cells. This hypothesis predicts that a drug will kill a certain percentage, rather than a constant number, of cancer cells. Why is this important?

Theoretically, every single cell in a malignant tumor must be eliminated from the body to cure a patient. Leaving even a single malignant cell could result in regrowth of the tumor. Eliminating every cancer cell with chemotherapy alone, however, is a very difficult task. As an example, consider that a small, 1-cm breast tumor may already contain 1 billion cancer cells before it can be detected during a manual examination. A drug that is able to kill 99% of these cells would be considered a very effective drug indeed. Yet even with this fantastic achievement, 10 million cancer cells would remain, any one of which could potentially cause the tumor to return and kill the patient. The relationship between cell kill and chemotherapy is illustrated in Figure 56.3. It is likely that no antineoplastic drug (or combination of drugs) has the ability to kill 100% of the tumor cells. The large burden of cancer cells, however, may be lowered sufficiently to permit the patient's immune system to control or eliminate the remaining cancer cells. Because the immune system is able to eliminate only a relatively small number of cancer cells, it is imperative that as many cancerous cells as possible be eliminated during treatment. This example reinforces the need to diagnose and treat tumors at an early stage when the number of cancer cells is smaller and to lower the tumor burden through surgical removal or radiation therapy whenever feasible.

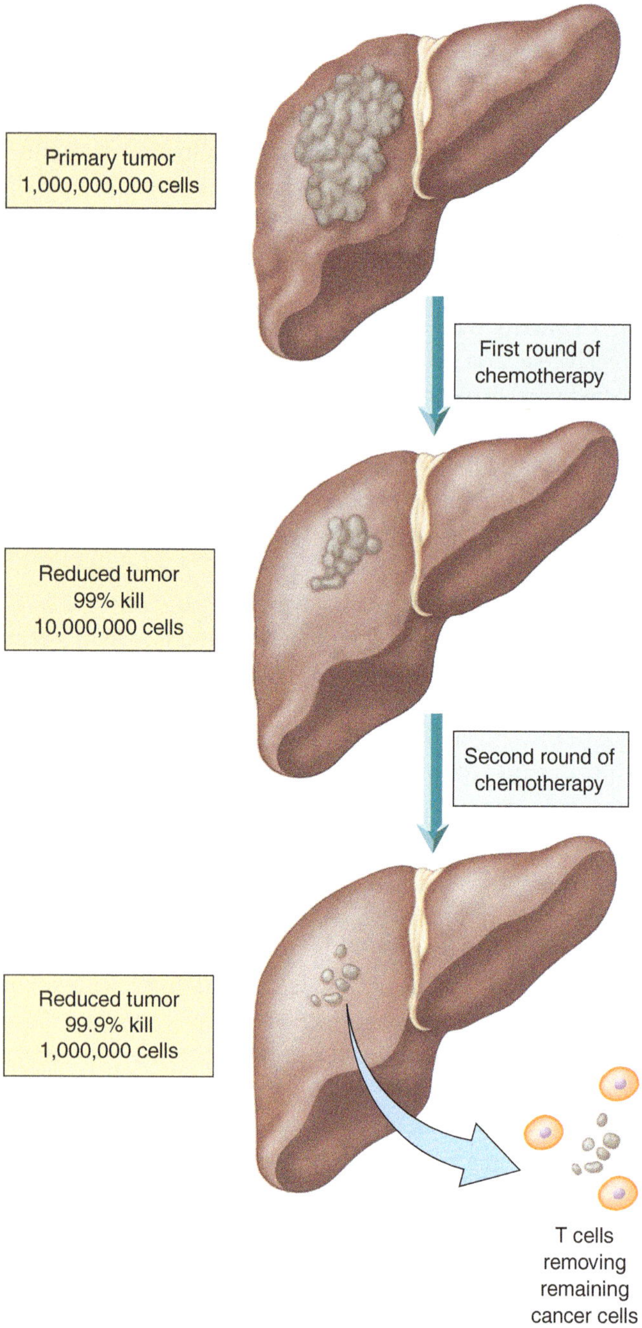

Figure 56.3 Cell kill and chemotherapy.

Because of their rapid cell division, tumor cells express a high mutation rate, which continually changes their genetic structure, resulting in a more heterogenous mass as the tumor grows. Essentially, the tumor becomes a mass of hundreds of different types of cancer cells with different growth rates and physiologic properties. Administration of an antineoplastic drug may kill only a small portion of the tumor, leaving some clones unaffected and able to repopulate the tumor with resistant cells. The appearance of cancer cells that are resistant to antineoplastic drugs complicates the chances for a pharmacologic cure because a therapy that was very successful in reducing the tumor mass at the start of chemotherapy may become less effective over time.

Improving the Success of Chemotherapy

56.8 Use of multiple drugs and intermittent dosing are strategies that allow for greater success of chemotherapy.

As has been seen throughout this text, the majority of pharmacotherapy is conducted with a single drug given in a constant amount over a specified time period. For most indications, the use of multiple drugs increases the expense of treatment and can cause additional adverse effects. Cancer chemotherapy is an important exception: The concurrent use of multiple drugs, combined with intermittent dosing, results in improved patient outcomes.

Combination Chemotherapy

Chemotherapy is conducted using established protocols that are specific to the type of cancer and its stage. A cancer treatment protocol describes the specific combination of antineoplastics that will be given, their doses, and the cycles in which they will be administered. The use of multiple drugs affects the different stages of the cancer cell's lifecycle and attacks the various clones within the tumor via several mechanisms of action, thus increasing the percentage of cell kill. Combination chemotherapy also allows for lower dosages of each individual drug, thereby reducing toxicity and slowing the development of resistance. Examples of established protocols using combination therapy include fluorouracil-epirubicin-cyclophoaphamide (FEC) for breast cancer and gemcitabine-cisplatin (GC) for lung cancer. Each type of cancer has its own individual protocol, which was established through clinical trials. These protocols are being refined and revised continually based on current research.

Dosing Schedules

Most chemotherapeutic medications are administered intermittently using specific dosing schedules that have been determined through research to increase the effectiveness of the antineoplastic drugs. For example, some of the anticancer drugs are given as a single dose or perhaps several doses over a few days. A few weeks may pass before the next series of doses begins. This gives normal cells time to recover from the adverse effects of the drugs and allows tumor cells that may not have been replicating at the time of the first dose to begin dividing and become more sensitive to the next round of chemotherapy. Sometimes the optimal dosing schedule must be delayed until the patient sufficiently recovers from the drug toxicities, especially bone marrow suppression. Delays or reductions in the planned dosages are likely to negatively affect treatment outcomes. The specific dosing schedule chosen depends on the type of tumor, stage of the disease, and overall condition of the patient.

Route of Administration

Antineoplastic drugs are available for administration by virtually any route. Whenever possible, the oral (PO) route is used because it is most acceptable to the patient and eliminates risks associated with intravenous (IV) administration, such as phlebitis or tissue necrosis. Antineoplastics may be given locally by topical application to the lesion or through direct instillation into the tumor region. Regional administration causes less systemic toxicity. The most common route for delivering antineoplastics is via the venous system.

Oral: The PO route is the easiest, most convenient, and least expensive route for chemotherapy administration. Patients can self-administer their PO chemotherapy medications at home. One problem associated with PO administration is the inconsistency of absorption. Chemotherapeutic medications that are administered PO produce many of the same adverse reactions as the injectable drugs, and the patient and caregivers must be aware of these. They must also be taught safe handling and disposal of these drugs. Examples of antineoplastics available as PO preparations include methotrexate, mercaptopurine, cyclophosphamide, and melphalan.

Intravenous: IV is the most common route for delivery of chemotherapy drugs. One advantage to the IV route is that a constant and consistent serum level of the drug can be obtained by fine adjustments to the infusion rate. A disadvantage is that **sclerosing**, or abnormal tissue hardening of the veins, may occur during prolonged administration. Another disadvantage to the patient is that chemotherapy administration is done in a cancer center, healthcare provider's office, or some other place away from the patient's home. This may require many miles of commuting and present a hardship to the patient and family. In addition, traveling out of the home may expose the patient to viruses and other infectious agents, which can be hazardous to those with diminished immune function. In some geographic areas, an oncology nurse will come to the patient's home and administer the chemotherapy.

Administration of chemotherapeutic drugs can be done through a centrally located access device such as a Groshong catheter, which is inserted by being tunneled under the skin on the chest into a major vein for long-term medication instillation or through a peripheral vein via a **peripherally inserted central catheter (PICC) line**. A PICC line is a central catheter that is threaded into the vena cava for administration of chemotherapy. The advantages of a central line are that it is less likely to infiltrate and it is inserted in a large vein, which less likely to become irritated during chemotherapy. A disadvantage of a central line is that it increases the patient's risk of acquiring an infection.

Because IV administration requires a free-flowing IV in a large vein, it is imperative for the nurse to constantly assess the insertion site of the IV for signs of infiltration or phlebitis. Some antineoplastics can cause extreme cellular damage if the solution is allowed to enter surrounding tissues. Because of the potential for tissue damage, most antineoplastics are not administered by the intramuscular (IM) or subcutaneous routes. Examples of IV antineoplastics are carmustine, cisplatin, doxorubicin, and mitomycin.

Intrathecal: Some antineoplastic medications may be delivered intrathecally into the subarachnoid space of the spinal cord. In intrathecal administration, the drug bypasses the blood–brain barrier and circulates with the cerebrospinal fluid (CSF) to expose central nervous system tumors to high concentrations of the drug. A specially trained individual must conduct the procedure because it requires a lumbar puncture or surgical placement of a reservoir or implanted pump for drug delivery. An advantage to intrathecal administration is that it provides a consistent drug level in the CSF. Potential adverse effects include headaches, confusion, lethargy, seizures, and nausea and vomiting, all of which are signs of increased intracranial pressure.

Intra-arterial: Occasionally the healthcare provider may choose to administer chemotherapeutic medications through an artery. Intra-arterial administration requires a surgical procedure for catheter placement and, often, special x-ray techniques. In most cases, a catheter is passed via the femoral or brachial artery so that its end lies close to the blood supply of the tumor. Injection delivers a high dose of drug directly to the tumor site. Although the drug subsequently distributes via the circulation to other tissues, the tumor area receives the highest dose.

Intraperitoneal: Intraperitoneal administration via a catheter or port is used to deliver antineoplastic drugs directly to intra-abdominal metastases. The drug is slowly absorbed into the systemic circulation, or it may be drained out of the peritoneum via a catheter after a few hours of treatment. A disadvantage of this method is that it requires the placing of a Tenckhoff catheter, which is a specialized catheter. One end is placed into the peritoneum and the other end has an external port, which provides an access area into which medication is instilled.

Intravesicular: The intravesicular route instills high doses of antineoplastics into the urinary bladder via a Foley catheter to treat tumors of the bladder mucosa. Only small amounts of the drugs are absorbed systemically. The patient retains the drug for a specified period, after which it is voided or removed via catheter.

Toxicity of Antineoplastic Drugs

56.9 Serious toxicity limits therapy with most antineoplastic drugs.

Although cancer cells are clearly abnormal in structure and function, much of their physiology is identical to that of normal cells. Because it is difficult to kill cancer cells selectively

Table 56.4 Examples of Adverse Effects of Anticancer Drugs

Common Expected Adverse Effects	Drug-Specific Adverse Effects	Dose-Limiting Adverse Effects
Alopecia	Cardiotoxicity (daunorubicin, doxorubicin)	Acute kidney injury
Anorexia	Fetal malformations (mercaptopurine, methotrexate, pemetrexed)	Bone marrow suppression
Fatigue	Peripheral-sensory neuropathy (cisplatin)	Diarrhea
Immunosuppression	Sterility (mechlorethamine)	Pulmonary fibrosis
Nausea and vomiting		
Stomatitis		

without profoundly affecting normal cells, all antineoplastic drugs have the potential to cause serious toxicity. These drugs are often pushed to their maximum dosages to obtain the greatest tumor cell kill. These high dosages always result in adverse effects in the patient, some of which are listed in Table 56.4. Because antineoplastic drugs primarily affect cells with a high growth fraction, normal cells that are replicating, such as cells in the hair follicles, GI tract, and hematologic system, are most susceptible to adverse effects.

Hematologic System

Many antineoplastic drugs produce a dose-dependent destruction of hematopoietic stem cells, resulting in bone marrow suppression (myelosuppression). Myelosuppression is the most common dose-limiting adverse effect of chemotherapy and the one that most often causes discontinuation or delays of chemotherapy. Severe bone marrow suppression is a contraindication to therapy with most antineoplastic drugs.

Chemotherapy causes erythrocyte, leukocyte, and platelet counts to decrease until they reach their lowest value, known as the **nadir**. Patients are most susceptible to the symptoms, such as anemia, infections, or bleeding, during the nadir. Following the nadir, blood counts begin their recovery back to normal values. The nadir is specific for each drug and for each type of blood cell. For example, antimetabolites produce rapid nadirs for neutrophils in 7 to 14 days after the initiation of chemotherapy, with recovery within 7 to 21 days following the nadir. Other drugs such as the nitrosoureas produce a delayed nadir for neutrophils at 26 to 63 days, with recovery at 35 to 89 days after the nadir.

Neutrophils are the type of white blood cells (WBCs) most affected by chemotherapy. This is primarily because the normal lifespan of a neutrophil is only 7 to 12 hours, and without continual replacement by stem cells the number of circulating neutrophils quickly falls. A patient is diagnosed with neutropenia when the neutrophil count is less than 1500 cells/mL. Patients are very susceptible to infections while they are neutropenic. Patients who are neutropenic are often placed in reverse isolation to protect them from exposure to any infections from family members or health-care providers. Even an infection from a mild cold could be fatal to patients with extremely low neutrophil counts. If a patient who is neutropenic and receiving chemotherapy acquires an infection, an increase in WBCs may not be evident. If a patient who is neutropenic does develop a fever, this may be an indication of sepsis, and antibiotics are indicated.

Colony-stimulating factors such as filgrastim (Neupogen) and sargramostim (Leukine) are administered to accelerate recovery of suppressed bone marrow cells and to increase the WBC count. The administration of these drugs shortens the time of neutropenia, thus lowering the risk of opportunistic infections and allowing the patient to maintain an optimal chemotherapy dosing schedule. Filgrastim is presented as a prototype drug in Chapter 39.

Because the lifespan of a platelet is only 7 to 8 days, these blood elements require constant replenishment by bone marrow stem cells. A patient is diagnosed with thrombocytopenia when the platelet count is less than 100,000 per milliliter of blood. Chemotherapy is often delayed if this occurs. In patients who are receiving chemotherapy, thrombocytopenia usually occurs concurrently with neutropenia. Thrombocytopenia can cause the patient to exhibit abnormal bleeding, with symptoms ranging from bruising to petechiae to serious hemorrhage. Bleeding precautions must be implemented if the platelet count falls below 50,000 per milliliter of blood. To prevent the platelet count from decreasing to a harmful level, platelet infusions may be necessary.

Because erythrocytes have a longer lifespan (90 to 120 days) than neutrophils or platelets, reductions in red blood cells (RBCs), or anemia, occur later in the course of chemotherapy. Hemoglobin carries oxygen to all tissues in the body; thus, anemia may affect every system in the body. An infusion of RBCs may be required to increase a patient's RBC count and hemoglobin value. A medication that the nurse may administer to help increase the number of RBCs is epoetin alfa (Epogen), which is presented as a prototype in Chapter 39. When assessing for anemia, remember that the etiology may be the result of nonchemotherapy-related causes, such as bleeding, iron deficiency, or kidney damage.

Gastrointestinal Tract

The vomiting center in the medulla is triggered by many antineoplastics. Acute nausea and vomiting often begin within minutes of chemotherapy administration and may last for 24 hours. Delayed nausea and vomiting begin 24 hours after chemotherapy and may continue for up to 6 days. Antineoplastics are sometimes classified by their capacity to induce vomiting or **emetogenic potential**. Highly emetogenic potential antineoplastics receive four antiemetics which frequently include ondansetron (Zofran) or palonosetron Aloxi), aprepitant (Emend), olanzapine

(Zyprexa), and dexamethasone. Antineoplastics with lower emetogenic potential may be treated. with prochlorperazine or metoclopramide. Antiemetic medications are presented in detail in Chapter 60.

The epithelial lining of the GI tract is very sensitive to the effects of chemotherapeutic drugs. The GI mucosa commonly becomes inflamed, a condition known as **mucositis**. Consequences of mucositis include painful ulcerations in the mouth and esophagus, difficulty eating or swallowing, GI bleeding, intestinal infections, or severe diarrhea. Some research has shown that eating popsicles during chemotherapy infusions can decrease the severity of mucositis. The nurse may also instruct the patient to eat a bland diet and to use a soft-bristle toothbrush for oral care. Some healthcare providers may order a "medical cocktail," which may include lidocaine viscous, liquid diphenhydramine, and Carafate to decrease the pain associated with mucositis. The patient should also be instructed to report any signs of thrush, which is an oral yeast infection.

Most patients receiving antineoplastics experience anorexia, usually due to a combination of nausea, vomiting, and mucositis. At times the patient's appetite is decreased such that tube feedings or parenteral feedings may be indicated. The body needs sufficient nutrients and calories for normal cells to repopulate and for repair of body tissues. When assessing for anorexia, remember that this symptom may be the result of direct effects from the tumor itself or from associated psychologic changes such as depression or anxiety.

The patient may experience constipation or diarrhea depending on the specific drugs administered. Some chemotherapeutic medications damage the intestinal lining, inhibiting the reabsorption of fluids and producing loose stools. Replacement of fluids and electrolytes as well as treatment with an antidiarrheal drug such as diphenoxylate with atropine (Lomotil), loperamide (Imodium), or bismuth salts (Pepto Bismol). Some chemotherapeutic medications decrease the motility of the GI tract, resulting in greater reabsorption of fluids, which leads to constipation. When assessing for constipation, note that other common reasons for this symptom include therapy with opioid analgesics and inadequate water and fiber intake.

Many patients with cancer experience a general wasting of muscle and other tissues, referred to as **cachexia**. Cachexia may be caused by toxic effects from the cancer itself or from its treatment. Chemotherapy symptoms such as anorexia, mucositis, and nausea and vomiting may contribute to cachexia, but other non-GI factors also contribute such as serious chronic pain, depression, and fatigue.

Cardiopulmonary System

Some of the chemotherapeutic medications can be toxic to the heart and lungs. For example, doxorubicin (Adriamycin) is specifically known for its cardiotoxicity and the nurse should monitor the patient for any changes in the electrocardiogram and assess for any signs of heart failure. This adverse effect can be serious enough to later cause the patient to need cardiac monitoring or a heart transplant. A cardioprotective drug such as dexrazoxane (Zinecard) is administered just prior to a doxorubicin infusion to prevent permanent heart damage.

Bleomycin is specifically known to cause pneumonitis in patients. Nursing care of the patient who is receiving bleomycin should include monitoring the patient's pulse oximeter and respiratory status. Auscultating crackles in the lung fields may be a sign of a developing pneumonitis. Chest x-rays may be necessary two to three times per week to assess for lung changes.

Urinary System

Some of the chemotherapeutic medications can exhibit considerable nephrotoxicity. For example, cisplatin can lead to acute kidney injury if the dosage limit is exceeded. When administering drugs that are nephrotoxic, the nurse should closely monitor intake and output and urine dipstick results for red cells. The patient should remain well hydrated during the treatment to help prevent kidney damage. Diuretics may be administered to help balance the intake and output of the patient. In addition, the drug mesna (Mesnex) is administered to prevent hemorrhagic cystitis during chemotherapy with cyclophosphamide or ifosfamide.

Reproductive System

Some antineoplastics, particularly the alkylating agents, affect the gonads and have been associated with infertility in both men and women. If a woman is pregnant while receiving treatment, the fetus may be severely damaged due to the high growth fraction of the fetus's cells or it may be killed during the treatment. Sexually active male and female patients should be instructed to use reliable contraception while receiving chemotherapy and for 3 to 6 months following treatment.

Antineoplastic medications are more likely to cause permanent sterility in men than in women. Some patients choose to have their sperm or eggs harvested prior to treatment in case the chemotherapy does affect their fertility.

Many hospitals have protocols specifying that female nurses and pharmacists not handle chemotherapeutic drugs if they are pregnant or are trying to become pregnant due to the toxic effects that the chemotherapy may have on the fetus.

Nervous System

Several chemotherapeutic drugs are toxic to the nervous system. For instance, vincristine (Marqibo) may cause muscle weakness and peripheral neuritis. It is important for the nurse to assess the patient's neurologic status frequently when administering this medication. Patients should also be informed of the potential adverse effects so that they may inform the nurse of any tingling or pain in their extremities or if changes occur in muscle strength.

Cisplatin has been known to cause hearing loss and deafness in some patients. The nurse should assess the patient's hearing throughout the course of treatment and document any changes noted in the patient's ability to hear.

Skin and Soft Tissue

Many antineoplastics are classified as **vesicants**, agents that can cause serious tissue injury if they escape from an artery or vein during an infusion or injection. Extravasation or infiltration from an injection site can produce severe tissue and nerve damage, local infection, and even loss of a limb. If a nurse is concerned that a peripheral IV is no longer working properly, the IV should not be used for chemotherapy administration. Although rare, extravasation can still occur with a central line so the nurse should continue to frequently assess the insertion site of a central line while administering chemotherapy. Rapid treatment of extravasation is necessary to limit tissue damage, and certain antineoplastics have specific antidotes. For example, extravasation of carmustine (BiCNU, Gliadel) is treated with injections of equal parts of sodium bicarbonate and normal saline into the extravasation site. Before administering IV antineoplastic drugs, the nurse should know the emergency treatment for extravasation. Antineoplastics with the strongest vesicant activity include busulfan, carmustine, dacarbazine, dactinomycin, daunorubicin, idarubicin, mechlorethamine, mitomycin, plicamycin, streptozocin, vinblastine, vincristine, and vinorelbine.

Other Adverse Effects

Fatigue is a common complaint during chemotherapy. The precise etiology of the fatigue is often difficult to determine. If the patient has anemia, the lack of hemoglobin to carry oxygen to the tissue can cause the patient to feel fatigued. The patient may be experiencing anxiety or depression due to the diagnosis of cancer, which may lead to sleep deprivation. The process of cellular regeneration after chemotherapy treatments may also cause feelings of fatigue. A nutritional consultation may be helpful in determining if the fatigue has a nutritional origin. Coping strategies for dealing with stress and scheduled periods of rest may benefit the patient.

Hair follicles are damaged by many chemotherapeutic drugs, resulting in hair loss, or **alopecia**. Hair loss usually begins within 1 to 2 weeks of the first treatment, and regrowth may take 3 to 5 months after the last chemotherapeutic treatment. The potential for alopecia should be discussed with patients before treatment begins so that they may choose to wear a hat, bandana, wig, or other accessory.

One of the ironies of chemotherapy is that the medications that are given to kill the cancer may cause a secondary cancer to develop elsewhere in the body. This is not a common adverse effect, but it has been clearly demonstrated in patients. The secondary malignancy usually occurs many years after the initial cancer; thus, this adverse effect is of most concern to children being treated with chemotherapy. It is estimated that pediatric cancer survivors have a 10 to 20 times greater risk than other children of developing a secondary malignancy. The most common secondary malignancy is nonlymphocytic leukemia.

Hyperuricemia is most frequently associated with chemotherapy for lymphomas and leukemias due to the rapid cell kill. A patient is diagnosed with hyperuricemia when uric acid levels in the blood are elevated, which can lead to renal failure if the uric crystals deposit in the renal tubules. Signs of hyperuricemia are nausea and vomiting and oliguria. Keeping the patient hydrated helps to preserve renal function by flushing microscopic crystals out of the kidney before they have a chance to form larger crystals. The nurse who is caring for a patient who is suspected of developing or has been diagnosed with hyperuricemia should monitor the patient's intake and output closely. Xanthine oxidase inhibitors such as allopurinol and be prescribed to prevent symptoms of gout.

Understanding Chapter 56

Key Concepts Summary

56.1 Cancer is characterized by rapid, uncontrolled growth of cells that eventually invade normal tissues and metastasize.

56.2 The etiology of cancer may be chemical, physical, or biologic.

56.3 The keys to successful cancer treatment are prevention and early detection.

56.4 The three primary goals of chemotherapy are cure, control, and palliation.

56.5 Cancers are described by their stage and grade.

56.6 Many antineoplastic drugs are more effective when given at specific stages of the cell cycle and in tumors with a high growth fraction.

56.7 The goal of chemotherapy is to kill as many cancer cells as possible while sparing normal cells.

56.8 Use of multiple drugs and intermittent dosing are strategies that allow for greater success of chemotherapy.

56.9 Serious toxicity limits therapy with most antineoplastic drugs.

CASE STUDY: Making the Patient Connection

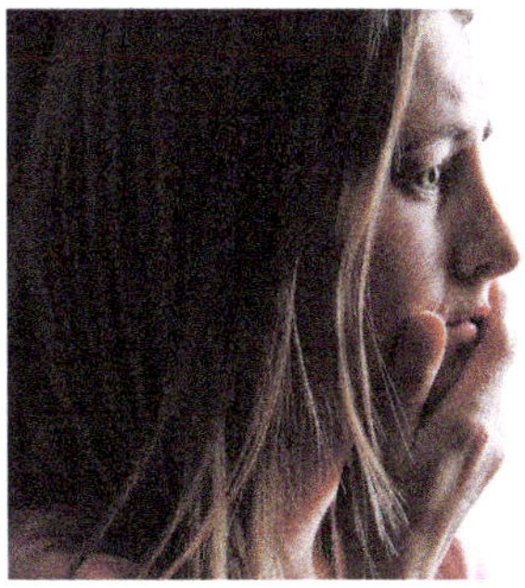

Remember the patient "Cheryl Ogen" at the beginning of the chapter? Now read the rest of the case study. Based on the information presented within this chapter, respond to the critical thinking questions that follow.

Cheryl Ogen is a 39-year-old woman who is employed as a kindergarten teacher. She has been married for 15 years and has never had any children. Her medical history confirms that both her mother and maternal grandmother died from breast cancer. Now Cheryl has been diagnosed with breast cancer. She is admitted to the hospital for tumor resection and chemotherapy. Cheryl's breast cancer is Stage T1, N0, M0, and G2. She has undergone a lumpectomy with regional lymph node biopsy and is now about to begin chemotherapy.

Critical Thinking Questions

1. Cheryl would like to know why she is receiving chemotherapy after the surgeon has removed the cancerous tumor. What would you tell her?
2. Why is it important to understand the staging and grading system used with cancer? How would you interpret the staging and grading of Cheryl's cancer?
3. Identify some of the hematologic changes that Cheryl may experience while receiving chemotherapy.

Additional Case Study

Patient Jonah Cooper has been newly diagnosed with acute lymphocytic leukemia. He is 28 years old and the father of two children ages 9 months and 2 years. Jonah is admitted to the hospital for his initial round of chemotherapy.

1. Will Jonah's children be allowed to visit him during his hospital admission?
2. Why is Jonah receiving more than one type of chemotherapy?
3. Why was Jonah's cancer not staged on diagnosis?

Chapter Review

1. The healthcare provider has written in the patient's chart that the cancer is at Stage I. The nurse knows that the implications for this staging are that the:
   1. Cancer is advanced and the patient has a poor prognosis.
   2. Cancerous cells are only moderately differentiated from the parent cells.
   3. Cancer has been detected at an early stage.
   4. Tumor is large and is invading surrounding tissue.
2. Which of the following statements by a patient who is undergoing chemotherapy would be of concern to the nurse? (Select all that apply.)
   1. "I attended a meeting of a cancer support group this week."
   2. "My husband and I are planning a short trip next week."
   3. "I try to eat six small meals plus two protein shakes each day."
   4. "I am taking my 15-month-old granddaughter to the pediatrician next week for her baby shots."
   5. "I am going to go shopping at the mall next week."

3. The nurse determines that the patient understands an important principle of chemotherapy when the patient makes which statement?
    1. "The use of multiple chemotherapy drugs affects different stages of the cancer cells' lifecycle."
    2. "Staging describes the process of determining how responsive the cancer is to the prescribed chemotherapy."
    3. "Antineoplastic drugs kill the entire tumor, including the clones, and prevent repopulation."
    4. "Combination chemotherapy requires higher dosages of each individual drug and increases toxicity."
4. Chemotherapy is being initiated for a patient with prostate cancer who is experiencing mucositis. Which health teaching would be most appropriate for this condition?
    1. Use an over-the-counter mouthwash to eliminate bacteria.
    2. Increase intake of citrus-containing foods and beverages.
    3. Eat a bland diet with low roughage and use a soft-bristle toothbrush or plain water rinses for oral care.
    4. This adverse effect is expected and will disappear within a few days.
5. The nurse is collaborating with other members of the healthcare team regarding the care of a patient with a brain tumor. The nurse knows that the most common reason that subsequent rounds of chemotherapy may be delayed is due to what condition?
    1. Myelosuppression
    2. Alopecia
    3. Mucositis
    4. Cachexia
6. A patient with cancer is started on a drug that is a known vesicant. The nurse performs which priority activity related to this drug? Monitor the patient's:
    1. Response to antinausea drugs.
    2. Intake of calcium-rich foods.
    3. Respiratory status for cough.
    4. IV port site for redness, swelling, and pain.

See Appendix A for answers to critical thinking questions, case study questions and review questions.

References

Siegel, R. L., Miller, K. D., & Jemal, A. (2020). Cancer statistics, 2020. *CA: A Cancer Journal for Clinicians*, *70*(1), 7–30. https://acsjournals.onlinelibrary.wiley.com/doi/full/10.3322/caac.21590

Selected Bibliography

American Cancer Society. (2020a). *American Cancer Society guidelines for the early detection of cancer.* http://www.cancer.org/healthy/findcancerearly/cancerscreeningguidelines/american-cancer-society-guidelines-for-the-early-detection-of-cancer

American Cancer Society. (2020b). *Cancer prevention & early detection: Facts and figures 2019–2020.* https://www.cancer.org/content/dam/cancer-org/research/cancer-facts-and-statistics/cancer-prevention-and-early-detection-facts-and-figures/cancer-prevention-and-early-detection-facts-and-figures-2019-2020.pdf

American Cancer Society. (2020c). *Cancer staging.* http://www.cancer.org/treatment/understandingyourdiagnosis/staging

Ashokkumar, R., Srinivasamurthy, S., Kelly, J. J., Howard, S. C., Parasuraman, S., & Uppugunduri, C. R. S. (2018). Frequency of chemotherapy medication errors: A systematic review. *Journal of Pharmacology and Pharmacotherapeutics*, *9*(2), 86–91. https://doi.org/10.4103/jpp.JPP_61_18.

National Cancer Institute (n.d.). *Cancer treatment.* https://www.cancer.gov/about-cancer/treatment

Wilkes, G. M., & Barton-Burke, M. (2020). *Oncology nursing drug handbook.* Jones & Bartlett.

Yarbro, C. H., Wujcik, D., & Gobel, B. H. (2018). *Cancer nursing: Principles and practice* (8th ed.). Jones & Bartlett.

"Being tired all the time isn't so bad; I get to play a lot of video games. And I'm used to wearing my bandana. I just wish people would stop staring at me."
—*Patient "Zack Amos"*

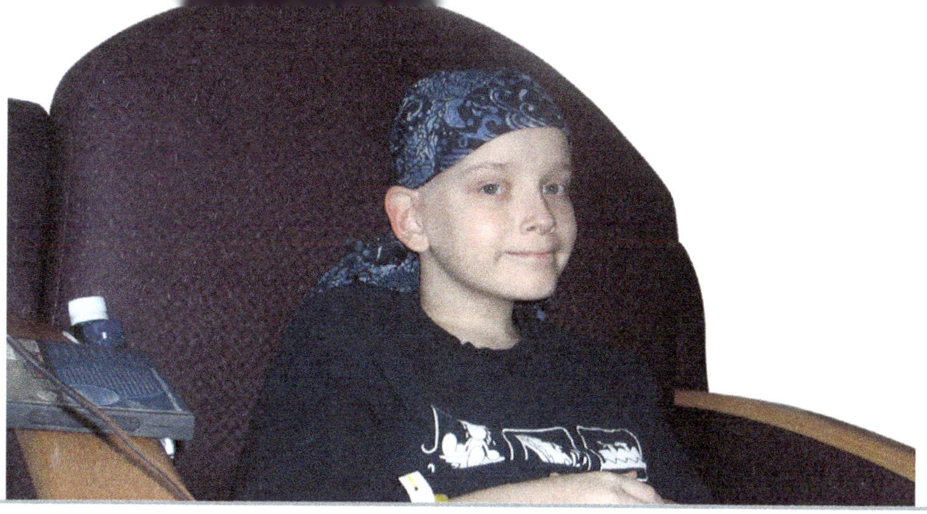

Chapter 57
Pharmacotherapy of Neoplasia

Chapter Outline

- Classification of Antineoplastic Drugs
- Antineoplastic Medications
  - Alkylating Agents
  - **PROTOTYPE** *Cyclophosphamide (Cytoxan), p. 997*
  - Antimetabolites
  - **PROTOTYPE** *Methotrexate (MTX, Trexall), p. 1003*
  - Antitumor Antibiotics
  - **PROTOTYPE** *Doxorubicin, p. 1007*
  - Hormones and Hormone Antagonists
  - **PROTOTYPE** *Tamoxifen, p. 1011*
  - Natural Products
  - **PROTOTYPE** *Vincristine (Marqibo), p. 1016*
  - Biologic Response Modifiers and Targeted Therapies
  - Miscellaneous Antineoplastics
- Drugs for Reducing Adverse Effects

Learning Outcomes

After reading this chapter, the student should be able to:

1. Explain why it is difficult to accurately classify antineoplastic drugs.
2. Describe the common and dose-limiting toxicities of antineoplastics.
3. Describe how the process of alkylation kills rapidly growing cells.
4. Describe how antimetabolites kill cancer cells.
5. Describe mechanisms by which antitumor antibiotics kill cancer cells.
6. Explain applications of hormones and hormone antagonists to cancer chemotherapy.
7. Identify natural products that have the ability to kill cancer cells.
8. Explain the use of biologic response modifiers and targeted therapies in cancer chemotherapy.
9. For each of the classes shown in the chapter outline, identify the prototype and representative drugs and explain the mechanism(s) of drug action, primary indications, contraindications, significant drug interactions, pregnancy data, and important adverse effects.
10. Apply clinical judgment to care for patients receiving cancer chemotherapy.

Key Terms

Definitions of the terms in bold may be found in the Glossary.

The decision to begin cancer chemotherapy is a collaborative one made by the patient, the family, and the healthcare provider. Although there have been some remarkable successes in treating cancer, patients will experience adverse effects that can challenge their resolve to complete the chemotherapy regimen. Healthcare providers must be prepared to assist patients and their families in dealing with the challenges of antineoplastic therapy and the psychologic impact of the decision to continue or discontinue treatment. This chapter examines the types of medications used in cancer chemotherapy and their applications to clinical practice.

Classification of Antineoplastic Drugs

57.1 Antineoplastic drugs kill or stop the growth of cancer cells and may be classified in multiple ways.

Drugs used in cancer chemotherapy come from diverse pharmacologic and chemical classes. Antineoplastics have been extracted from plants and bacteria as well as created entirely in a laboratory. Some of the drug classes attack cellular macromolecules in cancer cells, such as deoxyribonucleic acid (DNA) and proteins, whereas others poison vital metabolic pathways of rapidly growing cells. The common theme among all the antineoplastic drugs is their toxicity. They have the ability to kill or stop the growth of cancer cells.

Classification of the antineoplastics is difficult because some of these drugs kill cancer cells by multiple mechanisms and have characteristics from more than one class. For example, paclitaxel (Abraxane) can be classified as a natural product (it was derived from a plant), a taxane (its chemical structure), a mitotic inhibitor (its mechanism of action), or a cell cycle inhibitor. Furthermore, the mechanisms by which some antineoplastics act are incompletely understood. A simple method of classifying this complex group of drugs includes the following categories:

- Alkylating agents
- Antimetabolites
- Antitumor antibiotics
- Hormones and hormone antagonists
- Natural products
- Biologic response modifiers and targeted therapies
- Miscellaneous antineoplastic drugs.

PharmFACT

Because approximately 90% of all prostate cancer is diagnosed at the local and regional stages, the cure rate for cancer at this stage is nearly 100% (Prostate Cancer Foundation, n.d.).

Antineoplastic Medications

The antineoplastic medications include alkylating agents, antimetabolites, antitumor antibiotics, hormones and hormone antagonists, natural products, biologic response modifiers, targeted therapies, and miscellaneous antineoplastics.

Alkylating Agents

57.2 Alkylating agents change the shape of the DNA double helix and prevent cancer cells from dividing normally.

Alkylation, which is the transfer of a carbon group (alkyl group) from one molecule to another, is a common biochemical reaction. In the specific case of chemotherapy, alkylation involves covalent bonding of the antineoplastic drug to the DNA of the cancer cell. The drug may form a "bridge" or cross-link between the two DNA strands and markedly affect the function of the DNA.

Alkylating agents kill cancer cells by altering the shape of the DNA double helix and preventing the DNA from duplicating normally during cell division. Each alkylating agent attaches to DNA in a different manner; however, they all have the effect of inducing cell death or at least slowing the replication of tumor cells. Although the process of alkylation may occur at any time during the cell cycle, the killing action occurs when the affected cell attempts to duplicate the defective DNA strands. The alkylating agents are used against a broad range of malignancies, including certain types of lymphomas, myelomas, leukemias, and pancreatic cancers and some testicular, ovarian, and breast cancers. They are the oldest classification of antineoplastics, having been available since the 1940s, and are still the most widely used antineoplastic drugs. Alkylating agents are sometimes subdivided into chemical classes, which include the nitrogen mustards, nitrosoureas, and platinum compounds, as listed in Table 57.1. Figure 57.1 illustrates the process of alkylation.

Because blood cells are particularly sensitive to the actions of alkylating agents, myelosuppression (bone marrow suppression) is the primary dose-limiting toxicity of these drugs. Within days after administration, the numbers of erythrocytes, leukocytes, and platelets begin to decline, reaching a nadir at 9 to 14 days. These drugs are withheld if red blood cell (RBC), white blood cell (WBC), and platelet counts fall below a predetermined limit during therapy. Epithelial cells lining the gastrointestinal (GI) tract are also damaged by alkylating agents, causing nausea and vomiting and diarrhea. Alopecia may be expected from most of the alkylating agents. The nitrosoureas and mechlorethamine are also strong vesicants, and great care must be taken to avoid skin contact or extravasation. Like many other antineoplastics, secondary malignancies may occur with the alkylating agents. A small percentage of patients

Table 57.1 Alkylating Agents

Drug	Route and Adult Dose (Maximum Dose Where Indicated)	Adverse Effects
Nitrogen Mustards		*Headache, alopecia, nausea and vomiting, stomatitis, anorexia, rash, fluid retention*
bendamustine (Treanda)	IV: 100 mg/m² on days 1 and 2 of a 28-day cycle	Myelosuppression, severe nausea, vomiting, diarrhea, Stevens–Johnson syndrome (SJS), hemorrhagic cystitis (ifosfamide), neurotoxicity, ototoxicity (platinum agents), pulmonary toxicity, nephrotoxicity (platinum agents), hepatotoxicity (dacarbazine, lurbinectedin), anaphylaxis and other hypersensitivity reactions, tissue necrosis (due to extravasation), embryofetal toxicity
chlorambucil (Leukeran)	PO: 0.1–0.2 mg/kg/day for 3–6 wk	
cyclophosphamide (Cytoxan)	PO: 1–5 mg/kg/day	
estramustine (Emcyt)	PO: 14 mg/kg/day in 3–4 divided doses	
ifosfamide (Ifex)	IV: 1.2 g/m²/day for 5 consecutive days	
mechlorethamine (Mustargen)	IV: 0.4 mg/kg as a single or divided dose	
melphalan (Alkeran)	PO: 6 mg/day for 2–3 wk	
Nitrosoureas		
carmustine (BiCNU, Gliadel)	IV: 200 mg/m² once q6wk	
lomustine (CCNU, CeeNU)	PO: 130 mg/m² as a single dose, once q6wk	
streptozocin (Zanosar)	IV: 500 mg/m² for 5 consecutive days, q6wk	
Platinum Agents		
carboplatin (Paraplatin)	IV: 360 mg/m² once q4wk	
cisplatin	IV: 20 mg/m²/day for 5 days	
oxaliplatin (Eloxatin)	IV: 85 mg/m² for 2 h	
Miscellaneous Alkylating Agents		
busulfan (Busulfex, Myleran)	PO: 4–8 mg/day IV: 0.8 mg/kg qid for 4 days	
dacarbazine	IV: 2–4.5 mg/kg/day for 10 days, repeated q4wk	
lurbinectedin (Zepzelca)	IV: 3.2 mg/m² every 21 days	
procarbazine (Matulane)	PO: 2–4 mg/kg/day in single or divided doses for 1 wk, then 4–6 mg/kg/day	
temozolomide (Temodar)	PO: 75–150 mg/m²/day	
thiotepa	IV: 0.3–0.4 mg/kg q1–4wk	

Note: *Italics* indicate common adverse effects. Underline indicates serious adverse effects.

treated with alkylating agents develop acute myelogenous leukemia 4 years or more after chemotherapy has been completed.

When alkylating agents are taken for prolonged periods, cancer cells can develop resistance to them. The mechanism of resistance is incompletely understood. However, possible mechanisms include decreased drug uptake by cancer cells, increased cellular inactivation of the drug, and increased production of DNA repair enzymes.

CONNECTION Checkpoint 57.1

From what you learned in Chapter 43, explain why vaccinations are usually contraindicated in patients who are receiving antineoplastic drugs.

PROTOTYPE DRUG Cyclophosphamide (Cytoxan)

Classification **Therapeutic:** Antineoplastic
Pharmacologic: Alkylating agent, nitrogen mustard, disease-modifying antirheumatic drug, immunosuppressant

Therapeutic Effects and Uses: Approved in 1959 by the U.S. Food and Drug Administration (FDA), cyclophosphamide is available as an oral (PO) or injectable preparation. It has a very broad spectrum of action and is approved in combination with other antineoplastics in the chemotherapy of Hodgkin's and non-Hodgkin's lymphoma, acute and chronic lymphocytic and myelogenous leukemia, ovarian cancer, breast cancer, multiple myeloma, mycosis fungoides, neuroblastoma, sarcomas, and retinoblastoma. It may be used off-label to treat lung cancer, endometrial cancer, Ewing's sarcoma, osteogenic sarcoma, prostate cancer, rhabdomyosarcoma, and other neoplastic conditions. It is used in both children and adults. In children, it is also approved to treat nephritic syndrome when standard therapies have failed.

Cyclophosphamide is an effective immunosuppressant. Although immunosuppression is considered an adverse effect during cancer chemotherapy, this drug is used to intentionally cause it, often in combination therapy with corticosteroids. Off-label immunosuppressive indications include prophylaxis of organ transplant rejection, severe rheumatoid arthritis (RA), systemic lupus erythematosus (SLE), and scleroderma.

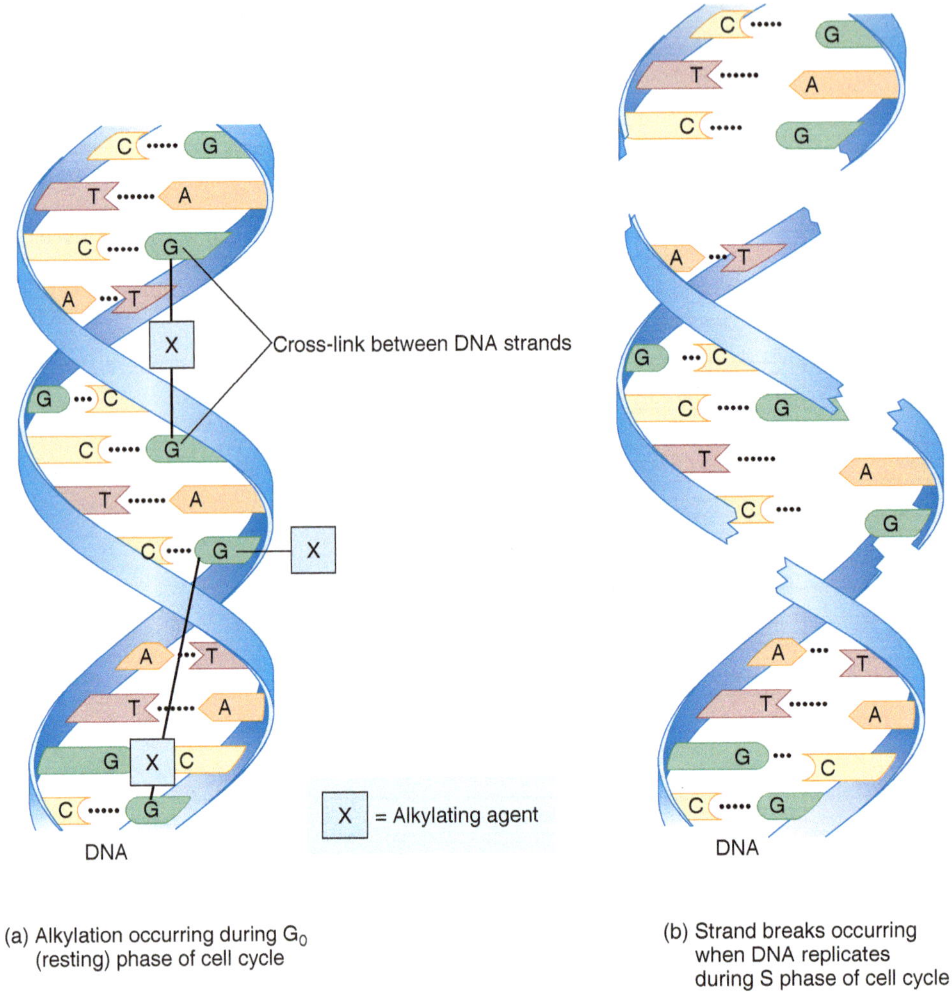

Figure 57.1 Mechanism of action of the alkylating agents.

Mechanism of Action: Cyclophosphamide is a prodrug that is converted to its active form (phosphoramide mustard) in the liver. Cyclophosphamide binds to DNA and forms cross-links, which prevent the synthesis of DNA, ribonucleic acid (RNA), and protein. It is a cell-cycle-nonspecific drug.

Pharmacokinetics:

Route(s)	PO, IV
Absorption	Well absorbed from the GI tract
Distribution	Widely distributed; crosses the placenta; secreted in breast milk; also found in brain tissue
Primary metabolism	Extensive hepatic metabolism by CYP2B6 and other CYP isozymes
Primary excretion	Renal
Onset of action	7 days
Duration of action	Half-life: 3–12 h; metabolites can still be identified in serum after 21 days

Adverse Effects: Adverse effects include those common to other antineoplastic drugs, such as anorexia, nausea, vomiting, weight loss, diarrhea, and mouth sores. Alopecia frequently occurs; 50% of patients will develop total baldness. Other common adverse effects are jaundice, acne, blistered skin, and darkened or thickened skin. Bone marrow suppression is a potentially life-threatening adverse reaction that occurs between days 9 and 14 of therapy; the patient is at dangerous risk for severe infection and sepsis during this period. Bone marrow recovery occurs by days 18 through 25. Other serious adverse effects include cardiotoxicity, and pulmonary fibrosis. Hematuria may signal hemorrhagic cystitis, which can be severe and even fatal. This drug is associated with an increased risk of secondary malignancies, including bladder cancer, lymphoma, and leukemia, that may occur several years after completion of chemotherapy.

Contraindications/Precautions: Contraindications to the use of cyclophosphamide include pregnancy, lactation, and severe myelosuppression. The drug must be used cautiously in patients with leukopenia, thrombocytopenia, previous radiation therapy, bone marrow infiltration of tumor cells, chronic kidney disease (CKD), impaired hepatic function, recent history of steroid use, or previous therapy that caused cytotoxicity.

Drug Interactions: Many drug interactions are possible with cyclophosphamide due to its extensive hepatic metabolism. This medication has additive immunosuppressive effects if administered with other drugs that cause bone marrow toxicity. There may be an increased anticoagulant effect if it is given with anticoagulants. Increased cardiotoxicity may result if it is given with doxorubicin. Insulin may increase hypoglycemia. Lower serum digoxin levels can be expected in the patient who takes digoxin. Phenobarbital use may lead to an increased rate of metabolism of cyclophosphamide, whereas phenytoin use may lead to an increased risk of toxicity. **Herbal/Food:** St. John's wort may increase the toxic effects of cyclophosphamide.

Pregnancy: Because this drug can cause fetal harm in laboratory animals and in humans, it is contraindicated during pregnancy and breastfeeding. Women of childbearing potential should use contraception during therapy and for up to 1 year after the last dose. Cyclophosphamide can cause infertility in both males and females.

Treatment of Overdose: Overdose can result in severe myelosuppression with the possibility of infection. General supportive measures are administered.

Clinician Responsibilities: Key clinical implications for patients receiving cyclophosphamide are included in Applied Clinical Judgment: Patients Receiving Cancer Chemotherapy.

Drugs Similar to Cyclophosphamide (Cytoxan)

Alkylating agents include other nitrogen mustards, including bendamustine, chlorambucil, estramustine, ifosfamide, mechlorethamine, and melphalan; the nitrosoureas, including carmustine, lomustine, and streptozocin; the platinum compounds, including carboplatin, cisplatin, and oxaliplatin; and miscellaneous alkylating agents, including busulfan, dacarbazine, lurbinectedin, procarbazine, temozolomide, and thiotepa. All the alkylating agents cause fetal harm in laboratory animals and are contraindicated during pregnancy and lactation. Use of contraception is recommended prior to, during, and following chemotherapy. Some may cause irreversible infertility in both male and female patients. Pregnant women and partners seeking to conceive a child should consult with their oncologist.

Bendamustine (Treanda): Approved in 2008, bendamustine is similar to mechlorethamine. Available by the IV route, bendamustine has two indications: chronic lymphocytic leukemia and non-Hodgkin's lymphoma that has not responded to rituximab therapy. Like many alkylating agents, the dose-limiting toxicity is myelosuppression. The most common nonhematologic adverse effects are pyrexia and nausea and vomiting. Rare, though serious, toxicity includes anaphylaxis, SJS, and tumor lysis syndrome.

Busulfan (Busulfex, Myleran): Approved in 1954, busulfan (Myleran) is a potent alkylating agent given PO for palliative treatment of chronic myelogenous leukemia for those patients who are no longer responsive to radiation therapy or other chemotherapeutic drugs. In combination with cyclophosphamide, busulfan (Busulfex) is given IV for bone marrow ablation prior to stem cell transplantation. Busulfan has a black box warning that myelosuppression is a serious adverse effect, and blood counts must be closely monitored. Pancytopenia occurs in 100% of patients who are taking high doses of this drug, and this condition may last as long as 2 years. Nausea, vomiting, stomatitis, and anorexia are common adverse effects. Because of the potential for infertility, men and women within childbearing years should be counseled regarding the drug's adverse reproductive effects.

Carboplatin (Paraplatin): Approved for the first-line palliative treatment of advanced ovarian cancer, carboplatin may be used off-label to treat acute lymphocytic leukemia, acute myelogenous leukemia, bladder cancer, breast cancer, and other tumors. Approved in 1989, carboplatin is administered by the IV route, is structurally similar to cisplatin, and works by the same mechanism but is less toxic. The drug carries a black box warning for anaphylaxis and severe myelosuppression, the dose-limiting toxicity. Neurotoxicity and nephrotoxicity occur less often than with cisplatin. Anaphylactic-like reactions may occur within minutes of carboplatin administration.

Carmustine (BiCNU, Gliadel): Carmustine, a nitrosourea alkylating agent, is one of the few drugs in its class that can penetrate the blood–brain barrier. Thus, it is used to treat brain tumors such as malignant glioma, astrocytoma, ependymoma, and brain metastases. In addition to brain tumors, carmustine is also given for Hodgkin's and non-Hodgkin's lymphomas and multiple myeloma. Carmustine is usually administered by the IV route. A wafer form of the drug (Gliadel) is available for implantation into the cavity created by removal of a brain tumor. The wafer dissolves over 2 to 3 weeks, delivering 1000 times the amount of carmustine to the tumor site than could be obtained through IV administration. Carmustine carries a black box warning that it can cause serious bone marrow suppression and pulmonary toxicity. Neurologic adverse effects include seizures and encephalopathy. Other adverse effects are those typical of other alkylating agents.

Chlorambucil (Leukeran): Chlorambucil, a nitrogen mustard alkylating agent, is used to treat chronic lymphocytic leukemia, lymphomas, and Hodgkin's disease. Because it is an immunosuppressant, chlorambucil is occasionally used off-label to treat nephrotic syndrome, RA, SLE, and other inflammatory disorders. Chlorambucil has a black box warning for severe myelosuppression, which is the major dose-limiting toxicity. Blood values usually return to baseline 3 to 4 weeks after administration. In general, chlorambucil produces less toxicity than most other alkylating agents and has a slower onset of action. Approved in 1957, it is available via the PO route.

Cisplatin: Cisplatin is a heavy metal complex containing platinum, chloride, and ammonia. It is cell cycle nonspecific and is usually used as combination therapy to treat metastatic testicular or ovarian tumors, bladder cancer, osteosarcoma, and soft tissue sarcomas and as adjuvant therapy in head, neck, esophageal, prostate, lung, and cervical cancers. It is available only as an injectable preparation. Cisplatin carries black box warnings for myelosuppression, ototoxicity, anaphylaxis, nausea and vomiting, and nephrotoxicity, which is the primary dose-limiting toxicity. Acute kidney injury may occur within 24 hours after administration, and permanent damage to renal tubular cells may eventually cause CKD. Peripheral neuropathy is another potentially serious adverse effect with symptoms that include numbness that begins in the fingers and toes and proceeds up the limbs toward the trunk. Ototoxicity is common and can result in permanent impairment. The nurse should be prepared for anaphylactic-like reactions that may occur within minutes of cisplatin administration.

Dacarbazine: Approved in 1998, dacarbazine is available by IV administration. It is approved to treat metastatic malignant melanoma and refractory Hodgkin's disease and is used off-label for sarcomas and neuroblastomas. Adverse GI effects occur in most patients, but tolerance to these adverse effects may develop over subsequent administrations. Myelosuppression occurs during therapy, although to a lesser extent than many other drugs in this class. Dacarbazine carries a black box warning that hepatic necrosis has occurred with the use of this drug.

Estramustine (Emcyt): Estramustine is unusual because it is a dual molecule. One portion is a nitrogen mustard alkylating agent, and the other is a molecule of estradiol. Thus, the drug may be classified as both an alkylating agent and a hormone. It is administered by the PO route for the palliative therapy of metastatic or advanced prostate cancer and may be used off-label to treat metastatic renal cell carcinoma. Unlike other alkylating agents, myelosuppression is infrequent. Nausea and vomiting are the dose-limiting toxicities. The estrogen component of the drug can cause gynecomastia, mastalgia, thromboembolic disease, and fluid retention.

Ifosfamide (Ifex): Ifosfamide is a nitrogen mustard alkylating agent approved in 1988 for the treatment of testicular cancer. Off-label indications include breast, lung, pancreatic, bladder, and cervical cancers; sarcomas; and non-Hodgkin's lymphoma. The drug has black box warnings for urotoxicity, central nervous system (CNS) toxicity, and myelosuppression. Myelosuppression is the primary dose-limiting toxicity, with blood count nadirs occurring after 5 days and recovering by 4 weeks. Nephrotoxicity also limits its use, and hematuria, hemorrhagic cystitis, and renal insufficiency occur in many patients. Signs of CNS toxicity such as confusion, drowsiness, hallucinations, and depression occur in about 12% of patients who are taking the drug. Cardiac toxicity may include dysrhythmias, heart failure, and myocarditis.

To prevent hemorrhagic cystitis in patients who are taking ifosfamide, the drug mesna (Mesnex) is administered at the time of chemotherapy by the IV route and 2 to 6 hours later by the IV or PO route. Mesna binds toxic metabolites in the urinary bladder, reducing the incidence of hematuria by 70 to 100%, depending on the dose of ifosfamide. Mesna may be used off-label for patients taking cyclophosphamide.

Lomustine (CCNU, CeeNU): Approved in 1976, lomustine is an oral nitrosourea alkylating agent that has actions similar to those of carmustine. It is used as palliative therapy in combination with other chemotherapeutic drugs or other treatment modalities in primary and metastatic brain tumors and as secondary therapy in Hodgkin's disease. The drug carries a black box warning for myelosuppression, which is its most serious dose-limiting toxicity. Delayed myelosuppression may occur up to 6 weeks following administration of the drug. Severe nausea and vomiting occur in most patients and require antiemetic therapy.

Lurbinectedin (Zepzelca): One of the newest alkylating agents, lurbinectedin was approved in 2020 for the treatment of metastatic small-cell lung cancer following platinum-based chemotherapy. Given by the IV route, the drug can cause significant myelosuppression and liver tests should be monitored for the potential development of hepatotoxicity. Common side effects include blood dyscrasias, increased creatinine, increased transaminase nausea, and increased glucose levels.

Mechlorethamine (Mustargen): Mechlorethamine is one of the oldest antineoplastics, approved in 1949. It is available by the IV, intrathecal, or topical routes. It is usually used to provide palliation in patients with Hodgkin's disease, lymphosarcoma, polycythemia vera, bronchogenic carcinoma, and chronic myelocytic or chronic lymphocytic leukemia. It may also be used for palliative treatment of metastatic cancer in intrapleural, intrapericardial, and intraperitoneal spaces when effusion has occurred as a result of the tumor. Nausea and vomiting are acute and require antiemetic therapy. Myelosuppression occurs in 8 to 14 days after drug administration and can be severe. Like cyclophosphamide, infertility is a potential adverse effect. This drug carries a black box warning to use extreme care when handling it because exposure to mucous membranes or inhaling the dust can cause toxicity. This drug is a vesicant; extravasation requires the administration of sodium thiosulfate to the injection site.

Melphalan (Alkeran): Melphalan is a nitrogen mustard approved for the palliative treatment of ovarian cancer and multiple myeloma. It may also be used off-label to treat breast or testicular cancer, osteogenic sarcoma, and non-Hodgkin's lymphoma. Because it has strong immunosuppressive and myelosuppressive effects, it has been used off-label for bone marrow ablation prior to stem cell transplantation in combination with other drugs. It is available as both a PO and an IV preparation. Melphalan carries black box warnings regarding myelosuppression, hypersensitivity reactions, and the possibility of secondary leukemia. Hematologic toxicity is the primary dose-limiting toxicity. Blood count nadirs usually occur 2 to 3 weeks after therapy starts, and recovery is seen 4 to 5 weeks after treatment. Unlike some of the other alkylating agents, melphalan is not highly emetogenic. Skin exposure can cause skin necrosis. Because of the potential for infertility, men and women with childbearing potential should be counseled regarding the drug's adverse reproductive effects.

Oxaliplatin (Eloxatin): Approved in 2002, oxaliplatin is a platinum drug that is approved only to treat advanced colorectal cancer in combination with fluorouracil and leucovorin, although it may be used off-label for other solid tumors. It acts by a different mechanism than cisplatin and exhibits little ototoxicity or nephrotoxicity. It does, however, cause significant levels of peripheral neuropathy, which can be dose limiting. An acute form of peripheral neuropathy begins within days of chemotherapy and resolves in 1 to 2 weeks. A more persistent form has a delayed onset and can cause functional impairment and discontinuation of therapy. The drug carries a black box warning for anaphylactic-like reactions that may occur within minutes of oxaliplatin administration.

Procarbazine (Matulane): Procarbazine is an oral alkylating agent that was approved in 1969 for the treatment of Hodgkin's disease. It may be used off-label for treating non-Hodgkin's lymphomas and CNS tumors such as medulloblastoma, malignant glioma, and astrocytoma. Because it has strong immunosuppressive effects, it may be used off-label for bone marrow ablation prior to stem cell transplantation in combination with other drugs. Myelosuppression is the primary dose-limiting toxicity. Blood count nadirs usually occur in week 4 after therapy starts, and recovery is seen 6 weeks after treatment. Nausea and vomiting are also common adverse effects that may be severe. CNS adverse effects are common and may include paresthesias, peripheral neuropathy, seizures, depression, and psychosis. When given by the IV route, neurotoxicity can be dose limiting.

Streptozocin (Zanosar): Approved in 1982, streptozocin is a nitrosourea alkylating agent that is more toxic than many other alkylating agents. A clinically effective response most likely will be accompanied by some evidence of serious toxicity. It is available IV to treat metastatic islet cell cancer of the pancreas either as monotherapy or in combination with fluorouracil. It may be used off-label to treat colorectal cancer and other solid tumors. Streptozocin carries black box warnings regarding nephrotoxicity, nausea and vomiting, diarrhea, hepatotoxicity, and hematologic toxicity. The most serious dose-limiting toxicity is nephrotoxicity, which occurs in more than half of patients taking the drug and can cause permanent impairment and death. Nausea, vomiting and diarrhea are also severe adverse effects of streptozocin.

Temozolomide (Temodar): Temozolomide is a prodrug that is metabolized to the same active compound as dacarbazine. Unlike dacarbazine, however, temozolomide can be administered by either the IV or PO route. Approved in 1999, it is indicated to treat malignant glioma concomitantly with radiotherapy and for refractory astrocytoma. It may also be used off-label to treat advanced metastatic melanoma. Adverse effects are similar to those of dacarbazine and include hepatotoxicity, myelosuppression, and nausea and vomiting.

Thiotepa: Thiotepa is an alkylating agent approved in 1994 to treat bladder, ovarian, and breast cancers and both Hodgkin's and non-Hodgkin's lymphomas. It is administered IV or by the intravesical route for bladder tumors. Myelosuppression is the primary dose-limiting toxicity, although neurotoxicity may also cause delay or discontinuation of therapy. Nausea and vomiting are uncommon. Injections and instillations of thiotepa can cause intense local pain. Intravesical administration causes bladder irritation, dysuria, and increased urgency. Note that the drug may be absorbed during intravesical administration and cause serious myelosuppression.

Antimetabolites

57.3 Antimetabolites disrupt the critical cellular pathways of cancer cells.

Rapidly growing cancer cells require large quantities of nutrients to construct proteins and nucleic acids. Antimetabolite drugs are structurally similar to these nutrients, but they do not perform the same functions as their natural counterparts. When cancer cells attempt to synthesize proteins, RNA, or DNA using the antimetabolites, metabolic pathways are disrupted and the cancer cells die or their growth is slowed. Some of these structural similarities are illustrated in Figure 57.2.

Some antimetabolites become incorporated into the DNA of cancer cells and interfere with DNA replication and function. Others inhibit the enzymes that synthesize the vital components of the cell. All antimetabolites are

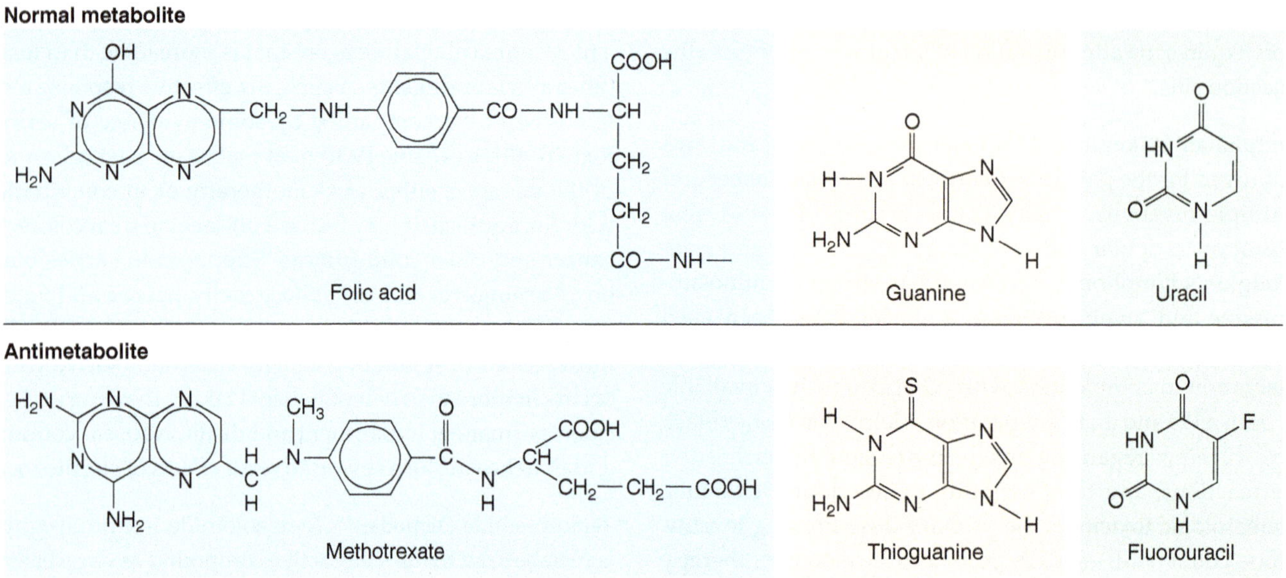

Figure 57.2 Structural similarities between antimetabolites and their natural counterparts.

cell cycle specific, with most of them affecting the S phase, although some can act during any of the active phases of the cell cycle. The three classes of antimetabolites are the folic acid analogs, the purine analogs, and the pyrimidine analogs. These drugs are listed in Table 57.2.

Folic acid analogs: Folic acid, or folate, is vitamin B_9, which is essential for the growth and maintenance of cells. It is especially important during periods of rapid cell growth because this vitamin is needed to replicate DNA. Lack of sufficient vitamin B_9 during pregnancy can cause neural

Table 57.2 Antimetabolites

Drug	Route and Adult Dose (Maximum Dose Where Indicated)	Adverse Effects
Folic Acid Analogs (Antifolates)		*Nausea and vomiting, stomatitis, anorexia, rash, fatigue, alopecia, headache* <u>Myelosuppression, severe nausea, vomiting, diarrhea, mucositis, hepatotoxicity, pulmonary toxicity, neurotoxicity (nelarabine), anaphylaxis and other hypersensitivity reactions, embryofetal toxicity</u>
methotrexate (MTX, Trexall)	PO: 10–30 mg/day for 5 days	
pemetrexed (Alimta)	IV: 500 mg/m² on day 1 of each 21-day cycle	
pralatrexate (Folotyn)	IV: 30 mg/m² once weekly for 6 wk in 7-wk cycles	
Purine Analogs		
cladribine	IV: 0.09 mg/kg/day as a continuous infusion for 7 days	
clofarabine (Clolar)	IV: 52 mg/m²/day over 2 h for 5 days	
fludarabine	IV: 25 mg/m²/day for 5 consecutive days	
mercaptopurine (6-MP, Purinethol)	PO: 1.5–2.5 mg/kg/day	
nelarabine (Arranon)	IV: 1500 mg/m² on days 1, 3, and 5; repeat every 21 days	
pentostatin (Nipent)	IV: 4 mg/m² every other wk	
thioguanine	PO: 2 mg/kg/day	
Pyrimidine Analogs		
azacytidine (Vidaza)	IV/subcutaneous: 75 mg/m² for 7 days every 4 wk PO: 300 mg once daily for days 1–14 of each 28-day cycle	
capecitabine (Xeloda)	PO: 1250 mg/m²/day bid for 2 wk	
cytarabine	IV: 100 mg/m² as a continuous infusion over 24 h	
floxuridine	Intra-arterial: 0.1–0.6 mg/kg/day as an intra-arterial infusion	
fluorouracil (5-FU, Carac, Efudex)	IV: 12 mg/kg/day for 4 consecutive days	
gemcitabine (Gemzar, Infugem)	IV: 1000–1250 mg/m² once weekly for 7 wk	
trifluridine/tipiracil (Lonsurf)	PO: 35 mg/m² bid on days 1–5 and days 8–12 of each 28-day cycle	

Note: *Italics* indicate common adverse effects. <u>Underline</u> indicates serious adverse effects.

tube defects in the fetus. Additional details on folic acid are presented in Chapter 61.

Three folic acid analogs (also called antifolates) are used as antineoplastic drugs. Methotrexate is the oldest and is prescribed for several autoimmune disorders in addition to cancer. Pemetrexed (Alimta) and pralatrexate (Folotyn) have very limited therapeutic applications. Trimethoprim and pyrimethamine (Daraprim) are folic acid analogs used as anti-infectives.

As antineoplastics, folic acid analogs are given at high doses, which can be toxic to normal cells as well as cancer cells. To "rescue" normal cells, the drug leucovorin is administered following chemotherapy with methotrexate. Leucovorin, or folinic acid, is a reduced form of folic acid that is able to enter normal cells but not cancer cells. The normal cells can thus continue metabolism and replication using leucovorin. Available by both the IV and PO routes, **leucovorin rescue therapy** must be initiated at very specific times following the methotrexate dose. Leucovorin is also used to treat overdose or prevent toxicity with other folic acid analogs such as pyrimethamine and trimethoprim. When used with fluorouracil in the treatment of colorectal cancer, leucovorin has been found to enhance cell killing. Levoleucovorin (Fusilev), given by IV infusion, is an isomer of leucovorin that is reported to have fewer adverse effects.

Purine and pyrimidine analogs: Purines and pyrimidines are bases used in the biosynthesis of DNA and RNA. The purine and pyrimidine analogs are drugs structurally similar to their naturally occurring counterparts that can act in several ways. They can inhibit the synthesis of purine or pyrimidine bases, thus limiting the precursors needed for DNA and RNA biosynthesis. The analogs can also become incorporated into the structures of DNA and RNA, resulting in a disruption of nucleic acid function.

Most of the purine and pyrimidine analogs used as antineoplastics are prodrugs that are converted to their active forms on entering the body. A few purine analogs are used for immunosuppression, gout, and antiviral therapy.

CONNECTION Checkpoint 57.2

Trimethoprim is a folic acid analog that is nearly always combined with another antibiotic medication. From what you learned in Chapter 50, name the antibiotic combination that contains trimethoprim and give its primary indications.

PROTOTYPE DRUG Methotrexate (MTX, Trexall)

Classification **Therapeutic:** Antineoplastic
Pharmacologic: Antimetabolite, folic acid analog, immunosuppressant, disease-modifying antirheumatic drug (DMARD)

Therapeutic Effects and Uses: Approved in 1953, methotrexate is a widely prescribed antifolate available by the PO, parenteral, and intrathecal routes. The PO route is preferred for low-dose therapy. It is approved for a large number of neoplasms, including osteosarcoma, acute lymphocytic and lymphoblastic leukemias, and lymphosarcomas in children; certain inoperable head, neck, and pelvic cancers; breast cancers; lung cancers; and advanced-stage non-Hodgkin's lymphoma. Its primary use as an antineoplastic is in combination therapy to maintain induced remissions in those individuals who have had surgical resection or amputation for a primary tumor.

Because of its powerful immunosuppressant properties, methotrexate is effective in treating severe RA in patients who have had inadequate response to nonsteroidal anti-inflammatory drugs (NSAIDs) and at least one or more antirheumatic drugs. It is also used to treat severe psoriasis that is unresponsive to other forms of therapy. Off-label uses include other autoimmune disorders such as active Crohn's disease, ulcerative colitis, and SLE. Methotrexate may be used to terminate pregnancy, usually in combination with misoprostol.

Mechanism of Action: Methotrexate is specific for the S phase of the cell cycle. It blocks an enzyme that is responsible for converting folic acid to reduced folate, which interferes with DNA synthesis, repair, and cellular replication mainly in actively proliferating tissues. This action is what enables it to be effective in treating psoriasis and arthritis in addition to treating cancer.

Pharmacokinetics:

Route(s)	PO, intramuscular (IM), IV, subcutaneous, intrathecal
Absorption	Variable absorption from the GI tract; well absorbed by the subcutaneous or IM routes
Distribution	Widely distributed; crosses the placenta and blood–brain barrier; secreted in breast milk; 60% bound to plasma protein
Primary metabolism	Hepatic, extensive first-pass metabolism
Primary excretion	Renal
Onset of action	Peak: 1–4 h PO; 0.5–2 h IM, IV
Duration of action	Half-life: 2–4 h

Adverse Effects: Methotrexate has many adverse effects, some of which can be serious. Nausea and vomiting are severe at high doses. **Black Box Warnings:** Methotrexate combined with NSAIDs may cause severe and sometimes fatal myelosuppression, which is the primary dose-limiting toxicity of this drug. The drug is hepatotoxic and may cause liver cirrhosis with prolonged use. Ulcerative stomatitis and diarrhea require suspension of therapy because they may lead to hemorrhagic enteritis and death from intestinal perforation. Potentially fatal opportunistic infections, including *Pneumocystis* pneumonia, may occur during therapy. Pulmonary toxicity may result in acute or chronic interstitial pneumonitis at any dose level. Severe, sometimes fatal, dermatologic reactions such as toxic epidermal necrolysis and SJS have been reported.

Contraindications/Precautions: The use of methotrexate as an antineoplastic is contraindicated in thrombocytopenia, anemia, leukopenia, concurrent administration of hepatotoxic drugs and hematopoietic suppressants, alcoholism, or lactation. Precautions must be taken in patients with CKD, impaired hepatic function, active infections, ulcerative colitis, and peptic ulcers; in patients with cancer who have preexisting bone marrow impairment; in the very young or old or debilitated; and in those with poor nutritional status. Caution should be used in handling this drug because it can cause severe skin reactions.

Drug Interactions: Methotrexate interacts with many drugs. Increased serum methotrexate levels can occur with the penicillins, vancomycin, cyclosporine, and para-aminobenzoic acid (PABA). Chloramphenicol may decrease the intestinal absorption of methotrexate. An increased methotrexate effect can occur with probenecid, ibuprofen, aspirin, and tetracyclines. Folic acid may alter the body's response to methotrexate. Sulfonamides can lead to an increased risk of methotrexate-induced immunosuppression. Methotrexate can cause decreased phenytoin effects, leading to increased seizure activity. Immunization during methotrexate therapy is not effective and any live vaccine use may lead to a severe reaction that is secondary to the immunosuppressant activity of methotrexate. **Herbal/Food:** Food delays the oral absorption of methotrexate. Echinacea may increase the risk of hepatotoxicity. More than 180 mg/day of caffeine (three to four cups of coffee) may decrease the effectiveness of methotrexate when taken for arthritis.

Pregnancy: There is evidence that methotrexate can cause teratogenic effects or fetal death when taken during pregnancy. Pregnancy should be avoided if either partner is receiving this drug. Breastfeeding is contraindicated.

Treatment of Overdose: Leucovorin or levoleucovorin is given as soon as possible after overdose to decrease the toxic effects of methotrexate. In some cases, leucovorin is given 24 to 36 hours after methotrexate chemotherapy to "rescue" normal cells from the adverse effects of the antineoplastic.

Clinician Responsibilities: Key clinical implications for patients receiving methotrexate are included in Applied Clinical Judgment: Patients Receiving Cancer Chemotherapy.

Drugs Similar to Methotrexate (MTX, Trexall)

Pemetrexed and pralatrexate are other folic acid analogs used in cancer chemotherapy. The purine analogs used for cancer chemotherapy include cladribine, clofarabine, fludarabine, mercaptopurine, nelarabine, pentostatin, and thioguanine. The pyrimidine analogs include azacitidine, capecitabine, cytarabine, floxuridine, fluorouracil, gemcitabine, and the combination drug trifluridine/tipiracil.

All the antimetabolites cause fetal harm in laboratory animals and are contraindicated during pregnancy and lactation. Some have been shown to cause birth defects in humans. Contraception is recommended prior to, during, and following chemotherapy. Pregnant women and partners seeking to conceive a child should consult with their oncologist.

Azacitidine (Onureg, Vidaza): Azacitidine (Vidaza) was originally approved in 2004 as parenteral medication for myelodysplastic syndrome, a group of cancers in which blood cells do not mature and many die before leaving the bone marrow. In 2020 an oral form of the drug (Onureg) was approved to treat acute myeloid leukemia. The parenteral and oral forms are not interchangeable. For both formulations, complete blood counts must be taken prior to each chemotherapy cycle to monitor response to treatment and possible toxicity. Common adverse effects include nausea and vomiting, diarrhea, thrombocytopenia, and neutropenia. Pretreatment with an antiemetic is required.

Capecitabine (Xeloda): Capecitabine is a pyrimidine analog that is converted into fluorouracil, another antimetabolite, by a series of three enzymatic steps. One of these enzymes, thymidine phosphorylase, is found in especially high amounts in cancer cells; thus, the drug is converted to a toxic form inside the cancer cell. Capecitabine blocks the synthesis of pyrimidines and can also be incorporated into nucleic acid molecules. It is available PO to treat metastatic breast cancer refractory to other treatments, colorectal cancer, or as adjuvant therapy for colon cancer following resection. Capecitabine causes less immunosuppression than many antineoplastics. Diarrhea is the dose-limiting toxicity; antidiarrheal therapy with loperamide is often indicated during chemotherapy. Nausea and vomiting, stomatitis, and abdominal pain are common adverse effects. An unusual adverse effect with this drug is palmar-plantar erythrodysesthesia (hand and foot syndrome), which can occur in over half the patients receiving the drug. Hand and foot syndrome is characterized by numbness, tingling, swelling, erythema, blistering, and severe pain. Capecitabine carries a black box warning that patients receiving warfarin (Coumadin) must be closely monitored to prevent serious or fatal bleeding.

Cladribine: Cladribine is an IV purine analog that is a preferred drug for active hairy cell leukemia. It may be used off-label to treat chronic lymphocytic leukemia, non-Hodgkin's lymphoma, acute and chronic myelogenous leukemia, and mycosis fungoides. Approved in 1993, cladribine differs from other purine analogs in that it is effective against both dividing (S phase) and nondividing cancer cells. Cladribine carries black box warnings regarding myelosuppression, neurotoxicity, and nephrotoxicity. Myelosuppression is the primary dose-limiting toxicity, with a nadir occurring in 14 days and recovery at 5 weeks. Lymphocyte counts may take up to a year to return to normal values, resulting in a high number of opportunistic infections. Fever and chills, which are often associated with infections, are common. Rash occurs in most patients but is not usually serious. Nausea and vomiting are mild compared to other antineoplastics. An oral form of cladribine (Mavenclad) was approved in 2019 to treat multiple sclerosis in patients who have not responded to safer medications.

Clofarabine (Clolar): Clofarabine is an IV purine analog that was approved in 2004. It only has one indication: the treatment of relapsed or refractory acute lymphocytic leukemia after at least two prior regimens have proven unsuccessful. It is approved for patients ages 1 to 21 years. Common adverse events include myelosuppression, opportunistic infections, nausea and vomiting, diarrhea, anorexia, fever, fatigue, abdominal pain, and edema.

Cytarabine: Approved in 1969, cytarabine is a pyrimidine antimetabolite available for IV, subcutaneous, or intrathecal administration. It is approved for remission induction in acute myelogenous leukemia. It may be used off-label for other hematologic malignancies, including acute lymphatic leukemia, chronic myelogenous leukemia, and Hodgkin's and non-Hodgkin's lymphoma. Cytarabine is specific for the S phase of the cell cycle. It is converted to its active form, Ara-CTP, and then becomes incorporated into DNA, where it suppresses further DNA synthesis. Cytarabine carries a black box warning regarding myelosuppression, which has a nadir occurring at week 1 and resolution by week 3 or 4. High-dose therapy can cause severe nausea and vomiting and other GI toxicities. A cluster of symptoms, called the cytarabine syndrome, can occur within 6 to 12 hours of treatment. Symptoms include bone pain, fever, myalgia, rash, and fatigue. Other serious adverse effects include peripheral neuropathy, respiratory distress, encephalopathy, palmar-plantar erythrodysesthesia, and hepatotoxicity. In 2017 a fixed-dose liposome encapsulated combination of cytarabine and daunorubicin (Vyxeos) was approved to treat adult myelocytic leukemia.

Floxuridine: Floxuridine is a pyrimidine analog antimetabolite that was approved in 1970. Because it is nearly entirely removed by hepatic first-pass metabolism, it has very limited applications. Its only approved indication is as a continuous intra-arterial infusion via a hepatic artery catheter for the palliative treatment of metastatic liver cancer. Due to its high concentration in the liver, floxuridine can cause elevated liver function enzymes and serious hepatotoxicity. This drug carries a black box warning regarding myelosuppression. Other adverse effects, such as nausea, vomiting, anorexia, diarrhea, rash, and alopecia, are common to other antineoplastics.

Fludarabine: Approved in 1991, fludarabine is an IV purine analog with a similar action to cladribine. It is approved only to treat chronic lymphocytic leukemia that has not responded to at least one alkylating agent, but it may be used off-label to treat other leukemias and non-Hodgkin's lymphoma. It is cell cycle specific for the S phase, where it inhibits DNA replication. Fludarabine carries black box warnings regarding myelosuppression, severe CNS toxicity, autoimmune complications, and pulmonary toxicity. Severe myelosuppression is the most common dose-limiting toxicity. Like cladribine, lymphocyte levels may take up to a year to return to normal levels. Rare instances of life-threatening autoimmune hemolytic anemia have been reported. High doses of fludarabine are neurotoxic and can result in blindness, coma, and death. Fever and infections are common, including serious interstitial pneumonitis. Nausea and vomiting are mild compared to other antineoplastics but may be severe at high doses.

Fluorouracil (5-FU, Carac, Efudex): Approved in 1962, fluorouracil is an antimetabolite that inhibits DNA and RNA synthesis in the S phase of the cell cycle. It is available as an injection, a topical solution, and a topical cream. The IV form is used to treat solid tumors, including inoperable breast, ovarian, cervical, urinary bladder, liver, colon, rectal, stomach, and pancreatic cancers. As a topical preparation it is used to treat superficial basal cell carcinomas and multiple actinic keratoses. A formulation of fluorouracil cream using a microsponge delivery system (Carac) allows for once-daily dosing and a sustained release of the drug. Fluorouracil carries a black box warning regarding myelosuppression, which may be dose limiting with a nadir at 9 to 14 days and recovery by 30 days. Palmar-plantar erythrodysesthesia occurs in up to 40% of patients receiving a prolonged IV infusion of this drug. Serious GI toxicity, including ulceration, stomatitis, diarrhea, anorexia, and vomiting, is common. Topical applications may cause local photosensitivity, burning, erythema, swelling, and desquamation.

Gemcitabine (Gemzar, Infugem): Gemcitabine is an IV pyrimidine analog approved in 1996 that kills cancer cells during the S phase of the cell cycle. Indications include locally advanced or metastatic solid tumors of the pancreas, breast, ovary, or lung. Gemcitabine is one of the most effective drugs for treating advanced pancreatic cancer, a disease that has a very low 5-year survival rate. The dose-limiting toxicity for gemcitabine is myelosuppression, which occurs in nearly all patients taking the drug. Serious pulmonary, renal, and hepatic toxicity has been reported. Fever, nausea and vomiting, and infection are common adverse effects.

Mercaptopurine (6-MP, Purinethol): Mercaptopurine is an older purine analog, approved in 1953, that is cell cycle specific to the S phase. It is a prodrug that has very similar actions, indications, and adverse effects to thioguanine. Mercaptopurine is indicated for acute lymphocytic and myelogenous leukemia in both adults and children. It is less effective in treating adults than children but remains a preferred drug. It can produce a temporary remission in patients with chronic granulocytic leukemia. Due to its powerful immunosuppressant activity, it may be used off-label to produce temporary remissions in patients with ulcerative colitis and Crohn's disease. The most frequent dose-limiting toxicity of mercaptopurine is myelosuppression, which results in leukopenia, thrombocytopenia, and anemia in nearly every patient. Nausea and vomiting are not severe, but diarrhea may require fluid replacement therapy.

Nelarabine (Arranon): Approved in 2005, nelarabine is an IV purine analog approved to treat T-cell acute lymphoblastic leukemia and T-cell lymphoblastic lymphoma in both adults and children. Its use is limited to patients who have not responded to or have relapsed during treatment with at least two chemotherapy regimens. The drug carries a black box warning for neurotoxicity, which is the major dose-limiting adverse effect with nelarabine. Neurologic signs and symptoms may include impaired cognition, severe somnolence, seizures, peripheral neuropathies, ataxia, tremor, dizziness, and cerebral hemorrhage. Myelosuppression occurs in most patients; fatigue, fever, and infection occur frequently. Nausea and vomiting and other GI complaints are usually not a major cause of discontinuation.

Pemetrexed (Alimta) and Pralatrexate (Folotyn): Pemetrexed and pralatrexate are antifolates given by IV injection that have very specific therapeutic applications. Approved in 2004, pemetrexed is approved to treat malignant pleural mesothelioma and advanced or metastatic non-small-cell lung cancer. It is administered along with cisplatin in these patients. Pralatrexate was approved in 2009 for the treatment of refractory T-cell lymphoma.

Myelosuppression is the primary dose-limiting toxicity for these drugs. GI adverse effects may be serious and include nausea, vomiting, anorexia, and mucositis. Patients may experience serious and even fatal skin reactions. Caution must be used to ensure adequate kidney function because impairment may cause pemetrexed to accumulate to fatal levels in the blood. To reduce toxicity from pemetrexed and pralatrexate, patients receive folic acid and vitamin B_{12} supplements preceding therapy.

Pentostatin (Nipent): Pentostatin is an IV purine analog approved in 1991 to treat hairy cell leukemia that has not responded to interferon (IFN) alfa. It may be used off-label to treat other leukemias and lymphomas. It is cell cycle specific in the S phase. Pentostatin has black box warnings regarding renal, liver, and pulmonary toxicities. Hematologic toxicity is dose limiting and patients experience a high rate of fever, chills, and infections. Rash and other skin reactions occur in most patients and may be severe. Neurologic toxicity is a serious problem at high doses.

Thioguanine: Approved in 1966, thioguanine is very similar to mercaptopurine in its actions and adverse effects. Like other antimetabolites, it is active in the S phase of the cell cycle. It is available PO to treat acute nonlymphocytic leukemia. Off-label indications include chronic myelogenous leukemia, psoriasis, refractory ulcerative colitis, and Crohn's disease. Myelosuppression is the most common dose-limiting toxicity. Long-term, continuous use of thioguanine is not recommended due to the risk for serious hepatotoxicity. Adverse GI effects are generally not severe at normal doses.

Trifluridine/Tipiracil (Lonsurf): One of the newer therapies in this class, Lonsurf is a combination drug approved in 2015 to treat metastatic colorectal cancer when at least two other therapies have failed to achieve successful results. The active ingredient is trifluridine, which is a pyrimidine that is incorporated into the DNA of the cancer cell. Tipiracil is added as a pharmacokinetic booster to increase the levels of trifluridine in the blood. The most serious adverse effect is myelosuppression. As eyedrops, trifluridine is available to treat ocular herpes (see Chapter 54).

Antitumor Antibiotics

57.4 The antibiotic antineoplastics contain substances obtained from bacteria that have the ability to kill cancer cells.

Antitumor properties have been identified in a number of chemicals isolated from microorganisms. These substances are more cytotoxic than traditional antibiotics, and their use is restricted to treating a few specific types of cancer. The antitumor antibiotics are listed in Table 57.3.

The antitumor antibiotics bind to DNA and affect its function by a mechanism similar to that of the alkylating agents; therefore, their general actions and adverse effects are like those of the alkylating agents. Unlike the alkylating agents, however, all the antitumor antibiotics must be administered IV or through direct instillation via a catheter into a body cavity or organ. As with many other antineoplastics, the primary dose-limiting toxicity of drugs in this class is myelosuppression. These drugs can cause major damage to the skin, subcutaneous tissue, and nerves should extravasation occur.

The antitumor antibiotics are divided into two groups, the anthracyclines and nonanthracyclines. The

Table 57.3 Antitumor Antibiotics

Drug	Route and Adult Dose (Maximum Dose Where Indicated)	Adverse Effects
bleomycin	IV: 0.25–0.5 units/kg q4–7days	*Nausea and vomiting, stomatitis, anorexia, headache, rash, alopecia*
dactinomycin (Cosmegen)	IV: 400–600 mcg/m²/day for 5 days	
daunorubicin (Cerubidine)	IV: 30–45 mg/m²/day for 3–5 days	Myelosuppression, severe nausea, vomiting, diarrhea, mucositis, pulmonary or cardiac toxicity, anaphylaxis and other hypersensitivity reactions, tissue necrosis (due to extravasation), hemolytic uremic syndrome (mitomycin), hepatotoxicity (dactinomycin)
doxorubicin	IV: 40–60 mg/m² as a single injection q21–28days	
doxorubicin liposomal (Doxil)	IV: 20 mg/m² q3wk	
epirubicin (Ellence)	IV: 100–120 mg/m² as a single dose	
idarubicin (Idamycin)	IV: 8–12 mg/m²/day for 3 days	
mitomycin	IV: 20 mg/m² as a single dose	
mitoxantrone	IV: 12 mg/m² q3days	

Note: *Italics* indicate common adverse effects. Underline indicates serious adverse effects.

anthracyclines include daunorubicin, doxorubicin, epirubicin, idarubicin, and mitoxantrone. The anthracyclines are closely related in structure, and all exhibit cardiotoxicity, a major limiting adverse effect. Cardiotoxicity may occur within minutes of administration, or it may be delayed for months or years after chemotherapy has been completed. The nonanthracyclines, which include bleomycin, dactinomycin, and mitomycin, tend to cause less cardiotoxicity than the anthracyclines.

The cardioprotective drug dexrazoxane (Zinecard) is administered to specifically treat doxorubicin cardiotoxicity. Started by slow IV infusion 30 minutes before doxorubicin, dexrazoxane reduces the incidence and severity of cardiomyopathy from the antitumor antibiotic. In 2007, a second form of dexrazoxane (Totect) was approved to treat the pain, inflammation, and tissue necrosis associated with extravasation of anthracyclines. For this indication, IV dexrazoxane is administered as soon as possible after confirmation of anthracycline extravasation, with subsequent doses at 24 and 48 hours. Dexrazoxane may add to the myelosuppression caused by anthracyclines.

PROTOTYPE DRUG Doxorubicin

Classification **Therapeutic:** Antineoplastic
Pharmacologic: Antitumor antibiotic, anthracycline

Therapeutic Effects and Uses: Approved in 1975, doxorubicin is a cytotoxic antibiotic obtained from *Streptomyces* that has a wide spectrum of antitumor activity and is considered one of the most effective single drugs against solid tumors. Doxorubicin is highly toxic to rapidly proliferating cells as well as slowly developing tumors. It is approved to treat neuroblastoma and solid tumors of the bone, bladder, breast, ovary, GI tract, lung, and thyroid. It is also part of many chemotherapy regimens for other tumors, such as acute lymphoblastic and myeloblastic leukemias, Wilms' tumor, soft tissue sarcomas, and multiple myeloma. Given by the IV route, it may also be instilled into the bladder for bladder cancer. It is also effective as a preradiation therapy to sensitize superficial tumors.

Doxorubicin liposomal (Doxil) is a form of the drug incorporated into liposomes, closed, spherical molecules that encase the drug. Administered IV, the liposomes have a long half-life and produce a prolonged duration of action. In addition, the liposomes tend to stay in the circulation until they reach tumors, which often have leakier capillaries than normal tissues. Once inside the tumor, the drug is released from its carrier. Doxorubicin liposomal is approved for use in patients with acquired immunodeficiency syndrome (AIDS)–related Kaposi's sarcoma, ovarian cancer (after failure of platinum-based chemotherapy), and relapsed multiple myeloma.

Mechanism of Action: Doxorubicin binds to DNA, causing strand splitting and inhibition of DNA synthesis. It is cell cycle nonspecific.

Pharmacokinetics:

Route(s)	IV
Absorption	N/A
Distribution	Widely distributed; crosses the placenta but does not cross the blood–brain barrier; secreted in breast milk; 75% bound to plasma protein
Primary metabolism	Hepatic
Primary excretion	Bile
Onset of action	Peak: 1/2–2 h
Duration of action	Triphasic half-life: 12 min, 3.3 h, and 30–40 h

Adverse Effects: Doxorubicin has many adverse effects, some of which are serious. These include severe nausea, vomiting, mucositis, rash, excessive lacrimation, hepatotoxicity, anaphylaxis, complete alopecia, and radiation recall phenomenon (a skin reaction due to prior radiation therapy).

Doxorubicin turns urine and tears a red color, which is harmless but anxiety provoking. Temporary decreased fertility is likely in both men and women. **Black Box Warnings:** Severe myelosuppression may occur, which is the major dose-limiting toxicity. It may manifest as thrombocytopenia, leukopenia, and anemia. The neutropenia nadir occurs at 7 days and recovers by 14 days. Doxorubicin exhibits significant cardiotoxicity, which may be either acute or chronic. Cardiac adverse effects can be life-threatening and may include sinus tachycardia, bradycardia, delayed heart failure, acute left-ventricular failure, and myocarditis. Heart failure may occur months or years after the termination of chemotherapy. Acute, infusion-related reactions may occur, including anaphylaxis. Severe local necrosis may result if extravasation occurs. Secondary malignancies, especially acute myelogenous leukemia, may occur 1 to 3 years following therapy.

Contraindications/Precautions: Contraindications to the use of doxorubicin include myelosuppression, thrombocytopenia, preexisting cardiac disease, obstructive jaundice, lactation, or previous treatment with complete cumulative doses of doxorubicin or daunorubicin. Precautions include CKD, impaired hepatic function, history of atopic dermatitis, and patients who have received cyclophosphamide or pelvic radiation therapy to areas surrounding the heart. Doxorubicin is a severe vesicant and precautions must be taken to avoid contact with the skin or soft tissue. Skin contact or extravasation should be treated immediately with local ice packs to reduce absorption of the drug.

Drug Interactions: Increased toxicity may occur with other antineoplastics, radiation therapy, or mercaptopurine. Cyclophosphamide may increase the risk of hemorrhagic cystitis or cardiac toxicity. Paclitaxel may decrease the clearance of doxorubicin, leading to more profound neutropenia and stomatitis. Phenobarbital and other barbiturates increase the elimination of doxorubicin. Possible decreased phenytoin levels may occur. Concurrent use with verapamil can raise the serum levels of doxorubicin, thus increasing the risk for cardiotoxicity. Use with paclitaxel will result in an increased incidence of stomatitis, neutropenia, and heart failure. Because doxorubicin causes thrombocytopenia, concurrent use with NSAIDs, anticoagulants, or platelet inhibitors may cause excessive bleeding. **Herbal/Food:** Unknown.

Pregnancy: Doxorubicin causes embryofetal harm in laboratory animals and is contraindicated during pregnancy and lactation. Contraception is recommended during therapy and for at least 6 months following the last dose. Doxorubicin may cause irreversible infertility in both male and female patients

Treatment of Overdose: If myelosuppression occurs, administration of antibiotics, platelets, and granulocytes may be necessary. Symptoms of mucositis and heart failure must be treated symptomatically.

Clinician Responsibilities: Key clinical implications for patients receiving doxorubicin are included in Applied Clinical Judgment: Patients Receiving Cancer Chemotherapy.

Drugs Similar to Doxorubicin

The anthracyclines include daunorubicin, epirubicin, idarubicin, and mitoxantrone. The nonanthracyclines are bleomycin, dactinomycin, and mitomycin. Both anthracyclines and nonanthracyclines cause fetal harm in laboratory animals and are contraindicated during pregnancy and lactation. Contraception is recommended prior to, during, and following chemotherapy. Some of these antineoplastics may cause infertility in both male and female patients. Pregnant women and partners seeking to conceive a child should consult with their oncologist.

Anthracyclines:

Daunorubicin (Cerubidine): Approved in 1979, daunorubicin is an IV antitumor antibiotic obtained from *Streptomyces*. Cell cycle specific for the S phase, daunorubicin binds to DNA, causing strand splitting and inhibition of DNA synthesis. Closely related structurally to doxorubicin, daunorubicin is approved to induce remission in acute myelogenous leukemia in adults and acute lymphocytic leukemia in children and adults. It is less effective than doxorubicin in treating solid tumors. Daunorubicin carries black box warnings regarding tissue necrosis following extravasation, cardiotoxicity, and myelosuppression. Myelosuppression is the major dose-limiting toxicity, and the drug exhibits the same types of cardiotoxicity as doxorubicin, although to a lesser extent. Other adverse effects, such as nausea, vomiting, alopecia, urine discoloration, and vesicant properties, are the same as those of doxorubicin.

Epirubicin (Ellence): Approved in 1999, epirubicin is an IV antitumor antibiotic closely related to doxorubicin in both structure and function. Epirubicin is approved only for adjuvant therapy for axillary node–positive breast cancer but may be used off-label for bladder, gastric, lung, head, neck, and liver cancers. Carrying black box warnings for extravasation, cardiotoxicity, myelosuppression, and secondary malignancies, epirubicin exhibits the same types of adverse effects as doxorubicin. Myelosuppression is the major dose-limiting toxicity, with a nadir occurring at 10 to 14 days and recovery at 21 days. Cardiotoxicity, including fatal heart failure, has been reported. Moderate to severe nausea, vomiting, and alopecia occur in many patients. Severe local tissue necrosis can occur with extravasation. Secondary acute myelogenous leukemia has been reported in patients treated with epirubicin.

Idarubicin (Idamycin): Approved in 1990, idarubicin is an IV antitumor antibiotic structurally similar to daunorubicin. Its only approved indication is for acute myelogenous leukemia, although it may be used off-label for other leukemias, advanced metastatic breast cancer, and refractory non-Hodgkin's lymphoma. Idarubicin carries black box warnings regarding tissue necrosis following extravasation, cardiotoxicity, and myelosuppression. Like other drugs in this class, myelosuppression is the primary dose limitation, with a nadir by day 15 and recovery by day 25. Idarubicin is a vesicant, and care must be taken to not allow extravasation or exposure to skin. Other common adverse effects include alopecia, cardiotoxicity, and moderate nausea and vomiting.

Mitoxantrone: Although not an anthracycline, mitoxantrone is structurally similar to the anthracyclines and shares some common properties. Approved in 1987, it is approved to treat acute myelogenous leukemia and for the palliation of severe pain associated with advanced prostate cancer. Off-label antineoplastic indications include other leukemias, breast cancer, metastatic ovarian cancer, liver cancer, and non-Hodgkin's lymphoma. It is also approved for reducing neurologic disability associated with chronic multiple sclerosis. It is administered by IV infusion. Mitoxantrone carries black box warnings regarding extravasation, cardiotoxicity, myelosuppression, and secondary malignancies. The dose-limiting toxicity is myelosuppression, with a nadir at 10 to 14 days and recovery by 2 to 3 weeks. It is less cardiotoxic than the anthracyclines, but this is still a significant adverse effect of mitoxantrone. Other adverse effects include stomatitis, moderate nausea, vomiting, alopecia, injection-site reactions, and secondary malignancy (leukemia).

Nonanthracyclines:

Bleomycin (Blenoxane): Approved in 1973, bleomycin is an antitumor antibiotic obtained from *Streptomyces* that is cell cycle specific to the G2 phase. Bleomycin is used for palliative therapy for many different cancers, including Hodgkin's and non-Hodgkin's lymphomas, testicular cancer, vulvar cancer, cervical cancer, and squamous cell carcinoma. It can be administered by the IM, IV, subcutaneous, and intrapleural routes. Bleomycin causes less myelosuppression than other drugs in this class. A black box warning states that the drug can cause severe and potentially fatal lung injury, with signs such as pulmonary fibrosis or pleural effusions. Patients who have received radiation treatment to the chest or cumulative doses of bleomycin are at increased risk for lung injury. The warning also states that bleomycin can cause a severe idiosyncratic reaction, similar to anaphylaxis, consisting of hypotension, mental confusion, fever, chills, and wheezing. Serious dermatologic reactions may require lower doses or discontinuation of the drug. Nausea and vomiting are generally mild; however, anorexia and weight loss are common.

Dactinomycin (Cosmegen): Approved in 1973, dactinomycin is an IV antitumor antibiotic obtained from *Streptomyces* that binds to DNA to inhibit RNA synthesis and is cell cycle nonspecific. Its primary indication is to treat Wilms' tumor and rhabdomyosarcoma, but it is also approved for choriocarcinoma, Ewing's sarcoma, and testicular carcinoma. Off-label indications include Kaposi's sarcoma, malignant melanoma, and osteogenic sarcoma. Dactinomycin has several dose-limiting toxicities. Myelosuppression can be severe and lead to serious infections with a nadir at 7 to 21 days. Nausea and vomiting are severe and require antiemetic therapy. Other GI effects include oral or esophageal ulceration, anorexia, and diarrhea. Hepatotoxicity, including hepatomegaly, ascites, hepatitis, and hyperbilirubinemia, can be serious, especially at high doses. Alopecia and dermatologic reactions are common. This drug carries a black box warning that special handling is required because the powder, dust, and solution are extremely irritating to soft tissue and mucous membranes.

Mitomycin: Mitomycin is an IV antitumor antibiotic extracted from *Streptomyces* that was approved in 1974. It is effective against both slowly developing and rapidly proliferating cells in solid tumors, including some tumors unresponsive to radiation and other chemotherapeutic drugs. Mitomycin is approved only for gastric and pancreatic cancers but may be used off-label for bladder cancer, colorectal cancer, breast cancer, and squamous cell carcinoma of the head, neck, lung, or cervix. Mitomycin carries black box warnings regarding myelosuppression and hemolytic uremic syndrome. The primary dose-limiting toxicity is bone marrow suppression with a nadir at 3 weeks. Recovery may take 4 to 8 weeks. Hemolytic uremic syndrome is a serious complication involving hemolytic anemia, thrombocytopenia, and irreversible renal failure. Severe skin reactions such as ulceration and cellulitis can occur, especially following extravasation. Lung toxicity is rare, but occurrences of interstitial pneumonitis can be fatal. Nausea and vomiting, anorexia, and fatigue may be persistent during therapy.

Hormones and Hormone Antagonists

57.5 Hormones and hormone antagonists block the substances necessary for continued growth of tumors.

A number of hormones are used in cancer chemotherapy, including corticosteroids, progestins, estrogens, and androgens. In addition, several hormone *antagonists* have been found to exhibit antitumor activity. Endocrine, or hormonal, therapy is limited to treating hormone-sensitive tumors of the breast, ovary or prostate. The antitumor hormones and hormone antagonists are listed in Table 57.4.

Table 57.4 Hormone and Hormone Antagonists Used for Neoplasia

Drug	Route and Adult Dose (Maximum Dose Where Indicated)	Adverse Effects
Selective Estrogen Receptor Modifiers		
fulvestrant (Faslodex)	IM: 500 mg once monthly	*Hot flashes, leg cramps, atrophic vaginitis, menstrual changes* Venous thromboembolism (including stroke, deep vein thrombosis (DVT), and pulmonary embolism), retinal changes, cataracts, fetal toxicity
raloxifene (Evista)	PO: 60 mg once daily	
tamoxifen	PO: 20–40 mg/day (treatment) or 20 mg/day (prophylaxis)	
toremifene (Fareston)	PO: 60 mg/day	
Androgen Blockers (Antiandrogens)		
abiraterone (Yonsa, Zytiga)	PO: 1 g once daily in combination with prednisone or methylprednisolone	*Joint swelling, hypokalemia, muscle weakness, back pain, diarrhea, hot flashes, gynecomastia, urinary tract infection, asthenia* Hepatotoxicity, fetal toxicity, fractures due to falls
apalutamide (Erleada)	PO: 240 mg once daily	
bicalutamide (Casodex)	PO: 50 mg/day	
darolutamide (Nubeqa)	PO: 600 mg bid	
enzalutamide (Xtandi)	PO: 160 mg once daily	
flutamide (Eulexin)	PO: 250 mg tid	
nilutamide (Nilandron)	PO: 150–300 mg once daily	
Aromatase Inhibitors		
anastrozole (Arimidex)	PO: 1 mg/day	*Hot flashes, vasodilation, fatigue, mood disturbances, nausea and vomiting* Fetal toxicity, fracture, ischemic heart disease, serious hypertension (HTN)
exemestane (Aromasin)	PO: 25 mg/day after a meal	
letrozole (Femara)	PO: 2.5 mg/day	
Gonadotropin-Releasing Hormone Analogs and Related Drugs		
degarelix (Firmagon)	Subcutaneous: 240-mg loading dose followed by 80 mg q28days	*Hot flashes, hyperglycemia (increased risk for diabetes mellitus), mood disturbances, bone pain, injection-site pain, fatigue* Seizures, spinal cord compression, QT interval prolongation
goserelin (Zoladex)	Subcutaneous: 1 implant q12wk (10.8 mg)	
histrelin (Supprelin LA, Vantas)	Subcutaneous (Supprelin LA): 1 implant every 12 months (50 mg)	
leuprolide (Eligard, Lupron)	Subcutaneous: 1 implant every 12 months (65 mg) IM depot: 22.5–45 mg every 3–6 months	
relugolix (Orogovyx)	PO: 350 mg loading dose followed by 120 mg once daily	
triptorelin (Trelstar, Triptodur)	IM (Trelstar): 3.75 mg once monthly or 22.5 mg q24wk	
Hormones		
dexamethasone	PO: 2 mg bid–qid	*Weight gain, insomnia, abdominal distention, sweating, flushing, diarrhea, nervousness, gynecomastia, hirsutism (testosterone)* Thrombophlebitis, muscle wasting (dexamethasone, prednisone), osteoporosis, hepatotoxicity
ethinyl estradiol (Estinyl, others)	PO: 1 mg tid for 2–3 months (breast cancer); 0.15–3 mg/day (prostate cancer)	
fluoxymesterone	PO: 10 mg tid	
medroxyprogesterone	IM: 400–1000 mg every wk	
megestrol	PO: 40–160 mg bid–qid	
prednisone	PO: 20–100 mg/day	
testosterone	IM: 200–400 mg q2–4wk	

Note: *Italics* indicate common adverse effects. Underline indicates serious adverse effects.

Hormones are essential signaling molecules in both normal and cancer cells. In certain types of cancer cells, the hormone stimulates the abnormal cells to divide rapidly. Thus, the mechanism by which most hormonal antineoplastic therapies act is to block the hormone from reaching its target receptors in the cancer cell. This can be done by either preventing the production of the hormone or by blocking its receptors. In some cases, the actual mechanism of action is unclear.

Because hormonal therapy is not cytotoxic, it produces few of the life-threatening toxic effects of antineoplastics from other classes. They can, however, produce significant adverse effects when given at high doses for prolonged periods. Because they rarely produce cancer cures when used singly, these drugs are normally given along with radiation, other antineoplastics or for palliation. The four general classes of hormone antagonists are:

- Selective estrogen receptor modifiers
- Aromatase inhibitors
- Gonadotropin-releasing hormone analogs
- Androgen blockers.

Selective estrogen receptor modifiers: Produced by the ovary and the adrenal gland, estrogen is a hormone that has profound metabolic actions on many organs. Estrogen produces its actions by activating estrogen receptors (ERs). ERs are widely distributed throughout the body, including the reproductive organs, heart, lungs, and bone. They are also found in many breast cancers, which are known as ER-positive tumors. Estrogen promotes the growth of ER-positive breast tumors.

Selective estrogen receptor modifiers (SERMs) are drugs that either activate or inhibit ERs, depending on the tissue. These medications have the ability to activate ERs in some tissues (such as bone), while blocking ERs in other tissues (such as breast). SERMs such as tamoxifen block ERs located in the breast, exerting an antiestrogen effect that slows tumor growth of ER-positive breast cancer. On the other hand, raloxifene (Evista) is a SERM that activates ERs in bone, increasing bone mass in patients with osteoporosis (see Chapter 72). Tamoxifen is the most widely prescribed SERM and serves as the prototype for antineoplastic hormones.

Aromatase inhibitors: Aromatase is the enzyme that catalyzes the last step in the synthesis of estrogen. During this step, aromatase converts androgens (testosterone and androstenedione) to estrogens (estradiol) in peripheral tissues such as fat and muscle. Blocking this step reduces the level of estrogen in the blood, starving ER-positive tumors of their primary growth stimulus.

Unfortunately, the aromatase inhibitors cannot prevent estradiol formation in the ovary, which is the primary site of estrogen synthesis in premenopausal women. Because of this, the drug is effective only in postmenopausal women, who secrete almost no estrogen from their ovaries.

Aromatase inhibitor therapy has become a first-line treatment for postmenopausal women with ER-positive breast cancer. Aromatase inhibitors can be started as primary therapy or instituted after the completion of 2 to 3 years of tamoxifen therapy. Extending treatment for up to 10 years has been shown to significantly reduce the risk of breast cancer recurrence (Goss et al., 2016).

Gonadotropin-releasing hormone (GnRH) analogs: Gonadotropin-releasing hormone analogs mimic the actions of endogenous GnRH and provide feedback to the pituitary gland. Initially, the effect is to increase the production of interstitial cell–stimulating hormone (ICSH), which increases the secretion of testosterone by the testes. ICSH is also known as follicle-stimulating hormone. With continued therapy, the pituitary becomes insensitive to the effects of GnRH, and the production of testosterone falls. In fact, testosterone secretion declines to near-zero levels such that treatment with a GnRH analog is considered a type of chemical castration. All are approved for the management of prostate cancer. The loss of testosterone "starves" prostate cancer cells of the hormone essential for their growth. Some drugs in this class are also approved to treat endometriosis and uterine leiomyomata and for the palliative treatment of advanced breast cancer. The GnRH analogs are administered by the IM route or subcutaneous implants.

Androgen blockers: Growth of prostatic carcinoma is highly androgen dependent. The androgen blockers prevent testosterone and other androgens from reaching their receptors in cancer cells, thus depriving these cells of an important growth promoter. Drugs in this group are administered PO and are indicated to treat prostate cancer. They have an additive or synergistic effect when used in combination with GnRH analogs. Androgen blockers slow the growth of prostate cancer, but they are not curative. Castration, either through surgery or the use of GnRH inhibitors, is often used with antiandrogens to lower androgens to their lowest possible level.

PROTOTYPE DRUG Tamoxifen

Classification **Therapeutic:** Antineoplastic
Pharmacologic: Hormonal agent, estrogen receptor blocker

Therapeutic Effects and Uses: Approved in 1985, tamoxifen is an oral SERM that has an antiestrogen effect on ER-positive tumors. It has no effect on ER-negative cancers. Tamoxifen is approved for the treatment of ER-positive breast cancer in both men and women; adjuvant treatment of breast cancer after patients have completed their primary treatment of surgery and radiation; treatment of women with ductal carcinoma in situ (noninvasive breast cancer) following surgery and radiation to the reduce the risk of invasive cancer; and reduce the risk of breast cancer in women at high risk. There are many off-label indications, some of which include meningioma, bone metastases, metastatic melanoma, and advanced ovarian cancer.

Tamoxifen and raloxifene are the only antineoplastics approved for the *prophylaxis* of breast cancer in women who have a high risk of developing the disease. In addition, it is approved as adjunctive therapy in women following a mastectomy to decrease the potential for cancer in the contralateral breast. It is not to be used for prophylaxis in women at low risk of acquiring breast cancer because the risks of adverse drug effects may outweigh the benefits in this population. Factors that may qualify a woman for tamoxifen prophylactic therapy include age, age at first menses, age at the time of birth of first child (if any), close family history of breast cancer, number of past breast biopsies showing atypical hyperplasia, history of carcinoma in situ, presence of *BRCA* mutation, and race/ethnicity.

Tamoxifen has several nonneoplastic indications, all of which are off-label. For the treatment of infertility, it may be used to induce ovulation in women who do not ovulate but desire to become pregnant. It may also be used to reduce the pain associated with gynecomastia in both women and men.

Mechanism of Action: Tamoxifen binds to ERs, producing agonist effects in some tissues (bone) and antagonist effects in other tissues (breast). The binding in breast tissue inhibits DNA replication and affects other growth factors in cancer cells.

Pharmacokinetics:

Route(s)	PO
Absorption	Slowly from the GI tract
Distribution	Widely distributed; crosses the placenta; unknown if secreted in breast milk
Primary metabolism	Hepatic by CYP3A, CYP2C9, and CYP2D6
Primary excretion	Feces
Onset of action	Peak serum concentration: 5 h
Duration of action	Half-life: 5–7 days

Adverse Effects: Tamoxifen has few serious adverse effects other than nausea and vomiting, which occurs in 12 to 25% of patients who are taking the drug. This can be controlled with antiemetics as necessary. Other common adverse effects include hot flashes, vaginal discharge, irregular menses, vaginal bleeding, fluid retention, headaches, lightheadedness, and rash. **Black Box Warnings:** The most serious potential adverse effect associated with tamoxifen is the increased risk of endometrial cancer and uterine sarcoma. The benefits of tamoxifen justify the risks of adverse effects in women taking tamoxifen to *treat* breast cancer. The benefit versus risk is not as clear in women who are taking tamoxifen to *prevent* breast cancer. There is also an increased risk of thromboembolic events, including stroke, pulmonary embolism, and DVT with the use of tamoxifen. The risk of a thromboembolic event is believed to be about the same as for oral contraceptives.

Contraindications/Precautions: Contraindications to the use of tamoxifen include anticoagulant therapy, preexisting endometrial hyperplasia, history of thromboembolic disease, pregnancy, and lactation. Precautions should be observed in patients with leukopenia, thrombocytopenia, visual disturbances, cataracts, bone marrow suppression, hypercalcemia, and hypercholesterolemia.

Drug Interactions: Tamoxifen is extensively metabolized by hepatic CYP enzymes and may interact with inducers or inhibitors of these enzymes. Use with warfarin increases the risks of bleeding. Cytotoxic antineoplastics may increase the risk of thromboembolism. Bromocriptine may increase tamoxifen levels, whereas aminoglutethimide, medroxyprogesterone, or rifamycin may decrease tamoxifen levels. Selective serotonin reuptake inhibitors (SSRIs) may decrease the effectiveness of tamoxifen. This drug should not be used concurrently with oral contraceptives. **Herbal/Food:** Black cohosh should not be taken unless approved by the healthcare provider.

Pregnancy: Tamoxifen causes fetal harm in laboratory animals and limited data confirms this effect in humans. Because it inhibits lactation and has the potential to cause serious adverse effects, breastfeeding is not recommended. Women of childbearing potential should be advised to use barrier contraception during therapy and for 3 months after the last dose.

Treatment of Overdose: Seizures, neurotoxicity, and QT-interval changes may occur with overdose. The patient is treated symptomatically.

Clinician Responsibilities: Key clinical implications for patients receiving tamoxifen are included in Applied Clinical Judgment: Patients Receiving Cancer Chemotherapy.

Drugs Similar to Tamoxifen

The drugs in this broad category of antineoplastics are divided into SERMs, aromatase inhibitors, gonadotropin-releasing hormone analogs, and androgen receptor blockers. Dexamethasone, diethylstilbestrol, medroxyprogesterone, prednisone, and testosterone are hormones used for nonneoplastic indications. Information on these drugs may be found in other chapters of this text. Abarelix (Plenaxis) is a hormone antagonist that has been discontinued in the United States.

Selective estrogen receptor modifiers: Because all the SERMs show fetal harm in laboratory animals, these drugs are not recommended during pregnancy and lactation. Raloxifene, fulvestrant, and toremifene are only indicated for use in postmenopausal women.

Fulvestrant (Faslodex): Approved in 2002, fulvestrant selectively binds to the ERs of breast cancer cells and inhibits cell division. It is used to treat metastatic breast cancer in ER-positive, postmenopausal women with disease progression following antiestrogen therapy. Fulvestrant is a pure estrogen antagonist and, unlike tamoxifen, it has no estrogen agonist activity. Administered by IM injection once a month, it appears to be as effective as the aromatase inhibitors. It is well tolerated, with the most common adverse effects being nausea and vomiting, constipation, diarrhea, headache, abdominal pain, hot flashes, back pain, and pharyngitis. Temporary injection-site pain and inflammation are possible.

Raloxifene (Evista): Raloxifene is an oral SERM that has antagonist effects on the ERs in the breast. It activates ERs in bone, which decreases bone resorption and increases bone mineral density. Unlike tamoxifen, it does not have agonist actions on the ERs in the uterus. Originally approved in 1997 for osteoporosis, its indications were expanded to include prophylaxis of breast cancer in postmenopausal women who are at high risk for developing the disease. It is used off-label to treat uterine leiomyomata in postmenopausal women. Raloxifene is associated with an increased risk of thromboembolic disorders such as DVT, pulmonary embolism, and retinal thrombosis. Hot flashes and leg cramps are common adverse effects. A prototype feature for raloxifene is presented in Chapter 72.

Toremifene (Fareston): Approved in 1997, toremifene is a PO medication closely related to tamoxifen that exerts antiestrogenic effects at ERs in the breast. Toremifene is indicated for the treatment of metastatic breast cancer in postmenopausal women with ER-positive or unknown tumors. Common adverse effects include hot flashes, vaginal discharge, diaphoresis, and fluid retention. Serious adverse effects are uncommon but may include stroke, angina, and increased intraocular pressure. Toremifene carries a black box warning that the drug prolongs the QT interval, resulting in dysrhythmias. It should not be given to patients with preexisting QT prolongation or uncorrected hypokalemia or hypomagnesemia.

Aromatase inhibitors: Because all the aromatase inhibitors show fetal harm in laboratory animals, these drugs are not recommended during pregnancy or lactation. Use of anastrozole, exemestane, and letrozole is contraindicated in premenopausal women.

Anastrozole (Arimidex): Anastrozole is an oral hormone antagonist highly specific for the aromatase enzyme. Anastrozole restricts tumor growth by inhibiting the biosynthesis of estrogens, thus depriving the tumor of necessary estrogen. First approved in 1995 for the treatment of advanced breast cancer, indications were expanded to include the adjuvant treatment of early breast cancer in postmenopausal women with ER-positive disease. An off-label indication of anastrozole is for the treatment of uterine leiomyomata. Serious adverse effects are uncommon during anastrozole therapy. The most common adverse effects are hot flashes, asthenia, arthritis, pharyngitis, bone pain, nausea and vomiting, and depression. Osteoporosis during therapy may lead to an increased incidence of spinal fractures. Women with preexisting ischemic heart disease have an increased incidence of ischemic cardiovascular events. As an antiestrogen, anastrozole will block the effects of estrogen-containing medications.

Exemestane (Aromasin): Exemestane is an oral aromatase inhibitor that reduces serum estradiol concentrations by binding irreversibly to the aromatase enzyme. Exemestane has greater antiestrogen actions than tamoxifen or anastrozole and is effective when tumors develop resistance to other drugs in this class. First approved in 1999 for the treatment of advanced breast cancer, indications now include the adjuvant treatment of early breast cancer in postmenopausal women with ER-positive disease. Adverse effects are the same as those of other aromatase inhibitors and include hot flashes, nausea and vomiting, arthralgia, and fatigue. Bone mineral density often decreases during exemestane use. An increase in ischemic heart disease has been reported during therapy.

Letrozole (Femara): Letrozole is an oral aromatase inhibitor that reduces serum estrogen levels. First approved in 1997, its indications include the adjuvant treatment of early breast cancer in patients who have received 5 years of adjuvant tamoxifen therapy; first-line treatment of patients with ER-positive or unknown, locally advanced, or metastatic cancer; advanced breast cancer with disease progression following antiestrogen therapy; and the adjuvant treatment of patients with hormone receptor–positive early breast cancer. Off-label indications include the treatment of infertility in anovulatory women who wish to become pregnant and to increase the height of boys with idiopathic short stature or delayed puberty. This drug is generally well tolerated, with the most common adverse effects being nausea and vomiting, asthenia, fatigue, headache, and bone and other musculoskeletal pain. Like other drugs in this class, bone mineral density decreases during therapy.

Gonadotropin-releasing hormone analogs and related drugs: Because all the GnRH analogs show fetal harm in laboratory animals, these drugs are not recommended during pregnancy or lactation. Degarelix, histrelin (Vantas), leuprolide, and triptorelin (Triptodur) are only indicated for use in men.

Degarelix (Firmagon): Approved in 2008, degarelix acts by a different mechanism than other drugs in this class. Rather than being an analog of GnRH, it is an antagonist, blocking the receptors for GnRH in the pituitary. Although its mechanism differs, the pharmacologic indications, actions, and adverse effects are similar to those of the GnRH agonists. It is given by the IM route for the treatment of patients with advanced prostate cancer. The most common adverse effects are pain and swelling at the injection site, hot flashes, increased weight, and increases in serum levels of transaminases and gamma-glutamyltransferase. Long-term use can prolong the QT interval. Another GnRH antagonist, relugolix (Orgovyx) was approved in 2020. This drug has the same indications and adverse effects as degarelix, except it is given by the PO route.

Goserelin (Zoladex): Approved in 1989, goserelin is a GnRH analog that is administered as a depot implant into the abdominal wall every 28 days. By inhibiting pituitary GnRH secretion, goserelin reduces testosterone levels in men to castration levels and lowers estrogen levels in women to postmenopausal levels. In men, the drug is approved for the treatment of early prostate cancer in combination with flutamide and radiotherapy and for the palliative management of advanced prostate cancer. In women, indications for goserelin include endometriosis and the palliative treatment of advanced breast cancer in pre- and postmenopausal women. It may be used off-label to treat uterine leiomyomata or benign prostatic hyperplasia. Hot flashes occur in most patients. Men experience sexual dysfunction and gynecomastia, whereas women experience amenorrhea, decreased libido, and breast atrophy. Bone pain and irritation at the injection site are common. Tumor flare phenomenon may occur, which includes a transient worsening of tumor symptoms during the first few weeks of treatment. Men have an increased risk of sudden cardiac death when using GnRH analogs.

Histrelin (Supprelin LA, Vantas): Approved in 2004, histrelin is a GnRH analog that is given subcutaneously as an implant, usually in the inner aspect of the upper arm. This drug is slowly released over a period of 12 months, at which time the implant is removed. Histrelin (Vantas) is approved for the palliation of advanced prostate cancer. Hot flashes occur in the majority of patients and inflammation may occur at the site of implantation. Men may experience impotence, gynecomastia, and testicular atrophy. Tumor flare phenomenon may occur during the first few weeks of treatment. Men have an increased risk of sudden cardiac death when using GnRH analogs.

Histrelin (Supprelin LA) uses the same implant technology to treat central precocious puberty in children. This condition is defined by the premature development of pubertal body characteristics earlier than age 8 in boys or age 9 in girls. Children with this disorder may have reduced adult height and psychosocial problems. Supprelin LA reduces estradiol levels (in girls) and testosterone levels (in boys) and stabilizes the condition. The most common adverse effect in is implant-site soreness and pain. Supprelin LA is contraindicated in females who are, or may become, pregnant while receiving the drug.

Leuprolide (Eligard, Lupron): The GnRH analog leuprolide is an effective androgen antagonist for treating hormone-dependent tumors. It reduces testosterone levels in men to castration levels and lowers estrogen levels in women to postmenopausal levels. It is used as a palliative treatment for advanced prostate cancer as an alternative to orchiectomy or estrogen therapy. It may be used off-label to induce ovarian ablation in premenopausal women with ER-positive breast cancer. Off-label nonneoplastic indications include the treatment of endometriosis, uterine leiomyomata (fibroids), and central precocious puberty. It is occasionally used to treat female infertility by hyperstimulating the ovary (see Chapter 70). Eligard is a subcutaneous implant for prostate cancer that releases the drug over a period of 1 to 12 months, depending on the formulation. Lupron Depot is an IM formulation that releases the drug over 1 to 6 months, depending on the dose. Leuprolide causes nausea, vomiting, hot flashes, and diaphoresis in both men and women. Women develop amenorrhea and men experience testicular atrophy due to reduced testosterone levels. CNS effects such as migraines, depression, insomnia, asthenia, and dizziness may occur. Injection-site reactions are frequent.

Triptorelin (Trelstar, Triptodur): Triptorelin (Trelstar) is a GnRH analog that was approved in 2000 for the palliative management of advanced prostate cancer. This drug is administered once monthly by the IM route, and most patients achieve castration levels of androgens in less than a month. Off-label uses include advanced breast cancer, uterine leiomyomata, and precocious puberty. Adverse effects are similar to those of other GnRH analogs.

Like histrelin (Supprelin LA), triptorelin (Triptodur) is approved to treat central precocious puberty in children age 2 years and older. It is given as an intramuscular suspension every 24 weeks. This drug reduces estradiol levels (in girls) and testosterone levels (in boys) and stabilizes the condition. The most common adverse effect in these children is implant-site soreness and pain. Children may experience an initial rise in gonadotropins that may worsen signs of puberty during the first 2 to 4 weeks of therapy. Triptodur is contraindicated in females who are, or may become, pregnant while receiving the drug.

Androgen blockers: Because androgen blockers cause fetal harm in laboratory animals, these drugs are not recommended during pregnancy or lactation. All drugs in this class are indicated only for use in men, however, they may be used off-label in women. All are given by the PO route. The primary side effect of all antiandrogens is feminization due to the loss of testosterone. This includes gynecomastia, decreased muscle mass, infertility, and sexual dysfunction.

Abiraterone (Yonsa, Zytiga): Abiraterone, approved in 2011, is indicated for the treatment of castration-resistant prostate cancer in patients. Either prednisone or methylprednisolone is given concurrently with abiraterone. Abiraterone is the only antiandrogen that lowers testosterone levels by inhibiting enzymes required for the biosynthesis of androgens. Abiraterone must be taken on an empty stomach because the presence of food results in increased risk of toxicity. Common adverse effects for abiraterone include joint swelling, peripheral edema, hypokalemia, HTN, and urinary tract infection.

Apalutamide (Erleada): Approved in 2018, apalutamide is approved to treat nonmetastatic, castration-resistant prostate cancer. Common adverse effects are fatigue, HTN, diarrhea, nausea, hot flashes, and weight loss. Fractures related to falls have occurred with this drug; thus, bone density should be periodically monitored. A small number of patients experience seizures. Patients should take a GnRH analog concurrently or have had a bilateral orchiectomy.

Bicalutamide (Casodex), Flutamide (Eulexin), and Nilutamide (Nilandron): These three antiandrogen agents are all closely related in structure and function. They are older drugs indicated for metastatic prostate cancer. Bicalutamide and flutamide are used in combination with a GnRH analog such as goserelin or leuprolide. Nilutamide is given following an orchiectomy. Adverse effects are mild to moderate and are those expected of blocking androgen secretion such as hot flashes, mastalgia, impotence, decreased libido, and gynecomastia. Flutamide carries a black box warning regarding the potential for serious hepatotoxicity. A black box warning for nilutamide states that 2% of patients receiving the drug develop pulmonary fibrosis. Patients taking bicalutamide should have periodic liver function tests because it may cause hepatic injury.

Darolutamide (Nubeqa): One of the newest antiandrogens, darolutamide was approved in 2019 to treat nonmetastatic, castration-resistant prostate cancer. Common side effects include fatigue, extremity pain, and rash. Patients should take a GnRH analog concurrently or have had a bilateral orchiectomy.

Enzalutamide (Xtandi): Enzalutamide was approved in 2012 for metastatic castration-resistant prostate cancer in men who have recently received docetaxel. Common adverse effects are fatigue, back pain, diarrhea, arthralgia, hot flashes, peripheral edema, headache, respiratory infection, dizziness, and insomnia. A small number of patients experience seizures.

Natural Products

57.6 Natural products that are derived from plants include the vinca alkaloids, taxanes, and topoisomerase inhibitors.

Agents with antineoplastic activity have been isolated from several plants, including the common periwinkle (*Vinca rosea*), Pacific yew (*Taxus baccata*), mandrake (May apple), and the shrub *Camptotheca acuminata*. Although structurally very different, medications in this class have the common ability to arrest cell division; thus, some of them are called mitotic inhibitors. The natural products, are listed in Table 57.5. The three primary subdivisions of this group of antineoplastics are:

- Vinca alkaloids
- Taxanes
- Topoisomerase inhibitors.

Vinca alkaloids: The vinca alkaloids vincristine (Marqibo) and vinblastine are older drugs derived from the periwinkle plant. The medicinal properties of this plant were described in folklore in several regions of the world long before their antineoplastic properties were discovered. Despite being derived from the same plant, vincristine, vinblastine, and the semisynthetic vinorelbine exhibit different effects and toxicity profiles.

Table 57.5 Natural Products Used as Antineoplastic Therapy

Drug	Route and Adult Dose (Maximum Dose Where Indicated)	Adverse Effects
Vinca Alkaloids		*Nausea and vomiting, stomatitis, anorexia, rash, alopecia, fatigue* Myelosuppression, severe nausea, vomiting, diarrhea, mucositis, pulmonary or cardiac toxicity, nephrotoxicity (vincristine), neurotoxicity (docetaxel, vincristine), anaphylaxis and other hypersensitivity reactions, severe fluid retention (docetaxel), severe diarrhea with electrolyte imbalances (topoisomerase inhibitors), hemorrhage (omacetaxine), interstitial pneumonia (cabazitaxel), fetal harm
vinblastine	IV: 3.7–18.5 mg/m^2 every 7–10 days	
vincristine (Marqibo)	IV: 1.4 mg/m^2 every wk (max: 2 mg/m^2) IV (Marqibo): 2.25 mg/m^2 once every wk	
vinorelbine	IV: 30 mg/m^2 every wk	
Taxanes		
cabazitaxel (Jevtana)	IV: 25 mg/m^2 q3wk	
docetaxel (Taxotere)	IV: 60–100 mg/m^2 q3wk	
paclitaxel (Abraxane)	IV: 100–260 mg/m^2 q3wk	
Topoisomerase Inhibitors		
etoposide	IV: 35–100 mg/m^2/day for 5 days	
irinotecan (Camptosar)	IV: 125 mg/m^2 once every wk for 4 wk	
topotecan (Hycamtin)	IV: 1.5 mg/m^2/day for 5 days PO: 2.3 mg/m^2/day for 5 days	
Miscellaneous Natural Products		
eribulin (Halaven)	IV: 1.4 mg/m^2 on days 1 and 8 of a 21-day cycle	
omacetaxine (Synribo)	Subcutaneous: 1.25 mg/m^2 for 14 days	

Note: *Italics* indicate common adverse effects. Underline indicates serious adverse effects.

PROTOTYPE DRUG Vincristine (Marqibo)

Classification **Therapeutic:** Antineoplastic
Pharmacologic: Vinca alkaloid, mitotic inhibitor, natural product

Therapeutic Effects and Uses: Vincristine is an antineoplastic obtained from the periwinkle plant that is specific for the M phase of the cell cycle where it inhibits cell division. It is approved to treat acute lymphocytic leukemia, Hodgkin's and non-Hodgkin's lymphomas, lymphosarcoma, malignant glioma, neuroblastoma, rhabdomyosarcoma, soft tissue sarcoma, and Wilms' tumor. It may be used off-label for breast, colorectal, and lung cancers. It is administered only by the IV route. A newer form of vincristine (Marqibo), encased in a liposomal carrier, is approved for acute lymphoblastic leukemia that has failed to respond to at least two other therapies for the disease.

Mechanism of Action: Vincristine binds to tubulin, which is a protein that makes up the microtubules of the cell that are necessary for cell division. This disrupts the process whereby chromosomes are distributed to the daughter cells during mitosis, resulting in cell death. Paclitaxel and colchicine also produce pharmacologic actions by binding to tubulin, but they bind at a different location than vincristine.

Pharmacokinetics:

Route(s)	IV
Absorption	N/A
Distribution	Widely distributed; does not cross the blood–brain barrier; crosses the placenta; unknown if secreted in breast milk
Primary metabolism	Hepatic
Primary excretion	Bile and feces (80%); renal (20%)
Onset of action	15–20 min
Duration of action	Triphasic half-life: 0.85 min, 7.4 min, and 164 min

Adverse Effects: Vincristine is a toxic medication, and even therapeutic doses may result in serious adverse effects. The major dose-limiting toxicity of vincristine is neurotoxicity. This manifests as motor difficulties, peripheral neuropathy, paresthesias (especially of the hands and feet), weakness, cranial nerve palsies (diplopia, hoarseness, deafness, trigeminal neuralgia, vocal cord paralysis), and decreased reflexes. Neurotoxicity may take several months to resolve. CNS effects may include seizures, depression, hallucinations, and coma. GI-related adverse effects include nausea, vomiting, anorexia, stomatitis, severe constipation, and abdominal pain. Other adverse reactions include hepatotoxicity, rash, paralytic ileus (especially in children), and alopecia. **Black Box Warnings:** Myelosuppression may be severe and predispose the patient to opportunistic infections. Extravasation can cause intense pain, inflammation, and tissue necrosis. If extravasation occurs, treatment with warm compresses and hyaluronidase is implemented; cold compresses will significantly increase the toxicity of vinca alkaloids.

Contraindications/Precautions: Contraindications to the use of vincristine include obstructive jaundice, men and women of childbearing age, active infection, adynamic ileus, radiation of the liver, and infants. Cautions must be taken when administering vincristine to patients with leukopenia, preexisting neuromuscular or neurologic disease, HTN, CKD, or hepatic impairment; those who are taking drugs with neurotoxic properties; and older adults. Doses should be reduced in patients with hepatic or biliary disease. Vincristine is a vesicant and caution must be used to avoid exposure of the skin to this drug.

Drug Interactions: Vincristine is a substrate for CYP3A4, and drugs that induce CYP3A4 (such as carbamazepine or phenytoin) may increase the metabolism of vincristine and decrease the effects of the medication. Vincristine will increase the action of methotrexate, bleomycin, and anticoagulants. Decreased digoxin and phenytoin levels will occur. Administration of L-asparaginase just prior to vincristine will cause additive neurotoxicity. Concurrent administration with mitomycin may cause acute dyspnea and severe bronchospasm. Neurotoxicity may occur with peripheral nervous system drugs. **Herbal/Food:** Unknown.

Pregnancy: This drug caused fetal harm in laboratory animals and use during pregnancy and lactation is contraindicated. Contraception use is recommended during therapy.

Treatment of Overdose: Overdose may cause life-threatening symptoms or death. Symptoms are extensions of the adverse effects of vincristine. There is no antidote and patients are treated symptomatically.

Clinician Responsibilities: Key clinical implications for patients receiving vincristine are included in Applied Clinical Judgment: Patients Receiving Cancer Chemotherapy.

Drugs Similar to Vincristine

The two additional vinca alkaloids are vinblastine and vinorelbine. Both drugs can cause fetal harm and use during pregnancy and lactation is contraindicated.

Vinblastine: Vinblastine is obtained from the periwinkle plant and has a chemical structure and mechanism of action very similar to those of vincristine. However, the toxicities and spectrum of actions of the two drugs differ. Vinblastine has traditionally been used to treat Hodgkin's disease and testicular tumors. Off-label uses include treatment of prostate, bladder, and lung cancers and metastatic malignant melanoma. It is administered only by the IV route. Unlike vincristine, neurotoxicity with vinblastine is infrequent. Instead, myelosuppression is the dose-limiting toxicity (especially neutropenia) with a nadir at 4 to 10 days and recovery between days 7 and 21. Extravasation can cause intense pain, inflammation, and tissue necrosis. This drug carries the same black box warnings as vincristine. Nausea and vomiting are generally mild. Other potential adverse effects include HTN, stroke, dyspnea, and Raynaud's phenomenon.

Vinorelbine: Vinorelbine is a semisynthetic drug derived from vinblastine to which it shares structural and functional similarities. In addition to having the same mechanism of action as the vinca alkaloids, vinorelbine also inhibits RNA synthesis and blocks the cellular use of glutamic acid that is needed for purine synthesis. Its only approved use is to treat non-small-cell lung cancer but it may be used off-label to treat metastatic breast cancer, head and neck cancers, ovarian cancer, and Hodgkin's disease. The primary dose-limiting toxicity is myelosuppression (especially neutropenia) with a nadir at 7 to 14 days and recovery between days 14 and 24. Like vinblastine, neurotoxicity is infrequent. Extravasation can cause intense pain, inflammation, and tissue necrosis. This drug carries the same black box warnings as vincristine and vinblastine. Other adverse effects include mild nausea, vomiting, thromboembolic events, asthenia, fatigue, and pulmonary hypersensitivity.

Taxanes: The taxanes, which include cabazitaxel (Jevtana), paclitaxel (Abraxane), and docetaxel (Taxotere), were originally isolated from the bark of the Pacific yew, an evergreen found in forests throughout the western United States. Although the taxanes are mitotic inhibitors like the vinca alkaloids, they act by a different mechanism. Myelosuppression is usually the dose-limiting factor for the taxanes. All taxanes may cause fetal harm and are contraindicated during pregnancy and lactation. Patients should use contraception during therapy and for 6 months following the last dose.

Cabazitaxel (Jevtana): Approved in 2010, cabazitaxel is a mitotic inhibitor indicated for hormone-refractory metastatic prostate cancer that has not responded to a docetaxel-containing regimen. Cabazitaxel carries black box warnings regarding severe hypersensitivity reactions and neutropenia. Deaths due to severe neutropenia have been reported and the drug is contraindicated in patients with neutrophil counts of less than 1500 cells/mm^3. To reduce the incidence of severe hypersensitivity reactions, patients are premedicated with dexamethasone, diphenhydramine, and ranitidine at least 30 minutes prior to cabazitaxel administration. Diarrhea may be extreme and requires premedication with antidiarrheals. Nonhematologic adverse effects include fatigue, nausea and vomiting, constipation, asthenia, abdominal pain, hematuria, and peripheral neuropathy.

Docetaxel (Taxotere): Approved in 1996, docetaxel is a semisynthetic taxane that is administered only by the IV route. It disrupts normal microtubule function and is a mitotic inhibitor. Docetaxel is approved to treat solid tumors, including advanced gastric cancer, head and neck cancers, metastatic breast or refractory prostate cancer, and non-small-cell lung cancer that has failed to respond to therapy with platinum antineoplastics. Off-label indications include metastatic malignant melanoma and advanced ovarian cancer. Docetaxel is a toxic drug that carries multiple black box warnings regarding increased mortality in patients with hepatic impairment, myelosuppression, skin toxicity, severe hypersensitivity reactions, and fluid retention. To reduce the incidence and severity of fluid retention and hypersensitivity reactions, patients receiving docetaxel are administered dexamethasone for 3 days prior to chemotherapy. Without premedication, a hypersensitivity reaction occurs in about 20% of patients within minutes of the injection. Severe fluid retention occurs in some patients and may include peripheral or generalized edema, dyspnea, pleural effusion, cardiac tamponade, and ascites. The major dose-limiting toxicity is myelosuppression, especially neutropenia, which occurs in nearly all patients. The nadir occurs at 7 days with recovery at 14 days. This drug is contraindicated in patients with neutrophil counts of less than 1500 cells/mm^3. Skin reactions, primarily erythema, rash, and pruritus on the feet and hands, occur in the majority of patients. Severe skin toxicity occurs in about 5% of patients. Neurologic toxicity such as paresthesias and peripheral neuropathy occur in half the patients taking this drug.

Paclitaxel (Abraxane): Approved in 1992, paclitaxel is a semisynthetic taxane that is administered by the IV route and approved to treat solid tumors, including metastatic breast cancer, ovarian cancer, Kaposi's sarcoma, and non–small-cell lung cancer in combination with cisplatin. Off-label indications include the chemotherapy of bladder, head, and neck cancers. Paclitaxel carries black box warnings regarding severe hypersensitivity reactions and low neutrophil counts. The major dose-limiting toxicity is myelosuppression, which occurs in nearly all patients. The nadir occurs at 11 days. This drug is contraindicated in patients with neutrophil counts of less than 1500 cells/mm^3. Anaphylaxis and severe hypersensitivity reaction may occur, usually within an hour after the start of the infusion. To reduce the incidence of severe hypersensitivity reactions, patients are premedicated with dexamethasone and diphenhydramine prior to paclitaxel administration. A protein-bound form of this drug (Abraxane) approved in 2013 does not require premedication. Abraxane is approved to treat late-stage pancreatic cancer (in combination with gemcitabine), non-small-cell lung cancer (in combination with carboplatin), and metastatic breast cancer. Extravasation of paclitaxel can result in an acute and delayed injection-site reaction. A local hyaluronidase injection may be beneficial in treating severe extravasation symptoms. Other common adverse events include musculoskeletal pain, asthenia, hypotension, rash, peripheral neuropathy, mild to moderate nausea, vomiting, diarrhea, and stomatitis. Alopecia occurs in nearly every patient.

Topoisomerase inhibitors: DNA exists in a double-stranded supercoiled state. The two strands must be separated if the macromolecule is to replicate or serve as a template for RNA synthesis (see Chapter 56). Topoisomerase is an enzyme that cuts the DNA strand, thus changing it to a more relaxed structure that can be used for DNA and RNA synthesis. The topoisomerase enzyme exists in two closely related forms: Topoisomerase I causes breaks in one strand of the DNA molecule, and topoisomerase II causes breaks in both DNA strands.

Topoisomerase inhibitor medications bind to the enzyme, preventing it from causing the strand breaks necessary for DNA to perform its functions. The cancer cell is unable to properly uncoil its DNA, and DNA replication prematurely terminates. Topoisomerase inhibitors are natural products, and they are available for IV administration only.

Native Americans described uses of the May apple or wild mandrake (*Podophyllum peltatum*) long before pharmacologists isolated podophyllotoxin, which is the primary active ingredient in the plant. As a botanical, podophyllum has been used as an antidote for snakebites, as a cathartic, and as a topical treatment for warts. Etoposide is a semisynthetic product of podophyllotoxin that inhibits topoisomerase II.

The topoisomerase I inhibitors include topotecan (Hycamtin) and irinotecan. These drugs are sometimes called camptothecins because they were first isolated from *Camptotheca acuminata*, a tree native to China. The camptothecins are administered IV, and their indications are limited. As with many other cytotoxic natural products, myelosuppression is the dose-limiting toxicity for the camptothecins.

All topoisomerase inhibitors may cause fetal harm and are contraindicated during pregnancy and lactation. Patients should use contraception during therapy and for 3 to 6 months following the last dose.

Etoposide: Approved in 1983, etoposide is one of the few antineoplastic natural products that is administered by both PO and IV routes. It is approved for patients with small-cell lung cancer and for testicular tumors in patients who have already received surgery, chemotherapy, and radiation without success. Off-label indications may include acute leukemia, Hodgkin's and non-Hodgkin's lymphoma, refractory ovarian cancer, gastric cancer, neuroblastoma, and malignant glioma. Etoposide carries a black box warning for severe, dose-limiting myelosuppression that has a nadir at day 16 and recovery by days 20 through 22. Alopecia occurs in a majority of patients. Anaphylaxis has been reported in up to 2% of patients who are receiving this drug. Secondary malignancies, especially acute nonlymphocytic leukemia, may occur in children who are treated with this drug.

Irinotecan: Approved in 1996, irinotecan is a cytotoxic alkaloid obtained from *Camptotheca acuminata* that acts by inhibiting topoisomerase I. Irinotecan is indicated for the treatment of metastatic colorectal cancer that has progressed despite treatment with fluorouracil. Off-label uses include advanced breast, cervical, ovarian, gastric, and lung cancers. Hematologic toxicity is dose limiting, with anemia, leukopenia, and neutropenia occurring in most patients. Irinotecan carries a black box warning about diarrhea, which can be severe and dose limiting. Early diarrhea occurs during or immediately after the infusion and may be accompanied by cholinergic symptoms such as rhinitis, increased salivation, miosis, lacrimation, diaphoresis, and abdominal cramping. Late diarrhea occurs more than 24 hours after the infusion and may be life-threatening due to prolonged dehydration and electrolyte imbalances. Nausea and vomiting are common and severe enough to require pretreatment with antiemetics. Other adverse events that occur at a high rate include asthenia, fever, dyspnea, abdominal pain, anorexia, and dizziness. Onivyde is a liposomal form of irinotecan approved to treat advanced pancreatic cancer in combination with fluorouracil and leucovorin.

Topotecan (Hycamtin): Approved in 1996, this drug is a topoisomerase I inhibitor very similar to irinotecan, although its indications are different. Topotecan is approved to treat small-cell lung cancer after failure of traditional chemotherapy and inoperable cervical cancer. It may be used off-label to treat rhabdomyosarcoma in children. Topotecan carries a black box warning regarding myelosuppression, which is a dose-limiting toxicity. The drug is contraindicated in patients with neutrophil counts of less than 1500 cells/mm^3. Nausea and vomiting are usually mild. Topotecan can cause infertility in both males and females. Other common adverse events include alopecia, fatigue, asthenia, fever, musculoskeletal pain, dyspnea, interstitial lung disease, and headache.

CONNECTIONS: APPLIED CLINICAL JUDGMENT

Patients Receiving Cancer Chemotherapy

Key Assessment Data

- History of current condition; baseline height, weight, and vital signs; physical exam findings; immunizations; respiratory, neurologic, hepatic, or renal disease; signs and symptoms of current infections and for history of herpes zoster or chickenpox; immunization history, especially recent vaccinations with live vaccines, particularly varicella; pregnancy or breastfeeding. Obtain a drug history, including over-the-counter drugs and alcohol use.
- Assess level of fatigue and presence of nausea or pain. Assess DTRs.
- Ongoing assessment during drug therapy should include monitoring appropriate laboratory findings (e.g., complete blood count [CBC], absolute neutrophil count [ANC; WBC count multiplied by total percentage of neutrophils, segmented plus banded], platelet count, urinalysis, hepatic and renal function studies, uric acid, electrolytes, glucose), diagnostic tests specific to type of antineoplastic therapy regimen planned (e.g., audiology or cardiac testing, electrocardiogram [ECG], electromyography).

Desired Therapeutic Outcomes

Improvement is observed and measurable by evidence of diminished tumor mass, decreased production of abnormal cell growth with absence of signs and symptoms of infection, maintenance of appetite, food and fluid intake, nausea and vomiting are decreased or absent, able to perform acceptable levels of activities of daily living, absence of signs and symptoms of concurrent infections.

Minimizing Adverse Effects

- Increasing fever, even low-grade temperatures less than 38.3°C [101°F], may be a sign of infection. Significant myelosuppression may allow infections to occur and disseminate rapidly and patients are at high risk for infection. Prophylactic therapy with antifungal and antibacterial mouth rinses or protective isolation may be required depending on the level of neutropenia.
- Nausea and vomiting are common adverse effects and usually require antiemetic therapy to manage. Dietary consultation may be required to maintain optimal nutrition.
- Pain may result from advanced disease or adverse drug effects. In advanced disease, pain medication is not withheld. Assess possible drug-related causes for pain and treat the cause when possible.
- Fatigue related to anemia and adverse drug effects is common, especially around the nadir and immediately after. Fatigue may continue after cell counts return to normal and may persist for several years after chemotherapy.
- Alkylating agents such as cyclophosphamide and natural product antineoplastics such as vincristine have neurologic adverse effects. Monitor DTRs, neurologic status, and level of consciousness.
- Alkylating agents such as cyclophosphamide, antitumor antibodies such as doxorubicin, natural product antineoplastics such as vincristine, and hormone and hormone antagonists such as tamoxifen have cardiovascular adverse effects such as pericarditis and effects on the cardiac conduction system. Monitor cardiovascular status including ECG, heart and breath sounds, presence of edema, angina, or chest wall pain.
- Alkylating agents such as cyclophosphamide, antimetabolites such as methotrexate, antitumor antibodies such as doxorubicin, natural product antineoplastics such as vincristine, and biologic response modifiers such as IFN alpha-2 have respiratory adverse effects such as interstitial pneumonitis. Monitor respiratory status including breath sounds and pulmonary function tests.
- Antineoplastic drugs may cause significant hepatotoxicity and nephrotoxicity. Alkylating agents such as cyclophosphamide may cause hemorrhagic cystitis. Monitor hepatic and renal status and for urinary tract dysfunction, including hepatic and renal function tests, urinalysis, and signs and symptoms such as jaundice, decreased urine output, or hematuria.
- Periodic audiology testing may be ordered. Alkylating agents such as cyclophosphamide and antimetabolites such as methotrexate may cause ototoxicity, affecting hearing or balance, or both.
- Hormone and hormone antagonists such as tamoxifen may cause ocular toxicity. Periodic ophthalmology examinations may be required.
- Alkylating agents such as cyclophosphamide may cause significant skin reactions including SJS.
- Antineoplastic drugs may cause significant mucositis related to the effects of rapidly dividing GI endothelial cells.
- Antineoplastic drugs may cause significant hypersensitivity and allergic responses, including anaphylaxis. Because reactions may not always be predictable, caution and frequent monitoring are essential to ensure prompt treatment.

Lifespan Considerations

- Be particularly cautious with older adults who are at increased risk for falls due to neurologic effects of drug therapy or from fatigue and weakness.
- Monitor infants and children for growth or developmental delays.
- Age-related physiologic changes increase the risk of hepatotoxicity and nephrotoxicity in the older adult.

Diversity Considerations

- Because some antineoplastics (e.g., tamoxifen, vincristine) are metabolized through the CYP450 system, monitor ethnically diverse patients frequently to ensure optimal therapeutic effects and minimize adverse effects.

Patient Education

- Take a temperature every 4 hours if behavior or symptoms indicate the need (e.g., increased body warmth, general malaise, lethargy). Report three temperatures taken every 4 hours over 38.1°C (100.5°F) or any single temperature over 38.3°C (101°F) or as directed by the oncology team.
- Antipyretics are not to be used unless explicitly approved by the oncology provider. Antipyretics may mask the symptoms of an infection, allowing rapid dissemination.
- Alert outpatient laboratory personnel of chemotherapy use.
- Take antiemetic therapy routinely during administration of drugs with high and moderate emetic potential. Notify the oncology team if nausea continues.
- Rinse the mouth with plain water, especially after eating, applying lip balm, and avoid alcohol-based mouthwash, which can be drying to the mucosa. Use prescription antifungal and antibiotic rinses as directed.
- Increase fluid intake, up to 2 L/day, taken in small amounts throughout the day. Eliminate alcohol use.
- If pain is present, discuss pain control measures with the oncology team. In end-stage therapy, pain relief is the goal.
- For home chemotherapy, consult the oncology team or local pharmacies if the drug is no longer needed or if additional dosing remains; many will accept unused drugs for proper disposal. Chemotherapy drugs should *never* be flushed down the toilet, poured in a drain, or thrown away in the trash.

Prescribing Considerations

- Myelosuppression and resulting blood dyscrasias are expected adverse effects and will be monitored by ANC, CBC, and platelet counts. Continued therapy will be based on the nadir and may be altered or withheld until blood counts are within acceptable limits.
- All chemotherapy and targeted therapy should be prescribed on the basis of a documented, referenced protocol and a treatment plan documented for all patients. Protocols should outline all therapy, dosages and scheduling relevant to the treatment.
- Prescribers should avoid the use of handwritten prescriptions (drugs *and* doses) and the use of pre-printed or computer-generated orders is preferable.

Biologic Response Modifiers and Targeted Therapies

57.7 Biologic response modifiers and targeted therapies enhance the body's ability to kill tumor cells.

Other than the hormones described in Section 57.5, most antineoplastics are cytotoxic and will kill rapidly growing cells indiscriminately, regardless of the type of cell or tissue. Biologic response modifiers and targeted therapies are an attempt to more selectively treat cancers without producing widespread, serious adverse effects throughout the body.

Biological response modifiers: In the context of pharmacology, a biologic response modifier (BRM) is a drug that modifies the body's immune defenses to treat a disease. In some cases, a BRM may be used to *suppress* an overactive immune response, such as the case in autoimmune diseases or prevention of transplant rejection. In chemotherapy, BRMs are given to *enhance* body defenses to more effectively remove cancer cells. Biologic response modifiers may produce their effects directly, by binding to cancer cells and destroying them, or indirectly, by activating general aspects of the immune response. The most frequently used cytokines that act as BRMs include the following:

- Interferons are natural proteins produced by T cells in response to viral infection and other antigens. They bind to specific receptors on cancer cell membranes and suppress cell division, enhance the phagocytic activity of macrophages, and promote the cytotoxic activity of T lymphocytes. PegIFN alfa-2a (Pegasys, Sylatron) and IFN alfa-2b (Intron A) are approved to treat hairy cell leukemia, chronic myelogenous leukemia, Kaposi's sarcoma, and melanoma with nodal involvement. Doses of the interferons and a prototype feature for IFN alfa-2b are provided in Chapter 42.
- Interleukin-2 activates cytotoxic T lymphocytes and promotes other actions of the immune response. Marketed as aldesleukin (Proleukin), this drug is indicated for metastatic renal cell carcinoma and malignant melanoma. A prototype feature for aldesleukin is provided in Chapter 42.

Targeted therapies: Although cancer cells originate from normal cells, researchers have identified a significant number of differences between the two. These differences are due to genetic changes or mutations that have allowed the cancer cell to rapidly divide, evade body defenses, invade normal tissues, and perhaps travel to distant sites. Scientists have been successful at identifying many of these mutations.

Targeted therapies are drugs that block specific gene products involved in the growth, progression, and survival of cancer cells. The targeted therapy may block signals telling the cancer cell to divide, program the cancer cell to undergo apoptosis (cell death), or directly destroy cancer cells. Targeted therapies differ from standard chemotherapy in that they attack *one specific aspect* of the cancer cell. Indeed, these drugs have been deliberately engineered to interact with their molecular target. Traditional chemotherapy drugs are designed to be cytotoxic, usually killing rapidly dividing cells of all types. A primary goal of targeted therapy is to attack cancer cells with greater precision, theoretically causing fewer side effects.

For a targeted therapy to be effective, the tumor cells must have the specific genetic mutation (target) and that mutation must be responsible for causing the characteristics of the cancer (e.g., growth, invasion, metastasis). Genetic testing is performed to determine if the patient's cancer contains the specific mutation for the targeted therapy. For example, about half of melanomas contain a gene known as a *BRAF* mutation. Targeted therapies such as dabrafenib are most effective in tumors that contain the *BRAF* mutation.

Targeted therapies are classified as monoclonal antibodies (MABs) or as small molecules. Monoclonal antibodies are large molecules that attack antigens present on the *surface* of the cancer cell. They are too large to cross the plasma membrane and are usually given IV. Table 57.6 lists selected MABs approved for oncology indications. Pharmacotherapy 57.1 illustrates the mechanisms of monoclonal antibodies. **Small-molecule therapies** can cross the plasma membrane and inhibit processes *inside* the cancer cell, as well as extracellular targets. Some can be given by the oral route, offering greater patient convenience. Table 57.7 lists selected small-molecule therapies approved for oncology indications

New targeted therapies are being developed at a very rapid pace, with several dozen approved each year. Examples of targeted therapies include the following:

- Tyrosine kinase (TK) is an enzyme that activates certain proteins in internal signaling pathways that regulate cell growth. In normal cells, the TK enzyme is turned on and off, depending on the cell's need for growth. Certain types of cancer cells turn on the TK enzyme permanently, leading to uncontrolled cell growth. Imatinib (Gleevec), dasatinib (Sprycel), alectinib (Alecensa), and crizotinib (Xalkori) are examples of drugs that are able to inhibit TKs, thus stopping this unchecked cell growth. Everolimus (Afinitor, Zortress) inhibits a different type of kinase and is approved as an antineoplastic drug as well as for the prophylaxis of transplant rejection (see Chapter 42). Vemurafenib (Zelboraf), midostaurin (Rydapt), and cobimetinib (Cotellic) are designed to specifically inhibit multiple types of kinases and are indicated for malignant melanoma.
- The epidermal growth factor receptor (EGFR) is a cell-surface receptor that, when activated, results in cell growth. Mutations of the EGFR can result in

Table 57.6 Selected Monoclonal Antibodies in Oncology

Drug	Indication	Drug	Indication
atezolizumab (Tecentriq)	Urothelial cancer, metastatic lung cancer	necitumumab (Portrazza)	Metastatic lung cancer
avelumab (Bavencio)	Merkel cell, urothelial, renal cancers	nivolumab (Opdivo)	Metastatic melanoma, lung cancer, renal cell carcinoma, Hodgkin's lymphoma, others
belantamab-mafodotin (Blenrep)	Multiple myeloma	obinutuzumab (Gazyva)	Chronic lymphocytic leukemia
bevacizumab (Avastin, Mvasi)	Metastatic colorectal cancer	ofatumumab (Arzerra, Kesimpta)	Chronic lymphocytic leukemia
blinatumomab (Blincyto)	Acute lymphoblastic leukemia	panitumumab (Vectibix)	Metastatic colorectal cancer
brentuximab (Adcetris)	Hodgkin's lymphoma, large-cell lymphoma	pembrolizumab (Keytruda)	Advanced melanoma, head and neck cancer, advanced non-small-cell cancer, Hodgkin's lymphoma, advanced urothelial carcinoma, advanced gastric cancer
cemiplimab (Libtayo)	Metastatic squamous cell carcinoma		
cetuximab (Erbitux)	Head and neck cancer, metastatic colorectal cancer		
daratumumab (Darzalex)	Multiple myeloma	pertuzumab (Perjeta)	Metastatic breast cancer
dinutuximab (Unituxin)	Neuroblastoma	polatuzumab (Polivy)	B-cell lymphoma
durvalumab (Infinzi)	Urothelial, lung cancers	ramucirumab (Cyramza)	Advanced gastric cancer, metastatic lung cancer
elotuzumab (Empliciti)	Multiple myeloma	rituximab (Rituxan)	Non-Hodgkin's lymphoma, chronic lymphocytic leukemia
enfortumab-vedotin (Padcev)	Metastatic urothelial cancer		
ibritumomab (Zevalin)	Non-Hodgkin's lymphoma	sacituzumab govitecan (Trodelvy)	Metastatic breast cancer
inotuzumab (Besponsa)	Acute lymphoblastic leukemia	tafasitamab (Monjuvi)	B-cell lymphoma
ipilimumab (Yervoy)	Metastatic melanoma	trastuzumab (Herceptin)	Metastatic breast cancer, metastatic gastric cancer
isatuximab (Sarclisa)	Multiple myeloma		
mogamulizumab (Poteligeo)	Mycosis fungoides	trastuzumab deruxtecan (Enhertu)	Metastatic breast cancer
moxetumomab (Lumoxiti)	Hairy cell leukemia	tucatinib (Tukysa)	Advanced breast cancer

uncontrolled cell growth and cancer. Antineoplastic drugs known as EGFR inhibitors are targeted to shut down this activation and slow the growth of certain neoplasms. Cetuximab (Erbitux), erlotinib (Tarceva), necitumumab (Portrazza), osimertinib (Tagrisso), and trastuzumab (Herceptin) are examples of drugs that target the EGFR.

- Vascular endothelial growth factor (VEGF) is a protein that signals the formation of new blood vessels during embryonic development or following injury or blockage to tissues. VEGF, also called *angiogenesis inhibitors*, prevents the formation of new blood vessels that are vital to the formation of new tumors. These drugs do not kill cancer cells, but they are able to slow tumor growth. Bevacizumab (Avastin, Mvasi) was the first drug to specifically target angiogenesis. An additional VEGF inhibitor, ramucirumab (Cyramza), was approved in 2014 to treat advanced gastric cancer. Thalidomide (Thalomid) and lenalidomide (Revlimid) are miscellaneous drugs, shown in Table 57.8, that possess antiangiogenic properties.
- CD20 is a protein located on the surface of B lymphocytes. While the normal function of CD20 is not completely understood, it is found in high concentrations in certain lymphomas and leukemias. Monoclonal antibody drugs have been developed that target CD20 and kill the cancer cells expressing this protein. Examples of CD20 antibody medications include rituximab (Rituxan), ofatumumab (Arzerra, Kesimpta), and ibritumomab (Zevalin).
- Since 2017, a new type of targeted therapy has received significant attention. Pembrolizumab (Keytruda), larotrectinib (Vitrakvi), and entrectinib (Rozlytrek) are called **tumor agnostic therapies**. Rather than approved for a specific type of cancer, these drugs are approved to treat certain genomic mutations or molecular features regardless of where the tumor is located. For example, pembrolizumab blocks the PD-1 receptor, a protein that allows tumor cells to "hide" from the immune system. The PD-1 receptor is common to many types of cancer cells. Indeed, pembrolizumab is approved to treat 10 very different types of cancers. Although they work by a different mechanism, larotrectinib and entrectinib are approved to treat specific gene mutations, rather than a specific type of cancer.

Miscellaneous Antineoplastics

57.8 Several miscellaneous antineoplastics act by unique mechanisms.

Some antineoplastics are classified as miscellaneous because they are structurally dissimilar to any of the previously discussed groups. Because these medications are unique, their

Pharmacotherapy Illustrated 57.1

Monoclonal Antibodies and Cancer Cells

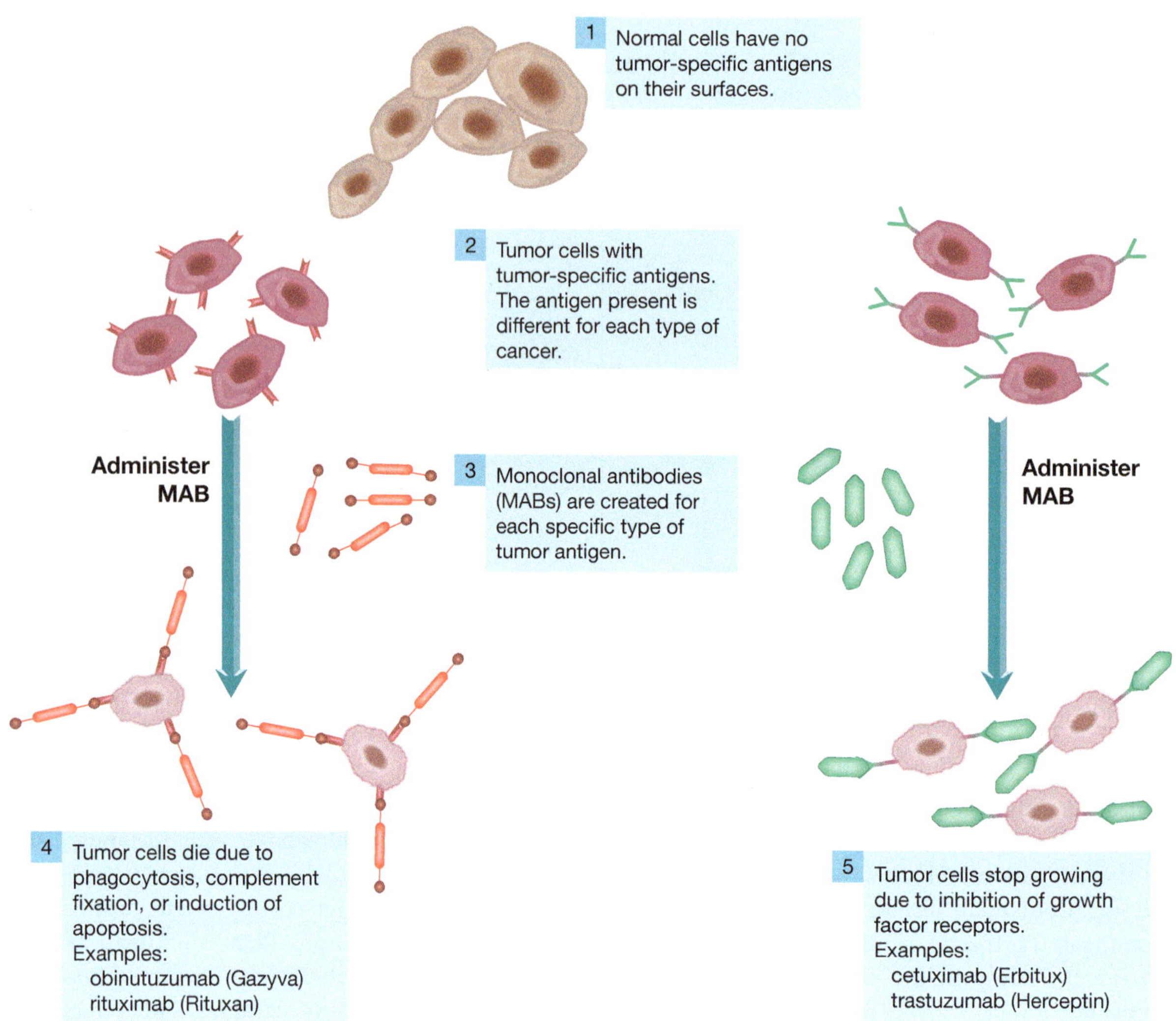

adverse reactions vary. Doses for the miscellaneous antineoplastics are listed in Table 57.8.

Arsenic Trioxide (Trisenox): Approved in 2000, arsenic trioxide is a toxic metal that has only one indication: acute promyelocytic leukemia. Its mechanism of action is incompletely understood but it appears to cause DNA fragmentation that is characteristic of apoptosis, or programmed cell death. It is administered by IV infusion. Leukocytosis, thrombocytopenia, nausea, vomiting, abdominal pain, diarrhea, and constipation are common adverse effects. Neurotoxicity is relatively common and manifests as headache, insomnia, paresthesias, anxiety, dizziness, and tremors. Because arsenic trioxide can cause QT-interval prolongation and complete atrioventricular block, other drugs that prolong the QT interval should be discontinued during therapy. This drug is a human carcinogen and can cause secondary malignancies. Arsenic trioxide can cause fetal harm in humans and use during pregnancy and lactation is contraindicated.

Asparaginase (Erwinaze, Oncaspar): Asparaginase is an enzyme that deprives cancer cells of asparagine, an essential amino acid, causing a marked reduction in protein, RNA, and DNA synthesis. It is approved only to treat acute lymphocytic leukemia in combination with other antineoplastics. It is administered by the IM or IV routes. Pretreatment with corticosteroids reduces the incidence of hypersensitivity reactions which occur in many patients with symptoms ranging from urticaria to anaphylactic shock. Asparaginase may cause fatal pancreatitis. This drug showed embryofetal toxicity in laboratory animals. It is not known if this drug enters milk or if it causes adverse effects in a breastfed neonate.

Table 57.7 Selected Small-Molecule Drugs in Oncology

Drug	Indication	Drug	Indication
abemaciclib (Verzenio)	Metastatic breast cancer	lapatinib (Tykerb)	Advanced or metastatic breast cancer
acalabrutinib (Calquence)	Mantle cell lymphoma	larotrectinib (Vitrakvi)	Solid tumors with *NTRK* gene fusion
alectinib (Alecensa)	Metastatic lung cancer	lenvatinib (Lenvima)	Metastatic thyroid cancer, renal cell carcinoma
alpelisib (Piqray)	Advanced breast cancer	lorlatinib (Lorbrena)	Lung cancer
avapritinib (Ayvakit)	Metastatic GI cancer	lutetium Lu177 (Lutathera)	Neuroendocrine tumors
axicabtagene (Yescarta)	B-cell lymphoma	nilotinib (Tasigna)	Chronic myeloid leukemia
axitinib (Inlyta)	Advanced renal cell carcinoma	niraparib (Zejula)	Ovarian cancer
binimetinib (Mektovi)	Metastatic melanoma, metastatic colon cancer	olaparib (Lynparza)	Ovarian cancer
bortezomib (Velcade)	Multiple myeloma, mantle cell lymphoma	osimertinib (Tagrisso)	Metastatic lung cancer
bosutinib (Bosulif)	Chronic myelogenous leukemia	palbociclib (Ibrance)	Advanced breast cancer
brexucabtagene (Tecartus)	Mantle cell lymphoma	panobinostat (Farydak)	Multiple myeloma
brigatinib (Alunbrig)	Metastatic lung cancer	pazopanib (Votrient)	Advanced renal cell carcinoma, advanced soft tissue sarcoma
cabozantinib (Cabometyx, Cometriq)	Renal cell carcinoma, metastatic thyroid cancer	pemigatinib (Pemazyre)	Cholangiocarcinoma
calaspargase (Asparlas)	Acute lymphoblastic leukemia	pexidartinib (Turalio)	Tenosynovial giant cell tumor
capmatinib (Tabrecta)	Metastatic lung cancer	regorafenib (Stivarga)	Metastatic colorectal cancer, metastatic GI stromal tumor
carfilzomib (Kyprolis)	Multiple myeloma	ribociclib (Kisqali)	Breast cancer
ceritinib (Zykadia)	Lung cancer	ripretinib (Qinlock)	Advanced GI cancer
cobimetinib (Cotellic)	Metastatic melanoma	rucaparib (Rubraca)	Ovarian cancer
copanlisib (Aliqopa)	Lymphoma	selpercatinib (Retevmo)	Lung, thyroid cancer
crizotinib (Xalkori)	Metastatic lung cancer	selumetinib (Koselugo)	Neurofibromatosis
dacomitinib (Vizimpro)	Lung cancer	selinexor (Xpovio)	Multiple myeloma
dasatinib (Sprycel)	Chronic myeloid or acute lymphoblastic leukemia	sonidegib (Odomzo)	Recurrent basal cell cancer
duvelisib (Copiktra)	Lymphocytic leukemia, lymphoma	sorafenib (Nexavar)	Hepatic cancer, advanced renal cell carcinoma, metastatic thyroid cancer
enasidenib (IDHIFA)	Acute myeloid leukemia	sunitinib (Sutent)	GI stromal tumor, advanced renal cell carcinoma, pancreatic cancer
encorafenib (Braftovi)	Metastatic melanoma	tagraxofusp (Elzonris)	Dendritic cell neoplasm
entrectinib (Rozlytrek)	Lung cancer, solid tumors	talazoparib (Talzenna)	Advanced breast cancer
erdafitinib (Balversa)	Advanced urothelial carcinoma	talimogene (Imlygic)	Recurrent melanoma
erlotinib (Tarceva)	Metastatic lung cancer, metastatic pancreatic cancer	tazemetostat (Tazverik)	Sarcoma, lymphoma
fedratinib (Inrebic)	Myelofibrosis	tisagenlecleucel (Kymriah)	Acute lymphoblastic leukemia
gefitinib (Iressa)	Advanced or metastatic lung cancer	tucatinib (Tukysa)	Advanced breast cancer
gilteritinib (Xospata)	Acute myeloid leukemia	vandetanib (Caprelsa)	Thyroid cancer
glasdegib (Daurismo)	Acute myeloid leukemia	vemurafenib (Zelboraf)	Metastatic melanoma
ibrutinib (Imbruvica)	Mantle cell lymphoma, chronic lymphocytic leukemia	venetoclax (Venclexta)	Chronic lymphocytic leukemia
imatinib (Gleevec)	Chronic myeloid leukemia, acute lymphoblastic leukemia, others	vismodegib (Erivedge)	Advanced or metastatic basal cell carcinoma
ivosidenib (Tibsovo)	Acute myeloid leukemia	zanubrutinib (Brukinsa)	Mantle cell lymphoma
ixazomib (Ninlaro)	Multiple myeloma	ziv-aflibercept (Zaltrap)	Metastatic colorectal cancer

Pegaspargase (Oncaspar) is asparaginase with a molecule of PEG bonded to it. Pegylation increases the half-life of the drug and allows for less frequent dosing. Erwinaze is a form of the drug made from chrysanthemums for patients who are allergic to *E. coli* proteins that may be found in vials of Oncaspar. The two drugs share the same adverse effects and indications.

Belinostat (Beleodaq), Romidepsin (Istodax), and Vorinostat (Zolinza): These three drugs induce apoptosis in cancer cells by inhibiting the activity of the enzyme histone deacetylase. They are approved for the treatment of cutaneous or peripheral T-cell lymphoma in patients who have progressive, persistent, or recurrent disease. Fatigue, diarrhea, nausea, anorexia, and blood dyscrasias are common

Table 57.8 Miscellaneous Antineoplastics

Drug	Route and Adult Dose (Maximum Dose Where Indicated)	Adverse Effects
arsenic trioxide (Trisenox)	IV: 0.15 mg/kg/day (max: 60 doses)	*Fever, leukocytosis, nausea, vomiting, diarrhea, abdominal pain, rash, fatigue, edema* Acute promyelocytic differentiation syndrome, QT prolongation, secondary malignancies
asparaginase *E. chrysanthemum* (Erwinaze), pegaspargase (Oncaspar)	IV/IM (Oncaspar): 2500 international units/m^2 IV/IM (Erwinaze): 10,000 international units/m^2	*Hyperglycemia, elevated transaminases, thrombosis, hemorrhage* Hypersensitivity, pancreatitis
belinostat (Beleodaq)	IV: 1000 mg/m^2 on days 1–5 of 21-day cycle	*Nausea, vomiting, fatigue, pyrexia, anemia* Serious infections, hepatotoxicity, tumor lysis syndrome, embryofetal toxicity, thrombocytopenia
bexarotene (Targretin)	PO: 100–400 mg/m^2/day Topical: 1% gel applied to lesion 1–4 times/day	*Hyperlipidemia, leukopenia, rash, headache, asthenia, nausea* Acute pancreatitis, elevated hepatic enzymes, hypothyroidism, embryofetal toxicity
hydroxyurea (Droxia, Hydrea)	PO: 80 mg/kg q3days or 30 mg/kg/day	*Nausea, vomiting, diarrhea, stomatitis, rash* Myelosuppression, secondary malignancies, embryofetal toxicity
ixabepilone (Ixempra)	IV: 40 mg/m^2 infused over 3 h q3wk	*Alopecia, diarrhea, fatigue, musculoskeletal pain, peripheral neuropathy, mucositis, nausea and vomiting* Myelosuppression, hypersensitivity, embryofetal toxicity
lenalidomide (Revlimid)	PO: 25 mg/day	Same as thalidomide
midostaurin (Rydapt)	PO: 50 mg bid	*Febrile neutropenia, nausea, mucositis, musculoskeletal pain* Pulmonary toxicity, embryofetal toxicity
mitotane (Lysodren)	PO: 9–10 g/day in divided doses tid or qid	*Anorexia, nausea, vomiting, diarrhea, rash, lethargy, drowsiness* Adrenal crisis, embryofetal toxicity
pomalidomide (Pomalyst)	PO: 4 mg/day on days 1–21 of repeated 28-day cycles	Same as thalidomide
romidepsin (Istodax)	IV: 14 mg/m^2 on days 1, 8, and 15 of a 28-day cycle	*Nausea, vomiting, fatigue, infections, anorexia* Blood dyscrasias, anemia, QT prolongation
sipuleucel-T (Provenge)	IV: 3 doses at 2-wk intervals; each dose contains 50 million autologous CD54 cells	*Chills, fatigue, fever, back pain, nausea, joint ache* Acute infusion-related reactions
thalidomide (Thalomid)	PO: 200–400 mg/day	*Fatigue, constipation, nausea, diarrhea, dyspnea, respiratory infections, back pain, pyrexia* Neutropenia, venous thromboembolism
vorinostat (Zolinza)	PO: 400 mg once daily	*Diarrhea, nausea, vomiting, anorexia, fatigue, chills, taste disorders* Blood dyscrasias, pulmonary embolism, QT prolongation
zoledronic acid (Zometa)	IV: 4 mg infused over at least 15 min	*Flulike symptoms, bone, muscle pain* Dysrhythmias, electrolyte imbalances, osteonecrosis of jaw, fetal harm

Note: *Italics* indicate common adverse effects. Underline indicates serious adverse effects.

adverse effects. Pulmonary embolism is a rare, though serious, adverse effect of vorinostat. These drugs may cause teratogenicity or embryotoxicity. Breastfeeding is not recommended.

Bexarotene (Targretin): Approved in 1999, bexarotene is a retinoid, a group of drugs related to vitamin A that are usually used for skin conditions such as psoriasis and acne (see Chapter 73). This drug is approved by the PO and topical routes to treat cutaneous T-cell lymphoma that has not responded to other therapies. Off-label indications include lung cancer, Kaposi's sarcoma, metastatic breast cancer, and severe psoriasis. Adverse effects of the oral formulation include hyperlipidemia, hypothyroidism, acute pancreatitis, leukopenia, headache, asthenia, anemia, anorexia, and photosensitivity. Topical bexarotene can cause rash, erythema, and pruritus. This drug may cause birth defects in humans and is contraindicated during pregnancy and lactation. Negative pregnancy tests should be obtained prior to and monthly during therapy.

Hydroxyurea (Droxia, Hydrea): Hydroxyurea is an oral antineoplastic approved in 1967 for chemotherapy of chronic myelogenous leukemia, head and neck cancers, malignant melanoma, and ovarian cancer. It may be used off-label for acute myelogenous leukemia, astrocytoma, lung cancer, and malignant glioma. Sickle cell disease is a nonneoplastic indication for the drug. Hydroxyurea causes myelosuppression, especially neutropenia. This drug carries a black box warning that long-term use may cause secondary leukemias. Nausea, vomiting, stomatitis, and diarrhea are common. Skin ulcers and gangrene have been reported. This drug showed embryofetal toxicity in laboratory animals and is contraindicated during pregnancy or lactation. Hydroxyurea may cause infertility. Contraception should be used in both male and female patients during and after therapy.

Ixabepilone (Ixempra): Approved in 2007, ixabepilone acts by the same mechanism as the taxanes but it has different pharmacokinetic properties. It is used in combination with capecitabine to treat metastatic or advanced breast cancer resistant to treatment with first-line medications such as the taxanes. At least 20% of patients experience alopecia, diarrhea, fatigue, asthenia, musculoskeletal pain, peripheral neuropathy, stomatitis, mucositis, nausea and vomiting. More than 40% of patients experience anemia, neutropenia, and thrombocytopenia. Ixabepilone carries a black box warning that it must not be given to patients with elevated serum aspartate aminotransferase, alanine transaminase, or bilirubin levels due to increased risk of toxicity and neutropenia-related death. Pretreatment with diphenhydramine is required to reduce the risk for hypersensitivity reactions. This drug showed embryofetal toxicity in laboratory animals and is contraindicated during pregnancy and lactation.

Midostaurin (Rydapt): Midostaurin was approved in 2017 for the treatment of acute myeloid leukemia that is *FLT3* mutation positive in combination with cytarabine and daunorubicin. It is also indicated for aggressive systemic mastocytosis, a potentially life-threatening accumulation of mast cells associated with leukemia or sarcoma. Midostaurin acts by inhibiting tyrosine kinases. The most frequent serious adverse reactions are febrile neutropenia and interstitial lung disease. This drug causes embryofetal toxicity in laboratory animals and is contraindicated during pregnancy and lactation. Pregnancy status should be verified before therapy and contraception is recommended during therapy and for 4 months following the last dose.

Mitotane (Lysodren): Mitotane, which is similar to the insecticide DDT, poisons cancer cells by forming links to proteins. Given by the PO route, its only indication is for the chemotherapy of advanced, inoperable adrenocortical cancer. Because the drug is cytotoxic to the adrenal gland, symptoms of acute adrenal insufficiency may emerge. Mitotane carries a black box warning that the drug should be temporarily stopped if shock or severe trauma occurs due to its adrenal suppression effects. Most patients experience adverse GI effects such as nausea, vomiting and diarrhea. CNS effects such as lethargy, drowsiness, and vertigo are observed in up to 40% of patients who are taking the drug. Because limited human data suggests that mitotane causes fetal harm, it is contraindicated during pregnancy and lactation.

Sipuleucel-T (Provenge): Approved in 2010, sipuleucel-T is very different from other antineoplastic medications. Three days prior to sipuleucel-T administration, the patient undergoes leukapheresis during which antigen-presenting cells (APCs) are collected. The APCs are then incubated with granulocyte-macrophage colony-stimulating factor (GM-CSF) and a prostate cancer antigen, which activates the collected cells. The product, consisting of GM-CSF mature and activated APCs, is reinfused into the patient to cause an immune response against prostate cancer cells. The product can be used only for the patient from whom the APCs were collected. Because acute infusion-related effects such as chills and fever have been reported, the patient is usually premedicated with acetaminophen and an antihistamine. The drug is not indicated for women.

Zoledronic Acid (Zometa): Approved in 2001, zoledronic acid is a bisphosphonate, a drug class commonly used to treat osteoporosis. The primary action of the drug is to inhibit bone resorption by osteoclasts. In addition to its use in managing osteoporosis, this drug is approved to treat multiple myeloma in patients with documented bone metastases, severe hypercalcemia caused by malignancy, and prostate cancer that has progressed after hormonal therapy. It is given by IV infusion. Adverse effects include flulike symptoms, nausea, fever, fatigue, headache, anemia, anorexia, severe bone pain or joint pain, and osteonecrosis of the jaw. it should not be used for patients with severe renal impairment. Because this drug is fetotoxic and teratogenic in laboratory animals and has a half-life of months to years, it is contraindicated during pregnancy or lactation.

Understanding Chapter 57

Key Concepts Summary

57.1 Antineoplastic drugs kill or stop the growth of cancer cells and may be classified in multiple ways.

57.2 Alkylating agents change the shape of the DNA double helix and prevent cancer cells from dividing normally.

57.3 Antimetabolites disrupt the critical cellular pathways of cancer cells.

57.4 The antibiotic antineoplastics contain substances obtained from bacteria that have the ability to kill cancer cells.

57.5 Hormones and hormone antagonists block the substances necessary for continued growth of tumors.

57.6 Natural products that are derived from plants include the vinca alkaloids, taxanes, and topoisomerase inhibitors.

57.7 Biologic response modifiers and targeted therapies enhance the body's ability to kill tumor cells.

57.8 Several miscellaneous antineoplastics act by unique mechanisms.

CASE STUDY: Making the Patient Connection

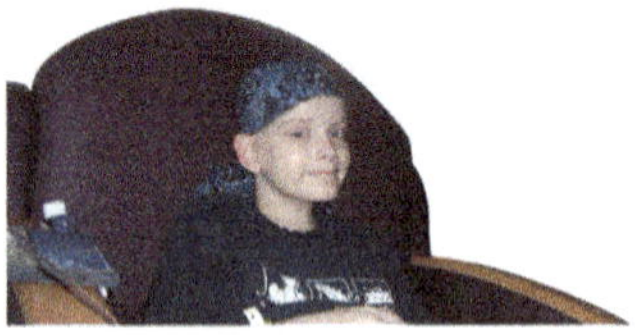

Remember the patient "Zack Amos" at the beginning of the chapter? Now read the remainder of the case study. Based on the information presented within this chapter, respond to the critical thinking questions that follow.

Zack is a 12-year-old boy who had been in good health with no significant medical history until 6 months ago. At that time, he began to experience episodic migraine-like headaches, and with a paternal family history of migraines, Zack was evaluated for possible antimigraine therapy if the headaches continued. After 3 months of increasing severity of the headaches, he was diagnosed by CT scan with a brain tumor. Zack underwent craniotomy for evacuation of a malignant tumor and began chemotherapy 1 month after surgery, prior to planned radiation therapy treatments. He has completed one cycle of chemotherapy over 2 months and will have a second cycle prior to radiation. He visits the oncology clinic today for evaluation prior to his second round of chemotherapy.

Physical examination on this clinic visit reveals a pleasant young boy in no obvious distress. Zack weighs 43.6 kg (96 lb) and is 157.5 cm (62 in.) in height. Blood pressure is 92/40 mmHg, pulse rate is 92 beats/min, respirations of 24 breaths/min, and temperature of 37.1°C (98.8°F). Zack denies having any pain and his neurologic examination is unremarkable except for diminished patellar DTRs, graded at 1 (decreased but present; normal of 2). His WBC count is 3420/mm^3; ANC, 1800; hemoglobin (Hgb), 13 g/dL; hematocrit (Hct), 36.5%; and platelet count, 225,000. CBC is within the range expected post-chemotherapy. Zack will be hospitalized for approximately 2 days for administration of cyclophosphamide (Cytoxan), carboplatin (Paraplatin), and vincristine and will continue to receive doses of vincristine as an outpatient and start etoposide in several weeks. Because he experienced significant nausea and vomiting with the last round of chemotherapy, he will also be given ondansetron (Zofran) regularly with supplemental corticosteroids IV as needed.

Critical Thinking Questions

1. Why are four antineoplastic drugs used for Zack? What is the pharmacologic classification of each of the drugs used?
2. What overlapping toxicities might Zack experience with these drugs? Considering his physical assessment findings from today, what system toxicities would be of most concern?
3. Fifteen days after the start of the second cycle of chemotherapy, Zack experiences his nadir. At this time his WBC count is 340/mm^3; ANC, 98; Hgb, 9.3 g/dL; Hct, 25.7%; and the platelet count is 55,000. Zack has been receiving filgrastim (Neupogen) subcutaneously since discharge and will continue until the WBC count begins to rise. Considering these laboratory values, what would be of most concern to the oncology team? What teaching should Zack and his family receive?

Additional Case Study

Ansen Rosenthal is a 25-year-old man who has recently begun chemotherapy at the local oncology center for treatment of Hodgkin's lymphoma. He has tolerated the chemotherapy fairly well but has experienced mild, daily nausea with occasional vomiting, usually controlled by granisetron (Kytril). His main concern is the fatigue he experiences and the impact it has on his work as a computer science engineer. Ansen also admits that he has been experiencing anorexia and "just doesn't feel like eating much," something that may be contributing to his fatigue. He has lost 2 kg (more than 4 lb) since his last clinic visit 2 weeks ago.

1. If you were Ansen's nurse, how might you manage his chemotherapy-related nausea and anorexia?
2. What suggestions might assist Ansen in managing his fatigue?

Chapter Review

1. The nurse is preparing to administer cyclophosphamide (Cytoxan) and knows that the patient will experience a nadir in approximately 9 to 14 days. Which laboratory value(s) will indicate to the nurse that the patient has reached the nadir?

1. Blood urea nitrogen and creatinine
2. WBC count and absolute neutrophil count
3. Ionized calcium
4. Serum albumin

2. A patient has been receiving vincristine as one of the drugs in a chemotherapy regimen. What important findings will the nurse monitor to prevent or limit the main dose-related toxicity for this patient? (Select all that apply.)

1. Numbness of the hands or feet
2. Angina and dysrhythmias
3. Constipation
4. Diminished reflexes
5. Dyspnea and pleuritis

3. A nurse is caring for a patient who is receiving tamoxifen for treatment of breast cancer. The nurse will teach the patient that postchemotherapy monitoring will be necessary to detect or treat which drug-associated adverse effect?

1. Paralytic ileus
2. Alopecia
3. Pulmonary fibrosis
4. Endometrial cancer

4. A patient with acute lymphoblastic leukemia has started therapy with doxorubicin. The nurse will assist the patient with what important intervention during the course of this treatment?

1. Perform active or assisted range-of-motion (ROM) exercises to maintain strength.
2. Participate in relaxation therapy to control pain.
3. Use daily mouth rinses as prescribed.
4. Maintain bedrest during treatment.

5. The patient will continue to take methotrexate (MTX, Trexall) for treatment of osteosarcoma. When teaching the patient prior to discharge, what over-the-counter drugs must not be taken concurrently with methotrexate?

1. Nonsteroidal anti-inflammatory drug pain relievers
2. Antihistamines
3. Laxatives
4. Cough suppressants

6. A patient receiving carboplatin (Paraplatin) is also receiving filgrastim (Neupogen). The nurse will explain to the patient that the filgrastim is used for what effect?

1. It boosts the effects of the carboplatin, so a decreased dosage is needed.
2. It prevents the development of secondary cancers related to the carboplatin.
3. It shortens the duration of neutropenia and associated infection risk related to the carboplatin.
4. It prevents bone loss and osteoporosis.

See Appendix A for answers to critical thinking questions, case study questions and review questions.

Reference

Prostate Cancer Foundation. (n.d.). *Prostate cancer FAQs.* http://www.pcf.org/site/c.leJRIROrEpH/b.5800851/k.645A/Prostate_Cancer_FAQs.htm

Selected Bibliography

Aleksakhina, S. N., Kashyap, A., & Imyanitov, E. N. (2019). Mechanisms of acquired tumor drug resistance. *Biochimica et Biophysica Acta (BBA) - Reviews on Cancer, 1872*(2), 188310. https://doi.org/10.1016/j.bbcan.2019.188310

American Cancer Society. (2020). *Cancer prevention & early detection: Facts and figures 2019–2020.* https://www.cancer.org/content/dam/cancer-org/research/cancer-facts-and-statistics/cancer-prevention-and-early-detection-facts-and-figures/cancer-prevention-and-early-detection-facts-and-figures-2019-2020.pdf

Badrinath, N., & Yoo, S. Y. (2019). Recent advances in cancer stem cell-targeted immunotherapy. *Cancers, 11*(3), 310. https://doi.org/10.3390/cancers11030310

Baldwin, A., & Rodriguez, E. S. (2016). Improving patient safety with error identification in chemotherapy orders by verification nurses. *Clinical Journal of Oncology Nursing, 20*, 59–65. https://doi.org/10.1188/16.CJON.59-65

Brazil, R. (2020). *Are tumor agnostic approaches the future for oncology?* Cancerworld. https://cancerworld.net/spotlight-on/are-tumour-agnostic-approaches-the-future-for-oncology/

Breastcancer.org. (2020). *U.S. breast cancer statistics.* https://www.breastcancer.org/symptoms/understand_bc/statistics

Kruger, S., Ilmer, M., Kobold, S., Cadilha, B. L., Endres, S., Ormanns, S., et al. (2019). Advances in cancer immunotherapy 2019 – latest trends. *Journal of Experimental & Clinical Cancer Research, 38*, 268. https://doi.org/10.1186/s13046-019-1266-0

National Cancer Institute (n.d.). *Cancer treatment.* https://www.cancer.gov/about-cancer/treatment

Seebacher, N. A., Stacy, A. E., Porter, G. M., & Merlot, A. M. (2019). Clinical development of targeted and immune based anti-cancer therapies. *Journal of Experimental & Clinical Cancer Research, 38*, 156. https://doi.org/10.1186/s13046-019-1094-2

Spring, L. M., Gupta, A., Reynolds, K. L., Gadd, M. A., Ellisen, L. W., Isakoff, S. J., et al. (2016). Neoadjuvant endocrine therapy for estrogen receptor–positive breast cancer: A systematic review and meta-analysis. *JAMA Oncology, 2*, 1477–1486. https://doi.org/10.1001/jamaoncol.2016.1897

Waks, A. G., & Winer, E. P. (2019). Breast cancer treatment: a review. *Journal of the American Medical Association, 321*(3), 288–300. https://doi.org/10.1001/jama.2018.19323

Wilkes, G. M., & Barton-Burke, M. (2020). *Oncology nursing drug handbook.* Jones & Bartlett.

Yarbro, C. H., Wujcik, D., & Gobel, B. H. (2018). *Cancer nursing: Principles and practice* (8th ed.). Jones & Bartlett.

Unit 9

Pharmacology of the Gastrointestinal System

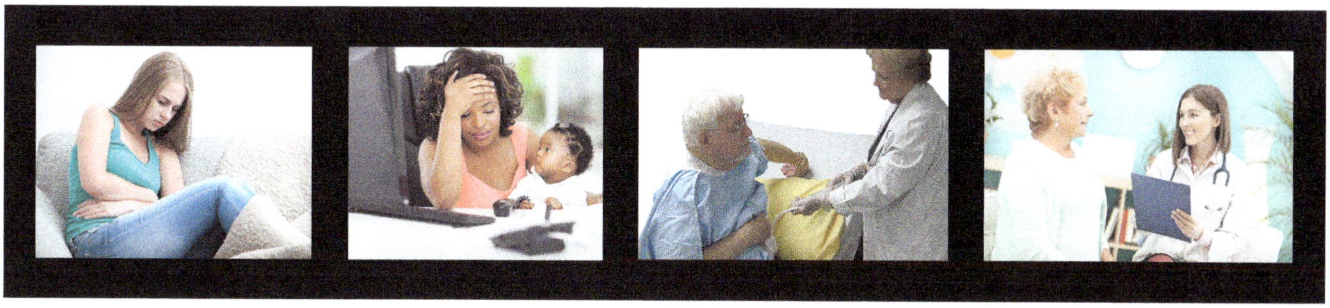

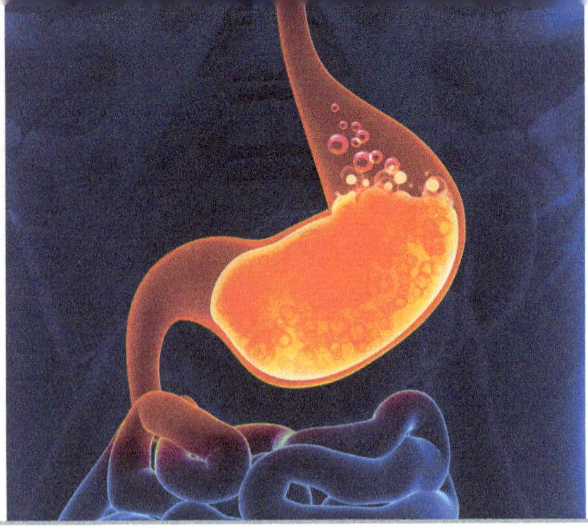

Chapter 58
Review of the Gastrointestinal System

Chapter Outline

- Overview of the Digestive System
- Physiology of the Upper Gastrointestinal Tract
- Physiology of the Lower Gastrointestinal Tract
- Physiology of the Accessory Organs of Digestion
- Regulation of Digestive Processes
- Nutrient Categories and Metabolism

Learning Outcomes

After reading this chapter, the student should be able to:

1. Describe the major anatomic structures of the digestive system.
2. Outline the steps in the process of digestion.
3. Describe the primary functions of the stomach.
4. Analyze how the anatomic structures of the small intestine promote the absorption of nutrients and drugs.
5. Describe the primary structures and functions of the large intestine.
6. Describe the functions of the liver and their relevance to drug therapy.
7. Explain the hepatic portal system and its importance to drug therapy.
8. Explain the nervous control of digestion.
9. Explain the enzymatic breakdown of nutrients by the digestive system.

Key Terms

Definitions of the terms in bold may be found in the Glossary.

Very little of the food we eat is directly available to body cells. Food must be broken down, absorbed, and chemically modified before it is in a form that is useful to cells. The digestive system performs these functions and many more. This chapter focuses on the aspects of digestion and physiology that are applicable to pharmacotherapy. For a complete review of the digestive system, the student should refer to an anatomy and physiology textbook.

Overview of the Digestive System

58.1 The function of the digestive system is to extract nutrients from food to fuel metabolic processes in the body.

The digestive system consists of two basic anatomic divisions: the alimentary canal and the accessory organs. The **alimentary canal**, or gastrointestinal (GI) tract, is a long, continuous, hollow tube that extends from the mouth to the anus. The **accessory organs of digestion** include the salivary glands, liver, gallbladder, and pancreas. The major structures of the digestive system are illustrated in Figure 58.1.

The overall function of the digestive system is to extract nutrients from food so that they may be used to fuel the metabolic processes in the body. Because food is a complex substance, multiple steps are necessary before cells can use its components. These steps are ingestion, propulsion, digestion, absorption, and defecation.

Ingestion is taking food into the body by mouth. In some patients, ingestion bypasses the mouth and delivers nutrients directly into the stomach or small intestine via a feeding tube.

Substances are propelled along the GI tract by **peristalsis**, which is the rhythmic contractions of layers of smooth muscle. The speed at which substances move through the GI tract is critical to the absorption of drugs, nutrients, and water and for the removal of wastes. If peristalsis is too fast, substances will not have sufficient contact with the GI mucosa to be absorbed. In addition, the large intestine will not have enough time to absorb water, and diarrhea may result. Abnormally slow transit may result in constipation or even obstructions in the small or large intestine.

Digestion is the mechanical and chemical breakdown of food into a form that may be absorbed into the systemic circulation. To chemically break down ingested food, a large number of enzymes and other substances are required. Digestive enzymes are secreted by the salivary glands, stomach, small intestine, and pancreas. The liver makes bile, which is stored in the gallbladder until it is needed for lipid emulsification.

Absorption is the movement of nutrients and other substances from the alimentary canal to the circulation. The mucosa layer lining of the alimentary canal provides a surface area on which the various acids, bases, and enzymes can break down food. In many parts of the alimentary canal, the mucosa is folded and contains deep grooves and pits. The small intestine is lined with tiny villi and microvilli that provide a huge surface area for the absorption of nutrients and medications.

Not all components of ingested food are useful to the human body or can be digested. The elimination of indigestible substances from the body is called **defecation**.

PharmFACT

Most people believe that people with obesity have larger stomachs. However, people who are naturally thin have the same size as or even larger stomachs than people who have problems with weight control. Weight has nothing to do with the size of the stomach (Bouchez, n.d.).

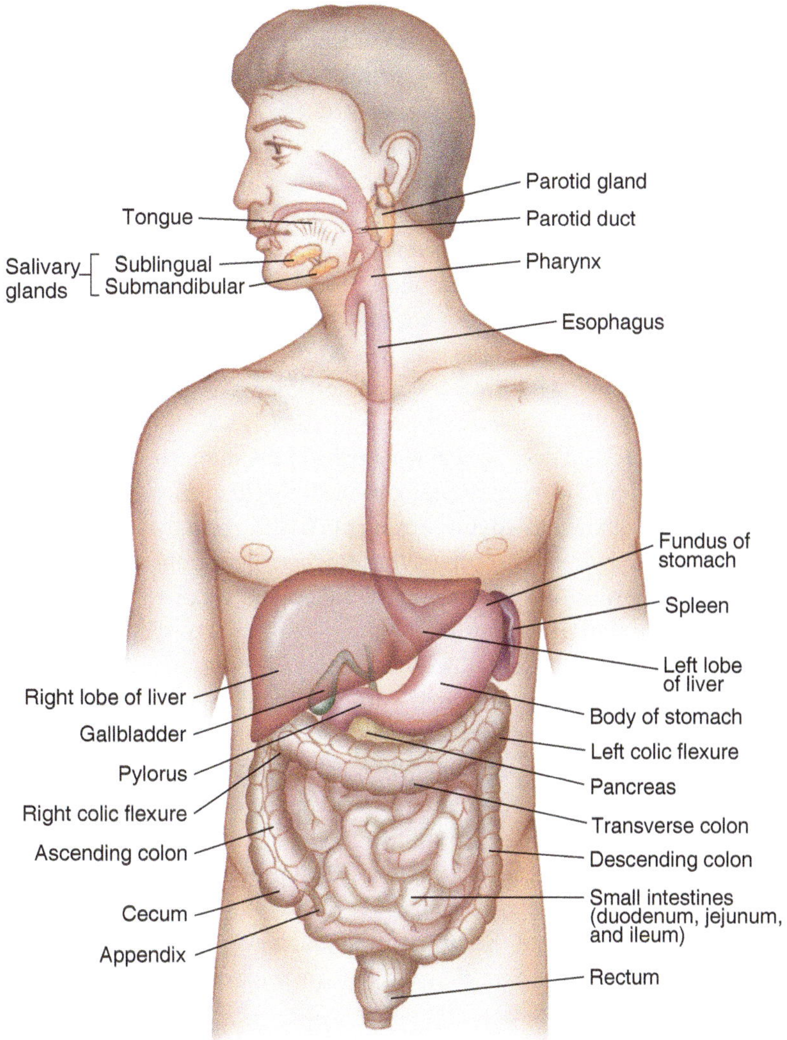

Figure 58.1 The digestive system.

Physiology of the Upper Gastrointestinal Tract

58.2 The upper gastrointestinal tract is responsible for mechanical and chemical digestion.

The upper GI tract consists of the mouth, pharynx, esophagus, and stomach. From a pharmacologic perspective, the most important regions of the upper GI tract are the buccal and sublingual areas of the mouth and the stomach.

The epithelial mucosa of the buccal and sublingual regions is very thin, being only 40 to 50 cells in thickness. The mucosal layer, along with the salivary glands, secretes mucus, which lubricates and moistens the oral cavity. The mucus also serves as a liquid medium for drug administration inside the mouth. The oral mucosa in the sublingual region is relatively permeable, and drugs are rapidly absorbed. The buccal region is less permeable, and drug absorption is slower. The buccal region, however, has less salivary flow and drugs can be retained longer, making it better suited for sustained-release delivery systems. For example, Fentora is a buccal form of fentanyl that is designed to dissolve and relieve pain in about 30 minutes.

The pharynx and esophagus serve as passageways for ingested food and liquids. Obstruction of these areas, or a loss of the swallowing reflex, precludes the administration of oral drugs. Little absorption occurs across the pharyngeal or esophageal mucosa because drugs travel quickly through these regions of the alimentary canal.

Food passes from the esophagus to the stomach by traveling through the lower esophageal (cardiac) sphincter. This ring of smooth muscle usually prevents the stomach contents from moving backward, a condition known as gastroesophageal reflux. The stomach has both mechanical and chemical functions. The muscular squeezing of the stomach churns and mixes the food, breaking it down mechanically to a semisolid known as **chyme**. Strong peristaltic contractions push the chyme toward the pylorus, where it encounters a second ring of smooth muscle called the pyloric sphincter. Located at the entrance to the small intestine, this sphincter regulates the flow of substances leaving the stomach. Chyme moves in "spurts" through the sphincter into the small intestine. Large pieces of food are refluxed back into the body of the stomach, where they are subjected to more churning to reduce them in size to about 2 mm so that they may pass through the sphincter.

The stomach also secretes substances that promote the processes of chemical digestion. Gastric glands extending deep into the mucosa of the stomach contain several cell types that are critical to digestion and that are important to the pharmacotherapy of digestive disorders:

- **Chief cells** secrete pepsinogen, an inactive form of the enzyme pepsin that chemically breaks down proteins.
- **Parietal cells** secrete 1 to 3 liters of hydrochloric acid each day. This strong acid helps to break down food, activates pepsinogen, and kills microbes that may have been ingested. Parietal cells also secrete intrinsic factor, which is essential for the absorption of vitamin B_{12}.
- **Enteroendocrine cells** secrete hormones that modify the digestive processes. In the stomach, the most important secretion is gastrin, which stimulates acid production by the parietal cells.

The combined secretion of the chief and parietal cells, known as gastric juice, is the most acidic fluid in the body, having a pH of 1.5 to 3.5. A number of natural defenses protect the stomach mucosa against this extremely acidic fluid. Certain cells that line the surface of the stomach secrete a thick, mucous layer and bicarbonate ion to neutralize the acid. These form such an effective protective layer that the pH at the mucosal surface is nearly neutral. On reaching the duodenum, the stomach contents are further neutralized by bicarbonate from pancreatic and biliary secretions.

The pharmacologic importance of the stomach lies in its capacity to absorb drugs. For most oral medications, the stomach is not the primary site of absorption because the drug does not stay long in the organ. Stomach acidity (pH 1 to 2) can either assist in the absorption process or destroy the drug entirely. Drugs that are weak acids tend to be absorbed in the stomach. Protein drugs are destroyed by pepsin in the stomach before they are absorbed or have a chance to reach the small intestine.

CONNECTION Checkpoint 58.1

Nitroglycerin is the most frequently prescribed sublingual medication. From what you learned in Chapter 35, what is the primary indication for nitroglycerin and what is the time for onset of action of the drug when it is given by the sublingual route?

Physiology of the Lower Gastrointestinal Tract

58.3 The small intestine is the longest portion of the alimentary canal and is the primary organ for absorption.

The lower GI tract consists of the small and large intestines. With its many folds and finger-like projections of villi and microvilli, the small intestine is highly specialized for absorption. The lining of each villus is composed of a single layer of epithelial cells and contains blood capillaries, as illustrated in Figure 58.2. Essentially, only a single cell separates a nutrient or drug molecule from the intestinal lumen of the body's circulatory system.

The duodenum, the first 10 inches of the small intestine, is the site where chyme mixes with bile from the gallbladder and digestive enzymes from the pancreas.

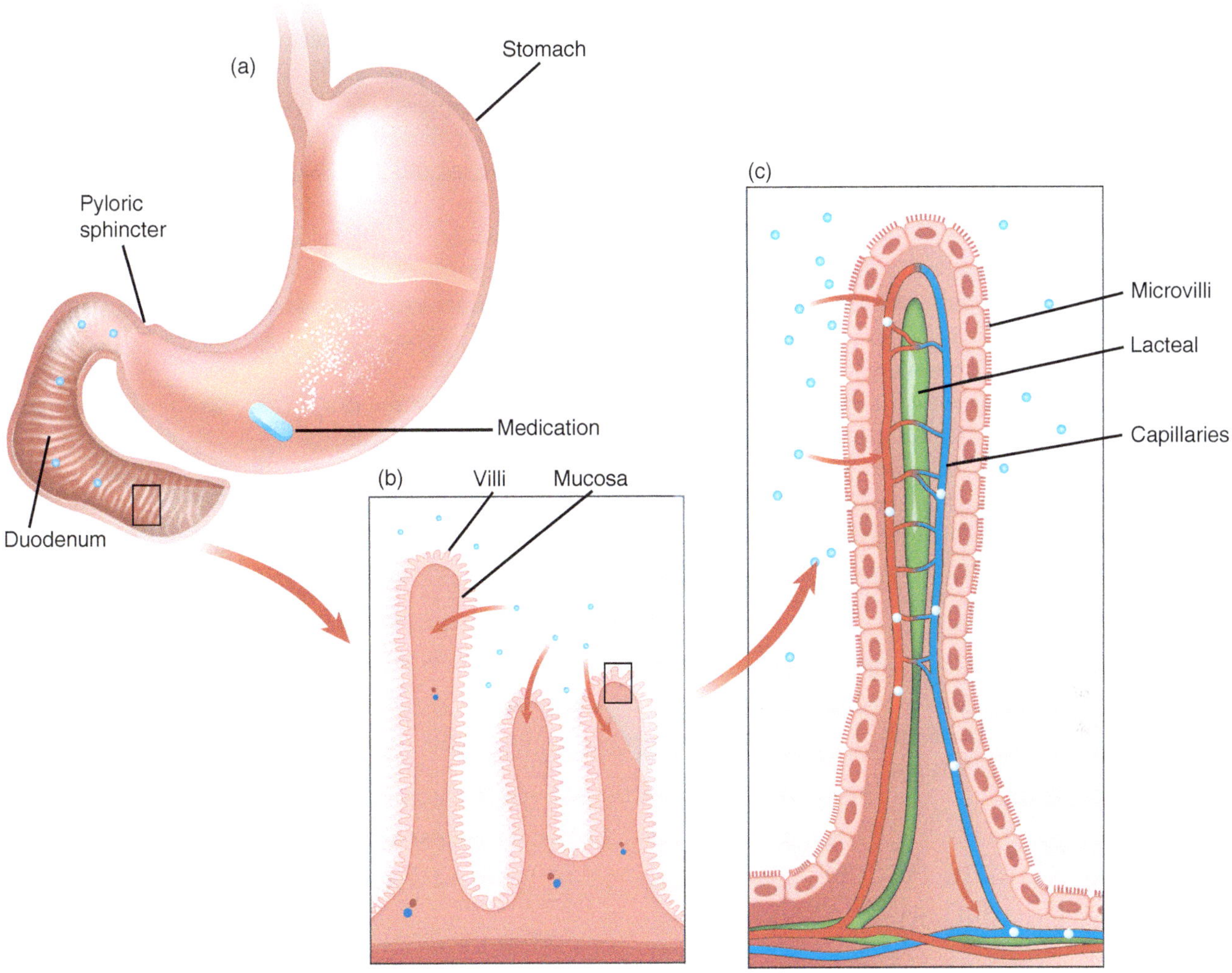

Figure 58.2 Villi and microvilli of the small intestine: (a) Tablet dissolves in the stomach. (b) Medication reaches the villi of the duodenum. (c) Drug molecules are absorbed into the microvilli capillaries.

Bile and pancreatic juice enter through an opening in the duodenum known as the duodenal papilla. The duodenum is sometimes considered part of the upper GI tract because of its proximity to the stomach. Peptic ulcer, the most common disorder of the duodenum, is discussed in Chapter 59.

The remainder of the small intestine consists of the jejunum and ileum. Because of its length and enormous absorptive surface, the first 1 to 2 meters (3 to 6.5 feet) of the jejunum is the site of the majority of nutrient and drug absorption. As the jejunum becomes the ileum, the diameter of the intestinal lumen diminishes and the villi become fewer in number. The terminal ileum is a primary site for the absorption of vitamin B_{12}, long-chain fatty acids, and fat-soluble vitamins. The ileum empties its contents into the large intestine through the ileocecal valve. Travel time for chyme through the entire small intestine varies from 3 to 6 hours.

The mucosa of the small intestine secretes intestinal juice, which is a mixture of mucus and digestive enzymes. The mucus has an alkaline pH, which neutralizes the acidity from the stomach. The small intestine also secretes cholecystokinin, a hormone that promotes pancreatic enzyme secretion, and secretin, which stimulates bicarbonate production to make the small intestine more alkaline.

CONNECTION Checkpoint 58.2

Many oral drugs have enteric coatings. From what you learned in Chapter 3, what is the purpose of the enteric coating and why are these drugs not to be split or crushed?

58.4 The large intestine contains host flora and is a major site of water reabsorption.

The large intestine, or colon, receives chyme from the ileum in a fluid state. The large intestine does not secrete digestive enzymes nor does it secrete hormones. With few exceptions, little reabsorption of nutrients occurs during the 12- to 24-hour journey through the colon. The large intestine does secrete a large amount of mucus, which helps lubricate the fecal matter. The major functions of the colon are to reabsorb water and electrolytes from the waste material and excrete the remaining fecal material from the body.

The colon harbors a substantial amount of bacteria and fungi, called the host flora, which serve a useful purpose by synthesizing B-complex vitamins and vitamin K. Disruption of the normal host flora can lead to diarrhea.

From a pharmacologic perspective, the large intestine may be the site of therapeutic or adverse drug effects. A large number of drugs cause either diarrhea or constipation. These effects are usually self-limiting and can be prevented or managed through nursing interventions. When bowel patterns are significantly disrupted, drugs may be given to slow the activity (antidiarrheals) or increase the activity (laxatives) of the large intestine.

Of additional pharmacologic importance are the drugs given by the rectal route. The mucosa of the rectum provides an excellent and rapid absorptive surface for drugs. It is a common route in children and in patients who are unable to take oral medications due to nausea, vomiting or other pathology that prevents oral administration. The onset of action is usually slower than the oral route, and drug action is limited by the length of time the patient can retain the drug without defecation.

Physiology of the Accessory Organs of Digestion

58.5 The liver is the most important accessory digestive organ.

The accessory organs of digestion include the teeth, tongue, salivary glands, pancreas, gallbladder, and liver. Of these, the pancreas and liver have the most pharmacologic importance. The endocrine functions of the pancreas, which include the secretion of insulin and glucagon, are presented in Chapter 66.

The liver is one of the most important organs in pharmacology. Along with the kidneys, any drug that reaches the systemic circulation, regardless of its route of administration, will pass through the liver. The overall function of the liver is to filter and process the nutrients and drugs delivered to it. Substances may be stored, chemically altered, or removed from the blood before they reach the general circulation. The following are some of the primary functions of the liver:

- *Regulation.* It stabilizes the serum levels of glucose, triglycerides, and cholesterol.
- *Protection.* It removes toxic substances and waste products such as ammonia.
- *Synthesis.* It synthesizes bile, plasma proteins, and certain clotting factors.
- *Storage.* It stores iron and fat-soluble vitamins.

When most drugs reach the liver, they are metabolized to less toxic substances that are more easily excreted by the kidney. The cytochrome P450 (CYP450) enzyme system in liver cells is especially active at metabolizing drugs; the various isozymes of CYP450 are discussed in Chapter 3. In a few cases, the liver changes the drug to a more active form. It is important to note that the handling of drugs and toxic substances by the liver can cause liver injury. This is especially true if the hepatocytes are chronically exposed to harmful substances such as alcohol. Hepatic impairment is a relatively common adverse effect of certain drugs. Whereas drug-induced hepatic impairment is often transient and asymptomatic, some drugs can cause severe, permanent, and even fatal liver damage.

PharmFACT

Acetaminophen (Tylenol) overdose is the leading cause of acute liver failure in the United States. Normal doses of the drug can cause acetaminophen poisoning in malnourished patients or those with chronic alcohol abuse (Farrell, 2020).

The unique structure of the vascular system serving the liver is important to digestion as well as pharmacology. The liver receives both oxygenated and deoxygenated blood. The **hepatic portal system**, shown in Figure 58.3, is a network of venous vessels that collects blood draining from the stomach, small intestine, and most of the large intestine. This blood is extremely rich in nutrients because it contains substances absorbed during digestion. It is important to know that this blood is delivered to the liver via the hepatic portal vein before it reaches the arterial circulation. The liver then can remove, store, excrete, or perform metabolic functions on these substances before they are sent into the inferior vena cava to reach the heart and be distributed to other organs.

The hepatic portal system serves as an important homeostatic mechanism, allowing a relatively stable composition of blood to circulate through the body. In terms of drug therapy, nearly all oral medications enter the hepatic portal vein for processing by the liver before they reach their target tissue. In some cases, the liver inactivates a substantial percentage of the drug before it reaches the inferior vena cava, a phenomenon called the *first-pass effect*. Drugs that have a significant first-pass effect may be given by other routes, such as intramuscular, intravenous, subcutaneous, or topical. Although a drug will still eventually reach the liver by these routes, it will have an opportunity to also reach its target tissue. Note that the venous systems serving the head and the lower rectum are not parts of the hepatic portal system. Thus, drugs that are given by the buccal, sublingual, or rectal routes bypass the first-pass effect of the liver.

After the liver makes bile, it is sent to the gallbladder for storage. When lipids enter the small intestine, the

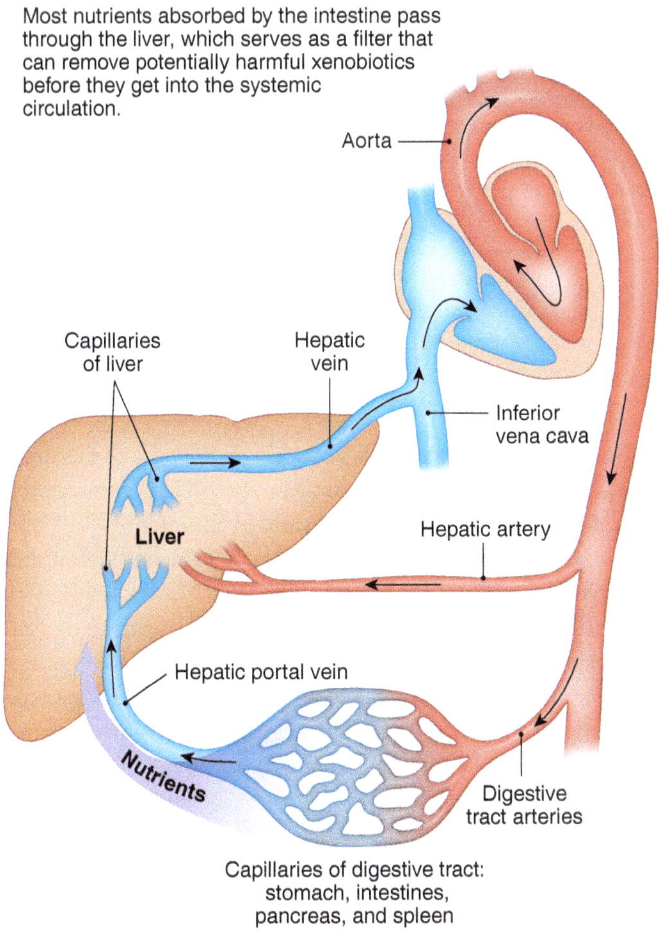

Figure 58.3 The hepatic portal system.

gallbladder contracts and sends its contents into the duodenum. The bile salts emulsify the lipids, making them easier to digest enzymatically. When bile salts reach the terminal portion of the ileum, 95% are reabsorbed back into the hepatic portal circulation by a process called *enterohepatic recirculation*. This process has direct implications to pharmacotherapy. Certain drugs, including digoxin, morphine, and estrogens, are eliminated in the bile and are reabsorbed by enterohepatic recirculation. Enterohepatic recirculation recycles the drug multiple times and can significantly extend a drug's half-life. Interactions can occur if one drug interferes with the enterohepatic recycling of another drug. Preventing this recycling can speed the elimination of a drug and reduce its therapeutic effectiveness. An example of such an interaction is when cholestyramine (Questran) interferes with the recycling of lorazepam (Ativan) and increases the clearance of lorazepam from the body.

The pancreas is an essential accessory digestive organ, secreting about a quart of pancreatic fluid into the duodenum each day. This fluid is alkaline (pH 7.5 to 8.8) and contains digestive enzymes to chemically break down carbohydrates, lipids, proteins, and nucleic acids. From a pharmacologic perspective, the pancreas is relatively protected from drugs and there are only a few therapies for pancreatic digestive disorders.

CONNECTION Checkpoint 58.3

The tricyclic antidepressant imipramine is a substrate for the CYP2D6 enzyme, and the selective serotonin reuptake inhibitor fluoxetine is a potent inhibitor of this enzyme. From what you learned in Chapter 5, predict the type of drug interaction that will occur in a patient stabilized on imipramine therapy when fluoxetine is added to the regimen.

Regulation of Digestive Processes

58.6 Digestion is regulated by numerous hormonal and nervous factors.

Digestion is controlled through a large number of hormonal and nervous factors that influence the speed of peristalsis and the amount of saliva, mucus, acid, and enzyme secretions. Various negative feedback loops help to regulate these activities so that digestion is a normally a smooth, continuous process. Disruption of homeostatic mechanisms can cause cramping, due to excessive peristalsis, or peptic ulcers, due to the overproduction of gastric acid.

The nervous control of digestion is provided at several levels. Chapter 12 discusses the role of the autonomic nervous system (ANS) in controlling the contraction of smooth muscle and glandular secretion. Activation of the parasympathetic nervous system stimulates the digestive processes by increasing peristalsis, salivation, and digestive gland secretion. The sympathetic nervous system has opposite effects, with beta$_2$-adrenergic receptors in the intestinal wall and alpha$_1$-adrenergic receptors in the salivary glands. Drugs that affect the ANS often affect the digestive processes.

The GI tract is also regulated by local reflexes called the **enteric nervous system**. This system consists of a vast network of neurons in the submucosa of the alimentary canal that has sensory and motor functions. Chemoreceptors and stretch receptors sense the presence and amount of food in the GI tract and respond accordingly by changing motility without sending signals to the ANS.

The GI tract functions at an automatic level; no conscious thought is required as the system goes about its daily tasks of secretion and digestion. The central nervous system, however, can greatly influence the activity of digestive functions. For example, merely thinking of food can evoke powerful responses. These may be positive, such as perhaps thinking of a steak sizzling on the grill or bread baking in the oven, and increase salivation and peristalsis. Images may also be negative and evoke feelings of nausea and vomiting at the sight or smell of food. Mental health conditions such as depression, anxiety, excessive stress, or bipolar disorder can affect the appetite and digestive processes.

Nutrient Categories and Metabolism

58.7 The chemical breakdown of food is accomplished by digestive enzymes.

The three basic nutrients are carbohydrates, lipids, and proteins. In food these nutrients are large molecules that cannot be absorbed across the mucosa of the alimentary canal. Chemical digestion must break down these complex food molecules into simpler substances so that they can be absorbed and used by the body for metabolic processes.

The breakdown of complex carbohydrates, lipids, and proteins requires digestive enzymes to be delivered when food is present at various parts of the alimentary canal, primarily the stomach and small intestine. These enzymes and their locations are listed in Table 58.1. Secretion of digestive enzymes is regulated by hormones and the nervous system, as described in Section 58.6. Patients who secrete insufficient quantities of digestive enzymes may be administered these substances as drugs.

In addition to the three basic nutrients, the body requires a host of other vitamins and minerals for proper metabolism. Deficiency symptoms will be observed if a patient has insufficient intake of these substances. The pharmacotherapy of vitamins and minerals is presented in Chapter 61.

The intake of various nutrients in sufficient amounts is necessary to maintain good health and to allow the body to heal during periods of illness or injury. The intake of sufficient amounts of proteins, carbohydrates, fats, vitamins, and minerals can often be achieved by eating a well-balanced diet of foods and fluids. When this does not occur, enteral or parenteral therapy may be indicated, as presented in Chapter 62.

Table 58.1 Major Digestive Enzymes

Nutrient	Enzyme	Source
Carbohydrates and starches	Salivary amylase	Saliva
	Pancreatic amylase	Pancreatic juice
	Maltase, sucrase, lactase	Small intestine
Lipids	Pancreatic lipase	Pancreatic juice
Proteins and polypeptides	Pepsin	Gastric glands
	Trypsin, chymotrypsin, carboxypeptidase	Pancreatic juice
	Aminopeptidase	Small intestine

Understanding Chapter 58

Key Concepts Summary

58.1 The function of the digestive system is to extract nutrients from food to fuel metabolic processes in the body.

58.2 The upper gastrointestinal tract is responsible for mechanical and chemical digestion.

58.3 The small intestine is the longest portion of the alimentary canal and is the primary organ for absorption.

58.4 The large intestine contains host flora and is a major site of water reabsorption.

58.5 The liver is the most important accessory digestive organ.

58.6 Digestion is regulated by numerous hormonal and nervous factors.

58.7 The chemical breakdown of food is accomplished by digestive enzymes.

References

Bouchez, C. (n.d.). *9 surprising facts about your stomach.* WebMD. http://www.webmd.com/women/features/stomach-problems

Farrell, S. E. (2020). *Acetaminophen toxicity*. Medscape. https://emedicine.medscape.com/article/820200-overview

Silverthorn, D. U. (2019). *Human physiology: An integrated approach* (8th ed.). Pearson.

Selected Bibliography

Krogh, D. (2014). *Biology: A guide to the natural world, technology update* (5th ed.). Benjamin Cummings.

Marieb, E. N., & Hoehn, K. N. (2019). *Human anatomy and physiology* (11th ed.). Pearson.

Martini, F. H., Nath, J. L., & Bartholomew, E. F. (2017). *Fundamentals of human anatomy and physiology* (11th ed.). Pearson.

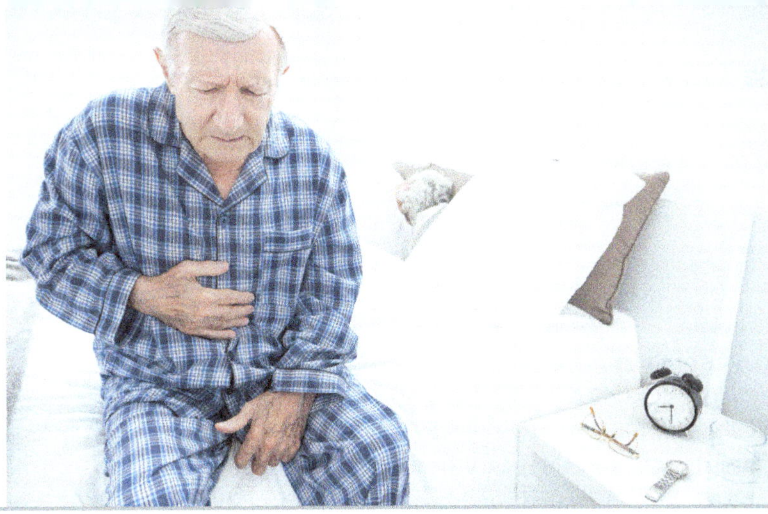

"I was diagnosed with a duodenal ulcer yesterday. Why do I need to take these antibiotics if I don't have an infection?"
—*Patient "Hugh Marshall"*

Chapter 59
Pharmacotherapy of Peptic Ulcer Disease

Chapter Outline

Learning Outcomes

After reading this chapter, the student should be able to:

1. Explain the physiologic regulation of gastric acid secretion.
2. Describe factors that suppress and those that promote the formation of peptic ulcers.
3. Compare and contrast duodenal ulcers and gastric ulcers.
4. Identify the etiology, signs, and symptoms of peptic ulcer disease and gastroesophageal reflux disease.
5. Outline the treatment goals for the pharmacotherapy of peptic ulcer disease and gastroesophageal reflux disease.
6. Identify the classification of drugs used to treat peptic ulcer disease and gastroesophageal reflux disease.
7. Explain the pharmacologic strategies for eradicating *Helicobacter pylori*.
8. Describe the nurse's role in the pharmacologic management of patients with peptic ulcer disease and gastroesophageal reflux disease.
9. For each of the classes shown in the chapter outline, identify the prototype and representative drugs and explain the mechanism(s) of drug action, primary indications, contraindications, significant drug interactions, pregnancy data, and important adverse effects.
10. Apply clinical judgment to care for patients receiving pharmacotherapy for peptic ulcer disease and gastroesophageal reflux disease.

Key Terms

Definitions of the terms in bold may be found in the Glossary.

Acid-related diseases of the upper gastrointestinal (GI) tract are some of the most common medical conditions. Because drugs for these disorders are available over the counter (OTC), many patients attempt self-treatment before seeking assistance from their healthcare provider. Signs and symptoms of acid-related conditions of the upper GI tract, however, may indicate more serious disease. This chapter examines the pharmacotherapy of two common disorders of the upper digestive system: peptic ulcer disease (PUD) and gastroesophageal reflux disease (GERD).

Physiology of Gastric Acid Secretion

59.1 The stomach secretes acid, enzymes, and hormones that are essential to digestive physiology.

Gastric glands contain several cell types that are critical to digestion and important to the pharmacotherapy of digestive disorders. Chief cells secrete the enzyme pepsinogen, which is then activated to become **pepsin**, which breaks down proteins from food. Parietal cells secrete gastric (hydrochloric) acid in the stomach, which provides a strongly acidic environment that promotes the conversion of pepsinogen to pepsin, helps to break down food, and kills microbes that may have been ingested. Parietal cells also secrete intrinsic factor, which is essential for the absorption of vitamin B_{12} (see Chapter 58). Parietal cells are targets for many of the drugs used to reduce acid secretion. The cell types present in gastric glands are shown in Figure 59.1.

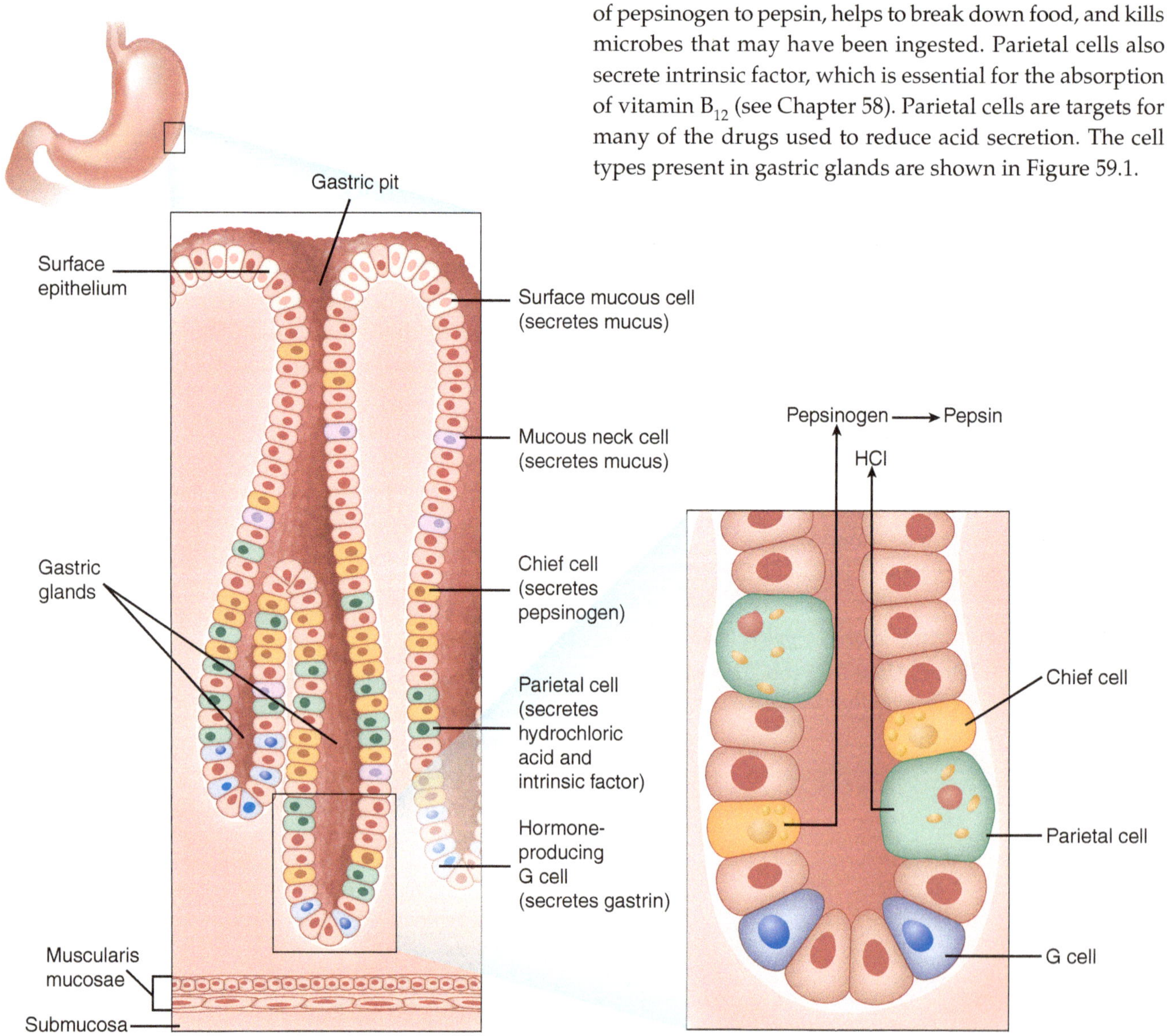

Figure 59.1 The stomach lining: gastric glands and the secretion of hydrochloric acid.

Several sources provide messages to parietal cells to increase or decrease acid production. parietal cells contain receptors for the hormone gastrin, histamine (H_2), and the neurotransmitter acetylcholine, which are the three principal physiologic stimuli that regulate acid secretion from the proton pump, or H^+, K^+-ATPase, located on the surface of parietal cells.

Ingestion of food and distention of the stomach stimulate the secretion of the hormone gastrin into the bloodstream. The target cells for gastrin are enteroendocrine cells in the gastric glands. When gastrin binds to their cell surface, the enteroendocrine cells produce and secrete histamine. Histamine then binds to the H_2 receptor on the parietal cell to stimulate acid secretion. In addition to promoting acid secretion, gastrin signals the chief cells to secrete pepsin, promotes the production of pancreatic enzymes, and increases gastric blood flow.

Like most hormones, gastrin is regulated by negative feedback. As the stomach contents reach pH 3 or lower, the hormone **somatostatin** is released by cells in the stomach, small intestine, and pancreas. This hormone suppresses the secretion of gastrin, thus lowering acid secretion. Interestingly, somatostatin is also released by the anterior pituitary gland and is known as growth hormone–inhibiting hormone. However, the nervous system secretion and actions are independent of its digestive actions.

Cells lining the stomach mucosa secrete a thick mucous layer that provides a continuous, protective physical barrier against acid and pepsin. Bicarbonate ion is also secreted by the epithelial cells in the stomach and serves to neutralize gastric acid on the mucosal surface. The mucus and bicarbonate ion form such an effective protective layer that the pH at the mucosal surface is nearly neutral. Once the stomach contents reach the duodenum, they are further neutralized by the bicarbonate ion from pancreatic and biliary secretions.

Another protective substance is the hormone **prostaglandin E_2**. This hormone stimulates the secretion of mucus and bicarbonate, promotes repair of damaged gastric mucosal cells, and increases blood flow to the mucosa to help maintain optimal mucosal conditions. Several frequently prescribed drugs, including corticosteroids and nonsteroidal anti-inflammatory drugs (NSAIDs), cause peptic ulcers because they are prostaglandin antagonists. The natural defenses of the stomach are shown in Figure 59.2.

Etiology and Pathogenesis of Peptic Ulcer Disease

59.2 Peptic ulcer disease is associated with a number of etiologic risk factors.

A **peptic ulcer** is a lesion or erosion located in either the stomach (gastric) or small intestine (duodenal) mucosa that is usually associated with acute inflammation. PUD was an uncommon condition until the 19th century. Thus, it is considered to be a "disease of civilization." Although PUD occurs most often in middle age, it may occur at any time, including infancy and childhood.

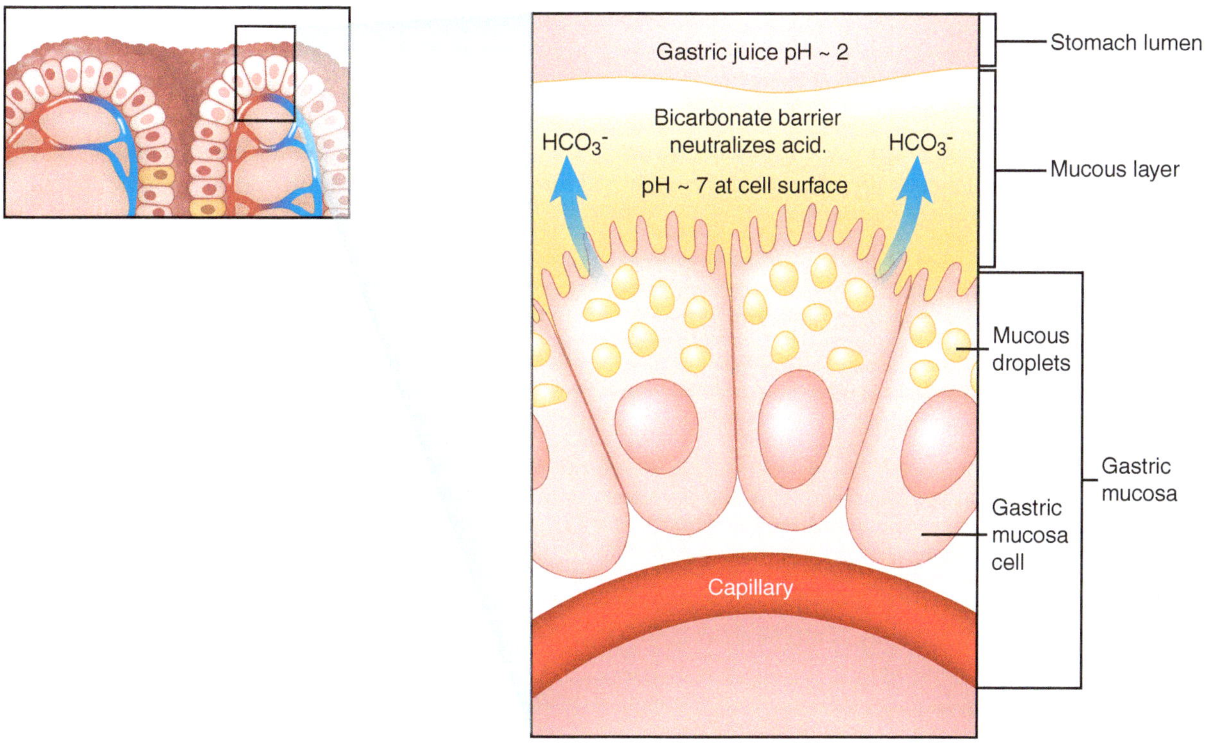

Figure 59.2 Natural defenses against stomach acid.

PUD occurs when there is an *imbalance* of protective factors versus aggravating factors: The levels of mucus and bicarbonate ion secretions are unable to protect the mucosa against the aggravating factors of pepsin and gastric acid. Complications of PUD include bleeding, perforation, penetration, and GI obstruction due to scarring. The incidence of PUD is associated with the following risk factors:

- Infection with the bacterium *Helicobacter pylori*
- Close family history of PUD
- Use of certain medications, particularly corticosteroids, NSAIDs, and platelet inhibitors such as aspirin and clopidogrel
- Blood group O (the intestinal epithelial cells bind to *H. pylori* more strongly in these individuals)
- Smoking tobacco (increases gastric acid secretion and reduces bicarbonate production)
- Consumption of beverages and foods that contain excessive caffeine
- Excessive psychologic stress.

PharmFACT

Approximately 4.6 million Americans are affected by PUD, and about 10% of Americans will experience an ulcer in their lifetime (Anand, 2020).

For many decades, it was thought that mental and physiologic stress, smoking, and spicy foods were the primary causes of PUD. It was theorized that bacteria could not survive the acidic environment of the stomach. Evidence now shows that 90% of all duodenal ulcers are associated with infection by the gram-negative bacterium *H. pylori*. Treatment of PUD as an infectious disease is now widely acknowledged. The pharmacotherapy of *H. pylori* is described in Section 59.8.

Drug therapy with NSAIDs is responsible for a large number of peptic ulcer cases. Gastric and duodenal ulcers occur in about 20% of patients using NSAIDs on a regular basis, with 4% experiencing serious bleeding.

NSAIDs promote ulcer formation and inflammation both topically and systemically. Topically, NSAIDs cause direct cellular damage to GI mucosal cells. Systemically, NSAIDs interfere with prostaglandin synthesis via the enzyme cyclooxygenase (COX) in the stomach, which normally aids in the production of mucus and bicarbonate. NSAIDs decrease gastric blood flow and slow cellular repair. NSAIDs are also weak acids that are nonionized in gastric acid and able to diffuse across the mucous barrier into the gastric epithelial cells, which leads to further cellular damage.

Risk factors for NSAID-induced PUD include long-term use of NSAIDs, advanced age, history of ulcers, concomitant use of corticosteroids or anticoagulants, or alcohol and cigarette smoking. In addition, *H. pylori* infection and NSAIDs act synergistically to promote ulcers. The combination poses a 3.5-fold greater risk of ulcers than either factor alone.

The characteristic symptom of duodenal ulcer is a gnawing or burning, upper abdominal pain that occurs 1 to 3 hours after a meal. The pain is usually worse when the stomach is empty and often disappears with ingestion of food. This is because the presence of food closes the pyloric sphincter and allows the acid to remain in the stomach, rather than to come into contact with the duodenal ulcer. Nighttime pain may awaken the patient. If the erosion progresses deeper into the mucosa, bleeding occurs and may be evident as either bright red blood in vomit or black, tarry stools. Many duodenal ulcers heal spontaneously, although scar tissue remains, predisposing the mucosa to future ulceration, and they frequently recur after months of remission. Perforation and hemorrhage are sometimes the first signs of a duodenal ulcer in infants. Many patients with PUD are asymptomatic.

Gastric ulcers are less common than the duodenal type and have different symptoms. Pain is often caused by or exacerbated with eating. Anorexia, weight loss, and vomiting are more common with gastric ulcers. Remissions may be infrequent or absent. Medical follow-up of gastric ulcers should continue for several years because a small percentage of the erosions become cancerous. The most severe ulcers may penetrate the wall of the stomach and cause death. Whereas duodenal ulcers most frequently occur in men age 30 to 50, gastric ulcers are more common in women over age 60. NSAID-related ulcers are more likely to produce gastric ulcers, whereas *H. pylori*–associated ulcers are more likely to be duodenal.

Patients who are experiencing physiologic stress resulting from severe trauma, surgery, burns, illness, or shock may experience stress ulcers. Stress ulcers are typically asymptomatic initially, and about 25% of patients present with painless upper GI bleeding. Vasoconstriction secondary to sympathetic nervous system involvement causes decreased blood flow to the small intestine, which may play a role in the development of stress ulcers. Patients who are placed on mechanical ventilation and other seriously ill patients are sometimes administered prophylactic antiulcer drugs to prevent complications due to PUD.

Zollinger-Ellison syndrome (ZES) is a rare cause of PUD. It is caused by a gastrinoma, a tumor of the pancreas or duodenum that secretes large amounts of the hormone gastrin. Because the presence of gastrin is the hormonal signal for increasing hydrochloric acid secretion, the huge amounts of acid easily overcome the protective defenses, leading to multiple gastric and duodenal ulcers. Peptic ulcers are persistent, difficult to treat, and slow to heal. Symptoms of ZES are the same as those of PUD. The acid also irritates the GI tract, resulting in diarrhea. Treatment involves aggressive acid suppression with drugs or surgical removal of the gastrinoma.

Ulceration in the distal small intestine is known as Crohn's disease, and erosions in the large intestine are called ulcerative colitis. These diseases, together categorized as inflammatory bowel disease, are discussed in Chapter 60.

Etiology and Pathogenesis of Gastroesophageal Reflux Disease

59.3 Gastroesophageal reflux disease is a chronic condition characterized by persistent heartburn.

Gastroesophageal reflux disease (GERD) results when acidic stomach contents enter the esophagus. Although most often considered a disease of people older than age 40, GERD can also occur in infants. The prevalence of the disease is increasing among both children and adults.

In adults, the cause of GERD is transient weakening or relaxation of the lower esophageal sphincter (LES), a specialized muscle segment at the end of the esophagus. The sphincter may no longer close tightly, allowing movement of gastric contents upward into the esophagus when the stomach contracts. The acidic gastric contents cause an intense burning (heartburn) and, in some cases, injury to the esophagus. In addition, the pathogenesis of GERD involves decreased salivary secretions and diminished esophageal motility. The pathophysiology of GERD is shown in Pharmacotherapy Illustrated 59.1.

Pharmacotherapy Illustrated 59.1

Treatment of Gastroesophageal Reflux Disease

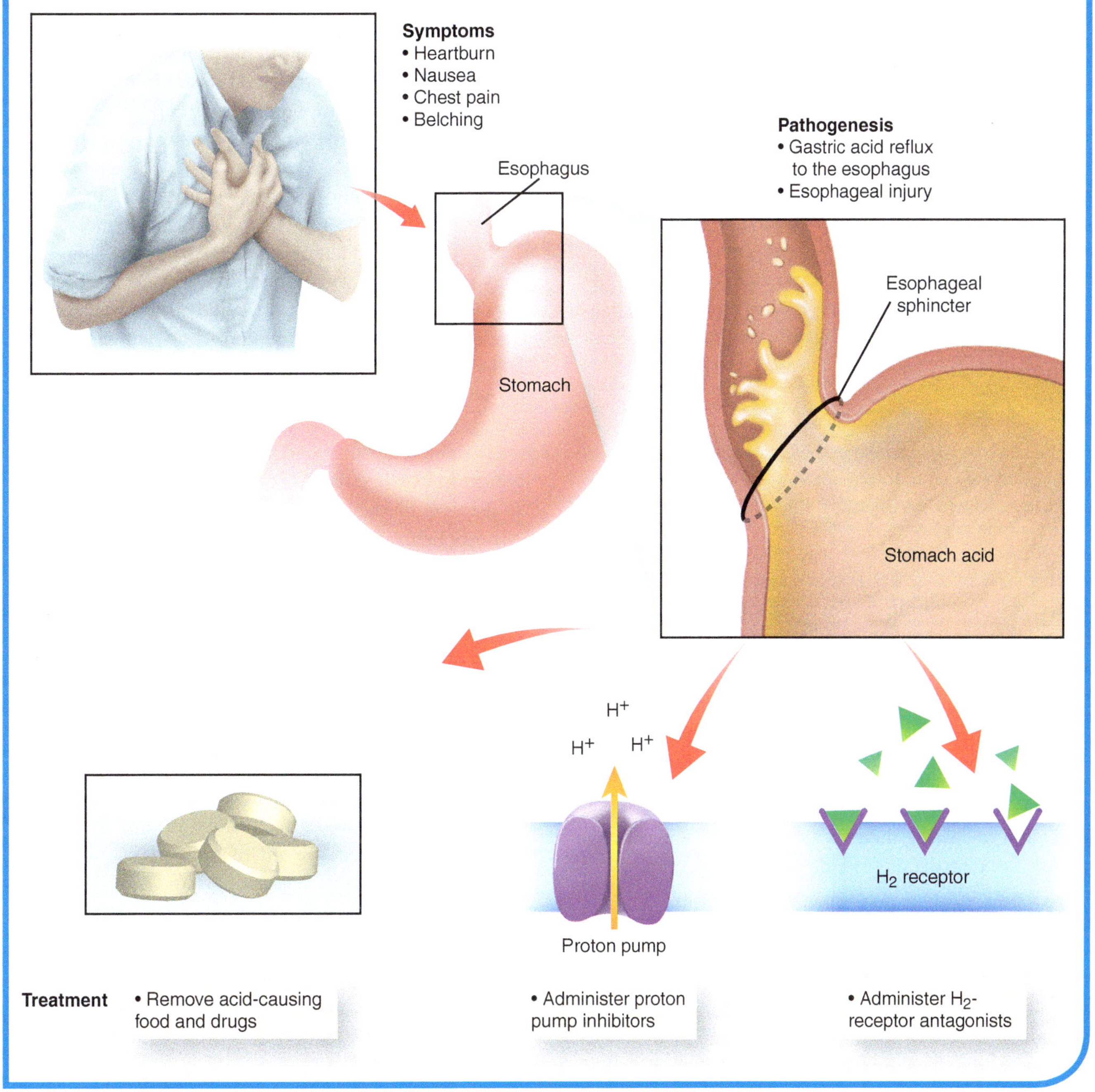

Symptoms of GERD include heartburn, dysphagia, dyspepsia, chest pain, nausea, and belching. Symptoms worsen following large meals, exercise, or when in a reclining or recumbent position. There is growing evidence that patients with GERD may also present with symptoms such as chronic cough, wheezing, bronchitis, sore throat, or hoarseness. GERD is a chronic condition with alternating periods of exacerbation and remission.

A large number of substances and conditions can worsen GERD symptoms. These include caffeine, alcohol, citrus fruits, tomato-based products, onions, carbonated beverages, spicy food, chocolate, smoking, pregnancy, and obesity. Certain medications may also contribute to or worsen GERD. They include nitrates, benzodiazepines, anticholinergics, beta blockers, alpha blockers, estrogen, progesterone, iron, calcium channel blockers, NSAIDs, tricyclic antidepressants, opioids, levodopa, bisphosphonates, and some chemotherapy drugs.

Left untreated, GERD can lead to complications such as esophagitis, esophageal ulcers, or strictures. Approximately 10% of patients diagnosed with GERD will develop **Barrett's esophagus**, a condition that is associated with an increased risk of esophageal cancer. Warning signs and symptoms of GERD that suggest a more complicated disease may include unexplained weight loss, early satiety, anemia, vomiting, initial onset of GERD symptoms after age 50, and prolonged anorexia or dysphagia. Patients who are experiencing these symptoms should notify their healthcare provider.

PharmFACT

Twenty-five to 40% of adults in the United States have GERD. Men are two to three times more likely to have the condition than women (Patti, 2019).

If a patient's GERD is associated with obesity, losing weight may eliminate the symptoms. Other lifestyle changes that can improve GERD symptoms include elevating the head of the bed, avoiding fatty or acidic foods, eating smaller meals at least 3 hours before sleep, and eliminating tobacco and alcohol use. Because patients often self-treat this disorder with OTC drugs, a good medication history may give clues to the presence of GERD. Also, patients should be informed that some medications can provoke GERD and reviewing their medication history may prove helpful. Because drugs provide only symptomatic relief, surgery may become necessary to eliminate the cause of persistent GERD.

Acid suppression currently remains the mainstay in the treatment of GERD. The presence of GERD does not warrant testing for *H. pylori* infection. Large studies have shown that neither the presence nor absence of *H. pylori* has any influence on the development of GERD.

Pharmacotherapy of Peptic Ulcer Disease and Gastroesophageal Reflux Disease

59.4 Peptic ulcer disease and gastroesophageal reflux disease are best treated with a combination of pharmacotherapy and lifestyle changes.

Before initiating pharmacotherapy, patients are usually advised to change lifestyle factors that may be contributing to the severity of PUD or GERD. For example, eliminating tobacco and alcohol use and reducing stress often allow healing of the ulcer and cause it to go into remission. Avoiding certain foods and beverages can lessen the severity of symptoms. For patients with GERD, losing weight may alleviate symptoms of the disorder.

The goals of PUD pharmacotherapy are to provide immediate relief from symptoms, promote healing of the ulcer, prevent complications, and prevent future recurrence of the disease. Eradication of *H. pylori* and discontinuing NSAIDs or other ulcer-promoting medications when possible are key factors.

For patients who are taking NSAIDs, the initial approach to PUD is to switch to an alternative medication, such as acetaminophen or another analgesic. This is not always possible, however, because NSAIDs are first-line drugs for treating chronic arthritis and other disorders associated with pain and inflammation. Those with a history of PUD should be advised to avoid NSAIDs in the future to prevent ulcer recurrences. If discontinuation of the NSAID is not possible, concurrent antiulcer drugs are indicated. Platelet inhibitors such as aspirin or clopidogrel should be used cautiously in patients at risk for ulcer complications.

Because the bacterium is strongly associated with PUD, diagnostic testing for *H. pylori* is conducted for all patients with active PUD or for those with chronic PUD who have never been tested. Various tests can be used, including a urea breath test, fecal antigen test, and tissue biopsy obtained during endoscopy. If PUD treatment includes only antiulcer drugs without eradicating *H. pylori*, a very high recurrence rate is observed. Some practitioners recommend *H. pylori* testing prior to initiating chronic NSAID therapy because eradicating *H. pylori* infection decreases the risk for peptic ulcers in many patients.

Once NSAIDs and *H. pylori* have been addressed, suppressing or neutralizing gastric acid is the aim of the pharmacologic treatment of both PUD and GERD. A wide variety of both prescription and OTC drugs are available to suppress acid secretion. The mechanisms of action of the major drug classes for PUD are shown in Pharmacotherapy Illustrated 59.2. These drugs fall into three primary classes and one miscellaneous group:

- Proton pump inhibitors
- H_2-receptor antagonists

- Antacids
- Miscellaneous drugs.

Because medications used to treat GERD and PUD suppress acid, keep in mind that certain nutrients and drugs need an acidic environment for complete absorption. For example, long-term acid suppression could lead to deficiencies in folic acid, iron, and vitamin B_{12}. Also, the effects of certain drugs such as fluconazole, tetracyclines, and indomethacin may be decreased because these drugs require an acidic environment for complete absorption.

Pharmacotherapy with Proton Pump Inhibitors

59.5 Proton pump inhibitors block gastric acid secretion and are preferred drugs for the therapy of peptic ulcer disease and gastroesophageal reflux disease.

The **proton pump inhibitors (PPIs)** act by blocking **H^+, K^+-ATPase**, the enzyme that is responsible for secreting hydrochloric acid in the stomach. PPIs are indicated for

Pharmacotherapy Illustrated 59.2

Mechanisms of Action of Antiulcer Drugs

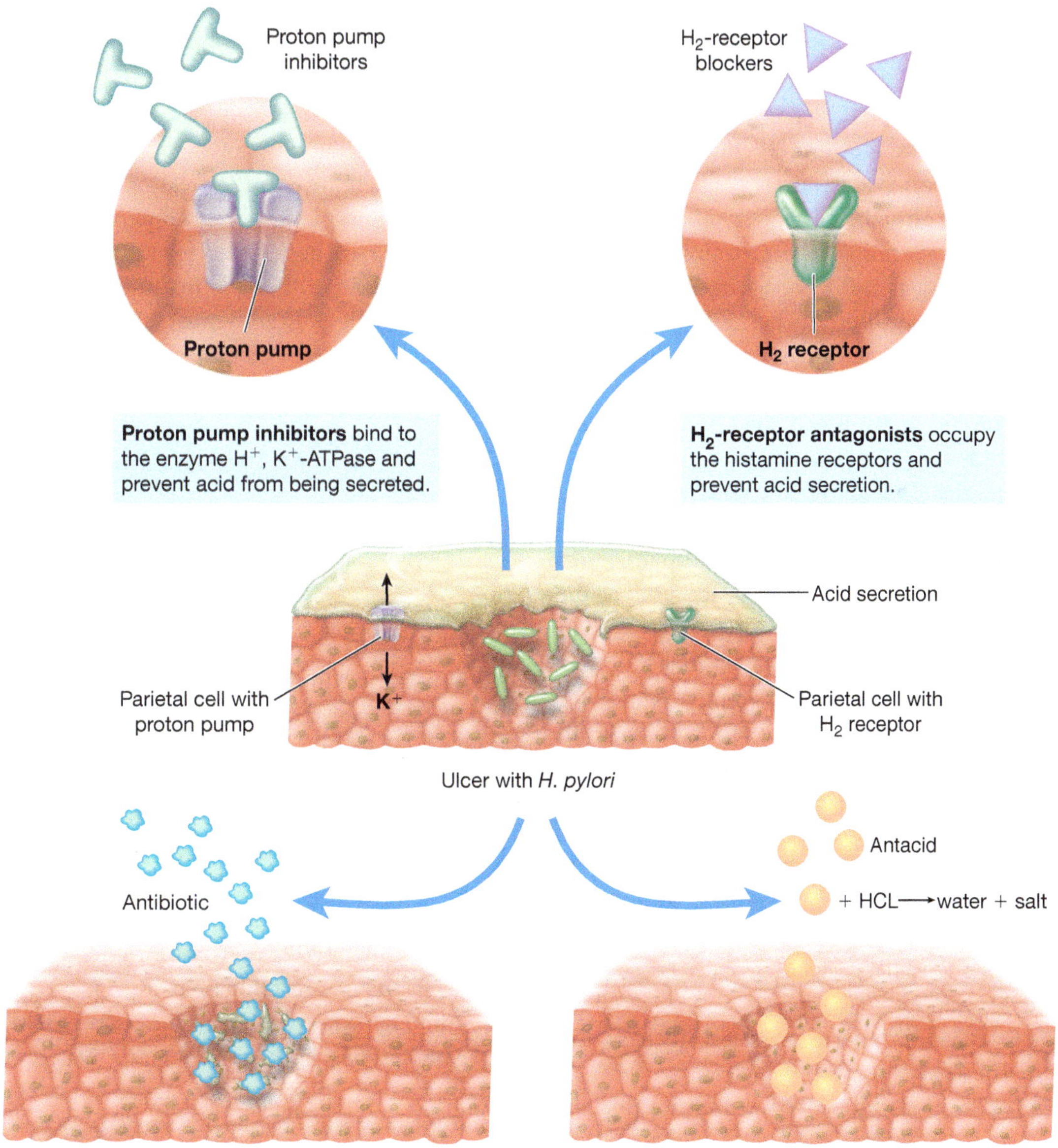

Proton pump inhibitors bind to the enzyme H^+, K^+-ATPase and prevent acid from being secreted.

H_2-receptor antagonists occupy the histamine receptors and prevent acid secretion.

Antibiotics eradicate *H. pylori*, the primary cause of peptic ulcers.

Alkaline antacids chemically combine with acids to increase stomach pH.

Table 59.1 Proton Pump Inhibitors

Drug	Route and Adult Dose (Maximum Dose Where Indicated)	Adverse Effects
esomeprazole (Nexium)	PO/IV: 20–40 mg once daily	*Diarrhea, headache, nausea, rash, abdominal pain* <u>Increased risk for osteoporosis-related fractures of the hip, wrist, or spine; acute interstitial nephritis</u>
lansoprazole (Prevacid) and dexlansoprazole (Dexilant)	PO (lansoprazole): 15–30 mg/day PO (dexlansoprazole): 60 mg once daily	
omeprazole (Prilosec)	PO: 20–60 mg daily or bid	
pantoprazole (Protonix)	PO: 20–40 mg daily IV: 40 mg daily for up to 7–10 days	
rabeprazole (AcipHex)	PO: 20–60 mg once daily	

Note: *Italics* indicate common adverse effects. <u>Underline</u> indicates serious adverse effects.

treatment of gastric and duodenal ulcers for 4 to 8 weeks, treatment of GERD, maintenance therapy to prevent recurrence, and treatment of ZES. Omeprazole, esomeprazole, and lansoprazole are available OTC. These and other PPIs are listed in Table 59.1.

PPIs reduce acid secretion in the stomach by binding irreversibly to the H^+, K^+-ATPase enzyme at the surface of the parietal cell, thereby blocking the final step in acid production. This enzyme acts as a pump to release acid (also called H^+, or protons) onto the surface of the GI mucosa. The PPIs reduce acid secretion to a greater extent than the H_2-receptor antagonists and have a longer duration of action. About 95% of the acid production is blocked, making the PPIs the most effective drugs for the maintenance therapy of acid-related disease.

Because the proton pump is activated by food intake, the PPI should be taken 20 to 30 minutes before the first major meal of the day. This allows the peak serum drug levels to coincide with the time at which the proton pumps are activated. PPIs are formulated in a delayed-release formation because the drug would be destroyed in the acidic environment of the stomach.

Although the PPIs have a short serum half-life, they continue to suppress acid for about 24 hours because the inactivation of the proton pump is irreversible. Because not all of the proton pumps are inactivated with the first dose, several days of PPI therapy are needed to achieve maximal acid inhibition. Beneficial effects continue for 3 to 5 days after the drugs have been discontinued. The PPIs are highly protein bound, metabolized in the liver, and excreted in the urine (80%) and feces (20%). Doses do not need to be adjusted for patients with renal insufficiency because there is negligible renal clearance.

All drugs in this class have similar effectiveness and adverse effects. The incidence of adverse effects with PPIs is very low, with headache, abdominal pain, diarrhea (including that associated with *Clostrioides difficile*), and nausea and vomiting being the most commonly reported ones. Rashes and blood dyscrasias are rare. Rebound hypersecretion of acid does not appear to occur after the drugs are discontinued. PPIs can mask an *H. pylori* infection because of the marked reduction in the bacterial load that they initiate. Long-term therapy with PPIs increases the risk for osteoporosis-related fractures, perhaps due to their interference with calcium absorption. Some healthcare providers recommend calcium supplements during therapy to prevent these types of fractures.

PPIs heal more than 90% of duodenal ulcers within 4 weeks and about 90% of gastric ulcers in 6 to 8 weeks. GERD may require 8 to 12 weeks of therapy for symptoms to diminish, and long-term maintenance therapy may be needed. PPIs are best suited for the long-term prevention of heartburn rather than the treatment of acute symptoms. In patients with PUD who must take NSAIDs for a chronic pain or inflammatory condition, PPIs taken once daily are effective in reducing the incidence of ulcers.

PROTOTYPE DRUG Omeprazole (Prilosec)

Classification **Therapeutic:** Antiulcer drug
Pharmacologic: Proton pump inhibitor

Therapeutic Effects and Uses: Omeprazole was the first PPI to be approved by the U.S. Food and Drug Administration in 1989 and is available by prescription and OTC. By prescription it is approved for the short-term, 4- to 8-week therapy of active duodenal and gastric ulcers, GERD, and maintenance of erosive esophagitis. OTC, it is indicated for the relief of heartburn. Most patients are symptom free after 2 weeks of therapy. It is used for longer periods and in higher doses in patients who have ZES. It is combined with antibiotics in regimens for eliminating *H. pylori*. Omeprazole may be prescribed off-label to prevent PUD in patients taking NSAIDs.

Although omeprazole can take 2 hours to reach therapeutic levels, its effects last up to 72 hours. Omeprazole is available by the oral (PO) route and is approved for pediatric use in children age 2 years and older. Zegerid is a combination drug that contains omeprazole and the antacid sodium bicarbonate. Yosprala is a drug containing omeprazole with aspirin.

Mechanism of Action: Omeprazole reduces acid secretion in the stomach by binding irreversibly to the enzyme

CONNECTIONS: Advanced Practice Application

Treating GERD

Case

Ginny McCarthy is a self-employed child care provider without health insurance. She is a 42-year-old mother of two who has been in good health, has never smoked, and rarely (less than once a month) drinks. She has no change in diet and no change in bowel habits. She exercises three times a week and is active with her own children and the children she watches in her home. Three months ago, she began experiencing episodes of chest pain that occur mostly after meals and during the night, when she lies down. During the past month she has experienced worsening symptoms and noticed a bad taste in her mouth. Ginny presented to the community clinic for care.

Ginny's medical history and physical examination were consistent with GERD. However, because of the complaints of chest pain, she should undergo a cardiac stress test to look for signs of coronary artery disease. Because she is under the age of 50 and does not have a history of weight loss, endoscopy to rule out cancer of the stomach or esophagus is not the standard of care and would not be indicated for Ginny. When Ginny asked about the cost of the cardiac stress test, you told her it would be $500 or more. She looked worried and stated that she could not afford to pay that. A discussion ensued, and although the standard approach for managing such a presentation involved ruling out cardiac disease, Ginny's symptoms were highly suggestive of being GI and not cardiac in nature.

The decision was to treat Ginny for GERD by starting a PPI, omeprazole 20 mg/day, at a cost of $15 per month and educating her about foods that would worsen her symptoms. You also taught her that she should elevate the head of her bed at night and should sit upright for 30 minutes after eating or drinking. You tell Ginny that she requires a follow-up in 2 weeks to make sure symptoms are improving. Additionally, you educated Ginny about cardiac symptoms that would require an immediate visit to the emergency department.

Discussion

With nearly 28 million uninsured people and even more people who are underinsured in the United States, many providers are confronted with patients who cannot afford the high cost of healthcare. When patients lack sufficient healthcare insurance, financial matters become intertwined in the process of clinical decision making. Providers should explicitly ask patients about financial concerns and be knowledgeable about the community resources available for the medically indigent.

Treating Ginny with a PPI, diet education, and environmental considerations such as elevation of the head of the bed and sitting upright for 30 minutes after eating or drinking, combined with medical follow-up and instructions on when to seek additional emergency care, is appropriate in this particular case. Clinical judgment using medical history and physical examination considerations is needed on a case-by-case basis.

H^+, K^+-ATPase. It inhibits the final pathway involved in acid secretion and effectively inhibits the active proton pumps.

Pharmacokinetics:

Route(s)	PO
Absorption	Rapidly absorbed; food does not influence bioavailability
Distribution	Bioavailability after oral dosing: 50–60%; crosses the placenta; secreted in breast milk; 95% bound to plasma protein
Primary metabolism	Hepatic; significant first-pass effect due to metabolism by CYP2C19
Primary excretion	Renal with small amounts in bile
Onset of action	0.5–3.5 h
Duration of action	3–4 days; half-life: 0.5–1.5 h

Adverse Effects: PPIs are generally well-tolerated with the most common adverse effects being headache, nausea, diarrhea, rash, and abdominal pain. Long term therapy is associated with atrophic gastritis and an increased risk for osteoporosis-related fractures. Delayed-release omeprazole has been associated with an increased risk of *C. difficile*–associated diarrhea (CDAD) in hospitalized patients.

Contraindications/Precautions: The only contraindication is hypersensitivity to the drug. It is not recommended for children under 1 year of age. Patients with hepatic impairment should be treated with caution.

Drug Interactions: Clinically significant interactions with PPIs are uncommon. Omeprazole has been shown to both inhibit and induce certain hepatic CYP450 enzyme systems. Therefore, concurrent use with other drugs using the CYP450 system—including warfarin, carbamazepine, diazepam, and phenytoin—may inhibit or delay metabolism and cause increased blood levels of these drugs. Concurrent use of omeprazole and clopidogrel reduces the conversion of clopidogrel to its active metabolite, thus reducing its effectiveness. Thus, concurrent use with warfarin may increase the likelihood of bleeding. Coadministration of omeprazole and clarithromycin has been shown to increase plasma levels of both omeprazole and clarithromycin.

PPIs increase gastric pH and have the potential to affect the bioavailability of medications that depend on a lower pH for absorption (e.g., iron salts, digoxin, ampicillin, ketoconazole, atazanavir, rilpivirine). Because an acidic environment promotes mineral absorption, mineral deficiencies could occur with long-term PPI use. Decreased vitamin B_{12} absorption may occur because an acid is optimal for vitamin B_{12} absorption. **Herbal/Food:** Ginkgo and St. John's wort may decrease the plasma concentration of omeprazole.

Pregnancy: Some animal studies showed increased embryofetal lethality, whereas others did not. Human data does not show increased teratogenicity above baseline levels. Small amounts of omeprazole are secreted in human milk but adverse effects on the breastfed neonate are unknown.

Treatment for Overdose: Overdose is uncommon and is treated symptomatically.

Clinician Responsibilities: Key clinical implications for patients receiving omeprazole are included in Applied Clinical Judgment: Patients Receiving Pharmacotherapy for Peptic Ulcer Disease.

Drugs Similar to Omeprazole (Prilosec)

The other PPIs include esomeprazole, lansoprazole, pantoprazole, and rabeprazole. Pregnancy data for these PPIs are the same as for omeprazole.

Esomeprazole (Nexium): Approved in 2001, this drug is an isomer of omeprazole, making the two medications very similar in structure, effectiveness, and safety. It is available by the PO and intravenous (IV) routes. Adverse effects include headache, diarrhea, and nausea. Similar to other PPIs, esomeprazole is available as once-daily dosing for uncomplicated PUD and GERD and twice-daily dosing for complicated conditions such as ZES. It is approved for the prophylaxis of ulcers in patients who are taking NSAIDs. Esomeprazole capsules can be opened and the pellets mixed with soft foods and swallowed without chewing. With all PPIs there is a risk of pneumonia due to the elevation in gastric pH. Long-term use (more than 3 years) may lead to vitamin B_{12} deficiency.

Lansoprazole (Prevacid) and dexlansoprazole (Dexilant): Approved in 1995, lansoprazole has a similar effectiveness and safety profile to omeprazole and is available by the PO route. Its antisecretory effects can last up to 24 hours. Similar to other PPIs, its adverse effects include headache, diarrhea, and nausea. As with other PPIs, lansoprazole offers once-daily dosing for uncomplicated PUD and GERD and twice-daily dosing for ZES. With lansoprazole, as with other PPIs, there is a risk of pneumonia due to the elevation in gastric pH. This drug is eliminated from the body by the biliary system. It is available by prescription as well as OTC.

For patients who have difficulty swallowing capsules, lansoprazole is available in an oral liquid suspension or as a PO disintegrating tablet (Prevacid SoluTab) that is placed under the tongue and disintegrates within 1 minute. Capsules of lansoprazole should be swallowed whole and not crushed or split. Dexlansoprazole (Dexilant) is a stereoisomer of lansoprazole that has identical effects to its parent drug.

Pantoprazole (Protonix): Approved in 2000, pantoprazole has a similar efficacy and safety profile to omeprazole and is available by PO and IV routes. Adverse effects include headache, diarrhea, and nausea. Because pantoprazole does not inhibit CYP450 enzymes, it is less likely to affect the metabolism of other drugs.

As with the other PPIs, pantoprazole offers once-daily dosing for uncomplicated PUD and GERD and twice-daily dosing for ZES. With all PPIs, there is a risk of pneumonia due to the elevation in gastric pH. Pantoprazole may be prescribed off-label to prevent ulcers in patients taking NSAIDs.

Rabeprazole (AcipHex): Although rabeprazole is similar to omeprazole, it causes reversible inhibition of the proton pump; thus, its effects are of shorter duration. Approved in 1999, rabeprazole is available by the PO route. The tablets should be swallowed whole and not crushed or chewed. Like other PPIs, rabeprazole accentuates the eradication of *H. pylori* when used with appropriate antibiotics. Although rabeprazole is metabolized by the hepatic CYP450 drug-metabolizing system, it exhibits few significant drug interactions. Adverse effects are mild and transient and include headache, diarrhea, nausea, malaise, dizziness, and rash.

CONNECTIONS: Lifespan Considerations

Use of Proton Pump Inhibitors in the Older Adult

PPIs have been associated with an increased risk for osteoporosis, decreased kidney function, and an increased risk of CDAD in older adults (Huntsberry et al., 2019; Pezeshkian & Conway, 2018). Long-term use has also been considered as a possible cause of iron and vitamin B_{12} deficiencies. Because age-related changes in the gastric acid levels of older adults may also explain these conditions, the links are not always conclusive. Risk-reduction strategies to avoid long-term complications such as osteoporosis, iron and vitamin B_{12} deficiencies, and kidney-related adverse effects in the older adult include increasing the intake of calcium and magnesium, increasing fluid intake and reducing the intake of carbonated soft drinks, increasing weight-bearing exercise to a minimum of three times weekly, and increasing intake of iron and vitamin B_{12}–rich foods such as meats, fish, fortified cereals, and green leafy vegetables. It is recommended that PPIs be prescribed for the shortest amount of time possible at the lowest dose possible (Pezeshkian & Conway, 2018).

Pharmacotherapy with H_2-Receptor Antagonists

59.6 The H_2-receptor antagonists suppress gastric acid secretion and are widely prescribed for treating peptic ulcer disease and gastroesophageal reflux disease.

The discovery of the **H_2-receptor antagonists**, or H_2 blockers, marked a major breakthrough in the treatment of PUD. Once available only by prescription, they are now OTC and are used extensively in the treatment of mild to moderate hyperacidity disorders of the GI tract. H_2-receptor antagonists are indicated for treatment of PUD and GERD to promote healing and prevent recurrence. Duodenal ulcers usually heal in 6 to 8 weeks, but gastric ulcers may require up to 12 weeks of therapy. All of the H_2-receptor antagonists are available OTC for the short-term (2 weeks) treatment of heartburn. These drugs are listed in Table 59.2.

Histamine has two types of receptors: H_1 and H_2. Activation of the H_1 receptors produces the classic symptoms of inflammation and allergy, whereas the H_2 receptors, which are located on the parietal cells in the stomach, promote gastric acid secretion when activated. The H_2-receptor antagonists effectively reduce both fasting and food-stimulated secretion and are also helpful in decreasing nocturnal acid secretion, which is largely dependent on histamine.

Pharmacokinetic properties of drugs in this class include rapid absorption from the small intestine, which is not affected by food, and a 30-minute onset of action. These drugs undergo hepatic metabolism and renal excretion, and their half-lives range from 1 to 4 hours. Although there are no known harmful effects on the fetus, these drugs cross the placenta and are secreted in breast milk. All drugs in this class have similar safety profiles: Their adverse effects are minor and rarely cause discontinuation of therapy. Patients who are receiving higher doses, those with chronic kidney disease (CKD) or hepatic disease, or older adults may experience confusion, restlessness, hallucinations, or depression. With moderate to severe kidney disease, doses of H_2-receptor antagonists should be cut in half to avoid toxicity. Antacids should not be taken at the same time as H_2-receptor antagonists because absorption is diminished.

PROTOTYPE DRUG Famotidine (Pepcid AC)

Classification **Therapeutic:** Antiulcer drug
Pharmacologic: H_2-receptor antagonist

Therapeutic Effects and Uses: Approved in 1986, famotidine has a higher potency than cimetidine, which allows it to be administered PO, once daily, usually at bedtime. It is approved to treat active PUD and gastric ulcers, GERD, erosive esophagitis, and hypersecretory disorders. Adequate healing of the ulcer takes 4 to 8 weeks, although those at high risk for PUD may continue on drug maintenance for prolonged periods to prevent recurrence. Gastric ulcers heal more slowly than duodenal ulcers and thus require longer therapy. An IV form is available for the treatment of acute stress-induced bleeding ulcers or hypersecretory conditions in hospitalized patients. Chewable tablets available OTC combine famotidine with calcium and magnesium salts.

Mechanism of Action: Famotidine acts by blocking H_2 receptors on the parietal cells in the stomach to decrease acid production. Both daytime and nocturnal basal gastric acids are suppressed.

Pharmacokinetics:

Route(s)	PO, IV
Absorption	Rapid absorption following PO administration; both routes achieve comparable blood levels
Distribution	PO bioavailability is approximately 50%; very little enters the central nervous system (CNS); crosses the placenta; secreted in breast milk; 20% bound to plasma protein
Primary metabolism	Minimal hepatic metabolism

Table 59.2 H_2-Receptor Antagonists

Drug	Route and Adult Dose (Maximum Dose Where Indicated)	Adverse Effects
cimetidine (Tagamet)	Active ulcers: PO: 300 mg q6h or 800 mg at bedtime IV: 300 mg q6h or 37.5 mg/h by continuous infusion GERD: 400 mg q6h or 800 mg bid	*Diarrhea, constipation, headache, fatigue, nausea, gynecomastia* Rare: hepatitis, blood dyscrasias, anaphylaxis, dysrhythmias, skin reactions, galactorrhea, confusion, or psychoses
famotidine (Pepcid)	Active ulcers: PO: 20–40 mg/day GERD: PO: 20 mg bid for 6 wk IV: 20 mg q12h	*Headache, nausea, dry mouth* Rare: musculoskeletal pain, tachycardia, blood dyscrasias, blurred vision
nizatidine	Active ulcers: PO: 150–300 mg once daily GERD: PO: 150 mg bid	

Note: *Italics* indicate common adverse effects. Underline indicates serious adverse effects.

Primary excretion	Renal (mostly unchanged)
Onset of action	30–60 min; peak effect: 2–4 h
Duration of action	6–12 h; half-life: 2–4 h

Adverse Effects: Adverse effects are uncommon and transient. Although rare, blood dyscrasias, especially neutropenia and thrombocytopenia, have been reported; thus, periodic blood counts should be performed. Confusion may occur rarely and is usually in the older patient or with IV dosing. High doses may result in gynecomastia, impotence, or loss of libido in men, although these effects are more common with cimetidine.

Contraindications/Precautions: Contraindications include hypersensitivity to H_2-receptor antagonists. The drug should be used with caution in patients with CKD. If dosages are not reduced, patients with CKD may experience prolonged QT intervals and episodes of confusion, hallucinations, or agitation.

Drug Interactions: Because famotidine has much less affinity for CYP450 enzymes, it is less likely to participate in drug–drug interactions than cimetidine. Famotidine may reduce the absorption of cefpodoxime, ketoconazole, and itraconazole because of the increase in gastric pH induced by H_2-receptor antagonists. Concurrent use can increase the effects of alcohol, sulfonylureas, salicylates, and warfarin. Antacids should not be given within 1 hour of H_2-receptor antagonists because their effectiveness may be decreased due to reduced absorption. Smoking decreases the effectiveness of famotidine. **Herbal/Food:** Absorption of vitamin B_{12} depends on an acidic environment, so deficiency may occur. Iron is also better absorbed in an acidic environment.

Pregnancy: Animal studies showed no evidence of fetal harm. Small amounts are secreted in human milk although adverse effects on the breastfed infant are unknown.

Treatment of Overdose: Overdose is uncommon and is treated symptomatically.

Clinician Responsibilities: Key clinical implications for patients receiving famotidine are included in Applied Clinical Judgment: Patients Receiving Pharmacotherapy for Peptic Ulcer Disease.

Drugs Similar to Famotidine (Pepcid AC)

Other H_2-receptor antagonists include cimetidine and nizatidine. The former prototype for this class was ranitidine (Zantac). In 2019, all medications containing ranitidine were withdrawn from the United States and Canadian markets because a probable carcinogen, N-nitrosodimethylamine was found in these products. Drugs in this class have not shown evidence of fetal harm in laboratory animals. Small amounts are secreted in human milk, but adverse effects on the breastfed neonate are unknown.

Cimetidine (Tagamet): Approved in 1977, cimetidine was the first of the H_2 blockers. It is used less frequently than other drugs in this class because (1) it inhibits hepatic drug-metabolizing enzymes and exhibits numerous drug–drug interactions, (2) it has a high incidence of adverse effects, and (3) it must be taken up to four times a day. Because cimetidine interacts with CYP450 enzymes, it may affect the metabolism of many drugs metabolized in the liver, including warfarin, phenytoin, diazepam, and opioids. Cimetidine also acts as an antiandrogen and may cause gynecomastia or sexual dysfunction in men. Cimetidine crosses the blood–brain barrier and therefore is more likely to cause CNS depression and confusion than the other H_2-receptor antagonists. A low-dose OTC preparation is available. Routes of administration include PO, IM, and IV.

Nizatidine: Although thought to have a safety and adverse effect profile similar to that of famotidine, nizatidine is not metabolized by the liver CYP450 enzyme system and therefore causes fewer drug–drug interactions. Adverse effects are infrequent and transient. Nizatidine is available PO and indicated for up to 8 weeks of PUD therapy or 12 weeks for GERD. Prescription nizatidine was approved in 1988 and an OTC preparation (Axid AR) is also available.

CONNECTION Checkpoint 59.1

From what you learned in Chapter 3, how is the excretion of drugs affected when they are metabolized through the hepatic CYP450 system?

Pharmacotherapy with Antacids

59.7 Antacids are alkaline substances that neutralize stomach acid to treat symptoms of heartburn.

Prior to the development of H_2-receptor antagonists and PPIs, antacids were the mainstay of peptic ulcer and GERD pharmacotherapy. Indeed, many patients still use these inexpensive and readily available OTC drugs. Antacids may provide temporary relief from heartburn or indigestion, but they are no longer recommended as the primary drug class for acid-related disorders. Although antacids relieve symptoms of heartburn, they do not promote ulcer healing or help to eliminate *H. pylori*. These drugs are listed in Table 59.3.

Antacids are inorganic compounds containing aluminum, magnesium, sodium, or calcium that neutralize gastric acid and inactivate pepsin. They are also thought to stimulate prostaglandin production in the mucosa and increase LES tone, which reduces gastroesophageal reflux. These drugs do not protect the stomach by coating the stomach wall. To be considered therapeutic, the dose of antacids should increase the gastric pH to a minimum of 3.5.

Table 59.3 Antacids

Drug	Route and Adult Dose (Maximum Dose Where Indicated)	Adverse Effects
aluminum hydroxide (AlternaGEL, others)	PO: 600 mg tid–qid	*Constipation, nausea* Fecal impaction, hypophosphatemia with chronic use
calcium carbonate (Titralac, Tums)	PO: 1–2 g bid–tid	*Constipation, flatulence* Fecal impaction, metabolic alkalosis, hypercalcemia, renal calculi
calcium carbonate with magnesium hydroxide (Mylanta Supreme, Rolaids)	PO: 2–4 capsules or tablets prn (max: 12 tablets/day)	
magaldrate (Riopan)	PO: 540–1080 mg/day (5–10 mL suspension or 1–2 tablets) (max: 20 tablets or 100 mL/day)	*Diarrhea, nausea and vomiting, abdominal cramping* Hypermagnesemia (in patients with CKD), dysrhythmias (when given parenterally)
magnesium hydroxide (Milk of Magnesia)	PO: 5–15 mL or 2–4 tablets up to 4 times daily	
magnesium hydroxide and aluminum hydroxide with simethicone (Mylanta, Maalox Plus, others)	PO: 10–20 mL (max: 120 mL/day) or 2–4 tablets (max: 24 tablets/day)	
magnesium trisilicate and aluminum hydroxide (Gaviscon)	PO: 2–4 tablets (max: 16 tablets/day)	
sodium bicarbonate (Alka-Seltzer, baking soda)	PO: 325 mg–2 g 1–4 times/day	*Abdominal distention, belching* Metabolic alkalosis, fluid retention, edema, hypernatremia

Note: *Italics* indicate common adverse effects. Underline indicates serious adverse effects.

Self-medication with antacids is safe when taken in doses as directed on the labels. Although antacids act within 10 to 15 minutes, their duration of action is only 2 hours; thus, they must be taken often during the day. Combinations of aluminum hydroxide and magnesium hydroxide, the most common types, are capable of rapidly neutralizing stomach acid.

All the antacids are equally effective at neutralizing acid and reducing symptoms of heartburn when given in therapeutic doses. Each type has certain disadvantages that may preclude their use:

- *Sodium.* Antacids that contain sodium should not be taken by patients on sodium-restricted diets or by those with hypertension (HTN), heart failure, or CKD because they may promote fluid retention.
- *Magnesium.* Absorption of magnesium from high doses of magnesium-containing antacids can cause symptoms of hypermagnesemia (fatigue, hypotension, and dysrhythmias). Magnesium also acts as a laxative when it reaches the large intestine.
- *Calcium.* Antacids that contain calcium can cause constipation and may cause or aggravate kidney stones. When absorbed, hypercalcemia is possible, and kidney failure may occur at very high doses. Administering calcium carbonate antacids with milk or any items with vitamin D can cause **milk-alkali syndrome** to occur. Early symptoms are the same as those of hypercalcemia and include headache, urinary frequency, anorexia, nausea, and fatigue. Milk-alkali syndrome may result in permanent kidney damage if the drug is continued at high doses.
- *Aluminum.* Aluminum antacids are not absorbed to any great extent, but they can cause constipation. The constipation effect is balanced when aluminum is combined with magnesium salts. Aluminum carbonate and aluminum hydroxide may interfere with dietary phosphate absorption to cause hypophosphatemia.
- *Bicarbonate.* Being a base, antacids that contain bicarbonate may provoke metabolic alkalosis (e.g., fatigue, mental status changes, muscle twitching, depressed respiratory rate) in patients at risk. Bicarbonate combines with gastric acid to form carbon dioxide, which causes bloating and belching.

Drug interactions with antacids occur by several mechanisms. Because antacids increase stomach pH, they affect the solubility and absorption of many oral drugs. Drugs that are weak acids are nonionized in the acidic environment of the stomach and are thus readily absorbed. If an antacid is given concurrently with a weak acid, the pH of the stomach will rise and result in a more ionized drug that is less readily absorbed. On the other hand, a drug that is a weak base is absorbed in a more alkaline medium. In other words, when taken with antacids, acidic drugs may have less therapeutic effect, and basic drugs may exhibit a greater effect. Examples of acidic drugs include NSAIDs, sulfonylureas, salicylates, warfarin, barbiturates, isoniazid, and digoxin. Basic drugs include morphine sulfate, antihistamines, tricyclic antidepressants, amphetamines, and quinidine.

Enteric-coated or delayed-release drugs are designed to dissolve when they reach the alkaline environment in the small intestine. By raising the pH of the stomach, antacids may "fool" enteric-coated tablets into dissolving early and releasing their contents into the stomach. The drug may either irritate the stomach lining, causing nausea or vomiting, or be inactivated.

Drug interactions may also occur if the antacid physically binds to other drugs. For example, certain antacids form chemical complexes with tetracyclines, preventing the antibiotic from being absorbed. Digoxin is another drug whose absorption is affected by binding to antacids.

A third mechanism of drug interaction is due to the effects of antacids on urine pH. Making the urine pH more alkaline increases the excretion of acidic drugs such as aspirin and inhibits the excretion of basic drugs such as amphetamines.

Because antacids are widely used OTC by patients for self-treatment, nurses must emphasize that these drugs should be used only as directed on the label due to the potential for adverse effects. To decrease the potential for antacid–drug interactions, nurses should advise that other medications be taken at least 1 hour before or 2 hours after giving an antacid.

PROTOTYPE DRUG **Aluminum Hydroxide (AlternaGEL, Others)**

Classification **Therapeutic:** Antiheartburn drug
Pharmacologic: Antacid

Therapeutic Effects and Uses: Aluminum hydroxide is an inorganic drug used alone or in combination with other antacids such as magnesium hydroxide. Combining aluminum compounds with magnesium (Gaviscon, Maalox, Mylanta) increases their effectiveness and reduces the potential for constipation. Unlike calcium-based antacids that can be absorbed and cause systemic effects, aluminum compounds are minimally absorbed. Their primary action is to neutralize stomach acid by raising the pH of the stomach contents. Unlike H_2-receptor antagonists and PPIs, aluminum antacids do not reduce the volume of acid secretion. They are most effectively used in combination with other antiulcer drugs for the symptomatic relief of heartburn due to PUD or GERD. A second aluminum salt, aluminum carbonate (Basaljel), is also available to treat heartburn.

Mechanism of Action: Aluminum hydroxide combines with gastric (hydrochloric) acid to produce aluminum chloride and water. This raises the pH of the stomach contents and inactivates pepsin.

Pharmacokinetics:

Route(s)	PO
Absorption	17–30% absorbed
Distribution	Widely distributed
Primary metabolism	Hepatic
Primary excretion	Renal
Onset of action	20–40 min
Duration of action	2 h when taken with food; 3 h when taken 1 h after meals

Adverse Effects: Aluminum antacids frequently cause constipation. At high doses aluminum products bind with phosphate in the GI tract and long-term use can result in phosphate depletion. Those at risk include people who are malnourished, those who have alcoholism, and those with CKD. The antacids are often combined with magnesium compounds, which counteract the constipation commonly experienced with aluminum antacids.

Contraindications/Precautions: Prolonged use in patients with low serum phosphate levels should be avoided. This drug should not be used in patients with suspected bowel obstruction.

Drug Interactions: Aluminum compounds should not be taken with other medications because they may interfere with their absorption. Concurrent use decreases the absorption of cimetidine, ciprofloxacin and other fluoroquinolones, digoxin, isoniazid, chloroquine, NSAIDs, iron salts, phenytoin, tetracycline, and thyroxine. Use with sodium polystyrene sulfonate may cause systemic alkalosis. Use of anticholinergic drugs can increase the effects of antacids. **Herbal/Food:** Aluminum antacids may inhibit the absorption of dietary iron.

Pregnancy: At clinically relevant doses, aluminum hydroxide has not shown fetal harm or adverse effects on breastfeeding.

Treatment of Overdose: There is no specific treatment for overdose.

Clinician Responsibilities: Key clinical implications for patients receiving aluminum hydroxide are included in Applied Clinical Judgment: Patients Receiving Pharmacotherapy for Peptic Ulcer Disease.

Drugs Similar to Aluminum Hydroxide (AlternaGEL, Others)

All aluminum salts have similar effects to those of aluminum hydroxide.

Pharmacotherapy of *Helicobacter pylori* Infection

59.8 The bacterium *H. pylori* is associated with approximately 70% of patients with peptic ulcer disease.

It is estimated that 60 to 80% of patients with duodenal ulcers are infected with *H. pylori* and that the majority of patients with gastric ulcers have the bacterium. Research has shown that the eradication of *H. pylori* decreases the recurrence of PUD. Risk factors for *H. pylori* include residing in a developing country, domestic crowding, unclean water, and exposure to the gastric contents of an infected individual.

H. pylori is the only known microorganism that has been found to survive the hostile conditions in the stomach. In fact, it has adapted well to the stomach's acidic environment. It has devised ways to neutralize the high acidity surrounding it and make chemicals called **adhesins** that allow the organism to penetrate the GI mucosa and alter the epithelial cell structure, which initiates inflammation. The inflammatory and immune responses lead to the chronic production of inflammatory cells, including lymphocytes, plasma cells, and macrophages. This response then leads to the formation of immunoglobulin G antibodies and increased production of cytokines, including interleukins and tumor necrosis factor, all of which contribute to the inflammation of the gastric mucosa. Increased gastrin secretion and decreased bicarbonate production also play a role in ulcer formation caused by *H. pylori*.

Another mechanism involves ammonia. *H. pylori* produces large amounts of urease, an enzyme that breaks down urea to ammonia and carbon monoxide. Ammonia neutralizes the acid around the bacterium and allows *H. pylori* to survive in the acidic environment of the stomach. Unfortunately, the ammonia is toxic to mucosal cells and erodes the mucous barrier. *H. pylori* then finds its home in the submucosal layer of the stomach, producing damage to the gastric and duodenal mucosae, which allows pepsin and gastric acid to further damage the mucosae. There may also be a genetic predisposition that determines one's susceptibility to *H. pylori* infection.

Prior to the identification of the link between *H. pylori* and ulcers, the first-line therapy for PUD was acid-reducing drugs. Although acid-reducers are effective at treating symptoms, the majority of patients experience relapses. This is because the acid-reducing drugs have little effect on *H. pylori*, which can remain active for life if not treated appropriately. Thus, for infected patients, elimination of this bacterium is the prime pharmacologic objective. Eradication of *H. pylori* allows ulcers to heal more rapidly and remain in remission longer, often permanently.

A combination of antibiotics is used concurrently to eradicate *H. pylori* and help decrease antibiotic resistance. A PPI or bismuth compound is usually included in the regimen. Once eliminated from the stomach, reinfection with *H. pylori* is uncommon. Suggested regimens include the following (Chey et al., 2017):

- **Initial regimen.** Omeprazole, clarithromycin, and amoxicillin
- **Alternative regimens.**
  - Omeprazole (or other PPI), clarithromycin, and metronidazole, or
  - Omeprazole (or other PPI), bismuth subsalicylate (Pepto-Bismol), metronidazole, and tetracycline.

Although technically not antibiotics, bismuth compounds inhibit bacterial growth by disrupting their cell wall and preventing *H. pylori* from adhering to the gastric mucosa. The PPI further suppresses *H. pylori*, and the increased pH that results from PPI administration creates a hostile environment for *H. pylori*, thus enhancing the effectiveness of the antibiotics.

H. pylori therapy continues for 10 to 14 days. Should resistance occur, rifabutin (Mycobutin) and fluoroquinolones may be used as part of the regimen. Drug regimens continue to evolve as antibiotic resistance patterns change.

Indiscriminate use of antibiotics can lead to antibiotic resistance; thus, patients should be tested for *H. pylori* before initiating treatment for infection. Patient adherence is vital to the successful eradication of *H. pylori*. Patients should be instructed on the importance of completing the drug regimen because discontinuing the anti-infectives too soon may result in reinfection. Four weeks after completion of therapy, patients are retested for the presence of *H. pylori* to confirm the success of the treatment.

CONNECTION Checkpoint 59.2

From what you learned in Chapter 46, explain why antibiotic resistance has become a major public health problem throughout the world.

Miscellaneous Drugs Used for Peptic Ulcer Disease and Gastroesophageal Reflux Disease

59.9 Several miscellaneous drugs, including sucralfate, bismuth subsalicylate, and misoprostol, are beneficial in treating peptic ulcer disease.

A few additional drugs are used in the pharmacotherapy of PUD and GERD. These drugs act by mechanisms other than the ones described for PPIs, H_2-receptor blockers, or antacids.

Sucralfate: Sucralfate (Carafate) is a PO medication that consists of sucrose (a sugar) plus aluminum hydroxide (an antacid). This drug stimulates mucus, bicarbonate, and prostaglandin secretion, all of which enhance mucosal defenses. Sucralfate also acts locally to produce a thick protective barrier that coats and binds to the ulcer, protecting it against further erosion from acid and pepsin to promote healing. It does not affect the secretion of gastric acid. It is intended for short-term therapy (up to 8 weeks). It is sometimes used in critically ill patients to prevent bleeding from stress-related gastritis. Sucralfate is not effective in preventing NSAID-related ulcers.

Other than constipation, the adverse effects of sucralfate are minimal because little of the drug is absorbed from the GI tract. Because sucralfate requires an acid medium to work effectively, concurrent use of antacids, H_2-receptor antagonists, and PPIs will reduce its effectiveness. Sucralfate may bind to other drugs and decrease their absorption, especially digoxin, warfarin, the quinolones and tetracyclines, and phenytoin. Antacids and other medications should be taken 2 hours before or after a dose of sucralfate. A major disadvantage of sucralfate is that it must be taken four times daily.

Bismuth compounds: Bismuth subsalicylate (Kaopectate, Pepto-Bismol) is a nonprescription formula containing both bismuth and salicylate. Bismuth subsalicylate stimulates mucosal bicarbonate and prostaglandin production and inhibits *H. pylori* from adhering to the ulcerated tissue. It has been shown to have local antimicrobial actions to *H. pylori* by causing cell wall death to the bacterium. Bismuth is often included as a component of a multidrug regimen containing tetracycline and metronidazole (Pylera) to eradicate *H. pylori* infection. As monotherapy, it is approved to treat dyspepsia, heartburn, and diarrhea.

Therapeutic doses of bismuth produce no significant adverse effects. This drug can cause stools to turn black, which is a normal side effect. In stomach acid bismuth subsalicylate is converted to salicylic acid, which is absorbed. Patients who are taking other salicylates, such as aspirin, may experience adverse effects such as tinnitus, headache, nausea and vomiting, and dizziness. In addition, it is not recommended for use in pediatric patients under the age of 19 because of the increased risk of Reye's syndrome associated with salicylate use. A "Children's Pepto" is available that contains the antacid calcium carbonate but no salicylates.

Misoprostol: Misoprostol (Cytotec) is a synthetic form of prostaglandin E_2 that stimulates the production of protective mucus and inhibits gastric acid secretion. Normally, the stomach synthesizes a number of prostaglandins, which suppress acid, promote bicarbonate secretion, and maintain blood flow to the gastric mucosa. The primary use of misoprostol is for the prevention of gastric ulcers in patients who are taking high doses of NSAIDs or corticosteroids. It has a serum half-life of less than 30 minutes and is administered three to four times per day. Diarrhea and abdominal cramping are relatively common with misoprostol. Arthrotec is a combination drug containing misoprostol and diclofenac, an NSAID. The use of misoprostol as an antiulcer drug is rare because of the availability of safer, more effective drugs. As an antiulcer drug, misoprostol is contraindicated for use during pregnancy or in women of childbearing potential. This drug is combined with mifepristone for pregnancy termination (see Chapter 70).

Metoclopramide: Approved in 1985, metoclopramide is occasionally used for the short-term (4 to 12 weeks) therapy of symptomatic GERD or PUD in patients who fail to respond to first-line drugs. It is more commonly prescribed to treat nausea and vomiting associated with surgery or cancer chemotherapy. Metoclopramide is available by the PO, IM, or IV routes. It causes muscles in the upper intestine to contract, resulting in faster emptying of the stomach. It also decreases esophageal relaxation and blocks food from entering the esophagus, which is of benefit in patients with GERD.

CNS adverse effects such as drowsiness, fatigue, confusion, and insomnia may occur in a significant number of patients. Metoclopramide carries a black box warning that it can cause tardive dyskinesia. Because the risk of this serious condition increases with duration of treatment, therapy should be limited to a maximum of 12 weeks. Due to the availability of safer, more effective drugs, metoclopramide is rarely prescribed to treat peptic ulcer.

CONNECTIONS: APPLIED CLINICAL JUDGMENT

Patients Receiving Pharmacotherapy for Peptic Ulcer Disease

Key Assessment Data

- History of current condition, baseline vital signs, physical exam findings; ulcers or GI bleeding, hepatic or renal disease; medication history, caffeine, nicotine, and alcohol use; pregnancy status.

Desired Therapeutic Outcomes

Improvement is observed and measurable by redused gastric area pain and lessened bloating or belching.

Minimizing Adverse Effects

- Continued symptoms may indicate ineffectiveness of the current drug therapy or the need to test for *H. pylori*.
- Drugs for PUD decrease gastric acidity, making the gastric environment less favorable for ulcer development, but they do not heal existing ulcers. Severe abdominal pain or blood in emesis or stools may indicate a worsening of the disease or a more serious condition.
- Drugs for PUD raise the gastric pH and impact the body's normal defense mechanisms against respiratory pathogens. Antibacterial therapy may be needed if respiratory infections develop.
- Some research studies have linked PPIs to an increase in osteoporosis-related fractures. Calcium and magnesium supplements or other preventive drug therapy may be needed.
- Drugs that raise gastric pH have been associated with an increased risk for CDAD. Severe diarrhea may indicate the presence of CDAD or pseudomembranous colitis.
- Decreased red blood cells, white blood cells, or platelets have been noted with long-term H_2-receptor antagonist therapy, and excessive use of antacids may affect electrolyte levels.
- PPIs, H_2 blockers, and antacids may significantly impair the effects of other drugs (e.g., clopidogrel), affecting therapeutic effects.

CONNECTIONS: APPLIED CLINICAL JUDGMENT *(continued)*

Patients Receiving Pharmacotherapy for Peptic Ulcer Disease

Lifespan Considerations

- Age-related physiologic changes increase the risk of adverse renal and hepatic effects in the older adult.

Diversity Considerations

- Some drugs used in PUD therapy (e.g., omeprazole, cimetidine) are metabolized through the CYP450 system. Monitor ethnically diverse patients frequently to ensure optimal therapeutic effects and minimize adverse effects.

Patient Education

- Some easing of discomfort may be noticed after beginning drug therapy; full effects may take several days to weeks or longer. Consistent treatment will provide the best results. If gastric discomfort or pain continue or worsen after several weeks of therapy, the healthcare provider should be notified. Immediately report severe abdominal pain or any blood in emesis or stools.
- Report symptoms of respiratory infection and report lung congestion or dyspnea accompanied by fever.
- Immediately report any diarrhea that increases in frequency or amount or that contains mucus, blood, or pus. Consult the healthcare provider before taking any antidiarrheal drugs, which cause the retention of harmful bacteria.
- Increase intake of dairy products containing live active cultures, such as yogurt, kefir, or buttermilk, to help restore normal intestinal flora. Eliminate alcohol use and reduce or eliminate smoking.
- Do not use aspirin or salicylates. Read labels on all OTC medications and avoid formulations with aspirin or salicylate on the label.
- Take the drug following appropriate guidelines:
  - **PPIs:** Take 30 minutes before meals. If once-daily dosing is ordered, take the drug in the morning before breakfast. Antacids may be used concurrently. Do not continue taking beyond 3 to 4 months unless directed by the healthcare provider.
  - **H_2-receptor blockers:** Take the drug with or immediately after meals unless otherwise instructed. Do not take concurrently with antacids unless using a combination product (e.g., famotidine with calcium and magnesium-based antacids such as Pepcid-Complete). Exceeding the recommended dose increases the risk of adverse effects such as dizziness or drowsiness.
  - **Antacids:** Take 2 hours before or after meals with a full glass of water. Do not take other medications concurrently unless available as a combination product or directed to do so by the healthcare provider. If relief is not achieved after several weeks of therapy, consult the healthcare provider for additional treatment recommendations.

Prescribing Considerations

- Ongoing assessment during drug therapy should include monitoring appropriate laboratory findings (e.g., complete blood count, electrolytes, hepatic or renal function studies); symptoms, including correlations between onset and presence of any pain related to meals, sleep, positioning, or other medications; what measures have been successful to relieve the pain (e.g., eating); assessment for GI bleeding (dark or tarry stools, hematemesis, coffee-ground emesis, or blood in the stool) and abdominal pain. Testing for *H. pylori* may be needed if symptoms fail to resolve.
- Tolerance to the effects of H2 receptor antagonists can occur within 7 to 14 days of continued treatment. Intermittent, or as needed, use may help prevent the development of tolerance.
- Famotidine, and nizatidine require dose adjustment for patients with a creatine clearance less than 50 mL/min, while cimetidine doses should be reduced for patients with a creatine clearance less than 30 mL/min.

Understanding Chapter 59

Key Concepts Summary

59.1 The stomach secretes acid, enzymes, and hormones that are essential to digestive physiology.

59.2 Peptic ulcer disease is associated with a number of etiologic risk factors.

59.3 Gastroesophageal reflux disease is a chronic condition characterized by persistent heartburn.

59.4 Peptic ulcer disease and gastroesophageal reflux disease are best treated with a combination of pharmacotherapy and lifestyle changes.

59.5 Proton pump inhibitors block gastric acid secretion and are preferred drugs for the therapy of peptic ulcer disease and gastroesophageal reflux disease.

59.6 The H_2-receptor antagonists suppress gastric acid secretion and are widely prescribed for treating peptic ulcer disease and gastroesophageal reflux disease.

59.7 Antacids are alkaline substances that neutralize stomach acid to treat symptoms of heartburn.

59.8 The bacterium *H. pylori* is associated with approximately 70% of patients with peptic ulcer disease.

59.9 Several miscellaneous drugs, including sucralfate, bismuth subsalicylate, and misoprostol, are beneficial in treating peptic ulcer disease.

CASE STUDY: Making the Patient Connection

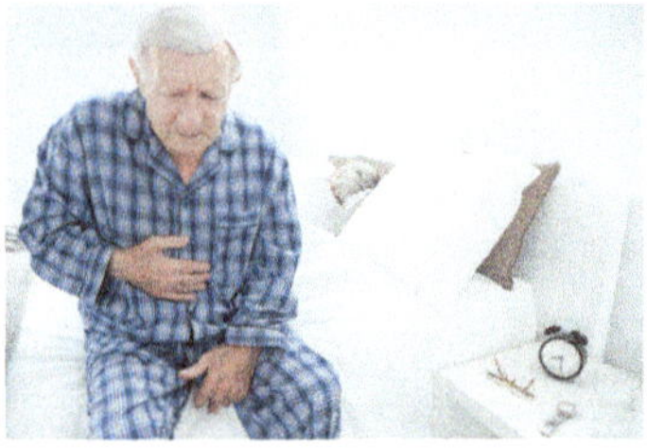

Remember the patient "Hugh Marshall" at the beginning of the chapter? Now read the remainder of the case study. Based on the information presented within this chapter, respond to the critical thinking questions that follow.

Hugh Marshall is a 71-year-old man who has been taking ibuprofen (Motrin) for a shoulder injury and assumed that this was the cause of his stomach pain. He is a one-pack-per-day smoker and drinks one glass of wine every night with dinner. His medical history includes HTN for which he takes a combination diuretic and angiotensin-converting enzyme (ACE) inhibitor. He stopped taking his ibuprofen, but the stomach pain did not subside. Because of worsening symptoms, an endoscopy was performed, which confirmed the presence of *H. pylori*. He is worried about taking antibiotics because he has been allergic to penicillin in the past.

Critical Thinking Questions

1. Based on the scenario above, what risk factors for PUD does Hugh have?
2. How would you as the nurse describe the recommended treatment for *H. pylori*–induced PUD to him?
3. Why would you be concerned about this patient with a history of HTN using NSAIDs?

Additional Case Study

Sara Gaggi is a 51-year-old woman who is overweight and has HTN. She presents for an evaluation of heartburn that has been increasing in both intensity and frequency during the past 18 months. She reports epigastric burning after eating. It is worse after eating spicy foods or drinking red wine. Sara is occasionally awakened at night with symptoms. OTC antacids and H_2-receptor antagonists relieved her symptoms initially, but lately they have provided only minimal relief. Her only routine medication is amlodipine, a calcium channel blocker for her HTN. Because the symptoms are increasing and Sara's current therapy is not relieving her symptoms, an endoscopy was performed, which revealed the presence of GERD.

1. How would you describe to Sara the dangers of self-medicating GERD symptoms with OTC medications?
2. What three risk factors in this case predispose Sara for the development of GERD?
3. What medications will her healthcare provider likely prescribe?

Chapter Review

1. The patient has developed severe diarrhea following 4 days of self-administered antacid preparation. The nurse suspects that the diarrhea may be caused by which type of antacid?

1. Aluminum compounds
2. Magnesium compounds
3. Calcium compounds
4. Sodium compounds

2. Omeprazole (Prilosec) is prescribed for a patient with GERD. The nurse would monitor a reduction in which symptom to determine if the drug therapy is effective? (Select all that apply.)

1. Dysphagia
2. Dyspepsia
3. Appetite
4. Nausea
5. Belching

3. The nurse is scheduling the patient's daily medication. When would be the most appropriate time for the patient to receive PPIs?

1. At night
2. After fasting at least 2 hours
3. About 1/2 hour before a meal
4. About 2 to 3 hours after eating

4. A patient who has duodenal ulcers is receiving long-term therapy with famotidine. The nurse includes in the care plan that the patient should be monitored for which adverse effects?

1. Photophobia and skin irritations
2. Neutropenia and thrombocytopenia
3. Dyspnea and productive coughing
4. Urinary hesitation and fluid retention

5. A patient has been diagnosed with *H. pylori* as the causative factor for a gastric ulcer. Which of the following drug orders would be considered first-line therapy? (Select all that apply.)

1. Omeprazole
2. Metronidazole
3. Sucralfate
4. Bismuth subsalicylate
5. Fluconazole

6. The nurse who is caring for a patient with GERD should question the order for which drug?

1. H_2-receptor antagonists
2. Proton pump inhibitors
3. Antibiotics
4. Antacids

See Appendix A for answers to critical thinking questions, case study questions and review questions.

References

Anand, B. S. (2020). *Peptic ulcer disease*. Medscape. http://emedicine.medscape.com/article/181753-overview#a0101

Chey, W. D., Leontiadis, G. I., Howden, C. W., & Moss, S. F. (2017). ACG clinical guideline: treatment of Helicobacter pylori infection. *American Journal of Gastroenterology, 112*(2), 212–239. https://doi.org/10.1038/ajg.2016.563

Huntsberry, A. M., Linnebur, S. A., Fixen, D. R., Saba, S. M. & Saseen, J. J. (2019). Effects of chronic proton-pump inhibitor use on kidney function in older adults. *The Senior Care Pharmacist, 34*(5), 325–333.

Patti, M. G. (2019). *Gastroesophageal reflux disease*. Medscape. https://emedicine.medscape.com/article/176595-overview

Pezeshkian, S., & Conway, S. E. (2018). Proton pump inhibitor use in older adults: Long-term risks and steps for deprescribing. *The Consultant Pharmacist, 33*, 497–503. https://doi.org/10.4140/TCP.n.2018.497

Selected Bibliography

Boyanova, L., Hadzhiyski, P., Kandilarov, N., Markovska, R., & Mitov, I. (2019). Multidrug resistance in Helicobacter pylori: Current state and future directions. *Expert Review of Clinical Pharmacology, 12*(9), 909–915. https://doi.org/10.1080/17512433.2019.1654858

Chapman, W., Siau, K., Thomas, F., Ernest, S., Begum, S., Iqbal, T., & Bhala, N. (2019). Acute upper gastrointestinal bleeding: a guide for nurses. *British Journal of Nursing, 28*(1), 53–59. https://doi.org/10.12968/bjon.2019.28.1.53

Dunlap, J. J., & Patterson, S. (2019). Peptic ulcer disease. *Gastroenterology Nursing, 42*(5), 451–454. https://doi.org/10.1097/SGA.0000000000000478

Jaynes, M., & Kumar, A. B. (2019). The risks of long-term use of proton pump inhibitors: A critical review. *Therapeutic Advances in Drug Safety, 10*, 2042098618809927. https://doi.org/10.1177/2042098618809927

Willis, T., & Duff, E. (2020). Optimizing prescribing and deprescribing of proton pump inhibitors. *Journal for Nurse Practitioners, 16*(4), 258–261. https://doi.org/10.1016/j.nurpra.2020.01.004

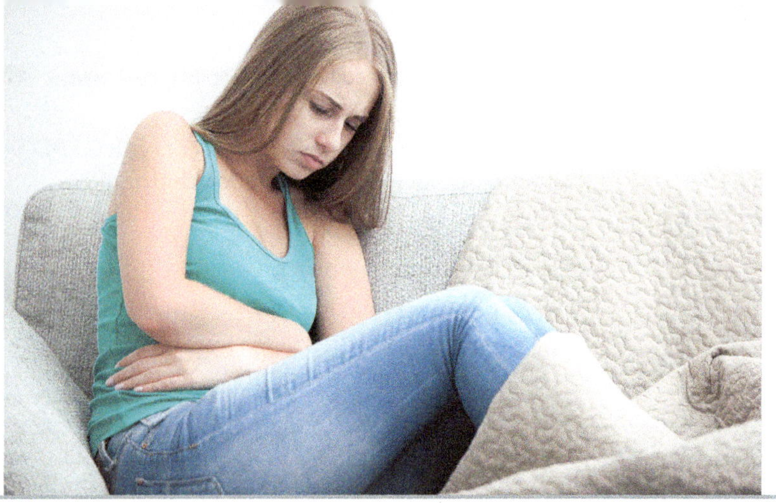

"This is ruining my life! I can't go to class; I can't go out with friends! I wish I'd never heard the term 'irritable bowel syndrome'!"
—*Patient "Kerry O'Grady"*

Chapter 60
Pharmacotherapy of Bowel Disorders and Other Gastrointestinal Conditions

Chapter Outline

Learning Outcomes

After reading this chapter, the student should be able to:

1. Compare and contrast the definition of constipation used by patients to that used for diagnosis by healthcare providers.
2. Compare and contrast the different mechanisms of action of laxatives.
3. Explain the pathogenesis of constipation and diarrhea.
4. Compare and contrast the types of drugs used to treat inflammatory bowel disease and irritable bowel syndrome.
5. Explain conditions for which the pharmacotherapy of nausea and vomiting is indicated.
6. Identify drugs that are used to treat acute and chronic pancreatitis.
7. Describe the nurse's role in the pharmacologic management of bowel disorders, nausea and vomiting, and other gastrointestinal conditions.
8. For each of the classes shown in the chapter outline, identify the prototype and representative drugs and explain the mechanism(s) of drug action, primary indications, contraindications, significant drug interactions, pregnancy data, and important adverse effects.
9. Apply clinical judgment to care for patients who are receiving pharmacotherapy for bowel disorders, nausea and vomiting, and other gastrointestinal conditions.

Key Terms

Definitions of the terms in bold may be found in the Glossary.

Bowel disorders, nausea, and vomiting are among the most common complaints for which patients seek medical consultation. Nonspecific symptoms of gastrointestinal (GI) distress may be caused by a large number of infectious, metabolic, inflammatory, neoplastic, or neuropsychologic disorders. In addition, nausea, vomiting, constipation, and diarrhea are the most common adverse effects of oral (PO) medications. Although symptoms often resolve without the need for pharmacotherapy, when severe or prolonged, these conditions may lead to serious consequences unless drug therapy is initiated. This chapter examines the pharmacotherapy of these and other conditions associated with the GI tract. The anatomy and physiology of the lower GI tract are reviewed in Chapter 58.

Pathophysiology of Constipation

60.1 Constipation is characterized by infrequent or difficult bowel movements.

A large percentage of the water we drink is reabsorbed as it travels through the large intestine. Reabsorption of the proper amount of water results in stools of a normal, soft-formed consistency. If feces remain in the colon for an extended period, too much water will be reabsorbed, leading to small, hard stools that are difficult to evacuate from the rectum without straining. Abdominal distention, discomfort, and flatulence may result.

Patients often define **constipation** as the infrequent passage of abnormally hard and dry stools. This definition, however, is not entirely satisfactory for diagnosis because the normal frequency of bowel movements varies widely among individuals, from two to three per day to as few as one per week. Constipation occurs more frequently in older adults because fecal transit time through the colon slows with aging. This population also exercises less, has diminished food intake, and is more likely to take certain drugs that cause constipation at a higher rate than in younger adults. Variations in frequency are normal and a daily bowel movement is not a requirement for good health.

Constipation is not a disease but a symptom of an underlying disorder or condition, some of which are shown in Table 60.1. A diagnosis of chronic constipation includes at least two of the following symptoms without the use of laxatives over the course of a year:

- Fewer than three bowel movements per week
- Lumpy or hard stools at least 25% of the time
- Straining to pass stools at least 25% of the time
- A feeling of incomplete evacuation at least 25% of the time.

Table 60.1 Etiology of Constipation

Condition	Causes
Dietary	Inadequate fiber intake
	Inadequate fluid intake
	Inadequate food intake
	Specific foods: alcoholic beverages, products with a high content of refined white flour, dairy products, and chocolate
GI disorders	Bowel obstruction
	Diverticulitis
	Irritable bowel syndrome
	Tumors
Lifestyle	Lack of exercise
Medications	Antacids containing bismuth, calcium, or aluminum
	Barium sulfate
	Calcium channel blockers
	Drugs with anticholinergic action: antihistamines, phenothiazines, tricyclic antidepressants, some antiparkinsonism drugs
	Iron supplements
	Nonsteroidal anti-inflammatory drugs (NSAIDs)
	Opioids
Metabolic disorders	Diabetes
	Hypercalcemia or hypocalcemia
	Hypothyroidism
Neurogenic/central nervous system (CNS) disorders	Clinical depression
	Diminished peristalsis
	Head or spinal trauma
	Parkinson's disease
	Stroke
Pregnancy	Diminished exercise, change in diet, pressure of fetus on the colon

Occasional constipation is self-limiting and does not require drug therapy. Lifestyle modifications that incorporate increased dietary fiber, fluid intake, and physical activity should be considered before drugs are utilized for constipation. Chronic, infrequent, and painful bowel movements that are accompanied by severe straining may justify initiation of treatment. Excessive straining may lead to anorectal pathology such as anal fissures, hemorrhoids, or rectal prolapse. In its most severe form, constipation can lead to a fecal impaction and complete obstruction of the bowel.

Constipation that is accompanied by acute pain and abdominal distention is a sign of a potential bowel obstruction or paralytic ileus. These conditions are medical emergencies, and laxatives, enemas, and other therapies are absolutely contraindicated until the patient receives a full medical evaluation.

Pharmacotherapy with Laxatives

60.2 Laxatives are drugs that increase the frequency and quality of bowel movements.

Laxatives, drugs that promote defecation (evacuation of the bowel), are commonly used to prevent and treat constipation. **Cathartic** is a related term that implies an accelerated, stronger, and more complete bowel emptying. A variety of prescription and over-the-counter (OTC) laxatives, including tablet and liquid formulations, are available. Suppositories are used for infants or patients who are unable to take PO drugs. Laxatives and their doses are listed in Table 60.2.

Laxatives have several important indications. These may be divided into prophylaxis of constipation and treatment of constipation:

Prophylaxis

- Patients who have had a myocardial infarction (MI) or those with rectal pathology who should not be straining
- Patients receiving drug therapies that have constipation as a known adverse effect, such as opioids
- Patients who are bedridden or otherwise unable to exercise
- Patients who are pregnant
- Older patients with weak abdominal or perineal muscles.

Table 60.2 Laxatives and Cathartics

Drug	Route and Adult Dose (Maximum Dose Where Indicated)	Adverse Effects
Bulk Forming		
calcium polycarbophil (Equalactin, FiberCon, others)	PO: 1 g daily	*Abdominal fullness or cramping, fainting*
methylcellulose (Citrucel)	PO: 5–20 mL tid in 8–10 oz liquid	Esophageal or GI obstruction if taken with insufficient fluid
psyllium (Metamucil)	PO: 2.5 g in 8 oz liquid daily prn	
Saline/(Osmotic)		
lactitol (Pizensy)	PO: 20 mg once daily	*Diarrhea, abdominal cramping, upper respiratory tract infection (lactitol)*
magnesium hydroxide (Milk of Magnesia)	PO: 20–60 mL or 6–8 tablets daily prn	
polyethylene glycol (MiraLAX)	PO: 17 g/day in 8 oz liquid daily for 2–4 days	Hypermagnesemia (magnesium hydroxide), dysrhythmias, respiratory failure
sodium biphosphate (Fleet Phospho-Soda)	PO: 15–30 mL mixed in liquid daily prn	
Stimulants		
bisacodyl (Correctol, Dulcolax, others)	PO: 10–15 mg daily prn	*Abdominal cramping, nausea, fainting, diarrhea*
castor oil (Emulsoil, Neoloid)	PO: 15–60 mL daily prn	Fluid and electrolyte loss
prucalopride (Motegrity)	PO: 2 mg/day	*Diarrhea, headache, abdominal pain, nausea* Suicidal ideation
Surfactants (Stool Softeners)		
docusate (Colace, DulcoEase)	PO: 50–500 mg daily	*Abdominal cramping, diarrhea* No serious adverse effects
Herbal Products		
castor oil	PO: 15–60 mL daily	*Abdominal cramping, diarrhea*
senna (Ex-Lax, Senokot, others)	PO: 8.6–17.2 mg daily	No serious adverse effects
Opioid Antagonists		
alvimopan (Entereg)	PO: 12 mg prior to surgery followed by 12 mg bid beginning the day after surgery for up to 7 days (maximum: 15 doses)	*Dyspepsia, nausea, abdominal pain, hyperhidrosis (methylnaltrexone)* GI perforation, opioid withdrawal, MI (alvimopan)
methylnaltrexone (Relistor)	Subcutaneous: 8 or 12 mg every other day PO: 450 mg once daily	
naloxegol (Movantik)	PO: 25 mg in the morning	
Miscellaneous Laxatives		
mineral oil	PO: 15–30 mL bid	*Diarrhea, nausea* Nutritional deficiencies
plecanatide (Trulance)	PO: 3 mg once daily	*Diarrhea* Serious dehydration in pediatric patients

***Note:** Italics* indicate common adverse effects. Underline indicates serious adverse effects.

Treatment

- Relieve simple, chronic constipation.
- Accelerate the removal of ingested toxic substances following overdose or poisoning.
- Accelerate the removal of dead parasites following anthelminthic drug therapy.
- Cleanse the bowel prior to diagnostic or surgical procedures of the colon or genitourinary tract, including colonoscopy or barium enema.

The most common adverse effects of laxatives include abdominal distention and cramping. Diarrhea may result from excessive use. When cleansing the bowel prior to a colonoscopy or purging the bowel of toxic substances or parasites, forceful, frequent bowel movements are expected outcomes. Care must be taken to rule out acute abdominal pathology, such as bowel obstruction prior to administration, because the drugs will increase colon pressure and possibly cause bowel perforation.

Laxatives may be classified into six primary groups and a miscellaneous category. The choice of a particular drug depends on the reason for use (treatment or prophylaxis), the onset of action desired (rapid or slow), and the completeness of evacuation needed (cathartic or laxative).

Bulk-forming laxatives: Bulk-forming drugs absorb water, thus adding size to the fecal mass. Because fiber absorbs water and expands to provide bulk, these drugs must be taken with plenty of water. Bulk-forming laxatives are first-line drugs for the treatment and prevention of chronic constipation and may be taken on a regular basis without ill effects. Because of their slow onset of action, they are not used when a rapid and complete bowel evacuation is necessary. Their onset of action is 24 to 48 hours.

Saline (osmotic) cathartics: Saline cathartics, also called osmotic laxatives, are poorly absorbed in the intestine. They pull water into the fecal mass to create a more watery stool. These drugs can produce a bowel movement very quickly but should not be used on a regular basis due to the possibility of dehydration and fluid and electrolyte depletion. Saline laxatives are highly effective and are an important component of colonoscopy prep and for purging toxins from the body. Their onset of action is 1 to 6 hours in high doses. Lactitol (Pizensy) is a saline laxative approved in 2020 to treat chronic idiopathic constipation.

Stimulant laxatives: Stimulant laxatives promote peristalsis by irritating the bowel. They are rapid acting and are more likely to cause diarrhea and cramping than the bulk-forming type of laxatives. They should not be used routinely because they may cause laxative dependence, abdominal cramping, and depletion of fluid and electrolytes. These products are often used to prepare the bowel prior to colon examination or surgery, sometimes in combination with other laxatives and enemas. Stimulant laxatives have an onset of action of 6 to 12 hours (PO) or 1 to 6 hours (rectal). Prucalopride (Motegrity) was approved in 2018 as daily oral therapy to treat chronic idiopathic constipation. This drug is a highly selective 5-HT_4 agonist that stimulates colon contractions and propulsion of bowel contents.

Surfactant (stool softener) laxatives: Surfactants, commonly called stool softeners, cause more water and fat to be absorbed into the stools. They are ineffective at treating constipation but are most often used to prevent the condition. Stool softeners are generally prescribed for patients who have a condition that puts them at risk for constipation, such as a surgery, an injury, or an MI where straining during defecation should be avoided. Their onset of action is 24 to 48 hours.

Herbal laxatives: Herbal laxatives are natural products that are available OTC and are widely used for self-treatment of constipation. The most commonly used herbal laxative is senna, a potent herb that stimulates the bowel and increases peristalsis. Other natural laxatives include rhubarb, cascara sagrada, aloe, flaxseed, and dandelion. Patients should be advised to exercise caution when using herbal products because many have not been evaluated through controlled studies for safety or effectiveness. Their onset of action varies.

Opioid antagonists: Opioids relieve pain by occupying mu receptors in the brain. Opioids, however, also occupy mu receptors at peripheral sites such as the large intestine, producing constipation. This constipation may be severe, resulting in a potential ileus following surgery. The drugs in this class block the opioid mu receptors in the large intestine, but they do not pass through the blood–brain barrier in any significant amount. This allows the patient to experience central pain relief from the opioids without peripheral side effects on the large intestine.

Approved by the U.S. Food and Drug Administration (FDA) in 2008, methylnaltrexone (Relistor) is specifically used to treat chronic constipation in patients with advanced illness who are receiving opioids for palliative care. Approved in 2014, naloxegol (Movantik) is indicated specifically for constipation induced by opioid medications. Alvimopan (Entereg) is available only for short-term, hospital use due to an increased risk for MI.

Miscellaneous drugs: Mineral oil is a miscellaneous drug that acts by lubricating the stool and the colon mucosa. The use of mineral oil should be discouraged because it interferes with the absorption of fat-soluble vitamins and can cause other potentially serious adverse effects. Its onset of action is 24 to 48 hours. Approved in 2017, plecanatide (Trulance) is an oral drug that treats chronic idiopathic constipation. Its mechanism of action is unique: It activates the enzyme guanylate cyclase in the intestine. This causes increased secretion of chloride and bicarbonate ion into the intestinal lumen, resulting in increased amounts of intestinal fluid and accelerated fecal transport. Plecanatide carries a black box warning that it is contraindicated in patients younger than age 6 and should be avoided in children ages 6 through 17 due to the potential for serious dehydration.

PROTOTYPE DRUG Psyllium (Metamucil)

Classification **Therapeutic:** Drug for constipation
Pharmacologic: Bulk-type laxative

Therapeutic Effects and Uses: Psyllium is derived from a natural product—the seeds of the plantain plant. Like other bulk-forming laxatives, psyllium is an insoluble fiber that is indigestible and not absorbed from the GI tract. When taken with a sufficient quantity of water, psyllium swells and increases the size of the fecal mass. The larger the size of the fecal mass, the greater will be the neural stimulus for defecation.

Several doses of psyllium may be needed over 1 to 3 days to produce an optimal therapeutic effect. Several 2.5-g doses may be taken each day. Frequent use of psyllium (7 g/day) may effect a small reduction in blood cholesterol level. This drug is available as granules, powder, and wafers.

Mechanism of Action: Psyllium expands the size of the stool and promotes colon peristalsis that closely resembles a natural bowel movement.

Pharmacokinetics:

Route(s)	PO
Absorption	Not absorbed; remains in the GI tract
Distribution	Not distributed
Primary metabolism	Not metabolized
Primary excretion	Feces
Onset of action	12–24 h
Duration of action	Unknown

Adverse Effects: Psyllium is the safest laxative and rarely produces adverse effects. It generally causes less cramping than the stimulant-type laxatives and results in a more natural bowel movement. If taken with insufficient water, psyllium may swell in the esophagus and cause obstruction.

Contraindications/Precautions: Psyllium should not be administered to patients with undiagnosed abdominal pain, suspected intestinal obstruction, or fecal impaction.

Drug Interactions: Psyllium may decrease the absorption and effects of warfarin, digoxin, nitrofurantoin, antibiotics, and salicylates. **Herbal/Food:** Unknown.

Pregnancy: Animal reproduction studies have not been conducted on this medication. Women should check with their health care provider regarding use during pregnancy or lactation.

Treatment of Overdose: Overdose from psyllium is unlikely.

Clinician Responsibilities: Key clinical implications for patients receiving psyllium are included in Applied Clinical Judgment: Patients Receiving Pharmacotherapy for GI Conditions.

Drugs Similar to Psyllium (Metamucil)

Other popular laxatives include bisacodyl, castor oil, docusate, and magnesium hydroxide.

Bisacodyl (Correctol, Dulcolax, others): Bisacodyl is the most frequently used stimulant-type laxative. It acts by irritating the mucosa in the colon and by altering intestinal and electrolyte absorption. Only 15% of the drug is absorbed after oral administration. Onset of action is 8 to 12 hours (PO) if taken at bedtime or 15 to 60 minutes per rectal suppository. Bisacodyl should not be taken with milk or other dairy products because these can dissolve the enteric coating and cause dyspepsia. The enteric-coated tablets should not be crushed or chewed. Minor adverse effects include abdominal pain and cramping. Prolonged use may lead to laxative dependence and fluid and electrolyte loss. Animal reproduction studies have not been conducted on this medication. Women should check with their healthcare provider regarding use during pregnancy or lactation.

Castor oil (Emulsoil, Neoloid): Castor oil is one of the oldest and worst-tasting laxatives. It was approved in 1939. A stimulant-type laxative, castor oil acts on the small intestine and produces a bowel movement in 2 to 6 hours. It causes more adverse effects than other laxatives, including diarrhea, cramping, nausea and vomiting, and dizziness. This drug is not recommended for use during pregnancy or lactation because it may stimulate uterine contractions and cause diarrhea in breastfed neonates.

Docusate (Colace, DulcoEase): Docusate is the most frequently prescribed surfactant-type laxative or stool softener. This drug permits additional water and lipids to penetrate the stool, making it softer. Docusate takes several days to act and therefore is not effective when a rapid and complete bowel evacuation is necessary. Only small amounts are absorbed systemically. Adverse effects are rare. Docusate sodium (Colace) should not be given to patients on sodium restriction. Docusate potassium (Dialose) should not be given to patients with chronic kidney disease. This drug increases the systemic absorption of mineral oil, so these two medications should not be given concurrently. Docusate should not be taken with certain herbal products such as senna, cascara, rhubarb, or aloe because it will increase their absorption and the risk of liver toxicity. Animal reproduction studies have not been conducted on this medication. Women should check with their healthcare provider regarding use during pregnancy or lactation.

Magnesium hydroxide (Milk of Magnesia): Magnesium hydroxide has two effects on the GI tract. Taken PO it exerts an antacid effect because it neutralizes gastric hydrochloric acid to form magnesium chloride. About 30% of the magnesium chloride is absorbed systemically. The remainder continues along the GI tract and reaches the colon, where it exerts a laxative effect by drawing water and electrolytes to form a larger and softer fecal mass. This drug has a chalky taste and has a small incidence of nausea and vomiting and abdominal cramping. Patients with impaired renal function should be monitored for hypermagnesemia. Magnesium hydroxide can bind to other drugs, delaying their absorption; thus, it should be taken at least 2 hours apart from other medications. Drugs that may result in decreased absorption include H_2-receptor antagonists, iron salts, phenytoin, digoxin, and tetracyclines. Magnesium citrate and magnesium sulfate are other saline-type laxatives with rapid onsets of action (30 minutes to 4 hours). Occasional use of OTC magnesium products has not been shown to adversely affect pregnancy outcomes or lactation.

CONNECTIONS: Using Research in Practice

Fecal Microbiota Transplant

The role that normal intestinal flora, or *intestinal microbiota*, plays in maintaining body health and immunity is becoming more apparent—and appreciated. Multiple organisms populate the intestinal tract. Their functions include boosting immune protection against toxins produced by some pathogenic bacteria and guarding against septic shock. In addition, they may play a role in preventing obesity.

When normal intestinal flora is disrupted, such as by antibiotic therapy, the pathogenic bacteria may overgrow and cause serious infection. *Clostridioides difficile*–associated diarrhea (CDAD) is a serious bowel infection that most often results from antibiotic therapy. It results in watery diarrhea that contains blood and pus, and rapid dehydration may occur because of fluid loss. The standard treatment for CDAD includes fluid replacement; for severe and recurrent cases, PO vancomycin may be prescribed. Recent research, however, has supported the process called fecal microbiota transplant (FMT), which involves transplanting small amounts of healthy intestinal flora from a donor into a recipient who has CDAD. The outcomes have been positive.

In FMT, donors are prescreened for serious viral diseases (e.g., HIV, hepatitis), syphilis, ova and parasites, and colon cancer. The donor stool is suspended in liquid and then instilled into the patient by enema or colonoscopy or during endoscopy. Studies also suggest that frozen fecal microbiota may be administered orally through capsules with positive results, including for Crohn's disease (Caldeira et al., 2020). What is not yet determined is the potential for long-term complications from diseases that may not be apparent in young healthy donors at the time of donation (Talley & Irani, 2020), and risks must be weighed against potential benefits.

CONNECTION Checkpoint 60.1

From what you learned in Chapter 22, describe the indications for using magnesium to treat seizure disorders.

Pathophysiology of Diarrhea

60.3 Diarrhea is an abnormal increase in the frequency and fluidity of bowel movements.

The small intestine receives about 9 L of fluid, or chyme, daily. Most is reabsorbed, such that only about 1 L reaches the colon. Travel through the colon results in even more reabsorption, and only about 100 mL remains to form stools. Should the small or large intestines fail to reabsorb sufficient fluids, diarrhea may occur. **Diarrhea** is an increase in the frequency and fluidity of bowel movements.

Like constipation, occasional diarrhea is a self-limiting disorder that does not warrant drug therapy. In some cases, diarrhea is a type of body defense, rapidly and completely eliminating toxins and pathogens. When prolonged or severe, especially in children, diarrhea can result in a significant loss of body fluids, and pharmacotherapy is indicated. In underdeveloped countries, diarrhea is a major cause of illness and death in young children. Prolonged diarrhea may lead to fluid, acid–base, or electrolyte imbalances.

Because diarrhea is a nonspecific symptom of an underlying condition or disease, a primary treatment goal is to identify and treat the cause. Assessing the patient's recent travels, dietary habits, immune system competence, and drug history may provide important clues about the etiology. Because such a large number of conditions can cause diarrhea, pinpointing an exact cause may be difficult. Therefore, symptomatic therapy is provided for the diarrhea while identifying its cause. Common etiologies include the following:

- **Infection.** Viral and bacterial infections are the most common cause of diarrhea. Intestinal protozoans and helminths are less common causes. The most frequently encountered diarrhea-producing organisms are *Campylobacter*, *Salmonella*, *Cryptosporidium*, *Giardia*, *Shigella*, *Escherichia coli* (traveler's diarrhea), and *Staphylococcus*.
- **Drugs.** Antibiotics often cause diarrhea by killing normal intestinal flora, thereby allowing an overgrowth of opportunistic pathogenic organisms. Laxatives, magnesium antacids, digoxin, orlistat, and NSAIDs are also common causes.
- **Inflammation.** Ulcerative colitis, Crohn's disease, and irritable bowel syndrome (IBS) cause inflammation of the bowel mucosa, leading to periods of intense diarrhea.

- **Foods.** Various foods can cause diarrhea, such as dairy products in lactose-intolerant patients, foods with capsaicin (hot pepper), and chronic alcohol ingestion.
- **Malabsorption.** Diseases of the small intestine and pancreas can cause insufficient absorption of foods and fluid.

Pharmacotherapy of Diarrhea

60.4 Opioids are the most effective drugs for controlling severe diarrhea.

Pharmacotherapy related to diarrhea depends on the severity of the condition and any identifiable etiologic factors. If the cause is an infectious disease, then an antibiotic or antiparasitic drug is indicated. Should the etiology be inflammatory, then anti-inflammatory drugs are warranted. When the cause appears to be due to an adverse effect of pharmacotherapy, the healthcare provider should discontinue the offending medication, lower the dose, or substitute an alternative drug.

The most effective drugs for the symptomatic treatment of diarrhea are the opioids, which dramatically slow peristalsis in the colon. The most common opioid antidiarrheals are codeine and diphenoxylate with atropine (Lomotil). Diphenoxylate is a Schedule V drug that acts directly on the intestine to slow peristalsis, thereby allowing for more fluid and electrolyte absorption in the large intestine. The opioids cause CNS depression at high doses and are generally reserved for the short-term therapy of acute diarrhea because of their potential adverse effects and the potential for dependence. Details on the indications and adverse effects of opioids are found in Chapter 25.

OTC drugs for diarrhea act by a number of different mechanisms. Loperamide (Imodium) is an analog of meperidine (Demerol), although it has no narcotic effects and is not classified as a controlled substance. Low-dose loperamide is available OTC; higher doses are available by prescription. Other OTC treatments include bismuth subsalicylate (Pepto-Bismol), which acts by binding and absorbing toxins. Psyllium preparations may also slow diarrhea because they absorb large amounts of fluid, which helps to form bulkier stools. Probiotic supplements containing *Lactobacillus*, a normal inhabitant of the human gut and vagina, are sometimes taken to correct the altered GI flora following a serious diarrhea episode. A good source of healthy *Lactobacillus* is yogurt with active cultures, although a freeze-dried form of the bacteria is available in tablets. The antidiarrheals are listed in Table 60.3.

In general, antidiarrheal medications should not be used to treat diarrhea caused by poisoning or infection by toxin-producing organisms. For these patients, it is important for the toxic substances and organisms to be expelled from the body. Use of antidiarrheals will retain these harmful substances. Antidiarrheal use is contraindicated in cases of diarrhea caused by pseudomembranous colitis that is caused by *C. difficile*. This infection can cause toxic megacolon. In this rare condition, the colon is unable to expel gas and stool, which causes it to become greatly distended and at risk of rupturing. An enlarged or ruptured colon requires emergency surgery and may be fatal.

Table 60.3 Antidiarrheals

Drug	Route and Adult Dose (Maximum Dose Where Indicated)	Adverse Effects
Opioids		
camphorated tincture of opium (Paregoric)	PO: 5–10 mL 1–4 times daily	*Drowsiness, lightheadedness, nausea, dizziness, dry mouth (from atropine), constipation* Paralytic ileus with toxic megacolon, respiratory depression, CNS depression
difenoxin with atropine (Motofen)	PO: 1–2 mg after each diarrhea episode (max: 8 mg/day)	
diphenoxylate with atropine (Lomotil)	PO: 5 mg 4 times daily (max: 20 mg/day)	
loperamide (Imodium)	PO: 4 mg as a single dose, then 2 mg after each diarrhea episode (max: 16 mg/day)	
Miscellaneous Antidiarrheals		
bismuth subsalicylate (Kaopectate, Pepto-Bismol)	PO: 2 tablets or 30 mL prn	*Constipation, nausea, tinnitus* Impaction, Reye's syndrome
octreotide (Sandostatin)	Subcutaneous/intravenous (IV): 100–600 mcg/day in 2–4 divided doses	*Nausea, diarrhea, abdominal pain* Hypo- or hyperglycemia, gallstones, cholestatic hepatitis
rifamycin (Aemcolo)	PO: 388 mg (two tablets) bid for 3 days	*Headache, constipation* Hypersensitivity to rifamycin antimicrobials
telotristat (Xermelo)	PO: 250 mg tid with food	*Nausea, headache, depression, flatulence, decreased appetite* Severe constipation, persistent abdominal pain

Note: *Italics* indicate common adverse effects. Underline indicates serious adverse effects.

PROTOTYPE DRUG **Diphenoxylate with Atropine (Lomotil)**

Classification **Therapeutic:** Antidiarrheal
Pharmacologic: Opioid

Therapeutic Effects and Uses: Approved in 1960, diphenoxylate is an oral opioid available by liquid or tablet that is a Schedule V controlled substance. Like other opioids, diphenoxylate slows peristalsis, allowing time for additional water reabsorption from the intestine and the formation of solid stools. It acts within 45 to 60 minutes. It is effective for moderate to severe diarrhea, but it is not recommended for infants. The atropine in Lomotil is not added for its anticholinergic effect but to discourage patients from taking too much diphenoxylate. At recommended doses the effects of atropine are negligible.

Diphenoxylate is discontinued as soon as the diarrhea symptoms resolve. A low-maintenance dose may be continued for up to 10 days if additional diarrhea is anticipated. Lomotil is approved for use in children 2 years and older.

Mechanism of Action: Diphenoxylate acts on the smooth muscle of the intestine to slow peristalsis.

Pharmacokinetics:

Route(s)	PO
Absorption	90% absorbed
Distribution	Small amounts are secreted in breast milk
Primary metabolism	Hepatic; metabolized to active metabolite
Primary excretion	Bile and feces
Onset of action	45–60 min
Duration of action	3–4 h

Adverse Effects: Unlike most opioids, diphenoxylate has no analgesic properties and has an extremely low potential for abuse. The drug is well tolerated at normal doses. Some patients experience dizziness, lethargy, or drowsiness, and care should be taken not to drive or operate machinery until the effects of the drug are known. At higher doses the anticholinergic effects of atropine, which include drowsiness, flushing, dry mouth, and tachycardia, may be observed.

Contraindications/Precautions: Contraindications to diphenoxylate include hypersensitivity to the drug, severe hepatic impairment, obstructive jaundice, and diarrhea associated with pseudomembranous colitis. Dehydration or electrolyte imbalances should be corrected before diphenoxylate therapy is initiated.

Drug Interactions: Other CNS depressants, including alcohol, will cause additive sedative effects. Opiate antagonists such as naloxone will reduce the effectiveness of diphenoxylate. When taken with monoamine oxidase inhibitors (MAOIs), diphenoxylate may cause hypertensive crisis. **Herbal/Food:** Unknown.

Pregnancy: Animal studies did not show evidence of teratogenicity. Because both diphenoxylate and atropine are secreted in human milk, caution is advised if breastfeeding.

Treatment of Overdose: Overdose with Lomotil may be serious. Narcotic antagonists such as naloxone may be administered parenterally to reverse respiratory depression within minutes.

Clinician Responsibilities: Key clinical implications for patients receiving diphenoxylate with atropine are included in Applied Clinical Judgment: Patients Receiving Pharmacotherapy for GI Conditions.

Drugs Similar to Diphenoxylate with Atropine (Lomotil)

Other antidiarrheal drugs include bismuth subsalicylate, difenoxin with atropine, loperamide, octreotide, opium tincture, rifamycin, and telotristat.

Bismuth subsalicylate (Kaopectate, Pepto-Bismol): Bismuth subsalicylate is an oral OTC drug approved for indigestion, heartburn, and diarrhea. Its more recent use is in the treatment of *Helicobacter* infections in patients with peptic ulcer disease. Doses may be taken every 30 to 60 minutes (max: 4 doses/day) until the diarrhea resolves. Adverse effects do not occur at recommended doses. Stools may become discolored, but this is not harmful. In stomach acid, bismuth subsalicylate forms salicylic acid, which is absorbed systemically. Thus, this drug should be used with caution by patients using aspirin; otherwise, salicylate toxicity may result. In addition, this drug should not be used in children with chickenpox or flu symptoms due to the possibility of Reye's syndrome. A "Children's Pepto" is available that contains calcium carbonate without salicylates. Animal reproduction studies have not been conducted on this medication; however, salicylates have been shown to cause fetal harm in laboratory animals. Bismuth subsalicylate is secreted in human milk.

Difenoxin with atropine (Motofen): Difenoxin is an opioid that is an active metabolite of diphenoxylate; thus, the two drugs have the same actions, contraindications, pregnancy data, and adverse effects. Like Lomotil, atropine is added to Motofen to discourage substance abusers from using the drug. It is a Schedule IV controlled substance.

Loperamide (Imodium): Approved in 1976, loperamide is an oral, first-line drug for the symptomatic treatment of acute diarrhea and the maintenance therapy of chronic diarrhea. Chemically related to the opioids, it shares the antidiarrheal properties of the opioids but has no analgesic action and does not produce dependence. This drug slows peristalsis, increasing the transit time, thus allowing for better-formed stools. If diarrhea is not controlled after 48 hours of loperamide therapy, the patient should seek medical attention. Adverse effects are rare. A dose may last up to 24 hours. Safety has been established in children less than 2 years of age. Animal studies did not show evidence of fetal harm. Because loperamide is secreted in human milk, breastfeeding is not recommended.

Octreotide (Sandostatin): Approved in 1988, octreotide is closely related to somatostatin (growth hormone–inhibiting hormone). It is approved to treat acromegaly and severe diarrhea associated with cancer. Octreotide is used off-label to treat a variety of other conditions including acquired immunodeficiency syndrome (AIDS)–related diarrhea, ileostomy-related diarrhea, and childhood diarrhea. It also directly inhibits intestinal secretions and enhances absorption. It is given by the intramuscular (IM) or IV route and a long-acting depot form (Sandostatin LAR) is available. The most frequent adverse effects are GI related, such as nausea, diarrhea, and abdominal pain. During long-term therapy, more than half the patients who are taking octreotide experience gallbladder pathology, including gallstones, or cholestatic hepatitis. Octreotide did not show evidence of fetal harm in laboratory animals. Because this drug is secreted in animal milk and has the potential to cause serious adverse effects, breastfeeding is not recommended.

Opium tincture (Paregoric): Paregoric contains opium, which includes morphine and codeine as active ingredients. Although once widely used in the treatment of severe diarrhea, it can cause opioid-related adverse effects and is a Schedule III controlled substance. This drug may also be used to prevent withdrawal symptoms in newborns of opioid-dependent mothers. Safer drugs have largely replaced Paregoric. Medication errors due to name confusion: Camphorated tincture of opium (Paregoric) contains only 0.4 mg/mL of morphine, whereas opium tincture contains 10 mg/mL of morphine.

Rifamycin (Aemcolo): Rifamycin is an antibacterial medication that is indicated for the treatment of traveler's diarrhea caused by noninvasive strains of *E. coli*. It should not be used for diarrhea complicated with fever and bloody stools. If diarrhea does not resolve after 3 days of therapy, the patient should be evaluated for a possible *C. difficile* infection. Rifamycin is not absorbed, therefore no fetal harm would be expected during pregnancy and negligible amounts should enter milk.

Telotristat (Xermelo): Approved in 2017, telotristat is an oral drug for treating adults experiencing diarrhea from carcinoid syndrome. This syndrome is caused by carcinoid tumors, which are rare and generally occur in the GI tract. Telotristat is administered concurrently with a somatostatin analog, such as octreotide. This medication caused fetal harm in laboratory animals and no data are available on breastfeeding.

Pharmacotherapy of Inflammatory Bowel Disease

60.5 Inflammatory bowel disease is treated with immunosuppressants and anti-inflammatory drugs.

Inflammatory bowel disease (IBD) is characterized by the presence of ulcers in the intestinal tract. Crohn's disease or Crohn's lesions typically appear in the distal small intestine (terminal ileum), although they can affect any region of the GI tract from the mouth to the anus. Crohn's lesions are usually discontinuous: Affected areas of the intestinal mucosa alternate with normal areas. The mucosal erosions characteristic of ulcerative colitis begin in the rectum and progress in an uninterrupted manner throughout the rest of the large intestine. It is estimated that 3 million Americans have IBD.

The etiology of IBD remains largely unknown. Several genes involved with immune responses are associated with the disorder. It is hypothesized that these defective genes cause hyperactivity of T-cell responses to normal flora in the terminal ileum and colon. These hyperactive responses result in chronic intestinal inflammation.

In addition to genetic susceptibility, certain environmental triggers exacerbate symptoms of IBD. Smoking, infections, the use of NSAIDs, and a high level of stress are additional environmental factors that have been identified. Less well known are triggers for ulcerative colitis; in many patients, triggers cannot be identified. It is known that symptoms of ulcerative colitis tend to peak between age 15 and 30 and again between age 50 and 70.

Symptoms of IBD range from mild to acute, and the condition is characterized by alternating periods of remission and exacerbation. The most common clinical presentation of ulcerative colitis is abdominal cramping with frequent bowel movements. Severe disease may lead to weight loss, bloody diarrhea, high fever, and dehydration. The patient with Crohn's disease also presents with abdominal pain, cramping, and diarrhea, which may have been present for years before seeking treatment. Symptoms of Crohn's disease are often similar to those of ulcerative colitis. Patients with IBD have an increased risk of acquiring GI cancer.

The expected outcomes for the pharmacotherapy of IBD are as follows:

- Reduce the acute symptoms of active disease by induction therapy and place the disease in remission.
- Keep the disease in remission with maintenance therapy.
- Change the natural course or progression of the disease.

Multiple medications are utilized to treat IBD, and pharmacotherapy is conducted in a stepwise manner, starting with the safest and most established medications for the disorder, as shown in Pharmacotherapy Illustrated 60.1. The first step of IBD treatment usually involves 5-aminosalicylic acid (5-ASA) drugs that include sulfasalazine, olsalazine (Dipentum), balsalazide (Colazal), and mesalamine (Canasa, Lialda, others). These medications act rapidly and exhibit a higher safety profile than the second-line drugs. While effective at initially reducing symptoms, the 5-ASA medications are not as effective in maintaining remission. Doses for the 5-ASA drugs are listed in Table 60.4. In some cases, a short course of antibiotics may benefit the patient experiencing mild symptoms.

When IBD symptoms are more intense or when patients have not responded well to the 5-ASA drugs, oral corticosteroids such as prednisone are used. Because of their potentially serious long-term adverse effects, however, they are prescribed for the shortest length of time needed to send the disease into remission. In hospitalized patients, IV corticosteroids may be used to put IBD into remission. For a detailed discussion of corticosteroid therapy, refer to Chapter 68.

Budesonide (Entocort-EC) is a corticosteroid with interesting properties that allow it to be used as a first-line therapy for IBD. Entocort-EC is encapsulated to avoid significant absorption in the stomach or duodenum. This drug is released slowly and reaches a high concentration in the terminal ileum and proximal colon—the two most frequently affected sites for IBD. Thus, budesonide is in direct contact with the GI mucosa and produces a topical anti-inflammatory effect. In addition, when budesonide is absorbed, it is almost entirely removed by first-pass metabolism in the liver. Thus, this drug shows few of the adverse effects seen with the long-term use of the other corticosteroids. It is approved for mild to moderate Crohn's disease. In 2012, a delayed-release form of budesonide (Uceris), administered once daily, was approved to treat ulcerative colitis.

Should therapy with corticosteroids fail, step 3 of IBD therapy includes immunosuppressive drugs, such as azathioprine (Azasan), mercaptopurine (Purinethol), or methotrexate (MTX, Rheumatrex, Trexall). These medications are normally not used for induction therapy because they have a 3-month onset of action. They are, however, effective at

Pharmacotherapy Illustrated 60.1

Inflammatory Bowel Disease

Mild Symptoms

Aminosalicylates
- Balsalazide
- Mesalamine
- Olsalazine
- Sulfasalazine

Antibiotics
- Ciprofloxacin
- Metronidazole

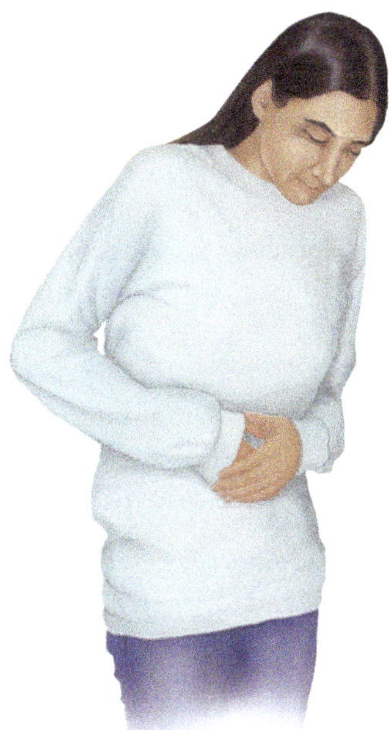

Moderate Symptoms

Oral corticosteroids
- Budesonide
- Dexamethasone
- Prednisolone
- Prednisone

IV corticosteroids
- Hydrocortisone
- Methylprednisolone

Severe Symptoms

Immunomodulators
- Azathioprine
- Cyclosporine
- Mercaptopurine
- Methotrexate
- Tacrolimus

Biologic therapies
- Adalimumab
- Certolizumab
- Infliximab
- Natalizumab

Table 60.4 Selected Drugs for Inflammatory Bowel Disease and Irritable Bowel Syndrome

Drug	Route and Adult Dose (Maximum Dose Where Indicated)	Adverse Effects
First-Line Drugs for Inflammatory Bowel Disease		
balsalazide (Colazal)	PO (Colazal): 2.25 g tid for 8–12 wk	*Headache, abdominal pain, diarrhea, nausea and vomiting, rash, flulike illness, allergic reactions* Hepatotoxicity, blood dyscrasias, renal impairment, salicylate hypersensitivity, crystalluria (sulfasalazine)
mesalamine (Canasa, Lialda, others)	PO (delayed-release tablets): 800 mg tid for 6 wk PO (delayed-release capsules): 1 g qid for 8 wk	
olsalazine (Dipentum)	PO: 500 mg bid (max: 3 g/day)	
sulfasalazine (Azulfidine)	PO: 1–2 g/day in 4 divided doses (max: 8 g/day)	
Drugs for Irritable Bowel Syndrome		
alosetron (Lotronex)	PO: Begin with 1 mg daily for 4 wk; may increase to 1 mg bid (max: 2 mg/day)	*Constipation, abdominal discomfort, nausea, rash* Ischemic colitis, ileus
dicyclomine (Bentyl) and hyoscyamine (Anaspaz, Gastrosed, Levsin)	PO/IM (dicyclomine): 20–40 mg qid (max: 160 mg/day PO; 80 mg/day IM) PO (hyoscyamine): 0.15–0.3 mg 1–4 times/day	*Dry mouth, blurred vision, drowsiness, constipation, urinary hesitancy, tachycardia* Confusion, paralytic ileus
eluxadoline (Viberzi)	PO: 100 mg taken with food	*Constipation, nausea, abdominal pain* Pancreatitis
linaclotide (Linzess)	PO (idiopathic constipation): 72–145 mcg once daily PO (IBS with constipation): 290 mcg once daily	*Abdominal pain and distention, flatulence* Severe diarrhea
lubiprostone (Amitiza)	PO (idiopathic constipation): 24 mcg bid PO (IBS with constipation): 8 mcg bid	*Diarrhea, nausea, headache, abdominal pain* Allergic reaction, dyspnea
rifaximin (Xifaxan)	PO: 550 mg tid	*Nausea, elevated alanine transaminase* No serious adverse effects
tenapanor (Ibsrela)	PO: 50 mg bid	*Abdominal distension, flatulence, dizziness* Severe diarrhea, dehydration

Note: *Italics* indicate common adverse effects. Underline indicates serious adverse effects.

extending the time between relapses. For a detailed discussion of immunosuppressant therapy, refer to Chapter 42.

The introduction of biologic therapies in the late 1990s gave clinicians another valuable tool in the pharmacotherapy of IBD. The biologic therapies for IBD comprise three primary classes:

- *Tumor necrosis factor (TNF) inhibitors:* The TNF inhibitors, such as infliximab (Remicade), have been shown to effectively reduce the acute symptoms of and provide maintenance therapy for both Crohn's disease and ulcerative colitis. Other anti-TNF drugs include adalimumab (Humira), certolizumab pegol (Cimzia), and golimumab (Simponi).
- *Integrin receptor inhibitors:* The two drugs in this class are monoclonal antibodies that bind integrins, which are receptors that mediate cell-to-cell communication. This binding impedes the ability of T lymphocytes to migrate to inflamed lymphoid tissue in the intestinal tract. Natalizumab (Tysabri) was approved in 2008 to treat severe Crohn's disease. This drug was previously approved for multiple sclerosis (see Chapter 21). Natalizumab has adverse effects that limit its use, the most serious of which is an increased risk for progressive multifocal leukoencephalopathy (PML), an often-fatal opportunistic viral infection of the brain. In 2014, a second integrin inhibitor, vedolizumab (Entyvio), was approved to treat IBD. No cases of PML have been recorded with vedolizumab. Both natalizumab and vedolizumab are administered by the IV route for patients who have not responded to immunomodulators or TNF inhibitors.
- *Interleukin antagonists:* Ustekinumab (Stelara) was originally approved in 2009 to treat moderate to severe psoriasis and psoriatic arthritis. Subsequently, it was approved for moderate to severe Crohn's disease and active ulcerative colitis. Ustekinumab is a monoclonal antibody targeted against IL-12 and IL-23. These interleukins promote abnormal inflammatory and immune processes that contribute to Crohn's disease and ulcerative colitis. For Crohn's disease and ulcerative colitis, IV infusions are given once every 8 weeks. This medication did not show evidence of fetal harm in laboratory animals. Ustekinumab is secreted in animal milk but effects on the breastfed neonate are unknown.

The biologic therapies are expensive, often costing thousands of dollars per injection, and some patients experience a high rate of serious infections due to their immunosuppressive actions. Biologic therapies are usually recommended only when first-line drugs are unable to control symptoms. Because they cause healing of the GI mucosa, it is possible that early use of these drugs could change the progressive course of IBD. For additional information on biologic therapies used for immunomodulation and doses of these drugs, refer to Chapter 42.

PROTOTYPE DRUG Sulfasalazine (Azulfidine)

Classification **Therapeutic:** Drug for inflammatory bowel disease, disease-modifying antirheumatic drug (DMARD)
Pharmacologic: 5-aminosalicylate, anti-inflammatory, sulfonamide

Therapeutic Effects and Uses: Approved in 1950, sulfasalazine is a PO drug with anti-inflammatory properties that is approved to treat mild to moderate symptoms of ulcerative colitis for adults and children age 6 years and older. It is approved as an alternate drug in the pharmacotherapy of rheumatoid arthritis and is classified as a DMARD (see Chapter 72). Sulfasalazine is used off-label to treat Crohn's disease.

Colon bacteria metabolize sulfasalazine to two active metabolites: sulfapyridine and 5-ASA. These metabolites are responsible for its anti-inflammatory properties.

Mechanism of Action: Sulfasalazine and its metabolites inhibit the mediators of inflammation in the colon such as prostaglandins and leukotrienes.

Pharmacokinetics:

Route(s)	PO
Absorption	Sulfasalazine is only 10–15% absorbed, but its metabolites in the colon produce therapeutic effects
Distribution	Crosses the placenta; secreted in breast milk; 93% bound to plasma protein
Primary metabolism	Hepatic; intestinal metabolism to the active metabolites sulfapyridine and 5-ASA
Primary excretion	Renal; active metabolites excreted in the feces
Onset of action	Peak: 1.5–6 h
Duration of action	Half-life: 5–10 h

Adverse Effects: The most common adverse effects of sulfasalazine are GI related and include nausea, vomiting, diarrhea, dyspepsia, and abdominal pain. Dividing the total daily dose evenly throughout the day and using the enteric-coated tablets may improve adherence. Headache is common. Blood dyscrasias occur infrequently during therapy. Skin rashes are relatively common and may be a sign of a more serious adverse effect such as Stevens–Johnson syndrome (SJS). Sulfasalazine can cause photosensitivity.

Contraindications/Precautions: Sulfasalazine is contraindicated in patients with sulfonamide or salicylate (aspirin or 5-ASA) hypersensitivity. Patients with preexisting anemia, folate, or other hematologic disorders should use this drug with caution because it may worsen blood dyscrasias. Sulfasalazine should be used with caution in patients with hepatic impairment because it can cause hepatotoxicity. This drug is contraindicated in patients with urinary obstruction and should be used with caution in dehydrated patients because it may cause crystalluria. Patients with diabetes or hypoglycemia should use sulfasalazine with caution because it can increase insulin secretion and worsen hypoglycemia.

Drug Interactions: Sulfasalazine may worsen bone marrow suppression caused by methotrexate and also result in additive hepatotoxicity. Absorption of digoxin may be decreased. The drug is a folic acid antagonist and will inhibit absorption of this vitamin. Sulfasalazine can displace warfarin from its protein-binding sites, causing increased anticoagulant effects. **Herbal/Food:** Unknown.

Pregnancy: Animal studies and limited human data did not show evidence of fetal harm. Sulfonamides are secreted in human milk and have the potential to cause kernicterus in a breastfed neonate.

Treatment of Overdose: Overdose will cause abdominal pain, anuria, drowsiness, gastric distress, seizures, nausea and vomiting. Treatment is mostly supportive with gastric lavage, emesis, and alkalinization of urine.

Clinician Responsibilities: Key clinical implications for patients receiving sulfasalazine are included in Applied Clinical Judgment: Patients Receiving Pharmacotherapy for GI Conditions.

Drugs Similar to Sulfasalazine (Azulfidine)

Other 5-aminosalicylates include balsalazide, mesalamine, and olsalazine.

Balsalazide (Colazal): Approved in 2000, balsalazide is a PO anti-inflammatory drug approved for the symptomatic treatment of ulcerative colitis in patients age 5 and above. Like sulfasalazine, balsalazide is metabolized in the intestinal mucosa to 5-ASA, which is responsible for its therapeutic effects. Almost 100% of this drug reaches the colon without being absorbed; thus, the primary action of the drug is topical rather than systemic. The drug is well tolerated, with headache, abdominal pain, diarrhea, nausea and vomiting being the most common adverse effects. Patients with salicylate hypersensitivity should not take this drug. Rare cases of hepatotoxicity have occurred. Animal studies did not show fetal harm. It is not known if this drug enters human milk and adverse effects on the breastfed neonate are unknown.

Mesalamine (Canasa, Lialda, others): Approved in 1987, mesalamine is sometimes referred to by its chemical name, 5-ASA. It is approved for the treatment of active ulcerative colitis and used off-label for Crohn's disease. A delayed-release formulation (Lialda) was developed for maintenance therapy, and a rectal suppository (Canasa) is available to treat ulcerative proctitis. Like other drugs in this class, mesalamine tablets and capsules are designed to release the drug in the terminal ileum and colon to produce its effects topically in the intestinal mucosa. Headache, abdominal pain, diarrhea, and nausea and vomiting are the most common adverse effects. Rectal irritation may be caused by the suppository forms of the drug. Patients with salicylate hypersensitivity should not take mesalamine. Animal studies and limited human data have not shown evidence of fetal harm. This drug is secreted in human milk although adverse effects on the breastfed neonate are unknown.

Olsalazine (Dipentum): Like other medications in this class, olsalazine is an oral drug that is metabolized in the intestinal mucosa to 5-ASA, which produces a topical anti-inflammatory effect. Nearly 100% of this drug reaches the colon without being absorbed systemically. Approved in 1990, the only indication for olsalazine is for the maintenance of remission of ulcerative colitis in patients who are unable to tolerate sulfasalazine. The most commonly reported adverse effects are diarrhea, abdominal pain, and rash. Rare cases of hepatotoxicity have occurred. Animal studies showed evidence of fetal harm and this drug is secreted in human milk. Olsalazine should be used during pregnancy or lactation only if the potential benefits to the mother justify the potential risks to the fetus.

PharmFACT

Irritable bowel syndrome affects 10 to 20% of adults. Women are two to three times more likely than men to have the disorder (Lehrer, 2016).

Pharmacotherapy of Irritable Bowel Syndrome

60.6 Irritable bowel syndrome is treated with dietary management, symptomatic therapy, and drugs that regulate intestinal motility.

Irritable bowel syndrome (IBS), also known as *spastic colon* or *mucous colitis*, is a common disorder of the lower GI tract characterized by symptoms that include abdominal pain, visible bloating, excessive gas, and colicky cramping. Bowel habits are altered, with diarrhea alternating with constipation, and there may be mucus in the stool. Pain is usually relieved by defecation, although the patient usually feels as if the evacuation is incomplete. Symptoms of IBS are likely caused by altered GI motility, increased peristalsis, and increased pain sensitivity of the GI tract.

The diagnosis of IBS is sometimes one of exclusion, ruling out other diseases such as colon cancer, ulcerative colitis, intestinal infections, Crohn's disease, and diverticulitis. It is not a precursor of more serious disease, and symptoms such as bleeding, anorexia, weight loss, or fever are not usually experienced by patients with IBS. IBS is considered a functional bowel disorder, meaning that the normal operation of the digestive tract is impaired without the presence of detectable organic disease. A diagnosis of IBS requires that the patient has experienced recurrent abdominal pain or discomfort for at least 3 days per month during the previous 3 months that is associated with two or more of the following:

- Relieved by defecation
- Onset associated with a change in stool frequency
- Onset associated with a change in stool form or appearance.

Treatment of IBS is supportive, with drug therapy targeted at *symptomatic treatment* depending on whether constipation or diarrhea is the predominant symptom. There is no single treatment that is effective for all, or even most, patients.

Lifestyle changes, diet, and aggravating medications: Stress is not a cause of IBS, but it can influence the condition. Attempts should be made to identify stressors and develop positive coping strategies. Psychotherapy, relaxation techniques, and hypnosis may benefit some patients. Because food-specific triggers are not always apparent, the patient should keep a food diary to help recognize and avoid foods that appear to worsen the condition. Dietary restriction of caffeine, wheat, or lactose-based products may be attempted. Foods that cause bloating and flatulence such as beans, cabbage, and peas should be avoided.

Part of a medical history for IBS should include drugs that may be contributing to the symptoms of IBS. Common drugs that may cause constipation include NSAIDs, calcium channel blockers, anticholinergics, and opioids. Diarrhea may result from the use of laxatives, magnesium-containing antacids, or antibiotics. Sometimes a change in medication can help reduce IBS symptoms.

Dietary fiber and laxatives: Constipation, diarrhea, cramping, painful bowel movements, and rectal urgency occur frequently in patients with IBS. Because constipation and diarrhea often alternate, pharmacotherapy can be challenging. Fiber supplementation with nonprescription bulk laxatives such as psyllium has long been recommended as a treatment for IBS and can help regulate bowel movements to bring relief to some patients. Unfortunately, increased fiber intake will worsen the symptoms in some patients. Loperamide is effective at relieving symptoms of diarrhea in patients with IBS.

Antidepressant therapy: For many years the tricyclic antidepressants such as amitriptyline, desipramine (Norpramin), and doxepin (Sinequan) have been used to treat patients with IBS who have pain as a major symptom. In some IBS patients, these medications exert a positive effect on GI motility and reduce pain. Selective serotonin reuptake inhibitors such as paroxetine (Paxil) have fewer side effects than the tricyclics and may show benefit in patients with constipation-dominant IBS. While antidepressants are effective for some patients, they are not first-line drugs for IBS. No antidepressants are FDA-approved for IBS.

Drug-specific therapies: Drugs used to treat IBS do not alter the course of the disease and, in some cases, may actually worsen the symptoms. These drugs may not be significantly more effective than nonpharmacologic treatments such as IBS support groups, relaxation therapy, or dietary changes. There is no prototype drug for this condition. Drugs that provide symptomatic relief for some patients include alosetron, antispasmodic drugs (dicyclomine and hyoscyamine), eluxadoline, linaclotide, lubiprostone, rifaximin, and tenapanor.

Alosetron (Lotronex): By inhibiting serotonin (5-HT_3) receptors, alosetron reduces GI-related sensitivity and slows peristalsis in patients with diarrhea-predominant IBS. Alosetron was approved in 2000 but was withdrawn later that same year due to several deaths from ischemic colitis. This drug was allowed to return to the market in 2002 but with severe restrictions on its use. It is approved only for severe diarrhea-predominant IBS in women who have not responded to conventional therapy. No refills are allowed without a follow-up examination by the prescribing healthcare provider. A risk–benefit statement must be signed by the patient and healthcare provider that they agree to adhere to therapy plans. A black box warning states that alosetron can cause adverse GI reactions, including ischemic colitis and serious complications of constipation that can cause death. The warning also states that healthcare providers who wish to prescribe alosetron must receive special training and testing to learn to appropriately diagnose and treat IBS. Furthermore, other therapies must have been attempted (and failed) prior to alosetron use. Other adverse effects include abdominal discomfort, nausea, and rash. Alosetron did not show evidence of fetal harm in laboratory animals. It is not known if the drug is secreted in milk or if it has adverse effects on the breastfed neonate.

Antispasmodic drugs: Antispasmodic drugs are those that relax smooth muscle and slow peristalsis. Dicyclomine (Bentyl) and hyoscyamine (Anaspaz, Gastrosed, Levsin) are older anticholinergic drugs that are used to reduce bowel spasms in patients with IBS (see Chapter 14). Dicyclomine was approved in 1950 for diarrhea-predominant IBS and other functional disorders of GI motility. Dicyclomine may be administered PO or by IM injection. Frequent adverse effects include typical anticholinergic effects such as dry mouth, blurred vision, drowsiness, urinary hesitancy, and tachycardia. Dicyclomine did not show evidence of fetal harm in laboratory animals. Because this drug is secreted in human milk, breastfeeding is not recommended.

Available since the FDA was established in 1938, hyoscyamine is an anticholinergic drug that is usually administered PO, but parenteral forms are available. It is approved to treat peptic ulcer disease and diarrhea-predominant IBS because the drug decreases acid secretion of the stomach and slows peristalsis. It has also been used to reverse bradycardia, to relieve symptoms of allergic rhinitis, and to dry respiratory and salivary secretions prior to surgery. Whereas in 1938 hyoscyamine may have been a preferred drug for these conditions, it has been replaced by safer and more effective drugs for nearly every indication. Animal reproduction studies have not been conducted on hyoscyamine. Because this drug is secreted in human milk, breastfeeding is not recommended.

Eluxadoline (Viberzi): Eluxadoline was approved in 2015 for the treatment of diarrhea-dominant IBS in adults. Given PO, it acts by activating the mu and kappa opioid receptors. It is contraindicated in patients with biliary tract obstruction or those with a history of alcohol abuse. An FDA safety warning states that serious pancreatitis may occur when eluxadoline is given to patients without a gallbladder. Eluxadoline is a Schedule IV controlled substance and should be used cautiously in patients with a history of substance use disorder. Eluxadoline did not show evidence of fetal harm in laboratory animals. Because this drug is secreted in animal milk, breastfeeding is not recommended.

Linaclotide (Linzess): Linaclotide was approved in 2012 for chronic idiopathic constipation and for constipation-dominant IBS. It is an oral drug that acts by the same mechanism as plecanatide: increasing the secretion of chloride and bicarbonate ion into the intestinal lumen, resulting in increased amounts of intestinal fluid and accelerated fecal transport. The most common adverse effects are diarrhea, abdominal pain, flatulence, and abdominal distention. The drug carries a black box warning that it is contraindicated in children up to age 6 and should be avoided in children age 6 through 17 due to the potential for serious dehydration. At clinically relevant doses, linaclotide did not show fetal harm in laboratory animals. It is not known if the drug is secreted in milk or if it has adverse effects on the breastfed neonate.

Lubiprostone (Amitiza): Lubiprostone is approved for the treatment of chronic idiopathic constipation, opioid-induced constipation in adults with chronic non-cancer pain and constipation-predominant IBS in women over age 18. Lubiprostone increases fluid secretion by activating chloride channels in the intestinal luminal cells, thereby altering stool consistency and promoting regular bowel movements. The most common adverse effect is nausea, which can be reduced by taking the drug with food. Lubiprostone should not be administered to patients with severe diarrhea or suspected GI obstruction. Because lubiprostone causes fetal loss in laboratory animals, it should be used during pregnancy only if the potential benefits to the mother justify the possible risks to the fetus. This drug caused fetal harm in laboratory animals when given at very high doses. There are no data regarding effects of lubiprostone during breastfeeding.

Rifaximin (Xifaxan): Rifaximin is an antibiotic similar in structure to rifampin, a first-line therapy for tuberculosis. Originally indicated for traveler's diarrhea, rifaximin was approved to treat diarrhea-dominant IBS in 2015. Given PO for 2 weeks, the mechanism by which it improves IBS symptoms is unclear. The drug is also a first-line therapy for the prevention hepatic encephalopathy, a disorder in which toxic byproducts of liver metabolism (primarily ammonia) accumulate to cause serious neuropsychiatric symptoms and potentially coma. Rifaximin alters the normal bacteria flora in the colon, resulting in less production of ammonia. The drug is minimally absorbed and concentrated in the GI tract. The most common adverse effects include nausea and elevations in alanine transaminase. Rifaximin is teratogenic in laboratory animals. There are no data regarding effects of rifaximin during breastfeeding.

Tenapanor (Ibsrela): One of the newer drugs for IBS, tenapanor was approved in 2019 for constipation-dominant IBS in adults. It acts by reducing absorption of sodium in the small intestine and colon. This results in more sodium in the colon and, because water always follows sodium, the intestinal contents have a softer consistency. Taking tenapanor 5 to 10 minutes prior to the morning and evening meal increases its effectiveness. Side effects are minor and include diarrhea and abdominal distension. It is contraindicated in children under age 6 due to an increased risk for dehydration. Tenapanor is minimally absorbed, therefore fetal harm would not be expected during pregnancy and negligible amounts enter milk.

Pathophysiology of Nausea and Vomiting

60.7 Nausea and vomiting occur when the vomiting center in the medulla is stimulated.

Nausea is an unpleasant feeling of the need to vomit that is accompanied by weakness, diaphoresis, dizziness, and hyperproduction of saliva. Intense nausea often leads to **vomiting**, or emesis, in which the stomach contents are forced upward into the esophagus and out of the mouth. Vomiting is a defense mechanism used by the body to rid itself of toxic substances.

Vomiting is a reflex primarily controlled by a portion of the medulla of the brain known as the **vomiting center**, which receives sensory signals from the digestive tract, the inner ear, and the **chemoreceptor trigger zone (CTZ)** in the cerebral cortex. Interestingly, the CTZ is not protected by the blood–brain barrier, as is the vast majority of the brain; thus, these neurons can directly sense the presence of toxic substances in the blood. Once the vomiting reflex is triggered, wavelike contractions of the stomach quickly propel its contents upward and out of the body.

The treatment outcomes for nausea or vomiting should focus on removal of the cause whenever feasible. Nausea and vomiting are common symptoms associated with a wide variety of conditions. Some conditions originate in the GI tract itself, such as peptic ulcer disease, GI obstruction, gallbladder disease, food poisoning, or ingestion of a toxic substance that irritates the mucosa. The nausea and vomiting may originate from systemic sources such as those caused by cancer, pregnancy, radiation sickness, migraine headache, trauma to the head or abdominal organs, inner ear disorders, extreme pain, diabetes, or systemic drug use. In addition to the CTZ, other parts of the nervous system may promote nausea and vomiting in response to nervousness, emotional imbalances, changes in body position (motion sickness), extreme stress, or when confronted with unpleasant sights, smells, or sounds.

The nausea and vomiting experienced by many women during the first trimester of pregnancy is referred to as *morning sickness*. The cause of nausea and vomiting during pregnancy is not completely understood but is probably due to hormonal changes, especially in levels of estrogen and human chorionic gonadotropin (hCG). All women of childbearing years who present with nausea and vomiting should receive a pregnancy test because this is a common explanation for these symptoms. Should this condition become acute, such as continual vomiting, it may lead to **hyperemesis gravidarum**, a situation in which the health and safety of the mother and developing baby can become severely compromised. Complications may include dehydration, electrolyte imbalances, and significant weight loss. Pharmacotherapy with fluid and electrolyte solutions and antiemetics is initiated after other antinausea measures have proven ineffective.

PharmFACT

Morning sickness occurs in 70 to 85% of pregnancies. Morning sickness has a peak incidence at 8 to 12 weeks of pregnancy but usually ends by week 20 (Khan, 2016).

Nausea and vomiting are the most frequently listed adverse effects for oral medications. The nurse should remember that because the vomiting center lies in the brain, nausea and vomiting occur just as frequently with parenteral formulations as with oral drugs. The most extreme example of this occurs with the antineoplastic drugs, most of which cause intense nausea and vomiting regardless of the route by which they are administered. The capacity of a chemotherapeutic drug to cause vomiting is called its **emetogenic potential**. Nausea and vomiting are common reasons for lack of adherence to the therapeutic regimen and for discontinuation of drug therapy.

When large amounts of fluids are vomited, dehydration and significant weight loss may occur. Because the contents lost from the stomach are strongly acidic, vomiting may cause a change in the pH of the blood, resulting in metabolic alkalosis. With excessive loss, severe acid–base disturbances can lead to vascular collapse, resulting in death if medical intervention is not initiated. Electrolytes such as sodium, potassium, and chloride are also lost during vomiting and may need to be replaced, especially in the infant, child, and older adult. Dehydration is especially dangerous for infants, small children, and the older adult and is evidenced by dry mouth, sticky saliva, and reduced urine output that is dark yellow-orange to brown in color.

Pharmacotherapy of Nausea and Vomiting

60.8 Antiemetics are prescribed to treat nausea and vomiting and motion sickness.

Drugs from at least eight different classes are used to prevent or treat nausea and vomiting. Most of these drugs were originally developed for other indications, and their antiemetic characteristics were discovered later. Selection of a specific drug depends on the cause of the nausea and vomiting and its severity.

Patients who are seeking self-treatment have access to several available OTC options. For example, simple nausea and vomiting are sometimes relieved by antacids or diphenhydramine (Benadryl). Peppermint and ginger are the most popular herbal therapies for nausea and vomiting.

Relief of serious nausea and vomiting requires prescription medications. Patients who are receiving antineoplastic drugs may receive three or more antiemetics concurrently to reduce the nausea and vomiting from chemotherapy. In fact, therapy with antineoplastics is one of the most common reasons for prescribing antiemetic drugs. Many antiemetics are available through the IM, IV, or suppository route to prevent loss of the medication due to vomiting. Pharmacotherapy Illustrated 60.2 shows the mechanisms of action of antiemetic medications. Doses for selected antiemetics are listed in Table 60.5.

Anticholinergics and antihistamines: These medications are effective for treating simple nausea, with some being available OTC. For example, nausea due to motion sickness is effectively treated with anticholinergics or antihistamines. Motion sickness is a disorder that affects a portion of the inner ear that is associated with significant nausea. The most common drug used for motion sickness is scopolamine (Transderm-Scop), an anticholinergic that is usually administered as a transdermal patch. Antihistamines such as dimenhydrinate (Dramamine), doxylamine, and meclizine (Antivert) are also effective but may cause significant drowsiness in some patients. Drugs that are used to treat motion sickness are most effective when taken 20 to 60 minutes before travel is expected.

When nonpharmacologic measures such as ginger are unable to control hyperemesis gravidarum, therapy with antihistamines may be initiated. Diclegis, a combination drug containing doxylamine (an antihistamine) and pyridoxine (vitamin B_6), has been found to be effective for the mother and safe for the fetus. It is the only FDA-approved medication for the condition, although other antihistamines, metoclopramide, promethazine, and ondansetron (Zofran) have been used off-label for patients with severe symptoms.

Serotonin (5-HT_3) receptor antagonists: The serotonin antagonists include granisetron (Sancuso, Sustol), ondansetron (Zofran, Zuplenz), and palonosetron (Aloxi). There are no significant differences in effectiveness or toxicity of the serotonin receptor antagonists in treating acute nausea and vomiting. They are available by the PO or parenteral route. Since the 1990s they have become the most widely prescribed drugs for chemotherapy-induced nausea and vomiting. For severe symptoms, the serotonin receptor antagonists are combined with a corticosteroid such as dexamethasone. The serotonin antagonists are most effective in the management of acute nausea and vomiting but are less effective at treating delayed symptoms. The few adverse effects they cause include headache, constipation or diarrhea, and dizziness. The combination drug Akynzeo (palonosetron with netupitant) is available to treat nausea and vomiting caused by highly emetogenic chemotherapy.

Phenothiazines and dopamine antagonists: Phenothiazines act by inhibiting the dopamine-2 (D2) receptor. The primary indication for phenothiazines is the treatment of psychoses (see Chapter 20), but they are also very effective antiemetics. Phenothiazines inhibit dopaminergic receptors in the CTZ, and the severe nausea and vomiting associated with antineoplastic therapy are often treated with these drugs. Some of the phenothiazines may cause sedation, and EPS are a concern with long-term therapy. Promethazine (Phenergan) is an older phenothiazine that is available by the PO, rectal, and parenteral routes that also has significant anticholinergic properties. In 2020, a nonphenothiazine D2 antagonist, amisulpride (Barhemsys), was approved as a single infusion to treat postoperative nausea and vomiting.

Cannabinoids: Cannabinoids are drugs that contain the same active ingredient as marijuana. Dronabinol (Marinol, Syndros) and nabilone (Cesamet) are given PO to reduce

Table 60.5 Selected Antiemetics

Drug	Route and Adult Dose (Maximum Dose Where Indicated)	Adverse Effects
Anticholinergics-Antihistamines		
dimenhydrinate (Dramamine, others)	PO: 50–100 mg q4–6h (max: 400 mg/day)	*Drowsiness, dry mouth, blurred vision (scopolamine)* Hypersensitivity reaction, sedation, tremors, seizures, hallucinations, paradoxical excitation (more common in children), hypotension
diphenhydramine (Benadryl, others)	PO: 25–50 mg tid–qid (max: 300 mg/day)	
doxylamine and pyridoxine (Diclegis)	PO: 20–40 mg daily	
hydroxyzine (Atarax)	PO: 25–100 mg tid or qid (max: 400 mg/day)	
meclizine (Antivert, Bonine, others)	PO: 25–50 mg daily, take 1 h before travel (max: 50 mg/day)	
scopolamine (Transderm-Scop)	Transdermal: 0.5 mg (patch) q72h	
Cannabinoids		
dronabinol (Marinol, Syndros)	PO: 5 mg/m^2 1–3 h before administration of chemotherapy, then q2–4h after chemotherapy for a total of 4–6 doses	*Dizziness, drowsiness, euphoria, confusion, ataxia, asthenia, increased sensory awareness* Paranoia, decreased motor coordination, hypotension
nabilone (Cesamet)	PO: 1–2 mg bid	
Corticosteroids		
dexamethasone	PO: 0.25–4 mg bid–qid	*Mood swings, weight gain, acne, facial flushing, nausea, insomnia, sodium and fluid retention, impaired wound healing, menstrual abnormalities, insomnia* Peptic ulcer, hypocalcemia, osteoporosis with possible bone fractures, loss of muscle mass, decreased growth in children, masking of infections
methylprednisolone (Medrol, Solu-Medrol, others)	PO: 4–48 mg/day in divided doses	
Neurokinin Receptor Antagonist		
aprepitant (Cinvanti, Emend Capsules) and fosaprepitant (Emend for Injection)	PO (Emend capsules): 125 mg 1 h prior to chemotherapy IV (Cinvanti, Emend for injection): 115–150 mg 30 min prior to chemotherapy	*Fatigue, constipation, diarrhea, anorexia, hiccups* Dehydration, peripheral neuropathy, blood dyscrasias, pneumonia
Phenothiazines and Dopamine Antagonists		
amisulpride (Barhemsys)	IV: 5–10 mg single infusion	*Increased prolactin, chills, hypokalemia, hypotension, infusion site pain* QT prolongation
metoclopramide (Reglan)	PO: 10–15 mg qid prior to meals	*Dry eyes, blurred vision, dry mouth, constipation, drowsiness, photosensitivity* extrapyramidal symptoms (EPS), neuroleptic malignant syndrome, agranulocytosis, orthostatic hypotension, tardive dyskinesia
perphenazine	PO: 8–16 mg bid–qid	
prochlorperazine (Compro, ProComp)	PO: 5–10 mg tid or qid Rectal: 25 mg bid IM: 5–10 mg tid or qid IV: 2.5–10 mg tid or qid (max: 10 mg/dose or 40 mg/day)	
promethazine (Phenergan, others)	PO: 12.5–25 mg q4h or qid	
trimethobenzamide (Tigan)	PO: 300 mg once daily IM: 200 mg 3–4 times/day	
Serotonin (5-HT$_3$) Receptor Antagonists		
granisetron (Sancuso, Sustol)	PO: 2 mg/day 1 h prior to chemotherapy IV: 10 mcg/kg 30 min prior to chemotherapy Transdermal (Sancuso): 1 patch 24–48 h prior to chemotherapy Subcutaneous (Sustol): 10 mg at least 30 min prior to chemotherapy	*Headache, drowsiness, fatigue, constipation, diarrhea, flulike symptoms, injection-site reactions* Dysrhythmias, EPS, hepatic failure, serotonin syndrome
ondansetron (Zofran, Zuplenz)	PO: 8 mg bid or tid IV: 32 mg 30 min prior to chemotherapy	
palonosetron (Aloxi)	PO: 0.5 mg single dose 1 h prior to chemotherapy IV: 0.25 mg 30 min prior to chemotherapy	

Note: *Italics* indicate common adverse effects. Underline indicates serious adverse effects.

Pharmacotherapy Illustrated 60.2

Mechanisms of Action of Antiemetic Medications

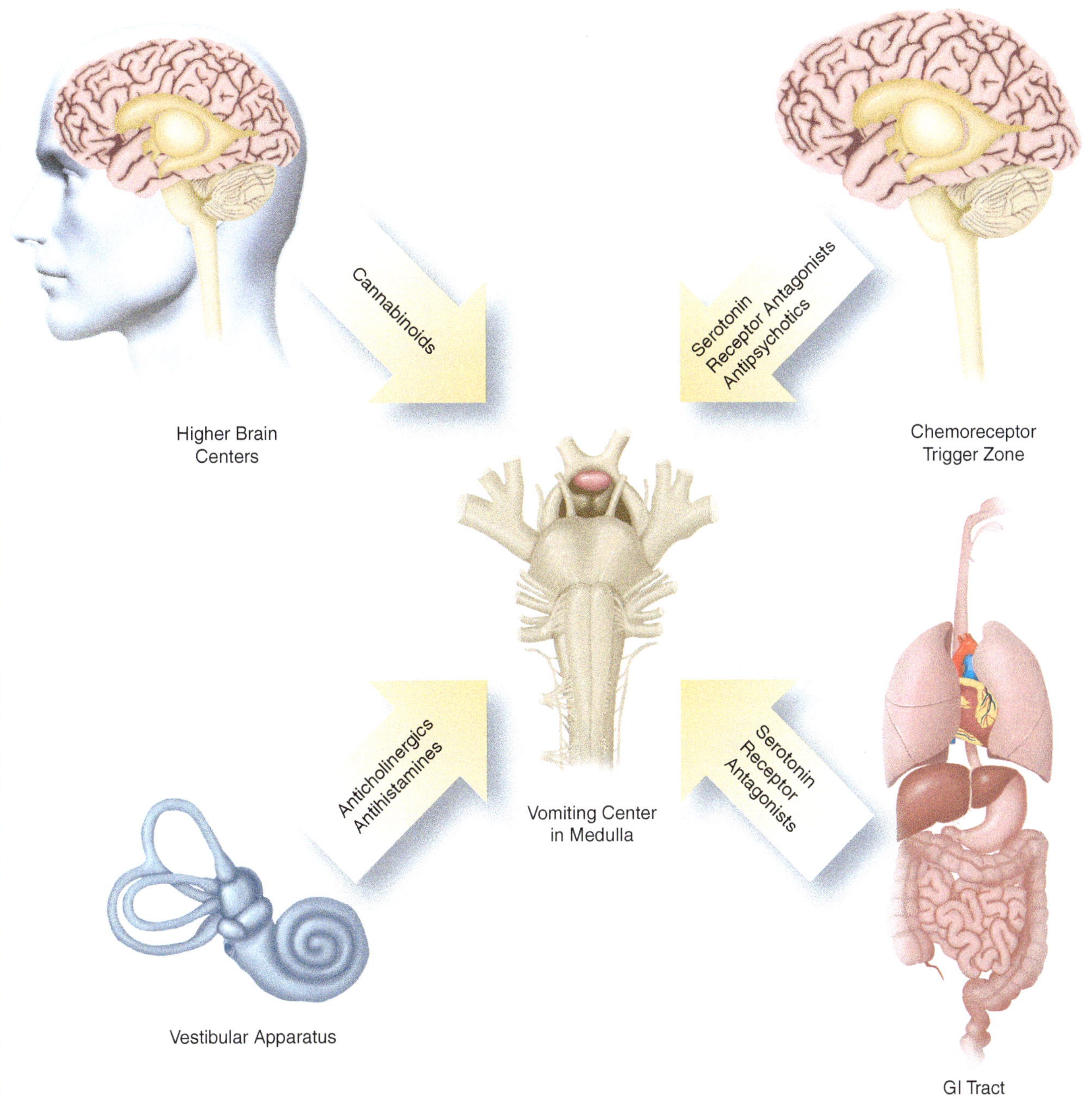

post-chemotherapy nausea and vomiting, with less euphoria compared to marijuana. Dronabinol is also indicated for the treatment of anorexia and weight loss in patients with AIDS. Cannabinoids are not as effective as other antiemetics.

Corticosteroids: Dexamethasone (Decadron) and methylprednisolone (Solu-Medrol) are used to prevent chemotherapy-induced and postsurgical nausea and vomiting. They are reserved for acute cases due to the possibility of serious adverse effects and are most often used in combination with other antiemetics. Dexamethasone is used for the treatment of delayed nausea and vomiting, which are common problems with certain antineoplastic drugs.

Other drugs: Aprepitant (Emend) belongs to a class of antiemetics called the neurokinin (NK) receptor antagonists that reduce the level of substance P, which is involved in the emesis reflex. Aprepitant was FDA-approved in 2003 as part

CONNECTIONS: Complementary and Alternative Therapies

Probiotics for Diarrhea

Description

Probiotics are live microorganisms that are taken in specified amounts to confer a health benefit on the host. Most commercial probiotics are bacteria from the genera *Lactobacillus* and *Bifidobacterium*; however, yeast such as *Saccharomyces* are also sometimes used.

History and Claims

Although probiotics have been used for thousands of years, only in the past 20 years has research begun to confirm their health benefits. Probiotics are claimed to improve immune function, decrease cancer risk, lower blood cholesterol, reduce blood pressure, and prevent vaginal infections. Probiotics are available in yogurts, fermented foods, added to some drinks, and as tablets. Although probiotics are safe, care must be taken not to exceed recommended doses.

Standardization

Supplements include capsules, tablets, and granules, as well as cultured dairy products that contain the probiotic bacteria. Doses are not standardized. Tablet doses range from 50 to 500 mg, and not all dairy products contain active cultures.

Evidence

Most of the evidence supporting the efficacy of probiotics is related to their effects on the intestinal tract microbiome. Both *Lactobacillus* and *Bifidobacterium* are normal nonpathogenic inhabitants of a healthy digestive tract. These are considered to be protective flora, inhibiting the growth of potentially pathogenic species such as *E. coli*, *Candida albicans*, *Helicobacter pylori*, and *Gardnerella vaginalis*. Probiotics are useful in restoring the normal flora of the intestine following diarrhea, particularly diarrhea resulting from antibiotic therapy, and have shown positive effects for a wide variety of other conditions such as allergies, dental problems, and some infections (National Center for Complementary and Integrative Health, 2019).

Although probiotics have been used for many years, they are not without risk. Infections (including sepsis), lactic acidosis, and other serious adverse effects have been noted and probiotic supplements should be used with caution in critically ill patients.

of a 3-day antiemetic regimen for antineoplastic chemotherapy in conjunction with a corticosteroid (dexamethasone) and a serotonin receptor antagonist (ondansetron). It is also approved to treat postoperative nausea and vomiting. The IV form of this drug, fosaprepitant, was approved in 2008. In 2015 a new NK receptor antagonist, rolapitant (Varubi), was approved to reduce nausea and vomiting associated with chemotherapy. Neither aprepitant nor rolapitant showed evidence of fetal harm in laboratory animals.

On some occasions, it is desirable to *stimulate* the vomiting reflex with drugs called emetics. Indications for emetics include ingestion of poisons and overdoses of oral drugs. Ipecac syrup, given PO, or apomorphine, given subcutaneously, will induce vomiting in about 15 minutes.

CONNECTION Checkpoint 60.3

From what you learned in Chapter 20, define *extrapyramidal adverse effects* and provide examples of symptoms that a patient might exhibit.

PROTOTYPE DRUG Ondansetron (Zofran, Zuplenz)

Classification **Therapeutic:** Antiemetic
Pharmacologic: Serotonin (5-HT_3) receptor antagonist

Therapeutic Effects and Uses: Ondansetron and other drugs in the serotonin receptor antagonist class have replaced older drugs for the treatment of serious nausea and vomiting due to their superior effectiveness and safety. To prevent chemotherapy-induced nausea and vomiting, the medication is started at least 30 minutes prior to chemotherapy and continued for several days after. For radiation-induced nausea and vomiting, ondansetron is administered 1 to 2 hours before therapy and continued for 1 to 2 days. It is available by the PO, IV, IM, oral disintegrating tablet, and oral soluble-film routes. Initially approved in 1991, the drug may be used off-label to treat cholestatic pruritus or opioid-induced pruritus.

Mechanism of Action: Ondansetron acts by blocking serotonin receptors in the chemoreceptor trigger zone, an area of the brain responsible for nausea and vomiting.

Pharmacokinetics:

Route(s)	PO, IV
Absorption	Rapidly absorbed
Distribution	Widely distributed; secreted in breast milk; over 70% bound to plasma proteins
Primary metabolism	Extensive hepatic metabolism by multiple CYP450 enzymes
Primary excretion	Renal (44–60%) and feces (25%)
Onset of action	PO: 1–1.5 h
Duration of action	Unknown

Adverse Effects: Ondansetron is well tolerated, with the most common adverse effects being headache, dizziness, drowsiness, and constipation or diarrhea.

Contraindications/Precautions: This drug should not be used in patients with hypersensitivity to other serotonin receptor antagonists. Caution should be used when treating patients with cardiac abnormalities because ondansetron can prolong the QT interval and cause dysrhythmias. If used following abdominal surgery, ondansetron may mask signs of progressive ileus.

Drug Interactions: Ondansetron exhibits few clinically significant drug interactions. However, serotonin syndrome may occur if used concurrently with other serotonergic drugs such as serotonin and norepinephrine reuptake inhibitors. Because the drug is extensively metabolized by hepatic CYP450 enzymes, inhibitors or inducers of these enzymes may affect the availability of ondansetron. **Herbal/Food:** Unknown.

Pregnancy: This drug did not show evidence of fetal harm in laboratory animals. Human data were inconclusive but did not show clear evidence of birth defects from ondansetron. This drug is secreted in animal milk, although effects on the breastfed neonate are unknown.

Treatment of Overdose: There is no specific therapy for ondansetron overdose and general supportive measures should be used.

Clinician Responsibilities: Key clinical implications for patients receiving ondansetron are included in Applied Clinical Judgment: Patients Receiving Pharmacotherapy for GI Conditions.

Drugs Similar to Ondansetron (Zofran, Zuplenz)

Other serotonin receptor antagonists include granisetron (Sancuso, Sustol) and palonosetron (Aloxi). All drugs in this class have similar effectiveness and safety profiles.

Pharmacotherapy of Pancreatitis

60.9 Pancreatic enzymes are administered as replacement therapy for patients with chronic pancreatitis.

The pancreas secretes insulin as well as essential digestive enzymes. The enzymatic portion of pancreatic juice contains carboxypeptidase, chymotrypsin, and trypsin, which are converted to their active forms once they enter the small intestine. Three other pancreatic enzymes—lipase, amylase, and nuclease—are secreted in their active form but require the presence of bile for optimal activity. When lack of pancreatic enzyme secretion results in malabsorption disorders, replacement therapy is warranted.

PharmFACT

The United States has the second-highest incidence of acute pancreatitis in the world. African Americans have a 10 times greater incidence than any other ethnic group (Tang, 2019).

Pancreatitis results when digestive enzymes remain in the pancreas rather than being released into the duodenum. Upon becoming activated and escaping into the surrounding tissue, the enzymes cause inflammation in the pancreas, which can lead to hemorrhage and necrosis. The backed-up enzymes and enteric bacteria may leak into the peritoneum, causing a severe systemic reaction and, possibly, death. Pancreatitis can be either acute or chronic. The two types of pancreatitis have different symptoms, mortality rates, and treatments.

Acute pancreatitis: Acute pancreatitis occurs most frequently in middle-aged adults and is often associated with gallstones in women and alcoholism in men. Symptoms of acute pancreatitis present suddenly, often after eating a fatty meal or consuming excessive amounts of alcohol. The most common symptom is a continuous severe pain in the epigastric area, often radiating to the back. Fever, tachycardia, abdominal tenderness, and muscular guarding (involuntary spasm of the abdominal muscles when palpated) are common. Although most patients recover from the illness and regain normal pancreatic functions, a small percentage of patients experience recurring attacks and progress to chronic pancreatitis.

Many patients with acute pancreatitis require only bedrest, fasting, and adequate fluid and electrolyte therapy for a few days for the symptoms to subside. There are no medications specific to acute pancreatitis. For patients with acute pain, an opioid such as hydromorphone (Dilaudid) brings effective relief. To reduce gastric and pancreatic juice secretions, H_2-receptor blockers, such as cimetidine (Tagamet), or proton pump inhibitors, such as omeprazole (Prilosec), may be prescribed. To decrease the amount of pancreatic enzymes secreted, carbonic anhydrase inhibitors, such as acetazolamide (Diamox), or antispasmodics, such as dicyclomine (Bentyl), may be used. In severe cases where enteral nutrition is not tolerated, total parenteral nutrition may be necessary.

Cases of pancreatitis accompanied by a high fever and infection have a very high mortality rate. Pharmacotherapy with an antibiotic from the imipenem class is usually begun immediately if there is evidence of pancreatic necrosis.

Chronic pancreatitis: Seventy to 80% of chronic pancreatitis cases are associated with alcohol use disorder. Other causes include pancreatic cancer and stones. Alcohol is thought to promote the formation of insoluble proteins that occlude the pancreatic duct. Pancreatic juice is prevented from flowing into the duodenum and remains in the pancreas, damaging cells and causing inflammation. Symptoms include chronic epigastric or left upper quadrant pain, anorexia, nausea and vomiting, and weight loss. **Steatorrhea**, the passing of bulky, foul-smelling fatty stools, occurs late in the course of the disease. Chronic pancreatitis causes permanent structural damage to the organ and may cause scarring of the pancreatic duct system. Chronic pancreatitis is a risk factor for the development of pancreatic cancer. The disease eventually leads to pancreatic insufficiency that may necessitate insulin therapy as well as replacement of pancreatic enzymes.

There is no curative treatment for chronic pancreatitis and the patient is treated symptomatically. Fasting, IV fluids, and opioid analgesics may be necessary. The chronic, severe pain may lead to high doses of opioids and a possibility of drug dependence. In addition, the patient with chronic pancreatitis may require insulin and antiemetics.

Pancreatic enzyme supplementation is often used in patients with chronic pancreatitis. Supplementation sends a negative feedback message to stop secreting endogenous pancreatic enzymes, which can reduce pain. These supplements are given orally. Pancrelipase (Creon, Pancreaze, Zenpep) is a pancreatic enzyme supplement that helps to digest fats and prevent steatorrhea.

PROTOTYPE DRUG Pancrelipase (Creon, Pancreaze, Zenpep)

Classification **Therapeutic:** Pancreatic enzymes
Pharmacologic: None

Therapeutic Effects and Uses: Pancrelipase contains lipase, protease, and amylase of pork origin and is used as replacement therapy for patients with insufficient pancreatic exocrine secretions, including those with pancreatitis and cystic fibrosis. Given PO the capsule dissolves in the alkaline environment of the duodenum and releases its enzymes. The enzymes act locally in the GI tract and are not absorbed. Pancrelipase is available in powder, tablet, and delayed-release capsule formulations.

The different trade names of pancrelipase are not interchangeable because the amounts of pancreatic enzymes in each product may vary. Dose is based on the amount of fat in the diet. Doses are taken just prior to meals or with meals.

Mechanism of Action: This drug facilitates the breakdown and conversion of lipids into glycerol and fatty acids, starches into dextrin and sugars, and proteins into peptides.

Pharmacokinetics:

Route(s)	PO
Absorption	Not absorbed
Distribution	Not distributed
Primary metabolism	Metabolized in the small bowel
Primary excretion	Feces
Onset of action	Immediate
Duration of action	Unknown

Adverse Effects: Adverse effects of pancrelipase are uncommon because the enzymes are not absorbed. The most common adverse effects are GI symptoms of nausea and vomiting and diarrhea. Very high doses are associated with a risk for hyperuricemia. A rare condition known as fibrosing colonopathy may occur when very high doses of pancreatic enzyme replacements are given to patients with cystic fibrosis.

Contraindications/Precautions: Pancrelipase is contraindicated in patients who are allergic to this drug or to pork products. The delayed-release products should not be given to patients with acute pancreatitis.

Drug Interactions: Pancrelipase interacts with iron, which may result in decreased absorption of iron. Calcium and magnesium antacids may diminish the drug's effectiveness. **Herbal/Food:** Unknown.

Pregnancy: Studies on the effects of this drug on pregnancy and lactation have not been conducted. Because pancreatic enzymes act locally and are not absorbed, no adverse effects are expected.

Treatment of Overdose: High levels of uric acid may occur with overdose. Patients are treated symptomatically.

Clinician Responsibilities: Key clinical implications for patients receiving pancrelipase are included in Applied Clinical Judgment: Patients Receiving Pharmacotherapy for GI Conditions.

Drugs Similar to Pancrelipase (Creon, Pancreaze, Zenpep)

There are no drugs similar to pancrelipase. Several unapproved forms of pancreatic enzyme products were removed from the market in 2010, per a directive from the FDA.

CONNECTIONS: APPLIED CLINICAL JUDGMENT

Patients Receiving Pharmacotherapy for GI Conditions

Key Assessment Data

- History of current condition, baseline vital signs, physical exam findings, especially abdominal assessment; ulcers or gastrointestinal bleeding, hepatic or renal disease; medication history and caffeine, nicotine, and alcohol use; pregnancy status.

Desired Therapeutic Outcomes

Improvement is observed and measurable by adequate pattern of elimination, normal stool consistency and volume, nausea is decreased, no vomiting present, able to tolerate fluids and increasing solids, abdominal pain has eased.

Minimizing Adverse Effects

- Constipation, diarrhea, and nausea are usually symptoms of other underlying conditions; treat the cause if a definitive cause for the current symptoms can be identified.
- Bowel obstruction must be ruled out in the presence of hypoactive or absent bowel sounds and laxatives should not be given until determined. If infection is a possible cause of diarrhea, giving antidiarrheal drugs may decrease peristalsis, giving the infection an opportunity to increase and spread. Any significant change in bowel sound activity or increased discomfort or pain may signal the development of worsening bowel disease or adverse drug effects.
- Vomiting, excessive use of laxatives, or continued diarrhea may affect electrolyte levels and replacement therapy may be needed.
- Antiemetics are most effective when taken before nausea occurs. Ensuring adequate hydration decreases the risk of dehydration should vomiting occur.
- Adverse reactions to sulfasalazine generally occur within a few days to 12 weeks after the start of therapy and are most likely to occur in patients who are receiving high doses.

Lifespan Considerations

- The older adult is at increased risk of hypotension, dizziness, injury, and falls. Diphenoxylate with atropine may cause agitation, confusion, or hallucinations in the older adult, particularly if dementia is a preexisting condition. Excessive vomiting may cause dehydration and decreased blood pressure or hypotension. Antiemetics such as anticholinergics, antihistamines, and phenothiazine or phenothiazine-like drugs may also cause dizziness or a decrease in blood pressure.
- Alternative antinausea measures should be used to control or ease nausea when possible. Drug effects in pregnancy and the trimester will be considered by the healthcare provider before prescribing the drug to avoid detrimental effects.
- Men may experience a decreased production of sperm and infertility if sulfasalazine is used; this is reversed with the discontinuation of this drug.

Patient Education

- Increasing abdominal pain, nausea and vomiting, especially if accompanied by fever, should be reported to the healthcare provider. Immediately report any diarrhea that increases in frequency or amount or that contains mucus, blood, or pus. Consult the healthcare provider before taking any antidiarrheal drugs, which cause the retention of harmful bacteria.
- Rise slowly from lying or sitting to standing to avoid dizziness or falls. If dizziness occurs, sit or lie down and not attempt to stand or walk until the sensation passes.
- Take antiemetics 30 to 60 minutes if nausea is anticipated (e.g., administration of chemotherapy, travel).
- Pregnant patients, or if pregnancy is suspected, should consult with the healthcare provider before taking any antiemetic drug for morning sickness.
- Increase intake of dairy products containing live active cultures, such as yogurt, kefir, or buttermilk, to help restore normal intestinal flora. Eliminate alcohol use and reduce or eliminate smoking.
- Patients taking sulfasalazine should avoid prolonged sun exposure because the skin may be more sensitive. Wear sunscreen, protective clothing, and sunglasses if exposed to direct sunlight. Report any sunburn or other skin rashes to the provider.
- Examine stools and report to the healthcare provider if enteric-coated sulfasalazine tablets have passed intact in feces. If this occurs, a conventional tablet form can be ordered.
- Increase fluid intake to 2 to 3 L/day because sulfasalazine may cause crystals in the urine. Be aware that this drug may color urine and skin orange-yellow.
- Take the drug following appropriate guidelines:
  - **All laxative drugs:** Take the drug with additional fluids and increase fluid intake throughout the day. Increase the intake of dietary fiber, especially whole grains, fruits, and vegetables. Exceeding the recommended dose or frequent laxative use increases the risk of adverse effects and decreases normal peristalsis over time, resulting in laxative dependence.
  - **Bulk-forming laxatives:** Take other medications 1 hour before or 2 hours after the laxative. Powdered formulations should be mixed with a full glass of liquid and taken immediately, followed by an additional full glass of liquid. Powders should never be swallowed dry or esophageal obstruction may result.
  - **Pancrelipase:** Take the drug just before, during, or immediately after meals. Capsules may be opened and sprinkled over food but avoid chewing or crushing the microspheres inside the capsules. Continue to take pancrelipase even if feeling well. Pancrelipase may control symptoms but will not cure the condition. Do not take the drug with iron supplements or with calcium or magnesium antacids unless directed by the provider because they may diminish the effectiveness of this drug.

Prescribing Considerations

- Ongoing assessment during drug therapy should include monitoring appropriate laboratory findings (e.g., electrolytes, hepatic or renal function studies); symptoms, including what measures have been successful to relieve the symptoms (e.g., increased fluids, fiber, dietary changes); and assessment for GI bleeding, abdominal pain.
- Monitor electrolyte levels frequently in the infant and older adult, who are at greater risk for the development of electrolyte imbalances secondary to the diarrhea.

Understanding Chapter 60

Key Concepts Summary

60.1 Constipation is characterized by infrequent or difficult bowel movements.

60.2 Laxatives are drugs that increase the frequency and quality of bowel movements.

60.3 Diarrhea is an abnormal increase in the frequency and fluidity of bowel movements.

60.4 Opioids are the most effective drugs for controlling severe diarrhea.

60.5 Inflammatory bowel disease is treated with immunosuppressants and anti-inflammatory drugs.

60.6 Irritable bowel syndrome is treated with dietary management, symptomatic therapy, and drugs that regulate intestinal motility.

60.7 Nausea and vomiting occur when the vomiting center in the medulla is stimulated.

60.8 Antiemetics are prescribed to treat nausea and vomiting and motion sickness.

60.9 Pancreatic enzymes are administered as replacement therapy for patients with chronic pancreatitis.

CASE STUDY: Making the Patient Connection

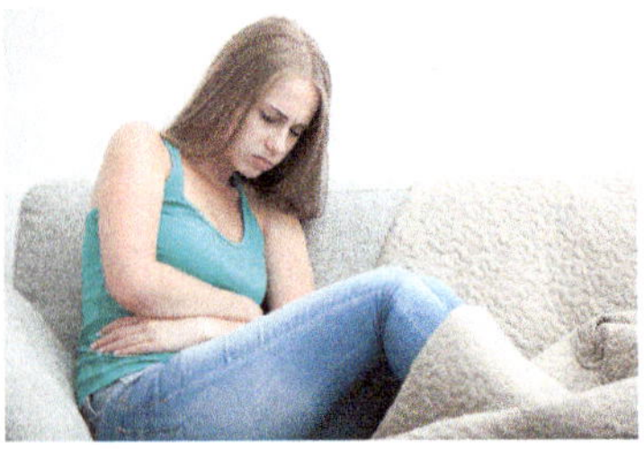

Remember the patient "Kerry O'Grady" at the beginning of the chapter? Now read the remainder of the case study. Based on the information presented within this chapter, respond to the critical thinking questions that follow.

Kerry O'Grady is a 20-year-old college sophomore studying to be a middle-school teacher. She was diagnosed with IBS at the end of her freshman year after enduring multiple bouts of abdominal cramping, diarrhea, constipation, gas, and bloating. She thought it was just the stress of her first year of college because her symptoms eased over the summer break. Now it has returned, and the diarrhea occurs more often than constipation. Some days Kerry finds that she is unable to sit through an entire class without having to leave for the restroom. She is increasingly worried about her grades and she is sure that the stress is not helping her condition either.

The nurse practitioner in the Student Health Services office has prescribed several weeks of dicyclomine (Bentyl) to be followed by loperamide (Imodium) after the diarrhea has slowed from the dicyclomine.

Critical Thinking Questions

1. How will the dicyclomine (Bentyl) and loperamide (Imodium) help treat Kerry's symptoms?
2. Considering the adverse effects of dicyclomine and loperamide, what should you as the nurse teach Kerry about her college course schedule?
3. What other nondrug measures might Kerry try to ease her symptoms?

Additional Case Study

Scott Mobley is a 25-year-old man with a diagnosis of ulcerative colitis. He currently reports having three to five loose bowel movements per day, associated with gas, cramps, and urgency of evacuation. He was diagnosed with ulcerative colitis 2 years earlier. Once he is stabilized, he will be placed on sulfasalazine.

1. Scott has asked you, his nurse, how this medication works. What is your response?
2. What adverse effects of this medication should you share with Scott?
3. What contraindications would you teach Scott about the drug sulfasalazine?

Chapter Review

1. The patient is taking diphenoxylate with atropine (Lomotil). What does the nurse assess when monitoring for therapeutic effects?

1. Reduction of abdominal cramping
2. Minimal passage of flatus
3. Decrease in loose, watery stools
4. Increased bowel sounds

2. The patient who is taking sulfasalazine (Azulfidine) develops a sore throat, bruising, and severe fatigue. The nurse determines that the patient is most likely experiencing drug-induced:

1. Stevens–Johnson syndrome.
2. Blood dyscrasias.
3. Idiosyncratic reaction.
4. Hypersensitivity response.

3. Ondansetron (Zofran) has been ordered prior to chemotherapy for a patient receiving treatment for lymphoma. Prior to administering this drug, the nurse will review the patient's past medical history for what condition?

1. Allergy to soy or soy products
2. History of chronic constipation
3. Glaucoma
4. Cardiac dysrhythmias

4. A nurse should question the order for pancrelipase (Pancreaze) for which patient?

1. The patient with allergy to pork products
2. The patient with hypertension
3. The patient with coronary artery disease
4. The patient with hypersensitivity to iodine products

5. A healthcare provider orders magnesium hydroxide (Milk of Magnesia) for a patient with constipation secondary to postoperative opioid use. Before administering the drug, the nurse would assess:

1. Blood pressure.
2. Dosage of the opioid drug prescribed.
3. The patient's ability to ambulate to the bathroom.
4. Bowel sounds.

6. A patient asks the nurse about giving an OTC drug, bismuth subsalicylate (Pepto-Bismol), to treat her daughter's diarrhea. On which of the following will the nurse base the recommendation? (Select all that apply.)

1. Cause of diarrhea
2. Normal activity level
3. Age
4. Weight
5. School schedule

See Appendix A for answers to critical thinking questions, case study questions and review questions.

References

Caldeira, L. F., Borba, H. H., Tonin, F. S., Wiens, A., Fernandez-Llimos, F., & Pontarolo, R. (2020). Fecal microbiota transplantation in inflammatory bowel disease patients: A systematic review and meta-analysis. *PLoS One*, *15*, e0238910. https://doi.org/10.1371/journal.pone.0238910

National Center for Complementary and Integrative Health. (2019). *Probiotics: What you need to know*. https://www.nccih.nih.gov/health/probiotics-what-you-need-to-know

Talley, N. J., & Irani, M. (2020). In irritable bowel syndrome, fecal microbiota transplantation improved symptoms at 3 months. *Annals of Internal Medicine*, *172*, JC52. https://doi.org/10.7326/ACPJ202005190-052

Tang, J. C. (2019). *Acute pancreatitis*. Medscape. http://emedicine.medscape.com/article/181364-overview

Selected Bibliography

Basson, M. D. (2020). *Constipation*. Medscape. http://emedicine.medscape.com/article/184704-overview

Billings, W., Mathur, K., Craven, H. J., Xu, H., & Shin, A. (2020). Potential benefit with complementary and alternative medicine in irritable bowel syndrome: A systematic review and meta-analysis. *Clinical Gastroenterology and Hepatology*. https://doi.org/10.1016/j.cgh.2020.09.035

Fejzo, M. S., Trovik, J., Grooten, I. J., Sridharan, K., Roseboom, T. J., Vikanes, Å., et al. (2019). Nausea and vomiting of pregnancy and hyperemesis gravidarum. *Nature Reviews Disease Primers*, *5*(1), 62. https://doi.org/10.1038/s41572-019-0110-3

Hesketh, P. J., Kris, M. G., Basch, E., Bohlke, K., Barbour, S. Y., Clark-Snow, R. A., et al. (2020). Antiemetics: ASCO guideline update. *Journal of Clinical Oncology*, *38*(24), 2782–2797. https://doi.org/10.1200/JCO.20.01296

Huffman, J. L. (2019). *Chronic pancreatitis*. Medscape. http://emedicine.medscape.com/article/181554-overview

Moayyedi, P., Andrews, C. N., MacQueen, G., Korownyk, C., Marsiglio, M., Graff, L., et al. (2019). Canadian Association of Gastroenterology clinical practice guideline for the management of irritable bowel syndrome (IBS). *Journal of the Canadian Association of Gastroenterology*, 2(1), 6–29. https://doi.org/10.1093/jcag/gwy071

Picardo, S., Altuwaijri, M., Devlin, S. M., & Seow, C. H. (2020). Complementary and alternative medications in the management of inflammatory bowel disease. *Therapeutic Advances in Gastroenterology*, *13*, 1756284820927550. https://doi.org/10.1177/1756284820927550

Pinto, C., Oliveira, P., Fernandes, O., Padilha, J., Machado, P., Ribeiro, A., & Ramos, J. (2020). Nonpharmacological clinical effective interventions in constipation: A systematic review. *Journal of Nursing Scholarship*, *52*(3), 261–269. https://doi.org/10.1111/jnu.12555

Rowe, W. A. (2020). *Inflammatory bowel disease*. Medscape. http://emedicine.medscape.com/article/ 179037-overview#a0156

Singh, S., Murad, M. H., Fumery, M., Dulai, P. S., & Sandborn, W. J. (2020). First-and second-line pharmacotherapies for patients with moderate to severely active ulcerative colitis: An updated network meta-analysis. *Clinical Gastroenterology and Hepatology*. https://doi.org/10.1016/j.cgh.2020.01.008

Vijayvargiya, P., Camilleri, M., Vijayvargiya, P., Erwin, P., & Hassan Murad, M. (2020). *Efficacy and safety of treatments for opioid-induced constipation*. Medscape. https://www.medscape.com/viewarticle/932498

"I still have some prenatal vitamins left over. I've been feeling pretty stressed and tired lately. Maybe they'll give me more energy."
—*Patient "Charlene Garrett"*

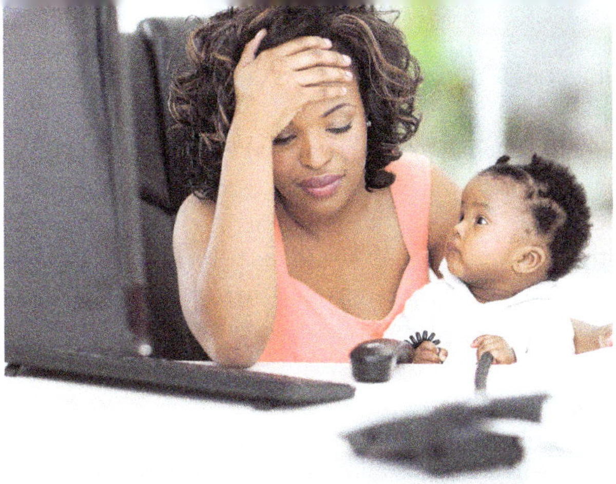

Chapter 61
Vitamins and Minerals

Chapter Outline

- Role of Vitamins in Health and Disease
- Regulation of Vitamins
- Recommended Dietary Allowance
- Fat-Soluble Vitamins
- Water-Soluble Vitamins
- Minerals
  - Macrominerals
  - Microminerals

Learning Outcomes

After reading this chapter, the student should be able to:

1. Describe the role of vitamins in maintaining wellness.
2. Identify conditions for which vitamin and mineral therapy may be indicated.
3. Explain the governmental regulation of vitamins and minerals.
4. Discuss the role of the recommended dietary allowance in determining the standardized requirement of various vitamins and minerals.
5. Compare and contrast fat-soluble and water-soluble vitamins.
6. For each of the major vitamins, identify the mechanism(s) of action, primary indications, contraindications, significant drug interactions, pregnancy data, and important adverse effects.
7. Identify the major functions of macrominerals and microminerals.
8. Apply clinical judgment to care for patients receiving vitamin and mineral supplementation therapy.

Key Terms

Definitions of the terms in bold may be found in the Glossary.

More than half of all Americans take vitamin supplements. Recognition of the health benefits of food nutrients dates back 3500 years ago when the Egyptians discovered that eating certain foods such as liver helped night blindness. Today, this nutrient is known as vitamin A. Through subsequent years the relationship of nutrients in food to disease was largely ignored. Many blamed the occurrence of disease on displeased gods, bad air, or witchcraft. Centuries would pass before a connection was made between vitamins and health. This chapter examines the rationales for vitamin and mineral pharmacotherapy.

Role of Vitamins in Health and Disease

61.1 Although the importance of nutrition has been known for centuries, the specific vitamins were discovered in the 1900s.

When ocean voyages became a preferred way of travel in the Renaissance, extended periods onboard a ship often meant limited access to fresh fruits and vegetables. People began to develop scurvy, a disease that causes bleeding of the gums, loss of teeth, ulcers on the lower legs, loss of hair, aching joints, fatigue, depression, hallucinations, blindness, and open wounds with decreased ability to heal. In 1774, James Lind, a Scottish surgeon in the Royal Navy, made a major discovery that saved the lives of many sailors. Lind had surmised that more men died from scurvy than from war injuries. Although he was not the first person to suspect that citrus fruit was important to health, he was the one who performed experiments to address this illness. He divided the affected sailors into groups and added different substances, such as cider, vinegar, barley water, oranges, or lemons, to their diets. Those who ate citrus fruit recovered from scurvy. Lind was ahead of his time because about 40 years passed before authorities accepted the connection between disease and nutrition.

Even in the early 1900s, most people believed that diseases like beriberi and pellagra were infectious processes. Beriberi is now known as a nutritional disease characterized by progressive neuropathy and accompanying dysfunction of the sensory process and an unsteady gait. In the late 1880s, Christiaan Eijkman studied beriberi in the West Indies and determined the cure for beriberi to be rice. He did not understand that it was a specific substance within the rice that caused the cure. In 1905, Dr. William Fletcher observed inmates who had beriberi at a mental asylum and found that ingesting unpolished rice could prevent the disease. This English physician determined that the rice husks contained some substance (thiamine) that treated beriberi. In 1907, Sir Frederick Gowland, an English biochemist, confirmed the positive relationship of food to health. He later joined with Eijkman to win the 1929 Nobel Prize for his work with food nutrients and vitamins. In 1911, a Polish chemist named Casimir Funk coined the term *vitamines*, meaning "nutrients vital for life."

In the 1920s and 1930s, scientists determined that small amounts of specific food substances (vitamins) prevented certain diseases. More than 160 years after Lind's discovery to prevent scurvy, Dr. Albert Szent-Györgyi, a Hungarian researcher, received the Nobel Prize in medicine by isolating and naming vitamin C.

61.2 Vitamins are essential for optimal health.

Today **vitamins** are defined as substances that are required in small amounts for normal growth and nutrition. These naturally occurring organic substances are critical for metabolism as well as regulation of cell function and human growth and development. They contain carbon, are found in living organisms such as plants and animals, and function primarily as catalysts that speed up biochemical processes. Vitamins must be taken into the body from the external environment, usually through the diet, and are not manufactured by the body in adequate amounts to maintain health (with the exception of vitamin D). Lack of sufficient amounts of vitamins results in symptoms of deficiency. People must consume vitamin supplements when their diet is lacking in these necessary nutrients or when they have health conditions that cause vitamin deficiencies. The vitamins and their functions are summarized in Table 61.1.

Vitamins are divided into two basic groups: those that dissolve in water (water soluble) and those that dissolve in lipids (fat soluble). Vitamin C and the B-complex vitamins are the primary **water-soluble vitamins**. This group of vitamins is stored briefly in the body and then excreted in the urine. The body's supply of water-soluble vitamins must be replenished on a daily basis. One exception is B_{12}, which is stored in the liver. In contrast, **fat-soluble vitamins** are stored in the liver and fatty tissue of the human body and need only periodic renewal. Because they are stored and not readily excreted, the possibility of toxicity from overdosing is greater with the fat-soluble group, which includes vitamins A, D, E, and K.

Most people who eat a well-balanced diet receive all the vitamins and minerals they need to maintain proper health. However, many Americans rely on nutrient-poor fast foods and processed edibles as their main diet. Although a healthy diet is the best way to maintain adequate and balanced nutrient intake, supplements are available as an additional way to meet the minimum daily requirements. It is important to remember that vitamin and mineral products should *supplement* a healthy balanced diet; they are not substitutes for good nutrition. Doses for the fat-soluble vitamin supplements are listed in Table 61.2. The water-soluble vitamin doses are listed in Table 61.3.

Table 61.1 Essential Vitamins

Vitamin	Function(s)	Common Cause(s) of Deficiency
A	Visual pigments, epithelial cells	Prolonged dietary deprivation, particularly when rice is the main food source; pancreatic disease; cirrhosis
B vitamins		
B_1: thiamine	Coenzyme in metabolic reactions, red blood cell (RBC) formation	Prolonged dietary deprivation, particularly when rice is the main food source; hyperthyroidism, pregnancy, liver disease, alcoholism
B_2: riboflavin	Coenzyme in oxidation–reduction reactions	Inadequate consumption of milk or animal products, chronic diarrhea, liver disease, alcoholism
B_3: niacin	Coenzyme in oxidation–reduction reactions	Prolonged dietary deprivation, particularly when Indian corn (maize) or millet is the main food source; chronic diarrhea; liver disease; alcoholism
B_6: pyridoxine	Coenzyme in amino acid metabolism and RBC production	Alcoholism, oral contraceptive use, malabsorption diseases
B_9: folic acid/folate	Coenzyme in amino acid and nucleic acid metabolism	Pregnancy, alcoholism, cancer, oral contraceptive use
B_{12}: cyanocobalamin	Coenzyme in nucleic acid metabolism	Lack of intrinsic factor, inadequate intake of foods with animal origin
C (ascorbic acid)	Coenzyme and antioxidant	Inadequate intake of fruits and vegetables, pregnancy, chronic inflammatory disease, burns, diarrhea, alcoholism
D	Calcium and phosphate metabolism	Low dietary intake, inadequate exposure to sunlight
E	Antioxidant	Prematurity, malabsorption diseases
K	Cofactor in blood clotting	Newborns, liver disease, long-term parenteral nutrition, certain drugs such as cephalosporins and salicylates

Regulation of Vitamins

61.3 Government regulations and consumer knowledge about vitamins are limited.

A 2019 survey by the Council for Responsible Nutrition, a Washington-based trade association representing ingredient suppliers and manufacturers in the dietary supplement industry, reported that 77% of adults in the United States take dietary supplements. The survey confirmed a trend in increased supplement usage among younger adults age 18 to 34. Ninety-six percent of those surveyed expressed confidence in the safety, effectiveness, and quality of supplements (Council for Responsible Nutrition, 2019).

Most people are unaware that taking too much of a vitamin or mineral can cause serious adverse effects. **Hypervitaminosis**, or toxic levels of vitamins, has been reported for vitamins A, C, D, E, B_6, niacin, and folic acid. In the United States, it is actually more common to observe syndromes of vitamin *excess* than of vitamin *deficiency*.

Consumers may assume that the U.S. Food and Drug Administration (FDA) regulates and approves nutritional supplements, as it does prescription and over-the-counter

Table 61.2 Fat-Soluble Vitamins for Treating Nutritional Disorders

Drug	Route and Adult Dose (Maximum Dose Where Indicated)	Adverse Effects
Vitamin A (Aquasol A)	PO: 100,000 units/day for 3 days, followed by 50,000 units/day for 2 wk; then 10,000–20,000 units/day for 2 months IM: 100,000 units/day for 3 days followed by 50,000 units/day for 2 wk	*Uncommon at recommended doses* High doses: nausea and vomiting, fatigue, irritability, night sweats, alopecia, dry skin
Vitamin D (Calcijex, Rocaltrol)	PO: 0.25 mcg/day (increased for patients with hypoparathyroidism or receiving dialysis); 800–1000 units/day or 50,000 units monthly for severe deficiency	*Uncommon at recommended doses, metallic taste* High doses: nausea and vomiting, fatigue, headache, polyuria, weight loss, hallucinations, dysrhythmias, muscle and bone pain
Vitamin E (Aquasol E, Vita-Plus E, others)	PO/IM: 60–75 units/day	*Uncommon at recommended doses* High doses: nausea and vomiting, fatigue, headache, blurred vision
Vitamin K (AquaMEPHYTON)	PO/IM/subcutaneous: 2.5–10 mg (max: 25 mcg)	*Facial flushing, pain at the injection site* IV route may result in dyspnea, hypotension, shock, cardiac arrest

Note: *Italics* indicate common adverse effects. Underline indicates serious adverse effects.

Table 61.3 Water-Soluble Vitamins for Treating Nutritional Disorders

Drug	Route and Adult Dose (Maximum Dose Where Indicated)	Adverse Effects
Vitamin B_1: thiamine	IV/IM: 50–100 mg tid PO: 5–30 mg/day	*Pain at the injection site* IV route may result in angioedema, cyanosis, pulmonary edema, GI bleeding, and cardiovascular collapse
Vitamin B_2: riboflavin	PO: 5–10 mg/day	*Adverse effects have not been reported*
Vitamin B_3: niacin (Niaspan, Nicobid, others)	PO: 100 mg/day for niacin deficiency or 1.5–3g/day for hyperlipidemia	*Uncommon at doses recommended for vitamin therapy* High doses: flushing, rash, diarrhea, hepatotoxicity
Vitamin B_6: pyridoxine (Hexa-Betalin, Nestrex)	PO/IM/IV: 2.5–10 mg/day for 3 wk; then may reduce to 2.5–5 mg/day	*Pain at the injection site* High doses: neuropathy, ataxia, seizures
Vitamin B_9: folic acid/folate (Folvite)	PO/IM/IV/subcutaneous: 0.4–1 mg/day	*Uncommon at recommended doses* Parenteral routes: allergic hypersensitivity
Vitamin B_{12}: cyanocobalamin (Nascobal)	IM/deep subcutaneous: 100–200 mcg/month Intranasal: 500 mcg (1 spray) in one nostril once weekly	*Headache, diarrhea, arthralgia* High doses: thrombosis, hypokalemia, pulmonary edema, heart failure, nasopharyngitis (intranasal route)
Vitamin C: ascorbic acid (Ascorbicap, Cebid, Vita-C, others)	PO/IV/IM/subcutaneous: 150–500 mg/day in 1–2 doses	*Uncommon at recommended doses* High doses: deep vein thrombosis (IV route), crystalluria

Note: *Italics* indicate common adverse effects. Underline indicates serious adverse effects.

(OTC) drugs. However, the legislative regulation of supplements is much more limited than that of drugs. The FDA regulates herbal, vitamin, and mineral products as dietary supplements. In 1994, the Dietary Supplement Health and Education Act required labeling of supplements. In 2007, the FDA passed the "current Good Manufacturing Practice" (cGMP) regulations, which mandated that manufacturers evaluate supplements for purity, strength, and composition (see Chapter 7).

The FDA's Office of Dietary Supplement Programs offers guidelines and tips for consumer safety. The best advice is to be knowledgeable about the purchase and use of supplements. This agency encourages consumers to consult with their healthcare providers before using supplements and to be leery of false claims. Supplements can be expensive and choosing foods with needed vitamins and minerals is a more natural way to reach nutritional health goals.

PharmFACT

Vitamin toxicity is responsible for over 60,000 calls to poison control centers each year in the United States (Rosenbloom, 2020).

Recommended Dietary Allowance

61.4 The recommended dietary allowance is the dietary intake level that is sufficient to meet the nutrient requirements for most people.

The Food and Nutrition Board of the National Academy of Sciences has established **recommended dietary allowances (RDAs)** for healthy adults. These values represent the minimum amount of vitamins and minerals needed to prevent disease and are based on scientific nutritional research. A newer value, the dietary reference intake (DRI), is based on four parameters: the estimated average requirement, RDA, adequate intake, and tolerable upper intake level.

Although a well-balanced diet provides the necessary vitamins and minerals for most people, the amount of vitamins and minerals needed varies based on certain factors. For example, infants, pregnant women, nursing mothers, older adults, vegans, vegetarians, and those with chronic diseases often require larger amounts of vitamins and minerals to maintain optimal health. Men and women can have different vitamin and mineral needs as do people who participate in vigorous exercise. With normal aging, the absorption of food diminishes and the quantity of ingested food is often reduced, leading to a higher risk of vitamin deficiencies in older adults. Vitamin deficiencies in patients with chronic liver and kidney disease are well documented. In cases where dietary needs are increased, the RDAs will need adjustment and supplements are indicated to achieve optimal wellness.

Certain drugs have the potential to affect vitamin metabolism. Alcohol is known for its ability to inhibit the absorption of thiamine and folic acid; alcohol abuse is the most common cause of thiamine deficiency in the United States. Folic acid levels may be reduced in patients who are taking phenothiazines, oral contraceptives, phenytoin (Dilantin), or barbiturates. Vitamin D deficiency can be caused by therapy with certain anticonvulsants. Inhibition of vitamin B_{12} absorption has been reported with a number of drugs, including omeprazole (Prilosec) and metformin (Glucophage), alcohol, and oral contraceptives. Nurses must be aware of these drug interactions and recommend vitamin supplements when appropriate.

Vitamin deficiencies follow certain patterns. The following are general characteristics of vitamin deficiency disorders:

- Patients more commonly present with multiple vitamin deficiencies than with a single vitamin deficiency.
- Symptoms of deficiency are nonspecific and often do not appear until the deficiency has been present for a long period.
- Deficiencies in the United States are most often the result of poverty, fad diets, chronic alcohol or drug abuse, or prolonged parenteral feeding.

Fat-Soluble Vitamins

61.5 Fat-soluble vitamins include vitamins A, D, E, and K.

The fat-soluble vitamins A, D, E, and K are found in fatty foods and oils. Because they are stored in lipid tissue, the body may go several weeks or months with insufficient dietary intake before signs of deficiency are noted. Excessive intake of these vitamins may be harmful. All fat-soluble vitamins are safe when taken at the recommended RDA levels during pregnancy and breastfeeding.

Vitamin A (Aquasol A)

Therapeutic Effects and Uses: Vitamin A is essential for the normal growth and development of bones and teeth, immune function, integrity of epithelial and mucosal surfaces, and for the synthesis of rhodopsin, or visual purple, necessary for adaptation to the dark. Beta-carotene is a plant pigment that is converted to vitamin A after ingestion of food.

Vitamin A deficiency is rare in the United States; however, certain people have an increased need for the vitamin. Vitamin A replacement therapy is used when metabolic needs are increased such as in pregnancy and during lactation. Vitamin A can be used in replacement therapy for conditions affecting the absorption, mobilization, or storage of vitamin A such as steatorrhea, severe biliary obstruction, liver cirrhosis, or total gastrectomy. Vitamin A has antioxidant properties and can be used as a screening test for fat malabsorption.

Mechanism of Action: As a fat-soluble vitamin, vitamin A acts as a cofactor in the synthesis of mucopolysaccharides, synthesis of cholesterol, and metabolism of steroids. It is easily absorbed through the gastrointestinal (GI) tract with bile salts, pancreatic lipase, and dietary fat, and it is stored in the liver. Small amounts may also be stored in the kidney and body fat. Vitamin A passes to the newborn through breast milk. It is metabolized in the liver and excreted in feces and urine.

Adverse Effects: Adverse effects with vitamin A are uncommon but the healthcare provider should be notified of difficulty breathing; hives; swelling of the lips, face, or tongue; or closing of the throat. Overdose of dietary supplements may result in hypervitaminosis syndrome symptoms that include fatigue, nausea and vomiting, decreased appetite, headache, gingivitis, dryness or cracking of the lips or skin, irritability, or loss of hair. Rare adverse effects include increased intracranial pressure, jaundice, leukopenia, anemia, and elevated prothrombin time (PT).

Contraindications/Precautions: Contraindications to vitamin A therapy include a history of sensitivity to vitamin A or to any ingredient in the formulation or hypervitaminosis. Oral (PO) administration to patients with malabsorption syndrome is also contraindicated. Vitamin A may falsely increase serum cholesterol determinations or falsely elevate bilirubin determination. Very high doses of vitamin A during pregnancy can cause birth defects.

Drug Interactions: Caution should be used if the patient is taking vitamin A analogs such as isotretinoin because their actions are additive. The patient should consult with the healthcare provider if using mineral oil because this can deplete fat-soluble vitamins. Cholestyramine may decrease the absorption of vitamin A. Oral contraceptives can increase serum levels of vitamin A.

Recommended Intake: *RDA:* 2500 international units for children, 5000 international units for males, and 4000 international units for females. The FDA has mandated that, starting in 2018, vitamin A labels must list units in micrograms (mcg) of retinol activity equivalents (RAEs). The RDA values converted to RAEs are 300 to 600 mcg/day for children (age 1 to 13), 900 mcg/day for males (age 14 and above), and 700 mcg/day for females (age 14 and above). Values are 750 to 770 mcg/day during pregnancy and 1200 to 1300 mcg/day during lactation.

Clinician Responsibilities: Key clinical implications for patients receiving vitamin A are included in Applied Clinical Judgment: Patients Receiving Pharmacotherapy with Vitamin or Mineral Supplements.

Vitamin D (Calcijex, Rocaltrol, Others)

Therapeutic Effects and Uses: Vitamin D maintains normal blood calcium and phosphate electrolyte levels by enhancing their intestinal absorption and by promoting mobilization of calcium from bone and the renal reabsorption of phosphate. This fat-soluble vitamin is necessary to

CONNECTIONS: Advanced Practice Application

Vitamins during Pregnancy

Case

Ana and her husband, Tyler, were thrilled to find out they were pregnant with their second baby. They have an almost 5-year-old girl, Maddie and had been trying to get pregnant again with a second one for over 3 years. When she comes to her first prenatal appointment at 11 weeks, she has mild morning sickness and reports occasional periods of dizziness and shortness of breath with exercise. Her family and medical histories are unremarkable. She reports healthy behaviors including taking an OTC prenatal supplement daily, exercising three times a week, and refraining from caffeine, tobacco products, and drugs. She has been a vegan for the past 10 years and is able to verbalize food sources that are rich in iron and high in protein. Her vital signs and physical examination are all normal and the fetal heart tones are strong. Her body mass index is 23. Her initial prenatal laboratory tests revealed mild anemia (hematocrit, 33%; hemoglobin, 10.5 g/dL). What additional vitamins does Ana need because she is anemic as well as vegan?

Discussion

Because birth defects can take place early in pregnancy, taking prenatal vitamins while the mother is trying to conceive is recommended. Vegan diets often are low in vitamin B_{12}, vitamin D, calcium, protein, iron, and iodine. Women of childbearing years prior to conceiving should consider adding additional folic acid (vitamin B_9), calcium, and iron. Folic acid prevents birth defects such as spina bifida, other neural tube problems, and congenital heart conditions. Consuming adequate amounts of calcium during pregnancy can be challenging for the vegan or vegetarian mother. Supplementation can stop the loss of bone density in the mother as the fetus absorbs calcium for bone growth. Iron is a central component in hemoglobin that carries oxygen for both mother and baby. Anemia can occur with insufficient iron intake and is a common issue for vegans. Iron supplements should be taken separately from calcium-rich food and caffeine because they interfere with iron absorption. Vitamin C enhances the absorption of iron, so the two can be taken concurrently. Because high amounts are extremely toxic, iron supplements should be kept away from children to avoid unintentional poisoning.

develop and maintain strong bones. Vitamin D is used to treat skeletal diseases that weaken the bones such as familial hypophosphatemia (vitamin D–resistant rickets), osteomalacia (adult rickets), osteoporosis, renal osteodystrophy, and hypocalcemia associated with hypoparathyroidism. Vitamin D is used as prophylaxis for and treatment of nutritional rickets and hypophosphatemia in Fanconi's syndrome. Sometimes vitamin D is helpful in treating psoriasis, rheumatoid arthritis, and lupus vulgaris. A drug prototype feature for calcitriol, the active form of vitamin D, is included in Chapter 72.

Patients at risk for vitamin D deficiency include breastfed infants; older adults; people with limited sun exposure, dark skin, or malabsorption disorders or those who have had gastric bypass surgery; and women who wear head scarves (e.g., hijabs) and body coverings (e.g., burqas) for extended periods of time.

Mechanism of Action: Vitamin D is a fat-soluble vitamin that is found in food and that is also made by the body after exposure to ultraviolet (UV) rays from the sun. Sunlight is a significant source of vitamin D because UV rays trigger vitamin D synthesis in the skin. Vitamin D is readily absorbed from the GI tract and distributed in the lymph. The body stores vitamin D in the liver, skin, brain, spleen, and bones. About half of each vitamin D dose is excreted in bile but it may be stored in tissues for months.

Adverse Effects: Adverse effects of vitamin D therapy are uncommon at therapeutic doses. At higher doses possible adverse effects include fatigue, weakness, dizziness, ataxia, muscle and joint pain, hypotonia (infants), pruritus, headache, drowsiness, photophobia, or convulsions. GI symptoms include anorexia, nausea and vomiting, diarrhea, metallic taste, dry mouth, constipation, and abdominal cramps. Some patients present with anemia. Musculoskeletal symptoms include calcification of soft tissues in the kidneys, myocardium, lungs, or skin. Acute kidney injury could occur with symptoms such as polyuria, polydipsia, albuminuria, and hematuria. Vitamin D is rarely but possibly implicated in hypertension and some cardiac dysrhythmias. Chronic hypervitaminosis with vitamin D can occur in children, resulting in mental and physical retardation or suppression of linear growth.

Contraindications/Precautions: Precautions should be taken in patients with a known hypersensitivity to vitamin D, hypervitaminosis, hypercalcemia, hyperphosphatemia, renal osteodystrophy with hyperphosphatemia, malabsorption syndrome, or decreased kidney function. Use cautiously in patients with coronary disease, arteriosclerosis (especially in older adults), history of kidney stones, or biliary tract disease or during lactation.

Drug Interactions: Consult with the healthcare provider if using mineral oil because it can deplete the supply of fat-soluble vitamins in the body. Cholestyramine may decrease the absorption of vitamin D. Patients should avoid OTC calcium supplements, other than those prescribed by the healthcare provider, because they may cause hypercalcemia. Oral corticosteroids can reduce calcium absorption and impair vitamin D metabolism.

Recommended Intake: *RDA:* Children (age 1 and above), men, and women until age 70 need 600 international units of vitamin D per day. Men and women age 71 and older need 800 international units per day. The RDA during pregnancy and lactation is 600 international units per day.

Clinician Responsibilities: Key clinical implications for patients receiving vitamin D are included in Applied Clinical Judgment: Patients Receiving Pharmacotherapy with Vitamin or Mineral Supplements.

PharmFACT

Indoor tanning has become increasingly popular with claims that it increases the level of vitamin D. However, most indoor tanning devices also emit UVA radiation, which is carcinogenic. If one wishes to safely increase vitamin D levels, vitamin supplements should be used, not tanning beds (Pierret et al., 2019).

Vitamin E (Aquasol E, Vita-Plus E, Others)

Therapeutic Effects and Uses: Vitamin E has many therapeutic uses. It prevents cell membrane and protein damage, protects against blood clot formation by decreasing platelet aggregation, enhances vitamin A utilization, and promotes the normal growth and development and tone of muscles. As an antioxidant, vitamin E prevents the damaging effects of free radicals, which are highly reactive chemical structures that damage cell membranes and alter nuclear proteins. Free radicals are associated with various conditions such as aging and disease.

Vitamin E supplementation can reverse or prevent hemolytic anemia in premature neonates caused by vitamin E deficiency. It is also used to prevent retinopathy associated with vitamin E deficiency in neonates and to treat diseases with secondary erythrocyte membrane abnormalities (e.g., sickle cell disease and G6PD deficiency). Vitamin E is used as a supplement in malabsorption syndromes. Topical vitamin E is used for dry or chapped skin and minor skin disorders.

Vitamin E deficiency is rare. People with lipid-absorption disorders may have deficiencies because fats are required for vitamin E absorption. This includes people who have an inability to secrete bile.

Mechanism of Action: When fat absorption is adequate, 20 to 60% of vitamin E is absorbed across the GI tract. It enters blood through the lymph and is stored in adipose (fat) tissue. Vitamin E is metabolized in the liver and is eliminated primarily in bile. Vitamin E crosses the placenta.

Adverse Effects: No adverse reactions have been found to consuming vitamin E in food. With excessive supplementation, symptoms may include fatigue, headache, skeletal muscle weakness, nausea, diarrhea, intestinal cramps, thrombophlebitis, contact dermatitis, blurred vision, or abnormal bleeding. With toxic levels laboratory tests may reveal increased serum creatine kinase, cholesterol, and triglycerides; decreased serum thyroxine and triiodothyronine; increased urinary estrogens and androgens; and creatinuria.

Contraindications/Precautions: Vitamin E should be used with caution in bleeding disorders and thrombocytopenia or during pregnancy. Vitamin E can prolong the PT by inhibition of vitamin K–dependent clotting factors. Large doses may worsen iron deficiency anemia because it may impair the hematologic response to iron.

Drug Interactions: Mineral oil should be avoided because it can deplete fat-soluble vitamins. Cholestyramine may decrease absorption of vitamin E. High doses of vitamin E may enhance the anticoagulant activity of warfarin, thus increasing the risk for bleeding.

Pregnancy: Some observational evidence suggests that high doses of vitamin E increases the risk for congenital heart defects. Vitamin E supplements should not be taken during pregnancy without approval of the healthcare provider.

Recommended Intake: *RDA:* Although the nutrient requirements for vitamin E have traditionally been listed as international units, the FDA has mandated that this be changed to milligrams (mg). From age 1 to 13, the RDA ranges from 6 to 11 mg and 15 mg for individuals age 14 through adult. The RDA during pregnancy is 15 mg and during lactation is 19 mg.

Clinician Responsibilities: Key clinical implications for patients receiving vitamin E are included in Applied Clinical Judgment: Patients Receiving Pharmacotherapy with Vitamin or Mineral Supplements.

Vitamin K (AquaMEPHYTON)

Therapeutic Effects and Uses: Vitamin K promotes the liver synthesis of clotting factors and is used in the production of RBCs. It helps maintain healthy bones, assists in healing fractures, and minimizes osteoporosis. Vitamin K is the antidote for warfarin overdose. Vitamin K reverses hypoprothrombinemia secondary to the administration of PO antibiotics, quinidine, salicylates, sulfonamides, and excessive vitamin A, and secondary to inadequate absorption and synthesis of vitamin K (as in obstructive jaundice, biliary fistula, ulcerative colitis, intestinal resection, or prolonged hyperalimentation). Vitamin K is used as prophylaxis of and therapy for neonatal hemorrhagic disease.

Most people receive adequate amounts of this vitamin in their diets. Those at risk for deficiency include newborns not treated with vitamin K at birth and those with malabsorption disorders.

Mechanism of Action: The body receives most of its needed vitamin K through the metabolism of bacterial flora in the GI tract. Phytonadione (also called phylloquinone) is a fat-soluble substance that is chemically identical to naturally occurring vitamin K. It is readily absorbed in the intestinal lymph when bile is present. Vitamin K is essential for the hepatic biosynthesis of blood clotting Factors II, VII, IX, and X. Hemorrhage is usually controlled within 3 to 8 hours, with normal PT obtained in 12 to 14 hours after vitamin K administration. Phytonadione is concentrated briefly in the liver after absorption, crosses the placenta, and is secreted in the breast milk of nursing mothers. It is metabolized quickly in the liver and eliminated in the urine and bile.

Adverse Effects: Reported effects after PO dosing include headache, GI upset, paradoxical hypoprothrombinemia (in patients with severe liver disease), severe hemolytic anemia, hyperbilirubinemia, kernicterus, bronchospasm, and dyspnea. Possible pain at the injection site, hematoma and nodule formation, erythematous skin eruptions (with repeated injections), and peculiar taste sensations may occur. **Black Box Warning:** Severe reactions such as shock, anaphylaxis, and cardiac arrest have occurred when vitamin K is given by the intravenous (IV) or intramuscular (IM) route. These routes should be used only when subcutaneous or oral routes are not feasible.

Contraindications/Precautions: Caution should be used in patients with biliary tract disease, obstructive jaundice, or severe liver disease. Patients should be monitored for hypersensitivity to phytonadione, benzyl alcohol, or castor oil. Some interference may occur with diagnostic tests such as falsely elevated urine steroids.

Drug Interactions: Vitamin K decreases the anticoagulant effects of warfarin. Patients may have decreased absorption with the use of cholestyramine, colestipol, or mineral oil.

Recommended Intake: *RDA:* 30 to 75 mcg for age 1 to 18, and 120 mcg for age 19 and older. Values for pregnancy and lactation are 75 to 90 mcg.

Clinician Responsibilities: Key clinical implications for patients receiving vitamin K are included in Applied Clinical Judgment: Patients Receiving Pharmacotherapy with Vitamin or Mineral Supplements.

CONNECTION Checkpoint 61.1

From what you learned in Chapter 38, describe how vitamin K reverses the effects of warfarin overdose (Coumadin).

Water-Soluble Vitamins

61.6 Water-soluble vitamins include the B-complex vitamins and vitamin C.

The water-soluble vitamins are found in rich abundance in fresh fruits and vegetables. Unlike the fat-soluble vitamins, vitamin C and most B-complex vitamins are not stored to any great extent, and signs of deficiency may be noted quickly if they are omitted from the diet. Excessive intake of these vitamins is usually not harmful because they are rapidly excreted. All water-soluble vitamins are safe when taken at the recommended RDA levels during pregnancy and breastfeeding.

Thiamine (Vitamin B_1)

Therapeutic Effects and Uses: Thiamine (vitamin B_1) functions as an essential coenzyme in the metabolism of carbohydrates and has a role in converting tryptophan to nicotinamide. Thiamine deficiency is called beriberi. Early symptoms of thiamine deficiency include anorexia, weight loss, and nervous system signs such as confusion, memory impairment, and depressed sensory and motor reflex functions. Severe beriberi can lead to heart failure and encephalopathy.

Because of its abundance in food, thiamine deficiency in the United States is uncommon. People at risk for deficiency include those with chronic alcohol dependence, chronic liver disease, human immunodeficiency virus (HIV) infection or diabetes; older adults; and patients following bariatric surgery. Therapy generally includes other members of the B-complex vitamins because thiamine deficiency rarely occurs alone. Thiamine is sometimes used in combination with other B vitamins to reduce depression and anxiety as well as to prevent motion sickness.

Mechanism of Action: Thiamine is necessary for the conversion of carbohydrates to energy and is essential in maintaining the proper functioning of the heart, nervous system, and muscles. Thiamine is absorbed from the GI tract and widely distributed, and it is secreted in breast milk. This vitamin is eliminated in the urine.

Adverse Effects: Thiamine has few adverse effects. Excessive doses may cause a feeling of warmth, weakness, sweating, restlessness, tightness of the throat, angioneurotic edema, cyanosis, pulmonary edema, cardiovascular collapse, or hypotension after rapid IV administration. Other adverse effects may include GI hemorrhage, nausea, urticaria, and pruritus.

Contraindications/Precautions: There are no contraindications if the dosage is within the RDA.

Drug Interactions: Antibiotics such as erythromycin and azithromycin may decrease thiamine levels by altering intestinal flora.

Recommended Intake: *RDA:* 0.5 to 0.9 mg (children age 1 to 13), 1.2 mg (males age 14 and above), 1.0 to 1.1 mg (females age 14 and above), and 1.4 mg during pregnancy and lactation.

Clinician Responsibilities: Key clinical implications for patients receiving thiamine (vitamin B_1) are included in Applied Clinical Judgment: Patients Receiving Pharmacotherapy with Vitamin or Mineral Supplements.

Riboflavin (Vitamin B_2)

Therapeutic Effects and Uses: Vitamin B_2, or riboflavin, is a component of coenzymes that participate in a number of different oxidation–reduction reactions. As with thiamine, a deficiency of riboflavin is most commonly observed in people with chronic alcoholism. Vegetarians, vegans, those who do not drink milk, and pregnant and lactating women are also at risk. Clinical symptoms of deficiency include digestive disturbances, headache, burning sensation of the skin (especially "burning" feet), cracking at the corners of the mouth (cheilosis), glossitis, seborrheic dermatitis (and other skin lesions), mental depression, corneal vascularization (with photophobia, burning and itchy eyes, lacrimation, roughness of eyelids), anemia, and neuropathy. Riboflavin therapy is used to prevent riboflavin deficiency and microcytic anemia and to supplement other B vitamins in the treatment of pellagra and beriberi.

Mechanism of Action: As a component of the flavoprotein enzymes, riboflavin works together with a wide variety of proteins to catalyze many cellular respiratory reactions by which the body derives its energy. The vitamin is readily absorbed from the GI tract. Little riboflavin is stored, and excess amounts are excreted in urine.

Adverse Effects: Riboflavin is nontoxic. It may discolor urine bright yellow. In large doses, riboflavin may produce yellow-green fluorescence in urine, which can cause false elevations in certain determinations of urinary catecholamines.

Contraindications/Precautions: Unknown.

Drug Interactions: Unknown.

Recommended Intake: *RDA:* 0.5 to 0.9 mg (children age 1 to 13), 1.3 mg (males age 14 and above), 1.0 to 1.1 mg (females age 14 and above), and 1.4 to 1.6 mg (pregnancy and lactation).

Clinician Responsibilities: Key clinical implications for patients receiving riboflavin (vitamin B_2) are included in Applied Clinical Judgment: Patients Receiving Pharmacotherapy with Vitamin or Mineral Supplements.

Niacin (Vitamin B_3)

The primary use for niacin is for the medical management of elevated cholesterol levels in patients at risk for atherosclerotic disease. It may be used as monotherapy or in combination with other antihyperlipidemic drugs. Additional details about niacin are provided in Chapter 29.

Pyridoxine (Vitamin B_6)

Therapeutic Effects and Uses: Pyridoxine is a coenzyme that participates in over 100 metabolic reactions in the body, most of them related to protein metabolism. Pyridoxine deficiency is uncommon in the United States and usually occurs concurrently with deficiencies of other B vitamins. Pyridoxine deficiency occurs with inadequate dietary intake due to alcoholism, drug-induced deficiency (e.g., isoniazid [INH], oral contraceptives), and congenital errors of metabolism (vitamin B_6–dependent convulsions or anemia). People with chronic kidney disease (CKD) or autoimmune disorders are also at risk for deficiency. Deficiency symptoms include nausea and vomiting, cheilosis, edema, and central nervous system (CNS) symptoms. Pyridoxine is administered to treat acute toxicity caused by overdosage of cycloserine, hydralazine, or INH; alcoholic polyneuritis; and sideroblastic anemia associated with high serum iron concentration. Pyridoxine has been used to manage many other conditions, including nausea and vomiting in radiation sickness and pregnancy, suppression of postpartum lactation, and diabetes; to decrease the symptoms of premenstrual syndrome (PMS); to minimize joint pain caused by some types of arthritis; and to treat carpal tunnel syndrome.

Mechanism of Action: Pyridoxine is usually available as part of a water-soluble complex of three closely related compounds with vitamin B_6 activity. Pyridoxine is converted in the body to pyridoxal, a coenzyme that functions in protein, fat, and carbohydrate metabolism and in facilitating the release of glycogen from the liver and muscle. In protein metabolism, pyridoxine participates in many enzymatic transformations of amino acids and in the conversion of tryptophan to niacin and serotonin. It aids in energy transformation in the brain and nerve cells and is thought to stimulate heme production. Pyridoxine is readily absorbed from the GI tract. It is distributed and stored in the liver and crosses the placenta. Metabolism of this vitamin takes place in the liver. Pyridoxine is eliminated in urine.

Adverse Effects: Adverse events are few, but the patient could experience paresthesias, slight flushing or feeling of warmth, temporary burning or stinging pain at the injection site, somnolence seizures (particularly following large parenteral doses), low folic acid levels, insomnia, or anxiety.

Contraindications/Precautions: Pyridoxine should be used with caution in patients with CKD, neonatal prematurity with renal impairment, or cardiac disease.

Drug Interactions: Use of INH, cycloserine, penicillamine, hydralazine, and oral contraceptives may increase pyridoxine requirements. This vitamin may reverse or antagonize the therapeutic effects of the antiparkinsonism drug levodopa because it reduces the amount of dopamine entering the brain by facilitating the breakdown of levodopa in peripheral circulation.

Recommended Intake: *RDA:* 0.5 to 1.0 mg (children age 1 to 13), 1.3 mg (males age 14 to 50), 1.9 mg (men over 50 years), 1.2 to 1.5 mg (females ages14 and above), and 1.9 to 2.0 mg (pregnancy and lactation).

Clinician Responsibilities: Key clinical implications for patients receiving pyridoxine (vitamin B_6) are included in Applied Clinical Judgment: Patients Receiving Pharmacotherapy with Vitamin or Mineral Supplements.

CONNECTION Checkpoint 61.2

From what you learned in Chapter 51, how does the antitubercular drug isoniazid affect levels of pyridoxine (vitamin B_6)?

Folic Acid (Folate; Vitamin B_9)

Therapeutic Effects and Uses: Folate and folic acid are forms of vitamin B_9. Folate is the form that is found naturally in food, whereas folic acid is the synthetic form of the vitamin found in supplements. Folate deficiency is rare in the United States. Those at increased risk for deficiency include people with alcohol dependence or malabsorption disorders and women of childbearing age or who are pregnant. Folic acid is used to treat folate deficiency, macrocytic anemia, and megaloblastic anemias, which are associated with inadequate dietary intake, alcoholism, primary liver disease, malabsorption syndromes, pregnancy, infancy, and childhood. Up to 80% of neural tube defects in newborns can be prevented with supplementation of folic acid prior to pregnancy.

Mechanism of Action: Vitamin B_9 is essential for the synthesis of nucleoproteins and the maintenance of RBCs, neurons, and proteins. It stimulates production of RBCs, white blood cells, and platelets in patients with megaloblastic anemias. Folic acid counters folic acid deficiency, which can result in the production of defective deoxyribonucleic acid, leading to megaloblast formation and arrest of bone marrow maturation. Folic acid is readily absorbed in the proximal small intestine, is distributed to all body tissues, crosses the placenta in pregnancy, and is secreted in breast milk in lactating women. It is metabolized in the liver and excreted in urine.

Adverse Effects: The patient may feel warmth or flushing with IV doses. Although rare, the possible adverse effects include irritability, depression, loss of appetite, rash, itching, nausea, or dyspnea.

Contraindications/Precautions: Folic acid should not be used in patients with allergic sensitivity to B vitamins. It should be administered with caution if using folic acid alone to correct pernicious anemia or other vitamin B_{12} deficiency states as well as normocytic, refractory, aplastic, or undiagnosed anemia. Caution should be used with neonates. Folic acid can cause false low serum folate levels in patients who are receiving antibiotics such as tetracyclines.

Drug Interactions: Folic acid inhibitors such as methotrexate can antagonize the effects of folate therapy. Folic acid therapy increases the metabolism of phenytoin (Dilantin), possibly causing increased seizure activity.

Recommended Intake: The recommended intakes for folic acid are based on units called dietary folate equivalents (DFEs). These units reflect the fact that not all folic acid in food is absorbed or bioavailable. *RDA:* 150 to 300 DFE (children age 1 to 13), 300 to 400 DFE (adults age 14 and above), and 500 to 600 DFE (pregnancy and lactation).

Clinician Responsibilities: Key clinical implications for patients receiving folic acid (vitamin B_9) are included in Applied Clinical Judgment: Patients Receiving Pharmacotherapy with Vitamin or Mineral Supplements.

Cyanocobalamin (Vitamin B_{12})

Therapeutic Effects and Uses: Cyanocobalamin is used to treat vitamin B_{12} deficiency and anemia due to malabsorption syndrome, such as in pernicious anemia; sprue; GI pathology, dysfunction, or surgery; fish tapeworm infestation; and gluten enteropathy. This drug is also used in vitamin B_{12} deficiency caused by increased physiologic requirements or inadequate dietary intake and in the vitamin B_{12} absorption (Schilling) test. It may be used to prevent and treat toxicity associated with sodium nitroprusside, to treat asthma, and possibly to aid in healing following surgery. A prototype drug feature for this vitamin is presented in Chapter 39.

Mechanism of Action: Vitamin B_{12} is a cobalt-containing B-complex vitamin that is essential for normal growth, cell reproduction, maturation of RBCs, synthesis of nucleoproteins, and maintenance of the nervous system (myelin synthesis). It is believed to be involved in protein and carbohydrate metabolism as well. Vitamin B_{12} deficiency results in megaloblastic anemia, dysfunction of the spinal cord with paralysis, and GI lesions. Intestinal absorption requires the presence of intrinsic factor in the terminal ileum. It is widely distributed and is principally stored in the liver, kidneys, and adrenals. It crosses the placenta and is excreted in breast milk. In metabolism this vitamin is converted in the tissues to active coenzymes and is enterohepatically cycled. Vitamin B_{12} is eliminated in urine in 48 hours.

Adverse Effects: Adverse effects are rare but may include the feeling of a swelling body, anaphylactic shock, peripheral vascular thrombosis, pulmonary edema, heart failure, mild transient diarrhea, unmasking of polycythemia vera (with correction of vitamin B_{12} deficiency), hypokalemia, itching, rash, flushing, severe optic nerve atrophy, and sudden death.

Contraindications/Precautions: Contraindications include a history of sensitivity to vitamin B_{12}, other cobalamins, or cobalt; early Leber's disease (hereditary optic nerve atrophy); and indiscriminate use in folic acid deficiency. Caution should be used in patients with heart disease, anemia, or pulmonary disease.

Drug Interactions: Alcohol, aminosalicylic acid, neomycin, and colchicine may decrease the absorption of PO cyanocobalamin. Chloramphenicol may interfere with the therapeutic response to cyanocobalamin.

Recommended Intake: *RDA:* 2.4 mcg/day for age 14 and older, 2.6 mcg/day during pregnancy, and 2.8 mcg/day during lactation. *DRI:* 0.9 to 1.2 mcg/day for children (age 1 to 13) and 2.4 mcg/day for adults (age 14 and above).

Clinician Responsibilities: Key clinical implications for patients receiving cyanocobalamin (vitamin B_{12}) are included in Applied Clinical Judgment: Patients Receiving Pharmacotherapy with Vitamin or Mineral Supplements.

Vitamin C (Ascorbic Acid)

Therapeutic Effects and Uses: Vitamin C is essential for the synthesis and maintenance of collagen and intercellular ground substance of body tissues, blood vessels, cartilage, bones, teeth, skin, and tendons. It helps maintain the functions of the immune system for improved wound healing and increased resistance to infection. Vitamin C is used for both prophylaxis and treatment of scurvy and as a dietary supplement. Off-label uses include acidification of urine, prevention and treatment of cancer, treatment of idiopathic methemoglobinemia, and use as an adjuvant during deferoxamine therapy for iron toxicity. In megadoses vitamin C may possibly reduce the severity and duration of the common cold. It is used as an antioxidant in formulations of parenteral tetracycline and other drugs.

Mechanism of Action: Vitamin C is readily absorbed and widely distributed to body tissues. It crosses the placenta and is secreted in breast milk. Vitamin C is metabolized in the liver and eliminated rapidly in urine when the plasma level exceeds the renal threshold of 1.4 mg/dL. Unlike most mammals, humans are unable to synthesize ascorbic acid in the body; thus, it must be consumed daily.

Adverse Effects: Possible adverse effects from large doses include nausea and vomiting, heartburn, diarrhea or abdominal cramps, acute hemolytic anemia, sickle cell crisis, headache, insomnia, urethritis, dysuria, crystalluria, hyperoxaluria, or hyperuricemia. With rapid IV administration temporary dizziness and soreness at the injection site may occur. Vitamin C may produce false-negative tests for occult blood in stools if taken within 48 to 72 hours of testing.

Contraindications/Precautions: Sodium ascorbate should not be used in patients on sodium restriction; calcium ascorbate is contraindicated in patients who are receiving digoxin (Lanoxin). Excessive doses should be avoided in patients with G6PD deficiency, hemochromatosis, thalassemia, sideroblastic anemia, or sickle cell disease or in patients prone to gout or renal calculi.

Drug Interactions: Large doses may attenuate the hypoprothrombinemic effects of PO anticoagulants. Aspirin and other salicylates may inhibit ascorbic acid uptake by leukocytes and tissues, and ascorbic acid may decrease elimination of salicylates. Chronic high doses of ascorbic acid may diminish the effects of disulfiram.

Recommended Intake: *RDA:* 60 mg/day. *DRI:* 15 to 45 mg/day for children (age 1 to 14) and 75 to 90 mg/day for adults (above age 14).

Clinician Responsibilities: Key clinical implications for patients receiving ascorbic acid (vitamin C) are included in Applied Clinical Judgment: Patients Receiving Pharmacotherapy with Vitamin or Mineral Supplements.

Minerals

Minerals are essential substances that constitute about 4% of the body's weight and serve many diverse functions. Some are essential ions or electrolytes in body fluids; others are bound to organic molecules such as hemoglobin, phospholipids, or metabolic enzymes. Those minerals that function as critical electrolytes in the body, most notably sodium and potassium, are covered in detail in Chapter 33.

Because minerals are needed in very small amounts for human metabolism, a balanced diet will supply the necessary quantities for most patients. Like vitamins, excess amounts of minerals can lead to toxicity, and patients should be advised not to exceed the recommended doses. Mineral supplements are, however, indicated for certain disorders. Iron deficiency anemia is the most common nutritional deficiency in the world and is a common indication for iron supplements. Women at high risk for osteoporosis are advised to consume extra calcium, either in their diet or as a dietary supplement.

61.7 Macrominerals are inorganic substances needed in amounts of at least 100 mg per day for normal body functioning.

Macrominerals are major inorganic substances that must be consumed daily in amounts of 100 mg or higher. Included in this group are calcium, chloride, magnesium, phosphorus, potassium, sodium, and sulfur. Two of the body's most important minerals affecting fluid and electrolyte balance, sodium and potassium, are presented in Chapter 33, with prototype features for sodium bicarbonate, sodium chloride, and potassium chloride. Each macromineral is listed in Table 61.4 along with its RDA and function. Brief descriptions of some of the common macrominerals and their therapeutic uses are given next.

Calcium: Calcium is primarily stored in the teeth and bones to provide strength. Calcium may also be found in blood, muscle, and body fluid between cells. A consistent level of calcium is needed for vital body processes and functions such as bone matrix construction, muscle contraction, hormone and enzyme secretion, hemostasis, and nerve conduction. When a calcium deficiency occurs, the patient may become irritable and restless, with muscular cramps, spasms, and cardiac abnormalities. Fractures may result from continued hypocalcemia. Calcium compounds are available for pharmacotherapy in many PO salts such as calcium carbonate, calcium citrate, calcium gluconate, or calcium lactate. IV preparations are administered in severe cases. Calcium salts are featured as a prototype drug for hypocalcemia and osteoporosis in Chapter 72.

Chloride: Chloride is a chemical that the human body needs for metabolism and to maintain acid–base balance. In the CNS the inhibitory actions of certain neurotransmitters rely on the entry of chloride into specific neurons. The amount of chloride in the blood is carefully controlled by the kidneys. Isolated imbalances of chloride are due to fluid, electrolyte, or acid–base imbalances. Chloride imbalances are corrected by treating the underlying pathology.

Magnesium: Magnesium is required for more than 300 biochemical reactions in the body. This mineral helps maintain normal muscle and nerve function, keeps cardiac rhythm steady, supports a healthy immune system, and maintains bone strength. The pharmacologic use of magnesium includes multiple pathologic conditions. For example, magnesium citrate is used for bowel evacuation, as is magnesium hydroxide, which can also be used as an antacid. Magnesium salicylate is used for the relief of pain and inflammation in rheumatoid arthritis. The mineral can also be used as a CNS depressant because magnesium sulfate is frequently used as an anticonvulsant in labor and delivery. Magnesium sulfate is featured as a drug prototype in Chapter 33.

Table 61.4 Minerals: RDAs and Functions

Mineral	RDA (adults)	Function
Macrominerals		
Calcium	1.0–1.2 g	Forms bony matrix; regulates nerve conduction and muscle contraction
Chloride	1.8–2.3 g	Major anion in body fluids; part of gastric acid secretion
Magnesium	Men: 400–420 mg Women: 310–320 mg	Cofactor for many enzymes; necessary for normal nerve conduction and muscle contraction
Phosphorus	700 mg	Forms bone matrix; part of ATP and nucleic acids
Potassium	4.7 g	Necessary for normal nerve conduction and muscle contraction; principal cation in intracellular fluid; essential for acid–base and electrolyte balance
Sodium	1.2–1.5 g	Necessary for normal nerve conduction and muscle contraction; principal cation in extracellular fluid; essential for acid–base and electrolyte balance
Sulfur	Not established	Component of proteins, B vitamins, and other critical molecules
Microminerals		
Chromium	20–35 mcg	Potentiates insulin; necessary for proper glucose metabolism
Cobalt	0.1 mcg	Cofactor for vitamin B_{12} and several oxidative enzymes
Copper	900 mcg	Cofactor for hemoglobin synthesis
Fluoride	3–4 mg	Influences tooth structure and possibly affects growth
Iodide	150 mcg	Component of thyroid hormones
Iron	Men: 8 mg Women: 8–18 mg	Component of hemoglobin and some enzymes of oxidative phosphorylation
Manganese	1.8–2.3 mg	Cofactor in some enzymes of lipid, carbohydrate, and protein metabolism
Molybdenum	45 mg	Cofactor for certain enzymes
Selenium	55 mcg	Antioxidant cofactor for certain enzymes
Zinc	5–13 mg	Cofactor for certain enzymes, including carbonic anhydrase; needed for proper protein structure, normal growth, and wound healing

Most recently, magnesium has been used to help regulate blood sugar levels, promote normal blood pressure, and assist in energy metabolism and protein synthesis. The metabolism of magnesium is important to insulin sensitivity and blood pressure regulation. Magnesium deficiency is common in people with diabetes. Several epidemiologic studies indicate that magnesium may play an important role in regulating blood pressure. Furthermore, magnesium assists in the metabolism of carbohydrates and may influence the release and activity of insulin, which is the hormone that helps control blood glucose (sugar) levels.

Phosphorous: Phosphorus, another essential macromineral, binds to calcium to form calcium phosphate in bones. In addition to playing a role in bone structure, phosphorus is a component of protein, adenosine triphosphate (ATP), and nucleic acids. Dietary sources of phosphorus are widely available; thus, hypophosphatemia is most often seen in patients with severe malnutrition, intestinal malabsorption disorders, or kidney impairment that results in excess phosphorus loss in the urine. When serum phosphorus levels fall below 1.5 mEq/L, phosphate supplements are usually administered. Sodium phosphate and potassium phosphate are available for treating phosphorus deficiencies.

61.8 Microminerals are inorganic substances needed in amounts of at least 20 mg per day for normal body functioning.

Commonly called trace minerals, the **microminerals** are required daily in amounts of 20 mg or less. Although they are needed in minute amounts, their functions should not be underestimated. Profound illness may result with deficits of some of the microminerals. Each micromineral is listed in Table 61.4 along with its RDA and function. Brief descriptions of some of the common microminerals and their therapeutic uses are given next.

Fluoride: Fluoride, a trace mineral, is best known as the mineral that is helpful for bone and teeth health. Dental professionals may apply concentrated fluoride topically to the teeth to prevent cavities, especially in children. Many cities have added fluoride to the municipal water supply to improve dental health. Because high amounts of fluoride can be quite toxic to children, the use of fluoride-containing products should be closely monitored.

Iodide: Iodide is a micromineral needed to synthesize thyroid hormone. The most common source of dietary iodide is iodized salt. When dietary intake of iodide is low, hypothyroidism occurs and enlargement of the thyroid gland results. At high concentrations iodide suppresses thyroid function. Lugol's solution, a mixture containing 5% elemental iodine and 10% potassium iodide, is given to patients with hyperthyroidism prior to thyroidectomy or during a thyrotoxic crisis. Sodium iodide is a drug that acts by rapidly suppressing the secretion of thyroid hormone and is indicated for patients who are having an acute thyroid crisis. Radioactive iodine (^{131}I) is given to destroy overactive thyroid glands (see Chapter 67). As an expectorant, the iodine ion increases mucous secretion formation in the bronchi and decreases viscosity of the mucus. Iodine salts such as iothalamate and diatrizoate are very dense and serve as diagnostic contrast agents in radiologic procedures of the urinary and cardiovascular systems.

Iron: Iron is essential to normal human physiology as an integral part of many proteins and enzymes that maintain good health. Iron is an essential component of proteins involved in oxygen transport; a deficiency limits oxygen delivery to cells, resulting in fatigue, poor work performance, and decreased immune function. It is also essential for the regulation of cell growth and differentiation. Dietary sources include meat, shellfish, nuts, and legumes.

Iron can be supplemented using various pharmacologic preparations, which often have ascorbic acid added to improve the absorption of PO iron. Generally, iron supplementation therapy is a PO therapy, and parenteral IV or IM iron therapy is given only when absorption is seriously compromised by illnesses or when the patient cannot swallow. A prototype drug feature for ferrous sulfate is presented in Chapter 39.

Zinc: Zinc is found in at least 100 enzymes and has a role in regulating nucleic acid synthesis as well as wound healing, bone formation, cell-mediated immunity, and male fertility. Sources of zinc include protein foods, beans, lentils, nuts, seeds, and whole-grain cereals. Zinc sulfate, zinc acetate, and zinc gluconate are available to prevent and treat deficiency states at doses of 60 to 120 mg/day. Lozenges that contain zinc can be purchased OTC for treating sore throats and cold symptoms.

Those at highest risk for zinc insufficiency include vegans and vegetarians, pregnant and lactating women, patients with alcohol dependence, older infants who are exclusively breastfed, and people with GI disorders.

CONNECTION Checkpoint 61.3

From what you learned in Chapter 39, what are the most common adverse effects experienced by patients taking iron salts such as ferrous sulfate by the oral route?

CONNECTIONS: APPLIED CLINICAL JUDGMENT

Patients Receiving Pharmacotherapy with Vitamin or Mineral Supplements

Key Assessment Data

- History of current condition, baseline vital signs, physical exam findings, history of any current symptoms that may indicate vitamin deficiencies or hypervitaminosis (e.g., dry and itchy skin, alopecia, sore and reddened gums or tongue, tendency to bleed easily or excessive bruising, nausea and/or vomiting, or excessive fatigue), dietary history, sun exposure; endocrine, hepatic, or renal disease; medication history, caffeine, nicotine, and alcohol use; pregnancy status.

Desired Therapeutic Outcomes

Improvement is observed and measurable by symptoms of deficiency are diminished or absent, electrolyte levels are maintained within normal limits.

Minimizing Adverse Effects

- If a definitive cause of vitamin or mineral deficiency is identified, correct the deficiency using natural sources of the nutrient when possible.
- In the United States, hypervitaminosis from excessive vitamin and mineral intake is more common than deficiencies for most nutrients. Excessive intake of vitamins A, C, D, E, B_6, niacin, and folic acid may cause toxic effects.
- Fat-soluble vitamins are stored in the body and may accumulate and result in toxic levels. Monitor liver function studies and for symptoms such as nausea and vomiting, headache, fatigue, dry and itchy skin, blurred vision, or palpitations.
- Large doses of vitamins, particularly vitamin C, may cause adverse effects such as renal calculi.

Lifespan Considerations

- Folic acid supplementation reduces the incidence of neurologic birth defects, and adequate folic acid intake should ideally begin before conception. Excessive vitamin intake may have deleterious effects on the developing fetus and prenatal vitamin use should be monitored by the healthcare provider.
- Poisonings with vitamins and iron are common in children and supplements should be kept out of reach of young children.

Patient Education

- Discuss the need for nutritional supplements with the healthcare provider if a normal diet is unable to supply these or if disease conditions (e.g., pernicious anemia) prevent absorption or utilization of essential nutrients.
- Keep prenatal vitamins in a secure location if young children are in the household to prevent unintentional ingestion and poisonings.
- Never take higher doses of vitamins or minerals than that recommended on the label, unless directed to do so by the healthcare provider.

Prescribing Considerations

- Ongoing assessment during drug therapy should include monitoring appropriate laboratory findings (e.g., complete blood count, electrolytes, hepatic and renal function studies, and ferritin and iron levels).
- Before prescribing vitamin or mineral supplements, discuss current dietary patterns to be certain the patient is not at risk for adverse effects due to hypervitaminosis.
- If taking antifolates such as methotrexate, trimethoprim, dapsone, or sulfasalazine, the patient will need folic acid supplementation to prevent adverse effects.
- Postmenopausal patients may need calcium and vitamin D supplements to prevent osteoporosis.

Understanding Chapter 61

Key Concepts Summary

61.1 Although the importance of nutrition has been known for centuries, the specific vitamins were discovered in the 1900s.

61.2 Vitamins are essential for optimal health.

61.3 Government regulations and consumer knowledge about vitamins are limited.

61.4 The recommended dietary allowance is the dietary intake level that is sufficient to meet the nutrient requirements for most people.

61.5 Fat-soluble vitamins include vitamins A, D, E, and K.

61.6 Water-soluble vitamins include the B-complex vitamins and vitamin C.

61.7 Macrominerals are inorganic substances needed in amounts of at least 100 mg per day for normal body functioning.

61.8 Microminerals are inorganic substances needed in amounts of at least 20 mg per day for normal body functioning.

CASE STUDY: Making the Patient Connection

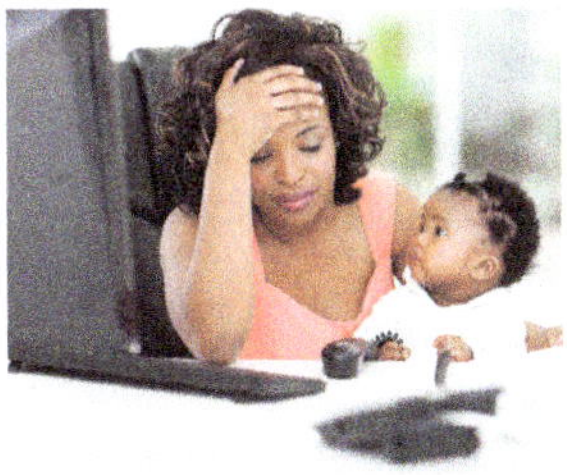

Remember the patient "Charlene Garrett" at the beginning of the chapter? Now read the remainder of the case study. Based on the information presented within this chapter, respond to the critical thinking questions that follow.

Charlene Garrett is a 32-year-old mother of a 1-year-old baby girl. She returned to work part time 3 months ago as a special-education instructor working with a group of preschoolers with special needs. Her husband watches their daughter two evenings a week so that Charlene can resume work toward a master's degree in special education at the local university.

Lately Charlene has begun feeling more stressed and tired. It is almost the end of the semester and papers are due; the holidays arrive in another month and both sides of the family will be coming to visit; and they have delayed celebrating the baby's birthday this month so that the families can enjoy the celebration when they visit.

Charlene lives next door and asks you, a nurse and the "reference for the neighborhood," about vitamin therapy to help her through this stressful period and to increase her energy level. She tells you that she still has some prenatal vitamins and wonders if she should take them.

Critical Thinking Questions

1. What other assessment data might you want to gather from Charlene before recommending vitamin therapy?
2. Should Charlene take the prenatal vitamins? Why or why not?
3. What other recommendations would you give to Charlene regarding vitamin therapy?

Additional Case Study

Jerrod is a 16-year-old Hispanic youth with moderate to severe developmental and intellectual disabilities. He is cared for by his mother in their home. Jerrod has been admitted for possible seizure activity after his mother reported that he began atypical twitching and jerking of the extremities. The mother reports that he was unresponsive to her commands throughout the episode, which lasted approximately 4 to 5 minutes.

On further questioning, Jerrod's mother discloses that until approximately 6 months ago he attended a daycare center for individuals with disabilities. However, due to his increased unpredictable irritability and combative behavior, his mother feared Jerrod venturing outside of the home. Typically, he spends his days watching television in a dark room or staring endlessly at a fish tank. Additionally, Jerrod is extremely selective about food intake and refuses to consume any dairy products, eggs, fish, or cereals. His daily intake consists mostly of chicken tenders and French fries.

1. One notable laboratory finding is Jerrod's elevated calcium and phosphate levels. What vitamin deficiency is most likely present given these findings and the patient's previous history?
2. What adverse effects should you monitor in Jerrod once the vitamin supplement therapy is initiated?
3. What environmental changes would you recommend to Jerrod's caregivers?

Chapter Review

1. A healthcare provider has ordered oral vitamin A (Aquasol A) supplements for a patient. The level of vitamin A may be increased if the patient is also taking:
   1. Vitamins D and E.
   2. Oral contraceptives.
   3. Mineral oil.
   4. Antibiotics.
2. Vitamin C (ascorbic acid) may cause a false-negative result in ____________ if taken within 48 to 72 hours of testing.
3. Pyridoxine (vitamin B_6) may cause antagonistic drug effects for the patient taking:
   1. Isoniazid (INH).
   2. Oral contraceptives.
   3. Hydralazine.
   4. Antiparkinsonism drugs.

4. The nurse is teaching the patient about the need for adequate intake of zinc in the diet. The nurse will teach the patient to increase consumption of:

   1. Protein foods such as beans, lentils, and nuts.
   2. Vegetables such as leafy greens, carrots, and squash.
   3. Citrus such as grapefruit, oranges, and lemons.
   4. Cruciferous vegetables such as broccoli, cauliflower, and Brussels sprouts.

5. A nurse should anticipate the administration of vitamin K (AquaMEPHYTON) for which of the following patients? (Select all that apply.)

   1. A newborn infant
   2. The patient with visual disturbances
   3. The patient who received an overdose of certain oral anticoagulants
   4. The patient with hypothyroidism
   5. A teenager with chronic acne

6. The nurse would suspect a calcium deficiency in the patient exhibiting:

   1. Night blindness.
   2. Anemia.
   3. Muscle cramping and spasms.
   4. Bleeding abnormalities.

See Appendix A for answers to critical thinking questions, case study questions and review questions.

References

Council for Responsible Nutrition. (2019). *Dietary supplement use reaches all time new high.* https://www.crnusa.org/newsroom/dietary-supplement-use-reaches-all-time-high

Pierret, L., Suppa, M., Gandini, S., Del Marmol, V., & Gutermuth, J. (2019). Overview on vitamin D and sunbed use. *Journal of the European Academy of Dermatology and Venereology, 33*, 28–33. https://doi.org/10.1111/jdv.15316

Rosenbloom, M. (2020). *Vitamin toxicity*. Medscape. https://emedicine.medscape.com/article/819426-overview

Selected Bibliography

Biesalski, H. K., & Tinz, J. (2017). Multivitamin/mineral supplements: Rationale and safety—a systematic review. *Nutrition, 33*, 76–82. https://doi.org/10.1016/j.nut.2016.02.013

Brown, B., & Wright, C. (2020). Safety and efficacy of supplements in pregnancy. *Nutrition Reviews, 78*(9), 782. https://doi.org/10.1093/nutrit/nuaa009

Office of Dietary Supplements. (n.d.). *Dietary supplement fact sheets.* National Institutes of Health. https://ods.od.nih.gov/factsheets/list-all/

U.S. Department of Health and Human Services and U.S. Department of Agriculture. (2015). *Dietary guidelines for Americans 2015–2020* (8th ed.). https://health.gov/our-work/food-nutrition/2015-2020-dietary-guidelines/guidelines/

"They say this might just be temporary and I sure hope so. Being fed through a tube is no way to live."
—Patient "Christopher Jones"

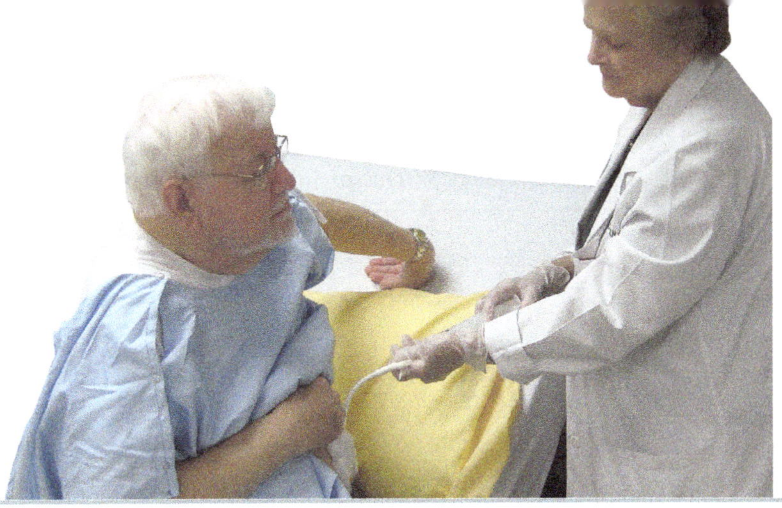

Chapter 62
Enteral and Parenteral Nutrition

Chapter Outline

Learning Outcomes

After reading this chapter, the student should be able to:

1. Identify conditions that may benefit from parenteral or enteral nutrition.
2. Compare and contrast enteral and parenteral methods of nutrition.
3. Distinguish among polymeric, elemental, semi-elemental, and modular formulas for enteral nutrition.
4. Identify the basic classes of nutrients contained in enteral formulas and their functions.
5. Identify the possible complications and adverse effects of enteral nutrition administration.
6. Describe the types of drug interactions that can occur when enteral nutrition formulas are given.
7. Explain the differences between delivering parenteral nutrition through a peripheral line versus a central line.
8. Describe the components of total parenteral nutrition solutions and the function of each element in attaining the body's daily requirements.
9. Describe the possible complications of parenteral nutrition therapy.
10. Identify drugs that may be incompatible with parenteral nutrition solutions.
11. Apply clinical judgment to care for patients receiving enteral or parenteral nutrition.

Key Terms Definitions of the terms in bold may be found in the Glossary.

To maintain good health and to allow healing during periods of illness, the body needs to receive various nutrients in predetermined amounts or in combinations. The intake of sufficient amounts of amino acids (proteins), carbohydrates, fats, vitamins, and minerals can often be achieved by eating a balanced diet of foods and fluids. In some circumstances, however, the daily nutritional needs of the body may require supplementation. Furthermore, certain diseases and conditions prevent feeding by the normal oral (PO) route. This chapter examines the methods and types of products available for providing enteral and parenteral nutrition.

62.1 Nutritional supplementation is required for patients with certain medical conditions.

Ensuring that patients have the necessary nutritional intake for proper health and wellness is a primary responsibility of the nurse. This responsibility extends to all patients, regardless of age, condition, or disease status. Although healthy patients can maintain their required caloric and nutritional requirements by eating a balanced diet, certain disease states, such as the following, may require nutritional intervention:

- Severe infections, such as human immunodeficiency virus
- States of malnutrition
- Bowel rest for inflammatory bowel disease and disorders of the gastrointestinal (GI) tract
- Coma
- Postsurgical complications
- Major burns and trauma
- Neuromuscular and central nervous system disorders
- Advanced age or premature birth
- Eating disorders
- Cancer-related chemotherapy or radiation therapy.

Although mechanical causes such as the inability to chew or swallow properly may limit caloric or nutritional intake, psychologic and social reasons also play a role in inadequate nutrition. For example, stress related to a hospitalization may alter a patient's normal eating habits or regimen. Unfamiliar foods and generalized malaise or fear associated with a patient's medical condition may also result in a decreased appetite. For the older patient, ill-fitting dentures or issues with dysphagia may lead to nutritional deficits. Younger patients may be on a fad diet with limited intake of specific nutrients or may have an eating disorder such as bulimia or anorexia nervosa.

Clinical nutritional support is utilized in all settings, including hospitals and extended or long-term care facilities, as well as in the individual patient's home. Pediatric patients are now provided various forms of nutritional support by specially trained providers at daycare facilities and schools.

Malnutrition in hospitalized patients or residents of nursing homes may present as dry, flaky skin and hair loss. More serious complications of malnutrition may include delayed wound healing, muscle atrophy, impaired immune function, infection, and even death. Secondary complications may include peripheral edema caused by a reduction in plasma proteins and a decreased oncotic pressure.

62.2 Supplemental nutrition may be provided by the oral or parenteral route.

Two basic routes are used to administer nutritional support: enteral and parenteral. **Enteral nutrition (EN)** is used for patients who have a functioning GI tract but are unable to orally ingest an adequate amount of nutrients to meet their metabolic needs. **Parenteral nutrition** involves the administration of high-caloric nutrients via a central vein, such as the subclavian vein.

Before initiating any form of nutritional support therapy, the medical team of healthcare providers, dietitians, and nurses must thoroughly evaluate the patient and determine which is the best method of treatment. It is also important to examine which route of nutritional support will achieve the desired optimal result. Areas that must be addressed include the amount of weight lost by the patient, the percentage of meals consumed, the patient's albumin level, and the patient's overall health and appearance. Other factors to consider when planning nutritional support are the patient's primary diagnosis, the ability to swallow, any anticipated diagnostic testing and treatments (e.g., nothing by mouth [NPO] for more than 3 days), and the overall prognosis. Socioeconomic factors of convenience, feasibility, and cost play a role in the decision-making process as well.

Enteral Nutrition

62.3 Various methods are utilized to administer enteral feedings to the patient.

Enteral nutrition includes products that are administered via the GI tract, either PO or through a feeding tube. When the patient's condition permits, EN is best administered by the PO route. Administering nutrition this way allows the natural digestive process to occur and requires less direct nursing supervision. Oral administration requires cooperation of the patient to adhere to the feeding regimen and an ability to safely swallow substances.

If the patient is unable to swallow properly, a feeding tube is passed either through the nose to the GI tract or surgically inserted directly into the stomach or small intestine. A nasogastric (nose to stomach) tube is more commonly used for short-term therapy and is often inserted by the nurse. If the patient displays symptoms of decreased gastric motility, a nasoduodenal or nasojejunal tube may be inserted by the healthcare provider. If therapy is expected to last longer than 4 weeks, surgical or percutaneous endoscopic insertion of a gastrostomy or jejunostomy tube may be appropriate. A percutaneous endoscopic gastrostomy (PEG) tube remains the preferred route for long-term therapy and is usually better tolerated than a nasogastric tube.

An advantage of providing nutritional support via a feeding tube is that the amount of enteral solution can be precisely controlled and measured and calories can be recorded. Contraindications to total enteral nutrition include peritonitis, intestinal obstruction, intractable vomiting, paralytic ileus, intractable diarrhea, and GI ischemia.

Enteral Formulations

62.4 Several types of liquid nutrition formulas are commercially available for enteral feedings.

Enteral solutions differ according to the various nutrients, the caloric values, and the osmolality of the solutions. The four basic groups of solutions for EN are as follows:

- **Polymeric formulas** contain various mixtures of intact proteins, lipids, and carbohydrates and are considered the most common type of enteral preparation. Typical composition includes 30% fat, 50 to 55% carbohydrate, and 15 to 20% protein. These formulas are used for patients who are generally undernourished but have a fully functioning GI tract. Polymeric formulas include blenderized diets and meal replacement formulas. Blenderized diets are generally high-residue, highly viscous products. Meal replacement formulas are either milk based or lactose free. These preparations are nutritionally complete, generally meet the recommended dietary allowance (RDA) for vitamins and minerals (see Chapter 61) and are palatable for oral ingestion. Examples include Osmolite and Promote.
- **Elemental (monomeric) formulas** include products that are usually lactose free and contain only a small percentage (1–3%) of calories from fats. The nutrient building blocks are broken down into small subunits (such as individual amino acids) that are able to be absorbed without the aid of digestive enzymes. These formulas are used for patients who have malabsorption disorders. Examples include Criticare HN and Vivonex T.E.N.
- **Semi-elemental (oligomeric) formulas** contain slightly larger molecules than those in elemental products, such as small peptides that require little or no digestion and are easily absorbed into the body. They contain a higher percentage of fats than elemental products, but they are in the form of medium-chain triglycerides (MCTs) that can be directly absorbed by the intestine without digestive enzymes or bile salts. They are used in patients with digestive disorders such as malabsorption syndrome, partial bowel obstruction, inflammatory bowel disease, short bowel syndrome, bowel fistulas, and antibiotic- or radiation-induced intestinal damage. Because there is little stimulation of digestive secretions, these products are also useful for patients with chronic pancreatitis. Oligomeric formulas are more expensive than polymeric preparations, with the main caloric source coming from carbohydrates. They are usually low in fat, which allows for rapid gastric emptying, and many of these preparations are designed for administration directly into the intestines. Flavor packets are available to improve the taste, but they are generally unpalatable and best suited for tube feedings. Examples of oligomeric products include Pepti-2000, Vital HN, Peptamen, and Subdue.
- **Modular formulas** or disease-specific supplements contain nutrients that are designed to meet a specific nutrient deficiency or disease state. For example, protein modules can be utilized to meet the extra nitrogen needs of patients with burns or severe trauma. Other conditions include chronic kidney disease (CKD), hepatic failure, pulmonary disease, and a specific genetic enzyme deficiency. They are not designed to meet 100% of a patient's nutritional needs.

Elements of Enteral Nutrition

62.5 Most enteral nutrition formulas contain four basic classes of nutrients.

There are many different enteral products, each containing various amounts of nutritional substances. The four basic nutrient classes and their functions are discussed next.

Carbohydrates: Carbohydrates are the major source of energy in the diet and function to spare body protein, prevent ketosis, and regulate blood glucose levels. Carbohydrate sources in enteral formulas must be soluble, digestible, and have a low osmolality. Commonly used sources of carbohydrates include corn syrup solids, hydrolyzed corn starch, maltodextrin, and other glucose polymers. Some special formulas include various types of fiber, fructose, and fructo-oligosaccharides. Simple sugars—such as sucrose, glucose, dextrose, and lactose—enhance the palatability of the oral preparations but increase the product's osmolality. These simple sugars retain water in the intestinal tract and can therefore promote diarrhea in the patient. The percentage of total calories derived from carbohydrates varies from 30 to 90%, depending on the particular preparation and the specific condition it was designed to treat. Most available EN products do not contain lactose and thus should not pose a problem for patients experiencing lactose intolerance.

Proteins: Proteins are essential to the diet because they support cellular growth as well as maintain and repair body tissues. They may be delivered as intact proteins, partially digested (hydrolyzed) proteins, or free amino acids. The selection of a particular protein product is based on the patient's medical condition and his or her ability to absorb the protein. Soy protein and caseinates are common sources of intact proteins and are found in polymeric formulas. Oligomeric formulas contain enzymatically hydrolyzed casein or whey. Elemental formulas contain free amino acids. Proteins may make up approximately 4 to 32% of the total calories of enteral formulas, depending on the specific product. Products that are designed for patients with CKD may contain no protein, whereas patients who are receiving immune-enhancing formulas may receive as much as 80 g of protein per 1000 kcal.

Lipids: Lipids provide an isotonic, high-caloric source of energy for the body. Soybean and corn oil are common lipid sources, and canola and safflower oils are also available. Long-chain triglycerides provide essential fatty acids, limit the osmolality, and enhance the palatability of the product. The fat content of the enteral product can vary from 1 to 55% of the total calories. Products that are designed for patients with glucose intolerance or pulmonary disease are generally high in fat, whereas products that are designed for patients with intestinal malabsorption contain lower amounts of total fat.

Other nutrients: Most commercially prepared enteral formulas are fortified with vitamins and minerals. When given in adequate volume, they provide most of the elements needed to maintain body functioning. However, the volume required to provide the RDA varies greatly among the numerous products available to the consumer. Fiber such as cellulose and pectin is added to enteral formulas to improve stool consistency but can create complications in patients who are fluid restricted or have delayed GI motility. Because most enteral formulas do not provide enough water in solution to maintain adequate hydration, additional free water (water without solutes) is needed to meet the minimum fluid requirements.

Complications of Enteral Therapy

62.6 Total enteral nutrition can predispose the patient to various complications.

Total enteral nutrition therapy poses a risk of mechanical complications such as aspiration, gastroesophageal reflux, diarrhea, metabolic and electrolyte disturbances, and procedural-related problems, such as tube clogging, migration, and dislodgment. Localized infections and sepsis are also potential problems during treatment. The most serious complications are related to potential electrolyte or fluid imbalances from the tube feeding solution or lack of supplementation or to mechanical complications such as aspiration and nasal or esophageal irritation and damage.

Aspiration: The most serious potential complication for patients receiving enteral feedings is tracheobronchial aspiration of gastric contents. Symptoms of aspiration may include dyspnea, tachypnea, wheezing, rales, tachycardia, agitation, and cyanosis. Aspiration of a small amount of enteral formula may not produce immediate symptoms, but a subsequent fever may suggest the development of aspiration pneumonia. The risk for aspiration is increased if the patient is fed while lying flat or if the patient is unconscious. The head of the bed should be elevated at least 30 degrees during the administration of the feeding and should remain elevated for at least 30 minutes after the feeding. The nurse should check for gastric residual volume by gently aspirating the stomach contents before administering the next feeding, or every 4 to 6 hours if the patient is on a continuous infusion. Other risk factors for aspiration include a diminished gag reflex, neurologic injury, gastroesophageal reflux, and the use of large-bore feeding tubes.

Nausea and vomiting: A small percentage of patients who receive enteral tube feedings experience nausea and vomiting, which increase the risk of aspiration. The most common cause for this problem is delayed gastric emptying. If this cause is suspected, the following steps should be considered:

- Reduce the doses of opioid or other medications that slow GI motility.
- Switch to a low-fat preparation.
- Administer the feeding at room temperature.
- Reduce the rate of administration.
- Administer a promotility medication such as metoclopramide (Reglan).
- Consider antiemetic medications if gastric residues are low yet nausea persists.

Diarrhea: One of the major problems in patients who require tube feeding is diarrhea, which is commonly due to the rapid administration of the feeding, high-caloric solutions, or bacterial contamination of the feeding formula or equipment. A patient who develops diarrhea while receiving EN should be evaluated for *Clostrioides difficile*, which usually results secondary to antibiotic therapy. Drugs that contain magnesium, such as antacids, may contribute to the problem of diarrhea, as well as drugs containing sorbitol, liquid cimetidine (Tagamet), and various multivitamin preparations. Diarrhea frequently coincides with the initiation of the enteral treatments because many of the medications that had been given by the intravenous (IV) route are changed to the PO route when enteral feeding is begun. If diarrhea develops during enteral therapy, the following should be considered:

- Add insoluble fiber, such as psyllium (see Chapter 60).
- Switch to a formula containing fiber.
- Decrease the rate of infusion.
- Dilute the solution.
- Administer an antidiarrheal drug.
- If *C. difficile* is confirmed, administer an appropriate antibiotic.

Metabolic complications: **Refeeding syndrome** can occur when nutritional support, including EN therapy, is introduced to severely malnourished patients. This syndrome consists of metabolic complications, such as dehydration, electrolyte imbalances, and hyperglycemia. In severe cases, nervous system complications such as confusion, seizures, and coma may occur.

Careful monitoring can minimize or prevent metabolic complications. To prevent refeeding syndrome, those at high risk should first be identified, including patients with anorexia nervosa, kwashiorkor, chronic alcohol abuse, prolonged fasting, and prolonged IV hydration. Any electrolyte abnormalities should be corrected before starting nutritional support therapy, and vital signs, intake and output (I&O), and laboratory values should all be carefully monitored.

Clogged feeding tube: Tube clogging is more likely to occur with the use of intact protein and highly viscous products. Routine flushing of the feeding tube with 20 to 30 mL of warm water every 4 hours during continuous feedings and before and after each intermittent feeding and drug administration can prevent most clogs. Aseptic technique should be utilized in order to minimize formula contamination, and extreme care should be maintained when administering medications via the feeding tube (Table 62.1).

Various methods are used to unclog a blocked feeding tube. The first is to instill warm water via a syringe, using slight manual pressure. If this fails, a sodium bicarbonate solution may be instilled in order to break down the clog. Pancrelipase (Creon, Pancreaze, Zenpep) crushed and instilled along with the sodium bicarbonate solution and left in place up to an hour may also break down the clog. These techniques may be repeated two to three times. If the tube remains clogged, the primary healthcare provider should be contacted.

Interrupted infusions: In the hospitalized patient, EN is sometimes interrupted for various diagnostic tests and procedures. These may include feedings held due to drug–food incompatibilities, hemodialysis treatment, "NPO after midnight" orders for surgery or procedures, physical or occupational therapy sessions, transportation from the unit, or GI intolerance (diarrhea, nausea and vomiting). When frequent interruptions are expected, recalculating the goal flow rate on a 22- or 23-hour basis instead of 24 hours may be more practical.

Drug and Food Interactions

62.7 Most medications that are administered orally can also be delivered to the patient via an enteral tube.

Medications that are delivered via an enteral tube must be in a liquid form (elixir or suspension) or finely crushed and dissolved in a liquid vehicle. Drugs that must not be

Table 62.1 Drug Administration Guidelines with Enteral Feedings

The following are guidelines for administering medications to patients who are receiving enteral nutrition:

- If the patient is able to take medications by mouth, the PO route is preferred over administration through the tube.
- Alternate routes of administration (IV, intramuscular [IM], rectal, sublingual, or transdermal) should be considered for certain medications that cannot be crushed, are not available in liquid form, or that repeatedly clog or block the tubing.
- Sterile technique is usually not required when administering enteral feedings or medications. Sterile technique, however, may be required for severely immunocompromised patients.
- Check the compatibility of the medication with the tube feeding formula first before administering it through the tube.
- If a tablet is to be administered through the feeding tube, check with the pharmacist first to make sure that crushing the medication will not alter its effectiveness. Then crush the tablet into a fine powder and mix it with warm water before administering. Enteric-coated drugs are never crushed and alternative formulations or a different drug may need to be ordered.
- For individual doses of most medications, the tube should be flushed with at least 30 mL of water before and after administration. This will clear the tube for the drug delivery, facilitate the transport of the drug to the intestine, and indicate if the tube is patent.
- When several medications are to be administered, all medications should be given separately and the feeding tube flushed with at least 5 mL of water after each one.
- Most drugs in elixir form are hypertonic. Highly concentrated drug solutions or suspensions should be diluted with at least 60 mL of water before administration in order to decrease gastric mucosal irritation and to prevent osmotic diarrhea.
- Medications should never be added directly to the feeding formula. This may result in a decrease in the potency of the medication as well as a decrease in the stability of the feeding formula.
- For most medications enteral feedings should be stopped for at least 15 minutes before and after the administration of a drug.

crushed or dissolved are enteric-coated pills, time-release forms, sublingual medications, and bulk-forming laxatives. If a tablet must be administered through the feeding tube, the nurse should check with the pharmacist to make sure that crushing the medication will not alter its effectiveness.

When liquid forms of drugs are mixed with enteral preparations, physical incompatibilities can cause the mixture to thicken and clog the feeding tube. Hyperosmolar liquid medications can also be poorly tolerated by the GI tract, resulting in abdominal distention and cramping, vomiting, and diarrhea. Both of these problems can be avoided by simply flushing the feeding tube with water and by diluting the medication first with warm water before instilling it into the feeding tube.

Enteral feeding products are usually delivered as a constant infusion and contain high concentrations of proteins and certain metals such as calcium, magnesium, and iron. These important nutrients can bind with certain medications, hindering the bioavailability of the drug and, in turn, reducing the total delivered dose of the medication. The fluoroquinolone antibiotics, such as ciprofloxacin (Cipro), are a frequently prescribed class of drugs that can interact with these metals. The effectiveness of liquid phenytoin (Dilantin) is often reduced by the drug's ability to bind with proteins in the enteral formula, resulting in subtherapeutic levels of the medication. Likewise, therapeutic levels of warfarin (Coumadin) may also be affected due to protein binding and the presence of vitamin K in the feeding preparation. Holding the enteral feeding for 1 hour before and after an antibiotic dose and 2 hours before and after giving phenytoin or warfarin will help minimize the drug's interaction with the enteral feeding. Table 62.2 lists the various drugs that interact with enteral formulas.

CONNECTION Checkpoint 62.1

From what you learned in Chapter 3, explain why drugs that have an enteric coating and those that are extended release should not be crushed and used in enteral feeding.

Table 62.2 Interaction of Drugs with Enteral Formulas

Interaction with Enteral Formula	Drugs
Decreased drug effect	carbamazepine (Tegretol), ciprofloxacin (Cipro), digoxin, levodopa (L-dopa), lithium, phenytoin, theophylline, warfarin (Coumadin)
Increased osmolality	digoxin (Lanoxin), furosemide (Lasix), methyldopa, phenytoin (Dilantin), theophylline
Physically incompatible	Antacids, cimetidine (Tagamet), dicyclomine (Bentyl), Dimetapp elixir, iron preparations, KCl liquid, MCT oil, Robitussin, thioridazine

Parenteral Nutrition

62.8 Parenteral nutrition is used when patients are unable to tolerate enteral feedings.

Parenteral nutrition is utilized for patients who are unable to eat or tolerate any form of EN or when there is inadequate oral intake to meet nutritional needs. It is frequently given to patients with severe GI disorders such as diseases of the small bowel (Crohn's disease, fistulas, adhesions, postoperative ileus), necrotizing pancreatitis, hyperemesis gravidarum (maternity patients), and pediatric patients with congenital anomalies or prolonged diarrhea. It is also used for patients with demonstrated undernutrition (less than 50% of the metabolic needs met for more than 7 days) as well as patients with AIDS, cancer chemotherapy or radiation-induced enteritis, burns, severe trauma, or anorexia.

Total parenteral nutrition (TPN), or *hyperalimentation*, will provide the patient with all the calories, glucose, proteins, fats, minerals, and trace elements needed by the body to sustain growth and to promote weight gain and wound healing. **Partial parenteral nutrition** lacks at least one essential element, usually fats or lipids, and supplies only part of the patient's daily nutritional requirements. Because these parenteral solutions are so concentrated, they can cause irritation and thrombosis of peripheral veins; therefore, a central venous catheter is usually required. Common central venous catheter sites include the subclavian and the internal jugular veins, and peripherally inserted central catheters (PICC lines) are often inserted in patients who require home therapy with TPN. TPN is always administered using an infusion pump in order to precisely monitor the amount of solution given. Figure 62.1 shows the locations of a central venous catheter for TPN therapy.

Peripheral parenteral nutrition (PPN) is used when a central vein cannot be accessed or when a central venous catheter is not appropriate for the patient. These situations may include patients in whom the subclavian vein is inaccessible due to scar tissue from repeated IV punctures or in patients with extensive trauma, severe burns, or cancer in the region of the upper torso or chest. These patients may be relatively healthy with only a slight nutritional deficit that cannot be met with enteral therapy. PPN is considered a temporary measure until a central venous catheter can be placed, and the solution administered is usually lower in osmolality than the solution delivered through a central venous catheter. PPN is advantageous because fewer risks are associated with the catheter placement, care of the infusion site is simpler, and the complications associated with hyperosmolar solutions can be avoided.

Problems associated with PPN include the need for several large peripheral veins because the catheter site is routinely rotated to prevent infection. The vein must also be able to accommodate the larger-sized venous catheter. PPN

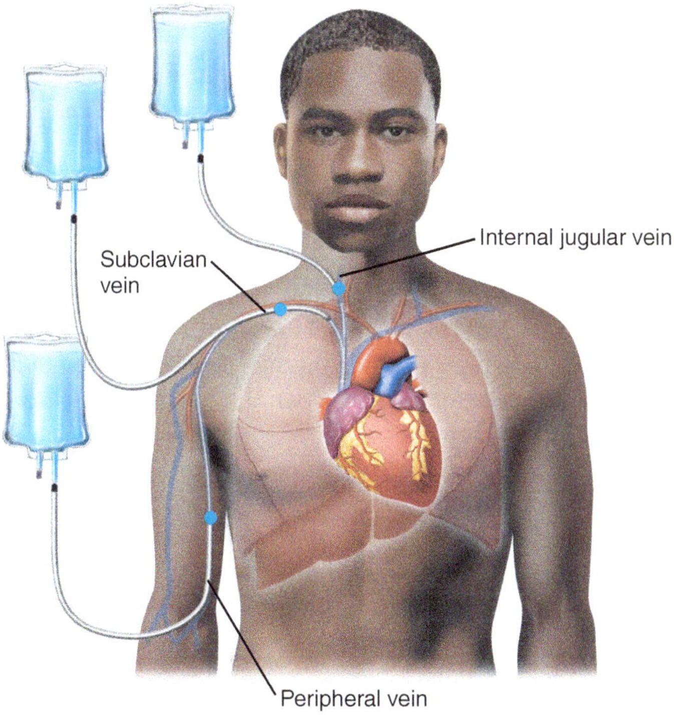

Figure 62.1 Routes of administration for parenteral nutrition.

is associated with a high risk of phlebitis and is therefore reserved for patients with robust veins.

PharmFACT

When assessing undernourished patients for potential enteral therapy, the nurse should consider that the lack of dietary intake may be caused by drugs that cause bleeding gums (anticoagulants), altered taste (captopril), candidiasis (broad-spectrum antibiotics), or nausea and vomiting (antineoplastics and many other drugs) (Dawodu, 2018).

Components of Total Parenteral Nutrition Solutions

62.9 The basic total parenteral nutrition solution consists of carbohydrates, lipids, amino acids, electrolytes, minerals, and vitamins.

TPN solutions may be modified daily based on the patient's laboratory results, the underlying disorder, the rate of metabolism, and other factors. Like the enteral products, the basic components include carbohydrates, lipids, amino acids (proteins), electrolytes, minerals, and vitamins.

Carbohydrates: Carbohydrates and lipids are the primary sources of calories for the patient on TPN. Dextrose is the most common carbohydrate source because it is inexpensive and readily available from cornstarch, beet, or cane sugar. The RDA of carbohydrates for adult patients ranges from 25 to 35 kcal/kg. When administered through a central line, the concentration of dextrose in the TPN solution usually comprises 25 to 35% of the overall solution.

When dextrose is administered as the primary calorie source (without lipids added), hyperglycemia can occur. Because insulin is required for dextrose utilization, a combination of dextrose and lipids may help reduce the risk of hyperglycemia and the patient's need for supplemental insulin injections. Dextrose increases the metabolic rate and the production of carbon dioxide, which may increase the demands placed on the patient's respiratory system. The addition of lipids will also decrease this risk. Abruptly stopping the TPN solution can result in hypoglycemia due to the continued release of endogenous insulin. This problem can be avoided by substituting a dextrose 10% solution until the new TPN solution bag is available or by gradually tapering the solution over a 24-hour period when discontinuing parenteral therapy.

CONNECTION Checkpoint 62.2

From what you learned in Chapter 36, what are the primary indications for an infusion of dextrose in water (D_5W)? Why should a patient with severe heart failure not receive D_5W?

Lipids: Unlike amino acids and concentrated dextrose solutions, fat emulsions are isotonic, which means that they can be infused through either a peripheral or central line. They are often a requirement for patients who are receiving TPN therapy for longer than 5 days. Currently available lipid preparations are produced from either safflower oil (Liposyn) or soybean oil (Intralipid). The principal fatty acids used in these preparations are linoleic, linolenic, oleic, palmitic, and stearic acids.

Fat emulsions can be hazardous for patients with liver disease, pulmonary disease, anemia, or blood coagulation disorders, with the most common adverse effect being hyperlipidemia. Fat emboli and death can occur when lipids are administered to premature, preterm, or low-birth-weight infants.

Amino acids: Amino acids are needed by the body to synthesize proteins, to conserve lean body mass, and to help promote wound healing. The RDA for infants and children ranges from 1.4 to 2.5 g/kg per day, whereas adults require 0.8 to 1 g/kg daily. Essential amino acids cannot be produced by the body, whereas nonessential amino acids can be synthesized from a nitrogen source, such as ammonium salts or urea. Amino acids must be closely monitored in patients with CKD because the blood urea nitrogen (BUN) level can become elevated. For the patient with liver failure, the administration of amino acids may result in hepatic coma due to the liver's inability to process nitrogen.

Electrolytes and minerals: Electrolytes—including sodium, potassium, magnesium, calcium, phosphorus, chloride, and acetate—can be added to the TPN formula as salts. Specific electrolyte amounts are ordered daily by the healthcare provider, based on preexisting deficiencies and the patient's current medical condition. To prevent interactions between specific elements and crystallization of the solution, the pharmacist should add the electrolytes.

Trace mineral mixtures typically contain copper, chromium, manganese, selenium, and zinc and are commercially available to meet the specific nutritional needs of the patient. Trace minerals are metabolic cofactors that are essential for the proper functioning of several enzyme systems.

Although it is routine to monitor electrolyte levels, serum levels of the trace minerals are generally not monitored. Trace mineral administration should be decreased or withheld in patients with a limited capacity to excrete them. For example, selenium and chromium should not be used in patients with CKD whereas copper and manganese should be withheld in patients with severe hepatic disease.

Vitamins: Vitamins are essential components of the TPN regimen. Most commercially prepared vitamin formulas can be given on alternate days in order to meet the patient's need for both fat-soluble vitamins as well as the water-soluble vitamins, and they can be added to the existing TPN solution. Vitamin K is usually administered weekly by subcutaneous or IM injection.

CONNECTION Checkpoint 62.3

Vitamin K is used as an antidote for overdose from a coagulation modifier. From what you learned in Chapter 38, what is the specific coagulation modifier and what would be the symptoms of an overdose from that drug?

Complications of Parenteral Therapy

62.10 As with enteral therapy, patients who are receiving parenteral nutrition therapy can experience various complications.

Despite improvements made in the delivery of parenteral nutrition during the past decade, patients may encounter certain problems during TPN therapy. It is important for the nurse to assess the TPN solution prior to hanging the bag for any signs of cloudiness, particles, or a change in color. If lipids have been added to the bag, then the nurse should assess for fat globules or separation of the lipids from the solution. If any of the above conditions are noted, the nurse should replace the solution with a different container of solution.

Other patient-specific complications can be classified as mechanical, metabolic, or infectious in nature. Selected complications of TPN therapy are summarized in Table 62.3.

Regular monitoring is important during TPN therapy. The patient's individual nutritional requirements should be reviewed regularly, taking into account the patient's current condition, drug therapy, nutritional status, concurrent treatments (e.g., hemodialysis), response to TPN, and supporting laboratory data.

Mechanical complications: Improper or incorrect placement of the catheter can result in subclavian artery puncture, pneumothorax, hemothorax, carotid artery injury, thromboembolism, catheter malposition, brachial plexus injury, subcutaneous emphysema, endocarditis, cardiac arrhythmias and tamponade, and phrenic nerve paralysis. Venous thrombosis is the most common

Table 62.3 Selected Complications of Total Parenteral Nutrition

Complication	Cause	Symptom
Mechanical		
Pneumothorax	Puncture of the pleural cavity by the catheter during insertion.	Sharp chest pain, decreased breath sounds
Hemothorax	Catheter damages a vein with blood entering the chest cavity.	Same as above
Hydrothorax	Catheter perforates a vein, releasing TPN solution into the chest. Clot in the subclavian vein.	Same as above
Venous thrombus	IV tubing is disconnected. Catheter is not clamped. Infusion cap fell off.	Distended neck veins, swelling of the face and arm
Air embolism	Same as above	Cough, shortness of breath, chest pain, and cyanosis
Metabolic		
Hyperglycemia	Fluid is infused too quickly. Insufficient insulin coverage.	Nausea, headache, weakness, thirst, increased blood glucose level
Hypoglycemia	Fluid stopped abruptly. Too much insulin administered.	Pallor, cold and clammy skin, increased pulse, headache, tremors, blurred vision
Fluid overload	Increased IV rate. Fluid shifts from the cellular to the vascular space due to hyperosmolar solution.	Cough, dyspnea, distended neck veins, rales, weight gain
Infection		
Sepsis	Poor aseptic technique when the catheter is inserted. Contamination of the catheter when changing tubing or when the TPN solution is mixed. Contamination when dressing is changed.	Fever, chills, tachycardia, drainage from the insertion site, lethargy, increased white blood cells, positive blood cultures

problem and is associated with significant morbidity rates. Signs of venous thrombosis include distended neck veins as well as swelling of the face and arm on the side of the IV catheter.

Metabolic complications: Metabolic complications of parenteral nutrition therapy fall into two broad categories: early complications or late complications. Early complications can usually be anticipated and include fluid volume overload, refeeding syndrome, and various electrolyte and mineral imbalances. Hypertriglyceridemia can lead to pancreatitis and altered pulmonary function if left untreated. The early complications can be prevented by carefully monitoring the patient and adjusting the composition of the TPN formula or the rate of infusion.

Late metabolic complications are less predictable and may be caused by the exacerbation of preexisting conditions, inadequate solution composition, or failure to monitor the patient adequately. Late complications can include fatty acid, mineral, and vitamin deficiencies and metabolic bone disease or bone demineralization, which may develop in patients who receive TPN for periods extending beyond 3 months. Although the exact mechanism is not known, metabolic bone disease can cause severe pain in the lower extremities and the back. The only known treatment is to temporarily or permanently discontinue the TPN infusion. Hepatic steatosis (fatty liver) and gallbladder complications (cholelithiasis and cholecystitis) are also late complications of TPN therapy.

Infectious complications: Parenteral nutrition therapy creates a chronic breach in the patient's physiologic line of defense. The IV infusion system from the solution container to the tip of the catheter may serve as a source for the introduction of bacterial or fungal organisms into the patient's bloodstream. The healthcare provider inserting the venous catheter, the pharmacist mixing the TPN solution, or the nurse hanging the IV bag or changing the central venous catheter dressing may inadvertently contaminate the patient's "lifeline."

Peripheral IV lines are at high risk for infection and infiltration, and the site of the peripheral line should be changed, if possible, every 48 hours in order to eliminate that risk. Unfortunately, severely debilitated patients often have few robust veins available for selection, necessitating the eventual placement of a central line.

Strict asepsis should be maintained when changing the IV tubing and dressings at the IV insertion site. TPN is an excellent medium for the growth of organisms; thus, most TPN solutions are prepared by the pharmacist with the use of a laminar airflow hood. Whenever possible, the central line should be used exclusively for the infusion of the TPN solution. Other preventive measures to reduce the patient's risk for infection include the following:

- Change the dressing routinely (every 48 to 72 hours, per institutional policy) or when it becomes soiled, wet, or loose. The caregiver should wear a mask and gloves while changing the dressing.
- Extend the application of antimicrobial solution (e.g., iodine) at least 1 inch beyond the edges of the final dressing.
- Place a sterile sponge over the catheter, then cover with an occlusive, waterproof dressing.
- Inspect the site for signs of tenderness, redness, edema, loose sutures, or any bleeding or drainage.
- Change the TPN tubing every 24 hours with the first bag of the day. A 0.22-micron inline filter should be used to reduce the introduction of bacteria from the TPN solution.
- Avoid the use of the TPN catheter for central venous pressure monitoring or the administration of IV medications or blood products.

Drug and Food Interactions

62.11 Certain drugs are incompatible and should not be added to parenteral nutrition solutions.

The major issue associated with the addition of medications to the parenteral formula is the potential for drug incompatibilities. A significant risk is that of a precipitate forming in the solution that is obscured by the opaque fat emulsion. Therefore, drug additions to the TPN solution should never be undertaken unless sufficient data exist to ensure the stability of the solution. Medications that are routinely added to parenteral preparations and are physiologically stable in solution are the H_2-receptor antagonists, such as famotidine and insulin.

When there is no other option but to administer a medication through the same access site as the TPN, it is best to use a separate lumen in a multilumen catheter to avoid the potential for incompatibility. The use of a Y site or piggyback drug delivery has helped to decrease the risk of drug compatibility problems. Flushing the IV line prior to and after the medication administration, along with temporarily turning off the TPN infusion during the drug administration for 15 to 30 minutes, will help lower the possibility of interactions.

Drugs with demonstrated physical incompatibilities with TPN include ampicillin, tetracycline, and amphotericin B. For administration of these medications, a second IV line should be sought. Medications that have a decreased therapeutic drug effect when given to patients who are receiving TPN with lipids include kanamycin and warfarin. It is important for the nurse to always check with the pharmacist to confirm compatibility and drug effectiveness when administering TPN with any medication.

CONNECTIONS: Community-Oriented Practice

Home Care of Patients on Total Parenteral Nutrition Therapy

Patients may be sent home on TPN. The patient and the patient's family should have the opportunity to practice the procedure for delivering TPN therapy while they are in the hospital setting under the supervision of the nurse.

Review the procedure for the storage of the solution. Instruct the patient to keep the containers refrigerated and to allow the container to come to room temperature before administering the solution. Instruct the patient never to warm the TPN in the microwave or the oven. Advise the patient to check the expiration date, label of contents, and the appearance of the solution. The patient should not use the solution if the TPN is cloudy, discolored, or has solid pieces floating in it. The solution should not be used if any separation (oil and water) is visible. The patient should check the integrity of the bag by gently squeezing it in order to detect any leakage.

The dressing should be changed at least every 2 days. Teach the patient, family, or caregiver how to use aseptic technique when changing the dressing. The supplies for the dressing and the infusion should be kept in a clean, dry place when not in use. The IV site should be inspected for any signs of swelling, redness, or drainage, which should be reported to the healthcare provider immediately. Demonstrate to the family how to irrigate the catheter and how to change the bags and the tubing. Instruct the patient about the various settings of the infusion pump, paying particular attention to reviewing what to do if the alarm goes off during the infusion. Review the local Environmental Protection Agency (EPA) policy regarding the proper disposal of used syringes and IV equipment.

Explain that the patient should be weighed daily and that the patient's I&O should be closely monitored. Ask the family to observe the patient for signs of edema. Demonstrate how to check the glucose level and ensure that all supplies needed are available. Review the potential complications of TPN, such as chills, fever, dyspnea, chest pain, coughing, reaction to lipid infusion, air embolism, nausea and vomiting, and hypo- or hyperglycemia. Instruct the patient never to stop the TPN infusion without conferring first with the healthcare provider. Recommend that the family keep the telephone numbers of the healthcare provider, the nursing service, and the community emergency services readily available in case an emergency or other need should arise. Whenever possible, provide written instructions for the patient and family to use as a reference before the patient is discharged.

CONNECTIONS: APPLIED CLINICAL JUDGMENT

Patients Receiving Pharmacotherapy with Enteral and Parenteral Nutrition

Key Assessment Data

- History of current condition, baseline vital signs, physical exam findings, history of any current symptoms that may indicate vitamin deficiencies or hypervitaminosis (e.g., dry and itchy skin, alopecia, sore and reddened gums or tongue, tendency to bleed easily or excessive bruising, nausea and/or vomiting, or excessive fatigue), dietary history, sun exposure; endocrine, hepatic, or renal disease; medication history and caffeine, nicotine, and alcohol use; pregnancy status.

Desired Therapeutic Outcomes

Improvement is observed and measurable by weight is maintained and electrolyte, glucose, protein, and lipid levels remain within normal limits.

Minimizing Adverse Effects

- Nutritional replacement solutions contain high glucose, protein, and lipid sources that may serve as a reservoir for infection. Tube insertion and access sites may also serve as points of entry for infection. Solutions must be refrigerated to inhibit bacterial growth.
- Blood glucose levels may be affected if the nutrition feeding is stopped or the rate is reduced or is dependent on other medications the patient takes. Supplemental insulin may be required.
- Solutions are hypertonic can create fluid shifting with resulting decreased intravascular fluid. Monitoring for a noticeable increase in the pulse rate and quality, changes in blood pressure from the baseline, dyspnea, or edema will assist in noting adverse effects quickly.
- I&O ratio, daily weight, and laboratory studies such as serum creatinine and BUN should be monitored to assess renal function.
- Venous thrombosis may occur in or around the catheter tubing. Signs and symptoms include the inability to obtain blood on aspiration from the catheter, inability to run fluids through the catheter, neck vein distention, and facial and neck edema on the side of the catheter. The infusion should be stopped immediately and the healthcare provider contacted.
- Proper central line insertion must be confirmed radiographically before any feeding is initiated.
- Proper gastric tube insertion should be confirmed radiographically before any feeding is initiated. Dependent on agency policy, confirmation of placement by observing the characteristics of the gastric aspirate or pH may be used. If any doubt exists about placement, hold the feeding and confirm the placement site. Excessive residual amounts of 50% or greater of the last bolus feeding, or two times the hourly amount by continuous feeding may indicate decreased absorption of the feeding or other conditions and increase the risk of aspiration. Return aspirated amounts unless agency policy requires otherwise.
- Diarrhea or constipation may occur with enteral feedings. Patients on enteral feeding, particularly with elemental formulas, are at increased risk of *C. difficile*–associated diarrhea or from other pathogens.
- Oral medications may be crushed for administration via enteral tube in most cases. Enteric-coated, sustained-release, gel capsules, and others may not be crushed and an alternative form or drug may be required.

CONNECTIONS: APPLIED CLINICAL JUDGMENT *(continued)*

Patients Receiving Pharmacotherapy with Enteral and Parenteral Nutrition

Patient Education

- If allowed, maintain small, frequent oral intake or have the caregiver assist the patient with oral nutrition and hydration. Monitor for dry mouth or lips, dry skin, or tenting of the skin as signs that insufficient water is being given.
- Immediately report any fever, chills, unusual changes to the insertion site, or changes in level of consciousness.
- Weigh self daily at the same time each day and record. An increase or loss in weight of over 1 kg (2 lb) per 24 hours should be reported. Immediately report any edema, shortness of breath, heart palpitations, swelling, decreased urine output, dizziness, disorientation, or confusion.
- Immediately report a stoppage in the infusion, neck vein distention, or swelling of the face or neck on the side of the IV placement.
- Follow appropriate technique (aseptic or clean) as instructed by the healthcare provider if the nutrition is to be continued at home. For enteral feedings, check placement prior to feeding, flush tubing as directed, and follow aspiration technique for residual amounts. The patient or family should provide a teach-back session on technique, dressing changes, and equipment changes.
- Promptly report signs of hyperglycemia (excessive thirst, copious urination, insatiable hunger) or hypoglycemia (nervousness, irritability, and dizziness).
- Report diarrhea or constipation. Immediately report any diarrhea that is profuse, watery, or contains blood or mucus.
- Discuss any changes in medications with the healthcare provider to ensure the medication may be given through the enteral tube or if alternative forms are needed.

Prescribing Considerations

- Ongoing assessment during drug therapy should include monitoring appropriate laboratory findings (e.g., complete blood count, electrolytes, hepatic and renal function studies, and ferritin and iron levels).

Understanding Chapter 62

Key Concepts Summary

62.1 Nutritional supplementation is required for patients with certain medical conditions.

62.2 Supplemental nutrition may be provided by the oral or parenteral route.

62.3 Various methods are utilized to administer enteral feedings to the patient.

62.4 Several types of liquid nutrition formulas are commercially available for enteral feedings.

62.5 Most enteral nutrition formulas contain four basic classes of nutrients.

62.6 Total enteral nutrition can predispose the patient to various complications.

62.7 Most medications that are administered orally can also be delivered to the patient via an enteral tube.

62.8 Parenteral nutrition is used when patients are unable to tolerate enteral feedings.

62.9 The basic total parenteral nutrition solution consists of carbohydrates, lipids, amino acids, electrolytes, minerals, and vitamins.

62.10 As with enteral therapy, patients who are receiving parenteral nutrition therapy can experience various complications.

62.11 Certain drugs are incompatible and should not be added to parenteral nutrition solutions.

CASE STUDY: Making the Patient Connection

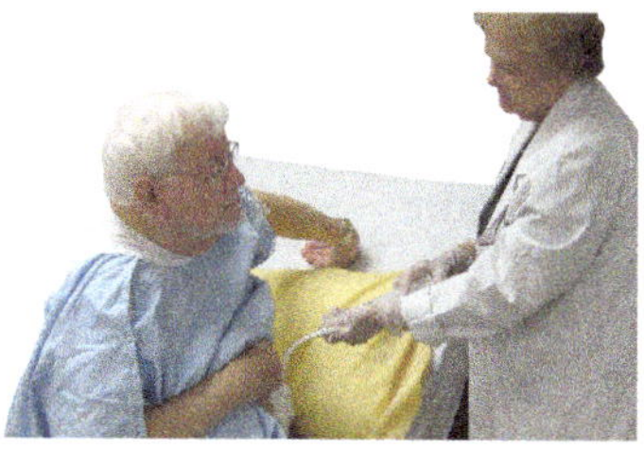

Remember the patient "Christopher Jones" at the beginning of the chapter? Now read the remainder of the case study. Based on the information presented within this chapter, respond to the critical thinking questions that follow.

Christopher Jones is a 62-year-old man with a long-standing history of diabetes, the past 20 years as an insulin-dependent diabetic. During the past few months, he has been having increasing difficulty eating. At first, he noticed that he felt full almost immediately and then nausea began in waves, eventually resulting in vomiting. Christopher began to lose weight and had trouble controlling his blood glucose levels, experiencing more frequent bouts of hypoglycemia. He visited his healthcare provider, and after an upper GI series, esophagogastroduodenoscopy, and a gastric emptying study, Christopher was diagnosed with gastroparesis diabeticorum. His provider has told him that it is most likely due to his diabetes and may be temporary. He has been started on a prokinetic drug (metoclopramide [Reglan]) and erythromycin in an attempt to increase gastric emptying.

The provider inserted a jejunostomy tube for feedings until the outcomes of drug therapy can be determined. Christopher has returned to the provider's office for his first postoperative visit and will need teaching about his feeding tube.

Critical Thinking Questions

1. Christopher wants to know if he can still eat foods "normally." Give a rationale for your answer.
2. The patient does not know how to take care of his feeding tube and wants to know if any special care is required. What would you teach him?
3. Create a list of potential complications to which Christopher and his family should be alerted.

Additional Case Study

Misty Moore is a 36-year-old woman who was admitted to the hospital with a complete bowel obstruction, multiple abdominal adhesions, and a flare-up of Crohn's disease. She stands 5 ft 5 in. and weighs 65 kg (143 lb). Her usual weight is 75 kg (165 lb). Misty's past medical condition includes Crohn's disease since age 16, as well as a 10-year history of type 2 diabetes. Exploratory surgery is scheduled to remove the diseased portion of her small bowel as well as to perform lysis of the adhesions, which occurred as a result of her previous bowel operations. Because of her depleted nutritional state and the 10% drop in her weight, nutritional support is indicated. Misty's GI tract is not expected to be accessible for at least 10 to 14 days.

1. What type of nutritional support do you think will be ordered for Misty? Why?
2. Considering the patient's condition, what metabolic problem would you suspect she is at risk for developing?
3. How can the risk of developing this problem be reduced?

Chapter Review

1. To meet his nutritional goals, the patient is placed on enteral feedings via a nasogastric (NG) tube. Which intervention should the nurse perform in order to ensure that the patient is maintaining a proper fluid balance?

1. Weigh the patient every other day.
2. Maintain a strict record of intake and output and flush the nasogastric tube once a day.
3. Provide additional free water in addition to that used for irrigating the tube.
4. Assess the skin around the tube insertion site for any drainage or irritation.

2. Before hanging a bag of TPN, the nurse checks the various components of the solution. Which elements would the nurse expect to see on the solution label? (Select all that apply.)

1. Electrolytes
2. Diuretic
3. Trace minerals
4. Isophane (NPH) insulin
5. Multivitamins

3. The nurse is making rounds at the beginning of the shift and notes that the patient's TPN bag is empty. Which solution should the nurse hang until the TPN solution can be properly prepared and delivered to the nursing unit?

1. 5% dextrose in water (D_5W)
2. 5% dextrose in Ringer's lactate (D_5RL)
3. 5% dextrose in 0.9% sodium chloride (D_5NS)
4. 10% dextrose in water ($D_{10}W$)

4. The patient has been discharged home on TPN therapy. When making the home visits, which assessments should the home care nurse closely monitor?

1. Temperature and blood pressure
2. Temperature and weight
3. Pulse and blood pressure
4. Pulse and weight

5. The nurse is preparing to hang a lipid solution and notes that fat globules are visible at the top of the bag. Which action should be taken?
   1. Roll the solution container gently.
   2. Shake the solution container vigorously.
   3. Run the solution container under warm water.
   4. Obtain a different container of solution.

6. The patient who is receiving enteral nutrition via a PEG tube suddenly spikes a fever of 38.6°C (101.5°F). The nurse notifies the healthcare provider who orders the solution and tubing to be changed immediately. Preventive measures to limit the risk of infection from enteral feedings include which of the following? (Select all that apply.)
   1. Refrigerate unused portions of feeding.
   2. Hang a feeding solution no longer than 4 hours.
   3. Wash feeding bags and tubes before reusing.
   4. Use plain water to irrigate the tube between feedings.
   5. Maintain sterile technique whenever initiating a new feeding solution.

See Appendix A for answers to critical thinking questions, case study questions and review questions.

Reference

Dawodu, S. T. (2018). *Nutritional management in the rehabilitation setting*. Medscape. http://emedicine.medscape.com/article/318180-overview#a2

Selected Bibliography

Akçay, K., Suluhan, D., Kesik, G., Uzunoğlu, K., Kartal, E., & Şahna, (2020). Nursing practices in enteral nutrition. *Clinical Science of Nutrition*, 2. https://doi.org/10.5152/ClinSciNutr.2020.984

da Silva, J. S., Seres, D. S., Sabino, K., Adams, S. C., Berdahl, G. J., Citty, S. W., et al. (2020). ASPEN consensus recommendations for refeeding syndrome. *Nutrition in Clinical Practice*, *35*(2), 178–195. https://doi.org/10.1002/ncp.10474

Hellerman Itzhaki, M., & Singer, P. (2020). Advances in medical nutrition therapy: Parenteral nutrition. *Nutrients*, *12*(3), 717. https://doi.org/10.3390/nu12030717

Zoeller, S., Bechtold, M. L., Burns, B., Cattell, T., Grenda, B., Haffke, L., et al. (2020). Dispelling myths and unfounded practices about enteral nutrition. *Nutrition in Clinical Practice*, *35*(2), 196–204. https://doi.org/10.1002/ncp.10456

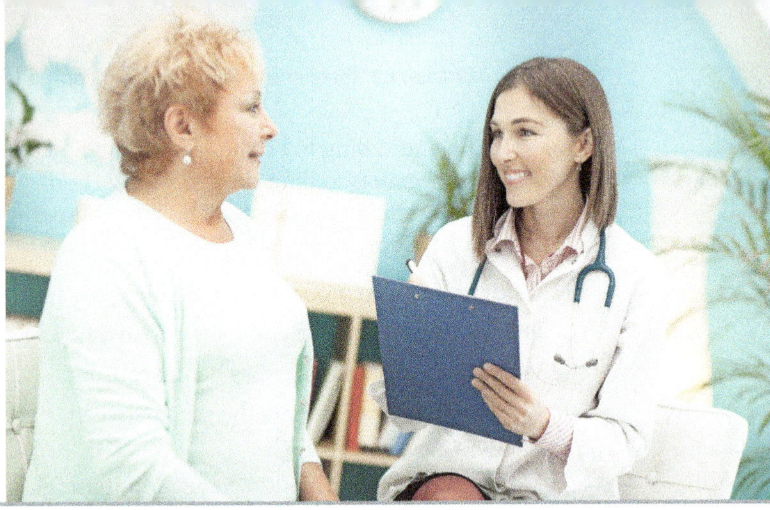

"I was shocked when the nurse weighed me in the office today: 30 pounds more! I didn't think I'd changed my habits all that much. Where did all that weight come from? I need to do something about this."
—*Patient "Rosemary Goodman"*

Chapter 63
Weight Reduction Strategies and the Pharmacotherapy of Obesity

Chapter Outline

Learning Outcomes

After reading this chapter, the student should be able to:

1. Identify genetic and lifestyle factors that contribute to obesity.
2. Explain how energy imbalances can cause weight gain or loss.
3. Describe the role of the hypothalamus in regulating appetite.
4. Explain how leptin and brain neurotransmitters regulate appetite.
5. Describe how obesity is measured.
6. Outline the major components of a successful weight management program.
7. Identify several weight loss agents that were removed from the market due to their adverse effects.
8. Describe the nurse's role in the pharmacologic management of obesity.
9. For each class shown in the chapter outline, identify the prototype and representative drugs and explain the mechanism(s) of drug action, primary indications, contraindications, significant drug interactions, pregnancy data, and important adverse effects.
10. Apply clinical judgment to care for patients receiving antiobesity therapy.

Key Terms

Definitions of the terms in bold may be found in the Glossary.

Americans spend about $72 billion each year in attempts to lose weight. In the majority of cases, people experience little long-term success in sustaining weight loss. Obesity is closely associated with increased health risks that include premature death, hypertension (HTN), hyperlipidemia, diabetes mellitus, heart disease, sleep apnea, osteoarthritis, and some cancers. In addition, the healthcare costs associated with treating obesity-related illness in the United States are estimated to be $193 billion per year. This chapter examines the etiology, pathogenesis, and treatment of obesity.

Etiology of Obesity

63.1 Genetic and lifestyle factors contribute to the etiology of obesity.

Obesity is a growing epidemic in the United States: More than 36% of the adult population over age 20 is obese. Along with the increase in adult obesity, infant and childhood obesity have also become concerns. About 20 to 25% of children and adolescents are either overweight or obese. Both these percentages have doubled or tripled since the mid-1980s. The trend is expected to continue because studies have shown that those who were obese as children are more likely to be obese as adults.

Despite considerable research, the specific causes of obesity have not been identified. The etiology is likely a complex combination of genetic, lifestyle, and physiologic factors. In a few cases, weight gain can be attributed to medical conditions, the most common being hypothyroidism. Certain rare disorders of the hypothalamus can also cause overeating. In addition, drugs such as corticosteroids clearly cause weight gain.

PharmFACT

Although obesity is increasing in the total population, the incidence is not uniform. The highest incidences (37% or higher) in adults are in Arkansas, Kentucky, Mississippi, and West Virginia. The lowest incidences (28% or less) are in California, Colorado, Florida, Hawaii, Massachusetts, and Vermont (Centers for Disease Control and Prevention, 2019).

Studies of family histories and twins support a strong genetic component to obesity. Researchers have identified a few genetic mutations that lead to obesity, although these are rare and likely contribute only a fraction of the total extent of obesity currently in the population. While a family history does not cause someone to be obese, it predisposes that individual to weight gain. The predisposition is best overcome by preventing weight gain. This is particularly important in identifying children at risk of adult obesity and implementing interventions aimed at prevention.

Lifestyle factors play a key role in the development of obesity, the two most obvious factors being diet and physical activity. The fundamental shift in obesity levels in the past three decades is likely due to the consumption of high-fat, calorie-dense diets combined with sedentary lifestyles.

Various theories have been proposed about the relationship between specific dietary practices and obesity, many of which are fueled by fad diets rather than research. While it is certainly true that the body metabolizes and stores carbohydrates, lipids, and proteins differently, no specific dietary nutrient limitation has been clearly demonstrated to prevent obesity or to result in more sustainable weight loss.

Despite the ongoing debate on the "best" diet, the fact remains that body weight is largely determined by energy (calorie) balance. Simply stated, if the number of calories consumed equals the number of calories expended, the individual will maintain (balance) body weight at the current level. Changes in weight occur when there is an energy imbalance. For example, an imbalance of as little as 10 surplus calories per day can lead to a 1-lb weight gain each year. While this seems insignificant, if the imbalance persists over several decades it can lead to obesity in older adults. Of course, this calculation also holds true for losing weight, but few people are patient enough to wait an entire year to lose a single pound.

Therefore, to lose weight people have to expend more calories than they consume. In terms of weight loss or gain, the source of the calories, carbohydrates, proteins, or lipids probably does not matter. Of course, the source is indeed important in terms of overall health and wellness, and the medical community continues to debate which of the energy sources (carbohydrate, protein, or lipid) contributes the most to adult obesity.

The second half of the energy equation is energy expenditure. Physical activity expends calories and can result in either prevention of weight gain or a faster loss of weight. The most successful diet plans always combine a reduction in calories with an increase in physical activity.

Pathogenesis of Obesity

63.2 Appetite is regulated by the satiety center in the hypothalamus and is influenced by various hormones.

Hunger occurs when the hypothalamus recognizes the levels of certain chemicals (glucose) or hormones (insulin) in the blood. Hunger is a normal physiologic response that drives people to seek nourishment. Appetite is somewhat different than hunger. **Appetite** is a psychologic response that drives food intake based on associations and memory. For example, people often eat not because they are experiencing hunger but because it is a particular time of day or because they find the act of eating pleasurable or social. The psychologic feeling of fullness or satisfaction following a meal is called **satiety**. The degree of satiety is directly recognized by a region of the hypothalamus known as the **satiety center**.

CONNECTION Checkpoint 63.1

The hypothalamus is part of the limbic system of the brain. From what you learned in Chapter 17, what are the primary functions of the limbic system?

In addition to glucose and insulin, another substance that regulates hunger and weight balance is **leptin**, a hormone secreted by **adipocytes** (fat cells). Adipocytes are metabolically active cells that are central to overall weight gain (and loss). After adipocytes have stored a certain amount of fat, they notify the brain of their energy status by secreting leptin. Leptin then binds to receptors in the satiety center in the hypothalamus, signaling the brain that the body now has sufficient energy stores. Body temperature (thermogenic) and energy expenditure increase. The body now "feels full"; leptin thus serves as a natural appetite suppressant.

It would seem that administering leptin would be a natural method for suppressing appetite and promoting weight loss. However, patients who are obese already have high levels of leptin circulating in the blood. Leptin receptors in these patients appear to have become desensitized and developed resistance to the satiety effects of leptin. The unfortunate result is an increase in appetite. At this time, the experimental administration of leptin does not have any effect on obesity.

Binding of the leptin receptors in the hypothalamus creates a signal cascade that leads to the secretion of a number of different hormones. Of primary interest is the action of neuropeptide Y (NPY), a hormone concentrated in the hypothalamus that has been associated with increased appetite. When the adipocytes are full, the hypothalamus inhibits NPY release, thus decreasing appetite. Unfortunately, experimental drugs that block NPY receptors have not been found to promote weight loss in patients with obesity.

Another important finding in the pathogenesis of obesity is the role of neurotransmitters in appetite suppression. Activation of certain subreceptors of the neurotransmitter serotonin ($5\text{-}HT_{1B}$ and $5\text{-}HT_{2C}$) reduces appetite and the consumption of calories at meals. In addition, activation of $alpha_1$- or $beta_2$-adrenergic receptors and the release of norepinephrine seem to decrease appetite. Antiobesity drugs are currently available that promote the release of these neurotransmitters.

Lipids are the most energy-dense nutrients for fueling long-term metabolic processes; more calories can be obtained from lipids than from any other molecule. While the body can store only small amounts of protein and carbohydrate, fat stores are nearly unlimited. The ability of adipocytes to increase in size and store a nearly unlimited quantity of fat is likely a consequence of evolutionary adaptation. For most of human history, starvation has been a major cause of death, and hard physical activity was necessary to survive. Those who had more efficient lipid-storage capacity survived the times of famine. Although starvation is still a problem in parts of the world, it is no longer a major cause of death in developed countries. Unfortunately, human metabolic systems are still programmed for low-fat diets, combined with lots of physical exercise. What was once a survival mechanism becomes a liability when individuals consume a high-fat diet and choose a sedentary lifestyle.

Measurement of Obesity

63.3 Obesity is measured by using the body mass index and waist circumference.

Obesity is defined by several different measures. In simple terms, obesity is being more than 20% above the ideal weight. The ideal weight fluctuates depending on the individual's gender, height, and general build.

The most commonly accepted measurement of obesity is the **body mass index (BMI)**. BMI is determined by dividing body weight (in kilograms) by the square of height (in meters). In adults, a BMI of 25 to 29 kg/m^2 indicates the individual is overweight. Obesity is defined by a BMI of 30 kg/m^2 and above. Figure 63.1 illustrates a simple graph of BMI for estimating obesity. BMI measurement is not accurate in athletes due to the higher proportion of muscle to fat in these individuals.

Another clinical measure of obesity is waist circumference, as measured by a simple tape measure. Waist circumference values of 80 cm (32 in.) for women and 94 cm (37 in.) for men are associated with increased health risk. Waist measurements greater than 88 cm (35 in.) for women and 102 cm (40 in.) for men have the greatest health risks. Waist circumference correlates well with BMI and also provides an estimate of abdominal (visceral) fat, which is more strongly associated with health risk than fat stored in other regions of the body.

PharmFACT

Obesity rates vary considerably by ethnic group and gender. From 2013 to 2014, the highest rates of obesity in adults over age 20 were found in Hispanic men (46%) and non-Hispanic Black women (57%). The lowest rates were found in Asian men and women (both 17%) (National Center for Health Statistics, 2020).

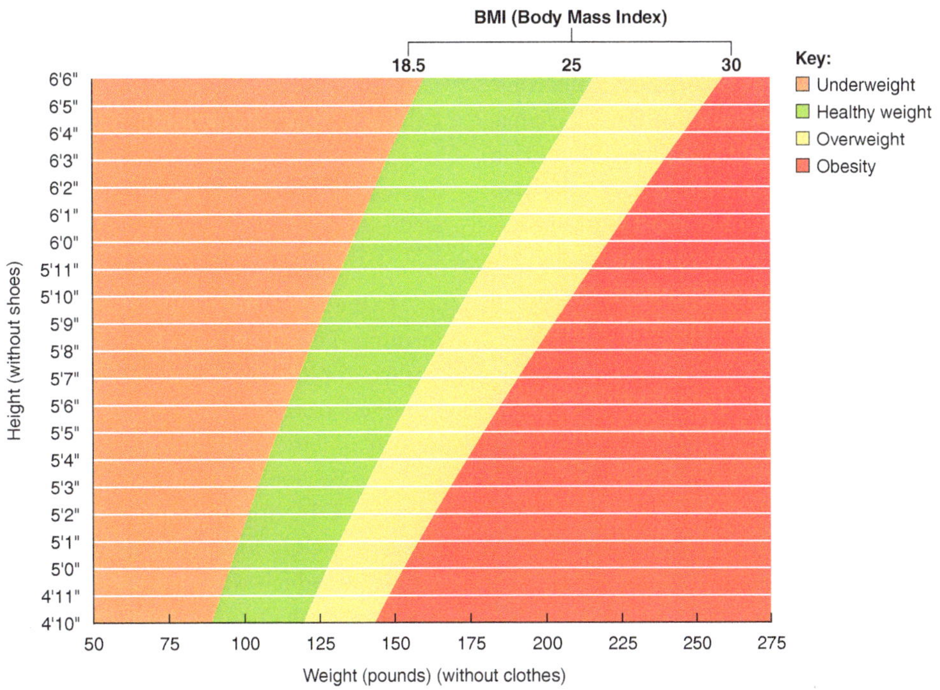

Figure 63.1 Calculation of body mass index. To determine your BMI, find the value for your height on the left and follow this line to the right until it intersects with the value for your weight on the bottom axis. The area in the graph where the two points intersect is your BMI.

Source: From Thompson and Manore (2017). Reprinted and electronically reproduced by permission of Pearson Education, Inc., Upper Saddle River, NJ.

Nonpharmacologic Therapies for Obesity

63.4 Nonpharmacologic treatment of obesity should be attempted prior to initiating pharmacotherapy.

Prior to initiation of drug therapy, the healthcare provider and patient must first attempt to achieve weight management through nonpharmacologic means. This involves making three major lifestyle changes: diet, exercise, and behavior modification. To obtain successful, sustained weight loss, lifestyle changes can be physically and emotionally demanding for a patient who is obese.

Choosing a sustainable nutritional plan (diet) is often the biggest hurdle for patients. Although it may have taken decades or longer to become obese, no one wants to take decades to lose weight. Weight loss schemes and fad diets that claim rapid weight loss while making few changes in dietary habits are very attractive to patients with obesity who are desperate to lose weight. The nurse should assist patients in setting realistic goals and steer them away from fad diets that may be unhealthy as well as unsuccessful. Severe restriction of any of the food groups—proteins, carbohydrates, or lipids—is not necessary or recommended by most nutritionists. The initial weight loss goal should be to lose 10% of the baseline weight, although smaller, progressive steps may be needed in patients who are accustomed to consuming two to six times the recommended daily calorie values. Weight loss of 0.5 to 1 kg (1 to 2 lb) per week is usually a physically safe and realistic goal.

Exercise is an essential component of any weight management program. Many patients with obesity, however, have chronic health problems that could impact an exercise program, the most common being diabetes, HTN, and heart disease. The patient should receive a thorough medical workup to be certain there are no physical contraindications to starting an exercise program. The patient who is obese should begin with very modest exercise goals and proceed to more challenging physical activity under the guidance of a healthcare provider. Exercise should be combined with calorie restriction because increased physical activity, by itself, is not an efficient method for losing weight.

Behavior modification is another essential component of successful weight management programs. The patient likely became obese due to poor eating habits and behaviors, which must be changed for the remainder of the individual's life. For patients with extreme obesity, the weight loss program will extend a year or longer; therefore, support groups should be encouraged. Breaking learned habits of eating is challenging and relapses always occur. Support groups can provide valuable help in adjusting to new lifestyle patterns.

Patients should be cautioned about taking over-the-counter (OTC) supplements that claim to promote weight loss. Many contain vitamins and minerals that can be obtained through a healthy diet, while others contain herbs and botanicals that have never been tested for weight loss. These products are costly as well as potentially dangerous. The U.S. Food and Drug Administration (FDA; 2017) has posted a warning that certain weight loss products contain hidden ingredients not included on their label. Over three dozen products were found to be tainted, most with sibutramine, a controlled substance removed from the market for safety reasons (see Section 63.5). Several products contained fluoxetine (an antidepressant) and sildenafil (a drug for erectile dysfunction).

Bariatric surgery is an option for patients with extreme obesity who have a BMI over 30 and who have been unsuccessful in conventional weight loss programs. The most common types of bariatric surgery involve placing a gastric band around the stomach, creating a smaller stomach (sleeve gastrectomy), or bypassing the stomach altogether. These operations create a smaller region for food storage so less food is consumed at each meal. Most patients having obesity surgery experience significant weight loss: 40 to 70% of their excess weight within 1 year. Although some patients eventually regain weight, most of the weight loss is maintained. The bariatric surgeries require strict adherence to dietary recommendations and vitamin and mineral supplementation to maintain health.

Pharmacotherapy of Obesity

63.5 Drugs used for weight management affect appetite or the absorption of fats.

Because of the prevalence of obesity in society and the difficulty most patients experience maintaining weight management plans for extended periods, drug manufacturers have long sought to develop safe drugs that induce sustainable weight loss. The quest for the "magic weight loss pill," however, has been very disappointing. Indeed, many of the prescription weight loss products have been discontinued due to health concerns. A brief history of these discontinued products is included because the nurse may still receive questions from patients regarding their use.

In the 1970s, amphetamine and dextroamphetamine (Dexedrine) were widely prescribed to reduce appetite. Although these drugs have strong appetite-suppressant actions, their effects are short lived due to the development of tolerance, which leads to the use of higher and higher doses. Although methamphetamine and dextroamphetamine are still available, they have high abuse potential and are rarely used for the therapy of obesity. A new formulation of amphetamine (Evekeo) was approved by the FDA in 2015 for narcolepsy, attention-deficit/hyperactivity disorder (ADHD), and the short-term treatment of obesity. Evekeo ODT is approved only for ADHD. Amphetamine is featured as a prototype central nervous system (CNS) stimulant in Chapter 24.

CONNECTION Checkpoint 63.2

Methylphenidate (Ritalin) is an amphetamine-like drug. From what you learned in Chapter 24, what are the primary indications for amphetamine and methylphenidate?

In the 1990s, the combination of fenfluramine and phentermine (Fen-Phen) was found to be effective at promoting weight loss. However, fenfluramine was subsequently removed from the market because it causes heart valve defects. Phentermine is still used as an adjunct to weight loss (see Section 63.7).

Two OTC appetite suppressants were widely used to promote weight loss in the 1980s and 1990s. Phenylpropanolamine, which was also used as a decongestant in cold remedies, was removed from the market in 2000 due to an increased incidence of stroke and adverse cardiac events. Until 2004, alternative weight loss products contained ephedra alkaloids, but these have also been removed from the market due to an increased incidence of adverse cardiovascular events.

Rimonabant (Acomplia, Zimulti) was the first of a new class of antiobesity drugs known as cannabinoid (CB1) receptor blockers. The CB1 receptors are primarily found in the brain, and their activation is responsible for the psychoactive effects of marijuana. Overeating activates CB1 receptors in the CNS; blocking them reduces appetite. Tobacco has a similar effect on cannabinoid receptors; thus, rimonabant was also used to promote tobacco cessation. Although approved in 2006, concerns about adverse effects, especially depression and suicidal ideation, prevented the drug from being marketed in the United States. Approval was subsequently withdrawn.

From 2007 until 2010, sibutramine (Meridia) was prescribed for the adjunctive treatment of obesity. The drug was able to produce a 5 to 10% loss of body weight within 6 to 12 months of treatment. Although well tolerated by most patients, sibutramine was found to produce an unacceptable incidence of serious cardiac events and stroke and was voluntarily removed from the market.

Given all these pharmacologic disappointments, current pharmacologic strategies for weight management focus on two sites of action. The lipase inhibitors act by reducing the absorption of fats in the small intestine. The approved antiobesity drugs produce only modest effects, and pharmacotherapy must be combined with a calorie-restricted diet. The appetite suppressants (also called anorexiants or anorectics) act centrally by increasing the amounts of norepinephrine, serotonin, and dopamine in the regions of the brain that affect appetite. Current drugs used as adjuncts in the treatment of obesity are shown in Table 63.1.

Table 63.1 Drugs for Treating Obesity

Drug	Route and Adult Dose (Maximum Dose Where Indicated)	Adverse Effects
amphetamine (Evekeo)	PO: 30 mg/day in divided doses	*Agitation, blurred vision, dizziness, tremor, insomnia, restlessness, HTN* Psychoses, tachycardia, drug abuse, dependence
benzphetamine	PO: 25–50 mg 1–3 times daily	*Agitation, blurred vision, dizziness, tremor, insomnia, restlessness, HTN* Psychoses, ischemic cardiac events, drug abuse, dependence
bupropion and naltrexone (Contrave)	PO: Begin with 1 tablet in wk 1 (90 mg bupropion/8 mg naltrexone); increase by 1 tablet/day each subsequent wk until maintenance dose of 2 tablets bid is achieved by wk 4	*Nausea and vomiting, constipation, headache* Suicidal behavior, seizures, HTN, liver impairment, hypoglycemia
diethylpropion	PO (regular release): 25 mg tid PO (extended release): 75 mg once daily	*Vomiting, diarrhea, dry mouth, changes in libido, nervousness, dizziness* Dysrhythmia, HTN, psychotic episodes, euphoria
liraglutide (Saxenda)	Subcutaneous: Start with 0.6 mg once daily and gradually increase to 3 mg daily	*Nausea and vomiting, diarrhea, constipation, headache, dyspepsia, fatigue, dizziness* Thyroid tumors, acute pancreatitis, acute gallbladder disease, serious hypoglycemia, suicidal behavior
methamphetamine (Desoxyn)	PO: 5 mg 30 min before each meal	*Agitation, blurred vision, dizziness, tremor, insomnia, restlessness, HTN* Psychoses, tachycardia, drug abuse, dependence
orlistat (Alli, Xenical)	PO: 60–120 mg with each meal containing fat	*Flatus with discharge, fatty or oily stool, increased defecation, and fecal urgency or incontinence* Hepatic toxicity, increased renal oxalate
phendimetrazine (Bontril)	PO (regular release): 35 mg bid or tid PO (extended release): 105 mg once daily	*Restlessness, insomnia, dry mouth* Valvular heart disease, pulmonary HTN, psychoses
phentermine (Adipex-P, Lomaira)	PO (capsule): 37.5 mg daily PO (orally disintegrating tablet): 15–37.5 mg daily	*Paresthesia, dizziness, dysgeusia, insomnia, constipation, dry mouth* Fetal toxicity, increased heart rate, suicidal behavior, acute myopia, glaucoma, mood and sleep disorders, cognitive impairment, metabolic acidosis
phentermine and topiramate (Qsymia)	PO: 3.75–15 mg phentermine and 23–92 mg topiramate once daily in the morning	*Paresthesia, dizziness, dysgeusia, insomnia, constipation, dry mouth* Suicidal behavior, fetal toxicity, increased heart rate, metabolic acidosis, cognitive impairment

Note: *Italics* indicate common adverse effects. Underline indicates serious adverse effects.

63.6 Lipase inhibitors cause weight loss by interfering with the absorption of fats.

One strategy to reduce weight is to block the absorption of dietary fats. Most of the accumulated fat in patients is derived from dietary sources.

Chemical digestion of lipids occurs through the enzymatic action of pancreatic lipase, which splits dietary triglycerides into glycerol and free fatty acids. Once absorbed, the fatty acids can be recombined with glycerol and stored in adipocytes. Attempts to produce antiobesity drugs that block lipid absorption have resulted in one approved drug: orlistat (Alli, Xenical).

PROTOTYPE DRUG Orlistat (Alli, Xenical)

Classification **Therapeutic:** Antiobesity drug
Pharmacologic: Lipase inhibitor

Therapeutic Effects and Uses: Approved in 1999, orlistat is indicated for the treatment of obesity in combination with a reduced-calorie diet and exercise. Orlistat is indicated for patients with a BMI of 30 or greater, or a BMI of 27 or greater if the patient has other risk factors such as HTN, hyperlipidemia, or diabetes. This drug produces only a modest weight reduction compared to placebos. A second indication is to reduce the risk for weight gain after prior weight loss.

CONNECTIONS: Complementary and Alternative Therapies

Green Tea and Weight Loss

Description

Green tea is a natural substance made from the leaves of the plant *Camellia sinensis*, which is native to mainland China but is cultivated worldwide. There are many varieties and types of green tea.

History and Claims

In China, green tea has been used for thousands of years for ceremonial functions as well as to treat a diverse variety of ailments. In modern times, the health effects of green teas have focused on improving cardiovascular function, weight loss, and preventing cancer. Some research has examined the role of green tea for improving symptoms or treatment of neurodegenerative diseases such as multiple sclerosis, Parkinson's disease, and Alzheimer's disease.

Standardization

Green tea extracts contain large amounts of catechins (also called polyphenols), a group of chemicals that have strong antioxidant properties as well as antihypertensive, anti-inflammatory, antiproliferative, antithrombogenic, and lipid-lowering effects. Green tea itself contains caffeine, although this is sometimes removed during processing. Extracts are sometimes standardized to percent polyphenols, which varies widely from 14 to 98%, depending on the product. Some products report the amount of epigallocatechin gallate (EGCG), which is the most abundant catechin in green tea extracts.

Evidence

After extensive study, there is little evidence that the ingestion of green tea or administration of green tea extract has any significant effect in a weight loss regimen. While there is some evidence that the polyphenols and compounds in green tea may have effects on the gut microbiome (Henning et al., 2018), green tea was not found to decrease satiety, promote weight loss, or help to maintain weight loss (Stuby et al., 2019; van Baak & Mariman, 2019; Wharton et al., 2020). Research is ongoing into the effects of green tea on inflammatory bowel conditions (Li et al., 2020). Adverse effects of high-dose green tea extract include GI symptoms (e.g., diarrhea) and potential hepatic toxicity. It is also known to interact with the beta-blocker nadolol and may reduce the effectiveness of other medications (National Center for Complementary and Integrative Health, 2020).

The prescription form of orlistat (Xenical) is available at 120 mg and is given three times daily, during or up to 1 hour after a meal containing fat. An OTC dosage form (Alli) is approved at 60 mg taken a maximum of three times daily. Orlistat is effective only if taken with meals containing lipids; the dose may be omitted if the meal contains no fat. Orlistat is not approved for individuals under age 12 (Xenical) or age 18 (Alli).

Mechanism of Action: Orlistat inhibits pancreatic lipase and acts by blocking lipid absorption in the gastrointestinal (GI) tract. It primarily lowers the absorption of free fatty acids but also has an effect on cholesterol absorption. The decreased lipid absorption lowers calories and promotes weight loss. Orlistat inhibits fat absorption by approximately 30%.

Pharmacokinetics:

Route(s)	PO
Absorption	Minimal absorption
Distribution	Not distributed; remains in the GI tract; does not cross the placenta; is not secreted in breast milk
Primary metabolism	Wall of the GI tract
Primary excretion	Feces
Onset of action	24–48 h
Duration of action	Half-life: 1–2 h

Adverse Effects: Some of the adverse effects of orlistat are directly related to its inhibition of lipid absorption. As more lipids reach the large intestine, flatus with discharge, oily stool, and fecal urgency are common, especially during the first 4 weeks of therapy. To avoid serious adverse GI effects, patients should restrict their fat intake. Rare cases of liver toxicity have been reported with this drug.

Contraindications/Precautions: Orlistat should be used with caution in patients with cholestasis because the drug inhibits gallbladder contractions. Orlistat is contraindicated for patients who have a known cause of obesity, such as hypothyroidism, and in patients with severe malabsorption disorders. The drug is contraindicated in patients with anorexia nervosa or bulimia because it may worsen these disorders. Orlistat is contraindicated during pregnancy because the benefits of weight loss do not outweigh the potential risks to the fetus.

Drug Interactions: Because orlistat inhibits the absorption of the lipid-soluble vitamins A, D, and E, a supplement containing these vitamins should be taken at least 2 hours before or after a dose of orlistat. Vitamin K levels may decrease in patients taking orlistat, which can affect anticoagulation produced by warfarin. Orlistat decreases the absorption of cyclosporine and the two drugs should not be used concurrently. Orlistat may also decrease the absorption of warfarin (Coumadin); therefore, coagulation values in these patients should be monitored closely. **Herbal/Food:** Unknown.

Pregnancy: Orlistat did not show evidence of fetal harm in laboratory animals. It is not known if this drug is secreted in milk or if it causes adverse effects on the breast-fed neonate. Orlistat is contraindicated during pregnancy because weight loss during pregnancy offers no benefit to the patient.

Treatment of Overdose: Overdose with orlistat is not a clinical problem because the effects of the drug are rapidly reversible.

Clinician Responsibilities:

- Obtain a complete health history, physical assessment including vital signs and apometric measurements such as BMI and body weight, and hepatic and renal function studies. Monitor weight and BMI periodically during use. Provide for dietary consult as needed.

Patient Education:

- Take a daily multivitamin containing fat-soluble vitamins at least 2 hours before or after orlistat. Adverse GI effects are common but typically resolve after 4 weeks of therapy. Avoid high-fat meals to minimize adverse GI effects. Distribute fat calories over three main meals daily. Do not skip meals.
- Monitor weight several times weekly. If diabetic, monitor blood glucose carefully following any weight loss.
- Immediately notify the healthcare provider of any known or suspected pregnancy.

Drugs Similar to Orlistat (Alli, Xenical)

Orlistat is the only lipase inhibitor indicated for obesity.

63.7 Anorexiants are drugs used to induce weight loss by suppressing appetite and hunger.

A second strategy to reduce weight is to block parts of the nervous system responsible for recognizing and reacting to hunger. All the anorexiants have the potential to produce serious adverse effects; thus, their use is limited to short-term therapy. Like the lipase inhibitors, anorexiants are prescribed for patients with a BMI of at least 30 or greater or a BMI of 27 or greater if the patient has other risk factors such as HTN, hyperlipidemia, or diabetes. The anorexiant lorcaserin (Belviq) was withdrawn from the U.S. market in 2020 due to an increased risk for cancer.

Bupropion and naltrexone (Contrave): In 2014, the FDA approved Contrave for the short-term pharmacotherapy of obesity. Bupropion is also approved as an atypical antidepressant and naltrexone as an opioid agonist. Contrave reduces appetite by increasing dopamine activity

CONNECTIONS: Advanced Practice Application

Obesity in Primary Care

Case

Sydney is a 42-year-old woman with a 9-year history of type 2 diabetes. She comes to the clinic with her husband, Frank, with complaints of fatigue, difficulty losing weight, and lack of motivation. Her PHQ-9, the depression screening, is 0. On physical exam, her height is 1.5 m (5 ft 2.5 in.) and her weight is 124 kg (275 lb) with a BMI of 50.3 kg/m^2. Her blood pressure is 160/88 mmHg. The remaining physical findings are all within age-appropriate range. During her first visit, Sydney was counseled on a low-calorie, high protein, low-fat, and low-carbohydrate diet and was asked to exercise at least five times a week. She was also instructed on behavioral triggers and coping mechanisms. At a 4-week follow-up appointment, she had lost 2.7 kg (6 lb) and her blood pressure was down to 146/85 mmHg. She did not seem happy with that and insisted that she be prescribed the diet pill that her sister was given. Sydney's diet and exercise plan was reviewed and it was recommended that she continue with the plan for another 6 weeks. Although she seemed frustrated and asked why her sister did not have to do all of this, she agreed to the plan. At her 6-week follow-up appointment she was down an additional 4 pounds! The diet and exercise plan was continued, and because the lifestyle plan had been followed and Sydney had shown positive lifestyle changes, she was started on phentermine/topiramate (Qsymia) for appetite suppression and canagliflozin (Invokana) was added to her medication regimen to help with glucose control. Sydney returned 6 weeks later with increased energy and was ecstatic with her 12-pound weight loss. Her blood pressure and blood sugar were also well controlled, and she let us know that she has reduced her snacking. Is this treatment plan appropriate for Sydney?

Discussion

The U.S. Preventive Services Task Force (USPSTF) recommends that clinicians screen all adults for obesity. Lifestyle and behavioral changes are considered first-line therapies and it is important for patients to maintain them for sustained weight management. Diet and exercise should remain the gold standard of care; however, systematic reviews of clinical trials have concluded that the use of pharmacologic therapies when compared with placebo are superior in reducing weight, reducing fasting blood glucose, HbA1c, total cholesterol, triglycerides, and systolic and diastolic blood pressure (Khalil, 2020). Clinicians should consider patient comorbidities and risk of adverse events when recommending medications for weight loss, but healthcare providers should consider adding pharmacologic management to weight loss treatment plans and should feel safe in prescribing these medications.

and blocking opioid receptors in the brain. Like other anti-obesity drugs, treatment should include a reduced-calorie diet and increased physical activity. Contrave should be discontinued after 4 months if a weight loss of less than 5% is observed. The drug carries a black box warning that antidepressants such as bupropion may increase the risk for suicidal behavior. It is contraindicated in patients with uncontrolled HTN because Contrave may increase blood pressure, especially early in therapy. Naltrexone is an opioid antagonist and may precipitate withdrawal in chronic opioid users. Naltrexone and bupropion both may cause fetal harm in laboratory animals. Use of Contrave during pregnancy and lactation is not recommended.

Liraglutide (Saxenda): Liraglutide (Victoza) was approved in 2010 for type 2 diabetes. Subsequently, liraglutide (Saxenda) was approved in 2014 for weight management in patients with obesity who have a comorbid condition such as HTN or type 2 diabetes. Although Saxenda and Victoza contain the same exact molecule, they have different indications. Like other anorexiants, Saxenda should be used with a reduced-calorie diet and increased physical activity. Liraglutide is a glucagon-like peptide-1 (GLP-1) receptor agonist. GLP-1 helps to regulate appetite by increasing feelings of satiety. Liraglutide has the potential to produce serious adverse effects such as pancreatitis, hypoglycemia, and gallbladder disease. The drug carries a black box warning that it may cause thyroid tumors. Animal studies show that liraglutide causes embryonic death and fetal malformations. This drug is secreted in animal milk although adverse effects on the breastfed neonate are unknown.

Sympathomimetic amines (SAs): The SAs are the oldest drugs for treating obesity. The prototype for this group is amphetamine. Adderall, commonly used to treat ADHD, is a 75:25 mixture of dextroamphetamine and levoamphetamine. Evekeo, indicated for weight loss and ADHD, is a 50:50 mixture of the two amphetamines. Other SAs approved for weight management include phentermine, phendimetrazine, methamphetamine, benzphetamine, and diethylpropion. For effective weight loss, the SAs should be combined with a calorie-restriction plan and a physical exercise regimen.

All of the SAs are CNS stimulants with the ability to suppress appetite. All are controlled substances that can cause physiologic and psychologic dependence. Methamphetamine is a Schedule II drug that carries a black box warning regarding its high potential for abuse. Typical weight loss is less than 0.5 kilogram (1 pound) per week and the effects tend to diminish over time due to tolerance. The SAs have limited clinical usefulness because they are only for short-term therapy (several weeks), whereas successful treatment of obesity may require years. Long-term therapy, or abuse, may cause HTN, cardiac abnormalities, bipolar illness, and other psychoses. Sympathomimetic stimulants may cause fetal harm and are contraindicated during pregnancy or lactation.

Gelisis (Plenity): Approved in 2020, gelisis is a unique product consisting of thousands of hydrogel particles made of cellulose and citric acid. When consumed with several glasses of water, the particles swell, rapidly making the person feel full. The particles are not absorbed and pass through the GI tract unchanged. Gelisis is approved for people with a BMI of 25 to 40 who are expected to follow a weight management program of nutrition, diet, and exercise. What truly makes this product unique is that the FDA approved gelisis as a transient, space-occupying *device*, not a drug. Weight loss products are not recommended during pregnancy because they offer no benefit to the patient.

CONNECTION Checkpoint 63.3

Orlistat may decrease the absorption of fat-soluble vitamins. From what you learned in Chapter 61, describe the types of effects that could result from deficiencies in the fat-soluble vitamins A and D.

Adjuncts to Obesity Therapy

63.8 Artificial sweeteners and fat substitutes are sometimes used as adjuncts to weight management programs.

A primary component of any weight management program is reduction of caloric intake. In an attempt to reduce total calories, many people have turned to artificial sweeteners and fat substitutes.

Artificial sweeteners include saccharin (Sweet'N Low®, Sugar-Twin®), aspartame (NutraSweet®, Equal®), acesulfame (ACK, Sweet One®, Sunett®), and sucralose (Splenda®). These agents are 200 to 600 times sweeter than table sugar, or sucrose, and thus less quantity is needed for sweetening food and beverages. Artificial sweeteners are regulated by the FDA because they are classified as food additives. Safety studies suggest that these substances are safe when used in usual amounts. Consumers should be aware that "sugar-free" foods that contain artificial sweeteners may have just as many calories and have a higher fat content than regular foods. Patients who have diabetes or are pregnant should consult with their healthcare providers before consuming artificial sweeteners.

Stevia (Truvia) is a genus of a plant in the sunflower family from which natural sweeteners are extracted. More than 30 times sweeter than sucrose, stevia is recognized by the FDA as a dietary supplement, not as a food additive. It has gained wide acceptance as an artificial sweetener in the United States. Stevia has a bitter taste when used in large amounts. Safety concerns have caused it to be banned in several countries.

Fats give food a smooth texture as well as calories. It is easy to identify fat-free or low-fat foods because they generally lack the taste and texture of normal fat. Fat substitutes attempt to simulate the texture of normal fat without the calories or effects of raising lipid levels in the blood. These products are categorized into the following types:

- The most common fat replacers are *carbohydrate*-based substances such as cellulose, gelatin, dextrin and modified dietary fibers.
- Simplesse is a *protein*-based fat substitute that is derived from natural whey protein or egg whites and is used in baked goods and dairy products.
- Olestra is a *fat*-based substitute that consists of a sucrose molecule surrounded by fatty acids. Olestra interferes with the absorption of fats, including lipid-soluble vitamins. It has the taste and texture appeal of fat but passes through the digestive tract undigested. It offers zero calories and zero fat but has the unpleasant adverse effects of loose stools and anal leakage. It is primarily restricted to use in snack foods.

Do artificial sweeteners and fat substitutes actually help patients lose weight? The answer depends on the dietary habits of the consumer. Certainly, drinking a liter of a regular soft drink gives one many more calories than drinking the same amount of a diet soft drink. Likewise, eating 8 ounces of potato chips using olestra gives fewer calories and fat than eating 8 ounces of regular chips. However, patients with serious weight problems should probably make better food choices than soft drinks and chips. A few studies have suggested that the body compensates by craving sucrose and high-fat meals. Note that the FDA has evaluated these food additives only for safety, not for their effectiveness in maintaining or losing body weight. Just as there are no miracle pills for weight loss, there are no miracle foods that will promote weight loss. The answer lies in the simple rules of limiting calorie intake, proper nutrition, and exercise.

Understanding Chapter 63

Key Concepts Summary

63.1 Genetic and lifestyle factors contribute to the etiology of obesity.

63.2 Appetite is regulated by the satiety center in the hypothalamus and is influenced by various hormones.

63.3 Obesity is measured by using the body mass index and waist circumference.

63.4 Nonpharmacologic treatment of obesity should be attempted prior to initiating pharmacotherapy.

63.5 Drugs used for weight management affect appetite or the absorption of fats.

63.6 Lipase inhibitors cause weight loss by interfering with the absorption of fats.

63.7 Anorexiants are drugs used to induce weight loss by suppressing appetite and hunger.

63.8 Artificial sweeteners and fat substitutes are sometimes used as adjuncts to weight management programs.

CASE STUDY: Making the Patient Connection

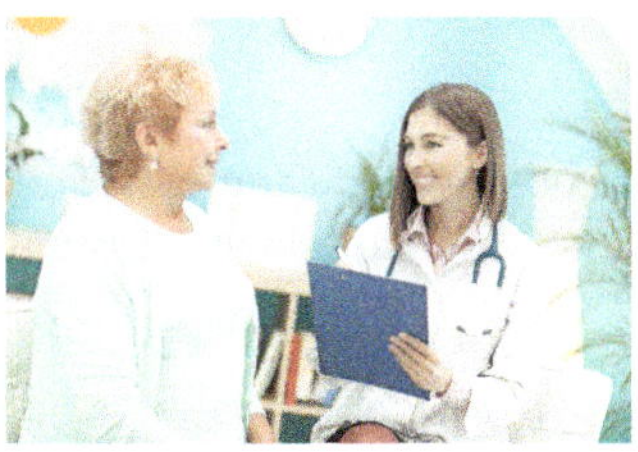

Remember the patient "Rosemary Goodman" at the beginning of this chapter? Now read the remainder of the case study. Based on the information presented within this chapter, respond to the critical thinking questions that follow.

Rosemary, a 58-year-old woman, has just had her annual physical examination with the nurse practitioner. She was shocked to learn that she has gained just under 13.6 kg (30 lb) since her office visit 2 years ago, 7.7 kg (17 lb) in the last year alone. She went through menopause 2 years ago and thought that some of the mild edema and resulting weight gain she experienced around the time of her menses was over. Rosemary has always been under or at normal weight except for the last office visit. At the time she was going through a personally stressful time and was not concerned about the weight gain. She works in an office as a financial manager, spending most of her day at her desk. Although Rosemary tries to take lunchtime walks, on most days there is just too much to do in the office.

The rest of Rosemary's physical examination was unremarkable except for a borderline hypertensive blood pressure reading of 138/82 mmHg. Her height is 1.6 m (5 ft 6 in.), and she now weighs 79.5 kg (175 lb). She states that she "watches what she eats" and normally eats three meals per day: a hurried breakfast of "something from the local fast-food place" on the drive to work, a sandwich at her desk or "whatever the rest of the office is ordering from take-out" for lunch, and a "regular dinner" at home with her husband. On the evenings when her husband is not home for dinner, Rosemary picks up something at the local supermarket from the prepared food aisle. She also enjoys a glass of wine with dinner. When the nurse and Rosemary add up the approximate number of calories she consumes, the average total is over 2000 per day. She is upset and asks the nurse about weight loss strategies.

Critical Thinking Questions

1. Rosemary asks about diet pills because her mother used to take them on occasion. What would you tell her about the availability of these drugs today?
2. Rosemary would like to try orlistat (Alli), which she has noticed on the shelf in the supermarket. What does Rosemary need to know about orlistat before deciding to take it? What teaching does she need about taking orlistat?
3. What factors have contributed to Rosemary's weight gain during the past 2 years? What general health teaching would be appropriate to aid in her weight reduction?

Additional Case Study

Kathryn is a 52-year-old woman who has been grossly overweight for more than 15 years. In that time, she has tried many diets, exercise regimens, diet clubs, and drug therapies, but all to no avail. She weighs 143 kg (315 lb) and has a BMI of 48. Her healthcare provider has prescribed orlistat (Xenical). Kathryn informs you that she has tried diet pills in the past. She has heard that amphetamines cause people terrible problems and is fearful that she will become dependent on orlistat or experience serious complications.

1. How would you address Kathryn's fears about diet drugs and the use of orlistat?
2. How is prescription-strength orlistat different from the OTC dosage? What adverse effects may occur at the higher dosage?
3. What effect does orlistat have on vitamin absorption? If Kathryn's provider prescribes a multivitamin, what should Kathryn know about taking it?

Chapter Review

1. A patient is prescribed bupropion and naltrexone (Contrave) for the treatment of obesity and is concerned about the risks involved with the drug. Which of the following should the nurse consider when teaching this patient? (Select all that apply)
   1. If less than a 5% weight loss has been achieved after 3 months, a different weight loss regimen may be needed.
   2. There are no long-term effects when the drug is taken as prescribed.
   3. The drug is known to increase blood pressure, potentially causing severe HTN, and BP will be monitored periodically.
   4. If opioids are currently used, the drug will initiate a withdrawal syndrome.
   5. The drug has been linked to suicidal behavior and the presence of depression or suicidal thoughts should be reported immediately.
2. A patient asks the provider about a prescription for phentermine (Adipex-P) for obesity. Which of the following would be considered a contraindication for the use of this drug?
   1. Extreme obesity
   2. A history of type 2 diabetes managed with oral antidiabetic drugs
   3. A history of HTN managed with beta blockers
   4. Pregnancy
3. The patient has been started on orlistat (Xenical). The nurse would teach this patient to take this medication:
   1. Once in the morning.
   2. When a feeling of hunger is noticed.
   3. Before daily exercise.
   4. Just prior to each meal containing fats.

4. Liraglutide (Saxenda) has been prescribed for a patient with obesity and prediabetes. Liraglutide has beneficial effects on which of the following conditions?

1. Hypothyroidism.
2. Gallbladder disease.
3. Pancreatitis.
4. Type 2 diabetes.

5. A nurse is instructing a patient taking orlistat (Xenical) about adverse effects of the medication. Which symptoms indicate the presence of an expected adverse effect?

1. Flatus with discharge and oily stool
2. Heartburn and dyspepsia
3. Constipation with fecal impaction
4. Nausea with projectile vomiting

6. Which of the following measures is used to assess the presence of obesity? (Select all that apply.)

1. Body weight
2. Body mass index
3. Waist circumference
4. Treadmill test
5. Buoyancy analysis

See Appendix A for answers to critical thinking questions, case study questions, and review questions.

References

Centers for Disease Control and Prevention. (2019). *Adult obesity maps.* https://www.cdc.gov/obesity/data/prevalence-maps.html

Henning, S. M., Yang, J., Hsu, M., Lee, R. P., Grojean, E. M., Ly, A., et al. (2018). Decaffeinated green and black tea polyphenols decrease weight gain and alter microbiome populations and function in diet-induced obese mice. *European Journal of Nutrition, 57*, 2759–2769. https://doi.org/10.1007/s00394-017-1542-8

Khalil, E. (2020). Pharmacological treatment for obesity in adults: An umbrella review. *Annals of Pharmacotherapy, 54*(7), 691–705. https://doi.org/10.1177/1060028019898912

Li, Y., Rahman, S.U., Huang, Y., Zhang, Y., Ming, P., Zhu, L., et al. (2020). Green tea polyphenols decrease weight gain, ameliorate alteration of gut microbiota, and mitigate intestinal inflammation in canines with high-fat-diet-induced obesity. *Journal of Nutritional Biochemistry, 78*, 108324. https://doi.org/10.1016/j.jnutbio.2019.108324

National Center for Complementary and Integrative Health. (2020). *Green tea.* https://www.nccih.nih.gov/health/green-tea

National Center for Health Statistics. (2020). *Prevalence of obesity and extreme obesity among adults: United States, 2073–2018.* https://www.cdc.gov/nchs/data/databriefs/db360-h.pdf

Stuby, J., Gravestock, I., Wolfram, E., Pichierri, G., Steurer, J., & Burgstaller, J. M., (2019). Appetite-suppressing and satiety-increasing bioactive phytochemicals: A systematic review. *Nutrients, 11*(9), 2238. https://doi.org/10.3390/nu11092238

Thompson, J. J., & Manore, M. (2017). *Nutrition: An applied approach* (5th ed.). Pearson.

van Baak, M. A., & Mariman, E. C. M. (2019). Dietary strategies for weight loss maintenance. *Nutrients, 11*(8), 1916. https://doi.org/10.3390/nu11081916

Wharton, S., Bonder, R., Jeffery, A., & Christensen, R. A. G. (2020). The safety and effectiveness of commonly-marketed natural supplements for weight loss in populations with obesity: A critical review of the literature from 2006 to 2016. *Critical Reviews in Food Science and Nutrition, 60*, 1614–1630. https://doi.org/10.1080/10408398.2019.1584873

Selected Bibliography

American Society for Metabolic and Bariatric Surgery. (2020). *Bariatric surgery procedures.* https://asmbs.org/patients/bariatric-surgery-procedures

Barrea, L., Pugliese, G., Muscogiuri, G., Laudisio, D., Colao, A., & Savastano, S. (2020). New-generation anti-obesity drugs: naltrexone/bupropion and liraglutide. An update for endocrinologists and nutritionists. *Minerva Endocrinologica, 45*(2), 127–137. https://doi.org/10.23736/s0391-1977.20.03179-x

Centers for Disease Control and Prevention. (2020). *Overweight and obesity.* https://www.cdc.gov/obesity/index.html

Hamdy, O. (2020). *Obesity guidelines.* Medscape. https://emedicine.medscape.com/article/123702-guidelines

Higgins, K. A., & Mattes, R. D. (2019). A randomized controlled trial contrasting the effects of 4 low-calorie sweeteners and sucrose on body weight in adults with overweight or obesity. *American Journal of Clinical Nutrition, 109*(5), 1288–1301. https://doi.org/10.1093/ajcn/nqy381

Heymsfield, S. B., & Wadden, T. A. (2017). Mechanisms, pathophysiology, and management of obesity. *New England Journal of Medicine, 376*(3), 254–266. https://doi.org/10.1056/NEJMra1514009

Izquierdo, A. G., Crujeiras, A. B., Casanueva, F. F., & Carreira, M. C. (2019). Leptin, obesity, and leptin resistance: Where are we 25 years later? *Nutrients, 11*(11), 2704. https://doi.org/10.3390/nu11112704

Laviada-Molina, H., Molina-Segui, F., Pérez-Gaxiola, G., Cuello-García, C., Arjona-Villicaña, R., Espinosa-Marrón, A., & Martinez-Portilla, R. J. (2020). Effects of nonnutritive sweeteners on body weight and BMI in diverse clinical contexts: Systematic review and meta-analysis. *Obesity Reviews, 21*(7), e13020. https://doi.org/10.1111/obr.13020

Schwarz, S. M. (2019). *Obesity in children.* Medscape. http://emedicine.medscape.com/article/ 985333-overview

Tronieri, J. S., Wadden, T. A., Chao, A. M., & Tsai, A. G. (2019). Primary care interventions for obesity: review of the evidence. *Current Obesity Reports, 8*(2), 128–136. https://doi.org/10.1007/s13679-019-00341-5

Walbolt, J., & Koh, Y. (2020). Non-nutritive sweeteners and their associations with obesity and type 2 diabetes. *Journal of Obesity and Metabolic Syndrome, 29*(2), 114–123. https://doi.org/10.7570/jomes19079

Unit 10

Pharmacology of the Endocrine System

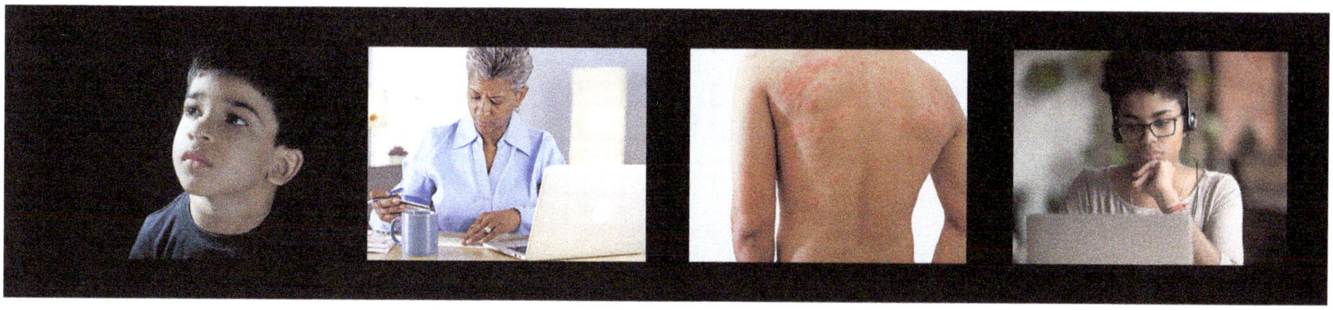

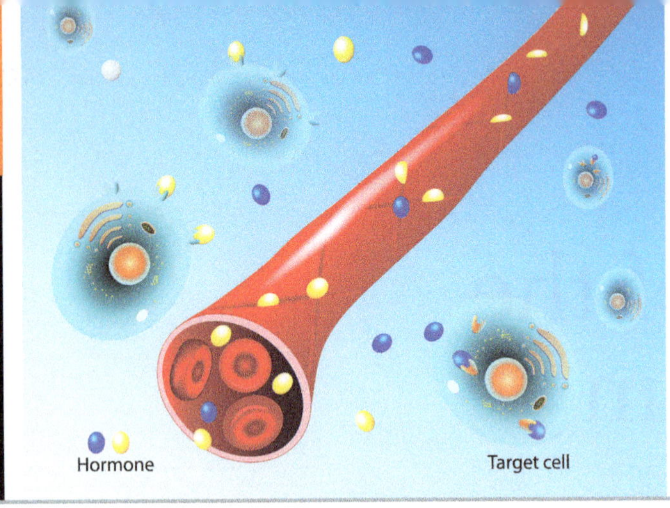

Chapter 64
Review of the Endocrine System

Chapter Outline

- Overview of the Endocrine System
- Hormone Receptors
- Negative Feedback Mechanisms
- Hormone Pharmacotherapy

Learning Outcomes

After reading this chapter, the student should be able to:

1. Describe the general structure and functions of the endocrine system.
2. Compare and contrast the nervous and endocrine systems in the control of homeostasis.
3. Explain circumstances in which hormone receptors may be up-regulated or down-regulated.
4. Through the use of a specific example, explain the concept of negative feedback in the endocrine system.
5. Explain the three primary types of stimuli that regulate hormone secretion.
6. Identify indications for hormone pharmacotherapy.

Key Terms

Definitions of the terms in bold may be found in the Glossary.

Like the nervous system, the endocrine system is a major controller of homeostasis. Whereas a nerve exerts instantaneous control over a single muscle fiber or gland, a hormone from the endocrine system may affect all body cells and take as long as several days to produce an optimal response. Hormonal balance is kept within a narrow range: Too little or too much of a hormone can produce profound physiologic changes. This chapter reviews endocrine anatomy and physiology and its relevance to pharmacotherapy. For a more detailed review of the endocrine system, the student should refer to an anatomy and physiology textbook.

Overview of the Endocrine System

64.1 The endocrine system controls homeostasis through the secretion of hormones.

The **endocrine system** consists of glands that secrete **hormones**, chemical messengers released in response to a change in the body's internal environment. The role of hormones is to maintain homeostasis in the body. For example, when the level of glucose in the blood rises above normal, the pancreas secretes insulin to return glucose levels to normal. The various endocrine glands and their hormones are illustrated in Figure 64.1.

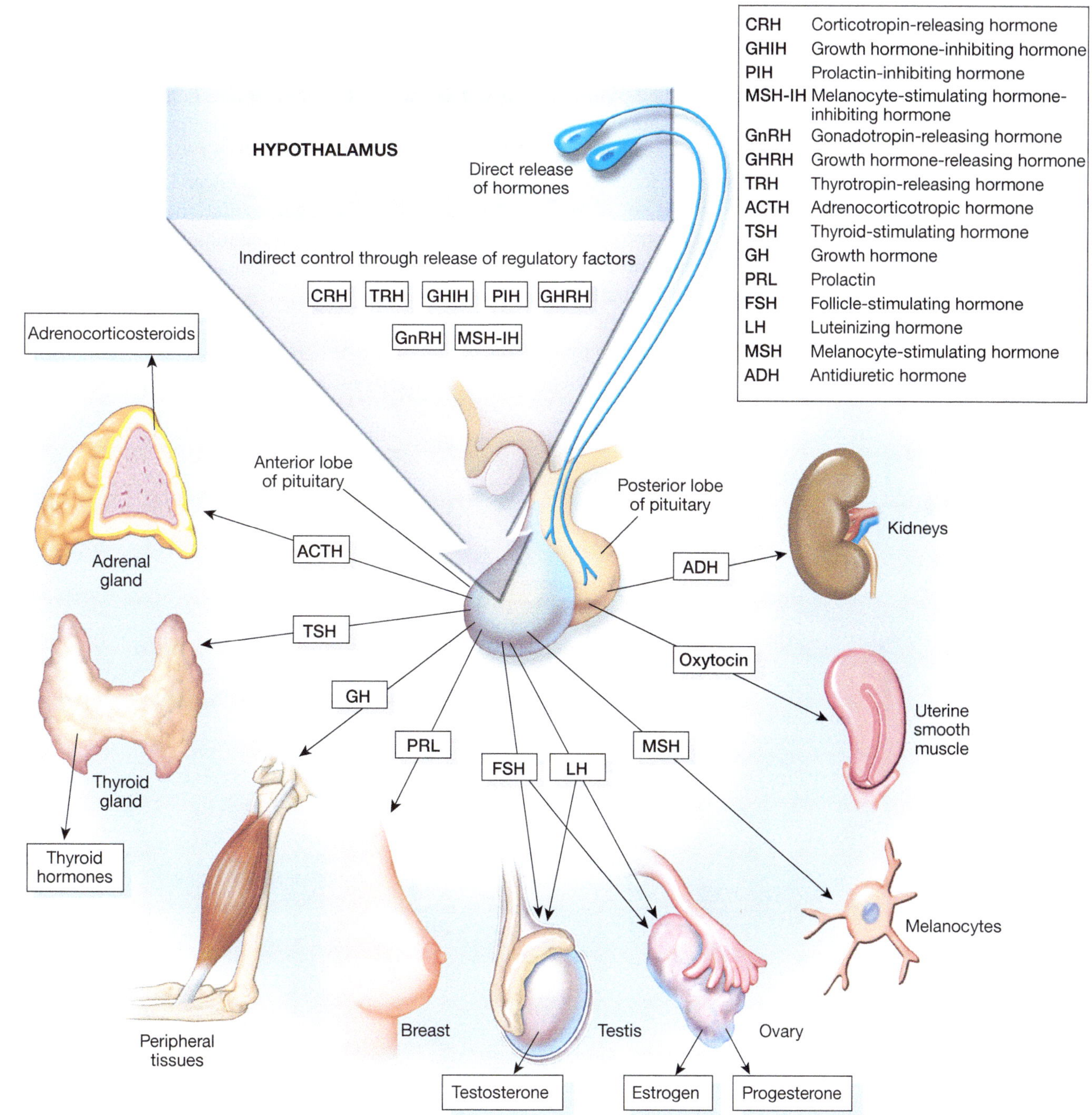

Figure 64.1 Hormones and the endocrine system.

After secretion from an endocrine gland, hormones enter the blood and are transported throughout the body. Compared to the nervous system, which reacts to body changes within milliseconds, the endocrine system responds relatively slowly. A few hormones, such as epinephrine, act within seconds, whereas others, such as testosterone, may take several days or even months to produce noticeable changes. Although slower in onset, the effects of hormones have a longer duration than those of the nervous system.

Hormone Receptors

64.2 Hormones must bind to specific receptors to cause physiologic changes.

The cells affected by a hormone are called its target cells. **Target cells** have specific protein receptors on their plasma membrane that bind to the hormone. For some hormones, the receptors are in the cytoplasm or nucleus of the target cell. Once binding occurs, a change is produced in the cell, resulting in an action that is characteristic for the hormone. For example, when epinephrine binds to receptors on smooth muscle cells, they contract. When prolactin binds to secretory cells in the breast, milk production occurs.

Although a hormone travels throughout the body via the circulation, it only affects cells that have receptors for that specific hormone. Epinephrine does not affect breast secretory cells because these cells have no epinephrine receptors. Prolactin does not cause muscular contraction because smooth muscle cells do not have prolactin receptors. This concept is illustrated in Figure 64.2.

In some cases, the target cells for a hormone are limited and specific. For example, the only receptors for thyroid-stimulating hormone are in the thyroid gland. However, some hormones, such as insulin and cortisol, have receptors on nearly every cell in the body; thus, these hormones have widespread effects.

The number of protein receptors for a hormone is dynamic and changes with the needs of the body. Cells can create more receptors on their plasma membrane to capture hormone molecules as they pass by, a process called **up-regulation**. This may occur if the cell is receiving signals that a hormone action is needed, such as the need for production of more breast milk or additional secretion of thyroid hormone. Once the hormone is up-regulated (secreted in large quantities), the cell no longer needs to capture every hormone molecule so it makes fewer receptors on its surface, a process called **down-regulation**. Receptors are very efficient at capturing hormone molecules; although most hormones are secreted only in small amounts, they produce profound changes.

Down-regulation has important implications for pharmacotherapy. When a hormone is administered as pharmacotherapy for long periods, the body recognizes an

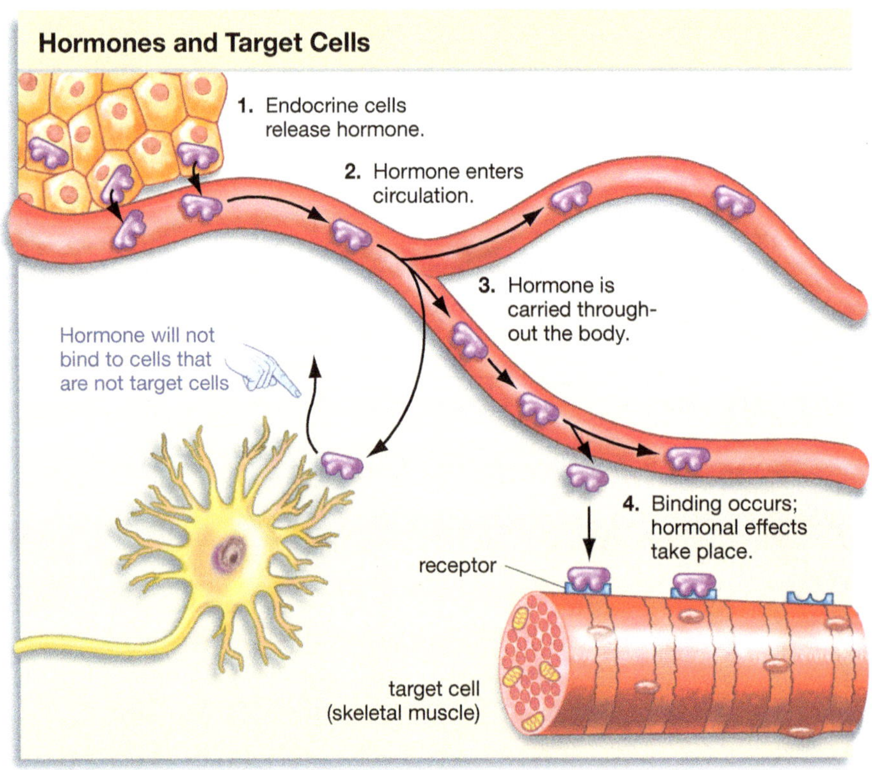

Figure 64.2 Hormones and their target cells.

From Krogh (2011). Reprinted and electronically reproduced by permission of Pearson Education, Inc., Upper Saddle River, New Jersey.

abundance of the hormone, and cells will down-regulate the number of receptors for that hormone. This causes a desensitization of the target cells; that is, they are less responsive to the effects of the hormone. When therapy is discontinued, the cells will need time, usually several days, to synthesize more protein receptors and adjust to the new hormone level.

It is important to understand that the amount of hormone secreted by an endocrine gland is only partially responsible for the therapeutic response. Other critical components include the number of receptors and their sensitivity. During pharmacotherapy, increasing the dose of a hormone will produce little additional pharmacologic effect if all the receptors are already occupied or if they are no longer sensitive to the hormone.

PharmFACT

Although it does not appear in most textbooks as an endocrine organ, adipose tissue secretes hormones that affect energy balance. Endocrine-disrupting chemicals, called obesogens, have been discovered that alter normal adipose tissue endocrine secretions and could possibly lead to obesity (Janesick & Blumberg, 2016).

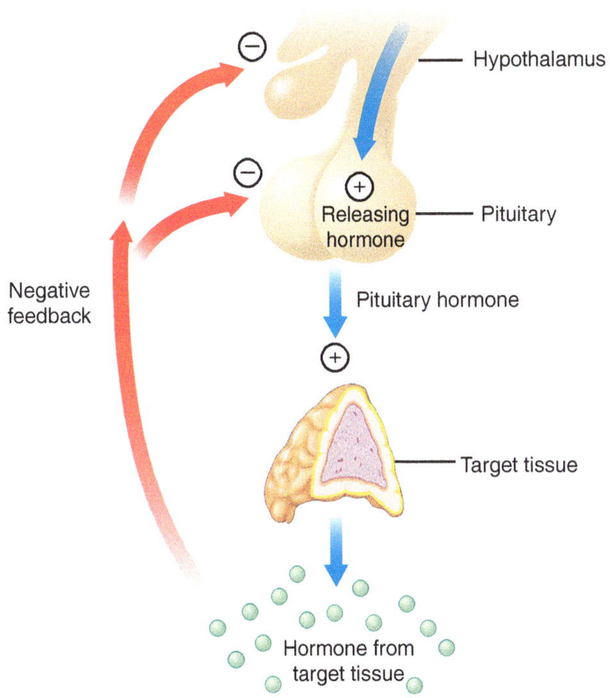

Figure 64.3 Negative feedback mechanism.

Negative Feedback Mechanisms

64.3 Most hormone action is regulated through negative feedback.

Because hormones can produce profound effects on the body, their secretion and release are carefully regulated by several levels of control. The most important mechanism is **negative feedback**, which is illustrated in Figure 64.3. A hormone causes an output or action in its target cell or tissue. As the level of a hormone rises, so does the hormone's action. The increased output or action is monitored by sensors. Once homeostasis is restored, the sensor signals the endocrine tissue to stop secreting the hormone; that is, the target tissue provides negative feedback.

Depending on the specific hormone, the negative feedback mechanism may be based on three primary types of stimuli: neuronal, humoral, and hormonal. In some cases, regulation involves multiple stimuli. The various hormones and their regulation are summarized in Table 64.1.

Neuronal stimuli: A few hormones are regulated by nerve impulses. The best example is epinephrine, which is released when a neuronal impulse from the sympathetic nervous system reaches the adrenal medulla. Another example is the release of oxytocin from the pituitary gland.

Humoral stimuli: Some endocrine glands sense the levels of specific substances in the blood and release the hormone when the substance rises above or falls below the normal range. For example, pancreatic islet cells can sense the level of glucose in the blood. If glucose levels become too high, insulin is secreted. Another example is the release of parathyroid hormone when blood calcium levels fall.

Hormonal stimuli: In the endocrine system, it is common for one hormone to control the secretion of another hormone. In some cases, the sequence involves three hormones. For example, thyrotropin-releasing hormone (TRH; from the hypothalamus) stimulates thyroid-stimulating hormone (TSH; from the pituitary), which causes the release of thyroid hormone (TH; from the thyroid gland). In a loop typical of the endocrine system, the last hormone in the pathway (TH) provides negative feedback to shut off secretion of the initial hormone (TRH).

CONNECTION Checkpoint 64.1

From what you learned in Chapter 15, identify indications for epinephrine pharmacotherapy.

Hormone Pharmacotherapy

64.4 Hormone pharmacotherapy is indicated for a diverse variety of conditions.

The goals of hormone pharmacotherapy vary widely. In many cases, a hormone is administered as **replacement therapy** for patients who are unable to secrete sufficient quantities of their own endogenous hormones. Examples of replacement therapy include administering thyroid hormone after the thyroid gland has been surgically removed,

Table 64.1 Selected Hormones and Their Regulation

Hormone	Target Organ(s) and Action	REGULATION	
		Stimulation	**Inhibition**
Adrenocorticotropic hormone (ACTH)	Adrenal cortex: stimulates release of glucocorticoids	Corticotropin-releasing hormone	Negative feedback from corticosteroids
Aldosterone	Kidneys: promotes reabsorption of sodium and water	Renin-angiotensin-aldosterone pathway, decreased blood volume, hypotension	Increased blood volume or hypertension
Antidiuretic hormone (ADH)	Kidneys: increases water reabsorption	Increased osmolarity of blood or decreased blood volume	Adequate hydration
Corticosteroids (glucocorticoids)	Most tissues: increases protein breakdown and glucose metabolism, provides resistance to stress, suppresses inflammation and immune response	ACTH	Negative feedback from corticosteroids
Follicle-stimulating hormone (FSH)	Ovaries: promotes maturation of ovarian follicles and estrogen production Testes: increases sperm production	Gonadotropin–releasing hormone (GnRH)	Negative feedback from estrogen (women) or testosterone (men)
Growth hormone (GH)	Most tissues, including bone, muscle, liver: stimulates growth and mobilizes lipids	Growth hormone–releasing hormone (GHRH)	Negative feedback from GH or growth hormone-inhibiting hormone (GHIH)
Insulin	Most tissues: promotes movement of glucose into cells, lowers blood glucose, decreases glycogen synthesis, and increases lipogenesis and protein synthesis	Hyperglycemia	Hypoglycemia
Luteinizing hormone (LH)	Ovaries: stimulates ovulation and production of estrogen Testes: produces testosterone	GnRH	Negative feedback from estrogen and progesterone (women) or testosterone (men)
Oxytocin	Uterus: stimulates contractions Breasts: ejects milk	Stretching of uterus or infant suckling	Lack of stretching of the uterus or discontinuation of breastfeeding
Parathyroid hormone	Kidneys, gastrointestinal tract, bone: increases calcium levels in blood	Hypocalcemia	Hypercalcemia
Prolactin	Breasts: promotes lactation	Prolactin-releasing hormone	Prolactin-inhibiting hormone
Thyroid hormone	Most tissues: increases basal metabolic rate and growth	Thyroid-stimulating hormone	Negative feedback from thyroid hormone

supplying insulin to patients whose pancreas is not functioning, or administering growth hormone to children with short-stature disorder. The pharmacologic goal of replacement therapy is to supply the same physiologic, low-level amounts of the hormone that would normally be present in the body. Selected endocrine disorders and their drug therapy are summarized in Table 64.2.

Some hormones are used in cancer chemotherapy to shrink the size of hormone-sensitive tumors. For example, certain breast cancers are highly dependent on estrogen for their growth. Giving the male hormone testosterone will lower the amount of estrogen in the body, thus depriving the breast cancer of its major growth stimulus. In a similar manner, high doses of estrogen are given to shrink the size of prostate cancer, which is dependent on testosterone for its growth. Hormones are nearly always used in combination with other antineoplastic medications.

Another goal of hormonal pharmacotherapy may be to produce an exaggerated response that is part of the normal action of the hormone. Administering hydrocortisone to suppress inflammation takes advantage of the normal action of the corticosteroids but at higher amounts than would normally be present in the body. Hydrocortisone is indicated for acute inflammatory disorders such as lupus or rheumatoid arthritis. As another example, supplying estrogen or progesterone at specific times during the uterine cycle can prevent ovulation and pregnancy. In this example, the patient is given natural hormones; however, they are taken at a time when levels in the body are normally low.

Endocrine pharmacotherapy also involves the use of "antihormones." These hormone antagonists block the actions of endogenous hormones. For example, PTU is given to block the effects of an overactive thyroid gland. Tamoxifen is given to block the actions of estrogen in estrogen receptor–dependent breast cancers (see Chapter 57).

CONNECTION Checkpoint 64.2

Glucocorticoids, or corticosteroids, are important drugs in treating inflammation. From what you learned in Chapter 42, explain their role in treating autoimmune disease.

Table 64.2 Selected Endocrine Disorders and Their Pharmacotherapy

Gland	Hormone(s)	Disorder	Drug Therapy Examples
Adrenal cortex	Corticosteroids	Hypersecretion: Cushing's syndrome	ketoconazole and mitotane (Lysodren)
		Hyposecretion: Addison's disease	hydrocortisone, prednisone
Gonads	Ovaries: estrogen	Hyposecretion: menstrual and metabolic dysfunction	conjugated estrogens and estradiol
	Ovaries: progesterone	Hyposecretion: dysfunctional uterine bleeding	medroxyprogesterone (Provera, others) and norethindrone
	Testes: testosterone	Hyposecretion: hypogonadism	testosterone
Pancreatic islets	Insulin	Hyposecretion: diabetes mellitus	insulin and oral antidiabetic drugs
Parathyroid	Parathyroid hormone	Hypersecretion: hyperparathyroidism	surgery (no drug therapy)
		Hyposecretion: hypoparathyroidism	vitamin D and calcium supplements
Pituitary	ADH	Hyposecretion: diabetes insipidus	desmopressin (DDAVP) and vasopressin
		Hypersecretion: syndrome of inappropriate antidiuretic hormone	conivaptan (Vaprisol) and tolvaptan (Samsca)
	GH	Hyposecretion: small stature	somatropin (Genotropin, others)
		Hypersecretion: acromegaly (adults)	octreotide (Sandostatin)
	Oxytocin	Hyposecretion: delayed delivery or lack of milk ejection	oxytocin (Pitocin)
Thyroid	Thyroid hormone (T_3 and T_4)	Hypersecretion: Graves' disease	propylthiouracil (PTU) and ^{131}I
		Hyposecretion: myxedema (adults), cretinism (children)	thyroid hormone and levothyroxine (T_4)

Understanding Chapter 64

Key Concepts Summary

64.1 The endocrine system controls homeostasis through the secretion of hormones.

64.2 Hormones must bind to specific receptors to cause physiologic changes.

64.3 Most hormone action is regulated through negative feedback.

64.4 Hormone pharmacotherapy is indicated for a diverse variety of conditions.

References

Janesick, A. S., & Blumberg, B. (2016). Obesogens: An emerging threat to public health. *American Journal of Obstetrics & Gynecology, 214*, 559–565. https://doi.org/10.1016/j.ajog.2016.01.182

Krogh, D. (2011). *Biology: A guide to the natural world* (5th ed.). Pearson.

Selected Bibliography

Chawla, J. (2016). *Endocrine system anatomy*. Medscape. http://emedicine.medscape.com/article/1948709-overview

Colbert, J. B., Ankney, J., & Lee, K. T. (2020). *Anatomy and physiology for health professionals: An interactive journey* (4th ed.). Pearson.

Hall, J. E. (2020). *Guyton & Hall textbook of medical physiology* (14th ed.). Elsevier.

Marieb, E., & Hoehn, K. (2019). *Human anatomy and physiology* (11th ed.). Pearson.

Martini, F. H., Nath, J. L., & Bartholomew, E. F. (2018). *Fundamentals of human anatomy and physiology* (11th ed.). Pearson.

Molina, P. (2014). *Endocrine physiology* (5th ed.). McGraw-Hill.

Silverthorn, D. U. (2019). *Human physiology: An integrated approach* (8th ed.). Pearson.

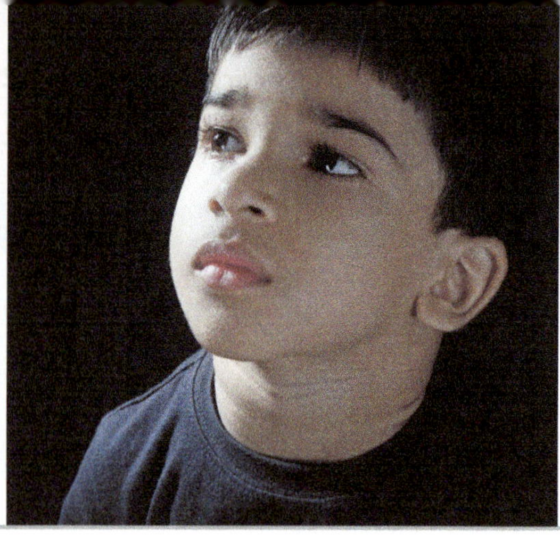

"I'm really worried about Raj. He's always been small, and today the pediatrician told me he is only at the fifth percentile for height and weight for his age. The doctor is referring us to a pediatric endocrinologist. Could it be something serious?"

—*"Jasdeep Singh," mother of 8-year-old patient "Raj"*

Chapter 65
Hypothalamic and Pituitary Drugs

Chapter Outline

Learning Outcomes

After reading this chapter, the student should be able to:

1. Explain the principal actions of the hormones secreted by the hypothalamus and pituitary gland.
2. Identify indications for hypothalamic hormone therapy.
3. Explain the pharmacotherapy of growth hormone disorders in children and adults.
4. Explain the pharmacotherapy of antidiuretic hormone disorders.
5. For each of the classes shown in the chapter outline, identify the prototype and representative drugs and explain the mechanism(s) of drug action, primary indications, contraindications, significant drug interactions, pregnancy data, and important adverse effects.
6. Apply clinical judgment to the care of patients receiving pharmacotherapy for disorders related to the hypothalamus and pituitary gland.

Key Terms

Definitions of the terms in bold may be found in the Glossary.

In the specialty of endocrinology, understanding the complex relationships between the hypothalamus and pituitary gland is important because these organs regulate so many homeostatic functions. For example, the two organs collaborate to secrete hormones that control functions of the gonads, adrenal glands, thyroid gland, kidneys, and the milk-producing tissues of the breast. The functioning of these two glands serves as the control center that provides integration between the nervous and endocrine systems. This chapter examines drugs that directly affect the functions of the hypothalamus and pituitary gland.

Functions of the Hypothalamus

65.1 The hypothalamus controls many diverse body processes and secretes hormones that influence pituitary function.

Roughly the size of an almond, the hypothalamus lies in the center of the diencephalon of the brain, just superior to the brainstem. The general purpose of the hypothalamus is to maintain homeostasis. To achieve this, the hypothalamus receives input from numerous vital regions of the nervous system, recognizes imbalances, and makes adjustments to bring the body back to homeostasis. Examples of the multiple and diverse functions of this organ include control of body temperature, thirst, appetite, fatigue, circadian rhythms, anger, and the rate of overall body metabolism. The hypothalamus also controls vital functions of the autonomic nervous system such as heart rate, vasoconstriction, digestion, and sweating. For the purposes of this chapter, only the endocrine functions of the hypothalamus are presented.

Every hormone has target cells that possess receptors for that specific hormone. For the hormones secreted by the hypothalamus, there is only one target organ: the pituitary gland. All hypothalamic hormones travel by the blood a short distance to the pituitary, which lies immediately below the hypothalamus. Upon reaching their receptors, the hypothalamic hormones simply increase or decrease the release of hormones by the pituitary gland. Because of this, hormones from the hypothalamus are called releasing hormones or inhibiting hormones. The major hypothalamic hormones and their actions on the pituitary gland are given in Table 65.1.

There are very few indications for the administration of hormones secreted by the hypothalamus. Rather than give hypothalamic hormones, it is more effective (and less expensive) to administer pituitary hormones or the secretions of a target endocrine organ such as thyroid hormone, estrogen, testosterone, or corticosteroids.

The hypothalamic hormones that do have clinical applications are analogs or antagonists of gonadotropin-releasing hormone (GnRH). Initially the effect of the GnRH analogs is to increase the production of interstitial cell-stimulating hormone (in men) or follicle-stimulating hormone (in women), which increases the secretion of sex hormones. With continued therapy, however, the pituitary becomes insensitive to the effects of GnRH and the production of sex hormones falls to near castration levels. Indications for these drugs are shown in Table 65.2. Doses and additional information may be found in Chapters 57 and 69.

CONNECTION Checkpoint 65.1

Target tissues can up-regulate or down-regulate the number of receptors for a specific hormone. From what you learned in Chapter 64, which of the two processes occurs when a hormone is administered as pharmacotherapy for long periods?

Functions of the Pituitary Gland

65.2 The pituitary gland secretes hormones that control many diverse body functions.

Although the pituitary gland is often referred to as the "master gland," its function is largely controlled by releasing or inhibiting hormones from the hypothalamus.

Table 65.1 Hormones Secreted by the Hypothalamus and Pituitary Glands

Hypothalamic Hormone	Pituitary Hormone	Target Organ	Principal Actions
Corticotropin-releasing hormone	Adrenocorticotropic hormone	Adrenal cortex	Stimulates release of corticosteroids
Gonadotropin-releasing hormone	Follicle-stimulating hormone Luteinizing hormone	Ovaries, testes Ovaries, testes	Stimulates release of estrogen and ovarian follicle development in women and sperm production in men Triggers ovulation and secretion of estrogen and progesterone in women, increases testosterone secretion in men
Growth hormone–inhibiting hormone Growth hormone–releasing hormone	Growth hormone	Most body cells	Regulates growth and development of bones, muscles, cartilage, organs; general body metabolism
None	Melanocyte-stimulating hormone	Skin	Stimulates pigmentation
Prolactin-inhibiting hormone Prolactin-releasing hormone	Prolactin	Mammary glands	Regulates lactation
Thyrotropin-releasing hormone	Thyroid-stimulating hormone	Thyroid gland	Stimulates release of thyroid hormone

Table 65.2 Hypothalamic Medications

Drug	Action	Indication (s)
cetrorelix (Cetrotide)	GnRH antagonist	Female infertility
degarelix (Firmagon)	GnRH antagonist	Advanced prostate cancer
ganirelix	GnRH antagonist	Female infertility
goserelin (Zoladex)	GnRH analog	Stage 2 prostate cancer and palliation of advanced prostate cancer
histrelin (Supprelin LA, Vantas)	GnRH analog	Palliation of advanced prostate cancer (Vantas) and precocious puberty (Supprelin LA)
leuprolide (Eligard, Fensolvi, Lupron depot)	GnRH analog	Palliation of advanced prostate cancer (Eligard, Lupron depot), endometriosis and leiomyomata (Lupron depot) and precocious puberty (Fensolvi)
nafarelin (Synarel)	GnRH analog	Endometriosis and precocious puberty
triptorelin (Trelstar Triptodur)	GnRH analog	Palliation of advanced prostate cancer (Trelstar) and precocious puberty (Triptodur)

The pituitary gland is divided into anterior and posterior lobes, which have very different structures and functions.

The **anterior pituitary gland** (adenohypophysis) comprises glandular tissue that manufactures and secretes hormones that control major body functions and systems. Four of these are called **tropic hormones**, a term that refers to the ability of these hormones to regulate the secretory actions of other endocrine glands. The anterior pituitary hormones are synthesized and stored in the pituitary until they receive a message from the hypothalamus. The message from the hypothalamus is usually to *enhance* the release of hormones, as is the case for growth hormone–releasing hormone (GHRH), thyrotropin-releasing hormone (TRH), prolactin-releasing hormone (PRH), corticotropin-releasing hormone (CRH), and gonadotropin-releasing hormone (GnRH). Two of the hypothalamic secretions, growth hormone–inhibiting hormone (GHIH) and prolactin-inhibiting hormone (PIH), *prevent* the release of pituitary hormones.

The **posterior pituitary gland** (neurohypophysis), by contrast, consists of nervous tissue and is basically an extension of the hypothalamus. It secretes two hormones: antidiuretic hormone (ADH) and oxytocin. These hormones are manufactured in the hypothalamus and travel down neurons to the posterior pituitary where they are stored until factors stimulate their release. The primary stimulus causing ADH secretion is an increased serum osmolality, or a high concentration of solutes in the blood. Oxytocin release is stimulated by touch receptors in the nipples of lactating women. Pharmacotherapy with oxytocin is presented in Chapter 69.

Regulation of hormone levels is an essential function because too little or too much of any of these endocrine secretions can cause profound symptoms. Many are controlled by negative feedback loops. As circulating levels of a hormone rise above normal, a message is sent to the hypothalamus, pituitary, or other endocrine gland to shut down the manufacture and secretion of the hormone. This prevents excess hormone levels. When hormones are administered as drug therapy, they can influence this normal negative feedback mechanism. One of the most important examples of this phenomenon is the negative feedback suppression of the adrenal glands caused by administration of corticosteroid medications. The student should review the information on negative feedback in Chapter 64 before proceeding.

Because of the widespread effects of the hormones secreted and controlled by the hypothalamus and pituitary glands, disorders of these glands are quite complex. In general, the pathologies of endocrine glands can be categorized as causing hypofunction or hyperfunction of the particular gland. Pituitary disorders can be the result of tumors, surgery, radiation therapy, infection, injury, infarction (loss of blood supply), or bleeding (hemorrhage) in the area. Congenital defects may also result in absent or impaired function of a hormone or the lack of an enzyme necessary for hormone production.

Pharmacotherapy of Growth Hormone Disorders

Growth Hormone Analogs

65.3 Growth hormone deficiency in adults and children can be treated by administering recombinant growth hormone.

Growth hormone (GH), also called *somatotropin* or *somatropin*, is produced and secreted by the anterior pituitary gland. This hormone was once believed to be of importance only during periods of active growth, but it is now recognized that adults produce nearly as much GH as children. Although its major targets are bone and skeletal muscle, GH stimulates many types of body cells to increase in size and replicate. It is considered an anabolic (tissue-building) hormone. The primary effects of GH, illustrated in Figure 65.1, are as follows:

- Increases length and width of bone
- Stimulates the growth and development of most visceral and endocrine organs, skeletal and cardiac muscle, cartilage, skin and connective tissue
- Enhances cellular uptake of amino acids and increased protein synthesis
- Breaks down adipose tissue to release fatty acids for use as fuel
- Decreases use of glucose; impairs glucose tolerance and induces insulin resistance in peripheral tissues.

Many of the effects of GH are dependent on **insulin-like growth factor (IGF)**, a family of peptides that promote cartilage and bone growth. IGFs are produced in the liver and are released when hepatic cells become activated by GH. Secretion of GH fluctuates during the day, peaking 1 to 4 hours following the onset of sleep. These nighttime bursts in GH are greater in children than in adults.

The overall regulation of serum GH levels resides in the hypothalamus, with the secretion of GHRH and GHIH.

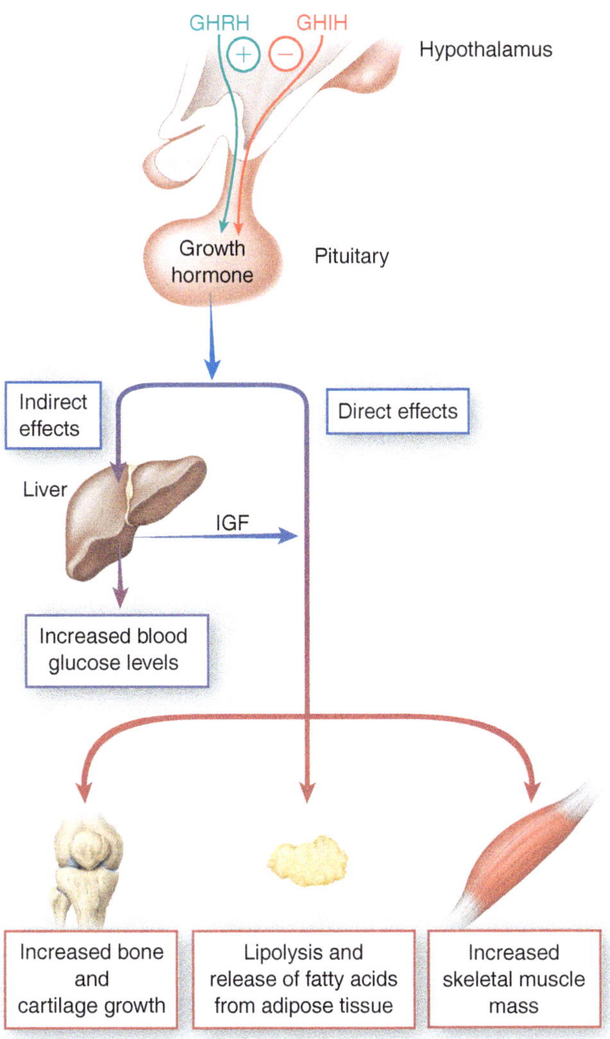

Figure 65.1 Physiologic and pharmacologic effects of growth hormone.

A large number of secondary factors, such as exercise and sleep, influence the release of GH, and these are listed in Table 65.3.

In children, GH deficiency results in dwarfism. **Dwarfism** is associated with normal birth length followed by a slowing of the growth rate. These children have normal intelligence, short stature, immature facial features, obesity, and delayed skeletal maturation. In this context, **short stature** is defined as well below the fifth percentile for age and gender, or more than two standard deviations below the mean (average) height for age and gender. Acquired GH deficiency develops later in childhood and can be caused by a hypothalamic-pituitary tumor or an infection. Children who have been severely neglected or emotionally deprived can develop a psychosocial dwarfism, with poor growth, a potbelly, and poor nutritional habits. GH levels often return to normal once the child is removed from the dysfunctional environment.

When GH deficiency is the cause of short stature, replacement therapy is the preferred treatment. Until 1985, GH was obtained from the pituitary glands of human cadavers, a practice that was halted following the deaths of several recipients who developed Creutzfeldt–Jakob disease. GH is now obtained using recombinant DNA technology. GH obtained through recombinant technology is called somatropin. Doses for the GH analogs are listed in Table 65.4.

Therapy with recombinant GH is expensive, with a cost of approximately $50,000 per inch of growth. The hormone is administered subcutaneously, several times a week during the period of active growth, and therapy may continue until adulthood. Females with Turner's syndrome and children with chronic kidney disease (CKD) may also be treated with GH. Often, treatment with GH produces only modest gains in final adult height, but these gains are considered beneficial to the psychologic well-being of the patient.

Table 65.3 Selected Factors Affecting the Release of Growth Hormone

Factors Increasing Release of GH	Factors Decreasing Release of GH
Amino acids: leucine, arginine	Beta-adrenergic agonists
Androgens and estrogens	Carbohydrate-rich diet
Clonidine	Cortisol
Elevated body temperature	Free fatty acids
Gamma-hydroxybutyrate	Increased serum glucose level
Growth hormone–releasing hormone	Obesity
Hypoglycemia, fasting, starvation	Somatostatin (GHIH)
L-dopa	
Stress, trauma	
Vigorous exercise	

Table 65.4 Drugs Acting on the Pituitary Gland and Target Tissues

Drug	Route and Adult Dose (Maximum Dose Where Indicated)	Adverse Effects
bromocriptine (Cycloset, Parlodel)	PO (Cycloset): 0.8 mg daily, increased weekly to achieve 1.6–4.8 mg daily PO: 1.25–2.5 mg/day for 3 days, then increase dose every 3–7 days to 30–60 mg/day	*Orthostatic hypotension, nausea and vomiting, fatigue, dizziness, headache* Shock, acute MI, cerebral ischemia, confusion, agitation, psychosis
cabergoline	PO: 0.25–1.0 mg twice/wk	*Nausea, constipation, headache* Cardiac valve disease, extracardiac fibrosis
desmopressin (DDAVP, Nocdurna)	IV/subcutaneous: 2–4 mcg in 2 divided doses PO: 0.2–0.4 mg/day Intranasal: 1 spray in either right or left nostril 30 min before bedtime	*Headache, nasal congestion or irritation, nausea* Water intoxication, coma, thromboembolic disorder, hyponatremia
lanreotide (Somatuline Depot)	Subcutaneous: 60–120 mg q4wk	*Pain at the injection site, nausea and vomiting, diarrhea, itching* Gallstones, abdominal pain, bradycardia, hyper- or hypoglycemia
mecasermin (Increlex)	Subcutaneous: 0.04–0.08 mg/kg bid; must be administered within 20 min of a meal or snack (max: 0.12 mg/kg bid)	*Injection-site reaction, iron deficiency anemia, goiter, antibody development, headache, hypertrophy of tonsils* Hypoglycemia, increased intracranial pressure
octreotide (Sandostatin)	Subcutaneous/IV: 100–600 mcg/day in 2–4 divided doses; after 2 wk may switch to IM depot, 20 mg q4wk	*Nausea and vomiting, diarrhea, headache, flushing, injection-site pain, cholelithiasis* Dysrhythmia, worsening heart failure, sinus bradycardia
pasireotide (Signifor LAR)	IM: 40 mg once q4wk	*Diarrhea, cholelithiasis, hyperglycemia, QT prolongation, bradycardia* Diabetes
pegvisomant (Somavert)	Subcutaneous: 40 mg loading dose, then 10 mg/day (max: 30 mg/day)	*Nausea, diarrhea, injection-site pain, flulike symptoms* Liver damage, elevated transaminase levels
somatropin (Genotropin, Humatrope, Norditropin, Nutropin, Saizen, others)	Subcutaneous (Humatrope): 0.006 mg/kg daily (max: 0.0125 mg/kg/day) Subcutaneous (Serostim): Weight more than 55 kg: 6 mg at bedtime; 45–55 kg: 5 mg at bedtime; 35–45 kg: 4 mg at bedtime; less than 35 kg: 0.1 mg/kg at bedtime Child: Subcutaneous (Genotropin): 0.16–0.24 mg/kg/wk in 6–7 divided doses Norditropin: 0.024–0.034 mg/kg 6–7 times/wk	*Pain at injection site, hyperglycemia, arthralgia, myalgia, abdominal pain, otitis media, headache, bronchitis, hypothyroidism, hypertension (HTN), flulike symptoms* Severe respiratory impairment in patients with severe obesity and Prader-Willi syndrome, diabetes, pancreatitis, scoliosis of the spine, papilledema, intracranial tumor
vasopressin (Vasostrict)	IM/subcutaneous: 5–10 units aqueous solution 2–4 times/day IV: 0.2–0.4 units/min up to 1 unit/min	*Tremor, pallor, nausea and vomiting, water retention, intoxication* Angina, acute MI, gangrene, anaphylaxis, cardiac arrest

Note: *Italics* indicate common adverse effects. Underline indicates serious adverse effects.

Adult GH deficiency is associated with reduced muscle mass, increased cardiovascular mortality, central adiposity and increased visceral fat, insulin resistance, and dyslipidemia. This hormonal deficiency may develop during adulthood or it may be a continuation of childhood deficiency. Several forms of recombinant human GH formulations (Humatrope and Genotropin) have been approved for use in adults with body-wasting-type disorders. Treatment can result in increased lean body mass, decreased fat mass, increased bone mineral density, and decreased lipid levels.

Human GH has been abused for its anabolic effects. Athletes have used the drug to build muscle, increase strength, and maintain less body fat. It has also been called an antiaging drug because it promotes younger-looking skin, improved memory, and reduced wrinkles. The administration of GH for these purposes is illegal, and prolonged use may lead to long-term adverse effects in patients. Despite potential adverse health effects, products advertised as "human growth hormone supplements" are readily marketed without a prescription. These do not contain any GH (which must be administered parenterally) but instead contain a mixture of oral (PO) supplements that are claimed to stimulate the pituitary gland. The safety and effectiveness of these products have not been evaluated adequately.

PROTOTYPE DRUG **Somatropin (Genotropin, Humatrope, Norditropin, Nutropin, Saizen)**

Classification **Therapeutic:** Human growth hormone
Pharmacologic: Pituitary hormone

Therapeutic Effects and Uses: Approved by the U.S. Food and Drug Administration (FDA) in 1987, somatropin is prepared through recombinant DNA technology and is identical to endogenous human GH. It is available in several different formulations that vary by dose and regimen. The preferred route of administration is subcutaneous, although some forms may be given via the intramuscular (IM) route. Somatropin produces growth of long bones in children prior to epiphyseal closure. The gain in growth is very rapid at the initiation of therapy but slows over time. Treatment may continue until the desired height is achieved, epiphyseal closure occurs, or the patient fails to respond to treatment. If treatment does not result in growth, it is stopped and the diagnosis is reevaluated. The metabolic effects of the drug include increased protein synthesis, reduced carbohydrate utilization, and increased use of fatty acids for energy.

Somatropin is used in the management of a number of growth-related disorders, including the following:

- Growth failure in children due to GH deficiency or Prader-Willi syndrome
- Growth failure in children due to CKD (Nutropin)
- Short stature associated with Turner's syndrome (Genotropin, Humatrope, Norditropin, Nutropin)
- Adult GH deficiency (Genotropin, Humatrope, Norditropin, Nutropin, Saizen, Sogroya)
- Acquired immunodeficiency syndrome (AIDS) wasting, cachexia, and severe thermal injuries (Serostim)
- Short bowel syndrome in patients receiving specialized nutrition support (Zorbtive).

Although the various brand-name products of somatropin have the same effectiveness, they differ in potency and are not interchangeable. Some are available in prefilled syringes, whereas others are longer acting. The nurse should check the package insert for specific dosing instructions.

Mechanism of Action: Somatropin has the same amino acid sequence as endogenous human GH and produces the same effects as the naturally occurring form of the hormone. The effects of GH are mediated by IGF.

Pharmacokinetics:

Route(s)	Subcutaneous, IM
Absorption	Well absorbed following injection
Distribution	Distributed to highly perfused organs (liver, kidneys); circulates bound to GH binding protein
Primary metabolism	Hepatic; some metabolism in kidneys
Primary excretion	Renal
Onset of action	Peak action variable: days to weeks
Duration of action	Half-life: 3.8–5 h

Adverse Effects: Adverse effects of somatropin include hyperglycemia and insulin resistance, which is made worse in patients with preexisting diabetes mellitus. It can also cause hypothyroidism. Edema of the hands and feet, headache, and HTN often occur initially but may resolve with continued therapy. Joint pain, muscle aches, and pain at the injection site are common. Carpal tunnel syndrome may occur with use of Serostim. Development of antibodies to GH may rarely occur. Hypercalciuria, possibly asymptomatic, may occur in the first few months of therapy.

Contraindications/Precautions: Somatropin is contraindicated for use in patients with closed epiphyses. It is also contraindicated in patients with severe obesity, respiratory impairment, or sleep apnea due to potentially fatal respiratory impairment. Somatropin should not be used in patients with active malignancy due to the risk for increased growth of tumor. The drug is contraindicated in patients who are sensitive to glycerin. Somatropin should be used with caution in patients with severe renal or hepatic disease due to reduced clearance and in patients with diabetes mellitus due to hyperglycemia and insulin resistance.

Drug Interactions: Corticosteroids interfere with the bone growth–promoting action of GH; thus, the two should not be given concurrently. Concurrent use with anabolic steroids, androgens, estrogens, or thyroid hormone may increase the rate of epiphyseal closure. Patients receiving insulin should be monitored carefully because somatropin decreases the actions of insulin. **Herbal/Food:** Unknown.

Pregnancy: Animal studies did not show teratogenicity or significant fetal harm. Adverse effects during pregnancy or breastfeeding are not known.

Treatment of Overdose: Overdose with somatropin has not been reported.

Clinician Responsibilities: Key clinical implications for patients receiving somatropin are included in Applied Clinical Judgment: Patients Receiving Pharmacotherapy with Growth Hormone.

Drugs Similar to Somatropin (Genotropin, Humatrope, Norditropin, Nutropin, Saizen, Others)

Mecasermin is the only other drug that has actions similar to somatropin.

Mecasermin (Increlex): Approved in 2005, mecasermin is a solution of IGF produced through recombinant DNA technology. This drug is identical to endogenous IGF and therefore has the same actions as GH. Mecasermin is indicated for two specific indications: the long-term treatment of growth failure in children with severe primary IGF deficiency or for those who have developed neutralizing

CONNECTIONS: Advanced Practice Application

Traumatic Brain Injury and Hormones

Case

Emma is a typical 17-year-old high school Junior who is being seen for her annual sports physical examination. While conducting her health history, her only concerns were her lack of height and that she often felt tired. At 1.5 meters (5 ft 1 in.) she had not grown since she was 12 years old. Her family history showed that her father was nearly 1.8 meters (6 feet) tall, her mother was 1.7 meters (5 ft 10 in.), and both sets of grandparents were above average in height. Emma did not smoke or drink alcohol and denied using any illicit drugs. She had a history of three mild head injuries that she acquired while playing soccer. In fact, she was diagnosed twice with mild concussions 3 months apart when she was 12 years old. On physical examination, Emma displayed minimal breast tissue growth and was only at Tanner stage III. Other than the slow development, her physical examination was unremarkable. As a result of the history of head injuries and her small stature and unusual growth pattern, blood testing for hormone levels was done. The results showed that Emma had GH deficiency, adrenal insufficiency, and hypothyroidism.

Emma was started on growth hormone, cortisol, and replacement thyroid hormone. On her annual sports physical examination 1 year later, she had grown an additional 8.9 cm (3.5 in.). She feels less tired and is excited to have been offered the opportunity to play soccer at the local university. Is Emma's case unusual at such a young age?

Discussion

Traumatic brain injury (TBI) is a form of acquired brain injury that occurs when a sudden trauma causes damage to the brain. In Emma's case, it occurred after a soccer ball hit her in the head. Symptoms of a TBI can be mild, moderate, or severe, depending on the extent of damage to the brain. When minor head injuries occur back-to-back, it can cause compounding effects Previously, it was believed that brain injuries were related to a player's age. The younger the player, the shorter the recovery time, and for this reason, many high school protocols called for a player showing concussion symptoms to be sidelined for 24 hours. However, new research is showing that that may be entirely too short a time and that with one concussion, a player should have at least 30 days of recovery prior to returning. Because visual motor speed and reaction time scores decrease with recurrent concussions, even more recovery time for players with a history of greater than two concussions is recommended (Jildeh et al., 2020).

Additionally, even when mild, TBIs can have a negative effect on pituitary function and can cause low levels of several hormones, including (Briet, 2019):

- Adrenal insufficiency may occur with symptoms include weight loss, fatigue, vomiting, dehydration, and low blood pressure.
- Diabetes insipidus, with ADH loss resulting in symptoms include frequent urination and extreme thirst.
- Hypothyroidism may occur with smptoms include fatigue, constipation, weight gain, irregular menstrual periods, and cold intolerance.
- Growth hormone deficiency in adults, leads to increased fat, loss of muscle and bone, and decreased energy; in children, this leads to growth problems and small stature.

antibodies to GH. It is not intended to be used for any other forms of GH deficiency. It should not be used in adults after the epiphyses have closed or in patients with active malignancy. Adverse effects include hypoglycemia, local and systemic hypersensitivity, and tonsillar hypertrophy. Rare adverse effects include intracranial HTN, slipped capital epiphysis, and progression of scoliosis. Mecasermin use should be monitored carefully in patients taking insulin or oral antidiabetic drugs because mecasermin can increase the actions of these medications. This medication is not indicated for adult use: Adverse effects during pregnancy or breastfeeding are not known.

Growth Hormone Antagonists

65.4 Overproduction of growth hormone in adults can be treated by administering growth hormone antagonists.

Excessive GH secretion that occurs prior to puberty and the sealing of epiphyseal plates of the long bones results in **gigantism**, or unusual tallness. Gigantism is rare due to early recognition of the cause of the oversecretion: a benign pituitary adenoma. GH excess in children is usually treated with surgery as soon as the disorder is diagnosed.

Excessive GH secretion in adults causes a condition known as **acromegaly**. Excess levels of GH stimulate the secretion of IGFs from the liver, which then produce the clinical manifestations of the disorder. Because the epiphyseal plates are closed in adults, bones become deformed rather than elongated with this disorder. The onset is gradual, with enlargement of the bones of the hands, feet, face, and skull; a broad nose; protruding lower jaw; and slanting forehead. The cartilage of the larynx enlarges, deepening the voice. Spinal changes can lead to kyphosis. Arthralgias and degenerative arthritis may occur, and enlargement of organs, including the heart, can result in an early death due to atherosclerosis. Metabolic changes lead to insulin resistance and impaired glucose tolerance.

The preferred treatment of acromegaly is surgical removal of the pituitary tumor that is oversecreting GH. Medications that lower GH are considered if the patient is not a candidate for surgery or if the entire tumor cannot be removed. Standard pharmacotherapy includes:

- Drugs that *block secretion* of GH (octreotide, lanreotide, and pasireotide); sometimes called somatostatin analogs, these are the most frequently prescribed drugs for acromegaly
- Drugs that *block the actions* of GH (pegvisomant)
- Dopamine receptor agonists (bromocriptine and cabergoline) that are considered second-line drugs for acromegaly.

Doses of the medications for acromegaly are listed in Table 65.4.

PROTOTYPE DRUG **Octreotide (Sandostatin)**

Classification **Therapeutic:** Growth hormone antagonist; antidiarrheal
Pharmacologic: Somatostatin

Therapeutic Effects and Uses: Approved in 1988, octreotide, which is also called somatostatin, is a long-acting peptide that mimics the actions of GHIH. Octreotide is effective in both children and adults with GH excess. To treat acromegaly, the drug is initially given three times daily by the subcutaneous route. Mycapssa is a somatostatin analog approved in 2020 that is the first acromegaly treatment given by the PO route. Given by the subcutaneous route, Bynfezia Pen is approved to treat acromegaly, carcinoid tumor, and VIPomas (a type of pancreatic tumor). A long-acting IM form (Sandostatin LAR Depot) is available that reduces dosing to every 4 weeks.

Although GHIH is primarily secreted by the hypothalamus, small amounts are also secreted by the stomach, intestine, and pancreas. Thus, in addition to its effect of blocking GH secretion in the anterior pituitary, octreotide suppresses the release of multiple gastrointestinal (GI) hormones, including gastrin, cholecystokinin, secretin, vasoactive intestinal peptide, insulin, and glucagon. This has resulted in its use in treating multiple secretory and bleeding conditions of the intestinal tract. Because it stimulates the absorption of fluid and electrolytes from the GI tract and prolongs intestinal transit time, it is approved to treat severe diarrhea and flushing episodes associated with metastatic carcinoid tumors or vasoactive intestinal peptide tumors. Octreotide inhibits enzymes that cause vasodilation, decreases hepatic and GI blood flow, and reduces hepatic-portal venous pressure. These properties make the drug useful in treating portal HTN and upper GI bleeding caused by esophageal varices. It is also used off-label to reduce the output from pancreatic and other GI fistulas.

Mechanism of Action: Octreotide produces the same effects as the natural hormone somatostatin to suppress secretion of GH. It also suppresses secretion of serotonin, pancreatic peptides, gastrin, vasoactive intestinal peptides, secretin, motilin, insulin, and glucagon.

Pharmacokinetics:

Route(s)	Subcutaneous or IM (depot formulation)
Absorption	Absorbed rapidly following subcutaneous injection
Distribution	May cross the placenta; may be secreted in breast milk; 65% bound to lipoproteins
Primary metabolism	Liver
Primary excretion	Renal
Onset of action	15–30 min (subcutaneous); 60 min (IM)
Duration of action	12 h; half-life: 1.5 h

Adverse Effects: The most common adverse effects of octreotide are related to the GI system: nausea and vomiting, diarrhea, abdominal discomfort, development of gallstones, and elevated liver enzymes. The nausea and vomiting and abdominal pain diminish with continued therapy. It can also cause headache, fatigue, flushing, and edema. Because hypoglycemia or hyperglycemia can develop with long-term use, an adjustment in insulin doses in patients with diabetes may be necessary. It can also cause cardiac dysrhythmias, heart failure, and chest pain. Pain at the injection site is very common.

Contraindications/Precautions: Octreotide is contraindicated in patients who are sensitive to it. It is used with caution in patients with CKD, liver disease, cardiac disease, diabetes, and hypothyroidism. Because the drug can cause cholelithiasis, biliary obstruction, or cholecystitis, it should be used cautiously in patients with preexisting gallbladder disease. In addition, it is used with caution in older adult patients due to a significantly longer half-life and delayed clearance; dose adjustments are necessary for these patients.

Drug Interactions: Octreotide may decrease cyclosporine levels and may alter the absorption of other drugs and nutrients because it slows intestinal motility. Concurrent administration of octreotide with PO antidiabetic drugs or insulin can produce hypoglycemia. Additive bradycardia may occur when administered with cardiac drugs such as beta blockers and calcium channel blockers. Concurrent use of octreotide with antidiarrheals and opioids can lead to severe constipation, intestinal obstruction, or paralytic ileus. **Herbal/Food:** Octreotide decreases the absorption of dietary fat and vitamin B_{12}.

Pregnancy: Octreotide may retore fertility in women with acromegaly so patients should be notified of the increased potential for conception. Adverse effects of this drug during pregnancy or lactation are not known.

Treatment of Overdose: Overdose with octreotide has not been reported.

Clinician Responsibilities: Key clinical implications for patients receiving octreotide are included in Applied Clinical Judgment: Patients Receiving Pharmacotherapy with Growth Hormone and Antagonists.

Drugs Similar to Octreotide (Sandostatin)

Drugs with similar actions to octreotide include bromocriptine, lanreotide, pasireotide, and pegvisomant.

Bromocriptine (Cycloset, Parlodel): Approved in 1978, bromocriptine is a PO drug that is classified as a dopamine agonist and is indicated for multiple diverse conditions. Dopamine itself is not used for acromegaly due to an unacceptable incidence of adverse effects. Bromocriptine inhibits the secretion of GH as well as prolactin from the pituitary. It is primarily indicated for Parkinson's disease and infertility caused by prolactin excess, but it has been used in combination with octreotide in children with GH excess. In 2009, the FDA approved bromocriptine (Cycloset) as an adjunct to diet and exercise to improve glycemic control in adults with type 2 diabetes mellitus.

The most common dose-limiting adverse effects are psychologic reactions including confusion, agitation, hallucinations, paranoid delusions, or nightmares. Other adverse effects include orthostatic hypotension, headache, nausea and vomiting, anorexia, or rash on the face and arms. Limited observational studies in pregnant women have not shown an increase in abnormalities or direct effects on the fetus. Bromocriptine interferes with lactation and should not be used during breastfeeding.

Lanreotide (Somatuline Depot): Approved in 2007, lanreotide is a somatostatin analog indicated for the treatment of patients with acromegaly who have not responded to radiation therapy or who are unable to undergo surgical treatment. The drug lowers levels of GH, thus improving symptoms related to acromegaly. Lanreotide is a depot formulation that requires dosing only once per month. It is available in prefilled syringes and is delivered by deep subcutaneous injection. Lanreotide is also approved to treat advanced gastroenteropancreatic neuroendocrine tumors. Adverse effects associated with lanreotide include pain at the injection site, nausea and vomiting, diarrhea, gallstones, skin reactions such as itching, bradycardia, and changes in blood glucose levels (either hyper- or hypoglycemia). Studies in laboratory animals showed decreased embryofetal survival. Lanreotide should be used during pregnancy only if the potential benefits to the mother justify the potential risks to the fetus.

Pasireotide (Signifor LAR): Pasireotide is a somatostatin analog given once monthly by IM injection. The drug was approved in 2012 for Cushing's disease, which is caused by a tumor of the adrenal gland that secretes excess adrenocorticotropic hormone. Its indications were extended in 2014 for acromegaly in patients for which surgical treatment is not an option. The formulation for Cushing's disease (Signifor) is not interchangeable with that for acromegaly (Signifor LAR). The most common side effects are diarrhea and cholelithiasis. Hyperglycemia and diabetes may become severe during therapy. Studies in laboratory animals showed evidence of fetal harm. Pasireotide should be used during pregnancy only if the potential benefits to the mother justify the potential risks to the fetus.

Pegvisomant (Somavert): Approved in 1997, pegvisomant is a specific GH receptor antagonist that is a highly effective, first-line pharmacotherapy for acromegaly. The drug is structurally very similar to GH, although when it binds to GH receptors, it causes no cellular response. The multiple polyethylene glycol molecules attached to the drug prolong its half-life and allow for once-daily dosing. It is administered subcutaneously once daily and is supplied as a powder for reconstitution. Adverse effects include nausea and vomiting, elevated liver enzymes, angina, chest pain and myocardial infarction (MI), HTN, flulike syndrome, and injection-site pain. Patients with diabetes should be monitored regularly to avoid hypoglycemia. Therapy for this drug is expensive and is continued indefinitely. Studies in laboratory animals did not show evidence of fetal harm. It is not known if this drug is secreted in milk or if it has adverse effects on the breastfed neonate.

CONNECTIONS: APPLIED CLINICAL JUDGMENT

Patients Receiving Pharmacotherapy with Growth Hormone and Antagonists

Key Assessment Data

- History of current condition, baseline vital signs, physical exam findings, growth- and development-related history including congenital conditions such as Prader-Willi syndrome; hepatic or renal disease; medication history, allergies; pregnancy status. Obtain radiologic assessment of epiphyseal plates, if appropriate.

Desired Therapeutic Outcomes

Improvement is observed and measurable by increase in height, improved nutritional intake, weight (GH), or measurable decrease in bone growth or control of severe diarrhea (antagonists).

CONNECTIONS: APPLIED CLINICAL JUDGMENT *(continued)*

Patients Receiving Pharmacotherapy with Growth Hormone and Antagonists

Minimizing Adverse Effects

- Carpal tunnel syndrome may occur, and avascular necrosis is an adverse drug effect of GH. Increasing or severe pain in joints or changes in gait require follow-up evaluation.
- GH analogs and antagonists may cause changes in glucose level. Patients with diabetes may need alterations in their normal medication routines if hyper- or hypoglycemia occurs.
- Fluid retention with an increased intravascular volume, HTN, and peripheral edema may occur in early GH therapy but should resolve over time. Any continuing or worsening symptoms require reevaluation of therapy.
- Hypercalciuria may occur in early GH therapy, sometimes without symptoms. Renal calculi are a possible adverse effect. Fluid intake should be increased up to 2 L/day if appropriate.
- Wasting syndromes caused by conditions such as AIDS or CKD may result in nutritional deficits and dehydration until the GH antagonist drug therapy is effective. Dietary consultation may be required to reach and maintain optimal nutrition.
- Periodic hepatic and biliary function tests are needed for patients taking GH antagonists because gallbladder disease may occur or existing disease may worsen.
- Electrocardiograms (ECGs) should be assessed periodically for patients on GH antagonists because bradycardia and other dysrhythmias may occur.
- Supplementation with vitamin B_{12} may be needed because GH antagonists can reduce the absorption of this vitamin.

Patient Education

- Record height and weight weekly and bring the record to each clinical visit.
- Report any changes in walking, discomfort or pain in knee or hip joints, bone pain, or consistent muscle pain over joint areas to the healthcare provider.
- Patients with diabetes should monitor capillary glucose levels more frequently during therapy. Report any consistent elevations or hypoglycemia to the healthcare provider.
- Immediately report pounding headache, dizziness, palpitations, or syncope.
- Report changes in bowel habits, either diarrhea or constipation, or abdominal pain that is severe or that lasts more than 2 days. Pain localized in the upper right abdomen or yellowing of the whites of the eyes or skin should be reported promptly.
- Take the drug following appropriate guidelines:
    - Reconstitute the parenteral drug exactly per package directions and do not shake the vial; gently rotate it to avoid breaking down the drug. Follow the manufacturer's instructions if an automated pen injector is used.
    - Store any unused reconstituted solutions in the refrigerator; do not freeze the solution. Discard any discolored solution or if particulate matter is present.
    - Administer GH drugs in the evening to mimic the body's natural rhythms.
    - Administer subcutaneous injections in the abdomen, buttock, or thigh areas, rotating injection sites. Do not use gluteal sites for children under the age of 2; these muscles are not well developed until the child has been walking for a year or more.

Prescribing Considerations

- Ongoing assessment during drug therapy should include monitoring appropriate laboratory findings (e.g., complete blood count, electrolytes, glucose, hepatic and renal function studies, thyroid hormone panels, insulin-like growth factor-1, IGF binding protein).
- The high cost of growth hormone therapy in certain patient populations is a significant consideration for patients and their caregivers. Provide social service referrals as needed.

Pharmacotherapy of Antidiuretic Hormone Disorders

65.5 Pharmacotherapy is used to treat deficient or excess secretion of antidiuretic hormone.

It is essential for the amount of fluid in the body to be maintained within narrow limits. Loss of large amounts of water leads to dehydration, a serious condition that can lead to shock and death. Too much body fluid leads to congestion, edema, and water intoxication. ADH is one of the most important means the body uses to maintain fluid balance homeostasis. For a complete discussion of fluid balance and the drugs used as fluid replacement agents, see Chapter 33.

The hypothalamus senses fluid balance by recognizing the osmolarity of the blood. *Osmolarity* is the number of dissolved particles, or solutes, in a fluid. As water is lost, the osmolality, or concentration of the blood, increases and the hypothalamus directs the posterior pituitary gland to release ADH. This hormone acts on the renal tubules to enhance water reabsorption. The increased amount of water in the body reduces serum osmolality to normal levels and ADH secretion stops. Other factors stimulating release of ADH include hypotension, decreased fluid volume, dehydration, pain, nausea and vomiting. Factors inhibiting ADH release include decreased serum osmolality and increased fluid volume. ADH is also called vasopressin because it has the ability to cause vasoconstriction at high doses.

CONNECTION Checkpoint 65.2

In addition to ADH, the renin-angiotensin-aldosterone system (RAAS) is essential for maintaining fluid balance. From what you learned in Chapter 31, how does the RAAS affect sodium and water balance?

A deficiency in ADH results in **diabetes insipidus (DI)**, a condition characterized by the production of large volumes of very dilute urine, usually accompanied by increased thirst. DI may be either nephrogenic or neurogenic. Nephrogenic DI is caused by the inability of the kidneys to respond to ADH. Drugs, such as lithium (Lithobid), or electrolyte disturbances can cause nephrogenic DI. Because nephrogenic DI results from an inability to respond to ADH, replacement therapy is not effective.

Neurogenic or central DI results from a lack of adequate production or secretion of ADH in the brain. The etiology of neurogenic DI can be genetic or acquired following head injury, surgery, tumors, infections, or vascular lesions of the region. The preferred drug for treating chronic neurogenic DI is desmopressin (DDAVP, Nocdurna). Both forms of DI respond in part to thiazide diuretics such as hydrochlorothiazide.

The primary symptoms of DI are polyuria and polydipsia (excessive thirst). Extremely large volumes of fluid (up to 30 L/day) may be ingested and the urine will be very dilute. The intense thirst and frequent urination usually keep patients awake during the night. Failure to ensure adequate fluid intake will result in hypovolemia and dehydration due to the large renal water loss.

Excess secretion of ADH is the cause of the **syndrome of inappropriate antidiuretic hormone (SIADH)**, a condition characterized by marked fluid retention, elevated urine osmolality, low serum osmolality, and sodium loss in the urine. SIADH may occur as a transient or chronic condition. The resulting hyponatremia and water retention cause muscle cramps, weakness, headache, apprehension, nausea and vomiting, and lethargy, progressing to stupor and coma. Treatment involves fluid restriction and diuretics such as mannitol or furosemide (Lasix) to remove excess fluid. Conivaptan (Viprostol) and tolvaptan (Samsca) are vasopressin receptor antagonists that promote renal water excretion and increased serum sodium levels in patients with SIADH. The tetracycline antibiotic demeclocycline may be used off-label to treat SIADH due to its ability to cause diuresis through the inhibition of ADH-induced water reabsorption in the tubules and collecting ducts of the kidneys. In severe cases, IV infusion of a hypertonic sodium chloride solution may be necessary to raise serum osmolality.

PROTOTYPE DRUG Desmopressin (DDAVP, Nocdurna)

Classification **Therapeutic:** Antidiuretic hormone replacement, drug for nocturia
Pharmacologic: Pituitary hormone

Therapeutic Effects and Uses: Approved in 1978, desmopressin is a synthetic analog of human ADH that has a longer duration of action than the natural hormone. It controls the acute symptoms of polyuria and polydipsia in patients with neurogenic DI but not nephrogenic diabetes insipidus. For DI, the PO route is preferred, although IV and subcutaneous forms are available for SIADH.

Desmopressin has vasoconstrictor activity that causes contraction of smooth muscle in the vascular system, uterus, and GI tract. It produces fewer vasoconstrictive effects than natural vasopressin. Desmopressin also produces an increase in plasma Factor VIII and von Willebrand's factor and is thus indicated for the management of bleeding in patients with hemophilia A and von Willebrand's disease (type I). Desmopressin is available in IV and intranasal forms for these indications. The use of desmopressin in treating coagulation disorders is presented in Chapter 38. This drug is the most effective pharmacologic intervention for controlling enuresis (bedwetting) in children. For enuresis, desmopressin is administered 1 hour before bedtime in children age 6 and older for up to 6 months. Nocdurna is a sublingual tablet approved in 2018 to treat nocturnal polyuria in adults who awaken at least two times per night to void.

Mechanism of Action: Desmopressin increases the permeability of renal collecting tubules to water, thereby increasing the reabsorption of water. It produces vasoconstriction of blood vessels at higher doses. The vasoconstriction produced is greatest in portal vessels and less in cerebral, coronary, pulmonary, and peripheral vessels. Desmopressin enhances GI motility and tone through contraction of smooth muscle in the GI tract.

Pharmacokinetics:

Route(s)	Subcutaneous, IV, PO
Absorption	5% through GI mucosa
Distribution	Small amount may cross the blood–brain barrier; secreted in breast milk
Primary metabolism	Metabolized rapidly by the liver
Primary excretion	Renal
Onset of action	PO: 1 h, with a peak at 4–7 h; IV: 1 min with a peak at 30 min; intranasal: 30 min with a peak of 1.5 h
Duration of action	PO: 8–20 h; IV: 3 h

Adverse Effects: Desmopressin can cause water intoxication. Early signs include drowsiness, headache, and listlessness, progressing to convulsions and coma. Other adverse effects include transient headache, nausea, mild abdominal pain and cramping, facial flushing, HTN, or pain or swelling at the injection site. A rare adverse effect of desmopressin is a severe allergic reaction or anaphylaxis (IV administration). Tolerance to the effects of desmopressin develops when it is administered more frequently than every 48 hours or by the IV route. The intranasal route may cause local irritation, rhinitis, and congestion. **Black Box Warning:** Intranasal and sublingual tablets may cause hyponatremia, which can be severe and even life-threatening.

Contraindications/Precautions: Desmopressin is contraindicated in patients with nephrogenic DI. It is used with caution in patients with coronary artery disease or HTN and in patients with a history of hyponatremia or thrombi. The drug is contraindicated in patients with CKD because the drug can worsen fluid retention and overload. Young children and the older adult should be treated with caution because these patients are more prone to water intoxication and hyponatremia.

Drug Interactions: Increased antidiuretic action can occur with carbamazepine, chlorpropamide, and nonsteroidal anti-inflammatory drugs (NSAIDs). Decreased antidiuretic action can occur with lithium, alcohol, heparin, and epinephrine. **Herbal/Food:** Unknown.

Pregnancy: Human experience with desmopressin over many decades has not shown evidence of major birth defects or fetal harm. Small amounts are secreted in human milk, although it is not known if it has adverse effects on the breastfed neonate.

Treatment of Overdose: In case of overdose, or if water intoxication develops, symptomatic treatment with diuretics is recommended.

Drugs Similar to Desmopressin (DDAVP, Nocdurna)

The only drug that is similar to desmopressin is vasopressin.

Vasopressin (Vasostrict): A synthetic analog of antidiuretic hormone, vasopressin is given IM or subcutaneously for central or neurogenic DI. Approved in 1941, it has a shorter duration of action than desmopressin and a more pronounced vasoconstrictor action, which can result in serious adverse effects.

Because vasopressin is a potent vasoconstrictor, it is given IV as an alternative to epinephrine for many off-label indications. These include bleeding from esophageal varices or the upper GI tract, cardiac arrest, and the treatment of severe hypotension or shock. Vasopressin may precipitate MI or angina. It may cause water intoxication. When used for its vasopressor effects, possible adverse effects include tissue necrosis and gangrene. It is not known if vasopressin causes fetal harm or adverse effects in the breastfed neonate. Vasopressin should be used during pregnancy only if the potential benefits to the mother justify the potential risks to the fetus.

CONNECTION Checkpoint 65.3

Desmopressin is used to treat von Willebrand's disease, the most common inherited coagulation disorder. From what you learned in Chapter 38, what is the function of von Willebrand's factor?

Understanding Chapter 65

Key Concepts Summary

65.1 The hypothalamus controls many diverse body processes and secretes hormones that influence pituitary function.

65.2 The pituitary gland secretes hormones that control many diverse body functions.

65.3 Growth hormone deficiency in adults and children can be treated by administering recombinant growth hormone.

65.4 Overproduction of growth hormone in adults can be treated by administering growth hormone antagonists.

65.5 Pharmacotherapy is used to treat deficient or excess secretion of antidiuretic hormone.

CASE STUDY: Making the Patient Connection

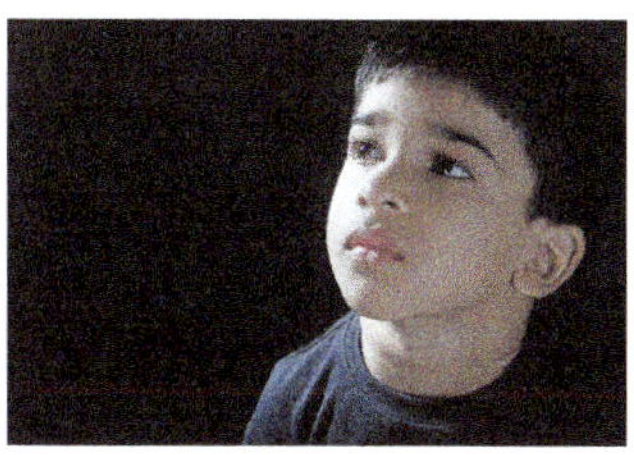

Remember the patient "Raj" at the beginning of the chapter? Now read the remainder of the case study. Based on the information presented in this chapter, answer the critical thinking questions that follow.

Raj, an 8-year-old boy, was referred to the pediatric endocrinology clinic for evaluation of his short stature. He had been healthy and developmentally normal until 3 years ago. Since that time, his growth has been extremely slow—in fact, almost imperceptible. On his initial examination, Raj's weight and height were 17 kg (37.4 lb) and 108 cm (42.5 in.), respectively. His height standard deviation score was –4.0

with a body mass index of 14.6. The remainder of his physical examination was normal.

When the pediatrician reviewed the results of hormonal tests with Raj's parents, everyone was relieved to find out that, although there is a problem, it is not due to a tumor or other life-threatening disorder. Raj has a congenital deficiency in GH, and the pediatrician discusses replacement therapy with the parents. They agree that he should have this therapy and want to start it as soon as possible. Somatropin (Humatrope) has been ordered. As the nurse working with Raj and his family, address each of the following questions.

Critical Thinking Questions

1. What teaching will you need to provide to Raj's parents regarding drug therapy for his disorder?
2. Raj's father states, "I hope my health insurance will cover this medication." What would you say in response to this comment?
3. The parents ask about the adverse effects that might occur with this therapy. How would you respond?

Additional Case Study

Edward Keithy, a 10-year-old boy, and his parents visit the pediatrician's office where you are a nurse. The parents are concerned with Edward's continuing nocturnal enuresis, or nighttime bedwetting. Increasingly, they see this condition as adversely affecting his self-image, self-esteem, and psychosocial well-being. Edward tells you that he is reluctant to take part in sleepovers at his friends' houses or to attend camping trips with his scouting troop.

1. What type of pharmacotherapy do you anticipate for Edward?
2. What information will Edward and his parents need as part of patient drug teaching?

Chapter Review

1. A teaching plan for a parent whose child is receiving somatropin should include what important information?
   1. The patient must adhere to therapy to prevent intellectual disability.
   2. The medication cannot be given orally; it can be given only parenterally.
   3. If growth hormone is begun in adolescence, it can add up to 15 cm (6 in.) in height.
   4. Growth hormone therapy requires frequent bloodwork.
2. Which of the following findings would the nurse consider to be effects of somatropin? (Select all that apply.)
   1. Increase in the length and width of long bones
   2. Organ, muscle, and connective tissue growth
   3. Increased synthesis of proteins
   4. Lowering of serum glucose levels
   5. Increase in fat deposits around the abdomen
3. The patient with neurogenic diabetes insipidus is being started on an oral dose of desmopressin (DDAVP). Which instruction should the nurse include in the teaching plan?
   1. Use the drug only if urine output is excessive.
   2. Use twice the prescribed dose if you miss a dose.
   3. Obtain and record your weight each morning.
   4. Use an NSAID such as ibuprofen if leg cramping occurs during walking.
4. A patient with metastatic colon cancer is experiencing bowel-related complications of the cancer and treatment. Octreotide (Sandostatin) has been ordered. The nurse will anticipate which therapeutic effect from this drug?
   1. Decrease in the number of diarrheal stools per day
   2. Slowing of the metastatic spread of the cancer
   3. Increase in lean body mass and fat deposits
   4. Episodes of hypo- or hyperglycemia
5. Prior to starting a patient on octreotide (Sandostatin) for control of esophageal varices, the nurse will obtain the patient's past health history. If present, what condition might indicate the need to verify the order with the prescriber?
   1. Glaucoma
   2. Alcoholism
   3. Chronic obstructive pulmonary disease (COPD)
   4. Diabetes

6. Which of the following assessment findings would indicate that therapeutic goals have been achieved for a patient with diabetes insipidus being treated with desmopressin (DDAVP)?
   1. Decreasing signs of dehydration
   2. Increasing pulse and urine output
   3. Decreasing urine specific gravity
   4. Decreasing hyperglycemia

See Appendix A for answers to critical thinking questions, case study questions, and review questions.

References

Briet, B. (2019). Should we assess pituitary function in children after a mild traumatic brain injury?: A prospective study. *Frontiers in Endocrinology*, *10*, 149. https://doi.org/10.3389/fendo.2019.00149

Jildeh, T. R., Okoroha, K. R., Denha, E., Eyers, C., Johnson, A., Shehab, R., & Moutzouros, V. (2020). Return to sport following adolescent concussion: Epidemiologic findings from a high school population. *Orthopedics*, *43*(4): e306–e310. https://doi.org/10.3928/01477447-20200521-03

Selected Bibliography

Campana, C., Corica, G., Nista, F., Cocchiara, F., Graziani, G., Khorrami, K., et al. (2020). Emerging drugs for the treatment of acromegaly. *Expert Opinion on Emerging Drugs*. https://doi.org/10.1080/14728214.2020.1819983

Collin, J., Whitehead, A., & Walker, J. (2016). Educating children and families about growth hormone deficiency and its management: Part 2. *Nursing Children and Young People*, *28*(2), 30–36. https://doi.org/10.7748/ncyp.28.2.30.s23

Khardori, R. (2020). *Diabetes insipidus*. Medscape. https://emedicine.medscape.com/article/117648-overview

Malanowski, S., & Baima, N. (2015). On treating athletes with banned substances: The relationship between mild traumatic brain injury, hypopituitarism, and hormone replacement therapy. *Neuroethics*, *8*, 27–38. https://doi.org/10.1007/s12152-014-9215-2

National Institute of Neurological Disorders and Stroke. (n.d.). *Traumatic brain injury information page*. National Institutes of Health. https://www.ninds.nih.gov/Disorders/All-Disorders/Traumatic-Brain-Injury-Information-Page

Peri, A., Grohé, C., Berardi, R., & Runkle, I. (2017). SIADH: Differential diagnosis and clinical management. *Endocrine*, 55, 311–319. https://doi.org/10.1007/s12020-016-0936-3

Robson, L. M. (2020). *Enuresis*. Medscape. http://emedicine.medscape.com/article/1014762-overview

Roth, K. S. (2017). *Pediatric diabetes insipidus*. Medscape. http://emedicine.medscape.com/article/919886-overview

Schwartz, R. A. (2020). *Gigantism and acromegaly*. Medscape. http://emedicine.medscape.com/article/925446-overview#a1

Teran, E., Chesner, J., & Rapaport, R. (2016). Growth and growth hormone: An overview. *Growth Hormone & IGF Research*, *28*, 3–5. https://doi.org/10.1016/j.ghir.2016.02.004

Thomas, C. P. (2019). *Syndrome of inappropriate antidiuretic hormone secretion SIADH)*. Medscape. http://emedicine.medscape.com/article/246650-overview

Yuen, K. C., Llahana, S., & Miller, B. S. (2019). Adult growth hormone deficiency: clinical advances and approaches to improve adherence. *Expert Review of Endocrinology & Metabolism*, *14*(6), 419–436. https://doi.org/10.1080/17446651.2019.1689119

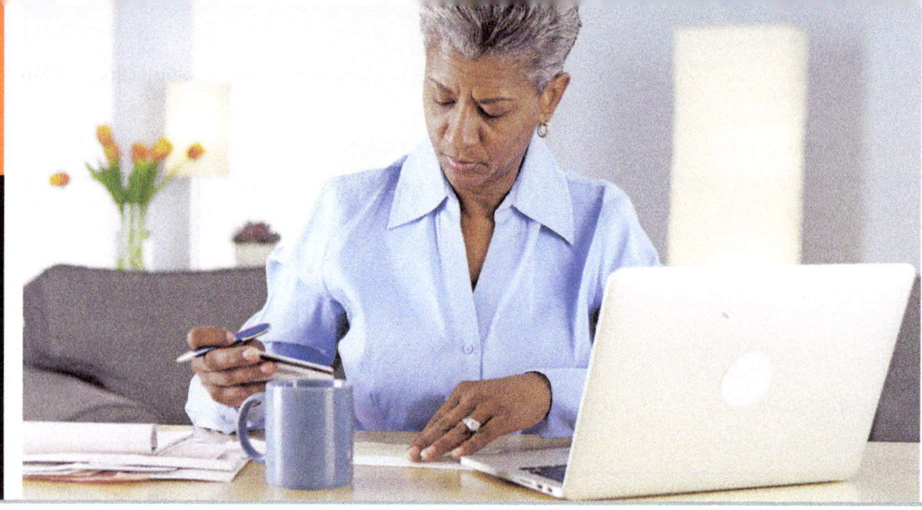

"Diabetes?! How can I have diabetes? I don't eat a lot of sugar; I try to watch my weight. And what is this type 2 thing about?"

—*Patient "Eileen Douglas"*

Chapter 66
Pharmacotherapy of Diabetes Mellitus

Chapter Outline

Learning Outcomes

After reading this chapter, the student should be able to:

1. Explain how blood glucose levels are maintained within narrow limits by insulin and glucagon.
2. Compare and contrast the etiology and pathogenesis of type 1, type 2, and gestational diabetes.
3. Describe the signs and diagnosis of diabetes.
4. Describe the acute complications of diabetes.
5. Identify the chronic complications of diabetes.
6. Compare and contrast the pharmacotherapy of the different types of diabetes.
7. For each type of insulin, identify the onset of action, peak action and duration of action, administration routes, when it is given related to meals, compatibility with other insulins, and adverse effects.
8. For each of the classes shown in the chapter outline, identify the prototype and representative drugs and explain the mechanism(s) of drug action, primary indications, contraindications, significant drug interactions, pregnancy data, and important adverse effects.
9. Apply clinical judgment to the care of patients receiving pharmacotherapy for diabetes.

Key Terms

Definitions of the terms in bold may be found in the Glossary.

It is estimated that over 34 million people in the United States have diabetes mellitus, with more than 7 million of those being undiagnosed. Mortality has risen in recent years, causing some public health officials to refer to it as an epidemic. Uncontrolled diabetes leads to serious acute and chronic complications, including heart disease, stroke, blindness, kidney failure, and amputations. Because nurses frequently care for patients with diabetes, it is imperative that they thoroughly understand the disorder, its treatment, and possible complications. An unrelated disorder, diabetes insipidus, results from a deficiency of antidiuretic hormone (see Chapter 65). When the term *diabetes* is used in this chapter, it is referring to diabetes mellitus.

Physiology of Serum Glucose Control

66.1 Serum glucose is maintained within a narrow range by the hormones insulin and glucagon.

Because diabetes is essentially a disorder of carbohydrate metabolism, it is important to understand the way the body obtains, metabolizes, and stores glucose. Of all the different molecules available, the body prefers to use glucose as its primary energy source. The brain relies almost exclusively on glucose for its energy needs because it is unable to synthesize glucose and it will exhaust its supply after just a few minutes of activity. Most other tissues can use fatty acids and proteins for energy production, if necessary, but they too prefer to use glucose. One of the most important roles of the liver and pancreas is to regulate the body's carbohydrate fuel supply so that all tissues of the body have sufficient energy to perform their functions.

Although the normal range for serum glucose is considered to be 60 to 100 mg/dL, it is usually tightly regulated by the body to remain between 80 and 90 mg/dL. Two pancreatic hormones contribute to maintaining a stable serum glucose level: **insulin**, which acts to decrease blood glucose levels, and glucagon, which acts to increase blood glucose levels.

Following a meal, glucose is rapidly absorbed from the gastrointestinal (GI) tract, and serum levels rise. Some of the glucose is taken up by cells and used for immediate energy needs, but about two-thirds is stored in liver and muscle cells as glycogen, the storage form of glucose. When glucose levels fall between meals, glycogen is broken down and glucose is released into the bloodstream. Maintaining a stable serum glucose level is simply a matter of storing glucose during times of excess and returning it to the bloodstream in times of deficiency. The importance of maintaining this delicate balance, however, cannot be overstated. Too much glucose or too little glucose can have lethal consequences.

Following a meal, the pancreas recognizes the rising serum glucose levels and releases insulin. Without insulin, glucose is not able to enter cells of the body. The cells may be surrounded by high amounts of glucose, but they are unable to use it until insulin arrives. It may be helpful to visualize insulin as a transporter or "gatekeeper." When present, insulin swings open the gate, transporting glucose inside cells—if there is no insulin, there is no entry. The physiologic actions of insulin are summarized as follows:

- It promotes the entry of glucose into cells.
- It provides for the storage of glucose, as glycogen.
- It inhibits the breakdown of fat and glycogen.
- It increases protein synthesis and inhibits **gluconeogenesis**, which is the production of new glucose from noncarbohydrate molecules.

Insulin is produced in beta cells of the pancreas known as islets of Langerhans, whereas alpha cells in the pancreas secrete glucagon. Glucagon maintains stable blood glucose levels between meals and during periods of fasting and has actions that are opposite to those of insulin. It removes glucose from its storage in the liver and sends it to the blood (glycogenolysis), raising serum glucose within minutes.

The level of glucose in the blood regulates the release of both insulin and glucagon. A hypoglycemic state (low serum glucose) stimulates the release of glucagon and inhibits the release of insulin, whereas a hyperglycemic state (high serum glucose) has the opposite effect: It stimulates the release of insulin and inhibits the release of glucagon. The physiologic dynamics of insulin and glucagon release are shown in Figure 66.1.

Additional factors that decrease blood glucose levels are fasting, exercise, and alcohol. Factors that increase blood glucose levels include stress from infection, injury, or surgery, which triggers release of epinephrine and norepinephrine; large meals or overconsumption of carbohydrates; growth hormone; and corticosteroids.

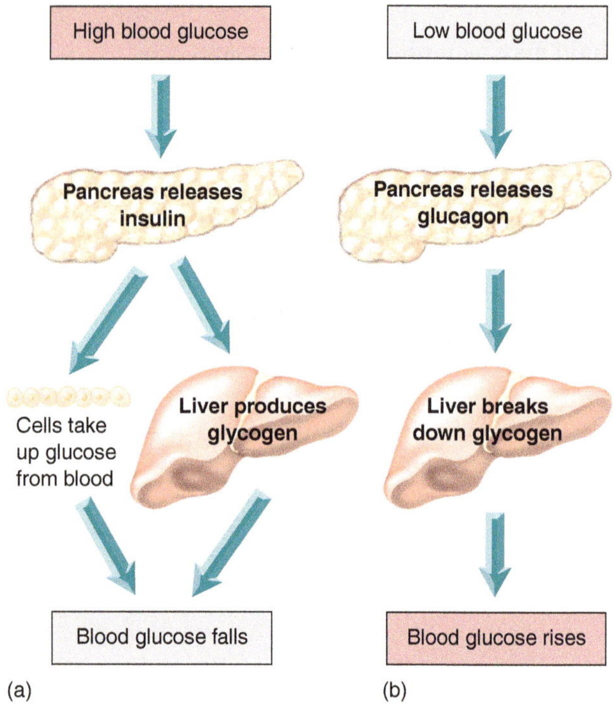

Figure 66.1 Insulin, glucagon, and blood glucose.

Pathophysiology of Diabetes Mellitus: Types of Diabetes

66.2 Type 1 diabetes is characterized by insufficient insulin synthesis by the pancreas, whereas type 2 diabetes is characterized by insulin resistance in the target cells.

Diabetes mellitus is a metabolic disorder characterized by an imbalance between insulin availability and insulin need. The two primary forms of diabetes are called type 1 and type 2. There are significant differences between the two types in terms of pathophysiology and disease management. A third form of the disease occurs during pregnancy and is known as *gestational diabetes*.

Type 1 diabetes results from an absolute lack of insulin secretion due to destruction of pancreatic beta cells. The destruction is believed to result from a combination of autoimmune, genetic, and environmental factors. Type 1 is the less common form of diabetes, accounting for 5 to 10% of all patients with the disorder. It is seen most frequently among children and young adults, but it may occur at any age.

Because of the lack of sufficient insulin in patients with type 1 diabetes, glucose cannot enter cells and fatty acids are used as the primary energy source. Metabolic byproducts of lipid metabolism known as ketones accumulate in the blood, producing diabetic ketoacidosis (DKA), a dangerous and potentially life-threatening condition (see Section 66.4).

Patients with type 1 diabetes must receive insulin therapy to survive. In the past, type 1 was called juvenile or insulin-dependent diabetes. Although these terms are still in use, they do not accurately reflect the nature of the disease.

Type 2 diabetes is the more common form of the disorder, representing 90 to 95% of people with diabetes. The primary physiologic characteristic of type 2 diabetes is hyperglycemia, caused by a relative deficiency of insulin. The disorder is characterized by **insulin resistance**, a condition in which cells become unresponsive to insulin due to a defect in insulin receptor function. The pancreas may be secreting sufficient amounts of insulin, but target cells do not recognize it.

As cells become increasingly resistant, blood glucose levels rise and the pancreas responds by secreting even more insulin. Eventually, the hypersecretion of insulin leads to beta cell exhaustion and, ultimately, to beta cell death. As type 2 diabetes progresses, it becomes a disorder characterized by insufficient insulin levels as well as insulin resistance. The activity of insulin receptors can be increased by exercise, which lowers the level of circulating insulin. In fact, adhering to a healthy diet and exercising regularly have been shown to reverse insulin resistance and to delay or prevent the development of type 2 diabetes.

Eighty percent of people with type 2 diabetes are overweight, and the degree of obesity directly affects the degree of insulin resistance. In particular, individuals with upper-body obesity (central or visceral obesity) are at increased risk for developing insulin resistance and type 2 diabetes. Although most patients with type 2 diabetes are older, this disease is increasingly being diagnosed in adolescents with obesity. Risk factors for type 2 diabetes are a family history of diabetes, obesity, and race and ethnicity. Hispanics/Latinos, non-Hispanic African Americans, and Asian Americans are at increased risk for type 2 diabetes (American Diabetes Association [ADA], 2020a). Other risk factors are age older than 45 years; a history of elevated fasting serum glucose levels or impaired glucose tolerance; hypertension (HTN); low levels of high-density lipoproteins; triglycerides above 250 mg/dL; and a history of gestational diabetes or delivery of a baby over 9 pounds, or both. Table 66.1 compares and contrasts type 1 and type 2 diabetes.

Most patients with type 2 diabetes do not require insulin administration, at least initially; their condition can be managed with oral or parenteraal antidiabetic drugs. Type 2 diabetes was formerly called adult-onset diabetes and non-insulin-dependent diabetes, but these are not accurate descriptions of the disorder because it occurs in children and may require insulin administration.

Gestational diabetes is a condition resulting from glucose intolerance with an onset, or first recognition, during pregnancy. This is a serious disorder that puts both the woman and fetus at risk for complications. In addition, women who develop gestational diabetes are at increased risk for developing diabetes 5 to 10 years after delivery.

Table 66.1 Comparison of Type 1 and Type 2 Diabetes Mellitus

Diabetes Mellitus	Type 1	Type 2
Cause	Destruction of beta cells causing lack of insulin	Insulin resistance in target cells; insulin deficiency may develop
Incidence	5–10%	90–95%
Age at onset	Children, young adults, usually younger than 35 years	Usually older than 35 years but incidence increasing in children
Symptom onset	Rapid	Gradual
Body weight	Usually underweight	Usually overweight or obese
Symptoms	Polyuria, polydipsia, polyphagia, weight loss	Same as type 1, plus blurred vision, fatigue, recurrent infections
Ketosis	Often present with poor control	Infrequent
Pharmacologic treatment	Insulin replacement	Antidiabetes drugs with or without insulin

It occurs most frequently in women with a family history of diabetes, a history of stillbirth or spontaneous abortion, a previous large-for-gestational-age baby, who are obese or of advanced maternal age, who have had five or more pregnancies, or who are members of a high-risk population (Hispanic, Native American, Asian, or African American). Insulin therapy is considered the standard therapy if careful nutritional management combined with an approved exercise plan is unable to normalize serum glucose levels. Metformin and glyburide may be prescribed off label by some practitioners.

Symptoms and Diagnosis of Diabetes

66.3 The classic signs and symptoms of diabetes include polyuria, polydipsia, and polyphagia.

The classic triad of signs and symptoms for either type of diabetes is known as the three "polys": **polyuria**, excessive urine production; **polydipsia**, excessive thirst; and **polyphagia**, excessive appetite.

Glucose is one of the body's most valuable energy molecules, and nondiabetic patients excrete very little. As glucose levels rise in the blood in patients with diabetes, however, the kidneys are unable to reabsorb the large amounts passing through the renal tubules, so glucose is eliminated in the urine (glucosuria). Glucose molecules create increased osmotic pressure in body fluids, pulling water along with it; thus, osmotic diuresis (polyuria) occurs. The glucose increases osmotic pressure in the bloodstream, pulling water out of tissue cells and causing cellular dehydration. This triggers thirst and causes the individual to increase fluid intake (polydipsia). The excess hunger (polyphagia) occurs primarily with type 1 diabetes, when nutrient stores become too depleted to meet the body's energy needs and weight is lost. Other signs and symptoms include blurred vision, fatigue, paresthesias, and skin infections. Nocturia, secondary to the polyuria, may occur.

Although symptomology is important for recognizing the possibility of diabetes, many patients with the disease have no symptoms. Laboratory tests are required for proper diagnosis. The primary blood tests for diagnosing diabetes are the **fasting plasma glucose (FPG) test**, **oral glucose tolerance test (OGTT)**, and **hemoglobin A1C test**.

- FPG: obtained following a fast of at least 8 hours. A value of 126 mg/dL or higher indicates diabetes.
- OGTT: A loading dose of 75 g of glucose is ingested and the plasma glucose level is obtained 2 hours later. A value of 200 mg/dL or higher indicates diabetes.
- A1C: As serum glucose increases, more glucose becomes bound to hemoglobin. A value of 6.5% or higher indicates diabetes. The advantage of the A1C test is that it does not require fasting and it provides an average measure of glucose control over the 8 to 12 weeks prior to the test.

Home monitoring of blood glucose is now commonplace and enables the patient with diabetes to maintain tighter control of glucose levels. Fingerstick testing involves placing a drop of capillary blood on a test strip, which is then read by a glucose meter.

Most patients who develop type 2 diabetes go through a period of impaired glucose tolerance referred to as **prediabetes**. In prediabetes, serum glucose levels are elevated but are not high enough to be diagnosed as diabetes. This condition increases the risk for developing diabetes, heart disease, and stroke. Prediabetes may result from impaired fasting glucose or impaired glucose tolerance, or both. Progression from prediabetes to diabetes is not inevitable. Careful management of nutrition, regular exercise, and weight management may prevent or delay progression to diabetes. Patients with prediabetes should be monitored on an annual basis for the potential development of diabetes and to evaluate the degree of success in managing comorbid conditions such as HTN, hyperlipidemia, and obesity.

Obesity-related insulin resistance can lead to **metabolic syndrome**, a cluster of biochemical changes that place the patient at increased risk for developing diabetes, heart disease, peripheral vascular disease, and stroke. Again, weight loss, exercise, and nutritional management enable people with this syndrome to delay or prevent the progression to type 2 diabetes. According to the American Heart Association (2016), metabolic syndrome is diagnosed by the presence of three or more of the following:

- Central (visceral) obesity, with waist circumference more than 88 cm (35 in.) for women or more than 102 cm (40 in.) for men

- Serum triglycerides equal to or greater than 150 mg/dL
- High-density lipoprotein cholesterol (HDL-C) less than 50 mg/dL in women or less than 40 mg/dL in men (or receiving drug therapy for hyperlipidemia)
- Blood pressure more than 130/85 mmHg (or receiving drug therapy for HTN)
- Fasting plasma glucose equal to or greater than 100 mg/dL (or receiving drug therapy for hyperglycemia).

Complications of Diabetes Mellitus

66.4 Acute complications of diabetes include diabetic ketoacidosis, hyperosmolar hyperglycemic state, and hypoglycemia.

Although most patients experience chronic diabetes, which develops over many years, acute episodes may occur suddenly in those with uncontrolled or poorly controlled diabetes. Diabetic ketoacidosis, hyperosmolar hyperglycemic syndrome (HHS), and hypoglycemia are the three primary acute conditions. The chronic complications are discussed in Section 66.5.

Diabetic ketoacidosis (DKA) is an acute condition that occurs primarily in patients with type 1 diabetes. The three major disturbances that occur with DKA are hyperglycemia, metabolic acidosis, and osmotic diuresis. DKA typically develops over several days with symptoms such as polyuria, polydipsia, nausea, vomiting, and severe fatigue, progressing to stupor and possibly coma. The patient may report having abdominal pain or tenderness, and the breath has a fruity smell as the lungs attempt to remove volatile ketoacids. As the acidosis worsens, Kussmaul's respirations may develop, with an increased rate and depth of respirations. Tachycardia and hypotension occur in response to dehydration and fluid depletion.

DKA may be the first presenting symptoms of an individual previously undiagnosed with diabetes. Treatment includes fluid replacement to improve circulating blood volume and tissue perfusion, normalization of blood glucose levels, and correction of electrolyte imbalances and metabolic acidosis. Insulin therapy is begun, usually with an IV loading dose, followed by a continuous low-dose infusion. Serum glucose levels must be lowered gradually because too rapid a drop can cause a fluid shift back into the cells that can lead to cerebral edema.

CONNECTION Checkpoint 66.1

From what you learned in Chapter 33, what is the clinical definition of acidosis? What is the preferred drug for reversing metabolic acidosis?

Hyperosmolar hyperglycemic syndrome (HHS) is a serious, acute complication of diabetes that carries a mortality rate of 20 to 40%. HHS is generally seen in people with type 2 diabetes and is characterized by extreme hyperglycemia (above 600 mg/dL), hyperosmolarity (above 310 mOsm/L) with dehydration, the absence of ketoacidosis, and central nervous system dysfunction. The typical patient is older, obese, and has comorbid medical problems, such as heart failure (HF) or chronic kidney disease (CKD). The elevated serum glucose levels and increased osmolarity produce a large osmotic diuresis with marked dehydration, confusion, and lethargy. Other possible neurologic symptoms are seizures, hemiparesis, abnormal reflexes, aphasia, and visual disturbances. Symptoms can progress to stupor and coma. Tachycardia and hypotension result from fluid depletion and poor tissue perfusion. Acidosis may develop, caused by an accumulation of lactic acid rather than ketoacids.

The onset of HHS is gradual and, because of the neurologic manifestations, may be mistaken for a stroke in older adults. Treatment consists of careful fluid replacement while avoiding cerebral and pulmonary edema and correction of electrolyte imbalances, particularly potassium. Low-dose insulin is given by continuous IV infusion to slowly lower glucose levels to 250 to 300 mg/dL. The nurse should closely monitor intake and output, blood pressure, heart rate, lung sounds, weight, peripheral pulses, and neurologic status. Finally, the underlying cause of the episode should be investigated and treated as needed.

A third acute complication of DM is hypoglycemia, which occurs most often in patients improperly treated with insulin and may occur during therapy with some oral antidiabetic drugs. The manifestations of hypoglycemia result from changes in mental status and by the activation of the sympathetic nervous system (SNS). Because the brain relies on a continuous supply of glucose, falling glucose levels may lead to headache, difficulty concentrating, confusion, and behavioral changes, progressing to seizures and coma. The SNS activation results from the body's attempt to increase serum glucose by the release of catecholamines (epinephrine and norepinephrine). These catecholamines cause symptoms that include tachycardia, anxiety, sweating, and the constriction of surface vessels, leading to cool, clammy skin. Severe hypoglycemia is considered a medical emergency and, if prolonged or severe, can lead to brain damage or death.

The symptoms of hypoglycemia may have a very rapid onset. Patients who have had diabetes for an extended time may develop the inability to recognize symptoms of hypoglycemia. Some drugs, such as beta-adrenergic blockers, interfere with the SNS symptoms of hypoglycemia, making it more difficult for the patient to recognize the condition and for the body to correct the low glucose levels.

Factors that cause hypoglycemia in patients with diabetes include errors in insulin dosage, failure to eat at regular intervals, increased exercise, or medication adjustments. The treatment for hypoglycemia is glucose, given in a concentrated source of 15 to 20 g. This can be repeated as necessary, while taking care not to overtreat the patient and cause hyperglycemia. If the individual is unconscious, or unable to swallow safely, a small amount of glucose gel or spray can be administered to the buccal mucosa. Intravenous (IV) glucose is immediately effective in treating hypoglycemia and glucagon may be administered.

PROTOTYPE DRUG | **Glucagon (GlucaGen)**

Classification **Therapeutic:** Antihypoglycemic drug
Pharmacologic: Pancreatic hormone

Therapeutic Effects and Uses: Glucagon is used for the emergency treatment of severe hypoglycemia in patients with diabetes who are unconscious or unable to eat sugar or drink a sweetened beverage. It is also used for radiographic studies to relax the smooth muscle of the GI tract. GlucaGen is obtained through recombinant deoxyribonucleic acid (DNA) technology and is identical in structure to human glucagon.

Given intramuscularly (IM), subcutaneously, or IV, glucagon will raise serum glucose levels in 10 to 20 minutes. Because glucagon raises glucose levels by stimulating breakdown of stored glycogen, it is not effective in patients who experience hypoglycemia due to starvation because their glycogen stores are depleted. In 2019 a prefilled autoinjector form of glucagon (Gvoke) was approved that offers rapid home treatment because it does not require premixing the ingredients. Also in 2019, an intranasal powder (Baqsimi) was approved that can be safely administered to patients experiencing a severe hypoglycemic episode. Peak effect occurs about 15 minutes after administration. In 2021 a new glucagon analog, dasiglucagon (Zegalogue) was approved to treat severe hypoglycemia. Dasiglucagon acts rapidly and is available by autoinjector or prefilled syringe.

Mechanism of Action: Glucagon increases glucose levels by increasing glycogenolysis; therefore, its actions are dependent on the presence of adequate liver glycogen stores. Glucagon stimulates the uptake of amino acids, increases their conversion to glucose, and promotes lipolysis in the liver with the release of fatty acids and glycerol.

Pharmacokinetics:

Route(s)	IM, IV, subcutaneous, intranasal
Absorption	Easily absorbed IM, subcutaneous or intranasal
Distribution	Throughout plasma
Primary metabolism	Liver, plasma, and kidneys
Primary excretion	Renal and through the bile
Onset of action	IV: 5–20 min; IM: 30 min; subcutaneous: 30–45 min
Duration of action	1–1.5 h

Adverse Effects: Glucagon is well tolerated. Adverse effects include nausea and vomiting, hypersensitivity reactions, transient changes in blood pressure (either hypotension or HTN), tachycardia, hyperglycemia, and hypokalemia.

Contraindications/Precautions: Glucagon is contraindicated in patients sensitive to protein compounds, in patients with depleted glycogen stores, or in patients with insulinoma or pheochromocytoma. It is used with caution in patients with coronary artery disease because it may affect blood pressure, heart rate, and myocardial oxygen demand. Administer supplemental oral carbohydrates once consciousness has been achieved to restore glycogen levels and prevent secondary hypoglycemia.

Drug Interactions: Glucagon increases serum glucose and will antagonize the effects of antidiabetic drugs. Beta-adrenergic blockers will inhibit the glucose-elevating effect of glucagon and will also increase the risk of blood pressure or heart rate adverse effects associated with glucagon. **Herbal/Food:** None known.

Pregnancy: Animal studies did not show evidence of significant fetal harm because glucagon does not cross the placenta. It is not known if glucagon is secreted in milk or has adverse effects on the breastfed neonate.

Treatment of Overdose: An overdose can cause hyperglycemia, which may be treated with insulin, IV fluids, and monitoring of electrolytes.

Drugs Similar to Glucagon (GlucaGen)

There are no drugs similar to glucagon.

66.5 Serious complications of chronic diabetes include neuropathy, nephropathy, retinopathy, and vascular disease.

Most patients with type 2 diabetes experience no symptoms of their illness for many years, perhaps even decades. However, while years may pass without symptoms, the effects of uncontrolled blood glucose levels are progressively producing major, irreversible changes on body systems, especially the nervous and circulatory systems.

Teaching patients about the long-term consequences of untreated diabetes can be a major challenge for the nurse. When diagnosed at an asymptomatic stage, it is difficult to convince patients to make radical changes to their lifestyle and to spend money on prescriptions when they do not feel ill. Patients must clearly understand that if they delay treatment until symptoms appear, it will likely be too late to prevent serious, chronic organ injury. Intensive management of blood glucose levels has been found to dramatically reduce the incidence of long-term complications of diabetes.

Neuropathies are common, affecting an estimated 60 to 70% of people with diabetes. Diabetic neuropathies affect both the somatic and autonomic nervous systems. Somatic neuropathies include paresthesias, numbness, tingling and pain, motor weakness, and muscle wasting. Autonomic neuropathies include postural hypotension, altered GI functioning including gastroparesis, or gastric atony, diarrhea, altered genitourinary functioning with difficulty voiding or erectile dysfunction, and possible cranial nerve impairment. Intensive management of blood glucose has been shown to reduce the occurrence of neuropathies.

Diabetic nephropathy is the leading cause of end-stage renal disease, which affects patients with both type 1 and type 2 diabetes. Most commonly, the renal glomeruli are damaged, and progressive loss of kidney function leads to eventual renal failure. Comorbid conditions that put the patient at high risk for nephropathy include HTN, poor glucose control, smoking, and hyperlipidemia.

Diabetic retinopathy is the leading cause of acquired blindness in the United States. Thirty years after the onset of diabetes, almost all people with type 1 diabetes, and over 60% of those with type 2 diabetes, show some degree of retinopathy (Bhavsar, 2017). Regular eye examinations are important for everyone who has diabetes.

Diabetes is a major risk factor for the development of vascular disease, including premature atherosclerosis, which leads to coronary artery disease, cerebrovascular disease, and peripheral vascular disease. Heart disease and stroke account for about 65% of deaths in individuals with diabetes. Preventive measures are directed toward reducing risk factors: control of blood pressure, smoking cessation, lowering of lipid levels, and optimal glucose control. In addition, antiplatelet drugs are often indicated.

Foot ulcers occur in patients with diabetes due to peripheral neuropathies and poor circulation. Neuropathies may impair sensation, so a small area of irritation may go unnoticed. Vascular insufficiency and elevated glucose levels inhibit healing of the ulcer. If the ulcer becomes infected, it is often resistant to treatment and may ultimately result in the need for amputation. Diabetes is the leading cause of nontraumatic amputations.

Insulin Therapy

66.6 Insulin is the cornerstone of therapy for patients with type 1 and gestational diabetes.

Because patients with type 1 diabetes are severely deficient in insulin production, insulin replacement therapy is required to survive. Insulin is also required for those with type 2 diabetes who are unable to manage their blood glucose levels with diet, exercise, and oral antidiabetic drugs. Among adults diagnosed with diabetes, 15% take only insulin, 14% take insulin with oral antidiabetic drugs, 52% take oral antidiabetic drugs only, and 19% take neither insulin nor antidiabetic drugs (ADA, 2020a).

The pharmacologic goal for patients with type 1 diabetes is to administer insulin as replacement therapy in normal physiologic amounts. Because insulin secretion varies greatly in response to daily activities, pharmacotherapy must be carefully planned in conjunction with proper meal planning and lifestyle habits. The desired outcome of insulin therapy is to prevent the long-term consequences of diabetes by maintaining blood glucose levels strictly within the normal range.

The fundamental principle to remember about insulin therapy is that the right amount of insulin must be available to cells when glucose is present in the blood. Administering insulin when glucose is not available can lead to hypoglycemia and, possibly, coma. This situation occurs when a patient administers insulin correctly but skips a meal. The insulin is available to cells, but glucose is not. In another example, the patient participates in strenuous exercise. The insulin may have been administered on schedule, and food eaten, but the active muscles quickly use up all the glucose in the blood, and the patient becomes hypoglycemic. Patients with diabetes who engage in competitive sports need to consume food or sports drinks just prior to and during the activity to maintain their blood glucose at normal levels. The nurse plays a key role in helping patients plan their meals, activities, and insulin dosages correctly. Figure 66.2 illustrates the management of type 1 diabetes and correct timing of the insulin dose with meals.

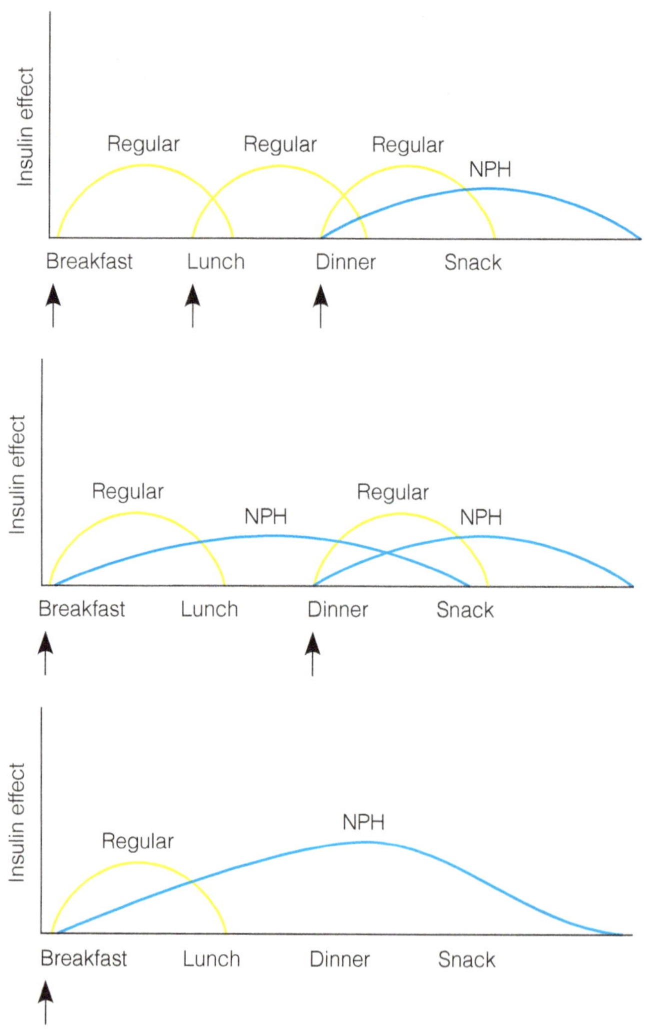

Figure 66.2 Insulin regimens.

Many types of insulin are available, differing in their source, time of onset, and peak effect and duration of action. Almost all insulin today is human insulin obtained through recombinant DNA technology. Pharmacologists have modified human insulin to create certain pharmacokinetic advantages, such as a more rapid onset of action (Humalog) or a more prolonged duration of action (Lantus). These modified forms are called insulin *analogs*. It is important for nurses and patients to know the time of peak action of any insulin because that is when the risk for hypoglycemic adverse effects is greatest. The different types of insulins available are listed in Table 66.2.

Doses of insulin are highly individualized for the precise control of blood glucose levels in each patient. Because the GI tract destroys insulin, it must be given by injection. Some patients require two or more injections daily for proper diabetes management. For ease of administration, two different compatible types of insulin may be mixed, using a standard method, to obtain the desired therapeutic effects. Some of these combinations are marketed in cartridges containing premixed solutions. A long-acting insulin may be taken daily to provide a basal blood level, with a supplemental rapid-acting insulin given shortly before a meal.

Rapid- or regular-acting insulin can be used in continuous subcutaneous infusion devices, often called insulin pumps. An infusion set, which holds a syringe of the drug, delivers insulin from the pump to a needle anchored in the subcutaneous tissue of the abdomen. The infusion set is replaced after 2 to 3 days, at which time the injection site should be moved at least 2 inches away from the old site. Many providers recommend checking blood glucose levels within 3 to 4 hours of replacement to ensure the system is working properly. The pump is programmed to release small subcutaneous doses of insulin into the abdomen at predetermined intervals, with larger boluses administered manually at mealtime, if necessary. Most pumps contain an alarm that reminds patients to take their insulin. They are generally worn on a belt or tucked into a pocket. Figure 66.3 shows an insulin pump.

The primary adverse effect of insulin therapy is overtreatment; insulin may remove too much glucose from the blood, resulting in hypoglycemia. This may occur when a patient with type 1 diabetes has more insulin in the blood than is needed to balance the amount of circulating blood

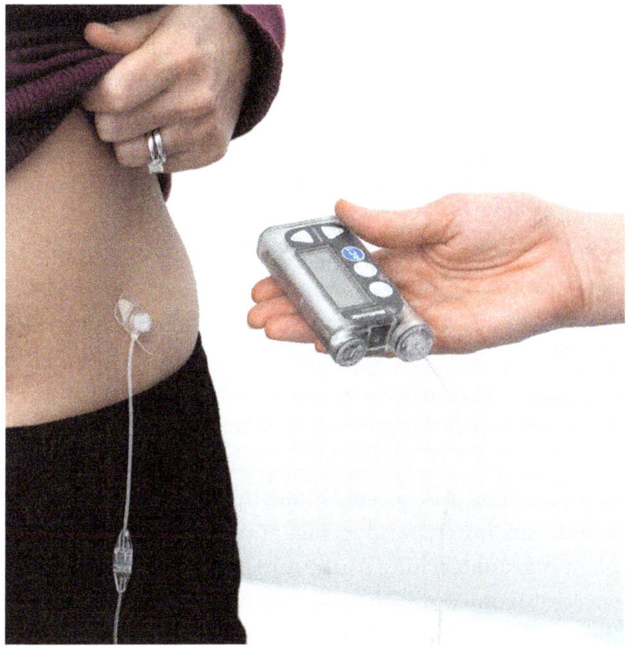

Figure 66.3 Insulin pump.
Ace Stock Limited/Alamy Stock Photo.

Table 66.2 Types of Insulin: Actions and Administration

Drug	Action	Onset	Peak	Duration	Administration and Timing	Compatibility
Insulin aspart (Fiasp, NovoLog)	Rapid	15 min	1–3 h	3–5 h	Subcutaneous: 5–10 min before meal	Can give with NPH; draw aspart up first, give immediately
Insulin degludec (Tresiba)	Long	Gradual	9 h	To 42 h	Subcutaneous: once daily, any time of day	Do not mix with any other insulin
Insulin detemir (Levemir)	Long	Gradual	6–8 h	To 24 h	Subcutaneous: 1–2 times daily	Do not mix with any other insulin
Insulin glargine (Basaglar, Lantus, Semglee, Toujeo)	Long	Gradual: begins at 1.1 h	No peak	To 24 h	Subcutaneous: once daily, same time each day	Do not mix with any other insulin
Insulin glulisine (Apidra)	Rapid	15–30 min	1 h	3–4 h	Subcutaneous: 15 min before meal	Can give with NPH; draw glulisine up first, give immediately
Insulin lispro (Admelog, Humalog)	Rapid	5–15 min	0.5–1 h	3–4 h	Subcutaneous: 15 min before or immediately after a meal	Can give with NPH; draw lispro up first, give immediately
Insulin regular (Humulin R, Myxredlin, Novolin R)	Short	30–60 min	2–4 h	5–7 h	Subcutaneous: 30–60 min before meal; IV	Can mix with NPH, sterile water, normal saline; do not mix with glargine
Isophane insulin suspension (Humulin N, NPH, ReliOn N)	Intermediate	1–2 h	4–12 h	18–24 h	Subcutaneous: mix (cloudy)	Can mix with aspart, lispro, reg; do not mix with glargine

glucose. Hypoglycemia may occur when the insulin level peaks, during exercise, when the patient receives too much insulin due to a medication error, or if the patient skips a meal. Some of the symptoms of hypoglycemia are the same as those of DKA. Those that differ and help to determine that a patient is hypoglycemic include pale, cool, and moist skin, with blood glucose less than 50 mg/dL and a sudden onset of symptoms. Left untreated, severe hypoglycemia may result in death.

Other adverse effects of insulin include injection-site reactions, generalized urticaria, and swollen lymph glands. Some patients will experience Somogyi phenomenon, a rapid decrease in blood glucose, usually during the night, which stimulates the release of hormones that elevate blood glucose (epinephrine, cortisol, and glucagon), resulting in an elevated morning blood glucose level. Administration of insulin above the patient's normal dose may produce a rapid rebound hypoglycemia. The hormone glucagon is administered as a replacement therapy for some patients with diabetes when they are in a hypoglycemic state and have impaired glucagon secretion.

Patients with diabetes who forget their insulin dose face equally serious consequences. Again, remember the fundamental principle of insulin pharmacotherapy: The right amount of insulin must be available to cells when glucose is present in the blood. Without insulin present, glucose from a meal can build up to high levels in the blood, causing hyperglycemia and possible coma. Proper planning and teaching by the nurse are essential to achieve successful outcomes and maximize patient adherence with therapy.

Pramlintide (Symlin) is an antihyperglycemic drug approved in 2005 that is used along with insulin in patients with type 1 or type 2 diabetes who are not able to achieve glucose control by the use of insulin alone. The drug is a synthetic analog of amylin, a natural hormone released by the beta cells of the pancreas at the same time as insulin. Its natural function is to act synergistically with insulin in glycemic control. The therapeutic actions of pramlintide are to slow gastric emptying time, reduce postprandial glucagon secretion, and increase satiety, thereby leading to reduced calorie intake. Pramlintide is administered subcutaneously immediately prior to major meals using a premeasured disposable injector called a SymlinPen. It cannot be mixed with insulin, and it must be injected into a different site than insulin. When initiating treatment, rapid- or short-acting insulin doses are usually reduced by 50%. Adverse effects include nausea and vomiting, abdominal pain, headache, dizziness, fatigue, coughing, allergic reaction, or arthralgia. The drug carries a black box warning that severe hypoglycemia may occur during therapy. Hypoglycemia may be prolonged and severe, usually occurring within 3 hours following an injection.

PROTOTYPE DRUG Human Regular Insulin (Humulin R, Myxredlin, Novolin R)

Classification **Therapeutic:** Antidiabetic drug, pancreatic hormone
Pharmacologic: Short-acting hypoglycemic drug

Therapeutic Effects and Uses: Human regular insulin is used to maintain blood glucose levels within normal limits. The primary effects of human regular insulin are promotion of cellular uptake of glucose, amino acids, and potassium; promotion of protein synthesis, glycogen formation and storage, and fatty acid storage as triglycerides; and conservation of energy stores by promoting the utilization of glucose for energy needs and inhibiting gluconeogenesis. Indications for insulin include the following:

- As monotherapy to lower blood glucose levels in patients with type 1 diabetes
- In combination with other antidiabetic drugs in patients with type 2 diabetes
- For the emergency treatment of DKA or hyperosmolar hyperglycemic state
- For gestational diabetes.

Because regular insulin is short acting, it is most often used in combination with intermediate- or long-acting insulin to achieve 24-hour glucose control. Nondiabetic indications for insulin include stimulation of growth hormone secretion in the evaluation of growth hormone deficiency and the treatment of hyperkalemia to promote a shift of potassium into cells.

Mechanism of Action: Regular insulin is identical to endogenous insulin. Insulin decreases blood glucose levels by increasing cellular uptake of glucose and stimulating storage of glucose as glycogen; it also inhibits the release of glucagon.

Pharmacokinetics:

Route(s)	Subcutaneous; IV (only regular insulin and Myxredlin are given IV)
Absorption	Rapidly absorbed following subcutaneous injection; absorption time can vary by site of injection
Distribution	Throughout extracellular fluids
Primary metabolism	Hepatic
Primary excretion	Liver and kidneys
Onset of action	Subcutaneous: 30–60 min; IV: 15 min
Duration of action	6–10 h

Adverse Effects: The most common adverse effect of insulin therapy is hypoglycemia. Rebound hyperglycemia

(Somogyi phenomenon) may occur. Irritation at injection sites may occur, including lipohypertrophy, the accumulation of fat in the area of injection. This effect is lessened with rotation of injection sites. Weight gain is a possible adverse effect. Because insulin facilitates the intracellular uptake of potassium, hypokalemia is possible.

Contraindications/Precautions: Insulin is used with caution in pregnancy, CKD, fever, and thyroid disease and among infants, children, and older adults. Insulin should not be administered to patients with hypoglycemia. Patients with hypokalemia should be monitored carefully because insulin may worsen this condition.

Drug Interactions: Caution must be used when insulin is concurrently administered with drugs that can produce hypoglycemia, including sulfonylureas, meglitinides, beta-adrenergic blockers, salicylates, anabolic steroids, monoamine oxidase inhibitors (MAOIs), and alcohol. Several drugs can antagonize the glucose-lowering effects of insulin including dextrothyroxine, corticosteroids, epinephrine or norepinephrine, furosemide, and thiazide diuretics. Angiotensin-converting enzyme inhibitors increase insulin sensitivity and may enhance the hypoglycemic effects of insulin. Many other drugs can influence blood glucose and the nurse should consult current drug references when treating patients who take high insulin doses or who have unstable diabetes. **Herbal/Food:** Garlic, chromium, black cohosh, bitter melon, bilberry, and ginseng may potentiate the hypoglycemic effects of insulin. Cocoa and rosemary may have a hyperglycemic effect.

Pregnancy: Human observational data have not associated insulin use with significant adverse fetal outcomes. However, poorly controlled diabetes in pregnant women is associated with major birth defects. No adverse effects have been associated with insulin use during breastfeeding.

Treatment of Overdose: An overdose of insulin can cause profound hypoglycemia, which is treated with a concentrated source of glucose (dextrose), such as D_5W or glucagon, by the parenteral route.

Clinician Responsibilities: Key clinical implications for patients receiving regular insulin are included in Applied Clinical Judgment: Patients Receiving Pharmacotherapy with Insulin.

Drugs Similar to Human Regular Insulin (Humulin R, Novolin R)

Many types of insulin are available. They are categorized by their onset of action and duration of action, as given in Table 66.2. Premixed formulations of insulin, such as Humulin 70/30, are also available. This type contains 70% NPH insulin and 30% regular insulin, so it can be given before a meal to help control postprandial glucose while also providing longer coverage of insulin needs. The combination insulins are shown in Table 66.3.

Insulin aspart (NovoLog): Insulin aspart is a rapid-onset drug, with a structure very similar to that of endogenous insulin. Insulin aspart has a more rapid onset of action than regular insulin, acting within about 15 minutes when given subcutaneously. Because insulin aspart acts rapidly, injections should be made 5 to 10 minutes before meals. It also has a short duration of action, 3 to 5 hours when compared to regular insulin. Because of its short duration, insulin aspart is usually given in combination with an intermediate- or long-acting form of insulin. Insulin aspart is available in 10-mL vials and 3-mL prefilled cartridges.

Insulin degludec (Tresiba): Insulin degludec is a newer long-acting insulin analog approved in 2015 for both type 1 and type 2 diabetes. Because it has a long duration of up to 42 hours, it may be taken at any time of day, regardless of meals. It is administered by the subcutaneous route. Ryzodeg 70/30 is a mixture of insulin degludec and insulin aspart, a rapid-acting human insulin analog.

Insulin detemir (Levemir): Insulin detemir is a long-acting insulin with a slow onset and dose-dependent duration of action. Detemir may be given once or twice a day, depending on the dose, which is individualized to the patient. At low doses (0.2 unit/kg), effects persist about 12 hours. At higher doses (0.4 unit/kg), effects last 20 to 24 hours. Because of its slow onset and prolonged duration, insulin detemir is used to provide basal glycemic control. It is not injected before meals to control postprandial hyperglycemia. It cannot be mixed with any other type of insulin and is only given by subcutaneous injection. Insulin detemir is supplied in 10-mL vials, 3-mL cartridges, a 3-mL pen, and a 3-mL InnoLet dosing device. The InnoLet dosing injection device is disposable and has an easy-to-read dial, large push

Table 66.3 Premixed Insulin Combinations

Drug	Description	Onset (min)	Peak (h)	Duration (h)	Adverse Effects
Humalog Mix 75/25	75% insulin lispro protamine/25% insulin lispro	15–20	1–2	10–16	*Pain and swelling at injection site* Hypoglycemia, DKA
Humulin 50/50	50% NPH insulin/50% regular insulin	30–60	2–12	10–16	
Humulin 70/30	70% NPH insulin/30% regular insulin	30–60	2–12	10–16	
Novolin 70/30	70% NPH insulin/30% regular insulin	30–60	2–12	Up to 24	
NovoLog Mix 70/30	70% insulin aspart protamine/30% insulin aspart	5–20	1–2	10–16	

Note: *Italics* indicate common adverse effects. Underline indicates serious adverse effects.

button for injection, and audible clicks that indicate each unit injected.

Insulin glargine (Basaglar, Lantus, Toujeo): Insulin glargine is a recombinant insulin analog that exhibits constant, long-duration insulin activity. It has no defined peak effect and provides for the maintenance of steady blood levels, leading to a lowered risk of hypoglycemia. Insulin glargine allows for once-daily dosing as basal insulin coverage. Although it can be given without regard to meals, it should be given at the same time each day to provide consistent blood levels. It cannot be mixed with any other type of insulin and is only given by subcutaneous injection. Insulin glargine may also help improve the lipid profiles and A1C levels of type 2 diabetes when added to therapy.

Insulin glulisine (Apidra): Insulin glulisine has a 10- to 15-minute onset and a short duration of 3 to 5 hours. Because of its rapid onset, the drug should be administered no sooner than 15 minutes before eating and no later than 20 minutes after starting a meal. Apidra is given by subcutaneous injection.

Insulin lispro (Humalog): Insulin lispro is a rapid-acting analog of regular insulin, with effects beginning within 15 to 30 minutes of subcutaneous injection. Insulin lispro acts faster than regular insulin but has a shorter duration of action, 5 hours or less. Because of its rapid onset, insulin lispro should be administered immediately before eating or shortly after eating. It is intended to help control the rise in blood glucose brought on by a meal and is normally given concurrently with an intermediate- or long-acting drug that provides a basal coverage of insulin. It is a clear insulin and does not require mixing prior to injecting. Lispro is often used with insulin infusion pumps and cannot be given IV.

Isophane insulin (Humulin N, NPH): Isophane insulin is the only intermediate-acting insulin. It has a slower onset of action (1 to 4 hours) than regular insulin and a duration of action of up to 18 to 24 hours. It is used to provide a basal level of insulin coverage between meals and at night. NPH insulin is normally administered 30 minutes before the first meal of the day, but in some instances a second, smaller dose is taken before the evening meal or at bedtime. Many patients are prescribed insulin that is premixed, such as 70% NPH with 30% regular or rapid acting. NPH is a cloudy suspension and requires mixing prior to drawing up a dose. NPH can be given with aspart, lispro, or regular insulin, but it cannot be mixed with glargine insulin. When mixed with another type of insulin, NPH should be drawn up after the other insulin, and the mixture should be administered immediately. The term *NPH* stands for neutral protamine Hagedorn, named for Hans Christian Hagedorn who was the scientist who developed the drug in the 1920s.

CONNECTIONS: Lifespan Considerations

Diabetes in the School Setting

Caring for the school-age child with diabetes in a school setting requires teamwork among the parents or caregiver, school nurse, school staff, the child's healthcare provider, and, most often, the child. For each child, an individual diabetes medical management plan (DMMP) should be established that addresses all aspects of diabetes care. The ADA (2020) recommends the following specific instructions be included in each child's DMMP:

- Blood glucose monitoring instructions, including the frequency and circumstances for requiring monitoring.
- Information on insulin injections, if used, to include type(s) of insulin, dose, times for administration, storage, and provider permission for adjustments in insulin dosage, if needed.
- Information on meals and snacks, including scheduling, the need for the child to be able to eat prn (as needed) to prevent hypoglycemia, and content and calories of school lunches.
- Symptoms and treatment for hypoglycemia and hyperglycemia. Specific levels of training should be provided to school personnel based on whether they will administer basic, intermediate, or advanced treatment in caring for the child.
- Information on participation in physical activity.
- Emergency plans for emergency evacuation, shelter-in-place, or school lockdowns.

By establishing a DMMP, routine daily care as well as emergency contingencies can be addressed. When all participants work as a team, a child with diabetes can participate fully and safely in the school setting.

CONNECTIONS: APPLIED CLINICAL JUDGMENT

Patients Receiving Pharmacotherapy with Insulin

Key Assessment Data

- History of current condition including duration and severity and other related signs or symptoms (e.g., paresthesias of hands or feet), baseline vital signs, physical exam findings, and endocrine, cardiovascular, hepatic, or kidney disease; pregnancy or breastfeeding; drug history including allergies, current prescription and over-the-counter (OTC) drugs and herbal preparations, and caffeine, nicotine, and alcohol use. Assess feet and lower extremities for possible injury, infection, or ulcerations.
- Obtain a dietary history including caloric intake if on an ADA diet, number of meals and snacks per day. Assess fluid intake and type of fluids consumed.

CONNECTIONS: APPLIED CLINICAL JUDGMENT *(continued)*

Patients Receiving Pharmacotherapy with Insulin

Desired Therapeutic Outcomes

Improvement is observed and measurable by glucose levels remaining within normal limits, electrolytes and osmolality remaining normal, A1C level demonstrates adequate glucose control.

Minimizing Adverse Effects

- Hypoglycemia is especially likely to occur around peak insulin activity, especially if food sources are inadequate. Insulin may be held if less than 70 mg/dL or per individual patient parameters.
- Insulin needs may increase or decrease during periods of illness or stress. Frequent monitoring during these times helps to prevent hypoglycemia and ensures adequate glucose control.
- Exercise assists muscles to use glucose more efficiently and increases insulin receptor sites in the tissues, lowering the blood sugar. Benefits of exercise and lowered blood sugar may continue for up to 48 hours, increasing the risk of hypoglycemia during this time. Frequent monitoring helps to prevent hypoglycemia and ensures adequate glucose control.
- Rotating injection sites weekly helps to prevent lipodystrophy. Insulin pump subcutaneous catheters should be changed every 2 to 3 days to prevent infections at the site of insertion.
- Unopened insulin may be stored at room temperature but avoid direct sunlight and excessive heat. Opened insulin vials may be stored at room temperature for up to 1 month. If noticeable change in solution occurs or if precipitate forms, discard the vial.
- Caloric needs and protein, carbohydrate, and fat percentages are calculated based on activity level and lifestyle and the need for weight loss. Alcohol use should be limited or eliminated. As alcohol is metabolized, it can raise and then precipitously lower blood sugar, increasing the risk of hypoglycemia.

Lifespan Considerations

- Age-related physiologic differences may place the older adult at greater risk for hypoglycemia.

Patient Education

- Observe for symptoms of hyper- and hypoglycemia and check capillary glucose levels routinely and if symptoms are present. If unsure whether symptoms indicate hypo- or hyperglycemia, treat as hypoglycemia and then check capillary glucose. If symptoms are not relieved in 10 to 15 minutes, or if capillary glucose is below 70 mg/dL (or parameters as ordered), immediately notify the healthcare provider.
- Monitor capillary glucose levels as ordered. Ensure that adequate food sources are consumed around peak insulin activity to avoid hypoglycemia, and carry a quick-acting carbohydrate, as well as a protein source, for times when food is not available and symptoms of hypoglycemia are present. Report any consistent elevations or hypoglycemia to the healthcare provider.
- Limit or eliminate alcohol use. If alcoholic beverages are consumed, limit to one per day and consume along with a complete meal to ensure that food intake balances alcohol metabolism.
- Notify the healthcare provider if unable to eat normal meals during periods of illness or stress for possible change in insulin dose.
- Exercise should occur an hour after a meal or after a 10- or 15-g carbohydrate snack to prevent hypoglycemia. If exercise is prolonged, small, frequent carbohydrate snacks can be consumed every 30 minutes during exercise to maintain blood sugar.
- Rotate insulin injection sites on a weekly basis to prevent tissue damage or rotate subcutaneous insulin pump catheter sites every 2 to 3 days.
- Take the insulin following appropriate guidelines:
  - Rotate vials gently between the palms and do not shake; if insulins are mixed, draw up the quickest-acting insulin and then the longer-acting one if insulins are compatible; insulin glargine or insulin detemir should not be mixed with any other type of insulin; use the appropriate syringe (100 unit) unless small amounts of insulin are ordered, then obtain syringes with smaller volumes to ensure accurate dosing.
  - Rotation of the site of injection should occur every week, inject at 90-degree angle, and apply a pad to the site after injection but do not massage the site.
  - Proper use of all equipment: blood glucose monitoring equipment, insulin pump.
- Carry a medical identification card or wear medical alert jewelry indicating diabetes.

Prescribing Considerations

- Ongoing assessment during drug therapy should include monitoring appropriate laboratory findings (e.g., complete blood count [CBC], electrolytes, glucose, A1C level, lipid profile, osmolality, and hepatic and renal function studies).
- Prescribers should follow the American Association of Clinical Endocrinologists and American College of Endocrinology practice guidelines (*https://pro.aace.com/disease-state-resources/diabetes/clinical-practice-guidelines/aaceace-clinical-practice-guidelines*).

CONNECTIONS: Patient Safety

Incorrect Insulin Dose

A patient with diabetes has 30 units of Humulin R (regular) insulin ordered for the morning dose. There are several patients with diabetes on the unit and the nurse has given many doses of insulin that morning. The nurse prepares the insulin but draws up Humalog 30 units instead. The patient begins experiencing symptoms of hypoglycemia within 15 minutes and is treated successfully.

What errors occurred and how could they be prevented in the future?

Antidiabetic Drugs for Type 2 Diabetes

66.7 Antidiabetic drugs from multiple classes are used to treat type 2 diabetes.

The primary classes of antidiabetic drugs used to treat type 2 diabetes are differentiated by their chemical structures and their mechanisms of action. Drug classes prescribed for patients with type 2 diabetes include alpha-glucosidase inhibitors, biguanides, incretin mimics, incretin enhancers, meglitinides, sodium-glucose co-transporter inhibitors, sulfonylureas, and thiazolidinediones. An additional group includes miscellaneous drugs from other classes. All the medications used to treat type 2 diabetes require some degree of endogenous insulin secretion. These antidiabetic medications are not effective in treating type 1 diabetes because these patients have a total lack of insulin secretion.

Most treatment goals are designed to target an A1C level of 6.5% or less. Although all of the antidiabetic drugs are similar in their ability to lower A1C levels in the short term, there are some differences in long-term control. For example, drugs in the thiazolidinedione class appear to maintain glycemic control for 5 to 6 years, whereas the sulfonylureas peak at 6 months and slowly decline in efficacy. The adverse effects observed for each class differ: Some cause hypoglycemia, whereas others cause weight gain or GI complaints such as diarrhea. Because there is no perfect drug for type 2 diabetes, choice of therapy is guided by the experiences of the prescriber and the results achieved by the individual patient. A comparison of the antidiabetic drug classes is presented in Table 66.4. Doses of the individual medications are listed in Table 66.5.

Therapy for type 2 diabetes is usually initiated with a single drug with metformin being a preferred agent. If glycemic control is not achieved with monotherapy, a second medication is added to the therapeutic regimen. Failure to achieve glycemic control with two oral antidiabetic drugs suggests the need for insulin to be added to the regimen.

Many fixed-dose combination products are available and frequently used for the treatment of type 2 diabetes. The main advantage of taking a combination drug is that it is more convenient than taking two separate drugs and may improve adherence to the therapeutic regimen. Doses for selected combination products are listed in Table 66.6.

Biguanides

Metformin (Glucophage) is the only drug in this class. It is a preferred drug for managing type 2 diabetes because of its superior effectiveness and safety.

PROTOTYPE DRUG **Metformin (Glucophage, Glumetza, Others)**

Classification **Therapeutic:** Antidiabetic drug
Pharmacologic: Biguanide

Therapeutic Effects and Uses: Approved in 1994, metformin lowers blood glucose levels in patients with type 2 diabetes who are unable to control glucose levels by diet and exercise. It can be used alone or in combination with sulfonylureas, alpha-glucosidase inhibitors, or insulin. It is approved for use in children age 10 and older. Several formulations of metformin are available:

- **Regular-release tablets.** Administered once or twice daily, absorption is decreased with food, and the peak plasma level is 2.5 hours.
- **Solution (Riomet).** Administered once or twice daily, absorption is slightly increased with food, and the peak plasma level is 2.3 hours.
- **Extended release (Fortamet, Glucophage XR, Glumetza, Riomet ER).** These are long-duration systems in which metformin is slowly released from a semipermeable membrane (Fortamet), gel (Glucophage XR), or gastric-retentive technology (Glumetza). Administered once daily, absorption is significantly increased with food and the peak plasma level is 6 to 8 hours.

Metformin reduces fasting and postprandial glucose levels. Because it does not promote insulin release, it does not

Table 66.4 Summary of Antidiabetic Drug Classes

Drug	Action(s)	Nursing Considerations
Alpha-Glucosidase Inhibitors	Interfere with carbohydrate breakdown and absorption; act locally in the GI tract with little systemic absorption	Common GI effects; hypoglycemia can occur if combined with another oral drug; if this occurs, treat with glucose, not sucrose; take with meals
Biguanides	Decrease production and release of glucose from the liver; increase cellular uptake of glucose; lower lipid levels; promote weight loss	Common GI adverse effects; risk for lactic acidosis (rare); avoid alcohol; low risk for hypoglycemia
Incretin enhancers	Slow the breakdown of insulin, keeping it circulating in the blood longer; slow the rate of digestion, which increases satiety	Well tolerated; minor nausea, vomiting and diarrhea; some weight loss is likely; low risk for hypoglycemia
Meglitinides	Stimulate insulin release	Can cause hypoglycemia, GI effects; well tolerated; administer shortly before meals
Sodium-glucose cotransporter-2 inhibitors	Inhibit reabsorption of glucose in the nephron, thus increasing its urinary excretion; promotes weight loss	Frequently cause increased urogenital infections; may also cause DKA and hypoglycemia
Sulfonylureas	Stimulate insulin release; decrease insulin resistance	Can cause hypoglycemia, GI disturbances, rash; cross sensitivity with sulfa drugs and thiazide diuretics; possible disulfiram response with alcohol
Thiazolidinediones	Decrease production and release of glucose from the liver; increase insulin sensitivity in fat and muscle tissue	Can cause fluid retention and worsening of HF; therapeutic effects take several weeks to develop

Table 66.5 Antidiabetic Drugs for Type 2 Diabetes

Drug	Route and Adult Dose (Maximum Dose Where Indicated)	Adverse Effects
Alpha-Glucosidase Inhibitors		
acarbose	PO: 25–100 mg tid (max: 300 mg/day)	*Flatulence, diarrhea, abdominal distention* Hypoglycemia (tremors, palpitations, sweating)
miglitol (Glyset)	PO: 25–100 mg tid (max: 300 mg/day)	
Biguanide		
metformin immediate release (Glucophage, Riomet) extended release (Fortamet, Glucophage XR, Glumetza, Riomet ER)	PO: 500 mg bid or 850 mg once daily; increase to 1000–2550 mg in 2–3 divided doses/day (max: 2.55 g/day) Glumetza: 1000–2000 mg once daily (max: 2 g/day) Glucophage XR: 500 mg once daily (max 2 g/day) Fortamet: 1000 mg once daily (max: 2.5 g/day)	*Flatulence, diarrhea, nausea, anorexia, abdominal pain, bitter or metallic taste, decreased vitamin B_{12} levels* Lactic acidosis
Incretin Enhancers (DPP-4 Inhibitors)		
linagliptin (Tradjenta)	PO: 5 mg once daily without regard to meals	*Headache, upper respiratory and urinary tract infections* Hypoglycemia (tremors, palpitations, sweating), anaphylaxis, peripheral edema, exfoliative dermatitis, Stevens–Johnson syndrome
saxagliptin (Onglyza)	PO: 2.5–5 mg once daily without regard to meals	
sitagliptin (Januvia)	PO: 100 mg once daily	
Incretin Mimetics (GLP-1 Receptor Agonists)		
dulaglutide (Trulicity)	Subcutaneous: 0.75–1.5 mg once weekly	*Nausea and vomiting, diarrhea, headache, nervousness* Hypoglycemia (tremors, palpitations, sweating), antibody formation, pancreatitis, worsening of CKD, thyroid C-cell tumors
exenatide (Bydureon, Byetta)	Subcutaneous: 5–10 mcg bid 60 min prior to morning and evening meals (Byetta) or 2 mg once weekly without regard to meals (Bydureon)	
liraglutide (Victoza)	Subcutaneous: 0.6–1.8 mg once daily, any time of day	
lixisenatide (Adlyxin)	Subcutaneous: 10–20 mcg once daily prior to morning meal	
semaglutide (Ozempic)	Subcutaneous: 0.25–1.0 mg/wk, without regard to meals	
Meglitinides		
nateglinide (Starlix)	PO: 60–120 mg tid, 1–30 min prior to meals	*Flulike symptoms, upper respiratory infection, back pain* Hypoglycemia (tremors, palpitations, sweating), anaphylaxis, pancreatitis
repaglinide	PO: 0.5–4 mg bid–qid, 1–30 min prior to meals (max: 16 mg/day)	
Sodium-Glucose Co-transporter Inhibitors		
canagliflozin (Invokana)	PO: 100 mg once daily (max: 300 mg/day) taken before first meal	*Female genital mycotic infections, urinary tract infection, nasopharyngitis* Hypotension, CKD, hyperkalemia, hypoglycemia (with use of insulin or sulfonylureas)
dapagliflozin (Farxiga)	PO: 5–10 mg once daily in the morning, with or without food	
empagliflozin (Jardiance)	PO: 10–25 mg once daily in the morning, with or without food	
ertugliflozin (Segluromet)	PO: 5–15 mg daily in the morning, with or without food	
Sulfonylureas		
glimepiride (Amaryl)	PO: 1–4 mg/day (max: 8 mg/day)	*Nausea, heartburn, dizziness, headache, drowsiness* Hypoglycemia (tremors, palpitations, sweating), cholestatic jaundice, blood dyscrasias
glipizide (Glucotrol)	PO: 2.5–20 mg 1–2 times/day (max: 40 mg/day)	
glyburide (DiaBeta) glyburide micronized (Glynase)	PO: 1.25–10 mg 1–2 times/day (max: 20 mg/day) PO: 0.75–12 mg 1–2 times/day (max: 12 mg/day)	
Thiazolidinediones		
pioglitazone (Actos)	PO: 15–30 mg/day (max: 45 mg/day)	*Upper respiratory infection, myalgia, headache, edema, weight gain* Hypoglycemia (tremors, palpitations, sweating), hepatotoxicity, bone fractures, HF, myocardial infarction (MI)
rosiglitazone (Avandia)	PO: 4–8 mg 1–2 times/day (max: 8 mg/day)	

Note: *Italics* indicate common adverse effects. Underline indicates serious adverse effects.

cause hypoglycemia, which is a major advantage of the drug. The drug actions do not depend on stimulating insulin release, so it is able to lower glucose levels in patients who no longer secrete insulin. In addition to lowering blood glucose levels, it lowers triglyceride levels, lowers total and low-density lipoprotein (LDL) cholesterol levels, and promotes weight loss.

Metformin may be used off-label to treat women with polycystic ovary syndrome. Women with this syndrome have insulin resistance and high serum insulin levels. Metformin reduces insulin resistance, which in turn lowers insulin and androgen levels, thus restoring normal menstrual cycles and ovulation.

Table 66.6 Selected Combination Oral Antidiabetic Drugs*

Trade-Name Drug	Generic Drug Combination	Route and Adult Dose (Maximum Dose Where Indicated)
Actoplus Met	pioglitazone/metformin	PO: 15 mg/500–850 mg bid (regular release) or 15–30 mg/1000 mg once daily (extended release)
Duetact	pioglitazone/glimepiride	PO: Start with 30 mg/2 mg once daily (max: 45 mg/8 mg daily)
—	glyburide/metformin	PO: 1.25–5 mg/250–500 mg once or twice daily with a meal (max: 20 mg/2000 mg daily)
Invokamet XR	canagliflozin/metformin	PO: 50–150 mg/500–1000 mg two tablets with the morning meal
Janumet	sitagliptin/metformin	PO: Starting dose 50 mg/500 mg bid (regular release) or 100 mg/1000 mg once daily (extended release) (max: 100 mg/2000 mg/day)
Jentadueto	linagliptin/metformin	PO: 2.5 mg/500–1000 mg bid (regular release) or 5 mg/1000 mg once daily (extended release) with meals
Kazano	alogliptin/metformin	PO: 12.5 mg/500 mg bid with meal
Kombiglyze XR	saxigliptin/metformin	PO: 2.5–5 mg/500–1000 mg once daily with the evening meal
Oseni	alogliptin/pioglitazone	PO: 25 mg/15 mg once daily with or without food
Qtern	dapagliflozin/saxagliptin	PO: 10 mg/5 mg once daily with morning meal
Segluromet	ertugliflozin/metformin	PO: 2.5–7.5 mg/500–1000 mg twice daily with meals
Synjardy	empagliflozin/metformin	PO: 12.5 mg/1000 mg bid with meals (regular release) or 25 mg/2000 mg once daily with morning meal (extended release)
Xigduo XR	dapagliflozin/metformin	PO: 2.5–10 mg/500–1000 mg once daily with the morning meal

*Dosage levels are determined individually according to patient response and glycemic laboratory results.

Mechanism of Action: Metformin reduces blood glucose levels by multiple mechanisms. The drug reduces gluconeogenesis, thereby suppressing hepatic production of glucose. In addition, the drug decreases the intestinal reabsorption of glucose and increases the cellular uptake of glucose.

Pharmacokinetics:

Route(s)	PO (regular-release tablets, solution, and extended-release preparations)
Absorption	Approximately 50–60% of a dose reaches systemic circulation; extended-release forms are absorbed very slowly
Distribution	Distributed to most tissues; crosses the placenta; secreted in breast milk; not protein bound
Primary metabolism	Not metabolized
Primary excretion	Kidneys
Onset of action	Less than 1 h; peak action: 1–3 h
Duration of action	12 h (regular release); 24 h (extended release)

Adverse Effects: The most common adverse effects that occur in 30% of patients taking metformin are GI related and include nausea and vomiting, abdominal discomfort, metallic taste, diarrhea, anorexia, and moderate weight loss. It may also cause headache, dizziness, agitation, and fatigue. Unlike the sulfonylureas, metformin rarely causes hypoglycemia or weight gain. **Black Box Warning:** Lactic acidosis is a rare, though potentially fatal, adverse effect of metformin therapy. The risk for lactic acidosis is increased in patients with CKD or any condition that puts them at risk for increased lactic acid production, such as liver disease, severe infection, excessive alcohol intake, shock, or hypoxemia.

Contraindications/Precautions: Metformin is contraindicated in patients with severe CKD because the drug can rise to toxic levels. It is also contraindicated in patients with HF, liver failure, history of lactic acidosis, concurrent serious infection, or with any condition that predisposes the patient to hypoxemia. It is contraindicated for 2 days prior to, and 2 days after, receiving IV radiographic contrast. Metformin is used with caution in patients with anemia, diarrhea, vomiting, dehydration, fever, gastroparesis, or GI obstruction; in older adults; and in those with hyperthyroidism, pituitary insufficiency, or trauma. Safety in children under age 10 has not been established.

Drug Interactions: Alcohol increases the risk for lactic acidosis and should be avoided. Captopril, furosemide, and nifedipine may increase the risk for hypoglycemia. Use with IV radiographic contrast may cause lactic acidosis and CKD. The following drugs may decrease renal excretion of metformin: amiloride, cimetidine, digoxin, dofetilide, midodrine, morphine, procainamide, quinidine, ranitidine, triamterene, trimethoprim, and vancomycin. Acarbose may decrease blood levels of metformin. Use with other antidiabetic drugs potentiates hypoglycemic effects. **Herbal/Food:** Metformin decreases the absorption of vitamin B_{12} and folic acid. Garlic and ginseng may increase hypoglycemic effects.

Pregnancy: Studies in laboratory animals as well as human data have not shown fetal harm. The drug is secreted in human milk although adverse effects on the breastfed neonate are not known.

Treatment of Overdose: Lactic acidosis can occur with metformin overdose. Hemodialysis can be used to correct the acidosis and remove excess metformin.

Clinician Responsibilities: Key clinical implications for patients receiving metformin are included in Applied Clinical Judgment: Patients Receiving Pharmacotherapy for Type 2 Diabetes.

Drugs Similar to Metformin (Glucophage, Glumetza, Others)

Metformin is the only biguanide available.

Sulfonylureas

This was the first oral antidiabetic drug class developed. Once divided into first- and second-generation categories, all the first-generation agents have since been discontinued.

The sulfonylureas act by stimulating the release of insulin from pancreatic islet cells and by increasing the sensitivity of insulin receptors on target cells. The most common adverse effect is hypoglycemia, which is usually caused by taking too much medication or not eating enough food. Hypoglycemia from these drugs may be prolonged and require administration of dextrose to return serum glucose to normal levels. Other adverse effects include weight gain, hypersensitivity reactions, GI distress, and hepatotoxicity. When alcohol is taken with sulfonylureas, some patients experience an uncomfortable disulfiram-like reaction, with flushing, palpitations, and nausea.

PROTOTYPE DRUG **Glyburide (DiaBeta, Glynase)**

Classification **Therapeutic:** Antidiabetic drug
Pharmacologic: Sulfonylurea

Therapeutic Effects and Uses: Approved in 1984, glyburide is a second-generation sulfonylurea used to lower blood glucose levels in patients with type 2 diabetes. Glyburide can be used alone or in combination with another oral hypoglycemic drug. It should be used only if diet and exercise have proven ineffective in controlling the elevated blood glucose levels.

Two types of glyburide are available: the conventional form (DiaBeta) and a micronized form (Glynase). Glynase allows for lower doses compared to the conventional forms. Glucovance is a combination product that contains glyburide and metformin.

Mechanism of Action: Glyburide stimulates the release of insulin from pancreatic beta cells and increases the sensitivity of peripheral tissues to insulin. The stimulation of insulin release relies on some residual beta cell functioning; therefore, the drug is not effective for type 1 diabetes.

Pharmacokinetics:

Route(s)	Oral (PO)
Absorption	Readily absorbed following PO administration
Distribution	Distributed widely to body tissues, with greatest concentrations in liver, kidneys, and intestines; crosses the placenta
Primary metabolism	Extensive hepatic metabolism
Primary excretion	Equal in urine and feces
Onset of action	15–60 min
Duration of action	Up to 24 h

Adverse Effects: The primary adverse effect of glyburide is hypoglycemia. Patients at increased risk for hypoglycemia include those with CKD or hepatic insufficiency, those consuming an improper diet, and patients who are older or malnourished. Excessive exercise or alcohol consumption also increases the risk for hypoglycemia. Other adverse effects of therapy include heartburn, nausea and vomiting, diarrhea, pruritus, erythema, urticaria, photosensitivity, and blurred vision. Rare, though serious, adverse effects include hepatotoxicity, cholestatic jaundice, aplastic anemia, leukopenia, thrombocytopenia, and agranulocytosis.

Contraindications/Precautions: Glyburide is contraindicated in patients with a known sensitivity to sulfa drugs or thiazide diuretics because sulfonylureas are chemically similar to sulfa drugs. It is contraindicated as the primary treatment for type 1 diabetes, diabetic coma, or DKA. The drug is used with caution in patients with CKD or hepatic disease because the drug may accumulate to toxic levels.

Drug Interactions: Many drug interactions are possible with sulfonylureas. Using alcohol with glyburide can interfere with glycemic control and has resulted in a disulfiram-type response, with severe nausea and vomiting, flushing, and palpitations. Drugs that can increase hypoglycemia when taken with glyburide are probenecid, sulfonamides, chloramphenicol, and salicylates. Increased risk of hyperglycemia can occur with use of rifampin and thiazides. Ciprofloxacin, ACE inhibitors, GLP-1 receptor agonists such as dulaglutide, SGLT2 inhibitors such as empagliflozin increase the toxicity of glyburide through a synergistic interaction. **Herbal/Food:** Ginseng, garlic, black cohosh, juniper berries, fenugreek, coriander, or dandelion root can cause hypoglycemia.

Pregnancy: Studies in laboratory animals did not show evidence of fetal harm. Glyburide should be discontinued at least 1 month before delivery because newborns exposed to sulfonylureas may develop severe hypoglycemia lasting several days. Due to the potential for hypoglycemia in the neonate, breastfeeding is not recommended.

Treatment of Overdose: Treatment is the same as for acute hypoglycemia: A concentrated source of glucose is administered.

Clinician Responsibilities: Key clinical implications for patients receiving glyburide are included in Applied Clinical Judgment: Patients Receiving Pharmacotherapy for Type 2 Diabetes.

Drugs Similar to Glyburide (DiaBeta, Glynase)

All first-generation sulfonylureas have been withdrawn from the market. The remaining second-generation sulfonylureas include glimepiride and glipizide. The pregnancy data on these two drugs is the same as for glyburide.

Glimepiride (Amaryl): Approved in 1995, glimepiride can be used alone or in combination with insulin for patients with type 2 diabetes. It is most often given once a day with the first meal of the day. More recently, glimepiride is included in a fixed-dose combination with pioglitazone (Duetact). Because of the increased risk for MI and HF (from rosiglitazone and pioglitazone), the fixed-dose combinations contain a black box warning regarding these risks.

Glipizide (Glucotrol): Approved in 1984, glipizide is available in a standard tablet form and an extended-release (XL) tablet, which should not be crushed or chewed. In addition to treating patients with type 2 diabetes who are unable to achieve glucose control with diet alone, it can be used for short-term therapy for those who normally can control their glucose levels by diet. Once-a-day dosing is given 30 minutes before the first meal of the day.

CONNECTION Checkpoint 66.2

Glyburide combined with alcohol can cause a disulfiram reaction. From what you learned in Chapter 27, what causes the symptoms of the disulfiram reaction and what are common symptoms of this reaction?

Meglitinides

The meglitinides act by stimulating the release of insulin from pancreatic islet cells in a manner similar to that of the sulfonylureas. Both drugs in this class have short durations of action of 2 to 4 hours. Their efficacy is equal to that of the sulfonylureas, and they are well tolerated. Hypoglycemia is the most common adverse effect.

PROTOTYPE DRUG Repaglinide

Classification **Therapeutic:** Antidiabetic drug
Pharmacologic: Meglitinide

Therapeutic Effects and Uses: Approved in 1997, repaglinide is used to lower blood glucose levels in patients with type 2 diabetes as an adjunct to diet and exercise. It may be used alone or in combination with metformin or a thiazolidinedione.

Because repaglinide is absorbed rapidly, it should be taken shortly before each meal. It is effective in lowering postprandial glucose levels and in reducing A1C levels but has little effect on fasting glucose levels. It undergoes almost no renal excretion, and so it can be used in patients with CKD.

Mechanism of Action: Repaglinide lowers glucose levels by stimulating insulin release from pancreatic beta cells. Patients must have some ability to secrete insulin for the drug to be effective.

Pharmacokinetics:

Route(s)	PO
Absorption	Rapidly absorbed following PO administration
Distribution	98% protein bound
Primary metabolism	Hepatic (CYP3A4)
Primary excretion	90% in feces
Onset of action	15–30 min; peak: 1 h
Duration of action	4 h

Adverse Effects: Repaglinide is generally well tolerated; the most common adverse effect is hypoglycemia. Other adverse effects include nausea and vomiting, diarrhea, and dyspepsia. Headache, paresthesias, upper respiratory infections, sinusitis, rhinitis, or bronchitis may also occur.

Contraindications/Precautions: Repaglinide is contraindicated in people with type 1 diabetes or DKA. It should be used with caution in patients with hepatic impairment, in older adults, or in those with systemic infection, surgery, or trauma. Its safety in children has not been established.

Drug Interactions: Drugs that induce hepatic CYP3A4 enzyme such as barbiturates, carbamazepine, rifampin, and pioglitazone may increase repaglinide metabolism and cause hyperglycemia. Drugs that inhibit CYP3A4 such as erythromycin, ketoconazole, and miconazole inhibit repaglinide metabolism and may cause hypoglycemia. Gemfibrozil is contraindicated because it increases the risk for hypoglycemia. Use with isophane insulin may cause myocardial ischemia. **Herbal/Food:** The concurrent intake of grapefruit juice inhibits metabolism and may result in increased repaglinide levels and hypoglycemia. Garlic and ginseng may increase hypoglycemic effects. St. John's wort will decrease the effectiveness of repaglinide.

Pregnancy: High doses caused fetal skeletal deformities in laboratory animals. This drug is secreted in animal milk. Breastfeeding is not recommended due to the potential for hypoglycemia in the neonate.

Treatment of Overdose: Severe hypoglycemia may occur with overdose. These patients should immediately receive a concentrated source of glucose, preferably by the IV route.

Clinician Responsibilities: Key clinical implications for patients receiving repaglinide are included in Applied Clinical Judgment: Patients Receiving Pharmacotherapy for Type 2 Diabetes.

Drugs Similar to Repaglinide

The only other meglitinide is nateglinide.

Nateglinide: Approved in 2000, nateglinide has actions and indications similar to those of repaglinide. It is used as monotherapy or in combination with metformin for managing glucose levels in patients with type 2 diabetes who have not achieved glycemic control through diet and exercise. It is not effective for type 1 diabetes. Like repaglinide, it is given 5 to 20 minutes before meals. An important difference between these drugs is that nateglinide is primarily excreted by the kidneys, so it should be used with caution in patients with CKD. Like repaglinide, nateglinide is well tolerated and hypoglycemia is usually mild. High doses caused fetal skeletal deformities in laboratory animals. The manufacturer recommends this drug not be used during pregnancy or breastfeeding.

Thiazolidinediones

The thiazolidinediones (TZDs), or glitazones, reduce blood glucose by decreasing insulin resistance and inhibiting hepatic formation of glucose. Optimal lowering of blood glucose may require 3 to 4 months of therapy. The most common adverse effects are fluid retention, headache, and weight gain. Hypoglycemia does not occur with drugs in this class. Because of their tendency to promote fluid retention, thiazolidinediones are contraindicated in patients with serious HF or pulmonary edema.

PROTOTYPE DRUG Rosiglitazone (Avandia)

Classification **Therapeutic:** Antidiabetic drug
Pharmacologic: Thiazolidinedione

Therapeutic Effects and Uses: Approved in 1999, rosiglitazone is used to lower blood glucose levels in patients with type 2 diabetes as an adjunct to diet and exercise. It can be used as monotherapy or in combination with metformin, a sulfonylurea, or insulin. It is effective in lowering fasting glucose and A1C levels. Optimal therapeutic effects take several weeks to occur.

Mechanism of Action: Rosiglitazone lowers blood glucose levels by increasing cellular sensitivity to insulin, thereby reducing insulin resistance. In addition, it decreases gluconeogenesis by the liver.

Pharmacokinetics:

Route(s)	PO
Absorption	Rapidly absorbed
Distribution	Greater than 99% protein bound
Primary metabolism	Hepatic (CYP2C8)
Primary excretion	Primarily renal, with approximately 25% in feces
Onset of action	Within 1 h; peak: 1 h
Duration of action	12–24 h

Adverse Effects: Rosiglitazone is generally well tolerated. The most prominent adverse effect is edema, including macular edema. Anemia, headache, back pain, fatigue, diarrhea, upper respiratory infection, or sinusitis may occur. The drug can also raise serum lipid levels, including HDL-cholesterol, triglycerides, and LDL-cholesterol. It is recommended that baseline liver function tests be obtained prior to initiating treatment and then assessed every 3 to 6 months. Patients should be informed of the signs of liver damage (nausea, fatigue, dark urine, jaundice) as well as the signs of HF (dyspnea, weight gain, edema, fatigue) while taking rosiglitazone. Drugs in this class are associated with an increased fracture risk among women. **Black Box Warning:** Drugs in this class can cause or worsen HF due to increased fluid retention. In addition, rosiglitazone may increase the risk of MI.

Contraindications/Precautions: Rosiglitazone is contraindicated in people with severe HF or active liver disease. Its safety in children has not been established. Rosiglitazone is contraindicated in patients with type 1 diabetes or DKA.

Drug Interactions: Inducers of hepatic CYP2C8 such as rifampin may decrease the effects of rosiglitazone. Inhibitors of CYP2C8 such as azole antifungals, fluvoxamine, gemfibrozil, and trimethoprim may elevate rosiglitazone plasma levels and increase the risk for adverse reactions. Concurrent use of rosiglitazone with insulin can increase edema and the risk for HF and myocardial ischemia. Other antidiabetic drugs, angiotensin II receptor antagonists, and gemfibrozil can increase the hypoglycemic effects. Use of rosiglitazone with nitrates is not recommended due to the potential for myocardial ischemia. Thiazide diuretics, phenothiazines, and atypical antipsychotic drugs can decrease the hypoglycemic effects of rosiglitazone by increasing blood glucose levels. **Herbal/Food:** Garlic and ginseng can increase the risk for hypoglycemia if used with rosiglitazone. Cocoa and rosemary may decrease the therapeutic effect and have a hyperglycemic effect.

Pregnancy: Rosiglitazone causes fetal harm in laboratory animals. The manufacturer recommends this drug not be used during pregnancy or lactation.

Treatment of Overdose: Standard treatment for hypoglycemia is initiated during overdose, along with symptomatic treatment of edema or fluid overload.

Clinician Responsibilities: Key clinical implications for patients receiving rosiglitazone are included in Applied Clinical Judgment: Patients Receiving Pharmacotherapy for Type 2 Diabetes.

Drugs Similar to Rosiglitazone (Avandia)

The only other drug in this class is pioglitazone.

Pioglitazone (Actos): Approved in 1999, pioglitazone has actions and uses similar to those of rosiglitazone. It is rapidly absorbed following PO administration, with peak effects occurring within 7 days of beginning therapy. Pioglitazone can decrease serum levels of oral contraceptives and can cause nonovulating premenopausal women to resume ovulation; therefore, a reliable form of contraception is recommended. Excessive alcohol consumption may affect glycemic control. Hepatic function should be assessed for a baseline and periodically thereafter as with rosiglitazone. Pioglitazone has been associated with an increased risk for bladder, prostate, and pancreatic cancer. The drug carries the same black box warnings regarding HF and myocardial ischemia as rosiglitazone. Pregnancy data are the same as for rosiglitazone.

Alpha-Glucosidase Inhibitors

The alpha-glucosidase inhibitors act by blocking enzymes in the small intestine responsible for breaking down complex carbohydrates into monosaccharides. Because carbohydrates must be in the monosaccharide form to be absorbed, digestion of glucose is delayed. These drugs have minimal adverse effects, with the most common being GI related, such as abdominal cramping, diarrhea, and flatulence. Although alpha-glucosidase inhibitors do not produce hypoglycemia when used alone, hypoglycemia may occur when these drugs are combined with insulin or a sulfonylurea.

PROTOTYPE DRUG Acarbose

Classification **Therapeutic:** Antidiabetic drug
Pharmacologic: Alpha-glucosidase inhibitor

Therapeutic Effects and Uses: Approved in 1995, acarbose lowers blood glucose levels in individuals with type 2 diabetes who cannot adequately manage glucose levels by diet and exercise alone. It may be used alone or in combination with a sulfonylurea, metformin, or insulin. By slowing the breakdown and absorption of carbohydrates, the rise in postprandial glucose level is reduced and A1C level is lowered.

Mechanism of Action: Acarbose lowers glucose levels by interfering with carbohydrate absorption from the GI tract. It acts locally in the GI tract to inhibit the enzyme responsible for carbohydrate breakdown.

Pharmacokinetics:

Route(s)	PO
Absorption	Only 2% absorbed (low absorption is desired because the drug acts locally in the GI tract); some metabolites are absorbed
Distribution	Acts locally in the digestive tract
Primary metabolism	Metabolized in the GI tract by intestinal bacteria and digestive enzymes
Primary excretion	Primarily in feces, 30% in urine
Onset of action	Peak: 1 h
Duration of action	2–4 h

Adverse Effects: The most common adverse effects of acarbose are diarrhea, flatulence, abdominal distention, borborygmi, anemia (iron deficiency), urticaria, and erythema. The GI-related effects may diminish as therapy progresses; however, they will worsen if the patient does not adhere to the prescribed diabetic diet. Hypoglycemia may occur if acarbose is combined with other hypoglycemic drugs. If hypoglycemia does develop, it must be treated with glucose and not sucrose (table sugar) because the drug inhibits the absorption of sucrose. Acarbose may cause elevation of liver enzymes (plasma transaminases), although liver damage has not been reported, and enzyme levels return to normal following drug withdrawal.

Contraindications/Precautions: Acarbose is contraindicated in patients with inflammatory bowel disease, bowel obstruction, or colon ulcers and in those predisposed to bowel obstructions. It is used with caution in patients with GI distress or liver disorders. Safety in children has not been established.

Drug Interactions: Use with sulfonylureas may increase the risk for hypoglycemia. Drugs that cause hyperglycemia such as thiazide diuretics, corticosteroids, phenothiazines, estrogens, phenytoin, or isoniazid may decrease the effectiveness of acarbose. **Herbal/Food:** Ginseng, garlic, black cohosh, juniper berries, aloe, or dandelion root can cause hypoglycemia. Cocoa and rosemary have a hyperglycemic effect and may decrease the therapeutic effect of acarbose.

Pregnancy: Studies in laboratory animals have not shown evidence of fetal harm. It is not known if this drug is secreted in human milk or if there are adverse effects on the breastfed neonate.

Treatment of Overdose: Unlike the sulfonylureas, overdose with acarbose will not cause hypoglycemia. Abdominal pain, flatulence, and diarrhea are treated symptomatically.

Clinician Responsibilities: Key clinical implications for patients receiving acarbose are included in Applied Clinical Judgment: Patients Receiving Pharmacotherapy for Type 2 Diabetes.

Drugs Similar to Acarbose

The only other drug in this class is miglitol.

Miglitol (Glyset): Approved in 1996, miglitol is an alpha-glucosidase inhibitor used as monotherapy or in combination with other antidiabetic drugs for the pharmacotherapy of type 2 diabetes. It acts by delaying the conversion of complex carbohydrates to monosaccharides (glucose), thereby lessening the rise in postprandial serum glucose levels. Like acarbose, the drug must be present in the intestine at the same time the carbohydrates are being digested; thus, the drug must be taken with a meal. The adverse effects are similar with the notable exception of not causing increased liver enzymes. Acarbose and miglitol both act locally in the intestine, although miglitol is completely absorbed and has the potential to produce systemic effects. Overdose does not cause hypoglycemia. Very high doses of this drug in laboratory animals caused fetal harm. Because small amounts are secreted in human milk, caution should be used if breastfeeding.

Incretin Therapies

66.8 Incretin therapies offer a different approach to treating type 2 diabetes.

Incretins are hormones released by the mucosa of the small intestine in response to meals. The most important incretin is glucagon-like peptide (GLP-1), which acts rapidly to produce the following effects:

- Lower blood glucose by increasing the amount of insulin secreted by the pancreas
- Decrease the amount of glucagon secreted by the pancreas
- Delay gastric emptying (slow glucose absorption)
- Decrease food intake by increasing the level of satiety.

Two groups of drugs have been developed that can influence incretin release. The first activates the GLP-1 receptor, causing essentially the same glucose-lowering actions as the natural hormone. Dulaglutide (Trulicity), exenatide (Byetta), liraglutide (Victoza), lixisenatide (Adlyxin), and semaglutide (Ozempic) are synthetic drugs that *mimic* the action of incretin, thus they are called incretin mimetics or GLP-1 receptor agonists. They are all administered by the subcutaneous route. Drugs in this class delay gastric emptying, which may impact the absorption of PO medications. Oral medications such as antibiotics, pain relievers, or oral contraceptives should be taken at least 1 hour prior to the GLP-1 agonist injection.

The second class of drugs that *enhance* incretin actions are the dipeptidyl peptidase 4 (DPP-4) inhibitors. Alogliptin (Nesina), linagliptin (Tradjenta), saxagliptin (Onglyza), and sitagliptin (Januvia) prevent the breakdown of incretins, allowing the hormone levels to rise and produce a greater response. These incretin enhancers (also called gliptins) are given orally and are effective at lowering blood glucose with few adverse effects. They work well with other antidiabetic drugs and do not cause hypoglycemia.

PROTOTYPE DRUG Sitagliptin (Januvia)

Classification **Therapeutic:** Antidiabetic drug
Pharmacologic: DPP-4 inhibitor, incretin enhancer

Therapeutic Effects and Uses: Approved in 2006, sitagliptin is an oral incretin enhancer that is used to help lower glucose levels in patients with type 2 diabetes who are unable to achieve normal glucose levels with diet and exercise alone. The drug is used as adjunct therapy along with diet and exercise and can be administered as monotherapy or in combination with other oral antidiabetic drugs.

The actions of sitagliptin are glucose dependent: They occur only in the presence of elevated serum glucose, and so the risk for hypoglycemia is reduced. Sitagliptin has the added benefit of increasing satiety, or the feeling of fullness following a meal, resulting in a lower calorie intake and improved weight control. Sitagliptin lowers both fasting and postprandial glucose levels. Janumet is a fixed-dose combination drug containing sitagliptin and metformin.

Mechanism of Action: Sitagliptin inhibits DPP-4, the enzyme responsible for breaking down incretins. Inhibition of DPP-4 reduces the destruction of incretins. Levels of incretin hormones increase, thus decreasing blood glucose levels in patients with type 2 diabetes.

Pharmacokinetics:

Route(s)	PO
Absorption	Rapidly absorbed
Distribution	Approximately 38% protein bound
Primary metabolism	20% metabolized in the liver by CYP3A4 and CYP2CB
Primary excretion	Renal
Onset of action	30–60 min; peak: 1–4 h
Duration of action	Half-life: 12 h

Adverse Effects: Sitagliptin is well tolerated by most patients and adverse effects are generally not serious. Possible adverse effects include headache, diarrhea, nasopharyngitis, and upper respiratory infection. Allergic skin reactions and anaphylaxis have been reported. As monotherapy, sitagliptin does not cause hypoglycemia; however, when used concurrently with a sulfonylurea or insulin, hypoglycemia may occur. Post marketing reports have shown suspected acute pancreatitis and acute kidney injury with sitagliptin.

Contraindications/Precautions: Sitagliptin is contraindicated in type 1 diabetes and DKA. It is used with caution in patients with CKD, those with a history of pancreatitis and in older adults. Safety for children under age 18 has not been established.

Drug Interactions: Sitagliptin may increase digoxin levels. **Herbal/Food:** Cinnamon increases the therapeutic effect and may cause hypoglycemia.

Pregnancy: Animal studies have not shown evidence of fetal harm. Because the drug is secreted in animal milk, caution should be used if breastfeeding.

Treatment of Overdose: Overdose is treated symptomatically. If used in combination with other glucose-lowering drugs and hypoglycemia occurs, a concentrated source of glucose should be administered by the IV route.

Clinician Responsibilities: Key clinical implications for patients receiving sitagliptin are included in Applied Clinical Judgment: Patients Receiving Pharmacotherapy for Type 2 Diabetes.

Drugs Similar to Sitagliptin (Januvia)

Other incretin modulators include the GLP-1 agonists dulaglutide, exenatide, liraglutide, and lixisenatide, and the DPP-4 inhibitors alogliptin, linagliptin, and saxagliptin. Albiglutide was discontinued in 2017.

Alogliptin (Nesina): Alogliptin was approved in 2013 for patients who are unable to control their blood glucose through exercise and diet alone. The drug works by the same mechanism and has the same effectiveness and side effects as the other DPP-4 inhibitors. When approving alogliptin, the U.S. Food and Drug Administration (FDA) simultaneously approved two fixed-dose combinations of alogliptin with metformin (Kazano) and pioglitazone (Oseni). Kazano carries a black box warning due to the possibility of lactic acidosis (from metformin) and Oseni due to the possibility of HF (from pioglitazone). Postmarketing reports have shown suspected acute pancreatitis and hepatic failure with alogliptin. Animal studies have not shown evidence of fetal harm. Because the drug is secreted in animal milk, caution should be used if breastfeeding.

Dulaglutide (Trulicity): Dulaglutide was approved in 2014 as an adjunct to diet and exercise in improving glycemic control in patients with type 2 diabetes. Given by the subcutaneous route once weekly, dulaglutide is a GLP-1 receptor agonist that causes increased insulin release by the pancreas. The drug may be used alone or in combination with metformin. The most common side effects include nausea, diarrhea, decreased appetite, and increased amylase and lipase levels. Dulaglutide carries a black box warning that it may increase the risk for thyroid gland tumors and thus is contraindicated in patients with a history of thyroid tumors or multiple endocrine neoplasia syndrome type 2. High doses of this drug in laboratory animals caused fetal harm. It is not known if this drug is secreted in human milk or if it has adverse effects on the breastfed neonate.

Exenatide (Bydureon, Byetta): Exenatide was approved in 2005 for patients with type 2 diabetes who are unable to achieve adequate glycemic control following metformin or sulfonylurea monotherapy. A GLP-1 receptor agonist, exenatide mimics the actions of the incretin hormones normally secreted by the intestines, which slow the absorption of glucose. It is effective in lowering fasting and postprandial glucose levels and causes a consistent, slow weight loss. Regular exenatide (Byetta) is given twice daily by the subcutaneous route, within 60 minutes before the morning and evening meals. Extended-release exenatide (Bydureon) is given once weekly and is available as a single-dose pen injector. Adverse effects include nausea and vomiting, diarrhea, dyspepsia, anorexia, and gastroesophageal reflux. It can also cause nervousness, dizziness, and diaphoresis. Patients with active or chronic pancreatitis should not take this medication. Exenatide showed fetal harm in laboratory animals. Because the drug is secreted in animal milk, caution should be used if breastfeeding.

Linagliptin (Tradjenta): Approved in 2011, linagliptin is a DPP-4 inhibitor. The drug is well tolerated and has the same actions and adverse effects as sitagliptin. Nasopharyngitis is the most common side effect. One potential advantage over the other DPP-4 inhibitors is that linagliptin is excreted through the liver rather than the kidneys. This allows the drug to be used in patients with significant CKD. Fixed-dose combinations include linagliptin with metformin (Jentadueto), empagliflozin (Glyxambi), and both metformin and empagliflozin (Trijardy XR). Linagliptin did not cause significant fetal harm in laboratory animals. It is not known if this drug is secreted in human milk or if it has adverse effects on the breastfed neonate

Liraglutide (Victoza): Approved in 2010 for glycemic control in patients with type 2 diabetes mellitus, liraglutide is a GLP-1 receptor agonist. Like exenatide, liraglutide is effective at reducing A1C levels as well as decreasing appetite and producing a desirable weight loss. An advantage over exenatide is that it can be given once daily. Because of its positive effects on weight loss, liraglutide (Saxenda) was subsequently approved for chronic weight management. Although Victoza and Saxenda have the same active ingredient, Saxenda is approved only for weight management. Liraglutide is well tolerated, with the most common adverse effects being headache, nausea, diarrhea, and antiliraglutide antibody formation. Hypoglycemia is not a problem with monotherapy, but it may occur if used in combination with other antidiabetic drugs. Patients with active or chronic pancreatitis should not take this medication. The drug carries a black box warning about the possibility of thyroid tumors. Patients with a personal or family history of thyroid cancer should not take this drug. In 2016, the FDA approved Xultophy, a combination containing liraglutide and insulin degludec for type 2 diabetes. Liraglutide showed fetal harm in laboratory animals and is not recommended for use during pregnancy or breastfeeding.

Postmarketing reviews determined that use of liraglutide reduced the rates of cardiovascular deaths and other adverse cardiovascular events. In 2017, the FDA added a new indication for liraglutide: to reduce the risk of major cardiovascular events in adult patients with type 2 diabetes mellitus and high cardiovascular risk.

Lixisenatide (Adlyxin): Approved in 2016, lixisenatide is a GLP-1 receptor agonist administered once daily by subcutaneous injection for glycemic control in patients with type 2 diabetes. Its actions, effectiveness, and safety are similar to other incretin mimetics. Common side effects include nausea and vomiting, headache, diarrhea, dizziness, and hypoglycemia. Patients with active or chronic pancreatitis should not take this medication. Soliqua is a combination containing lixisenatide and insulin glargine for type 2 diabetes. Lixisenatide showed fetal harm in laboratory animals and is not recommended for use during pregnancy. The drug is secreted in animal milk but adverse effects in the breastfed infant are not known.

Saxagliptin (Onglyza): Saxagliptin is a DPP-4 inhibitor approved in 2009 to improve glycemic control in patients with type 2 diabetes. The drug is well tolerated and has the same actions and adverse effects as sitagliptin. The most common side effects of saxagliptin are upper respiratory and urinary tract infections. Kombiglyze XR is a fixed-dose combination of saxagliptin and metformin. Qtern is a combination of saxagliptin with dapagliflozin. Saxagliptin was not teratogenic in laboratory animals. The drug is secreted in animal milk but adverse effects in the breastfed infant are not known.

Sodium-Glucose Co-transporter Inhibitors

66.9 Sodium-glucose co-transporter inhibitors are newer medications for treating diabetes and reducing the risk of cardiovascular disease.

In 2013, the FDA approved canagliflozin (Invokana), the first in a new class of oral antidiabetic drugs called the sodium-glucose co-transporter-2 (SGLT2) inhibitors. Additional drugs in this class, dapagliflozin (Farxiga), empagliflozin (Jardiance), and ertugliflozin (Segluromet), were subsequently approved with very similar actions and adverse effects. The SGLT2 inhibitors are sometimes combined with medications from other antidiabetic classes such as metformin and linagliptin.

The SGLT2 proteins are located in the proximal tubule of the nephron. After being filtered, the SGLT2 proteins "grab" glucose molecules and return them to the blood. Inhibiting the SGLT2 proteins allows more glucose to stay in the renal tubule and ultimately to be excreted in the urine. This ability to lower blood glucose is accomplished without stimulating insulin release. The SGLT2 inhibitors also have beneficial effects on weight loss and blood pressure reduction.

Considerable research has focused on the ability of the SGLT2 inhibitors to reduce cardiovascular mortality. Based on this research, canagliflozin and empagliflozin have been indicated to reduce the risk of cardiovascular death in adult patients with type 2 diabetes mellitus and cardiovascular disease. In 2019, dapagliflozin was approved to reduce the risk for hospitalization for HF patients with type 2 diabetes and multiple cardiovascular risk factors. Canagliflozin is also approved to reduce the risk of end-stage renal disease in patients with diabetic nephropathy.

These medications are contraindicated in patients with CKD. The added glucose in the urine serves as a substrate for bacterial and fungal growth, thus increasing the frequency of mycotic infections of the urinary tract and genitalia. DKA is a rare, though serious adverse effect. In 2019, the FDA issued an alert regarding another rare though serious adverse effect called necrotizing fasciitis of the perimeum (a type of gangrene). A black box warning states that use of SGLT2 inhibitors has been associated with a higher risk for lower limb amputations, most frequently the toe. Based on animal data, the SGLT2 inhibitors are not recommended during the second and third trimesters of pregnancy or while breastfeeding.

CONNECTIONS: APPLIED CLINICAL JUDGMENT

Patients Receiving Pharmacotherapy for Type 2 Diabetes

Key Assessment Data

- History of current condition including duration and severity and other related signs or symptoms (e.g., paresthesias of hands or feet), baseline vital signs, physical exam findings, and endocrine, cardiovascular, hepatic, or kidney disease; pregnancy or breastfeeding; drug history including allergies, current prescription and OTC drugs and herbal preparations, and caffeine, nicotine, and alcohol use. Assess feet and lower extremities for possible injury, infection, or ulcerations.
- Obtain a dietary history including caloric intake if on an ADA diet, number of meals and snacks per day. Assess fluid intake and type of fluids consumed.

(continued)

CONNECTIONS: APPLIED CLINICAL JUDGMENT *(continued)*

Patients Receiving Pharmacotherapy for Type 2 Diabetes

Desired Therapeutic Outcomes

Improvement is observed and measurable by glucose levels remaining within normal limits, A1C level demonstrates adequate glucose control.

Minimizing Adverse Effects

- Hypoglycemia is especially likely to occur with sulfonylureas or meglitinides, although it may occur with other types of oral antidiabetic drugs, especially if food sources are inadequate.
- Anaphylactic reactions are possible, although rare. As sensitivity occurs, reactions may continue to develop.
- Thiazolidinediones may cause edema and worsening of HF.
- For patients taking sulfonylureas, nausea and vomiting, yellowing of the skin or sclera, abdominal pain, light- or clay-colored stools, or darkening of urine may indicate hepatotoxicity.
- For patients taking biguanides, drowsiness, malaise, decreased respiratory rate, or general body aches may indicate lactic acidosis.
- Beta blockers may antagonize the action of some oral antidiabetic drugs and may mask the symptoms of a hypoglycemic episode, allowing the blood sugar to drop lower before it is perceived.
- Increased genital fungal and bacterial infections may occur with SGLT2 inhibitors, especially in women.
- Some oral antidiabetic drugs have teratogenic effects and must be discontinued during pregnancy. Monitor for pregnancy at each healthcare visit.
- Exercise assists muscles to use glucose more efficiently and increases insulin receptor sites in the tissues, lowering the blood sugar. Benefits of exercise and lowered blood sugar may continue for up to 48 hours, increasing the risk of hypoglycemia during this time.
- Caloric needs and protein, carbohydrate, and fat percentages are calculated based on activity level and lifestyle and the need for weight loss. Alcohol use should be limited or eliminated, especially if sulfonylureas are used. As alcohol is metabolized, it can raise and then precipitously lower blood sugar, increasing the risk of hypoglycemia.

Lifespan Considerations

- Age-related physiologic differences may place the older adult at greater risk for hepatic toxicity.
- Women who are pregnant or considering pregnancy should consult with their healthcare provider. Due to the increasing metabolic needs of pregnancy, supplemental insulin or switching to insulin coverage may be required for the duration of the pregnancy.

Patient Education

- Observe for symptoms of hyper- and hypoglycemia and check capillary glucose levels routinely and if symptoms are present. If unsure whether symptoms indicate hypo- or hyperglycemia, treat as hypoglycemia and then check capillary glucose. If symptoms are not relieved in 10 to 15 minutes, or if capillary glucose is below 70 mg/dL (or parameters as ordered), immediately notify the healthcare provider.
- Monitor capillary glucose levels as ordered. Carry a quick-acting carbohydrate, as well as a protein source, for times when food is not available and symptoms of hypoglycemia are present. Report any consistent elevations or hypoglycemia to the healthcare provider.
- Limit or eliminate alcohol use. If alcoholic beverages are consumed, limit to one per day and consume along with a complete meal to ensure that food intake balances alcohol metabolism.
- Notify the healthcare provider if unable to eat normal meals during periods of illness or stress for possible change in drug dose.
- Exercise should occur an hour after a meal or after a 10- or 15-g carbohydrate snack to prevent hypoglycemia. If exercise is prolonged, small, frequent carbohydrate snacks can be consumed every 30 minutes during exercise to maintain blood sugar.
- If taking SGLT2 drugs, monitor for perineal and/or vaginal yeast infections, burning, reddened or itching areas of the body, especially those in covered areas (e.g., feet, under breasts and armpits), and notify the healthcare provider if these occur.
- Take the drug following appropriate guidelines:
  - Most oral antidiabetic drugs are taken once or twice a day. For drugs given once a day, take approximately 30 minutes before the first meal of the day. Alpha-glucosidase inhibitors (e.g., acarbose) should be taken with meals.
  - Insulin injections may be required in addition to the oral antidiabetic drug on occasion. This does not necessarily signal a worsening of the disease condition but may be a temporary need.
- Carry a medical identification card or wear medical alert jewelry indicating diabetes.

Prescribing Considerations

- Ongoing assessment during drug therapy should include monitoring appropriate laboratory findings (e.g., CBC, electrolytes, glucose, A1C level, lipid profile, osmolality, and hepatic and renal function studies).
- The AACE and ACE publish annual updates to their joint algorithm for the management of type 2 diabetes. Prescribers should follow the most current AACE Comprehensive Type 2 Diabetes Management Algorithm (2020) (*https://pro.aace.com/disease-state-resources/diabetes/clinical-practice-guidelines-treatment-algorithms/comprehensive*).

Understanding Chapter 66

Key Concepts Summary

66.1 Serum glucose is maintained within a narrow range by the hormones insulin and glucagon.

66.2 Type 1 diabetes is characterized by insufficient insulin synthesis by the pancreas, whereas type 2 diabetes is characterized by insulin resistance in the target cells.

66.3 The classic signs and symptoms of diabetes include polyuria, polydipsia, and polyphagia.

66.4 Acute complications of diabetes include diabetic ketoacidosis, hyperosmolar hyperglycemic state, and hypoglycemia.

66.5 Serious complications of chronic diabetes include neuropathy, nephropathy, retinopathy, and vascular disease.

66.6 Insulin is the cornerstone of therapy for patients with type 1 and gestational diabetes.

66.7 Antidiabetic drugs from multiple classes are used to treat type 2 diabetes.

66.8 Incretin therapies offer a different approach to treating type 2 diabetes.

66.9 Sodium-glucose co-transporter inhibitors are newer medications for treating diabetes and reducing the risk of cardiovascular disease.

CASE STUDY: Making the Patient Connection

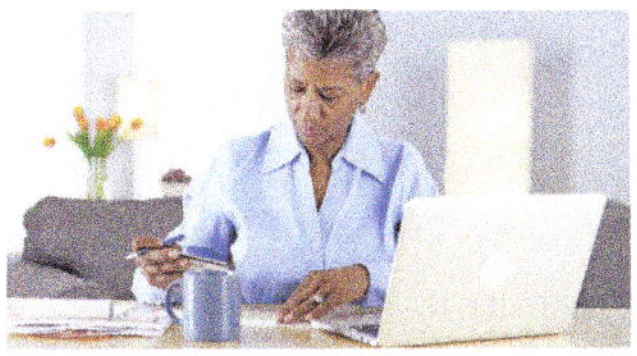

Remember the patient "Eileen Douglas" at the beginning of the chapter? Now read the remainder of the case study. Based on the information presented within this chapter, respond to the critical thinking questions that follow.

Eileen is a 54-year-old woman who works full time as an art teacher in a local high school. She also teaches art courses on the weekends at the local senior center. She visited her healthcare provider last week for her annual physical examination and to update her TB screening (PPD) for the coming school year. The office called Eileen back this morning and requested that she make an appointment to return tomorrow to discuss the results of her laboratory tests. Her serum glucose level was elevated at 224 mg/dL and she will need further testing to rule out type 2 diabetes.

Eileen has follow-up testing with the results of a fasting serum glucose level at 131 mg/dL and a 2-hour 75-g oral glucose test of 242 mg/dL. A diagnosis of new-onset type 2 diabetes is confirmed. Eileen expresses disbelief and tells you, the nurse, "I can't believe it! I watch what I eat; I don't eat a lot of sugar, cookies, or candy. I drink only diet soda. I don't have any of the symptoms you hear about. And no one in my family has ever had diabetes." A health history and the results of Eileen's recent physical examination confirm overall good health. Her height is 1.7 meters (5 ft 6 in.) and her weight is 79.5 kg (175 lb) with a BMI of 28.2 kg/m^2, placing her in the "overweight" category. Vital signs, physical examination, and all other laboratory work are within acceptable limits. Eileen admits that she has been thirstier lately, "But it's summertime and I always drink more when it's hot." She has also been urinating more frequently but attributes that to her increased fluid intake.

Eileen's provider will start her on glyburide (DiaBeta) and metformin (Glucophage) and will recheck her serum glucose in 1 month. In the meantime, she is to begin capillary blood glucose testing before meals and at bedtime and bring her log to the next visit. She is given dietary instructions and you will be providing instruction on her medications.

Critical Thinking Questions

1. Why are two oral antidiabetic drugs prescribed for Eileen?
2. What essential teaching does Eileen need about her glyburide (DiaBeta) and metformin (Glucophage)?
3. Eileen asks why she is not being started on insulin. Why is insulin not being used at this time?
4. Eileen tells you that she occasionally enjoys a glass of wine with her dinner and wants to know if this is allowed. How will you answer?

Additional Case Study

Nicholas Jefferson is 8 years old and has just been diagnosed with type 1 diabetes. After increasing symptoms during the past month, he was hospitalized for continuous nausea and vomiting and gradually increasing lethargy. His parents report that during the past month or two, Nicholas has had blurry vision and has been thirsty and hungry constantly. He has been eating frequently but does not seem to be gaining any weight. They also tell you that on several occasions, Nicholas has wet the bed, which is very unusual for him. On admission, his serum glucose level is 420 mg/dL with a urine sample positive for glucose and ketones. Nicholas is to remain NPO and will be started on an IV with 0.45 normal saline for fluid replacement, given an IV bolus of insulin, and then started on an insulin drip at 0.5 unit per hour. Glucose levels are to be checked every hour using fingerstick blood samples, and serum blood glucose samples are to be drawn every 4 hours. The IV insulin drip is to be discontinued when Nicholas's blood glucose level is 240 mg/dL and subcutaneous insulin will be started at that time.

1. What type of insulin do you anticipate using for the IV bolus dose and IV drip?
2. Why do you think the insulin IV will be stopped when the blood glucose level is 240 mg/dL and not at the normal level of 70 to 100 mg/dL?
3. What essential teaching will Nicholas and his family need at this time?

Chapter Review

1. A patient with type 1 diabetes will use a combination insulin that includes NPH and regular insulins. The nurse is explaining the importance of knowing the peak times for both insulins. Why is this important information for the patient to know?

1. The patient will be able to estimate the time for the next injection of insulin based on these peaks.
2. The risk of a hypoglycemic reaction is greatest around the peak of insulin activity.
3. It is best to plan activities or exercise around peak insulin times for the best utilization of glucose.
4. Additional insulin may be required at the peak periods to prevent hyperglycemia.

2. Before administering a morning lispro insulin (Humalog) injection, which activity should the nurse perform? (Select all that apply.)

1. Obtain a morning urine sample for glucose and ketones.
2. Check the patient's fingerstick glucose level.
3. Ensure that breakfast trays are present on the unit and that the patient eats.
4. Obtain the patient's pulse and blood pressure.
5. Assess for symptoms of hypoglycemia.

3. The nurse would consider which of the following assessment findings as adverse effects to metformin therapy?

1. Hypoglycemia
2. GI distress
3. Lactic acidosis
4. Weight loss

4. A patient was started on rosiglitazone for type 2 diabetes. He tells the nurse that he has been taking it for 5 days, but his glucose levels are unchanged. What is the nurse's best response?

1. "You should double the dose. That should help."
2. "You need to give the drug more time. It can take several weeks before it becomes fully effective."
3. "You will need to add a second drug since this one has not been effective."
4. "You most likely require insulin now."

5. A young woman calls the clinic and reports that her mother had an insulin reaction and was found unconscious. The young woman gave her a glucagon injection 20 minutes ago, and her mother woke up but is still groggy and "does not make sense." What should the nurse tell the daughter?

1. "Let her wake up on her own, then give her something to eat."
2. "Place some hard candies in her mouth."
3. "Just let her sleep. People are sleepy after hypoglycemic episodes."
4. "Give her another injection and call the paramedics."

6. The nurse explains the benefit of using the long-acting insulin glargine (Lantus) over other insulins. What will the nurse tell the patient about this insulin?

1. It does not need to be administered by injection.
2. It can be given by intramuscular or subcutaneous injection.
3. It does not require blood glucose monitoring.
4. It has no definite peak but maintains a steady state of insulin in the body.

See Appendix A for answers to critical thinking questions, case study questions, and review questions.

References

American Association of Clinical Endocrinologists (AACE) and American College of Endocrinology (ACE). (2015). Clinical guidelines for developing a diabetes mellitus comprehensive care plan–2015. *Endocrine Practice*, *21*(Suppl. 1), 1–87. Retrieved from https://www.aace.com/files/dm-guidelines-ccp.pdf

American Diabetes Association (ADA). (2020a). *Fast facts: Data and statistics about diabetes.* https://professional.diabetes.org/sites/professional.diabetes.org/files/media/sci_2020_diabetes_fast_facts_sheet_final.pdf

American Diabetes Association (ADA). (2020b). *Diabetes medical management plan.* https://www.diabetes.org/sites/default/files/2019-06/ADA%20Childcare%20DMMP.pdf

American Heart Association (AHA). (2016). *Symptoms and diagnosis of metabolic syndrome.* https://www.heart.org/HEARTORG/Conditions/More/MetabolicSyndrome/Symptoms-and-Diagnosis-of-Metabolic-Syndrome_UCM_301925_Article.jsp

Bhavsar, A. R. (2017). *Diabetic retinopathy.* Medscape. http://emedicine.medscape.com/article/1225122-overview#a4

Selected Bibliography

Bailey, C. J., & Day, C. (2019). The future of new drugs for diabetes management. *Diabetes Research and Clinical Practice*, *155*, 107785. https://doi.org/10.1016/j.diabres.2019.107785

Bonaventura, A., Carbone, S., Dixon, D. L., Abbate, A., & Montecucco, F. (2019). Pharmacologic strategies to reduce cardiovascular disease in type 2 diabetes mellitus: Focus on SGLT-2 inhibitors and GLP-1 receptor agonists. *Journal of Internal Medicine*, *286*(1), 16–31. https://doi.org/10.1111/joim.12890

Centers for Disease Control and Prevention (CDC). (2020). *National diabetes statistics report, 2020.* https://www.cdc.gov/diabetes/data/statistics-report/index.html

Chaudhury, A., Duvoor, C., Dendi, V. S. R., Kraleti, S., Chada, A., Ravilla, R., et al. (2017). Clinical review of antidiabetic drugs: Implications for type 2 diabetes mellitus management. *Frontiers in Endocrinology*, *8*, 6. https://doi.org/10.3389/fendo.2017.00006

Gamble, J. M., Clarke, A., Myers, K. J., Agnew, M. D., Hatch, K., Snow, M. M., & Davis, E. M. (2015). Incretin-based medications for type 2 diabetes: An overview of reviews. *Diabetes, Obesity and Metabolism*, *17*, 649–658. https://doi.org/10.1111/dom.12465

Horta, B. L., & de Lima, N. P. (2019). Breastfeeding and type 2 diabetes: Systematic review and meta-analysis. *Current Diabetes Reports*, *19*(1), 1. https://doi.org/10.1007/s11892-019-1121-x

Keresztes, P., & Peacock-Johnson, A. (2019). CE: Type 2 diabetes: A pharmacologic update. *American Journal of Nursing*, *119*(3), 32–40. https://doi.org/10.1097/01.NAJ.0000554008.77013.cf

Lew, K. N., & Wick, A. (2015). Pharmacotherapy of type 2 diabetes mellitus: Navigating current and new therapies. *Medsurg Nursing*, *24*(6), 413–419.

Longo, M., Bellastella, G., Maiorino, M. I., Meier, J. J., Esposito, K., & Giugliano, D. (2019). Diabetes and aging: from treatment goals to pharmacologic therapy. *Frontiers in Endocrinology*, *10*, 45. https://doi.org/10.3389/fendo.2019.00045

Nguyen, T. (2016). Keeping up with safety warnings of oral antidiabetic drugs. *Journal for Nurse Practitioners*, *12*, 61–62. https://doi.org/10.1016/j.nurpra.2015.10.002

Sattar, N., Petrie, M. C., Zinman, B., & Januzzi, J. L. (2017). Novel diabetes drugs and the cardiovascular specialist. *Journal of the American College of Cardiology*, *69*(21), 2646–2656. https://doi.org/10.1016/j.jacc.2017.04.014

Tomlinson, B., Hu, M., Zhang, Y., Chan, P., & Liu, Z. M. (2016). An overview of new GLP-1 receptor agonists for type 2 diabetes. *Expert Opinion on Investigational Drugs*, *25*, 145–158. https://doi.org/10.1517/13543784.2016.1123249

Wang, S. S. (2020). *Metabolic syndrome.* Medscape. http://emedicine.medscape.com/article/165124-overview

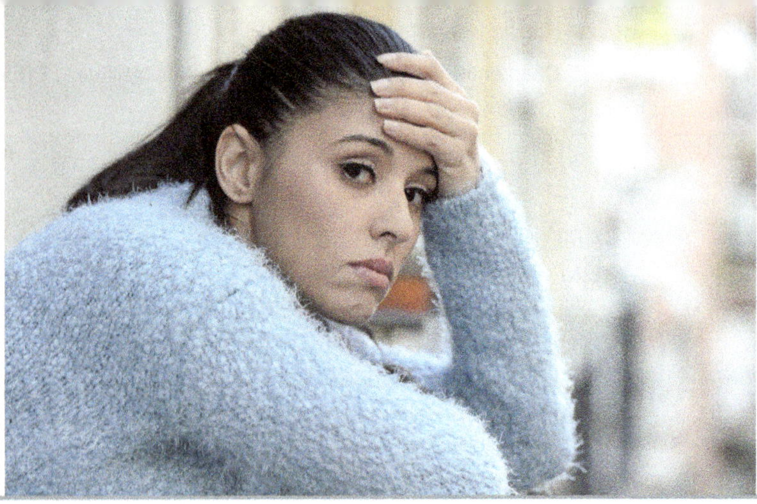

"I don't know why I've been so tired lately. Maybe it's just my hormones starting to change or keeping up with the kids. I feel like I'm cold all the time and barely have the energy to go to work. Maybe I should have it checked out."
—*Patient "Helen Mercado"*

Chapter 67
Pharmacotherapy of Thyroid Disorders

Chapter Outline

Learning Outcomes

After reading this chapter, the student should be able to:

1. Explain the functions of thyroid hormone.
2. Explain the negative feedback control of thyroid function.
3. Explain how thyroid disorders are diagnosed.
4. Describe the pathophysiology of thyroid disorders.
5. Describe the pharmacotherapy of thyroid disorders.
6. For each of the classes shown in the chapter outline, identify the prototype and representative drugs and explain the mechanism(s) of drug action, primary indications, contraindications, significant drug interactions, pregnancy data, and important adverse effects.
7. Apply clinical judgment to the care of patients receiving pharmacotherapy for thyroid disorders.

Key Terms

Definitions of the terms in bold may be found in the Glossary.

The thyroid gland affects the function of virtually every organ of the body. It synthesizes and secretes hormones that increase overall body metabolism and protein synthesis. Adequate secretion of these hormones is also necessary for normal growth and development in infants and children, including mental development and attainment of sexual maturity. The thyroid also affects functions of the cardiovascular, respiratory, gastrointestinal (GI), and neuromuscular systems. Thyroid disorders are common, affecting women 5 to 10 times more often than men. This chapter presents the pharmacotherapy of thyroid imbalances.

Physiology of the Thyroid Gland

67.1 Thyroid hormones contain iodine and stimulate the basal metabolic rate of nearly all tissues.

The thyroid gland lies on both sides of the trachea just below the larynx. The gland contains two distinct types of endocrine cell types: follicular cells and parafollicular cells. Follicular cells produce, store, and secrete thyroid hormone. Parafollicular cells produce calcitonin, a hormone totally unrelated to the structure or function of thyroid hormone. Calcitonin regulates calcium metabolism and is used as a drug in the pharmacotherapy of osteoporosis (see Chapter 72).

Thyroid hormone actually consists of two distinct hormones: **tri-iodothyronine (T_3)** and **thyroxine (T_4)**. Both T_3 and T_4 are synthesized from the amino acid tyrosine and iodine; the subscript numeral refers to the number of iodine molecules each hormone contains. Because the two have very similar actions, they are usually considered a single hormone.

When secreted into the bloodstream, more than 99% of T_3 and T_4 is bound to **thyroxine-binding globulin (TBG)**, a plasma protein manufactured by the liver. Any condition that causes decreased amounts of plasma proteins, such as protein malnutrition or liver impairment, can lead to a larger percentage of free thyroid hormone, with subsequent symptoms of hyperthyroidism.

Most circulating thyroid hormone is in the form of T_4. Upon entering target cells, however, T_4 is converted in peripheral tissues to T_3, which is three to five times more biologically active. This offers an additional level of control (tissue level) of thyroid hormone function.

The two thyroid hormones are metabolized by the liver and excreted by the kidneys, with small amounts excreted in the stool. Iodine is conserved in the process and returned to the thyroid gland for the production of more hormone molecules. Therefore, only a small daily intake of iodine is needed to meet the demands of the thyroid gland. High amounts of iodine are found in shellfish, but the main dietary source is the use of iodized salt. Thyroid hormones are the only known use for iodine in the body.

Thyroid hormone stimulates the basal metabolic rate of nearly all tissues. This increases the oxidation of energy sources (glucose, fats, and proteins), which in turn increases oxygen consumption and generates large amounts of heat. The rapid metabolic rate increases the body's demands for vitamins. Thyroid hormone affects GI function and motility, appetite, and body weight. Thyroid hormone increases the number of beta$_1$- and beta$_2$-adrenergic receptors and enhances their affinity to catecholamines (norepinephrine, epinephrine, and dopamine). The increase in sympathetic activity leads to increased heart rate and force of contraction, cardiac output, and cardiac demands for oxygen. Thyroid hormones also stimulate the secretion of growth hormone and are therefore essential for the normal growth and development of the skeletal and nervous systems. Thyroid hormone affects reflexes, thought processes, and overall level of consciousness. Signs and symptoms of thyroid hormone deficiency and excess are presented in Sections 67.3 and 67.5, respectively.

The secretion of thyroid hormone is regulated by the hypothalamus and anterior pituitary gland through a negative feedback loop, as shown in Figure 67.1. When blood levels of thyroid hormone are low, the hypothalamus secretes **thyrotropin-releasing hormone (TRH)**. Secretion of TRH stimulates the anterior pituitary to secrete **thyroid-stimulating hormone (TSH)**. TSH then stimulates the thyroid to produce and secrete T_3 and T_4. As blood levels of free, unbound thyroid hormone increase, negative feedback suppresses the secretion of TSH and TRH. High levels of iodine can also cause a temporary decrease in thyroid activity that can last for several weeks. One of the strongest stimuli for increased thyroid hormone production is exposure to cold.

Disorders of the thyroid result from a hypofunction or hyperfunction of the thyroid gland. Hormonal imbalances may occur due to disease within the thyroid gland itself or be caused by abnormalities of the pituitary or hypothalamus.

Thyroid disorders can be due to a congenital defect, or they may develop later in life. They may have an insidious or sudden onset. An increase in the size of the thyroid gland is referred to as a **goiter**. This can occur with normal, high, or low levels of thyroid hormone. Goiters may be diffuse, involving the entire gland, or nodular. When they become considerably enlarged, the goiter can compress the trachea and esophagus, causing difficulty swallowing, a choking sensation, and possibly inspiratory stridor (abnormal high-pitched sounds when breathing). They may also compress the superior vena cava, causing distention of the neck veins and facial edema.

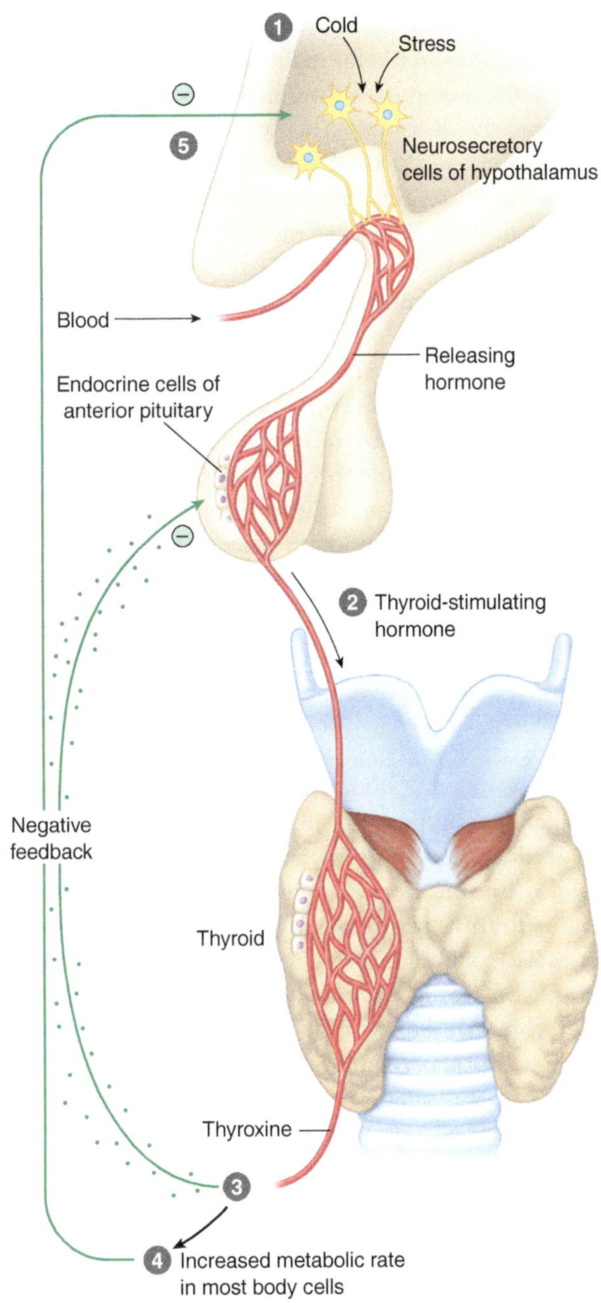

Figure 67.1 Feedback mechanisms of the thyroid gland.

Diagnosis of Thyroid Disorders

67.2 An accurate diagnosis of thyroid hormone dysfunction is based on the patient's symptoms and the results of diagnostic tests.

Because the thyroid gland is located close to the skin surface, palpation of the thyroid gland is conducted for routine screening of enlargements and nodules. Serum laboratory tests for T_3, T_4, and TSH levels are used for diagnosis, as listed in Table 67.1. TSH is the preferred laboratory value for diagnosing and monitoring the progression of thyroid disease. Primary hypothyroidism is characterized by a low serum T_4 level and an elevated TSH level.

Abnormal laboratory values must be carefully evaluated because a number of conditions, including stress in critically ill adults, can affect TSH and T_4 levels. In addition, these laboratory values are influenced by abnormalities in serum protein levels because both T_3 and T_4 are heavily protein bound. Any condition that affects protein levels requires careful analysis of these test results.

Antibodies to thyroglobulin or to thyroid peroxidase in the blood suggests the presence of an autoimmune disorder that is targeting the thyroid gland. Individuals without thyroid disease have minimal or none of these antibodies in their blood. However, most patients with Hashimoto's thyroiditis or Graves' disease will show elevated levels of antithyroid antibody titer. In the case of Hashimoto's, the elevated antibodies may lead to hypothyroidism; for Graves' disease, however, the elevated antibodies may indicate hyperthyroidism. Patients with other autoimmune disorders such as systemic lupus erythematosus or rheumatoid arthritis may have elevated antibody values without thyroid disease.

Ultrasonography can be used to assess masses, cysts, and enlargement of the thyroid gland. The radioactive iodine uptake test measures the rate of iodine uptake by the thyroid gland after administration of ^{123}I tracer. This test can detect areas of increased and decreased function. Computed tomography (CT) and magnetic resonance imaging (MRI) scans can be used to determine tracheal compression or pressure on neighboring structures caused by thyroid

Table 67.1 Serum Values for Thyroid Function Tests*

Thyroid Test	Reference Value	Hypothyroid	Hyperthyroid
T_3 (serum)	80–220 ng/dL	Decreased	Increased
Free T_4	0.8–1.8 ng/dL	Decreased	Increased
Total T_4	4.5–12.5 mcg/dL	Decreased	Increased
TSH (serum)	0.5–5.5 microinternational units/mL	Increased	Decreased
Antithyroglobulin antibody (TgAb)	Less than 20 international units/mL	–	–
Thyroid peroxidase antibody (TPOAb)	Less than 9.0 international units/mL	–	–

*Reference values vary somewhat among different laboratories.

gland enlargement. The diagnostic tool for detecting malignancy of a thyroid nodule is the fine needle biopsy.

An accurate diagnosis of thyroid hormone dysfunction is essential. Proper treatment of the disorder will depend on whether the abnormality lies within the thyroid gland itself or is the result of a defect in the negative feedback control by the hypothalamus or pituitary.

PharmFACT

The demands on the mother's thyroid gland increase during pregnancy. If women have too little iodine during pregnancy, the damage to the nervous system of the fetus may be irreversible (Harding et al., 2017).

Pathophysiology of Hypothyroid Disorders

67.3 Hypothyroidism, or thyroid deficiency, can occur as a congenital or acquired disorder.

Hypothyroidism may occur as a congenital disorder or it may be acquired in adulthood. Congenital hypothyroidism is a common, preventable cause of intellectual disability. The infant appears normal at birth due to hormones supplied by the mother while in utero. If untreated, congenital hypothyroidism results in a condition known as **cretinism**, marked by profound intellectual disability and impaired growth. Almost half of normal brain development occurs during the first 6 months of life, and thyroid hormone is essential for this to occur. If thyroid replacement therapy is begun in the first 6 weeks of life, normal growth and development take place and cretinism can be prevented. In the United States and Canada, screening for hypothyroidism is conducted for most neonates.

Hypothyroidism in older children and adults results in a general slowing of metabolic processes and **myxedema**, a mucous type of edema caused by an accumulation of hydrophilic substances in connective tissues. Primary hypothyroidism, the most common type in children and adults, results from dysfunction of the thyroid gland. Secondary hypothyroidism is due to pathology of the pituitary gland. Tertiary hypothyroidism is a result of a disorder of the hypothalamus. Causes of hypothyroidism include thyroidectomy or ablation of the thyroid gland with radiation, or treatment with antithyroid drugs. Large amounts of iodine or substances that contain iodine—such as kelp tablets, certain cough syrups, the cardiac drug amiodarone, or iodine-containing radiographic contrast media—can block thyroid hormone production and cause goiter and hypothyroidism. Iodine deficiency is rarely a cause of hypothyroidism in the United States due to the widespread use of iodized salt.

The most common cause of hypothyroidism is an autoimmune disorder known as **Hashimoto's thyroiditis**. This disease affects women 5 to 10 times more often than men.

Hypothyroidism affects nearly all major organ systems, with manifestations arising from two factors: a hypometabolic state and myxedematous changes in body tissues. The hypometabolic state is marked by a gradual onset of weakness and fatigue, a tendency to gain weight despite a decreased appetite, and cold intolerance. Hypotension, bradycardia, hypoventilation, and subnormal temperature may occur. In time, the skin becomes rough and dry and may have a yellowish cast; the hair becomes coarse and brittle; and GI motility slows, causing chronic constipation, flatulence, and abdominal distention. Mental dullness, lethargy, slowed reflexes, and memory problems may occur. Because of the importance of thyroid hormone to fetal development, women experiencing hypothyroidism should be treated with thyroid hormone during pregnancy. Women also experience a high incidence of postpartum thyroiditis, which occurs following about 10% of pregnancies.

As fluid accumulates in tissues, the face takes on a puffy look, especially around the eyes; the tongue enlarges; and the voice may be husky. Fluid can accumulate in the pericardial or pleural spaces, causing effusions, cardiac dilation, and bradycardia. **Myxedema coma** or crisis is a life-threatening end-stage condition of hypothyroidism, characterized by coma, hypothermia, cardiovascular collapse, hypoventilation, hyponatremia, hypoglycemia, and lactic acidosis. This condition occurs most often in older women. Even with early detection and treatment, the mortality rate is 30% for those who develop myxedema coma. Treatment consists of supportive measures, correction of electrolyte and acid–base imbalances, treatment of hypotension, and immediate thyroid replacement therapy. If hypothermia is present, active rewarming is contraindicated because this may precipitate vasodilation and lead to cardiovascular collapse. Features of thyroid emergencies are described in Table 67.2.

Table 67.2 Signs and Symptoms of Thyroid Emergencies

Thyroid Storm	Myxedema Coma
Tachycardia	Bradycardia
Hyperthermia	Hypothermia
Tachypnea	Hypoventilation
Hypercalcemia	Hyponatremia
Hyperglycemia	Hypoglycemia
Metabolic acidosis	Respiratory and metabolic acidosis
Cardiovascular collapse: cardiogenic shock, hypovolemia, arrhythmias	Cardiovascular collapse: decreased vascular tone
Depressed LOC	Depressed LOC
Emotional lability	Seizures, coma
Psychosis	Hyporeflexia
Tremors, restlessness	–

CONNECTION Checkpoint 67.1

Patients with hypothyroidism tend to have low rates of angina and myocardial infarction. From what you learned in Chapter 35, explain this link.

Pharmacotherapy of Hypothyroid Disorders

67.4 Hypothyroidism is treated by replacement therapy with thyroid hormone.

The standard replacement regimen for hypothyroidism consists of levothyroxine (T_4), although combined therapy with levothyroxine plus liothyronine (T_3) is an option. Although T_4 is less biologically active than T_3, it is readily converted to T_3 in peripheral tissues. In most cases, thyroid replacement therapy is lifelong.

In children with cretinism, therapy with levothyroxine should continue for 3 years, after which it should be stopped for 1 month. During this time, thyroid hormone levels are monitored to assess the status of the deficiency and to determine if further treatment is needed.

In adults, serum TSH levels are used to evaluate the progress of therapy. When initiating therapy in older adults, the precaution is to "go low and go slow" because there is a risk for inducing acute coronary syndromes in susceptible individuals. Table 67.3 lists the doses of the drugs used to treat hypothyroidism.

PROTOTYPE DRUG **Levothyroxine (Levoxyl, Synthroid, Unithroid)**

Classification **Therapeutic:** Thyroid hormone
Pharmacologic: Thyroid hormone replacement

Therapeutic Effects and Uses: Levothyroxine is a synthetic form of T_4, with actions identical to endogenous thyroid hormone. It is used for primary or secondary hypothyroidism, congenital hypothyroidism, hypothyroid state resulting from the surgical removal of the thyroid gland, radiation or antithyroid drugs, management of thyroid cancer, or treatment of myxedema coma. The drug is given by the oral (PO) route for routine replacement therapy and intravenously (IV) for myxedema coma.

To avoid adverse effects, doses of thyroid hormone are highly individualized for each patient. When given by the PO route, 1 to 3 weeks may be required to obtain full therapeutic benefits. Doses for patients with preexisting cardiac disease are usually increased at 4- to 6-week intervals to avoid the possibility of dysrhythmias or angina attacks.

Mechanism of Action: The actions of levothyroxine are identical to those of endogenous thyroid hormone. The drug increases the metabolic rate, thereby increasing oxygen consumption, respiration, and heart rate; increases the rate of fat, protein, and carbohydrate metabolism; and promotes growth and maturation. Because levothyroxine is converted to T_3, it is not necessary to also give T_3.

Pharmacokinetics:

Route(s)	PO, IV
Absorption	Variable; partial absorption from the GI tract (50 to 80%)
Distribution	Gradually released to peripheral tissues; crosses the placenta; secreted in breast milk; more than 99% bound to protein
Primary metabolism	Hepatic
Primary excretion	Kidneys, with some secreted in bile and excreted in feces
Onset of action	PO: Slow; IV: 6–8 h
Duration of action	1–3 weeks; half-life: 6–7 days

Adverse Effects: At therapeutic doses, adverse effects of levothyroxine therapy are rare. At high doses, treatment may cause central nervous system (CNS) excitability such as tremors, headache, nervousness, or insomnia. Cardiovascular adverse effects include palpitations, tachycardia, angina, and cardiac arrest. Other possible adverse events include allergic skin reactions, diarrhea, and nausea and vomiting. Synthroid 100-mcg and 300-mcg tablets contain tartrazine, a yellow dye that may cause an allergic reaction

Table 67.3 Drugs for Hypothyroidism

Drug Name	Dose for Adults (Maximum Dose Where Indicated)	Adverse Effects
levothyroxine (Levoxyl, Synthroid, Unithroid)	PO: 100–400 mcg/day IV: initial loading dose of 300–500 mcg followed by maintenance doses of 50–100 mcg	*Weight loss, headache, tremors, nervousness, heat intolerance, irritability, sweating, insomnia, menstrual irregularities* Dysrhythmias, hypertension (HTN), palpitations, angina
liothyronine (Cytomel, Triostat)	PO: 25–75 mcg/day IV: 25–100 mcg/day	
thyroid, desiccated (Armour thyroid, Thyroid USP)	PO: 60–180 mg/day	

Note: *Italics* indicate common adverse effects. Underline indicates severe adverse effects.

in some patients, especially those sensitive to aspirin. **Black Box Warning:** Use of thyroid hormone for weight loss or the treatment of obesity is contraindicated.

Contraindications/Precautions: The use of levothyroxine is contraindicated if the patient is hypersensitive to the drug, is experiencing thyrotoxicosis, or has severe cardiovascular conditions or acute myocardial infarction (MI). If thyroid hormone is given to patients with adrenal insufficiency, it may cause a serious adrenal crisis; thus, the insufficiency should be corrected prior to administration of levothyroxine. It should be used with caution in patients with cardiac disease, angina pectoris, cardiac dysrhythmias, HTN, and impaired kidney function and in older adults. Symptoms of diabetes mellitus may be worsened with administration of thyroid hormone, and doses of antidiabetic drugs may require adjustment.

Drug Interactions: A large number of medications can interact with thyroid hormone and result in either increased or decreased effects. Drugs that decrease the absorption of levothyroxine include cholestyramine, colestipol, calcium- or aluminum-containing antacids, sucralfate, and iron supplements. Several drugs are known to accelerate the metabolism of levothyroxine, including phenytoin, carbamazepine, rifampin, phenobarbital, and sertraline. Levothyroxine increases the effects of warfarin, resulting in an increased risk of bleeding. Digoxin decreases the effectiveness of levothyroxine. Thyroid hormone sensitizes cardiac responsiveness to catecholamines; therefore, administration of epinephrine or norepinephrine must be carefully monitored in these patients to prevent dysrhythmias. **Herbal/Food:** Soybean flour (infant formula), cottonseed meal, walnuts, and dietary fiber may bind and decrease the absorption of levothyroxine from the GI tract. Calcium or iron supplements should be taken at least 4 hours after taking levothyroxine to prevent interference with drug absorption. The patient should also avoid consuming large amounts of foods that can inhibit thyroid secretion, such as strawberries, peaches, pears, cabbage, turnips, spinach, kale, Brussels sprouts, cauliflower, radishes, and peas.

Pregnancy: Thyroid replacement therapy should be continued during pregnancy. Human data have not shown fetal harm. The drug is secreted in human milk, although adverse effects have not been found in breastfed neonates.

Treatment of Overdose: The treatment of levothyroxine overdose is the same as the treatment of thyroid crisis or thyroid storm, as discussed later in Section 67.6. Treatment is directed at reducing the level of circulating thyroid hormone with antithyroid drugs and decreasing sympathetic stimulation with corticosteroids and beta-adrenergic blockers.

Clinician Responsibilities: Key clinical implications for patients receiving levothyroxine are included in Applied Clinical Judgment: Patients Receiving Pharmacotherapy with Thyroid Hormone Replacement and Thyroid Antagonists.

Drugs Similar to Levothyroxine (Levothroid, Levoxyl, Synthroid, Unithroid)

Other thyroid replacement medications include liothyronine and desiccated thyroid. All thyroid drugs carry a black box warning stating they should not be used for weight loss or to treat obesity. All are considered safe to use during pregnancy and lactation. Liotrix, a synthetic mixture of T_4 and T_3, was discontinued in 2018.

Liothyronine (Cytomel, Triostat): Approved in 1954, liothyronine is a synthetic form of T_3 used in replacement therapy for hypothyroidism. Its actions, adverse effects, and contraindications are similar to those for endogenous thyroid hormone. It has a shorter onset, half-life, and duration of action than levothyroxine and is more expensive. Liothyronine is readily converted to T_3 in the bloodstream. The injectable form of liothyronine is a preferred drug for the treatment of myxedema coma. It is available in oral and IV formulations.

Thyroid, Desiccated (Armour Thyroid, Thyroid USP): Desiccated thyroid is an older formulation, approved in 1939, obtained from the dried thyroid glands of pigs. The drug contains T_3 and T_4 in their natural proportions. Desiccated thyroid is less pure and has less reliable content than synthetic formulations and has been replaced by levothyroxine. It is used only for patients who have taken it for years—newly diagnosed cases of hypothyroidism are treated with synthetic thyroid hormone.

CONNECTIONS: Treating the Diverse Patient

Ethnic Differences in Thyroid Hormone Replacement

As more is learned in the quest for personalized medicine, the influence of ethnic differences on replacement therapies is also being discovered. In a study of Jewish and non-Jewish children, Oron et al. (2020) discovered that the level of TSH was influenced by both body mass index (BMI) and ethnicity. While thyroid dosing is usually based on weight or BMI, TSH was found to be lower in those of Jewish ancestry that was studied than in the non-Jewish population. While BMI remains an appropriate consideration for thyroid replacement dosing, possible differences in TSH related to ethnic ancestry should also be considered to fine-tune the dose.

CONNECTIONS: APPLIED CLINICAL JUDGMENT

Patients Receiving Pharmacotherapy with Thyroid Hormone Replacement and Thyroid Antagonists

Key Assessment Data

- History of current condition including cardiovascular, GI, hepatic, and kidney disease, baseline vital signs, physical exam findings; T_3, T_4, and TSH levels; complete blood count; platelets, electrolytes, glucose, and lipid levels; pregnancy or breastfeeding; drug history including allergies, current prescription and over-the-counter (OTC) drugs, herbal preparations, and caffeine, nicotine, and alcohol use. Obtain ECG if dysrhythmias are present.

Desired Therapeutic Outcomes

Improvement is observed and measurable by T_3, T_4, and TSH levels return to normal, associated symptoms ease.

Minimizing Adverse Effects

- Daily fluctuations in symptoms may occur because thyroid replacement therapy may not precisely approximate the body's own levels. Significant increases in original symptoms may signal less-than-optimal therapeutic results. Dramatic "opposite" effect and hypo- or hyperthyroid symptoms may signal drug toxicity.
- When antithyroid drugs are used, significant return of hyperthyroid symptoms may indicate that inadequate therapeutic levels are being maintained; symptoms of hypothyroidism may signal drug toxicity.
- Thyroid replacement and thyroid antagonist therapy may cause changes in glucose levels and an adjustment in antidiabetic medications may be needed.
- Thyroid replacement drugs interact with many medications and may cause suboptimal or excessive responses. Drugs such as calcium and aluminum antacids decrease absorption of thyroid hormone.

Lifespan Considerations

- Older patients are more sensitive to thyroid replacement therapy. Minor changes in daily thyroid levels may cause a significant change in symptoms.
- Infants and children receiving thyroid replacement therapy should continue to display normal growth and development curves.
- The older adult is especially at risk for falls related to dizziness. Effects of thyroid hormone on bone remodeling may place the patient at risk for fractures.
- If radioactive iodine is used, women who are pregnant and young children should avoid contact with the patient and others should limit contact to no more than 1 hour per day.

Diversity Considerations

- Monitor ethnically diverse patients for effects of thyroid replacement as differences in TSH may affect the dose given per BMI or weight.

Patient Education

- The lowest dose of thyroid replacement will be started and gradually increased to find the optimal level. Any significant change in symptoms should be promptly reported to the healthcare provider. Full effects may take a week or longer to be realized. Use the same brand of drug each time the prescription is filled and contact the provider if the drug manufacturer is changed.
- Antithyroid drugs will help to stabilize thyroid hormone levels quickly, but other methods (e.g., surgery, radioactive iodine) may be required for long-term management.
- Weigh self two to three times per week, record the findings, and bring the record to each clinic visit.
- Small daily fluctuations may occur, especially during periods of stress or illness. Any significant or increasing changes in pulse rate, weight, nervousness or fatigue, intolerance to heat or cold, and diarrhea or constipation should be reported to the healthcare provider.
- Avoid excessive intake of iodine-containing foods (e.g., iodized salt, soy sauce, tofu, yogurt, milk, strawberries, eggs).
- Patients with diabetes should monitor capillary glucose levels more frequently during therapy. Report any consistent changes to the healthcare provider.
- If dizziness occurs, sit or lie down and do not attempt to stand or walk until the sensation passes.
- Take the drug following appropriate guidelines:
    - Take thyroid replacement therapy at the same time each morning to approximate normal body hormone levels. If night shift hours are worked, consult with the healthcare provider about scheduling appropriate time of drug administration.
    - Take antithyroid medication 1 hour before or 2 hours after the first meal of the day.
    - To ensure optimal therapeutic response from thyroid replacement therapy, take the same brand of drug and request the same manufacturer each time the prescription is filled. If the same drug is unavailable, consult with the healthcare provider about dosage or observe for adverse drug effects. Do not switch trade names until the provider has been consulted.
    - When radioactive iodine is used, increase fluid intake up to 2 L/day as allowed and void frequently to avoid irradiation to gonads from radioactivity in urine excretion. Do not expectorate and cover the mouth when coughing. Any contaminated tissues should be disposed of per instructions of the healthcare provider.
- Carry a medical identification card or wear medical alert jewelry indicating thyroid replacement therapy.

Prescribing Considerations

- In adult patients with primary hypothyroidism, monitor serum TSH levels after an interval of 6 to 8 weeks after any change in dose. In patients on a stable and appropriate replacement dose, evaluate clinical and biochemical response every 6 to 12 months and whenever there is a change in the patient's clinical status.
- During pregnancy for women with preexisting hypothyroidism, measure serum TSH and free-T4 as soon as pregnancy is confirmed and, at minimum, during each trimester of pregnancy.
- Start levothyroxine at the full replacement dose in otherwise healthy, nonelderly individuals who have been hypothyroid for only a short time (such as a few months). The average full replacement dose is approximately 1.6 mcg per kg per day (e.g., 100 to 125 mcg per day for a 70-kg adult).
- Adjust the dose by 12.5 to 25 mcg increments every 4 to 6 weeks until the patient is clinically euthyroid and the serum TSH returns to normal. Doses greater than 200 mcg per day are seldom required. An inadequate response to daily doses of greater than 300 mcg per day is rare and may indicate poor compliance, malabsorption, or drug interactions.
- For elderly patients or patients with underlying cardiac disease, start with a dose of 12.5 to 25 mcg per day. Increase the dose every 6 to 8 weeks, as needed, until the patient is clinically euthyroid and the serum TSH returns to normal. The full replacement dose of levothyroxine sodium may be less than 1 mcg per kg per day in elderly patients.

Pathophysiology of Hyperthyroid Disorders

67.5 Hyperthyroidism, or Graves' disease, is an autoimmune disorder accompanied by ophthalmopathy and goiter.

Symptoms of hyperthyroidism have been recorded in medical documents dating back to the 12th century. The most common cause of hyperthyroidism is **Graves' disease**, named after Irish doctor Robert Graves, who described the disorder in 1835. The condition is characterized by the excessive secretion of thyroid hormone.

The two most visible signs of Graves' disease are goiter and **exophthalmos**, an outward bulging of the eyes. Up to one-third of those with Graves' disease develop severe eye problems such as paralysis of the ocular muscles, damage to the optic nerve with some vision loss, and corneal ulceration due to the inability of the eyelids to close. These eye problems are aggravated by smoking, which should be strongly discouraged in patients with Graves' disease. Not all eye changes are reversible with therapy. A rare skin disorder, pretibial myxedema, may also occur, with thickening of the skin, plaques, and nodules over the shins and dorsal surface of the feet. Like the ophthalmic changes, these skin changes may persist despite effective treatment of the disease.

Causes of Graves' disease include adenoma and excessive treatment with thyroid hormone. The onset is usually between the ages of 20 and 40 years, and it occurs five times more often in women than in men. Graves' disease is an autoimmune disorder caused by the formation of **thyroid-stimulating immunoglobulin (TSI)** in the thyroid gland. The TSI stimulates the synthesis, secretion and actions of thyroid hormone.

The manifestations of hyperthyroidism are caused by the hypermetabolic state and the increase in sympathetic nervous system activity. The symptoms include nervousness, irritability, fatigue, insomnia, weight loss despite a large appetite, tachycardia, palpitations, HTN, shortness of breath, increased sweating, muscle cramps, hyperthermia, and heat intolerance. A fine-muscle tremor may occur. Approximately 15% of older adults with new-onset atrial fibrillation, a common cardiac dysrhythmia, have thyrotoxicosis.

Very high levels of circulating thyroid hormone may cause **thyrotoxicosis**. **thyroid crisis**, or **thyroid storm**, is a rare, life-threatening form of thyrotoxicosis. If untreated, it is associated with mortality rates of 80 to 90%. Even with treatment, mortality from thyroid storm exceeds 20%. It occurs most often in teenage and young adult women with undiagnosed or untreated cases of hyperthyroidism and can be precipitated by the stress of an acute infection, diabetic ketoacidosis, trauma, or manipulation of the thyroid gland during surgery. Manifestations include high fever, cardiovascular effects (tachycardia, heart failure, angina, and MI), and CNS effects (agitation, restlessness, delirium, progressing to coma). It is treated with supportive measures such as efforts to reduce body temperature without causing shivering; fluid, glucose, and electrolyte replacement; and beta-adrenergic blockers. Aspirin should not be used to lower the body temperature of an individual in thyroid storm because it displaces thyroid hormone from its protein-binding sites in the serum, increasing the level of free, or active, thyroid hormone, which worsens the condition. Antithyroid drugs may be used to decrease thyroid hormone production.

PharmFACT

Although Graves' disease most commonly occurs in adults, it also occurs in children. About 10% of infants born to women with Graves' disease have hyperthyroidism, but most are asymptomatic. Concordance for Graves' disease is 30 to 50% in identical twins (Levitsky, 2016).

Pharmacotherapy of Hyperthyroid Disorders

67.6 Hyperthyroidism is treated with surgery or drugs that reduce the production of thyroid hormone.

Large thyroid nodules and those with a possibility of thyroid cancer etiology require surgical removal of all or part of the thyroid gland. In less serious cases of the disorder, pharmacotherapy can be used to diminish the secretion of thyroid hormone.

One strategy to lower thyroid hormone secretion is to destroy part of the gland (ablation) by administering radioactive iodide (^{131}I). The goal of thyroid ablation is to use the ionizing radiation from the drug to destroy just enough of the thyroid gland to return the patient to a normal thyroid state. This therapy results in a permanent, long-term solution to hyperthyroidism, is contraindicated during pregnancy due to the risk of exposing the fetus to ionizing radiation.

Antithyroid drugs may be administered to manage hyperthyroidism. Propylthiouracil (PTU) and methimazole (Tapazole) prevent the incorporation of iodine into the thyroid hormone molecule and block the conversion of T_4 to T_3 in peripheral tissues. Doses of the antithyroid drugs are listed in Table 67.4.

Treatment of thyroid storm is a medical emergency. Methimazole or propylthiouracil are administered to prevent further synthesis of thyroid hormone. Propylthiouracil also blocks the conversion of T_4 to T_3 in peripheral tissues and is preferred for pregnant patients. Potassium iodide

Table 67.4 Antithyroid Drugs

Drug Name	Dose for Adults (Maximum Dose Where Indicated)	Adverse Effects
methimazole (Tapazole)	PO: 5–15 mg tid (max: 60 mg/day)	*Nausea, rash, pruritus, urticaria, fever, numbness in fingers, peripheral neuropathy, leukopenia, hypothyroidism* Agranulocytosis, bradycardia, hepatotoxicity
potassium iodide and iodine (Iosat, Lugol's solution, Thyro-Safe)	PO: 65 mg (Thyro-Safe) or 130 mg (Iosat) once daily	*Diarrhea, nausea and vomiting, stomach pain, fever, weakness, irregular heartbeat, hypothyroidism* Angioneurotic edema, iodine poisoning
propylthiouracil (PTU)	PO: 300–450 mg tid	*Nausea, rash, pruritus, headache, fever, numbness in fingers, diarrhea, myelosuppression, hypothyroidism* Agranulocytosis
radioactive iodide (^{131}I)	PO: 0.8–150 millicurie (a curie is a unit of radioactivity)	*Adverse effects are uncommon* Thyroiditis, hypothyroidism, hypersensitivity

Note: Italics indicate common adverse effects. Underline indicates severe adverse effects.

solution can be given to immediately block the release of thyroid hormone but should not be given until 1 hour after the administration of antithyroid medications.

Several drugs are used as adjuncts in the therapy of thyroid storm. During hyperthyroid states, beta-adrenergic blocking drugs such as propranolol (Inderal), esmolol (Brevibloc), or metoprolol (Toprol) are given to block the effects of the thyroid hormones on sympathetic receptors in the heart. The actions include a decrease in heart rate and strength of contraction, thereby decreasing myocardial oxygen demands. These effects occur quickly, while the actions of antithyroid drugs take longer to occur. Refer to Chapter 16 for the specific pharmacology of beta-adrenergic blockers.

IV corticosteroids such as hydrocortisone (Solu-Cortef) or dexamethasone may be ordered to treat acute hyperthyroid states. Corticosteroids block the conversion of T_4 to T_3 in peripheral tissues. In addition, severe hyperthyroid states create high levels of stress that deplete adrenal corticosteroids in the body, and administration of replacement doses is necessary. The pharmacology of the corticosteroids is presented in Chapter 68.

PROTOTYPE DRUG Propylthiouracil (PTU)

Classification **Therapeutic:** Antithyroid drug
Pharmacologic: Thyroid hormone inhibitor

Therapeutic Effects and Uses: Approved in 1947, propylthiouracil decreases thyroid hormone levels in hyperthyroid states that are caused by the overproduction of thyroid hormone. It is also used to establish the normal thyroid state prior to surgery or radioactive iodine treatment and for palliative control of toxic nodular goiter. Propylthiouracil is not effective in treating thyroiditis because this condition is due to overrelease, not overproduction, of thyroid hormone.

Mechanism of Action: Propylthiouracil inhibits the first step in the synthesis of thyroid hormone and suppresses the peripheral conversion of T_4 to T_3. It does not affect thyroid hormone that has already been synthesized, so therapeutic response may be delayed by 3 to 12 weeks, until existing supplies of thyroid hormone have been depleted.

Pharmacokinetics:

Route(s)	PO
Absorption	Rapidly absorbed
Distribution	Concentrated by the thyroid gland; crosses the placenta; secreted in breast milk; 60–80% bound to plasma protein
Primary metabolism	Hepatic
Primary excretion	Kidneys
Onset of action	Absorbed within 30 min, but therapeutic effects may take up to 3 weeks
Duration of action	Half-life: 1–2 h; peak: 1–1.5 h

Adverse Effects: Approximately 15 to 20% of patients taking this drug will experience leukopenia, which is normally asymptomatic. Serious hypersensitivity reactions are rare but may include agranulocytosis, aplastic anemia, thrombocytopenia, rash, urticaria, and glomerulonephritis. Arthralgias and joint swelling occur in 5% of patients. CNS effects include headache, vertigo, neuritis, and paresthesias. Propylthiouracil can also cause hypothyroidism and goiter at high doses. **Black Box Warning:** Severe liver injury and acute hepatic failure have been reported in patients taking propylthiouracil. This drug should be reserved for those unable to tolerate methimazole and in whom radioactive iodine therapy or surgery are not appropriate treatments for hyperthyroidism.

Contraindications/Precautions: The use of propylthiouracil is contraindicated if the patient has a hypersensitivity to the drug. It should be used with caution during active infection and bone marrow depression. Because propylthiouracil can cause liver impairment, caution should be used when treating patients with preexisting hepatic disease.

Drug Interactions: Propylthiouracil increases the actions of anticoagulants, which creates an increased risk of bleeding. Iodine-containing drugs (amiodarone, potassium iodide, sodium iodide, radioactive iodine) and thyroid hormones can inhibit the effectiveness of this drug. Altered serum levels of metoprolol, propranolol, and digoxin can occur as the patient moves from a hyperthyroid to a normal thyroid state. Cross hypersensitivity occurs in about 50% of patients who have experienced a hypersensitivity reaction to methimazole, the other major antithyroid medication. Propylthiouracil should not be used with carbamazepine or clozapine because this may increase the risk of agranulocytosis. **Herbal/Food:** Unknown.

Pregnancy: This drug crosses the placenta and may induce goiter or cause cretinism in the fetus. If an antithyroid drug is required, some practitioners recommend propylthiouracil during the first trimester, followed by methimazole for the remainder of the pregnancy. Because this drug is secreted in human milk, infant thyroid levels should be regularly monitored if breastfeeding.

Treatment of Overdose: When propylthiouracil is taken in high doses, it can induce hypothyroidism; the administration of thyroid hormone may be necessary.

Clinician Responsibilities: Key clinical implications for patients receiving propylthiouracil are included in Applied Clinical Judgment: Patients Receiving Pharmacotherapy with Thyroid Hormone Replacement and Thyroid Antagonists.

Drugs Similar to Propylthiouracil (PTU)

Drugs similar to propylthiouracil include Lugol's solution, methimazole, potassium iodide, and radioactive iodide.

Lugol's Solution (5% Elemental Iodine and 10% Potassium Iodide): This strong iodine solution is given orally to treat hyperthyroidism, as adjunctive therapy 10 to 14 days prior to thyroid surgery, or for the treatment of thyrotoxicosis. It has been used as a topical antiseptic. Although iodine is necessary for the synthesis of thyroid hormone, high levels inhibit both the synthesis and release of thyroid hormone. Chronic use can result in toxicity known as **iodism**, which is characterized by burning in the mouth and throat, a metallic taste, sore teeth and gums, increased salivation and nasal discharge, swollen eyelids, gastric irritation, and diarrhea. The distribution of Lugol's solution is regulated by the U.S. Drug Enforcement Administration because strong iodine solutions are used in the manufacture of crystal methamphetamine. Lugol's solution is contraindicated during pregnancy and lactation.

Methimazole (Tapazole): Approved in 1950, methimazole is given by the oral route to correct hyperthyroidism by inhibiting the synthesis of thyroid hormone. Like PTU, it does not affect existing stores of thyroid hormone; thus, it may take many weeks before a normal thyroid state is achieved. Its uses, contraindications, and adverse effects are similar to those for PTU, except that methimazole has a lower risk for liver injury and does not induce hypothyroidism. Other important differences are that methimazole does not inhibit conversion of T_4 to T_3; therefore, its effects may take longer to occur. Methimazole has a longer half-life, allowing for once-a-day dosing, while PTU must be taken three times a day. Methimazole is usually administered for 12 to 18 months, then tapered or discontinued if TSH levels are normal. This drug is teratogenic in laboratory animals and some evidence links it to human birth defects. Because this drug is secreted in human milk, infant thyroid levels should be regularly monitored if breastfeeding.

Potassium Iodide (Iosat, Thyro-Safe): Generic potassium iodide is given orally prior to thyroid surgery to reduce the vascularity (risk of bleeding), fragility, and size of the thyroid gland. It may also be used alone for hyperthyroidism or in combination with antithyroid drugs and beta-adrenergic blockers in the treatment of thyroid storm. Like other forms of iodide, it suppresses the synthesis and release of thyroid hormone. Iosat and Thyro-safe are OTC products used to protect the thyroid gland in instances of radiation exposure secondary to a nuclear incident. It is taken up by the thyroid gland, thereby blocking the uptake of radioactive iodide by the thyroid gland, reducing the risk for developing thyroid cancer. As a protective agent, it must be given immediately prior to, or within 3 hours following, radiation exposure. In high doses, potassium iodide causes fetal harm in laboratory animals. Prolonged use during pregnancy is not recommended. Because this drug is secreted in human milk and has the potential to suppress thyroid function in the neonate, caution should be used if breastfeeding.

Radioactive Iodide (^{131}I): Radioactive iodide is an isotope of iodine used for hyperthyroidism. Like all iodine, ^{131}I is taken up by the thyroid gland, where its radioactivity destroys thyroid tissue. The goal is to destroy part of the gland, thereby decreasing the amount of thyroid hormone produced and secreted. In some patients, too much thyroid gland is destroyed and hypothyroidism results, which is then treated with levothyroxine. Approximately two-thirds of patients treated with ^{131}I respond to a single treatment, whereas the rest require two or more treatments. Therapeutic effects develop slowly over 2 to 3 months, and the tissue damage is limited to the thyroid gland with no surrounding structures affected. Although it is contraindicated during pregnancy and breastfeeding, and usually not used in children, ^{131}I has not been known to cause cancer or other serious adverse effects to the thyroid gland or elsewhere in the body. It is used in patients wishing to avoid surgery or those who do not tolerate antithyroid drugs. It is administered PO and is also used to treat thyroid cancer (in high doses) and for the diagnosis of thyroid disorders. This drug is contraindicated during pregnancy or lactation. Many practitioners advise that pregnancy be delayed for at least 6 months following treatment with radioactive iodide.

Understanding Chapter 67

Key Concepts Summary

67.1 Thyroid hormones contain iodine and stimulate the basal metabolic rate of nearly all tissues.

67.2 An accurate diagnosis of thyroid hormone dysfunction is based on the patient's symptoms and the results of diagnostic tests.

67.3 Hypothyroidism, or thyroid deficiency, can occur as a congenital or acquired disorder.

67.4 Hypothyroidism is treated by replacement therapy with thyroid hormone.

67.5 Hyperthyroidism, or Graves' disease, is an autoimmune disorder accompanied by ophthalmopathy and goiter.

67.6 Hyperthyroidism is treated with surgery or drugs that reduce the production of thyroid hormone.

CASE STUDY: Making the Patient Connection

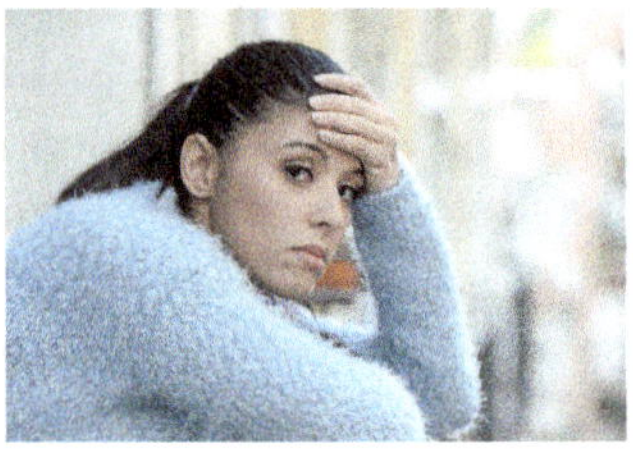

Remember the patient "Helen Mercado" at the beginning of the chapter? Now read the remainder of the case study. Based on the information presented within this chapter, respond to the critical thinking questions that follow.

Helen is a 38-year-old mother of three young children who works full time in a department store. She has been feeling extremely tired, has been gaining weight, and says she feels cold all the time. Acting on her feelings that something might be wrong, she goes to her healthcare provider. Helen's vital signs at that time are as follows: blood pressure, 94/60 mmHg; heart rate, 58 beats/min; temperature, 36.3°C (97.4°F). Her weight has increased 13.6 kg (30 lb) from when she was last seen 6 months ago. She confirms that her appetite has decreased. After completing a physical examination, the healthcare provider orders some laboratory tests including T_3, T_4, and TSH.

Critical Thinking Questions

1. Based on the patient's symptoms, what test results would you anticipate?
2. The healthcare provider orders levothyroxine (Synthroid) 200 mcg PO daily for Helen. What will you teach Helen about this drug and when to take it?
3. Helen asks you if she will need to be on the medication for very long. How will you answer her?
4. What symptoms should Helen report to the provider while she is taking the Synthroid?

Additional Case Study

The nurse receives a new patient admission onto a cardiac unit: Carolyn James, a 72-year-old woman, with new-onset atrial fibrillation with rapid ventricular response. The nurse connects the patient to a cardiac monitor and obtains the following vital signs: blood pressure, 168/96 mmHg; respirations, 28 breaths/min; heart rate, 162 beats/min; temperature, 38.7°C (101.6°F). The nurse learns from the patient's daughter that Carolyn was recently diagnosed with Graves' disease, but she has not been taking her medications.

1. What diagnostic tests do you expect to see ordered for this patient?
2. What drug therapy do you anticipate for Carolyn?
3. What long-term therapy do you believe is appropriate for this patient?

Chapter Review

1. The patient on replacement therapy with levothyroxine (Synthroid) reports feeling nervous and is having occasional palpitations and tremors. The nurse recognizes that these symptoms may indicate what effect is occurring?
   1. The patient is still experiencing hypothyroidism and the dose may need to be increased.
   2. The patient now has normal thyroid function and the levothyroxine is no longer needed.
   3. The patient has developed diabetes and needs further evaluation.
   4. The patient is experiencing symptoms of hyperthyroidism and the drug dosage may need to be decreased.

2. Which of the following assessment findings would the nurse expect to observe in an adult patient experiencing therapeutic effects from levothyroxine (Synthroid)? (Select all that apply.)
   1. Constipation and weight gain
   2. Decreased blinking and exophthalmos
   3. Decreased reports of fatigue
   4. Decreased blood cholesterol levels
   5. Pulse rate between 60 and 100 beats/minute

3. A patient will be treated with propylthiouracil (PTU) for hyperthyroidism. While the patient is taking this drug, which symptoms will the nurse teach the patient to report to the healthcare provider?
   1. Sore throat, low-grade fever, chills
   2. Increase in appetite and caloric intake
   3. Tinnitus, altered taste, thickened saliva
   4. Insomnia, nightmares, and night sweats

4. Which assessment finding would cause the nurse to withhold a regularly scheduled dose of levothyroxine?
   1. A 1-kg (2-lb) weight gain
   2. A blood pressure reading of 100/70 mmHg
   3. A heart rate of 110 beats/min
   4. A temperature of 37.9°C (100.2°F)

5. A patient is taking a solution of 5% iodine and 10% potassium iodide (Lugol's solution) prior to a thyroidectomy. The patient asks why iodine solution is used since iodine is needed to make thyroid hormone. What is the nurse's best answer?
   1. "The symptoms you were having indicate you were not receiving enough iodine."
   2. "High levels of iodine can temporarily reduce the amount of thyroid hormone your body makes and secretes."
   3. "High levels of iodine are always used prior to thyroidectomy to make up for the loss of iodine when the thyroid is removed."
   4. "The high levels of iodine help prevent diabetes from developing."

6. What should the nurse teach the patient who is newly diagnosed with hypothyroidism and will start taking levothyroxine (Synthroid)?
   1. Take the pill in the afternoon with a high-fiber snack to prevent stomach upset.
   2. Eat plenty of fruits and vegetables such as strawberries, spinach, and kale to replace vital nutrients.
   3. Take the dose in the morning before breakfast, as close to the same time each day as possible.
   4. The drug may be taken every other day if diarrhea occurs.

See Appendix A for answers to critical thinking questions, case study questions, and review questions.

References

Harding, K. B., Peña-Rosas, J. P., Webster, A. C., Yap, C. M., Payne, B. A., Ota, E., & De-Regil, L. M. (2017). Iodine supplementation for women during the preconception, pregnancy and postpartum period. *Cochrane Database of Systematic Reviews*, Issue 3, Article No. CD011761. https://doi.org/10.1002/14651858.CD011761.pub2

Oron, T., Lazar, L., Feldhamer, I., Manor, M., Koren-Morag, N., Tenenbaum, A., & Meyerovitch, J (2020). Pediatric reference values of TSH should be personalized according to BMI and ethnicity. *European Journal of Endocrinology*, *183*, 419–426. https://doi.org/10.1530/EJE-20-0239

Selected Bibliography

American College of Obstetrics and Gynecology. (2020). *ACOG update: Thyroid disease in pregnancy*. https://www.obgproject.com/2020/06/22/acog-update-thyroid-disease-in-pregnancy/

Azizi, F., & Malboosbaf, R. (2019). Safety of long-term antithyroid drug treatment?: A systematic review. *Journal of Endocrinological Investigation, 42*(11), 1273–1283. https://doi.org/10.1007/s40618-019-01054-1

Bekkering, G. E., Agoritsas, T., Lytvyn, L., Heen, A. F., Feller, M., Moutzouri, E., et al. (2019). Thyroid hormones treatment for subclinical hypothyroidism: A clinical practice guideline. *British Medical Journal, 365*, l2006. https://doi.org/10.1136/bmj.l2006

Eledrisi, M. S. (2020). *Myxedema coma or crisis*. Medscape. http://emedicine.medscape.com/article/123577-overview

Leung, A. M. (2016). Thyroid emergencies. *Journal of Infusion Nursing, 39*, 281–286. https://doi.org/10.1097/NAN.0000000000000186

Maraka, S., Ospina, N. M. S., O'Keeffe, D. T., Espinosa De Ycaza, A. E., Gionfriddo, M. R., Erwin, P. J., et al. (2016). Subclinical hypothyroidism in pregnancy: A systematic review and meta-analysis. *Thyroid, 26*, 580–590. https://doi.org/10.1089/thy.2015.0418

Misra, M. (2020). *Thyroid storm*. Medscape. http://emedicine.medscape.com/article/925147-overview

Nguyen, C. T., Sasso, E. B., Barton, L., & Mestman, J. H. (2018). Graves' hyperthyroidism in pregnancy: A clinical review. *Clinical Diabetes and Endocrinology, 4*(1), 4. https://doi.org/10.1186/s40842-018-0054-7

Ramdath, D. D., Padhi, E. M. T., Sarfaraz, S., Renwick, S., & Duncan, A. M. (2017). Beyond the cholesterol-lowering effect of soy protein: A review of the effects of dietary soy and its constituents on risk factors for cardiovascular disease. *Nutrients, 9*, 324. https://doi.org/10.3390/nu9040324

Ross, D. S., Burch, H. B., Cooper, D. S., Greenlee, M. C., Laurberg, P., Maia, A. L., et al. (2016). 2016 American Thyroid Association guidelines for diagnosis and management of hyperthyroidism and other causes of thyrotoxicosis. *Thyroid, 26*, 1343–1421. https://doi.org/10.1089/thy.2016.0229

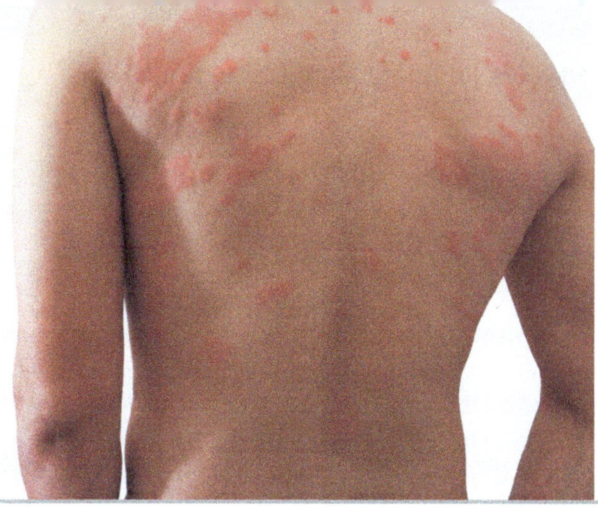

"I don't think this is poison ivy.
I've never had a problem with it and
I've been around it a lot.
But man, does this itch!"
—*Patient "Charlie Harness"*

Chapter 68
Corticosteroids and Drugs Affecting the Adrenal Cortex

Chapter Outline

- Physiology of the Adrenal Gland
- Overview of Corticosteroid Pharmacotherapy
- Adverse Effects of Corticosteroids
- Replacement Therapy with Corticosteroids

  PROTOTYPE *Hydrocortisone (Cortef, Solu-Cortef, Others), p. 1188*
- Corticosteroids for Nonendocrine Conditions
- Mineralocorticoids

  PROTOTYPE *Fludrocortisone, p. 1193*
- Antiadrenal Drugs

Learning Outcomes

After reading this chapter, the student should be able to:

1. Identify the functions of the three classes of hormones secreted by the adrenal gland.
2. Diagram the negative feedback regulation of corticosteroid secretion.
3. Identify common properties of the corticosteroid medications.
4. Describe the potential adverse effects of long-term corticosteroid therapy.
5. Compare and contrast the pharmacotherapy of acute and chronic adrenocortical insufficiency.
6. Explain how corticosteroids affect the inflammatory and immune responses.
7. Recognize nonendocrine disorders that respond to corticosteroid therapy.
8. Describe indications for pharmacotherapy with mineralocorticoids.
9. Explain the pharmacotherapy of Cushing's syndrome.
10. Describe the nurse's role in the pharmacologic management of adrenal disorders.
11. For each of the classes shown in the chapter outline, identify the prototype and representative drugs and explain the mechanism(s) of drug action, primary indications, contraindications, significant drug interactions, pregnancy data, and important adverse effects.
12. Apply clinical judgment to the care of patients receiving pharmacotherapy with corticosteroids and mineralocorticoids.

Key Terms

Definitions of the terms in bold may be found in the Glossary.

Though small, the adrenal glands secrete hormones that affect all body tissues. The primary secretions of the adrenal glands, the corticosteroids, are some of the most widely used drugs in medicine. They can be delivered by any route to treat conditions as diverse as dermatitis, lymphoma, ulcerative colitis, allergic rhinitis, and arthritis. This chapter examines the pharmacologic properties of corticosteroids that make them so important to pharmacotherapy.

Physiology of the Adrenal Gland

68.1 The adrenal glands secrete gonadocorticoids, mineralocorticoids, and corticosteroids.

Weighing only two-tenths of an ounce, each pyramid-shaped adrenal gland sitting atop each kidney is divided into two major portions: an inner medulla and an outer cortex. The secretions from these two portions have very different functions.

The adrenal medulla secretes 75 to 80% epinephrine, with the remainder of the secretion being norepinephrine. Adrenal release of epinephrine is triggered by activation of the sympathetic division of the autonomic nervous system. Symptoms of the fight-or-flight response resulting from the secretion of these hormones are described in Chapters 12 and 15.

The adrenal cortex secretes three essential classes of steroid hormones: mineralocorticoids, glucocorticoids, and gonadocorticoids. Collectively, the mineralocorticoids and glucocorticoids are called corticosteroids or adrenocortical hormones. Although the terms *corticosteroid* and *glucocorticoid* are sometimes used interchangeably in clinical practice, the term *corticosteroid* technically refers to a hormone or drug that has both glucocorticoid and mineralocorticoid activity. The hormones secreted by the adrenal gland are illustrated in Figure 68.1.

Mineralocorticoids: Aldosterone accounts for more than 95% of the **mineralocorticoids** secreted by the adrenal

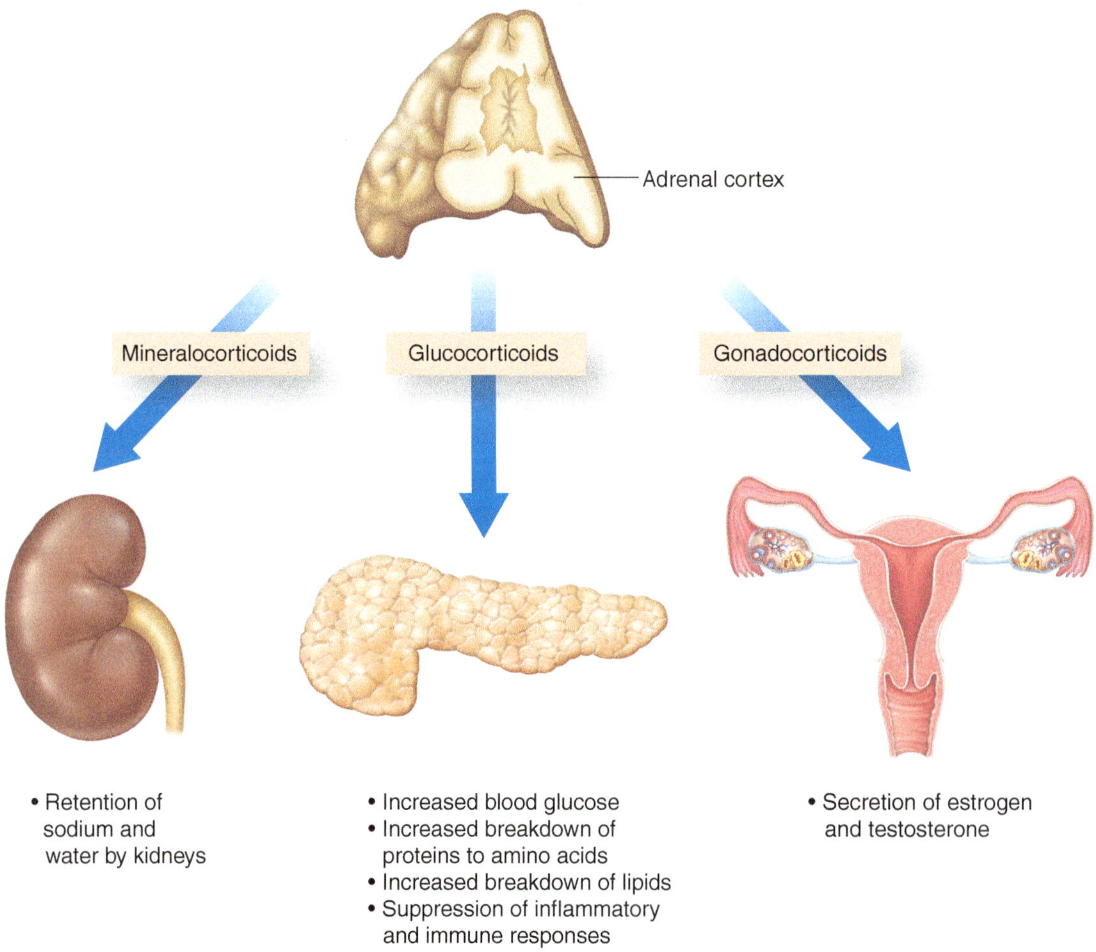

Figure 68.1 Hormonal secretions of the adrenal gland.

glands. The primary function of aldosterone is to conserve sodium and water and promote the excretion of potassium by the renal tubule, thus regulating plasma volume. Pharmacotherapy with mineralocorticoids is presented in Section 68.6.

Glucocorticoids: More than 30 different **glucocorticoids** are secreted from the adrenal cortex. Cortisol, also called hydrocortisone, is secreted in the highest amount and is the most important pharmacologically. The liver converts hydrocortisone into cortisone, an active metabolite that is also available as a medication. Corticosterone is an additional steroid secreted by the adrenal cortex.

Glucocorticoids prepare the body for long-term stress and affect the metabolism of nearly every cell. The effects of glucocorticoids are diverse and include the following:

- Increase the level of blood glucose (hyperglycemic effect) by inhibiting insulin secretion and promoting gluconeogenesis, which is the synthesis of carbohydrates from lipid and protein sources. This decreases glucose utilization by tissues and promotes the storage of glycogen in the liver.
- Increase the breakdown of proteins to amino acids. Amino acids are then converted to glucose and glycogen in the liver, resulting in protein depletion.
- Increase the breakdown of lipids (lipolysis). The fatty acids are then utilized as energy sources.
- Suppress the inflammatory and immune responses.
- Increase the sensitivity of vascular smooth muscle to the actions of norepinephrine and angiotensin II, thus modifying smooth muscle tone.
- Influence the central nervous system (CNS) by affecting mood and maintaining normal nerve excitability.
- Increase the breakdown of bony matrix, resulting in bone demineralization.
- Promote bronchodilation by making bronchial smooth muscle more responsive to sympathetic nervous system activation.
- Stabilize mast cells, inhibiting the release of inflammatory mediators.

As this list confirms, the glucocorticoids are essential hormones for maintaining homeostasis. When given as medications, some of the physiologic actions of glucocorticoids are considered therapeutic effects, whereas others are adverse effects. Unfortunately, it is impossible to totally separate therapeutic effects from adverse effects when drugs with such widespread actions are used in pharmacotherapy.

The physiologic levels of glucocorticoids vary based on a circadian rhythm. The lowest serum levels occur during early sleep. Secretion rises during the night, with levels peaking at awakening and declining during the day, depending on the needs of the body. Stress can cause a rapid increase in glucocorticoid levels; when faced with internal inflammatory or stressful conditions, the secretion of glucocorticoids can increase to 10 times their baseline level.

Regulation of glucocorticoid levels begins with corticotropin-releasing factor (CRF), secreted by the hypothalamus. CRF travels to the pituitary where it causes the release of **adrenocorticotropic hormone (ACTH)**. ACTH then travels via the blood to reach the adrenal cortex, causing it to release glucocorticoids. When the serum level of cortisol rises, it provides negative feedback to the hypothalamus and pituitary to shut off further release of glucocorticoids. This negative feedback mechanism is illustrated in Figure 68.2.

Gonadocorticoids: The **gonadocorticoids** or sex hormones secreted by the adrenal cortex are mostly androgens, though small amounts of estrogens are also produced. The amounts of adrenal sex hormones are far less than the levels secreted by the testes or ovaries during the reproductive years. Though their amount is small, the adrenal gonadocorticoids contribute to the onset of puberty and are the primary source of endogenous estrogen in postmenopausal women (see Chapter 69). Tumors of the adrenal cortex can cause hypersecretion of gonadocorticoids, resulting in hirsutism and masculinization, signs that are more noticeable in women than in men. The physiologic effects of androgens are discussed in Chapter 71.

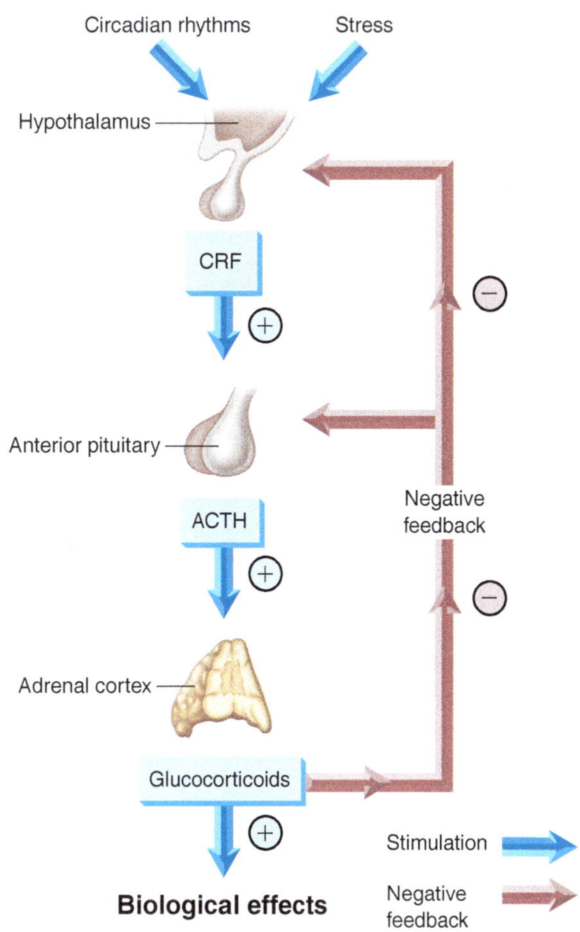

Figure 68.2 Feedback control of the adrenal cortex.

Overview of Corticosteroid Pharmacotherapy

68.2 Corticosteroids are widely used, and all drugs in the class have similar indications, actions, and adverse effects.

Corticosteroids are some of the most widely prescribed medications because they are useful in treating conditions affecting nearly every body system. Furthermore, some of their indications are for diseases common to all age groups and that occur frequently in the population. Some are available over the counter (OTC).

Corticosteroids can be classified in many different ways. One method is based on pathophysiology, such as grouping corticosteroids used for the treatment of inflammation, allergies, or neoplasias. Another method is to group the drugs by body system, such as corticosteroids used for skin conditions, immune disorders, or lung diseases. A third method is to look at corticosteroid use based on their pharmacologic actions, as listed in Table 68.1. In clinical practice, all methods are used.

Regardless of the method of classification, several general statements can be made about the corticosteroid medications:

- They all act by the same mechanism.
- All have the same basic adverse effects, which are dose dependent.
- Indications and adverse effects vary by the dose, length of use, and route of administration.
- They are well absorbed when administered orally or parenterally, and they are widely distributed to all body tissues. Topical administration (intra-articular, inhalation, skin products, and ocular drops) results in systemic absorption, although at a slow rate.
- Most are highly bound to plasma proteins.
- All are metabolized by the liver and excreted by the kidneys.
- All have the potential to cross the placenta and are secreted in breast milk. Use should be avoided during pregnancy and lactation.

More than 20 corticosteroids are available as medications, and the choice of a particular drug depends primarily on its pharmacokinetic properties. The duration of action, which is sometimes used to classify these drugs, ranges from short to long acting. Some, such as hydrocortisone, also have mineralocorticoid activity and may cause sodium and fluid retention; others, such as prednisone, have no such effect. Some corticosteroids are available by only one route, such as topical for dermal conditions or intranasal for allergic rhinitis. An overview of the indications for corticosteroid therapy is given in Table 68.1.

Table 68.1 Actions and Indications for Corticosteroids

Pharmacologic Action	Example Indications
Inhibit cell division	Lymphomas and other neoplasms
Reduce joint inflammation	Rheumatoid arthritis, osteoarthritis, bursitis, tendonitis
Reduce lung inflammation	Asthma, chronic obstructive pulmonary disease
Reduce skin inflammation	Dermatitis, psoriasis
Supply exogenous corticosteroids	Replacement therapy
Suppress allergic response	Allergic rhinitis; anaphylaxis
Suppress gastrointestinal (GI) inflammation	Inflammatory bowel disease
Suppress general inflammatory response	Systemic lupus erythematosus (SLE)
Suppress immune response	Prophylaxis of transplant rejection Autoimmune hemolytic anemia
Suppress ocular inflammation	Conjunctivitis

Adverse Effects of Corticosteroids

68.3 Long-term therapy with corticosteroids has the potential to cause serious adverse effects in multiple body systems.

Low-dose or brief-duration regimens of corticosteroids produce few clinically significant adverse effects. However, high doses taken for prolonged periods offer a significant risk for serious adverse effects. These adverse effects of corticosteroid therapy are well documented and can impact nearly any body system. The following list includes the most significant adverse events from long-term corticosteroid therapy:

- **Immune response.** Suppression of inflammation and immune responses increases patients' susceptibility to infections. Latent infections, such as herpesvirus or tuberculosis, may be reactivated during corticosteroid therapy. In addition, the anti-inflammatory actions of the corticosteroids may mask the signs of an existing infection.
- **Peptic ulcers.** Prolonged corticosteroid use is associated with the development of peptic ulcers, especially when these drugs are combined with nonsteroidal anti-inflammatory drugs (NSAIDs). Both classes of drugs reduce prostaglandin synthesis in the gastric mucosa, which normally provides protection from the high acidity in the stomach. Use of proton pump inhibitors may reduce the incidence of peptic ulcers in patients who are taking corticosteroids (see Chapter 59).
- **Osteoporosis.** Corticosteroids inhibit calcium absorption, suppress bone formation, and accelerate bone resorption—all actions that weaken the bony matrix. Up to 50% of patients on long-term corticosteroid therapy will sustain a fracture due to osteoporosis.

Treatment with a bisphosphonate may reduce the incidence of fractures in these patients (see Chapter 72).

- **Behavioral changes.** By an unknown mechanism, corticosteroids can induce psychologic changes. These may be minor, such as nervousness or moodiness, or may involve hallucinations and increased suicidal tendencies.
- **Eye changes.** Cataracts and open-angle glaucoma are potential adverse events of long-term corticosteroid therapy.
- **Metabolic changes.** Corticosteroids have a hyperglycemic action that raises serum glucose and can cause glucose intolerance, especially in patients with diabetes. Mobilization of lipids may cause hyperlipidemia and abnormal fat deposits. Electrolyte changes include hypocalcemia, hypokalemia, and hypernatremia. Fluid retention, weight gain, hypertension (HTN), and edema are other possible effects.
- **Myopathy.** Muscle wasting induced by corticosteroids may cause weakness and fatigue. The myopathy may involve ocular or respiratory muscles.

CONNECTION Checkpoint 68.1

From what you learned in Chapter 41, what drug class includes the preferred drugs for treating mild to moderate inflammation?

Corticosteroids also interact with many drugs. Their hyperglycemic effects may decrease the effectiveness of antidiabetic medications. Combining glucocorticoids with other ulcerogenic drugs such as aspirin and other NSAIDs markedly increases the risk of peptic ulcer disease. Administration with certain diuretics may lead to hypocalcemia and hypokalemia. Vaccines will have a diminished effect if administered during corticosteroid therapy. The nurse should always check for potential drug interactions when a patient is receiving prolonged corticosteroid therapy.

An important goal during long-term corticosteroid therapy is to prevent the development of serious adverse effects. The following strategies are often used to minimize the incidence of serious adverse effects:

- Doses are kept to the lowest amount that will achieve the therapeutic goal. In some cases, concurrent drug therapy with a noncorticosteroid may be implemented to produce additive therapeutic effects while keeping the corticosteroid dose low. Careful monitoring of the effectiveness of the drug is necessary.
- Corticosteroids are sometimes administered every other day (alternate-day dosing) to minimize adrenal atrophy (see Section 68.4). This prevents constant, negative feedback on the pituitary and forces the patient's adrenal glands to secrete endogenous corticosteroids every other day.
- For acute conditions, patients are administered large doses of corticosteroids for a few days and then the drug dose is gradually decreased until discontinued. This prevents the severe symptoms of adrenal atrophy from developing. For example, methylprednisolone (Medrol Dosepak) consists of twenty-one 4-mg tablets taken over 6 days. Six tablets are taken on day 1, five on day 2, four on day 3, three on day 4, two on day 5, and one on day 6.
- Whenever possible, corticosteroids should be administered locally by inhalation, intra-articular injections, or topical applications to the skin, eyes, or ears to diminish the extent of systemic effects. Local administration rarely produces systemic adverse effects.

CONNECTIONS: Complementary and Alternative Therapies

Turmeric for Inflammation

Description

Turmeric is a member of the ginger family and has been used for centuries in traditional Indian, East Asian, and Ayurveda medicine for skin, upper respiratory tract, joint, and digestive system conditions. The rhizome of the plant is dried and used to make dietary supplements or ground into paste for skin conditions. Curcumin is the major component of turmeric and the active substances are called curcuminoids. Turmeric is also a main ingredient in curry powder.

History and Claims

Turmeric has been used to treat a variety of inflammatory conditions including allergies, itching, arthritis, high cholesterol, cardiovascular conditions, and depression.

Standardization

There is no current standardized dose, but the capsules range between 400 and 1000 mg.

Evidence

Turmeric has low bioavailability and little reaches the bloodstream, and curcumin is unstable and changes into other substances (National Center for Complementary and Integrative Health, 2020). The substance shows promise in treating conditions associated with inflammation such as Parkinson's, Alzheimer's, and obesity and research is ongoing to determine the adequate dosage based on solubility of absorption and metabolism, active substances, and impact on body systems (Cavaleri, 2018).

Replacement Therapy with Corticosteroids

68.4 Adrenocortical insufficiency is treated by administering physiologic levels of corticosteroids.

Adrenocortical insufficiency (AI) is a lack of adequate secretion by the adrenal cortex. When pathology of the adrenal glands is the cause of the hyposecretion, it is called *primary* AI, or **Addison's disease**. The most common etiology of primary AI is the autoimmune destruction of both adrenal glands. Addison's disease is rare and includes a deficiency of all three cortex secretions: glucocorticoids, mineralocorticoids, and gonadocorticoids.

PharmFACT

One of the earliest symptoms of Addison's disease is hyperpigmentation of the oral and vaginal mucosas and the sun-exposed areas of the skin. This occurs because high ACTH levels stimulate melanocytes to produce excessive amounts of melanin (Griffing, 2020).

Secondary AI occurs when the adrenal glands are normal, but they are not receiving adequate stimulation due to lack of sufficient ACTH from the pituitary. Low serum levels of both ACTH and cortisol are diagnostic of secondary AI because this indicates that the adrenal gland is not receiving ACTH stimulation. The most common cause of secondary AI is prolonged use of glucocorticoid medication, which causes negative feedback to shut off production of ACTH by the pituitary. Patients taking more than 5 mg of corticosteroid for longer than 3 weeks are at risk for AI. Secondary AI is much more common than primary AI. Symptoms of primary and secondary AI are the same because both are characterized by inadequate corticosteroid secretion.

The onset of chronic AI is gradual, and it may take several months or even years before an accurate diagnosis is made. Symptoms include hypoglycemia, fatigue, muscle weakness, hypotension, increased skin pigmentation, and GI disturbances such as anorexia, vomiting, and diarrhea. Replacement therapy with corticosteroids is indicated, with the goal of achieving the same physiologic level of hormones that would be present if the adrenal glands were functioning properly. Patients requiring replacement therapy usually must take corticosteroids their entire lifetime, and concurrent therapy with a mineralocorticoid such as fludrocortisone may be necessary.

Acute AI has a sudden onset and usually occurs when corticosteroid medications are abruptly withdrawn from a patient who has been on long-term therapy. This is because constant, high amounts of corticosteroid medications provide continuous negative feedback to the hypothalamus and pituitary, shutting down the secretion of ACTH. Without stimulation by ACTH, the adrenal cortex shrinks and stops secreting endogenous corticosteroids, a condition known as **adrenal atrophy**. If the corticosteroid medication is abruptly withdrawn, the shrunken adrenal glands will not be able to secrete sufficient corticosteroids, and symptoms of **adrenal crisis** will appear. Symptoms of this condition include nausea and vomiting, lethargy, confusion, myalgia, arthralgia, fever, asthenia, acute abdominal pain, hypotension, seizures, kidney failure, and coma. Immediate administration of IV hydrocortisone is essential because shock may quickly result if symptoms remain untreated. To prevent adrenal crisis, corticosteroids should be discontinued gradually. The mechanism by which adrenal atrophy is induced by corticosteroid use is illustrated in Pharmacotherapy Illustrated 68.1.

The most frequently prescribed corticosteroid for treating AI is hydrocortisone. Hydrocortisone has some intrinsic mineralocorticoid activity; therefore, concurrent administration of fludrocortisone may not be necessary. Doses of hydrocortisone are individualized to the specific amount of replacement therapy needed by the patient, and doses will need to be increased during periods of high stress. Alternative corticosteroids include prednisone and dexamethasone. Because prednisone and dexamethasone have little or no mineralocorticoid activity, concurrent fludrocortisone therapy is necessary. Doses for selected corticosteroids are listed in Table 68.2.

Cosyntropin (Cortrosyn) is a drug structurally similar to ACTH that is used as a simple diagnostic test for AI. For this test, cosyntropin is injected IV and the plasma levels of cortisol are measured 30 to 60 minutes later. If the adrenal gland responds by secreting corticosteroids after the cosyntropin injection, the pathology lies at the level of the pituitary or hypothalamus (secondary AI). If plasma cortisol levels fail to rise after the injection, the pathology is at the level of the adrenal gland (primary AI).

CONNECTION Checkpoint 68.2

From what you learned in Chapter 43, explain why immunizations are sometimes contraindicated in patients receiving high-dose corticosteroid therapy.

PROTOTYPE DRUG **Hydrocortisone (Cortef, Solu-Cortef, Others)**

Classification **Therapeutic:** Adrenal hormone
Pharmacologic: Corticosteroid

Therapeutic Effects and Uses: Structurally identical to the natural hormone cortisol, hydrocortisone is a synthetic corticosteroid that is the preferred drug for treating adrenocortical insufficiency. When used for replacement therapy, it is given at physiologic doses. Once proper dosing has

Pharmacotherapy Illustrated 68.1

Corticosteroids and Adrenal Atrophy

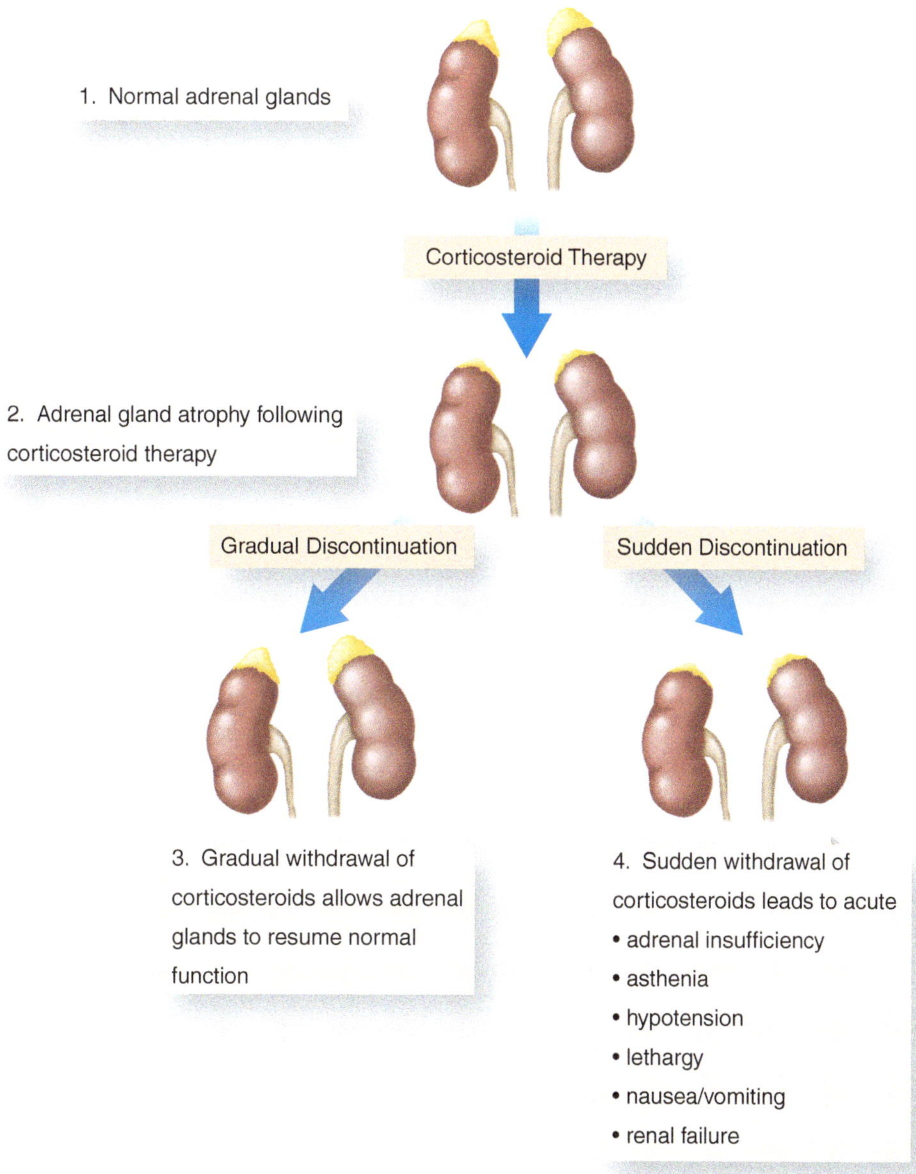

been achieved, its therapeutic effects should mimic those of endogenous corticosteroids. Hydrocortisone is also available for the treatment of inflammation, allergic disorders, and many other conditions. Intra-articular injections may be given to decrease severe inflammation in affected joints.

Hydrocortisone is available in eight different salts: base, acetate, butyrate, cypionate, probutate, sodium phosphate, sodium succinate, and valerate. Some of the salts, such as hydrocortisone acetate, are designed for topical use, whereas others such as hydrocortisone sodium succinate are for parenteral use only. When administering hydrocortisone, care should be taken to use the correct route for the prescribed formulation of this drug.

Mechanism of Action: The actions of hydrocortisone are complex, and the drug is thought to act by multiple mechanisms in different tissues. As a replacement drug, it restores deficient levels of glucocorticoids and, to a lesser extent, mineralocorticoids. As an anti-inflammatory drug, it blocks the actions of various chemical mediators in the inflammatory and allergic responses, including histamine, prostaglandins, and kinins.

Table 68.2 Selected Corticosteroids

Drug	Route and Adult Dose (Maximum Dose Where Indicated)	Adverse Effects
betamethasone	IM/IV: 0.5–9 mg/day Topical: Variable dosage	*Mood swings, weight gain, acne, facial flushing, nausea, insomnia, sodium and fluid retention, impaired wound healing, menstrual abnormalities* Peptic ulcer, hypocalcemia, osteoporosis with possible bone fractures, loss of muscle mass, decreased growth in children, possible masking of infections
budesonide (Entocort EC, Pulmicort Flexhaler, Rhinocort, Others)	Intranasal (Rhinocort): 1–2 sprays in each nostril/day (each spray: 32 mcg) PO (Entocort EC): 9 mg/day	
cortisone	PO: 20–300 mg/day in divided doses	
dexamethasone	PO: 0.25–9 mg/day in divided doses	
hydrocortisone (Cortef, Solu-Cortef, others)	PO: 10–320 mg/day in 3–4 divided doses IV/IM: 15–800 mg/day in 3–4 divided doses (max: 2 g/day)	
methylprednisolone (Depo-Medrol, Medrol, others)	PO: 4–48 mg/day in divided doses	
prednisolone	PO: 5–60 mg 1–4 times/day	
prednisone	PO: 5–60 mg 1–4 times/day	
triamcinolone (Aristospan, Kenalog, others)	IM: 60 mg q6wk Intra-articular: 2.5-40 mg depending on joint size	

Note: *Italics* indicate common adverse effects. Underline indicates serious adverse effects.

Pharmacokinetics:

Route(s)	PO, IV, IM, subcutaneous, rectal, intra-articular, topical
Absorption	Rapid
Distribution	Widely distributed when given PO or parenterally; crosses the placenta; secreted in breast milk; extensively bound to plasma protein
Primary metabolism	Hepatic
Primary excretion	Renal
Onset of action	PO: 1–2 h; IM: 20 min
Duration of action	1–1.5 days (PO or IM)

Adverse Effects: When used at low doses for replacement therapy, or by the topical or intranasal routes, adverse effects of hydrocortisone are uncommon. However, signs of Cushing's syndrome can develop with high doses or with prolonged use. Hydrocortisone possesses some mineralocorticoid activity, so sodium and fluid retention may be observed. A wide range of CNS effects have been reported, including insomnia, anxiety, headache, vertigo, confusion, and depression. Cardiovascular effects may include HTN and tachycardia. Long-term therapy may result in peptic ulcer disease, osteoporosis, hyperglycemia, cataracts, HTN, and impaired wound healing.

Contraindications/Precautions: Hydrocortisone is contraindicated in patients who are hypersensitive to the drug or who have known infections, unless the patient is being treated concurrently with anti-infectives. Patients with diabetes, osteoporosis, psychosis, liver disease, or hypothyroidism should be treated with caution. Patients with heart failure (HF) or HTN should be treated with caution due to the possibility of fluid retention with hydrocortisone. If taken for longer than 2 weeks, hydrocortisone should be discontinued gradually. Caution should be used in treating children because the drug may delay normal growth and development. PO corticosteroids must be used with caution in patients with preexisting GI disease such as peptic ulcers or ulcerative colitis because they may worsen these conditions. Use with potassium-wasting drugs such as thiazide or loop diuretics may increase the risk of hypokalemia. Anticholinesterase drugs may produce severe weakness. Hydrocortisone may cause a decrease in immune response to vaccines and toxoids. Patients on high doses of hydrocortisone should not receive live vaccines due to the possibility of infection. Because hydrocortisone can cause hyperglycemia, doses of insulin and oral hypoglycemic drugs may require adjustment. Vitamin D supplements are recommended to prevent corticosteroid-induced osteoporosis. **Herbal/Food:** Chronic use of aloe, senna, cascara, or buckthorn may cause potassium deficiency.

Pregnancy: Hydrocortisone has shown teratogenicity in laboratory animals. If the drug is required during pregnancy, doses should be kept as low as possible for short durations. If higher dosage is necessary, the fetus may develop AI. Low-potency, topical corticosteroids appear to be safe during pregnancy. Breastfeeding is not recommended if the mother is taking higher doses of corticosteroids.

Treatment of Overdose: Hydrocortisone has no acute toxicity and deaths are rare. No specific therapy is available, and patients are treated symptomatically.

Clinician Responsibilities: Key clinical implications for patients receiving hydrocortisone are included in Applied Clinical Judgment: Patients Receiving Pharmacotherapy with Systemic Corticosteroids.

Drugs Similar to Hydrocortisone (Cortef, Solu-Cortef, Others)

There are many other corticosteroids, all having the same actions. Pregnancy data are the same as for hydrocortisone.

Dexamethasone: Dexamethasone is a synthetic corticosteroid that has almost no mineralocorticoid activity. It is 20 to 30 times more potent than hydrocortisone and is available by PO, IV, IM, topical, aerosol, and ophthalmic routes. The parenteral formulations (dexamethasone sodium phosphate) are used for serious disorders such as anaphylaxis, reduction of cerebral edema, or acute AI or when PO therapy is not possible. Dexamethasone may be injected intra-articularly for the short-term therapy of inflamed joints, or intralesionally into acute inflamed lesions associated with discoid lupus, psoriatic plaques, and granulomatous disorders. It is also indicated for the palliative management of leukemias and lymphomas. Dexamethasone is sometimes found in fixed-dose combinations with antibiotics such as ciprofloxacin to treat otic or ocular infections that have significant inflammation. Systemic forms of the drug are metabolized by the liver to inactive metabolites. Dexamethasone has one of the longest durations of action of any corticosteroid.

Prednisone: Prednisone is rapidly absorbed and is the most frequently prescribed oral corticosteroids. It is about four times more potent than hydrocortisone and has a longer duration of action. It has little mineralocorticoid activity. Prednisone is a synthetic corticosteroid whose actions are the result of being metabolized to an active form, which is also available as the drug prednisolone. Although prednisone is available only by the PO route, prednisolone may be administered PO, parenterally, or topically and may be of value in patients with liver impairment because it does not require hepatic activation. Oral solutions (Prelone) and an orally disintegrating tablet (Orapred ODT) are primarily prescribed for treating childhood asthma. When used for inflammation, duration of prednisone therapy is commonly 4 to 10 days. For long-term therapy, alternate-day dosing is used. Prednisone is occasionally used to terminate acute bronchospasm in patients with asthma and as an antineoplastic drug for cancers such as Hodgkin's disease, acute childhood leukemias, and lymphomas. Prednisone has the same adverse effects and contraindications as hydrocortisone.

Corticosteroids for Nonendocrine Conditions

68.5 Corticosteroids are frequently used to suppress the inflammatory and immune responses.

One of the most important physiologic effects of corticosteroids is their natural ability to dampen the immune response and inhibit the synthesis of inflammatory mediators. When used to treat conditions characterized by hyperactive body defenses, the anti-inflammatory effects of the corticosteroids are therapeutic. When the drugs are administered as replacement therapy, however, suppression of the immune response can result in an increased incidence of infections.

Part of the reason for the effectiveness of the corticosteroids in reducing inflammation and the immune response is that they act by multiple mechanisms. These mechanisms include the following:

- Decreased numbers of circulating lymphocytes, eosinophils, monocytes, and basophils
- Inhibited movement of macrophages and leukocytes to areas of inflammation
- Decreased production of inflammatory cytokines, including histamine, bradykinin, interferons, interleukins, and granulocyte-macrophage colony-stimulating factor
- Decreased formation of prostaglandins.

It is important to note that the doses necessary to treat inflammatory and other nonendocrine diseases are much higher than those used to treat AI. For example, a daily maintenance dose of prednisone for a patient with Addison's disease is 7.5 mg/day. This amount approximates what would normally be secreted by the adrenal glands. Daily doses of prednisone for nonendocrine disorders range from 5 to 30 mg for transplant prophylaxis; 80 mg for chronic lymphocytic leukemia; 40 to 60 mg for Crohn's disease; and 20 to 300 mg for SLE. At these high doses, the adverse effects of corticosteroids will quickly manifest and the adrenal gland will begin to atrophy in only 2 to 4 weeks. Interventions should be planned to prevent anticipated adverse effects.

Arthritis: Arthritis is one of the most common diseases affecting older adults. Rheumatoid arthritis (RA) is a chronic autoimmune disease that causes inflammation of joints and is characterized by disfigurement and inflammation of multiple joints. Osteoarthritis is also a progressive joint disease, but it occurs with more advanced age and is characterized by less inflammation than RA. Both types of arthritis are treated with NSAIDs early in the course of the disease. Corticosteroids are administered when inflammation becomes severe, with therapy being limited to 1 to 2 weeks, or until the pain and inflammation subside. If the pain and inflammation are localized to one or two joints, intra-articular injections may be used. Corticosteroids offer only symptomatic treatment and do not alter the course of either type of arthritis. Arthritis pharmacotherapy is presented in Chapter 72.

Inflammatory bowel disease: Inflammatory bowel disease (IBD) is characterized by ulceration in the distal portion of the small intestine (Crohn's disease) or in the large intestine (ulcerative colitis). Various drugs, including the

5-aminosalicylic acid drugs, are used to control inflammation, cramping, and diarrhea. Exacerbations are treated with corticosteroids for brief time periods. Budesonide (Entocort-EC, Uceris) is a corticosteroid that has a delayed release and remains in the intestine to treat the inflammation locally, without causing significant systemic effects. IBD pharmacotherapy is presented in Chapter 60.

Asthma: Asthma is characterized by chronic inflammation that causes bronchoconstriction in the respiratory passages. Inhaled corticosteroids are preferred drugs for the prevention of asthmatic attacks and the management of chronic asthma. The inhaled drugs produce few systemic adverse effects. Oral corticosteroids are used for the short-term management of acute asthma exacerbations. Asthma pharmacotherapy is presented in Chapter 44.

Allergies: Allergic rhinitis is inflammation of the nasal mucosa caused by exposure to allergens. Intranasal corrticosteroids prevent symptoms of allergic rhinitis and have largely replaced antihistamines as preferred drugs for this condition. When administered intranasally, the corticosteroids do not exhibit systemic adverse effects. For acute allergies, corticosteroids may be administered parenterally. Because their onset of action is slow, however, they are always administered concurrently with other drugs, such as epinephrine, for this indication. The pharmacotherapy of allergic rhinitis is presented in Chapter 45.

Transplant rejection prophylaxis: Successful tissue transplantation requires the use of immunosuppressant drugs; otherwise, the patient's immune system would reject the transplant. One or more immunosuppressants are administered at the time of transplantation and are continued for several months following surgery. Corticosteroids are part of most therapeutic regimens to prevent transplant rejection. They may be used for several weeks or maintained for 3 to 6 months following surgery. The prophylaxis of transplant rejection is presented in Chapter 42.

Dermatologic conditions: Topical corticosteroids are the most effective therapy for treating the inflammation and itching of dermatitis. These corticosteroids are specially formulated to penetrate deep into the skin layers. Topical corticosteroids such as betamethasone and hydrocortisone acetate are also the primary, initial treatment for psoriasis. High-potency corticosteroids are used for 1 to 2 weeks, followed by moderate- to low-potency corticosteroids for maintenance therapy. The pharmacotherapy of dermatologic diseases is presented in Chapter 73.

Neoplasms: Corticosteroids such as prednisone and dexamethasone are used as adjuncts in the treatment of certain neoplasms, especially acute childhood leukemias and Hodgkin's disease. They are always used in combination with other antineoplastics. The pharmacotherapy of cancer is presented in Chapter 57.

Edema: Corticosteroids are occasionally used to treat disorders characterized by edema. They have been used for many years to reduce intracranial edema associated with trauma, tumors, and cerebral ischemia. These hormones tend to stabilize capillary membranes. Their effectiveness in treating edema is controversial.

CONNECTIONS: APPLIED CLINICAL JUDGMENT

Patients Receiving Pharmacotherapy with Systemic Corticosteroids

Key Assessment Data

- History of current condition; baseline vital signs and weight; physical exam findings; endocrine, cardiovascular, hepatic, or kidney disease; glucose level or history of diabetes; pregnancy or breastfeeding; drug history including allergies and current prescription and OTC drugs and herbal preparations.

Desired Therapeutic Outcomes

Improvement is observed and measurable by reduced signs and symptoms of inflammation such as redness or swelling.

Minimizing Adverse Effects

- Corticosteroids may cause increased blood pressure and tachycardia due to increased retention of fluids.
- Corticosteroids have effects on the complete blood count and may cause hyperglycemia, hypernatremia, hyperlipidemia, and hypokalemia. Patients with diabetes may require a change in antidiabetic medication if the glucose remains elevated.
- GI bleeding is an adverse drug effect and may manifest as hypotension if occult bleeding occurs.
- Corticosteroids suppress the body's normal immune and inflammatory response and may mask the signs and symptoms of infection.
- Corticosteroids affect bone metabolism and may cause osteoporosis and fractures. Weight-bearing exercise stresses bone and encourages normal bone remodeling.
- Fluid retention may occur but may need additional treatment if a weight gain of 1 kg (2 lb) or more in a 24-hour period, more than 2 kg (5 lb) per week, or increasing peripheral edema occurs.
- Corticosteroids may cause increased intraocular pressure and an increased risk for glaucoma and cataracts.
- Corticosteroids may cause increased or decreased mood, euphoria, depression, or severe mental instability.
- Mineralcorticoids may cause loss of potassium and hypokalemia.
- Adrenal insufficiency and crisis may occur with profound hypotension, tachycardia, and other adverse effects if the drug is stopped abruptly.

Lifespan Considerations

- Older patients are at increased risk of adverse effects in all body systems due to normal physiologic changes related to aging.
- Children receiving long-term corticosteroid therapy should continue to display normal growth and development curves.

CONNECTIONS: APPLIED CLINICAL JUDGMENT *(continued)*

Patients Receiving Pharmacotherapy with Systemic Corticosteroids

Patient Education

- Report any return of original symptoms or an increase in inflammation, allergic response, or generalized malaise.
- Report any signs or symptoms of infection (e.g., increasing temperature or fever, sore throat, redness or swelling at the site of injury, white patches in the mouth, vesicular rash).
- Immediately report any signs or symptoms of GI bleeding including abdominal pain, black or tarry stools, blood in the stool, hematemesis, coffee-ground emesis, dizziness, lightheadedness, and hypotension, especially if associated with tachycardia.
- Patients with diabetes should test blood glucose more frequently and notify the healthcare provider if a consistent elevation is noted.
- Weigh self daily, ideally at the same time of day. Report weight gain of more than 1 kg in a 24-hour period, more than 2 kg per week, or increasing peripheral edema.
- Eye examinations should be scheduled twice yearly or more frequently as instructed by the healthcare provider. Immediately report any eye pain, rainbow halos around lights, diminished vision, blurring, and inability to focus.
- Promptly report excessive mood swings or unusual changes in mood.
- If mineralocorticoids are used, immediately report symptoms of hypokalemia (e.g., nausea and vomiting, muscle cramps, and fatigue).
- Do not stop corticosteroids abruptly. Notify the healthcare provider if unable to take medication for more than 1 day due to illness.
- Patients on replacement therapy should obtain and carry replacement doses in both oral and parenteral forms for emergency use.
- Take the medication following appropriate guidelines:
  - Take the drug in the morning at the same time each day.
  - Take the drug with food, milk, or a meal to prevent GI upset.
  - Do not use household measuring spoons to measure liquid or pediatric doses. Use the measuring device included with the drug or obtain a dose syringe or other device from a pharmacy or the healthcare provider.
- Carry a medical identification card or wear medical alert jewelry indicating corticosteroid use, especially if needed for replacement therapy.

Prescribing Considerations

- Blood pressure, body weight, routine laboratory studies, including serum potassium and fasting blood glucose, should be obtained at regular intervals during prolonged therapy.
- Diagnostic studies should be performed in patients on prolonged therapy with known or suspected peptic ulcer disease and in patients at risk for reactivation of latent tuberculosis infections.
- Monitor for hypothalamic–pituitary–adrenal (HPA) axis suppression, Cushing's syndrome, and hyperglycemia; drug-induced secondary adrenocortical insufficiency may be minimized by gradual reduction of dosage.

Mineralocorticoids

68.6 Patients with adrenal insufficiency often require replacement therapy with mineralocorticoids.

Aldosterone is the primary hormone regulating sodium and potassium balance in the body. Regulation of aldosterone secretion is through activation of the renin-angiotensin-aldosterone system. When plasma volume falls, the kidney secretes renin, which results in the production of angiotensin II. Angiotensin II then promotes aldosterone secretion, which in turn acts on the renal tubules to promote sodium and water retention and increased excretion of potassium.

Lack of adequate aldosterone secretion, or **hypoaldosteronism**, may be caused by a number of disorders. The three broad categories of hypoaldosteronism are as follows:

- **Decreased stimulation of the adrenal cortex.** Beta blockers, NSAIDs, and calcium channel blockers may reduce renin serum levels and suppress the stimulation of aldosterone secretion. Angiotensin-converting enzyme inhibitors block the formation of angiotensin II, which is the normal signal for aldosterone secretion.
- **Hyposecretion of aldosterone.** Low aldosterone secretion may result from primary AI, which is usually a deficiency in the secretion of both glucocorticoids and mineralocorticoids. Heparin can also suppress aldosterone synthesis and secretion.
- **Aldosterone resistance.** The renal tubules may become resistant to the actions of aldosterone. Aldosterone resistance occurs during diseases of the renal tubules and may also result from therapy with spironolactone (Aldactone) or progestins.

Whenever possible, the cause of hypoaldosteronism is identified and treated. In some cases, replacement therapy with fludrocortisone is necessary.

Excessive secretion of aldosterone, or **hyperaldosteronism**, is usually caused by a benign tumor of the adrenal gland. Also known as Conn's syndrome, symptoms include HTN caused by fluid retention and muscle weakness due to hypokalemia. Surgical excision of the adrenal tumor is the preferred treatment for most patients; however, pharmacotherapy with spironolactone (Aldactone) may benefit patients whose surgical risk is high. Spironolactone is a potassium-sparing diuretic that blocks the actions of aldosterone in the renal tubule. Spironolactone is featured as a drug prototype in Chapter 32.

PROTOTYPE DRUG **Fludrocortisone**

Classification **Therapeutic:** Drug for hypoaldosteronism
Pharmacologic: Mineralocorticoid

Therapeutic Effects and Uses: Approved by the U.S. Food and Drug Administration in 1954, fludrocortisone is a synthetic oral mineralocorticoid that has actions similar to aldosterone. It exhibits minimal glucocorticoid activity. It is approved for the treatment of Addison's disease and for salt-losing forms of adrenogenital syndrome, a life-threatening congenital disorder that occurs during the first few weeks of life. Fludrocortisone has been used off-label to treat neurogenic orthostatic hypotension.

Mechanism of Action: Fludrocortisone has the same pharmacologic actions as aldosterone. It acts on the distal renal tubule to promote sodium and water reabsorption and increased urinary potassium excretion.

Pharmacokinetics:

Route(s)	PO
Absorption	Rapidly absorbed
Distribution	Distributed to most tissues; crosses the placenta; secreted in breast milk; highly bound to plasma protein
Primary metabolism	Hepatic to inactive metabolites
Primary excretion	Renal
Onset of action	Peak plasma level: 1.5 h
Duration of action	Half-life: 3.5 h

Adverse Effects: Most adverse effects of fludrocortisone are the result of excessive mineralocorticoid activity: sodium and fluid retention, edema, cardiomegaly, HTN, and HF. Excessive urinary loss of potassium may result in symptoms of hypokalemia: nausea and vomiting, prolongation of the QT interval, muscle cramps, and fatigue.

Contraindications/Precautions: Fludrocortisone must be used with caution if the patient has any disorders in which fluid accumulation could be hazardous, such as HF, HTN, chronic kidney disease, or hepatic impairment. Because the drug has glucocorticoid properties that could lead to immunosuppression, it should not be administered to patients with a known systemic fungal infection.

Drug Interactions: If used with drugs that cause potassium loss, fludrocortisone use will result in additive hypokalemia. Potassium-wasting drugs include thiazide and loop diuretics and amphotericin B. Fludrocortisone should be used with caution in patients taking digoxin due to the potential for hypokalemia-induced digoxin toxicity. Concurrent use with androgens may cause additive sodium retention and edema. Fludrocortisone may affect glycemic control in patients with diabetes; doses of antidiabetic drugs may need to be increased. **Herbal/Food:** Sodium intake should be monitored because high levels may lead to sodium retention.

Pregnancy: Animal studies have not been conducted and adverse effects during pregnancy and breastfeeding are not known. This drug enters animal milk and has the potential to cause hypoadrenalism in the neonate, therefore caution should be used if breastfeeding.

Treatment of Overdose: Overdosage results in HTN, edema, and hypokalemia. Treatment is symptomatic. Potassium supplements may be beneficial.

Clinician Responsibilities: Key clinical implications for patients receiving fludrocortisone are included in Applied Clinical Judgment: Patients Receiving Pharmacotherapy with Systemic Corticosteroids.

Drugs Similar to Fludrocortisone

Fludrocortisone is the only drug in its class.

Antiadrenal Drugs

68.7 Antiadrenal drugs may be administered to lower serum corticosteroid levels in patients with Cushing's syndrome.

Cushing's syndrome occurs when high levels of corticosteroids are present in the body over a prolonged time period. Although hypersecretion of these hormones can occur due to pituitary or adrenal tumors, the most common cause of Cushing's syndrome is long-term therapy with high doses of systemic corticosteroids. Signs and symptoms include adrenal atrophy, osteoporosis, HTN, increased risk of infections, delayed wound healing, acne, peptic ulcers, general obesity, and a redistribution of fat around the face (moon face), shoulders, and neck (buffalo hump). Mood and personality changes are common, and the patient may become psychologically dependent on the drug. Some corticosteroids, including hydrocortisone, also have mineralocorticoid activity and can cause retention of sodium and water. Because of their anti-inflammatory and immunosuppressant properties, corticosteroids may mask signs of infection. It is important to note that corticosteroids do not have anti-infective properties. Even though the patient may not exhibit signs and symptoms of infection, the microorganisms continue duplicating and spreading. This could result in a delay in the initiation of antibiotic therapy.

PharmFACT

Cushing's syndrome caused by adrenal or pituitary tumors is quite rare, has a peak incidence between the ages of 25 and 40 years, and afflicts five times as many women as men (Nguyen, 2020).

Because Cushing's syndrome has a high mortality rate, medical intervention is necessary. The primary therapeutic goal is to identify and treat the cause of the excess corticosteroids. If the patient is receiving high doses of a corticosteroid medication, gradual discontinuation of the drug is usually sufficient to reverse the syndrome. When the cause of the hypersecretion is an adrenal tumor or an ectopic tumor secreting ACTH, surgical removal is indicated.

When removal of the tumor is not possible, a secondary option is to administer medications to reduce the excess cortisol secretion. The antifungal drug ketoconazole has been the traditional drug for long-term therapy of Cushing's syndrome. Used off-label for this indication, ketoconazole rapidly blocks the synthesis of glucocorticoids, lowering serum levels. Unfortunately, the falling glucocorticoid level signals the pituitary to release more ACTH. Eventually, the very high levels of ACTH may overcome ketoconazole's inhibition of glucocorticoid synthesis. Although effective, ketoconazole carries a black box warning that it should be used only for fungal infections that have not responded to other medications due to the potential for serious hepatotoxicity.

The drug pasireotide (Signifor) was approved in 2012 to treat Cushing's syndrome in patients who are not candidates for pituitary surgery. Pasireotide is closely related to somatostatin (growth hormone–inhibiting hormone). Binding of pasireotide to somatostatin receptors causes inhibition of ACTH secretion by the pituitary and subsequently corticosteroid secretion from the adrenals. Given by the subcutaneous route, several weeks or months of therapy may be needed for optimal suppression of corticosteroid secretion. Studies in laboratory animals showed evidence of fetal harm. Pasireotide should be used during pregnancy only if the potential benefits to the mother justify the potential risks to the fetus.

In 2020, another medication was approved to treat Cushing's disease in patients who are unable to have pituitary surgery or in whom surgery was not curative. Osilodrostat (Isturisa) inhibits the enzyme 11-beta-hydroxylase, the enzyme that catalyzes the final step of cortisol synthesis in the adrenal gland. Taken orally twice daily, common adverse effects include AI, fatigue, nausea, headache, and edema. Animal studies did not show evidence of fetal harm. Breastfeeding is not recommended due to the potential for serious adverse effects in the neonate.

Understanding Chapter 68

Key Concepts Summary

68.1 The adrenal glands secrete gonadocorticoids, mineralocorticoids, and corticosteroids.

68.2 Corticosteroids are widely used, and all drugs in the class have similar indications, actions, and adverse effects.

68.3 Long-term therapy with corticosteroids has the potential to cause serious adverse effects in multiple body systems.

68.4 Adrenocortical insufficiency is treated by administering physiologic levels of corticosteroids.

68.5 Corticosteroids are frequently used to suppress the inflammatory and immune responses.

68.6 Patients with adrenal insufficiency often require replacement therapy with mineralocorticoids.

68.7 Antiadrenal drugs may be administered to lower serum corticosteroid levels in patients with Cushing's syndrome.

CASE STUDY: Making the Patient Connection

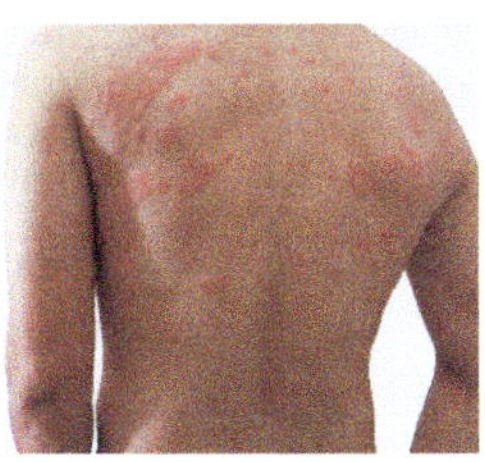

Remember the patient "Charlie Harness" from the beginning of the chapter? Now read the remainder of the story. Based on the information presented within this chapter, answer the critical thinking questions that follow.

Charlie Harness is a 36-year-old man who, while clearing out weeds and brush in his yard, pulled up a patch of poison ivy. He was not concerned about the incident because he had never reacted to poison ivy in the past. Later that afternoon, he experienced intense itching, first on his hands and arms, which then spread to his chest, shoulder, and back. A macular rash appeared on his arms and small blisters erupted on his hands. He is seen in the local urgent care clinic by the nurse practitioner, who diagnosed the rash as allergic dermatitis caused by poison ivy and prescribed prednisone 60 mg/day for 4 days, then tapering by 10 mg every 2 days for a 14-day treatment regimen.

Critical Thinking Questions

1. Why has Charlie reacted to the poison ivy now when he has had no reaction to previous exposures?
2. Why would the nurse practitioner use a 14-day prednisone taper and not a Medrol Dosepak for Charlie?
3. What would you teach this patient about not abruptly discontinuing this medication before completing the entire taper? Why?
4. Charlie asks you if there are any additional precautions that he should take related to his exposure. How would you respond?

Additional Case Study

Monica Hamric, a 53-year-old woman, is referred to the endocrinologist for evaluation after being seen by the advanced practice nurse. She has a history of SLE, managed with corticosteroids, and has begun to experience weight gain, facial hirsutism with thinning of the hair on her head, spontaneous bruising, muscle weakness, and a recent diagnosis of diabetes. She has been taking prednisone for the past 3 months. The physical examination reveals that Monica has developed a "buffalo hump" on her shoulder and red striae on her abdominal and underarm areas. Her blood pressure is also elevated, measuring 162/100 mmHg. The healthcare provider has diagnosed Monica with Cushing's syndrome related to her prednisone use. Monica will be withdrawn from the prednisone and started on immunosuppressant therapy. Because she has taken the prednisone for some time, how do you anticipate the drug will be stopped and why?

Chapter Review

1. A patient has been given a few prescriptions for acute bronchitis. One of the prescriptions is for methylprednisolone (Medrol Dosepak). The nurse will teach the patient to report which adverse effects to the healthcare provider? (Select all that apply.)
    1. Edema
    2. Tinnitus
    3. Eye pain or vision changes
    4. Dizziness upon standing
    5. Abdominal pain

2. A patient has been taking a thiazide diuretic for treatment of HTN and has been prescribed hydrocortisone (Cortef) for a significant allergic reaction to shellfish. Which symptom should be immediately reported to the provider?
    1. Irregular heart rate and rhythm
    2. Delayed wound healing
    3. Weight gain of 2 to 3 pounds in 1 week
    4. Elevated serum lipid levels

3. An older adult patient with chronic bronchitis has been receiving low-dose therapy with dexamethasone for several months to reduce the inflammation occurring secondary to the bronchitis. What teaching should this patient receive to reduce the risk of osteoporosis related to dexamethasone use? (Select all that apply.)
    1. Perform weight-bearing exercises at least three to four times weekly.
    2. Increase dietary intake of calcium- and vitamin D–rich foods.
    3. Remain sedentary except during periods of exercise.
    4. Increase fluid intake, including carbonated sodas, but avoid alcohol.
    5. Request a prescription for a bisphosphonate drug from the provider.

4. A patient with adrenocortical insufficiency has started therapy with fludrocortisone. What important intervention related to this drug therapy should the nurse teach the patient?
    1. "Report any abdominal pain or changes in your stool color."
    2. "Return monthly for laboratory work to assess blood lipid levels."
    3. "Report any unusual changes in your mood."
    4. "Weigh yourself daily, ideally at the same time each day."

5. A patient who has been taking dexamethasone for RA was unable to take the drug for several days due to an intestinal virus. The patient seeks treatment in the emergency department for complaints of severe nausea and vomiting, lethargy, fever, and hypotension. What drug does the nurse anticipate will be given to this patient?

1. Fludrocortisone
2. Ketoconazole (Nizoral)
3. Hydrocortisone (Solu-Cortef)
4. Pasireotide (Signifor)

6. A patient with chronic adrenal insufficiency taking hydrocortisone (Cortef) and fludrocortisone is planning a family vacation. What essential teaching does this patient need prior to taking this trip?

1. "Take your blood pressure once or twice while you're gone."
2. "Avoid crowded indoor areas to avoid infections."
3. "Have your vision checked before you leave."
4. "Carry an oral and injectable form of both drugs with you on your trip."

See Appendix A for answers to critical thinking questions, case study questions, and review questions.

References

Cavaleri, F. (2018). Presenting a new standard drug model for turmeric and its prized extract, curcumin. *International Journal of Inflammation, 2018*, 5023429. https://doi.org/10.1155/2018/5023429

Griffing, G. T. (2020). *Addison disease clinical presentation.* Medscape. http://emedicine.medscape.com/article/116467-clinical

National Center for Complementary and Integrative Health. (2020). *Turmeric.* https://www.nccih.nih.gov/health/turmeric

Nguyen, H. C. T. (2020). *Endogenous Cushing syndrome.* Medscape. http://emedicine.medscape.com/article/2233083-overview#a2

Selected Bibliography

Bornstein, S. R., Allolio, B., Arlt, W., Barthel, A., Don-Wauchope, A., Hammer, G. D., et al. (2016). Diagnosis and treatment of primary adrenal insufficiency: An Endocrine Society clinical practice guideline. *Journal of Clinical Endocrinology and Metabolism, 101*, 364–389. https://doi.org/10.1210/jc.2015-1710

Feelders, R. A., Newell-Price, J., Pivonello, R., Nieman, L. K., Hofland, L. J., & Lacroix, A. (2019). Advances in the medical treatment of Cushing's syndrome. *The Lancet Diabetes & Endocrinology, 7*(4), 300–312. https://doi.org/10.1016/S2213-8587(18)30155-4

Fleseriu, M., & Petersenn, S. (2015). Medical therapy for Cushing's disease: Adrenal steroidogenesis inhibitors and glucocorticoid receptor blockers. *Pituitary, 18*, 245–252. https://doi.org/10.1007/s11102-014-0627-0

Lonser, R. R., Nieman, L., & Oldfield, E. H. (2016). Cushing's disease: Pathobiology, diagnosis, and management. *Journal of Neurosurgery, 126*, 404–417. https://doi.org/10.3171/2016.1.JNS152119

Pivonello, R., De Martino, M. C., De Leo, M., Simeoli, C., & Colao, A. (2017). Cushing's disease: The burden of illness. *Endocrine, 56*(1), 10–18. https://doi.org/10.1007/s12020-016-0984-8

Simpson, H., Tomlinson, J., Wass, J., Dean, J., & Arlt, W. (2020). Guidance for the prevention and emergency management of adult patients with adrenal insufficiency. *Clinical Medicine, 20*(4), 371. https://doi.org/10.7861/clinmed.2019-0324

Störmann, S., & Schopohl, J. (2018). New and emerging drug therapies for Cushing's disease. *Expert Opinion on Pharmacotherapy, 19*(11), 1187–1200. https://doi.org/10.1080/14656566.2018.1504021

Tritos, N. A., & Biller, B. M. (2019). Current management of Cushing's disease. *Journal of Internal Medicine, 286*(5), 526–541. https://doi.org/10.1111/joim.12975

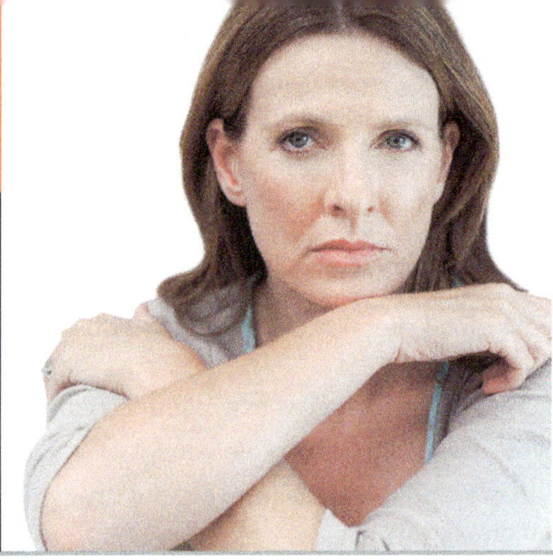

"I get fatigued so easily. I'm having mood swings, headaches, bouts of depression, and irritability; but my main concern is that I have absolutely no desire to have sexual intercourse. What's happening to me, and what can I do about it?"

—*Patient "Maureen John"*

Chapter 69
Estrogens, Progestins, and Drugs Modifying Uterine Function

Chapter Outline

- Hormonal Regulation of Female Reproductive Function
- Estrogens

  PROTOTYPE *Conjugated Estrogens (Premarin), p. 1200*
- Progestins

  PROTOTYPE *Medroxyprogesterone (Depo-Provera, Depo-SubQ-Provera, Provera), p. 1204*
- Hormone Therapy During Menopause
- Uterine Stimulants: Oxytocics

  PROTOTYPE *Oxytocin (Pitocin), p. 1208*
- Uterine Relaxants: Tocolytics
- Pharmacotherapy of Female Infertility and Female Sexual Desire Disorder

  Female Infertility

  Female Sexual Desire Disorder

  PROTOTYPE *Clomiphene, p. 1213*

Learning Outcomes

After reading this chapter, the student should be able to:

1. Describe the roles of the hypothalamus, pituitary, and ovaries in maintaining female reproductive function.
2. Identify indications for estrogen pharmacotherapy.
3. Identify indications for progestin pharmacotherapy.
4. Compare and contrast the advantages and disadvantages of hormone replacement therapy during menopause.
5. Explain the role of uterine stimulants and relaxants during labor and delivery.
6. Explain how drug therapy may be used to treat female infertility.
7. Describe the nurse's role in the pharmacologic management of disorders and conditions of the female reproductive system.
8. For each of the classes shown in the chapter outline, identify the prototype and representative drugs and explain the mechanism(s) of drug action, primary indications, contraindications, significant drug interactions, pregnancy data, and important adverse effects.
9. Apply clinical judgment to the care of patients receiving pharmacotherapy for disorders and conditions of the female reproductive system.

Key Terms

Definitions of the terms in bold may be found in the Glossary.

Estrogen and progesterone are steroid hormones responsible for the growth, development, and reproductive health of females throughout the lifespan. Deficiencies or excesses of these hormones can result in profound changes that extend beyond the reproductive system. These hormones impact virtually every body system including effects on coagulation, blood vessels, bone, muscles, overall body metabolism, and behavior. Stimulating hormones from the pituitary also affect reproductive function, including fertility, labor, delivery, and the production and ejection of breast milk. This chapter examines hormones and drugs used to treat conditions associated with the female reproductive system.

Hormonal Regulation of Female Reproductive Function

69.1 Regulation of the female reproductive system is achieved by hormones from the hypothalamus, pituitary gland, and ovary.

The two primary hormones of the female reproductive system are estrogen and progesterone. During a woman's childbearing years, nearly all estrogen and progesterone is secreted by the ovaries. Small amounts of estrogen are secreted by nonreproductive organs, including the adrenal glands, liver, kidney, skeletal muscle, and adipose tissue. In postmenopausal women, nearly all estrogen and progesterone are secreted by these nonreproductive tissues. In men, estrogen and progesterone are also secreted in small amounts by the testes.

Unlike men, who secrete steady and continuous levels of testosterone throughout adult life, secretion of the female sex hormones is variable and complex. Knowledge of these complexities is essential to understanding the pharmacotherapy of the female reproductive system. Although this section reviews physiology that is relevant to drug therapy, the student should refer to an anatomy and physiology textbook for more detailed information.

Secretion of female reproductive hormones varies on a 28-day menstrual cycle. The menstrual cycle is described by changes that occur in the ovaries (ovarian cycle) and in the lining of the uterus (uterine cycle). Both cycles are controlled by hormones from the hypothalamus and pituitary. The first day of menstruation is considered day 1 of the cycle. The hormonal changes that occur during the ovarian and uterine cycles are illustrated in Figure 69.1.

The hypothalamus secretes gonadotropin-releasing hormone (GnRH), which travels a short distance to the pituitary to stimulate the secretion of the gonadotropins: follicle-stimulating hormone (FSH) and luteinizing hormone (LH). Both of these anterior pituitary hormones act on the ovary and promote the development of immature ovarian follicles. Under the influence of FSH and LH, several ovarian follicles begin the maturation process each month during the reproductive lifespan. As ovarian follicles mature, they secrete increasing amounts of estrogen. On approximately day 14 of the ovarian cycle, a surge of LH (and to a lesser extent FSH) secretion causes one follicle to expel its oocyte (egg), a process called **ovulation**. The LH surge is an absolute requirement for ovulation and, thus, conception. The oocyte begins its journey through the uterine tube and eventually reaches the uterus.

The ruptured follicle, minus the oocyte, remains in the ovary and is transformed into the **corpus luteum**, an endocrine tissue that secretes steadily increasing amounts of progesterone for the next 12 days. Progesterone thickens the uterine mucosa, readying this organ for implantation and potential pregnancy.

High progesterone and estrogen levels in the final third of the uterine cycle provide negative feedback to shut off GnRH, FSH, and LH secretion, as illustrated in Figure 69.2. Without stimulation from FSH and LH, estrogen and progesterone levels fall sharply, the endometrium is shed, and menstrual bleeding begins a new monthly cycle.

Estrogens

69.2 Estrogens are administered as replacement therapy, to prevent conception, and for certain neoplasms.

Estrogen is a general term for three different steroid hormones: estradiol, estrone, and estriol. Estradiol is present in the body in the largest amount. Estrogens are responsible for the maturation of the reproductive organs and for the appearance of the secondary sex characteristics of the female during puberty. When women enter menopause around age 50 to 55, the secretion of estrogen by the ovaries diminishes and eventually stops.

Apart from its reproductive functions, estrogen also affects the heart, liver, blood vessels, and bones. Estrogen decreases the levels of low-density lipoprotein (LDL) and increases the amount of high-density lipoprotein (HDL) in the blood. These effects are cardioprotective and help lower the risk of myocardial infarction (MI) in premenopausal women. By blocking resorption of the bony matrix, estrogen causes bones to grow longer and stronger in younger women. As estrogen levels decrease in postmenopausal women, the risk of osteoporosis and bone fractures dramatically increases.

Estrogens are used as contraception and to treat menopausal symptoms, female hypogonadism, and primary ovarian failure. When used as replacement therapy following surgical removal of the ovaries, estrogen is usually combined with a progestin. The purpose of the progestin is to counteract some of the adverse effects of estrogen on the uterus. Estrogen drugs are listed in Table 69.1. The contraceptive uses of estrogen are presented in Chapter 70.

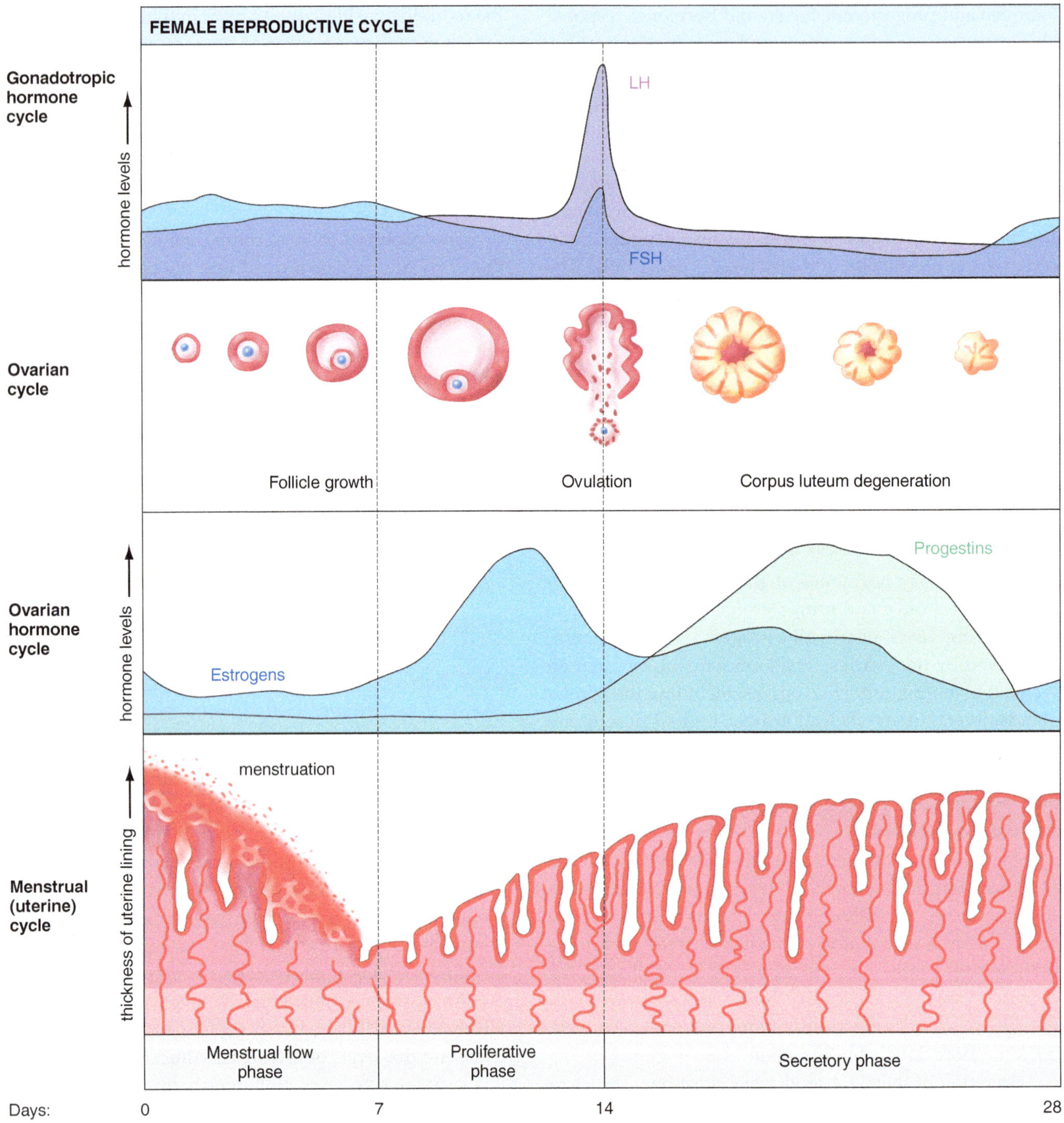

Figure 69.1 Hormonal changes during the ovarian and uterine cycles.

High doses of estrogens are sometimes used to treat advanced prostate and breast cancer. Prostate cancer is usually dependent on androgens for growth, and administration of estrogens will suppress androgen secretion. In the treatment of cancer, estrogen is nearly always used in combination with other antineoplastics.

PROTOTYPE DRUG **Conjugated Estrogens (Premarin)**

Classification **Therapeutic:** Hormone
Pharmacologic: Estrogen

Therapeutic Effects and Uses: Conjugated estrogen, equine (Premarin) was approved by the U.S. Food and Drug Administration (FDA) in 1938 and contains a mixture of different natural estrogens, traditionally obtained from pregnant mares' urine. The primary indication for conjugated estrogens is to treat moderate to severe vasomotor symptoms of menopause, such as hot flashes and night sweats, caused by diminished estrogen secretion. Topical preparations may be used to treat symptoms associated with menopause such as vulvar or vaginal atrophy and dyspareunia (pain during

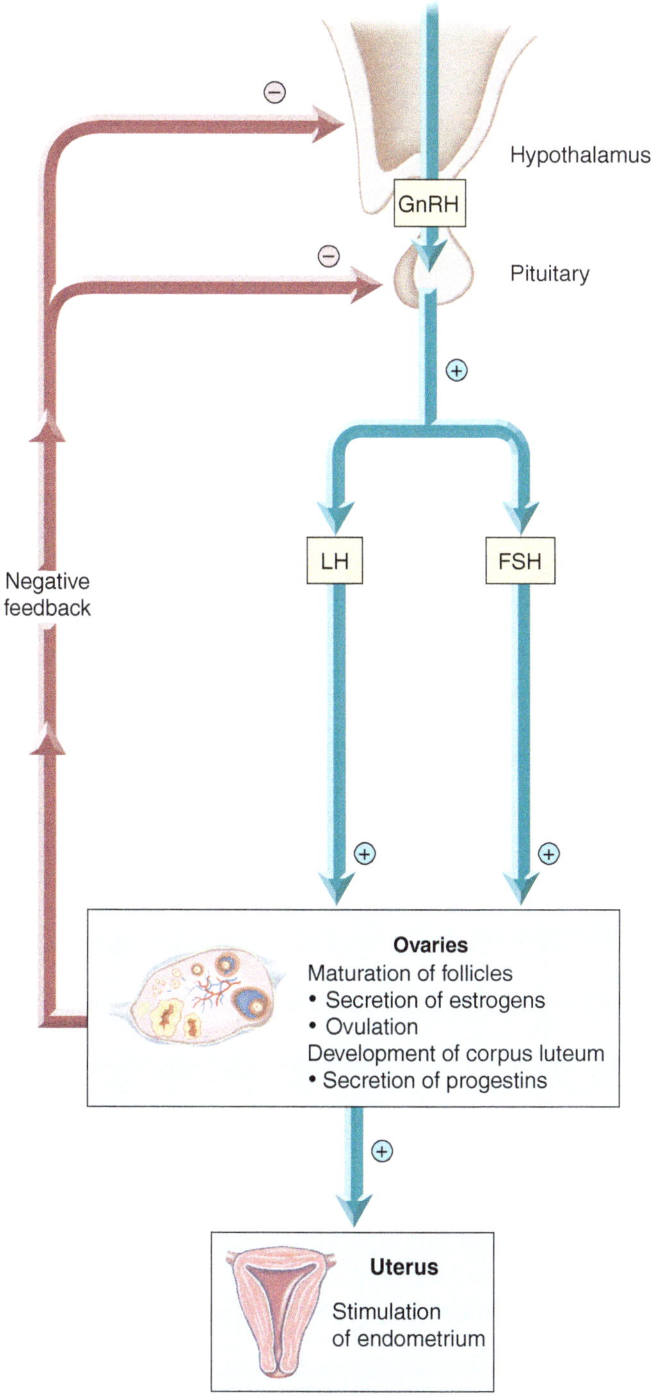

Figure 69.2 Negative feedback control of the female reproductive hormones.

intercourse). Replacement therapies include treatment of female hypogonadism and use following oophorectomy. Premarin is approved for the palliative treatment of prostate cancer and certain types of breast cancer. Conjugated estrogens have been used for osteoporosis prophylaxis in postmenopausal women.

Conjugated estrogens are usually administered by the oral (PO) or topical routes. For dysfunctional uterine bleeding, they may be administered by the intramuscular (IM) or intravenous (IV) routes.

Mechanism of Action: Conjugated estrogens bind to intracellular estrogen receptors that stimulate deoxyribonucleic acid (DNA) and ribonucleic acid to synthesize proteins responsible for the biologic effects of estrogens.

Pharmacokinetics:

Route(s)	PO, IM, IV, intravaginal
Absorption	Rapid absorption from the gastrointestinal (GI) tract, readily absorbed through the skin and mucous membranes, slow absorption through IM injections
Distribution	Widely distributed; crosses the placenta; secreted in breast milk; bound primarily to albumin
Primary metabolism	Hepatic metabolism by CYP3A4 to estrone, estradiol, and estriol
Primary excretion	Renal
Onset of action	PO: 30–60 min; IM: 15–30 min
Duration of action	Half-life: 4–18 h

Adverse Effects: The most frequent adverse effects of conjugated estrogens include headache, infections, abdominal cramps and bloating, breast tenderness, and vaginal bleeding. Other, less common adverse effects may include thromboembolic events, fluid retention, edema, acute pancreatitis, appetite changes, skin eruptions, mental depression, decreased or increased libido, fatigue, nervousness, and weight gain. The risks of adverse effects increase in patients over age 35. Effects are dose dependent. **Black Box Warnings:** Estrogens have been associated with a higher risk of endometrial cancer in postmenopausal women. Using conjugated estrogens with medroxyprogesterone increases the risk of breast cancer. Estrogens when used alone increase the risk of stroke, deep vein thrombosis (DVT), MI, and pulmonary emboli. They may also increase the risk for dementia.

Contraindications/Precautions: Estrogens should be avoided in patients who have a history of breast cancer, cervical cancer, endometrial cancer or hyperplasia, prostate cancer, and hepatic diseases or cancer. Additionally, because estrogens have been associated with thromboembolic disorders, hypercalcemia, and lupus, they should not be prescribed without a thorough investigation of these conditions. Estrogens should be used with caution in patients with lipid disorders because they may increase HDL cholesterol and triglycerides.

Drug Interactions: Estrogen is metabolized by CYP450 enzymes and may interact with other drugs metabolized

Table 69.1 Selected Estrogens and Progestins

Drug	Route and Adult Dose (Maximum Dose Where Indicated)	Adverse Effects
Estrogens		
estradiol (Alora, Climara, Divigel, Elestrin, Estrace, Estraderm, others)	PO (Estrace): 0.5–2 mg daily Transdermal patch: 1 patch (0.025–0.1 mg/day) once weekly (Climara) or twice weekly (Alora, Estraderm, Minivelle) Topical gel (Divigel, Elestrin): 0.25–1.0 g/day applied to skin of upper thigh or arm Vaginal cream (Estrace): 1 g 1–3 times/wk maintenance dose Vaginal ring (Estring, Femring): 1 ring every 90 days	*Breakthrough bleeding, spotting, breast tenderness, libido changes* Hypertension (HTN), gallbladder disease, MI, deep vein thrombosis, increased endometrial cancer risk, hypercalcemia, dementia, fetal toxicity (PO and parenteral forms)
estradiol valerate (Delestrogen)	IM: 10–20 mg q4wk	
estrogen, conjugated (Premarin)	PO: 0.3–1.25 mg daily for 21 days each month	
estropipate (Ogen 5)	PO: 0.75–6 mg daily for 21 days each month	
Progestins		
medroxyprogesterone (Depo-Provera, Depo-SubQ-Provera, Provera)	PO (Provera): 5–10 mg daily on days 1–12 of menstrual cycle IM (Depo-Provera): 400–1000 mg/wk Subcutaneous (Depo-SubQ-Provera): 104 mg every 3 months; give first dose during the first 5 days of the menstrual period	*Breakthrough bleeding, spotting, breast tenderness, weight gain* Amenorrhea, dysmenorrhea, depression, thromboembolic disorders, fetal toxicity (PO and parenteral forms)
progesterone (Crinone, Endometrin, Prometrium)	IM (amenorrhea or uterine bleeding): 5–10 mg/day Vaginal (assisted reproductive technology): 90-mg gel once daily or 100-mg tablets bid–tid	
Estrogen–Progestin Combinations		
conjugated estrogens with medroxyprogesterone (Premphase, Prempro)	PO (Premphase): Estrogen 0.625 mg/daily on days 1–28; add 5 mg medroxyprogesterone daily on days 15–28 PO (Prempro): Estrogen 0.3 mg and medroxyprogesterone 1.5 mg daily Vaginal cream: Insert 0.5–2 g daily for 3–6 months	*Breakthrough bleeding, spotting, breast tenderness, weight gain* Amenorrhea, dysmenorrhea, depression, thromboembolic disorders, HTN
estradiol with norgestimate	PO: 1 mg estradiol for 3 days, followed by 1 mg estradiol combined with 0.09 mg norgestimate for 3 days	
ethinyl estradiol with norethindrone acetate (Activella)	PO: 0.5–0.1 mg of estradiol and 0.5–1 mg norethindrone Transdermal patch: 1 patch, twice weekly	

Note: *Italics* indicate common adverse effects. Underline indicates serious adverse effects.

in the liver. The following drugs will decrease the effects of conjugated estrogens: corticosteroids, erythromycin, heparin, rifampin, tetracycline, and warfarin. Use with azole antifungals, diltiazem, or statins may increase the effects of conjugated estrogens. **Herbal/Food:** St. John's wort, red clover, and black cohosh have weak estrogenic effects and may interfere with estrogen therapy. Effects of estrogen may be enhanced if combined with ginseng. Estrogen may decrease the absorption of folic acid. If allergic to soy products, patients should not take Cenestin because it contains soy estrogens.

Pregnancy: Estrogens are contraindicated during pregnancy. Because estrogens decrease the quantity and quality of breast milk, breastfeeding is not recommended.

Treatment of Overdose: Overdose will cause nausea and vomiting and breakthrough bleeding, which are treated symptomatically.

Clinician Responsibilities: Key clinical implications for patients receiving conjugated estrogens are included in Applied Clinical Judgment: Patients Receiving Pharmacotherapy with Ps and Progestins.

Drugs Similar to Conjugated Estrogens (Premarin)

Other estrogens are listed in Table 69.1. These drugs have the same actions, adverse effects, and contraindications as those of conjugated estrogens.

CONNECTIONS: APPLIED CLINICAL JUDGMENT

Patients Receiving Pharmacotherapy with Estrogens and Progestins

Key Assessment Data

- History of current condition including cardiovascular, peripheral vascular, thyroid, hepatic, or kidney disease, migraine headaches, diabetes; baseline vital signs, physical exam findings; pregnancy or breastfeeding. Note personal or family history of thromboembolic disorders (e.g., MI, stroke, peripheral vascular disease) and of reproductive cancers (e.g., breast, uterine, or ovarian cancer); CBC, platelets, electrolytes, glucose, lipid, and thyroid function levels, Pap test, human papillomavirus screening, and pregnancy test results; medication history including allergies, current prescription and over-the-counter (OTC) drugs, herbal preparations, caffeine, nicotine, and alcohol use.

CONNECTIONS: APPLIED CLINICAL JUDGMENT *(continued)*

Patients Receiving Pharmacotherapy with Estrogens and Progestins

Desired Therapeutic Outcomes

Improvement is observed and measurable by reduction in symptoms of menopause or dysfunctional uterine bleeding.

Minimizing Adverse Effects

- Thromboembolic events may occur with estrogen and progestin drugs. The risk increases with age over 35, in women with a previous history of cardiovascular disease, and in women who smoke. Monitor for symptoms of peripheral thrombophlebitis, pulmonary embolism, MI, stroke, or other complications related to blood clots.
- Smoking greatly increases the risk of adverse effects of hormone therapy. Referral to smoking cessation programs may be helpful.
- Pap tests and breast examinations, including mammography as appropriate, are recommended to monitor for the development of breast tumors or of cervical cancer.
- Small amounts of spotting may occur, especially with low-dose hormone therapy, at midcycle. Any continuous, unusual, or heavy bleeding may indicate adverse effects or disease and should be reported because an increased risk of endometrial cancer has been noted.
- Estrogens are associated with increased risk of gallbladder disease and a rare risk of hepatotoxicity.
- Progestins are associated with an increased risk of loss of bone density. Bone density monitoring (e.g., DEXA scan) may be ordered periodically. Radiographic assessment should be used if bone pain or loss of function occurs.
- Many drugs decrease or alter the effectiveness of estrogens and progestins including drugs in the penicillin, barbiturate, antiseizure, antidepressant, and benzodiazepine classifications. Check for drug interactions that may affect hormone effectiveness before any new prescription is started.

Lifespan Considerations

- Progestins are associated with increased risk of dementia in women age 65 or older.

Diversity Considerations

- Because estrogens metabolize through the CYP450 system pathways, monitor ethnically diverse patients to ensure optimal therapeutic effects and to minimize adverse effects.

Patient Education

- Immediately report dyspnea, chest pain, or blood in sputum (possible pulmonary embolism); heaviness, chest pain, or overwhelming feeling of fatigue and weakness accompanied by nausea and diaphoresis (possible MI); sudden, severe headache, especially if associated with a preheadache aura; dizziness; difficulty with speech; numbness in arm or leg; and difficulty with vision (possible stroke).
- Keep routine age-appropriate gynecologic and breast examinations to ensure continued health. Frequency may be decreased after age 65 after consultation with the healthcare provider.
- Slight spotting may occur midcycle but report any unusual changes in the amount or if the bleeding continues.
- Immediately report any symptoms of abdominal or right upper quadrant discomfort or pain, yellowing of the skin or sclera, fatigue, anorexia, darkened urine, or clay-colored stools.
- Immediately report any sudden and severe pain or continuous moderate pain in joints or muscles, loss of motion, or difficulty with ambulation or movement.
- Promptly report any changes in behavior, depression, or mental status.
- Advise all healthcare providers of the use of estrogens or progestins before beginning any new prescription so that potential drug interactions may be assessed.
- Referrals to appropriate support groups and literature on smoking cessation programs should be offered.
- Take the drug following appropriate guidelines:
  - Take the drug at the same time daily to help with remembering to take it. Do not omit, increase, or decrease doses without consulting the healthcare provider. Omitting doses increases the chance of breakthrough bleeding. Take the drug with food or milk if nausea occurs.
  - Transdermal patches should be changed weekly or every other week per the healthcare provider's directions.
  - Apply topical gels or creams only to the area to be treated. Do not wear tampons after intravaginal application.

Prescribing Considerations

- Do not prescribe estradiol to patients who are pregnant or at increased risk for breast or endometrial cancer.
- No dosage adjustments are needed for renal impairment.
- Patients should be prescribed estrogen or estrogen-progestin hormone therapy (HT) for the shortest duration consistent with the treatment goals.
- Estrogen HT with or without a progestin is not indicated and should not be used to prevent coronary artery disease or other cardiovascular disease.
- The risks and benefits of HT must be determined for each woman individually.

Progestins

69.3 Progestins are administered to treat dysfunctional uterine bleeding, to prevent conception, and for certain neoplasms.

Progestins are synthetic hormones that have actions identical to natural, endogenous progesterone. In combination with estrogen, progesterone promotes breast development and regulates the monthly changes of the uterine cycle. Under the influence of estrogen and progesterone, the uterine endometrium becomes more vascular and thickens in preparation for receiving a fertilized egg. If implantation does not occur, levels of progesterone fall dramatically and menses begins. If pregnancy does occur, the ovary will continue to secrete progesterone, maintaining a healthy endometrium until the placenta develops sufficiently to begin producing the hormone.

Whereas the function of estrogen is to cause proliferation of the endometrium, progesterone limits and stabilizes endometrial growth. Progestins are preferred drugs for treating many uterine abnormalities. They are also a component of HT and are used as contraceptives (see Chapter 70).

The primary noncontraception indication for progestins is **dysfunctional uterine bleeding**, a condition in which hemorrhage occurs on a noncyclic basis or in abnormal amounts. Dysfunctional uterine bleeding is common in adolescents and menopausal women and is often associated with anovulatory menstrual cycles. **Anovulatory cycles** are those that occur without ovulation. Dysfunctional uterine bleeding is the health problem most frequently reported by women and a common reason for a hysterectomy.

PharmFACT

Dysfunctional uterine bleeding most commonly occurs at the extreme ages of the reproductive years. The most severe cases occur in adolescents during the first 2 years after the onset of menstruation. Abnormal bleeding also occurs in 50% of perimenopausal women (Estephan, 2018).

Ninety percent of dysfunctional uterine bleeding cases result from anovulation. Possible causes of uterine bleeding include early abortion, pelvic neoplasms, thyroid disorders, pregnancy, and infection. Types of dysfunctional uterine bleeding include the following:

- *Amenorrhea*. Absence of menstruation
- *Endometriosis*. Abnormal location of endometrial tissues
- *Oligomenorrhea*. Infrequent menstruation
- *Menorrhagia*. Prolonged or excessive menstruation occurring at regular intervals
- *Breakthrough (intermenstrual) bleeding*. Hemorrhage between regular menstrual periods
- *Premenstrual syndrome (PMS)*. Symptoms developed during the luteal phase
- *Postmenopausal bleeding*. Hemorrhage following menopause
- *Endometrial carcinoma*. Cancer of the uterine endometrium.

Dysfunctional uterine bleeding is often due to a hormonal imbalance between estrogen and progesterone. Although estrogen increases the thickness of the endometrium, bleeding occurs sporadically unless it is balanced by adequate progesterone secretion. Administration of a progestin in a regimen starting 5 days after the onset of menses and continuing for the next 20 days can sometimes help to reestablish a normal, monthly cyclic pattern. Oral contraceptives may also be prescribed for this disorder.

In patients experiencing heavy bleeding, high doses of conjugated estrogens may be administered for 3 weeks prior to adding medroxyprogesterone for the last 10 days of therapy. Treatment with nonsteroidal anti-inflammatory drugs helps to ease painful menstrual flow. If aggressive hormonal therapy fails to stop the heavy bleeding, dilation and curettage may be necessary.

Progestins are occasionally prescribed for the treatment of metastatic endometrial carcinoma. In these cases, they are used for palliation, in combination with other antineoplastics. Selected progestins and their dosages are shown in Table 69.1.

PROTOTYPE DRUG **Medroxyprogesterone (Depo-Provera, Depo-SubQ-Provera, Provera)**

Classification **Therapeutic:** Hormone, drug for dysfunctional uterine bleeding
Pharmacologic: Progestin

Therapeutic Effects and Uses: Approved in 1959, medroxyprogesterone is a synthetic progestin with a prolonged duration of action. Like progesterone, the primary target tissue for medroxyprogesterone is the uterine endometrium. It antagonizes the effects of estrogen on the uterus, thus restoring normal hormonal balance. It also inhibits the midcycle LH surge, which prevents ovulation and causes a thick cervical mucus plug that is resistant to the passage of sperm.

Medroxyprogesterone is given PO (Provera) to treat dysfunctional uterine bleeding or secondary amenorrhea. It is administered IM (Depo-SubQ-Provera) at high doses for the palliative treatment of inoperable metastatic endometrial or renal cell carcinoma. At low doses, the drug is given by the subcutaneous route (Depo-Provera) as a contraceptive. The use of medroxyprogesterone in contraception is presented in Chapter 70. The drug is used in combination with estrogen to treat the vasomotor symptoms of menopause.

Mechanism of Action: This drug is a synthetic derivative of progesterone with prolonged, variable duration of action and androgenic and antiestrogenic activity. The drug inhibits GnRH, thus preventing the LH surge and ovulation.

Pharmacokinetics:

Route(s)	PO, IM, subcutaneous, IV
Absorption	Readily absorbed from the GI tract or IM
Distribution	Crosses the placenta; secreted in breast milk; 90% bound to protein
Primary metabolism	Hepatic
Primary excretion	Feces
Onset of action	PO: 30–60 min; IM: 15–30 min
Duration of action	Half-life: 30 days (PO); 50 days (IM)

Adverse Effects: The most common adverse effects of medroxyprogesterone are breast tenderness, breakthrough bleeding, and other menstrual irregularities. Weight gain, depression, HTN, nausea, vomiting, fluid retention, and vaginal candidiasis may also occur. **Black Box Warning:** Progestins combined with conjugated estrogens may increase the risk of stroke, DVT, MI, pulmonary emboli, and invasive breast cancer. Women age 65 and older have an increased risk of dementia when treated with progestins. Women receiving injectable medroxyprogesterone are at significant risk for loss of bone mineral density.

Contraindications/Precautions: Patients with a history of thromboembolic disorders, or who are pregnant, should not take progestins. Doses should be reduced in patients with hepatic impairment. Patients with preexisting breast, uterine, or vaginal cancer should not receive medroxyprogesterone unless it is for palliation of advanced cancer. The drug should be discontinued at the first sign of mental depression or dementia. The drug is contraindicated in patients with undiagnosed vaginal bleeding.

Drug Interactions: Serum levels of medroxyprogesterone are decreased by barbiturates, carbamazepine, rifabutin, rifampin, and topiramate. Azole antifungals, carbamazepine, nicardipine, and protease inhibitors such as ritonavir will increase the effects of medroxyprogesterone. **Herbal/Food:** St. John's wort may cause intermenstrual bleeding and loss of efficacy. Grapefruit may increase the effects of medroxyprogesterone.

Pregnancy: Progestins are fetotoxic and teratogenic in laboratory animals and contraindicated during pregnancy. Progestins are secreted in human milk and caution should be used if breastfeeding.

Treatment of Overdose: Overdose is treated symptomatically.

Clinician Responsibilities: Key clinical implications for patients receiving medroxyprogesterone are included in Applied Clinical Judgment: Patients Receiving Pharmacotherapy with Estrogens and Progestins.

Drugs Similar to Medroxyprogesterone (Depo-Provera, Depo-SubQ-Provera, Provera)

Progestins used as contraceptives include desogestrel, dienogest, levonorgestrel, norethindrone, and norgestrel. These are presented in Chapter 70. Another progestin is progesterone.

Progesterone (Crinone, Endometrin, Prometrium): Approved in 1978, progesterone is available in a variety of formulations. As a vaginal suppository (Endometrin) or vaginal gel (Crinone), progesterone is used to treat infertile women with progesterone deficiency as part of an assisted reproductive technology system. The vaginal formulations may also be used as progesterone supplements to support embryo implantation and early pregnancy. When used intravaginally, the drug may be absorbed and cause systemic adverse effects such as breast tenderness, bloating, drowsiness, headaches, irritability, and mood swings.

Prometrium capsules contain micronized progesterone, approved to treat secondary amenorrhea and may be used off-label to ease symptoms of PMS. Prometrium is also indicated for the prevention of endometrial hyperplasia in postmenopausal women who are receiving conjugated estrogens. The drug has a transient hypnotic effect and should be taken at bedtime.

Progesterone IM injections are indicated for amenorrhea and to stop abnormal uterine bleeding. Adverse effects and contraindications are the same as those for medroxyprogesterone. The PO and IM progesterone formulations carry the same black box warnings as medroxyprogesterone and are contraindicated during pregnancy.

Hormone Therapy During Menopause

69.4 Hormone therapy provides relief from moderate to severe menopause symptoms.

Menopause is characterized by a progressive decrease in estrogen secretion by the ovaries resulting in the permanent cessation of menses. The mean age for the start of menopause is about 51 to 52. Menopause is neither a disease nor a disorder but is a natural consequence of aging that is often accompanied by the following symptoms:

- Vasomotor symptoms (VMS) include intense hot flashes, night sweats, anxiety, and sleep disruption.
- Genitourinary symptoms of menopause (GSM) include vulvovaginal atrophy and dryness resulting in pain during intercourse and adverse effects on health, sexuality, and quality of life.
- Osteoporosis and loss of bone mass may lead to increased risk for fractures.

PharmFACT

Women who enter menopause at an early age (40 to 45) are at increased risk for developing future HF. Smoking can increase this risk, even for women who enter menopause from age 46 to 49 (Rahman, Åkesson, & Wolk, 2015).

During the past 50 years, healthcare providers have commonly prescribed hormone therapy (HT), formerly called *hormone replacement therapy*, to treat distressing symptoms of menopause. HT supplies physiologic doses of estrogen, often combined with a progestin, to treat moderate to severe symptoms of menopause and to prevent the long-term consequences of estrogen loss.

The safety of HT during menopause has been a topic of intense study for at least 40 years. Two large, randomized, double-blind, placebo-controlled studies examined the safety of using HT during menopause. The Women's

Health Initiative (WHI) and the Heart and Estrogen/Progestin Replacement Study (HERS) enrolled more than 26,000 women. Hundreds of additional studies have added to the HT safety database.

The results of these studies are complex and based on the intensity of the symptoms and comorbid risk factors, such as history of breast cancer and thromboembolism. The decision to begin (and later, discontinue) HT is one to be thoroughly discussed with the healthcare provider.

Most treatment guidelines for HT include the following:

- The most effective therapy for VMS is either oral or transdermal estrogen. Because low doses reduce the risk of adverse effects, therapy is usually continued with low doses for 8 to 12 weeks to determine if the VMS have resolved.
- In women with an intact uterus, an estrogen–progestin combination is recommended. The progestin protects against endometrial neoplasia.
- Systemic HT is effective at treating both VMS and GSM. However, if GSM is the only symptom of menopause, low-dose vaginal estrogen is effective.
- HT is effective at preventing bone loss and reducing the risk of fractures.
- For women who request a nonhormonal alternative, or who have contraindications for the use of estrogens, the following have been prescribed to treat VMS: paroxetine, venlafaxine, citalopram, gabapentin, or pregabalin.

In recent years, several drugs have been marketed as alternatives to estrogen–progestin combinations. Duavee is a combination drug that contains conjugated estrogens with bazedoxifene, which belongs to a class of drugs called selective estrogen receptor modifiers (SERMs). Duavee offers the advantages of preventing intense hot flashes (the estrogen component) while reducing the risk of osteoporosis-related fractures that are common in postmenopausal women (the SERM component). Approved in 2013, Duavee was the first HT to include a SERM instead of a progestin. This drug carries the same black box warning as that for conjugated estrogens regarding an increased risk of endometrial cancer and DVT. Duavee is given by the oral route and has the same pregnancy data as conjugated estrogens.

Several drugs have been approved to treat dyspareunia, acute pain that occurs in the genital area during intercourse. Although dyspareunia can occur in both sexes and has many physical and psychological causes, it commonly occurs during menopause or postmenopause due to vaginal atrophy and dryness. Drugs for treating this condition include ospemifene (Osphena), prasterone (Intrarosa), and estradiol (Imvexxy).

Ospemifene is a SERM approved in 2013 that acts as an estrogen agonist on the vagina, increasing the thickness of the vaginal epithelium. Ospemifene is given by the oral route.

Prasterone is administered as a once-daily vaginal insert. This drug consists of dehydroepiandrosterone (DHEA), a natural hormone secreted primarily by the adrenal gland. Metabolically, DHEA is converted into androgens and estrogens. It is interesting to note that DHEA is a widely used dietary supplement that is claimed to produce a wide variety of positive effects, including increased muscle strength, memory, and bone density. Most of these claims have little scientific basis. Although DHEA tablets are available OTC in the United States, its use is banned by world sports organizations.

Imvexxy consists of estradiol inserts that are administered intravaginally several times weekly. The most frequent side effect is headache. Some systemic absorption does occur, therefore women with an intact uterus should also take a progestin to protect against endometrial cancer.

Uterine Stimulants: Oxytocics

69.5 Oxytocics are drugs used to stimulate the uterus and promote labor and delivery.

Oxytocics are drugs that stimulate uterine contractions and promote the induction of labor. The most widely used oxytocic is the natural hormone oxytocin, which is secreted by the posterior pituitary gland. The target organs for oxytocin are the uterus and the breast. Increasing amounts of oxytocin are secreted as the uterus is distended by the growing fetus. As pregnancy progresses, the number of oxytocin receptors in the uterus increases, making it even more sensitive to the effects of the hormone. As blood levels of oxytocin rise, uterine smooth muscle is stimulated to contract, thus promoting labor and the delivery of the baby and the placenta.

Oxytocin and other uterine stimulants are indicated only when there are demonstrated risks to the mother or fetus in continuing the pregnancy. Parenteral oxytocin (Pitocin) may be given to induce labor. Doses in an IV infusion are increased gradually, every 15 to 60 minutes, until a normal labor pattern is established. After delivery, IV oxytocin is administered to control postpartum uterine bleeding by temporarily restricting blood flow to this organ. Doses of these drugs are listed in Table 69.2.

In postpartum women, oxytocin is released in response to suckling, whereby it promotes the ejection (letdown) of milk from the mammary glands. Oxytocin does not increase the volume of milk production; this function is provided by the pituitary hormone prolactin, which increases the synthesis of milk. Although rare, deficiencies of prolactin can result in insufficient milk to conduct breastfeeding. The

Table 69.2 Uterine Stimulants and Relaxants

Drug	Route and Adult Dose (Maximum Dose Where Indicated)	Adverse Effects
Stimulants (Oxytocics)		
oxytocin (Pitocin)	To control postpartum bleeding: 10–40 units per infusion pump in 1000 mL of IV fluid at a rate to prevent uterine atony To induce labor: IV: 0.5–2 milliunits/min, gradually increasing the dose to no greater than 1–2 milliunits/min at 30- to 60-min intervals until contraction pattern is established	*Nausea and vomiting, maternal dysrhythmias* Fetal bradycardia, uterine rupture, fetal intracranial hemorrhage, water intoxication, fetal brain hemorrhage
Ergot Alkaloid		
methylergonovine (Methergine)	IM/IV: 1.0 mL (0.2 mg) q2–4h not to exceed 5 doses	*Nausea and vomiting, uterine cramping* Shock, severe HTN, severe dysrhythmias
Prostaglandins		
carboprost (Hemabate)	IM (initial): 250 mcg (1 mL) repeated at 1.5- to 3.5-h intervals if indicated by uterine response	*Nausea and vomiting, cramping, diarrhea, fever* Uterine laceration, rupture, or hemorrhage
dinoprostone (Cervidil, Prepidil, Prostin E_2)	Intravaginal insert (Cervidil): 10 mg (1 insert) Intravaginal gel (Prepidil): 0.5 mg Intravaginal suppository: 20 mg (1 suppository)	
Relaxants (Tocolytics)		
magnesium sulfate	IV: 1–4 g in 5% dextrose by slow infusion (initial max dose: 10–14 g/day, then no more than 30–40 g/day at a max rate of 1–2 g/h)	*Flushing, sweating, muscle weakness* Complete heart block, circulatory collapse, respiratory paralysis
nifedipine (Adalat, Procardia)	PO: Initial dose of 20 mg, followed by 20 mg after 30 min. If contractions persist, therapy can be continued with 20 mg q3–8h for 48–72 h with a maximum dose of 160 mg/day After 72 h, if maintenance is still required, long-acting nifedipine 30–60 mg daily can be used	*Flushing, sweating, muscle weakness* Complete heart block, circulatory collapse, respiratory paralysis
terbutaline (Brethine)	IV: 2.5–10 mcg/min; increase every 10–20 min; duration of infusion: 12 h (max: 17.5–30 mcg/min) PO (maintenance dose): 2.5–10 mg q4–6h as long as necessary to delay preterm labor	*Nervousness, tremor, drowsiness* Bronchoconstrictions, dysrhythmias, altered maternal and fetal heart rates

Note: *Italics* indicate common adverse effects. Underline indicates serious adverse effects.

actions of oxytocin during breastfeeding are illustrated in Figure 69.3.

Ergot alkaloids are obtained from a fungus that grows on rye plants. These drugs are used as alternatives to oxytocin to control postpartum hemorrhage. The primary drug in this class, methylergonovine (Methergine), is effective at promoting uterine contractions but is rarely prescribed due to the risk of serious HTN, especially when administered by the IV route. Ergot alkaloids are also second-line drugs in the pharmacotherapy of migraines.

Several prostaglandins are also used as uterine stimulants. Unlike most hormones that travel through the blood to affect distant tissues, prostaglandins act directly at the site where they are secreted. In the uterus, prostaglandins cause intense smooth muscle contractions. Carboprost (Hemabate) may be used to control postpartum hemorrhage. Dinoprostone (Cervidil, Prepidil, Prostin E_2) is used intravaginally to promote cervical ripening, a softening and dilation of the cervix that must occur prior to vaginal delivery. Misoprostol (Cytotec) is another prostaglandin that has been used off-label to promote cervical ripening. When used in high doses, the prostaglandins can induce pharmacologic abortion (see Chapter 70).

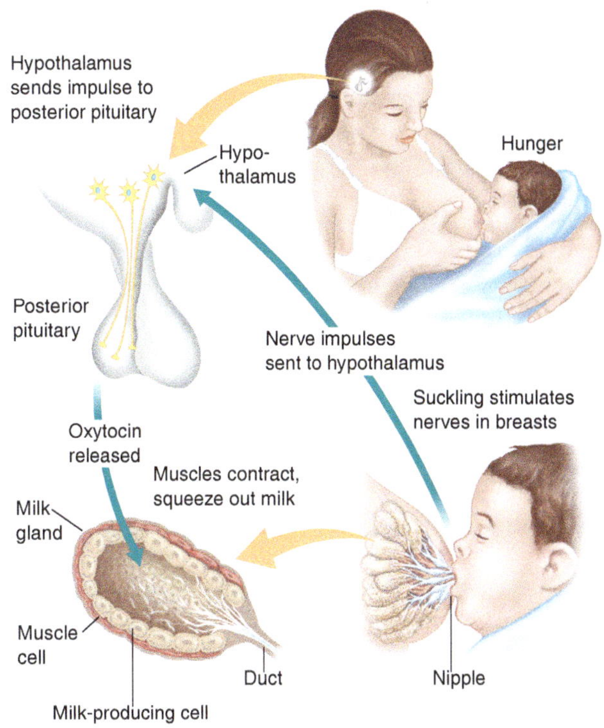

Figure 69.3 Oxytocin and breastfeeding.

CONNECTIONS: Patient Safety

Incomplete Medication Order

It has been a very busy morning on the obstetrics unit with multiple patient discharges and several new admissions. One patient is a 35-year-old woman with preeclampsia who is admitted for labor induction with an order that reads "Begin oxytocin infusion at 2 milliunits/min and increase by 2 milliunits/min every 30 min." The nurse places a call to the obstetrician to clarify this. What is missing from this order?

PROTOTYPE DRUG Oxytocin (Pitocin)

Classification **Therapeutic:** Drug to induce labor, uterine stimulant
Pharmacologic: Hormone, oxytocic

Therapeutic Effects and Uses: Oxytocin (Pitocin), identical to the natural hormone secreted by the posterior pituitary gland, is the preferred drug for inducing labor. Given by IV infusion antepartum, oxytocin induces labor almost immediately by increasing the frequency and force of contractions of uterine smooth muscle. It is administered during the final stages of labor, after the cervix is dilated, membranes have ruptured, and presentation of the fetus has occurred. It is also used to induce labor in cases of maternal diabetes, preeclampsia, eclampsia, and erythroblastosis fetalis. It should not be used for elective induction of labor, due to potential adverse effects to the mother or baby.

Oxytocin is also approved to reduce postpartum hemorrhage following expulsion of the placenta and to aid in returning normal muscular tone to the uterus. This drug is approved at higher doses for the adjunct management of incomplete or inevitable abortion. Intranasal forms once used to promote milk letdown are no longer available in the United States.

Mechanism of Action: Oxytocin increases the intensity and frequency of uterine smooth muscle contractions. When stimulated by sucking, oxytocin causes smooth muscle in alveolar ducts to contract, thus ejecting milk from the breast.

Pharmacokinetics:

Route(s)	IV or IM
Absorption	Destroyed in the GI tract
Distribution	Widely distributed in extracellular fluid; small amounts may cross the placenta; secreted in breast milk
Primary metabolism	Rapidly destroyed in the kidney and the liver
Primary excretion	Small amounts via the kidney
Onset of action	IV: immediate; IM: 3–5 min
Duration of action	Half-life: 3–5 min

Adverse Effects: The most common adverse effects of oxytocin are rapid, painful uterine contractions and fetal tachycardia. Uterine rupture or fetal trauma from too-rapid expulsion through the pelvis, seizure, and coma are regarded as the most serious adverse effects. The risk of uterine rupture is increased in women who have delivered five or more children. When given IV, vital signs of the fetus and mother must be monitored continuously to prevent fetal complications, such as dysrhythmias or intracranial hemorrhage. **Black Box Warning:** Oxytocin is not indicated for the elective induction of labor in a pregnant patient who has no medical indications for induction.

Contraindications/Precautions: Oxytocin has an antidiuretic effect and care must be taken to avoid water intoxication. Oxytocin is contraindicated when there is evidence of fetal distress, placenta previa, uterine prolapse, active herpes infection, abnormal fetal position, and cervical cancer. Breastfeeding should be delayed for at least 24 hours after the drug is discontinued.

Drug Interactions: Vasoconstrictors used concurrently with oxytocin may cause severe HTN. Oxytocin may cause adverse cardiovascular effects when administered with fibrinolysin, warfarin, and cyclopropane anesthesia. **Herbal/Food:** Ephedra used with oxytocin may lead to HTN.

Pregnancy: If given during pregnancy, oxytocin will cause uterine contractions and promote delivery or possible abortion. Caution should be used during lactation, although adverse effects in the breastfed neonate are not expected.

Treatment of Overdose: Overdose will cause severe cramping and possible damage to the uterus. Discontinuation of the infusion will result in a rapid resolution of symptoms due to the short half-life of the drug.

Clinician Responsibilities: Key clinical implications for patients receiving oxytocin are included in Applied Clinical Judgment: Patients Receiving Pharmacotherapy with Oxytocin (Pitocin).

Drugs Similar to Oxytocin (Pitocin)

Uterine stimulants also include prostaglandins (carboprost and dinoprostone) and the ergot alkaloid methylergonovine.

Carboprost (Hemabate): Carboprost, equivalent to endogenous prostaglandin F_2 alpha, is approved for controlling postpartum bleeding that has not responded to oxytocin and for inducing pharmacologic abortion between weeks 13 and 20 of gestation. For postpartum bleeding, it is administered by the IM route every 15 to 90 minutes until hemorrhage is controlled. Nausea and vomiting, diarrhea, and fever are common adverse effects. This drug is contraindicated during pregnancy and adverse effects during breastfeeding are not known.

Dinoprostone (Cervidil, Prepidil, Prostin E_2): Dinoprostone, or prostaglandin E_2, is approved to prepare the cervix for labor or to abort a fetus that has died. To promote cervical ripening, it is administered intravaginally. The gel form of the drug is placed into the cervical canal using prefilled syringes and doses may be repeated every 6 hours, as needed. The vaginal insert releases the drug slowly, over 12 hours. The insert may be quickly and easily removed once labor begins. Both the gel and the insert may stimulate the uterus to begin contracting. Like carboprost, GI effects and fever are very common adverse effects. Other than its use for cervical ripening, this drug is contraindicated during pregnancy. This drug is secreted in human milk but adverse effects on the breastfed neonate are not known.

Methylergonovine (Methergine): Ergonovine is an older drug, approved in 1946. It may be administered by the IM, or IV routes to control postpartum hemorrhage and restore uterine tone. The IV route is used only in emergency situations because it may produce serious HTN or stroke in the mother. Uterine contractions begin in 3 to 5 minutes after an IM dose. Cramping and GI-related adverse effects are common with this drug. The drug is contraindicated during pregnancy because it can cause immediate uterine contractions that could injure the fetus. Caution should be used if breastfeeding; for 12 hours after the last dose, milk should be discarded.

CONNECTION Checkpoint 69.1

Calcium channel blockers, including nifedipine, are widely used to treat cardiovascular disorders. From what you learned in Chapter 30, what effects would you expect nifedipine to have on vascular smooth muscle, myocardial oxygen demand, and myocardial conduction?

CONNECTIONS: APPLIED CLINICAL JUDGMENT

Patients Receiving Pharmacotherapy with Oxytocin (Pitocin)

Key Assessment Data

- Complete health history including current length of pregnancy duration; presence of preeclampsia or eclampsia; recent labor, type of delivery, history of labors or caesarean births; cardiovascular, neurologic, hepatic, or kidney disease; diabetes; or breastfeeding; CBC, platelets, coagulation studies, electrolytes, glucose, magnesium level, and hepatic and kidney function studies levels; allergies, current prescription and over-the-counter (OTC) drugs, herbal preparations, caffeine, nicotine, and alcohol use.
- Obtain fetal heart rate, intrauterine positioning; check for presence of cervical dilation and effacement and monitor quality and duration of any existing contractions. Monitor fetal response to contractions, noting any sign of fetal distress.
- Check for postpartum bleeding and note the number of pads saturated.

Desired Therapeutic Outcomes

Improvement is observed and measurable by strong, regular contractions supportive of labor, and control of postpartum bleeding.

Minimizing Adverse Effects

- Oxytocin may cause sustained uterine muscle contractions with potential uterine rupture. Uterine contractions must be monitored and any continuous, sustained contractions managed by stopping the drug infusion, infusing normal saline or solution as ordered if sustained contractions continue.
- Uterine contractions can affect the amount of blood flow through the placenta with diminished oxygenation to the fetus. Changes in fetal heart rate may signal fetal distress, and the patient should be placed on her side, oxygen administered unless otherwise ordered, and the infusion stopped.
- Oxytocin has vasoconstrictive and water-retention properties. Blood pressure and heart rate may increase, and water intoxication is a possible adverse effect. Blood pressure or pulse rate exceeding parameters, increasing disorientation or confusion, and diminished urine output may signify adverse drug effects or possible complications.
- Oxytocin may be given to control postpartum bleeding. Lochia that increases, or if two or more pads are saturated over a 2-hour period, should be immediately assessed.

Patient Education

- Labor contractions will gradually increase, and the drug will be decreased or stopped once contractions reach an optimal level to support cervical dilation.
- Immediately report any headache, dizziness, disorientation or confusion, palpitations, or chest pressure or pain.
- For postpartum care, immediately report any sudden increase in lochia, dizziness, lightheadedness, or if more than two pads are saturated after 2 hours.

Prescribing Considerations

- The initial dose should be 0.5 to 1 mU/min (equal to 3 to 6 mL of the dilute oxytocin solution per hour). At 30- to 60-minute intervals, the dose should be gradually increased in increments of 1 to 2 mU/min until the desired contraction pattern has been established. Once the desired frequency of contractions has been reached and labor has progressed to 5 to 6 cm dilation, the dose may be reduced by similar increments.
- To control postpartum uterine bleeding, administer 10 to 40 units of oxytocin intravenous infusion or 10 mg IM.

Uterine Relaxants: Tocolytics

69.6 Uterine relaxants are used to suppress preterm labor.

Preterm labor, the initiation of labor prior to week 37 of gestation, is a major cause of neonatal mortality. The most common cause is premature rupturing of membranes or infections of the chorion or uterus. If the organ systems of the fetus are determined to be immature, attempts may be made to delay labor because preterm infants have a high morbidity and mortality rate. Suppressing labor allows additional time for the fetal organs to develop and may permit the pregnancy to reach normal term. Bedrest is mandatory and corticosteroids may be administered to accelerate fetal lung maturity and reduce the incidence of neonatal respiratory distress syndrome. Antibiotics such as ampicillin or erythromycin are indicated if the preterm labor is due to a uterine or chorionic infection. Preterm labor can be stopped and delivery delayed in about 50% of women, if the membranes have not yet ruptured. The success rate is only 25% in patients with membrane rupture.

Tocolytics are uterine relaxants prescribed to suppress preterm labor contractions. Typically, the mother is given a monitor with a sensor that records uterine contractions and this information is used to determine the doses and timing of tocolytic medications. Tocolytics can generally delay labor by only 24 to 72 hours, but this is often enough time for the fetus to develop normal lung function. The benefits of these drugs must be carefully weighed against their potential adverse effects, which include tachycardia in both the mother and the fetus. There is no clear evidence that tocolytics reduce perinatal or neonatal mortality.

Only a few drugs are available as tocolytics, and none can be realistically considered a prototype. For over 30 years, magnesium sulfate was the preferred drug for delaying preterm labor, but some evidence suggests that it may be ineffective and that it poses undue risks to the fetus and mother. The only drug that is FDA approved for this indication is ritodrine (Yutopar), but it is no longer available in the United States. Calcium channel blockers and beta-adrenergic agonists appear to be effective and are used off-label for this indication. Doses for these drugs are listed in Table 69.2.

Magnesium sulfate: A traditional preferred tocolytic, magnesium sulfate is administered by continuous IV infusion via a controlled pump device until preterm contractions diminish, usually in about 30 minutes. It is used off-label for this indication. During therapy, careful monitoring of deep tendon reflexes, blood pressure, respirations, urinary output, and serum magnesium concentrations are necessary. Early signs of magnesium overdose include flushing of the skin, sedation, confusion, intense thirst, and muscle weakness. Extreme levels cause neuromuscular blockade with resultant respiratory paralysis, heart block, and circulatory collapse. In 2013, the FDA issues a safety warning that use for more than 5 to 7 days during pregnancy may cause fetal harm. This drug is featured as a prototype electrolyte in Chapter 33 for the treatment of magnesium deficiency.

Nifedipine (Adalat, Procardia): Nifedipine is a calcium channel blocker widely prescribed for the treatment of HTN and angina. The drug has been used off-label as a tocolytic as an option to magnesium sulfate. Nifedipine is given either by the PO or sublingual route. A typical regimen includes a loading dose followed by additional PO doses every 15 to 20 minutes until contractions diminish. Nifedipine appears to be as effective as magnesium sulfate and the beta-adrenergic agonists but exhibits fewer adverse effects. Adverse effects include acute pulmonary edema, dysrhythmias, and hypotension. A prototype feature for nifedipine is presented in Chapter 30.

Terbutaline (Brethine): Terbutaline is a beta$_2$-adrenergic agonist that is FDA approved to treat acute bronchospasm due to asthma. It has been used off-label to suppress preterm contractions due to its ability to relax smooth muscle. It is given by the subcutaneous route either by injection every 20 minutes or by using a continuous infusion device. It may also be administered orally. The FDA has issued a black box warning that administration of terbutaline for more than 48 to 72 hours during pregnancy can result in serious adverse reactions, including death of the fetus. The mother may experience increased heart rate, dysrhythmias, myocardial ischemia, transient hyperglycemia, hypokalemia, and pulmonary edema. The fetus may experience increased heart rate and neonatal hypoglycemia.

Pharmacotherapy of Female Infertility and Female Sexual Desire Disorder

69.7 Female infertility may be treated with drugs that promote oocyte maturation and ovulation.

Infertility is defined as the inability to become pregnant after at least 1 year of frequent, unprotected intercourse. Infertility is a common disorder: 25% of couples experience difficulty in conceiving children at some point during their reproductive lifetimes. It is estimated that female reproductive tract conditions contribute to approximately 60% of the infertility disorders. Drugs used to treat female infertility are listed in Table 69.3. Treatment of male infertility is presented in Chapter 71.

The three primary causes of female infertility are pelvic infections, physical obstruction of the uterine tubes, and lack of ovulation. Extensive testing is often necessary to determine the exact cause, and it is not uncommon to find multiple etiologies for the infertility. Prior to initiating

Table 69.3 Drugs for Female Infertility

Drug	Route and Adult Dose (Maximum Dose Where Indicated)	Adverse Effects
bromocriptine (Parlodel)	PO: 1.25–2.5 mg/daily (max: 2.5 mg bid–tid)	*Nausea and vomiting, cramping, constipation, drowsiness, headache, orthostatic hypotension, anorexia* GI bleeding, psychosis, seizures, syncope
clomiphene	PO first course: 50 mg/day for 5 days; start on fifth day of cycle following start of spontaneous or induced bleeding (with progestin) Second course if ovulation: Repeat first course until conception or for 3 cycles Second course if no ovulation: 100 mg/day for 5 days as above (max: 100 mg/day)	*Weight gain, symptoms of PMS, hot flashes, dermatitis* Blurred vision, ovarian hyperstimulation, cataracts, thrombosis of temporal arteries
danazol	PO: 200–400 mg bid for 3–6 months; may extend to 9 months	*Hirsutism, alopecia, voice deepening, weight gain, vaginal dryness, reduction in breast size, edema, emotional lability, hot flashes* Thromboembolic events, hepatotoxicity, intracranial HTN, fetal toxicity
FSH- and LH-Enhancing Drugs		
chorionic gonadotropin-HCG (Novarel, Ovidrel, Pregnyl)	IM: 5000–10,000 units 1 day following last dose of menotropins	Women: *Pelvic pain, depression, fatigue* Ovarian hyperstimulation syndrome Men: *Gynecomastia, acne* Aggressive behavior, depression
follitropin alfa (Gonal-F)	Subcutaneous: 75 international units/day initially, then increased by 37.5 international units at the end of 14 days. Further 37.5-unit dose increases may be made every 7 days (max: 300 international units/day)	*Headache, nausea, abdominal pain, diarrhea, increased infections* Ovarian hyperstimulation syndrome, thromboembolic disorders
follitropin beta (Follistim AQ)	Subcutaneous (for ovulation induction): 50 international units/day initially for 7 days, then increased by 25–50 international units at weekly intervals	
menotropins (Menopur)	Subcutaneous: 225 international units initially with 125 international unit dosage increases not more often than every 2 days	*Abdominal cramps, fullness, or pain, injection-site reaction, nausea* Ovarian hyperstimulation syndrome, thromboembolic disorders, respiratory disorders
GnRH Antagonists		
cetrorelix (Cetrotide)	Subcutaneous: 0.25 mg/day during the early to midfollicular phase of the cycle following the initiation of FSH	*Hot flashes, headache, menstrual irregularities* Fetal death, ovarian hyperstimulation syndrome
ganirelix	Subcutaneous: 250 mcg once daily during the early to midfollicular phase of the cycle following the initiation of FSH	
GnRH Analogs/Agonists		
goserelin (Zoladex)	Subcutaneous implant for endometriosis: 3.6 mg every 28 days Subcutaneous implant for advanced carcinoma: 10.8 mg every 3 months	Women: *Headache, depression, sweating, acne, vaginitis, vaginal dryness, menstrual irregularities, bone density loss, emotional lability* Tumor flare-up (goserelin, leuprolide) Men: *Erectile dysfunction, lethargy, gynecomastia* Heart failure All patients: *Pain at injection site, hot flashes, loss of libido* Bone density loss, fractures
leuprolide (Eligard, Lupron Depot)	IM for endometriosis: 3.75 mg every month or 11.25 mg every 3 months Subcutaneous for infertility: 0.5–1 mg/day. By day 3 of the menstrual cycle, the dosage is typically decreased by 50%	
nafarelin (Synarel)	Intranasal: 2 inhalations/day (200 mcg/inhalation), one in each nostril; begin between days 2 and 4 of menstrual cycle (may increase to 800 mcg/day as 2 inhalations)	

Note: *Italics* indicate common adverse effects. Underline indicates serious adverse effects.

therapy, other causes of infertility should be excluded, such as thyroid disorders, adrenal disorders, hyperprolactinemia, and male-factor infertility.

For women whose infertility is due to inadequate ovulation, pharmacotherapy may be of value. **Ovulatory dysfunction** is defined as the presence of abnormal, irregular, or absent ovulation. Signs and symptoms of ovulatory dysfunction include irregular or absent menses, excessive abdominal bloating, and mood lability. Confirmation of the disorder is made by measuring hormone levels.

Ovulatory dysfunction may occur at the level of the hypothalamus, pituitary, or ovary, and pharmacotherapy is targeted to the specific cause of the dysfunction. The most common etiology of ovulatory dysfunction is **polycystic ovary syndrome**, a condition in which the ovaries are filled with follicular cysts and the patient has elevated levels of androgens and estrogen. Hirsutism is commonly observed in these women due to the excessive androgen levels. Another cause of ovulatory dysfunction is hyperprolactinemia, excessive levels of the hormone prolactin, which is most frequently caused by a tumor of the pituitary gland.

Many women with ovulatory dysfunction can be successfully treated with drug therapy; restoring regular, monthly ovulation is an essential goal of fertility management. Ovulation induction protocols are sometimes divided into the following three medication groups, which are shown in Pharmacotherapy Illustrated 69.1:

- Drugs used to promote maturation of ovarian follicles
- Drugs used to trigger ovulation at the end of follicular maturation
- Drugs that promote ovulation to occur on a regular, monthly basis, at the midpoint of the menstrual cycle.

Promotion of follicle maturation: Ovulation cannot occur unless the ovarian follicles receive a hormonal signal to mature each month. This signal is normally supplied by

Pharmacotherapy Illustrated **69.1**

Mechanisms of Action of Drugs Used to Treat Female Infertility

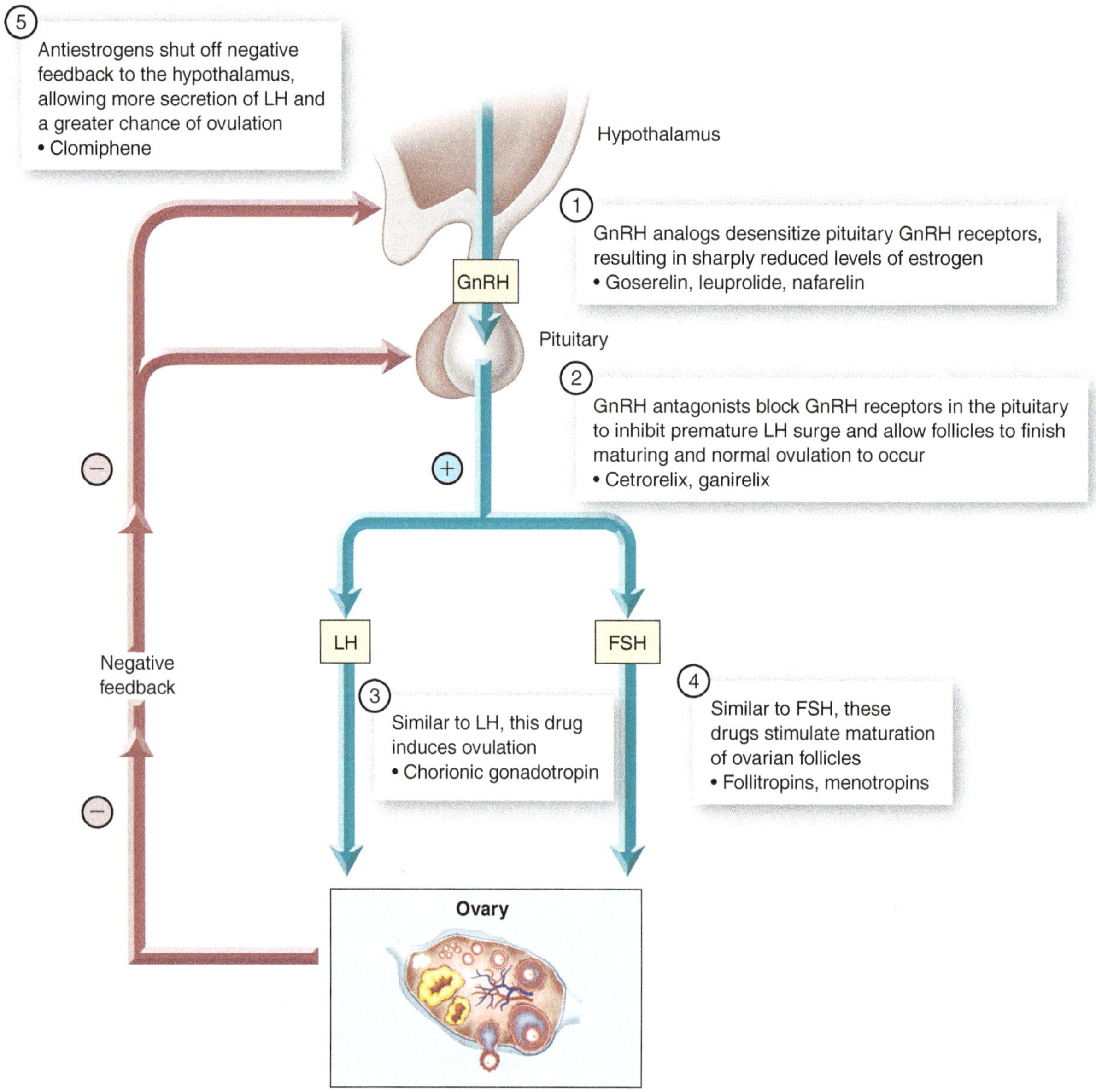

LH and FSH during the first few weeks of the menstrual cycle. Clomiphene is the traditional preferred drug for treating female infertility because it stimulates the release of LH, resulting in the maturation of more ovarian follicles than would normally occur. The rise in LH level induced by clomiphene is sufficient to induce ovulation in about 80% of treated patients. The use of clomiphene assumes that the pituitary gland is able to respond by secreting LH and that the ovaries are responsive to LH. If either of these assumptions is false, other treatment options must be considered.

If the infertility is a result of endocrine disruption at the pituitary level, therapy with human menopausal gonadotropin (HMG) or GnRH may be indicated. These therapies are generally indicated only after clomiphene has failed to induce ovulation. Also known as menotropins (Menopur, Repronex), HMG acts on the ovaries to increase follicle maturation and results in a 25% incidence of multiple pregnancies. Successful therapy with HMG assumes that the ovaries are responsive to LH and FSH. Newer formulations use recombinant DNA technology to synthesize gonadotropins containing nearly pure FSH, rather than extracting the FSH–LH mixture from urine.

Promotion of ovulation: Unless maturing follicles receive the final "burst" of LH, ovulation will not occur. HMG is similar in structure to natural LH and produces the same effect: ovulation.

Restoration of a normal monthly pattern of ovulation: The success of conception will be improved if a regular, monthly pattern of ovulation is established. Premature ovulation, the expulsion of the oocyte from the ovary before it has fully matured, is prevented by the use of two antagonists of GnRH: ganirelix and cetrorelix (Cetrotide).

Stimulation of the ovary by certain fertility drugs causes the ovaries to enlarge. Mild enlargement may cause pelvic pain but is generally benign and disappears when therapy is discontinued. One serious complication of certain fertility drugs is **ovarian hyperstimulation syndrome (OHS)**. The onset of OHS is characterized by rapid, massive enlargement of the ovaries accompanied by nausea and vomiting, rapid weight gain, ascites, respiratory difficulties, increased risk of thromboembolism, and progressive kidney impairment. Progressive symptoms call for discontinuation of drug therapy, fluid restriction, bedrest, and symptomatic treatment of nausea and vomiting and pain. Although OHS can be fatal, most cases resolve in 1 to 2 weeks.

Endometriosis is characterized by the presence of endometrial tissue that has implanted outside the uterus in locations such as the surface of pelvic organs or the ovaries. About 50% of infertile women have endometriosis. Being responsive to hormonal stimuli, this abnormal tissue can cause pain, dysfunctional uterine bleeding, and dysmenorrhea. The pain, discomfort, and infertility brought on by endometriosis may be treated by danazol, nafarelin, and leuprolide. These drugs suppress the production of estrogen and progesterone, resulting in a decrease in growth potential of endometrial tissues. Surgical removal of the abnormal endometrial lesions may be necessary, and women who have completed their childbearing or who are postmenopausal may consider a hysterectomy with oophorectomy.

Estrogen–progestin oral contraceptives are a first-line therapy in treating endometriosis. Leuprolide (Lupron Depot) and nafarelin (Synarel) are GnRH agonists that produce an initial release of LH and FSH, followed by suppression due to the negative feedback effect on the pituitary. Many women experience relief from the symptoms of endometriosis after 3 to 6 months of leuprolide therapy, and the benefits may extend well beyond the treatment period. As an alternative choice, danazol is an anabolic steroid that suppresses FSH production, which in turn shuts down both ectopic and normal endometrial activity. While leuprolide is given only by the parenteral route, danazol is given orally. The GnRH antagonist elagolix (Orilissa) is a newer medication indicated for relief of severe pain caused by endometriosis. The combination of elagolix, norethindrone, and estradiol (Oriahnn) was approved in 2020 to treat heavy menstrual bleeding in women with uterine fibroids.

PROTOTYPE DRUG Clomiphene

Classification **Therapeutic:** Infertility drug
Pharmacologic: Ovarian stimulant

Therapeutic Effects and Uses: Approved in 1967, clomiphene is a first-line drug for female infertility caused by ovulatory dysfunction. It acts by inducing ovulation in anovulatory women. The pregnancy rate of patients taking clomiphene is high, and twins occur in about 3 to 5% of treated patients. Therapy is usually begun with a low dose for 5 days following menses because this is the time of greatest follicle maturation. If ovulation does not occur, the dose is increased. If ovulation still is not induced, HCG is added to the regimen. If pregnancy has not occurred following six cycles of successful ovulation, the drug is usually discontinued and other means of restoring fertility are explored. The use of clomiphene does not permanently restore normal follicle maturation. Its effects diminish once the drug is discontinued.

Clomiphene is used off-label to treat low sperm counts (oligospermia) in men. Just as in women, the drug increases the secretion of LH. In men, LH stimulates the testes to produce testosterone and additional sperm.

Mechanism of Action: Clomiphene is a SERM that has both estrogen agonist and antagonist effects, depending on the tissue. In the pituitary and hypothalamus, clomiphene acts as an "antiestrogen," shutting off LH secretion, which is required for ovulation. Clomiphene competes for estrogen receptors in the hypothalamus by sending a message that estrogen levels are low; in response, LH is secreted, leading to ovarian stimulation.

Pharmacokinetics:

Route(s)	PO
Absorption	Readily absorbed
Distribution	Crosses the placenta; unknown if secreted in breast milk; 90% bound to protein
Primary metabolism	Hepatic
Primary excretion	Feces; small amounts in urine
Onset of action	30–60 min
Duration of action	Half-life: 5–7 days; peak effects: 4–10 days

Adverse Effects: Few serious adverse effects occur during clomiphene therapy. The most common are weight gain, symptoms of PMS, hot flashes, allergic dermatitis, and urticaria. The most serious adverse effects are blurred vision, ovarian hyperstimulation, cataracts and other visual impairments, and thrombosis of temporal arteries. The drug may cause ovarian enlargement with subsequent pelvic pain in about 14% of women taking the drug.

Contraindications/Precautions: Clomiphene should be avoided in patients with lactation, gynecomastia, fibrocystic breast disease, liver disease, ovarian cysts not due to polycystic ovary syndrome, and hepatic, thyroid, or adrenal dysfunction. The drug is contraindicated in patients with dysfunctional uterine bleeding until the cause can be determined.

Drug Interactions: Androgens will reduce the success of clomiphene therapy. **Herbal/Food:** Black cohosh and chasteberry have estrogen effects that may reduce the effectiveness of clomiphene.

Pregnancy: Clomiphene is teratogenic and fetotoxic in laboratory animals and is contraindicated during pregnancy. Prior to beginning therapy, a negative pregnancy test should be confirmed. It is not known whether clomiphene is secreted in human milk or if it has adverse effects on the breastfed neonate.

Treatment of Overdose: Symptoms of overdose include nausea, vomiting, visual blurring, hot flashes, and pelvic pain. The patient is treated symptomatically.

Drugs Similar to Clomiphene

Other drugs for female infertility include bromocriptine, cetrorelix, chorionic gonadotropin–HCG, danazol, follitropins, ganirelix, goserelin, leuprolide, menotropins, and nafarelin. Once pregnancy is confirmed, the infertility drugs are discontinued because they have been shown to cause fetal harm in laboratory animals.

Bromocriptine (Parlodel): Approved in 1978, bromocriptine is chemically related to the ergot alkaloids and is indicated for a large number of diverse conditions. The drug is a dopamine agonist, activating dopaminergic receptors in the hypothalamus. For infertility, its primary use is to treat prolactin-secreting tumors of the pituitary, which often cause amenorrhea and female infertility. Normal menses are usually restored after 6 to 8 weeks of therapy. This reduces elevated serum prolactin levels and restores ovulation and ovarian function in amenorrheic women. It is used as a short-term treatment for amenorrhea in the absence of pituitary tumors. It is also approved to treat acromegaly and Parkinson's disease and to improve glycemic control in patients with type 2 diabetes. Off-label indications include mastalgia associated with PMS, alcoholism, cocaine withdrawal, and neuroleptic malignant syndrome. Bromocriptine causes frequent adverse effects that include nausea and vomiting, cramping, constipation, drowsiness, headache, orthostatic hypotension, and anorexia.

Cetrorelix (Cetrotide): Approved in 2000, cetrorelix is a GnRH antagonist given by the subcutaneous route that blocks GnRH receptors in the pituitary. Women undergoing ovarian stimulation with FSH or menotropin therapy experience a sharp rise in estrogen levels due to the maturing follicles, which can trigger an early surge of LH and premature ovulation. Cetrorelix inhibits this premature LH surge in women who are undergoing controlled ovarian stimulation for assisted reproduction, thus allowing follicles to finish maturing and normal ovulation to occur. The only indication for cetrorelix is infertility. Adverse effects are minor and include hot flashes and headache. It is contraindicated for use in primary ovarian failure, chronic kidney disease (CKD), and pregnancy.

Chorionic gonadotropin–HCG (Novarel, Ovidrel, Pregnyl): This drug has two forms. HCG is secreted by the placenta and obtained and purified from the urine of pregnant women. Choriogonadotropin alfa (r-HCG, Ovidrel) is a recombinant form with actions identical to those of HCG. The chorionic gonadotropin drugs have the same actions as LH and can mimic the LH surge that normally causes ovulation. As part of an assisted reproductive program, chorionic gonadotropin is administered at midcycle, after clomiphene or FSH has been used to mature sufficient numbers of ovarian follicles. A single IM dose is sufficient to induce ovulation. The drug has few adverse effects when administered as a single dose in women.

In males, HCG is approved to treat prepubertal cryptorchidism, hypogonadism, and oligospermia. Therapy in males may continue for several months and gynecomastia, acne, and behavioral changes may occur.

Danazol: Danazol is a PO drug used to treat endometriosis. Approved in 1976, the drug exerts antiestrogenic and weak androgenic properties, which cause ectopic endometrial tissue to atrophy. After 6 weeks of therapy, danazol causes anovulation and amenorrhea, which are its therapeutic effects. When the drug is discontinued, normal ovulation and menstrual cycles return in about 2 to 3 months. Danazol is also approved to treat fibrocystic breast disease and for the prophylaxis of hereditary angioedema. The drug has androgenic actions that may cause permanent masculinization effects such as hirsutism, alopecia, voice deepening, and weight gain. Women may experience effects of estrogen deficiency such as vaginal dryness, reduction in breast size, emotional lability, and hot flashes. Serious adverse effects include thromboembolism, hepatic adenoma, and intracranial HTN.

Follitropins: The follitropins are two different drugs with the same actions. Follitropin alfa (Gonal-F) and follitropin beta (Follistim AQ) are identical to human FSH obtained through recombinant DNA technology. Both are given by the parenteral route to stimulate the maturation of ovarian follicles. The drugs are given early in the menstrual cycle, followed by a dose of chorionic gonadotropin, which provides the boost for ovulation. Multiple births, including triplets, quadruplets, and quintuplets, are common during therapy with follitropins. In men, follitropins are used to stimulate spermatogenesis in patients with hypogonadism and oligospermia. Minor adverse effects include headache, nausea, abdominal pain, diarrhea, and increased infections. The most serious potential adverse effects are OHS, thromboembolism, acute respiratory distress syndrome, and exacerbation of asthma.

Ganirelix: Like cetrorelix, ganirelix is a GnRH antagonist given by the subcutaneous route that blocks GnRH receptors in the pituitary. Approved in 1999, its only indication is for female infertility. Ganirelix inhibits the premature LH surge in patients undergoing controlled ovarian stimulation for assisted reproduction. Adverse effects are minor and include hot flashes, menstrual irregularities, and headache. It is contraindicated for use in primary ovarian failure, CKD, and pregnancy.

Goserelin (Zoladex): Goserelin is a GnRH hormone agonist. It has the same physiologic actions as endogenous GnRH; however, the way it is administered causes the opposite effect. Natural GnRH is released by the hypothalamus in an "on–off" pulsatile manner, which stimulates the release of LH and FSH (and eventually estrogen). Like GnRH, goserelin first stimulates LH and FSH secretion. With continuous administration, however, the pituitary receptors become insensitive to the effects of GnRH and the gland stops releasing LH and FSH. Without FSH or LH, the levels of estrogen in women and testosterone in men fall dramatically. This hypoestrogenic state relieves the symptoms of endometriosis. It is also approved for palliative treatment of estrogen-dependent breast cancer and for advanced prostate cancer. Goserelin is available subcutaneously as a once-monthly implant (for men or women) and a 3-month implant for men with prostate cancer. Women may experience hypoestrogenic effects such as vaginal dryness, depression, menstrual irregularities, bone density loss, emotional lability, and hot flashes. Men may experience erectile dysfunction, gynecomastia, and loss of libido. Pain at the injection site is common.

Leuprolide (Eligard, Lupron Depot, Viadur): Like goserelin, leuprolide is a GnRH agonist. The two drugs act by the same mechanism: desensitizing pituitary GnRH receptors, resulting in sharply reduced levels of estrogen and testosterone. For relief of endometriosis symptoms, a depot IM injection is given once monthly or once every 3 months, depending on the dose. Treatment of endometriosis is limited to 6 months. Like goserelin, it is also approved for the palliative treatment of advanced prostate cancer and used off-label for breast cancer. Leuprolide is an orphan drug for treating precocious (early) puberty in children less than 9 years old. The drug was once widely used to treat infertility by inhibiting premature LH surges, but the GnRH antagonists are now used for this indication. The adverse effects are the same as those for goserelin.

Menotropins (Menopur): Approved in 1975, menotropins is sometimes referred to as HMG. Menotropins is a product containing a combination of FSH and LH purified from the urine of postmenopausal women. The FSH activity of menotropins is significantly higher than its LH activity. Like the follitropins, menotropins is given by the parenteral route during the first half of the menstrual cycle to promote follicle maturation. At the end of therapy, HCG is often administered to supply the LH surge necessary for ovulation. Menotropins therapy is associated with a 20 to 35% possibility of multiple births. In men, menotropins is FDA approved to stimulate spermatogenesis in patients with hypogonadism and oligospermia. In men, gynecomastia, acne, and behavioral changes may occur. In women, the drug often causes ovarian enlargement and OHS is possible. Serious pulmonary conditions such as acute respiratory distress syndrome and exacerbation of asthma have been reported.

Nafarelin (Synarel): Like goserelin and leuprolide, nafarelin is a GnRH agonist. The three drugs act by the same mechanism: desensitizing pituitary GnRH receptors, resulting in sharply reduced levels of estrogen and testosterone. Unlike the other GnRH analogs, nafarelin is applied topically to the nasal mucosa, where the drug is rapidly absorbed. When used to treat endometriosis, the typical dose is one spray in each nostril daily. It is also approved to treat precocious puberty and used off-label for hirsutism. Nafarelin may be used off-label to prevent premature LH surges in women with infertility; however, ganirelix and cetrorelix are more frequently prescribed for this indication. Adverse effects are the same as those of the other GnRH agonists goserelin and leuprolide. This drug was approved in 1990.

69.8 Low sexual desire in women may be treated with pharmacotherapy.

Hypoactive sexual desire disorder (HSDD), also called *female sexual interest arousal disorder*, is a condition marked by a persistent lack of interest in sexual activity over a prolonged period. To be diagnosed with HSDD, the patient must be experiencing marked distress or interpersonal difficulty that negatively impacts her quality of life. Before implementing pharmacotherapy, the healthcare provider should investigate causes of HSDD such as relationship problems, coexisting medical or psychiatric conditions, or side effects of other medications such as selective serotonin reuptake inhibitors.

In 2015 the FDA approved the first drug for female HSDD. Flibanserin (Addyi) is approved to treat HSDD in premenopausal women who previously had no problems with sexual desire. It is administered PO, once daily at bedtime. The drug carries a black box warning that it can cause severe hypotension and syncope if taken concurrently with alcohol or moderate or strong inhibitors of CYP3A4, such as azole antifungals, ritonavir, telaprevir, or verapamil. Because of the potential for serious hypotension, the FDA requires prescribers to complete special training. In addition, pharmacies must be certified to dispense the medication, and patients must sign an agreement that they understand the adverse effects. Common adverse effects include dizziness, sleepiness, nausea, fatigue, and dry mouth. The mechanism by which flibanserin increases sexual desire is not known. Studies on laboratory animals showed fetal harm at high doses. Flibanserin is not recommended during lactation because it is secreted in animal milk and has the potential to cause sedation in the breastfed neonate.

A second drug for HSDD, bremelanotide (Vyleesi), was approved in 2019 for use in premenopausal women. It is not indicated to improve sexual performance or for men. It is administered subcutaneously by autoinjector at least 45 minutes prior to anticipated sexual activity. Nausea, flushing injection-site reactions and headache are common adverse reactions. This drug may cause transient increases in blood pressure and is contraindicated for women with uncontrolled HTN. Bremelanotide causes fetal harm in laboratory animals. Women of reproductive potential should use contraception and discontinue the drug if pregnancy is suspected. It is not known if this drug is secreted in milk or if it has adverse effects on the breastfed neonate. The mechanism by which bremelanotide increases sexual desire is not known.

Understanding Chapter 69

Key Concepts Summary

69.1 Regulation of the female reproductive system is achieved by hormones from the hypothalamus, pituitary gland, and ovary.

69.2 Estrogens are administered as replacement therapy, to prevent conception, and for certain neoplasms.

69.3 Progestins are administered to treat dysfunctional uterine bleeding, to prevent conception, and for certain neoplasms.

69.4 Hormone therapy provides relief from moderate to severe menopause symptoms.

69.5 Oxytocics are drugs used to stimulate the uterus and promote labor and delivery.

69.6 Uterine relaxants are used to suppress preterm labor.

69.7 Female infertility may be treated with drugs that promote oocyte maturation and ovulation.

69.8 Low sexual desire in women may be treated with pharmacotherapy.

CASE STUDY: Making the Patient Connection

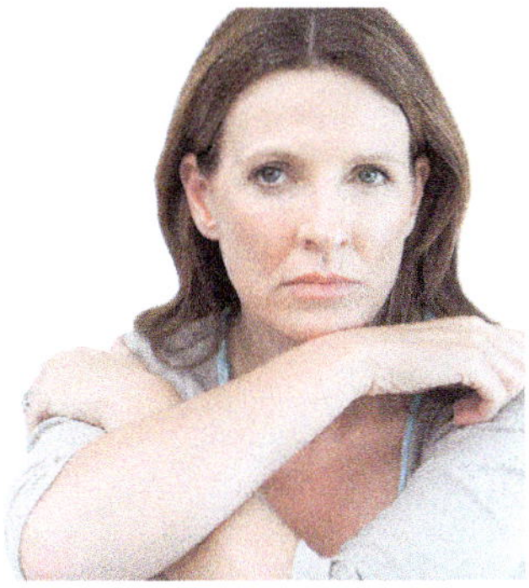

Remember the patient "Maureen John" at the beginning of the chapter? Now read the remainder of the case study. Based on the information presented within this chapter, respond to the critical thinking questions that follow the case study.

Maureen John is 46 years old and exhibiting signs of menopause. She reports a change in her menstrual cycle regularity. For the past year, her periods have occurred between 6 and 8 weeks apart and have lasted only 2 to 3 days. Previously, she experienced her periods approximately every 28 days and they lasted from 4 to 5 days. Maureen reports to the nurse that she is now feeling easily fatigued, has more mood swings, occasional headaches, hot flashes, insomnia, bouts of depression, and irritability. She is also concerned about her loss of libido. She admits to smoking half a pack of cigarettes a day and drinking several cups of coffee during work hours. She has a family history of HTN, cardiac disease, and diabetes, but she has never been diagnosed with any of those disorders.

A complete history and physical examination, along with a vaginal examination and a Pap smear, were performed.

Critical Thinking Questions

1. Do you think that Maureen is a candidate for hormone therapy? Why or why not?
2. Create a list of some treatment options for this patient.
3. Maureen asks about the precautions related to suggested treatment options. How would you respond?

Additional Case Study

Prithi Kaur, a 23-year-old woman, and her 25-year-old husband attend the infertility clinic for evaluation. Efforts at becoming pregnant naturally for the past 2 years have failed. They inform the nurse that the husband has a 3-year-old son from an earlier relationship. The wife has never conceived. Both denied any sexually transmitted infections. The patient is started on clomiphene (Clomid) 50 mg for 5 days.

1. Prithi asks you, the nurse, "What are some causes of infertility?" How would you respond?
2. What instructions would you give to the patient regarding the administration of this drug?

Chapter Review

1. A 52-year-old patient experiencing symptoms of menopause is interested in taking HT with conjugated estrogen (Premarin). Which conditions may be a contraindication for HT for this patient? (Select all that apply.)
    1. History of type 2 diabetes mellitus
    2. History of deep vein thrombosis
    3. History of breast cancer with "lumpectomy" treatment
    4. History of hyperlipidemia, controlled by drug therapy
    5. History of two cesarean births

2. The nurse is evaluating the effect of an oxytocin infusion in a laboring woman. Which of the following indicates that the drug is exerting therapeutic effects?
    1. Hemorrhage is controlled.
    2. Contractions are sustained at 60 seconds long.
    3. Contractions are occurring every 4 minutes and lasting 20 seconds.
    4. Milk letdown has begun in preparation for breastfeeding.

3. Which instruction about clomiphene (Clomid) will the nurse provide to a woman with infertility?
    1. "The drug will be taken for a year and then reevaluated for an increased dose."
    2. "The drug will be continued for the first 3 months of pregnancy to guard against miscarriage."
    3. "You may stay on this indefinitely until pregnancy occurs. There are few adverse effects."
    4. "If pregnancy does not occur within six cycles, other options for treatment will be explored."

4. A 48-year-old patient has received a prescription for medroxyprogesterone (Provera) for treatment of dysfunctional uterine bleeding. Because of related adverse effects, the nurse will teach the patient to monitor and report which symptoms?
   1. Insomnia or difficulty falling asleep
   2. Excessive mouth, eye, or vaginal dryness
   3. Joint pain or pain on ambulation
   4. Breakthrough spotting between menstrual periods

5. The patient informs the healthcare provider that she has been trying to become pregnant for more than 2 years and has not used any form of contraception. The healthcare provider prescribes clomiphene 50 mg/day for 5 days. The nurse should instruct the patient to begin taking the drug on the:
   1. First day of the menstrual cycle.
   2. Fifth day of the menstrual cycle.
   3. Fifth day after ovulation.
   4. Last day of the menstrual cycle.

6. A patient in preterm labor is receiving magnesium sulfate by IV infusion. Which early sign of magnesium toxicity would prompt the nurse to stop the infusion and notify the provider?
   1. Hyperactive patellar reflexes
   2. Chest congestion and coughing
   3. Seizure activity
   4. Sedation and intense thirst

See Appendix A for answers to critical thinking questions, case study questions, and review questions.

References

Estephan, A. (2018). *Dysfunctional uterine bleeding in emergency medicine*. Medscape. http://emedicine.medscape.com/article/795587-overview

Rahman, I., Åkesson, A., & Wolk, A. (2015). Relationship between age at natural menopause and risk of heart failure. *Menopause*, *22*(1), 12–16. https://doi.org/10.1097/GME.0000000000000261

Selected Bibliography

Chlebowski, R. T., Anderson, G. L., Sarto, G. E., Haque, R., Runowicz, C. D., Aragaki, A. K., et al. (2016). Continuous combined estrogen plus progestin and endometrial cancer: The Women's Health Initiative randomized trial. *Journal of the National Cancer Institute*, *108*(3), djv350. https://doi.org/10.1093/jnci/djv350

Davidson, M. R., London, M. L., & Ladewig, P. L. (2019). *Old's maternal-newborn nursing and women's health across the lifespan* (11th ed.). Pearson.

Ferrero, S., Evangelisti, G., & Barra, F. (2018). Current and emerging treatment options for endometriosis. *Expert Opinion on Pharmacotherapy*, *19*(10), 1109–1125. https://doi.org/10.1080/14656566.2018.1494154

Gompel, A., & Plu-Bureau, G. (2018). Progesterone, progestins and the breast in menopause treatment. *Climacteric*, *21*(4), 326–332. https://doi.org/10.1080/13697137.2018.1476483

Hanson, B., Johnstone, E., Dorais, J., Silver, B., Peterson, C. M., & Hotaling, J. (2017). Female infertility, infertility-associated diagnoses, and comorbidities: A review. *Journal of Assisted Reproduction and Genetics*, *34*, 167–177. https://doi.org/10.1007/s10815-016-0836-8

Kagan, R., Kellogg-Spadt, S., & Parish, S. J. (2019). Practical treatment considerations in the management of genitourinary syndrome of menopause. *Drugs & Aging*, *36*(10), 897–908. https://doi.org/10.1007/s40266-019-00700-w

Lamont, C. D., Jørgensen, J. S., & Lamont, R. F. (2016). The safety of tocolytics used for the inhibition of preterm labour. *Expert Opinion on Drug Safety*, *15*, 1163–1173. https://doi.org/10.1080/14740338.2016.1187128

Puscheck, E.E. (2020). *Infertility*. Medscape. https://emedicine.medscape.com/article/274143-overview

Ross, M. G. (2018). *Preterm labor*. Medscape. http://emedicine.medscape.com/article/260998-overview#a6

Saul, T. (2018). *Emergent treatment of endometriosis*. Medscape. https://emedicine.medscape.com/article/795771-overview

Venturella, R., Vaiarelli, A., Cimadomo, D., Pedri, S., Lico, D., Mazzilli, R., et al. (2019). State of the art and emerging drug therapies for female infertility. *Gynecological Endocrinology*, *35*(10), 835–841. https://doi.org/10.1080/09513590.2019.1603289

"I really don't want to ruin my chances of finishing college by becoming pregnant right now. What are my choices?"
—*Patient "Lila Bastian"*

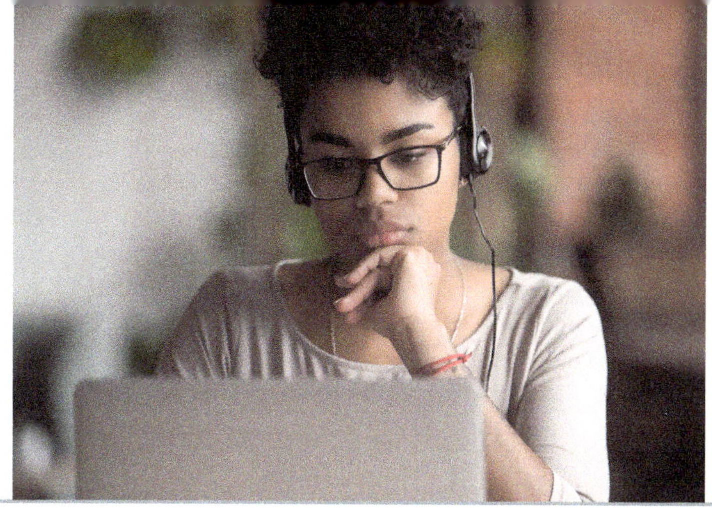

Chapter 70
Drugs for Modifying Conception

Chapter Outline

Learning Outcomes

After reading this chapter, the student should be able to:

1. Identify the choices available for birth control.
2. Delineate advantages and disadvantages of the different contraceptive options.
3. Explain the mechanisms by which estrogens and progestins prevent conception.
4. Compare the safety and effectiveness of different birth control methods.
5. Compare and contrast the options available for long-term contraception.
6. Explain the use of drugs for emergency contraception and for terminating pregnancy.
7. Describe the nurse's role in the pharmacologic management of patients who are taking oral contraceptives.
8. For each of the classes shown in the chapter outline, identify the prototype and representative drugs and explain the mechanism(s) of drug action, primary indications, contraindications, significant drug interactions, pregnancy data, and important adverse effects.
9. Apply clinical judgment to the care of patients receiving pharmacotherapy for contraception.

Key Terms

Definitions of the terms in bold may be found in the Glossary.

About 72 million women in the United States are of childbearing age (15–49 years). Of these women about 65% practice **contraception**, the use of devices, drugs, or surgery to prevent pregnancy (National Center for Health Statistics, 2018). This chapter discusses the female sex hormones that are used to modify conception, describes other widely used methods of contraception, and identifies the nursing connections to patient and family education.

Options and Choices for Birth Control

70.1 Selection of a contraceptive is based on effectiveness, safety, and personal choice.

The decision to engage in sexual activity is one of the most important decisions in life; the choice affects not just the partners but may impact generations to follow. A couple engaging in intercourse on a regular basis without contraceptive protection has a 90% probability of conceiving a child over the course of a year. Thus, the voluntary choice to use contraceptive measures is a critical decision faced by most women in the childbearing years.

Prior to the 1960s, the three primary methods of avoiding pregnancy were total abstinence, abstinence during periods of greatest fertility (rhythm or calendar method), and withdrawal prior to ejaculation (coitus interruptus). The discovery of oral contraceptives and the development of long-acting reversible contraceptives (LARCs) have given couples more effective choices for birth control. For women unable to take medication for contraception, intrauterine devices are safe and effective alternatives. Many contraceptive options are now available, each having specific advantages and disadvantages. The primary options, their effectiveness, and advantages and disadvantages are listed in Table 70.1.

Table 70.1 Effectiveness of Conception Modifiers

		PREGNANCY RATE (%/YEAR)*			
Type	Description	With Perfect Use	With Typical Use	Selected Advantages	Selected Disadvantages
Hormonal Methods					
Combination oral contraceptives (OCs)	Daily tablets	0.3%	9%	Very effective, decreased risk of ovarian and endometrial cancer	Fluid retention, venous thromboembolism, amenorrhea, nausea and vomiting, irregular bleeding, headache; must be taken daily
Progestin-only OCs	Daily tablets	0.5%	9%	No estrogen adverse effects; may be used in women with history of thromboembolic disease	Less effective than combination OCs; frequent spotting, amenorrhea, ectopic pregnancy
Progestin injections	Every 3 months	0.2%	6%	Do not have to take daily pills; long-term protection	Amenorrhea, irregular bleeding, headache, loss of bone density, may delay return of fertility when discontinued
Transdermal patches	Weekly patch	0.3%	9%	Do not have to take daily pills; easy to apply	Similar to OCs; higher risk of thromboembolic disease compared to OCs, irritation at application site
Subdermal progestin implants	Every 3 years	0.05%	1%	Do not have to take daily pills; long-term protection	Amenorrhea, irregular bleeding, headache
Barrier and Miscellaneous Methods					
Condoms (male), diaphragms	Coitus based	2–6%	12–18%	Inexpensive; some protection against sexually transmitted infections, no hormonal adverse effects; few significant adverse effects	Less convenient than hormonal methods
Spermicides	Coitus based	18%	28%	Inexpensive, no hormonal adverse effects	Ineffective if used without barrier protection; inconvenient; vaginal irritation
Intrauterine devices/systems	Mirena, Skyla, Copper T380A; every few years	0.2–0.6%	0.2–0.8%	Effective, long-term contraception; decreased menstrual flow and cramping; inexpensive; no hormonal adverse effects (Copper T380A), quick return of fertility	Irregular bleeding, pelvic pain, spontaneous expulsion, uterine perforation
Withdrawal method	Coitus based	4%	22%	Free; no adverse effects	Requires cooperation of partner, inconvenient and ineffective
Biologic	Calendar/rhythm	3–5%	24%	Free; no adverse effects	Requires cooperation of partner, inconvenient and ineffective

*Pregnancy rates from using the various methods listed vary considerably in the scientific literature.

Women make personal birth control decisions based on several factors. Their ability to prevent pregnancy and the safety of the medication or device are the highest priorities. Other factors, however, may be of personal concern. Women who engage in intercourse frequently or who are likely to forget to take their medication may prefer the convenience of the LARCs. For patients who have a history of thromboembolic disorders, barrier protection or the use of progestin-only types of contraceptives are safer options.

Women seeking to prevent conception should discuss the available options with their healthcare provider. Final decisions on choosing a contraceptive should be made with knowledge of its advantages and disadvantages, effectiveness, adverse effects, contraindications, and potential long-term risks. When the desire to have children in the future no longer exists, sterilization of either the male or female partner is the most common and effective option for birth control. Whatever the choice of birth control, personal motivation must be taken into consideration because it is important that the woman be consistent in using the chosen method if pregnancy is to be prevented.

Contraceptives act in different regions of the female reproductive tract. The student should refer to Pharmacotherapy Illustrated 70.1 often while reading this chapter to obtain an overall perspective on the sites and mechanisms of contraceptive action.

Combination Oral Contraceptives

70.2 The most effective oral contraceptives include combinations of low-dose estrogens and progestins.

The physiology and pharmacologic indications for the female sex hormones estrogen and progesterone are presented in Chapter 69. Because estrogen and progesterone are the two

Pharmacotherapy Illustrated 70.1

Mechanisms of Action of Contraceptives

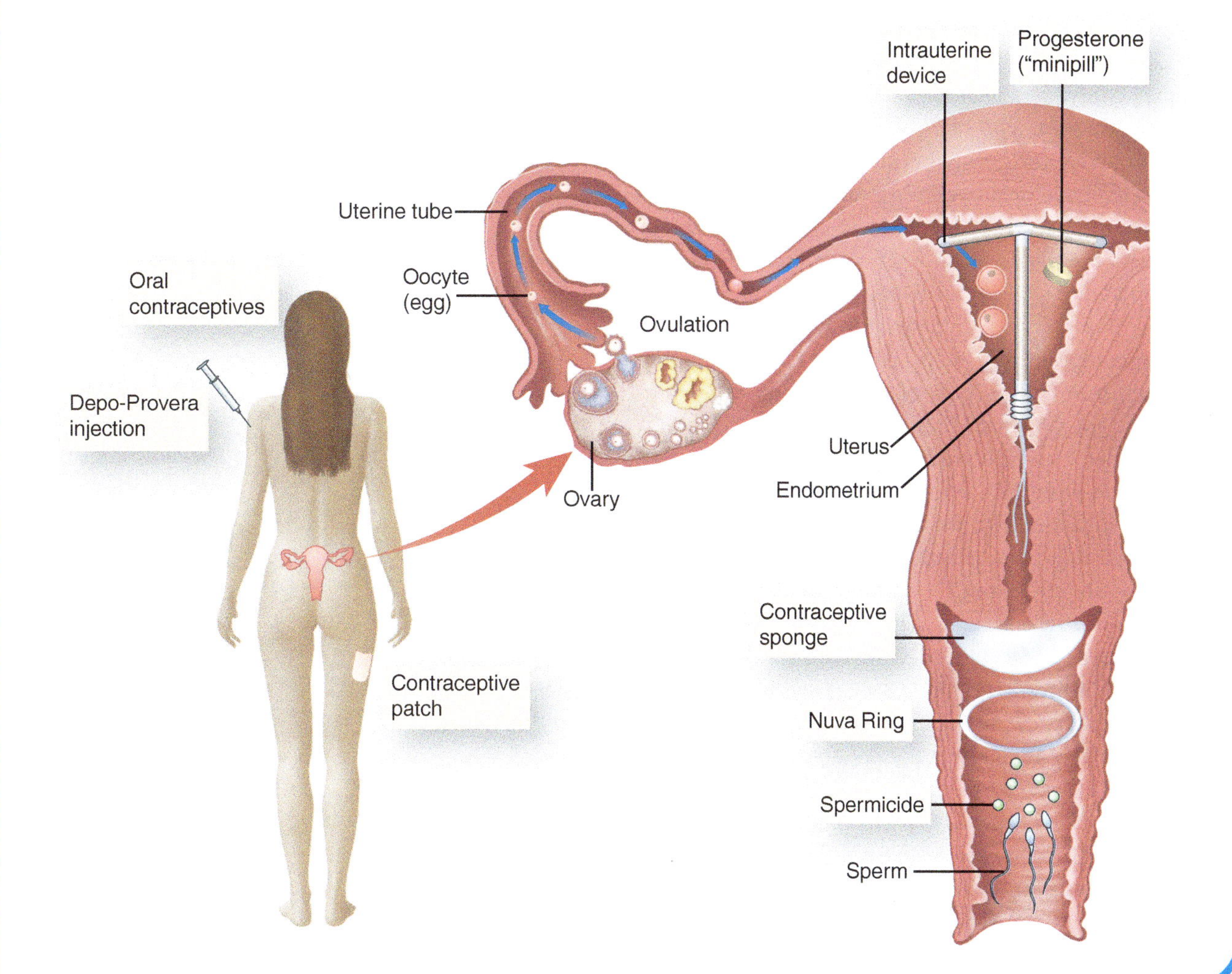

classes of drugs used most frequently for contraception, the student should review that chapter before proceeding.

The most widespread pharmacologic use of estrogen and progesterone combinations is to prevent pregnancy. *Estrogen* is a general term that refers to several female sex hormones. The ones used most frequently in oral contraceptives are the synthetic estrogens ethinyl estradiol and ethinyl valerate. In 2021 the FDA approved estetrol, the first new estrogen introduced in the United States in over 50 years. A naturally-occurring estrogen, estetrol is claimed to have more selective actions on reproductive tissues.

Progestin is a general term that refers to synthetic hormones that have actions identical to progesterone. Although **progesterone** is the natural progestin secreted by the corpus luteum, it is rarely used for contraception. Instead, synthetic progestins are used because they have a long half-life that allows for the convenience of once-daily dosing. All progestins have the same pharmacologic activity. Progestins used in contraceptives include desogestrel, dienogest, drospirenone, ethynodiol diacetate, etonogestrel, levonorgestrel, norethindrone, norgestimate and segesterone.

The first oral contraceptive (OC) was approved by the U.S. Food and Drug Administration (FDA) in 1960, and it was quickly recognized as a landmark discovery in reproductive medicine. Medications containing estrogen or progestin for the purpose of preventing pregnancy are sometimes called *hormonal contraceptives*. Approximately 30% of the women who choose contraceptive methods select OCs. These inexpensive, readily available drugs are up to 99% effective at preventing pregnancy when taken daily. They are excellent methods of contraception for women who are healthy and have no contraindications. One advantage of OCs is that they can be discontinued at any time without long-lasting adverse effects.

Many combination OC preparations are available, differing in dose and by type of estrogen and progestin. Selection of a specific drug is individualized for each patient and determined by which product gives the best contraceptive protection with the fewest adverse effects. Treatment is generally initiated with the lowest dose that effectively provides contraceptive protection. Daily doses of estrogen in OCs have declined from 150 mcg 50 years ago to about 20 mcg in newer formulations. This reduction has resulted in a significant decrease in estrogen-related adverse effects.

Typically, administration of an OC begins on day 5 of the menstrual cycle and continues for 21 days. During the other 7 days of the month, the patient takes a placebo. Although the placebo serves no pharmacologic purpose, it does encourage the patient to take the pills on a daily basis. Some of these placebos contain iron, which replaces iron lost due to menstrual bleeding.

The most frequent reason for treatment failure (pregnancy) is forgetting to take the medication daily. If one dose is missed, taking two pills the following day usually provides continuous contraception. If two consecutive doses are missed, two tablets should be taken on both the day the missed doses are remembered and the following day. The regular schedule should then be continued, but a second method of contraception should be used for at least 7 days after restarting the pills. If 3 or more consecutive days are missed, the patient should implement other means to prevent pregnancy until the regimen can be restarted in the next monthly cycle. Figure 70.1 shows a typical monthly OC packet with the 28 pills.

Estrogen–progestin combination OCs act by preventing ovulation. They accomplish this by providing negative feedback to the pituitary, which suppresses the secretion of luteinizing hormone (LH) and follicle-stimulating hormone (FSH) near the midpoint of the menstrual cycle. Without the influence of LH and FSH, the ovarian follicles cannot mature and ovulation is prevented. The estrogen–progestin combination drugs also make the uterine endometrium less favorable to receiving an embryo, thus reducing the likelihood of implantation. In addition, the hormones promote the formation of a thick cervical mucus that slows sperm transport and inhibits the process that allows sperm to penetrate the ovum. The student should refer to Figure 69.2 in Chapter 69 for a review of the negative feedback control of female reproductive hormones.

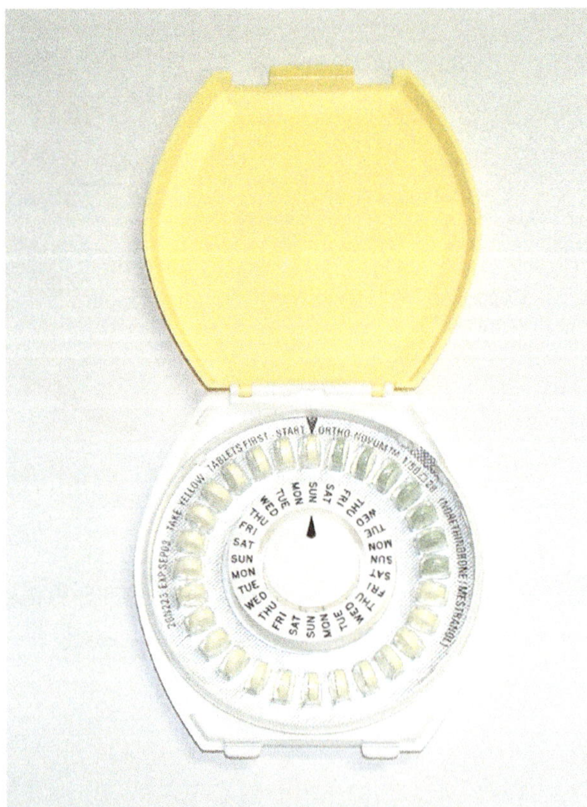

Figure 70.1 An oral contraceptive showing the daily doses and the different formulation taken in the last 7 days of the 28-day cycle. Pearson Education, Inc.

PharmFACT

In 2015 to 2017, 53% of sexually active female teens (age 15 to 19) used oral contraceptives to prevent pregnancy. Emergency contraception in this group was used by 19% (Martinez & Abma, 2020).

The four types of estrogen–progestin OC formulations are monophasic, biphasic, triphasic, and quadriphasic. The monophasic OC delivers a constant dose of estrogen and progestin throughout a 21-24 day treatment cycle. In biphasic drugs, the amount of estrogen in each pill remains constant, but the amount of progestin is increased toward the end of the treatment cycle to better nourish the uterine lining. In triphasic formulations, the amounts of both estrogen and progestin vary in three distinct phases during the treatment cycle. Natazia is a quadraphasic OC containing estradiol valerate and dienogest that provides four different doses over the 28-day cycle. Natazia was the first OC also approved by the FDA to treat heavy menstrual bleeding.

Extended-cycle OCs consist of tablets containing estrogen and progestin ("active pills") that are taken for 84 consecutive days, followed by seven "inactive pills" that contain either a placebo or very low-dose estrogen. This allows for continuous contraceptive protection while extending the time between menses; only four periods are experienced per year. Trade names for extended-cycle OCs include Seasonique, LoSeasonique, Seasonale, and Quartette.

When discontinuing OCs, it may take several months for ovulation to return to normal and for monthly menstrual periods to become regular. Some women can conceive in the first month, whereas others experience a delay for up to a year before fertility is restored. The length of contraceptive use does not appear to affect fertility. The incidence of miscarriage is not increased in women who conceive after having taken OCs.

CONNECTION Checkpoint 70.1

Certain drugs that are used to treat infertility block the negative feedback cycle by occupying the estrogen receptors in the hypothalamus. From what you learned in Chapter 69, name the class of drugs that can do this and explain how they are used to increase fertility.

Although the main purpose for taking combination OCs is to prevent pregnancy, there are several noncontraceptive indications, most of which are off-label. These include acne, dysmenorrhea, amenorrhea, menorrhagia, hirsutism, polycystic ovarian syndrome, and endometriosis.

PROTOTYPE DRUG Estradiol and Norethindrone

Classification **Therapeutic:** Combination oral contraceptive
Pharmacologic: Estrogen–progestin

Therapeutic Effects and Uses: The primary indication for this combination is to prevent pregnancy, for which it is up to 99% effective. It is available in monophasic, biphasic, and triphasic formulations. Off-label indications for the drug include acne vulgaris (in females who have achieved menarche), endometriosis, hypermenorrhea, dysfunctional uterine bleeding, and hirsutism related to hyposecretion of estrogen or oversecretion of androgens. Noncontraceptive benefits include improvement in menstrual cycle regularity and decreased incidence of dysmenorrhea.

Mechanism of Action: Combination OCs decrease the potential for conception by inhibiting ovulation. When the right combination of estrogens and progestins is present in the bloodstream, the release of FSH and LH is inhibited, thus preventing ovulation.

Pharmacokinetics:

Route(s)	Oral (PO)
Absorption	83% (norethindrone) and 47–73% (ethinyl estradiol)
Distribution	Widely distributed; secreted in breast milk
Primary metabolism	Hepatic and gastrointestinal mucosa; extensively metabolized
Primary excretion	Renal and feces
Onset of action	30–60 min
Duration of action	Half-life: 3–27 h

Adverse Effects: The adverse effects of OCs are presented in detail in Section 70.3. **Black Box Warning:** Cigarette smoking increases the risk of serious cardiovascular adverse effects in women taking hormonal contraceptives containing estrogen. This risk increases markedly with age (over age 35) and with heavy smoking (more than 15 cigarettes per day).

Contraindications/Precautions: There are many contraindications and precautions regarding the use of OCs. The risk of cancer following long-term OC use has been studied extensively. Because some studies have shown a small increase in the incidence of breast cancer, OCs are contraindicated in patients with known or suspected breast cancer. The incidences of endometrial and ovarian cancers, however, are significantly reduced after long-term OC administration. It is likely that the relationship between the long-term use of these drugs and cancer will continue to be a controversial and frequently researched topic. Obesity is a risk factor for treatment failure and for increased possibilities of thromboembolic events. OCs may significantly worsen symptoms of lupus. Mood disorders, including depression, may be worsened in patients taking OCs. All combination OCs are pregnancy category X and are contraindicated in pregnancy.

Drug Interactions: A number of anticonvulsants (phenobarbital, phenytoin, and carbamazepine) and antibiotics (tetracyclines, rifampin, and ampicillin) can reduce the effectiveness of OCs, thus increasing a woman's risk of pregnancy. Women who are taking these drugs should be advised to use additional means of birth control or to have their OC dosages revised. Because OCs can reduce the effectiveness of warfarin, heparin, insulin, and certain oral antidiabetic drugs, dosage adjustment may be necessary. Protease inhibitors (indicated for human immunodeficiency virus [HIV] infection) are contraindicated because they may result in contraceptive failure. Patients who are taking theophylline for asthma or imipramine as an antidepressant in conjunction with OCs should be evaluated often because these drugs may accumulate to toxic levels in these individuals. **Herbal/Food:** OCs have been shown to cause breakthrough bleeding when used concurrently with St. John's wort.

Pregnancy: Estrogens cause fetal harm and are contraindicated during pregnancy. However, human data show no significant evidence of fetal harm if OCs are taken inadvertently during early pregnancy. Once pregnancy is confirmed, the medication should be immediately discontinued. Because estrogen can decrease milk production and enter human milk, use during breastfeeding is not recommended.

Treatment of Overdose: There is no specific treatment for overdose. The patient is treated symptomatically.

Clinician Responsibilities: Key clinical implications for patients receiving conjugated estrogens are included in Applied Clinical Judgment: Patients Receiving Hormonal Contraceptives.

Drugs Similar to Estradiol and Norethindrone

Dozens of different estrogen–progestin combinations are available as OCs. All have the same indications and adverse effects. Those with higher doses may be expected to produce more adverse effects.

Adverse Effects of Combination Oral Contraceptives

70.3 The adverse effects of combined oral contraceptives are uncommon but may be serious in some women.

The adverse effects of combination OCs have been extensively studied, and various risk factors have been identified. These are summarized in Table 70.2. For the large majority of patients, OCs are safe and serious adverse effects are uncommon. A few of the adverse effects, however, may be serious. Because OCs are so widely prescribed, nurses should become familiar with the adverse effects and incorporate them into the teaching component of the treatment plan.

Much of the early research on OCs was performed on women who were taking high doses of estrogens and progestins. Most, and perhaps all, of the serious adverse effects

Table 70.2 Adverse Effects Associated with Combination Oral Contraceptives

Adverse Effect	Prevention
Breast milk reduction	OCs may reduce the quantity of breast milk and should not be taken until 6 weeks postpartum.
Cancer	Women who test positive for human papillomavirus (HPV) have an increased risk of cervical cancer. Because estrogens promote the growth of certain types of breast cancer, patients with a history of this cancer should not take OCs.
Glucose elevation	OCs may cause small increases in blood glucose. Patients with diabetes should monitor their serum glucose carefully during OC therapy.
Hypertension	Hypertensive risk increases with age, dose, and length of therapy. Blood pressure should be monitored periodically and antihypertensives prescribed as needed.
Increased appetite, weight gain, fatigue, depression, acne, hirsutism	These are common effects that are often caused by high amounts of progestin. The dose of progestin may need to be lowered.
Lupus exacerbation	Symptoms of systemic lupus erythematosus (SLE) may worsen in some patients. These patients are at increased risk for thromboembolism. A progestin-only OC may be an option for these patients.
Menstrual irregularities	Amenorrhea or hypermenorrhea is often caused by low amounts of progestin. The dose of progestin may need to be increased. Breakthrough bleeding and spotting are common with the low-dose OCs. The patient may need a higher dose.
Migraines	Estrogen may decrease or increase the incidence of migraines. Because migraines are a risk factor for stroke, patients with migraines should seek advice from their healthcare provider.
Nausea, edema, breast tenderness	These are common effects that are often caused by high amounts of estrogen. The dose of estrogen may need to be lowered.
Teratogenicity	Patients should be advised to discontinue OCs immediately if pregnancy is suspected or confirmed.
Thromboembolic disorders	Estrogens promote blood clotting. OCs should not be prescribed for patients with a history of thromboembolic disorders, stroke, or coronary artery disease or for those who are heavy smokers.

of OCs are dose dependent. The current low-dose formulations result in far less risk than the original OCs.

The Centers for Disease Control and Prevention and the World Health Organization have developed a comprehensive list of preexisting medical conditions as absolute contraindications for the use of estrogen–progestin contraceptives (Curtis et al., 2016). These include current breast cancer, severe hepatic disease, major surgery with prolonged immobilization, migraines (with aura), impaired cardiac function, complicated valvular heart disease, hypertension (HTN; systolic ≥ 160 mmHg or diastolic ≥ 100 mmHg), smoking (age ≥ 35, ≥15 cigarettes/day), history of stroke, SLE (positive or unknown antiphospholipid antibodies), and high risk for thromboembolic disorders. Relative contraindications exist when there are preexisting disorders such as depression, migraines (without aura), epilepsy, epilepsy therapy (with certain anticonvulsants), and controlled HTN. The nurse should discuss nonhormonal contraceptive choices for women who have serious medical conditions for which OCs are contraindicated.

CONNECTION Checkpoint 70.2

Thromboembolic events are a serious concern for many patients who are taking OCs. From what you learned in Chapter 38, identify the classes of drugs that may be used to reduce the risk of thromboembolic events in high-risk patients.

About 5% of women who are taking OCs will develop HTN because the drugs elevate angiotensin and aldosterone levels. Angiotensin is a vasopressor substance produced by the kidney, and aldosterone is a hormone secreted by the adrenal cortex of the kidney (see Chapter 31). The action of both substances can result in HTN. The mean elevation from high doses of OCs is about 3 to 6 mmHg systolic and 2 to 5 mmHg diastolic. Low-dose formulations do not pose a major risk for HTN.

OCs can mimic certain symptoms of pregnancy, including breast tenderness, nausea, bloating, and **chloasma**, which is a darkened pigmentation found on the forehead, temples, cheeks, and upper lips. If a woman suspects pregnancy while taking an OC, the drug should be discontinued immediately because estrogen and progestin can cause fetal harm.

Because estrogen and progesterone can stimulate the growth of some types of cancers, the incidence of cancer in women taking OCs has been studied for several decades in large numbers of women. Some studies have demonstrated that long-term use may pose a slightly higher risk of breast cancer, whereas others have shown no relationship. Cervical cancer is also slightly increased, and this has been closely associated with HPV infections. The risk of liver cancer may be increased. However, OCs appear to have protective effects for ovarian and endometrial cancers that continue for many years after the drugs are discontinued. A protective effect has also been observed for colorectal cancer. Conclusions of these studies are that women who have a personal or very close family history of breast cancer should explore nonhormonal means of contraception. All women taking OCs should be aware of the importance of routine scheduling of mammograms as appropriate for their age range and as recommended by their healthcare provider.

Other conditions associated with OCs are abnormal uterine bleeding, benign hepatic adenoma, multiple births, retinal disorders, and melanoderma. These conditions, though rare, have been reported and they normally resolve after discontinuing the use of OCs. OCs may accelerate the formation of gallstones in patients who have preexisting gallbladder disease. The drugs may increase glucose levels and suppress insulin responsiveness, although this can be prevented by adjustments in the insulin dose of patients with diabetes.

Although not an adverse effect, healthcare providers and their patients should be aware that some studies have indicated that the combined hormonal patch and oral levonorgestrel emergency contraception may have lower rates of effectiveness in women who are obese (Simmons & Edelman, 2016). The correlation between effectiveness and weight (or body mass index [BMI]) is an ongoing area of research.

When discussing the risks and benefits of hormonal contraception with patients, the nurse should place the drug in context with the health risks associated with pregnancy and delivery. Many patients do not understand that pregnancy itself may cause many challenging health conditions for the mother. Pregnancy-related mortality in the United States averages 16 deaths per 100,000 live births, with non-Hispanic black women having the highest incidence of death (Creanga et al., 2015). Maternal morbidity includes conditions such as hemorrhages, preeclampsia or eclampsia, obstetric trauma, infections, gestational diabetes, and HTN. Placed in the proper context, the risks of pregnancy for most patients (those without absolute contraindications for OC use) are likely as great, or greater, than hormonal contraception.

Progestin-Only Oral Contraceptives

70.4 Oral contraceptives that contain only progestin are often used when estrogen is contraindicated.

Although most OCs use a combination of estrogen and progestin, a few products contain only progestin. The progestin-only OCs, sometimes called minipills, are less effective at preventing ovulation. They prevent pregnancy primarily by causing a thick, viscous cervical mucus at the entrance to the uterus that discourages sperm penetration. They also tend to inhibit implantation of a fertilized egg.

Progestin-only oral contraceptives are taken daily throughout the month without the use of placebo tablets. Minipills are somewhat less effective than estrogen–progestin combinations, having a failure rate of 1 to 4%.

Their use also results in a higher incidence of irregular menstrual cycles, including amenorrhea, prolonged bleeding, or breakthrough spotting. Menstrual irregularity is the most frequently reported adverse effect. The risk of ectopic pregnancy is higher with progestin-only products. Progestin-only PO drugs are generally reserved for patients who are at high risk for estrogen-related adverse effects or who are lactating. Unlike estrogens, progestins are not associated with a higher risk of thromboembolic events, and they do not have any effect on breast cancer. The progestin-only products should not be taken during pregnancy.

Products that contain norethindrone only include Camila, Errin, Nor-QD, and Incassia. In addition to contraception, norethindrone therapy is approved to treat amenorrhea, dysfunctional uterine bleeding, and endometriosis. The doses used for contraception are only 0.35 mg/day, whereas those for uterine conditions are 2.5 to 10 mg/day. Detailed information on the contraindications, drug interactions, and adverse effects of progestins are included in Chapter 69, along with a prototype feature for medroxyprogesterone (Depo-Provera, Depot-SubQ-Provera, Provera).

Long-Acting Reversible Contraceptives

70.5 Long-acting contraceptives and novel delivery methods offer women additional birth control choices.

Delivery methods have been developed that are able to provide long-acting reversible contraception for periods lasting from weeks to years. The **long-acting reversible contraceptives (LARCs)** and novel delivery systems were developed to offer ease of use and improve adherence. They vary in efficacy, reversibility, and discreteness of use.

Transdermal patch: Transdermal hormonal contraception is a safe, effective, and easy-to-use birth control method. Twirla is a topical patch worn on the skin of the buttock, arm, or trunk that contains ethinyl estradiol and levonorgestrel. The patch slowly releases the hormones, which penetrate the skin and are distributed throughout the body. The patch is changed every 7 days for the first 3 weeks, followed by a patch-free week 4 (days 22 to 28). The patch may be worn during bathing, exercise, and other daily activities. Should the patch fall off it should be replaced as soon as possible. Used patches still contain significant hormone levels and must be discarded in a waste container away from children and pets. They should not be flushed down the toilet because residual estrogen can pollute wastewater, lakes, and streams. Xulane is another transdermal patch that offers a higher dose of medication than Twirla.

Adverse effects and contraindications are the same as those for OCs. Twirla contains a black box warning that women over age 35 who smoke cigarettes are at higher risk for serious cardiovascular events. The warning also states that the drug is contraindicated in women with a BMI equal to or greater than 30 because it has reduced effectiveness and a higher risk for thromboembolic events.

Vaginal ring: The NuvaRing, illustrated in Figure 70.2, is a flexible, soft vaginal ring impregnated with a low-dose, sustained-release, combined hormonal contraceptive. It is approximately 5 to 7.5 cm (2–3 in.) in diameter and contains ethinyl estradiol and etonogestrel. The ring is inserted

CONNECTIONS: Advanced Practice Application

Contraceptive Choices

Case

Lauren, a 33-year-old mother of four, is married and is looking for a reliable method of birth control. When asked about her plans for more children, she states that she is not interested in having another child right now but may want another child in the future. She insists on a contraceptive method other than condoms because her husband doesn't like using them. Lauren was taking "the pill" for a while, but had a difficult time remembering to take it every day and she would miss several days at a time. You conduct some basic screening and obtain the following information: blood pressure, 126/82 mmHg; pulse, 62 beats/min; and respiratory rate, 16 breaths/min; she does not smoke or drink and denies drug use. Her BMI is 22 (normal weight). You determine Lauren is a candidate for a transdermal patch and after discussion about potential risks and adverse effects, she is started on Twirla and is taught how to use it. Is this an appropriate birth control option for Lauren?

Discussion

Deciding on the right method of birth control is very personal and is a common reason women seek gynecologic care. Using the birth control patch is safe, simple, and convenient. Lauren's ability to become pregnant will return quickly when use of the patch is stopped, and because the patch works like the pill, it increases adherence for women who are concerned about forgetting to take a pill every day.

Lauren's BMI was within normal range. However, if it were above the normal range or she weighed over 90 kg (198 lb), the transdermal patch would not be a good option. Research shows that the transdermal patch has reduced effectiveness and a higher risk for thromboembolic events for women who are obese. Healthcare providers should offer patients an additional prescription for the contraceptive patch in case of detachment. The drug is mixed with the adhesive and, therefore, patches that do not stick must be replaced to maintain therapeutic levels of hormone.

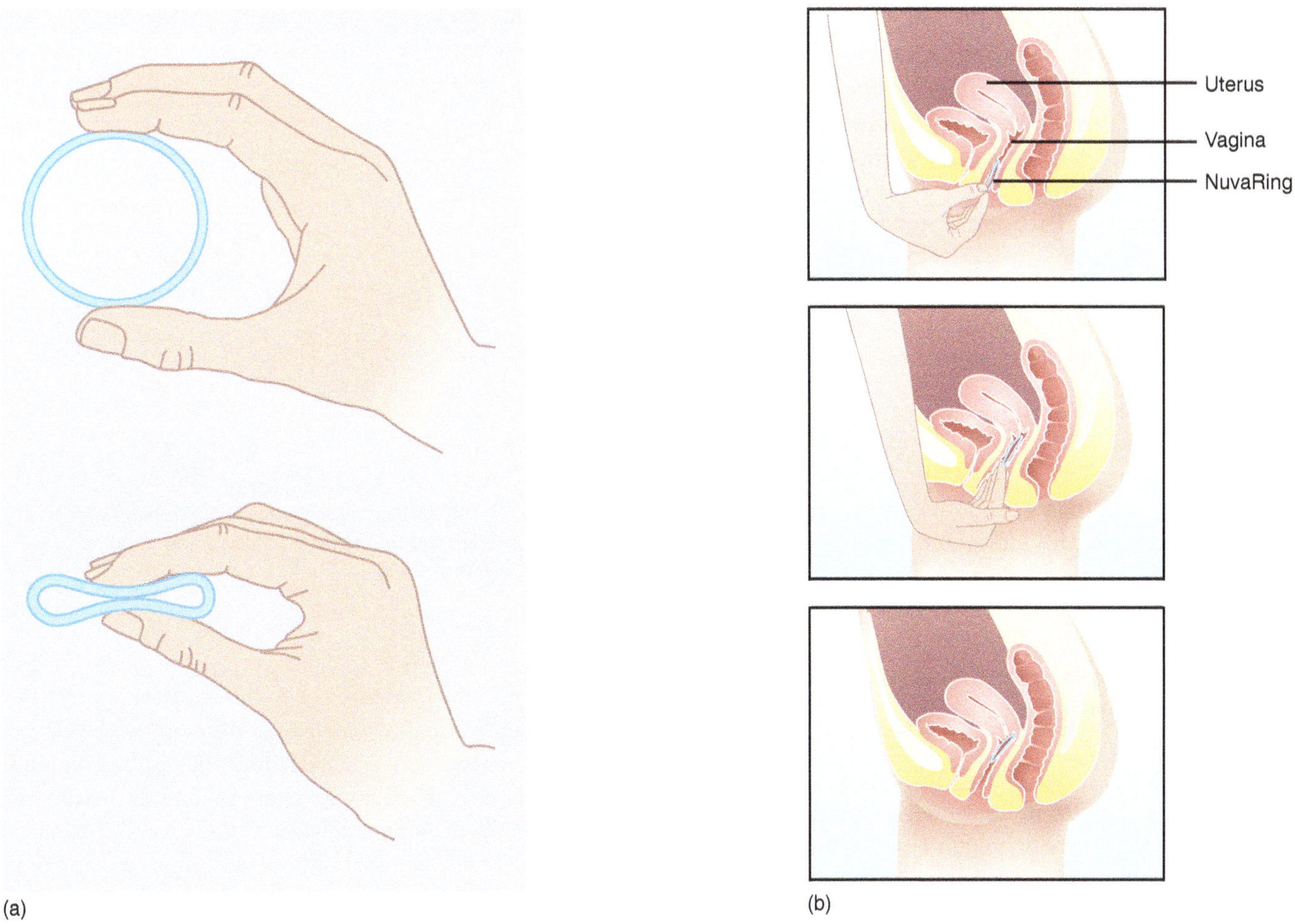

Figure 70.2 Vaginal medication administration: (a) The NuvaRing® contraceptive; (b) proper insertion of the NuvaRing.

into the vagina once a month to provide 3 weeks of contraceptive protection. The ring slowly releases the hormones, which are absorbed across the vaginal mucosa into the blood and distributed throughout the body. The contraceptive action is systemic in nature and not localized to the vagina. The ring is removed at the end of week 3, and a new ring is inserted a week later. If forgotten and left in place for more than 3 weeks, contraceptive action may be lost. In 2018 the FDA approved Annovera, a reusable ring that contains ethinyl estradiol and segesterone. The ring can be reused for 13 cycles (1 year).

The main adverse effects of the vaginal rings are similar to those of combination OCs. Women may discontinue using the vaginal delivery method due to discomfort of the device during intercourse. Women who are experiencing uterine prolapse must monitor the ring frequently because it may fall out. Adverse effects include nausea, vulvovaginal infections, bloating, headaches, breast tenderness, and breakthrough bleeding. If the ring is expelled from the vagina, it may be rinsed with water and replaced. Local effects may include vaginal irritation, sensation of a foreign body, and vaginitis. The NuvaRing should be discarded in a waste container away from children and not flushed down the toilet.

Depot injection methods: Intramuscular (IM) medroxyprogesterone acetate (Depo-Provera) was approved for contraceptive use in the United States in 2004. A single deep IM injection provides 3 months of contraceptive protection. The same drug may be injected subcutaneously (Depo-SubQ-Provera) with the same duration of action and effectiveness. Medroxyprogesterone suppresses ovulation, inhibits sperm from reaching the egg by thickening the cervical mucus, and prevents a fertilized egg from implanting in the uterus. Neither depot delivery method contains estrogen. The drug is usually given on days 1 through 5 of the menstrual cycle. The depot injection methods are very effective at preventing pregnancy.

Once injected the actions of the drug cannot be reversed and fertility may be delayed for up to 12 months after discontinuation. The most common adverse effects are menstrual disturbances, headache, acne, injection-site reactions, weight gain, and decreased libido. This drug carries a black box warning that long-term use causes significant loss of bone mineral density. Medroxyprogesterone is also approved to treat inoperable endometrial and renal cell carcinomas and menstrual disturbances. A prototype feature for medroxyprogesterone is found in Chapter 69.

Subdermal implant: Although several contraceptive subdermal implants have been approved since 1996, only Nexplanon is available. Formerly called Implanon, the implant consists of a single plastic tube about the size of a matchstick, containing 68 mg of the progestin etonogestrel. Inserted on the inner side of the upper arm, the device is highly effective at preventing pregnancy, releasing the progestin slowly, for up to 3 years. Although the device can be readily removed, some women may experience pain, inflammation, or hematoma at the removal site. Other adverse effects are the same as those of other progestins.

Intrauterine devices: Intrauterine devices (IUDs) are LARCs designed in a T shape that are safe, inexpensive, and reliable methods of contraception. They are placed by the healthcare provider and offer a major advantage for women who are likely to forget a daily pill or who prefer greater ease of use. Unlike OCs, these devices have no effect on ovulation. The IUD is not felt by the woman or her partner during intercourse and it can be removed at any time. Fertility returns quickly after removal of the device.

Liletta, Mirena, Kyleena, and Skyla are called hormonal IUDs because they contain levonorgestrel that is released very slowly to prevent conception for 3 to 6 years, depending on the product. Contraception results from a thickening of the endometrium and increased cervical mucus that slows down sperm motility. The most common adverse effects include uterine and vaginal bleeding, dysmenorrhea, intermenstrual bleeding and spotting, abdominal and pelvic pain, and ovarian cysts.

The oldest product, ParaGard, is a plastic device that is partially covered with copper. It is believed that the copper triggers a spermicidal-like reaction in the body that slows sperm motility and prevents the sperm from reaching the ovum. If fertilization does occur, implantation is not likely to happen because the copper causes endometrial changes to make the lining less favorable. It can be left in place for up to 10 years, and the main adverse effects are bleeding between menses, dysmenorrhea, and expulsion of the device. ParaGard is an effective, nonhormonal option for patients who have contraindications to using estrogen or progesterone.

Spermicides

70.6 Spermicides are safe but should be combined with barrier protection for maximum effectiveness.

Spermicides come in a variety of creams, foams, jellies, and suppositories that immobilize or destroy sperm when inserted into the vagina prior to intercourse. Spermicides are inexpensive and available over the counter (OTC).

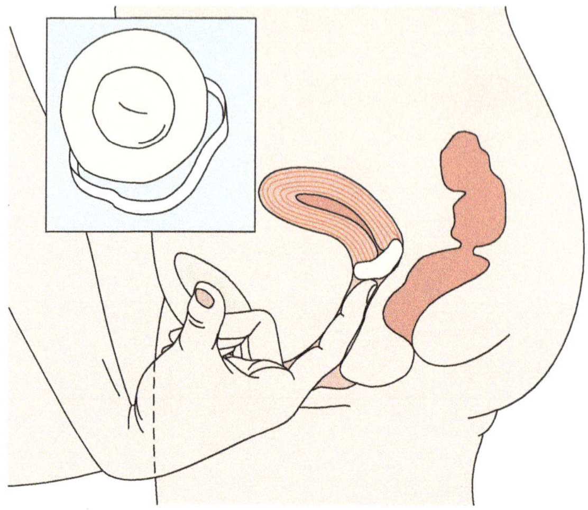

Figure 70.3 The contraceptive sponge is moistened well with water and inserted into the vagina with the concave portion positioned over the cervix.

To be effective, spermicides must be applied high into the vagina, as close to the cervix as possible, approximately 10 to 15 minutes before intercourse. Most spermicides have a duration of action of only 1 hour and must be reapplied if coitus extends beyond this time.

The contraceptive sponge, which is illustrated in Figure 70.3, is soft and absorbent and contains nonoxynol-9. The sponge is moistened with water to activate the spermicides and inserted into the vagina to cover the cervix. The sponge releases the drug slowly and may provide up to 24 hours of contraceptive protection. It is left in place for 6 hours after intercourse but must be removed by 30 hours after insertion. The sponge delivery system has the same effectiveness as spermicidal gels, creams, and suppositories. Adverse effects include local irritation and vaginal dryness.

Patients should be informed that spermicides have low levels of effectiveness when used alone and should therefore be used in conjunction with barrier methods such as condoms and diaphragms. Nonoxynol-9 does not offer any protection against chlamydia, gonorrhea, or HIV.

Adverse effects to spermicides are uncommon. Vaginal irritation and dryness, increase in vaginal infections, toxic shock syndrome, and irritation of the genitalia of the sexual partner have been reported. Women with cystocele, prolapsed uterus, sensitivity or allergy to nonoxynol-9, vaginitis, or toxic shock syndrome, or those who are pregnant, postabortion, or postpregnancy should avoid this drug.

CONNECTIONS: APPLIED CLINICAL JUDGMENT

Patients Receiving Hormonal Contraceptives

Key Assessment Data
- History of current condition including cardiovascular, peripheral vascular, thyroid, hepatic, or kidney disease, migraine headaches, diabetes; baseline vital signs, physical exam findings; pregnancy or breastfeeding. Note personal or family history of thromboembolic disorders (e.g., MI, stroke, peripheral vascular disease) and of reproductive cancers (e.g., breast, uterine, or ovarian cancer); CBC, platelets, electrolytes, glucose, lipid, and thyroid function levels, Pap test, HPV screening, and pregnancy test drug; medication history, including allergies, current prescription and OTC drugs, herbal preparations, caffeine, nicotine, and alcohol use.

Desired Therapeutic Outcomes
Improvement is observed and measurable by pregnancy prevention.

Minimizing Adverse Effects
- Thromboembolic events may occur with OCs. The risk increases with age over 35, in women with a previous history of cardiovascular disease, and in women who smoke. Monitor for symptoms of peripheral thrombophlebitis, pulmonary embolism, MI, stroke, or other complications related to blood clots.
- Smoking greatly increases the risk of adverse effects of hormone therapy. Referral to smoking cessation programs should be recommended.
- Pap tests and breast examinations, including mammography as appropriate, are recommended to monitor for the development of breast tumors or of cervical cancer.
- Small amounts of spotting may occur, especially with low-dose hormone therapy, at midcycle. Any continuous, unusual, or heavy bleeding may indicate adverse effects, pregnancy loss, or disease and should be assessed.
- OCs are associated with increased risk of gallbladder disease and a rare risk of hepatotoxicity.
- Transdermal patches, depot injections, or IUDs may be desirable for women who experience difficulty adhering to OCs or for those who prefer not to take daily medication.
- Many drugs decrease or alter the effectiveness of OCs including drugs in the penicillin, tetracycline, barbiturate, antiseizure, antidepressant, and benzodiazepine classifications.

Patient Education
- Immediately report dyspnea, chest pain, or blood in sputum (possible pulmonary embolism); heaviness, chest pain, or overwhelming feeling of fatigue and weakness accompanied by nausea and diaphoresis (possible MI); sudden, severe headache, especially if associated with a preheadache aura, dizziness, difficulty with speech, numbness in arm or leg, and difficulty with vision (possible stroke).
- Keep routine gynecologic and breast examinations to ensure continued health.
- Slight spotting may occur midcycle but report any unusual changes in the amount or if the bleeding continues.
- Immediately report any symptoms of abdominal or right upper quadrant discomfort or pain, yellowing of the skin or sclera, fatigue, anorexia, darkened urine, or clay-colored stools.
- Advise all healthcare providers of the use of OCs before beginning any new prescription so that potential drug interactions may be assessed.
- Referrals to appropriate support groups and literature on smoking cessation programs should be offered.
- Take the drug following appropriate guidelines:
  - *For estrogen–progestin combination OCs:* If a dose is missed, take it as soon as it is remembered, and take the next pill at its normally scheduled time. If two consecutive doses are missed, take two tablets on both the day the missed doses are remembered and on the following day. Follow the remaining schedule of pills, but a second method of contraception (e.g., a barrier method) should be used for at least 7 days after restarting the pills. If 3 or more consecutive days are missed, use another form of contraception until the pills can be restarted in the next monthly cycle.
  - *For progestin-only OCs:* If a dose is missed, take the pill as soon as remembered, but use an additional form of contraception until the next cycle of pills is started.
  - *Transdermal patches and vaginal rings:* Patches and rings are changed weekly for 3 weeks, followed by 1 week of being patch- or ring-free. If the patch falls off or the ring falls out, it should be replaced with a new patch or ring. Safely discard used patches or rings in the trash.

Prescribing Considerations
- Requiring prerequisite preventive services, such as cervical cytology; breast examination; or evaluation for sexually transmitted infections, diabetes mellitus, dyslipidemia, liver disease, or thrombophilia, can introduce unnecessary barriers to contraceptive care and are not necessarily required prior to prescribing contraceptives.
- Prescription of hormonal contraceptives should preferentially cover one year's supply to decrease barriers to care.
- Estrogen-containing contraceptives should be deferred until at least 3 or up to 6 weeks postpartum because of the risk of venous thromboembolism.

Emergency Contraception

70.7 Emergency contraception provides a reproductive option for women who have unprotected sex or contraceptive failure.

Emergency contraception (EC) is the prevention of implantation following unprotected intercourse or contraceptive failure. Statistics suggest that almost half the pregnancies in the United States are unplanned and some of these occur due to the inconsistent use or failure of contraceptive devices. EC, commonly referred to as the "morning-after pill," offers a means of protecting against unwanted pregnancies.

The treatment goal for these patients is to provide effective and immediate contraception. EC must be taken as soon as possible after intercourse. When used accordingly, these drugs act by preventing ovulation; they do not cause abortion. If implantation of an embryo has already occurred, the drugs used for EC will have no effect on the established pregnancy. Two different medications are approved for EC: Plan B and ulipristal (Ella). Table 70.3 lists drugs, routes,

Table 70.3 Drugs for Emergency Contraception and Pharmacologic Abortion

Drug	Route and Adult Dose (Maximum Dose Where Indicated)	Adverse Effects
Drugs for Emergency Contraception		
levonorgestrel (Plan B, Plan B One Step)	PO (Plan B): 1 tablet within 72 h of intercourse followed by 1 tablet 12 h later (0.75 mg in each pill) PO (Plan B One Step): 1 tablet (1.5 mg) within 120 h of intercourse	*Nausea, heavy menstrual bleeding, lower abdominal pain, headache, fatigue, and dizziness* Serious adverse effects are rare when only on or two doses are administered
ulipristal (Ella, Logilia)	PO: 1 tablet (30 mg) within 5 days of unprotected intercourse or contraceptive failure	*Headache, abdominal pain, nausea, dysmenorrhea, fatigue, dizziness* Serious adverse effects are rare when only one dose is administered
Drugs for Pharmacologic Abortion		
carboprost (Hemabate)	IM (initial): 250 mcg (1 mL) repeated at 0.5- to 3.5-h intervals if indicated by uterine response.	*Nausea and vomiting, cramping, diarrhea, fever* Uterine laceration, rupture, or hemorrhage, abdominal pain
dinoprostone (Cervidil, Prepidil, Prostin E_2)	Intravaginal: Insert 20-mg suppository high in the vagina; repeat q2–5h until abortion occurs or membranes rupture (max: total dose 240 mg)	
methotrexate with misoprostol	IM methotrexate (50 mg/m^2) followed 5 days later by intravaginal 800 mcg of misoprostol	
mifepristone (Mifeprex) with misoprostol	PO: 200 mg of mifepristone on first day, followed 24–48 h later with 800 mcg of misoprostol	

Note: *Italics* indicate common adverse effects. Underline indicates serious adverse effects.

and dosages for EC. These drugs are not intended to replace regular methods of contraception.

Plan B is approved for OTC purchase without age restriction. Plan B has largely been replaced by Plan B One Step, which offers the convenience of a single 1.5-mg dose.

The active drug in Plan B is levonorgestrel, which is the same progestin used for contraception in some IUDs (see Section 70.5). There is, however, a large difference in doses. Whereas the long-acting Mirena releases 20 mcg/day of levonorgestrel over a 5-year period, Plan B delivers a total of 1500 mcg of levonorgestrel in a single day. The drug is most effective when taken either within 72 hours (Plan B) or 120 hours (Plan B One Step) after unprotected intercourse.

Plan B is not 100% effective. The normal rate of pregnancy from a single unprotected sex act is 8%; Plan B is estimated to lower this risk to 1 to 2%. Serious adverse effects with Plan B are uncommon. Nausea and vomiting are the most common adverse effects, and abdominal pain, fatigue, headache, irregular (increased or decreased) menstrual bleeding, and dizziness are reported by a number of patients. Fertility returns quickly after taking Plan B; therefore, the patient should be encouraged to implement routine contraception measures as soon as possible.

In 2010, ulipristal (Ella) was approved as a single-dose product for EC. This drug is a mixed progesterone agonist–antagonist that acts by preventing ovulation. Unlike Plan B, which is available OTC, ulipristal requires a prescription. One advantage of ulipristal is that it retains its effectiveness for 5 days following unprotected sex.

Drugs for Pharmacologic Abortion

70.8 Abortifacients are drugs that are used to terminate pregnancy.

A woman who is in early pregnancy may decide that she is no longer able to carry the child to term. In some pregnancies, major abnormalities may be identified in the fetus that would prevent it from reaching term. Nurses should use their knowledge of the stages of fetal growth and development to counsel patients regarding the risks and benefits of available options. Nurses must, however, be aware of applicable state laws and regulations that restrict certain treatments.

One option for the patient may be a medical abortion. Pharmacologic (medical) abortion is the removal of an embryo by the use of drugs after implantation has occurred. Drugs used to induce abortion are called **abortifacients**.

Once the ovum has been fertilized, several drugs are available to terminate the pregnancy, as listed in Table 70.3. A single dose of mifepristone (Mifeprex) followed 24 to 48 hours later by a single dose of misoprostol is a frequently used regimen. Although the mifepristone–misoprostol combination should never be used as a substitute for an effective means of contraception, these drugs do offer women a safer alternative than surgical abortion. The actions of the two drugs are as follows:

- Mifepristone acts by blocking progesterone receptors, resulting in softening and dilation of the cervix and degeneration of the uterine endometrium. If given within 3 days of intercourse, mifepristone alone is almost 100% effective at preventing pregnancy. Given up to 9 weeks after conception, mifepristone aborts the implanted embryo.

- Misoprostol is a prostaglandin that induces strong uterine contractions, thus increasing the effectiveness of the pharmacologic abortion.

Pharmacologic abortion must be conducted under the close supervision of a healthcare provider. The patient may be required to sign consent forms after it has been determined that the pregnancy is under 49 days. The patient receives an assessment by the healthcare provider 2 days after dosing. If abortion has not occurred, additional misoprostol may be administered and the patient should return to the healthcare provider in 14 days to confirm that abortion is complete. The primary adverse effect of mifepristone–misoprostol is cramping that occurs soon after taking it. Nausea is common, and the most serious adverse effect is prolonged bleeding, which may continue for 1 to 2 weeks after dosing.

Methotrexate, an antineoplastic drug, is sometimes combined with intravaginal misoprostol. Methotrexate 50 mg/m^2 is given IM, followed in 5 days by 800 mcg of intravaginal misoprostol. If abortion does not occur within 24 hours, the misoprostol is repeated. The treatment is 96% effective at causing abortion. Most patients experience adverse effects such as nausea and vomiting, diarrhea, headache, dizziness, abdominal cramping, and hot flashes.

Prostaglandins may also be used to induce abortion. Prostaglandins are natural hormones that produce a diverse number of local actions in virtually every body system. In the uterus, the normal function of prostaglandins is to cause contraction of smooth muscle. They serve a valuable function in inducing contractions at the beginning of labor and in promoting cervical ripening.

The three approved prostaglandins include dinoprostone (Cervidil, Prepidil, Prostin E_2), carboprost (Hemabate), and misoprostol. All three may be used to induce uterine contractions that can expel an implanted embryo and result in abortion up to the second trimester. Dinoprostone is used early in pregnancy and comes in preparations of vaginal suppositories (Prostin E), vaginal inserts (Cervidil), and gel, which are inserted high into the vaginal canal. Carboprost is administered by deep IM injection and misoprostol by tablet. When used for abortion, misoprostol is administered with either mifepristone or methotrexate. Nausea, vomiting and diarrhea are common adverse effects of prostaglandins and uterine cramping is expected. Drug-induced fever occurs in the majority of patients and may last up to 6 hours. Because rare instances of uterine laceration and rupture have been reported, the patient is monitored closely for uterine activity, excessive pain, and vaginal bleeding. Indications for the prostaglandins are given in Table 70.4.

PROTOTYPE DRUG Mifepristone (Mifeprex)

Classification **Therapeutic:** Drug for pharmacologic abortion
Pharmacologic: Abortifacient, progesterone antagonist

Therapeutic Effects and Uses: Approved in 2000, mifepristone is indicated for terminating pregnancies of less than 70 days. In the United States, distribution is restricted and tightly controlled through a Risk Evaluation and Mitigation Strategy. It is not available in commercial pharmacies and must be obtained from an approved, registered clinic or hospital. Over half the states only allow physicians to prescribe mifepristone, whereas some allow other prescribers such as nurse practitioners, physician assistants or nurse-midwives. Furthermore, several states require the physical presence of a physician during the medical abortion and forbid the use of telemedicine. In Canada, the drug is available through commercial pharmacies and has not such restrictions.

Pharmacotherapy with mifepristone requires one 200-mg tablet of mifepristone followed 24 to 48 hours later by 800 mcg of misoprostol taken by the buccal route. Patients must return to their healthcare provider between 7 and 14 days to assess whether pregnancy termination has occurred.

Table 70.4 Indications for Prostaglandins

Drug	INDICATIONS				
	Abortifacient	Control of Postpartum Bleeding	Cervical Ripening Induction	Labor Induction	Other
carboprost (Hemabate) prostaglandin F_2	A	A	O	O	Hemorrhagic cystitis (O); hydatidiform mole (O)
dinoprostone (Cervidil, Prepidil, Prostin E_2) prostaglandin E_2	A	—	A	—	Hydatidiform mole (A)
misoprostol prostaglandin E_1	O	O	O	O	Nonsteroidal anti-inflammatory drug-induced ulcer prophylaxis (A); kidney transplant rejection prophylaxis (O)

Note: A, FDA-approved indication; O, off-label indication.

Mifepristone may be used off-label as a means of EC. Given as a single 600-mg dose, it has the same effectiveness and safety profile as Plan B. Other off-label indications include breast cancer, endometriosis, uterine leiomyomata, Cushing's syndrome, and termination of ectopic pregnancy (in combination with methotrexate).

Mechanism of Action: Mifepristone is a strong antagonist of progesterone that drug blocks the supportive actions of progesterone on the uterine lining. If given within 72 hours of intercourse, a fertilized ovum will not be able to implant in the uterus. During early pregnancy, mifepristone acts by increasing the synthesis of prostaglandins and sensitizing the uterus to the effects of prostaglandins. When misoprostol (a prostaglandin) is given 24 to 48 hours after mifepristone, the prostaglandin increases uterine contractions, which aids in expelling the embryo from the uterus.

Pharmacokinetics:

Route(s)	PO
Absorption	Rapidly absorbed
Distribution	Crosses the placenta; it is unknown if secreted in breast milk; 98% bound to plasma protein
Primary metabolism	Hepatic (CYP3A4)
Primary excretion	Mostly feces, small amounts in urine
Onset of action	Rapid
Duration of action	Half-life: 18 h

Adverse Effects: Nearly all patients who take the mifepristone–misoprostol combination experience adverse effects. The most frequent adverse effects of mifepristone are headache, dizziness, nausea and vomiting, fatigue, and abdominal pain or cramping. Vaginal bleeding and spotting will occur for about 16 days. **Black Box Warning:** Serious and sometimes fatal infections and prolonged heavy bleeding have occurred. Excessive or prolonged bleeding may be a sign of incomplete abortion and prompt medical intervention is required. Rare cases of septic shock have been reported.

Contraindications/Precautions: Because mifepristone is also a corticosteroid antagonist, its use in patients who are taking long-term corticosteroid therapy or who have chronic adrenal failure is contraindicated. The mifepristone–misoprostol combination is contraindicated in patients with ectopic pregnancy because the therapy will be ineffective. Those on anticoagulant therapy or who otherwise have an increased risk for bleeding should not receive mifepristone. Patients with an IUD in place should have the device removed before mifepristone is administered. The drug is contraindicated for use in patients who are unable to understand the implications of abortion or who may not comply with the established regimen. Safety in patients under age 18 has not been established. When administered for nonabortion indications, this drug is contraindicated in pregnancy (category X).

Drug Interactions: Because mifepristone is taken in only one or two doses, serious drug interactions are unlikely. This drug does, however, have an extended half-life that may cause interactions after it is discontinued. Mifepristone is metabolized by hepatic CYP450 enzymes and may interact with drugs that induce or inhibit this enzyme system. For example, phenytoin, phenobarbital, and carbamazepine induce CYP3A4, increasing the metabolism of mifepristone and lowering its serum levels. **Herbal/Food:** St. John's wort and grapefruit juice may decrease serum levels of mifepristone.

Pregnancy: Mifepristone causes pregnancy loss. Nonhormonal contraception should be used for at least one month after stopping treatment because this drug lowers the effectiveness of hormonal contraceptives.

Treatment of Overdose: Overdose has rarely occurred with mifepristone. Treatment is supportive.

Drugs Similar to Mifepristone (Mifeprex)

There are no drugs that are similar to mifepristone.

Understanding Chapter 70

Key Concepts Summary

70.1 Selection of a contraceptive is based on effectiveness, safety, and personal choice.

70.2 The most effective oral contraceptives include combinations of low-dose estrogens and progestins.

70.3 The adverse effects of combination oral contraceptives are uncommon but may be serious in some women.

70.4 Oral contraceptives that contain only progestin are often used when estrogen is contraindicated.

70.5 Long-acting contraceptives and novel delivery methods offer women additional birth control choices.

70.6 Spermicides are safe but should be combined with barrier protection for maximum effectiveness.

70.7 Emergency contraception provides a reproductive option for women who have unprotected sex or contraceptive failure.

70.8 Abortifacients are drugs that are used to terminate pregnancy.

CASE STUDY: Making the Patient Connection

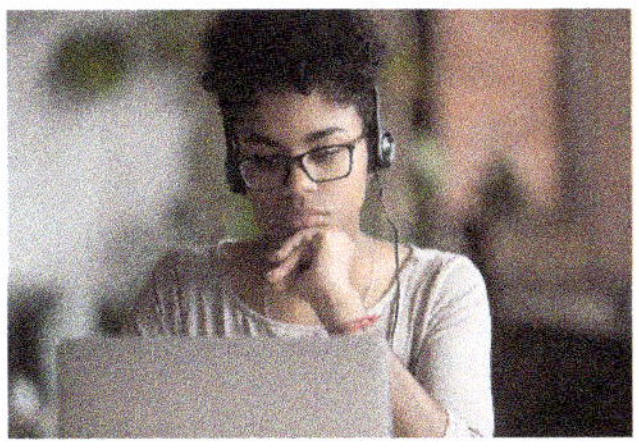

Remember the patient "Lila Bastian" from the beginning of the chapter? Now read the remainder of the case study. Based on the information presented within this chapter, respond to the critical thinking questions that follow.

Lila, a 19-year-old college student, comes to the clinic for renewal of her prescription for OC pills. She finished her last pack of pills (estradiol–norethindrone) 10 days ago. She has been unable to get to the clinic to have her prescription renewed before today. She remembers having unprotected intercourse 2 days ago, and now she is concerned that she will become pregnant. Lila asks the nurse, "How can you help me?"

A complete history and physical examination finds Lila in very good health. Her vital signs are temperature, 36.7°C (98°F); pulse, 68 beats/min; respiratory rate, 18 breaths/min; and blood pressure, 118/71 mmHg. Her weight is 62.6 kg (138 lb) and her height is 1.7 m (5 ft 7 in.). Her skin is dry and warm to the touch, mucous membranes are pink and moist, and there are no outward signs of distress. Her abdomen is soft and not tender, and there are no signs of bloating or distention. She has no vaginal bleeding at this time. Lila emphasizes that she only had sex once, 2 days ago. A urine pregnancy test is negative. Lila is prescribed the emergency contraceptive Plan B.

Critical Thinking Questions

1. Lila asks you, the nurse, if it is too late to prevent pregnancy. How would you respond to her question?
2. How does Plan B work to prevent pregnancy? What is another emergency contraceptive option that this patient could use?
3. What instructions would you give Lila regarding pregnancy and Plan B for emergency contraception?

Additional Case Study

Gina Martin, age 22, has been taking combination OCs for the past 2 years. Her healthcare provider orders antibiotics for a recurrent throat infection. As she is leaving the clinic, she asks you, the nurse, if she should temporarily discontinue her OC.

1. Explain the relationship between antibiotics and OCs.
2. What advice would you give Gina with regard to continuing the OC?

Chapter Review

1. Estradiol–norethindrone is prescribed for each of the following patients. Which patients would the nurse consider at highest risk for an adverse response to this therapy? (Select all that apply.)
   1. A 38-year-old with a BMI classified as overweight
   2. A 16-year-old athlete with asthma
   3. A 22-year-old who smokes two packs of cigarettes per day
   4. An 18-year-old with a history of chronic clinical depression
   5. A 42-year-old who has delivered four healthy children

2. The patient who is taking an oral contraceptive containing estradiol and drospirenone informs the nurse that she forgot to take her pills for the past 2 days. Which response by the nurse would be best when addressing this concern?
   1. "Take two pills today and tomorrow then resume your normal dosage."
   2. "Take one pill now and resume your normal dosage time tomorrow."
   3. "Skip another day and then resume the normal medication schedule."
   4. "Stop taking the pills and have a pregnancy test performed as soon as possible."

3. The patient is interested in taking levonorgestrel–estradiol (Seasonique) and asks how to take it. Which would be the correct response provided by the nurse?
   1. "Seasonique is taken one pill per day for 3 weeks, then 1 week of 'dummy pills' with inert ingredients."
   2. "Seasonique is taken year-round without a break and without a period."
   3. "Seasonique is taken for 2 months then off for 1 month using regular oral contraceptives."
   4. "Seasonique is taken for 84 days followed by 7 days of a lower dose that comes with the pack."

4. The nurse is teaching the patient who has received a prescription for mifepristone (Mifeprex) and misoprostol to terminate a pregnancy. When should the patient be instructed to take the misoprostol?
   1. Take it after taking one additional dose of mifepristone.
   2. Take it 1 week after taking the mifepristone.
   3. Take it 24 to 48 hours after taking mifepristone.
   4. Take it only if she is still bleeding in 3 days.

5. The nurse is providing health education about contraceptive methods to a group of young adults. Which of the following statements is correct about the use of spermicides?
   1. They are extremely effective in preventing pregnancy.
   2. They have relatively low levels of effectiveness when used alone.
   3. They are the main causes of HIV and pelvic inflammatory disease.
   4. They can prevent ectopic pregnancy.

6. Rank the following contraceptive methods in order of effectiveness from most to least effective:
   1. Depo-Provera
   2. Spermicides
   3. Calendar rhythm
   4. Oral contraceptives
   5. Transdermal

See Appendix A for answers to critical thinking questions, case study questions, and review questions.

References

Centers for Disease Control and Prevention (CDC). (2018). *Current contraceptive status among women aged 15–49: United States, 2015–2017.* https://www.cdc.gov/nchs/products/databriefs/db327.htm

Creanga, A. A., Berg, C. J., Syverson, C., Seed, K., Bruce, F. C., & Callaghan, W. M. (2015). Pregnancy-related mortality in the United States, 2006–2010. *Obstetrics & Gynecology*, *125*(1), 5–12. https://doi.org/10.1097/AOG.0000000000000564

Curtis, K. M., Jatlaoui, T. C., Tepper, N. K., Zapata, L. B., Horton, L. G., Jamieson, J. D., & Whiteman, M. K. (2016). U.S. selected practice recommendations for contraceptive use, 2016. *MMWR Recommendations and Reports*, *65*(4), 1–66. https://doi.org/10.15585/mmwr.rr6504a1

Martinez, G. M., & Abma, J.C. (2020). Sexual activity and contraceptive use among teenagers aged 15–19 in the United States, 2015–2017. Centers for Disease Control and Prevention. https://www.cdc.gov/nchs/products/databriefs/db366.htm

Simmons, K. B., & Edelman, A. B. (2016). Hormonal contraception and obesity. *Fertility and Sterility*, *106*, 1282–1288. https://doi.org/10.1016/j.fertnstert.2016.07.1094

Selected Bibliography

Bahamondes, L., Fernandes, A., Monteiro, I., & Bahamondes, M. V. (2020). Long-acting reversible contraceptive (LARCs) methods. *Best Practice & Research Clinical Obstetrics & Gynaecology*, *66*, 28–40. https://doi.org/10.1016/j.bpobgyn.2019.12.002

Centers for Disease Control and Prevention (CDC). (2020). *Pregnancy mortality surveillance system*. https://www.cdc.gov/reproductivehealth/maternal-mortality/pregnancy-mortality-surveillance-system.htm

Fok, W. K., & Blumenthal, P. D. (2016). Update on emergency contraception. *Current Opinion in Obstetrics and Gynecology*, *28*, 522–529. https://doi.org/10.1097/GCO.0000000000000320

Guttmacher Institute. (2017). *American teens' sexual and reproductive health*. https://www.guttmacher.org/fact-sheet/american-teens-sexual-and-reproductive-health

Haeger, K. O., Lamme, J., & Cleland, K. (2018). State of emergency contraception in the US, 2018. *Contraception and Reproductive Medicine*, *3*(1), 20. https://doi.org/10.1186/s40834-018-0067-8

Menon, S. (2020). Long-acting reversible contraception: Specific issues for adolescents. *Pediatrics*, *146*(2), e2020007252. https://doi.org/ https://doi.org/10.1542/peds.2020-007252

Saldanha, N. (2018). Use of short acting reversible contraception in adolescents: The pill, patch, ring and emergency contraception. *Current Problems in Pediatric and Adolescent Health Care*, *48*(12), 333–344. https://doi.org/10.1016/j.cppeds.2018.11.003

Sobel, L., Salganicoff, A., & Rosensweig, C. (2017). *The future of contraceptive coverage*. KFF. http://kff.org/womens-health-policy/issue-brief/the-future-of-contraceptive-coverage

Wu, J. P., Moniz, M. H., & Ursu, A. N. (2018). Long-acting reversible contraception—highly efficacious, safe, and underutilized. *Journal of the American Medical Association*, *320*(4), 397–398. https://doi.org/10.1001/jama.2018.8877

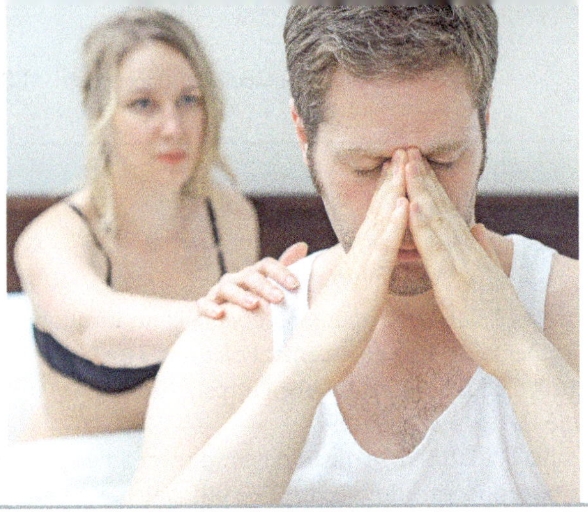

"What's wrong with me? Dana excites me so much, but when we get into bed, I just can't please her sexually."
—*Patient "Mike Mayhew"*

Chapter 71
Drugs for Disorders and Conditions of the Male Reproductive System

Chapter Outline

Learning Outcomes

After reading this chapter, the student should be able to:

1. Explain the physiologic effects of androgens.
2. Describe the roles of the hypothalamus, pituitary, and testes in regulating male reproductive function.
3. Explain the role of androgens in the treatment of male hypogonadism, delayed puberty, and breast cancer.
4. Describe the potential consequences associated with the use of anabolic steroids to enhance athletic performance.
5. Identify the types and causes of male sexual dysfunction disorders.
6. Explain the role of drugs in the management of male infertility.
7. Describe the etiology, pathogenesis, and pharmacotherapy of erectile dysfunction.
8. Describe the pathogenesis and pharmacotherapy of benign prostatic hyperplasia.
9. For each of the classes shown in the chapter outline, identify the prototype and representative drugs and explain the mechanism(s) of drug action, primary indications, contraindications, significant drug interactions, pregnancy data, and important adverse effects.
10. Apply clinical judgment to the care of patients receiving pharmacotherapy for disorders and conditions of the male reproductive system.

Key Terms

Definitions of the terms in bold may be found in the Glossary.

As in women, reproductive function in men is regulated by a small number of hormones from the hypothalamus, pituitary, and gonads. Because hormonal secretion in men is relatively constant throughout the adult lifespan, the pharmacologic treatment of reproductive disorders in men is less complex and more limited than in women. This chapter examines the drugs used to treat the disorders and conditions of the male reproductive system.

Regulation of Male Reproductive Function

71.1 Male reproductive function is controlled through the secretion of androgens.

Male reproduction function is controlled by **androgens**, which are hormones secreted by **interstitial endocrine (Leydig) cells** in the testes. Testosterone, the primary androgen, is responsible for maturation of the male reproductive system and the secondary sex characteristics of men. Other important androgens include androstenedione and dehydroepiandrosterone (DHEA). Androgens are sometimes referred to as anabolic steroids.

Androgens are responsible for the development of the male urogenital system in the fetus. After birth the interstitial endocrine cells are quiet until activated by the gonadotropins, which are hormones secreted by the pituitary gland. The resulting increased production of testosterone by the testes begins the cascade of changes that accompany the onset of puberty in the male adolescent. The increased testosterone levels are responsible for the process of **virilization**, or the development of the male sexual characteristics. During the next several years, the testes, scrotum, and penis enlarge until they reach adult proportions. Pubic, axillary, and facial hair grows and other body hair becomes more adult-like in nature. The production of sperm that are capable of fertilizing an ovum begins in the seminiferous tubules of the testes. The cartilage of the larynx grows, causing the deeper-toned male voice. Sebaceous gland activity is stimulated, resulting in an increase in the level of acne.

Testosterone also has profound metabolic effects in nonreproductive tissues. Of particular importance is its ability to build skeletal muscle mass and to stimulate bone growth, which contributes to the differences in muscle strength and body composition between men and women. Testosterone promotes the synthesis of erythropoietin, resulting in an increased production of red blood cells (RBCs) and accounting for the higher hemoglobin and hematocrit levels found in males.

Androgen secretion is regulated by the same pituitary hormones that control reproductive function in women. Although the name follicle-stimulating hormone (FSH) applies to its target in the female ovary, this same hormone influences testosterone secretion in men. Luteinizing hormone (LH), more accurately called interstitial cell–stimulating hormone in the male reproductive system, regulates the production of testosterone by the interstitial endocrine cells of the testes. Unlike the 28-day cyclic secretion of estrogen and progesterone in women, testosterone secretion is relatively constant in adult men. Beginning in puberty, testosterone production increases rapidly and continues to maintain a high level of production until late adulthood, after which it slowly declines. Normal plasma concentrations of testosterone are 250 to 1000 mg/dL. If the level of testosterone in the blood rises above normal, negative feedback to the pituitary shuts off the secretion of LH and FSH. The relationship among the hypothalamus, pituitary, and the male reproductive hormones is illustrated in Figure 71.1.

Precursor molecules of testosterone, androstenedione, and DHEA are secreted in small amounts by the adrenal glands and are controlled by the secretion of adrenocorticotropic hormone. These weaker androgens are converted to testosterone once they reach peripheral tissues. Adrenal androgens have a role in the growth of pubic hair and are thought to influence the skeletal growth spurt in adolescents. In adult men, the adrenal androgens have minimal effects due to the comparatively larger amount of testosterone secreted by the testes.

Pharmacotherapy with Androgens

71.2 Androgens are used to treat hypogonadism and delayed puberty in males and breast cancer in females.

Androgens are used to treat testosterone deficiency, delayed puberty, oligospermia, hypogonadism, anemia, muscle-wasting disorders, and certain cancers. These hormones are listed in Table 71.1.

Lack of sufficient testosterone secretion by the testes can result in male **hypogonadism**. Hypogonadism may be congenital or acquired later in life. When the condition is caused by a testicular disorder, it is called *primary* hypogonadism. Examples of disease states that may cause primary testicular failure include mumps, testicular trauma or inflammation, and certain autoimmune disorders.

A deficiency in FSH and LH secretion by the pituitary will result in a lack of stimulus to the testes to produce

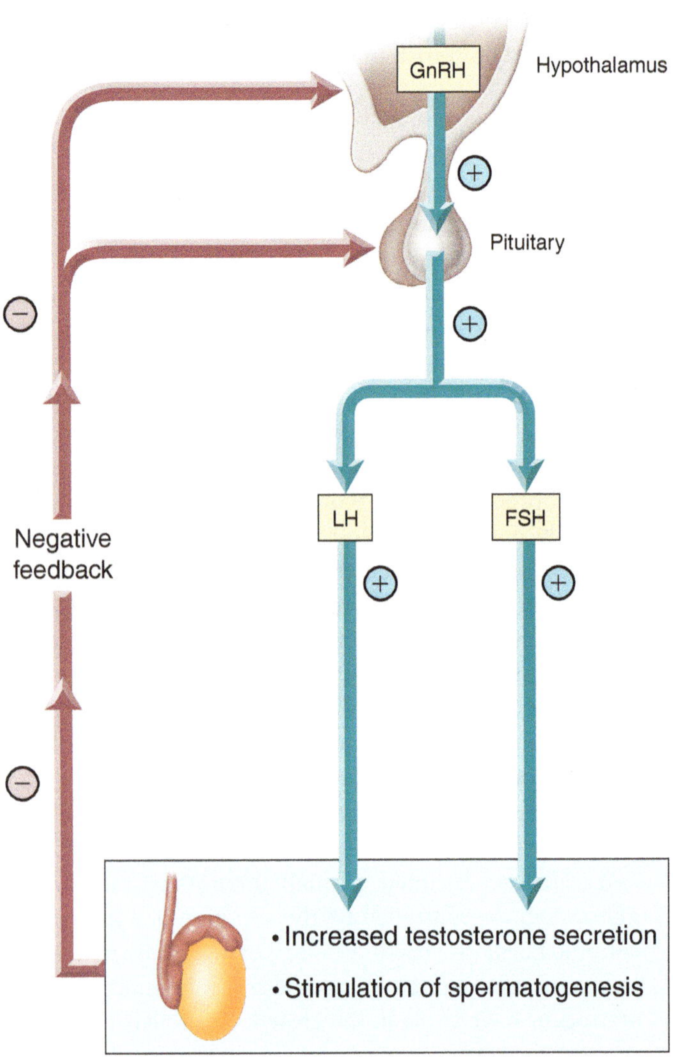

Figure 71.1 Hormonal control of the male reproductive hormones.

androgens. Lack of FSH and LH secretion may have a number of causes, including Cushing's syndrome, thyroid disorders, estrogen-secreting tumors, and therapy with gonadotropin-releasing hormone (GnRH) agonists such as leuprolide (Lupron). Hypogonadism that is caused by defects in the pituitary or hypothalamus is known as *secondary* hypogonadism.

Insufficient testosterone secretion may delay the onset of puberty. If total lack of testosterone secretion occurs, puberty will not occur. In adult men, symptoms of hypogonadism include diminished secondary sex characteristics such as sparse axillary, facial, and pubic hair; increased subcutaneous fat; reduced muscle mass; and smaller testes. The lack of testosterone can lead to erectile dysfunction (ED); low sperm counts (oligospermia); a decrease in the amount of ejaculate; and decreased **libido**, or a lack of interest in sexual intercourse. Nonspecific complaints may include behavioral and mood changes such as irritability, fatigue, depression, and a general loss of motivation.

Hypogonadism is confirmed by obtaining serum testosterone levels. Assessment of LH and FSH levels, as well as prolactin, estradiol, and thyroid hormone levels, may be useful in determining causation. Low serum levels of testosterone concurrent with normal or elevated levels of FSH and LH suggest that the testes are unresponsive to hormonal activation; thus, the patient has primary hypogonadism. If testosterone, FSH, and LH levels are all low, this would indicate secondary hypogonadism.

Pharmacotherapy of hypogonadism includes replacement therapy with testosterone or other androgens. For boys experiencing delayed puberty, puberty is generally induced when the boy reaches 15 to 17 years of age using

Table 71.1 Selected Androgens and Anabolic Steroids

Drug	Route and Adult Dose (Maximum Dose Where Indicated)	Adverse Effects
fluoxymesterone	PO: 5–20 mg/day	*Acne, gynecomastia, hirsutism and male sex characteristics (in women), sodium and water retention, emotional lability, amenorrhea, decreased libido, hypercholesterolemia* <u>Anaphylaxis, testicular atrophy, and oligospermia at high doses; priapism, peliosis hepatis, benign intracranial hypertension (HTN), thromboembolism, stroke, systemic HTN</u>
methyltestosterone (Android, Testred)	PO: 10–50 mg/day	
nandrolone	IM: 50–200 mg/wk	
oxandrolone	PO: 2.5–20 mg/day divided bid–qid for 2–4 wk	
oxymetholone (Anadrol-50)	PO: 1–5 mg/kg/day	
testosterone (buccal) (transdermal patch: Androderm) (topical gels: AndroGel, Fortesta, Testim, Vogelxo) (implantable pellets: Testopel) (nasal spray: Natesto)	Buccal: 30 mg q12h Transdermal: Apply one to two 2.5-mg patches daily (max: 5 mg/day) Gel: Apply 5–50 g daily, depending on product Pellets: 150–450 mg every 6 months (each pellet is 75 mg) Nasal spray: 1 spray in each nostril tid	
testosterone cypionate (Depo-Testosterone)	IM: 50–400 mg q2–4wk	
testosterone enanthate (Xyosted)	Subcutaneous: 50–100 mg q1/wk	
testosterone undecanoate (Aveed, Jatenzo)	IM (Aveed): 750 mg initially, followed by the same dose at 4 wk and q10wk thereafter PO (Jatenzo): 158—396 mg bid	

Note: *Italics* indicate common adverse effects. <u>Underline</u> indicates serious adverse effects.

a long-acting testosterone preparation. A 6-month period of androgen therapy is given, followed by 6 months without the drug. If further therapy is needed, then testosterone cypionate (Depo-Testosterone) may be administered every 2 to 4 weeks. Therapy may be continued for up to 4 years. Once appropriate physiologic hormonal levels have been attained, the normal progression of pubertal changes typically occurs.

A variety of testosterone replacement preparations are available for the adult patient. With appropriate therapy, the patient should experience improved libido, increased amount of ejaculate, and correction of ED within days or weeks of initiating therapy. Male sex characteristics become better defined, depression resolves, and muscle strength rapidly improves. Therapy with androgens is targeted to return serum testosterone to normal physiologic levels. Above-normal levels serve no therapeutic purpose and increase the risk of adverse effects.

Nonreproductive indications: Because androgens have widespread physiologic effects, they have been used to treat certain nonreproductive disorders. Testosterone promotes the synthesis of erythropoietin, which is essential for RBC production, and the drug may be used to correct anemia unresponsive to other treatments. These indications include aplastic anemia and anemias associated with chronic kidney disease (CKD) and chemotherapy. Taking advantage of the anabolic effects of testosterone on bone and skeletal muscle, the drug is sometimes given to debilitated patients who have muscle-wasting disease, such as that seen in patients with acquired immunodeficiency syndrome (AIDS).

High doses of androgens are occasionally used for the palliative management of certain types of breast cancer in combination with other antineoplastics. The high doses required for breast cancer treatment will cause virilization in women. Androgen therapy is contraindicated in males with breast cancer because it promotes the growth of the cancer. Similarly, because the growth of most prostate carcinomas is testosterone dependent, androgens should not be prescribed for older men unless the possibility of prostate cancer has been ruled out. Patients with prostate carcinoma are sometimes given a GnRH agonist such as leuprolide (Lupron depot) to reduce circulating testosterone levels, a process called androgen deprivation therapy.

Testosterone formulations: Testosterone is available in a wide variety of formulations. All are equally effective, and the choice is based on healthcare provider experience, ease of use, and the personal preference of the patient. Common to all dosage forms is the need for regular follow-up healthcare visits to ensure that the serum testosterone level is maintained within the designated range.

Intramuscular (IM) testosterone: Testosterone cypionate (Depo-Testosterone), testosterone enanthate, and testosterone undecanoate (Aveed) are IM forms of testosterone. These drugs are slowly absorbed, metabolized to free testosterone, and result in blood levels that will vary widely after administration. This variation in serum levels may cause patients to experience fluctuations in their libido and energy and experience mood swings. Patients tend to report soreness at the site of injection. IM injections are given deep in the gluteal muscle every 2 to 4 weeks.

Implantable testosterone pellets: Testopel is a long-acting form of testosterone that is implanted subcutaneously, usually on the anterior abdominal wall. One to six pellets are implanted depending on the dose required. Testosterone levels are obtained regularly during therapy and the number of pellets adjusted accordingly. To induce puberty, low doses are usually used for 4 to 6 months. For adult replacement therapy, higher doses are administered, with the effectiveness of the pellets lasting 3 to 4 months.

Transdermal testosterone patch: The Androderm patch is applied to the upper arm, thigh, back, or abdomen, rotating application sites. The patch is not to be applied to the scrotum or to damaged skin. A rash at the site of the application tends to be the only adverse effect noted. The patches are applied in the evening and changed daily. Because the used patches contain some testosterone, they should be disposed of safely, away from children and pets.

Transdermal and intranasal testosterone gel: AndroGel, Fortesta, Testim, and Vogelxo are testosterone gels that are indicated for the treatment of hypogonadism. The drug is applied once daily in the morning to clean and dry skin of the upper arms, shoulders, or abdomen (not the genitals). Showering or swimming should be avoided for several hours after application to avoid washing off the drug. The alcohol-based gels dry quickly. The testosterone is absorbed in the skin in about 30 minutes and released slowly to the blood. Many patients prefer the gels because they cause less local irritation, do not fall off like the patches, and deliver a more consistent level of testosterone. A disadvantage is that the gel can be transferred to another individual by skin-to-skin contact, causing virilization of female contacts and potential fetal harm. Testosterone levels should be measured after a few weeks of therapy and at regular intervals thereafter to ensure that physiologic levels have been achieved.

Natesto delivers testosterone gel via intranasal spray. Absorption is rapid across the nasal mucosa, but the drug needs to be applied three times daily. The most common side effects are nasal related and include nasopharyngitis, rhinorrhea, and epistaxis.

Testosterone buccal tablets: Buccal tablets are is a form of testosterone that produces a continuous supply of testosterone in the blood. Patients are instructed to place a tablet in the gum area just above the incisor, holding it in place for 30 seconds. Usual doses are one tablet every 12 hours, alternating sides of the cheek. Patients may eat, drink, and chew gum with the buccal tablet in place. This route exhibits only minor adverse effects such as local irritation to the area, bad taste, and altered taste perceptions.

PROTOTYPE DRUG Testosterone

Classification **Therapeutic:** Male sex hormone
Pharmacologic: Androgen, anabolic steroid, antineoplastic

Therapeutic Effects and Uses: The primary therapeutic use of testosterone is to treat delayed puberty and hypogonadism in boys by promoting virilization, including maturation of the sexual organs, growth of facial hair, and a deepening of the voice. In adult men testosterone administration will increase libido and restore masculine characteristics that may be deficient. Testosterone is approved to treat ED when the cause is associated with low androgen levels. The drug is also approved for the palliative treatment of inoperable breast cancer in women. Off-label indications for testosterone include treatment of postpubertal cryptorchidism, microphallus, anemia in patients with CKD, female-to-male gender change, and AIDS-associated wasting syndrome.

Testosterone base is administered by the IM route, although other salts are available for the transdermal, implantable pellet, and buccal routes. Testosterone is classified as a Schedule III controlled substance because it may be abused by body builders and other athletes.

Mechanism of Action: Testosterone binds to specific receptors located in the cell cytoplasm. The hormone-receptor complex then migrates to the nucleus where it acts on the deoxyribonucleic acid to promote the synthesis of specific messenger ribonucleic acid molecules. These form templates for the production of specific proteins that mediate testosterone effects.

Pharmacokinetics:

Route(s)	Buccal, transdermal, IM, implantable pellets
Absorption	Cypionate and enanthate are slowly absorbed from IM sites
Distribution	98% bound to sex hormone–binding globulin; unknown if secreted in breast milk
Primary metabolism	Hepatic
Primary excretion	90% renal, 6% feces
Onset of action	Steady-state levels are reached in 3–4 weeks
Duration of action	2–4 weeks cypionate and enanthate; half-life: 10–100 min

Adverse Effects: Androgens may cause either decreased or increased libido. Salt and water are often retained, causing edema, and a diuretic may be indicated. Liver damage and hepatic cancer are potentially serious adverse effects and are of special concern when high doses are taken for prolonged periods. Acne and skin irritation are common during therapy. High doses may suppress spermatogenesis, reduce ejaculatory volume, and cause oligospermia. **Black Box Warning:** Virilization in children and women may occur following secondary exposure. Children and women should avoid touching the application sites in men using testosterone gel. Signs of virilization in women include suppression of ovulation, lactation, or menstruation; hoarseness or deepening of the voice, which is often irreversible; hirsutism; oily skin; clitoral enlargement; regression of breasts; and male-pattern baldness.

Contraindications/Precautions: Testosterone is contraindicated in men with known or suspected breast or prostatic carcinomas because it can promote the growth of these tumors. Testosterone should be used with caution in patients with CKD or hepatic impairment. Caution must be used if testosterone is administered to patients with diabetes mellitus, history of myocardial infarction (MI), coronary artery disease, benign prostatic hyperplasia (BPH), and acute intermittent porphyria and in geriatric patients. Monitoring of serum cholesterol and electrolytes, as well as liver function tests, is needed throughout therapy because testosterone may increase these values.

Drug Interactions: Testosterone may potentiate the effects of oral (PO) anticoagulants and increase the risk of severe bleeding. Concurrent use of testosterone with corticosteroids may cause additive edema, which can be a serious concern for those with heart failure (HF). Hepatotoxic drugs should be avoided because their use with testosterone can cause additive liver damage. The 5-alpha reductase drugs (finasteride) used to treat prostatic hyperplasia are antiandrogenic and their use with testosterone will inhibit the therapeutic effects of both drugs. **Herbal/Food:** Insulin requirements may decrease, and the risk of hepatotoxicity may increase when used with echinacea. Evaluation of calcium levels is necessary because hypercalcemia may result.

Pregnancy: Testosterone is contraindicated during pregnancy because it may cause virilization of the female fetus. Women of childbearing potential are advised to use contraception during therapy. Testosterone is secreted in human milk although adverse effects on the breastfed neonate are unknown. High levels in milk have the potential to cause androgenic effects in the breastfed infant.

Treatment of Overdose: There is no specific treatment for overdose.

Clinician Responsibilities: Key clinical implications for patients receiving testosterone are included in Applied Clinical Judgment: Patients Receiving Pharmacotherapy with Androgens.

Drugs Similar to Testosterone

Other androgens include fluoxymesterone, methyltestosterone, and oxandrolone. All are contraindicated during pregnancy and breastfeeding is not recommended.

Fluoxymesterone: Approved in 1983, fluoxymesterone is a PO androgen that is indicated for male hypogonadism and for palliative therapy of inoperable breast cancer in women. This drug has the same adverse effects, contraindications, and actions as those of testosterone. Like other androgens, hepatitis and hepatic neoplasms may occur with long-term use. Fluoxymesterone should be used with caution in patients with preexisting cardiac or CKD because the edema caused by the drug can worsen these disorders. Older men have an increased risk for prostate cancer when taking androgens.

Methyltestosterone (Android, Testred): Methyltestosterone is available PO tablets and is indicated for male hypogonadism, delayed male puberty, and inoperable breast cancer in women. This drug has the same adverse effects, contraindications, and actions as those of testosterone. Caution must be used during long-term use because of the potential for hepatotoxicity and for the development of prostate cancer in older men.

Oxandrolone: Originally approved in 1964, oxandrolone is an anabolic steroid with actions and adverse effects that are the same as testosterone. It is approved to promote weight gain in patients who are severely ill, to decrease bone pain that accompanies osteoporosis, and to offset protein catabolism associated with prolonged administration of corticosteroids.

CONNECTIONS: APPLIED CLINICAL JUDGMENT

Patients Receiving Pharmacotherapy with Androgens

Key Assessment Data

- Health history including cardiovascular, peripheral vascular, thyroid, hepatic, or kidney disease, diabetes, prostatic hyperplasia, or breast cancer; baseline vital signs, physical exam findings; complete blood count (CBC), electrolytes, glucose, lipid levels.

Desired Therapeutic Outcomes

Improvement is observed and measurable by hormone levels normalized and normal signs of masculinization present.

Minimizing Adverse Effects

- Androgens cause sodium and water retention with resulting increases in weight, blood pressure (BP), and possible edema.
- Androgens may cause increases in cholesterol and calcium levels. Hepatotoxicity and hepatic neoplasms are rare but potential adverse effects.
- Androgens may affect carbohydrate metabolism, leading to increased glucose levels. Patients with diabetes may require an alteration in their usual regimen.
- Androgen administration may result in premature closure of epiphyseal bone endings and loss of normal growth patterns. Children prescribed androgens should have frequent height measurements to ensure adequate growth.
- Abuse of androgens and anabolic steroids may occur, along with resulting adverse effects.

Lifespan Considerations

- Age-related physiologic differences may place the older adult at greater risk for hepatotoxicity.
- Women and children should not come in contact with gels or creams as they may rub off and cause significant adverse effects.

Patient Education

- Monitor BP on a weekly basis. Report any BP over 140/90 mmHg, or as directed. Weigh self daily and report any weight gain of 1 kg (2 lb) in 24 hours or 2 kg (5 lb) in 1 week to the healthcare provider. Report any peripheral edema.
- Immediately report any symptoms of abdominal or right upper quadrant discomfort or pain, yellowing of the skin or sclera, fatigue, anorexia, darkened urine, clay-colored stools, weakness, lethargy, nausea or vomiting.
- Patients with diabetes should monitor capillary blood glucose more frequently while on the drug and should report consistent elevations.
- For children prescribed androgens, measure height once per month or as directed. Return for clinical assessments as needed, approximately every 6 months, to monitor bone growth.
- Take the drug following appropriate guidelines:
  - *Oral drugs* should be taken at the same time each day to help with remembering the dose.
  - *Transdermal patches* should be applied to the upper arm, thigh, back, or abdomen. Change the patch and rotate sites daily and report any skin irritation. Discard used patches safely in the trash. Do not apply the patch to the scrotal area or on broken or irritated skin.
  - *Buccal tablets* should be placed between the cheek and upper gum near the incisor and held in place for 30 seconds. Eating, drinking, and chewing gum may continue while the tablet is in place. Rotate doses from side to side, avoiding areas of irritation.
  - *Gels and creams* should be applied to the upper arms, shoulders, or abdomen. Do not apply to the scrotal area or to broken or irritated skin. Swimming and showering should be avoided for several hours following administration. Do not allow women or children to come in contact with the drug or application sites because the drug may rub off and cause adverse effects.
  - *Transdermal pellets* are implanted in the abdominal wall every 3 to 6 months.
  - *Injections* should be given into deep gluteal muscle. Instruction on how to administer the injection will be given, followed by opportunities to demonstrate the technique.

Prescribing Considerations

- Prior to starting testosterone replacement therapy, a baseline testosterone, estradiol, prostate-specific antigen (PSA), and hematocrit should be obtained. A baseline prostate exam should also be performed.
- After starting testosterone replacement therapy, labs should be checked at 3 and 6 months and then annually.
- Patients should be reevaluated 6 to 12 weeks after initiating treatment to determine if dosing adjustments are needed.
- Testosterone dosing should be carefully adjusted such that men achieve a serum total testosterone level of 450 to 600 ng/dL.

Anabolic Steroids

71.3 Often abused by athletes, anabolic steroids can cause serious adverse effects.

Testosterone has both androgenic and anabolic effects. Its androgenic effects are responsible for creating and maintaining the male sexual characteristics. The hormone's **anabolic effects** relate to its ability to accelerate the growth of RBCs, muscle, bone, and neural tissues.

Anabolic steroids also include testosterone-like substances that were originally developed to produce the anabolic effects of androgens while minimizing the androgenic effects. They are often taken inappropriately by athletes who hope to build muscle mass and strength, thereby obtaining a competitive edge. The use of anabolic steroids to improve athletic performance is illegal and all major athletic organizations prohibit the use of anabolic steroids by their participants. Many adolescents take these drugs to enhance their appearance, rather than to compete in athletics.

Interestingly, despite their regulation, some formulations of anabolic steroids can be purchased over the counter (OTC) or online. They are promoted as natural steroid alternatives for building muscle mass. FDA-approved anabolic steroids, including all testosterone products, oxandrolone, oxymetholone, and nandrolone, are classified as Schedule III drugs under the Anabolic Steroid Control Acts of 1990 and 2004 because of their abuse potential. The anabolic steroids are listed in Table 71.1.

When taken in large doses for prolonged periods, anabolic steroids can produce significant adverse effects, some of which may persist for months after discontinuation of the drugs. When given in higher doses, androgen suppresses the release of LH and FSH, resulting in oligospermia, testicular atrophy, and impotence in men. In female athletes menstrual irregularities are likely with an obvious increase in masculine appearance, such as hair growth and reduction in breast size. When administered to children and teens, androgens can promote premature epiphyseal plate closure, thereby reducing adult height. Anabolic steroids are hepatotoxic, and permanent liver damage or hepatic carcinoma may result with prolonged use. Accompanying salt and water retention can result in HTN. These drugs tend to raise low-density lipoprotein and lower high-density lipoprotein cholesterol levels, possibly accelerating atherosclerosis. Acne is common. Behavioral changes include an increase in aggressive behavior and psychologic dependence. Another unusual adverse effect is peliosis hepatis, which is a condition in which liver, and sometimes splenic, tissue is replaced with blood-filled cysts. These cysts are sometimes asymptomatic and may not be recognized until life-threatening hepatic failure or intra-abdominal hemorrhage occurs. Anabolic steroids are contraindicated during pregnancy.

The FDA requires warning labels on all testosterone products and other prescription anabolic steroids. The label is intended to alert prescribers to the abuse and dependence potential of these products and to the serious adverse effects that can result from abuse. It also advises healthcare providers of the importance of measuring serum testosterone when abuse is suspected.

CONNECTION Checkpoint 71.1

Anabolic steroids are often taken illegally by "stacking" or "pyramiding." From what you learned in Chapter 27, define the use of these terms in the abuse of these drugs.

Etiology of Male Sexual Dysfunction

71.4 Male sexual dysfunction may have both medical and psychologic etiologies.

Approximately 50% of men will experience some form of sexual dysfunction during their adult life. The primary types of male dysfunction disorders may be classified as follows:

1. *Diminished libido*: lack of interest in sexual activity
2. *Erectile dysfunction (ED)*: inability to obtain or maintain an erection
3. *Ejaculation disorder*: premature, delayed, or retrograde ejaculation
4. *Infertility*: inability to conceive a child.

Certain causes of male sexual dysfunction are treatable, either medically or surgically, or can be improved to the degree that a couple can achieve successful conception or maintain a satisfactory sexual lifestyle. For example, therapy with testosterone can rapidly increase libido in patients who have insufficient serum testosterone levels or hypogonadism. Many men with ED can now be successfully treated with medications.

A large number of drugs can cause or worsen male sexual dysfunction, as listed in Table 71.2. In most cases, the dysfunction is dose related and is much less evident when a single drug is taken at low doses. However, taking multiple drugs that have the potential to cause sexual adverse effects may result in additive sexual dysfunction. The two most common drug classes that cause sexual dysfunction are antihypertensives and antidepressants. Because sexual adverse effects are a potential cause of nonadherence, nurses should ask specific questions regarding changes in sexual function when their patients are taking these drugs.

Many comorbid medical conditions are associated with sexual dysfunction. Conditions that result in general debility, such as pain, muscle weakness, shortness of breath, or stroke, may cause dysfunction. Diabetes and

Table 71.2 Selected Drugs That May Cause or Worsen Male Sexual Dysfunction

Drug/Drug Class	Sexual Adverse Effect(s)
Antihypertensives	
alpha$_1$-adrenergic antagonists (e.g., alfuzosin, tamsulosin)	Retrograde ejaculation, priapism
angiotensin-converting enzyme (ACE) inhibitors (e.g., lisinopril)	ED
beta-adrenergic antagonists (e.g., propranolol)	Diminished libido, ED
methyldopa	Diminished libido, ED
spironolactone	Diminished libido, ED, gynecomastia
thiazide diuretics	ED
Nervous System Drugs	
antipsychotics (e.g., haloperidol, risperidone)	Diminished libido, ED, ejaculatory disorder
carbamazepine	ED
lithium carbonate	ED
phenothiazines (e.g., chlorpromazine)	Diminished libido, ED, inhibited ejaculation, priapism
selective serotonin reuptake inhibitors (e.g., fluoxetine)	Anorgasmia, inhibited ejaculation, diminished libido
trazodone	Priapism
tricyclic antidepressants (e.g., imipramine)	Diminished libido, ED, inhibited ejaculation
Other Drugs	
alcohol	ED
anabolic steroids	Infertility
antineoplastics (e.g., cyclophosphamide)	Infertility
digoxin	ED
finasteride	Diminished libido, ED, gynecomastia
methotrexate	Infertility

HTN are the two chronic medical conditions most frequently associated with male sexual dysfunction. Patients who present with psychologic conditions such as anxiety and depression have a high incidence of sexual dysfunction. Other factors associated with ED include obesity and cigarette smoking. Combining multiple risk factors—for example, a man who has diabetes, is obese, takes antihypertensive drugs, and smokes—will result in a high risk for sexual dysfunction.

Nurses play a key role in treating male sexual dysfunction by obtaining a thorough medical history and by recognizing factors that contribute to the disorder. Should patients experience unacceptable sexual adverse effects from their medications, alternative drugs can usually be substituted. Encouraging patients to receive treatment for anxiety, depression, and other comorbid conditions sometimes helps improve the sexual dysfunction. All men at risk for ED should be encouraged to maintain optimal weight, stop smoking, and limit their alcohol use.

Pharmacotherapy of Male Infertility

71.5 Male infertility is treated with endocrine drugs that boost sperm production.

Infertility affects approximately 6.1 million people in the United States, or roughly 10% of the reproductive age population. It is estimated that 30 to 40% of infertility among couples is due to difficulties with the male reproductive system.

Like female infertility, male infertility may have a number of complex causes. The most common congenital cause is Klinefelter's syndrome, which is the presence of an extra X chromosome. Acquired infertility may result from testicular trauma; pituitary or hypothalamus disorders; and infections such as mumps, chronic tuberculosis, and sexually transmitted infections. Infertility may occur with or without signs of hypogonadism. Rarely, life-threatening conditions such as testicular cancer and pituitary tumors may be the cause. In addition, the lack of ability to conceive may be caused by factors such as ED or ejaculation disorders. Identifying the etiology of infertility is important because not all causes can be successfully treated with pharmacotherapy.

The most obvious etiology of male infertility is lack of sufficient sperm production. **Oligospermia** is the presence of less than 20 million sperm per milliliter of ejaculate. **Azoospermia**, which occurs in 15% of men with infertility, is the complete absence of sperm in ejaculate. Azoospermia can be caused by severely reduced or absent sperm production, or it may indicate an obstruction of the vas deferens or ejaculatory duct that can be corrected surgically. Drug therapy with calcium channel blockers, colchicine, spironolactone, and cimetidine can lower sperm production.

Depending on the cause of the condition, one goal of pharmacotherapy for male infertility may be to increase sperm production. If the cause of the infertility is decreased testosterone secretion due to hypogonadism, administration of this hormone can increase sperm production and cure the condition.

Another method of increasing sperm production is to stimulate testosterone secretion in the testes by administering pituitary hormones. Pharmacotherapy often begins with IM injections of human chorionic gonadotropin (HCG) three times per week over 1 year. Although HCG is secreted by the placenta, its effects in men are identical to those of LH: increased testosterone secretion and spermatogenesis. Sperm counts are conducted periodically to assess therapeutic progress. If HCG is unsuccessful, therapy with menotropins (Menopur, Repronex) or newer recombinant forms of FSH may be attempted. Menotropins consists of a mixture of purified FSH and LH, which increases testosterone and sperm production.

Once testosterone levels rise, either through the administration of testosterone or HCG, the natural feedback mechanism of the body will signal the pituitary to shut down testosterone secretion in the testes. To boost testosterone levels, antiestrogen drugs such as tamoxifen and clomiphene have been used to block the negative feedback of adrenal estrogen to the pituitary and hypothalamus, thus increasing the levels of FSH and LH. Unfortunately, these drugs produce only a small increase in sperm count and can produce such adverse effects as gynecomastia, decreased libido, and weight gain. Clomiphene is presented as a prototype drug for female infertility in Chapter 69.

Other pharmacologic approaches to treating male infertility have been attempted. If retrograde ejaculation has been identified as a probable cause, sympathomimetics may be used to convert to normal, antegrade ejaculation. Various nutritional supplements—such as zinc to improve sperm production, L-carnitine to improve sperm motility and sperm count, and vitamins C and E as antioxidants to reduce reactive intermediates—have been tested. Unfortunately, these and other therapies have not conclusively been shown to have any positive effect on male infertility.

Drug therapy of male infertility is not as successful as pharmacotherapy in women because only about 5% of infertile men have an endocrine etiology for their disorder. Long-term therapy may be required. Because of the expense of pharmacotherapy, the large number of injections needed, and the relative lack of success, other means of conception for the infertile man should be explored. A wide range of assistive reproduction procedures, including *in vitro* fertilization or intrauterine insemination, may be pursued.

CONNECTION Checkpoint 71.2

Clomiphene is used for both male and female infertility. From what you learned in Chapter 69, how does this drug act to improve female fertility?

Pharmacotherapy of Erectile Dysfunction

71.6 Erectile dysfunction is a common disorder that may be successfully treated with inhibitors of the enzyme phosphodiesterase-5.

Erectile dysfunction (ED) is defined as the consistent inability to either attain an erection or to sustain an erection long enough to achieve satisfactory sexual intercourse. **Impotence**, a term often used interchangeably with ED, is the total inability to achieve an erection, an inconsistent ability to achieve an erection, or the ability to have only brief erections. An estimated 15 to 30 million men in the United States have ED. The incidence of ED increases with age, although it may occur in men of any age.

Penile erection is a complex event that has psychologic, neuromuscular, and vascular components. Sexual arousal results in the release of neurotransmitters, primarily nitric oxide and epinephrine, from the hypothalamus. This stimulation along the autonomic nerves results in the release of an enzyme that makes cyclic guanosine monophosphate (cGMP). cGMP causes dilation of the arterioles leading to the major erectile tissues of the penis, called the **corpora cavernosa**. Rigidity of the penis results when the increased local blood flow and pressure fill the vascular spaces within the corpora. This engorgement causes occlusion of the veins that drain blood from the corpora, allowing the penis to remain rigid long enough for successful coitus. When stimulation ends or after ejaculation, cGMP is removed by the enzyme phosphodiesterase-5 (PDE-5). At this point, the pressure in the penis decreases, the veins dilate, blood leaves the corpora, and the penis quickly loses its rigidity. The anatomy of the penis is illustrated in Figure 71.2.

A thorough health history and physical examination of male patients is usually sufficient to diagnose ED. Many chronic illnesses have the potential to damage the arteries, smooth muscle, and fibrous tissues of the penis, most notably atherosclerosis, diabetes, stroke, CKD, and HTN.

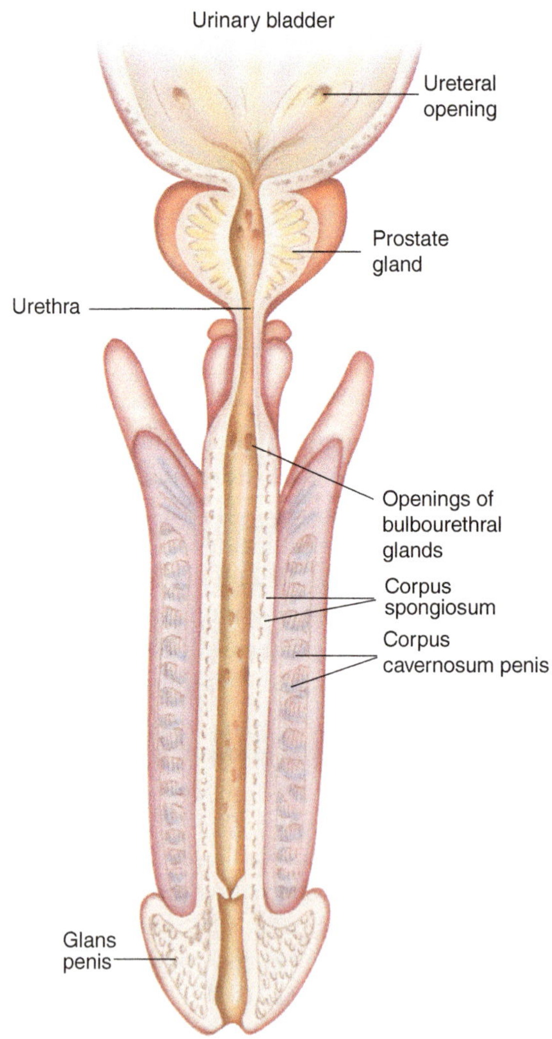

Figure 71.2 Anatomy of the penis.

Psychogenic causes may include depression, fatigue, stress, or fear of sexual failure. In some men, a number of common drugs cause sexual dysfunction as an adverse effect (see Table 71.2. Another potential cause of ED is hypogonadism, which can cause an inability to develop an erection, owing to the loss of libido. Nerve innervation and blood flow to the penis may be damaged by trauma or by surgery, particularly during procedures involving the prostate gland.

The treatment of ED is becoming more prevalent as the population ages because more men are becoming affected by the disorder. If hormones are the cause of the dysfunction, treatment is aimed at correcting the abnormality. In some, testosterone replacement therapy by IM injection or transdermal patches may assist with ED, particularly if associated with hypogonadism or low libido. If the cause is found to be psychologic, treatment will usually consist of a combination of psychotherapy and pharmacotherapy.

The approval of sildenafil (Viagra), the first PDE-5 inhibitor, revolutionized the treatment of ED. Three other PDE-5 inhibitors have since been approved by the FDA: avanafil (Stendra), vardenafil (Levitra, Staxyn), and tadalafil (Cialis). Drugs for ED are listed in Table 71.3.

The PDE-5 inhibitors do not cause an erection. They merely enhance the erection resulting from physical contact or other sexual stimuli by maintaining relaxation of the smooth muscle in the penis and increasing blood flow. These drugs are not as effective in promoting erections in men who do not have ED. Despite considerable research interest, PDE-5 inhibitors have no effects on female sexual function. These drugs are not approved for use by women.

The PDE-5 inhibitors are equally effective at promoting erections in 60 to 80% of male patients, and the adverse effects are similar. The most common adverse effects are nasal congestion, headache, facial flushing, and dizziness. These drugs produce a 5- to 10-mm fall in blood pressure, but this drop is usually not clinically important. In patients who are taking nitrates or multiple antihypertensive medications, however, this blood pressure change may produce symptoms of hypotension. Therefore, PDE-5 inhibitors are contraindicated in patients who are taking organic nitrates in any form. Organic nitrates include nitroglycerin and isosorbide mononitrate.

Alprostadil (Caverject, Edex, Muse) is an alternative for men who have contraindications to the use of PDE-5 inhibitors. Caverject and Edex formulations are self-injected directly into the corpora cavernosa just prior to intercourse. Muse is a pellet containing the drug that is inserted by an applicator into the urethra just prior to intercourse. Alprostadil by either method should not be used more than three times per week and not more than once in 24 hours. Penile pain, burning sensations, and priapism and, more rarely, penile fibrosis are adverse effects. The effectiveness of alprostadil is less than that of the PDE-5 inhibitors or intracavernosal injections, and the strength of the erection can be improved by using a constriction ring.

PROTOTYPE DRUG Sildenafil (Viagra)

Classification **Therapeutic:** Drug for treating impotence
Pharmacologic: Phosphodiesterase-5 inhibitor

Therapeutic Effects and Uses: Approved in 1998, sildenafil is a PO drug and was the first PDE-5 inhibitor approved for ED. The onset of action is relatively rapid (less than 1 hour), and its effects last up to 4 hours. The medication is taken 60 minutes prior to expected intercourse and should be used only once daily.

In 2005, sildenafil (Revatio) was approved for the treatment of pulmonary arterial HTN. For this indication, blocking PDE-5 in pulmonary vascular smooth muscle causes vasodilation and reduction in arterial HTN. The drug improves exercise capacity in these patients. The dosing for Revatio is 5 to 20 mg three times daily. Off-label indications include prevention of pulmonary HTN induced by altitude sickness and treatment of Raynaud's phenomena resistant to vasodilator therapy.

Mechanism of Action: Sildenafil inhibits PDE-5 and increases and preserves cGMP levels in the penis. This relaxes smooth muscle in the corpus cavernosa, allowing

Table 71.3 Drugs for Erectile Dysfunction

Drug	Route and Adult Dose (Maximum Dose Where Indicated)	Adverse Effects
avanafil (Stendra)	PO: 100 mg approximately 30 min before intercourse (max: 200 mg once/day)	*Nasal congestion, headache, facial flushing, dizziness, vision abnormalities, myalgia* Hypotension when taken with nitrates, priapism, hearing loss, nonarteritic anterior ischemic optic neuropathy
sildenafil (Viagra)	PO: 25–50 mg approximately 30–60 min before intercourse (max: 100 mg once/day)	
tadalafil (Cialis)	PO: 10 mg approximately 30 min before intercourse (max: 20 mg/day); once-daily dosing: 2.5–5 mg daily	
vardenafil (Levitra, Staxyn ODT)	PO: 10 mg approximately 1 h before intercourse (max: 20 mg once/day)	

Note: *Italics* indicate common adverse effects. Underline indicates serious adverse effects.

increased blood flow into the penis and allowing a harder and longer-lasting erection in about 70% of men taking the drug.

Pharmacokinetics:

Route(s)	PO
Absorption	Rapid; bioavailability: 40%
Distribution	96% protein bound
Primary metabolism	Hepatic (CYP3A4 and 2C9)
Primary excretion	80% feces, 12% renal
Onset of action	20–60 min
Duration of action	24 h; half-life: 4 h

Adverse Effects: Sildenafil is well tolerated and adverse effects are usually transient and mild. Common adverse effects include headache, dizziness, flushing, rash, and nasal congestion. The most serious adverse effect, hypotension, occurs in patients who are concurrently taking organic nitrates for angina and can result in MI and sudden cardiac death. Sildenafil can produce blurred vision, increased sensitivity to light, or changes in color perception in 10% of patients using it. Priapism, a sustained erection lasting longer than 6 hours, has been reported with sildenafil use and may lead to permanent damage of penile tissue.

Contraindications/Precautions: Sildenafil is contraindicated in patients who are taking nitrates and in those with hypersensitivity to this drug. It is contraindicated in patients with severe cardiovascular disease, recent MI, stroke, HF, or dysrhythmias, and in the presence of anatomic deformities of the penis. This drug should be used with caution in patients with CKD or hepatic impairment and periodic liver and kidney function tests should be evaluated. Patients with preexisting visual disturbances should not use sildenafil.

Drug Interactions: Cimetidine, erythromycin, and ketoconazole will increase serum levels of sildenafil and necessitate lower drug doses. Concurrent use with nitrates is contraindicated and will result in hypotension and possibly death. Protease inhibitors (amprenavir, ritonavir, others) will cause increased sildenafil levels, which may lead to toxicity. Rifampin may decrease sildenafil levels, leading to decreased effectiveness. Concurrent use of sildenafil with drugs that lower blood pressure, including $alpha_1$-adrenergic antagonists, should be avoided due to the potential for additive hypotension. **Herbal/Food:** Administration of sildenafil with high-fat meals should be avoided because absorption is decreased. Grapefruit juice increases the plasma concentrations of sildenafil and may cause adverse effects.

Pregnancy: Sildenafil did not show evidence of fetal harm in laboratory animals. Adverse effects on human pregnancy or breastfeeding are not known.

Treatment of Overdose: There is no specific treatment for overdose.

Drugs Similar to Sildenafil (Viagra)

The other PDE-5 inhibitors are avanafil, tadalafil, and vardenafil. Only sildenafil and tadalafil are indicated for use in women (for pulmonary arterial HTN). These drugs did not show evidence of fetal harm in laboratory animals. Adverse effects on human pregnancy or breastfeeding are not known.

Avanafil (Stendra): The newest ED drug, avanafil, was approved in 2012 and acts by the same mechanism as the other three PDE-5 inhibitors. It acts in 15 to 30 minutes, which is the fastest of the drugs in this class. It has a duration of about 6 hours, which is short compared to 36 hours for tadalafil. Avanafil may be taken twice daily. This drug's absorption is not affected by food. The adverse effects and contraindications are the same as those of other drugs in this class.

Tadalafil (Cialis): Initially approved in 2003, tadalafil acts by the same mechanism as sildenafil, which is relaxation of penile arterial and trabecular smooth muscle. This drug's absorption is not affected by food. It acts within about 60 minutes and has a longer duration of action than sildenafil: up to 36 hours. The longer duration allows for more spontaneity of sexual activity. Contraindications include patients who take nitrates, and dosing can be prescribed every 72 hours. Tadalafil produces less blood pressure decrease than the other drugs in this class, making it safer for patients with HF or a history of MI. It also results in a lower incidence of visual disturbances. Other adverse effects are similar to those of sildenafil. A daily dosing of 2.5-mg tadalafil for erectile dysfunction was approved in 2008.

Like sildenafil, tadalafil (Adcirca) is also approved to treat pulmonary arterial HTN. The dose for this indication is higher, at 40 mg/day. In 2011, tadalafil (Cialis) was

CONNECTIONS: Patient Safety

Increased Plasma Drug Concentrations

A 53-year-old man is prescribed sildenafil (Viagra) for treatment of erectile dysfunction. His medical history reveals no cardiovascular disease and no other medication use, and his blood pressure is within normal range. Later that evening, he is admitted to the emergency department with reports of chest pain and dizziness and has a blood pressure of 80/48 mmHg. The triage nurse notes in the electronic health record that the patient took two acetaminophen (Tylenol) tablets 4 hours before taking the sildenafil. A dietary history reveals that he follows a gluten-free diet and drinks three glasses of grapefruit juice daily. What is a potential cause of this patient's symptoms, and what should the nurse teach this patient?

approved for the symptomatic treatment of BPH. Although its exact mechanism is still being investigated, tadalafil is believed to reduce BPH symptoms by relaxing urinary smooth muscles and increasing blood perfusion and oxygenation of the bladder and prostatic tissue.

Vardenafil (Levitra, Staxyn ODT): Like other drugs in this class, vardenafil allows for relaxation of arterial and trabecular smooth muscle in the penis. Approved in 2003, vardenafil acts within 30 to 60 minutes and its effects continue for 4 to 5 hours. In 2010, an orally disintegrating tablet (ODT) form of this drug (Staxyn) was approved. Headache, flushing, rhinitis, and dyspepsia are the common adverse effects. Vardenafil may prolong the QT interval and is to be used with caution in patients who are taking nitrates. Administration with high-fat meals should be avoided because absorption is decreased.

Pathophysiology of Benign Prostatic Hyperplasia

71.7 Benign prostatic hyperplasia is an enlargement of the prostate that occurs in older men.

The prostate is a gland the size of a walnut that surrounds the male urethra. Its primary function is to contribute fluids to the ejaculate. The prostate contains two major types of tissues:

- *Epithelial tissue.* This is the glandular portion of the prostate that secretes fluids for the ejaculate. The growth of prostatic epithelial tissue is controlled by the presence of androgens. Testosterone is converted to its active metabolite, dihydrotestosterone (DHT), in the epithelial cells of the prostate by the enzyme 5-alpha reductase.
- *Stomal tissue.* This is smooth muscle tissue, which is controlled by alpha$_1$-adrenergic receptors. When activated, these receptors cause the smooth muscle to contract around the urethra.

Benign prostatic hyperplasia (BPH), an abnormal enlargement of the prostate, is the most common benign neoplasm in older men. The exact cause of BPH is unknown. It is present in 70% of men by age 60 and 90% by age 80. Other than age, the risk factors for BPH include a family history of the disorder, smoking, heavy alcohol consumption, HTN, diabetes, a diet high in meats and fats, and African American ancestry. BPH is not considered to be a precursor to prostate carcinoma, though it is well known that many men with BPH eventually experience prostate cancer.

The characteristic feature of BPH is an enlargement of the prostate gland that decreases the outflow of urine by obstructing the urethra, causing difficult urination. The pathogenesis of BPH involves two components: static and dynamic. The static factors are caused by the physical enlargement of the prostate gland due to the overgrowth of the epithelial cells. The gland can double or triple in size with aging, creating a blockage of urine outflow at the neck of the bladder. The dynamic factors are due to excessive numbers of alpha$_1$-adrenergic receptors located in stromal tissue in the neck of the urinary bladder and in the prostate gland. When activated, these receptors compress the urethra and provide resistance to urine outflow from the bladder. The two mechanisms of disease, static and dynamic, have led to two different classes of drugs for treating the symptoms of BPH. These mechanisms are shown in Pharmacotherapy Illustrated 71.1.

Certain frequently used medications may worsen symptoms of BPH. Alpha$_1$-adrenergic drugs, which include decongestants such as pseudoephedrine and phenylephrine, activate alpha$_1$-adrenergic receptors in the bladder neck, restricting urine flow. Drugs with anticholinergic effects such as antihistamines, TCAs, or phenothiazines may worsen the associated urinary retention. Testosterone and other anabolic steroids may increase prostate enlargement, which contributes to the physical obstruction of the urethra. Drugs that worsen symptoms of BPH should be avoided in older men.

There is no clear correlation between the symptoms experienced by patients and the size of the prostate. Some men may have minimal enlargement and experience moderate symptoms, whereas others may have extremely enlarged glands and be asymptomatic. This is because the smooth muscle in the urinary bladder has the ability to compensate for the obstruction by contracting with greater force to eject the urine stream. Over time, the bladder is no longer able to compensate and symptoms of BPH manifest, such as increased urinary frequency (usually with small amounts of urine), increased urgency to urinate, postvoid leakage, excessive nighttime urination (nocturia), decreased force of the urine stream, and a sensation that the bladder did not completely empty.

Some patients do not seek medical attention until complications caused by the long-standing obstruction at the neck of the urinary bladder arise. Serious complications include recurrent urinary infections, incontinence, gross hematuria, bladder stones, and CKD.

Pharmacotherapy of Benign Prostatic Hyperplasia

71.8 In its early stages, benign prostatic hyperplasia may be treated successfully with drug therapy.

The goal of treatment for patients with BPH focuses on minimizing the urinary obstruction and preventing complications. Drug therapy can only treat symptoms; it cannot reverse or cure BPH. Patients who are asymptomatic or who

Pharmacotherapy Illustrated 71.1

Mechanism of Action of Antiprostatic Drugs

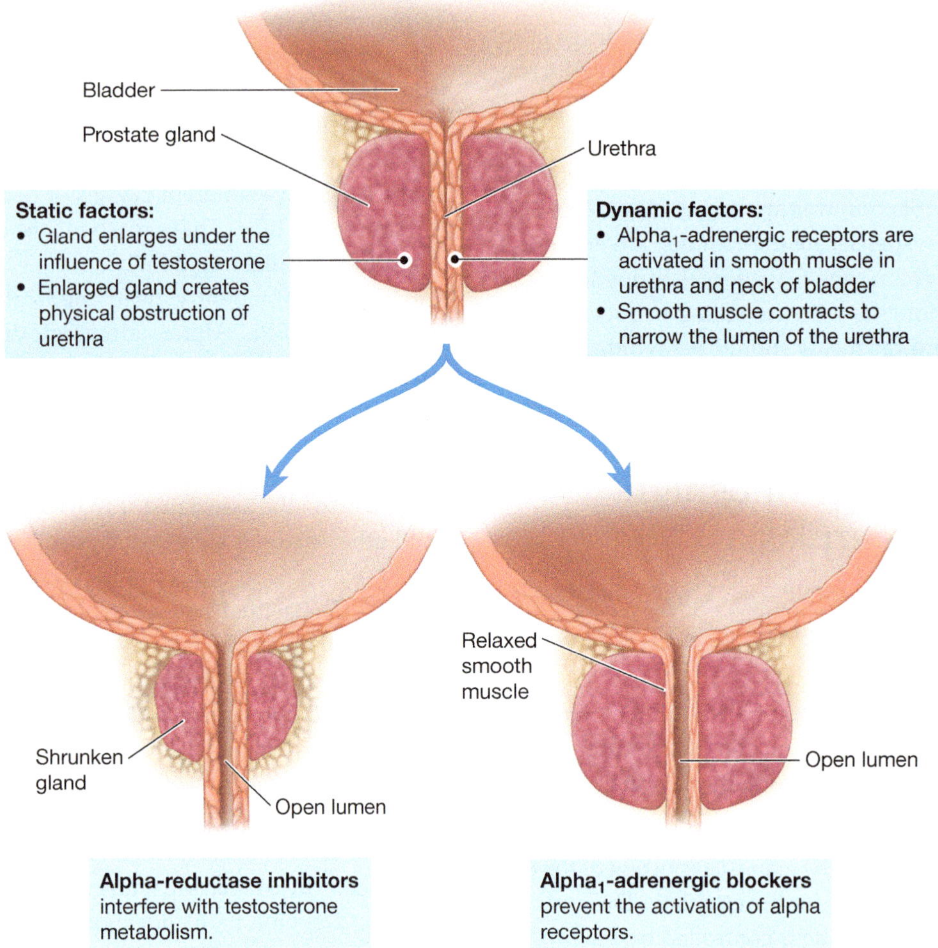

present with mild symptoms generally do not receive pharmacotherapy. Not all BPH is progressive, and many patients never experience moderate or advanced symptoms. Patient education such as avoiding caffeine or alcohol intake, eliminating drugs that worsen BPH, and restricting fluids close to bedtime may be sufficient to achieve symptomatic improvement. Morning diuretic therapy may be used to reduce nighttime diuresis. The patient is reevaluated at 6- to 12-month intervals to assess for worsening symptoms.

When symptoms of BPH worsen, pharmacotherapy is indicated. Only a few drugs are available for the pharmacotherapy of BPH, and these are listed in Table 71.4. Drugs that are used to treat BPH have limited effectiveness and have value only in treating mild to moderate disease as an alternative to surgery. Because pharmacotherapy does not cure the disease, these medications must be taken for the remainder of the patient's life or until surgery is indicated. If the drugs are discontinued, the prostate returns back to its enlarged state and symptoms of BPH return. In advanced cases, transurethral resection of the prostate or a laser prostatectomy is needed to restore the patency of the urethra.

The major drug classes for treating BPH are the alpha$_1$-adrenergic antagonists and the 5-alpha reductase inhibitors. Research has shown that combination therapy with an alpha$_1$ antagonist and a 5-alpha reductase inhibitor is more effective than therapy with either drug alone. This is the preferred treatment for patients with moderate symptoms of BPH. More recently, tadalafil (Cialis), a PDE-5 inhibitor, joined the list of approved drugs for BPH.

The alpha$_1$-adrenergic antagonists act on the stromal tissue of the prostate to relax smooth muscle in the prostate gland, bladder neck, and urethra, thus easing the urinary obstruction. Doxazosin (Cardura) and terazosin (Hytrin) are of particular value to patients who have both HTN and BPH; these two disorders occur concurrently in about 25% of men older than age 60. Three alpha$_1$ antagonists—silodosin

Table 71.4 Drugs for Benign Prostatic Hyperplasia

Drug	Route and Adult Dose (Maximum Dose Where Indicated)	Adverse Effects
Alpha$_1$-Adrenergic Antagonists		
alfuzosin (Uroxatral)	PO: 10 mg/day (max: 10 mg/day)	*Orthostatic hypotension, headache, dizziness, decreased libido, decreased ejaculate volume* First-dose phenomenon (severe hypotension and syncope), tachycardia
doxazosin (Cardura)	PO: 1–8 mg/day (max: 8 mg/day)	
doxazosin XL (Cardura XL)	Extended release: 4–8 mg/day (max: 8 mg/day)	
silodosin (Rapaflo)	PO: 8 mg once daily with a meal	
tamsulosin (Flomax)	PO: 0.4 mg 30 min after a meal (max: 0.8 mg/day)	
terazosin (Hytrin)	PO: Start with 1 mg at bedtime, then 1–5 mg/day (max: 20 mg/day)	
5-Alpha Reductase Inhibitors		
dutasteride (Avodart)	PO: 0.5 mg/day	*Sexual dysfunction, decreased libido, decreased ejaculate volume, gynecomastia* Possible increased risk for prostate cancer
finasteride (Proscar)	PO: 5 mg/day (max: 5 mg/day)	
Phosphodiesterase-5 Inhibitors		
tadalafil (Cialis)	PO: 5 mg once daily	See Table 71.3.

Note: *Italics* indicate common adverse effects. Underline indicates serious adverse effects.

(Rapaflo), tamsulosin (Flomax), and alfuzosin (Uroxatral)—are selective for the prostate and have no effect on blood pressure at normal doses. Drugs in this class improve urine flow and reduce other symptoms of BPH after 1 to 2 weeks of therapy. Common adverse effects include headache, fatigue, and dizziness. Doxazosin and terazosin are not associated with an increased risk of sexual dysfunction, but ejaculatory disorders have been reported with silodosin, tamsulosin, and alfuzosin. Reflex tachycardia due to stimulation of baroreceptors is common with alpha$_1$ antagonists. Additional information on the alpha$_1$ antagonists is presented in Chapter 16.

Some patients are unable to tolerate the cardiovascular adverse effects of the alpha$_1$-adrenergic antagonists. For these patients, the 5-alpha reductase inhibitors are used as monotherapy. These drugs act by blocking 5-alpha reductase, the enzyme responsible for converting testosterone to DHT, which is its active metabolite. Without DHT the hormonal signal for prostatic epithelial tissue growth is eliminated, thus causing the enlarged prostate to shrink in size. The most commonly prescribed drug in this class is finasteride (Proscar), which is featured below as a prototype for BPH. These drugs may take several months to shrink the size of the prostate; thus, they are not appropriate for severe disease. The 5-alpha reductase inhibitors produce few adverse effects, although they can cause sexual dysfunction and gynecomastia in some men.

CONNECTIONS: Complementary and Alternative Therapies

Saw Palmetto

Description

Saw palmetto (*Serenoa repens*) is a dwarf palm tree that grows in the coastal regions of the southern United States. The berries of the saw palmetto are used in supplements. More than 2 million men in the United States use saw palmetto each year in the hopes that it will treat their symptoms of BPH.

History and Claims

Like finasteride, saw palmetto is thought to help stop a cascade of prostate-damaging enzymes that may create BPH. In theory, it occupies binding sites on the prostate that are typically occupied by DHT, an enzyme that may trigger BPH, inhibiting growth of the prostate gland.

Standardization

Saw palmetto is available in capsule, tablet, and liquid dosage forms. PO saw palmetto products should be standardized to contain 80% or more of the active ingredients, which are fatty acids.

Evidence

Although several clinical studies have suggested that saw palmetto may be beneficial in treating BPH symptoms, two large well-conducted studies demonstrated no conclusive evidence to demonstrate that it is as effective as finasteride in treating mild to moderate BPH and does not have effects on PSA (National Center for Complementary and Integrative Health, 2020). Although considered a safe supplement, GI distress and headache are common adverse effects and saw palmetto may cause damage to the liver and pancreas. It is important that the nurse obtain a thorough health and supplement use history and advise the patient of its potential adverse effects.

CONNECTION Checkpoint 71.3

Alpha$_1$-adrenergic antagonists are very susceptible to causing the first-dose phenomenon. From what you learned in Chapter 16, define this phenomenon and describe what should be done to minimize its effects.

PROTOTYPE DRUG Finasteride (Proscar)

Classification **Therapeutic:** Drug for BPH
Pharmacologic: Antiandrogen, 5-alpha reductase inhibitor

Therapeutic Effects and Uses: Approved in 1992, finasteride is a PO drug that inhibits the metabolism of testosterone. The drug is sometimes called an antiandrogen. Finasteride shrinks enlarged prostates, helping to restore urinary function. It is most effective in patients with larger prostates. It is sometimes prescribed in combination with doxazosin to reduce the risk of symptomatic progression of BPH. This drug is also marketed as Propecia, which is prescribed to promote hair regrowth in patients with male-pattern baldness. Doses of finasteride are five times higher when prescribed for BPH than when prescribed for baldness.

Off-label indications for finasteride take advantage of its antiandrogen effects. It may be used to treat mild to moderate hirsutism in females. Although some clinical trials suggested the drug exerted a protective effect against prostate cancer, the drug insert from the manufacturer clearly states it is not to be prescribed for this purpose.

Mechanism of Action: Finasteride acts by inhibiting 5-alpha reductase, which is the enzyme responsible for converting testosterone to one of its metabolites, 5-alpha dihydrotestosterone. This active metabolite causes proliferation of prostate cells and promotes enlargement of the gland. Finasteride promotes regression of prostate epithelial tissue and decreases mechanical obstruction of the urethra.

Pharmacokinetics:

Route(s)	PO
Absorption	Well absorbed
Distribution	Crosses the blood–brain barrier; found in semen; 90% bound to plasma protein
Primary metabolism	Hepatic (CYP3A4)
Primary excretion	39% renal, 57% feces
Onset of action	Maximum effects take 3–6 months
Duration of action	2 weeks

Adverse Effects: Finasteride is well tolerated and adverse effects are generally mild and transient. Finasteride causes various types of sexual dysfunction in up to 16% of patients, including gynecomastia, impotence, diminished libido, and ejaculatory disorders such as decreased volume of ejaculate. The drug reduces sperm production and may impair fertility. The actual incidence of drug-induced sexual dysfunction is difficult to estimate because a large percentage of older men develop these symptoms as a consequence of aging or comorbid conditions. Other minor adverse effects include headache, nausea, rash, dizziness, and asthenia. Men over age 55 may have a slightly increased risk of developing high-grade prostate cancer.

Contraindications/Precautions: Contraindications to finasteride include hypersensitivity to the drug, and use in women and children. The pregnant nurse or pharmacist should avoid handling crushed medication because it may be absorbed through the skin and cause harm to a male fetus. Caution must be used when administering the drug to patients with CKD or hepatic impairment.

Drug Interactions: Use with anticholinergics may decrease the effects of finasteride. Use of finasteride with testosterone will result in a reduction in the effects of both drugs. **Herbal/Food:** Saw palmetto may potentiate the effects of finasteride.

Pregnancy: Finasteride is not approved for use in women.

Treatment of Overdose: There is no specific treatment for overdose.

Clinician Responsibilities: Key clinical implications for patients receiving finasteride are included in Applied Clinical Judgment: Patients Receiving Pharmacotherapy for Benign Prostatic Hyperplasia.

Drugs Similar to Finasteride (Proscar)

The only other 5-alpha reductase inhibitor is dutasteride.

Dutasteride (Avodart): Approved in 2001, dutasteride is a PO drug approved only for the treatment of BPH. Compared to finasteride, dutasteride causes a greater inhibition of 5-alpha reductase and thus is able to more effectively lower DHT levels. Dutasteride has a half-life of 5 weeks and it remains in the body for several months after the drug is stopped. Like finasteride, sexual adverse effects such as reduced ejaculate volume, diminished libido, and ED occur in some patients. Other warnings, contraindications, and actions are the same as those of finasteride. Jalyn is a fixed-dose combination drug that contains dutasteride with tamsulosin. Dutasteride is not indicated for use in women.

CONNECTIONS: APPLIED CLINICAL JUDGMENT

Patients Receiving Pharmacotherapy for Benign Prostatic Hyperplasia

Key Assessment Data

- Health history including cardiovascular, peripheral vascular, thyroid, hepatic, or kidney disease, diabetes, prostatic hyperplasia, or prostatic cancer; baseline vital signs, physical exam findings; CBC, electrolytes, glucose, lipid levels.

Desired Therapeutic Outcomes

Improvement is observed and measurable by increased urinary stream and lessened urinary retention.

Minimizing Adverse Effects

- 5-alpha reductase inhibitors may cause urinary frequency, nocturia, or hesitancy.

Lifespan Considerations

- Age-related physiologic differences may place the older adult at greater risk for hepatotoxicity.
- Be cautious with the older adult who has a greater risk for falls if $alpha_1$-adrenergic antagonists are used. Ensure patient safety.
- 5-alpha reductase inhibitors have teratogenic effects and handling by women of childbearing age should be avoided. Men should wear condoms during sexual activity and should not donate blood while taking the drug and up to 1 month after stopping the drug.

Diversity Considerations

- Because finasteride metabolizes through the CYP450 system pathways, monitor ethnically diverse patients to ensure optimal therapeutic effects and to minimize adverse effects.

Patient Education

- Full therapeutic effects from 5-alpha reductase inhibitors may take 3 to 6 months to be achieved. Consistent dosing is needed to ensure therapeutic effects.
- Promptly report urinary hesitancy, frequency, or an increase in nocturia.
- If 5-alpha reductase inhibitor drugs are prescribed, take the first dose of medication at bedtime and avoid driving for 12 to 24 hours after the first dose, or when the dosage is increased, until the effects are known. If dizziness occurs, sit or lie down and do not attempt to stand or walk until the sensation passes. Monitor blood pressure on a weekly basis and weigh self daily. Report any weight gain of 1 kg (2 lb) in 24 hours or 2 kg (5 lb) in 1 week or any peripheral edema. Do not stop the medication abruptly and call the healthcare provider for instructions if unable to take the medication for more than 2 days due to illness.
- Immediately report any symptoms of abdominal or right upper quadrant discomfort or pain, yellowing of the skin or sclera, fatigue, anorexia, darkened urine, clay-colored stools, weakness, lethargy, nausea or vomiting.
- Keep 5-alpha reductase inhibitor drugs in a secure location to guard against unintentional exposure to women of childbearing age or children. Use condoms consistently to avoid exposing women of childbearing age to semen, which may also contain the drug. Do not donate blood during the time the drug is taken and up to 1 month after the drug is stopped.

Prescribing Considerations

- Hepatotoxicity is a potential adverse effect and hepatic function tests should be assessed throughout drug therapy.
- $Alpha_1$-adrenergic antagonists may cause reflex tachycardia. At normal doses they do not cause significant hypotension but may induce a first-dose phenomenon and trigger sodium and water retention with resulting increases in weight, blood pressure, and possible edema. The drug should not be stopped abruptly as rebound HTN and tachycardia may occur.
- Finasteride is the most common 5-alpha reductase inhibitor and has a very low risk of adverse effects and few interactions with other medications. The dosage is 5mg/day with no dose modification needed for age or chronic renal failure.

Understanding Chapter 71

Key Concepts Summary

71.1 Male reproductive function is controlled through the secretion of androgens.

71.2 Androgens are used to treat hypogonadism and delayed puberty in males and breast cancer in females.

71.3 Often abused by athletes, anabolic steroids can cause serious adverse effects.

71.4 Male sexual dysfunction may have both medical and psychologic etiologies.

71.5 Male infertility is treated with endocrine drugs that boost sperm production.

71.6 Erectile dysfunction is a common disorder that may be successfully treated with inhibitors of the enzyme phosphodiesterase-5.

71.7 Benign prostatic hyperplasia is an enlargement of the prostate that occurs in older men.

71.8 In its early stages, benign prostatic hyperplasia may be treated successfully with drug therapy.

CASE STUDY: Making the Patient Connection

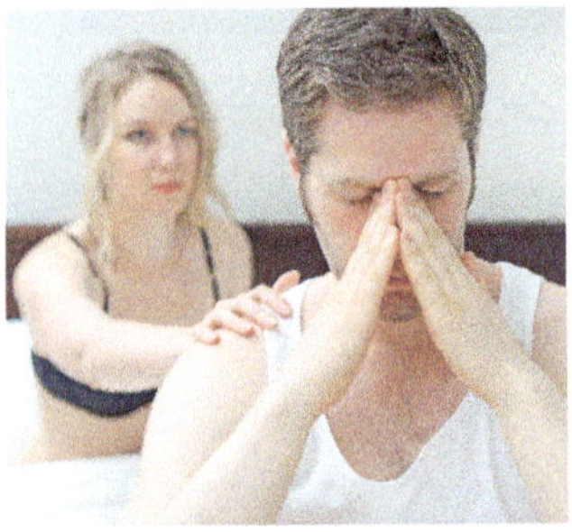

Remember the patient "Mike Mayhew" at the beginning of the chapter? Now read the remainder of the case study. Based on the information presented within this chapter, respond to the critical thinking questions that follow.

One year after his divorce, Mike, a 34-year-old man, began dating and soon met Dana. The couple found that they had a lot in common and enjoyed each other's company. As the relationship grew, the couple became more intimate and sexually involved. However, the emotional scars from his previous marriage were painful and affected him deeply.

After the divorce, Mike was depressed and had low self-esteem. The condition required short-term hospitalization, and he now follows up on an outpatient basis with a psychiatrist. He has been taking antidepressants and was recently prescribed tadalafil (Cialis) for a diagnosis of ED. Mike also has a past history of HTN and is taking nifedipine (Procardia).

Critical Thinking Questions

1. What factors in Mike's life and health history do you think are contributing to the diagnosis of ED?
2. If you were the nurse, what patient education instructions would you provide to Mike regarding administration of tadalafil along with nifedipine?
3. After considering both options, Mike would rather be prescribed sildenafil (Viagra) instead of tadalafil. What should the healthcare provider discuss with Mike about this request?

Additional Case Study

Morrie Jones, a 72-year-old man, has been having difficulty with urinary frequency and excessive nighttime urination. He scheduled an appointment with his healthcare provider and is diagnosed with BPH. He is prescribed finasteride (Proscar) and needs to see his healthcare provider again in 6 months.

1. How would you explain the purpose of finasteride in treating BPH?
2. What education would you provide Mr. Jones that he may find helpful in dealing with BPH?
3. What additional health history and physical assessment findings would be considered in diagnosing this condition?

Chapter Review

1. An adult patient has been receiving testosterone (Testoderm) for the treatment of primary hypogonadism. Which laboratory test would the nurse monitor to determine that this drug therapy is effective?
   1. RBC count
   2. Sperm count
   3. FSH
   4. LH
2. The patient with erectile dysfunction is being evaluated for pharmacotherapy. Which question should the nurse ask prior to initiating therapy with sildenafil (Viagra)?
   1. "Are you currently taking medications for angina?"
   2. "Do you have a history of diabetes?"
   3. "Have you ever had an allergic reaction to penicillin products?"
   4. "Have you ever been treated for gastric ulcers?"
3. The nurse is teaching a patient who has received a prescription testosterone gel for treatment of symptoms related to low androgen levels. What instructions should the nurse give the patient? (Select all that apply.)
   1. "Apply the gel to the scrotal and perineal area daily."
   2. "Avoid exposing women to the gel or to areas of skin where gel has been applied."
   3. "Report any weight gain over 2 kilograms (5 pounds) in 1 week's time."
   4. "Avoid showering or swimming for at least 12 to 14 hours after applying the gel."
   5. "Maintain a low-fat diet and return periodically for blood lipid laboratory studies."

4. The nurse is counseling a patient about the goal of therapy with sildenafil (Viagra). What will the nurse teach the patient about the drug's effects?
   1. It should always result in a penile erection within 10 minutes.
   2. It is not effective if sexual dysfunction is psychologic in nature.
   3. It will result in less intense feelings with prolonged use.
   4. It may heighten sexual response in female partners.

5. The nurse is teaching the patient about the use of silodosin (Rapaflo). What patient teaching related to this medication is needed? (Select all that apply.)
   1. Silodosin promotes shrinkage of an enlarged prostate and helps restore urinary function.
   2. The drug should not be handled by women who may be pregnant.
   3. Headache, fatigue, and dizziness are common adverse effects.
   4. The drug should not be stopped abruptly because rebound HTN may occur.
   5. The drug may cause dizziness, which can be avoided by making position changes slowly.

6. A patient who has taken finasteride (Proscar) for the past 8 months reports a sudden increase in urinary hesitancy, urinary retention, and slowing of the urinary stream. What will the nurse teach this patient to do?
   1. Continue to take the drug to achieve full effects.
   2. Decrease the intake of coffee, tea, and alcohol.
   3. Discuss the use of a low-dose diuretic with the healthcare provider.
   4. Return to the healthcare provider for a prostate exam.

See Appendix A for answers to critical thinking questions, case study questions, and review questions.

References

National Center for Complementary and Integrative Health. (2020). *Saw palmetto.* https://www.nccih.nih.gov/health/saw-palmetto

Selected Bibliography

Centers for Disease Control and Prevention (CDC). (2020). *Prostate cancer.* http://www.cdc.gov/cancer/prostate

Deters, L.A. (2019). *Benign prostatic hypertrophy*. Medscape. http://emedicine.medscape.com/article/437359-overview#a1

Duca, Y., Calogero, A. E., Cannarella, R., Condorelli, R. A., & La Vignera, S. (2019). Current and emerging medical therapeutic agents for idiopathic male infertility. *Expert Opinion on Pharmacotherapy, 20*(1), 55–67. https://doi.org/10.1080/14656566.2018.1543405

Dornbier, R., Pahouja, G., Branch, J., & McVary, K. T. (2020). The new American Urological Association Benign Prostatic Hyperplasia Clinical Guidelines: 2019 update. *Current Urology Reports, 21*(9), 32. https://doi.org/10.1007/s11934-020-00985-0

Kim, E. D. (2020). *Erectile dysfunction*. Medscape. http://emedicine.medscape.com/article/444220-overview

Matsui, H., Sopko, N. A., Hannan, J. L., & Bivalacqua, T. J. (2015). Pathophysiology of erectile dysfunction. *Current Drug Targets, 16*(5), 411–419. https://doi.org/10.2174/1389450116605150504114041

Morgentaler, A., Traish, A., Hackett, G., Jones, T. H., & Ramasamy, R. (2019). Diagnosis and treatment of testosterone deficiency: Updated recommendations from the Lisbon 2018 International Consultation for Sexual Medicine. *Sexual Medicine Reviews, 7*(4), 636–649. https://doi.org/10.1038/s41572-019-0087-y

Patel, D. P., Pastuszak, A. W., & Hotaling, J. M. (2019). Emerging treatments for erectile dysfunction: a review of novel, non-surgical options. *Current Urology Reports, 20*(8), 44. https://doi.org/10.1007/s11934-019-0908-2

Retzler, K. (2019). Erectile dysfunction: A review of comprehensive treatment options for optimal outcome. *Journal of Restorative Medicine, 8*(1). https://doi.org/10.14200/jrm.2019.0104

Unit 11
Additional Drug Classes

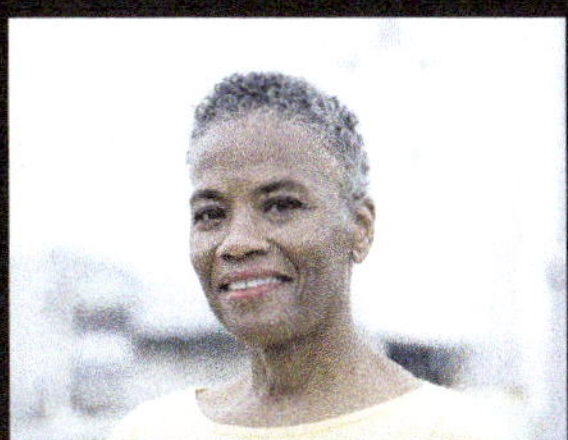
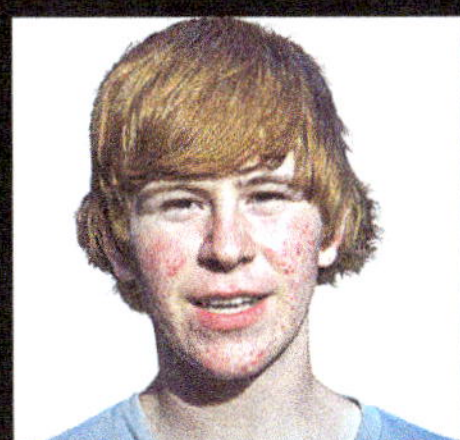
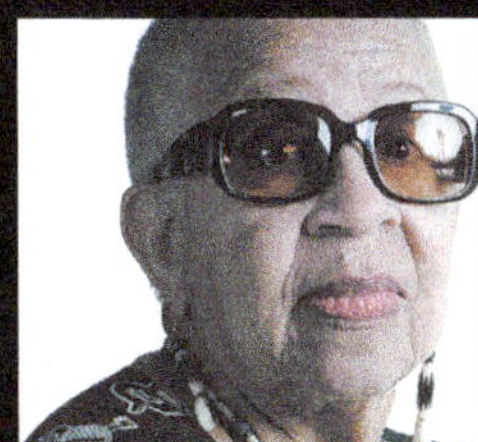
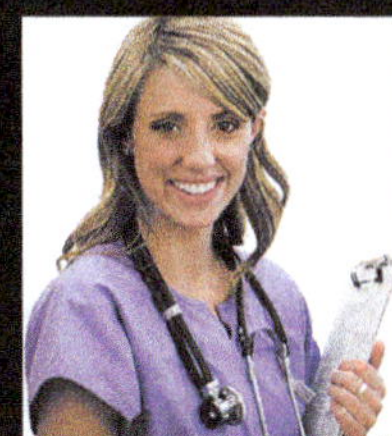

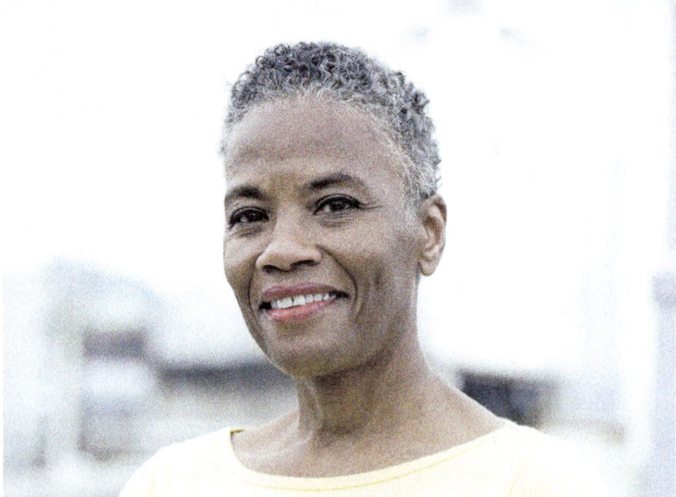

"My clothes just don't seem to fit right anymore. My pant legs are dragging on the ground. Is it possible that I'm getting shorter?"
—*Patient "Charlene Coleman"*

Chapter 72
Pharmacotherapy of Bone and Joint Disorders

Chapter Outline

- Role of Calcium in Body Homeostasis
- Regulation of Calcium Balance
- Pharmacotherapy of Calcium Imbalances
  - Treatment of Hypocalcemia
  - **PROTOTYPE** *Calcium Salts, p. 1260*
  - Treatment of Hypercalcemia
- Pathophysiology of Metabolic Bone Disease
  - Osteoporosis
  - Osteomalacia
  - Paget's Disease
- Pharmacotherapy of Metabolic Bone Disease
  - Vitamin D Therapy
  - **PROTOTYPE** *Calcitriol (Rocaltrol), p. 1265*
  - Bisphosphonates
  - **PROTOTYPE** *Alendronate (Fosamax), p. 1267*
  - Selective Estrogen Receptor Modulators
  - **PROTOTYPE** *Raloxifene (Evista), p. 1270*
  - Calcitonin and Miscellaneous Drugs
- Pathophysiology and Pharmacotherapy of Joint Disorders
  - Osteoarthritis
  - Rheumatoid Arthritis
  - **PROTOTYPE** *Adalimumab (Humira), p. 1277*
- Pharmacotherapy of Gout and Hyperuricemia
  - **PROTOTYPE** *Colchicine (Colcrys), p. 1282*
  - **PROTOTYPE** *Allopurinol (Lopurin, Zyloprim), p. 1284*

Learning Outcomes

After reading this chapter, the student should be able to:

1. Describe the role of calcium in maintaining homeostasis in the nervous, muscular, skeletal, and cardiovascular systems.
2. Identify the recommended dietary allowance and the normal serum levels of calcium.
3. Explain the roles of parathyroid hormone, calcitonin, and vitamin D in maintaining calcium balance.
4. Explain the etiology, pathogenesis, and pharmacotherapy for hypocalcemia, hypercalcemia, osteomalacia, osteoporosis, rickets, osteoarthritis, rheumatoid arthritis, and gout.
5. Describe the nurse's role in the pharmacologic management of bone and joint disorders.
6. For each of the classes shown in the chapter outline, identify the prototype and representative drugs and explain the mechanism(s) of drug action, primary indications, contraindications, significant drug interactions, pregnancy data, and important adverse effects.
7. Apply clinical judgment to the care of patients receiving pharmacotherapy for bone and joint disorders.

Key Terms Definitions of the terms in bold may be found in the Glossary.

Disorders associated with bones and joints can lead to immobility and affect a patient's ability to fulfill activities of daily living (ADLs). In addition, the skeletal system serves as the primary repository for calcium, which is one of the body's most important minerals.

This chapter focuses on the pharmacotherapy of important skeletal and joint disorders such as osteomalacia, osteoporosis, arthritis, and gout. The importance of calcium balance and the action of vitamin D are stressed because they are critical to the proper structure and function of bones.

Role of Calcium in Body Homeostasis

72.1 Adequate levels of calcium in the body are necessary to transmit nerve impulses, to prevent muscle spasms, and for proper bone health.

Calcium balance is critical to the proper functioning of the nervous, muscular, skeletal, and cardiovascular systems. In the nervous system calcium ions influence the release of neurotransmitters and the excitability of all neurons. Contraction is dependent on calcium ion movement in skeletal, smooth, and cardiac muscle cells. Calcium is important for the normal functioning of other body processes such as blood coagulation by converting prothrombin into thrombin and in activating enzymes that catalyze many essential chemical reactions.

Calcium is the major cation for the structure of the bones and teeth. Total body content of calcium is about 1200 g or approximately 2% of the total body weight. More than 99% of that calcium is in the skeletal system and is bound as a hard matrix known as hydroxyapatite crystals. Only about 1% of the calcium in bone is rapidly exchangeable with blood calcium; the remaining calcium is more stable and slowly exchanged.

Much of the calcium found outside of bone circulates in the blood. Calcium exists in plasma in three forms: ionized, bound, and complexed. About 50% of the serum calcium is in an active, ionized form that participates in intracellular functions, including neuromuscular activity and blood coagulation. This is the only physiologically and clinically significant form of calcium. An adequate amount of free or ionized calcium is required for normal body functions. Most of the remaining 50% of calcium in plasma is bound to plasma proteins, primarily albumin, and other substances and is unavailable for general use by the body.

To maintain homeostasis, the body must obtain sufficient amounts of calcium through proper nutrition and dietary supplements, if needed. Unfortunately, only 30 to 50% of dietary calcium is absorbed from the small intestine. The amount absorbed, however, is dynamic and changes with body conditions. Absorption is increased by moderate amounts of fat or high protein intake, high gastric acidity, and when certain hormones are secreted in response to low blood calcium. Decreased absorption occurs with vitamin D deficiency, high-fat diet, decreased gastric acidity, certain hormones secreted in response to high blood calcium, and conditions that increase gastrointestinal (GI) motility such as diarrhea. Dietary calcium that remains unabsorbed is excreted in feces. Calcium can also be lost through the nails, hair, sweat, and other body fluids. In lactating women, large amounts are lost through breast milk.

The recommended dietary allowance (RDA) of calcium for healthy adults is 1000 to 1200 mg/day. Higher amounts are needed by pregnant and lactating women, growing children, and postmenopausal women, as given in Table 72.1. The best dietary sources of calcium are dairy products. The calcium found in milk is the most readily available form because milk contains sufficient amounts of vitamin D, which is necessary for calcium absorption. Other rich sources of calcium include seafood, such as salmon, oysters, and clams, and green leafy vegetables, such as kale, broccoli, spinach, and mustard greens. If the body does not obtain enough dietary calcium, it will remove calcium from the bones, resulting in bones that become soft and weakened and that eventually develop osteoporosis. The importance of meeting the daily RDA for calcium is vital to both women and men. Although not as prevalent, men may develop bone conditions such as osteoporosis, and adequate calcium intake should be added to their list of preventive healthcare interventions.

Table 72.1 Recommended Dietary Allowances for Calcium

Age/Condition	U.S. RDA (mg)
0–6 months	200
7–12 months	260
1–3 years	700
4–8 years	1000
9–18 years	1300
19–50 years	1000
51–70 years	1000 (men) 1200 (women)
71+	1200
Pregnant and lactating women (14–18 years)	1300
Pregnant and lactating women (19–50 years)	1000

The normal serum calcium range varies widely and is dependent on gender, age, and season. A normal reference range may be considered 8.5 to 10.5 mg/dL. Serum calcium concentrations that exceed 11.5 mg/dL result in symptoms of hypercalcemia, which causes a decrease in sodium permeability across cell membranes. This is a dangerous state because nerve conduction depends on the proper influx of sodium into cells. When calcium levels in the bloodstream are below 8.0 mg/dL, a state of hypocalcemia develops and the cell membranes become hyperexcitable. If this situation becomes severe, convulsions or muscle spasms may result.

PharmFACT

In the United States, over 2 million osteoporotic fractures occur each year. It is estimated that almost 10 million individuals have osteoporosis (Bethel, 2020).

Regulation of Calcium Balance

72.2 Calcium balance is regulated by parathyroid hormone, calcitonin, and vitamin D.

Calcium balance is controlled by parathyroid hormone, calcitonin, and vitamin D. Acting together, these three substances regulate the rate of absorption of calcium from the small intestine, the excretion of calcium from the kidney, and the movement of calcium into and out of bone. Calcium balance is illustrated in Figure 72.1.

Parathyroid hormone: Parathyroid hormone (PTH) is secreted from the parathyroid gland, as illustrated in Figure 72.1. The parathyroid glands contain calcium receptors that are able to sense very small changes in serum calcium concentration. When the serum levels of ionized calcium decrease, the parathyroid glands secrete PTH. PTH directly increases calcium reabsorption in the renal tubule and releases calcium from bone (resorption). PTH indirectly increases serum calcium by promoting the formation of activated vitamin D, which then increases calcium absorption from the GI tract. The overall effect of these physiologic changes is to rapidly (within minutes) increase serum calcium, returning it to normal levels.

The parathyroid glands are regulated by a typical negative feedback loop. An increase in the ionized serum calcium is recognized by calcium receptors in the parathyroid gland, which suppress PTH secretion. A second piece of the negative feedback loop is that activated vitamin D also shuts down PTH secretion. Without PTH present, the absorption of calcium from the GI tract is diminished, the reabsorption in the kidney tubule decreases, and calcium remains deposited in bone.

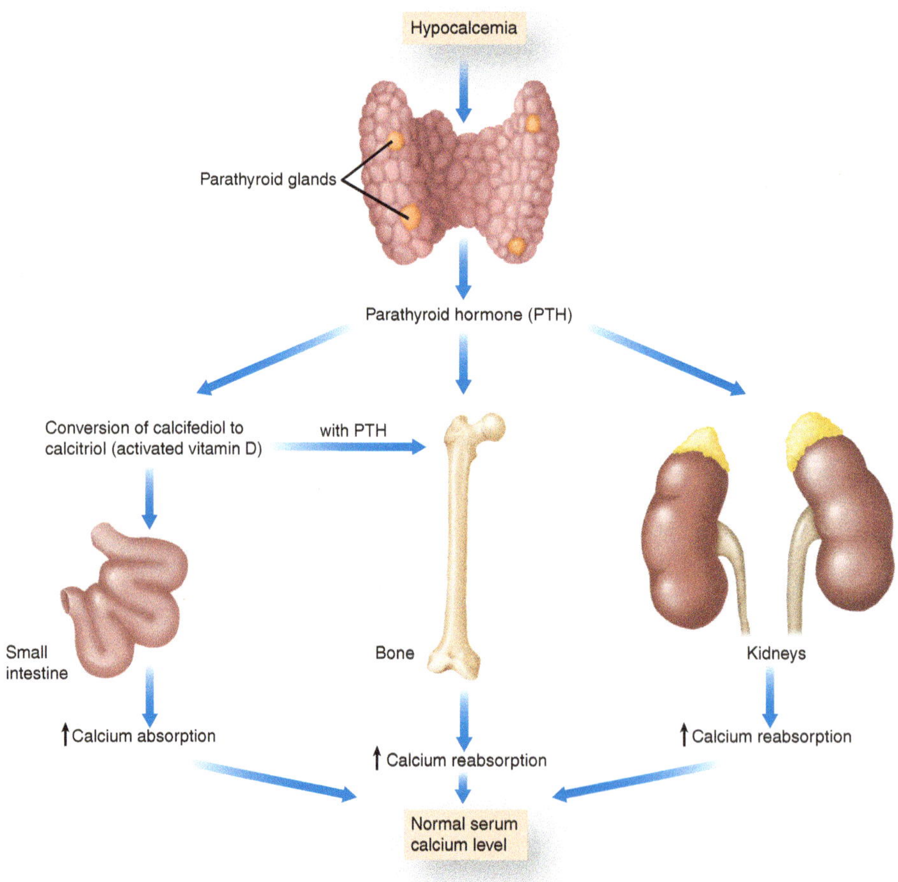

Figure 72.1 Calcium balance.

The exchange of calcium between the serum and bones is influenced by PTH and calcitonin. PTH stimulates bone cells called osteoclasts. These cells accelerate the process of **bone resorption**, or demineralization, which breaks down bone into its mineral components. Once bone is broken down (resorbed), calcium becomes available to be transported and used elsewhere in the body. The opposite of this process is **bone deposition**, or bone building, which is accomplished by cells called osteoblasts. This process, which removes calcium from the blood to be placed in bone, is stimulated by the hormone calcitonin. It is important to note that maintaining normal serum calcium levels takes precedence over the calcium requirements of the bone. If serum calcium levels are low, bone resorption will occur even if it compromises the structural integrity of the bone matrix.

Calcitonin: When serum calcium levels become elevated, the hormone **calcitonin** is released by the thyroid gland. Calcitonin acts in opposition to PTH and vitamin D to decrease the plasma levels of calcium by inhibiting the resorption of calcium from bone and increasing the excretion of calcium by the kidney, thus decreasing the concentration of serum calcium. It is important to note that calcitonin does not affect the rates of calcium absorption from the small intestine. Calcitonin is available as a medication for the treatment of osteoporosis.

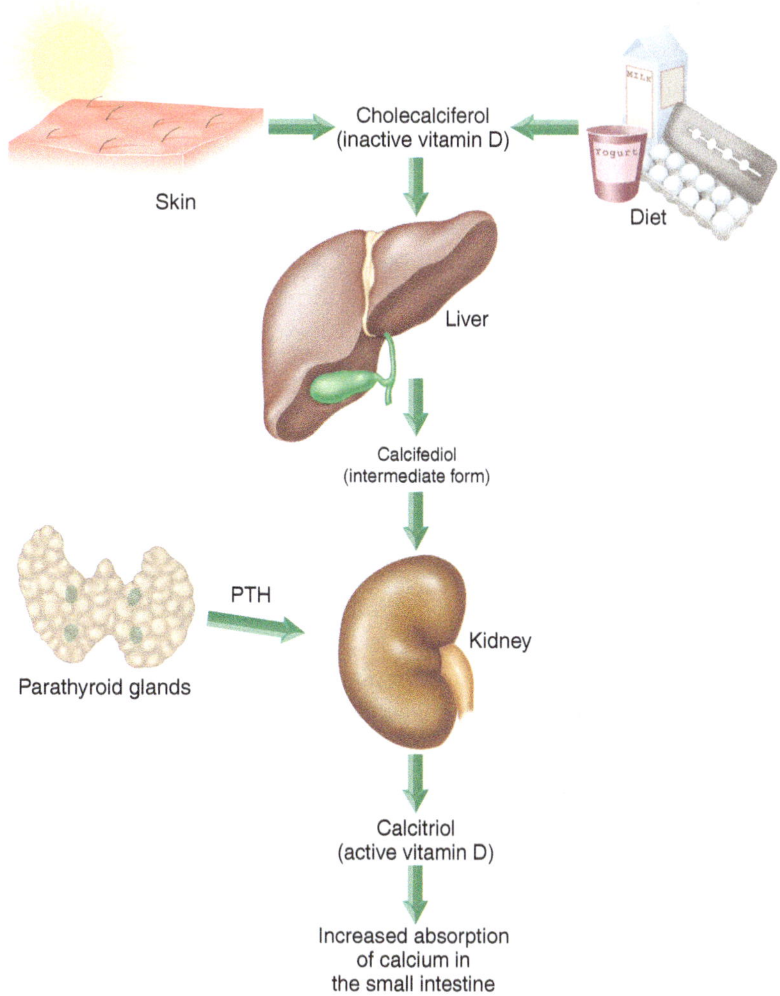

Figure 72.2 Pathway for vitamin D activation.

Vitamin D: Vitamin D and calcium metabolism are intimately related: Absorption of calcium is increased in the presence of vitamin D, and absorption is inhibited by vitamin D deficiency. Thus, calcium disorders are often associated with vitamin D disorders.

Vitamin D is unique among vitamins because it is the only vitamin that the body is able to synthesize from precursor molecules. Several steps, however, are required before vitamin D can act on target tissues, as illustrated in Figure 72.2. In the skin, **cholecalciferol**, the inactive form of vitamin D, is synthesized from cholesterol. Exposure of the skin to sunlight or ultraviolet light increases the level of cholecalciferol in the blood. Cholecalciferol can also be obtained from dietary products such as milk or other foods fortified with vitamin D.

Following its absorption from dietary sources or formation in the skin, cholecalciferol is converted to an intermediate vitamin form called calcifediol. Kidney enzymes metabolize calcifediol to **calcitriol**, the active form of vitamin D. PTH stimulates the formation of calcitriol at the level of the kidneys. Patients with extensive kidney disease are unable to adequately synthesize calcitriol and thus frequently experience calcium and vitamin D abnormalities. The primary function of calcitriol is to increase calcium absorption from the GI tract. Dietary calcium is absorbed more efficiently in the presence of active vitamin D and PTH, resulting in higher serum levels of calcium, which is then transported to bone, muscle, and other tissues.

CONNECTION Checkpoint 72.1

Inhibition of calcium transport into cells can have important physiologic effects. From what you learned in Chapter 30, what are the primary indications for pharmacotherapy with calcium channel blockers?

Pharmacotherapy of Calcium Imbalances

72.3 Hypocalcemia and hypercalcemia are treated with nutritional adjustments or with pharmacotherapy.

Calcium imbalances occur frequently. When minor, dietary adjustments are used to correct the imbalance; however, serious imbalances require pharmacotherapy.

Treatment of Hypocalcemia

Hypocalcemia is not a disease but is a sign of underlying pathology; thus, diagnosis of the cause of hypocalcemia is essential. Many factors can cause hypocalcemia. Lack of sufficient dietary calcium or vitamin D intake is a common cause and one that can be easily reversed by nutritional adjustments. If hypocalcemia occurs despite normal dietary intake, GI causes must be examined, such as excessive vomiting or the presence of malabsorption disorders. Damage to renal tubular cells may cause excessive loss of calcium in the urine. Most patients with chronic kidney disease (CKD) will require calcium and vitamin D therapy to prevent hypocalcemia.

Another etiology for hypocalcemia is hypoparathyroidism leading to decreased secretion of PTH, as occurs when the thyroid and parathyroid glands are diseased or surgically removed. A rare cause of hypocalcemia is pseudohypoparathyroidism, which is an uncommon group of genetic disorders where the target organs for PTH (bone and kidneys) become resistant to the hormone. Recombinant PTH (Natpara) is available as an adjunct to calcium and vitamin D therapy in controlling hypoglycemia in patients with hypoparathyroidism.

Drug therapy is occasionally a *cause* of hypocalcemia. Blood transfusions and certain anticonvulsants such as phenytoin and phenobarbital can lower serum calcium levels. In addition, overtreatment with drugs that are used to lower serum calcium can result in overshooting normal levels. Some of these include furosemide, phosphate therapy, or bisphosphonates. Of special concern is long-term therapy with corticosteroids, which is a very common cause of hypocalcemia and osteoporosis. To help prevent corticosteroid-induced osteoporosis, patients should receive daily supplements of calcium and vitamin D.

Hypocalcemia is frequently asymptomatic. Signs and symptoms of hypocalcemia are those of nerve and muscle excitability. The symptoms include confusion, paresthesias around the mouth and in the digits, carpopedal spasms, and hyperreflexia. Muscle twitching, tremors, or cramping may be evident. Two clinical signs are Chvostek's sign and Trousseau's sign. Chvostek's sign is elicited by tapping on the facial nerve just below the temple. A positive sign is a twitch of the nose or lip. Trousseau's sign is the contraction of the hand and fingers when the arterial blood flow in the arm is occluded for 5 minutes.

Intestinal cramping and hyperactive bowel sounds may be present because the low calcium levels affect the smooth muscle of the GI tract. Severe symptoms include convulsions, laryngeal spasms, and tetany. Tetany is a continuous muscle spasm that can interfere with breathing and even cause death. The characteristic electrocardiogram (ECG) change is a prolonged QT interval, indicating prolonged ventricular depolarization with characteristically weak cardiac muscle contractions.

Unless the hypocalcemia is especially severe or life-threatening, adjustments in diet may be attempted prior to initiating therapy with calcium supplements. Increasing the consumption of calcium-rich foods, especially dairy products, fortified orange juice, cereals, and green leafy vegetables, is often sufficient to restore calcium balance.

PROTOTYPE DRUG Calcium Salts

Classification **Therapeutic:** Calcium supplement
Pharmacologic: Drugs for hypocalcemia

Therapeutic Effects and Uses: Calcium salts are available in a wide variety of products and formulations. Calcium has two major forms: complexed and elemental. Most calcium supplements are in the form of complexed calcium. These products are often compared on the basis of their ability to release elemental calcium into the bloodstream. The greater the ability of complexed calcium to release elemental calcium, the more potent the supplement. Table 72.2 lists the doses for selected calcium supplements.

Table 72.2 Selected Calcium Salts

Drug	Calcium Content	Route and Adult Dose (Maximum Dose Where Indicated)	Adverse Effects
Calcium Supplements (All doses are in terms of elemental calcium)			*Constipation, nausea and vomiting, metallic taste* Hypercalcemia (drowsiness, lethargy, headache, anorexia, nausea and vomiting, increased urination, and thirst), dysrhythmias, cardiac arrest, confusion, delirium, stupor, coma
calcium acetate	25%	PO: 2–4 tablets with each meal (each tablet contains 169 mg elemental calcium)	
calcium carbonate (Os-Cal, Rolaids, Tums, others)	40%	PO: 1–2 g bid–tid	
calcium chloride	27 mg Ca/mL	IV: 0.5–4 g by slow infusion (1 mL/min)	
calcium citrate (Citracal)	21%	PO: 1–2 g bid–tid	
calcium gluconate (Kalcinate)	9% (PO); 9 mg Ca/mL (IV)	IV: 0.5–4 g by slow infusion (1 g/h)	
calcium lactate (Cal-Lac)	13%	PO: 325–650 mg bid–tid before meals	
calcium phosphate tribasic (Posture)	39%	PO: 1–2 g bid–tid	

Note: Italics indicate common adverse effects. Underline indicates serious adverse effects.

For mild, chronic hypocalcemia, effective and inexpensive calcium supplements are readily available over the counter (OTC). Calcium carbonate and calcium citrate are two common salts for routine supplementation. Many calcium supplements also contain vitamin D.

The administration of intravenous (IV) calcium salts may be necessary for severe cases of hypocalcemia or if the patient is in tetany. Repeated infusions are sometimes required to return the serum calcium level to normal. Constant monitoring of serum calcium is required during IV administration to prevent hypercalcemia.

In addition to preventing or treating hypocalcemia, calcium salts are administered for other conditions, including osteoporosis, Paget's disease, osteomalacia, chronic hypoparathyroidism, rickets, pregnancy, lactation, and rapid childhood growth. Calcium carbonate is a common antacid used to treat heartburn. It may also be used to bind excessive dietary phosphate in patients with hyperphosphatemia caused by end-stage renal failure.

IV calcium gluconate can protect the heart against the hyperexcitability of excessive potassium (hyperkalemia) and help to maintain cardiorespiratory function during magnesium sulfate toxicity (hypermagnesemia) situations. IV calcium salts have been administered during cardiac arrest due to their ability to increase cardiac muscle tone and the force of systolic contraction (positive inotropic effect). However, the use of calcium salts in cardiac resuscitation has declined and is limited to patients with cardiac disease who have hypocalcemia because calcium salts may cause dysrhythmias at high doses.

Mechanism of Action: Calcium salts restore the normal serum levels of calcium, which promotes deposition of the mineral in bone. This helps to restore bone strength and prevent fractures. Calcium also restores normal neuromuscular function and muscular contraction.

Pharmacokinetics: The pharmacokinetics of calcium salts varies by the route of administration and the specific formulation. They are widely distributed and excreted primarily in the feces, with about 20% in the urine. The duration of action of calcium salts is generally only a few hours.

Adverse Effects: Oral (PO) calcium products are safe and produce few adverse effects when used as directed. The most common adverse effect of calcium supplements is hypercalcemia, which is caused by taking too much of this supplement. This can be especially serious in the IV formulations. Symptoms of hypercalcemia include drowsiness, lethargy, weakness, headache, anorexia, constipation, increased gastric acid secretion, nausea and vomiting, a tingling sensation, increased urination, and thirst. IV administration of calcium may cause pain and burning at the IV site, severe venous thrombosis, necrosis, sloughing of the skin (with extravasation), hypotension, sensations of heat waves (peripheral vasodilation), fainting, bradycardia, cardiac dysrhythmias, and cardiac arrest. Large doses of supplemental calcium may lead to the formation of kidney stones.

Contraindications/Precautions: Calcium salts are contraindicated in patients with ventricular fibrillation, metastatic bone disease, renal calculi, hypercalcemia, predisposition to hypercalcemia, hyperparathyroidism, certain malignancies, and digoxin toxicity. Calcium salts should not be injected into the myocardium or administered by the subcutaneous or intramuscular (IM) route. Caution must be used with patients who have renal or cardiac insufficiency, dysrhythmias, dehydration, diarrhea, hyperphosphatemia, sarcoidosis, or history of kidney stones. Immobilized patients are at high risk for the development of hypercalcemia.

Drug Interactions: Concurrent use with digoxin increases the risk of dysrhythmias and enhances the inotropic effects of digoxin. Magnesium may compete for GI absorption. Calcium decreases the absorption of tetracyclines and fluoroquinolones, such as ciprofloxacin. Their use may antagonize the effects of verapamil and possibly other calcium channel blockers. **Herbal/Food:** Zinc-rich foods such as shellfish, dried beans, sesame seeds, pumpkin seeds, and many meats may decrease the absorption of calcium. Alcohol, caffeine, and carbonated beverages affect the absorption of calcium. Oxalic acid in spinach, rhubarb, Swiss chard, and beets can suppress calcium absorption. Phytic acid, which is present in bran and whole-grain cereals, depresses calcium absorption.

Pregnancy: As long as it is not taken in excess amounts, calcium supplements are safe during pregnancy. Women should discuss the amount that is safe to consume with their healthcare provider.

Treatment of Overdose: Measures may be taken to treat cardiac abnormalities caused by the hypercalcemia that results from overdose.

Clinician Responsibilities: Key clinical implications for patients receiving calcium supplementation are included in Applied Clinical Judgment: Patients Receiving Pharmacotherapy for Osteoporosis.

Drugs Similar to Calcium Salts

A large number of calcium salts are available. A summary of their indications is shown in Table 72.3.

Table 72.3 Indications for Selected Calcium Salts

Salt	Antacid	Management of Hyperkalemia	Management of Hypermagnesemia	Management of Hyperphosphatemia	Prevention and Treatment of Hypocalcemia	Cardiotonic	Mineral Supplement	Electrolyte Replenishment
calcium acetate				X				
calcium carbonate	X			X	X		X	
calcium chloride	X	X	X		X	X		X
calcium citrate				X	X		X	
calcium glubionate					X		X	
calcium gluconate injection		X	X		X	X		X
calcium lactate					X		X	
calcium phosphate, dibasic					X		X	

Treatment of Hypercalcemia

In patients with CKD, the kidneys are unable to control mineral metabolism. As a consequence, the parathyroid glands secrete large amounts of parathyroid hormone, which can cause serious hypercalcemia. This disorder is called secondary hyperparathyroidism (secondary HPT) because the condition is not a disease of the parathyroid gland itself but is a consequence of CKD.

The two drugs for treating secondary HPT, cinacalcet (Sensipar) and etelcalcetide (Parsabiv), are called calcimimetics because they mimic the effects of calcium in tissues. The drugs act on the calcium sensors in the parathyroid, in effect tricking the gland into thinking the body has plenty of calcium. The gland thus reduces its secretion of parathyroid hormone.

Cinacalcet was approved by the U.S. Food and Drug Administration (FDA) in 2004. Given PO, the dose is slowly escalated until serum PTH and calcium levels return to normal values. Overtreatment may cause hypocalcemia. Nausea, vomiting and diarrhea are common during therapy. This drug is a strong inhibitor of CYP450 enzymes and should be used with caution in patients who are receiving other drugs that are CYP450 substrates or inhibitors. Etelcalcetide, approved in 2017, is administered by the IV route, usually at the end of a hemodialysis session. The most common adverse effects are hypocalcemia, muscle spasms, diarrhea, nausea and vomiting, headache, and paresthesia. In animal studies, both cinacalcet and etelcalcetide decreased fetal growth. Breastfeeding is not advised due to the potential for hypocalcemia in the infant.

Pathophysiology of Metabolic Bone Disease

72.4 Metabolic bone disease is characterized by abnormal bone structure.

Metabolic bone disease (MBD) is a general term that refers to a cluster of disorders that have in common defects in the structure of bone. MBDs are caused by abnormal amounts of the minerals or hormones responsible for bone homeostasis, such as calcium, phosphate, vitamin D, or PTH. Some MBDs have a genetic etiology, whereas others are iatrogenic and caused by certain drugs and therapies.

Osteoporosis

Osteoporosis is an MBD characterized by bone demineralization, decreased bone density, and subsequent fractures. Osteoporosis is the most prevalent MBD in the United States. This disorder is usually asymptomatic until the bones become brittle enough to fracture or for vertebrae to collapse.

Normal bone remodeling requires a balance between bone deposition (gain) and bone resorption (loss). The exact pathophysiology of osteoporosis is unknown, but there are two major theories. In the first, osteoporosis may be caused by defective osteoblasts that have an abnormally short lifespan or work less efficiently, resulting in slow bone deposition. The second and more popular theory suggests that the osteoclasts have increased activity, resorbing bone at an increased rate. The common factor between the two theories is that normal bone turnover is altered, with the rate of resorption greater than bone formation, resulting in a decrease in total bone density and an altered bone structure.

Numerous risk factors have been identified for osteoporosis. Women are four times more likely than men to develop this condition, and the most common risk factor associated with the development of osteoporosis is the onset of menopause. When women reach menopause, estrogen secretion declines and bones become weak and fragile. In women with osteoporosis, fractures often occur in the hips, wrists, forearms, or spine. In some cases, a lack of dietary calcium and vitamin D contributes to bone deterioration. The metabolism of calcium in osteoporosis is illustrated in Figure 72.3.

Two methods are used to screen patients for osteoporosis. The fracture risk assessment tool (FRAX) is a simple method that uses readily available information to calculate a 10-year probability of hip fracture. Some of the factors include age, smoking, glucocorticoid use, weight, and family history of hip fracture and rheumatoid arthritis.

The second screening method is the measurement of bone mineral density (BMD) using dual-energy x-ray absorptiometry (DEXA). BMD at the spine and hip is measured and data are reported as T-scores. Positive T-scores represent the BMD values of a young adult between the ages of 30 and 35, which is the period of peak bone strength. Negative T-scores indicate some loss in BMD. Osteopenia, or a low bone mass, is present when the T-score is between –1 and –2.4. Osteoporosis is defined as a T-score of –2.5 or less.

Drug therapies for osteoporosis include calcium and vitamin D therapy, bisphosphonates, estrogen receptor modulators, parathyroid hormone analogs (abaloparatide [Tymlos] and teriparatide [Forteo]), denosumab, and calcitonin. Clinical considerations for treating osteoporosis are shown in Applied Clinical Judgment: Osteoporosis.

CONNECTIONS: APPLIED CLINICAL JUDGMENT

Patients Receiving Pharmacotherapy for Osteoporosis

Key Assessment Data

- History of current condition including musculoskeletal, GI, cardiovascular, neurologic, endocrine, hepatic, or kidney disease; baseline vital signs, physical exam findings; pregnancy or breastfeeding; complete blood count (CBC), electrolytes, calcium, phosphorus, and magnesium levels, and bone density studies; dietary and medication history including allergies, current prescription and OTC drugs, calcium, vitamin D, and magnesium intake, sunscreen use and sun exposure, herbal preparations, caffeine, nicotine, and alcohol use.
- Assess current symptoms and their effect on ADLs, muscle strength, and gait and note any pain or discomfort on movement or at rest.

Desired Therapeutic Outcomes

Improvement is observed and measurable by calcium, phosphate, and magnesium levels maintained within normal limits and bone density studies show improvement.

Minimizing Adverse Effects

- Bisphosphonates may cause esophageal irritation and erosion. Increasing nausea, gastric, or abdominal pain should be assessed for further treatment.
- An increased incidence of fractures has been noted in some patients taking bisphosphonates, particularly with long-term use or with concurrent corticosteroid use. Thigh or groin pain may occur prior to fracture and should be assessed.
- Excessive vitamin D intake may lead to toxic effects. Monitor liver function studies and for symptoms such as nausea and vomiting, headache, fatigue, dry and itchy skin, blurred vision, or palpitations.

Patient Education

- Adequate sun exposure, approximately 15 to 20 min/day without sunscreen, may assist in vitamin D formation.
- Adequate activity and exercise, especially weight-bearing exercise, three to five times per week will assist in maintaining bone mass.
- Increased fluid intake up to 2 L/day will assist in decreasing the risk of renal calculi formation from calcium supplement therapy.
- Avoid excessive soda and caffeine intake, which may diminish absorption of dietary calcium.
- Promptly report any new onset of groin or thigh pain, either unilaterally or bilaterally, if bisphosphonates are used. Bone density studies will be monitored on a regular basis.
- Immediately report any new onset of nausea or any increasing or severe chest or abdominal discomfort or pain if bisphosphonates are used.
- Immediately report symptoms of hypocalcemia (muscle spasms, facial grimacing, irritability, hyperreflexes) or hypercalcemia (increased bone pain, anorexia, nausea and vomiting, constipation, thirst, lethargy, or fatigue).
- Maintain consistent administration of drug therapy to ensure full effects. Therapeutic response may take 1 to 3 months and effects continue after the drug has been discontinued.
- Do not take additional or large amounts of vitamin D unless instructed by the provider as it may accumulate to cause adverse effects.
- Take the drug following appropriate guidelines:
    - *Bisphosphonates:* Take with a full glass of plain water and remain in an upright position for 30 minutes to 1 hour after taking.
    - *Calcium supplements:* Take with meals or immediately after meals. Do not take more than the amount recommended by the prescriber.

Prescribing Considerations

- Monitor adherence to the recommended regimen to ensure that the patient does not discontinue drug therapy because of a perceived lack of response. Bone remodeling occurs over several months and effects may not be noted immediately.

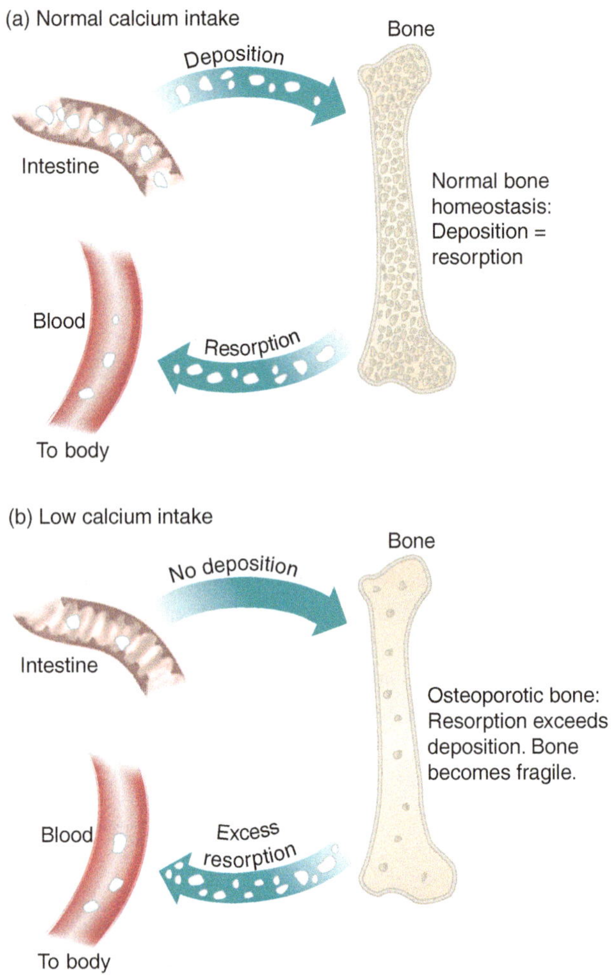

Figure 72.3 Calcium metabolism in osteoporosis.

Osteomalacia

Osteomalacia, referred to as *rickets* in children, is a disorder characterized by softening of bones without alteration of basic bone structure. Weight-bearing stress on the softened bones causes skeletal deformities. Many factors contribute to the development of osteomalacia and rickets, but the most important is a deficiency of vitamin D and calcium. This risk factor for the disease is extremely rare in the United States, being most prevalent in older adults, premature infants, and individuals on strict vegetarian diets. Other factors that may result in the development of osteomalacia include malabsorption disorders of the small bowel, damage to the renal tubules, adverse effects of anticonvulsant therapy, hepatic impairment, or a limited exposure to sunlight.

The promotion of breastfeeding over vitamin D–fortified formulas is thought to be responsible for some cases of osteomalacia, particularly in mothers who are vitamin D deficient. In addition, the increased use of sunscreens to prevent skin cancer inhibits the formation of adequate vitamin D by sunlight. The replacement of vitamin D–fortified milk with carbonated beverages by children and teens also contributes to the possibility of rickets. Nurses need to emphasize the importance of getting enough extra dietary vitamin D to children and pregnant women. Drug therapy for children and adults consists of calcium salts and vitamin D.

Symptoms of osteomalacia include hypocalcemia, muscle weakness, muscle spasms, and diffuse bone pain, especially in the hip area. Patients may also experience pain in the arms, legs, and spine. Classic signs of rickets in children include bowlegs and a pigeon breast. Children may also develop a slight fever and become restless at night.

The standard test for diagnosing osteomalacia is to determine vitamin D status by measuring the serum levels of 25-hydroxyvitamin D. Additional tests may include bone radiographs and computed tomography (CT) scans of the vertebral column.

Paget's Disease

Paget's disease, or osteitis deformans, is a chronic, progressive condition characterized by accelerated remodeling of the bone, producing enlarged and softened bones. With this disorder, the processes of bone resorption and bone formation occur simultaneously but at a very high rate. The rapid turnover causes new bone to be weak and brittle, resulting in deformities and fractures. Paget's disease can occur in any bone, but it most often affects the vertebrae, skull, sternum, pelvis, femur, and tibia. Paget's disease occurs with equal frequency in men and women over 40 years of age. The cause of Paget's disease is unknown.

Although many patients with Paget's disease are asymptomatic, approximately 10% experience vague, nonspecific complaints for many years. Symptoms include pain of the hips and femurs, joint inflammation, headaches, facial pain, and hearing loss if bones around the ear are affected. Nerves along the spinal column may be pinched because of the abnormal vertebral bone growth.

The evaluation of Paget's disease is based on radiographic and laboratory findings. The enzyme alkaline phosphatase (ALP) is elevated in the blood because of the extensive bone turnover. The disease is usually confirmed by early detection of this enzyme in the blood. Calcium is also liberated because of its close association with phosphate. If diagnosed early enough, symptoms can be treated successfully. If the diagnosis is made late in the progression of the disease, permanent skeletal abnormalities develop and other disorders may appear, including arthritis, kidney stones, and heart disease.

Bisphosphonates are the primary pharmacotherapy for Paget's disease. Calcitonin may be used as a second-line drug. Patients with Paget's disease should consume adequate amounts of calcium and vitamin D on a daily basis.

Pharmacotherapy of Metabolic Bone Disease

72.5 Vitamin D therapy is indicated for treating osteomalacia, hypoparathyroidism, and osteoporosis.

Inactive, intermediate, and active forms of vitamin D are available as medications. Patients' vitamin D needs vary depending on how much sunlight they receive. After age 70, the RDA of vitamin D increases from 400 units/day to 600 units/day. In severe cases of malabsorption disorders, patients may receive 50,000 to 100,000 units/day. Because vitamin D is needed to absorb calcium from the GI tract, many supplements combine vitamin D and calcium into a single tablet.

Several forms of vitamin D are available for therapy. Three of those products—ergocalciferol, cholecalciferol, and calcitriol—are identical to the forms of vitamin D that occur in nature. Each vitamin D product has a slightly different potency and pharmacokinetics. Indications for vitamin D products include the following:

- Hypocalcemia
- Hypophosphatemia
- Osteomalacia (rickets)
- Osteoporosis prophylaxis
- Parathyroid dysfunction
- Vitamin D deficiency.

Vitamin D is a fat-soluble vitamin that is stored by the body. It is possible to consume too much of this vitamin or to show signs of overdose from prescription medications. Excess vitamin D will cause calcium to leave bones and enter the blood. The signs and symptoms of hypercalcemia, such as anorexia, vomiting, excessive thirst, fatigue, and confusion, may become evident. Kidney stones may occur, and bones may fracture easily.

PROTOTYPE DRUG Calcitriol (Rocaltrol)

Classification **Therapeutic:** Vitamin D
Pharmacologic: Bone resorption inhibitor

Therapeutic Effects and Uses: Calcitriol is the active form of vitamin D. This medication is used in cases of hypocalcemia and for patients who have hypoparathyroidism. Calcitriol reduces bone resorption and is useful in treating rickets. Patients with CKD are unable to synthesize sufficient calcitriol and thus will receive this drug as replacement therapy.

The effectiveness of calcitriol depends on having an adequate amount of calcium; therefore, it is usually prescribed in combination with calcium supplements. It is available for administration via the oral (PO) route in the form of tablets and solutions. An IV solution for injection is available to treat dialysis-associated hypocalcemia.

Mechanism of Action: Calcitriol elevates serum calcium levels, decreases elevated blood levels of phosphate, and decreases bone resorption and demineralization by promoting the intestinal absorption and renal reabsorption of calcium. The rising calcium levels provide negative feedback to the parathyroid glands, reducing the secretion of PTH. Calcitriol itself also provides negative feedback to the parathyroid glands.

Pharmacokinetics:

Route(s)	PO (tablets, capsules, or solution), IV
Absorption	Readily absorbed from the GI tract
Distribution	Widely distributed; crosses the placenta; small amounts are secreted in breast milk; 99% bound to vitamin D–binding protein
Primary metabolism	Hepatic
Primary excretion	Mostly feces with small amounts in urine
Onset of action	2–6 h
Duration of action	3–5 days

Adverse Effects: The adverse effects of vitamin D therapy include symptoms of hypercalcemia, such as palpitations, anorexia, nausea and vomiting, blurred vision, photophobia, constipation, abdominal cramps, metallic taste, headache, weakness, dry mouth, thirst, increased urination, and muscle or bone pain.

Contraindications/Precautions: This drug should not be given to patients with hypercalcemia or those who have evidence of vitamin D toxicity. Caution must be used in patients with CKD who are at increased risk for vitamin D–induced hypercalcemia.

Drug Interactions: Thiazide diuretics may enhance the effects of vitamin D, causing hypercalcemia. Too much vitamin D may cause dysrhythmias in patients who are receiving digoxin. Magnesium antacids or supplements should not be given concurrently owing to an increased risk of hypermagnesemia. Orlistat (Xenical) may prevent the absorption of fat-soluble nutrients such as vitamin D. Corticosteroids inhibit the absorption of calcium, which is a major effect of vitamin D. **Herbal/Food:** Unknown.

Pregnancy: Calcitriol causes cause fetal harm in laboratory animals. Because this drug is secreted in human milk, the breastfed neonate should be monitored for possible hypercalcemia.

Treatment of Overdose: Vitamin D overdose results in hypercalcemia, hypercalciuria, and hyperphosphatemia. If the overdosage was recent, emesis should be induced to remove any remaining drug from the stomach. All vitamin D and calcium supplements are discontinued, and the patient is placed on a low-calcium diet until the hypercalcemia resolves.

Clinician Responsibilities: Key clinical implications for patients receiving calcitriol are included in Applied Clinical Judgment: Patients Receiving Pharmacotherapy for Osteoporosis.

Drugs Similar to Calcitriol (Rocaltrol)

Other forms of vitamin D for therapy include calcifediol, cholecalciferol, doxercalciferol, ergocalciferol, and paricalcitol. Pregnancy and lactation information is the same as for calcitriol. Doses for the vitamin D preparations are given in Table 72.4.

Calcifediol (Rayaldee): Calcifediol is an analog of vitamin D_3 that is converted to the active hormone, calcitriol, in the kidneys. Calcifediol was approved in 2016 for the treatment of secondary hyperparathyroidism in adult patients with CKD. It has the same adverse effects as calcitriol. Caution must be used to avoid overtreatment because this may cause severe hypercalcemia.

Cholecalciferol (Delta-D): Cholecalciferol (vitamin D_3) is the form of vitamin D that is produced in the skin after exposure to UV light. It is activated by the liver and kidneys to form calcitriol. Once activated, cholecalciferol produces the same actions and adverse effects as calcitriol. It is an oral dietary supplement for the prophylaxis and treatment of vitamin D deficiency. Fosamax plus D is a combination drug containing alendronate and cholecalciferol.

Doxercalciferol (Hectorol): Doxercalciferol is an analog of vitamin D that is given by either the PO or IV route. This drug is activated by the liver alone: No kidney metabolism is necessary. Adverse effects are the same as those of calcitriol. However, caution must be taken to avoid the rapid development of hypercalcemia when this drug is administered by the IV route. Its only approved indication is for the treatment of secondary hyperparathyroidism and resultant bone disease.

Ergocalciferol (Calciferol, Drisdol): Ergocalciferol (vitamin D_2) is a natural vitamin D analog found in plants, fortified milk, eggs, and cereals. Once activated, ergocalciferol produces actions and adverse effects identical to those of calcitriol. Bile is required for its absorption, and the drug requires adequate kidney function to be metabolized to its active form. Indications for therapy with ergocalciferol are the same as those for calcitriol.

Paricalcitol (Zemplar): Paricalcitol is an analog of vitamin D that is given by either the PO or IV route. Adverse effects are the same as those of calcitriol; however, caution must be taken to avoid the rapid development of hypercalcemia when this drug is administered by the IV route. The only indication for paricalcitol is for the treatment of secondary hyperparathyroidism and resultant bone disease.

72.6 Bisphosphonates increase bone density and are used to treat osteoporosis and Paget's disease.

The most frequently prescribed drug class for osteoporosis is the **bisphosphonates**. These drugs are structural analogs of pyrophosphate, which is a natural substance that inhibits bone resorption. Bisphosphonates bind to hydroxyapatite in bone and suppress osteoclast activity, thus increasing bone mass density and reducing the incidence of fractures by about 50%. Examples include alendronate (Fosamax),

Table 72.4 Vitamin D Preparations

Drug	Route and Adult Dose (Maximum Dose Where Indicated)	Adverse Effects
calcifediol (Rayaldee)	PO: 30–60 mcg once daily	*Diarrhea, infection, hypertension (HTN), dizziness* Hypercalcemia (bone pain, lethargy, anorexia, nausea and vomiting, increased urination), hallucinations, dysrhythmias, anemia
calcitriol (Calcijex, Rocaltrol)	PO: 0.25–0.50 mcg/day IV: Begin with 1–4 mcg 3 times/wk	
cholecalciferol (Delta-D)	PO: 400–1000 international units/day	
doxercalciferol (Hectorol)	PO: 10 mcg, 3 times/wk IV: 4 mcg, 3 times/wk (max: 60 mcg/wk [PO]; 18 mcg/wk [IV])	
ergocalciferol (Calciferol, Drisdol)	PO: 15–25 mcg once daily IV: 4 mcg 3 times/wk	
paricalcitol (Zemplar)	IV: 0.04–0.1 mcg/kg, every other day (max: 24 mcg/kg) PO: 1–4 mcg every other day or 3 times/wk	

Note: Italics indicate common adverse effects. Underline indicates serious adverse effects.

zoledronate (Reclast, Zometa), risedronate (Actonel, Atelvia), and pamidronate (Aredia), which is available as an injectable drug. In addition to treating postmenopausal osteoporosis, some of the bisphosphonates are approved to treat corticosteroid-induced osteoporosis. A summary of the indications for bisphosphonates is given in Table 72.5 and their doses are listed in Table 72.6.

The beneficial effects of bisphosphonates on bone mass density increase rapidly during the first year of therapy and plateau after 2 to 3 years. Even after discontinuation of therapy, bone density will remain increased for up to 1 year. For optimal effects, the patient must have adequate dietary consumption of calcium and vitamin D; any deficiencies should be corrected prior to initiating bisphosphonate therapy. Studies suggest that once-weekly dosing with bisphosphonates may give the same bone density benefits as daily dosing because of their extended duration of drug action.

Bisphosphonates are also preferred drugs for the pharmacotherapy of Paget's disease. For this disorder, therapy is usually cyclic, with bisphosphonates administered until serum ALP levels return to normal followed by several months without drugs. When the serum ALP level becomes elevated, therapy is begun again. The pharmacologic goals are to slow the rate of bone reabsorption and encourage the deposition of strong bone.

Several bisphosphonates are used to treat bone metastases and malignant hypercalcemia. Bone metastases are characterized by osteoclast hyperactivity, which creates "punched-out," osteolytic lesions that release large amounts of calcium into the blood. Bisphosphonates suppress osteoclast activity, thus slowing the rate of bone resorption and the rate of calcium release. Thus, some of these drugs are approved for treating hypercalcemia due to malignancy. It is important to note that bisphosphonates are not antineoplastics; they have no effect on tumor cells and are given only as a palliative measure.

The most frequent adverse effects of bisphosphonates include GI symptoms such as nausea and vomiting, abdominal pain, dyspepsia, and esophageal irritation. Because these drugs are poorly absorbed from the intestinal tract, they must be taken on an empty stomach with plain water, at least 30 minutes before any other fluid, food, or medications. To avoid esophageal irritation, the patient should stay in an upright position for at least 30 minutes following the dose. Bisphosphonates are not metabolized and are excreted in the urine.

Patients taking the bisphosphonates are evaluated on a regular basis to determine if the drug is still necessary. To avoid the possibility of long-term adverse effects, these drugs are usually discontinued after several years of therapy in patients who have a low risk for fracture.

One unusual adverse effect that may occur during bisphosphonate therapy is osteonecrosis of the jaw. Symptoms include local pain and swelling, loosening of teeth, and infection at the site of the lesion. It is not clear what causes the necrosis. Discontinuing the bisphosphonate does not resolve the lesion because the drugs are incorporated in bone for many months and perhaps years.

PROTOTYPE DRUG Alendronate (Fosamax)

Classification **Therapeutic:** Drug for osteoporosis and Paget's disease

Pharmacologic: Bisphosphonate, bone resorption inhibitor

Therapeutic Actions and Uses: First approved in 1995, alendronate is the best studied drug in this class. Alendronate is approved for the following indications:

- Prevention and treatment of osteoporosis in postmenopausal women
- Treatment of glucocorticoid-induced osteoporosis in both women and men
- Treatment to increase bone mass in men with osteoporosis
- Treatment of symptomatic Paget's disease in both women and men.

Table 72.5 Indications for Bisphosphonates

Drug	Osteoporosis in Postmenopausal Women	Osteoporosis in Men	Glucocorticoid-Induced Osteoporosis	Paget's Disease	Hypercalcemia of Malignancy	Breast Cancer Metastases	Multiple Myeloma/Bone Metastases
alendronate (Fosamax)	X	X	X	X			
ibandronate (Boniva)	X						
pamidronate (Aredia)				X	X	X	
risedronate (Actonel, Atelvia)	X	X	X	X			
zoledronate (Reclast, Zometa)	X	X		X	X		X

Table 72.6 Selected Drugs for Osteoporosis and Other Bone Disorders

Drug	Route and Adult Dose (Maximum Dose Where Indicated)	Adverse Effects
Bisphosphonates		
alendronate (Fosamax)	Osteoporosis: PO: 10 mg/day or 70 mg once weekly Paget's disease: PO: 40 mg/day for 6 months	*Nausea, dyspepsia, diarrhea, bone pain, back pain* Bone fractures, nephrotoxicity, hypocalcemia, hypophosphatemia, gastric ulcer, esophageal perforation, dysrhythmias, anemia, osteonecrosis of the jaw, atrial fibrillation
ibandronate (Boniva)	PO: 2.5 mg/day or one 150-mg tablet per month, taken on the same date each month IV: 3 mg every 3 months	
pamidronate (Aredia)	IV: 15–90 mg in 1000 mL normal saline or D_5W over 4–24 h	
risedronate (Actonel, Atelvia)	PO: 5 mg/day or 35 mg once weekly at least 30 min before the first drink or meal of the day	
zoledronate (Reclast, Zometa)	IV (Zometa): 4-mg single dose infused over at least 15 min; may be repeated q3–4wk for cancer IV (Reclast): one 5-mg single dose per year, infused over at least 15 min	
Miscellaneous Drugs		
abaloparatide (Tymlos)	Subcutaneous: 80 mcg/day using a prefilled pen	*Orthostatic hypotension, dizziness, nausea, headache, fatigue* Hypercalcemia, hypercalciuria, urolithiasis, risk for osteosarcoma
calcitonin-salmon (Miacalcin)	Subcutaneous/IM: salmon, 4–8 international units/kg bid for hypercalcemia; 100 international units every 1–3 days for osteoporosis or Paget disease	*Flushing of the face and hands, pain at the injection site* Anaphylaxis
cinacalcet (Sensipar)	PO: Start with 30 mg once daily; increase until target PTH of 150–300 mg/mL (max: 300 mg/day) for secondary hyperparathyroidism	*Dizziness, noncardiac chest pain, HTN, nausea, anorexia, myalgia* Hypocalcemia, seizures
denosumab (Prolia, Xgen)	Subcutaneous (Prolia): 60 mg every 6 months Subcutaneous (Xgen): 120 mg q4wk	*Fatigue, asthenia, hypophosphatemia, nausea, hypercholesterolemia, musculoskeletal pain, and cystitis* Hypocalcemia, serious infections, osteonecrosis of jaw
etelcalcetide (Parsabiv)	IV: 5-mg bolus	*Muscle spasms, diarrhea, headache, nausea and vomiting* Severe hypocalcemia, worsening heart failure (HF), GI bleeding
raloxifene (Evista)	PO: 60 mg/day	*Hot flashes, leg cramps, peripheral edema, flu syndrome, arthralgia, sweating* Breast pain, vaginal bleeding, pneumonia, chest pain, venous thromboembolism, stroke
romosozumab (Evenity)	Subcutaneous: 210 mg q4wk for 12 months	*Arthralgia, headache, hypersensitivity, injection-site reactions* Increased risk for MI, stroke and cardiovascular death, osteonecrosis of jaw
teriparatide (Forteo)	Subcutaneous: 20 mcg/day using a prefilled pen	*Dizziness, depression, insomnia, vertigo, rhinitis, increased cough, leg cramps, nausea, arthralgia* Syncope, angina, transient hypercalcemia, risk for osteosarcoma

Note: *Italics* indicate common adverse effects. Underline indicates serious adverse effects.

Alendronate is also used off-label for treating hypercalcemia due to malignancy. Several regimens for alendronate are available: once daily (10 mg), twice weekly (35 mg), or once weekly (70 mg). Although the once weekly is more convenient, higher doses can produce more GI-related adverse effects. All doses must be taken on an empty stomach, preferably in a fasting state 2 hours before breakfast.

Therapeutic effects of alendronate may take 1 to 3 months to appear and may continue for several months after therapy is discontinued. This drug lowers serum alkaline phosphatase, which is the enzyme associated with bone turnover, without major adverse effects.

The safety and effectiveness of long-term therapy with alendronate is still being investigated. Patients should be regularly evaluated to determine the need for continued therapy and the drug discontinued after 3 to 5 years of use in those at low risk for fractures.

Mechanism of Action: Alendronate inhibits osteoclast-mediated bone resorption to minimize loss of bone density. Its effects appear to be localized to resorption sites of active bone turnover and it does not interfere with bone mineralization.

Pharmacokinetics:

Route(s)	PO
Absorption	Less than 1% (significantly decreased by food or beverages)
Distribution	Rapid skeletal uptake; unknown if secreted in breast milk; 78% bound to plasma protein
Primary metabolism	Not metabolized
Primary excretion	50% excreted unchanged in the urine
Onset of action	3–6 weeks
Duration of action	12 weeks or more after discontinuation

Adverse Effects: The most common adverse effect of alendronate is hypocalcemia, which is usually transient and mild. Other adverse effects include diarrhea, constipation, flatulence, nausea and vomiting, GI irritation, a metallic or altered taste perception, hypocalcemia, hypophosphatemia, abdominal pain, dyspepsia, myalgia, and headache. Pathologic fractures may occur if the drug is taken longer than 3 months or in cases of chronic overdose. Although rare, this drug may cause serious esophagitis, which is why patients should remain in an upright position at least 30 minutes after receiving a dose. Osteonecrosis of the jaw has occurred spontaneously in patients taking bisphosphonates.

Contraindications/Precautions: Contraindications include patients with osteomalacia or who have hypersensitivity to this drug. Caution should be used in patients with CKD, HF, hyperphosphatemia, liver disease, fever or infection, active upper GI problems, and pregnancy. This drug is contraindicated in patients with abnormalities of the esophagus that delay esophageal emptying, such as stricture or achalasia, and in those who are unable to stand or sit upright for at least 30 minutes following administration of the drug.

Drug Interactions: Calcium, iron, antacids containing aluminum or magnesium, and certain mineral supplements interfere with the absorption of alendronate and have the potential to decrease its effectiveness. Patients should wait at least 30 minutes after taking alendronate before taking any other supplements or other medications. **Herbal/Food:** The patient's diet must have adequate amounts of vitamin D, calcium, and phosphates. Excessive amounts of calcium supplements or dairy products reduce alendronate absorption.

Pregnancy: Alendronate causes fetal harm in laboratory animals. There is not enough human data to determine pregnancy risk. It is not known if this drug is secreted in human milk or if it has adverse effects on the breastfed neonate.

Treatment of Overdose: Hypocalcemia is an expected effect of overdose and may be treated with PO or IV calcium compounds.

Clinician Responsibilities: Key clinical implications for patients receiving alendronate are included in Applied Clinical Judgment: Patients Receiving Pharmacotherapy for Osteoporosis.

Drugs Similar to Alendronate (Fosamax)

Other bisphosphonates include ibandronate, pamidronate, risedronate, and zoledronate. These drugs share the same pregnancy data as alendronate. Etidronate, the first bisphosphonate approved in the United States, has been discontinued.

Ibandronate (Boniva): Ibandronate was approved in 2003 for the prevention and treatment of postmenopausal osteoporosis. In addition to its oral formulation, it is the only IV bisphosphonate approved for the prophylaxis of postmenopausal osteoporosis. When administered IV, injections are spaced 3 months apart. Off-label indications include Paget's disease, bone metastases from prostate cancer, and malignant hypercalcemia. Adverse effects are similar to those of other drugs in this class.

Pamidronate (Aredia): Approved in 1991, pamidronate is available by slow IV infusion for hypercalcemia, moderate to severe Paget's disease, and bone metastases due to breast cancer or multiple myeloma. It may be used off-label to treat osteoporosis and osteogenesis imperfecta. Caution must be used when treating patients with CKD or those who are receiving nephrotoxic drugs because significant renal function deterioration can occur with pamidronate, even after a single dose. Other common adverse effects are nausea, fever, constipation, and dyspnea.

Risedronate (Actonel, Atelvia): Approved in 1998, risedronate is considered a first-line drug for the treatment of glucocorticoid-induced and postmenopausal osteoporosis, and it is also approved to treat symptomatic Paget's disease. It may be used off-label to treat osteolytic lesions due to multiple myeloma. Available by the PO route, it is reported to cause less GI distress than other bisphosphonates. Like other oral bisphosphonates, it is contraindicated in patients who are unable to sit upright for at least 30 minutes after drug administration or who have disorders that cause delayed esophageal emptying. Atelvia is a delayed-release form of the drug that can be taken once weekly. Arthralgia, back pain, diarrhea, abdominal pain, and dyspepsia are common adverse effects.

Zoledronate (Reclast, Zometa): Originally approved in 2001, zoledronate (also called zoledronic acid) is available by the IV route to treat hypercalcemia of malignancy, multiple myeloma, and bone metastases. One advantage of Zometa is that it can be infused over 15 to 20 minutes compared to 2 to 4 hours for pamidronate. Frequent adverse effects include nausea and vomiting, fatigue, anemia, bone pain, constipation, fever, and dyspnea.

In 2007, the FDA expanded the indications for zoledronate (Reclast) to include prevention or treatment of postmenopausal osteoporosis, osteoporosis in men, and Paget's disease. A major advantage of Reclast is that its prolonged duration of action results in a once-yearly dose for Paget's disease and osteoporosis prophylaxis. Reclast is available by IV infusion, administered over at least 15 minutes. Common adverse effects include bone pain, pyrexia, nausea, headache, arthralgia, fatigue, and constipation.

Reclast and Zometa are not interchangeable and the drugs should not be administered concurrently. Zoledronate is nephrotoxic and should be used with caution in patients with CKD.

72.7 Selective estrogen receptor modulators increase bone mass density and prevent fractures in postmenopausal women.

Selective estrogen receptor modulators (SERMs) are drugs that bind to estrogen receptors (ERs). Estrogen exerts its effects on target tissues by interacting with ERs and causing either activation or inhibition of specific cellular actions. ERs are found in the reproductive organs of both males and females where they enhance the development of reproductive tissues. But ERs are found in more than just reproductive tissues. In the cardiovascular system, ERs are responsible for lowering blood cholesterol, and in the brain, these receptors influence behavior and mood. In bone, ERs help to maintain BMD.

Certain estrogens are produced by plants. These substances, called phytoestrogens, mimic the effects of natural estrogen and are thought to exert beneficial effects on the cardiovascular system and possibly protection from cancer. For example, soybeans, flax seed, and tofu are rich sources of phytoestrogens.

SERMs are medications that may activate or inhibit ERs. Thus, SERMs may be estrogen agonists or antagonists, depending on the specific drug and the tissue involved. For example, raloxifene (Evista) blocks estrogen receptors in the uterus and breast; it has no estrogen-like proliferative effects on these tissues that might promote cancer. Raloxifene does, however, have estrogen-like effects that reduce bone resorption, thus increasing bone density and reducing the likelihood of fractures. It is most effective in preventing vertebral fractures. The dose for raloxifene is shown in Table 72.6.

The other SERMs include tamoxifen, toremifene (Fareston), and bazedoxifene (Duavee). Tamoxifen and toremifene are used to treat metastatic breast cancer in postmenopausal women (see Chapter 57). Bazedoxifene is formulated in a fixed-dose combination with conjugated estrogens to manage symptoms of menopause as well as to prevent bone fractures (see Chapter 69).

PROTOTYPE DRUG Raloxifene (Evista)

Classification **Therapeutic:** Drug for osteoporosis prophylaxis
Pharmacologic: Selective estrogen receptor modifier

Therapeutic Effects and Uses: Approved in 1997, raloxifene is primarily used for the prevention or treatment of osteoporosis in postmenopausal women. It is also approved for the prophylaxis (reduction of risk) of invasive breast cancer in postmenopausal women at high risk for breast cancer. High risk of breast cancer is defined as at least one breast biopsy showing carcinoma or atypical hyperplasia or having a first-degree relative with breast cancer. Other factors considered are current age, number of breast biopsies, age at menarche, nulliparity, or age of first live birth. It is important for nurses and patients to understand that this drug is for the prevention, not treatment, of breast carcinoma.

Raloxifene increases bone mass density, reducing vertebral fractures. It does not appear to reduce the incidence of fractures at nonvertebral sites. Raloxifene also reduces serum total cholesterol and low-density lipoproteins without lowering high-density lipoproteins or triglycerides. Unlike estrogen, which causes proliferation of uterine and breast tissue, causing adverse effects, raloxifene is an estrogen antagonist on these tissues. Raloxifene has been used off-label to treat uterine leiomyomas, for pubertal gynecomastia, and for the prevention of bone loss in men with prostate cancer.

Mechanism of Action: As a selective estrogen receptor antagonist or agonist, raloxifene decreases bone resorption while increasing bone mass and density by activating estrogen receptors.

Pharmacokinetics:

Route(s)	PO
Absorption	60% absorbed
Distribution	Crosses the placenta; unknown if secreted in breast milk; 95% bound to plasma protein
Primary metabolism	Hepatic; extensive first-pass metabolism
Primary excretion	Primarily in feces
Onset of action	8 weeks
Duration of action	Half-life: 28 h

Adverse Effects: The most common adverse effects of raloxifene therapy are hot flashes, leg cramps, and weight gain. Less common adverse effects include fever, arthralgia, myalgia, arthritis, depression, insomnia, chest pain, peripheral edema, decreased serum cholesterol, nausea and vomiting, dyspepsia, flatulence, GI disorders, gastroenteritis, cystitis, migraine, flulike symptoms, endometrial disorder, breast pain, and vaginal bleeding. **Black Box Warning:** Raloxifene increases the risk of venous thromboembolism and death from stroke. Women with a history of venous thromboembolism should not take this drug.

Contraindications/Precautions: This drug is contraindicated during lactation and pregnancy and in women who may become pregnant. Patients with a history of venous thromboembolism and those who are hypersensitive to raloxifene should not take this drug. Raloxifene should be discontinued 72 hours before prolonged immobilization is anticipated due to risk of thromboembolic events.

Drug Interactions: Concurrent use with warfarin may decrease prothrombin time. Decreased raloxifene absorption will result from concurrent use with ampicillin or cholestyramine. Use of raloxifene with other highly protein-bound drugs (e.g., ibuprofen, indomethacin, diazepam) may interfere with binding sites. Patients should not take cholesterol-lowering drugs or have enzyme replacement therapy concurrently with this medication. **Herbal/Food:** Black cohosh has estrogenic effects and may interfere with the actions of raloxifene.

Pregnancy: Raloxifene is only indicated for postmenopausal women. Because this drug causes fetal harm in laboratory animals, it is contraindicated during pregnancy, in women who may become pregnant, and in nursing mothers.

Treatment of Overdose: Overdose with raloxifene is uncommon and symptoms are given supportive treatment.

Clinician Responsibilities: Key clinical implications for patients receiving raloxifene are included in Applied Clinical Judgment: Patients Receiving Pharmacotherapy for Osteoporosis.

Drugs Similar to Raloxifene (Evista)

The other SERMs are discussed in previous chapters: tamoxifen and toremifene in Chapter 57 and bazedoxifene with conjugated estrogens in Chapter 69.

CONNECTION Checkpoint 72.2

From what you learned in Chapter 57, what are the indications for pharmacotherapy with tamoxifen?

72.8 Calcitonin and several miscellaneous drugs are used for osteoporosis and other metabolic bone diseases.

Several miscellaneous drugs are used to treat MBDs. Although they act by different mechanisms, they are presented together in this section because each is the only drug in its class.

Calcitonin-salmon (Miacalcin): Calcitonin is a hormone that is produced and secreted by the thyroid gland in response to elevated serum calcium levels. This hormone directly inhibits osteoclasts. The function of calcitonin is to lower serum calcium levels by decreasing bone resorption and increasing the urinary excretion of calcium. It acts in direct opposition to PTH and vitamin D.

As a drug, calcitonin is obtained from salmon and is approved for the treatment of osteoporosis in women who are more than 5 years postmenopause. Because calcitonin is less effective for reducing osteoporosis-related fractures than the bisphosphonates, it is considered a second-line treatment. The dose for calcitonin is given in Table 72.6.

In addition to treating osteoporosis, calcitonin is indicated for Paget's disease and hypercalcemia. In Paget's disease calcitonin slows the rate of bone turnover and decreases the incidence of bone pain. It is most effective in treating hypercalcemia caused by hyperparathyroidism or prolonged immobility or that accompanies certain malignancies.

Calcitonin is available by subcutaneous or IM injection and intranasal forms. Subcutaneous injections are initially given as a daily dose then decreased to two to three times per week. Adverse effects of calcitonin include nausea, injection-site inflammation, and generalized flushing of the face and hands. At clinically relevant doses, calcitonin showed no embryofetal toxicity in laboratory animals. It is not known if this drug is secreted in human milk or if it has adverse effects on the breastfed neonate.

Monoclonal antibodies: Researchers have found ways to disrupt the metabolic pathways associated with bone formation and resorption. Although they act by very different mechanisms, two monoclonal antibodies have been developed that attack proteins that normally cause bone resorption. By inhibiting resorption, BMD is maintained and fractures are prevented.

Approved in 2010, denosumab (Prolia, Xgen) has three indications: to prevent fractures in postmenopausal women with osteoporosis; to increase bone mass in women receiving adjuvant aromatase therapy for breast cancer; and to increase bone mass in men receiving antiandrogen therapy for nonmetastatic prostate cancer. Denosumab is given by

CONNECTIONS: Using Research in Practice

Carbonated Drink Consumption and Fractures

Multiple studies have attempted to determine if the consumption of carbonated drinks leads to an increase risk of fractures, particularly hip fractures in postmenopausal women. The results have been mixed and people who consume large amounts of carbonated beverages may simply consume less milk and calcium-containing drinks.

Kremer et al. (2019) studied participants in the Women's Health Initiative, their consumption of carbonated drinks, and evaluated BMD to determine risk for hip fracture. While there were no specific ingredients in carbonated beverages that could be determined to be a causative factor in increased risk, it was found that women who consumed more than two beverages per day (14 per week) had an increased risk of hip fracture based on BMD studies. The authors also posit that the carbonation process, which leads to carbonic acid, may alter gastric acidity, affecting nutrient absorption.

Limiting carbonated beverages to less than two servings per day and continuing other measures to promote bone health such as weight-bearing exercise and consumption of foods containing calcium and magnesium, may provide some protective effects against hip fracture, particularly for postmenopausal women.

subcutaneous injection, either every 4 weeks (Xgen) or every 6 months (Prolia). The drug is a monoclonal antibody classified as a RANKL inhibitor that prevents the removal of calcium from bone. Common adverse effects include fatigue, asthenia, hypophosphatemia, nausea, hypercholesterolemia, musculoskeletal pain, and cystitis. Because the drug can cause severe hypocalcemia, serum calcium levels should be monitored regularly and calcium supplements and vitamin D administered as necessary. Some patients also experience osteonecrosis of the jaw. This drug causes fetal harm in laboratory animals and is not recommended during pregnancy. It is not known if this drug is secreted in human milk or if it has adverse effects on the breastfed neonate.

Rosomosozumab (Evenity) is a monoclonal antibody approved for osteoporosis treatment in postmenopausal women at high risk for fracture. It is given subcutaneously once monthly. Because this drug slowly decreases in effectiveness, therapy is limited to 12 months. Rosomosozumab binds to and inactivates the protein sclerostin, a natural inhibitor of bone formation. Like denosumab, osteonecrosis of the jaw is a potential adverse effect. This drug carries a black box warning that it may increase the risk for major cardiovascular adverse events and death. It should not be administered to patients who have experienced an MI or stroke in the past 12 months. Rosomosozumab is only indicated for postmenopausal women.

Parathyroid hormone analogs: Abaloparatide (Tymlos) and teriparatide (Bonsity, Forteo) are forms of human PTH produced by recombinant DNA technology. Both are for the treatment of osteoporosis in postmenopausal women who are at high risk of bone fractures. Teriparatide has two additional indications: to increase bone mass in men with primary or hypogonadal osteoporosis at high risk for fracture and treatment of men or women with osteoporosis due to sustained glucocorticoid therapy.

The actions of the PTH analogs are identical to those of endogenous PTH. Unlike other medications that simply reduce bone resorption, the PTH analogs also stimulate the production of new bone. Both drugs are given daily by the subcutaneous route and are available as prefilled pen injectors. Both teriparatide (approved in 2002) and abaloparatide (approved in 2017) carry a black box warning that PTH analogs cause osteosarcomas in laboratory animals. Because of this, they should not be used in patients with an increased risk for osteosarcoma. The black box warning also states that the PTH analogs should not be used for more than 2 years total time during a patient's lifetime. Teriparatide is well tolerated, with dizziness and leg cramps being the most frequent adverse effects. Abaloparatide has no pregnancy data because it is only indicated for postmenopausal women. Teriparatide showed fetal harm in laboratory animals at very high doses. Because it is associated with osteosarcoma, breastfeeding is not recommended.

Pathophysiology and Pharmacotherapy of Joint Disorders

72.9 Osteoarthritis is treated with a combination of analgesics and nonpharmacologic therapies.

A simple classification of joint disorders places them into two categories: noninflammatory and inflammatory. The most common of the noninflammatory disorders is osteoarthritis. Common inflammatory joint disorders such as rheumatoid arthritis and gout are covered in Sections 72.10 and 72.11, respectively. These joint conditions are frequent indications for pharmacotherapy, with joint pain being common to all disorders. Analgesics and anti-inflammatory drugs are important components of pharmacotherapy. A few additional drugs are specific to the particular joint pathology. Pharmacotherapy Illustrated 72.1 shows the types of joint pathology and their drug therapy.

Pharmacotherapy Illustrated 72.1

Joint Disorders

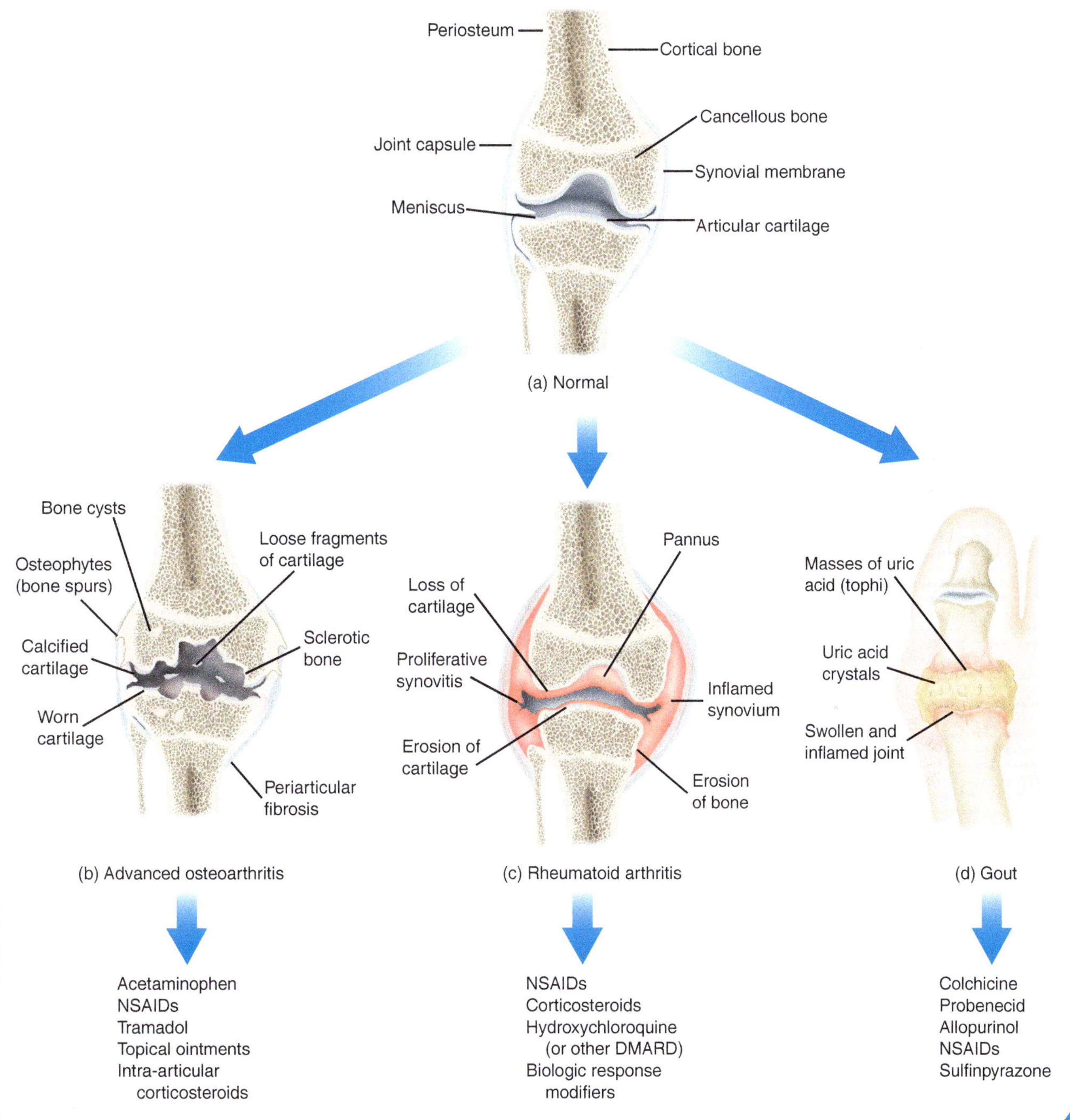

Osteoarthritis (OA) is a progressive, degenerative joint disease caused by the breakdown of articular cartilage. It is the most common cause of disability in the United States, affecting over 30 million people. Weight-bearing joints such as the knee, vertebral column, and hip are most commonly affected. The hands are also affected because they are frequently used. OA may be classified as idiopathic or secondary. Idiopathic OA, the most common type, has no known cause but is associated with increasing age. The causes of secondary OA include trauma, mechanical stress, inflammation of the joint structures, neurologic disorders, use of certain medications, and joint instability. Excessive weight contributes to the development of OA, particularly in the knee and hip jpoints. Other risk factors associated with OA include decreased estrogen in menopausal women, excessive growth hormone, and increased PTH.

As cartilage thins in the affected joints, there is less padding and, eventually, the underlying bone is affected. The bone thickens in the exposed areas, forming bone spurs and cysts that narrow the joint space. As these growths enlarge, small pieces may break off, leading to inflammation of the synovial membrane and a loss of lubricating fluid. This leads to further pain, inflammation, and destruction of the synovial membrane lining the joint. The affected joint becomes unstable and more susceptible to injury, with partial joint dislocations and other deformities that are common in advanced disease being seen.

The onset of OA is usually gradual, with pain and stiffness in one or more joints being the first manifestations. The patient with OA typically describes a deep, aching, localized pain, which is usually aggravated by movement and relieved by rest. Pain at night may be accompanied by paresthesias. As the disease advances, the range of motion (ROM) of the joint decreases; this is often accompanied by complaints of progressive pain. Bone enlargement can increase joint size; flexion contractures contribute to joint instability. It is important to note that OA is not accompanied by the degree of inflammation associated with other forms of arthritis. The joints of a patient with OA are characteristically hard and cool to palpation. A patient with OA is shown in Figure 72.4. The diagnosis of OA is typically made through a medical history, physical examination, and routine x-rays.

Nonpharmacologic therapies are an essential component of OA management. Walking, nonimpact aerobics, and passive ROM exercises are important to maintain joint flexibility. Improving muscle strength, especially of the quadriceps muscle, will help patients improve their ability to perform ADLs. Bracing may help keep joints positioned correctly and relieve pain. Patients who are obese should consider a weight loss program, especially if weight-bearing joints such as the hip and knee are affected. Weight loss has been associated with decreased pain and disability. Surgical procedures such as joint replacement and reconstructive surgery may become necessary when other methods are ineffective.

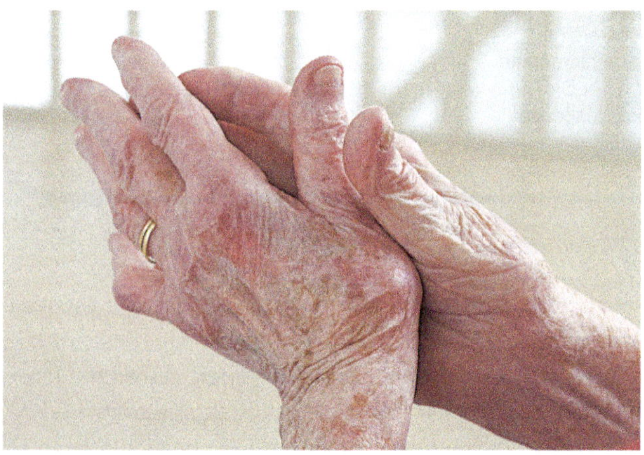

Figure 72.4 Patient with osteoarthritis.
JPC-PROD/Shutterstock.

The goals of pharmacotherapy for OA include reducing pain and inflammation and minimizing disability. The initial treatment for most patients is acetaminophen. Acetaminophen is inexpensive, participates in few drug–drug interactions, and has fewer serious adverse effects than other analgesics. For patients whose pain is unrelieved by acetaminophen, nonsteroidal anti-inflammatory drugs (NSAIDs), including naproxen and ibuprofen derivatives, are usually given. Because high doses of NSAIDs can result in GI bleeding and affect platelet aggregation, patients must be carefully monitored. Aspirin is no longer recommended because the high doses needed to produce pain relief in patients with OA may cause GI bleeding. Opioids such as tramadol (Ultram) or codeine may be combined with acetaminophen for more severe pain. The student should refer to Chapter 25 for a complete discussion of the actions and adverse effects of analgesics.

In acute cases, intra-articular corticosteroid injections may be used. With intra-articular injections, a long-acting corticosteroid such as triamcinolone is injected directly into the joint space of the affected joint. Pain relief generally lasts 3 months following the injection. Although this procedure relieves pain on a temporary basis, it can speed the destruction of cartilage if it is performed more frequently than every 4 to 6 months.

Many patients use topical medications—including salicylates (Aspercreme, Sportscreme), capsaicin (Capzasin), and counterirritants (Bengay, Icy Hot), which are sold OTC as creams, gels, sprays, patches, or ointments—to relieve OA pain. These therapies are well tolerated and produce few adverse effects. These products should not be used more than four times daily and should be discontinued if skin irritation occurs.

Another drug therapy option for patients with moderate OA who do not respond adequately to analgesics includes hyaluronate sodium (Hyalgan), a chemical normally found in high amounts within the synovial fluid. Administered by injection directly into the knee joint, this drug replaces or supplements the body's natural hyaluronic acid, which deteriorates as a result of the inflammation of OA. Treatment consists of one injection per week for three to five injections. Hyalgan helps provide a barrier that prevents friction and further inflammation of the joint by coating the articulating cartilage surface. Information that is given to the patient prior to administration should include adverse effects such as pain or swelling at the injection site and the avoidance of any strenuous activities for approximately 48 hours after injection.

CONNECTIONS: Complementary and Alternative Therapies

Glucosamine and Chondroitin for Osteoarthritis

Description

Many patients use OTC herbal medicines to relieve the pain and inflammation associated with OA. Two of the most commonly used agents are glucosamine and chondroitin.

History and Claims

Glucosamine is a natural substance that is an important building block of cartilage. With aging, glucosamine is lost with the natural thinning of cartilage. As cartilage wears down, the joints lose their normal cushioning ability, resulting in the pain and inflammation of OA. Chondroitin is another substance that forms part of the matrix between cartilage cells.

The use of glucosamine is thought to reduce cartilage breakdown and improve cartilage production and repair. Chondroitin is another dietary supplement purported to repair cartilage damaged by inflammation or injury.

Standardization

Glucosamine is made from the crushed shells of shrimp, lobster, and crab, although nonshellfish forms are available for patients allergic to shellfish. It is available as oral tablets, capsules, or in powder form, with a typical dose being 1.5 g/day. Chondroitin is derived from bovine or shark cartilage and is also taken orally, with doses in the range of 800 to 1200 mg/day.

Evidence

Typical of many other specialty supplements, research regarding the effectiveness of chondroitin and glucosamine has delivered mixed results. In the United States, large research trials have not demonstrated significant improvement in pain in patients who took glucosamine and chondroitin for osteoarthritis, although there is some evidence to suggest that the combination may improve function and ease pain as well as celecoxib, especially when combined with celecoxib or acetaminophen (Zhu et al., 2018). The Arthritis Foundation (n.d.) has given conditional approval for the use of the combination.

Glucosamine and chondroitin supplements are known to interact with warfarin (Coumadin), increasing the risk of bleeding, and some studies suggest that large doses may cause renal damage. As with all supplements, patients should be encouraged to talk with their healthcare provider about using the supplement and at what dosage.

72.10 Pharmacotherapy for rheumatoid arthritis includes analgesics, anti-inflammatory drugs, corticosteroids, and disease-modifying antirheumatic drugs.

Rheumatoid arthritis (RA) is a chronic, progressive autoimmune disease that causes inflammation of the joints. It is characterized by disfigurement and inflammation of multiple joints. RA is less common than OA, with RA affecting over 2 million people in the United States. Typically, RA occurs at an earlier age than OA, with the incidence of RA increasing up to age 70. It is important to differentiate between the two types of arthritis because the treatments are very different.

In RA, autoantibodies known as rheumatoid factors attack the individual's tissues, activating complement and drawing leukocytes into the area, where they attack the cells of the synovial membranes and blood. Inflammation first occurs in the synovial membranes, which line joint cavities, then progresses to the surrounding articular cartilage. The damaged synovial membrane swells and the persistent inflammation spreads and damages the surrounding blood vessels, ligaments, and tendons. The swelling also causes hemorrhage, coagulation, and deposits of fibrin within the joints. This ultimately leads to scar tissue formation that immobilizes the joint.

The exact etiology of RA is not known, but it is likely a combination of environmental and genetic factors. Genetic factors account for 50% of the risk for developing rheumatoid arthritis. Female reproductive hormones may influence the development of RA because it affects women about three times more frequently than men. Infectious organisms, such as the Epstein-Barr virus, may play a role in an individual developing the autoimmune processes seen with RA.

The course of RA and the rate at which joint deformities develop are variable. Disease progression is typically fastest during the first 6 years, slowing thereafter. The onset is typically insidious, though it may be acute if precipitated by a stressor, such as infection. The patient with early RA typically experiences morning joint stiffness, swelling, pain, and generalized fatigue. The joints may be slightly reddened, warm, and tender to palpation. The pattern of joints involved is usually symmetric. The upper extremity joints are often involved, beginning with the hands and wrists, as well as the joints of the toes, ankles, and knees. As the disease worsens, the morning stiffness can extend several hours into the day and occur with any periods of prolonged rest. The persistent inflammation causes deformities of the joints and the supporting ligaments, tendons, and muscles, making activity painful. Muscle weakness and decreased ROM may be apparent. Most or all synovial joints are eventually affected. A patient with RA is shown in Figure 72.5.

Joint manifestations in RA typically precede systemic manifestations, which are associated with advancing disease. Extreme fatigue, anorexia, weight loss, anemia, and low-grade fever are common. Rheumatoid nodules may

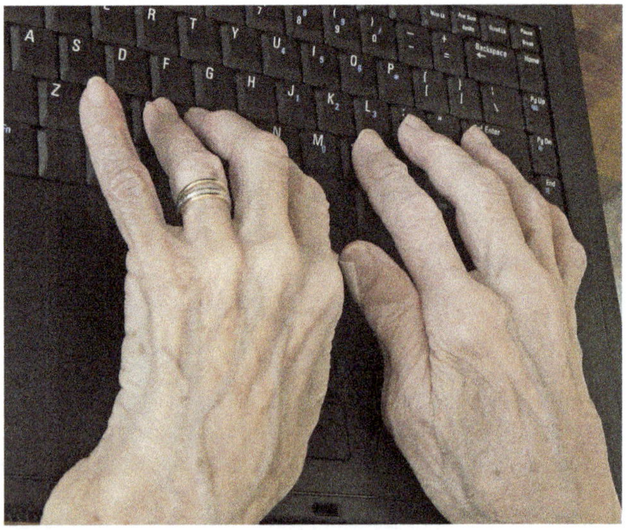

Figure 72.5 Patient with rheumatoid arthritis.
Lee319/Shutterstock.

develop in the subcutaneous tissue of the forearm, toes, and fingers and in the viscera surrounding the heart, lungs, dura, and intestinal tract. Inflammation of the blood vessels can result in vasculitis. Respiratory complications, including pleurisy, pneumonitis, and fibrosis, are common as well as cardiac complications such as pericarditis and myocarditis.

Diagnosis of RA is based on the patient's history, physical examination, and diagnostic tests. The two most-used diagnostic laboratory tests to support a diagnosis of RA include serum rheumatoid factor (RF) and the cyclic citrullinated peptide (CCP) antibody test. Whereas elevated RF values are found in several types of immune disorders, elevated CCP is specific for RA. Routine x-rays are used to determine the extent of structural joint damage.

Like OA, nonpharmacologic therapies are an essential component of RA management. ROM and joint and muscle strengthening exercises are important if the patient is to continue performing normal ADLs. Psychologic counseling may be helpful to help the patient deal with a potentially debilitating disease. Braces, splints, canes, and walkers can assist in ambulation. Loss of excess weight can help take the stress off inflamed joints. Proper rest helps reduce pain.

The primary goal of RA pharmacotherapy is to prevent or slow the progression of the disease. Pain management is important because the disease-modifying medications may take many months to achieve full effectiveness. Symptomatic pain management is usually achieved with NSAIDs because these drugs relieve both pain and inflammation. NSAIDs that are used to treat RA are usually given in doses that are higher than those for the patient with OA. Aspirin is not recommended for long-term therapy due to its adverse effects on the GI system and platelet aggregation. Acetaminophen is effective at relieving pain and fever but has no anti-inflammatory actions. Although the analgesics relieve symptomatic pain, they have no effect on disease progression.

Corticosteroids are frequently used because of their rapid onset of potent anti-inflammatory action. They are often administered as initial therapy and for RA flare-ups. They are not used for prolonged therapy because of their long-term adverse effects (see Chapter 68).

The progression of tissue damage characteristic of RA can be slowed or prevented with a diverse group of drugs called **disease-modifying antirheumatic drugs (DMARDs)**. These drugs, which modify immune and inflammatory responses, reduce mortality rates, improve symptoms, and enhance the quality of life in patients with RA. Doses of DMARDs are listed in Table 72.7. The medications are grouped as follows:

- Conventional DMARDs
- Biologic DMARDs (tumor necrosis factor [TNF] antagonists)
- Biologic DMARDS (non-TNF antagonists).

The choice of a specific DMARD depends on the experiences of the healthcare provider and the response of the patient to therapy. Many rheumatologists consider methotrexate to be the first-line therapy for the initial treatment of RA. It acts quickly, has a relatively favorable safety profile, is low in cost, and slows the progression of the disease. A once-weekly subcutaneous formulation of methotrexate (Otrexup) was approved in 2013 for severe RA that has not responded to other forms of therapy. Other nonbiologic DMARDs considered for initial therapy include hydroxychloroquine (Plaquenil) and sulfasalazine (Azulfidine). Risks of toxicity with these drugs is among the lowest associated with DMARDs. Nonbiologic DMARDs such as azathioprine (Azasan, Imuran) and leflunomide (Arava) have more adverse effects than other DMARDs but may be used in combination with some of the biologic therapies.

Biologic DMARDS are newer therapies for the treatment of RA. These drugs block steps in the inflammatory response, reduce joint inflammation, and slow the progression of joint damage. Adalimumab (Humira), etanercept (Enbrel), certolizumab pegol (Cimzia), golimumab (Simponi), and infliximab (Remicade) are TNF antagonists. TNF is a naturally occurring cytokine produced by macrophages and activated T cells that mediates inflammation and modulates cellular immune responses. Elevated levels of TNF are found in the synovial fluid of patients with RA. Certolizumab pegol (Cimzia) and golimumab (Simponi) are newer-generation TNF antagonists. Anakinra (Kineret) and abatacept (Orencia) are biologic drugs that block actions of interleukins in inflammatory pathways. The biologic drugs appear to be effective and relatively nontoxic, but they are very expensive; thus, they are normally not prescribed until conventional therapy has been attempted and failed. Combinations of biologic and nonbiologic drugs may be effective for patients unresponsive to monotherapy.

Table 72.7 Selected Disease-Modifying Antirheumatic Drugs

Drug	Route and Adult Dose (Maximum Dose Where Indicated)	Adverse Effects
Conventional DMARDs		
azathioprine (Azasan, Imuran)	PO: 1 mg/kg/day once or in divided doses bid for 6–8 wk (max: 2.5 mg/kg/day) Maintenance dose: 1–2.5 mg/kg/day as a single dose or divided	*Chills, fever, malaise, myalgia* Myelosuppression, hepatotoxicity, lymphoproliferative disorders
hydroxychloroquine (Plaquenil)	PO: 400–600 mg/day for 4–12 wk, then 200–400 mg once daily Maintenance dose: 10–20 mg/day	*Anorexia, nausea and vomiting, headache, personality changes* Retinopathy, agranulocytosis, aplastic anemia, seizures
leflunomide (Arava)	PO: 100-mg loading dose for 3 days, then 20 mg/day	*Diarrhea, elevated hepatic enzymes, alopecia, rash* Hepatotoxicity, immunosuppression
methotrexate (Otrexup, Rasuvo, Trexall)	PO: 7.5 mg once/wk or 2.5 mg q12h for 3 doses once/wk (max: 20 mg/wk) Subcutaneous (Otrexup): 10–25 mg once weekly	*Headache, glossitis, gingivitis, mild leukopenia, nausea* Ulcerative stomatitis, myelosuppression, aplastic anemia, hepatic cirrhosis, nephrotoxicity, sudden death, pulmonary fibrosis, teratogenicity
sulfasalazine (Azulfidine)	PO: 500–1000 mg/day (max: 3 g/day)	*Headache, anorexia, nausea and vomiting* Anaphylaxis, Stevens–Johnson syndrome (SJS), agranulocytosis, leukopenia, reversible oligospermia
Biologic DMARDs (TNF Antagonists)		
adalimumab (Humira)	Subcutaneous: 40 mg every other week	*Local reactions at the injection site (pain, erythema, myalgia), nasopharyngitis* Serious infection, sepsis, invasive fungal infections, lupus-like syndrome, positive antinuclear antibodies, tumor lysis syndrome, HF exacerbations, SJS, increased malignancies, neutropenia
certolizumab pegol (Cimzia)	Subcutaneous: 400 mg initially and at wk 2 and 4, followed by 200 mg every other week	
etanercept (Enbrel)	Subcutaneous: 25 mg twice weekly or 0.08 mg/kg or 50 mg once weekly	
golimumab (Simponi)	Subcutaneous: 50 mg once monthly (for RA) or 100 mg q4wk (for ulcerative colitis)	
infliximab (Remicade)	IV: 3 mg/kg at wk 0, 2, and 6, then q8wk	
Biologic DMARDs (Non-TNF Antagonists)		
abatacept (Orencia)	IV: 500–1000 mg given at 0, 2, and 4 wk, then q4wk thereafter	*Local reactions at the injection site (pain, erythema, myalgia), nasopharyngitis* Serious infection, sepsis, invasive fungal infections, tumor lysis syndrome, neutropenia, increased malignancies, anaphylaxis, hypotension (rituximab), bowel obstruction and perforation (rituximab, tocilizumab, tofacitinib)
anakinra (Kineret)	Subcutaneous: 100 mg/day	
baricitinib (Olumiant)	PO: 2 mg once daily	
rituximab (Rituxan)	IV: 1000 mg q2wk for a total of 2 doses (give a corticosteroid 30 min prior to infusion)	
sarilumab (Kevzara)	Subcutaneous: 150 mg/1.14 mL or 200 mg/1.14 mL using a prefilled syringe	
tocilizumab (Actemra)	IV: 4–8 mg/kg every other week Subcutaneous: 162 mg every week or every other week	
tofacitinib (Xeljanz)	PO: 5 mg bid	

Note: *Italics* indicate common adverse effects. Underline indicates serious adverse effects.

PROTOTYPE DRUG Adalimumab (Humira)

Classification **Therapeutic:** Disease-modifying antirheumatic drug
Pharmacologic: TNF antagonist

Therapeutic Effects and Uses: Initially introduced to treat RA in 2002, adalimumab was the first fully human monoclonal antibody approved by the FDA. Since then, it has become one of the bestselling drugs in history. Indications for the drug have expanded to include psoriatic arthritis, ankylosing spondylitis, polyarticular juvenile idiopathic arthritis, Crohn's disease, hidradenitis suppurativa, ulcerative colitis, chronic plaque psoriasis, and uveitis. Amjevita is a biosimilar drug approved in 2016 for seven indications of adalimumab. A biosimilar is a biologic drug that is substantially similar in clinical properties.

Adalimumab is administered by the subcutaneous route, usually every other week. Doses differ by indication. The drug is available in a single-use pen injection system for home administration.

Mechanism of Action: Adalimumab blocks the inflammatory activity of TNF. High levels of TNF are often found in patients with inflammatory disorders such as RA.

Pharmacokinetics:

Route(s)	Subcutaneous
Absorption	Peak levels occur in about 5 days
Distribution	Unknown
Primary metabolism	Unknown
Primary excretion	Unknown
Onset of action	4–5 weeks
Duration of action	10–20 days

Adverse Effects: The most common adverse effects are injection-site pain, upper respiratory infection, increased creatine phosphate, headache, and rash. **Black Box Warning:** Due to its ability to suppress the immune system, patients are at increased risk for the development of serious infections and malignancies. Latent infections such as tuberculosis and hepatitis B virus may become reactivated. Leukemias, lymphomas, and other malignancies have been reported with TNF blockers. Although rare, fatal cases of hepatosplenic T-cell lymphoma have been documented with TNF blockers.

Contraindications/Precautions: There are no contraindications. As a precaution, patients should be monitored for the development of infections or malignancies.

Drug Interactions: Adalimumab should not be administered concurrently with the TNF blockers anakinra or abatacept. Administration of live vaccines should be avoided. Concurrent use with other immunosuppressants should be avoided or carefully monitored to avoid an increased risk for serious infections. **Herbal/Food:** Echinacea should be avoided because it may decrease the immunosuppressive effects of adalimumab.

Pregnancy: This drug does not show evidence of fetal harm in laboratory animals. Adalimumab is secreted in human milk but has not shown adverse effects in breastfed neonates.

Treatment of Overdose: Treatment is supportive.

Clinician Responsibilities: Key nursing implications for patients receiving adalimumab are included in Applied Clinical Judgment: Patients Receiving Pharmacotherapy for Rheumatoid Arthritis and Osteoarthritis.

Other DMARDS for Rheumatoid Arthritis

Gold salts (Auranofin, Aurothioglucose, gold sodium thiomalate) and penicillamine (Cuprimine, Depen) are DMARDs that are rarely used and the student should refer to a drug guide for information. Cyclosporine and azathioprine are immunosuppressants that occasionally are used as DMARDs. They are described in Chapter 42.

Abatacept (Orencia): Approved in 2005, abatacept is indicated for the treatment of moderate to severe RA in adults. juvenile idiopathic RA in children ages 2 and older, and active psoriatic arthritis. The drug acts by inhibiting the actions of T cells, which are often hyperactive in patients with RA. It is administered as an IV infusion, usually every 2 to 4 weeks, or weekly by the subcutaneous route. Headache, upper respiratory tract infection, and nausea are common adverse effects. Like other immunosuppressants, there is an increased risk of serious infections or reactivation of latent TB infections. Although abatacept is sometimes used in combination with other DMARDs, it should not be administered concurrently with TNF blockers due to a high risk for serious infections. Abatacept does not show evidence of fetal harm in laboratory animals. This drug is secreted in animal milk but adverse effects on the breastfed neonate are not known.

Anakinra (Kineret): Approved in 2001, anakinra inhibits interleukin-1 (IL-1), an important chemical mediator of inflammation. It is approved for RA that has not responded to one or more DMARDs and for treatment of neonatal-onset multisystem inflammatory disease. Given daily by the subcutaneous route, injection-site reactions such as pain, swelling, edema, and bruising occur often. Ice and hydrocortisone cream are recommended to diminish the pain, along with site rotation. Upper respiratory infections and influenza symptoms occur in many patients. Anakinra is not administered concurrently with TNF inhibitors such as etanercept due to an increased risk of infections. Laboratory animal and limited human data do not show evidence of fetal harm. Limited studies do not show evidence of adverse effects on the breastfed neonate.

Baricitinib (Olumiant): Baricitinib was approved in 2018 for the treatment of severe RA that is unresponsive to TNF antagonists. In 2020, it received emergency-use authorization in combination with remdesivir to treat hospitalized patients on mechanical ventilators infected with the COVID-19 virus. This approval was temporary and based on preliminary efficacy data. Like many of the biologics, baricitinib carries a black box warning about the risk for serious infections and malignancy. The warning also includes an increased incidence of thrombosis. Very high doses showed fetal harm in laboratory animals. It is not known if this drug enters human milk or if it has adverse effects on the breastfed neonate.

Hydroxychloroquine (Plaquenil): Approved in 1955, hydroxychloroquine is indicated for the treatment of RA. This drug is also used for the prophylaxis and treatment of malaria, but chloroquine (Aralen) is the preferred drug for this parasitic infection (see Chapter 53). It may be used to treat systemic lupus erythematosus in patients who have not responded well to other anti-inflammatory drugs. Hydroxychloroquine therapy for 3 to 6 months is required to achieve therapeutic effects. For full effectiveness, hydroxychloroquine is most often prescribed concurrently with salicylates and glucocorticoids. The primary adverse effects of hydroxychloroquine are GI related, such as anorexia, weight loss, and nausea and vomiting. Possible ocular effects include blurred vision, photophobia, diminished ability to read, and blacked-out areas in the visual field. Human data have not shown evidence for an increase in adverse pregnancy outcomes or teratogenicity above the baseline rate. This drug is secreted in human milk, although adverse effects on the breastfed neonate are unknown.

Leflunomide (Arava): Approved in 1998, leflunomide is a DMARD with a unique mechanism of action. It inhibits an enzyme in mitochondria that is responsible for the synthesis of pyrimidines, which are building blocks for DNA and ribonucleic acid (RNA). The result is an inhibition in B-cell and T-cell function. Reduced cytokine and antibody production by these cells reduce inflammation and joint destruction. After a loading dose for 3 days, this drug is given PO once daily. Leflunomide has an exceptionally long half-life and it can be detected in the blood as long as 2 years after discontinuation. If toxicity occurs, the administration of cholestyramine for 11 days can clear most leflunomide from the body. Common adverse effects include diarrhea, nausea and vomiting, headache, and alopecia. Leflunomide is hepatotoxic and liver function must be regularly monitored during therapy. This drug is embryotoxic and teratogenic in laboratory animals. The possibility of pregnancy should be excluded before therapy is begun and women should wait 2 years after discontinuation of therapy to become pregnant. Breastfeeding is contraindicated.

Methotrexate (Otrexup, Rasuvo, Trexall): Methotrexate is prescribed for a number of proliferative and inflammatory diseases, including various carcinomas and leukemias, immunosuppression following kidney transplantation, severe psoriasis, and RA. Methotrexate is a folic acid antagonist and a potent immunosuppressant. Gastric irritation and stomatitis are the most frequent adverse effects; these are minimized by the concurrent use of folic acid. Patients, particularly those who are older, obese, or have diabetes or CKD, need to be monitored for hepatotoxicity, bone marrow suppression, and pneumonitis. Human data suggests that methotrexate can cause teratogenic effects or fetal death when taken during pregnancy. Pregnancy should be avoided if either partner is receiving this drug. The possibility of pregnancy should be excluded before therapy is begun. Breastfeeding is contraindicated. A prototype feature for methotrexate may be found in Chapter 57.

Rituximab (Rituxan): Rituximab is a monoclonal antibody originally approved in 1997 as an antineoplastic drug. The drug binds to CD20, a surface protein present on B lymphocytes involved in certain leukemias and lymphomas. Once bound, rituximab lyses the tumor cells. Later, it was discovered that B lymphocytes also play a major role in producing the severe inflammation associated with RA. In 2006, rituximab was approved to treat moderate to severe RA that has not responded to therapy with TNF blockers. For RA, the drug is administered concurrently with methotrexate. Other indications include non-Hodgkin's lymphoma, chronic lymphocytic leukemia, granulomatosis with polyangiitis, and pemphigus vulgaris. Rituximab carries a black box warning for severe mucocutaneous reactions, fatal infusion-related reactions, hepatitis B reactivation, and leukoencephalopathy. Rituximab can also produce adverse effects such as serious infections, life-threatening dysrhythmias, and tumor lysis syndrome. Based on human data, rituximab can cause fetal harm. Females of childbearing potential should use effective contraception during therapy and for at least a year after the last dose. Breastfeeding is not advised until at least 6 months postpartum.

Sarilumab (Kevzara): Approved in 2017, sarilumab acts by blocking receptors for interleukin-6 (IL-6), a cytoline secreted by immune cells that promotes inflammation and activates the immune response. It may be used as monotherapy or in combination with other DMARDs such as methotrexate to treat moderate to severe RA in patients who have not responded to one or more DMARDS. Sarilumab carries a black box warning that serious invasive and opportunistic infections can occur and to monitor all patients for TB during therapy. This drug may cause neutropenia; therefore, it should be avoided if an active infection is present. The drug is not recommended for patients with active hepatic disease. Sarilumab did not show evidence of fetal harm in laboratory animals. There are insufficient data regarding the safety of this drug during breastfeeding.

Sulfasalazine (Azulfidine): Sulfasalazine is a sulfonamide and, having been approved in 1950, one of the oldest drugs for RA. It is also approved for juvenile RA, Crohn's disease, and ulcerative colitis. It is available as an enteric-coated tablet that must be taken three to four times daily. Its beneficial effects are noted quickly, often after 4 weeks of therapy. GI complaints such as nausea and vomiting, anorexia, diarrhea, and abdominal pain occur in a significant number of patients taking this drug, and these may cause discontinuation of therapy. The adverse GI effects are better tolerated if therapy starts with a low dose that is gradually increased. Headache; blood dyscrasias, especially leukopenia; and skin rashes also occur frequently. Regular monitoring of CBCs for bone marrow suppression should be conducted. Patients with allergies to sulfur or other sulfonamides should not receive sulfasalazine. Concurrent administration with iron supplements or antibiotics should be avoided because doing so diminishes the absorption of this drug. Human data does not show significant evidence for fetal harm. Sulfasalazine is secreted in human milk. If breastfeeding, the neonate should be monitored for possible jaundice, hemolysis, and bloody diarrhea.

TNF Antagonists: In addition to the prototype adalimumab, the TNF blocker class includes certolizumab, etanercept, golimumab, and infliximab. Although each of these monoclonal antibodies is unique, they have similar actions and adverse effects. The most common adverse effects are injection-site reactions such as pain, swelling, and bruising. Other adverse effects include upper respiratory tract infection, neutropenia, and rare cases of central nervous system (CNS) demyelinating disorders such as multiple sclerosis. Also, some of these medications may worsen or cause HF. Because they are potent immunosuppressants, all pose an increased risk for serious infections and malignancy. These drugs carry a black box warning that reactivation of latent infections such as tuberculosis may occur. The warning also includes an increased risk for lymphoma and other malignancies, especially when used in children and adolescents treated for juvenile RA.

- *Certolizumab pegol (Cimzia):* Certolizumab was approved in 2008 and is indicated for the treatment of moderate to severe RA, ankylosing spondylitis, psoriatic arthritis, moderate to severe plaque psoriasis, inflammatory spondylitis, and Crohn's disease unresponsive to safer medications. The drug is given as a subcutaneous injection, usually every other week. Certolizumab does not show evidence of fetal harm in laboratory animals. This drug is secreted in human milk but has not shown adverse effects in breastfed neonates.
- *Etanercept (Enbrel):* Approved in 1998, etanercept is approved for the treatment of moderate to severe RA, psoriatic RA in adults, polyarticular juvenile RA in children age 2 and older, ankylosing spondylitis, and plaque psoriasis. Etanercept is administered by the subcutaneous route twice a week. Concurrent use of etanercept with sulfasalazine may result in leukopenia. Human observational studies in pregnancy are inconclusive but etanercept may increase the risk for birth defects. This drug is secreted in human milk but has not shown adverse effects in breastfed neonates.
- *Golimumab (Simponi):* Golimumab was approved in 2009 and is indicated for the management of moderate to severe RA, active psoriatic RA in adults, active ankylosing spondylitis in adults, and moderate to severe ulcerative colitis that cannot be managed by first-line medications. This drug is often combined with methotrexate and is given as a subcutaneous injection once a month. Golimumab does not show evidence of fetal harm in laboratory animals. This drug is secreted in animal milk but adverse effects on the breastfed neonate are not known.
- *Infliximab (Remicade):* Originally approved in 1998, infliximab is indicated for moderate to severe RA, psoriatic RA, ankylosing spondylitis, Crohn's disease, ulcerative colitis, and plaque psoriasis. For RA, infliximab is usually combined with methotrexate and is given as an IV infusion over several hours, followed by subsequent injections in weeks 2 and 6 and every 8 weeks thereafter. Acetaminophen and diphenhydramine (Benadryl) are given prior to infusion to decrease infusion reaction symptoms such as chest pain, tachycardia, shortness of breath, and lightheadedness. Human observational studies in pregnancy are inconclusive but infliximab may be associated with preterm delivery and low birth weight. This drug is secreted in human milk but has not shown adverse effects in breastfed neonates.

Tocilizumab (Actemra): Tocilizumab was approved in 2010 for the treatment of moderate to severe RA in adults and for polyarticular juvenile idiopathic arthritis in children age 2 and older. It was subsequently approved to treat giant cell arteritis and cytokine release syndrome. Like sarilumab, tocilizumab acts by inhibiting IL-6 and may be used as monotherapy for RA or in combination with other DMARDs such as methotrexate. It is administered by either the IV or subcutaneous route. Headache, upper respiratory tract infection, HTN, and increased liver enzymes are common adverse effects. Like other immunosuppressants, the risk of serious infections or reactivation of latent infections is increased. Tocilizumab therapy should not be initiated if the absolute neutrophil count is less than 2000/mm^3, if the platelet count is below 100,000/mm^3, or if liver enzymes are elevated (1.5 times normal). Tocilizumab carries a black box warning that serious invasive and opportunistic infections can occur and to monitor all patients for TB during therapy. This causes abortion and fetal death in laboratory animals. It is not known if this drug enters breast milk or if it has adverse effects on the breastfed neonate.

Tofacitinib (Xeljanz): Tofacitinib is a biologic DMARD, first approved in 2013. Indications include treating RA that has not responded adequately to methotrexate therapy, psoriatic arthritis, ulcerative colitis, and juvenile idiopathic arthritis. This drug acts by inhibiting Janus kinases (JAKs). JAKs are enzymes that signal the immune system to release certain cytokines that cause inflammation. By blocking the signaling pathway, JAK inhibitors (sometimes called Jakinibs) reduce the progress and clinical symptoms of RA. Like some other biologic therapies, tofacitinib carries a black box warning that its use may result in serious infections and that the existence of latent tuberculosis should be excluded prior to therapy. The black box warning also notes that lymphoma and other malignancies have developed in patients taking this drug. This drug is embryotoxic and fetotoxic in laboratory animals. It is not known if this drug enters human milk or if it has adverse effects on the breastfed neonate.

CONNECTIONS: APPLIED CLINICAL JUDGMENT

Patients Receiving Pharmacotherapy for Rheumatoid Arthritis and Osteoarthritis

Key Assessment Data

- History of current condition including musculoskeletal, GI, cardiovascular, neurologic, endocrine, hepatic, or kidney disease; baseline vital signs, physical exam findings; pregnancy or breastfeeding; CBC, sedimentation rate, hepatic and renal function studies, RF, CCP antibody test, coagulation panels, bleeding time, electrolytes, glucose, lipid profile; dietary and medication history including allergies, current prescription and OTC drugs, herbal preparations, caffeine, nicotine, and alcohol use.
- Assess for inflammation, nodules, and deformities, as well as their location, and note the presence of pain or discomfort, time of day of occurrence, on movement, or at rest. Assess effects on sleep. Obtain a dietary history and the effect of the disease on the ability to obtain food sources, cooking, and eating. Assess adequacy of fluid intake.

Desired Therapeutic Outcomes

Improvement is observed and measurable by diminished symptoms of acute inflammation, pain is diminished or absent, and increased ability to carry out ROM and ADLs.

Minimizing Adverse Effects

- Drugs for RA treat the symptoms and slow the progression of the disease but are not a cure. Acute exacerbations may require hospitalization and a change in the medication regimen.

Lifespan Considerations

- Age-related physiologic differences may place the older adult at greater risk for adverse hepatic, renal, or cardiac adverse effects.

Patient Education

- Promptly report increasing pain, stiffness, and decreased ability to carry out ADLs. Hospitalization may be required during acute exacerbations dependent on the severity of symptoms.
- Immediately report any signs or symptoms of GI bleeding. Alcohol use should be avoided or eliminated.
- Immediately report any signs or symptoms of ringing, humming, buzzing in ears, difficulty with balance, dizziness, vertigo, or nausea.
- If NSAIDs or salicylates are used, increase fluid intake, especially if fever is present, and report any changes in the quantity of urine output or darkening of urine promptly. Weigh self daily, ideally at the same time of day, and report a weight gain of more than 1 kg (2 lb) in a 24-hour period or more than 2 kg (5 lb) per week or increasing peripheral edema.
- If corticosteroids or DMARDs are used, immediately report any flulike symptoms, fever, mouth irritation or soreness, or skin rashes.
- If NSAIDs or DMARDs are used, obtain eye examinations twice yearly or as instructed by the provider. Immediately report any sudden changes in vision.
- If corticosteroids are used, patients with diabetes may need a change in insulin or oral medications. Report any consistent elevations in capillary glucose.
- Supplement drug therapy with nonpharmacologic measures (e.g., a balance between low-impact activity and rest, application of warm or cool compresses, or warm showers prior to activity).
- Immediately report pregnancy or suspected pregnancy because many of the DMARDS have the potential to cause fetal harm.
- If corticosteroids or DMARDs are ordered, carry a wallet identification card or wear medical identification jewelry indicating type of drug therapy.

Prescribing Considerations

- NSAIDs and salicylates may be nephrotoxic. Patients on long-term or high-dose therapy require close monitoring of dosage and have periodic renal function studies.
- Corticosteroids may affect electrolytes, glucose, and lipid levels. Patients with diabetes taking corticosteroids may need an alteration in their insulin or oral antidiabetic drugs.
- Monitor the patient closely for signs of GI irritation and bleeding when prescribing NSAIDs and glucocorticoids.
- NSAIDs and salicylates may be ototoxic and cause hearing loss.
- Bone marrow suppression may occur with corticosteroids or DMARDs. Monitor carefully for early signs of new infections or reactivation of latent infections such as herpes and TB and prescribe antiinfectives as appropriate.
- NSAIDs may cause blurred or diminished vision, decreased color sense, diplopia, or scotomas. DMARDs may cause significant retinal changes with blurred vision, difficulty reading, photophobia, or blacked-out areas of the vision field.

Pharmacotherapy of Gout and Hyperuricemia

72.11 Gout is caused by an accumulation of uric acid crystals in the joints.

Gout is a form of acute arthritis caused by an accumulation of uric acid (urate) crystals in the joints and other body tissues, causing inflammation. Between 1 and 3% of the U.S. population are affected by gout. Of patients with gout, 90% are men, who first manifest symptoms between the ages of 30 and 60; women are affected after menopause.

Gout may be classified as primary or secondary. Primary gout is caused by genetic errors in the metabolism of purines. Uric acid is a waste product created by the metabolic breakdown of the nucleic acids DNA and RNA. The kidneys are responsible for excreting uric acid. High levels of uric acid crystals may result from an increased metabolism of nucleic acids or the reduced excretion of uric acid by the kidneys. Primary gout may therefore be viewed as an imbalance in the handling of uric acid by the body. The production of uric acid crystals exceeds the excretion capability of the kidneys. Primary gout is inherited as an X-linked trait; males inherit the disorder through female carriers.

Secondary gout is caused by diseases or drugs that increase the metabolic turnover of nucleic acids or that interfere with the excretion of uric acid. Some examples of drugs that may cause gout include thiazide diuretics, aspirin, cyclosporine, and alcohol, when ingested on a chronic basis. Conditions that can cause secondary gout include diabetic ketoacidosis, hypothyroidism, multiple myeloma, CKD, and diseases associated with a rapid cell turnover such as leukemia, hemolytic anemia, and polycythemia.

The primary diagnostic criterion for gout is the serum uric acid level. **Hyperuricemia** is defined as a serum uric acid level of 7 mg/dL. Patients with mild hyperuricemia are asymptomatic. Once the level of uric acid rises to saturation levels in body fluids, urate crystals form and symptoms appear, usually with a sudden onset.

Acute gouty arthritis occurs when needle-shaped uric acid crystals accumulate in joints, resulting in extremely painful, red, and inflamed tissue. Attacks have a sudden onset, often occur at night, and may be triggered by ingestion of alcohol, dehydration, stress, injury to the joint, or fever. Gouty arthritis most often occurs in the big toes, heels, ankles, wrists, fingers, knees, or elbows and may be accompanied by an elevated temperature. With chronic gout, bumps called tophi, or deposits of sodium urate crystals in the subcutaneous tissue, may be present, particularly on the outer ear, arms, and fingers. Deposits of urate crystals in the kidneys may lead to the development of urinary calculi and kidney failure. Nephrolithiasis occurs in 10 to 25% of patients with gout and is more likely to occur in patients with low fluid intake and when the urine is acidic.

Gout may be difficult to diagnose because early symptoms may be vague. Although most people with gout have hyperuricemia, the serum levels of uric acid may be normal even during an acute attack. To confirm a diagnosis, a synovial fluid analysis may be performed to evaluate for the presence of uric acid crystals or to rule out synovial fluid infection as the cause of the symptoms.

In its early phases, treatment of gout is very successful. The goals of gout pharmacotherapy are threefold:

- Termination of acute episodes
- Prevention of future gout attacks
- Avoidance of the formation of gout complications, such as tophi and kidney stones.

NSAIDs are the preferred drugs for treating the pain and inflammation of acute episodes of gout. Commonly used NSAIDs include indomethacin (Indocin) and naproxen (Naprosyn), which are taken PO every day. Aspirin should be avoided because it can increase uric acid levels and worsen symptoms. Corticosteroids may be used to treat exacerbations of acute gout, particularly when the symptoms are in a single joint and the medication can be delivered intra-articularly. Commonly prescribed corticosteroids for gout include triamcinolone and prednisone. Most patients report that symptoms improve within a few hours of treatment and that an acute episode terminates within a week.

If a patient is unable to tolerate NSAIDs, oral colchicine (Colcrys) is highly effective at terminating gout flare-ups. Low doses may also be used for gout prophylaxis. Drugs for gout are listed in Table 72.8.

PROTOTYPE DRUG **Colchicine (Colcrys)**

Classification **Therapeutic:** Antigout drug
Pharmacologic: Anti-inflammatory drug

Therapeutic Effects and Uses: Colchicine is a natural product obtained from the autumn crocus, which is grown in gardens and found in meadows throughout the United States and Canada. It has been used for centuries as a natural product. Although first available by prescription prior to 1938, colchicine was not officially approved by the FDA

Table 72.8 Drugs for Gout

Drug	Route and Adult Dose (Maximum Dose Where Indicated)	Adverse Effects
allopurinol (Lopurin, Zyloprim)	PO (primary): 100 mg/day (max: 800 mg/day) PO (secondary): 200–800 mg/day IV: 200–400 mg/m²/day	*Drowsiness, skin rash, diarrhea* Severe skin reactions, bone marrow depression, hepatotoxicity, kidney failure
colchicine (Colcrys)	PO for prophylaxis: 0.5 mg once or twice daily PO for gout flare-up: 1.2 mg followed by another dose of 0.6 mg 1 h later	*Nausea and vomiting, diarrhea, GI upset* Bone marrow depression, aplastic anemia, leukopenia, thrombocytopenia, agranulocytosis, severe diarrhea, nephrotoxicity
febuxostat (Uloric)	PO: 40–80 mg once daily	*Liver enzyme elevation, nausea, arthralgia, rash, gout flare-up* Adverse cardiovascular events
pegloticase (Krystexxa)	IV: 8 mg q2wk	*Gout flare-up, nausea, ecchymosis, nasopharyngitis* Anaphylaxis, infusion reaction, worsening HF
probenecid (Probalan)	PO: 250 mg bid for 1 wk, then 500 mg bid (max: 3 g/day)	*Nausea and vomiting, headache, anorexia, flushed face* Anaphylaxis, severe skin reactions, hepatotoxicity, anemia, aplastic anemia, leukopenia

Note: *Italics* indicate common adverse effects. Underline indicates serious adverse effects.

until 2009. The trade-name form, Colcrys, is approved for the treatment and prophylaxis of acute gout flare-ups and for familial Mediterranean fever.

Colchicine is much more effective if taken within 24 hours of the onset of symptoms. Colchicine has several off-label indications that include amyloidosis, Paget's disease, and hepatic cirrhosis.

Although colchicine has no analgesic properties, patients experience pain relief due to the reduction in inflammation. Low doses of colchicine may be used as prophylactic therapy for gouty arthritis in patients with normal or slightly elevated serum uric acid levels. Should the patient note the onset of an acute episode, the dose can be increased until symptoms subside. It is important to understand, however, that colchicine does not inhibit uric acid synthesis and does not promote uric acid excretion. Thus, if the patient has escalating serum uric acid levels, allopurinol is the preferred drug for prophylaxis (see Section 72.12). Patients who are on colchicine prophylaxis therapy may discontinue the drug after they have been symptom free for a year and have normal serum uric acid levels. In some patients, discontinuation may precipitate an acute gout episode.

Mechanism of Action: Colchicine inhibits the migration of neutrophils into the area of inflammation. This drug reduces the inflammation associated with acute gouty arthritis by inhibiting the synthesis of microtubules, which are the subcellular structures responsible for helping white blood cells infiltrate an area.

Pharmacokinetics:

Route(s)	PO
Absorption	Rapidly absorbed
Distribution	Widely distributed; concentrated in leukocytes, kidney, liver, spleen, and intestinal tract
Primary metabolism	Hepatic
Primary excretion	Feces
Onset of action	12 h
Duration of action	Half-life: variable (1.7–20.9 h)

Adverse Effects: The most significant adverse effects of colchicine are GI related, and these may occur in up to 80% of patients. Adverse effects include nausea and vomiting, abdominal pain, anorexia, and diarrhea. This drug may cause bone marrow toxicity, and aplastic anemia, leukopenia, thrombocytopenia, or agranulocytosis may occur. Additional adverse effects include hepatotoxicity, mental confusion, azotemia, proteinuria, hematuria, and oliguria. Severe irritation and tissue damage may occur if the IV formulation leaks around the injection site.

Contraindications/Precautions: This drug is contraindicated in patients with a known hypersensitivity to colchicine and in those with CKD or GI, hepatic, or cardiac impairment. Patients with blood dyscrasias should not receive colchicine. This drug should be used with caution in older adults and debilitated patients, or in patients with an early manifestation of GI, renal, hepatic, or cardiac disease.

Drug Interactions: Concurrent use with NSAIDs may increase the risk of serious GI symptoms. Colchicine may exhibit additive bone marrow toxicity with cyclosporine, phenylbutazone, and other drugs that adversely affect bone marrow. Erythromycin may increase serum colchicine levels. Loop diuretics may decrease its effects. Alcohol or products that contain alcohol may cause skin rashes and result in additive liver damage. Colchicine may increase a patient's sensitivity to CNS depressants. It may also directly interfere with the absorption of vitamin B_{12}. **Herbal/Food:** Alcohol and foods that are rich in purines, including salmon, sardines, and organ meats, should be avoided. Foods that cause the urine to become more alkaline, such as milk, fruits, carbonated drinks, most vegetables, molasses, and baking soda, may increase the risk of kidney stones.

Pregnancy: Colchicine is teratogenic in laboratory animals. The drug is secreted in human milk although adverse effects on the breastfed neonate are unknown.

Treatment of Overdose: Overdoses (including unintentional ingestion of autumn crocus) may cause severe GI distress, shock, paralysis, delirium, respiratory failure, and death. Treatment is symptomatic and may include gastric lavage and hemodialysis.

Clinician Responsibilities: Key clinical implications for patients receiving colchicine are included in Applied Clinical Judgment: Patients Receiving Pharmacotherapy for Gout.

Drugs Similar to Colchicine (Colcrys)

Colchicine is the only drug in this class.

72.12 Long-term management of gout includes dietary modifications and drugs that reduce levels of uric acid.

Long-term prophylaxis of gout begins with lifestyle changes that include weight loss and dietary adjustments. Patients should avoid high-purine foods such as organ meats, legumes, alcoholic beverages, mushrooms, and oatmeal because these foods form nucleic acids when they are metabolized. Patients should avoid aspirin, niacin, and diuretics because their use can precipitate an acute episode of gout. Renal complications may be avoided by adequate fluid intake and consumption of a low-protein diet.

Pharmacotherapy is indicated if lifestyle changes prove unsuccessful or if patients continue to experience repeated gout flare-ups. The goal of long-term gout pharmacotherapy is to lower serum uric acid levels. Prophylaxis may be obtained by either blocking the *formation* of uric acid (allopurinol) or by increasing its *excretion* (probenecid)

Allopurinol (Lopurin, Zyloprim) is a preferred drug for gout *prophylaxis*. Allopurinol acts by inhibiting **xanthine oxidase**, which is the enzyme responsible for the formation of uric acid. Blocking the synthesis of uric acid will lower serum uric acid levels, thus preventing gout.

Uricosurics are drugs that increase the rate of excretion of uric acid by blocking its reabsorption in the kidney. These drugs are most effective in preventing hyperuricemia associated with chronic gout and are not effective for gout flare-ups. The uricosuric drugs have no analgesic or anti-inflammatory properties. Probenecid (Probalan) is the traditional uricosuric drug used to increase excretion of uric acid. This drug may precipitate acute gout during the period of initial therapy because it mobilizes uric acid that has been stored in the body. Concurrent administration of colchicine can help prevent this adverse effect.

Acute hyperuricemia can occur following antineoplastic therapy as part of a serious condition called tumor lysis syndrome when cancer cells are broken down. The massive load of uric acid crystals can result in acute kidney failure and possibly death. Rasburicase (Elitek) is a recombinant form of the enzyme urate oxidase, which can lower serum uric acid levels when given IV to patients receiving antineoplastic therapy.

PROTOTYPE DRUG Allopurinol (Lopurin, Zyloprim)

Classification **Therapeutic:** Antigout drug
Pharmacologic: Xanthine oxidase inhibitor

Therapeutic Effects and Uses: Allopurinol is an older drug that was approved in 1966 for gout and its complications. It controls the hyperuricemia that causes severe gout and reduces the possibility of gout flare-ups. It is also approved to prevent recurrent nephrolithiasis due to calcium oxalate stones in patients with elevated uric acid levels. It may be used prophylactically to reduce the severity of the hyperuricemia associated with antineoplastic and radiation therapies, both of which increase plasma uric acid levels by promoting nucleic acid degradation. This drug takes 1 to 3 weeks to bring serum uric acid levels to within the normal range.

Allopurinol is available by the PO and IV routes. IV administration is usually reserved for patients with high uric acid levels resulting from cancer chemotherapy.

Mechanism of Action: Allopurinol reduces uric acid formation by selectively inhibiting the action of xanthine oxidase, which is the enzyme responsible for the formation of uric acid. Lowering the formation of uric acid prevents hyperuricemia. Unlike the uricosuric drugs, allopurinol does not increase the renal excretion of uric acid.

Pharmacokinetics:

Route(s)	PO, IV
Absorption	80–90% absorbed in the GI tract
Distribution	Widely distributed; secreted in breast milk; less than 1% bound to plasma proteins
Primary metabolism	Hepatic to the active metabolite oxypurinol
Primary excretion	Primarily renal
Onset of action	24–48 h
Duration of action	1–3 weeks after drug is discontinued

Adverse Effects: The most frequent and serious adverse effects are dermatologic, including micropapular rash, rare cases of fatal toxic epidermal necrolysis, and SJS. A rare, sometimes fatal, hypersensitivity syndrome may occur and includes a skin rash, fever, hepatitis, leukocytosis, eosinophilia, and progressive kidney failure. Other adverse effects include drowsiness, headache, vertigo, nausea and vomiting, malaise, diarrhea, cataracts, retinopathy, and thrombocytopenia.

Contraindications/Precautions: Contraindications include hypersensitivity to allopurinol and idiopathic hemochromatosis. Use cautiously in patients with CKD or impaired hepatic function, history of peptic ulcers, lower GI tract disease, bone marrow depression, and pregnancy.

Drug Interactions: Alcohol may inhibit the renal excretion of uric acid. Ampicillin and amoxicillin may increase the risk of skin rashes. An enhanced anticoagulant effect may be seen with the use of warfarin, and toxicity risks increase for azathioprine, mercaptopurine, cyclophosphamide, and cyclosporine. The risk of ototoxicity is increased when allopurinol is used with thiazides and angiotensin-converting enzyme (ACE) inhibitors. Aluminum antacids taken concurrently with allopurinol may decrease its effects. An increased effect may be seen with phenytoin, theophylline, and anticancer drugs, necessitating the need for altered doses of these medications. **Herbal/Food:** Unknown.

Pregnancy: Allopurinol did not show evidence of fetal harm in laboratory animals. The drug is secreted in human milk although adverse effects on the breastfed neonate are unknown.

Treatment of Overdose: Overdose with allopurinol is rare. There is no specific treatment for an overdose and the patient is treated symptomatically.

Clinician Responsibilities: Key clinical implications for patients receiving allopurinol are included in Applied Clinical Judgment: Patients Receiving Pharmacotherapy for Gout.

Drugs Similar to Allopurinol (Lopurin, Zyloprim)

Additional drugs for gout prophylaxis and hyperuricemia include febuxostat, pegloticase, and probenecid. Sulfinpyrazone and lesinurad are uricosurics that have been discontinued in the United States.

Febuxostat (Uloric): Febuxostat was approved in 2009 for the chronic management of hyperuricemia in patients with gout. The drug acts by inhibiting xanthine oxidase and offers the convenience of once-daily dosing. Febuxostat exhibits little nephrotoxicity or dermatologic toxicity. Liver function tests should be monitored periodically to prevent the development of hepatotoxicity. It should not be administered concurrently with drugs metabolized by xanthine oxidase such as mercaptopurine or azathioprine because these drugs could accumulate to toxic levels. Febuxostat carries a black box warning that it may increase the risk for cardiovascular adverse effects. In addition, this drug should only be considered when allopurinol has proven ineffective. Febuxostat did not show evidence of fetal harm in laboratory animals. The drug is secreted in animal milk although adverse effects on the breastfed neonate are unknown.

Pegloticase (Krystexxa): Approved in 2010, pegloticase is a synthetic enzyme that metabolizes uric acid to an inert substance. It is used to lower uric acid levels in patients with chronic gout who have not responded to conventional therapies. Pegloticase is administered over a 2-hour period by IV infusion, once every 2 weeks. The drug has a black box warning that anaphylaxis may occur during and after the infusion, and emergency equipment should be readily available to address such a reaction. Patients should also be pretreated with antihistamines and corticosteroids. Other common adverse effects include gout flare-ups at the initiation of therapy, infusion reactions, nausea, ecchymosis, nasopharyngitis, and worsening of HF. Pegloticase did not show evidence of fetal harm in laboratory animals. It is not known if this drug is secreted in human milk or if it has any adverse effects on the breastfed neonate.

Probenecid (Probalan): Probenecid is an older drug approved in 1951 that inhibits the reabsorption of uric acid in the kidneys, thus increasing its renal excretion. Given PO, it is effective for prophylaxis but will not terminate acute gout episodes. However, tablets are available with a combination of probenecid and colchicine, which can terminate gout flare-ups. Probenecid should be taken with meals to decrease gastric irritation. Several combination drugs that contain probenecid and colchicine are available for long-term maintenance therapy. Adverse effects are generally minor and include headache, nausea and vomiting, and anorexia. It is not known if probenecid has adverse effects on the fetus or breastfed neonate.

Unrelated to its use in treating gout, probenecid blocks the transport of organic acids in the renal tubule. When given concurrently with antibiotics such as penicillins or cephalosporins, the serum levels of antibiotics will be boosted, making them more effective. Because of its effect on renal transport mechanisms, probenecid has the potential to interact with virtually any acidic drug. A drug guide should be consulted when administering probenecid to patients who are taking multiple medications.

The mobilization of uric acid may also cause or worsen kidney stones due to the increased amount of uric acid being excreted by the kidneys. To prevent these adverse effects of early therapy, the uricosurics are started at low doses and increased gradually over several weeks. During this initial therapy, the urine may be made more alkaline by the administration of sodium bicarbonate to prevent uric acid crystals from forming.

CONNECTIONS: APPLIED CLINICAL JUDGMENT

Patients Receiving Pharmacotherapy for Gout

Key Assessment Data

- History of current condition including musculoskeletal, GI, cardiovascular, neurologic, endocrine, hepatic, or kidney disease; baseline vital signs, physical exam findings; pregnancy or breastfeeding; uric acid level, CBC, hepatic and renal function studies, urinalysis; dietary and medication history including allergies, current prescription and OTC drugs, herbal preparations, caffeine, nicotine, and alcohol use.
- Assess for inflammation and location and note any pain or discomfort on movement or at rest. Obtain a dietary history, noting correlations between food intake and increase in symptoms. Assess adequacy of fluid intake.

Desired Therapeutic Outcomes

Improvement is observed and measurable by symptoms of acute inflammation are diminished or absent, with no return of symptoms.

Minimizing Adverse Effects

- Intake of high-purine foods and alcohol may increase production of uric acid. Large doses of vitamin C may acidify the urine, leading to formation of uric acid stones. Uric acid excretion may cause urate crystal formation in the kidneys with resulting kidney impairment. Flank pain may indicate the presence of renal calculi. Fluid intake should be increased to 2L/day or more.

Lifespan Considerations

- Age-related physiologic differences may place the older adult at greater risk for adverse hepatic or renal effects.

(continued)

CONNECTIONS: APPLIED CLINICAL JUDGMENT *(continued)*

Patients Receiving Pharmacotherapy for Gout

Patient Education

- Keep a food diary, noting any occurrence or increase of symptoms related to food or beverage intake. Bring the diary to each healthcare visit. Limit intake of high-purine foods and limit or eliminate alcohol consumption.
- Promptly report any continued inflammation, pain, increased joint involvement, or general worsening of symptoms.
- Increase fluid intake to 2 to 4 L/day, taken throughout the day. Report any diminished urine output or changes in urine appearance and return periodically for urinalysis. Weigh self daily at the same time and report any weight gain of over 1 kg (2 lb) in a 24-hour period. Immediately report any flank pain.
- Immediately report any flulike symptoms, fever, mouth irritation or soreness, or skin rashes.
- Avoid high-purine foods (e.g., salmon, sardines, organ meats, alcohol, mushrooms, legumes, oatmeal), decrease or eliminate alcohol consumption, and avoid increased vitamin C intake or supplementation.
- Colchicine should be taken on an empty stomach. Other antigout medications should be taken with food or meals.

Prescribing Considerations

- Bone marrow suppression may occur with colchicine. Monitor carefully for early signs of new infections and prescribe antiinfectives as appropriate.
- Severe dermatologic reactions are possible with allopurinol. Assess carefully for early skin rashes, especially with the appearance of blisters and discoloration.
- Maintain consistent drug dosing to ensure that uric acid levels are diminishing.

Understanding Chapter 72

Key Concepts Summary

72.1 Adequate levels of calcium in the body are necessary to transmit nerve impulses, to prevent muscle spasms, and for proper bone health.

72.2 Calcium balance is regulated by parathyroid hormone, calcitonin, and vitamin D.

72.3 Hypocalcemia and hypercalcemia are treated with nutritional adjustments or with pharmacotherapy.

72.4 Metabolic bone disease is characterized by abnormal bone structure.

72.5 Vitamin D therapy is indicated for treating osteomalacia, hypoparathyroidism, and osteoporosis.

72.6 Bisphosphonates increase bone density and are used to treat osteoporosis and Paget's disease.

72.7 Selective estrogen receptor modulators increase bone mass density and prevent fractures in postmenopausal women.

72.8 Calcitonin and several miscellaneous drugs are used for osteoporosis and other metabolic bone diseases.

72.9 Osteoarthritis is treated with a combination of analgesics and nonpharmacologic therapies.

72.10 Pharmacotherapy for rheumatoid arthritis includes analgesics, anti-inflammatory drugs, corticosteroids, and disease-modifying antirheumatic drugs.

72.11 Gout is caused by an accumulation of uric acid crystals in the joints.

72.12 Long-term management of gout includes dietary modifications and drugs that reduce levels of uric acid.

CASE STUDY: Making the Patient Connection

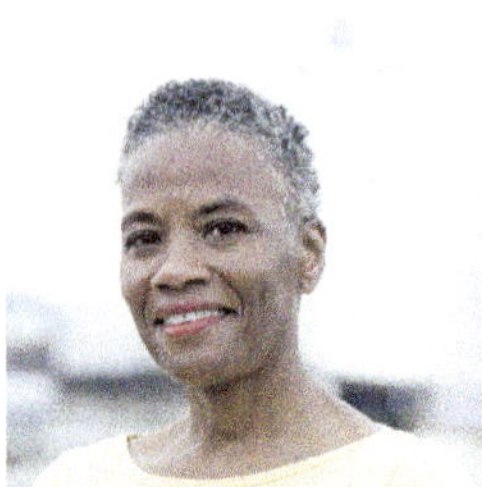

Remember the patient "Charlene Coleman" at the beginning of the chapter? Now read the remainder of the case study. Based on the information presented within this chapter, respond to the critical thinking questions that follow.

Charlene Coleman is a 65-year-old Black woman who is generally in good health. She has scheduled a routine checkup visit with her healthcare provider. While assessing Charlene's vital signs, height, and weight, the nurse notes a significant deviation from the data recorded during last year's visit. Apparently, the patient has lost 2.5 cm (1 in.) in height during the last year. When the nurse shares this information, Charlene states, "I have always been short.

You should see my mother who is much shorter than I am. But lately, my clothes just don't seem to fit. I haven't lost any weight, but my pant legs drag on the ground. Is it possible that I'm actually getting shorter?"

Critical Thinking Questions

1. As the nurse, how would you respond to the patient's statement?
2. As you talk with Charlene, she asks you, "Is there any way to slow my declining height?" What could you recommend?

Additional Case Study

A female patient, age 56, has been ordered methotrexate (Otrexup, Rasuvo, Trexall) and etanercept (Enbrel) for treatment of severe RA. She wants her daughter to administer the etanercept because of limitations due to arthritis-related deformities in her hands. The daughter is worried about giving her mother the medication.

1. How is etanercept (Enbrel) given? How often?
2. What instructions should the nurse give the daughter about administering this medication?
3. What potential adverse effects may occur in addition to those related to the injection itself?
4. What is the drug classification for methotrexate? What are potential adverse effects for this drug?

Chapter Review

1. The patient who has been prescribed alendronate (Fosamax) demonstrates an understanding of how to correctly take the medication when stating:

1. "I will take my medication prior to eating my lunch or dinner."
2. "I will take my medication immediately before bedtime or at 9:00 p.m."
3. "I will take my medication with a full glass of water 30 minutes before breakfast."
4. "I should lie flat for at least 30 minutes after I take this medication."

2. Which of the following symptoms would alert the nurse to the possibility of the development of toxicity to methotrexate (Otrexup, Rasuvo, Trexall)?

1. Headache, dizziness, and blurred vision
2. Hematuria, hiccoughs, and jaundice
3. Stomatitis, constipation, and dyspepsia
4. Jaundice, ascites, and edema formation

3. The patient asks the nurse to explain how colchicine (Colcrys) works. The nurse would base the response on which physiologic principle?

1. It increases the deposits of uric acid in the synovial spaces of the joints.
2. It reduces the pain associated with joint inflammation from gouty arthritis.
3. It prevents the accumulation of uric acid crystals in the joints.
4. It increases renal excretion of uric acid crystals.

4. Which laboratory findings would the nurse monitor to determine if pharmacotherapy is helping a patient taking calcium supplementation for osteomalacia?

1. Increasing serum calcium and increasing phosphate levels
2. Increasing serum calcium and decreasing phosphate levels
3. Decreasing serum calcium and increasing phosphate levels
4. Decreasing serum calcium and decreasing phosphate levels

5. Which assessment findings in a patient who is receiving calcitriol (Rocaltrol) should the nurse immediately report to the prescriber?

1. Muscle weakness and nausea and vomiting
2. Diarrhea, abdominal pain, and stomatitis
3. Bone pain, joint stiffness, and fever
4. Photosensitivity, tinnitus, and bone pain

6. A patient with rheumatoid arthritis will begin treatment with adalimumab (Humira). Which of the following statements related to this therapy is correct? (Select all that apply.) Adalimumab:

1. May lower immune response and increase the risk of infections and malignancies.
2. Is associated with osteoporosis and baseline and periodic DEXA scans should be conducted.
3. May reactivate latent TB.
4. May cause local injection-site irritations such as pain and bruising.
5. Must be taken daily for up to 6 months.

See Appendix A for answers to critical thinking questions, case study questions, and review questions.

References

Arthritis Foundation (n.d.). *Glucosamine and chondroitin for osteoarthritis pain*. https://www.arthritis.org/health-wellness/treatment/complementary-therapies/supplements-and-vitamins/glucosamine-chondroitin-osteoarthritis-pain

Bethel, M. (2020). *Osteoporosis*. Medscape. http://emedicine.medscape.com/article/330598- overview#a0156

Kremer, P. A., Laughlin, G. A., Shadyab, A. H., Crandall, C. J., Masaki, K., Orchard, T., et al. (2019). Association between soft drink consumption and osteoporotic fractures among postmenopausal women: The Women's Health Initiative. *Menopause, 26*, 1234–1241. https://doi.org/10.1097/GME.0000000000001389

Zhu, X., Wu, D., Sang, L., Wang, Y., Shen, Y., Zhuang, X., et al. (2018). Comparative effectiveness of glucosamine, chondroitin, acetaminophen or celecoxib for the treatment of knee and/or hip osteoarthritis: a network meta-analysis. *Clinical and Experimental Rheumatology, 36*(4), 595–602.

Selected Bibliography

Arthritis Foundation. (2019). *Arthritis by the numbers*. https://www.arthritis.org/getmedia/e1256607-fa87-4593-aa8a-8db4f291072a/2019-abtn-final-march-2019.pdf

Centers for Disease Control and Prevention (CDC). (2020a). *Gout*. https://www.cdc.gov/arthritis/basics/gout.html

Centers for Disease Control and Prevention (CDC). (2020b). *Rheumatoid arthritis*. https://www.cdc.gov/arthritis/basics/rheumatoid-arthritis.html

Cotts, K. G., & Cifu, A. S. (2018). Treatment of osteoporosis. *Journal of the American Medical Association, 319*(10), 1040–1041. https://doi.org/10.1001/jama.2017.21995

Eastell, R., Rosen, C. J., Black, D. M., Cheung, A. M., Murad, M. H., & Shoback, D. (2019). Pharmacological management of osteoporosis in postmenopausal women: An Endocrine Society clinical practice guideline. *Journal of Clinical Endocrinology and Metabolism, 104*(5), 1595–1622. https://doi.org/10.1210/jc.2019-00221

FitzGerald, J. D., Dalbeth, N., Mikuls, T., Brignardello-Petersen, R., Guyatt, G., Abeles, A. M., et al. (2020). 2020 American College of Rheumatology guideline for the management of gout. *Arthritis Care & Research, 72*(6), 744–760. https://doi.org/10.1002/acr.24180

Köhler, B. M., Günther, J., Kaudewitz, D., & Lorenz, H. M. (2019). Current therapeutic options in the treatment of rheumatoid arthritis. *Journal of Clinical Medicine, 8*(7), 938. https://doi.org/10.3390/jcm8070938

National Institutes of Health (NIH). (2020a). *Calcium: Fact sheet for health professionals*. https://ods.od.nih.gov/factsheets/Calcium-HealthProfessional

National Institutes of Health (NIH). (2020b). *Vitamin D Fact sheet for health professionals*. https://ods.od.nih.gov/factsheets/VitaminD-HealthProfessional/

Rothschild, B. M. (2020). *Gout and pseudogout*. Medscape. http://emedicine.medscape.com/article/329958-overview

Saadeh, C. K. (2020). *Calcium pyrophosphate deposition disease*. Medscape. http://emedicine.medscape.com/article/330936-overview#a5

Smith, H. R. (2020). *Rheumatoid arthritis*. Medscape. http://emedicine.medscape.com/article/331715-overview

Tangpricha, V. (2020). *Vitamin D deficiency and related disorders*. Medscape. http://emedicine.medscape.com/article/128762-overview

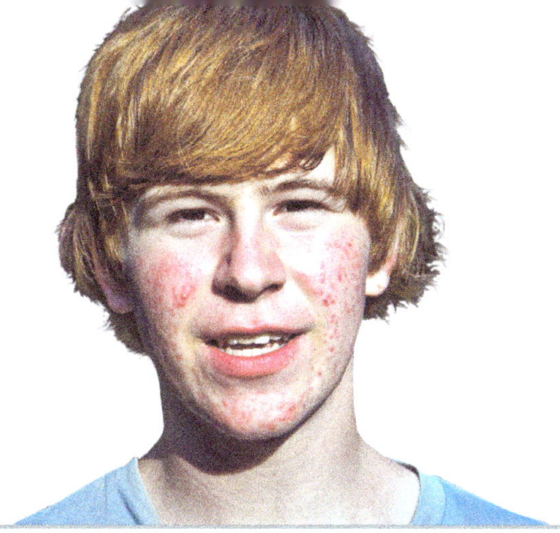

"I hate the way my skin looks. I know people are just staring at my face and not really listening to me."
—*Patient "Danny McBride"*

Chapter 73
Pharmacotherapy of Dermatologic Disorders

Chapter Outline

Learning Outcomes

After reading this chapter, the student should be able to:

1. Identify the structure and functions of the skin and associated structures.
2. Explain the process by which superficial skin cells are replaced.
3. Explain how skin diseases are classified.
4. Describe the drug therapies for bacterial, fungal, viral, and parasitic infections of the skin.
5. Explain the etiology, pathogenesis, and pharmacotherapy for acne vulgaris, rosacea, dermatitis, and psoriasis.
6. Outline the stepwise approach to treating psoriasis.
7. Describe the prevention and management of minor burns.
8. Explain the pharmacotherapy of alopecia.
9. Describe the nurse's role in the pharmacologic management of dermatologic disorders.
10. For each of the classes shown in the chapter outline, identify the prototype and representative drugs and explain the mechanism(s) of drug action, primary indications, contraindications, significant drug interactions, pregnancy data, and important adverse effects.
11. Apply clinical judgment to the care of patients receiving pharmacotherapy for dermatologic disorders.

Key Terms Definitions of the terms in bold may be found in the Glossary.

The integumentary system consists of the skin, hair, nails, and glands. The largest and most visible of all organs, healthy skin provides an effective barrier between the outside environment and the body's internal tissues, helps to regulate body temperature, and assists in maintaining fluid and electrolyte balance. At times, however, environmental conditions damage the skin or conditions within the body change, resulting in unhealthy skin. Some of these changes can even lead to systemic changes that affect tissues outside the integumentary system. When this occurs, pharmacotherapy may be utilized to improve the skin's condition. The purpose of this chapter is to examine the broad scope of skin disorders and the drugs used for skin pharmacotherapy.

Anatomy of the Integumentary System

73.1 Three layers of skin, the epidermis, dermis, and subcutaneous layers, provide effective barrier defenses for the body.

To understand the actions of dermatologic drugs, it is necessary to have a thorough knowledge of the structure of the skin. The skin comprises three primary layers: the epidermis, dermis, and subcutaneous layers, as illustrated in Figure 73.1. The epidermis is the visible, outermost layer that constitutes only about 5% of the skin depth. The middle layer is the dermis, which accounts for about 95% of the entire skin

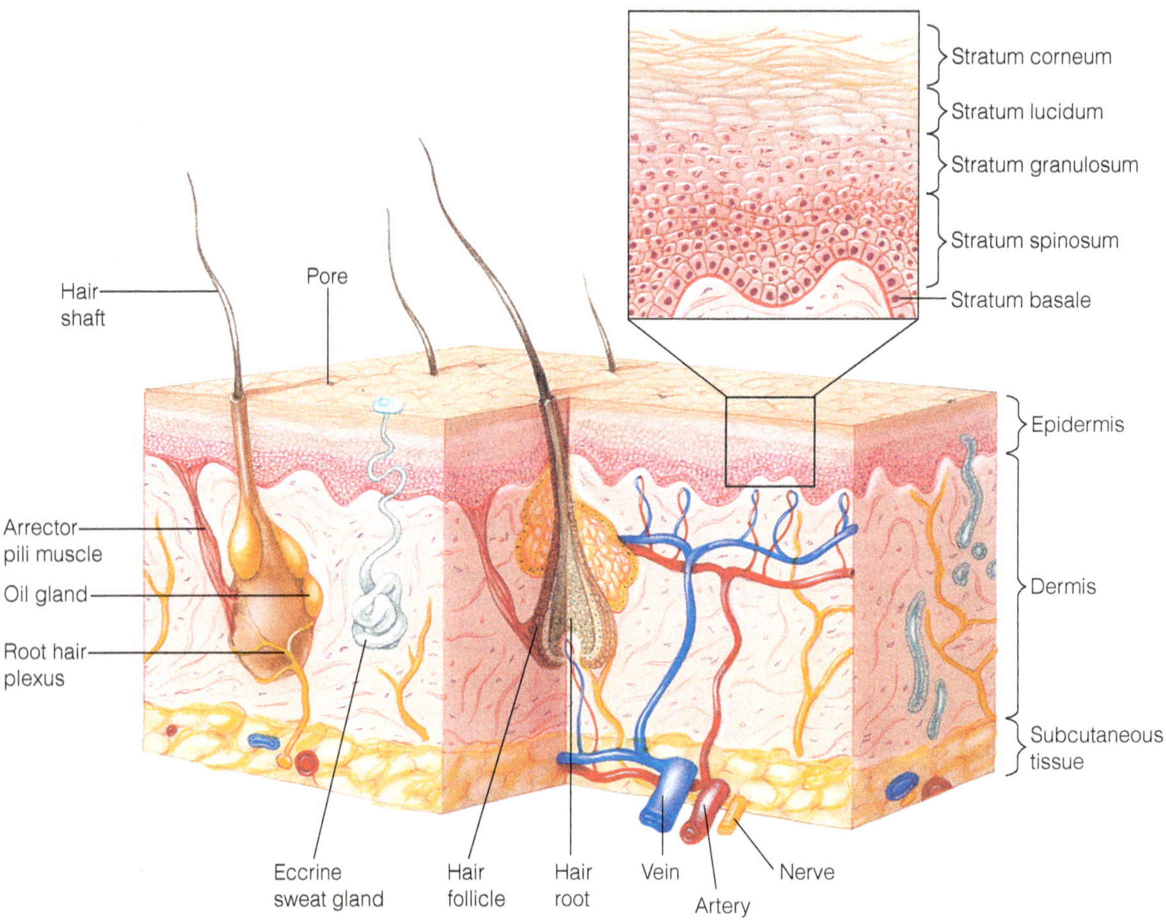

Figure 73.1 Anatomy of the skin.

thickness. The subcutaneous layer lies beneath the dermis. Some textbooks consider the subcutaneous layer as being separate from the skin and not one of its layers. Each layer of skin is distinct in form and function and provides the basis for how drugs are injected or topically applied.

Epidermis: The epidermis consists of epithelial cells with either four or five sublayers depending on its location. The five layers from the innermost to outermost are the stratum basale (also referred to as the stratum germinativum), stratum spinosum, stratum granulosum, stratum lucidum, and the strongest layer, the stratum corneum. The stratum corneum is referred to as the "horny layer" because of the abundance of the protein keratin, a water-insoluble material secreted by keratinocytes, which is also found in the hair, hooves, and horns of many mammals. Keratin gives the skin its tough, protective seal, forming a barrier that repels bacteria and foreign matter. Most substances cannot penetrate it. The largest amount of keratin is found in those areas subject to mechanical stress, for example, the soles of the feet and the palms of the hands.

The deepest epidermal sublayer, the stratum basale, supplies the epidermis with new cells after older superficial cells have been damaged or lost through normal wear. Over time, these newly created cells migrate from the stratum basale to the outermost layers of the skin. As these cells are pushed to the surface, they are flattened and covered with keratin. The outermost skin layer, called the stratum corneum, is composed of these dead cells. On average, it takes a cell about 2 to 3 weeks to move from the stratum basale to the body surface.

Melanocytes within the deeper layers of the epidermis secrete the dark pigment melanin. Melanin forms a protective shield, which protects the keratinocytes and the nerve endings in the dermis from the sun's ultraviolet (UV) rays. The number and type of melanocytes determine the overall pigment of the skin and determine racial differences in skin tone. Darker skin tones are not caused by an increased number of melanocytes, but by the amount of the pigment melanin that is contained in each cell. The more melanin, the darker the skin color. Freckles, birthmarks, and age spots are caused by the production of melanin. In areas where the melanocytes are destroyed, there are milk-white areas of depigmented skin referred to as vitiligo.

The epidermis does not have a separate blood supply. It receives its nutrients by diffusion from the many blood vessels in the dermis.

Dermis: The dermis is a layer of connective tissue lying deep to the epidermis that contains no cells. The dermis is composed of collagen fibers and elastic fibers that give the skin both flexibility and strength and provides a foundation for the epidermis and accessory structures such as hair and nails. Most sensory nerves that transmit the sensations of touch, pressure, temperature, pain, and itch are located within the dermis, as well as the oil glands and sweat glands. A vast network of lymph and capillary vessels is also found within the dermis.

Subcutaneous tissue: Beneath the dermis is the subcutaneous tissue, or hypodermis, which lies over muscle and bone. It consists mainly of adipose tissue, which cushions, insulates, and serves as an energy reserve in the event that extra calories are needed to fuel the body. The amount of subcutaneous tissue varies in an individual and is determined by body area, sex, age, nutritional status, and heredity. Many blood vessels pass through the fatty layer and extend into the dermis, forming capillary networks that supply nutrients and remove wastes.

Skin appendages: Hair follicles are located in the dermis. Hair growth varies by race, gender, age, and heredity. Individual hairs vary in both structure and rate of growth, depending on their location. Composed primarily of dead cells, hair consists of a root that begins in the bulb of the hair follicle and grows from the dermis outward. The hair shaft is the portion that projects through the epidermis and exits the skin. Stressors can alter the growth cycle and cause temporary hair loss. Permanent baldness is genetic in origin and is seldom influenced by stressors. Hair color is genetically determined by an individual's rate of melanin production within the hair shaft.

The sebaceous glands are distributed over the entire skin surface, except for the palms of the hands and the soles of the feet. Most sebaceous glands are directly connected to the hair follicles. Sebaceous glands produce sebum, which is emptied into the space between the hair follicle and shaft. Sebum lubricates and softens the skin and hair and reduces water loss from the skin surface in low humidity. Sebum is also mildly bacteriostatic. The secretion of sebum is stimulated by hormones, especially androgens.

The skin has two types of sweat glands: apocrine and eccrine. The apocrine glands are directly connected to the hair follicles and are mainly found in the axillary, perineal, nipple areolae, and umbilical areas. The interaction of skin bacteria with the milky secretions of apocrine glands causes distinct body odor. The eccrine glands are found over the entire skin surface. Their ducts open directly onto the skin surface and are not associated with hair follicles. The secretions of the eccrine glands are an important factor in the regulation of body temperature. Sweat is released from the eccrine glands in response to elevated body temperature or ambient temperature and is under the control of the sympathetic nervous system.

Classification of Skin Disorders

73.2 The etiology of skin disorders may be classified as infectious, inflammatory, or neoplastic.

Of the many types of skin disorders, some have vague, generalized signs and symptoms and others have specific and easily identifiable causes. **Urticaria** is a hypersensitivity response that is characterized by hives and is often accompanied by pruritus, or itching. Allergies to foods often manifest as urticaria. **Pruritus** is a general condition that is associated with dry, scaly skin or a parasite infestation. Pruritus may also be a sign of serious systemic pathology, such as cholestatic disease and uremia. A substantial number of drugs have urticaria or pruritus listed as adverse effects. Local **erythema** or redness accompanies inflammation and many other skin disorders. Inflammation is a characteristic of burns and trauma to the skin.

Skin disorders are diverse and difficult to classify because some conditions have overlapping components. For example, lesions that are characteristic of acne may be inflamed and become infected. One simple method, which is summarized in Table 73.1, is to group the disorders into the following categories:

- **Infectious.** Bacterial, fungal, viral, and parasitic infections of the skin and mucous membranes are relatively common and are frequent indications for anti-infective pharmacotherapy. A brief overview of anti-infectives most frequently prescribed for skin conditions is presented in Section 73.3, with further emphasis on parasitic infections in Section 73.4. Greater detail on the individual anti-infective drugs may be found in Chapters 46 through 54.
- **Inflammatory.** Inflammatory disorders encompass a broad range of pathology that includes acne, dermatitis, burns, and psoriasis. The pharmacotherapy of inflammatory skin disorders includes many of the drugs discussed in Chapter 41, such as corticosteroids.
- **Neoplastic.** Malignant tumors include malignant melanoma and basal cell carcinoma, which are treated with the therapies described in Chapter 57.

Systemic disease processes that occur in the body may cause dermatologic signs and symptoms. Skin abnormalities, including color, size, type, and character of surface lesions, and skin turgor and moisture may have systemic causes such as chronic kidney disease, liver impairment, cardiovascular insufficiency, metastatic tumors, recent injury, and poor nutritional status.

Although there are many skin disorders, some warrant only localized or short-term pharmacotherapy. Examples include lice infestation, sunburn, minor abrasions, and acne. Eczema, dermatitis, and psoriasis are more serious disorders that require more extensive therapy.

Pharmacotherapy of Skin Infections

73.3 When the integrity of the skin is compromised, microbes can gain entrance and cause infections that require anti-infective therapy.

The skin is normally populated with microorganisms or flora that includes a diverse collection of bacteria, fungi, and viruses. The skin is very dry, and keratin is a poor energy source for microbes. Although perspiration provides a wet environment, its high salt content discourages microbial growth. Furthermore, the outer layer is continually being sloughed off, and the microorganisms leave with the dead skin.

Bacterial skin diseases may occur when the skin is punctured or cut, or when the outer layer is deeply abraded through trauma or removed through severe burns. Some bacteria also infect hair follicles. The most common bacterial infections of the skin are caused by *Staphylococcus* and *Streptococcus*, which are normal skin inhabitants.

Table 73.1 Classification of Skin Disorders

Type	Examples
Infectious	Bacterial infections: boils, impetigo, infected hair follicles
	Fungal infections: ringworm, athlete's foot, jock itch, nail infection
	Parasitic infections: ticks, mites, lice
	Viral infections: cold sores, fever blisters (herpes simplex), chickenpox, warts, shingles (herpes zoster), measles (rubeola), and German measles (rubella)
Inflammatory	Injury and exposure to the sun
	Combination of overactive glands, increased hormone production, and/or infection such as acne and rosacea
	Disorders with itching, cracking, and discomfort such as atopic dermatitis, contact dermatitis, seborrheic dermatitis, stasis dermatitis, and psoriasis
Neoplastic	Skin cancers: squamous cell carcinoma, basal cell carcinoma, and malignant melanoma
	Benign neoplasms include keratosis and keratoacanthoma

Staphylococcus aureus is responsible for furuncles (boils), carbuncles (abscesses), and other pus-containing lesions of the skin. Both *S. aureus* and *Streptococcus pyogenes* can cause impetigo, which is a superficial skin disorder that commonly occurs in school-age children. Cellulitis is an acute skin and subcutaneous tissue infection caused by *Staphylococcus* and *Streptococcus*. Folliculitis, an infection of hair follicles usually caused by *S. aureus*, is often called a "hot-tub" infection because it is acquired when water in these types of tubs is not adequately treated with chlorine.

Although many skin bacterial infections are self-limiting, some are serious enough to require pharmacotherapy. When possible, topical drugs are applied directly to the infection site. Topical medications offer the advantage of causing fewer adverse effects, and many are available over the counter (OTC) for self-treatment. If the infection is deep within the skin, affects large regions of the body, or has the potential to enter the systemic circulation, oral (PO) or parenteral therapy is indicated. Some infections such as those caused by methicillin-resistant *S. aureus* (MRSA) may require pharmacotherapy with two or more antibiotics. Some of the more common topical antibiotics for skin infections include the following:

- Bacitracin ointment
- Erythromycin ointment
- Gentamicin cream and ointment
- Metronidazole cream and lotion
- Mupirocin (Centany)
- Neomycin with polymyxin B (Neosporin), cream and ointment
- Tetracycline.

Fungal infections of the skin or nails such as tinea pedis (athlete's foot) and tinea cruris (jock itch) commonly occur in warm, moist areas covered by clothing. Tinea capitis (ringworm of the scalp) and tinea unguium (ringworm of the nails) are also common. These pathogens are responsive to therapy with topical OTC antifungals such as undecylenic acid (FungiNail, Gordochom, others). More serious fungal infections of the skin and mucous membranes, such as *Candida albicans* infections that occur in immunocompromised patients, require systemic antifungals (see Chapter 52). Clotrimazole and miconazole (Monistat-3) are common antifungals available as creams and lotions that are used for a variety of dermatologic mycoses. Oral fluconazole (Diflucan) is indicated for more serious fungal infections of the skin.

Certain viral infections can manifest with skin lesions. Childhood viral infections that affect the skin include varicella (chickenpox), rubeola (measles), and rubella (German measles). Usually, these infections are self-limiting and nonspecific, so treatment is directed at controlling the extent of skin lesions. Viral infections with skin lesions in adults include herpes zoster (shingles) and herpes simplex (cold sores and genital lesions). Pharmacotherapy of severe or persistent viral skin lesions may include topical or PO antiviral therapy with acyclovir (Zovirax) or other antivirals.

CONNECTION Checkpoint 73.1

From what you learned in Chapter 52, what is onychomycosis and what types of drugs are used to treat it?

Scabicides and Pediculicides

73.4 Scabicides and pediculicides are used to treat parasitic skin infestations.

Common skin parasites include mites and lice. Scabies is an eruption of the skin caused by the female mite *Sarcoptes scabiei*, which burrows into the skin to lay eggs that hatch in about 5 days. Scabies mites are barely visible without magnification. Scabies lesions most commonly occur between the fingers, on the extremities, in axillary and gluteal folds, around the trunk, and in the genital area. The major symptom is intense pruritus; vigorous scratching may lead to secondary infections. Scabies is easily spread through skin-to-skin contact and from mites living in upholstery, shared beds, and bath linens. Diagnosis is made by visual inspection of the burrows and confirmed by microscopic scrapings of the mite's ova or fecal pellets.

Lice are larger than mites and are readily spread by sharing infected hats, hairbrushes, bedding, or clothes or by close personal contact. These parasites require human blood for survival and die within 24 hours without the blood of a human host. Lice (singular: louse) often infest the pubic area or the scalp and lay eggs, referred to as **nits**, which attach to body hairs. Head lice are referred to as *Pediculus humanus capitis*, body lice as *Pediculus humanus corporis*, and pubic lice as *Phthirus pubis*. The pubic louse is referred to as a "crab louse" because it looks like a tiny crab when viewed under a microscope. Individuals with pubic lice will sometimes say that they have "crabs." Pubic lice may produce sky-blue macules on the inner thighs or lower abdomen. The bite of the louse and the release of its saliva into the wound both lead to intense pruritus, followed by vigorous scratching. Secondary infections can result from scratching.

The treatment of skin parasites consists of using **scabicides**, which are drugs that kill mites, or **pediculicides**, which are drugs that kill lice. Some drugs are effective against both mites and lice. The choice of drug depends on where the infestation is located as well as other factors such as age, pregnancy, or breastfeeding.

The preferred drug for lice is permethrin, a chemical derived from chrysanthemum flowers and formulated as a 1% liquid (Nix). This drug is considered the safest agent, especially for infants and children. Pyrethrin (RID, others) is a related product that is also obtained from the chrysanthemum plant. Permethrin and pyrethrin, which are also widely used as insecticides on crops and livestock, kill lice and their eggs on contact. These drugs are effective in 97 to 99% of patients, although a repeat application may be needed. Adverse effects are generally minor and include stinging, itching, or tingling. If two treatments of pyrethrin-based medications fail to eliminate the infestation, lindane shampoo or malathion lotion may be prescribed. Resistant lice are most likely to appear in patients who have received multiple treatments with pyrethrin-based shampoos.

Permethrin is also a first-line drug for scabies. The 5% cream is applied to the entire skin surface and allowed to remain for 8 to 14 hours before bathing. A single application cures 95% of patients, although itching may continue for several weeks as the dead mites are eliminated from the skin. Crotamiton (Eurax) is an alternative scabicide that is available by prescription as a 10% cream. Abametapir (Xeglyze) was approved in 2020 for the topical treatment of head lice in patients 6 months of age and older. If the scabies is unresponsive to topical medications, the antiparasitic drug ivermectin (Stromectol) may be administered as a single oral dose.

All scabicides and pediculicides must be used strictly as directed because excessive use can cause serious systemic effects and skin irritation. Drugs for the treatment of lice or mites must not be applied to the mouth, open skin lesions, or eyes because this will cause severe irritation.

PROTOTYPE DRUG **Permethrin (Acticin, Elimite, Nix)**

Classification **Therapeutic:** Antiparasitic
Pharmacologic: Scabicide, pediculicide

Therapeutic Effects and Uses: Nix is marketed as a cream, lotion, or shampoo to kill head and crab lice and mites and to eradicate their ova. A 1% lotion is approved OTC for lice and a 5% lotion by prescription for mites. The medication should be allowed to remain on the hair and scalp 10 minutes before removal. Patients should be aware that penetration of the skin by mites causes itching, which lasts up to 2 or 3 weeks even after the parasites have been killed.

Successful elimination of parasitic infections should include removing the nits with a nit comb, washing bedding, and cleaning or removing objects that have been in contact with the head or hair.

Mechanism of Action: Permethrin affects the nervous system of the parasite, causing paralysis. Because lice are dependent on blood for survival, they die within 24 to 28 hours. It has ectoparasitic and ovicidal activity against *P. humanus capitis*, *P. pubis*, *S. scabiei* (scabies), ticks, mites, and fleas.

Pharmacokinetics:

Route(s)	Topical: 5% and 1% formulations
Absorption	Less than 2% is absorbed through intact skin
Distribution	Stored in body fat
Primary metabolism	Hepatic
Primary excretion	Urine
Onset of action	10 min
Duration of action	14 days

Adverse Effects: Permethrin causes few systemic effects. Local reactions may occur and include pruritus, rash, transient tingling, burning, stinging, erythema, and edema of the affected area.

Contraindications/Precautions: Contraindications include hypersensitivity to pyrethrins, chrysanthemums, sulfites, or other preservatives. Permethrin should be used cautiously on inflamed skin, in those with asthma, or in lactating women.

Drug Interactions: No clinically significant interactions have been documented.

Pregnancy: Permethrin did not show evidence of fetal harm in laboratory animals. No data are available regarding safety during human pregnancy or lactation.

Treatment of Overdose: No specific treatment for overdose with permethrin has been reported. Flush eyes well with water if the medicine unintentionally gets into the eyes.

Clinician Responsibilities: Key clinical implications for patients receiving permethrin are included in Applied Clinical Judgment: Patients Receiving Pharmacotherapy for Lice or Mite Infestation.

Drugs Similar to Permethrin (Acticin, Elimite, Nix)

Other drugs for parasitic skin infections include crotamiton, ivermectin, lindane, malathion, and pyrethrin.

Crotamiton (Eurax): Crotamiton is a scabicide and antipruritic that is used to eradicate *S. scabiei* and relieve itching. Available as a 10% cream or lotion, this drug should not be applied to skin that is acutely inflamed, raw, or has weeping surfaces. It should not be instilled into the eyes or mouth. If this drug comes in contact with the eyes, they must be flushed thoroughly with water. Adverse effects may include skin irritation, rash, and erythema. Data are not available regarding the safety of this drug during pregnancy or lactation.

Ivermectin (Sklice): Ivermectin is a drug first approved by the U.S. Food and Drug Administration (FDA) to treat helminthic infections. It is a preferred drug treating river blindness, a debilitating infection in many developing countries. In 2012, ivermectin (Sklice) was approved as a 0.5% lotion for head lice in patients 6 months of age and older. Sklice is applied to dry hair and rinsed off with water after

10 minutes. A single application is usually sufficient. Side effects are minor and include dry scalp and eye irritation if the eyes are exposed to the drug. Single doses of oral or topical preparations of ivermectin are unlikely to cause fetal harm; however, pregnant or lactating women should check with their healthcare provider before using.

Lindane: Lindane is a scabicide and pediculicide in a 1% lotion or shampoo form that is applied directly to the skin to be absorbed by parasites and ova (nits), resulting in their death. This drug is used for treatment of head and crab lice and scabies infestations. Lindane should not be applied to skin that has open cuts or to the mucous membranes, eyes, or face. It should be used cautiously in infants and patients with a history of seizures, human immunodeficiency virus infections, and alcoholism. Gloves should be worn when applying the medication to reduce exposure to the skin. Although effective, this drug penetrates the skin and may cause significant adverse effects. Lindane has a black box warning that states that the drug is indicated for patients who are unresponsive to safer therapies because seizures and deaths have been reported with repeated applications. The warning also states that the drug is contraindicated in premature infants and in individuals with uncontrolled seizure disorders. Lindane is not recommended during pregnancy or lactation.

Malathion: Available as a 0.5% lotion, malathion kills lice and ova by poisoning the nervous system of the parasite. It is contraindicated in children under the age of 6. Care must be taken to keep this drug out of the eyes during treatment because it can cause conjunctivitis. One treatment is all that is needed when using this medication. Because the solution contains alcohol, it is flammable and needs to be kept away from any heat source such as hair dryers or cigarettes. Malathion is very toxic if swallowed. Malathion did not show evidence of fetal harm in laboratory animals. No data are available regarding safety during human pregnancy or lactation.

Pyrethrin (RID): Pyrethrin is a pediculicide solution or shampoo that poisons the parasite's nervous system, resulting in paralysis and death. Pyrethrin may require a repeat application a week after the first dose. Contraindications include skin infections, abrasions, lactation, and sensitivity to the solution components. Pyrethrin is usually formulated with 4% piperonyl butoxide because this combination results in greater parasite killing. Pyrethrin should be used with caution in ragweed-sensitized patients, infants, and children. This medication is applied to infested areas that are wet, allowing it to stay in place for at least 10 minutes. The areas are then washed and rinsed with warm water. For shampoo applications, the hair is shampooed as usual then a fine-toothed comb is used to remove the lice and eggs from the hair. Single applications of topical pyrethrin are unlikely to cause fetal harm; however, pregnant or lactating women should check with their healthcare provider before using.

CONNECTIONS: APPLIED CLINICAL JUDGMENT

Patients Receiving Pharmacotherapy for Lice or Mite Infestation

Key Assessment Data

- History of current condition including dermatologic and social history of recent exposure; baseline vital signs, physical exam findings; pregnancy or breastfeeding; assess skin areas to be treated for signs of infestation (e.g., lice or nits in hair, reddened track areas between webs of fingers, around belt, or elastic lines), irritation, excoriation, or drainage.

Desired Therapeutic Outcomes

Improvement is observed and measurable by decreased visible infestation, nits are removed, skin healing is visible.

Minimizing Adverse Effects

- Monitor the affected area after treatment for 1 to 2 weeks to ensure that the infestation has been eliminated and that retreatment is not needed.
- Reinfestation may recur if those in close contact with the patient are infested. Close contacts should be treated at the same time as the patient.
- Skin reactions are relatively uncommon but may occur. Allergic reactions should be reported and assessed in case additional treatment is needed.

Patient Education

- Continue to assess the area daily for 1 to 2 weeks and contact the healthcare provider for a second prescription if reinfestation is noted. Promptly report any continued inflammation, pain, increased joint involvement, or general worsening of symptoms.
- Wash bedding, clothing used currently, combs, and brushes in soapy water and dry thoroughly. Vacuum furniture or fabric that cannot be cleaned to remove any errant vermin. Dry-clean hats or caps that cannot be washed. Seal children's toys in plastic bags for 2 weeks if they cannot be washed.
- Report any redness, swelling, itching, excoriation, or burning.
- Follow administration guidelines as follows:
  - Wash hair or shower to remove any residual creams or gels before applying the drug. Dry thoroughly.
  - Apply the drug per package directions and allow it to remain in the hair or on the skin for the prescribed length of time (usually 10 minutes). Most packages contain enough drug for one treatment, although a second package may be required if the hair is long. Do not allow the drug to come in contact with eyes.
  - Dry thoroughly after showering or shampooing the drug out of the hair or skin.
  - Comb through the hair with a small-toothed comb to remove any remaining dead lice, nits, or nit casings.
  - If eyelashes are infested, apply a thin coat of petroleum jelly to eyelashes once a day for 1 week. Comb through using a small-toothed comb to remove any dead lice, nits, or nit casings.
  - Check hair, webbings of fingers and toes, belt, or elastic waistbands for signs of reinfestation over the next week. If needed, a second application of the drug can be used after 1 week.

(continued)

CONNECTIONS: APPLIED CLINICAL JUDGMENT *(continued)*

Patients Receiving Pharmacotherapy for Lice or Mite Infestation

Prescribing Considerations

- Ensure that all household members and close contacts receive treatment.
- Topical medications are the treatment of choice due to their safety and ease of use. In persistent cases, oral ivermectin is prescribed.
- Pubic lice are transmitted through sexual contact and sexual partners will need treatment.

Pharmacotherapy of Acne and Rosacea

73.5 The pharmacotherapy of acne includes treatment with benzoyl peroxide, retinoids, and antibiotics; pharmacotherapy for rosacea includes retinoids and metronidazole.

Acne vulgaris and rosacea are two disorders that produce similar-appearing lesions on the face. Although the two conditions have some visual similarities and share a few common treatments, the pharmacotherapy of the disorders is very different.

Acne Vulgaris

Acne vulgaris, a disorder of the hair follicles and sebaceous glands, is a common condition that affects 80% of adolescents. Although acne occurs most often in teenagers, it is not unusual to find patients with acne who are older than age 30, which is a condition referred to as *mature acne* or *acne tardive*. Acne vulgaris is more common in men but tends to persist longer in women. Acne affects approximately 17 million people in the United States, making it one of the most common skin conditions encountered by the nurse.

Although the precise cause of acne is unknown, several factors that are associated with acne vulgaris include abnormal formation of keratin that blocks oil glands and **seborrhea**, the overproduction of sebum by oil glands. The bacterium *Cutibacterium acnes* (formerly *Propionibacterium acnes*) grows within oil gland openings and changes sebum to an acidic and irritating substance. As a result, small, inflamed bumps appear on the surface of the skin. Other factors associated with acne include androgens, which stimulate the sebaceous glands to produce more sebum. This is clearly evident in teenage boys and in patients who are administered testosterone. Studies have indicated that dietary factors do not promote acne. Remissions tend to occur in the summer, perhaps due to more exposure of the skin to the UV rays from sunlight.

PharmFACT

Although many young people believe that indoor tanning helps to clear up acne, there is no scientific evidence to support this claim. Indoor tanning is responsible for about 400,000 cases of skin cancer in the United States each year. A single tanning session can increase the risk of developing squamous cell carcinoma by 67% and basal cell carcinoma by 29% (American Academy of Dermatology, n.d.).

Acne lesions are most frequently distributed on the face, chest, and back and include open and closed **comedones**. Blackheads, or open comedones, occur when sebum has plugged the oil gland, causing it to become black because of the presence of melanin granules. Whiteheads, or closed comedones, develop just beneath the surface of the skin and appear white rather than black. Some closed comedones may rupture, resulting in an inflammatory response. The result is seen as papules, inflammatory pustules, and cysts. Mild papules and cysts drain on their own without treatment. Deeper lesions can cause permanent scarring of the face. Acne is graded as mild, moderate, or severe, depending on the number and type of lesions present.

The goals of acne therapy are to treat existing lesions and to prevent or lessen the severity of future recurrences. The regimen used depends on the extent and severity of the acne and the response of each individual patient. Mechanisms of action of antiacne medications include the following:

- Inhibit sebaceous gland overactivity
- Reduce bacterial colonization
- Prevent follicles from becoming plugged with keratin
- Reduce inflammation of lesions.

Many of the medications used for acne are available OTC. Mild acne is treated by topical therapy with drugs such as benzoyl peroxide, topical antibiotics, and salicylic acid. Moderate to severe acne is treated with increasing strengths of tretinoin and the use of systemic antibiotics. Because of their increased toxicity, prescription medications are reserved for more severe, persistent cases. These drugs are listed in Table 73.2.

Benzoyl peroxide (Clearasil, Fostex, others) is the most common topical OTC medication for acne. Benzoyl peroxide has a **keratolytic** effect, which helps to treat acne by loosening dry skin and causing an increased shedding of the outer layer of the epidermis. In addition, this drug suppresses sebum production and exhibits antibacterial effects against *C. acnes*. Benzoyl peroxide is available as a topical lotion, cream, or gel in various percentage concentrations. Typically, the patient applies benzoyl peroxide once daily

Table 73.2 Drugs for Acne

Drug	Remarks
adapalene (Differin)	Retinoid-like compound used to treat acne formation
azelaic acid (Azelex, Finacea)	For mild to moderate inflammatory acne
benzoyl peroxide	Keratinolytic sometimes combined with adapalene (Epiduo), erythromycin (Benzamycin), or clindamycin (Benzaclin, Duac) for acne caused by *C. acnes*
clascoterone (Winlevi)	A newer topical medication for acne vulgaris that acts by blocking androgen receptors.
clindamycin and tretinoin (Veltin, Ziana)	Combination product with an antibiotic and a retinoid in a gel base; for mild to moderate acne
dapsone (Aczone)	Topical medication for acne vulgaris; oral formulations are indicated for other disorders, including leprosy
ethinyl estradiol (Estinyl)	Oral contraceptives are sometimes used for acne; for example, ethinyl estradiol plus norgestimate
isotretinoin (Absorica, Zenatane, others)	For severe acne with cysts or acne formed in small, rounded masses; contraindicated during pregnancy
sulfacetamide (Klaron)	For sensitive skin; sometimes combined with sulfur to promote peeling, as in the condition rosacea; also used for conjunctivitis
tazarotene (Avage, Tazorac)	A retinoid drug that may also be used for plaque psoriasis; has antiproliferative and anti-inflammatory effects
tetracyclines	Antibiotics; refer to Chapter 48
tretinoin (Avita, Retin-A, others)	To prevent clogging of pore follicles; also used for the treatment of acute promyelocytic leukemia and wrinkles
trifarotene (Aklief)	A newer retinoid approved for the topical treatment of acne vulgaris

and, in many instances, this is the only treatment needed. The drug is very safe, with local redness, irritation, and drying being the most common adverse effects. Although the symptoms might worsen during the early weeks of therapy, the skin usually adjusts quickly to its use. Other keratolytic drugs that are available by prescription are used for severe acne and include benzoyl peroxide with erythromycin (Benzamycin) and benzoyl peroxide with sulfur (Sulfoxyl).

The use of OTC acne products containing benzoyl peroxide and salicylic acid may cause rare, but potentially life-threatening allergic reactions. Symptoms of this reaction include throat tightness; difficulty breathing; feeling faint; or swelling of the eyes, face, lips, or tongue. The allergic reaction may occur immediately or several days after initiating therapy. New users are urged to test the product on a small patch of skin for 3 days. If no discomfort occurs, the drug may be safely applied.

Retinoids are a class of drug closely related to vitamin A. They are used in the treatment of inflammatory skin conditions, dermatologic malignancies, and acne. The topical formulations are often the first-line drugs for mild to moderate acne characterized by inflammatory cysts. Drugs in this class are called **comedolytics** because they prevent and break up the formation of clogged pores. Tretinoin (Avita, Retin-A, others) is an older drug with comedolytic action that decreases comedone formation and increases extrusion of comedones from the skin. Tretinoin also has the ability to improve photodamaged skin and is used for wrinkle removal. Other retinoids include isotretinoin (Absorica, Zenatane, others), a PO vitamin A metabolite medication that aids in reducing the size of sebaceous glands, thereby decreasing oil production and the occurrence of clogged pores. Therapy with retinoids may require 8 to 12 weeks to achieve maximum effectiveness. Common reactions to retinoids include burning, stinging, and sensitivity to sunlight. Adapalene (Differin) is a third-generation retinoid that causes less irritation than the older drugs. Epiduo is a topical drug that contains both adapalene and benzoyl peroxide. Additional retinoid-like drugs and the related compounds that are used to treat acne are listed in Table 73.2.

Antibiotics are prescribed to reduce the severe redness and inflammation associated with moderate to severe acne, especially when the acne is inflammatory and results in cysts and pustules. Oral doxycycline, minocycline, sarecycline (Seysara), and tetracycline, administered in low doses over a long period, have been the traditional antibiotics used in acne therapy. Due to their effects on teeth formation, tetracyclines should not be used in children younger than age 8. Erythromycin and clindamycin are frequently used topically and have a low incidence of adverse effects. Antibiotics are not comedolytic and resistance can develop with continued therapy. Benzamycin is a prescription product that contains erythromycin and benzoyl peroxide.

Oral contraceptives (OCs) that contain ethinyl estradiol and norgestimate are also used in pubertal girls to help clear the skin of acne by suppressing sebum production and reducing skin oiliness. Hormonal therapy is used when antibiotic therapy has proved ineffective. OCs are most effective for young women when the acne begins somewhat later than usual and tends to flare up at certain times in the menstrual cycle. Estrogen is not administered to male patients because of undesirable adverse effects, such as breast enlargement and decrease in body hair. For the actions and contraindications of oral contraceptives, see Chapter 70.

Rosacea

Rosacea is an inflammatory skin disorder of unknown etiology with lesions affecting mainly the face. Unlike acne, which most commonly affects teenagers, rosacea is a progressive disorder with an onset between 30 and 50 years of age. Rosacea is characterized by small papules or inflammatory bumps without pus that swell, thicken, and become painful. These lesions typically occur in the middle third of the face, including the forehead, nose, cheeks, and chin. The face takes on a reddened or flushed appearance with accompanying telangiectasia (dilation of small blood vessels). With time the redness becomes more permanent, and lesions resembling acne appear. The soft tissues of the nose may thicken, resulting in a reddened, bulbous, irregular swelling called **rhinophyma**. Disorders of the eye frequently accompany rosacea, particularly conjunctivitis, itching, edema, and keratitis.

Rosacea is exacerbated by factors such as sunlight, stress, increased temperature, and medications that dilate facial blood vessels, including alcohol, spicy foods, skin care products, and hot beverages. Rosacea affects more women than men, although men more often develop rhinophyma. Learning and avoiding the environmental triggers that worsen the symptoms of the condition may prevent rosacea flare-ups.

The two most effective treatments for rosacea are topical metronidazole (MetroCream, MetroGel) and azelaic acid (Azelex, Finacea). Benzoyl peroxide may be applied as needed. Alternative medications include topical tretinoin (Avita, Retin-A, others), clindamycin (Cleocin-T, Clindagel), and sulfacetamide. Tetracycline antibiotics such as minocycline are of benefit to patients with rosacea who have multiple pustules or ocular involvement. Severe, resistant cases may respond to isotretinoin (Absorica, Zenatane). Newer topical therapies include brimonidine (Mirvaso), oxymetazoline (Rhofade), and ivermectin (Soolantra), which are used to reduce the persistent redness of facial rosacea.

PROTOTYPE DRUG Tretinoin (Avita, Retin-A, Others)

Classification **Therapeutic:** Antiacne drug
Pharmacologic: Retinoid

Therapeutic Effects and Uses: Approved as a topical drug in 1971, tretinoin is a natural derivative of vitamin A. This drug is indicated for the early treatment and control of mild to moderate acne vulgaris. Renova is a topical form of tretinoin that is approved to treat fine facial wrinkles and hyperpigmentation associated with photodamaged skin. Altreno was approved in 2018 as the first lotion form of tretinoin. Tretinoin has antineoplastic actions; a PO form is approved to treat acute promyelocytic leukemia (APL) and may be prescribed off-label for skin malignancies.

Symptoms take 4 to 8 weeks to improve, and maximum therapeutic benefit may take 5 to 6 months. Because of potentially serious adverse effects, this drug is most often reserved for cystic acne or severe keratinization disorders.

Mechanism of Action: The principal action of tretinoin is regulation of skin growth and turnover. As cells from the stratum germinativum grow toward the surface, skin cells are lost from the stratum pore openings and their replacement is slowed. Tretinoin reverses retention hyperkeratosis and comedone formation, which are the primary events in acne pathology. The drug increases the permeability of the skin and supports conversion of follicular epithelium into a less sturdy and almost fragile condition. Tretinoin also decreases oil production by reducing the size and number of oil glands.

Pharmacokinetics:

Route(s)	Topical, PO
Absorption	Minimally absorbed from intact skin; well absorbed PO
Distribution	Secreted in breast milk; more than 95% bound to plasma protein
Primary metabolism	Hepatic
Primary excretion	Renal; small amounts in feces
Onset of action	Unknown
Duration of action	Half-life: 0.5–2 h

Adverse Effects: Nearly all patients who use topical tretinoin will experience local effects such as redness, scaling, erythema, crusting, and peeling of the skin with temporary hypopigmentation or hyperpigmentation. Skin irritation can be severe and cause discontinuation of therapy; a lower-strength solution may be necessary to limit the severity of these adverse effects. Dermatologic adverse effects resolve once therapy is discontinued. Oral therapy can also cause adverse skin effects.

For treatment of APL, very high oral doses are used and adverse effects are more serious than with topical therapy. The most common effects with PO therapy include bone pain, fever, headache, nausea and vomiting, rash, stomatitis, pruritus, sweating, and ocular disorders. Other adverse effects may include hyperlipidemia, shivering, hemorrhage, pain, dizziness, paresthesias, anxiety, insomnia, depression, cerebral hemorrhage, intracranial hypertension (HTN), hallucinations, dysrhythmias, flushing, hypotension or HTN, heart failure (HF), visual disturbances, abdominal pain, diarrhea, constipation, dyspepsia, gastrointestinal hemorrhage, kidney impairment, dysuria, and acute kidney failure. **Black Box Warning:** Patients with APL are at high risk for serious adverse effects. About 25% of patients develop retinoic acid–APL syndrome, which is a serious condition characterized by fever, weakness, fatigue, dyspnea, weight gain, peripheral edema, respiratory insufficiency, and pneumonia. About 40% of patients develop a rapidly evolving leukocytosis, which is associated with a high risk of life-threatening complications.

Contraindications/Precautions: Contraindications for topical administration include eczema, exposure to sunlight or UV rays, sunburn, hypersensitivity to this drug or vitamin A preparation, and children less than 12 years of age. This drug should be used cautiously in patients who are in an occupation necessitating considerable sun exposure or weather extremes or in patients with hepatic disease. Oral tretinoin is contraindicated in patients who have hepatic disease, leukopenia, or neutropenia or who are hypersensitive to the drug.

Drug Interactions: Topical acne keratinolytics (sulfur, resorcinol, benzoyl peroxide, and salicylic acid) may increase inflammation and peeling; topical products that contain alcohol or menthol may cause stinging. Additive phototoxicity can occur if tretinoin is used concurrently with other phototoxic drugs such as tetracyclines, fluoroquinolones, or sulfonamides. Use of this medication with hypoglycemic drugs may lead to a loss of glycemic control and cardiovascular risk because tretinoin raises serum triglyceride levels. Hepatotoxic drugs may cause additive liver impairment if used concurrently with PO tretinoin. **Herbal/Food:** The PO absorption of tretinoin is increased if taken with a high-fat meal.

Pregnancy: Tretinoin is a known teratogen and therapy is contraindicated during pregnancy. Pregnancy testing is required for women of childbearing potential prior to, during, and for 1 month after discontinuation of therapy.

Treatment of Overdose: Overuse of the topical drug will lead to excessive skin drying and peeling. Symptoms of PO overdose are nonspecific and resolve with symptomatic treatment.

Clinician Responsibilities: Key clinical implications for patients receiving tretinoin are included in Applied Clinical Judgment: Patients Receiving Pharmacotherapy for Acne and Related Skin Conditions.

Drugs Similar to Tretinoin (Avita, Retin-A, Others)

Other antiacne drugs include adapalene, azelaic acid, clascoterone, isotretinoin, and tazarotene.

Adapalene (Differin): Approved in 1996, adapalene is a topical acne drug that modulates the inflammation, epithelial keratinization, and differentiation of follicular cells. It is very similar to the retinoids but is reported to produce less skin irritation. Optimal results may take up to 12 weeks of therapy. Patients must be cautious with sun exposure because this drug can increase the potential for sunburn. Other adverse effects include local burning, pruritus, scaling, and peeling. Only minimal amounts of adapalene are absorbed through the skin. Safety of this drug in patients under age 12 has not been established. This drug is a teratogen in laboratory animals. Adapalene is not recommended during pregnancy or lactation.

Azelaic acid (Azelex, Finacea): Approved in 1995, azelaic acid is a natural product found in wheat, rye, and barley. Azelaic acid is a topical therapy that is effective for the treatment of mild to moderate acne by suppressing the growth of *P. acnes* and decreasing the proliferation of keratinocytes. It is also approved for the topical treatment of inflammatory pustules associated with rosacea. Only 4% is absorbed systemically. Adverse effects are typical of other topical antiacne drugs: local burning, pruritus, scaling, and peeling. Safety of this drug in patients under age 12 has not been established. Large dermal doses showed fetal harm in laboratory animals. Azelaic acid is secreted in human milk although adverse effects on breastfed neonates are unknown.

Clascoterone (Winlevi): Approved in 2020, clascoterone acts by a new mechanism for the treatment of acne vulgaris. This drug is a synthetic steroid that acts as an antagonist at androgen receptors in sebaceous glands. This decreases sebum production and inflammation. The cream is administered twice daily with the most common side effects being local skin irritation, burning, or peeling. Data regarding the safety of topical clascoterone during pregnancy or lactation are not available.

Isotretinoin (Absorica, Zenatane, others): Approved in 1982, isotretinoin is a PO retinoid that is the most effective drug for severe, inflammatory acne. Therapy may require several months for optimal benefit. Off-label uses include rosacea, psoriasis, and the treatment of squamous cell carcinoma of the skin. Because of potentially serious adverse effects, this drug is usually used when other therapies fail to produce satisfactory results. Isotretinoin carries a black box warning that it causes birth defects, which can occur after even short courses of therapy. The warning further states that the drug has special requirements for distribution that require patients, healthcare providers, and pharmacists to register and adhere to the iPledge Program, a pregnancy risk management program. Before starting therapy, the patient must submit to two negative pregnancy tests and sign a statement of understanding about the drug's adverse effects. Each subsequent month, the pharmacist must document receipt of a negative pregnancy test and verify that two forms of effective contraception are being utilized by the patient. Males must also register with the iPledge

Program because small amounts of isotretinoin are found in semen and could potentially cause birth defects in a pregnant partner. Other common adverse effects include cheilitis, epistaxis, xerostomia, hair loss, eczema, elevated serum lipid levels, myalgia, and arthralgia. Clinical depression, psychosis, and aggression have been reported.

Tazarotene (Avage, Tazorac): Approved in 1997, tazarotene is a topical retinoid derivative of vitamin A that is used for the treatment of acne, fine facial wrinkles, and psoriasis. Patients become sensitive to the sun's UV light and need to wear protective sunscreen and clothing when using this drug. Adverse effects are similar to those of topical tretinoin: local burning, stinging, erythema, and general skin irritation. This drug is metabolized in the skin to an active metabolite; small amounts are absorbed systemically. Safety of this drug in patients under age 12 has not been established. Tazarotene is a known teratogen and therapy is contraindicated during pregnancy. Women of childbearing potential should submit a negative pregnancy test prior to therapy and use effective contraception during treatment.

Pharmacotherapy of Dermatitis

73.6 The most effective treatment for dermatitis is topical corticosteroids, which are classified by their potency.

Dermatitis is a general term that refers to superficial inflammatory disorders of the skin. General symptoms include local redness, pain, and pruritus. Intense scratching may lead to **excoriation**, which are scratches that break the skin surface and fill with blood or serous fluid to form crusty scales. A wide variety of factors can cause dermatitis, with different types of symptoms occurring depending on the causative agent. The three most common types that respond to topical pharmacotherapy are atopic, contact, and seborrheic. Dermatitis may be acute or chronic.

Atopic dermatitis, or **eczema**, is a chronic, inflammatory skin disorder with a genetic predisposition. Patients who present with eczema often have a family history of asthma and hay fever as well as allergies to a variety of irritants such as cosmetics, lotions, soaps, pollens, food, pet dander, and dust. About 75% of patients with atopic

CONNECTIONS: APPLIED CLINICAL JUDGMENT

Patients Receiving Pharmacotherapy for Acne and Related Skin Conditions

Key Assessment Data

- History of current condition, dermatologic, hepatic, or kidney disease; psychiatric disorders; baseline vital signs, physical exam findings; pregnancy or breastfeeding; medication history including allergies, current prescription and OTC drugs. Evaluate appropriate laboratory tests (e.g., complete blood count [CBC], lipid profiles, hepatic or renal function tests).
- Assess for inflammation and location and note any pain or discomfort on movement or at rest. Obtain a dietary history, noting correlations between food intake and increase in symptoms.

Desired Therapeutic Outcomes

Improvement is observed and measurable by skin is clear of acne lesions.

Minimizing Adverse Effects:

- Overcleansing or overdrying of the skin may make the condition worse. If drying products such as benzoyl peroxide were used before treatment with retinoids, a brief recovery period may be needed to avoid excessive skin irritation. Protection from sun exposure is essential to prevent increasing skin damage.
- Severe allergic reactions are possible from topical benzoyl peroxide and salicylic drugs. Test a small area of skin for three days before full use.
- Corneal opacities or cataracts are an adverse effect of some oral antiacne medications. Dryness of eyes during treatment is common. Night vision may be diminished during treatment.

Patient Education

- Topical treatment areas should show signs of improvement within 2 to 4 weeks but may require up to 3 to 4 months of treatment. Oral treatment is usually successful within one course and a second course may be delayed for several weeks to monitor continuing improvement.
- Gently cleanse the skin using a nonoily soap and avoid vigorous scrubbing. If excessive dryness occurs, use a nonoily lotion to areas of dryness.
- If oral medications are used, report any symptoms of abdominal or right upper quadrant discomfort or pain, yellowing of the skin or sclera, fatigue, anorexia, darkened urine, or clay color stools.
- Oral drugs may cause eye dryness and adverse effects. Maintain regular eye examinations and report any changes in visual acuity, especially with night driving. Artificial tear solutions may assist in relieving eye dryness.
- Use sunscreens of SPF 15 or higher and wear protective clothing and hats to avoid sun exposure to areas under treatment for acne or wrinkles. Tanning beds should not be used.
- Follow appropriate administration guidelines:
  - Apply a thin layer of topical cream or lotion to the affected area after cleansing the skin. Keep the drug out of the eyes. Allow to dry and avoid contact with clothing, towels, or bedding to avoid staining or bleaching.
  - For oral medications, take in the morning, and if twice-a-day dosing is ordered, take the second dose approximately 8 hours after the first.

Prescribing Considerations

- iPledge is required of all patients on isotretinoin before receiving a prescription or refills of the drug. It includes educational information and requires the patient to ensure that all requirements to prevent teratogenic effects have been met.
- Assess lipid levels, which may increase in up to 70% of patients on PO acne therapy. Adjust dose or change medication accordingly.
- If depression or suicidal ideation occurs during therapy with isotretinoin, adjust dose or change medication.
- Some acne and rosacea drugs are contraindicated during pregnancy. Caution should be used when prescribing these medications for females of childbearing potential.

dermatitis have had an initial onset before 1 year of age. In those babies predisposed to eczema, breastfeeding seems to offer protection because it is rare for a breastfed child to develop eczema before the introduction of other foods. In infants and small children, lesions usually begin on the face and scalp and then progress to other parts of the body. A frequent and prominent symptom in infants is the appearance of red cheeks.

Contact dermatitis can be caused by a hypersensitivity response resulting from exposure to specific natural or synthetic allergens such as plants, chemicals, latex, drugs, metals, or foreign proteins. Accompanying the allergic reaction may be various degrees of cracking, bleeding, or small blisters. See Figure 73.2.

Seborrheic dermatitis is a form of eczema that can affect patients at any age. The exact cause of seborrheic dermatitis is unknown, but hormone levels, coexisting fungal infections, nutritional deficiencies, and immunodeficiency states are associated with the disease. Seborrheic dermatitis presents as greasy, not dry, scales that affect the scalp, central face, and anterior chest, often presenting as scalp scaling, or dandruff. Other symptoms may include redness of the nasolabial fold, particularly during times of stress; blepharitis; otitis externa; and acne vulgaris. In infants, thick, greasy scales on the vertex of the scalp, commonly known as cradle cap, are seen. These scales can become more widespread, with the central face, forehead, and ears being affected.

Pharmacotherapy of dermatitis is symptomatic and involves lotions and ointments to control itching and skin flaking. Antihistamines may be used to control inflammation and reduce itching, and analgesics or topical anesthetics may be prescribed for pain relief. Atopic dermatitis can be controlled, but not cured, by medications. Part of the management plan must include the identification and elimination of allergic triggers that cause flare-ups.

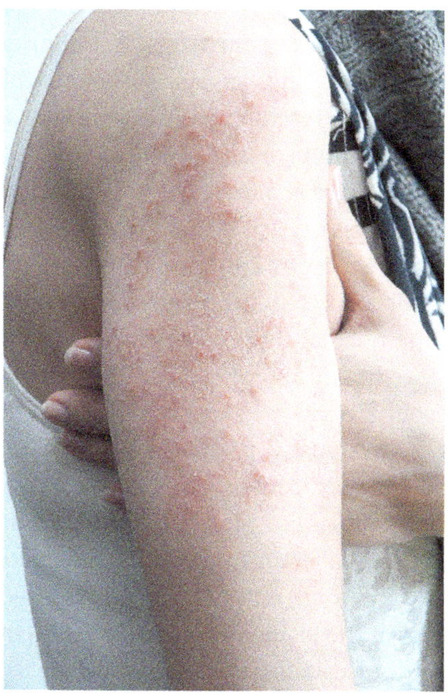

Figure 73.2 Dermatitis.
librakv/123rf.

Topical corticosteroids are the most effective treatment for controlling the inflammation and itching of dermatitis. Creams, lotions, solutions, gels, and pads that contain corticosteroids are specially formulated to penetrate deep into the skin layers. These dermatologic drugs are classified by potency, as listed in Table 73.3. The high-potency medications are used to treat acute flare-ups and are limited to 2 to 3 weeks of therapy. The medium-potency formulations are for more prolonged therapy of chronic dermatitis. The low-potency corticosteroids are prescribed for children or minor inflammation.

Because long-term corticosteroid use can lead to irritation, redness, hypopigmentation, and thinning of the skin, high-potency formulations are not advised for the head or regions with thin skin. Absorption of topical corticosteroids may produce undesirable systemic effects, including adrenal insufficiency, mood changes, serum imbalances, and loss

Table 73.3 Selected Topical Corticosteroids for Dermatitis and Related Symptoms

Generic Name	Strength (%)	Trade Name
Very High Potency		
betamethasone dipropionate, augmented, cream	0.05	Diprolene
clobetasol propionate	0.05	Olux
diflorasone diacetate	0.05	—
halobetasol	0.05	Ultravate
High Potency		
amcinonide	0.1	—
fluocinonide	0.025	Lidex
halcinonide	0.1	Halog
Medium Potency		
betamethasone valerate	0.1	Beta-val
clocortolone pivalate	0.1	Cloderm
desoximetasone, cream	0.025	Topicort
flurandrenolide, cream	0.025	Cordran
fluticasone propionate, cream	0.05	Cutivate
hydrocortisone valerate	0.2	—
mometasone furoate	0.1	Elocon
prednicarbate	0.1	—
triamcinolone acetonide	0.025–0.1	Kenalog
Low Potency		
alclometasone dipropionate	0.05	—
desonide	0.05	Desonate, DesOwen
dexamethasone	0.1	—
hydrocortisone	0.25–1	Cortizone

of bone mass, as discussed in Chapter 68. To avoid serious adverse effects, careful attention must be given to the amount of corticosteroid applied, the frequency of application, and how long it should be used. For most patients with dermatitis, topical corticosteroids have minimal adverse effects.

Patients with persistent atopic dermatitis that does not respond to corticosteroids may benefit from PO immunosuppressants, such as cyclosporine. This drug is generally used for the short-term treatment of severe disease. The topical calcineurin inhibitors pimecrolimus 1% (Elidel) and tacrolimus 0.03%, 0.1% (Protopic) are available for patients older than 2 years of age. These medications may be used on all skin surfaces (including the face and neck) because they have fewer adverse effects than the topical corticosteroids. Adverse effects include burning and stinging on broken skin. Pimecrolimus and tacrolimus are not approved for long-term therapy because of a small risk of skin cancer and lymphoma. When using these drugs, occlusive dressings should not be used because this promotes absorption of the drug and can increase the risk of systemic toxicity. The immunosuppressants are presented in Chapter 42.

Other alternatives to corticosteroids for atopic dermatitis include doxepin (Zonalon), crisaborole (Eucrisa), and dupilumab (Dupixent). When given PO doxepin is used to treat depression; however, Zonalon cream is indicated for atopic dermatitis. Some of the drug is absorbed across the skin, causing drowsiness in about 20% of patients. Applied topically, crisaborole is an anti-inflammatory drug approved in 2016 to treat atopic dermatitis.

The approval of dupilumab in 2017 led to a new approach to treating persistent atopic dermatitis. This drug is a monoclonal antibody that targets the interleukin-4 (IL-4) receptor pathway. By blocking the binding of IL-4 (and to some extent IL-13), the drug prevents the release of inflammatory cytokines. It is administered by the subcutaneous route every other week. The most common adverse effects are injection-site reactions and conjunctivitis. Subsequently, dupilumab was approved as an adjunct to treat severe asthma and for chronic rhinosinusitis with nasal polyposis.

Topical therapy for seborrheic dermatitis primarily consists of antifungals and low-dose topical corticosteroids, depending on the location affected. The first-line therapy for seborrheic dermatitis that affects the scalp should be topical corticosteroids. These may be administered as a shampoo, topical solution, or a lotion applied to the scalp. A typical regimen for an adult would be to use a topical corticosteroid once or twice daily with the use of a medicated shampoo two to three times per week. Shampoos that contain selenium sulfide (Selsun), salicylic acid, zinc pyrithione, or an antifungal azole are most often used. Once-daily antifungal medication with fluconazole, ketoconazole, or ciclopirox combined with 2 weeks of once-daily desonide is recommended for seborrheic dermatitis of the face and ears.

CONNECTION Checkpoint 73.2

Topical applications of corticosteroids are used for a variety of conditions. What are some indications for corticosteroids given by the following routes of administration: aerosol inhalation (see Chapter 44), intranasal (see Chapter 45), and intra-articular (see Chapter 72)?

Pharmacotherapy of Psoriasis

73.7 Psoriasis is a chronic, inflammatory disease that is treated with topical and systemic medications.

Psoriasis is a chronic, inflammatory skin disorder that affects 1 to 2% of the population and appears with greater frequency in people of European ancestry. The onset of psoriasis is generally established by 20 years of age, although it may occur throughout the lifespan.

Although the etiology of psoriasis is incompletely understood, it appears to have both genetic and autoimmune components. About 33 to 50% of the cases have a genetic basis, with a close family member also having the disorder. When one identical twin presents with psoriasis, the other twin has a 70% probability of also acquiring the disease. The immune nature of psoriasis is supported by the discovery that activated T lymphocytes (T cells) migrate to the dermis and release cytokines such as tumor necrosis factor (TNF) that increase the production of skin cells and cause inflammation. Furthermore, suppressing T-cell function through the use of immunosuppressants or biologic therapies improves symptoms of psoriasis.

Specific environmental triggers worsen psoriasis, including stress, smoking, alcohol, climate changes, and infections. In addition, certain drugs, including angiotensin-converting enzyme inhibitors, beta-adrenergic blockers, tetracyclines, and nonsteroidal anti-inflammatory drugs, act as triggers. People with psoriasis seem to improve in warmer climates, where there is more exposure to sunlight.

When psoriasis occurs, both the dermis and epidermis become thickened from an extremely fast skin turnover rate, with skin cells reaching the surface in 4 to 7 days instead of the normal 2 to 3 weeks. This rapid proliferation time does not allow for cell maturation and keratinization to occur, giving the skin lesions their characteristic appearance. The typical psoriatic lesions are characterized by red, raised patches of skin covered with flaky, thick, silver scales called **plaques**. Plaques are ultimately shed from the surface while the underlying skin becomes inflamed and irritated. If the scales are scraped away, the dark-red base of the lesion is exposed, producing multiple bleeding points. Lesions vary in size and are usually present on the scalp, elbows, knees, extensor surfaces of the arms and legs, sacrum, hands, and occasionally around the nails (Figure 73.3). The face is rarely affected. When

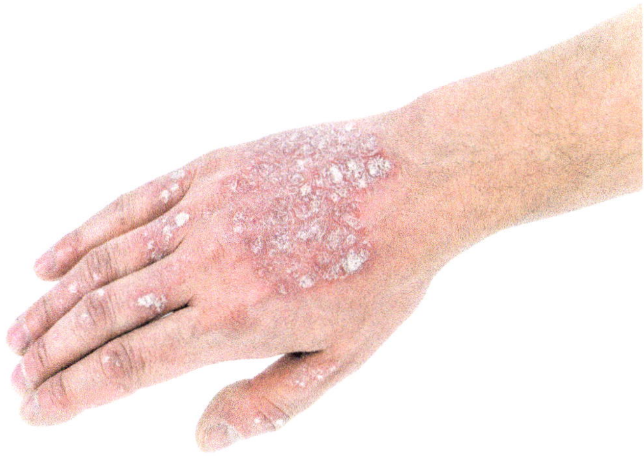

Figure 73.3 Psoriasis.
Casi/Fotolia.

psoriasis affects the nails, a yellow or brown discoloration may result, and the nail itself may separate from the nail bed, thicken, and crumble. The various forms of psoriasis are described in Table 73.4.

The goal of psoriasis pharmacotherapy is to reduce erythema, plaques, and scales to improve the cosmetic appearance of the patient, leading to the ability to perform normal lifestyle activities. This is accomplished by reducing epidermal cell turnover and promoting healing of the psoriatic lesions. The choice of therapy depends on the type and extent of the disease and the history of response to a previous treatment of psoriasis. A number of prescription and OTC drugs are available for the treatment of psoriasis and are listed in Table 73.5. Therapy is often conducted in a stepwise manner. Psoriasis is a lifelong disease and there is no pharmacologic cure.

Topical Drugs

Corticosteroids: Topical corticosteroids are a first-line therapy for the initial treatment of psoriasis. These drugs are effective, inexpensive, and relatively safe. When they are applied to psoriatic lesions, topical corticosteroids suppress cell division, reduce inflammation, relieve pruritus, and delay the movement of keratinocytes that are associated with fast skin turnover. Choosing the correct strength of corticosteroid and the most effective vehicle base are important aspects of treatment because the effectiveness of a topical steroid depends on its potency and ability to be absorbed into the skin. Initial therapy may begin with a high-potency drug to obtain rapid clearing of the lesions. High-potency medications are also used for acute flare-ups for 2 to 3 weeks. The high-potency formulations are best applied to the areas thickest with plaque, such as the hands or feet, and should not be used on the face and genital areas. For chronic maintenance therapy, the patient is switched to moderate- and low-potency corticosteroids because they have a lower potential for adverse effects.

Plastic occlusive dressings may be applied to increase the effectiveness of the corticosteroid. A simple way to enhance drug penetration is to apply the steroid directly to the skin followed by warm, moist dressings and an occlusive outer wrap. Care should be taken that the wraps are not left in place longer than 8 hours. The skin should be inspected for atrophy, striae, hypopigmentation, and telangiectasias, which are all adverse effects of topical corticosteroid therapy.

Repeated use of topical corticosteroids will result in tolerance. To delay tolerance, doses of the high-potency drugs are kept as low as possible. Some healthcare providers discontinue corticosteroids after an adequate response has been obtained and switch to a different therapy for several weeks.

Table 73.4 Types of Psoriasis

Form of Psoriasis	Description	Most Common Location of Lesions	Comments
Guttate (droplike) or eruptive psoriasis	Lesions smaller than those of psoriasis vulgaris	Upper trunk and extremities	More common in early-onset psoriasis; can appear and resolve spontaneously a few weeks following a streptococcal respiratory infection
Psoriasis vulgaris	Lesions are papules that form into erythematous plaques with thick, silver or gray plaques that bleed when removed; plaques in dark-skinned individuals often appear purple	Skin over scalp, elbows, and knees; lesions possible anywhere on the body	Most common form; requires long-term specialized management
Psoriatic arthritis	Resembles rheumatoid arthritis	Fingers and toes at the distal interphalangeal joints; can affect the skin and nails	About 20% of patients with psoriasis also have arthritis
Psoriatic erythroderma or exfoliative dermatitis	Generalized scaling; erythema without lesions	All body surfaces	Least common form
Pustular psoriasis	Eruption of pustules; presence of fever	Trunk and extremities; can appear on the palms, soles, and nail beds	Average age of onset is 50 years

Table 73.5 Selected Drugs for Psoriasis and Related Disorders

Drug	Route and Adult Dose (Maximum Dose Where Indicated)	Adverse Effects
Topical Medications		
calcipotriene (Dovonex)	Topical: Apply a thin layer to the lesions 1–2 times/day up to 8 wk	*Burning, stinging, folliculitis, itching, dry skin, hyperpigmentation* No serious adverse effects
coal tar (Balnetar, Cutar, others)	Topical: Apply to affected areas 1–4 times/day	*Folliculitis, irritation, photosensitivity* No serious adverse effects
salicylic acid (Neutrogena, Salex, others)	Topical: Apply to affected areas tid–qid in concentrations ranging from 2 to 10%	*Erythema, pruritus, stinging of the skin* No serious adverse effects
tazarotene (Tazorac)	Acne: Apply a thin film to the clean, dry area daily Plaque psoriasis: Apply thin film daily in the evening	*Pruritus, burning, stinging, skin irritation, transient worsening of psoriasis, skin peeling, photosensitivity* Hypertriglyceridemia, teratogenicity
Systemic Medications		
abatacept (Orencia)	Subcutaneous: 125 mg once weekly	*Headache, upper respiratory infection, nausea* Serious infections, hypersensitivity, TB reactivation,
acitretin (Soriatane)	PO: 25–50 mg/day with the main meal	*Dry mouth, alopecia, cheilitis, dry skin, dry mucous membranes* Increased triglycerides and cholesterol, paresthesias, rigors, arthralgia, skin peeling, pseudotumor cerebri, depression, elevated liver function tests, teratogenicity
adalimumab (Humira)	Subcutaneous: 40 mg every other week	*Upper respiratory infection, local reactions at the injection site* Malignancies, serious infections, worsening HF
alefacept (Amevive)	IM: 15 mg once weekly for 12 wk	*Nausea and vomiting, diarrhea, pharyngitis, dizziness, cough, pruritus* Malignancies, serious infection, hepatotoxicity, lymphopenia
apremilast (Otezla)	PO: Begin with 10 mg/day and increase over a 6-day period to 30 mg bid	*Diarrhea, nausea, headache* Depression, weight loss
brodalumab (Siliq)	Subcutaneous: 210 mg at wk 0, 2, and 4 followed by 210 mg q2wk	*Arthralgia, headache, fatigue, diarrhea, injection-site reactions* Neutropenia, serious infections, suicidal ideation
cyclosporine (Gengraf, Neoral, Sandimmune)	PO: 1.25 mg/kg bid (max: 4 mg/kg/day)	*Hirsutism, tremor, nausea and vomiting, pruritus, diarrhea* HTN, myocardial infarction, nephrotoxicity, hyperkalemia, paresthesias, hepatotoxicity, infection
etanercept (Enbrel)	Subcutaneous: 50 mg twice weekly (given 3–4 days apart) Maintenance dose: 50 mg/wk	*Local reactions at the injection site (pain, erythema, myalgia), abdominal pain, vomiting, nasopharyngitis* Serious infections, lupus-like syndrome, positive antinuclear antibodies, HF exacerbations
golimumab (Simponi)	Subcutaneous: 50 mg once monthly	*Upper respiratory infection, injection site reaction, diarrhea, serious infections* Hypersensitivity, infections, lupus-like syndrome, HF, lymphoma
guselkumab (Tremfya)	Subcutaneous: 100 mg at wk 0 and 4 followed by 100 mg q8wk	*Upper respiratory infection, headache, arthralgia, diarrhea, injection-site reactions* Serious infections
infliximab (Remicade)	IV: 5 mg/kg given as an induction dose at 0, 2, and 6 wk followed by a maintenance dose of 5 mg/kg q8wk thereafter	*Infections, headache, abdominal pain* Infusion-related reactions, invasive fungal infections, malignancies, hepatotoxicity, lupus-like syndrome
ixekizumab (Taltz)	Subcutaneous: 160 mg at wk 0, followed by 80 mg at wk 2, 4, 6, 8, 10, and 12 followed by 80 mg q4wk	*Local reactions at the injection site, upper respiratory infections, nausea* Serious infections, hypersensitivity, worsening of inflammatory bowel disease
methotrexate (Otrexup, Trexall)	PO: 2.5–5 mg bid for 3 doses each week (max: 25–30 mg/wk) Subcutaneous (Otrexup): 10–25 mg once weekly	*Headache, glossitis, gingivitis, mild leukopenia, nausea* Ulcerative stomatitis, myelosuppression, aplastic anemia, hepatic cirrhosis, nephrotoxicity, sudden death, pulmonary fibrosis, acute renal failure, teratogenicity

Table 73.5 (Continued)

Drug	Route and Adult Dose (Maximum Dose Where Indicated)	Adverse Effects
secukinumab (Cosentyx)	Subcutaneous: 150–300 mg at wk 0, 1, 2, 3, and 4 followed by 300 mg q4wk	*Nasopharyngitis, diarrhea, upper respiratory tract infection* Serious infections, hypersensitivity reactions
tildrakizumab (Ilumya)	Subcutaneous: 100mg at weeks 0, 4 and followed by q12wk thereafter	*Upper respiratory infection, injection site reaction, diarrhea* Hypersensitivity, infections, TB reactivation
ustekinumab (Stelara)	Subcutaneous: 45–90 mg initially and 4 wk later, followed by 45–90 mg q12wk	*Nasopharyngitis, upper respiratory tract infection, headache, and fatigue* Malignancies, serious infections

Note: *Italics* indicate common adverse effects. Underline indicates serious adverse effects.

When large areas of the body have psoriatic lesions, topical corticosteroid therapy can be expensive and involve some systemic risk. The larger the area treated, the greater the absorbed doses. The student should refer to Chapter 68 for a discussion of the adverse effects of systemic corticosteroid therapy.

Coal tar: Coal tar may be used as monotherapy or in combination with other psoriasis medications. The drug inhibits DNA synthesis, arrests abnormal cell growth, and reduces inflammation. Coal tar is inexpensive and available as a solution, gel, lotion, and shampoo. Coal tar preparations, however, are messy, staining, and have a foul odor. The use of coal tar is considered a second-line therapy except for shampoos, which can treat scalp lesions.

Calcipotriene (Dovonex): Approved in 1993, calcipotriene is a derivative of vitamin D that is available as a cream for use on the body and as a solution for the scalp. The drug binds to vitamin D receptors in the skin, suppresses cellular proliferation, and decreases cellular turnover in the psoriatic plaques. Symptomatic improvement is seen in 2 to 3 weeks, but optimum effect may take 8 weeks. Calcipotriene is an effective alternative to topical corticosteroids. Only about 6% of a topical dose is absorbed systemically. Its most common adverse effect is local irritation. It is not recommended for use by patients over age 65, who have an increased incidence of adverse effects with the drug. Its use may produce hypercalcemia if applied over large areas of the body or if used in higher than recommended doses. Phototherapy of excessive exposure to UV light should be avoided due to the potential for increased tumor incidence. Enstilar and Wynzora are combination drugs containing calcipotriene and betamethasone. This drug caused fetal abnormalities in laboratory animals. There are no data regarding risks during human pregnancy or lactation.

Salicylic acid: Salicylic acid is a keratinolytic that has been used as an OTC remedy to treat various skin conditions, including psoriasis, acne, dandruff, warts, and dermatitis. It is the active metabolite of aspirin and has been available for over 100 years. Salicylic acid removes the outer layers of skin, allowing improved penetration of other dermatologic drugs. Topical salicylic acid at strength 2% or less is considered safe to use during pregnancy, following directions given by the healthcare provider.

Tazarotene (Tazorac): Approved in 1997, tazarotene (Tazorac) is a vitamin A retinoid that causes sloughing of the scales covering the psoriatic plaques. Available as an ointment or gel, this drug is applied once daily in the evening. Tazarotene is also approved for facial wrinkles and acne. Its use is contraindicated during pregnancy (see Section 73.5).

Systemic Drugs

Some patients have severe psoriasis that is resistant to topical therapy. Because systemic drugs have the potential to cause serious adverse effects, they are generally used when topical drugs and phototherapy fail to produce an adequate response. In some cases, they may be used for a few weeks to produce a rapid improvement in symptoms before beginning topical therapy.

Acitretin (Soriatane): Acitretin is a PO retinoid that is approved for severe, resistant psoriasis. Two to 3 months of therapy may be required for significant symptomatic improvement. Approved in 1997, acitretin acts like other retinoids to inhibit keratin formation and skin inflammation. This drug is very effective at eliminating psoriatic lesions; however, the lesions return soon after therapy is discontinued. Many adverse effects occur frequently during therapy, including cheilitis, hair loss, dry skin, pruritus, rash, epistaxis, bleeding gums, and joint pain. The patient should refrain from drinking alcohol during acitretin therapy because this converts more of the drug to its toxic metabolite. Acitretin is teratogenic in both laboratory animals and humans. In women with childbearing potential, at least two negative pregnancy tests should be obtained prior to and during treatment. The patient should use effective birth control for 3 years after discontinuing the drug.

Apremilast (Otezla): Approved in 2014, apremilast is used to treat psoriatic arthritis and plaque psoriasis. The drug inhibits the enzyme phosphodiesterase-4, which results in a reduction in several different proinflammatory mediators. It is the first drug approved for psoriasis that acts by this mechanism. Apremilast is considered an option for patients who have not responded to phototherapy or systemic therapy with other drugs. Patients with a history of depression, suicidal behavior, or weight loss should be monitored regularly while on apremilast therapy. This drug causes abortion and embryofetal death in laboratory animals. Apremilast is secreted in animal milk but adverse effects on the breastfed neonate are unknown.

Biologic therapies: An understanding of the role of the immune system in the pathogenesis of psoriasis has led to the use of biologic therapies to treat patients with moderate to severe disease. Biologic drugs suppress the hyperactive inflammatory and immune responses characteristic of psoriasis by several different mechanisms. Adalimumab (Humira), etanercept (Enbrel), golimumab (Simponi), and infliximab (Remicade) are TNF blockers. Brodalumab (Siliq), guselkumab (Tremfya), ixekizumab (Taltz), risankizumab (Skyrizi), secukinumab (Cosentyx), tildrakizumab (Ilumya) and ustekinumab (Stelara) are newer drugs that inhibit interleukins. Abatacept (Orencia) and alefacept (Amevive) inhibit T-cell activation. Upadacitinib (Rinvoq) is a Janus kinase (JAK) inhibitor.

Because the biologic therapies induce general immunosuppression, patients are at increased risk for infection, including reactivation of latent infections such as tuberculosis, as well as possible malignancies. Major disadvantages of biologic drugs are that they are not available in PO formulations and their annual costs may exceed $40,000 per year. Most biologics are contraindicated or used with caution during pregnancy and lactation.

Cyclosporine (Gengraf, Neoral, Sandimmune): Cyclosporine is effective at providing rapid relief from the symptoms of psoriasis and is often combined with other drugs, such as calcipotriene, to provide for a lower dose and reduced toxicity. See Chapter 42 for a prototype feature on this drug.

Methotrexate (Otrexup, Trexall): Methotrexate is one of the most frequently prescribed systemic drugs for severe psoriasis. Methotrexate inhibits the rapid proliferation of cells in the skin. It is administered either once weekly or twice daily for 3 days each week. Otrexup permits a once-weekly subcutaneous injection for patients with severe psoriasis. Improvement is noted after several weeks of therapy, but maximum effects may take 2 to 3 months. Methotrexate is discussed as a prototype drug in Chapter 57.

Nonpharmacologic therapy: Phototherapy with ultraviolet-A (UVA) and ultraviolet-B (UVB) light is used in cases of severe debilitating psoriasis. Phototherapy with UVA is combined with methoxsalen, a drug from a chemical family known as the psoralens. The concurrent use of UVA and the drug is called PUVA therapy. **Psoralens** are PO or topical drugs that produce a photosensitive reaction when exposed to UV light. This reaction reduces the number of psoriatic lesions, but unpleasant adverse effects such as headache, nausea, and skin sensitivity occur that may limit the effectiveness of PUVA therapy. Treatments are limited to two to three times per week, and an interim period of 48 hours between treatments is necessary. Because of the strong photosensitizing properties of the psoralens, patients must wear dark glasses during treatment and for the remainder of the day. The use of PUVA has been associated with an increased risk for cataract development.

The second type of phototherapy is with narrow-band UVB light, which is less hazardous than UVA therapy. The wavelength of UVB is similar to that of sunlight, and it reduces the lesions that cover a large area of the body that normally resist topical treatments. It is usually used in conjunction with topical coal tar. If access to a light treatment unit is not feasible, natural sunlight may be used. The use of commercial tanning beds is not recommended for the patient with psoriasis.

All UV treatments may cause acute sunburn reactions, including generalized redness with edema and tenderness as well as the development of long-term effects of actinic keratosis, premature aging of the skin, and skin cancers. Immunosuppressant drugs such as cyclosporine are not used in conjunction with PUVA therapy because they increase the risk of skin cancer.

Pharmacotherapy of Minor Skin Burns

73.8 The pharmacotherapy of sunburn includes prevention with sunscreens and treatment with lotions, topical anesthetics, and analgesics.

Sunburn results from overexposure of the skin to UV light and is associated with light skin complexions, prolonged exposure to the sun during the more hazardous hours of the day (10:00 a.m. until 3:00 p.m.), and lack of protective clothing when outdoors. Chronic sun exposure can result in serious conditions, including eye injury, cataracts, and skin cancer.

Minor, first-degree burns affect only the outer layers of the epidermis. Excessive exposure to UV light, however, injures the dermis and dilates the capillaries, leading to redness, tenderness, edema, and occasional blister formation. In addition to producing local skin damage, sun overexposure releases toxins that may produce systemic effects. The signs and symptoms of sunburn include erythema, intense pain, nausea and vomiting, chills, edema, and headache. Once sunburn has occurred, medications can only alleviate the symptoms; they do not speed recovery time.

The best treatment for sunburn is prevention. Sunscreens are liquids or lotions applied for chemical or physical protection. Chemical sunscreens absorb the spectrum of UV light that is responsible for most sunburns. Chemical sunscreens include those that contain benzophenone for protection against UVA rays and those that work against UVB rays such as cinnamates, para-aminobenzoic acid (PABA), and salicylates. Physical sunscreens such as zinc oxide, talc, and titanium dioxide reflect or scatter light to prevent the penetration of both UVA and UVB rays. Parsol is another sunscreen product that is being used more frequently as a key ingredient in lip balm.

The effectiveness of a sunscreen is indicated by its SPF. An SPF of 8 means the product offers eight times more protection than using no sunscreen. Patients with skin that sunburns easily should use products with an SPF of 15 or greater. Waterproof sunscreens are meant to withstand 8 minutes of exposure to water. People tend to apply sunscreen too infrequently and in layers that are too thin. To be effective, sunscreen must be applied generously and often during the exposure period.

Treatment for sunburn consists of addressing symptoms with soothing lotions, rest, prevention of dehydration, and topical anesthetics, if needed. Treatment is usually done on an outpatient basis. Topical anesthetics for minor burns include benzocaine (Solarcaine), lidocaine (Xylocaine), and tetracaine. Aloe vera is a popular natural therapy for minor skin irritations and burns. Hydrocortisone cream may decrease pain and swelling and assist in the healing of damaged tissue. These same drugs may also provide relief from minor pain due to insect bites and pruritus. In more severe cases, PO analgesics and anti-inflammatory medications such as aspirin or ibuprofen may be indicated.

PROTOTYPE DRUG **Benzocaine (Americaine, Anbesol, Others)**

Classification **Therapeutic:** Topical anesthetic
Pharmacologic: Local anesthetic (ester type), antipruritic

Therapeutic Effects and Uses: Approved in 1938, benzocaine inhibits the conduction of nerve impulses from sensory nerve endings, producing surface anesthesia. It is indicated for the temporary relief of pain and discomfort in patients with pruritic skin problems, minor burns and wounds, and insect bites. It is available in a variety of delivery forms, including sprays, lotions, gels, and lozenges. Several products are available OTC to treat pain due to toothaches, dentures, or canker sores. Because of its short duration of action, it must be applied three to four times a day.

Mechanism of Action: Benzocaine produces surface anesthesia by inhibiting the conduction of nerve endings.

Pharmacokinetics:

Route(s)	Topical
Absorption	Minimally absorbed from intact skin
Distribution	Unknown
Primary metabolism	Hepatic
Primary excretion	Renal
Onset of action	1 min
Duration of action	15–20 min

Adverse Effects: Adverse effects include sensitization in susceptible individuals, allergic reactions, and anaphylaxis.

CONNECTIONS: Complementary and Alternative Therapies

Aloe Vera

Description

Numerous products on the market, including soaps, lotions, creams, and sunscreens, are aimed at the consumer who is seeking the healing properties of aloe vera gel. Healthcare providers have also recommended aloe vera gel to treat dermatitis, burns, and a variety of skin disorders.

History and Claims

Aloe vera is derived from the gel inside the leaf of the aloe plant, which is a member of the lily family. Aloe vera contains over 70 active substances, including antioxidants, minerals, vitamins, and enzymes. These substances are supposed to kill a variety of microorganisms, decrease pain, and reduce localized inflammation. Aloe vera also has value for its moisturizing and wound healing properties. It has been used medicinally for thousands of years. Early mention is made of aloe's use in ancient Sumer in 2200 BC, where it was proclaimed a plant of great healing power.

Standardization

Aloe vera has not been evaluated by the FDA for safety, effectiveness, or purity.

Evidence

Like other herbal products, controlled research studies demonstrating the effectiveness of aloe vera are lacking. The gel is most often used topically, although it may be taken orally. The yellow latex component of aloe produces a strong laxative effect and intense cramping may occur; the drug is not recommended to be taken orally for this reason (National Center for Complementary and Integrative Health, 2020). While it is known that whole-leaf aloe vera extract has demonstrated carcinogenic outcomes, less is known about the long-term effects of the gel, used topically or orally. Until more rigorous clinical trials have been conducted, nurses should advise patients wanting to use aloe vera, particularly the PO form, to discuss it with their healthcare provider.

Because it is poorly absorbed, systemic adverse effects are rarely observed. Caution should be used if applying benzocaine to large areas of abraded skin or skin that has evidence of infection.

Contraindications/Precautions: Contraindications include hypersensitivity to benzocaine or other PABA derivatives or to any of the components in the formulation. Caution should be used in patients with a history of drug sensitivity to ester-type anesthetics, denuded skin, or severely traumatized mucosa and in children under age 6 years.

Drug Interactions: Benzocaine may antagonize the antibacterial activity of sulfonamides.

Pregnancy: Animal studies have not been conducted on the safety of this drug during pregnancy or lactation.

Treatment of Overdose: Overdose with topical benzocaine is unlikely.

Drugs Similar to Benzocaine (Americaine, Anbesol, Others)

Benzocaine is the only drug in its class that is used for minor burns.

Pharmacotherapy of Alopecia

73.9 Several drugs are able to stimulate moderate hair regrowth in patients with male- and female-pattern alopecia.

Alopecia is the loss of hair, resulting in baldness. Male-pattern baldness is the most common cause of hair loss in men and is genetically determined. Men affected by this type of alopecia typically experience a loss of hair at the temples, followed by a recession of the hairline and baldness at the crown.

Two drugs are currently available to promote hair regrowth in patients with male-pattern baldness: topical minoxidil (Rogaine) and PO finasteride (Propecia, Proscar). Neither drug was originally developed for baldness. Although their exact mechanisms of action are unknown, it is thought that these drugs work by stimulating the epithelial cells within the hair follicle. They are most successful in patients with recent onset of symptoms or who are less than 50 years of age. About 40% of patients who are treated two to three times daily for a year will experience moderate regrowth of hair. For both drugs, hair regrowth stops when the drug is discontinued.

Hair loss in women differs from hair loss in men and varies by ethnicity. A common type of alopecia in Caucasian women, female-pattern hair loss, typically begins in the early 20s and 30s, with progressive thinning and loss of hair on the top of the scalp but not the back. These women typically do not have a receding hairline. The hair also becomes finer as individual hairs become smaller, resulting in less dense hair. Some women with this pattern of hair loss may have elevated androgen levels or diabetes that requires treatment. Topical minoxidil is currently the only hair regrowth treatment approved for women by the FDA. Applied to the scalp twice daily, it stimulates hairs that are actively growing to have more robust growth.

Women of African descent have a different type of alopecia called *central centrifugal alopecia*. This type also results in hair loss on the top of the scalp, but it is different from the female-pattern hair loss in that the hair follicles are destroyed. Topical minoxidil is used in this group to stimulate growth in the unaffected hair follicles, whereas anti-inflammatory medications are used to decrease the destruction of the hair follicles.

Minoxidil (Rogaine): Oral minoxidil (Loniten) was first approved for HTN in 1979. Approval to market the topical solution for hair loss occurred in 1996. The drug is rubbed onto the scalp twice daily. Although minoxidil is a potent vasodilator, this mechanism is likely not involved in its effectiveness as a hair regrowth agent. Only 2% of a topical dose is absorbed systemically; therefore, this route does not affect blood pressure. An off-label use is to treat chemotherapy-induced alopecia. In patients who are receiving chemotherapy, hair regrowth occurs at a faster rate with minoxidil use. Response rates vary, however, and over half of patients treated do not experience significant regrowth. The drug has no significant adverse effects. Caution should be taken to keep the solution out of the reach of children because one teaspoon contains the amount of a daily adult antihypertensive dose. This drug is absorbed through the skin and not recommended during pregnancy or lactation.

Finasteride (Propecia, Proscar): Proscar was approved for benign prostatic hyperplasia (BPH) in 1992. Propecia was later approved to treat male-pattern baldness in 1997. The dose used for treating BPH is five times higher than that used for baldness. Unlike minoxidil, finasteride is a PO medication. This drug is thought to act by reducing the amounts of dihydroxytestosterone in hair follicles, thus slowing hair loss. It is less effective than minoxidil at promoting hair regrowth. At the low doses used for hair regrowth, adverse effects are uncommon. It is not approved for use in women. This drug is contraindicated during pregnancy because it may cause abnormalities in the genitalia of male fetuses. Pregnant women should not handle this drug because it is absorbed in the skin.

CONNECTION Checkpoint 73.3

From what you learned in Chapter 71, describe the mechanism by which finasteride reduces symptoms of BPH.

Understanding Chapter 73

Key Concepts Summary

73.1 Three layers of skin, the epidermis, dermis, and subcutaneous layers, provide effective barrier defenses for the body.

73.2 The etiology of skin disorders may be classified as infectious, inflammatory, or neoplastic.

73.3 When the integrity of the skin is compromised, microbes can gain entrance and cause infections that require anti-infective therapy.

73.4 Scabicides and pediculicides are used to treat parasitic skin infestations.

73.5 The pharmacotherapy of acne includes treatment with benzoyl peroxide, retinoids, and antibiotics; pharmacotherapy for rosacea includes retinoids and metronidazole.

73.6 The most effective treatment for dermatitis is topical corticosteroids, which are classified by their potency.

73.7 Psoriasis is a chronic, inflammatory disease that is treated with topical and systemic medications.

73.8 The pharmacotherapy of sunburn includes prevention with sunscreens and treatment with lotions, topical anesthetics, and analgesics.

73.9 Several drugs are able to stimulate moderate hair regrowth in patients with male- and female-pattern alopecia.

CASE STUDY: Making the Patient Connection

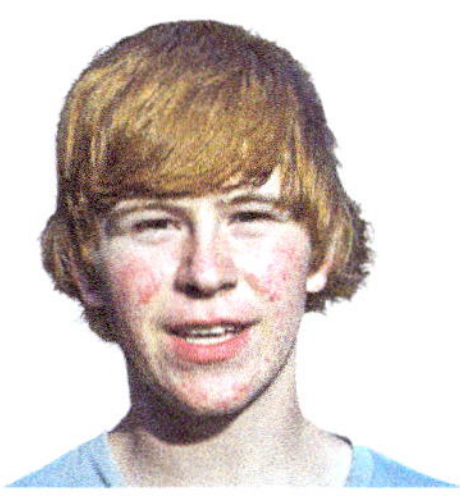

Remember the patient "Danny McBride" at the beginning of the chapter? Now read the remainder of the case study. Based on the information presented within this chapter, respond to the critical thinking questions that follow.

Danny McBride is a 17-year-old high school student in his senior year. He is active in lacrosse and baseball but is finding that his skin is breaking out more often lately and is becoming discouraged at the frequency. He feels it has started to affect his social life, so his parents make an appointment with a dermatologist. The healthcare provider diagnoses Danny's skin condition as acne vulgaris and prescribes tretinoin (Retin-A).

Critical Thinking Questions

1. What would you tell Danny about his condition? Include what acne is, who is prone to develop it, and what methods of treatment have been found to be beneficial.
2. What are some reasons why Danny's acne outbreaks may have increased at this time?
3. What will you teach Danny about the application of tretinoin and adverse effects that may occur?

Additional Case Study

Stephanie Caldera, age 36, is seen by her healthcare provider for scaling patches on her forearms, elbows, and lower legs. She is diagnosed with psoriasis vulgaris and the provider prescribes betamethasone cream. Stephanie asks the nurse, "What is psoriasis? I look so awful! Is it contagious?"

1. How should the nurse respond?
2. What specific instructions should Stephanie be given about the application of the betamethasone cream?
3. Stephanie's psoriasis has not been responsive to betamethasone and she is prescribed calcipotriene (Dovonex). What teaching does Stephanie receive about this new prescription?

Chapter Review

1. An important inclusion in a teaching plan prepared for the patient who is taking permethrin (Nix) is:

1. Nix can be applied after body lotion is applied.
2. All body hair, including eyelashes and eyebrows, can be treated with lindane.
3. Lice cannot live outside the body.
4. In addition to hair shafts, examine the inner thigh areas, gluteal folds, and pubic areas for lice.

2. A patient is being treated with a course of topical desoximetasone (Topicort) for atopic dermatitis. In planning teaching for this patient, which adverse effects would the nurse anticipate?

1. Burning and stinging of the skin in the affected area
2. Development of localized pruritus and hives
3. Hair loss in the application area
4. Worsening of acne vulgaris

3. The patient reports using benzoyl peroxide (Benzac) for treatment of acne. The nurse notes that the action of this drug includes which of the following? (Select all that apply.)

1. Sebum suppression
2. Antimicrobial effect
3. Keratolytic effect
4. Microdermal abrasion
5. Sunscreen activity

4. A patient has been prescribed topical tretinoin (Retin-A) for treatment of acne unresponsive to OTC products. What essential information should the nurse include in the patient's teaching?

1. Wash the face thoroughly three times a day with an antiacne soap while using this medication.
2. Plan to expose the involved skin areas to sunlight for a minimum of 15 minutes each day.
3. Use only mild soaps, warm water, and pat the skin dry to avoid excessive irritation.
4. Alternate the topical tretinoin with benzoyl peroxide on an every-other-day rotation for best results.

5. Benzocaine has been recommended to a 17-year-old patient for treatment of a mild sunburn. What should the patient be taught about using this product?

1. It may be used on superficial and partial-thickness sunburns.
2. Warming the lotion under warm water will prevent a chilled sensation when applied.
3. A small test area should be used if the drug has not been used before to assess for allergy.
4. Cover the treated area with a light dressing wrapped in plastic wrap to keep it from rubbing off.

6. A patient who has been prescribed isotretinoin (Absorica, Zenatane) must comply with the iPledge Program because of the risk of ________________ effects.

See Appendix A for answers to critical thinking questions, case study questions, and review questions.

References

American Academy of Dermatology. (n.d.). *Indoor tanning*. https://www.aad.org/media/stats-indoor-tanning

National Center for Complementary and Integrative Health. (2020). *Aloe vera*. https://www.nccih.nih.gov/health/aloe-vera

Selected Bibliography

American College of Allergy, Asthma and Immunology. (n.d.). *Eczema (atopic dermatitis)*. https://acaai.org/allergies/types-allergies/skin-allergy/eczema-atopic-dermatitis

Banasikowska, A. K. (2020). *Rosacea*. Medscape. http://emedicine.medscape.com/article/1071429-overview

Barry, M. (2020). *Scabies*. Medscape. http://emedicine.medscape.com/article/1109204-overview

Del Rosso, J. Q., Tanghetti, E., Webster, G., Gold, L. S., Thiboutot, D., & Gallo, R. L. (2019). Update on the management of rosacea from the American Acne & Rosacea Society (AARS). *Journal of Clinical and Aesthetic Dermatology, 12*(6), 17–24.

Habashy, J. (2020). *Psoriasis*. Medscape. http://emedicine.medscape.com/article/1943419-overview

National Psoriasis Foundation. (n.d.). *About psoriasis*. https://www.psoriasis.org/about-psoriasis/

Ogé, L. K., Broussard, A., & Marshall, M. D. (2019). Acne vulgaris: Diagnosis and treatment. *American Family Physician, 100*(8), 475–484.

Rao, J. (2020). *Acne vulgaris*. Medscape. http://emedicine.medscape.com/article/1069804-overview

Singh, J. A., Guyatt, G., Ogdie, A., Gladman, D. D., Deal, C., Deodhar, A., et al. (2019). 2018 American College of Rheumatology/National Psoriasis Foundation guideline for the treatment of psoriatic arthritis. *Arthritis & Rheumatology, 71*(1), 5–32. https://doi.org/10.1002/art.40726

Toussi, A., Maverakis, N., Le, S. T., Sarkar, S., Raychaudhuri, S. K., & Raychaudhuri, S. P. (2020). Updated therapies for the management of psoriatic arthritis. *Clinical Immunology, 220*, 108536. https://doi.org/10.1016/j.clim.2020.108536

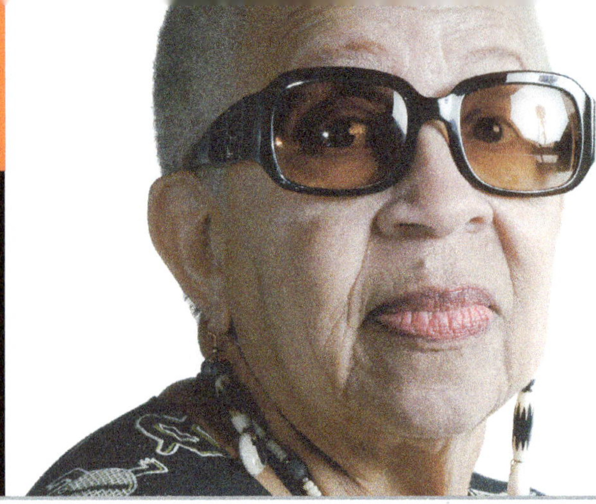

"I just cannot see clearly while driving at night anymore. All I see are halos around the other cars' headlights."
—*Patient "Therese Duclos"*

Chapter 74
Pharmacotherapy of Eye and Ear Disorders

Chapter Outline

Learning Outcomes

After reading this chapter, the student should be able to:

1. Identify the major anatomic structures of the eye.
2. Identify the primary risk factors associated with glaucoma.
3. Compare and contrast open-angle and closed-angle glaucoma.
4. Explain the two major mechanisms by which drugs reduce intraocular pressure.
5. Identify examples of drugs that dilate or constrict pupils, relax ciliary muscles, constrict ocular blood vessels, or moisten eye membranes.
6. Identify the types of ear conditions that could benefit from pharmacotherapy.
7. Describe the nurse's role in the nonpharmacologic and pharmacologic management of eye and ear disorders.
8. For each of the classes shown in the chapter outline, identify the prototype and representative drugs and explain the mechanism(s) of drug action, primary indications, contraindications, significant drug interactions, pregnancy data, and important adverse effects.
9. Apply clinical judgment to the care of patients receiving pharmacotherapy for eye and ear disorders.

Key Terms

Definitions of the terms in bold may be found in the Glossary.

The senses of vision and hearing are the primary means for us to communicate with the world around us. Disorders that affect the eye and ear can result in problems with self-care, mobility, safety, and communication. The eye is vulnerable to a variety of conditions, many of which can be prevented, controlled, or reversed with proper pharmacotherapy. The first part of this chapter covers drugs that are used for the treatment of glaucoma and those used routinely by ophthalmic healthcare providers. The remaining part of this chapter presents drugs that are used for the treatment of common ear disorders, including infections, inflammation, and the buildup of earwax.

Anatomy of the Eye

74.1 Knowledge of basic eye anatomy is fundamental to understanding eye disorders and their pharmacotherapy.

Knowledge of basic ocular anatomy is key to understanding eye disorders and their pharmacotherapy. The important structures of the eye are shown in Figures 74.1 and 74.2.

The wall of the eye contains three layers, known as tunics. The outermost fibrous tunic is composed of the cornea and the sclera. The cornea is the transparent layer that covers the anterior portion of the eye. It has no blood vessels

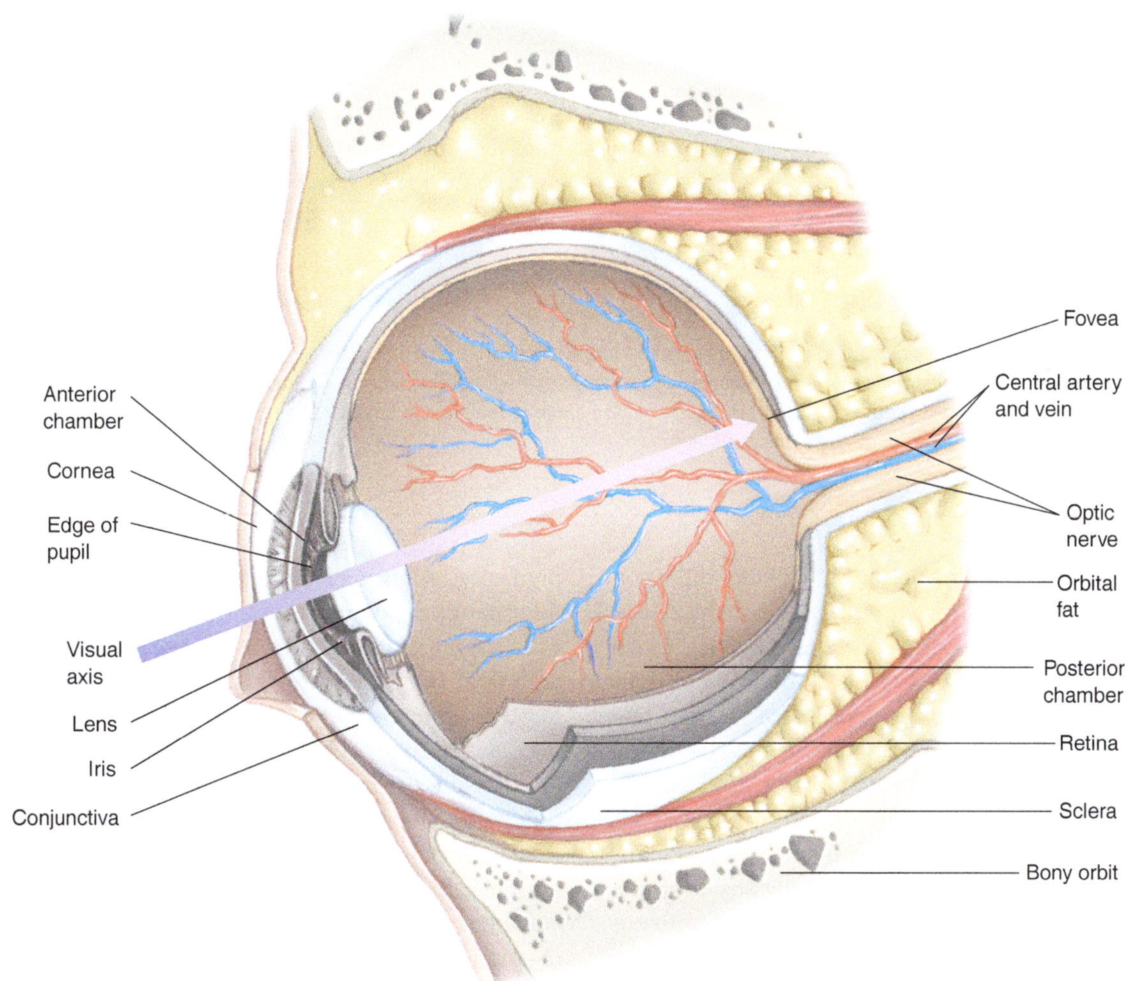

Figure 74.1 Anatomy of the interior of the eye.

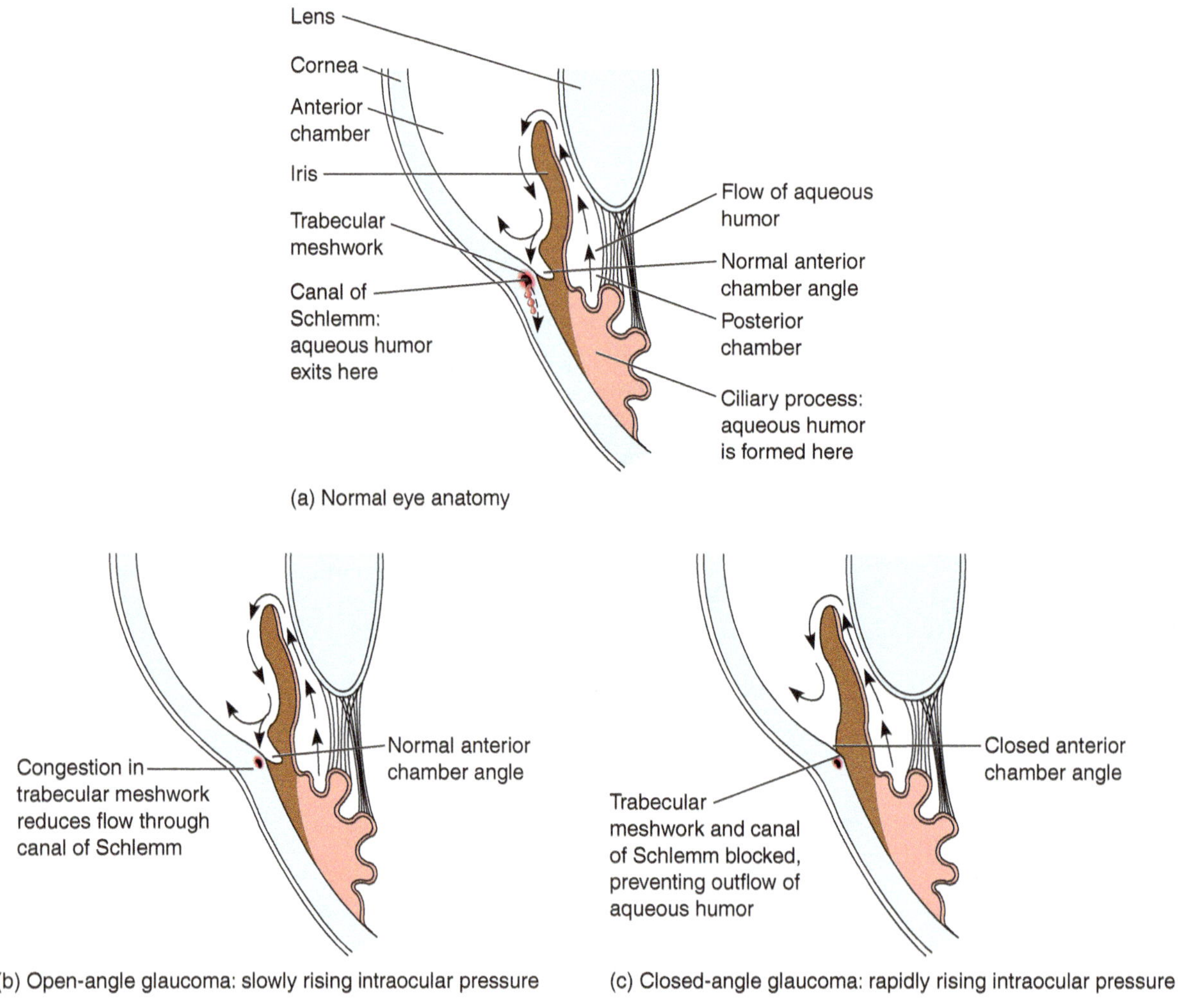

Figure 74.2 (a) In a healthy eye, aqueous humor is formed in the ciliary process and drains through the canal of Schlemm. (b) In chronic open-angle glaucoma, the anterior chamber angle remains open, but drainage of aqueous humor through the canal of Schlemm is impaired. (c) In acute closed-angle glaucoma, the angle of the iris and anterior chamber narrows, obstructing the drainage of aqueous humor through the canal of Schlemm.

and receives nutrients from the fluid lying behind the cornea, or aqueous humor. It is continuous with the sclera, which is the thick, white, opaque portion covering the posterior portion of the eye. The vascular tunic is the middle layer of the eye, which is rich in blood vessels. The vascular tunic contains specialized structures that include the iris and ciliary body. The innermost layer is the neural tunic or retina, which contains the photoreceptors for vision.

The interior of the eye is divided into two cavities. The largest portion of the interior of the eye is the posterior cavity, which is filled with a gel-like substance called vitreous humor that helps the eyeball to maintain its shape and keep the retina in place.

The anterior cavity is smaller but is very important from a pharmacologic perspective. This cavity is separated into two chambers by the lens. The anterior chamber extends from the cornea to the iris; the posterior chamber lies between the iris and the lens. In front of the lens is the pigmented iris, which is made up of smooth muscle fibers that change the diameter of the pupil. The pupil is the central opening that allows light to enter. These muscle fibers are under the control of the sympathetic nervous system. Pupil constriction is the result of parasympathetic stimulation, and its dilation is a sympathetic response.

The anterior cavity is filled with **aqueous humor**, a thin fluid that slowly circulates to bring nutrients to the area and remove wastes. The aqueous humor is secreted by cells in a muscular structure called the ciliary body. Once secreted, the aqueous humor flows from the posterior chamber through the pupil and into the anterior chamber. Within the anterior chamber and around the periphery is a network of spongy connective tissue, or trabecular meshwork, that contains an opening called the canal of Schlemm (scleral venous sinus). The aqueous humor drains into the canal of Schlemm and out of the anterior chamber into the venous system, thus completing its circulation. Under normal circumstances, the rate of aqueous humor production is equal to its outflow, maintaining intraocular pressure (IOP) within a normal range. Interference with either the production or outflow of aqueous humor, however, can lead to an increase in IOP.

The conjunctiva, eyebrows, eyelashes, eyelids, and lacrimal apparatus that produce tears all serve to protect the eye. Infection and inflammatory responses are common conditions in these supporting structures. Redness, edema, and itching are common indications for medications.

Pathophysiology of Glaucoma

74.2 The two principal types of glaucoma, closed-angle glaucoma and open-angle glaucoma, are characterized by increased intraocular pressure.

Glaucoma is a condition that is characterized by gradual loss of peripheral vision, usually accompanied by increased IOP. Glaucoma occurs when the IOP becomes high enough to cause optic nerve damage, leading to visual field loss and possible progression to blindness. Although the median IOP in the population is 15 to 16 mmHg, this pressure varies greatly with age, daily activities, and even time of day. As a rule, IOPs that are consistently above 21 mmHg are considered abnormal. Many patients, however, tolerate IOPs in the mid to high 20s without damage to the optic nerve. IOPs that are above 30 mmHg require treatment because they are associated with a high risk for permanent vision changes. Some patients of Asian descent may experience glaucoma at "normal" IOP values, below 21 mmHg.

PharmFACT

Blindness from glaucoma is six to eight times higher in African Americans than in Caucasians. After cataracts, it is the leading cause of blindness among African Americans (Glaucoma Research Foundation, 2017).

Glaucoma affects more than 3 million Americans over the age of 40 and is the leading cause of preventable blindness worldwide. Primary glaucoma usually occurs without an identifiable cause and is most frequently found in people older than 60 years of age. In some cases, glaucoma is associated with genetic factors; it can be congenital in infants and children. Glaucoma can also be secondary to eye trauma, infection, diabetes, inflammation, hemorrhage, tumor, or cataracts. Some medications may contribute to the development or progression of glaucoma, including the long-term use of corticosteroids, some antihypertensives, antihistamines, and antidepressants. Other major risk factors associated with glaucoma include hypertension (HTN), migraines, refractive disorders with high degrees of nearsightedness or farsightedness, and normal aging.

Diagnosis of glaucoma can be difficult because it sometimes occurs so gradually that patients do not experience symptoms or seek medical attention until late in the disease process. **Tonometry** is a primary ophthalmic technique that tests for glaucoma by measuring IOP. Patients with unusually thick or thin corneas may have false negatives or false positives during tonometry. Patients who have had Lasik surgery, which removes corneal tissue to correct myopia, may appear to have normal IOPs, yet have glaucoma. Gonioscopy uses a gonioscope to measure the angle in the eye where the iris meets the cornea and is useful in distinguishing between open-angle and closed-angle glaucoma. Visual field testing (perimetry) assesses the degree of central visual field narrowing and peripheral vision loss. Funduscopic examinations look at retinal field changes that accompany glaucoma.

The two major types of primary glaucoma are closed-angle glaucoma and open-angle glaucoma, as shown in Figure 74.2. Both disorders result from the same problem: a buildup of aqueous humor in the anterior cavity. This buildup is caused either by an excessive production of aqueous humor or by a blockage of its outflow. In either case, IOP increases, leading to progressive damage to the optic nerve. As the optic nerve degenerates, the patient will first notice a loss of visual field, then a loss of central visual acuity, and eventually total blindness. The major differences between closed-angle glaucoma and open-angle glaucoma include how quickly the IOP develops and whether there is narrowing of the anterior chamber angle between the iris and cornea.

Closed-angle glaucoma, also called *acute-* or *narrow-angle glaucoma,* accounts for only 5% of all primary glaucoma. The incidence is higher in older adults and in individuals of Asian descent. It is typically caused by the normal thickening of the lens and may develop gradually over several years. This type of glaucoma is usually unilateral and is often associated with conditions that result in dilation of the pupil, such as stress, impact injury, or medications. Closed-angle glaucoma occurs when the pressure inside the anterior chamber increases suddenly because the iris is being pushed over the area where the aqueous humor normally drains into the trabecular network and the canal of Schlemm. The displacement of the iris is due in part to the dilation of the pupil or accommodation of the lens, causing the angle between the posterior cornea and the anterior iris to narrow or close.

Signs and symptoms of closed-angle glaucoma are caused by acute obstruction of the outflow of aqueous humor from the eye and include dull to severe eye and facial pain, headaches, seeing colored halos around bright lights, a bulging iris, and a sudden change in visual acuity. The affected eye may appear reddened and the pupil may be nonreactive. Ocular pain may be so severe that it causes nausea and vomiting. If the outflow is totally closed,

closed-angle glaucoma constitutes a medical emergency and laser or conventional surgery is indicated for the preservation of sight. Surgical options include iridectomy, laser trabeculoplasty, trabeculectomy, and drainage implants.

Open-angle glaucoma is the most common type of glaucoma, accounting for more than 90% of the cases. Its cause is unknown, and many patients are asymptomatic. It is usually bilateral, with the elevated IOP developing over years. Open-angle glaucoma is named as such because the anterior chamber angle is normal; the iris does not completely cover the trabecular meshwork and canal of Schlemm. They remain open with their flow being partially obstructed. This leads to the gradual development of increased IOP with slow degeneration of the optic nerve, resulting in a gradual loss of vision. Most patients with open-angle glaucoma can be successfully treated with medications.

Pharmacotherapy of Glaucoma

74.3 The primary goal of glaucoma pharmacotherapy is to prevent damage to the optic nerve by lowering intraocular pressure.

When glaucoma is diagnosed and treated early in the course of the disease, permanent vision disability can usually be prevented. Some healthcare providers initiate pharmacotherapy in all patients with an IOP greater than 21 mmHg. Because of the expense of pharmacotherapy and potential adverse drug effects, other healthcare providers will instead carefully monitor the patient through regular follow-up examinations and wait until the IOP rises to 28 to 30 mmHg before initiating treatment. If signs of optic nerve damage or visual field changes are evident, the patient is treated regardless of the IOP.

Once pharmacotherapy has been initiated, reevaluation is performed after 2 to 4 months to assess for therapeutic effectiveness. Some of the antiglaucoma drugs take 6 to 8 weeks to reach peak effect. If the therapeutic goals are not achieved with a single drug, it is common to add a second medication from a different class to the regimen to produce an additive decrease in IOP. Some of the drugs may continue to have effects on the eye for 2 to 4 weeks after being discontinued.

Maintaining patient adherence with the medication regimen is a key factor in preventing progressive vision impairment. It is essential for the nurse to determine any factors that could decrease adherence, such as insufficient financial resources, lack of knowledge about the disease, inability to properly instill the medication, or difficulty remembering the dosing schedule. The patient diagnosed with glaucoma may experience fear and anxiety about potential blindness and disability. Accurate and thorough teaching for the patient and family or caregiver should be directed at how the disease can be managed with the correct use of the medications.

Many drugs are available to treat glaucoma. These medications work by one of two mechanisms: increasing the outflow of aqueous humor at the canal of Schlemm or decreasing the formation of aqueous humor at the ciliary body. Many antiglaucoma drugs produce these effects by modifying actions of the autonomic nervous system.

Although topical drugs are most commonly prescribed, oral (PO) medications may be used for severe glaucoma. Drugs for glaucoma, which are listed in Table 74.1, include the following classes:

- Prostaglandin analogs
- Autonomic drugs, including beta-adrenergic blockers, alpha$_2$-adrenergic agonists, cholinergic agonists, and nonselective sympathomimetics
- Carbonic anhydrase inhibitors
- Osmotic diuretics.

Prostaglandins

74.4 Prostaglandin analogs are the first-line drugs for treating high intraocular pressure because of their long durations of action and high safety profiles.

Prostaglandin analogs are often the preferred drugs for glaucoma because they have long durations of action, allowing for once-daily dosing, and produce fewer adverse effects than the beta-adrenergic blockers. They may be used as monotherapy or combined with drugs from other classes to produce an additive reduction in IOP in patients with resistant glaucoma.

Prostaglandin analogs lower IOP by increasing the outflow of aqueous humor. Latanoprost (Xalatan), which is available as a 0.005% eyedrop solution, is one of the most commonly used prostaglandin analogs. Other ocular prostaglandins include bimatoprost (Lumigan) and travoprost (Travatan Z). An occasional adverse effect of these medications is heightened pigmentation, which turns a blue iris to a browner color. Many patients experience thicker and longer eyelashes. These drugs cause local irritation, stinging of the eyes, and redness during the first month of therapy. Because of these effects, prostaglandins are normally administered just before bedtime.

PROTOTYPE DRUG **Latanoprost (Xalatan)**

Classification **Therapeutic:** Drug for glaucoma and intraocular HTN
Pharmacologic: Prostaglandin analog

Therapeutic Effects and Uses: Approved by the U.S. Food and Drug Administration (FDA) in 1996, latanoprost

Table 74.1 Selected Drugs for Glaucoma

Drug	Route and Adult Dose (Maximum Dose Where Indicated)	Adverse Effects
Prostaglandin Analogs		
bimatoprost (Lumigan)	1 drop of 0.03% solution daily in the evening	*Increased length and thickness of eyelashes, darkening of the iris, stinging, sensation of foreign body in the eye* Respiratory infection, flu, angina, muscle or joint pain
latanoprost (Xalatan)	1 drop of 0.005% solution daily in the evening	
tafluprost (Zioptan)	1 drop of 0.0015% solution daily in the evening	
travoprost (Travatan Z)	1 drop of 0.004% solution daily in the evening	
Beta-Adrenergic Blockers		
betaxolol (Betoptic)	1 drop of 0.5% solution bid	*Local burning and stinging, blurred vision, headache* Conjunctival hyperemia, angina, anxiety, bronchoconstriction, hypotension, dysrhythmias
carteolol	1 drop of 1% solution bid	
levobunolol (Betagan)	1–2 drops of 0.25–0.5% solution 1–2 times/day	
timolol (Betimol, Timoptic, others)	1–2 drops of 0.25–0.5% solution 1–2 times/day Gel (salve): apply daily	
Alpha$_2$-Adrenergic Agonists		
apraclonidine (Iopidine)	1 drop of 0.5% solution bid	*Local itching and burning, blurred vision, dry mouth, headache, eye discharge* Allergic conjunctivitis, conjunctival hyperemia, hypotension, bulbar conjunctival follicles
brimonidine (Alphagan P)	1 drop of 0.1–0.15% solution in the affected eye tid, 8 h apart	
Cholinergic Agonists		
carbachol (Miostat)	Intraocular: 0.5 mL injected into the aqueous humor to produce miosis and lower IOP prior to ocular surgery	*Induced myopia, reduced visual acuity in low light, eye redness, headache* Salivation, tachycardia, hypotension, bronchospasm, sweating, nausea and vomiting, retinal detachment (pilocarpine)
echothiophate iodide (Phospholine Iodide)	1 drop of 0.03–0.25% solution 1–2 times/day	
pilocarpine (Isopto Carpine)	Acute glaucoma: 1 drop of 1–2% solution every 5–10 min for 3–6 doses Chronic glaucoma: 1 drop of 0.5–4% solution q4–12h	
Sympathomimetics		
epinephrine	1 drop of solution in affected eye 1–2 times/day	*Local burning and stinging, blurred vision, headache, photosensitivity* Tachycardia, HTN
Carbonic Anhydrase Inhibitors		
acetazolamide (Diamox)	PO: 250 mg 1–4 times/day	*For topical medications: blurred vision, bitter taste, dry eye, blepharitis, local itching, sensation of foreign body in the eye, headache* For PO medications: diuresis, electrolyte imbalances, blood dyscrasias, flaccid paralysis, hepatic impairment
brinzolamide (Azopt)	1 drop of 1% solution tid	
dorzolamide (Trusopt)	1 drop of 2% solution in the affected eye(s) tid	
methazolamide (Neptazane)	PO: 50–100 mg bid–tid	
Osmotic Diuretic		
mannitol (Osmitrol)	IV: 1.5–2 mg/kg as a 15–25% solution over 30–60 min	*Orthostatic hypotension, facial flushing, headache, palpitations, anxiety, nausea* Severe headache, electrolyte imbalances, edema

Note: *Italics* indicate common adverse effects. Underline indicates serious adverse effects.

is a prostaglandin analog that reduces IOP by increasing the outflow of aqueous humor for patients with open-angle glaucoma and ocular HTN. The recommended dose is one drop in the affected eye(s) in the evening. It is used to treat open-angle glaucoma.

In 2018, the FDA approved Rocklatan, a combination ophthalmic drug that contains latanoprost and netarsudil. Netarsudil is a Rho kinase (ROCK) inhibitor that repairs the diseased trabecular meshwork, allowing latanoprost to better increase the outflow of aqueous humor.

Mechanism of Action: Latanoprost reduces elevated IOP in patients with open-angle glaucoma. Latanoprost is a prodrug that is metabolized to its active form in the cornea, reaching its peak effect in about 12 hours.

Pharmacokinetics:

Route(s)	Ophthalmic solution
Absorption	Through the cornea
Distribution	Enters systemic distribution in small amounts

Primary metabolism	Metabolized in the aqueous humor to its active form
Primary excretion	Renal
Onset of action	3–4 h with peak effect at 8–12 h
Duration of action	Unknown

Adverse Effects: Adverse effects include ocular symptoms such as conjunctival edema, tearing, dryness, burning, pain, irritation, itching, sensation of a foreign body in the eye, photophobia, or visual disturbances. The eyelashes on the treated eye may grow thicker or darker. Changes may occur in the pigmentation of the iris of the treated eye and in the periocular skin. Rare, systemic adverse effects include headaches, rashes, flulike symptoms, and abnormal liver function tests.

Contraindications/Precautions: Contraindications include hypersensitivity to the drug or another component in the solution, pregnancy, lactation, intraocular infection, or conjunctivitis. It should not be administered to patients with closed-angle glaucoma. The safety of this drug has not been demonstrated in children.

Drug Interactions: Latanoprost interacts with the preservative thimerosal: If used concurrently with other eyedrops that contain thimerosal, precipitation may occur. **Herbal/Food:** Unknown.

Pregnancy: Some prostaglandin analogs are used as uterine stimulants (see Chapter 70). In ophthalmic solutions, small amounts are absorbed into the systemic circulation; however, human observational studies have not shown evidence of fetal harm during pregnancy. Women should consult with their healthcare provider before using this drug during pregnancy or lactation.

Treatment of Overdose: Overdose with the ophthalmic solution is unlikely.

Clinician Responsibilities: Key clinical implications for patients receiving latanoprost are included in Applied Clinical Judgment: Patients Receiving Pharmacotherapy for Glaucoma.

Drugs Similar to Latanoprost (Xalatan)

Bimatoprost, tafluprost, and travoprost are other prostaglandin analogs used for glaucoma. All the analogs have the same pregnancy data as latanoprost.

Bimatoprost (Lumigan): Approved in 2001, bimatoprost is a synthetic prostaglandin analog indicated for the treatment of open-angle glaucoma. In 2008, a newer formulation of this drug, Latisse, was approved to treat hypotrichosis, a condition of having too few eyelashes. Use of bimatoprost can cause a gradual increase in the development of brown pigmentation in the iris, which may be irreversible, and includes an increase in pigmentation of the eyelid. Other adverse effects include blurred vision, eye discomfort, ocular pruritus, conjunctivitis, dry eye, light intolerance, and tearing. It is available as a 0.01% or 0.03% solution applied once daily in the evening. In 2020, a bimatoprost implant (Durysta) was approved. The tiny implant is placed into the anterior chamber of the eye, slowly releasing bimatoprost over a 6-month period. Daily medication drops are no longer necessary once the implant is inserted.

Tafluprost (Zioptan): When approved in 2012, tafluprost became the first antiglaucoma prostaglandin completely free of preservatives. Preservatives sometimes cause allergic reactions in susceptible patients and may worsen ocular surface disorders such as dry eye syndrome. The actions, effectiveness, and side effects of tafluprost are equivalent to those of other prostaglandin analogs.

Travoprost (Travatan Z): Approved in 2001, travoprost is approved for the treatment of open-angle glaucoma. Travoprost has been found to be more effective in Blacks than in non-Blacks. Use of this drug can cause a gradual increase in the development of brown pigmentation in the iris, which may be irreversible, and includes an increase in pigmentation of the eyelid and growth of the eyelashes. Conjunctival hyperemia has been reported in 35 to 50% of patients treated with travoprost. Some other adverse effects include blurred vision, eye discomfort, ocular pruritus, dry eye, light intolerance, and tearing. It is available as a 0.004% solution, applied once daily in the evening.

CONNECTION Checkpoint 74.1

Several prostaglandins are used for their actions on uterine smooth muscle. From what you learned in Chapter 70, what are the primary indications for the prostaglandins carboprost (Hemabate), dinoprostone (Cervidil), and mifepristone (Mifeprex)?

Autonomic Drugs

74.5 Drugs that affect the autonomic nervous system are sometimes prescribed to treat glaucoma.

Several structures within the eye are activated by the sympathetic and parasympathetic divisions of the autonomic nervous system. As such, a significant number of autonomic drugs have been used to treat glaucoma and to aid in ophthalmic examinations of the eyeball.

- Sympathetic activation (or parasympathetic division blockade): Muscles of the iris contract to dilate the pupil; the ciliary muscle relaxes to enhance distance vision.
- Parasympathetic activation (or sympathetic division blockade): Muscles of the iris contract to constrict the pupil; the ciliary muscle contracts to enhance near vision.

The most frequently used autonomic drugs are the beta-adrenergic antagonists or blockers. Alpha$_2$-adrenergic agonists, cholinergic agonists, and nonselective sympathomimetics play minor roles. Prior to reading this section, the student may want to review Chapter 12 to brush up on the terminology and anatomy of the autonomic nervous system.

Beta-adrenergic blockers: Prior to the discovery of the prostaglandin analogs, beta-adrenergic blockers were the preferred drugs for open-angle glaucoma. These drugs decrease the production of aqueous humor by the ciliary body in the affected eye and can lower IOP by 20 to 30%. Four beta-adrenergic blockers are available as ophthalmic solutions: betaxolol (Betoptic), carteolol, levobunolol (Betagan), and timolol (Betimol, Timoptic, others). These drugs generally produce fewer adverse ocular effects than cholinergic agonists or sympathomimetics. In most patients, the topical administration of beta blockers does not result in significant systemic absorption. Should absorption occur, however, adverse systemic effects may include bronchoconstriction, dysrhythmias, and hypotension. Because of the potential for adverse systemic effects, these drugs should be used with caution in patients with asthma, bradycardia, or heart failure (HF). Tolerance will develop with long-term use in about 25% of patients who take these drugs.

Alpha$_2$-adrenergic agonists: Alpha$_2$-adrenergic agonists lower IOP by decreasing the production of aqueous humor and increasing its absorption. Only two alpha$_2$-adrenergic agonists are currently approved: apraclonidine and brimonidine. Apraclonidine (Iopidine) is infrequently used but may be prescribed for the prevention or short-term therapy of postoperative increases in IOP. Brimonidine (Alphagan P) is more commonly prescribed, either as monotherapy or as an adjunct in combination with a beta-adrenergic blocker, for the long-term treatment of open-angle glaucoma or glaucoma secondary to uveitis, which is an inflammation of the middle layer of the eyeball. Alpha$_2$-adrenergic agonists may be used in combination with other antiglaucoma drugs to cause additive reduction in IOP. Combigan is an ophthalmic solution that consists of brimonidine and timolol.

Alpha$_2$-adrenergic agonists are contraindicated in closed-angle glaucoma because the pupil dilation that results would worsen the condition. The most significant adverse effect, and one that is a frequent cause for discontinuation of therapy, is an allergic-type reaction that causes sensation of a foreign body, itching, and hyperemia. Other adverse effects include headache, drowsiness, dry mucosal membranes, blurred vision, and irritated eyelids. These drugs produce few cardiovascular or pulmonary adverse effects. Rare systemic adverse effects may occur, including nervousness, anxiety, and muscle tremors.

Cholinergic agonists (miotics): Drugs that directly activate cholinergic receptors in the eye produce **miosis**, or constriction of the pupil, and contraction of the ciliary muscle. These actions physically stretch the trabecular meshwork to allow greater outflow of aqueous humor and a lowering of IOP. Pilocarpine (Isopto Carpine) is the most commonly prescribed antiglaucoma drug in this class. The cholinergic agonists are applied topically to the eye up to four times daily. Because of their greater toxicity and frequent dosing, these drugs are normally used only in patients with open-angle glaucoma who do not respond to other drugs. Local effects include headache, induced myopia, and decreased vision in low light. Systemic absorption can result in hypotension, vomiting, diuresis, bronchoconstriction, diaphoresis, and abdominal pain with diarrhea. Toxic effects include vertigo, bradycardia, tremors, syncope, and cardiac dysrhythmias. Echothiophate is rarely used because it exhibits a high incidence of adverse effects, including cataracts Other actions of the cholinergic agonists are presented in Chapter 13.

CONNECTION Checkpoint 74.2

Cholinergic agonists such as pilocarpine activate muscarinic receptors. From what you learned in Chapter 13, what effect do muscarinic agonists have on lacrimation and how is this used therapeutically?

Nonselective sympathomimetics: Nonselective sympathomimetics activate the sympathetic nervous system to produce **mydriasis** (pupil dilation) and increase the outflow of aqueous humor, resulting in a lower IOP. They are not as effective as the beta-adrenergic blockers or the prostaglandin analogs and are rarely used. Epinephrine, the only ophthalmic drug in this class, is administered topically for open-angle glaucoma and contraindicated in closed-angle glaucoma. Epinephrine will increase blood pressure and the heart rate if it reaches the systemic circulation; thus, the drug is contraindicated in patients with unstable cardiovascular disease. Sympathomimetics also produce a high frequency of ocular adverse effects, including tearing, burning, hyperemia, and stenosis of the nasolacrimal duct.

PROTOTYPE DRUG Timolol (Betimol, Timoptic, Others)

Classification **Therapeutic:** Drug for glaucoma
Pharmacologic: Miotic, beta-adrenergic antagonist

Therapeutic Effects and Uses: Approved in 1978, timolol is a nonselective beta-adrenergic blocker available as a 0.25% or 0.5% ophthalmic solution. Its primary indication is chronic open-angle glaucoma. It may also be used for aphakic glaucoma (high IOP in patients with no lens), secondary glaucoma, and ocular HTN. The usual dose is one drop in the affected eye(s) twice a day. Timoptic XE allows for once-daily dosing. Treatment may require 2 to 4 weeks to reach the maximum therapeutic effect.

Timolol is available in several formulations. Cosopt is an antiglaucoma drug that combines timolol with dorzolamide, a topical carbonic anhydrase inhibitor. Combigan is an ophthalmic solution of timolol with brimonidine, an alpha-adrenergic agonist. Timolol is also available in tablets, which are prescribed to treat mild HTN.

Mechanism of Action: Timolol topically lowers the elevated and normal IOP by reducing the formation of aqueous humor and possibly increasing outflow. It affects both $beta_1$ and $beta_2$ receptors.

Pharmacokinetics:

Route(s)	Eye solution or gel
Absorption	Small amounts reach the systemic circulation from topical application
Distribution	Secreted in breast milk
Primary metabolism	80% metabolized in the liver to inactive metabolites
Primary excretion	Renal
Onset of action	30 min
Duration of action	12–24 h

Adverse Effects: The most common adverse effects from ophthalmic administration are local burning and stinging on instillation. Vision may become temporarily blurred. In most patients absorption is not significant enough to cause adverse systemic effects as long as timolol is applied correctly. If absorption occurs, hypotension, HF, or dysrhythmias are possible.

Contraindications/Precautions: Although little is absorbed through ocular administration, this drug should be used with caution in certain patients. Timolol is contraindicated in patients with asthma, severe chronic obstructive pulmonary disease (COPD), sinus bradycardia, second- or third-degree atrioventricular block, HF, cardiogenic shock, or hypersensitivity to the drug. Safety in children has not been established.

Drug Interactions: Drug interactions may result if significant systemic absorption occurs. Timolol should be used with caution in patients who are taking other beta blockers owing to additive cardiac effects. Concurrent use with anticholinergics, nitrates, reserpine, methyldopa, or verapamil could lead to hypotension and bradycardia. Epinephrine use could lead to HTN followed by severe bradycardia. When given by the ocular route, timolol will produce additive lowering of IOP when given concurrently with other antiglaucoma drugs. **Herbal/Food:** There are no known herbal or food interactions with this drug.

Pregnancy: Ophthalmic timolol does not show fetal harm in laboratory animals. Because this drug is secreted in human milk and has the potential to cause systemic adverse effects in a breastfed neonate, women should consult with their healthcare provider before using this drug during lactation.

Treatment of Overdose: Overdose could result in systemic symptoms such as reduced heart rate and bronchospasm. Treatment is supportive.

Clinician Responsibilities: Key clinical implications for patients receiving timolol are included in Applied Clinical Judgment: Patients Receiving Pharmacotherapy for Glaucoma.

Drugs Similar to Timolol (Betimol, Timoptic, Others)

Other beta-adrenergic blockers with external ophthalmic indications include betaxolol and levobunolol. Levobetaxolol (Betaxon) metipranolol are ophthalmic beta blockers that have been discontinued in the United States.

Betaxolol (Betoptic): Approved in 1985, betaxolol is a selective $beta_1$-adrenergic receptor blocker. This drug reduces IOP by decreasing the production of aqueous humor. Betaxolol is indicated for intraocular HTN and chronic open-angle glaucoma. A tablet form of this drug (Kerlone) is available to treat HTN. Although only small amounts are absorbed from ophthalmic administration, this drug should be used cautiously in patients with HF and if used concurrently with a systemic beta-adrenergic blocker. Ocular irritation and tearing are frequent adverse effects. High doses of ophthalmic betaxolol showed postimplantation loss but no teratogenicity in laboratory animals. It is not known if this drug is secreted in milk or if it has adverse effects on the breastfed neonate.

Levobunolol (Betagan): Approved in 1985, levobunolol is a nonselective beta-adrenergic blocker that is indicated for the treatment of intraocular HTN and chronic open-angle glaucoma. Because small amounts may reach the systemic circulation, caution needs to be practiced when using this drug in patients with asthma, COPD, bradycardia, thyroid conditions, diabetes, and abnormal blood glucose levels. Tolerance can develop with long-term use. Ocular irritation is a frequent, transient adverse effect. High doses of ophthalmic levobunolol showed signs of beta blockade (bradycardia, hypotension, and respiratory distress) in the fetus and newborn. It is not known if this drug is secreted in milk or if it has adverse effects on the breastfed neonate.

Miscellaneous Drugs for Treating Glaucoma

74.6 Carbonic anhydrase inhibitors and osmotic diuretics are occasionally used for treating glaucoma.

Although prostaglandin analogs and beta-adrenergic blockers are the two most frequently prescribed classes for lowering IOP, some patients may experience adverse effects from these drugs or have particularly resistant glaucoma. Two additional classes, the carbonic anhydrase inhibitors and the osmotic diuretics, are not routinely prescribed.

Carbonic anhydrase inhibitors: Carbonic anhydrase inhibitors interfere with the synthesis of carbonic acid, which decreases the production of aqueous humor and reduces IOP. They are used as long-term therapy in patients with open-angle glaucoma when prostaglandin inhibitors, beta blockers, and other autonomic drugs have not been effective.

Drugs in this class are divided into topical or oral formulations. Dorzolamide (Trusopt) is used topically to treat open-angle glaucoma, either as monotherapy or in combination with other medications. Dorzolamide and other topical carbonic anhydrase inhibitors, including brinzolamide (Azopt), are well tolerated and produce few significant adverse effects other than photosensitivity. PO formulations such as acetazolamide (Diamox) are very effective at lowering IOP in both open-angle and closed-angle glaucoma but are rarely used because they produce more adverse systemic effects than drugs from other classes. These adverse effects include lethargy, nausea and vomiting, depression, paresthesias, and drowsiness. Patients must be cautioned when taking these medications because they contain sulfur and may cause allergic reactions. Because the oral formulations are diuretics and can reduce IOP quickly, serum electrolytes should be monitored during treatment. A prototype feature for acetazolamide is presented in Chapter 32.

Osmotic diuretics: Mannitol (Osmitrol) is an osmotic diuretic occasionally used preoperatively and postoperatively with ocular surgery or as emergency treatment of acute closed-angle glaucoma attacks. Given by IV infusion 60 to 90 minutes prior to ocular surgery, mannitol has the ability to quickly reduce the formation of aqueous humor, thereby reducing IOP. A prototype feature for mannitol is presented in Chapter 32.

CONNECTIONS: APPLIED CLINICAL JUDGMENT

Patients Receiving Pharmacotherapy for Glaucoma

Key Assessment Data

- History of current condition, ophthalmologic, respiratory, cardiovascular, and endocrine disease; baseline vital signs, physical exam findings; pregnancy or breastfeeding; medication history including allergies, current prescription and over-the-counter (OTC) drugs.
- Assess visual acuity and visual fields. Assess for the presence of eye pain, visual disturbances such as halos around lights, diminished foggy vision, loss of peripheral vision, recent eye trauma or infection.

Desired Therapeutic Outcomes

Improvement is observed and measurable by IOP remains below 21 mmHg, with no abnormal changes in visual acuity or fields.

Minimizing Adverse Effects

- Eye redness, pain, light sensitivity, or changes in visual acuity may indicate worsening disease, infection, or adverse drug effects.
- Nonadherence with drug therapy may result in the total loss of vision.
- Contact lenses may hinder eye medications from fully reaching all eye surfaces or may absorb solution, resulting in higher-than-expected amounts in the eye over time. Remove contact lenses before administering ophthalmic solutions. Avoid use of other eyedrops or ointments as they may interact with or counteract the effects of the prescribed solution.

Lifespan Considerations

- Monitor older adults frequently for hypotension related to systemic absorption of the eye drops to prevent falls. Ensure patient safety.

Patient Education

- Immediately report changes in vision, eye pain, light sensitivity, halos around lights, or headache.
- Assess blood pressure once per week and report any blood pressure less than 90/60 mmHg or per parameters set by the healthcare provider. Immediately report any dizziness, lightheadedness, headache, palpitations, syncope, or difficulty breathing.
- Exercise caution when driving or other activities in low-light conditions or at night until the effects of the drug are known.
- Maintain all regular eye examinations. Seek the healthcare provider's advice before using any OTC eye solutions.
- Follow appropriate administration guidelines:
  - Remove contact lenses if worn. Do not reinsert lenses for a minimum of 15 minutes after eyedrop instillation, or as directed.
  - Gently pull down on the lower eyelid, anchoring the hand against the cheekbone.
  - Tilt the head back; steadying the hand on the forehead as needed, drop prescribed numbers of drops into the conjunctival sac. Do not drop solution directly onto the eye surface or touch the dropper to the eye.
  - Close the eye gently. Hold light pressure on the tear duct for 1 full minute to retain the solution.

Prescribing Considerations

- Immediate onset of acute eye pain is an indicator of angle closure and is treated as a medical emergency.
- Consistent IOP readings above 21 mmHg may indicate worsening disease or ineffective drug therapy and should be promptly evaluated by an ophthalmologist.
- Early diagnosis and treatment of glaucoma is essential. Once vision loss occurs, medications can prevent, but not reverse, vision loss.
- Emphasize the importance of keeping all appointments and taking the medication as directed.

Pharmacotherapy for Eye Examinations

74.7 Drugs that are routinely used for eye examinations include mydriatics, cycloplegics, diagnostic dyes, and local anesthetics.

Various drugs are used as adjuncts to diagnostic eye examinations and during ophthalmic surgery. **Mydriatic** drugs cause sympathetic activation that relaxes the ciliary muscle, causing dilation of the pupil and thus allowing for better visualization of retinal structures. **Cycloplegic** drugs not only dilate the pupil but also paralyze the ciliary muscle and prevent the lens from moving during assessment. Mydriatics and cycloplegics are often used in combination to achieve the maximum pupil dilation needed for surgery or during funduscopic examinations. Examples of drugs used for eye examinations include anticholinergics, such as atropine (Isopto Atropine) and tropicamide (Mydriacyl, Tropicacyl), and sympathomimetics, such as phenylephrine. Mydriatic, cycloplegic, and other drugs for eye conditions are listed in Table 74.2.

Mydriatics cause intense photophobia and pain in response to bright light. Mydriatics can worsen glaucoma by impairing aqueous humor outflow and thereby increasing IOP. In addition, strong concentrations of anticholinergics have the potential to have systemic effects on the central nervous system (CNS) and cause confusion, unsteadiness, or drowsiness. Cycloplegics can cause severe blurred vision and loss of near vision. Scopolamine, an anticholinergic often used to prevent motion sickness, can cause blurred vision due to cycloplegia, as well as angle-closure glaucoma attacks. The response to mydriatics and cycloplegics can last from 3 hours up to several days. The patient should be taught to wear sunglasses and that the ability to drive, read, and perform visual tasks may be affected during treatment.

Diagnostic drugs are used to help locate lesions or foreign bodies within the eye and to provide some local anesthesia. Fluorescein sodium is a dye used in assessing the cornea and fitting contact lenses. Scratches may turn bright green; foreign bodies are surrounded by a green halo. Areas where the conjunctiva is damaged show an orange-yellow discoloration. Fluorescein sodium with benoxinate (Altafluor Benox) adds local anesthesia, making it useful

Table 74.2 Miscellaneous Drugs Used for the Eye

Drug	Route and Adult Dose (Maximum Dose Where Indicated)	Adverse Effects
Mydriatics: Sympathomimetics		
phenylephrine	1 drop of 2.5% or 10% solution before eye examination	*Eye pain, photosensitivity, eye irritation, headache* HTN, tremor, dysrhythmias
Cycloplegics: Anticholinergics		
atropine (Isopto Atropine)	Uveitis: 1–2 drops of 1% solution up to 4 times daily; also give 1–2 drops 1 h prior to eye examination	*Eye irritation and redness, dry mouth, local burning or stinging, headache, blurred vision, photosensitivity, eczematoid dermatitis (tropicamide)* Somnolence, tachycardia, convulsions, mental changes, keratitis
cyclopentolate (Cyclogyl, Pentolair)	1 drop of 0.5–2% solution 40–50 min before eye examination	
tropicamide (Mydriacyl, Tropicacyl)	1–2 drops of 0.5–1% solution before eye examination	
Anesthetics		
lidocaine (Akten)	2 drops of 3.5% gel in affected eye, reapplied as needed	*Stinging, corneal erosion, headache, slowed healing of corneal abrasions* Anaphylactic reactions
proparacaine (Alcaine)	1 drop of 0.5% solution in affected eye q5–10min for 5–7 doses	
tetracaine	1–2 drops of a 0.5% solution or 1.25–2.5 cm of ointment in the lower conjunctival sac	
Lubricants		
lanolin alcohol (Lacri-Lube)	Apply a thin film to the inside of the eyelid	*Temporary burning or stinging, eye itching or redness, headache* No serious adverse effects
polyvinyl alcohol (Liquifilm, others)	1–2 drops tid–qid prn	
Vasoconstrictors		
naphazoline (Allerest, Clear Eyes, others)	1–3 drops of 0.1% solution q3–4h prn	*Temporary burning or stinging, eye itching or redness, headache* No serious adverse effects
oxymetazoline (OcuClear, Visine LR)	1–2 drops of 0.025% solution qid	
phenylephrine	1–2 drops of 0.12% solution up to 4 times/day	
tetrahydrozoline (Murine Plus, Visine, others)	1–2 drops of 0.05% solution bid–tid	

Note: *Italics* indicate common adverse effects. Underline indicates serious adverse effects.

for the identification and removal of foreign bodies from the cornea.

Local anesthetics are used to prevent the pain associated with diagnostic and surgical procedures, suturing and removal of foreign bodies, and ocular injections. The drugs used include proparacaine (Alcaine) and tetracaine. Application consists of one to two drops applied to the affected eye. Anesthesia typically occurs within 20 seconds and lasts for 10 to 20 minutes. Adverse effects of their use include local irritation, including conjunctivitis. Systemic effects are rarer, but CNS excitation has been known to occur. The nurse must be careful to protect the patient's eye from injury while anesthetized or corneal damage may occur.

Pharmacotherapy for Other Eye Conditions

74.8 Numerous pharmacologic drugs are used to treat minor eye irritation and redness.

Drugs for minor eye irritation and dryness come from a broad range of classes. Some drugs lubricate only the eye's surface, whereas others are designed to penetrate and affect a specific area of the eye.

Dry eye disease (or syndrome) is a condition in which the patient secretes either an insufficient amount of tears or poor-quality tears. Common in older adults, this condition is worsened by certain medications such as decongestants or antihistamines or by environmental conditions such as wind or dry climate. Long-term use of contact lenses and refractive surgeries (Lasik) can decrease tear production.

Minor dry eye disease is treated with lubricants such as artificial tears. Artificial tear drugs are topical preparations of methyl or vinyl cellulose. These drops can be instilled as often as every hour. A wide variety of OTC preparations are available, including eyedrop solutions, ointments, and inserts.

Two prescription drugs are available to treat dry eye disease. Cyclosporine ophthalmic emulsion (Restasis) stimulates the production of tears in patients whose tear production is suppressed by ocular inflammation. It is most effective when used in combination with artificial tear replacement and is administered as one drop in the affected eye(s) twice daily. Cyclosporine is presented as a prototype immunosuppressant in Chapter 42.

Approved in 2016, lifitegrast (Xiidra) is an ophthalmic solution that blocks certain inflammatory cytokine interactions on the surface of the eye. This reduces dry eye discomfort. It is administered as one drop daily in each eye. Side effects are minor and include local irritation, dysgeusia (distorted sense of taste), and decreased visual acuity.

Minor eye irritation is a frequent condition that is often treated with vasoconstrictors. Common vasoconstrictors include phenylephrine, naphazoline, and tetrahydrozoline. The adverse effects of the vasoconstrictors are usually minor and include blurred vision, tearing, headache, and rebound vasodilation with redness.

Infection and inflammatory responses are common conditions in the supporting structures of the eye and may result from foreign bodies, bacteria, or viruses. Allergies and irritants such as tobacco smoke are also common sources of inflammation. Redness, edema, and itching are common symptoms. The anti-infectives used to treat eye infections are the same drugs used to treat infections in other areas of the body. Applied topically they carry the common adverse effects of conjunctivitis and local skin and eye irritation. Examples of eye infections that are treated with anti-infective medications include:

- **Blepharitis.** Inflammation of the edges of the eyelids that is commonly seen in older adults and those with dry eyes.
- **Conjunctivitis.** Inflammation or infection of the lining of the eyelids. Bacterial conjunctivitis is often caused by *Staphylococcus aureus*, *Streptococcus pneumoniae*, and *Haemophilus influenzae*. Viral conjunctivitis is highly contagious, and treatment is symptomatic.
- **Chalazion and styes.** A chalazion is a lump or cyst along the edge of an eyelid. Hordeolum, or an external stye, is a blockage of the sebaceous glands at the base of the eyelashes. A chalazion or hordeolum may become infected and require the use of ocular antibiotics.
- **Keratitis.** An inflammation of the cornea that may also be caused by trauma or dryness of the cornea from decreased lubrication. If left untreated, corneal scarring with impaired vision may result.

Nonsteroidal anti-inflammatory drugs (NSAIDs), such as ketorolac (Acular, Acuvail), can be used to treat conjunctivitis and other inflammatory conditions. They are also used to reduce inflammation postoperatively and the symptoms associated with seasonal allergies. Topical corticosteroids are also very effective at reducing inflammation in the eye, although they should not be administered if an infection is suspected. The most common adverse effects of topical corticosteroids are cataracts, glaucoma, mydriasis, and ptosis. Cycloplegics can also be used to treat ocular pain caused by almost any inflammatory condition, except glaucoma.

Several medications, including antihistamines, mast cell stabilizers, and combination antihistamine–mast cell stabilizers, are used to decrease the redness and itching associated with allergic conjunctivitis. Systemic antihistamines may be used but they may cause ocular dryness, which could aggravate symptoms. Topical mast cell stabilizers, with or without an antihistamine, are the preferred treatment for allergic conjunctivitis because they do not cause further drying of the eyes. Olopatadine (Pataday) and ketotifen (Alaway, Zaditor) are combination antihistamine–mast cell stabilizers. Ketotifen is available OTC. Drugs for the treatment of allergic conjunctivitis are listed in Table 74.3.

Table 74.3 Drugs for the Treatment of Allergic Conjunctivitis

Drug	Route and Adult Dose (Maximum Dose Where Indicated)	Adverse Effects
Mast Cell Stabilizers		
cromolyn	1–2 drops of 4% solution q4–6h	*Dry mouth, headache, nausea, sneezing, nasal symptoms, and transient eye stinging and burning* Bronchospasm, angioedema, anaphylaxis
lodoxamide (Alomide)	1–2 drops of 0.1% solution qid	
nedocromil (Alocril)	1–2 drops of 2% solution bid	
Antihistamines		
alcaftadine (Lastacaft)	1 drop of 0.25% solution once daily	*Fatigue, dizziness, dry mouth, headache, pharyngitis, cough, bitter taste, rhinitis* No serious adverse effects
azelastine	1 drop of 0.05% solution bid	
bepotastine (Bepreve)	1 drop of 1.5% solution bid	
cetirizine (Zerviate)	1 drop of 0.24% solution bid	
epinastine (Elestat)	1 drop of 0.05% solution bid	
ketotifen (Alaway, Zaditor)	1 drop of 0.025% solution q8–12h	
olopatadine (Pataday)	1 drop of 0.1% solution bid	

Note: *Italics* indicate common adverse effects. Underline indicates serious adverse effects.

Anatomy of the Ear

74.9 Knowledge of basic ear anatomy is fundamental to understanding ear disorders and pharmacotherapy.

The ear has two major sensory functions: hearing and maintenance of equilibrium and balance. The three structural areas of the ear—the external, middle, and inner ear—carry out these functions, as shown in Figure 74.3.

The external ear consists of the pinna and the external auditory canal, which transmits sound waves to the tympanic membrane, or eardrum. This canal is lined with numerous ceruminous glands that protect the canal and help keep the tympanic membrane pliable. The tympanic membrane separates the external ear from the middle ear. The middle ear consists of a bony cavity containing the three ossicles, called the malleus, incus, and stapes, that transmit sound waves to the inner ear. The eustachian tube

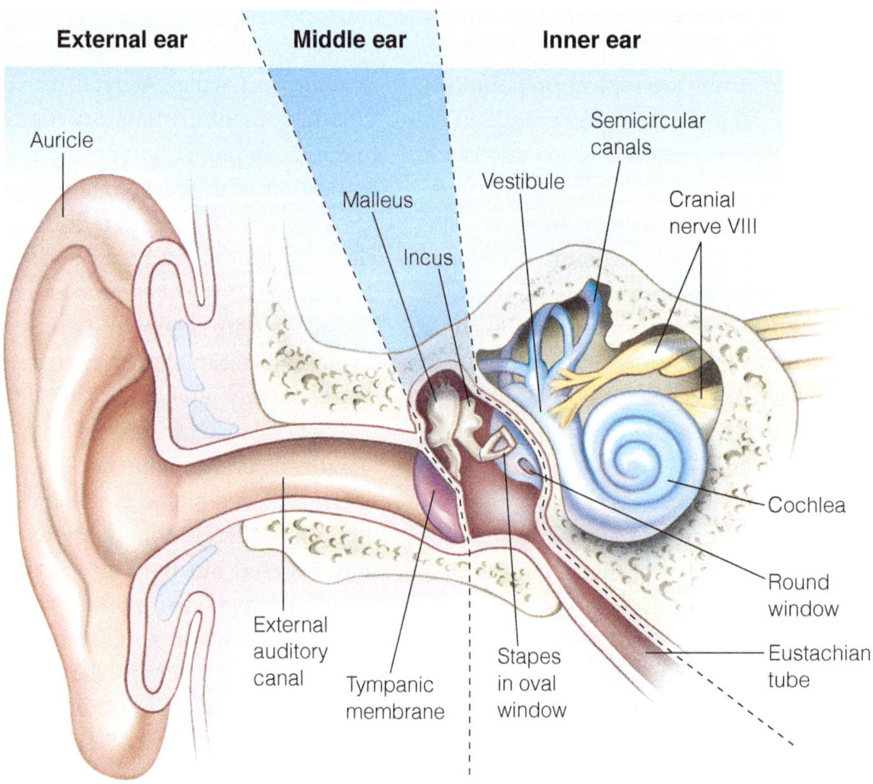

Figure 74.3 Anatomy of the ear.

provides a connection between the middle ear and the nasopharynx. It permits equalization of pressure in the middle ear by allowing air to enter or leave the middle ear cavity and for the drainage of secretions. Its mucosa is continuous with the mucosal lining of the throat, providing a means for infectious organisms to enter the middle ear from the nose and throat. The inner ear consists of the semicircular canals, the vestibule, and the cochlea. The cochlea is the main organ of hearing, whereas the semicircular canals and vestibule are responsible for balance and equilibrium.

Pharmacotherapy with Otic Preparations

74.10 Otic preparations treat infections, inflammation, and earwax buildup.

Otic medications commonly used to treat ear infections, inflammation, and wax buildup are shown in Table 74.4. Otitis, or inflammation of the ear, is a common indication for pharmacotherapy. **Otitis externa**, commonly called swimmer's ear, is an inflammation with or without infection of the skin in the external auditory canal. The acute form is bacterial in origin and most often due to *Pseudomonas aeruginosa* or *S. aureus*. It is associated with water exposure, high humidity, and a history of ear trauma generally from sharp or small objects. Chronic otitis externa is most often caused by a fungal infection or an allergic response usually associated with cosmetics, hair products, or devices placed within the ear canal. The typical presentation is that of acute-onset ear pain associated with pruritus, swelling, and tenderness to the touch or with movement. A greenish white drainage may accompany symptoms. Hearing impairment may result if the swelling is sufficient to obstruct the auditory canal.

Treatment of otitis externa focuses on reducing pain and inflammation, usually with topical corticosteroids, antibiotics, and analgesics, as needed. Neomycin, gentamicin, and ciprofloxacin (Cipro otic) are the most commonly used topical otic antibiotics. Mild fungal infections can be treated with a 90% to 95% alcohol solution; more advanced disease may be treated with topical 1% clotrimazole (Lotrimin) or tolnaftate (Tinactin). If swelling obstructs the external canal, an ear wick may be placed past the blockage and the drops applied to the end. The use of systemic antibiotics may be necessary in cases when outer ear infections are extensive, such as with cellulitis or lymph node involvement.

PharmFACT

Otitis externa has a peak incidence of 7 to 12 years of age and occurs most commonly in the summer months. Although called swimmer's ear, the condition may also be caused by cleaning and scratching the ear canal with cotton swabs or paper clips (Waltzman, 2020).

Otitis media, which is inflammation of the middle ear, is a common disorder that affects infants and young children, although people of any age may be affected. Among children, 75% experience at least one episode of otitis media by their third birthday, and almost half of these children will have three or more ear infections during that time.

There are three common types of otitis media: acute, chronic, and serous. Acute otitis media and chronic otitis media are similar. An infectious agent, most often a viral upper respiratory infection, results in pathogens being introduced into the middle ear through the eustachian tube, leading to swelling and inflammation of the ossicles of the middle ear. Bacterial infection with *S. pneumoniae*, *H. influenzae*, and *Streptococcus pyogenes* causes most cases. Otitis media may also be associated with allergies or eustachian tube dysfunction. Acute otitis has a duration of less than 3 weeks; chronic otitis follows repeated episodes and has a longer duration of symptoms. Sometimes the eardrum ruptures, and pus drains out of the ear. More commonly, the pus and mucus remain in the middle ear due to the swollen and inflamed eustachian tube. This is called middle ear effusion or serous otitis media. After the acute infection has passed, the effusion may remain and become chronic, lasting for weeks, months, or even years.

Table 74.4 Otic Preparations

Drug	Route and Adult Dose (Maximum Dose Where Indicated)	Adverse Effects
acetic acid and hydrocortisone (Acetasol HC, Vosol HC)	3–5 drops q4h–qid for 24 h, then 5 drops tid–qid	*Ear irritation, local stinging or burning, dizziness* Allergic reactions (antibiotics)
carbamide peroxide (Debrox)	1–5 drops of 6.5% solution bid for 4 days	
ciprofloxacin-dexamethasone (Ciprodex)	4 drops in the affected ear bid for 7 days	
ciprofloxacin-hydrocortisone (Cipro HC)	3 drops of the suspension instilled into the affected ear bid for 7 days	
ofloxacin (Floxin otic)	5–10 drops in the affected ear once daily for 7 days	
polymyxin B, neomycin, and hydrocortisone (Cortisporin) colistin, neomycin, thonzonium bromide, and hydrocortisone (Cortisporin TC)	3–5 drops in the affected ear tid–qid	

Note: *Italics* indicate common adverse effects. Underline indicates serious adverse effects.

Otitis media is treated with a course of systemic, rather than topical, antibiotics. Amoxicillin, at a dose of 80 to 90 mg/kg/day, is prescribed for most children. For patients who have symptoms of a more severe illness and in those for whom additional coverage for β-lactamase–positive *H. influenzae* and *Moraxella catarrhalis* is desired, therapy is initiated with high-dose amoxicillin-clavulanate. For patients with mild penicillin allergy, a cephalosporin may be considered. If the penicillin allergy is more severe, azithromycin or clarithromycin can be used. In the patient who is vomiting or cannot otherwise tolerate oral medication, a single dose of parenteral ceftriaxone has been shown to be effective.

Otitis interna, or labyrinthitis, is an inner ear infection that may occur as the result of chronic otitis media or as part of a viral systemic infection, including mononucleosis or an upper respiratory infection. Of all ear infections, otitis interna is the most difficult to treat because the blood–labyrinth barrier makes it difficult for systemic medications to reach the affected areas. **Mastoiditis**, or inflammation of the mastoid sinus, is frequently the result of chronic or inadequately treated bacterial otitis media or an otitis interna infection. The infection moves into the bone and surrounding structures of the ear. Symptoms of pain, hearing loss, and tenderness typically appear 2 to 3 weeks after an episode of otitis media. Mastoiditis can be a serious problem. If left untreated, it can result in hearing loss.

The treatment of acute mastoiditis involves aggressive antibiotic therapy. IV gentamicin or ticarcillin may be used initially. Therapy may be adjusted once culture and sensitivity results have been obtained. Therapy is continued for at least 14 days. If the antibiotics are not effective and symptoms persist, surgery such as a mastoidectomy or meatoplasty may be indicated.

Cerumen (earwax) softeners are also used for proper ear health. When cerumen accumulates, it narrows the ear canal and may interfere with hearing. **Cerumenolytics** may be needed to loosen and remove impacted cerumen from the ear canal. Use of these agents usually involves the instillation of an earwax softener and then a gentle lavage of the wax-impacted ear with tepid water using an irrigating syringe to gently insert the water. An instrument called an ear loop may be used to help remove earwax but should be

CONNECTIONS: Advanced Practice Application

Otitis Media

Case

Aadila, a 3-year-old, is brought to the clinic by her mother because she has been experiencing a low-grade fever of 38°C (100.5°F) for 2 days. The fever is accompanied by reports of left ear pain that has been awakening her. Mom tells you that Aadila has had rhinorrhea, nasal congestion, and a nonproductive cough for 1 week. She denies any changes in eating or elimination patterns. Mom has not tried any home medications, but has been putting warm compresses over the ear, which seems to relieve some pain. Aadila has no significant medical history and has had only one other ear infection when she was 9 months old. She is fully immunized. On exam in the office, her temperature is 37.7°C (100°F) and her physical examination revealed slight redness of the throat, a nose full of thick green mucus, a pearly gray right tympanic membrane with positive light reflex and visible bony landmarks; an erythematous and bulging left tympanic membrane with diminished light reflex and bony landmarks not visualized. No drainage was observed and no pain on palpation of the mastoid bone was noted. How should Aadila be treated?

Discussion

Although one of the best indicators for otitis media is otalgia (ear pain), many children with otitis media also present with nonspecific signs and symptoms such as pulling or tugging at the ears, irritability, headache, disturbed or restless sleep, poor feeding, anorexia, vomiting, or diarrhea. Approximately two-thirds of the patients also present with a low-grade fever.

In the last 20 years, management guidelines have evolved to recommend a period of watchful waiting in children with mild to moderate AOM rather than initiation of antibiotic therapy at the time of diagnosis. The American Academy of Pediatrics released revised clinical practice guidelines for the diagnosis and management of uncomplicated AOM intended as a clinical decision-making framework for primary care providers (Lieberthal et al., 2013). The decision to place a patient on antibiotics or to observe is based on the child's age, diagnostic certainty, and illness severity, remembering that viruses are the most common cause of upper respiratory tract infection in children. Deferring antibacterial treatment for children over 6 months of age with mild illness for 48 to 72 hours and limiting management to symptomatic relief is appropriate. All children under 6 months of age should receive antibiotic therapy regardless of illness severity. Amoxicillin remains the first-line therapy for children who have not received amoxicillin within the past 30 days. Amoxicillin/clavulanate is recommended if amoxicillin has been taken within the past 30 days, if concurrent conjunctivitis is present, or if the child has a history of recurrent AOM unresponsive to amoxicillin.

Symptomatic pain management, especially during the first 24 hours of an episode of AOM, should be part of the care plan, regardless of the use of antibiotics. Symptomatic relief involves the use of analgesics, such as acetaminophen or ibuprofen (for children over 6 months of age), to relieve pain and reduce fever. Patients with severe pain may require therapy with opioid analgesics such as codeine. A 7-day course of a corticosteroid is often combined with antibiotics when severe inflammation is present. Antihistamines or decongestants may be used to decrease mucus production and fluid levels in the middle ear (Lieberthal et al., 2013).

used only by healthcare providers who are skilled in using it. There are three types of cerumen-softening preparations: water based, oil based, and nonwater oil based. Water-based preparations include solutions of triethanolamine, 3% hydrogen peroxide, 10% sodium bicarbonate, and saline or water. The nonwater oil-based preparation available in the United States includes the OTC drug carbamide peroxide (Debrox). Oil-based preparations include household olive, mineral, and almond oils and commercially prepared combinations, such as Cerumol, Earex, and Otocerol. Research has shown that the water-based and nonwater oil-based agents have equal effectiveness.

CONNECTIONS: APPLIED CLINICAL JUDGMENT

Patients Receiving Pharmacotherapy for Otitis

Key Assessment Data

- History of current condition, complete health history and history of neurologic disease; baseline vital signs, physical exam findings; pregnancy or breastfeeding; medication history including allergies and current prescription and OTC drugs.

Desired Therapeutic Outcomes

Improvement is observed and measurable by infection is clearing or hearing is maintained.

Minimizing Adverse Effects

- Otitis media with effusion may lead to hearing loss and speech or language impairment, especially in young children.
- Dizziness or vertigo may cause intolerance to activity and increase the risk for falls.
- Eardrops should be administered into the ear canal without dropping the solution directly on the tympanic membrane, which may induce vertigo.

Lifespan Considerations

- Monitor older adults frequently for dizziness to prevent falls. Ensure patient safety.

Patient Education

- Immediately report severe ear pain, increased drainage, fever, increasing dizziness, vertigo, nausea and vomiting, or tenderness in or around the ear.
- Promptly report any increasing dizziness or vertigo. If dizziness occurs at home, sit or lie down and do not attempt to stand or walk until the sensation passes.
- Maintain regular hearing examinations.
- Apply warm but not hot compresses to the external ear for approximately 15 to 20 minutes as needed for discomfort
- Follow appropriate administration guidelines:
    - Warm eardrop solution by placing in or under warm but not hot water. The bottle may be placed in a plastic bag to protect the label before warming. *Never* warm eardrops in the microwave.
    - Lie down with the ear to be treated uppermost. Gently pull the outer ear down and back for children under age 3, up and back for children over age 3, adolescents, and adults.
    - Instill the number of drops ordered into the ear canal, taking care not to drop the solution directly onto the eardrum, but allowing it to slide down the side of the ear canal.
    - Gently massage the area in front of the ear to promote thorough administration of the drop unless pain is severe.
    - Continue to lie down for 5 to 10 minutes to ensure complete absorption of the medication. A small piece of cotton may be placed at the entrance to the ear canal if any solution returns upon arising.

Prescribing Considerations

- In mild cases, watchful waiting for 24-48 hours is appropriate.
- Evidence of suppurative inflammation is treated immediately with oral antibiotics, usually amoxicillin.
- Four or more episodes of AOM within 12 months should be referred for placement of a tympanostomy tube.

Understanding Chapter 74

Key Concepts Summary

74.1 Knowledge of basic eye anatomy is fundamental to understanding eye disorders and their pharmacotherapy.

74.2 The two principal types of glaucoma, closed-angle glaucoma and open-angle glaucoma, are characterized by increased intraocular pressure.

74.3 The primary goal of glaucoma pharmacotherapy is to prevent damage to the optic nerve by lowering intraocular pressure.

74.4 Prostaglandin analogs are the first-line drugs for treating high intraocular pressure because of their long durations of action and high safety profiles.

74.5 Drugs that affect the autonomic nervous system are sometimes prescribed to treat glaucoma.

74.6 Carbonic anhydrase inhibitors and osmotic diuretics are occasionally used for treating glaucoma.

74.7 Drugs that are routinely used for eye examinations include mydriatics, cycloplegics, diagnostic dyes, and local anesthetics.

74.8 Numerous pharmacologic drugs are used to treat minor eye irritation and redness.

74.9 Knowledge of basic ear anatomy is fundamental to understanding ear disorders and pharmacotherapy.

74.10 Otic preparations treat infections, inflammation, and earwax buildup.

CASE STUDY: Making the Patient Connection

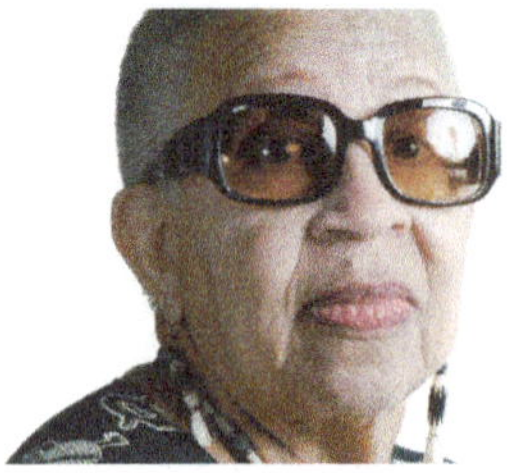

Remember the patient "Therese Duclos" from the beginning of the chapter? Now read the remainder of the case study. Based on the information presented within this chapter, respond to the critical thinking questions that follow.

Therese Duclos, a 65-year-old African American woman, visits her ophthalmologist with reports of blurry vision and not being able to see well at night while driving. Her health history includes adult-onset diabetes for the past 10 years and osteoporosis since age 55. Her medical regimen includes diet control for the diabetes and Boniva monthly. She denies any injury to her eyes and last had an eye checkup 1 year ago.

Critical Thinking Questions

1. What factors are present in Mrs. Duclos's health history that you identify as predisposing conditions for the development of primary open-angle glaucoma?
2. Therese needs to learn the proper administration of eyedrops. What teaching would you provide to ensure that the skill will be performed correctly?
3. What would be possible effects from systemic absorption if the patient were taking beta-adrenergic drops (e.g., timolol)? Prostaglandin drops (e.g., latanoprost, bimatoprost)? Cholinergic agonists (e.g., pilocarpine)?

Additional Case Study

Zachary, a 4-year-old boy, is experiencing pain in his right ear. His mother takes him to the healthcare provider, and he is diagnosed with otitis media. Zachary is prescribed ciprofloxacin with dexamethasone (Ciprodex) otic drops to be instilled in his right ear twice a day for a week. To ensure that the mother is knowledgeable in this form of administration, the nurse will teach her about the proper technique. Create a patient information sheet for a parent who needs to administer eardrops.

Chapter Review

1. The nurse is teaching a patient about a new eyedrop prescription for timolol (Timoptic) for treatment of open-angle glaucoma. The patient has a history of seasonal allergies and HTN. What is an important administration technique to stress for this patient?
    1. Take any eyedrops for allergies 5 minutes before administering the timolol drops.
    2. Do not use the timolol drops while concurrently taking allergy medication.
    3. The timolol drops may temporarily worsen seasonal allergies.
    4. Gently put pressure on the inner canthus (tear duct) for 1 minute after instilling the timolol drop.

2. The nurse is providing health teaching to a patient who has been prescribed latanoprost (Xalatan) for open-angle glaucoma. While harmless, the nurse would caution the patient about which potential non-ocular effects of the drug? (Select all that apply.)
    1. Darkening and thickening of the upper eyelid
    2. Darkening and thickening of eyelashes
    3. A lightening of iris color and a slight darkening of the sclera
    4. A slight darkening of the iris color
    5. A permanent bluish tint to the conjunctiva

3. Pilocarpine (Isopto Carpine) has been ordered for a patient with closed-angle glaucoma who has not responded well to other drugs. Pilocarpine causes ______________________________, which stretches the trabecular meshwork, allowing a greater outflow of aqueous humor and lowering intraocular pressure.

4. The nurse is teaching a 25-year-old patient about the administration of ciprofloxacin with hydrocortisone (Cipro) for otitis. In which order will the nurse instruct the patient to use the drug?
   1. Gently massage the area in front of the ear.
   2. Pull the earlobe upward and back.
   3. Allow the drop to fall into the ear canal flowing down the side.
   4. Remain with the treated ear in an uppermost position for 5 minutes.

5. The nurse is teaching a patient with otitis about a prescription for polymyxin B, neomycin, with hydrocortisone (Cortisporin). The patient should be instructed to immediately report which symptom?
   1. Mild itching in the outer ear canal
   2. Gradually decreasing pain
   3. Slight dizziness after instilling the eardrop
   4. Increasing pain, particularly in the area around the ear

6. The nurse is instilling drops of phenylephrine into the patient's eye before cataract surgery. Phenylephrine is used prior to cataract surgery because it causes ________________, allowing visualization of the operative area.

See Appendix A for answers to critical thinking questions, case study questions, and review questions.

References

Glaucoma Research Foundation. (2017). *Glaucoma facts and stats.* http://www.glaucoma.org/glaucoma/glaucoma-facts-and-stats.php

Lieberthal, A. S., Carroll, A. E., Chonmaitree, T., Ganiats, T. G., Hoberman, A., Jackson, M. A., et al. (2013). The diagnosis and management of acute otitis media. *Pediatrics, 131*(3), e964–e999. https://doi.org/10.1542/peds.2012-3488

Waltzman, A. A. (2020). *Otitis externa.* Medscape. http://emedicine.medscape.com/article/994550-overview#a5

Selected Bibliography

Falkland, M. (2019). Practice update: Dry eye syndrome. *Australian Journal of Pharmacy, 100*(1188), 76.

Foster, C.S. (2019). *Dry eye disease (keratoconjunctivitis sicca).* Medscape. https://emedicine.medscape.com/article/1210417-overview

Harasymowycz, P., Birt, C., Gooi, P., Heckler, L., Hutnik, C., Jinapriya, D., et al. (2016). Medical management of glaucoma in the 21st century from a Canadian perspective. *Journal of Ophthalmology, 2016,* Article ID 6509809. https://doi.org/10.1155/2016/6509809

Schwartz, S. R., Magit, A. E., Rosenfeld, R. M., Ballachanda, B. B., Hackell, J. M., Krouse, H. J., et al. (2017). Clinical practice guideline (update) earwax (cerumen impaction). *Otolaryngology–Head and Neck Surgery, 156*(Suppl. 1), S1–S29. https://10.1177/0194599816671491

Stainsby, H. (2016). Management of patients with chronic open angle glaucoma. *Nursing Standard, 30*(37), 52–60. https://doi.org/10.7748/ns.30.37.52.s42

Strelow, B., & Fleischman, D. (2020). Glaucoma in pregnancy: an update. *Current Opinion in Ophthalmology, 31*(2), 114–122. https://doi.org/10.1097/ICU.0000000000000641

Ventocilla, M. (2019). *Allergic conjunctivitis.* Medscape. http://emedicine.medscape.com/article/1191467-overview#a4

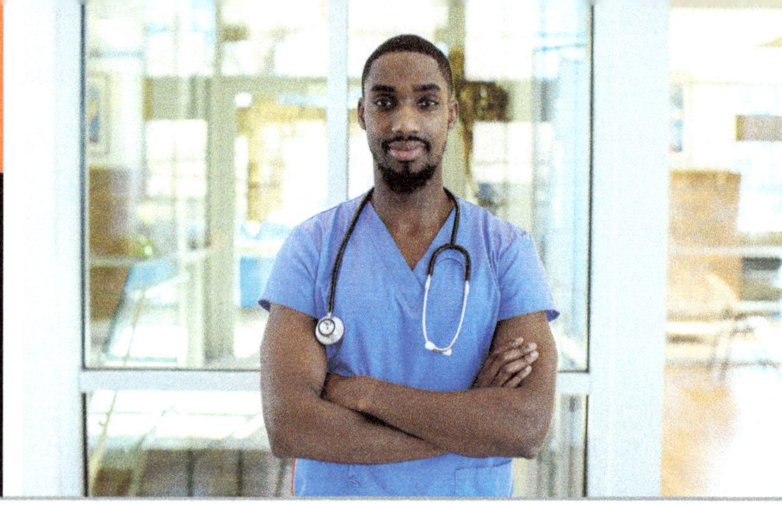

"I don't know if you can ever be completely prepared, but that's why we keep practicing and running drills. If something occurs, we'll be ready."

—*"C. Richard Drew," emergency department nurse*

Chapter 75

Emergency Preparedness: Bioterrorism and Management of Poisoning

Chapter Outline

Learning Outcomes

After reading this chapter, the student should be able to:

1. Discuss the role of professional nursing in emergency preparedness and the management of poisoning.
2. Discuss the purpose, function, and components of the Strategic National Stockpile.
3. Identify the types of agents that might be used for a bioterrorist attack.
4. Compare and contrast the various chemical agents that can be used as poisons.
5. Explain the risks associated with ionizing radiation emitted from a nuclear terrorist attack.
6. Describe the five general principles for treating acute poisoning.
7. Identify the drugs important in emergency preparedness and management of poisoning.
8. Compare the pharmacologic management of biologic, chemical, radiologic, nuclear, and explosive agents in emergency preparedness.
9. Discuss the management of poisoning by the poison control center, including minimizing poison absorption and enhancing poison removal.
10. Apply clinical judgment to the care of patients receiving pharmacotherapy for poisoning or overdose.

Key Terms

Definitions of the terms in bold may be found in the Glossary.

Emergency preparedness is the ability to respond swiftly and effectively to an unexpected event that may impact human health. The unexpected event may be a natural disaster caused by severe weather, an unintentional chemical spill, a purposeful terrorist attack, or a national infectious disease outbreak. Nurses have an essential role in assessing and recognizing emergency situations and taking appropriate interventions to save lives. Sometimes, specific drugs are necessary to counter the effects of biologic hazards and minimize the loss of life in emergency situations. This chapter focuses on the role of pharmacology in emergency preparedness as related to bioterrorism and management of poisoning.

Emergency Preparedness, Bioterrorism, and Nursing

75.1 Emergency preparedness has become an essential competency for all healthcare professionals.

Emergency preparedness has been an emerging role of professional nursing for many years. In the past, however, most training focused on emergency management for natural disasters, catastrophic incidents, or infectious epidemics. Often nurses responded to victims at the location of the disaster or incident. Today, nurses must learn how to respond to mass casualty incidents and potential disasters that can result from agents that are biologic, chemical, radiologic, nuclear, or explosive in nature. Standard emergency triage may be reversed, focusing on patients with the best chance to live.

Nurses are among the first responders to victims who arrive at emergency departments (EDs), clinics, healthcare provider offices, or school health settings. They must be prepared to assess and recognize when someone has been exposed to potential hazards and to take appropriate actions. Failure to do so could lead to an epidemic or major loss of life. Examples include patients who present to the healthcare setting with symptoms of anthrax, avian flu, severe acute respiratory syndrome, or COVID-19.

Since the terrorist attacks of September 11, 2001, Americans are more concerned with threats of terrorism and are more aware of emergency preparedness than ever before. Increased efforts to safeguard the general populace remain at an all-time high. Healthcare providers must continually update their knowledge of emergency management and think more globally in dealing with patients whose illness presents in a less typical way. Knowledge of treatment modalities related to bioterrorism has become a basic competency required of all healthcare providers.

75.2 Bioterrorism is the intentional release of a virus or microorganism to cause human harm.

The past two decades have brought the acts and effects of terrorism to the forefront of discussion in this and other countries. Terrorism is generally defined as the systematic use of terror, violence, or intimidation to achieve a desired purpose or end. The U.S. Federal Criminal Code describes terrorism as activities that involve life-threatening acts intended to coerce or intimidate a given population. Terrorists use chemical, nuclear, radiologic, explosive, or biologic hazards to commit violent and intimidating crimes against general and special targeted populations.

Bioterrorism is the intentional release of an infectious agent for the purpose of causing harm to a large number of people. In the United States, governmental agencies such as the Centers for Disease Control and Prevention (CDC) and the Department of Defense provide education to prepare the general public for possible bioterrorism events. In the wrong hands, simple and easily obtained toxic agents could be disseminated for public harm. However, of greatest concern is the use of highly infectious diseases such as anthrax, smallpox, hemorrhagic viruses, and plague; toxic agents such as nerve gas and cyanide; and chlorinated agents, as well as nuclear and radiation threats. Table 75.1 provides the CDC list of biologic threats and their potential impact on the health of the general public.

75.3 Nurses may have the first opportunity to recognize and initiate a response to bioterrorism.

Nursing has a rich history in emergency preparedness. Florence Nightingale began defining the role of nursing in emergency preparedness as early as the Crimean War. Throughout many wars and disasters, nurses have honed their assessment and critical care skills to support people in need and improve healthcare outcomes. The Civil War was a time when nurses worked together with leaders like Clara Barton to establish the American Red Cross, with nursing becoming a special service in 1909. In World War II, nurses became a defined group within the military, and the Cadet Nurse Corps was established. These wartime nurses learned triage, provided trauma care, and administered penicillin to save many lives. Nurses have played a major

Table 75.1 Categories of Infectious Agents

Category	Description	Examples
A	Agents that pose a significant risk to national security because they • can easily be disseminated or transmitted person to person; • result in high mortality rates with potential for major public health impact; • might cause public panic and social disruption; and • require special action for public health preparedness.	Anthrax (*Bacillus anthracis*) Botulism (*Clostridium botulinum* toxin) Plague (*Yersinia pestis*) Smallpox (*Variola major*) Tularemia (*Francisella tularensis*) Viral hemorrhagic fevers such as Marburg, Ebola, Lassa, and Machupo
B	Second highest priority agents include those that • are moderately easy to disseminate; • result in moderate morbidity and low mortality rates; and • require specific enhancements of CDC's diagnostic capacity and enhanced disease surveillance.	Brucellosis (*Brucella* species) Epsilon toxin of *Clostridium perfringens* Food safety threats such as salmonella, Shigella, and *Escherichia coli* Glanders (*Burkholderia mallei*) Melioidosis (*Burkholderia pseudomallei*) Psittacosis (*Chlamydia psittaci*) Q fever (*Coxiella burnetii*) Ricin toxin from *Ricinus communis* Staphylococcal enterotoxin B Typhus fever (*Rickettsia prowazekii*) Viral encephalitis Water safety threats such as *Vibrio cholerae* and *Cryptosporidium parvum*
C	Third highest priority agents include emerging pathogens that could be engineered for mass dissemination in the future because of • availability; • ease of production and dissemination; and • potential for high morbidity and high mortality rates and major health impact.	Hantaviruses Nipah virus (NiV)

From Centers for Disease Control and Prevention (n.d.)

role in providing emergency assistance in natural disasters such as earthquakes, tornados, hurricanes, floods, and tsunamis. The challenges have now expanded to include bioterrorism, toxins, radiation, mass casualty emergencies, and infectious pandemics.

Emergency preparedness has come to the forefront of professional nursing practice. Established through a grant in 2004 in collaboration with the U.S. Department of Homeland Security, the National Nurse Emergency Preparedness Initiative advances the education and policy related to emergency preparedness for professional nurses.

In 2001, the International Nursing Coalition for Mass Casualty Education was established, defining emergency preparedness competencies for registered nurses responding to mass casualty incidents (MCIs). Now known as the Nursing Emergency Preparedness Education Coalition, the coalition identified a set of general core competencies that provides guidelines for the role of professional nurses in responding to MCIs. Competencies identified included the ability to adequately assess the situation and victims of an MCI and to have the technical and communication skills required to function as an effective member of the response team. Under technical skills, nurses must demonstrate safe administration of medications and immunizations and have knowledge of nursing interventions for adverse medication events. This is but one area of professional nursing practice where knowledge of pharmacology is important to nursing emergency preparedness.

For more than 40 years, The Joint Commission has required accredited hospitals to meet standards in disaster planning. In the late 1990s, The Joint Commission added standards that address possible bioterrorism and emergency management. State and federal agencies have developed updated emergency preparedness plans that include bioterrorism. Nurses are part of the collaborative developed by healthcare professionals to respond immediately to a community emergency. Key roles for nurses include education, resources, referrals, diagnosis, treatment, and planning. Pharmacology for emergency preparedness has a role in each of these.

75.4 The Strategic National Stockpile has large quantities of medicine to protect the public if a health emergency arises.

When a health emergency such as a biologic or chemical attack, viral outbreak, or earthquake occurs, the response must be rapid to minimize health consequences and protect the American public. Due to the unexpected nature of such an incident, shortages in medical supplies, equipment, and drugs may occur. The **Strategic National Stockpile (SNS)** is a national repository of antibiotics, chemical antidotes, antitoxins, antiviral drugs, life support medications, intravenous (IV) administration equipment, airway maintenance supplies, and personal protective equipment for use in a declared biologic or terrorism incident or other major health emergency. The CDC manages the SNS to ensure immediate availability and deployment of essentials to any state.

One of the two components of the SNS is a Push Package, which includes preassembled caches of drugs, antidotes, and medical supplies that broadly cover a nonspecific emergency for use in the early hours. Stored strategically, deployment can be accomplished within 12 hours. The SNS program ensures that the medical materials stock is rotated and kept within potency shelf-life limits. The second component is vendor-managed inventory (VMI) packages that contain additional supplies that can be more event specific and ship within 24 to 36 hours. This plan is designed to minimize local hospital stockpiling of bioterrorism pharmaceuticals that have expiration dates and can be costly.

Parts of the SNS were deployed for relatively recent health threats. In 2005, SNS response teams were sent to support state efforts in responding to hurricanes Rita and Katrina on the Gulf Coast. Part of the SNS antiviral inventory was used to help state efforts to control the H1N1 swine influenza outbreak in 2009. In 2020, many of the materials in the SNS were used to support response to the COVID-19 pandemic.

Biologic Agents

75.5 Highly infectious bacteria or viruses could be used as bioterrorist threats.

The U.S. government takes the threat of bioterrorism seriously and has implemented a program to prepare the public for such catastrophes. Six biologic agents are considered category A threats (see Table 75.1), meaning they could cause enough mortality and morbidity damage to interfere with the social functioning of a large city or populated area. These six threats are anthrax, botulism toxin, pneumonic plague, smallpox, tularemia, and viral hemorrhagic fevers. Knowing the agents most likely to be used in a terrorist event allows the professional nurse to plan and to prepare for emergencies of this nature. The nurse can be an effective member of the emergency team who is responding to the widespread panic and life-threatening illnesses caused by an attack of bioterrorism.

Anthrax is an acute infectious disease that results from exposure to the spore-forming bacterium *Bacillus anthracis*. The spore produces a toxin that can be fatal to the host. Although microbiologist Robert Koch confirmed the bacterial nature of anthrax in 1876, anthrax has plagued the world for many centuries, even in biblical times. Anthrax infection is found among hoofed animals such as cattle, sheep, goats, pigs, bison, antelopes, and elephants. It was recognized as a potential biologic weapon in World War I, and several countries were suspected of experimenting with its use as a weapon in World War II. In 1995, Iraq admitted producing anthrax as a biologic weapon. U.S. military personnel were vaccinated before deployment to the Gulf War areas.

In the fall of 2001, following the terrorist attacks on the World Trade Center, five people died from exposure to anthrax in what most believe were purposeful acts of bioterrorism. In total, 19 confirmed and four suspected cases occurred across the United States and over 32,000 people were treated for possible exposure, many of whom were postal workers. Lives were lost, government workers and U.S. citizens were critically threatened, and agency operations such as the U.S. Postal Service were interrupted for weeks.

Anthrax poisoning can occur by ingestion, absorption through an open wound on the skin, or inhalation, which is the most dangerous route. The method of transmission affects the symptoms demonstrated. Table 75.2 summarizes the clinical picture of anthrax. Anthrax infects by releasing two toxins, edema toxin and lethal toxin. Both cause necrosis and exudate accumulation and symptoms such as pain, edema, and restricted activity. The anthrax-binding receptor binds with a human cell, allowing the bacterial toxins to enter. Anthrax produces heat and chemically resistant spores, which can remain viable in soil for many years. These are dangerous because they have the potential for inhalation infection for humans. Left untreated, inhalation

Table 75.2 Clinical Manifestations of Anthrax

Type	Description	Symptoms
Cutaneous anthrax	Most common but least complicated form of anthrax; almost always curable if treated within the first few weeks of exposure; results from direct contact of contaminated products with an open wound or cut	Small skin lesions develop and turn into black scabs; inoculation takes less than 1 week; cannot be spread by person-to-person contact
Gastrointestinal anthrax	Rare form of anthrax; without treatment, can be lethal in up to 50% of cases; results from eating anthrax-contaminated food, usually meat	Sore throat, difficulty swallowing, cramping, diarrhea, and abdominal swelling
Inhalation anthrax	Least common but the most dangerous form of anthrax; can be successfully treated if identified within the first few days after exposure; results from inhaling anthrax spores	Initially, fatigue and fever for several days, followed by persistent cough and shortness of breath; without treatment, death can result within 4–6 days

anthrax is usually deadly. In the anthrax attacks in the United States in fall 2001, anthrax was delivered as a fine powder. This form is easily inhaled and adheres to almost any surface.

Several drugs can be used to treat anthrax. Ciprofloxacin (Cipro) is the primary antibiotic used with a prophylaxis oral (PO) dose of 500 mg every 12 hours for 60 days. If anthrax exposure is confirmed, the patient is immediately administered IV treatment with 400 mg every 12 hours. Anthrax can also be treated with other antibiotics such as penicillin, ampicillin, vancomycin, erythromycin, tetracycline, and doxycycline. Inhalation anthrax exposure may necessitate the combined use of ciprofloxacin and doxycycline but must be done immediately to avoid death. The public should be discouraged from seeking the prophylactic use of antibiotics in cases where anthrax exposure has not been confirmed. Indiscriminate, unnecessary use of antibiotics can be expensive, can cause significant adverse effects, and can promote the appearance of resistant bacterial strains. A prototype feature for ciprofloxacin can be found in Chapter 49.

Two newer medications have been developed to treat inhalation anthrax. In 2015, the U.S. Food and Drug Administration (FDA) approved Anthrasil, an immune globulin preparation prepared from the plasma of people vaccinated against anthrax. The globulin preparation contains antibodies that neutralize toxins produced by the anthrax bacteria. Anthrasil carries a black box warning that thrombosis may occur when using immune globulin products. In 2016, the FDA approved obiltoxaximab (Anthim), the first monoclonal antibody for treating inhalational anthrax. Obiltoxaximab neutralizes toxins secreted by the anthrax bacteria. The drug carries a black box warning that it may cause hypersensitivity reactions, including anaphylaxis. Neither Anthrasil nor Anthim have antibacterial activity; therefore, they must be used in combination with antibacterial drugs.

CONNECTION Checkpoint 75.1

From what you learned in Chapter 49, name the antibiotic class to which ciprofloxacin belongs and describe its mechanism of bactericidal action.

Although anthrax immunization was approved by the FDA 40 years ago, it has not been widely used because of the extremely low incidence of this disease in the United States. The vaccine is effective only if given prior to exposure. The anthrax vaccine causes the body to make protective antibodies, thus preventing the onset of disease and its symptoms. At this time, the CDC recommends vaccination for only select populations who might be exposed to large amounts of anthrax on the job. This includes certain laboratory or remediation workers, some military personnel, and those handling animals or animal products (CDC, 2017a).

Controversy is ongoing regarding the safety of the anthrax vaccine and whether it is truly effective in preventing the disease. Until these issues are resolved, the use of anthrax immunization will likely remain limited to select groups. Vaccines and the immune response are discussed in more detail in Chapter 43.

Botulism is caused by *Clostridium botulinum*, an organism that secretes a potent toxin that paralyzes the muscles after an individual is poisoned. Respiratory failure and paralysis may force a patient to be on a ventilator for weeks or months. As a biologic weapon, botulism could be transmitted in air, food, or water. Treatment includes immediate administration of an antitoxin and assisted ventilation until patients are able to function independently. The antitoxin should be given as soon as possible and never delayed pending the microbiologic testing. Trivalent botulinum antitoxin is available through state departments of health or the CDC. A pentavalent toxoid vaccine for botulism prophylaxis is available as an investigation drug through the Department of Defense.

Pneumonic plague is a life-threatening infectious lung disease that occurs after breathing *Yersinia pestis*, a bacterium found on rodents and their fleas that is responsible for the bubonic plague. It is highly contagious and can be deadly if untreated within 24 hours of contact. As a biologic agent, *Y. pestis* could be spread by aerosol over the population. Within 1 to 6 days of exposure, the patient would be infectious to everyone coming into contact during that time. This makes the plague difficult to contain. Symptoms include fever and weakness, rapid development of pneumonia, chest pain with shortness of breath, cough, and bloody sputum. Without immediate treatment, respiratory failure will result followed by shock and death. Treatment with antibiotics must occur within 24 hours and last for at least 7 days to prevent death from the infection. The primary antibiotic for *Y. pestis* infection is doxycycline 100 mg twice a day or ciprofloxacin 500 mg twice a day for 7 days. There is no vaccine approved in the United States for this bacterium at the present time.

Caused by the organism *Francisella tularensis*, **tularemia** is a serious infectious disease found in rodents, rabbits, and hares. Cases have been reported in almost every state, although overall the infection is rare in the United States. *F. tularensis* is one of the most infectious bacteria known and survives at low temperatures for weeks in hay, straw, and moist soil or in the bodies of decaying animals. As a biologic weapon the most casualties would be with aerosol release in an area of high population, causing hemorrhagic inflammation of the respiratory airway. Treatment includes IV therapy with streptomycin as the preferred drug, with parenteral gentamicin being an alternative. Aminoglycosides should be used for 10 days. Tetracyclines and chloramphenicol can be used for at least 14 days but have a higher rate of relapse and treatment failure. In mass casualty incidents, oral doxycycline for 14 to 21 days and ciprofloxacin for 10 days are preferred for adults and children. Antibiotics for treating tularemia are included in the SNS. An attenuated (live) vaccine is available as an investigational drug and is under review by the FDA.

A major viral biologic threat is the variola virus, better known as **smallpox**. This serious, contagious disease is fatal in up to 30% of cases. Although believed to be eradicated, with the last case in the United States occurring in 1949 and in Somalia in 1977, the virus may still be stockpiled in laboratories across the world for use as a biologic weapon. Generally, personal contact is needed to spread this disease, but only a few viral droplets spread through the air or on contaminated objects are needed to produce the disease. Humans are the only carriers. Unvaccinated populations are at risk.

Vaccination gives immunity for 3 to 5 years and is effective if given prior to exposure to the virus or up to 3 days postexposure. Smallpox vaccinations are contraindicated for certain groups such as pregnant or lactating women; children under 1 year old; people with impaired immune systems, such as those with human immunodeficiency virus or leukemia; people with atopic dermatitis or eczema; or anyone with an allergy to a component in the vaccine. Although serious adverse effects are very rare, vaccines can cause death. A mutation in the virus would render the vaccine ineffective, so mass vaccinations for smallpox are not considered prudent at this time. The SNS maintains enough smallpox vaccinations for the public in the event of an outbreak. In 2018, tecovirimat (TPOXX) was developed for treatment of smallpox infection, should a bioterrorism event occur.

Viral hemorrhagic fevers, which are caused by a number of virus families, can cause severe physical damage affecting multiple organ systems. Usually, these viruses damage the circulatory system, resulting in hemorrhage. The host can be the cotton rat and deer mouse but some, such as Ebola or Marburg, have unknown hosts. There is no cure or vaccine for these viruses and patients are treated with supportive therapy, such as fluid and electrolytes, and management of complications. Ribavirin is an antiviral drug that has shown some success in treating Lassa fever. CDC researchers in the Viral Special Pathogens Branch work with these hemorrhagic fever viruses, which are considered a biosafety level 4. This class consists of exotic agents that can be transmitted by aerosol and pose a high risk of life-threatening disease.

Chemical and Physical Agents

75.6 There are 13 categories of toxic chemicals that could cause mass casualties if released into the environment.

Chemical warfare agents have been used since World War I, but few drug antidotes exist today. Many treatments provide minimal help other than to relieve some symptoms and provide comfort following exposure. Whether a chemical is released by terrorists, enemy military, or by industry in a chemical release accident, the result is the same: A hazardous chemical is released into the environment that may harm the health of the public. The CDC has classified hazardous chemicals into the following categories:

- *Biotoxins*. Poisons from plants or animals
- *Vesicants and blister agents*. Agents that severely blister the skin, respiratory tract, or eyes on contact
- *Blood agents*. Poisons that are absorbed into the circulation
- *Acids and caustics*. Chemicals that burn the eyes, skin, or lining of the respiratory tract on contact
- *Pulmonary and choking agents*. Chemicals that irritate the lungs and cause swelling and choking
- *Incapacitating agents*. Chemicals that alter consciousness, making it difficult for the patient to think clearly
- *Long-acting anticoagulants*. Chemicals that produce uncontrolled bleeding by preventing clotting
- *Metals*. Agents that are metallic poisons
- *Nerve agents*. Poisons that impair nervous system functioning
- *Organic solvents*. Chemicals that damage living tissue by dissolving fats and oils
- *Tear gas or mace*. Agents used for riot or crowd control by law enforcement or for self-defense; irritate the eyes and the respiratory tract, resulting in incapacitation
- *Toxic alcohols*. Chemicals that damage vital organs such as the heart, kidneys, and nervous system
- *Vomiting agents*. Chemicals that induce nausea and vomiting.

Table 75.3 lists well-known chemical agents and their symptoms and treatments. The primary chemical hazards related to pharmacology are nerve agents. Individuals who breathe nerve gas experience convulsions and loss of consciousness, which result in respiratory failure within minutes. The antidote for nerve gas is the anticholinergic drug atropine.

75.7 Ionizing radiation produces immediate and long-term effects on human tissue.

Bioterrorists may use nuclear bombs or attack nuclear facilities that could cause mass casualty deaths at the point of impact and create residual ionizing radiation for miles around the site. Some radioisotopes emit radiation for decades and even centuries. Smaller-scale radiation could occur with the release of solid or liquid nuclear material into public areas or a dirty bomb, which explodes with radioactive powder or pellets, contaminating the area.

Radiation sickness occurs after exposure to ionizing radiation and can last from hours to days. Initial symptoms include nausea and vomiting and diarrhea with later

Table 75.3 Chemical Agents and Treatments

<table>
<tr><th>Agent</th><th>Signs and Symptoms</th><th>Decontamination</th><th>Persistence</th></tr>
<tr><td colspan="4">Nerve Agents</td></tr>
<tr><td>Tabun (GA)</td><td rowspan="4">Salivation, lacrimation, urination, defecation, gastric disturbances, emesis</td><td rowspan="4">Remove contaminated clothing.
Flush with a soap and water solution for patients.
Flush with large amounts of a 5% bleach and water solution for objects.</td><td>1–2 days if heavy concentration</td></tr>
<tr><td>Sarin (GB)</td><td>1–2 days will evaporate with water</td></tr>
<tr><td>Soman (GD)</td><td>Moderate, 1–2 days</td></tr>
<tr><td>V agents (VX)</td><td>High, 1 wk if heavy concentration; as volatile as motor oil</td></tr>
<tr><td colspan="4">Vesicants (Blister Agents)</td></tr>
<tr><td>Sulfur mustard (H)</td><td rowspan="4">Acts first as a cell irritant, then as a cell poison. Conjunctivitis, reddened skin, blisters, nasal irritation, inflammation of throat and lungs.</td><td rowspan="6">Remove contaminated clothing.
Flush with soap and water solution for patients.
Flush with large amounts of a 5% bleach and water solution for objects.</td><td rowspan="3">Very high, days to weeks</td></tr>
<tr><td>Distilled mustard (HD)</td></tr>
<tr><td>Nitrogen mustard (HN 1, 3)</td></tr>
<tr><td>Mustargen (HN 2)</td><td>Moderate</td></tr>
<tr><td>Lewisite (L)</td><td>Immediate pain with blisters later.</td><td>Days, rapid hydrolysis with humidity</td></tr>
<tr><td>Phosgene oxime (CX)</td><td>Immediate pain with blisters later—necrosis equivalent to second- and third-degree burns.</td><td>Low, 2 h in soil</td></tr>
<tr><td colspan="4">Chemical Asphyxiants (Blood Agents)</td></tr>
<tr><td>Hydrogen cyanide (AC)</td><td rowspan="3">Cherry red skin or ~30% cyanosis. Patients may appear to be gasping for air. Seizures prior to death. Effect is similar to asphyxiation but is more sudden.</td><td rowspan="3">Remove contaminated clothing.
Flush with a soap and water solution for patients.
Flush with large amounts of 5% bleach and water solution for objects.</td><td>Extremely volatile, 1–2 days</td></tr>
<tr><td>Cyanogen chloride (CK)</td><td>Rapidly evaporates and disperses</td></tr>
<tr><td>Arsine (SA)</td><td>Low</td></tr>
</table>

From Homeland Defense Information Products (n.d.).

symptoms of weight loss, anorexia, fatigue, and suppression of the bone marrow. When exposed to large amounts of radiation or to small amounts over many decades, patients tend to develop certain malignancies such as leukemia or thyroid cancer.

Except for supportive therapies, the only recognized treatment available to counter the thyroid uptake of radiation is ingestion of potassium iodine (KI) before or immediately after exposure. One of the radioisotopes produced by a nuclear explosion is iodine-131 (^{131}I). Because iodine is naturally concentrated in the thyroid gland, ^{131}I will immediately enter the thyroid and damage thyroid cells. For example, following the Chernobyl nuclear disaster, the incidence of thyroid cancer in the Ukraine jumped from four to six cases per million people to 45 cases per million. If taken prior to, or immediately following, a nuclear incident, KI can prevent up to 100% of the radioactive iodine from entering the thyroid gland. It is effective even if taken 3 to 4 hours after radiation exposure. Generally, a single 130-mg dose is necessary for adults.

Unfortunately, KI protects only the thyroid gland from ^{131}I. It has no protective effects on other body tissues, and it offers no protection against the dozens of other harmful radioisotopes generated by a nuclear explosion. As with vaccines and antibiotics, the stockpiling of KI by local healthcare agencies or individuals is not recommended.

CONNECTION Checkpoint 75.2

From what you learned in Chapter 67, describe the therapeutic use of ^{131}I in treating thyroid disease.

Management of Poisoning

75.8 The general management of poisoning includes contacting the poison control center or emergency medical services as soon as possible.

Virtually any chemical may cause poisoning if taken in excessive amounts. The body has a remarkable capacity to tolerate a wide variety of chemicals and has physiologic mechanisms to detoxify and rapidly eliminate many of them. Toxicity results when the body's detoxification and excretion abilities are exceeded. Toxic effects may appear immediately, or they may appear decades after the initial exposure.

Medications are the most frequently involved substances in poisonings for all age groups. Household cleaning compounds comprise a second large group of poisonings, with cosmetics being close behind. Although exposure to poisons may occur by any route, ingestion accounts for over 75% of all poisoning cases. Swallowing dangerous substances is common among children with curious minds who put strange substances into their mouths. Most poisonings present with low levels of toxicity, but some can result in fatalities, such as the ingestion of gun-bluing agents used to maintain the color of gun barrels. Signs and symptoms of ingested poisons include abdominal cramping or stomach pain, nausea and vomiting, diarrhea, sleepiness or loss of consciousness, bottles or containers of poisons close by, or odor, stains, or burns around the mouth.

Poisoning from medications may be unintentional or intentional (suicide). Acetaminophen is a common toxin because so many analgesic medications contain this drug. Although legal for adults, alcohol is a potential poison and its abuse is a major health problem in the United States. Ingestion of alcohol, along with certain prescribed medications, amphetamines, hallucinogens, or inhaled substances such as solvents or glue can create life-threatening situations. Symptoms of drug overdose include confusion, elevated heart rate, drowsiness, enlarged or dilated pupils, and hallucinations. Other medications that cause frequent poisonings include iron, calcium channel blockers, and tricyclic antidepressants.

When a specific antidote is available, it is administered as soon as the poisoning is diagnosed (Table 75.4). In the vast majority of poisoning cases, there is no specific antidote. General therapies such as activated charcoal, peritoneal dialysis, hemodialysis, and gastric lavage have only limited effectiveness. In some cases, they are totally ineffective. Emergency physicians and nurses are generally faced with treating individual symptoms either because the poison is unknown or because there is no antidote. The strategy for treatment of acute poisoning consists of five general principles:

- *Topical decontamination.* Removal of contaminated clothing, flushing of the skin or eyes
- *Prevention of absorption.* Administration of adsorbents (activated charcoal), whole-bowel irrigation, induction of vomiting, and gastric lavage
- *Neutralization.* Administration of acids or bases
- *Increase in the rate of excretion.* Administration of diuretics, peritoneal or hemodialysis, and ion trapping
- *Antidotes and symptomatic therapy.* Administration of specific antidotes and support of vital functions.

Treatment for ingested poisons depends on the age and physical size of the patient and the time between swallowing and presenting for medical intervention. Any information about the poisoning that can be obtained from the patient, family, or caregiver can be helpful, such as the type of poison that was swallowed, when it was ingested, and how much was taken. Following are some specific interventions for managing the patient poisoned by ingestion:

- Do not implement the package instructions for poisoning without consulting the American Association of Poison Control Centers or an appropriate healthcare provider. Preferred therapy may have changed since the packaging was printed.
- Contact the poison control center if the poisoning is the result of taking too much or the wrong medication was taken.

Table 75.4 Specific Antidotes

Drug or Poison	Antidote
acetaminophen	acetylcysteine (Acetadote)
acetylcholinesterases, organophosphates	pralidoxime (Protopam); atropine with pralidoxime (DuoDote)
anticholinergic drugs	neostigmine, physostigmine
benzodiazepines	flumazenil
beta-adrenergic blockers	glucagon
calcium channel blockers	calcium, IV insulin in high doses with IV glucose
coumadin	vitamin K (phytomenadione)
digoxin (Lanoxin)	digoxin immune Fab (Digibind)
ethylene glycol (antifreeze, brake fluid, coolants) and methanol	ethanol, fomepizole
heavy metals	chelating drugs such as edetate calcium disodium
heparin	protamine sulfate
iron	deferoxamine (Desferal)
isoniazid (INH)	pyridoxine (vitamin B_6)
methemoglobin-forming drugs (some local anesthetics, nitrates, nitrites, phenacetin, sulfonamides)	methylene blue
methotrexate	leucovorin
opioids	naloxone (Evzio, Narcan)
organophosphates	atropine, pralidoxime (Protopam)
tricyclic antidepressants	sodium bicarbonate

- Provide fresh air to the individual if the poison was inhaled.
- Remove contaminated clothes if the poison came in contact with the individual's skin. Take care not to spread contamination from the poisoned clothes to the surrounding environment. Flush the skin with water for 15 to 20 minutes to dilute or remove the poison.
- Rinse the eyes with running water for 15 to 20 minutes if in contact with poison.
- Do not induce vomiting by gagging or tickling the back of the throat.
- Do not give ipecac syrup. Though once considered a routine procedure, this method of poison management is now considered ineffective. Discourage parents from keeping ipecac syrup in the home. There is no evidence that syrup of ipecac actually helps improve the outcome in poisoning cases. Furthermore, the administration of syrup of ipecac can delay the administration of more effective treatments, such as activated charcoal or antidotes.
- Do not give milk or water unless directed to do so by the poison center. Though once thought to dilute the poison, fluids can liquefy dry poison and send it more rapidly to the small intestine. The exception to this is caustic or corrosive poisons.

CONNECTIONS: Lifespan Considerations

Intentional Poisonings in Children and Adolescents

Suicide by poisoning is an increasing health problem for children and adolescents In this age population, intentional poisoning is much more common than adult suicide methods such as firearms. Gonzalez-Urdiales et al. (2020) determined that suicide attempts by the intentional ingestion of drugs accounts for 50% of poisonings seen in the ED in children age 12 and older. Analgesic drugs such as acetaminophen, ibuprofen, and opioids accounted for almost 50% of suicide attempts, with psychotropic drugs representing another 36%. Females attempted suicide almost five times more often than males, and over 87% of the attempts occurred at home. In 2018, the suicide rate of adolescents age 15 to 24 was 14.45% per 100,000 (American Foundation for Suicide Prevention, 2020).

Suicide is the third leading cause of death in youths age 10 to 14 and the second for those age 15 to 24 (CDC, 2017b). With as many as 50% of poisonings seen in the ED being intentional, any adolescent who is brought to the ED for treatment should have a mental health evaluation by a qualified professional in addition to therapies to treat the actual poisoning.

75.9 Activated charcoal is effective at adsorbing (binding) most poisons if administered within 60 minutes of ingestion.

Activated charcoal has been used as an adsorbent for acute poisoning for almost 200 years. Activated charcoal is the only FDA-approved poison-adsorbent drug. Although it is effective in the treatment of many poisons, it is not beneficial when given to individuals with lithium, iron, or cyanide poisoning or strong acid or alkali ingestion.

PROTOTYPE DRUG | **Activated Charcoal (CharcoAid)**

Classification **Therapeutic:** Antidote
Pharmacologic: Adsorbent drug

Therapeutic Effect and Uses: Activated charcoal consists of organic material such as coal, wood, or vegetables that have been carbonized, reduced, and dried to a charcoal-like substance. It is then activated by exposing it to steam, carbon dioxide, or other oxidizing chemicals at extremely high temperatures. The activation drives off impurities and reduces the particle size so that the surface area of the charcoal is very large.

This drug effectively adsorbs toxins in the intestinal tract, thus preventing their systemic absorption. Adsorption is the process of a drug physically binding to the charcoal. As a general-purpose emergency antidote, it is used in the treatment of poisonings from most drugs and chemicals. To be most effective, the charcoal should be administered within 1 hour of oral ingestion. Normally, a single dose is administered, although some poisons benefit from multiple doses. The general dosage is 5 to 10 times the estimated weight of the poison ingested.

Activated charcoal can also be used off-label to adsorb intestinal gases in the treatment of dyspepsia, flatulence, and distention. It is sometimes used topically as a deodorant for foul-smelling wounds and ulcers.

Mechanism of Action: Activated charcoal (carbon) is a chemically inert, odorless, tasteless, fine black powder. It acts by binding (adsorbing) toxic substances, thereby inhibiting their gastric absorption, enterohepatic circulation, and bioavailability.

Pharmacokinetics:

Route(s)	PO or via nasogastric tube
Absorption	Not absorbed
Distribution	Not distributed systemically
Primary metabolism	Not metabolized
Primary excretion	Fecal
Onset of action	Rapid
Duration of action	Unknown

Adverse Effects: Vomiting may occur when given by rapid ingestion and at high doses. Constipation and diarrhea have also been reported.

Contraindications/Precautions: Activated charcoal is not effective for poisonings by cyanide, mineral acids, caustic alkalis, organic solvents, iron, ethanol, or methanol ingestion. This drug should not be used in patients at a decreased level of consciousness or with a diminished gag reflex due to the risk of pulmonary aspiration. Activated charcoal should also not be used in individuals with central nervous system depression, coma, or gastrointestinal (GI) obstruction.

Drug Interactions: Activated charcoal will decrease absorption of all other oral medications. Oral medication should not be given for at least 2 hours after administration of activated charcoal. **Herbal/Food:** Milk and dairy products may decrease the effectiveness of activated charcoal.

Pregnancy: This drug has not shown teratogenicity in laboratory animals. Data are not available regarding safety during lactation.

Clinician Responsibilities: Key clinical implications for patients receiving activated charcoal are included in Applied Clinical Judgment: Patients Receiving Pharmacotherapy for Poisoning or Overdose.

Drugs Similar to Activated Charcoal (CharcoAid)

Activated charcoal is the only drug in this class.

75.10 Ion trapping with forced diuresis may be helpful for some poisonings.

One procedure that is occasionally used in acute poisoning is ion trapping through forced diuresis. Because most drugs are either weak acids or weak bases, changing the urine pH can be used to enhance the elimination of some drugs. For example, if the urine is made alkaline, the acidic drugs are trapped in the renal tubules and their elimination in urine is increased. The opposite effect applies for alkaline drugs.

Forced alkaline diuresis may be used to increase the excretion of acidic drugs like salicylates and phenobarbital and forced acid diuresis has been used to eliminate amphetamines, quinine, and strychnine. When forced alkaline diuresis is employed, a diuretic such as furosemide along with IV sodium bicarbonate will make the urine more alkaline. Forced alkaline diuresis is specifically recommended when rhabdomyolysis (the rapid breakdown of skeletal muscle tissue) occurs.

Ascorbic acid is used for forced acid diuresis. In past decades, ammonium chloride was used for forced acid diuresis; however, due to its toxicity its use has greatly diminished. Research studies indicate that ion trapping through forced diuresis produces only a slight increase in the renal clearance of the drug and is rarely done in practice.

75.11 Chelating agents are capable of forming bonds with heavy metals.

Human exposure to metals has risen dramatically in the past 50 years as a result of an increase in the use of heavy metals in industrial processes and products. **Chelation therapy** is the use of drugs to detoxify poisonous metals such as mercury, arsenic, and lead by converting them to a chemically inert form that can be easily excreted. The compound formed by a chelating drug and a metal is called a chelate. Chelating drugs are most frequently administered intravenously or intramuscularly depending on the agent and the type of poisoning. Chelation was introduced during World War I originally as an antidote to arsenic-based poison gas.

The mechanism of action of chelation therapies involves the chelating drug "latching onto" and removing positively charged metals from the body. Once the amino acid binds with the metal or poison, it can be eliminated from the body by the kidneys. Two chelating drugs are described in this chapter. Both medications are often given to the individual who is experiencing heavy metal poisoning.

PROTOTYPE DRUG Edetate Calcium Disodium (Calcium EDTA)

Classification **Therapeutic:** Drug for heavy metal poisoning
Pharmacologic: Chelating drug

Therapeutic Effects and Uses: Approved in 1953, edetate calcium disodium is a chelating drug that binds with heavy metals such as lead to form a soluble complex that can be excreted by the kidneys, thereby ridding the body of the poisonous substance. Although usually used for acute poisoning, this drug can also remove lead that is stored in fat, bone, or other locations. Edetate calcium disodium is administered by the IV or intramuscular (IM) routes. This drug is generally used in combination with dimercaprol (BAL) in the treatment of lead encephalopathy or when the blood lead level exceeds 100 mcg/dL.

The off-label uses of edetate calcium disodium include the treatment of poisoning from other heavy metals such as chromium, manganese, nickel, zinc, and possibly vanadium and removal of radioactive and nuclear fission products such as plutonium, yttrium, and uranium. However, this drug is not effective in treating poisoning from arsenic, gold, or mercury.

Mechanism of Action: As a chelating drug, Calcium EDTA combines with metals to form stable, nonionizing soluble complexes that can be readily excreted by the kidneys. Action is dependent on the ability of the heavy metal to displace the weakly bound calcium in the drug molecules.

Pharmacokinetics:

Route(s)	IV/IM
Absorption	Rapidly absorbed
Distribution	Distributed to extracellular fluid; does not enter the cerebrospinal fluid
Primary metabolism	Not metabolized
Primary excretion	Chelated lead is excreted in urine; 50% is excreted in 1 h
Onset of action	Peak chelation: 24–48 h
Duration of action	Half-life: 20–60 min IV, 90 min IM

Adverse Effects: Calcium EDTA may produce kidney injury such as proteinuria and microscopic hematuria. Treatment-induced nephrotoxicity is dose dependent and may be reduced by ensuring adequate diuresis before therapy begins. Patients should be monitored for cardiac rhythm irregularities and other electrocardiogram (ECG) changes during IV therapy. Additional cardiovascular effects include hypotension and thrombophlebitis.

Many patients experience febrile reaction (excessive thirst, fever, chills, severe myalgia, arthralgia, GI distress) or histamine-like reactions (flushing, throbbing headache, sweating, sneezing, nasal congestion, lacrimation, postural hypotension, tachycardia). **Black Box Warning:** Patients with lead encephalopathy and cerebral edema may experience a lethal increase in intracranial pressure if the drug is given by IV infusion. The IM route is preferred for these patients.

Contraindications/Precautions: Edetate calcium disodium is contraindicated in patients with severe kidney disease, anuria, or oliguria. IV administration is contraindicated in patients with lead encephalopathy because of a possible increase in intracranial pressure.

Drug Interactions: No clinically significant interactions have been identified. **Herbal/Food:** None known.

Pregnancy: The safety of this drug during pregnancy is not definitively known. However, removal of heavy metals from the mother after poisoning likely justifies the potential risks to the fetus.

Clinician Responsibilities: Key clinical implications for patients receiving edetate calcium disodium are included in Applied Clinical Judgment: Patients Receiving Pharmacotherapy for Poisoning or Overdose.

PROTOTYPE DRUG Dimercaprol (BAL in Oil)

Classification **Therapeutic:** Antidote
Pharmacologic: Chelating drug

Therapeutic Effects and Uses: Given by the IM route, dimercaprol is a chelating drug that neutralizes the effects of various heavy metals such as arsenic, gold, and mercury. The drug forms stable, nontoxic intermediates with these metals so they are more easily excreted in the urine and bile. Dimercaprol is also used as an adjunct to EDTA in the treatment of lead encephalopathy. Off-label uses include chromium dermatitis and ocular and dermatologic manifestations of arsenic poisoning. Dimercaprol may be used as an adjunct to penicillamine to increase the rate of copper excretion in Wilson's disease. Wilson's disease is a rare genetic disorder in which copper builds up in the liver and is released into other parts of the body.

Mechanism of Action: Dimercaprol forms ring complexes with some heavy metals, such as arsenic, gold, and mercury, preventing or reversing the binding of metallic cations to body proteins.

Pharmacokinetics:

Route(s)	IM only
Absorption	Well absorbed
Distribution	Distributed mainly in intracellular spaces, including the brain; highest concentration is in the liver and kidneys
Primary metabolism	Unknown
Primary excretion	Urine and feces
Onset of action	Peak: 30–60 min
Duration of action	Half-life: unknown

Adverse Effects: About 50% of patients who receive high therapeutic doses have adverse reactions, including nausea and vomiting, fatigue, restlessness, apprehension, headache, lacrimation, blepharospasm, salivation, tingling of extremities, a feeling of constriction in the chest muscle, diffuse pain and muscle spasm, hypertension, tachycardia, and a burning sensation of the mouth, throat, and eyes. Most patients report pain at the injection site.

Contraindications/Precautions: Dimercaprol is contraindicated in individuals with hepatic insufficiency (with the exception of postarsenic jaundice); severe kidney disease; or poisoning due to cadmium, iron, selenium, or uranium. Because dimercaprol is formulated in peanut oil, patients with a hypersensitivity to peanut products should not receive this drug. This drug should be used cautiously in patients with hypertension, oliguria, G6PD deficiency, and preexisting chronic kidney disease.

Drug Interactions: Dimercaprol should not be given when iron, cadmium, selenium, or uranium poisoning is suspected. When this drug is given in the presence of these poisonings, it forms toxic complexes. **Herbal/Food:** Unknown.

Pregnancy: Pregnancy and lactation data are not available for this drug.

Clinician Responsibilities: Key clinical implications for patients receiving dimercaprol are included in Applied Clinical Judgment: Patients Receiving Pharmacotherapy for Poisoning or Overdose.

CONNECTIONS: APPLIED CLINICAL JUDGMENT

Patients Receiving Pharmacotherapy for Poisoning or Overdose

Key Assessment Data

- History of current condition including musculoskeletal, GI, cardiovascular, neurologic, endocrine, hepatic, or kidney disease; baseline vital signs, physical exam findings, laboratory findings (e.g., hepatic and renal function studies, complete blood count, and urinalysis); pregnancy or breastfeeding; medication history including allergies, current prescription and over-the-counter drugs.

Desired Therapeutic Outcomes

Improvement is observed and measurable by cardiopulmonary status is maintained, symptoms related to poison or drug overdose are diminishing, level of consciousness is improving.

Minimizing Adverse Effects

- Observe for changes in urine character and color. Myoglobin may be present if rhabdomyolysis occurs as a result of overdose, causing a cola-colored or rust-brown appearance to the urine.
- A mental health consultation should be ordered for patients who demonstrate suicidal ideations or behaviors.

Lifespan Considerations

- Age-related physiologic differences or undetected cardiac disease may place the older adult at greater risk for adverse effects from calcium EDTA.

Patient Education

- To allay possible anxiety, teach the patient, family, or caregiver the rationale for all procedures. Emergency treatment is rapid and may seem confusing or frightening to the bystander.
- Stools may become temporarily black if activated charcoal has been used.
- Frequently evaluate the home environment and medication storage to prevent accidental poisonings.

Prescribing Considerations

- After an acute poisoning or overdose with agents such as ethanol and salicylates, order lab tests to assess for poisoning-related nephrotoxicity and hepatotoxicity.
- Cardiac dysrhythmias and pulmonary edema may result from overdose of many poisons, including barbiturates, sedatives, hypnotics, and tranquilizers. Continuous ECG and ACLS may be needed.
- Review nutritional status following chelation because this therapy removes vital minerals as well as toxins.

Understanding Chapter 75

Key Concepts Summary

75.1 Emergency preparedness has become an essential competency for all healthcare professionals.

75.2 Bioterrorism is the intentional release of a virus or microorganism to cause human harm.

75.3 Nurses may have the first opportunity to recognize and initiate a response to bioterrorism.

75.4 The Strategic National Stockpile has large quantities of medicine to protect the public if a health emergency arises.

75.5 Highly infectious bacteria or viruses could be used as bioterrorist threats.

75.6 There are 13 categories of toxic chemicals that could cause mass casualties if released into the environment.

75.7 Ionizing radiation produces immediate and long-term effects on human tissue.

75.8 The general management of poisoning includes contacting the poison control center or emergency medical services as soon as possible.

75.9 Activated charcoal is effective at adsorbing (binding) most poisons if administered within 60 minutes of ingestion.

75.10 Ion trapping with forced diuresis may be helpful for some poisonings.

75.11 Chelating agents are capable of forming bonds with heavy metals.

CASE STUDY: Making the Patient Connection

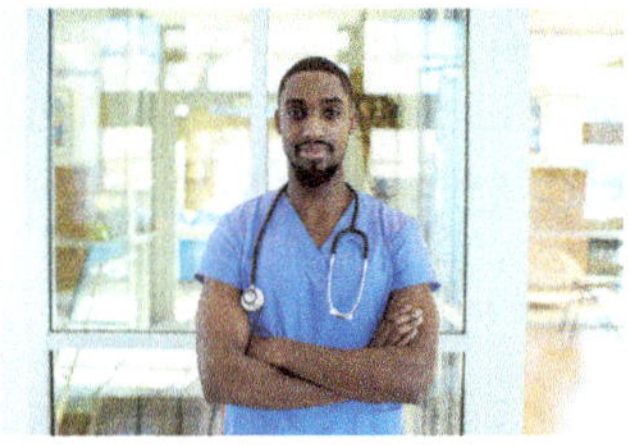

Remember the ED nurse "C. Richard Drew" at the beginning of the chapter? Now read the remainder of the case study. Based on the information presented within this chapter, respond to the critical thinking questions that follow.

As an ED nurse in a busy urban hospital, C. Richard Drew participates in frequent emergency practice drills to be prepared for mass casualty events and acts of bioterrorism. Although there have been no incidents yet, he knows that with a military base nearby, there is a chance that such an incident could occur, and they often participate in joint disaster drills. He is working with unit staff to plan a series of staff education meetings to discuss bioterrorism threats.

Critical Thinking Questions

1. When discussing the bioterrorism threat with a group of staff nurses, which information regarding smallpox should be included?
2. Identify the nursing assessments and interventions that the nurse should initiate when a patient is exposed to anthrax.
3. Discuss the mode of transmission and symptoms associated with *Y. pestis* exposure.

Additional Case Study

As a school nurse, you have been asked to speak to a group of mothers about unintentional poisonings in young children.

1. Outline the information you need to present to this audience.
2. What recommendations should you give to the group about the use of ipecac syrup?

Chapter Review

1. The patient is suspected of having been exposed to ionizing radiation. Which nursing intervention would have the greatest priority?

1. Provide supportive care for nausea and vomiting and diarrhea.
2. Limit the patient's exposure to ultraviolet light.
3. Avoid contamination of self through limited exposure to the patient.
4. Administer antiradiation medications as indicated.

2. The patient is exhibiting the symptoms of *Yersinia pestis* exposure. Which pharmacologic therapy would most likely be used in the treatment of this patient?

1. Doxycycline
2. Trivalent botulinum antitoxin
3. Ribavirin
4. Atropine sulfate

3. The nurse has received a telephone call from an anxious mother of an 18-month-old child. In a panicked voice, the mother states, "I just discovered that my baby has swallowed an unknown amount of household cleanser." Which instruction would be appropriate for the nurse to give?

1. "Consult the package instructions for information concerning poisoning."
2. "Force your child to vomit using a mixture of warm water and raw eggs."
3. "Call 911 to take your child immediately to the nearest emergency department or healthcare agency."
4. "If your child develops seizures or difficulty breathing, call the healthcare provider."

4. Activated charcoal is ordered for a patient who unintentionally overdosed on prescription medications. The nurse would question the order for activated charcoal for the patient with which condition?

1. Acute hepatitis and cirrhosis
2. Chronic kidney disease
3. Decreased level of consciousness
4. Anxiety and nervousness

5. The nurse knows that the mechanism of action for chelating therapy is:

1. Removal of positively charged metals.
2. Deactivation of chemical reaction.
3. Increased liver metabolism.
4. Decreased glomerular filtration.

6. Which of the preadministration assessment parameters would the nurse consider before administering edetate calcium disodium (Calcium EDTA) to a patient?

1. Bowel sounds
2. Urinary output
3. Visual acuity
4. Skin turgor

See Appendix A for answers to critical thinking questions, case study questions, and review questions.

References

American Foundation for Suicide Prevention. (2020). *Suicide statistics*. https://afsp.org/suicide-statistics/.

Centers for Disease Control and Prevention (CDC). (n.d.). *Emergency preparedness & response: CDC bioterrorism agents/diseases*. https://fas.org/biosecurity/resource/documents/CDC_Bioterrorism_Agents.pdf

Centers for Disease Control and Prevention (CDC). (2017a). *Anthrax vaccine*. https://www.cdc.gov/vaccines/hcp/vis/vis-statements/anthrax.html

Centers for Disease Control and Prevention (CDC). (2017b). *Preventing suicide: A technical package of policy, programs, and practices*. https://www.cdc.gov/violenceprevention/pdf/suicideTechnicalPackage.pdf

Gonzalez-Urdiales, P., Kuppermann, N., Dalziel, S. R., Prego, J., Benito, J., & Mintegi, S. (2020). Pediatric intentional self-poisoning evaluated in the emergency department: An international study. *Pediatric Emergency Care*, *36*. https://doi.org/10.1097/PEC.0000000000002141

Homeland Defense Information Products. (n.d.) *Biological and chemical agent quick reference*. https://www.hsdl.org/?view&did=483529

Selected Bibliography

Andersen, O., & Aaseth, J. (2016). A review of pitfalls and progress in chelation treatment of metal poisonings. *Journal of Trace Elements in Medicine and Biology*, *38*, 74–80. https://doi.org/10.1016/j.jtemb.2016.03.013

Chugh, T. (2019). Bioterrorism: Clinical and public health aspects of anthrax. *Current Medicine Research and Practice*, *9*(3), 110–111. https://doi.org/10.1016/j.cmrp.2019.05.004

Golden, P., Lindblad, L., Kim, H., Lee, K. L., & Lamas, G. A. (2019). The effect of EDTA-based chelation on patients with diabetes and peripheral artery disease in the Trial to Assess Chelation Therapy (TACT). *Journal of Diabetes and Its Complications*, *33*(7), 490–494. https://doi.org/10.1016/j.jdiacomp.2019.04.005

Green, M. S., LeDuc, J., Cohen, D., & Franz, D. R. (2019). Confronting the threat of bioterrorism: realities, challenges, and defensive strategies. *The Lancet Infectious Diseases*, *19*(1), e2–e13. https://doi.org/10.1016/S1473-3099(18)30298-6

Griffin, K. M., Karas, M. G., Ivascu, N. S., & Lief, L. (2020). Hospital preparedness for COVID-19: a practical guide from a critical care perspective. American Journal of Respiratory and Critical Care Medicine, *201*(11), 1337–1344. https://doi.org/10.1164/rccm.202004-1037CP

Spain, K. M., Clements, P. T., DeRanieri, J. T., & Holt, K. (2012). When disaster happens: Emergency preparedness for nurse practitioners. *Journal for Nurse Practitioners*, *8*(1), 38–44. https://doi.org/10.1016/j.nurpra.2011.07.024

Veenema, T. G., Griffin, A., Gable, A. R., MacIntyre, L., Simons, R. N., Couig, M. P., et al. (2016). Nurses as leaders in disaster preparedness and response—a call to action. *Journal of Nursing Scholarship*, *48*, 187–200. https://doi.org/10.1111/jnu.12198

Villarreal, J., Kahn, C. A., Dunford, J. V., Patel, E., & Clark, R. F. (2015). A retrospective review of the prehospital use of activated charcoal. *American Journal of Emergency Medicine*, *33*, 56–59. https://doi.org/10.1016/j.ajem.2014.10.019

Wilkinson, A. M., & Matzo, M. (2015). Nursing education for disaster preparedness and response. *Journal of Continuing Education in Nursing*, *46*(2), 65–73. https://doi.org/10.3928/00220124-20150126-01

Appendix
Answers to Chapter Review

Chapter 1

Patient Safety: A potentially dangerous drug interaction may occur if paroxetine and St. John's wort are taken concurrently. Symptoms such as headache, sweating, confusion, and agitation may occur and may worsen, with hypertension and hyperpyrexia occurring. The patient should be taught to stop taking the St. John's wort while using paroxetine and to consult with their healthcare provider before taking any over-the-counter medication.

Making the Patient Connection

1 A therapeutic classification describes what the drug is treating. These drugs are often identified by the prefix *anti-* such as antiseizure, anti-inflammatory, and antihypertensive. The pharmacologic classification describes how the drug acts within the body. A drug's pharmacologic classification is more specific than a therapeutic classification.

2 A barbiturate is the pharmacologic classification for a major sedative. A macrolide is the pharmacologic classification for a major type of antibiotic. Although the words "birth control pills" do not begin with "anti," this classification describes what the drug is being used for (anti-conception). Laxative denotes a therapeutic classification of drugs that enhance peristalsis to cause bowel emptying. Folic acid antagonist is a therapeutic classification for drugs that treat autoimmune disorders such as rheumatoid arthritis and in the treatment of some cancers. An antianginal agent is the therapeutic class of drugs that treat chest pain.

3 A prototype drug is representative of a group, classification, or category of medication. By learning about a prototype drug, students can apply this knowledge to the actions and adverse effects of other drugs in the same class.

4 The nurse is a critical member of the healthcare team who has tremendous responsibility for a patient's drug therapy. The nurse not only administers medication but also closely monitors the patient for the desired outcome and adverse effects. Nurses provide patients with essential drug-related education.

Additional Case Study

1 Although generic drugs are less expensive than their trade-name equivalent, they may vary in their bioavailability. In most cases, this difference does not affect the therapeutic effect of the drug and therefore can be safely substituted. However, in certain critical situations, the onset time of the drug may be important. In such situations, such as heart attack, stroke, or shock syndromes, generic forms of a medication may not be recommended.

2 To be safe, you should advise Sarah to talk with her healthcare provider about prescribing generics. Explain how important it is for her to inform her healthcare providers that her income status is limited. This information will assist the prescriber in determining the best and most cost-effective treatment modalities for her.

Chapter Review

1 Answer: 3 Rationale: Indications are the conditions for which a particular drug is approved. Options 1, 2, and 4 are incorrect. A description of how a drug works on its target organs and cells is called the mechanism of action. The dosage is the amount of the drug that is given. The conditions whereby the drug should be avoided are contraindications.

2 Answer: 3 Rationale: Like the original reference product drug, biosimilars are derived from living cells, such as yeast or bacteria. They are not exact, duplicate copies of the original medication, but have comparable effectiveness and safety. Options 1, 2, and 4 are incorrect. Because it is not an exact duplicate copy of the original drug, it cannot be considered a generic drug. It is not in a different therapeutic or chemical class because it differs little from the reference product. It must still be evaluated by the FDA and demonstrate that the biosimilar differs very little from the approved reference product, before it is approved.

3 Answers: 1, 2, 4 Rationale: Monitoring patient response to drug therapy, teaching the patient about self-administration and how to monitor drug effects, and verifying drugs currently being used by the patient are all key nursing responsibilities. Options 3 and 5 are incorrect. The prescribing provider weighs alternative treatment options but may not consider all available options due to many variables such as cost or complexity of treatment. Whereas the best option to treat a patient's condition will be chosen, the "ideal drug" does not exist because each patient's outcomes from drug therapy will be affected by many variables.

4 Answer: 1, 2, 3, 4 Rationale: Physiological responses to drug therapy are affected by a patient's age, gender, race, body mass, and health status. Many diseases such as diabetes have genetic origins. Familial history of disease conditions may reflect potential problems in the patient. Option 5 is incorrect because not having medical insurance is not a physiological variable that would affect drug therapy.

5 Answer: 2 Rationale: Antihypertensive indicates the therapeutic classification of the drug by describing its usefulness in lowering blood pressure. Options 1, 3, and 4 are incorrect. Beta-adrenergic antagonists, diuretics, and calcium channel blockers all focus on how the drug works, rather than on what therapeutic effects occur.

6 Answer: 2 Rationale: Under most state laws, a prescription for a reference product must be filled without substitution of a biosimilar. However, an interchangeable product can be substituted for the reference product. Options 1, 3, and 4 are incorrect. The term generic is not used to describe biosimilar products, federal laws for substitution do not apply to biosimilars and biosimilars are not exact copies of their reference product.

Chapter 2

Making the Patient Connection

1 Many people think OTC drugs are harmless. Any drug can have dangerous properties if taken inappropriately, and adverse effects can vary from person to person. OTC drugs may produce

toxic results if not used as directed. OTC drugs should be used as a temporary measure for minor problems. Individuals who use OTC drugs for recurrent and persistent problems should see a healthcare provider.

2 OTC medications have several advantages: (1) They do not require a visit to a healthcare provider. (2) Cost; in many cases, OTC drugs are reasonably priced. Many prescription medications are costly and may create financial hardship for individuals. (3) Easy administration; most OTC medications are created so that the administration is fairly simple and does not require any advanced medical knowledge. (4) OTC medications are sold in a variety of places from grocery stores to vending machines.

The disadvantages of OTC drugs include the following: (1) Some individuals take OTC medications in improper amounts and frequencies. OTC medications should only be used as described in the directions. (2) When patients diagnose themselves, the potential for misdiagnosis of serious and life-threatening illnesses arises. Using OTC medications is not a substitute for a physical examination and care by a healthcare provider. (3) When health problems are persistent or intense in nature, individuals should seek medical care. Individuals with conditions such as chest pain, chronic cough, or abdominal pain who prolong seeking medical care by taking OTC medications may increase the risk of disability and mortality.

3 Gertrude can obtain correct information about OTC drugs by asking a pharmacist or healthcare provider. Most pharmacists and healthcare providers will be happy to talk with individuals about possible drug–drug interactions, adverse effects, and contraindications for OTC medications.

Additional Case Study

1 The FDA is a federal agency whose function is to protect the public by validating the safety and efficacy of drugs, medical devices, food, and cosmetics. This organization works to provide the public with accurate and scientific-based information related to pharmaceutical products.

2 While the FDA does not require testing of herbal or dietary supplements prior to marketing, it monitors the administration of herbal products, dietary supplements, and cosmetics through the Center for Food Safety and Applied Nutrition (CFSAN).

3 The FDA has developed four categories to accelerate the process of drug review and approval: fast tracks, breakthrough therapies, priority reviews and accelerated approval.

Chapter Review

1 Answer: 2 Rationale: The FDA requires that drug manufacturers demonstrate both the safety and effectiveness of pharmaceutical products. Options 1, 3, and 4 are incorrect. All drugs have potential reactions and adverse effects. Many factors determine the cost of a drug and newly approved drugs may be the most expensive and not fully covered by healthcare insurance plans. Not all drugs have been tested in diverse populations and women, minority ethnic groups, children, and older adults are often underrepresented in drug research studies.

2 Answer: 2 Rationale: Phase 2 of the clinical investigation relies on studying patients with the disease to be treated. Options 1, 3, and 4 are incorrect. Phase 1 studies use small groups of healthy subjects. Phase 3 studies use large numbers of subjects with the condition being treated by the drug. Phase 4 is considered postmarketing surveillance after the drug has been approved.

3 Answer: 2 Rationale: A new drug is approved for a specific indication, but after several years of clinical experience, healthcare providers may find that the drug is also useful for indications not approved by the FDA. Once initially approved by the FDA, healthcare providers may legally prescribe the drug for any indications they feel are appropriate, despite the fact that the drug was never tested or approved for these additional conditions. Options 1, 3, and 4 are incorrect. The drug may be available in Europe or Canada but is regulated by those countries' laws and not the FDA. The approval of a drug for specific indications applies whether the drug is approved under normal or expedited review processes. A generic name is assigned by the U.S. Adopted Names Council and does not refer to the drug's use.

4 Answer: 4 Rationale: Telephone orders are not permissible under federal law for Schedule II controlled substances. Options 1, 2, and 3 are incorrect. Refill prescriptions are usually not more or less expensive than the original prescription. The number of listeners is irrelevant. Prescriptions are not confirmed or verified by the DEA.

5 Answer:

Fast Track: The drug under development has the *potential* to meet an unmet need for a condition in which there is no current therapy, or the drug may offer significant improvement over existing therapies.

Breakthrough therapy: Research trials suggest there is *clinical evidence* that the drug may demonstrate substantial improvement over existing therapies for a serious or life-threatening condition.

Priority review: A NDA is received, and the FDA makes the decision to perform a priority review (average 6 months) rather than a standard review (average 10 months), based on the drug offering the potential for significant improvement over existing therapies for a serious condition.

Accelerated approval: The FDA approves a drug based on "intermediate clinical endpoints" before the drug has demonstrated that it provides real clinical benefit (e.g., improved patient survival or how a patient feels or functions), which may take many years. For example, a new anticancer drug may show positive evidence of tumor shrinkage in clinical trials. The new drug can be marketed although the company must perform follow-up studies, known as confirmatory trials. If the confirmatory trials show the drug did not improve survival, the FDA may withdraw the accelerated approval.

6 Answer: 1, 2, 3 Rationale: Adverse drug reactions may continue to be discovered after the FDA approval process as larger groups of patients take the drug. Any reaction should be noted in the patient's chart, the provider notified, and an Adverse Event Report filed with the FDA when adverse reactions are noted. Options 4 and 5 are incorrect. Healthcare providers are responsible for reporting adverse reactions as they occur and should not wait for the FDA to send a recall notice. Many factors influence a patient's reaction to medications and each patient may not have the same exact reaction to the medication.

Chapter 3

Making the Patient Connection

1 John Kessler's deteriorating condition will affect drug metabolism in several ways. First, the condition of diabetes is an alteration in metabolism and therefore the nurse must always consider that drug therapies given to a patient with diabetes may be influenced by this pathology. Additionally, John's heart disease and hepatic function are directly related to cardiovascular function. When perfusion to the liver is less than optimal, it can disturb the hepatic metabolism of drugs and nutrients. Another consideration regarding metabolism involves his lifestyle and ultimately his hepatic function with his habitual use of alcohol. Chronic alcohol abuse is destructive to the liver.

2 The patient has preexisting kidney disease and requires renal dialysis. Pathologic states such as kidney disease can increase the duration and intensity of drug action when drugs are not excreted

as expected. The nurse must be particularly vigilant in monitoring the patient for signs of drug toxicity.

3 Both IV and inhalation routes of administration allow the drug to be immediately absorbed and circulated to the target organs. Therapeutic responses to drugs given by these routes are frequently rapid in onset, as are toxic effects. Although these are the preferred routes of administration for this patient, the nurse must not forget that the patient has other factors that will affect both the metabolism and excretion of these drugs.

4 When it is desirable to achieve the target plasma level rapidly, a loading dose (also known as a bolus dose) is necessary. This large dose of medication is used to achieve the therapeutic range quickly. Because the patient is critically ill, there is no time to wait several days for the drug level to reach a therapeutic range. He will be given maintenance doses to maintain a steady plasma level of the drug.

Additional Case Study

1 There is no way to memorize the half-lives of all drugs. However, this is important information that will guide the nurse in effectively managing the patient's drug therapy. Plasma half-life is the time it takes for half a given amount of a substance, such as a drug, to be removed from the blood plasma. Liver and kidney function may affect the half-life. Drugs with a short half-life leave the body quickly and require more frequent dosing intervals; drugs with long half-lives leave the body more slowly and present a greater risk for medication accumulation and toxicity.

2 The use of drugs with short half-lives is indicated with conditions or procedures that are brief in duration. Patients with chronic illness such as renal and hepatic disease may benefit from the use of drugs with shorter half-lives to prevent toxicities related to the existence of higher drug levels, but most need the benefits of a long half-life drug and the dosage may need to be adjusted.

3 Drugs with long half-lives are particularly useful when the maintenance of a constant and consistent level of a drug in the body is critical. Such conditions include hypertension and heart disease.

Chapter Review

1 Answer: 2 Rationale: Although taking a larger dose of a medication usually results in a greater therapeutic response, the response also depends on the drug's plasma concentration. If a toxic level is reached from too large a dose, the drug will have adverse effects instead of a better therapeutic response. Options 1, 3, and 4 are incorrect because they are true statements. The liquid form of a drug will be absorbed faster than its tablet form. Food decreases the absorption rate of most drugs. Patients should always consult a healthcare provider if unexpected adverse effects develop.

2 Answer: 1 Rationale: Infants do not develop a mature microsomal enzyme system until they are a year old and therefore do not metabolize drugs very efficiently. Options 2, 3, and 4 are incorrect. Pregnancy does not significantly affect drug metabolism. The concern with pregnant patients is primarily focused on alterations in distribution due to the fetal–placental barrier. The presence of kidney stones would not influence drug metabolism. Hypertension is not a factor that directly results in abnormal metabolism.

3 Answer: 3 Rationale: An increase in peristalsis would decrease the time that drugs would remain in the GI system and therefore decrease absorption. Options 1, 2, and 4 are incorrect. Excretion for most drugs occurs through the kidneys, lungs, and glands. Peristalsis would not reduce excretions of medications. A delay in peristalsis would prolong absorption time, and peristalsis is not involved in the distribution of drugs to their target sites.

4 Answer: 3 Rationale: Inhaled drugs produce an immediate therapeutic response. Options 1, 2, and 4 are incorrect. Most inhaled medication can be used at any time during the day. Doses for inhaled drugs are small compared to orally ingested medications, and because these drugs go directly to the lung surface area and are readily absorbed, very little of the substance is lost due to metabolism.

5 Answer: 4 Rationale: Patients with hepatic impairment do not effectively metabolize drugs, which increases the duration of action. Options 1, 2, and 3 are incorrect. In patients with hepatic disease, the duration of action most likely will increase since drug metabolism is impaired. Although the duration of action is extended, the effects of the drug are not improved.

6 Answer: 2, 4 Rationale: A therapeutic drug level that is in the acceptable range indicates that the drug is at a minimally effective concentration but not at a toxic level. Because each patient response to a drug is unique, the nurse should continue monitoring the patient throughout the drug's use. Options 1, 3, and 5 are incorrect. Because individual patient responses to drugs can he highly variable, adverse effects, toxicities or even no effect may occur at levels within the therapeutic range. For that reason, the dose may be adjusted throughout therapy.

Chapter 4

Making the Patient Connection

1 Potency refers to the amount of drug (usually expressed in milligrams) needed to produce an effect. Efficacy refers to the potential maximum therapeutic response that a drug can produce.

2 In most cases efficacy is more important than potency. When judging the relative merits of drugs for a patient, other factors should be considered, such as adverse effects, potential toxicity, duration of effect (which determines the number of doses needed each day), and cost.

3 Comparing drugs is not always a simple process. Generally, higher doses produce more intense adverse effects. However, when two drugs are compared, one cannot assume that the drug with the lower dose produces fewer adverse effects.

Additional Case Study

1 Most drugs work through a mechanism that is similar to a lock and key. Drugs interact with cellular receptors and bind to specific sites to produce actions. When drugs are manufactured, companies attempt to create a drug for a specific receptor that will produce a specific response. This is not always possible, however, because receptors are located everywhere in the body. Drugs without a specific receptor site produce more adverse effects than those with specific receptors.

2 Several factors produce variation in drug effects among people. Such factors include an individual's unique metabolism rate, age, weight, sex, and hereditary influences.

3 A drug that is an agonist is a drug that initiates activity in the cell and triggers a response. An antagonist acts to block a cellular response.

Chapter Review

1 Answer: 1, 2, 3, 5 Rationale: One of the critical determinants of the effectiveness of drug therapy is a physical examination. Nurses will utilize assessment skills to ascertain whether the drug is effective. A patient's vital signs may indicate the effectiveness of a drug such as a decrease in body temperature, a change in blood pressure and pulse, or improved respiratory status. The effects of

many drugs are monitored by diagnostic laboratory values such as white blood cell counts, cultures, and various electrolyte values. Efficacy describes the ability of a drug to produce the desired therapeutic effect. Option 4 is incorrect. The dosage time does not directly evaluate the effectiveness of drug therapy

2 Answer: 1 Rationale: Therapeutic index is the ratio between the therapeutic dose of a drug and the toxic dose and is used as a measure of the relative safety of the drug. The higher the therapeutic index, the safer the drug. Options 2, 3, and 4 are incorrect. A drug may be labeled dangerous for many reasons other than the therapeutic index, including potential for abuse. The higher the therapeutic index, the less risk of drug toxicity. A high degree of safety does not signify the degree of effectiveness.

3 Answer: 1 Rationale: A dose–response curve is a graphic representation that shows the relation between the amount of a drug administered and the extent of response it produces. Options 2, 3, and 4 are incorrect. A dose–response curve does not illustrate the toxic effects related to a drug or any specific population or graphically present the duration of action of a drug. Serum drug levels must be measured to determine the peak serum drug level. It is unique to each patient and the dose–response curve only represents a maximum (toxic) dose level.

4 Answer: 4 Rationale: The TD_{50} level measures the median toxicity dose. This information indicates the dose that will produce a given toxicity in 50% of a group of patients. Options 1, 2, and 3 are incorrect. Effectiveness, dose response, and receptor subtypes are not represented by the TD_{50} level.

5 Answer: 2 Rationale: Antagonists bind to receptors and block the effects of an endogenous chemical or another drug by competing with receptor binding sites or inhibiting the drug effect. As an antagonist, benztropine would block the effects of neostigmine and the neostigmine would exhibit a lesser effect. Options 1, 3, and 4 are incorrect. A drug that produces an effect after binding with a receptor is an agonist.

6 Answer: 1 Rationale: Potency is a reflection of a drug's ability to bind to a receptor. Options 2, 3, and 4 are incorrect. Efficacy and the affinity of a drug to bind to a receptor are separate variables from potency. Metabolism is a function of pharmacokinetics, not pharmacodynamics. First-pass effect is a phenomenon that occurs during enteral absorption and does not affect drug affinity.

Chapter 5

Making the Patient Connection

1 There are several steps a nurse can take to help Elizabeth minimize adverse drug effects. First, with the advent of computerized medical records, a summary list of multiple medical diagnoses and medications can be created. For institutions that still use paper documents, including clinics that treat lower-socioeconomic-status patients, the nurses in the clinic may consider proposing a "medical summary page" to be added to the medical record that could include medical diagnoses, hospital admissions, and prescribed drug therapies.

Second, Elizabeth should be advised to carry a list of her medications with her at all times. When patients are on multiple medications, it is easy to forget one or two when asked about drug therapies. Listing the purpose and dosage for each medication would also be helpful for Elizabeth and the healthcare provider. The nurse could assist Elizabeth if she is unable to do this herself or encourage her family's participation. The nurse should review the list with her each time she comes to the clinic.

Elizabeth should be taught to report any symptoms that "just don't feel right." In addition, the nurse should encourage Elizabeth to become more assertive when healthcare providers suggest a new drug. Assure Elizabeth that it is acceptable to question healthcare providers when it concerns her health and her drug therapy.

2 Several conditions make Elizabeth more susceptible to a drug reaction. The aging process makes the metabolism and excretion of drugs less predictable. Additionally, as the number of drugs a patient takes increases, the risk of adverse drug reactions increases. Alterations in pharmacokinetics will influence the reactions expected from a given drug. The speed of absorption of enteral drugs may enhance or reduce the effect of a drug. The distribution of a drug can be altered through modification in protein binding and may produce an unpredicted reaction. Elizabeth has also experienced a stroke, suggesting that vascular changes may be present that may affect the distribution of her medications or her hepatic and renal blood flow (thus metabolism and excretion).

3 Pharmacokinetics is the movement of drugs from the point of administration to the target cell. Drug reactions can affect each element of pharmacokinetics. Drug–drug reactions that increase or decrease gastric motility may influence the absorption time for enteral drugs. Examples include laxatives and antacids. Additionally, when drugs compete for binding ability to plasma proteins or change the pH of the plasma, drug distribution can be altered. Any drug-generated modification in hepatic enzymes has the ability to cause a drug–drug interaction. Lastly, if a drug changes the rate of renal filtration, a drug interaction may occur.

4 An additive effect occurs when two drugs from a similar therapeutic class generate a combined response. A synergistic effect is the interaction of two or more drugs so that their combined effect is greater than the sum of their individual effects. An antagonistic effect is described as the interaction of two or more drugs that produces a reduced pharmacologic response.

Additional Case Study

1 Patients are often confused when determining the difference between an adverse effect and a drug allergy. Ask the patient to describe the symptoms that occurred related to the medication and ask how the adverse symptoms were treated. It is questionable whether the patient received sufficient drug education or that she understood the possible adverse effects associated with this medication. Adverse effects from codeine almost always include nausea and sleepiness.

2 First, the term drug allergy (also known as hypersensitivity reaction) is a reaction that occurs due to an overactive response from the immune system. In an allergic response, the drug is recognized as the antigen and the body produces antibodies as a defense mechanism. Side effects are usually predictable and characterized by an unwanted effect produced by a medication. An adverse effect is an abnormal, often harmful, undesired, and unintended result of a drug. Adverse effects are not necessarily unexpected. Sometimes, the terms side effect and adverse effect are used interchangeably.

3 The patient is not experiencing an idiosyncratic reaction. This type of reaction is defined as an unusual or exaggerated reaction to a drug that is not caused by an allergy. Many of these responses are related to the genetic differences between individuals. Nausea and sleepiness are expected adverse (side) effects to codeine.

Chapter Review

1 Answer: 1 Rationale: Collecting additional information will provide the prescriber with knowledge about the type and severity of the reaction to that specific drug and will assist in determining the appropriateness of the order. Options 2, 3, and 4 are incorrect. The nurse should gather additional information from the patient before notifying the prescriber. A medication is never administered to a patient when allergic sensitivity is suspected

until investigation into the type and severity of the reaction has been completed. Although documentation of the event may be in the patient's medical record, the reaction may not have been documented or may have occurred after the last healthcare visit.

2 Answer: 1 Rationale: As the dose increases, the risk for adverse effects also increases. The patient should be closely observed for the onset of adverse effects whenever the dose of the drug is increased. Options 2, 3, and 4 are incorrect. Although adverse effects are sometimes noted after the first dose, they may occur at any time during drug administration. Although some adverse effects are common when a drug is given PO, others are more common when given by other routes, such as IV or IM. The timing of medication is not a factor associated with dose-related adverse effects.

3 Answer: 4 Rationale: Promoting adequate hydration may significantly reduce the risk of kidney damage produced by drug therapies. Options 1, 2, and 3 are incorrect. Avoiding direct sunlight is appropriate teaching to provide to patients receiving drugs that cause photosensitivity. The consumption of potassium-enriched foods will not reduce the risk of drug-induced nephrotoxicity, nor will avoiding alcohol consumption.

4 Answer: 3 Rationale: Urticaria or hives, with raised, itchy areas of skin, is often a sign of an allergic reaction. Options 1, 2, and 4 are incorrect. Angioedema is a notable swelling around the eyes and lips and sometimes of the hands and feet that occurs beneath the skin instead of on the surface. SJS is characterized by a flulike period of fever, sore throat, and headache followed by the sudden development of circular lesions that cover the majority of the skin. Photosensitivity occurs when a drug renders the skin susceptible to damage by sunlight.

5 Answer: 2 Rationale: The function of the bone marrow is to produce blood cells. When drugs cause bone marrow toxicity, the condition manifests as a decrease in all blood cell types. Options 1, 3, and 4 are incorrect. Muscle and bone pain are most often associated with muscle toxicity. Bone marrow toxicity is not related to a decline in an individual's range of motion. Liver enzymes are not typically affected by bone marrow toxicity.

6 Answer: 3 Rationale: The presence of right upper quadrant pain and anorexia are early symptoms often associated with drug-induced liver damage. Options 1, 2, and 4 are incorrect. Black, "furry" tongue or infections elsewhere are not related to liver damage. A sudden drop in BP is orthostatic hypotension. Unusual and uncontrolled movements are neurologic-related effects.

Chapter 6

Making the Patient Connection

1 All members of the healthcare team are responsible for safe medication administration. The nurse failed to follow the standard routines designed to safeguard a patient from medication errors. It is not unusual for patients to forget some part of their health history, and nurses must always consider that patient information may not always be totally accurate. The healthcare provider should have indicated the route of administration at the time the order was given, and the nurse failed to clarify the complete order before administration. Nurses should look up all unfamiliar drug orders in a pharmacology reference and consult the pharmacist if further clarification as to administration techniques is needed. When any one part of the normal routine for drug administration is overlooked, medication errors can occur, sometimes with disastrous consequences.

2 First, the nurse must always be certain that the route of administration is clearly specified and never assume to know the route or dose of a medication. Second, when unfamiliar with a drug, the nurse should look it up in a drug handbook. Doing so would have alerted the nurse to a typical dose, possible adverse reactions to monitor, and the dilution required by the drug. It is impossible to know everything about every drug. To ensure safety, the nurse must rely on quick resources, including consultation with the agency's pharmacist, to verify any unknowns. Lastly, reading a label or dilution guidelines is another step in the process of administration and must not be skipped.

3 A nurse can employ multiple strategies to decrease the chances a medication error will occur. The nurse always clarifies a medication order and never assumes dose or route. Drug references and the agency's pharmacist can be consulted. The nurse also learns to take into consideration environmental factors such as noise or the stress of an emergency situation and the impact they have on drug administration. In this scenario, the nurse may have been anxious about the stat order. Remember that *stat* means immediately but with all required procedures and caution included.

4 Healthcare facilities have taken multiple steps to reduce medication errors. In most hospitals, medications that require premixing or preparation are done within the hospital pharmacy. When this is not the case, the medication is packaged with the solution to be used for dilution. Regular updates and education by pharmacists, nurse educators, and unit staff can also assist all personnel involved in medication administration to prevent medication errors.

5 When a medication error occurs, the nurse and healthcare providers should follow the institution's protocol for reporting it. Because this is considered a sentinel event, The Joint Commission should be notified. Additionally, several other national and international reporting programs have been established to allow healthcare providers to report adverse drug reactions and medication errors. Reporting these medication-related problems helps to alert other providers of potential problems. The ISMP operates a confidential, national, voluntary medication error reporting program. To report a medication error, visit ISMP Medication Errors Reporting Program (MERP). The FDA also operates a program, called *MedWatch*, for reporting medication errors.

Additional Case Study

1 Administering medications to children can be frightening and should never be taken lightly. Chaanges associated with both pharmacokinetics and pharmacodynamics are influenced by children's physiologic growth and development. This scenario provides the nurse with an opportunity to develop rapport with the parent. The nurse can discuss the child's health problems and gather other pertinent information while the child is at school. Also, the nurse needs to determine exactly what this parent's concern is. Is it administration, adverse effects, or something else? As the nurse talks with this parent, specific concerns may be addressed.

2 Several strategies can help parents avoid medication errors. Parents should make sure:

- the child's healthcare provider knows the child's current weight and has a list of every prescription, OTC medicine, and dietary supplement the child is taking.
- the healthcare provider knows about any allergies and how the child reacts to medicines, including reactions that have occurred since the last healthcare visit.
- they can read the prescriptions written by the healthcare provider or ask the provider to read it to them.
- to ask for information about the child's medicines including questions about the directions on the child's medicine labels
- to ask the pharmacist for the best advice to measure the child's liquid medicine.
- to ask for written information about any adverse effects associated with the child's medicine.
- they know when to call the provider for any unusual reactions or concerns the parent may have.

3 Parents use many resources to gain information about medication for their children such as the internet, drug guides, and friends and family. These sources may or may not provide correct information. Parents should be encouraged to consult with the child's healthcare provider who is knowledgeable about the child's health status and any medications prescribed for the child.

Chapter Review

1 Answer: 4 Rationale: When medication orders are given via telephone, it is critical for the nurse to repeat the order verbatim to the prescriber. Options 1, 2, and 3 are incorrect. Whenever possible it is best for the prescriber to write an order for medication, but this is not always possible. It is correct for the nurse to attempt to comfort the patient using nursing interventions for pain. However, the nurse is required to consult the prescriber when a change in the patient's status occurs, regardless of the time. The nurse is responsible for contacting the prescriber and relaying clinical findings and assessment.

2 Answer: 1 Rationale: Whenever a medication order is unclear, the nurse should always contact the prescriber, and then have the order rewritten to prevent errors. Options 2, 3, and 4 are incorrect. Having another nurse read the order will not necessarily ensure that the dosage is correct. Whereas the pharmacist or a drug guide may provide the nurse with the usual dose for most patients, they do not take into consideration the patient's weight, disease condition, and other variables that influence the drug's pharmacokinetic and pharmacodynamic actions.

3 Answer: 2 Rationale: Pharmacies maintain records of medication dispensed to patients. If a pharmacist conducts a medication reconciliation by reviewing the patient's drug history on each subsequent visit, serious drug–drug interactions may be identified. Options 1, 3, and 4 are incorrect. Insisting on acquiring a trade-name drug rather than a generic does not ensure the safety of a medication. For safety reasons, drugs are dispensed in containers that are sometimes difficult to open. Unless there is a specific reason (such as impaired hand dexterity), medications should be stored in their original safety bottles. Information found on the internet may vary in quality and accuracy. When in doubt, the prescriber or pharmacist can provide the most accurate information about expected effects.

4 Answer: 3 Rationale: The nurse should always validate a questionable order when a patient verbalizes concern. Options 1, 2, and 4 are incorrect. Medications purchased by a clinical agency vary in appearance depending on the manufacturer. The nurse should withhold the medication and then confirm that it is the correct drug before administering. If a patient questions a change in medication or procedure, the nurse should verify the order and obtain validation from the prescriber.

5 Answer: 1 Rationale: The nurse's first priority is always the patient. The nurse should first assess the patient's baseline assessment data in order to determine if any adverse effects are occurring. Options 2, 3, and 4 are incorrect. The healthcare provider should be notified of the medication error; however, it is also important to report the patient's assessment data at the same time. All healthcare agencies have protocols for drug errors, and the nurse is responsible for completing this process after assessing the patient and notifying the provider. If the patient experiences an adverse reaction to the drug, further investigation is needed before confirming that the drug itself, rather than a patient variable (e.g., allergy), was behind the reaction before filing an Adverse Drug Reaction report (see Chapter 5).

6 Answer: 3 Rationale: Returning when the patient is available ensures that the patient takes the medication correctly and offers opportunity for the nurse to provide teaching related to the medication. Options 1, 2, and 4 are incorrect. A nurse must ensure that the patient takes the medication. By leaving the medication at the bedside or with visitors, the nurse will not know with certainty that the patient took the medication. When a patient refuses a medication, the nurse should document reasons for the refusal so that appropriate follow-up may be carried out. In this situation, the patient did not refuse the medication but was not available to take it at that moment.

Chapter 7

Making the Patient Connection

1 Ginkgo is reported to interact with anticoagulants. This supplement will increase the time required for coagulation and therefore place the patient at risk for bleeding. Although his vital signs do not indicate active bleeding, the bruises on his arms indicate that localized bleeding has occurred in the tissue.

2 Larry should stop taking the ginkgo immediately because further doses will exacerbate his potential for bleeding. Furthermore, the prescriber may inform the patient to temporarily stop taking the anticoagulant until the risk of hemorrhage subsides. Larry should also be informed not to take any OTC medications that will increase his risk for bleeding, such as aspirin and NSAIDs such as ibuprofen (Motrin, Advil).

3 Many complementary and alternative therapies, if used correctly, are considered safe products and are gaining in popularity. However, there are some risks involved in taking these preparations. Patients should be told that dietary supplements do not require testing prior to marketing and, additionally, safety does not need to be demonstrated by the manufacturer. Although dietary supplement labels must state that the product is not intended to diagnose, treat, cure, or prevent any disease, it is acceptable for the manufacturer to use statements such as "helps to promote a healthy immune system."

4 Larry's forgetfulness should not be minimized. Several abnormalities can contribute to changes in a patient's mental status including electrolyte disturbances, lack of mental stimulation, diet, and brain pathologies such as a microemboli from the episode of atrial fibrillation. Larry should receive a diagnostic evaluation to rule out physiologic reasons for his forgetfulness. There are also some psychosocial conditions that can influence a patient's cognitive ability. The nurse should assess the patient for sources of stress or anxiety. In either case, appropriate referral is critical to aid the patient with this problem.

Additional Case Study

1 OTC supplements are usually safe if used as directed on the instructions. However, if the patient has preexisting health problems or is taking other drugs, then OTC medications and herbal supplements can be potentially harmful. Nurses should teach patients to consult a healthcare professional before taking these products.

2 When a product is classified as "all natural," it usually implies that the substance is derived from or obtained from ingredients found in nature and is not synthetic or man-made. Just because a substance comes from a natural product, however, does not mean it is safe or effective.

3 The role of the nurse is to be sensitive to the patient's need for alternative treatment. Presenting a judgmental attitude about a patient's health practices will reduce open and honest communication. The nurse can provide the patient with information about the advantages and the limitations of complementary and alternative methods so the patient can make rational and informed decisions about treatment choices.

Chapter Review

1 Answer: 1 Rationale: Although CAM therapies have been used for thousands of years, most of these substances lack adequate scientific clinical studies to verify their effectiveness. Most healthcare providers are hesitant to recommend a substance that has questionable effectiveness. Options 2, 3, and 4 are incorrect. CAM has a rich history of use over thousands of years in treating certain conditions. To imply that all alternative therapies are nothing more than fable is incorrect. There is no evidence that response to CAM therapies is related to the placebo effect. In many cases the CAM therapy may be less expensive than prescription medications.

2 Answer: 3 Rationale: It is best to advise the patient to take small amounts of a new supplement to determine any initial intolerance or allergy. Options 1, 2, and 4 are incorrect. Doubling dosages can be extremely dangerous and is seldom, if ever, advisable. There is no indication that fluid intake should be reduced with echinacea. Allergic reactions are possible with natural supplements. Patients should be taught to read the label carefully and avoid any supplement that contains any known allergy-provoking substances.

3 Answer: 1 Rationale: Older adults with hepatic disease are at higher risk of developing serious drug reactions when taking dietary supplements. Options 2, 3, and 4 are incorrect. Patients with cardiac irregularities, pneumonia, or acne may require traditional medications and should be encouraged to consult their healthcare provider. If the patient prefers to use CAM, this can also be discussed with the provider at the time of the healthcare visit.

4 Answer: 1, 2, 3, 5 Rationale: Dietary supplements can be found in almost every supermarket, pharmacy, and health food store. Due to aggressive marketing, herbal supplements are also extremely popular. Most dietary supplements are less expensive than prescribed medications and are therefore more appealing to individuals for whom cost is a critical issue. Older patients may also seek therapeutic alternatives for chronic health conditions. Option 4 is incorrect. Natural substances are not necessarily safer than synthetic products and do not undergo the same rigorous testing as synthetic products.

5 Answer: 1 Rationale: The USP-verified dietary supplement mark is awarded to dietary supplements that pass verification processes. The mark represents that USP has tested the supplement to verify that the label accurately reflects the product in the bottle and that the supplement does not contain harmful levels of contaminants. Options 2, 3, and 4 are incorrect. A DEA number is assigned to a healthcare provider and allows him or her to write prescriptions for controlled substances. The FDA does not control herbal supplements and this code does not exist. U.S. Customs is not responsible for ensuring that herbal supplements are pure.

6 Answer: 4 Rationale: Changes in liver or kidney function in the older adult may lead to changes in metabolism or excretion for herbal as well as synthetic medications. Options 1, 2, and 3 are incorrect. Older adults are no more likely to have difficulty taking herbal medications or to spend more money on these products than the younger adults. These difficulties are patient specific at any age. Due to aggressive marketing by the herbal and dietary supplement industry, all age groups are as likely to hold unrealistic expectations for herbal products.

Chapter 8

Making the Patient Connection

1 Once it has been established that May is indeed pregnant, the nurse's first task is to talk with her about the pregnancy and any concerns she may have. She may be very happy, ambivalent, or not wish to continue the pregnancy. If May plans to continue the pregnancy, then the nurse should consider the antiseizure medications or any other medications she may be taking, including the herbal products she has mentioned. A thorough drug history should be taken at this time if it was not included in an earlier assessment. The provider will use the information to assist in determining if the benefits of taking the drug justify the risks to the fetus and to consider alternative strategies.

2 At this early stage of pregnancy, the nurse would provide May with the necessary prenatal teaching regarding caring for herself and her baby during pregnancy. She should be taught to avoid all medications and herbal supplements unless prescribed by the healthcare provider and to discuss any concerns with her provider regarding her current medications. Once the nurse has established a rapport with May, a discussion about the effects that smoking and illicit drug or alcohol use have on the developing baby should occur; if necessary, strategies to help her avoid these substances should be developed. If May requires any medications during her pregnancy, the healthcare provider will make any adjustments necessary so that the effects on the developing baby are minimized as much as possible. The nurse would teach May that it is important that she continue with the prescribed drug regimen as directed by her provider to keep her and the developing baby healthy.

3 Although the FDA no longer uses the pregnancy categories A, B, C, D, and X, the manufacturer is still required to supply data regarding the risks of each medication during pregnancy, labor, delivery and lactation. Also included are recommendations regarding effects of the drug on fertility, pregnancy testing and the use of contraception while taking the drug. The healthcare provider needs to share this information, in terms the patient can understand.

4 Nicotine and smoking may double the risk of having a low-birth-weight baby. Low birth weight can result from poor growth before birth, preterm delivery, or a combination of both. The American Congress of Obstetricians and Gynecologists (ACOG) recommends that healthcare providers counsel their pregnant patients on smoking-cessation techniques. Many women convert to nicotine replacement therapy (NRT) during pregnancy. The safety and efficacy of NRT during pregnancy have not been established. Therefore, ACOG's position is that NRT should only be used under the close supervision of a healthcare provider.

Additional Case Study

1, 2 The nurse would explain to Irina the effects that using illicit drugs while breastfeeding can have on the baby and help her develop strategies for managing her stress, anxiety, or depression. Irina may need to obtain a referral to other healthcare professionals such as a mental health counselor to deal with her depression. Because marijuana enters breast milk, it may cause her baby to become sleepy and unable to take in an adequate amount of milk. Insufficient nutrition may alter its growth and development. The nurse will be concerned for both mother and baby and will consider the needs of both when planning teaching and interventions.

3 The most common antidepressants, the selective serotonin reuptake inhibitors, have been shown to increase the risk of preterm labor and may cause withdrawal symptoms in newborns that include agitation, irritability, trouble feeding, sleep disturbances, and convulsions. Additionally, there is evidence linking SSRI usage, especially in the third trimester, with an increased risk of neonatal persistent pulmonary. Healthcare providers have been advised to taper dosages of SSRIs during the third trimester so that the fetus receives no drug through the placenta for at least 7 to 10 days prior to birth.

Chapter Review

1 Answer: 2 Rationale: It is recommended that all drugs be avoided as much as possible during pregnancy due to the potential effect on the fetus or infant. Options 1, 3, and 4 are incorrect. Drugs that are available OTC may also be hazardous and may affect the unborn fetus and nursing infant. Drugs used for treating medical conditions such as asthma, hypertension, diabetes, and epilepsy should be continued throughout pregnancy after review by the healthcare provider for the safety of both mother and infant. In such cases the benefits may justify the risks. The woman should consult with her healthcare provider regarding any drugs taken during pregnancy and lactation.

2 Answer: 2, 3, 4 Rationale: The Pregnancy and Lactation Labeling Rule (PLLR) updated the information about drugs used in pregnancy and lactation to include information about risks to the expectant mother and fetus, possible drug effects in the breastfed infant, and information about pregnancy testing, birth control, and a medication's effect on fertility. Options 1 and 5 are incorrect. The former alphabetical pregnancy risk categories are no longer used. The new PLLR does not include lists of "safe" drugs and each drug carries a safety profile during pregnancy and lactation.

3 Answer: 1 Rationale: Although multiple factors affect the transfer of drugs across the placenta, highly lipid-soluble drugs will cross the placenta more easily than water-soluble drugs. Options 2, 3, and 4 are incorrect. Small molecules such as alcohol easily cross the placenta, whereas larger molecules are slower to cross. When drugs are highly protein bound, they are too large to cross the placental membrane.

4 Answer: 1 Rationale: Weeks 1–2 of the first trimester is the preimplantation phase. Before implantation, the developing embryo has not yet established a blood supply with the mother. This is sometimes called the "all-or-none" period because exposure to a teratogen either causes death of the embryo or has no effect. Drugs are less likely to cause congenital malformations during this period because the baby's organ systems have not yet begun to form. Options 2, 3, and 4 are incorrect because the embryonic period is 3 to 8 weeks postconception. During the embryonic period there is rapid development of internal structures and maximum sensitivity to teratogens. Teratogenic agents taken during this phase can lead to structural malformation and spontaneous abortion. The specific abnormality depends on which organ is forming at the time of exposure.

5 Answer: 1, 3, 4, and 5 Rationale: OTC drugs are generally safe when taken as directed but any drug taken by the mother should be discussed with the healthcare provider first. Lowering the dose will not alter the safety profile of an unsafe OTC drug. Medications are found in breast milk and may be ingested by the infant. The provider will review any prescription medications the mother is taking and will plan for alternatives if any are unsafe during breastfeeding. The form of the medication does not affect the passage of the drug into the breast milk. Option 2 is incorrect. It is true that the higher the dose, the more likely it is that the drug will enter the breast milk and the patient has understood that part of the teaching.

6 Answer: 3 Rationale: Increased levels of progesterone cause a decrease in gastric tone and intestinal motility, resulting in delayed gastric emptying. This leads to extended time for drug absorption. Options 1, 2, and 4 are incorrect. Medications may take a longer time to be absorbed and distributed, thus delaying their onset and prolonging their duration of action. Due to the changes in body fluid volume associated with pregnancy, there is greater hemodilution, not hemoconcentration, of drugs. Of all pharmacokinetic factors, drug metabolism is least affected by pregnancy.

Chapter 9

Patient Safety: This case provides an example of a "tenfold error" caused by misinterpretation of the location of a decimal point. On reviewing the chart, the nurse noted that the original order was written as "15.0 mg/kg/day" and that the decimal point had been omitted during transcription and processing. To avoid such tenfold errors, the use of "trailing zeroes," zeroes placed after the whole number, should be avoided and, ideally, computerized order entry rather than handwritten orders should be encouraged.

Making the Patient Connection

1 An infant's fluid and electrolyte balance is easily altered by vomiting and diarrhea. An infant has a very high percentage (80%) of total body fluid compared to mass. Compared to adults, who have a 6% water turnover daily, infants lose and replace up to 25% of their total body water over a period of 24 hours. When an infant stops taking in fluids over a 48-hour period, and is also experiencing diarrhea, the potential for severe dehydration is very high. Also, the infant has a high metabolic rate, which causes increased water loss. Another reason for fluid and electrolyte imbalance is the fact that the infant's immature renal system prevents concentration and retention of fluid.

2 When the body is no longer able to compensate for fluid loss, the total circulating volume is diminished, and peripheral vessels constrict. When assessing the dehydrated infant, you will expect to find weak to absent peripheral pulses, slow capillary filling, mottled skin color, tenting of the skin when pinched between the thumb and forefinger, rapid respiration, depressed anterior fontanel, and dry sunken eyes. The temperature increase to 39.1°C (102.4°F) may also be a sign of dehydration because less body water is present to cool the body even though the metabolic rate is increased.

3 Acute gastroenteritis is usually attributed to viral infections. The virus alters the balance of fluid and electrolytes in the bowels, causing stool and water loss. This patient was being treated with an oral antibiotic for an ear infection. It is possible that the antibiotic could have caused the diarrhea.

4 Inserting and maintaining an IV line on an infant can be challenging. The nurse must accurately calculate the volume of fluid the child needs and set the rate of flow accordingly on the infusion pump. Tiny veins are sometimes hard to find under normal circumstances, and when the patient is dehydrated, it can be even more difficult. Choosing a site that can be stabilized, easily observed, and does not restrict the infant's movement is of utmost importance. The nurse would choose superficial veins of the hand, forearm, foot, or ankle. In the infant a 22-gauge needle is usually appropriate but the nurse will choose the smallest gauge and shortest length catheter that can deliver the prescribed fluid and medication. The IV site must be monitored at least every 15 minutes for redness, swelling, and discoloration. The IV should be removed if there is a doubt about its patency.

Additional Case Study

1 The first nursing action is to render emergency airway care to ensure proper breathing. This includes placing the patient in a sitting position to maintain an open airway and administering oxygen as needed.

2 The nurse would next carry out a full assessment of vital signs including temperature, pulse, respiration, blood pressure, and chest examination for cardiopulmonary status. Vital signs most likely will be elevated with hyperresonance present over the lung fields.

3 The expected outcome of treatment for status asthmaticus is that the patient will have improved ventilation and respiratory status with vital signs within the normal expected range.

Chapter Review

1 Answer: 1, 3 Rationale: In young children, delayed gastric emptying causes oral medications to remain in the stomach longer, resulting in slowed absorption and an increased risk for adverse drug reactions. Between age 3 and 5, the liver's metabolic rate reaches adult levels. Before age 5, extra caution and dosage adjustments may be required, particularly for drugs that are metabolized primarily in the liver. Options 2, 4, and 5 are incorrect. Before 6 months of age, there are very small amounts of plasma proteins, and drugs that are normally protein bound remain as free drugs, increasing drug distribution and increasing the risk for adverse effects. Drug excretion through the kidneys increases with age, and standard pediatric doses may be used between 3 and 5 months of age. Cautious monitoring should be continued even after this age, especially with nephrotoxic drugs . The blood–brain barrier is not well developed at birth and drugs can easily penetrate the CNS, causing heightened effects.

2 Answer: 1 Rationale: The poison control center will have an exact plan of action for this child. Options 2, 3, and 4 are incorrect. Whenever poisoning is suspected, the poison control center and the 911 EMS system should be called immediately. Treatment should begin as soon as possible. Waiting to observe the child for symptoms or driving the child to the hospital, delays appropriate treatment. Syrup of ipecac is not to be used, especially in cases where a caustic substance is suspected, because it may increase damage or lead to aspiration.

3 Answer: 1 Rationale: IM injections in infants are absorbed slowly due to low blood flow to skeletal muscles. Options 2, 3, and 4 are incorrect because children experience delayed absorption and distribution of IM drugs and IM medications may be absorbed slowly and erratically in children. Children have very weak muscle contractions that contribute to this delayed absorption and distribution.

4 Answer: 3 Rationale: Giving the patient a choice of liquid with which to combine the medicine will give the child a feeling of control and independence and at the same time encourage cooperation. Options 1, 2, and 4 are incorrect. At age 3 years the child does not yet associate medicine with getting better. Threatening patients to get them to take medicine is never appropriate. Three-year-olds do not imitate actions unless they want to, and saying that a roommate took the medicine may not result in the child doing the same.

5 Answer: 3 Rationale: Two or more drugs with extensive protein binding compete for binding sites, resulting in increased absorption and high potential for drug interactions. Options 1, 2, and 4 are incorrect. Low-potency drugs, drugs with a wide therapeutic index, and drugs applied to the skin are at low risk for drug interactions.

6 Answer: 1 Rationale: Children and their parents are most likely to adhere if their medication regimen is simple and inexpensive. Options 2, 3, and 4 are incorrect. Patients are less likely to adhere to the regimen if the medications are costly, they have to be taken over an extended period of time, or they have to be taken at varying times during the day.

Chapter 10

Making the Patient Connection

1 Older adults are at increased risk for dehydration because of age-related physiologic changes, including altered thirst perception, reduced total body water, increased proportion of fat to muscle, impaired renal conservation of water, and increased prevalence of multiple chronic diseases. Mary Smith's risk factors for dehydration are that she is functionally independent; has poor fluid and nutritional intake; is taking a diuretic (hydrocholorothiazide), which will increase fluid loss; and has a fever. Her depression could be related to her inability to fully care for herself and neglect of her fluid intake.

2 The nurse will focus on providing frequent reassurance and reorienting the patient to her surroundings; maintaining patient safety; administering the rehydration fluid as ordered; and continuing to assess the patient's level of dehydration. Mary is mildly confused and may need frequent reminders of place and time. The nurse would also ensure that all safety precautions are taken and arrange for directly observed therapy if the neighbor is unable to stay at the patient's bedside. Vital signs should be monitored frequently during rehydration and urine output, and color and consistency should be assessed hourly. The use of urinary catheters is discouraged to avoid infection risk. The nurse would arrange for toileting facilities (e.g., bedside commode or bedpan) so that the patient does not try to ambulate without assistance. The IV site should also be frequently monitored for extravasation.

3 A complete physical assessment including temperature, pulse, respiration (TPR), and blood pressure should be obtained. Altered TPR readings may indicate hyperthermia due to dehydration or infection, tachycardia due to hypovolemia, and tachypnea secondary to acidosis. The condition of the skin may reveal tenting secondary to severe dehydration. There may be hypotension secondary to both hypovolemia related to lack of oral intake or increased fluid loss due to diuretic use or response to the antihypertensive drug atenolol. Altered mental status or confusion should be assessed frequently and may be unrelated to the dehydration. Chronic dehydration may also be manifested by urinary tract infections, respiratory infections, and constipation.

4 Expected patient outcomes include an increase in urine output and decreased urine concentration as evidenced by clear, light yellow-amber urine with urine specific gravity within normal limits (1.005 to 1.025); improved skin turgor without evidence of tenting; an increase in mentation and alertness; decreased pulse rate and increased BP; and moist mucous membranes of the oral cavity and eyes.

Additional Case Study

1 The nurse would ask Ms. Haynes if she has been taking her medication and if she has any concerns about the drugs. If Ms. Haynes has been keeping a diary account of her fingerstick blood glucose levels and her blood pressure, the nurse should also review these records to determine whether the information suggests Ms. Haynes has been adhering to her medications. If she has not been keeping records, an easy-to-follow plan should be implemented to help her record this information. Ms. Haynes should be encouraged to record her glucose level right before going to the group dining hall and her blood pressure before eating in the mornings. Because Ms. Haynes is extremely independent, asking her input into which strategies would work best for her may have the best outcomes. A hemoglobin A1C should be drawn. Hemoglobin A1C provides an average blood sugar control over the past 2 to 3 months and is used along with home blood sugar monitoring to assess glucose control.

2 If Ms. Haynes has not been taking her medications, a thorough assessment of possible reasons should be evaluated. Is she just forgetting the medications or deliberately not taking them? Are there any signs of forgetfulness or confusion? Does Ms. Haynes express concern about side or adverse effects and their impact on her ADLs? Are there cost concerns? Investigating the reasons for nonadherence will help in planning strategies to help Ms. Haynes take her medications.

3 Depending on the outcomes of the assessment from question 2, the nurse would discuss her findings with Ms. Haynes's daughter and include the patient in developing joint strategies with her daughter. Perhaps her daughter could check with her mother in the evening and Ms. Haynes could report on her day, her blood

sugar and blood pressure, and whether she had any difficulty taking her medication. A personalized medication record could be established so that she could record her medications and any symptoms she has, along with questions to ask the healthcare provider. Her daughter could review it with her mother during each visit. Maintaining Ms. Haynes's level of independence is important, and the best strategies will be the ones that are mutually derived among the patient, nurse, caregivers, and the patient's daughter.

Chapter Review

1 Answer: 1, 2 Rationale: Increased gastric pH is a common physiological condition of aging that can affect absorption by increasing the time it takes for oral medications to dissolve. Decreased blood flow to the GI tract decreases the amount of absorption as well as distribution. Options 3, 4, and 5 are incorrect. GI motility slows in the older adult and increased body surface area does not directly impact the area of absorption of oral drugs. The older adult may have decreased cardiac output, but this will not affect the absorption of a drug.

2 Answer: 2 Rationale: A patient who is functioning independently in all ADLs should be encouraged to take full responsibility for self-administering medications. Options 1, 3, and 4 are incorrect. Teaching the daughter to administer the insulin may become an option if the patient does not want to or cannot self-administer the drug, but that is not noted at this time. There is no reason for recommending a home health aide if the patient is competent in self-administering. Since the provider's original order was to treat the patient's condition with insulin, there may be a reason that an oral antidiabetic medication is not appropriate for this patient.

3 Answer: 2 Rationale: In the older adult, kidney blood flow decreases and excretion of drugs also decreases, requiring dosage or frequency adjustments for many drugs. Options 1, 3, and 4 are incorrect. Total body fat increases rather than decreases, which may increase storage of fat-soluble drugs. Liver function declines and the amount of plasma proteins decreases. There is a decrease in total body water, and water-soluble drug concentration may increase.

4 Answer: 1, 2, 3 Rationale: Excessive prescribing, multiple drug therapy, and increased drug sensitivity are all reasons for adverse effects in older adults. As a person ages, renal function decreases, leading to alterations in pharmacokinetics and pharmacodynamics. Coupled with multiple drug therapy and increased sensitivity, it is not unusual for adverse effects to develop. Options 4 and 5 are incorrect. Body mass decreases as age increases. Exercise engagement does not influence the frequency of adverse effects.

5 Answer: 2 Rationale: Thirty-one percent of older adult patients report that they did not take their medication because they did not have it on hand when it was time to take it. Options 1, 3, and 4 are incorrect. These are other reasons cited for nonadherence, but they are not the most frequently cited answer.

6 Answer: 1 Rationale: Making the statement "It doesn't matter if the medication works as long as the doctor prescribed it" indicates that the patient is not aware of how to monitor the drug's effectiveness or for its adverse effects, and more teaching is required. Options 2, 3, and 4 are positive responses by the patient that indicate that teaching has been effective toward increasing the potential for adherence.

Chapter 11

Making the Patient Connection

1 It is critical for nurses to strive to understand their patients' cultural beliefs about health and the attainment of wellness. Nurses must remain nonjudgmental about cultural practices that may seem different or unusual from their own. Open communication will establish a rapport with the patient and will allow the nurse to better understand the patient's beliefs and practices. If patients experience prejudicial responses from healthcare providers, they are likely to be selective in what they are willing to talk about, resulting in an increased risk of potentially harmful drug interactions between conventional and nonconventional healthcare practices.

2 Most patients are willing to share cultural beliefs and practices. Often the nurse can engage the patient in casual conversation, which may reveal valuable information. In addition, reference materials found in libraries and on the internet may also provide further information about specific cultural beliefs or practices.

3 It is impossible for healthcare providers to totally understand all cultures. Cultural competence is an ongoing process for all healthcare providers. Healthcare providers who support holistic health will clearly understand and respect the cultural differences of their patients. As providers, the opportunity to work with a variety of patients from all cultures increases this competence and a willingness to be open to learning about other cultures will foster increased understanding.

Additional Case Study

1 Caring for her diabetes adequately will be a challenge and Marjorie can benefit from assistance by the nurse. The nurse's critical roles are to provide the patient with health information, to connect her to community resources, and to monitor her ability to manage her condition. Without this support, it is unlikely that she will be capable of managing a chronic disease such as diabetes.

2 Multiple psychosocial factors will influence the patient's ability to care for herself. Being a single mother of three children is a critical factor in this case. Marjorie may be more likely to neglect her own care as she struggles to meet the demands of three small children. Her limited income may also prevent her from purchasing needed supplies and medications that she needs to manage her diabetes. Limited education is also a strong indicator of one's ability to manage chronic disease conditions. Lastly, fear is a psychologic factor that will influence the pharmacologic treatment of her disease.

3 Self-care of a chronic illness is difficult, especially when the patient believes that he or she is dealing with the disease alone. Establishing a therapeutic nurse and patient rapport will be one of the most important components of this patient's care. The nurse can serve a pivotal role in helping the patient understand how to live effectively with diabetes. The nurse should ensure that this patient has been referred to other healthcare providers (such as a dietitian and medical social worker) who can be helpful in securing needed community resources.

Chapter Review

1 Answer: 2 Rationale: The statement reflects an attempt to understand the patient holistically. The nurse understands that multiple contributing factors may contribute to illness and involving the patient helps elicit possible factors. Options 1, 3, and 4 are incorrect. Tylenol should not be recommended initially because it may not address the possible causative factors related to the headaches. Monitoring the patient's pupil response to light, although eventually appropriate, should not be performed initially. An ophthalmology referral should be done after ruling out other possible sources of the headaches.

2 Answer: 3 Rationale: Factors associated with a drug's expense and the patient's ability to purchase are psychosocial variables that may influence adherence to drug therapy. Options

1, 2, and 4 are incorrect. Unpleasant taste or medications that are difficult to swallow may hinder patient adherence; however, the problem is physiological rather than psychosocial. Liver damage (hepatotoxicity) is also a physiological factor.

3 Answer: 2 Rationale: Cultural beliefs refer to the cumulative ideas of knowledge, experiences, values, attitudes, meanings, and roles acquired by a group of people. A preference for traditional healers, such as a Shaman, reflects these beliefs. Options 1, 3, and 4 are incorrect. Ethnicity is a population of human beings whose members identify with each other either on the basis of common genealogy or ancestry. Genetic polymorphisms are changes in enzyme structure and DNA function that occur within a specific subset of the population. A health-related bias is a prejudice for one particular point of view and is not specifically culturally related.

4 Answer: 1 Rationale: Patients who are known to have the genetic variant affecting acetyltransferase are known as slow acetylators and have reduced hepatic metabolism of many drugs. These patients have a greater potential for drug toxicity. Options 2, 3, and 4 are incorrect. Acetylation is a metabolic process that does not influence absorption. The route or form of administration is not associated with acetylation, and protein intake does not affect the rate of acetylation.

5 Answer: 1, 2, 3, 4 Rationale: All of these factors—fat-to-muscle ratio, cerebral blood flow, limited drug research on women, and health beliefs—may be considered gender factors that influence pharmacotherapy. Option 5 is incorrect. Dietary considerations are a potential cultural consideration.

6 Answer: 4 Rationale: Drug response is unique to each individual. The nurse should observe the responses and exercise caution with all medications. Options 1, 2, and 3 are incorrect. Patient self-report may not be a reliable method, and the patient may not have taken a particular drug before. Learning more about genetic effects on pharmacotherapy is important, but each patient response is unique. Other patients' responses to a drug will not help predict the response in another patient and there are wide genetic variations, even within ethnic or cultural groups.

Chapter 13

Connections to Practice

1 The nurse should inform Patricia that it is common to experience some urinary retention after surgery, and the drug she has been prescribed will assist her in returning to normal voiding patterns. Instruct her to take the medication 1 hour before or 2 hours after meals to avoid nausea and vomiting. Dizziness, lightheadedness, or fainting may occur with bethanechol, especially when rising from a lying or sitting position. Patients receiving this medication should be instructed to rise gradually from a lying or sitting position to standing, not to drive or engage in activities that require alertness until the effects of this drug have been determined, and to be cautious in low-light conditions. The nurse would also want to explore Patricia's home situation, whether a caregiver is available to assist her, and whether any home modifications (e.g., safety hazards that may cause tripping or falls) should be made. If she experiences difficult breathing, chest tightness, or pain, she should immediately contact her healthcare provider.

2 Patricia may be assisted in remembering to take her medication by providing the following tips:

- Place your medication next to something you use frequently. It is not recommended to keep medication at the bedside because additional doses may be taken when drowsy and lead to overdosage.
- Post reminder notes on the refrigerator or the bathroom mirror.
- Take the medication the same time every day.
- Set an alarm clock, watch, or cell phone alarm to notify you when it is time to take the medication.
- Keep a medication diary or checklist of when you have taken your pills each day
- Carry medication in your purse or pocket if you leave your house.
- If you miss a dose, take the missed dose as soon as you remember it. However, if it is almost time for the next dose, skip the missed dose and continue your regular dosing schedule. Do not take a double dose to make up for a missed one.

3 B bethanechol is being prescribed to relieve urinary retention. Continue to monitor the patient's voiding patterns to determine the drug effectiveness. If the therapy is not effective, the patient may complain of a sensation of being unable to empty the bladder even though she feels a strong urge to urinate. Additionally, many people with acute urinary retention feel pain in the lower abdomen or experience a small amount of urine leaking out of the bladder. If urinary retention is allowed to continue, Patricia may demonstrate symptoms of urinary tract infection, which include back pain, fever, and painful urination.

Additional Case Study

1 Although nicotine replacement therapy will reduce the physical dependence on nicotine, it does not eliminate the psychologic dependence. Successful smoking cessation is often dependent on additional assistance such as behavior modification and support groups.

2 Helpful websites include the following: How to Quit—Quit Tips—sponsored by the Centers for Disease Control and Prevention (https://www.cdc.gov/tobacco/quit_smoking/how_to_quit/index.htm) and Smoking Cessation Support—sponsored by the American Lung Association (https://www.lung.org/quit-smoking/i-want-to-quit/how-to-quit-smoking).

Chapter Review

1 Answer: 1 Rationale: Muscarinic agonists may cause reflex tachycardia, which is precipitated by a drop in the patient's blood pressure. When this occurs, the baroreceptors recognize the decline in pressure and alert the medulla to increase the heart rate as a compensatory mechanism. Options 2, 3, and 4 are incorrect. Although the heart rate increases, muscarinic agonists do not directly affect the sinoatrial node. Hypertension is not a problem with this drug therapy; however, hypotension may occur. Muscarinic agents stimulate bronchial smooth muscles; however, this does not impact the heart rate.

2 Answer: 3 Rationale: Pyridostigmine is used primarily for myasthenia gravis, a neurologic disorder characterized by muscle weakness and ptosis. A decrease in these symptoms is an expected therapeutic outcome for this drug. Options 1, 2, and 4 are incorrect because the symptoms listed are not usual problems faced by the patient with myasthenia gravis and would therefore be inappropriate outcome statements.

3 Answer: 4 Rationale: Bethanechol acts on the muscles needed for urination by increasing ureteral peristalsis and promoting urinary bladder elimination. Options 1, 2, and 3 are incorrect. Bethanechol does not cause changes to urinary structures, nor does it increase urine production or renal blood flow.

4 Answer: 1, 2, 3, 5 Rationale: Common adverse effects of bethanechol include abdominal discomfort, sweating, flushed skin, and blurred vision. Option 4 is incorrect because bethanechol increases GI peristalsis and promotes bowel evacuation.

5 Answer: 3 Rationale: Because of the potential for bronchoconstriction, patients with COPD should be treated cautiously

with cholinergic agonists. Options 1, 2, and 4 are incorrect. Neostigmine is used to reduce postoperative abdominal distention. Urinary retention may also be relieved with the administration of neostigmine. Neostigmine may be used to reverse the effects of nondepolarizing muscle relaxants.

6 Answer: 4 Rationale: Symptoms of a cholinergic crisis include tachycardia, hyperglycemia, and muscle weakness progressing to paralysis, which may require intubation and mechanical ventilation if profound. Options 1, 2, and 3 are incorrect. Nausea and vomiting, miosis, drooling, and involuntary muscle twitching are common adverse effects and may be treated with atropine. Atropine is the antidote for cholinergic crisis.

Chapter 14

Patient Safety: The PACU nurse can decrease the chance of medication errors by thoroughly reviewing the patient's chart before transfer to a surgical unit. A process known as a *discharge time-out* may also be used where one nurse compares the medications ordered with the electronic medical record while a second nurse compares the medications against the admission record. At a minimum, a review of the medication information should include the admission record and list of home medications, medication administration record from any previous inpatient unit, and a review of postoperative orders compared to preoperative orders to note any omissions of previously ordered medications or for appropriateness (e.g., antihypertensives if blood pressure is low). This information should be communicated clearly to the nurse on the receiving unit and any omissions noted for further follow-up. The use of written checklists so that all information is reviewed and no information is omitted is also recommended.

Making the Patient Connection

1 Atropine blocks acetylcholine effects on cholinergic receptors in smooth muscle, cardiac muscle, exocrine glands, urinary bladder, and the sinoatrial and atrioventricular nodes of the heart. Due to its diverse action, atropine has multiple uses that include certain types of bradycardia, spastic disorders of the GI system, and ophthalmic examinations.

2 In Pete's case, the adverse effect of atropine (suppression of exocrine secretions) becomes a therapeutic effect. Atropine is useful in controlling the copious secretions associated with organophosphate poisoning.

3 As the nurse, you would anticipate that Pete will probably experience dry mouth, constipation, urinary retention, increased heart rate, and blurred vision.

Additional Case Study

1 Neuromuscular blocking agents are drugs that interfere with the neural transmission between motor neurons and skeletal muscles. These drugs produce paralysis of all muscles, including those used for breathing.

2 Neuromuscular blocking agents such as succinylcholine are sometimes used during short medical–surgical procedures. Frequently, when patients are placed on a mechanical ventilator, a neuromuscular drug is given to paralyze the patient during the procedure of inserting the endotracheal tube.

3 The major problem associated with these drugs is their effect on the respiratory system. Patients will be unable to maintain their own respirations due to the paralysis. The nurse will closely monitor the patient for the absence of respirations and assist the patient mechanically, if necessary. Emergency equipment should be in close proximity. Another associated problem with the administration of neuromuscular blocking agents is that these drugs do not produce a decrease in the patient's level of consciousness. Although paralyzed, patients are very aware of their surroundings. An important nursing consideration is communication. Nurses should continue to communicate with the patient by reassuring the patient while in the paralyzed state.

Chapetr Review

1 Answer: 2 Rationale: Anticholinergic drugs such as tolterodine can cause constipation by slowing GI motility. Therefore, increases in dietary fiber and water intake will help avoid constipation. Options 1, 3, and 4 are incorrect. Daily exercise helps in avoiding muscle atrophy and anticholinergic drugs are not related to muscle atrophy. Consuming foods high in iron to increase red blood cell production is not related to the effects of anticholinergic drugs. Anticholinergic drugs cause tachycardia, not bradycardia.

2 Answer: 1, 2, 3, 4 Rationale: These drugs cause mydriasis and paralysis of the ciliary muscle, which is useful in ophthalmic examinations. These drugs are therapeutic in correcting cardiac rhythm abnormalities such as bradycardia. Muscarinic antagonists, most notably ipratropium and tiotropium, are useful in treating asthma due to their ability to dilate the bronchi. These drugs are used to reverse the symptoms of overdose of organophosphate insecticides. Option 5 is incorrect. Urinary retention is an adverse effect of these drugs.

3 Answer: 2 Rationale: Atropine can worsen urinary retention in patients with BPH. Options 1, 3, and 4 are incorrect because these are not contraindications for using atropine.

4 Answer: 1 Rationale: Muscarinic drugs affect intraocular pressure by causing mydriasis and paralysis of the ciliary muscle. Options 2, 3, and 4 are incorrect because the drug does not promote infections, cause miosis, or affect the retina.

5 Answer: 3 Rationale: Cholinergic antagonists typically cause dry eyes and the patient should be encouraged to use lubricating eyedrops. Options 1, 2, and 4 are incorrect. These statements suggest that the patient has understood the teaching. Patients receiving anticholinergic antagonists frequently complain of extreme dry mouth discomfort and increased fluid intake may ease this symptom. Many anticholinergic antagonists may cause drowsiness initially. Women receiving anticholinergic therapy should be advised to avoid breastfeeding until the medication is discontinued.

6 Answer: 1 Rationale: The therapeutic effect of succinylcholine is to paralyze skeletal muscles. However, this drug does not produce anesthesia or a loss of consciousness. Options 2, 3, and 4 are incorrect. Succinylcholine produces no change in the patient's sensorium (consciousness) and the patient can still experience pain. The effect of succinylcholine is total muscle paralysis, not muscle relaxation.

Chapter 15

Making the Patient Connection

1 Albuterol is a sympathomimetic drug that selectively stimulates beta$_2$-adrenergic receptors. The therapeutic responses associated with this drug are bronchodilation and vasodilation. Therefore, albuterol expands constricted bronchial tubes and enhances the passage of airflow into the lungs.

2 Albuterol is used to relieve and prevent bronchospasms in patients with obstructive diseases such as asthma. The patient is receiving the medication via the inhalation route because it is one of the fastest and most effective routes to administer respiratory medications. Administration of an adrenergic agonist by the parenteral or inhalation routes causes immediate bronchodilation.

3 Alexia is experiencing typical adverse effects associated with the administration of an adrenergic agonist. These include CNS stimulation, such as tremor, anxiety, and irritability. Tachycardia is another common adverse effect related to these medications.

Additional Case Study

1 Both epinephrine and pseudoephedrine directly affect alpha receptors by causing additional vasoconstriction. In Bill's case, the combination of drugs is creating medication-induced HTN.

2 First, you should inform Bill that the combination of drugs may be causing his blood pressure to be dangerously high. He should be encouraged to stop using the medication immediately and to have his blood pressure rechecked within the next 24 hours. It is essential that you instruct him to not use any OTC medications for sinus relief until seen by his healthcare provider. Lastly, inform him that new medications for seasonal allergies are available that are safer and more effective. Encourage him to ask his healthcare provider to recommend one.

Chapter Review

1 Answer: 1 Rationale: Epinephrine is a preferred drug in cardiac arrest because of its ability to immediately restore heart rhythm and prevent circulatory collapse. Options 2, 3, and 4 are incorrect. While the drug does cause bronchodilation, the highest priority is to restore heart rhythm and circulation. Because of peripheral vasoconstriction, renal blood flow may be restricted and not improved. Epinephrine is a nonselective adrenergic agonist.

2 Answer: 1, 2, 4 Rationale: Adrenergic agonist nasal sprays should not be shared among individuals due to the risk of spreading infection. Individuals should be taught the dangers of using adrenergic nasal sprays for longer than 3 days. These medications can increase blood pressure, increase heart rate, and cause insomnia. Habitual use of nasal adrenergic drugs can also cause rebound congestion as well as necrosis of the nasal mucosa due to the severe vasoconstriction caused by the drug. Due to the CNS stimulation, nasal adrenergic agents are not indicated in children and infants. Options 3 and 5 are incorrect. The drug causes CNS stimulation rather than depression. People with diabetes must use caution when using adrenergic drugs and must monitor their blood glucose levels more frequently for hyperglycemia. They are also at higher risk for adverse cardiac effects.

3 Answer: 4 Rationale: Epinephrine is used during anaphylaxis to prevent hypotension and bronchoconstriction. Options 1, 2, and 3 are incorrect because the administration of epinephrine for anaphylaxis does not prevent the formation of histamine or antibodies in response to an invading antigen nor does it affect white blood cell function.

4 Answer: 1 Rationale: When $beta_2$-adrenergic agonists such as albuterol are taken too close to bedtime, the patient may experience insomnia. Options 2, 3, and 4 are incorrect because all adrenergic agonists act as stimulators, and urticaria and tinnitus are not adverse effects associated with this drug.

5 Answer: 2 Rationale: At high dosage, dopamine stimulates $alpha_1$-adrenergic receptors, causes vasodilation and increases blood pressure. Options 1, 3, and 4 are incorrect. Dopamine does not affect the reflexes responsible for pupillary response or the patient's gag reflex, and it does not directly affect the patient's level of consciousness.

6 Answer: 1, 4 Rationale: The nurse should consult with the prescriber when adrenergic drugs are prescribed for individuals with hyperthyroid disease or dysrhythmias. The medication can further increase the already overactive metabolic system in hyperthyroidism and may increase the risk for dysrhythmias due to the cardiac stimulation caused by these medications. Options 2, 3, and 5 are incorrect. These are therapeutic indications for the administration of adrenergic agonists.

Chapter 16

Making the Patient Connection

1 Prazosin works by decreasing peripheral resistance (relaxing blood vessels) so that blood may flow through the vessels more easily. This lowers blood pressure. The mechanism of action is based on the drug's ability to block $alpha_1$-adrenergic receptors.

2 Some antihypertensive medications can induce impotence. The physiologic mechanism that creates this situation in men is related to the muscle contraction in the vas deferens, which is the main duct through which semen is carried from the epididymis to the ejaculatory duct. When these smooth muscles are inhibited, ejaculation becomes difficult.

3 Men may be reluctant to report medication-induced impotence. Clinicians must determine exactly what the patient means by "sexual problem". Healthcare providers sometimes must be frank and candid about such matters. A nurse could say "Do you mean problems with erection or problems with ejaculation?" Chris should be informed that not all antihypertensive medications will have the same effect and that a different medication may be prescribed.

Additional Case Study

1 There are two reasons why Mr. Perry should not take pseudoephedrine for his allergic symptoms. First, adrenergic agonists such as Sudafed antagonize the antihypertensive action of propranolol, thereby causing the medication to be less effective. Second, adrenergic agonists create vasoconstriction, which will elevate Mr. Perry's blood pressure.

2 A safer medication for this patient would be OTC diphenhydramine. This drug blocks the histamine receptors and reduces allergic symptoms without increasing blood pressure.

Chapter Review

1 Answer: 1 Rationale: With beta-adrenergic blockers such as propranolol, the most important action is to monitor the patient for cardiovascular adverse such as changes in pulse and blood pressure. Options 2, 3, and 4 are incorrect. Elevation of the head of the bed is not specifically required for this drug regimen. Inderal can be taken anytime regardless of meals, and its therapeutic action is not contingent on serum K^+ levels.

2 Answer: 4 Rationale: Beta-adrenergic antagonists may cause hypoglycemia in patients with diabetes. The patient should monitor blood glucose levels frequently and to notify the prescriber of any persistent decrease. Options 1, 2, and 3 are incorrect. Insulin dosages are never arbitrarily increased without checking with a healthcare provider. Patients with diabetes should remain on their normal diabetic diets even though they may be taking antihypertensive medications. Elevation of the extremities is not relevant to a patient with diabetes taking beta-adrenergic blocker drugs.

3 Answer: 1 Rationale: Initial doses of drugs that cause a "first-dose phenomenon" should be very low and administered at bedtime. The decline in blood pressure due to prazosin is marked when beginning pharmacotherapy and when increasing the dose. This can lead to syncope due to reduced blood flow to the brain. Options 2, 3, and 4 are incorrect. Doses of antihypertensive medications should never be doubled but should be gradually increased to avoid hypotension, and the best time to give prazosin in the initial phases of therapy is at bedtime.

4 Answer: 1 Rationale: The patient is likely describing orthostatic hypotension induced by the medication. Patients find it helpful to move slowly from a recumbent position to avoid dizziness and syncope. Options 2, 3, and 4 are incorrect. Although drinking a full glass of water with the medication is a healthy suggestion, this action does not eliminate orthostatic hypotension. Sleeping positions do not influence orthostatic hypotension. The patient should never abruptly stop taking antihypertensive medication. Such action could result in hypertensive crisis, stroke, or heart attack.

5 Answer: 4 Rationale: Tachycardia is an adverse effect of alpha$_1$-adrenergic antagonists. Patients experiencing tachycardia should not receive alpha$_1$-adrenergic antagonists. Options 1, 2, and 3 are incorrect. Alpha$_1$-adrenergic antagonists are often prescribed for BPH because they relax muscles in the prostate. A pheochromocytoma is a benign tumor of the adrenal medulla that secretes catecholamines. Alpha$_1$-adrenergic antagonists help to reduce the HTN associated with these tumors. Alpha$_1$-adrenergic antagonists diminish the vasospasms associated with Raynaud's disease.

6 Answer: 2, 3, 4 Rationale: Beta-adrenergic blockers can have metabolic effects that increase serum triglycerides and cause hypoglycemia. Additionally, these drugs can cause decreased libido in men. Options 1 and 5 are incorrect. Anorexia and thrombocytopenia are not adverse effects associated with beta-adrenergic antagonists.

Chapter 18

Making the Patient Connection

1 Seraphina and Joe's plans for their retirement may have to be changed because they have financial concerns now. Raising teenagers is costly, and it might be difficult if their income is limited to Social Security and pensions. Seraphina may feel resentful toward her grandchildren and may also feel guilty for being resentful because she recognizes that they did not cause the situation.

2 The healthcare provider may order antianxiety medications, such as alprazolam, buspirone, diazepam, or lorazepam. She may also be prescribed a medication such as zolpidem for short-term treatment of insomnia, while receiving psychotherapy for assistance in resolving her current difficulties.

3 Herbal remedies may influence the effects of traditional drug therapy. Herbs that are commonly used include kava, which promotes muscle relaxation and sleep and acts as an antidepressant. It may be used in combination with St. John's wort and valerian to promote relaxation. St. John's wort is used for mild depression. If taken with a prescription antidepressant, St. John's wort may increase the risk of suicide. Valerian is a mild sedative that induces sleep. Its effects are similar to those of the benzodiazepines. Special care must be taken when combining herbal remedies with prescription medications. Herbals can enhance or decrease the actions of the prescription medications. Encourage Seraphina to notify her healthcare provider of all herbs she is taking so the interactions among them and her ordered medications can be determined.

Additional Case Study

1 Adverse effects associated with lorazepam include dizziness, ataxia, drowsiness, blurred vision, vertigo, sedation, and confusion. These effects are dose related and tolerance to them may develop as therapy progresses.

2 Craig should be instructed to avoid performing potentially hazardous activities (e.g., driving) that require alert mental status until the effects of the drug are known. The drug should not be stopped abruptly, and other CNS depressants such as alcohol and antihistamines must be avoided while the drug is used.

3 The nurse can make several suggestions to Craig: Encourage nonpharmacologic strategies for stress reduction such as daily walking or moderate exercise; refer Craig to the appropriate social service agency (e.g., local workforce development) for possible employment opportunities; and encourage group or individual behavioral therapy.

Chapter Review

1 Answer: 3 Rationale: Ataxia, weakness, restlessness, dizziness, and other motor problems can occur with lorazepam. Options 1, 2, and 4 are incorrect. These are not adverse effects associated with lorazepam.

2 Answer: 4 Rationale: Sleeping for 7 hours is the desired effect of temazepam. Options 1, 2, and 3 are incorrect. The client should experience periods of sleep lasting longer than 3 hours and should obtain a full night's sleep. The client will be taking temazepam to assist with insomnia, not to treat anxiety related to everyday stress or to help control panic attacks.

3 Answer: 3 Rationale: This medication must be gradually reduced, not abruptly terminated. Abrupt termination may cause withdrawal symptoms (nausea and vomiting, abdominal cramps, diaphoresis, confusion, tremors, seizures). Options 1, 2, and 4 are incorrect. These are appropriate statements and indicate that the client understands the teaching.

4 Answer: 2 Rationale: Panic disorder is not an appropriate use for phenobarbital. Options 1, 3, and 4 are incorrect. Treatment of status epilepticus, use prior to diagnostic testing, and use prior to receiving general anesthesia are all appropriate for phenobarbital.

5 Answer: 3 Rationale: Client safety is the major concern with sedative–hypnotics, so prevention of falls is the highest priority. Options 1, 2, and 4 are incorrect. The client may experience urinary incontinence, activity intolerance, or poor nutritional intake related to drug therapy or other reasons. Safety, however, is the priority concern.

6 Answer: 1 Rationale: Smoking enhances the metabolism of benzodiazepines, so the medication is broken down and removed from the body more quickly. Therefore, a smoker may require a larger dose of a benzodiazepine to get the same effect as that of a nonsmoker. Options 2, 3, and 4 are incorrect. A smaller or half dose, or a single extra dose, may not adequately help relieve the client's symptoms.

Chapter 19

Making the Patient Connection

1 The priority is for Adelphia to receive complete physical and mental assessments. Any physical cause for the changes in her behavior must be ruled out, and the recent weight gain may be caused by other disorders, such as hypothyroidism. After this has been done, a mental status examination must be performed, with emphasis on suicidal ideation.

2 Antidepressants are drugs used to enhance, elevate, or stabilize mood. Most antidepressants act by restoring normal neurotransmitter balances of primarily norepinephrine, serotonin, and, to a lesser degree, dopamine.

3 To determine if antidepressants are achieving a therapeutic effect, the nurse can monitor the patient's interest in personal appearance and the performance of normal ADLs. In Adelphia's case, the clues that demonstrate improvment include a renewed interest in her personal appearance and in her children and their activities, a return to her normal day-to-day activities, and resumption of contact with friends and social activities.

Additional Case Study

1 Andrew is at risk for possible suboptimal effects of lithium if his diet or activity level causes changes in his sodium or fluid balance, which in turn affects his serum lithium level. The nurse should assess Andrew's electrolytes and serum drug level on each office visit. Routine weights will also be monitored. The nurse would also teach Andrew important signs and symptoms that suggest a change in lithium level that should be reported immediately.

2 The nurse can explain the importance of normal fluid and sodium balance with Andrew. They can discuss the need to stay hydrated during games and the need to report signs and symptoms of dehydration such as weakness, thirst, and dizziness. The nurse should assess Andrew's normal post-game menu choices and work with him as needed to develop healthy eating habits that allow him to participate fully in team activities.

3 The nurse can encourage Andrew to remain close with his parents while also experiencing the freedom they have provided him for self-care by including his parents in game-day preparation or planning menu choices when eating out. The nurse can also discuss with Andrew and his parents the need for monitoring drug levels, sodium level and intake, and signs and symptoms to be reported to the provider along with plans for notifying his parents if any of these symptoms develop during or after games.

Chapter Review

1 Answer: 1 Rationale: Imipramine should not be used by clients with seizure disorders because it lowers the seizure threshold. Options 2, 3, and 4 are incorrect. Imipramine is a drug that is effective in treating depression and is one of only a few drugs approved for enuresis (bedwetting) in children. Like other TCAs, imipramine has a number of off-label indications. These include the adjuvant treatment of cancer or neuropathic pain.

2 Answer: 3 Rationale: Full therapeutic effects of fluoxetine may take up to 1 month. Options 1, 2, and 4 are incorrect. Normal water and sodium intake do not affect fluoxetine. The client cannot take an MAOI or other CNS depressant concurrently. The use of other drugs or CNS depressants such as alcohol could increase the risk of adverse effects or increased depression.

3 Answer: 1, 2 Rationale: Persistent GI upset and confusion are signs of elevated lithium levels between 1.5 and 2.0, which signify early toxicity. Options 3, 4, and 5 are incorrect. Polyuria is an adverse effect that may occur in early therapy but is not associated with early toxicity. Convulsions may occur at serum levels above 2.5, but not in early stages of toxicity. Ataxia is also not a sign of early lithium toxicity.

4 Answer: 1 Rationale: The client taking lithium must be conscious of maintaining normal sodium intake. Because lithium is a salt, if sodium intake is low the body will replace the sodium with lithium, leading to lithium toxicity. Options 2, 3, and 4 are incorrect. The client taking lithium must have regular blood studies and toxicity is a very real concern, hence the necessity for routine blood studies. Women should refrain from breastfeeding while taking lithium.

5 Answer: 3 Rationale: A typical antidepressant such as venlafaxine may take 3 weeks or longer to reach full therapeutic effect, so the client must continue taking the medication as ordered so that therapeutic drug levels can be reached and maintained. Options 1, 2, and 4 are incorrect. It is not within a nurse's scope of practice to suggest changes in medication routine without consulting the prescriber, and these comments are not helpful to maintaining a therapeutic nurse–client relationship.

6 Answer: 2, 3 Rationale: Fluoxetine causes weight loss in some clients, while other clients experience weight gain or fluctuations in weight. A healthy diet and adequate exercise will help maintain normal weight. While rare, an increased risk of suicide has been noted in clients up to age 24, and the client should be carefully monitored, especially during the early initiation of therapy. Options 1, 4, and 5 are incorrect. Fluoxetine may cause insomnia but not sedation. Abrupt withdrawal of fluoxetine may lead to withdrawal symptoms. If the drug needs to be discontinued, gradually tapering the dose is recommended. Fluoxetine is not known to cause excessive thirst.

Chapter 20

Making the Patient Connection

1 Persons with schizophrenia and other serious mental disorders may feel normal while taking their medications as prescribed. These patients often believe they no longer need the medications. George is functioning as any adult does—he goes to work, coaches his children's sports teams, provides for his family, and cares for his wife. Because he views all of these activities as normal, he convinces himself he no longer has schizophrenia and stops taking his medications.

2 There are many clues, probably subtle at first, then becoming more obvious: George quit coaching his children's sports teams, exhibited a decline in personal hygiene and appearance, and, finally, quit his job without reason.

3 Sheri can assist George by working with him to develop a schedule for taking his medications and helping him keep track on a calendar. She may need to count his remaining pills to ensure that he is taking his medication. She can intervene at the first sign of negative symptoms (e.g., decline in personal hygiene, decreased interest in usual activities, or delusions). Other family members can tell Sheri if they notice unusual changes in George's behavior or thought patterns. Sheri is the appropriate person to tell because George will be reluctant to admit that he has stopped taking his medication or will not recognize that behaviors or thoughts are abnormal. George, Sheri, and other family members may benefit from a comprehensive behavioral health treatment plan, developed in collaboration with the healthcare provider and other members of the health team, to ensure long-term success in George's treatment.

Additional Case Study

1 Haloperidol is a nonphenothiazine antipsychotic medication that can be used to calm agitation and to decrease psychotic manifestations. Because Suzette is becoming more and more out of control, she would probably refuse to take an oral medication, so an IM preparation is the best choice. Haloperidol will calm her down, slowing her thoughts and activity so she does not harm herself or others. The onset of the medication is 30 to 45 minutes, so Suzette must be watched closely during that time. She should be lying down for the entire time (which may be difficult, depending on her level of agitation) and up to 1 hour following administration.

2 Common adverse effects to haloperidol are drowsiness and EPS, which include involuntary movements, tremors, rigidity, body restlessness, muscle contractions, and changes in breathing and heart rate.

3 Suzette most likely will be hospitalized for less than 1 week. Returning the patient to the least restrictive environment possible for treatment is advisable as soon as possible to minimize further stress and adverse effects of the hospital stay. Her psychiatric medication will be started, and she will be stabilized before discharge. Suzette will also have several chances to speak with a counselor or psychiatric nurse who can try to assist her to gain insight into the reasons behind this hospitalization. She will be given patient education about her disorder, her medication, and

the importance of continuing to take the medication even though she feels better. Family members will also be involved in Suzette's care and education so they are alert to signs that would suggest nonadherence to the medication regimen or worsening psychiatric illness.

Chapter Review

1 Answer: 4 Rationale: Antipsychotic medications treat the symptoms associated with mental illness but do not cure these disorders. Without the medication, the symptoms will return. Options 1, 2, and 3 are incorrect. These are not symptoms associated with abrupt withdrawal of an antipsychotic medication.

2 Answer: 2 Rationale: Grapefruit or grapefruit juice are known to interact with drugs and may increase drug levels of aripiprazole to potentially toxic concentrations. Options 1, 3, and 4 are incorrect. Social withdrawal is a symptom of the disease and slowed activity may occur as a result of the medication. Tardive dyskinesia is not commonly noted with aripiprazole. SSRIs such as fluoxetine inhibit CYP2D6, which can cause reduced metabolism of aripiprazole and raised serum levels and potentially cause toxicity.

3 Answer: 1 Rationale: Benztropine is classified as an autonomic nervous system drug and an anticholinergic. It suppresses tremor and rigidity by decreasing the excess cholinergic effect associated with dopamine deficiency. Options 2, 3, and 4 are incorrect. Diazepam and lorazepam are antianxiety medications that will not improve the patient's symptoms. Haloperidol is an antipsychotic medication that may cause these symptoms.

4 Answer: 2, 4 Rationale: EPS occurs frequently, especially at the beginning of therapy with haloperidol. A person with Parkinson disease, seizure disorders, alcoholism, or severe mental depression should not take haloperidol because they are all disorders that affect the CNS. Dementia, seizures, depression, and severe CNS depression are known to occur with the use of haloperidol in these patients. Options 1, 3, and 5 are incorrect. Haloperidol and antacids may be given simultaneously; there are no known interactions between these two medications. Haloperidol must be taken as ordered, on a regular schedule. Taking the drug prn will not reduce symptoms of psychosis because it takes several weeks of regular administration before therapeutic levels are reached. Sustained-release medications should never be crushed. If the patient cannot take the medication, another form should be used.

5 Answer: 4 Rationale: The patient taking risperidone or any antipsychotic medication should refrain from consuming alcohol. Concurrent use of alcohol with antipsychotic medications will increase CNS depression. Because there is an increased risk of hyperglycemia or diabetes in patients taking risperidone, alcohol should also be avoided because it may affect blood sugar levels. Options 1, 2, and 3 are incorrect. Weight gain may occur and obtaining a weekly weight will help the patient track any gain. Increasing fluids and fiber may help to limit GI adverse effects. Hypotension is related to adverse reactions the patient may experience and must be monitored and reported if it occurs.

6 Answer: 1 Rationale: Fever, tachycardia, stupor, and incontinence are symptoms of neuroleptic malignant syndrome (NMS), a potentially fatal adverse effect of antipsychotics that must be diagnosed and treated immediately. Options 2, 3, and 4 are possible adverse reactions but are not life-threatening and therefore do not need to be reported with the same urgency as symptoms of NMS.

Chapter 21

Making the Patient Connection

1 The four types of MS are relapsing-remitting MS (RRMS), secondary-progressive MS (SPMS), primary-progressive MS (PPMS), and progressive-relapsing MS (PRMS). RRMS is the most common. Diagnosis of MS is made after other neurologic disorders have been ruled out, with imaging studies such as MRI used to identify areas of demyelination in the brain.

2 The goals of drug therapy in MS are to modify the progression of the disease, treat acute exacerbations, and to manage symptoms. The DMDs are used to prevent irreversible neuronal damage in patients with MS to delay the progressive phase of MS and prolong the ability of patients to remain active. Additional drugs such as antianxiety drugs, antidepressants, and analgesics for chronic pain may be needed to manage symptoms.

3 While Althea works in a relatively low-risk environment as it relates to the adverse effect of increased risk of infection with the DMDs, she should take precautions to minimize her risk, especially outside of the work environment. She should also be aware of activities that may aggravate her symptoms, including fatigue, hot environments, overexertion, and stress, and take measures to avoid or mitigate these. Because the drugs do not cure the disease but lessen its effects by delaying progression, Althea may need to try several different drugs before one works well for her. With adequate drug therapy, Althea should be able to continue the job she loves and manage the family with alterations to her daily routines as needed.

Additional Case Study

1 Idiopathic PD, the most common type, has no known cause. It is characterized by a progressive loss of neurons from a region of the brain called the substantia nigra. Physiologic defects with PD occur in the amounts of neurotransmitters of dopamine and acetylcholine in specific regions of the brain. A nurse could describe the disease as a gradual lack of a brain chemical, dopamine, that results in the physical symptoms that cause difficulty with movement and with tremors. It is not known why the brain stops making sufficient dopamine, but once the chemical is depleted, it must be replaced by drug therapy. Other newer therapies may be available, and Michael should discuss treatment with his healthcare provider.

2 Drug therapy attempts to restore the functional balance of dopamine and acetylcholine in the striatum of the brain. Levodopa is a precursor in the synthesis of dopamine and helps to restore the imbalance. Levodopa is nearly always combined with carbidopa because the combination increases the effectiveness of levodopa. Carbidopa inhibits the breakdown of levodopa in the intestine and peripheral tissues, which makes more levodopa available to the CNS. Without carbidopa, only 1% of the dose of levodopa reaches the CNS.

3 Patients receiving prolonged antiparkinson pharmacotherapy may periodically experience a loss of drug effect. This "wearing-off effect" appears gradually near the end of a dosing interval. Symptoms worsen at this time because the concentration of the drug has fallen below the therapeutic level. Assess the timing of the dose in respect to the symptoms and encourage Michael to keep a symptom diary. Because the drugs may also be affected by high protein or vitamin B_6 taken concurrently, assessing Michael's diet and other medications may help to rule out this cause. Adjusting the dosing interval to provide for more frequent dosing can help to reduce the wearing-off effect.

Chapter Review

1 Answer: 2 Rationale: Benztropine, a cholinergic antagonist, is frequently used as combination therapy with other antiparkinson drugs to decrease tremors. Options 1, 3, and 4 are incorrect. Amantadine acts to increase dopamine's release, but only as long as dopamine is available. Haloperidol is a phenothiazine antipsychotic that may lead to pseudo-Parkinson's disease in many persons. Donepezil prolongs the time between diagnosis and the institutionalization of the patient with Alzheimer's disease and is not used for Parkinson's disease.

2 Answer: 3 Rationale: Being independent with ADLs shows an improvement in physical abilities. Options 1, 2, and 4 are incorrect. Drowsiness is a common adverse effect of anti-Parkinson's medications. Anorexia or loss of appetite is a common adverse effect, not an expected therapeutic effect. Itchy skin is not directly related to PD symptoms or to the medications used.

3 Answer: 3 Rationale: It is important that the caregivers understand that there is no cure for AD but that the medication may delay the worsening of symptoms. Options 1, 2, and 4 are incorrect. The medication should be given continuously and not only when the symptoms are present. The patient may become constipated but does not require emergency treatment. The drug may cause bradycardia or atrial fibrillation and the pulse rate should be checked weekly, but it is not necessary to take the patient's vital signs before each dose of medication.

4 Answer: 1, 2, 5 Rationale: Alzheimer's patients and their families may struggle with complex medication routines, and it is difficult to remember to take a medication multiple times a day. Donepezil has not been associated with hepatotoxicity. Donepezil requires once per day dosing, usually at bedtime. While it does not cure AD, donepezil may lengthen the time between when the patient is diagnosed and when memory care in a skilled facility is needed. Options 3 and 4 are incorrect. There is a risk of GI bleeding, especially in patients with a history of peptic ulcers or chronic NSAID use. Potentially life-threatening dysrhythmias, including atrial fibrillation and sinus bradycardia, are possible adverse effects associated with donepezil.

5 Answer: 1 Rationale: Rivastigmine has no significant drug interactions. This is thought to be true because there is no interaction with enzymes in the liver that metabolize drugs. Options 2, 3, and 4 are incorrect because they do not apply to rivastigmine.

6 Answer: 1, 2, 4 Rationale: Flulike symptoms with general malaise, body aches, fever, and headache are common. Insomnia and rashes may also occur and may be treated symptomatically after conferral with the provider. Options 3 and 5 are incorrect. Depression should never be ignored and should be reported immediately. Significant pain with darkening or blackening of the skin at the injection site indicates that tissue necrosis may be occurring and requires prompt treatment.

Chapter 22

Making the Patient Connection

1 Even with multiple medications, Jorge may still continue to experience seizure activity. The family should be told that their primary concern is to protect him from injury. It is important for Jorge's mother to look closely at the home setting for potential hazards. Here are just a few considerations: pad sharp corners, do not leave the patient unattended in a bathtub or swimming pool, avoid climbing activities high off the ground (rock or rope climbing), avoid sleeping in a top bunk, place screen guards around fireplaces, and wear a helmet and other protective gear when bicycling.

2 Jorge's mother should be instructed on the action, adverse effects, administration guidelines, and nursing implications regarding carbamazepine and phenytoin. It is important that she understand that a medication dose should not be missed, and if it is, to administer it immediately. Instruct her that missing doses of antiepileptic medications could result in status epilepticus. Instruct her to keep using the same brand of phenytoin. Neither of the medications should be stopped abruptly.

Additional Case Study

1 Valproic acid increases the brain's concentrations of the inhibitory neurotransmitter gamma-aminobutyric acid (GABA). Abnormal electrical impulses in the brain are suppressed, leading to decreased seizure activity.

2 The most common adverse effects are GI related, such as nausea and vomiting, diarrhea, abdominal pain, and diminished appetite. These effects are usually transient and not severe. An enteric-coated formulation of valproic acid can be used to reduce these uncomfortable effects.

3 One potential adverse effect of valproic acid is an increased tendency to bleed. Before any dental procedure, Matt should inform his dentist that he is taking valproic acid.

Chapter Review

1 Answer: 3 Rationale: GI effects such as nausea, anorexia, and abdominal pain are common with ethosuximide. Improper nutrition may affect normal growth. Monitoring height and weight weekly will assist in tracking normal growth. Options 1, 2, and 4 are incorrect. Physical activity will not affect the drug's metabolism and activity is normal and needed for healthy growth and development. Ethosuximide is not known to cause bone loss or dehydration.

2 Answer: 4 Rationale: Oxcarbazepine is excreted by the kidneys, and laboratory studies will be monitored to detect adverse renal effects. Because hyponatremia may develop during treatment, serum sodium levels should also be monitored. Options 1, 2, and 3 are incorrect. Oxcarbazepine does not affect CBC, platelets, sedimentation rate, or albumin or serum glucose levels.

3 Answer: 4 Rationale: Sedation and an increased risk of falls are associated with carbamazepine. Options 1, 2, and 3 are incorrect. Carbamazepine is used off-label to treat dementia with aggressiveness and agitation. The drug is not associated with insomnia and has not been demonstrated to increase the risk of stroke.

4 Answer: 2 Rationale: Slurred speech, diplopia, sedation, and dyspnea are symptoms of gabapentin overdose. Options 1, 3, and 4 are incorrect. Seizure activity may recur if the drug is stopped abruptly. Neither grapefruit juice nor smoking are known to affect drug level.

5 Answer: 1 Rationale: High doses of phenytoin can cause nystagmus, confusion, ataxia, coma, and seizures and the dosage should be reduced. Options 2, 3, and 4 are incorrect. Increasing or maintaining the same dose will continue or exacerbate the symptoms of toxicity. The drug should not be discontinued abruptly because seizure activity may occur.

6 Answer: 3 Rationale: Carbamazepine is associated with an increased risk of SJS and toxic epidermal necrosis in genetically susceptible individuals. Sunburning and a reddish-purple rash, especially associated with blisters, are possible symptoms of severe dermatologic reactions and should be evaluated immediately. Options 1, 2, and 4 are incorrect. Blurred vision, leg cramping, and lethargy are all possible side effects of carbamazepine but tolerance to these effects usually develops over time.

Chapter 23

Making the Patient Connection

1 Andrew's back pain is a likely a result of excessive use and local injury to the lower back. This is a common complaint, and one of the leading reasons why patients go to emergency departments. Other possible causes of muscle spasm include hypocalcemia, debilitating neurologic disorders, seizure disorders, and overmedication with antipsychotic agents. Muscle spasms are involuntary contractions of a muscle group or group of muscles. The muscles become tight with a fixed pattern of resistance, which results in diminished function.

2 Cyclobenzaprine is used to relieve muscle spasms associated with acute and painful musculoskeletal disorders. It has been

prescribed to relax the muscles of the lumbosacral region and decrease muscle spasms.

3 Cyclobenzaprine produces muscle relaxation and CNS depression. Andrew should be instructed to protect himself from injury, not to engage in the operation of machinery while taking the medication, and not to consume alcoholic beverages or mood-altering drugs. He should also be warned against taking OTC medications. He should be instructed on all adverse effects and advised to notify the prescriber if therapeutic effects do not occur within 2 to 3 weeks. Due to its anticholinergic effects, the patient should be instructed to notify the provider of any difficulties in urination and to sip water or ice chips to relieve dry mouth.

Additional Case Study

1 OnabotulinumtoxinA is a preferred drug to treat cervical dystonia and is used to improve the severity of abnormal head position. The toxin binds to the motor nerve receptor sites to block neuromuscular conduction and inhibit the release of acetylcholine. The result of this action is the reduction of painful muscle activity.

2 Possible adverse effects include injection reactions, headache, dysphagia, muscle weakness, pain, tenderness, bruising, flulike symptoms, dry mouth, upper respiratory infection, and ptosis.

Chapter Review

1 Answer: 1, 4, 5 Rationale: Cyclobenzaprine may cause tachycardia, and any palpitations or rapid heart rate should be reported. Drowsiness may also occur and driving or other hazardous activities should be avoided until the effects of the drug are known. Swelling of the face or tongue may occur and must be reported immediately to the provider. Options 2 and 3 are incorrect. Patients with severe muscle spasms are encouraged to rest affected muscle groups until acute spasms subside. Cyclobenzaprine may cause dry mouth, and alcohol-based mouth rinses may exacerbate the condition.

2 Answer: 3 Rationale: Abruptly discontinuing baclofen may result in fever, seizures, rebound spasticity, and hallucinations. Options 1, 2, and 4 are incorrect. Baclofen may cause weakness and, like other muscle relaxants and antispasmodics, may cause constipation. Being cautious with activities and increasing fluid and fiber intake will help to limit the adverse effects. It may take several months before the full effects of baclofen are reached.

3 Answer: 2 Rationale: Capsaicin should be applied to the site of pain with a gloved hand to prevent irritation of the skin and to avoid introducing the capsaicin to the eyes or other parts of the body not under treatment. Options 1, 3, and 4 are incorrect. Capsaicin should only be applied to the site of pain, not proximal or distal to the pain. If capsaicin begins to irritate and cause redness and inflammation, it should be discontinued. Capsaicin should not be applied with a bare hand.

4 Answer: 2 Rationale: Dysphagia, blurred vision, and ptosis are all symptoms of possible botulism toxicity and should be reported immediately. Options 1, 3, and 4 are incorrect. Fever, aches, and chills are not anticipated adverse effects of this drug, and while they should be evaluated, they do not require immediate reporting. Moderate levels of muscle weakness may occur after the drug is administered and strengthening exercises may be needed on the affected side. Continuous muscle spasms and pain should not occur because the drug blocks muscle contraction.

5 Answer: 4 Rationale: Physostigmine may be administered to reverse serious anticholinergic adverse effects. Options 1, 2, and 3 are incorrect. Naloxone is used to decrease the effects of opioids on the CNS but is not a the drug for the treatment of CNS depression with cyclobenzaprine. Meperidine is a CNS depressant and should not be administered with cyclobenzaprine. Diazepam is a skeletal muscle relaxant and should not be administered with cyclobenzaprine.

6 Answer: 2, 3, 5 Rationale: Dantrolene may cause hepatotoxicity, with the greatest risk occurring in women over age 35. Estrogen taken concurrently with dantrolene may increase this risk. The drug may cause xerostomia and sucking on hard candy or sipping water or ice chips may relieve the dryness. Options 1 and 4 are incorrect. Fluids and fiber may also help diarrhea, but dantrolene may cause diarrhea, not constipation. Dantrolene may cause photosensitivity, so patients should avoid direct sun exposure.

Chapter 24

Making the Patient Connection

1 ADHD is characterized by inattention and hyperactivity. It is four times more common in males than females. A child who is diagnosed with ADHD has difficulty completing tasks, is frequently loud, and interrupts others. Females with ADHD show less aggression but suffer from greater anxiety and mood swings. Jonathon is exhibiting the symptoms of ADHD and may be experiencing more difficulty now that he is in middle school because of the compartmentalized classes or because of the different teaching styles of the instructors he has had for each course. Prepuberty hormonal changes may also be contributing to Jonathon's symptoms.

2 Amphetamine sulfate may increase Jonathon's attention and alertness and assist him to focus on schoolwork, class activities and lessons.

3 Jonathon and his parents should be taught that the drug should be taken in the morning to avoid nighttime insomnia. Because the drug causes anorexia, Jonathon should eat an adequate breakfast before the drug is taken. If anorexia at lunch is a problem, high-calorie, nutrient-dense foods can be packed in his lunch sack and an afternoon snack after school. Weekly weights should be taken to ensure adequate growth is continuing. Insomnia, heart palpitations, and excessive anxiety or nervousness should be reported to the provider. The drug should be kept secured in the home and if it is to be taken at school, the school's protocols for dosages and labeling should be followed.

4 Cognitive-behavioral therapy and neurofeedback are non-pharmacologic treatments. Changes to lifestyle and diet have also been suggested as possible approaches to the treatment of ADHD (e.g., increasing levels of physical activity and removing or adding certain foods to the diet). Educating patients, their families, and teachers about ADHD is important to ensure appropriate management. This can include teaching parents and teachers about strategies to cope with disruptive behavior and problematic behavioral habits at home or at school.

Additional Case Study

1 Modafinil is known to increase extracellular dopamine to enhance alertness. It increases wakefulness in patients with narcolepsy, excessive sleepiness, and with shift work sleep disorder.

2 The patient should be taught to use a barrier contraceptive if she is of childbearing age. She should not take OTC medications unless approved by her healthcare provider. She should notify her provider if she develops any signs and symptoms of hypersensitivity to the medication. It is important for her to have periodic liver function tests.

3 The patient should be instructed to change positions slowly to reduce the potential for the occurrence of orthostatic hypotension.

Chapter Review

1 Answer: 4 Rationale: Many ADHD medications are Schedulesd drugs that require tight controls. Because they can be abused, they should be kept under lock and tightly monitored with only the minimal number of doses kept at the school as per school policy. Options 1, 2, and 3 are incorrect. Keeping the drug in a lunch bag may lead to the child forgetting to take it or to other children taking the drug. Because it is a highly regulated drug, additional prescriptions or dosages are not allowed under the Schedule because they could result in the misuse of the drug by people other than the student for whom it is prescribed.

2 Answer: 2 Rationale: Atomoxetine should decrease hyperactivity. Options 1, 3, and 4 are incorrect. Atomoxetine should increase attention, not decrease it. Mydriasis and elevated liver enzymes are adverse effects associated with atomoxetine; they are not therapeutic effects.

3 Answer: 1 Rationale: Chlorpromazine is the preferred drug to assist in counteracting amphetamine overdosage. It has strong alpha-adrenergic blocking actions that treat the effects of amphetamine. Options 2, 3, and 4 are incorrect. Phenytoin is an antiepileptic drug; propofol is a nonbarbiturate sedative–hypnotic; and dexamethasone is a corticosteroid. None of these drugs would counteract the effects of an amphetamine overdose.

4 Answer: 3 Rationale: Atomoxetine has been linked to suicidal ideations and an increased risk of suicide. These symptoms should be reported immediately to the family for assessment and treatment by the healthcare provider. Options 1, 2, and 4 are incorrect. The need for drug withdrawal will be determined by the provider after assessing the patient. The drug may take up to 4 weeks to achieve maximum therapeutic effects, but this patient is experiencing an adverse effect linked to the drug. Caffeine will not counteract depressive effects and may increase the risk of CNS adverse effects.

5 Answer: 1, 2 Rationale: Modafinil is a Schedule IV drug with prescribing and refill restrictions, similar to other drugs in that class. Modafinil may cause psychoactive symptoms such as euphoria, similar to other stimulant drugs. Options 3, 4, and 5 are incorrect. Unlike other stimulant drugs, modafinil does not suppress appetite or promote weight loss. Similar to other stimulants, it may cause hyperactivity and nervousness and should not be used in the presence of cardiovascular disease.

6 Answer: 3 Rationale: Taking the medication before 4:00 p.m. ensures that peak drug activity will occur during waking hours. Options 1, 2, and 4 are incorrect. Drinking wine with dinner should not have a noticeable effect on sleep unless taken directly before bedtime when the metabolism of the alcohol may actually diminish sleep as the blood glucose rises and falls. Chocolate contains caffeine, and also sugar, which may cause additional wakefulness. Decaffeinated coffee will limit the intake of the additional stimulant of caffeine but will not significantly improve the patient's sleep if the methylphenidate is taken later in the afternoon or evening.

Chapter 25

Making the Patient Connection

1 Given the complexity of Larry's situation, the best solution would be referral to the hospital pain management team. In most instances, baseline opioid analgesics would be continued, and acute surgical pain management would be superimposed on that baseline. The nurse caring for Larry after surgery should consider several interventions related to pain management. His age puts him at higher risk for hypotension, respiratory depression, and increased incidence of adverse CNS effects. The nurse would monitor for these problems and should consider supplemental interventions such as frequent repositioning, relaxation techniques, and distraction.

2 Depending on the type of documentation used in the agency, the nursing plan of care should include a note about Larry's chronic pain history. An alert might be placed on the physical chart if electronic medical records are not used. Pain management should be included in all nurse hand-off reporting and, if possible, the same nurses should be assigned to his care.

3 Hypotension, with unsafe ambulation, and constipation are the most likely adverse effects that Larry will experience. In addition to monitoring vital signs, including respiratory rate and BP, position changes should be made gradually with assisted ambulation. A high-fiber diet would be started with stool softeners and laxatives as needed. He should walk three or four times a day for increasing distances. In addition, nausea from the hydromorphone would need to be assessed and managed if it occurs.

Additional Case Study

1 Use of IV opioid analgesia with separate antiemetic therapy would be appropriate. Morphine would most likely be the initial preferred drug.

2 Initially the nurse should assess Rita, including pain and vital signs every 2 hours or more frequently if her condition warrants. An initial dose of IV morphine should be based on her current pain rating, followed by doses every 2 hours within the ordered range. She should be monitored for respiratory depression while keeping pain at tolerable levels. The nurse would need to regularly medicate with an IV agent that effectively manages Rita's nausea and vomiting without additional sedation.

3 Adverse effects might include respiratory depression, orthostatic hypotension, nausea, and constipation.

4 Dexamethasone, a corticosteroid, is ordered to reduce swelling and pressure on the spinal nerves from the metastases; reducing pressure helps relieve the back pain.

Chapter Review

1 Answer: 1, 3, 4, 5 Rationale: Common adverse effects of opioids include respiratory depression, urinary retention, constipation, and nausea. Option 2 is incorrect. Hypotension, not hypertension, is an adverse effect of opioids.

2 Answer: 4 Rationale: Opioids decrease peristalsis, and bowel surgery may produce a temporary cessation of peristalsis (paralytic ileus). Both lead to constipation. Once bowel function has returned enough for the patient to start eating, constipation is still likely and needs to be prevented by increased dietary fiber and fluids as well as taking a stool softener. Options 1, 2, and 3 are incorrect. Respiratory depression and urinary retention are not likely after several days with decreasing opioid use. Addiction is not a concern in the treatment of acute pain in this scenario.

3 Answer: 3 Rationale: Chest pain is a serious adverse effect of sumatriptan and needs to be differentiated from angina, which can also be caused by the drug. Options 1, 2, and 4 are incorrect. The patient should not use the drug again until being evaluated by the provider and should report the chest pain immediately. Reclining in a quiet room with cold packs is a nondrug treatment for migraines but reporting the chest pain is most important at this time.

4 Answer: 2 Rationale: The patient is describing neuropathic pain, which is most likely to respond to the adjuvant analgesic gabapentin, an antiseizure drug used for neuropathic pain. Options 1, 3, and 4 are incorrect. Nonopioids such as ibuprofen, or opioids such as methadone, are less effective at relieving pain that is of neurologic origin. Naloxone is an opioid antagonist and will not relieve the patient's pain.

5 Answer: 2 Rationale: Ergot alkaloids such as dihydroergotamine are one of the two drug classes for aborting migraines. Options 1, 3, and 4 are incorrect. Morphine is an opioid agonist and is not effective in aborting migraines. Propranolol is a beta blocker and is used to prevent migraines. Ibuprofen is a nonopioid analgesic that is used to treat mild to moderate pain.

6 Answer: 4 Rationale: Older adult patients are at highest risk for hypotension, respiratory depression, and increased incidence of adverse CNS effects such as confusion. Options 1, 2, and 3 are incorrect. Most 23-year-old patients can tolerate opioids without adverse effects. Individuals who suffer from traumatic injury may receive opioids. However, caution should be taken if the individual has also experienced any type of head injury. Opioids are often used with patients who suffer MI. No adverse effects such as hypotension or respiratory depression are usually present if the dose is appropriate for the size of the patient.

Chapter 26

Making the Patient Connection

1 Balanced anesthesia is the use of a combination of medications to produce general anesthesia. Balanced anesthetics provide for a rapid and smooth induction. The agents administered include neuromuscular blocking agents, short-acting barbiturates, opioids, and nitrous oxide. The purpose of the combination of these medications is to provide muscle relaxation and analgesia along with sedation and loss of sensation.

2 The main actions of nitrous oxide are analgesia and reduction in anxiety. Nitrous oxide suppresses the pain mechanism of the CNS. This agent has a low potency and does not produce loss of consciousness or profound skeletal muscle relaxation. Because nitrous oxide does not induce stage 3 surgical anesthesia, it is commonly combined with other surgical anesthetic agents.

3 The patient should be educated on the action and effect of balanced anesthesia and the agent to be used to induce and maintain anesthesia. Propofol is administered to induce and maintain anesthesia throughout the procedure, which will prevent her from awakening during surgery. The patient should also be aware that the medication may cause shivering when she awakens and that she will be provided with warm blankets to ensure her comfort.

Additional Case Study

1 Lidocaine blocks the conduction of electrical impulses by reducing the sodium permeability at the cellular level. This prevents pain transmission to the CNS.

2 Lidocaine is a local anesthetic agent with a prompt and intense anesthetic action that lasts longer than procaine and exhibits a lower incidence of adverse effects.

Chapter Review

1 Answer: 2 Rationale: In stage 2 the patient becomes excitable with hyperactivity and irregular heart and respiratory rates. Options 1, 3, and 4 are incorrect. In stage 1, the patient loses general sensation but remains awake. In stage 3, the patient's skeletal muscles become relaxed, and delirium stabilizes. In stage 4, the patient has paralysis of the medulla with possible adverse effects on respiratory and cardiac function.

2 Answer: 1 Rationale: Patients who have an allergy to eggs or soy products may have an allergic reaction to the propofol emulsion, which contains these products. Options 2, 3, and 4 are incorrect. Patients with allergies to iodine, kidney disease, or Addison's disease may be administered propofol cautiously.

3 Answer: 4 Rationale: Anxiety, excitement, and combativeness are signs that the dose of nitrous oxide is excessive and the patient is exhibiting signs of the stage 2 anesthesia. Lowering the dose will reduce these symptoms. Options 1, 2, and 3 are incorrect. The dose of nitrous oxide would be lowered, not increased. Propofol would cause additional CNS depression and is not advised. Succinylcholine is a neuromuscular blocking agent that will increase the risk of significant respiratory adverse effects due to its muscle-paralyzing actions.

4 Answer: 3 Rationale: Ketamine produces dissociation anesthesia, which is a feeling of being separated from the environment. Options 1, 2, and 4 are incorrect because anxiety and dry mouth are not significant adverse effects of ketamine. Ketamine may cause decreased energy.

5 Answer: 1 Rationale: Epinephrine is administered with lidocaine to increase the duration of the anesthetic action around the injection site by causing vasoconstriction, keeping the anesthetic localized. Options 2, 3, and 4 are incorrect because epinephrine will cause vasoconstriction, not vasodilation; may increase blood pressure if the drug enters the systemic circulation; and neither lidocaine nor epinephrine has any antibacterial properties.

6 Answer: 2, 3, 4 Rationale: Alfentanil is a parenteral opioid agent that promotes general anesthesia. Sufentanil is also a parenteral opioid agent. Regimental is an opioid agent that is used to induce and maintain general anesthesia. Options 1 and 5 are incorrect. Nitrous oxide is not an opioid and it is administered by inhalation. Succinylcholine is a neuromuscular blocking agent.

Chapter 27

Making the Patient Connection

1 Jamie's substance use is classified as both physical and a psychologic dependence. She said that when she is unable to obtain drugs, she feels sick with symptoms of trembling and diaphoresis. This describes a physiologic state that results in a withdrawal syndrome when addictive drug use is stopped. Her comments about needing drugs just to "get through the night" is characteristic of psychologic dependence, a condition in which an individual feels that they need drugs in order to cope with problems.

2 Here are the drugs that Jamie reports using, along with the associated withdrawal symptoms:

Drug Reported	Withdrawal Symptoms
Alcohol	Tremors, anxiety, confusion, and seizures
Heroin	Diaphoresis, agitation, dilated pupils (mydriasis), goose bumps (piloerection), and tremors
Crack	Agitation, depression, intense craving for the drug, and extreme fatigue
Valium	Rapid heartbeat, tremor, insomnia, sweating, irritability, anxiety, blurred vision, and decreased concentration

3 Drug use can trigger serious complications during pregnancy and possibly damage the fetus. Heavy consumption of drugs such as alcohol, tobacco, heroin, and tranquilizers can lead to premature birth, low birth weight, and increased risk of stillbirth. It is usually advisable for a pregnant woman to stop using drugs during pregnancy. However, this is not always the case when heroin use because sudden discontinuation during pregnancy can be dangerous to the fetus. Some healthcare professionals believe that it is safer for the mother to continue using the drug until the baby is born.

4 Essential to dealing with a pregnant patient with a substance use disorder is the development of a nonjudgmental attitude. The effect of the substance use on the unborn child evokes strong

emotions with most people, including nurses. However, little can be accomplished if a patient feels that the healthcare provider views them as evil or unworthy of healthcare. Obviously, Jamie needs a stabilizing force within her life. The nurse has an opportunity to assist this patient to seek a healthy lifestyle that will be a positive influence for both mother and baby. A nurse who is open and willing to accept the patient will have a greater chance of referring this patient to critical resources. The nurse should consider referrals to social services and substance abuse counselors.

5 Jamie's life has all the variables that trap her in a web of addiction. First, the drug factor in this case may include the quickness of the substance to relieve her psychologic pain. Second, the user factors involve her risk-taking behavior (prostitution) and prior history of drug abuse. Lastly, Jamie's limited opportunities for education and for the development of healthy social norms put her at risk. Her peer influences were most likely individuals in similar living situations.

Additional Case Study

1 Delirium tremens is a severe condition that occurs in chronic alcoholism due to sudden withdrawal from alcohol. This condition is complicated by physical and psychologic deterioration that can progress from disorientation, hallucinations, and seizures to death. Whole-body tremors are associated with DTs. Mortality for this condition is reported at 20%. The treatment priority for this condition is prevention of seizure activity. Multiple drug therapies will be initiated to prevent seizure activity including antiseizure medications, sedatives, and vitamin therapy.

2 The key to the level of alcohol intoxication is directly related to the rate of excretion. There are no foods or beverages that will increase the excretion rate. The consumption of coffee, for example, does not produce a sobering effect.

3 Alcohol consumption depresses the CNS. The effects are dose related and produce varying degrees of sedation, relaxation, loss of motor coordination, reduced judgment, and decreased inhibition.

Chapter Review

1 Answer: 1 Rationale: When narcotic analgesia is used for the shortest amount of time and the lowest dose possible to adequately control pain, addiction is usually not a problem for the majority of patients in the postoperative period. The nurse should administer the dose to treat the pain. Options 2, 3, and 4 are incorrect. Reviewing the patient's past medical history is an important assessment that should guide nursing practice, but past tendencies toward substance abuse are not appropriate criteria to consider in the nurse's decision to provide analgesia. Pain is best treated in the early stage. If a nurse waits to treat pain until it becomes intolerable, the patient will require a higher dose of analgesia. There is no evidence that patients request medication when it is not needed.

2 Answer: 3 Rationale: Patients with a substance use disorder tend to revert back to drug-seeking behavior when they return to the company of other substance abusers. Options 1, 2, and 4 are incorrect. A good support system can be extremely beneficial when an individual is attempting to withdraw from addictive substances. Patients with substance use disorder may experience the desire to use drugs long after the drug has physiologically cleared the body. Generally speaking, individuals who share a common experience will be perceived as being most helpful to an individual undergoing the same or a similar experience.

3 Answer: 1, 4, 5 Rationale: Varenicline doses are increased over an 8-day period and maintained for 12 to 24 weeks, reducing withdrawal symptoms and craving for smoking. Serious dermatologic reactions or angioedema should be reported to the provider immediately and the drug stopped. Varenicline carries a black box warning for serious neuropsychiatric events, and any changes in behavior, depression, hostility, or thoughts of suicide should be immediately reported. Options 2 and 3 are incorrect. Varenicline activates nicotinic acetylcholine receptors in the brain and blocks nicotine from reaching the receptors. It does not prevent nicotine's harmful effects on body systems from occurring. It has several adverse effects, including serious dermatologic and neuropsychiatric effects.

4 Answer: 2 Rationale: Sedatives cause suppress the respiratory system through direct action with the CNS and patients who have experienced an overdose of sedatives are at high risk for respiratory arrest. Options 1, 3, and 4 are incorrect. Sedatives do not typically cause any type of stimulation. Long-term effects of overdose will most likely manifest through liver and kidney dysfunction, but the immediate need is to determine the current status of the patient. Level of consciousness is one of the assessments to be made with a patient receiving sedatives, but the nurse would expect a decrease in consciousness with an overdose of sedatives.

5 Answer: 4 Rationale: Typical symptoms of heroin withdrawal include chills, dilated pupils, diarrhea, runny nose, muscle spasms, goose bumps, abdominal pain, sweating, and agitation. Options 1, 2, and 3 are incorrect. Heroin is an opiate that depresses the CNS, and the patient may exhibit hyperactive behavior during withdrawal. Dermatologic effects are not common during heroin withdrawal. Paranoia, delusions, or hallucinations are more typical effects.

6 Answer: 1 Rationale: Disulfiram is used in the rehabilitation of alcoholism. When patients are taking this drug, even small amounts of alcohol can induce flushing, throbbing in the head and neck, respiratory difficulty, nausea and vomiting, sweating, thirst, chest pain, blurred vision, and confusion. Options 2, 3, and 4 are incorrect. There is no reason for a patient to avoid dairy products or foods high in iron. Disulfiram should not directly impact driving or level of alertness.

Chapter 29

Making the Patient Connection

1 The etiology of hyperlipidemia may be inherited or acquired. Diets high in saturated fats, lack of exercise, smoking, and excessive alcohol intake contribute significantly to hyperlipidemia and resulting cardiovascular diseases. However, genetics determines one's ability to metabolize lipids and contributes to high lipid levels in a substantial number of patients. For most patients, dyslipidemias are the result of a combination of genetic and environmental (lifestyle) factors.

2 The patient should be taught the following health concepts related to lowering her LDL level:
Maintain weight at an optimal level; implement a medically supervised exercise plan; reduce dietary saturated fats and cholesterol; increase soluble fiber in the diet; eliminate tobacco use; eliminate alcohol use or consume no more than one 4-oz glass per day (for women; no more than two for men); monitor blood lipid levels regularly; as recommended by the healthcare provider.

3 Back pain, asthenia, hypersensitivity reaction, myalgia, headache, abdominal pain, constipation, diarrhea, dyspepsia, and flatulence are potential adverse effects.

Additional Case Study

1 David needs to understand all the routine concepts related to lowering LDL levels (e.g., weight control or low-fat diet). However, for David the problem may not be deficient knowledge. The nurse and the patient need to explore ways in which he can be more consistent with his medication and exercise regimen.

2 Adverse associated with cholestyramine include constipation, fecal impaction, hemorrhoids, abdominal pain and distention, flatulence, bloating sensation, and belching.

3 David may be switched to a statin drug such as atorvastatin if his triglyceride levels continue to increase or are consistently elevated.

Chapter Review

1 Answer: 1 Rationale: Rhabdomyolysis is a serious adverse effect of the statins. Early signs include unexplained fatigue or muscle weakness, pain in joints or muscles, and an increase in CK level. Options 2, 3, and 4 are incorrect. The weakness, fatigue, and pain that the patient is experiencing are not symptoms of renal failure or hepatic insufficiency. In rheumatoid arthritis, pain is often present but tends to be greatest in the mornings and associated with red, hot, swollen joints.

2 Answer: 2 Rationale: One of the most serious adverse effects of cholestyramine is obstruction of the GI tract. Options 1, 3, and 4 are incorrect. Cholestyramine does not cause orange urine, sore throat, and fever or affect capillary refill.

3 Answer: 1 Rationale: Although there are few contraindications to using bile acid sequestrants such as colestipol, they should be used cautiously in patients with GI disorders such as peptic ulcer disease. Options 2, 3, and 4 are incorrect. MI is not a contraindication for the use of bile acid sequestrants. Bile acid sequestrant agents do not affect serum sodium levels, and patients allergic to foods high in tyramine may be prescribed these drugs.

4 Answer: 2, 3 Rationale: Intense flushing and hot flashes occur in most patients taking niacin. Tingling of the extremities may also occur. Options 1, 4, and 5 are incorrect. Neither fever and chills nor dry mucous membranes are associated adverse effects of niacin therapy. Niacin may cause an increase in fasting blood glucose, especially in people with diabetes.

5 Answer: 4 Rationale: Grapefruit juice inhibits the metabolism of statins allowing them to reach high serum levels. Options 1, 2, and 3 are incorrect. Most patients with lipid disorders are asymptomatic. A patient should be instructed that maintenance of optimal body weight will help reduce unhealthy lipid levels. Because cholesterol biosynthesis in the liver is higher at night, statins are usually best taken in the evening.

6 Answer: 1, 4, 5 Rationale: Fibric acid agents (fibrates) such as gemfibrozil may cause or worsen gallbladder disease and may enhance the hypoglycemic effects of antidiabetic drugs. Because it is excreted through the kidneys, it may be used cautiously in patients with renal impairment, but the order should be validated with the provider before giving if the patient has a history of kidney disease. Options 2 and 3 are incorrect. Angina and hypertension may indicate the existence of atherosclerosis and arteriosclerosis, both of which are indications for a lipid-lowering drug.

Chapter 30

Making the Patient Connection

1 CCBs slow the rate at which calcium passes into the heart muscle and into the vessel walls. This relaxes the vessels which will then let blood flow more easily, thereby lowering blood pressure.

2 There is no cure for primary HTN. However, patients with this chronic disease can live normal lives if they adopt lifestyle changes and adhere to a therapeutic regimen.

3 Adverse effects of CCBs include hypotension, dizziness, constipation, dysrhythmias, and HF.

Additional Case Study

1 Even though Mabel is not having any symptoms, HTN is often a "silent" disease and, if left untreated, can lead to significant organ damage. Consistent use of her amlodipine is essential for maintaining blood pressure control.

2 The peripheral vasodilation caused by amlodipine may trigger flushed skin, headache, dizziness, and lightheadedness.

3 Reminders are often helpful when scheduling a patient's medication doses. Some suggestions that the nurse might offer include: take medications around daily activities, such as setting an alarm clock, brushing teeth, eating meals, or going to work; place reminder notes in visible places such as on the bathroom mirror or on the refrigerator; a medication box that holds an entire day's supply of all medications is helpful. If use of such a device is desired, ensure that the patient notes the names of all drugs included, as well as the color, size, and dose of each pill, on a separate list; if the patient continues to have problems remembering, Mabel should speak to the prescriber to see if her medication schedule can be simplified.

Review Questions

1 Answer: 1 Rationale: A major complication associated with the administration of CCBs such as nifedipine is HF. Daily weighing will help identify signs of fluid retention, which may indicate cardiac dysfunction. A weight gain of 1 kg or more in 24 hours suggests possible fluid retention and may signal impending HF. Options 2, 3, and 4 are incorrect. Nifedipine does not affect the immune system, and there is no reason to avoid crowds. The intake of oral or dietary calcium and CCBs has not been shown to be problematic. HTN is asymptomatic, and patients should be instructed to take the medication even when feeling healthy.

2 Answer: 4 Rationale: Felodipine may cause hypotension with associated reflex tachycardia. Options 1, 2, and 3 are incorrect. Rash and chills, increased urine output, and weight loss are not adverse effects of CCBs.

3 Answer: 4 Rationale: An adverse effect of verapamil is HF, which will be reflected in the patient's intake and output ratio and weight gain of more than 1 kg per 24 hours. Options 1, 2, and 3 are incorrect. Verapamil does not affect coagulation or thrombocytes. Verapamil is usually given during hours that the patient is awake; however, it can be administered at any time.

4 Answer: 2 Rationale: Grapefruit juice will enhance the absorption of nifedipine. Options 1, 3, and 4 are incorrect. Nifedipine should not be taken with antacids since this will affect the absorption rate of the drug. Patients should never double the dose of nifedipine because life-threatening hypotension could result. Nifedipine does not affect the efficacy of birth control pills.

5 Answer: 1, 2, 3, 4 Rationale: Diltiazem reduces the patient's blood pressure, which may result in syncope or dizziness. Until the effects of the medication are known the patient should avoid driving or other activities requiring mental alertness. One of the adverse effects associated with diltiazem and CCBs is constipation, which can be reduced by increasing fluid and dietary fiber intake. Diltiazem may cause orthostatic hypotension. To ensure safety, patients should be instructed to rise slowly from sitting or lying positions. Patients should be taught to report a weight gain of 1 kg per day or 2 kg per week. Option 5 is incorrect. Sudden discontinuation could cause the patient to experience hypertensive crisis.

6 Answer: 3 Rationale: Nifedipine is a negative inotropic drug and symptoms of pulmonary edema call for discontinuation of the drug. The nurse should also monitor a patient more closely for congestive HF and pulmonary edema if a medical history of pulmonary edema is noted. Options 1, 2, and 4 are incorrect.

An appendectomy does not warrant additional monitoring of the patient. Patients receiving renal dialysis should be closely monitored during therapy with nifedipine due to a reduction in renal function. However, these patients are not as high risk as a patient with pulmonary edema. Psychotropic drugs are not known to interact negatively with this drug.

Chapter 31

Making the Patient Connection

1 Losartan is an ARB and acts by blocking the action of angiotensin II at its receptors. Angiotensin II causes the blood vessels to narrow and makes the blood pressure increase. When this chemical is blocked, vasodilation occurs and blood pressure falls.

2 Common adverse effects associated with losartan include headache and dizziness. Carlos should be informed that typically these adverse effects disappear after a few days of therapy. However, if these symptoms continue after 1 week, he should notify his healthcare provider. Severe effects include angioedema and acute kidney failure. You should inform Carlos to immediately report edema, decreased urinary output, difficulty breathing, skin rash, and hives to the prescriber.

3 Carlos should receive dietary instruction including the need to reduce salt and fat intake, avoid salt substitutes that contain potassium, and increase the amount of fresh fruits and vegetables in his diet. Regular exercise, including daily walking, will also help reduce his blood pressure.

Additional Case Study

1 Lisinopril binds to and inhibits the action of ACE, thus preventing the conversion of angiotensin I to angiotensin II. Spironolactone acts by blocking aldosterone receptors in the kidney tubules. Both help to reduce blood pressure.

2 Spironolactone is used for its mild diuretic effects and as an antihypertensive medication. It causes the kidneys to eliminate excess water and sodium but reduces the loss of potassium from the body. The patient should avoid potassium-containing salt substitutes while taking this medication. Ella should also talk with her healthcare provider about the amount of potassium-rich foods (e.g., bananas, prunes, tomatoes, potatoes, citrus fruits and juices) that she may eat.

Review Questions

1 Answer: 4 Rationale: Lisinopril does not affect serum calcium levels and, thus, would not cause an elevated blood pressure. Options 1, 2, and 3 are incorrect. Common adverse effects for lisinopril are cough, headache, dizziness, orthostatic hypotension, and rash. These symptoms should be reported to the prescriber. Salt substitutes usually contain potassium chloride and should be avoided to reduce the risk of hyperkalemia. If a dose is missed, the patient take it as soon as possible but not too close to the next dose and to never take a double dose.

2 Answer: 1 Rationale: Lisinopril should be stored in a dry place at room temperature because heat and moisture may cause drug breakdown. Options 2, 3, and 4 are incorrect. Heat and moisture do not enhance the strength of the drug, crystallize the medication, or convert the medication to toxic metabolites.

3 Answer: 3 Rationale: ACE inhibitors such as enalapril also prevent the breakdown of bradykinin. Accumulation of bradykinin in the lungs can cause a nonproductive cough which may require an antihistamine for treatment. Options 1, 2, and 4 are incorrect. Dry mucous membranes are not adverse effects related to ACE inhibitors. The expected outcome associated with ACE inhibitors is a decline in blood pressure, and the nurse should expect both systolic and diastolic pressures to be reduced.

4 Answer: 2 Rationale: Common adverse effects of losartan are headache, dizziness, nasal congestion, and insomnia. Options 1, 3, and 4 are incorrect. Irritability, tremors, sleepiness, slurred speech, pruritus, or rash are not common adverse effects associated with losartan.

5 Answer: 1 Rationale: Patients with severe dehydration may experience hypovolemia and are at high risk of life-threatening hypotension. Options 2, 3, and 4 are incorrect. Irbesartan may be prescribed for the prevention of diabetic nephropathy, HTN, and as an off-label use for heart failure.

6 Answer: 3 Rationale: Patients receiving benazepril should avoid driving or engaging in other hazardous activities until the effects of the drug are known. Benazepril may cause adverse effects that impair thinking and reaction time. Options 1, 2, and 4 are incorrect. The patient should be taught methods of home blood pressure measurement and maintenance of a blood pressure log. OTC medications for colds, sinus, fever, asthma, or appetite control should be avoided because they may increase blood pressure. The consumption of alcohol while taking benazepril can lower blood pressure, which could lead to dizziness and fainting.

Chapter 32

Making the Patient Connection

1 a) Loop diuretics act on the ascending loop of Henle in the kidney. They are primarily used to treat HTN and edema, often due to HF or renal insufficiency. Although all electrolytes may be lost due to diuretic therapy, it is potassium that is most affected and presents the greatest problem to patients receiving loops diuretics. b) Thiazide diuretics also deplete potassium levels and cause the body to lose magnesium. Are frequently used in combination with other drugs to treat HTN. c) Potassium-sparing diuretics do not promote the excretion of potassium into the urine. They are also used as adjunctive therapy in the treatment of HTN and HF. d) Osmotic diuretics work through the diffusion of fluid through semipermeable membranes by creating a shift in fluid from intercellular and interstitial areas to the intravascular space. Due to the increase in the circulating volume, the nurse should monitor the patient for fluid overload, and electrolyte levels should be monitored frequently.

2 Most diuretics potentially create a deficit of potassium. Hypokalemia predisposes the patient to digoxin toxicity.

3 The patient taking diuretics should be instructed to: take the medication exactly as prescribed, watch for electrolyte imbalances and dehydration and take steps to prevent such from occurring, weigh weekly and report significant changes such as weight gain of 1 kg in 24 hours, consult the prescriber before consuming OTC medications, rise slowly to minimize orthostatic hypotension.

Additional Case Study

1 Spironolactone inhibits the action of aldosterone, causing the kidneys to excrete sodium and water while retaining potassium. Spironolactone is classified as a potassium-sparing medication that promotes the output of urine (diuretic).

2 Foods high in potassium include apricots, avocado, banana, cantaloupe, honeydew, kiwi, lima beans, milk, oranges, orange juice, potatoes, prunes, spinach, tomatoes, and vegetable juice; they should be eaten sparingly.

3 Often hyperkalemia is asymptomatic. Vague symptoms that include nausea, fatigue, muscle weakness, or tingling. Serious signs include slow heartbeat and weak pulse.

Review Questions

1 Answer: 2 Rationale: Furosemide may dramatically reduce circulating blood volume, thus producing episodes of orthostatic hypotension. Patients may minimize this effect by rising slowly from sitting or lying positions. Options 1, 3, and 4 are incorrect. Cabbage, cauliflower, and kale are high in vitamin K, but furosemide does not require restricted consumption of these foods. Monitoring pulse rate during administration of furosemide for reflex tachycardia secondary to hypotension is advised, but it is not required that it be taken before the dose or for 1 full minute. Due to the potential for significant diuresis, fluids should not be restricted unless ordered by the healthcare provider.

2 Answer: 2 Rationale: Loop diuretics such as bumetanide cause a significant loss of potassium with the possibility of hypokalemia. Options 1, 3, and 4 are incorrect. Hypernatremia is unlikely with the administration of bumetanide because it promotes sodium loss. Hyperkalemia is inconsistent with the administration of bumetanide due to the increase in potassium excretion. Bumetanide does not cause hypocalcemia but may cause hypercalciuria with an increased risk of calcium-based kidney stones.

3 Answer: 3 Rationale: Muscle cramps and weakness may indicate hypokalemia and should be reported to the healthcare provider. Options 1, 2, and 4 are incorrect. Many patients taking diuretic therapy are instructed to monitor the intake of both sodium and water to maintain adequate but not excessive amounts. Patients should ingest foods high in potassium, not vitamin K. Thiazide diuretics and antihypertensive drugs are not known to cause sleepiness when taken together.

4 Answer: 1 Rationale: Spironolactone is a potassium-sparing diuretic and may cause hyperkalemia. Options 2, 3, and 4 are incorrect. This drug does not have a direct effect on magnesium and does not cause hypokalemia. It does not have calcium-binding effects.

5 Answer: 4 Rationale: Mannitol causes fluid to be drawn into extracellular spaces and vascular compartments. Pulmonary and peripheral edema may occur and increased intracranial pressure may also occur along with an early change in level of consciousness. Options 1, 2, and 3 are incorrect. Keeping a urinal or bedpan nearby; monitoring electrolytes, including potassium; and recording input and output and daily weight are important nursing interventions but are not the main nursing priority in the early administration of mannitol.

6 Answer: 1 Rationale: Patients receiving acetazolamide are at risk for metabolic acidosis due to excess bicarbonate loss. Options 2, 3, and 4 are incorrect. Metabolic alkalosis is characterized by a deficit of bicarbonate and is not an adverse effect of acetazolamide. Acetazolamide does not cause respiratory acidosis or respiratory alkalosis.

Chapter 33

Patient Safety: Serious patient injury or death may result from concentrated electrolyte solutions such as potassium chloride. The Joint Commission, the accrediting body for many healthcare organizations, considers potassium to be a "high-alert medication." While policies may vary at different healthcare agencies, it is recommended that potassium supplies be removed from the patient care units and be under pharmacy controls, premixed concentrations be used when possible, and requests for unusual concentrations be clarified. As an added precaution, some agencies may require that the potassium dosage be checked with another nurse.

Making the Patient Connection

1 Because Peggy has been in good health, an IV is not required to replace lost fluids but to serve as an IV route to administer other drugs during surgery. The dextrose 5% in water (D_5W) solution will provide only minimal calories and, at the rate of 15 mL/h, will not prevent dehydration. It is anticipated that Peggy will return home that afternoon and should be able to resume oral fluids soon thereafter. You would explain this to Peggy and also tell her that should additional fluids or drugs be required during or after surgery, they may be administered through her existing IV line.

2 The two main categories of IV fluids are colloids and crystalloids. Blood products is the third category but is not indicated in this scenario. Colloids are proteins, starches, or other large molecules that have the same effect as hypertonic solutions. Crystalloids are the most commonly used IV fluids and are solutions that contain electrolytes or other agents, such as dextrose. Peggy has an order for dextrose 5% in water (D_5W), which is a crystalloid solution.

3 Dextrose 5% in water (D_5W) is an isotonic solution that will supply a small number of calories through metabolism of the glucose and will provide an IV route should drugs or additional fluids be required during or after surgery. The nurse should question Peggy about a possible history of diabetes or cardiac or renal conditions before administering the fluids and notify the provider if any are noted.

Additional Case Study

1 Loop diuretics can cause potassium loss, resulting in hypokalemia. Usually, the amount of potassium loss is greater than the amount a patient can consume through daily dietary intake.

2 Patients taking potassium supplementation should be taught symptoms of both hyperkalemia and hypokalemia. Symptoms associated with hyperkalemia include dysrhythmias, fatigue, paresthesias, muscle twitching, dyspnea, nausea, cramping, and diarrhea. Symptoms of hypokalemia include muscle weakness, lethargy, irregular heartbeat, and anorexia.

3 Because the patient is taking potassium supplements, he should be taught to avoid an intake of foods with high potassium levels. Salt substitutes should be avoided because most contain high amounts of potassium.

Chapter Review

1 Answer: 1 Rationale: The serum pH is a measure of alkalinity or acidity in the blood. The administration of bicarbonate neutralizes acidic conditions and causes the patient's serum to become more alkaline. Options 2, 3, and 4 are incorrect. Administration of sodium bicarbonate will not influence the number of circulating RBCs. The liver does not metabolize sodium bicarbonate and liver function tests are not indicators of the drug's effectiveness. Although sodium bicarbonate excretion occurs in the kidneys, the blood urea nitrogen level will not reflect the effectiveness of this drug.

2 Answer: 2 Rationale: Liquid preparations are KCl are irritating to the gastric mucosa and should always be diluted with juice or water. Options 1, 3, and 4 are incorrect. Salt substitutes are high in potassium and should be avoided by patients on potassium supplementation. Symptoms such as weakness or fatigue may be the first indicators of potassium imbalances. The GI secretions are rich in potassium. Episodes of persistent vomiting may lead to hypokalemia and should be reported to the healthcare provider.

3 Answer: 4 Rationale: Dextran 40 interferes with coagulation and reduces blood viscosity. Bleeding, potentially severe, is associated with these effects. Options 1, 2, and 3 are incorrect. Dextran solutions are used to correct low circulating blood volume states. This solution does not cause dehydration. Dextran increases the circulating volume and thereby increases urine output, which is a therapeutic effect of the solution. Dextran is used for shock (hypovolemia); it does not cause shock.

4 Answer: 2 Rationale: D_5W is often used to dilute (reconstitute) powdered forms of drugs that to be given parenterally. Options 1, 3, and 4 are incorrect. This solution can cause hyperglycemia in the patient with diabetes due to the dextrose content. D_5W is considered a crystalloid solution. One liter of this solution supplies only 170 calories, which is not enough to supply the metabolic nutritional needs of adult patients.

5 Answer: 4 Rationale: Magnesium sulfate toxicity may cause significant neuromuscular depression as noted by changes in LOC and diminished deep tendon reflexes. Options 1, 2, and 3 are incorrect. Pupillary constriction to bright light is a normal physiological response. The nurse should notify the prescriber if the patient develops chest congestion and coughing, but they are not directly associated with magnesium sulfate toxicity. Elevated blood pressure is common in preeclampsia, but it is not associated with magnesium toxicity.

6 Answer: 1, 3, 4 Rationale: Normal serum albumin is a product derived from blood. Although rare, transfusion reactions can still occur with normal serum albumin. Albumin causes intercellular and interstitial fluid to move into the intravascular compartment. This movement of fluid will cause increases in the patient's blood pressure and heart rate. The nurse should monitor the patient for fluid overload with this solution. As the circulating fluid volume is corrected, the patient's urinary output will increase. Options 2 and 5 are incorrect. Patients receiving normal serum albumin typically do not have any dietary restrictions while receiving this solution. Serum albumin is not administered for potassium imbalances.

Chapter 34

Making the Patient Connection

1 Elmer is on the right track. Although lifestyle changes aid in high blood pressure reduction, they take time. Plus, even with dietary changes, exercise, and smoking cessation, HTN may still be present. Inform Elmer that controlling HTN sometimes requires more than one medication and that it may take some time to find the right combination to effectively treat his condition.

2 HTN is complex and may be caused by a series of physiologic factors. It is not unusual for multiple medications to be prescribed before the right type and right dosage brings high blood pressure under control.

3 Elmer should be praised for his efforts. There is a good chance his blood pressure reading would have been much higher had he not initiated the lifestyle changes. HTN is a chronic disease that can cause some individuals to feel hopeless. Providing the patient with support and encouragement is an important nursing intervention. It may be the determining factor in the patient choosing to adhere to the therapeutic regimen.

Additional Case Study

1 Nitroprusside acts directly on vascular smooth muscle to produce peripheral vasodilation, thereby lowering arterial blood pressure. It is used for short-term, rapid reduction of blood pressure in hypertensive emergencies.

2 Nitroprusside is only given in critical care or ED settings. Adverse effects include profound hypotension, palpitation, bradycardia, and ECG changes.

3 Helen has multiple factors that predispose her to HTN-E: Black, history of HTN, poor adherence to hypertensive management, and obesity.

Review Questions

1 Answer: 1 Rationale: Black patients are often resistant to the antihypertensive effects of beta blockers, ACE inhibitors, or ARBs. Thiazide diuretics or calcium channel blockers are preferred for the treatment of HTN in Black patients. Options 2, 3, and 4 are incorrect. While extended-release formulations may make adherence easier with a once- or twice-daily dosing, other drug classifications also have these formulations. The cost of a drug has no relation to its effectiveness. Beta blockers have been shown to have less effect in Black patients and may not adequately control HTN.

2 Answer: 4 Rationale: Orthostatic hypotension is a common adverse effect of vasodilators such as hydralazine. Options 1, 2, and 3 are incorrect. Hydralazine does not typically cause atelectasis. Crystalluria is not an adverse effect of hydralazine and it does not cause photosensitivity.

3 Answer: 2, 3, 4, 5 Rationale: Adverse effects of ACE inhibitors such as enalapril include persistent cough and orthostatic hypotension. Hyperkalemia can be a major concern for patients with renal impairment and in patients taking potassium-sparing diuretics. Though rare, the most serious adverse effect of ACE inhibitors is the development of angioedema. Option 1 is incorrect. Hypotension with reflex *tachycardia* is a possibility depending on how low or how fast the blood pressure decreases.

4 Answer: 4 Rationale: The nurse will titrate the rate of infusion based on the patient's blood pressure. Options 1, 2, and 3 are incorrect. Listening for bowel sounds in the patient with hypertensive crisis is not a nursing priority. Urine specific gravity and glucose levels may be obtained but are not associated with hypertensive crisis or the administration of this drug. Observing skin pressure points is a nursing intervention that does not directly relate to hypertensive crisis or nitroprusside therapy.

5 Answer: 2, 3, 4 Rationale: ACE inhibitors or ARBs, CCBs, and thiazide diuretics are the primary treatment options for most patients. Options 1 and 5 are incorrect. Beta blockers may still be used for some patients but are no longer recommended for primary treatment of HTN. Direct-acting vasodilators are used to treat hypertensive crisis and for patients who have not responded adequately to other antihypertensive drugs.

6 Answer: 1, 2, 4 Rationale: Thiocyanate poisoning may develop more quickly in patients with impaired renal function. Renal function and creatinine levels should be evaluated before starting the drug. Signs of thiocyanate poisoning include hypotension, lethargy, unconsciousness, and faint heart sounds. Options 3 and 5 are incorrect. Past alcohol use will not determine whether thiocyanate poisoning develops or influences its symptoms. While flushing of the skin may occur with nitroprusside administration, skin color and turgor are not reliable indicators of thiocyanate poisoning.

Chapter 35

Making the Patient Connection

1 Myocardial cells require a steady supply of oxygen. When the supply is decreased or stopped, these cells begin to die. The chest pain that he was having is a symptom of the lack of adequate blood supply to his heart. The treatment is aimed at supplying the myocardium with adequate oxygen-enriched blood.

2 Nitroglycerin dilates both arteries and veins. This allows the coronary arteries to supply more blood to oxygen-deprived myocardial tissue. Additionally, the venous dilation decreases cardiac afterload and reduces the oxygen demand of the myocardium. Together, the nonselective vasodilation helps to restore the supply–demand balance to the myocardium.

3 Adverse effects associated with nitroglycerin infusions include hypotension, tachycardia, flushing, and headache.

4 IV nitroglycerin infusions are typically titrated based on the patient's pain and other hemodynamic indicators such as blood pressure and heart rate. Also, IV nitroglycerin must be

administered using specialized IV tubing and should always be delivered via infusion pump.

Additional Case Study

1 Variant angina is caused by spasms of the coronary arteries and is sometimes called vasospastic angina. Because the narrowing and decreased blood flow is caused by spasms and not a clot or narrowing of the artery, drugs such as nifedipine are used to relax the artery and improve blood supply.

2 Drugs such as sildenafil are not to be used with nitroglycerine because they may cause a significant and severe drop in blood pressure. They may be used with caution when nifedipine and other calcium channel blockers are used. Consult the healthcare provider as to the appropriate erectile dysfunction drug to use.

Review Questions

1 Answer: 4 Rationale: A decline in blood pressure is an expected adverse effect. The nurse should assess blood pressure prior to and 5 minutes after administering nitroglycerin. Options 1, 2, and 3 are incorrect. Photosensitivity, vomiting, and diarrhea are not expected adverse effects. Nitroglycerin causes a decline in blood pressure, not an increase

2 Answer: 4 Rationale: Skin irritation can occur if the same site is used repeatedly. Options 1, 2, and 3 are incorrect. Patients should be instructed to rotate the site of application when using nitroglycerin patches. Repeated use of the same application site may actually decrease absorption. Rebound phenomenon is not an expected occurrence with nitroglycerin, but tolerance may occur if the patches are not removed for a period of time each day.

3 Answer: 3 Rationale: Patients may experience lightheadedness or dizziness as a result of the hypotensive effects of isosorbide. Options 1, 2, and 4 are incorrect. Because the oral form of isosorbide has a slower onset than sublingual forms, a flushing sensation and headache are not usually experienced as they are with sublingual nitroglycerin. Tremors and anxiety are not associated adverse effects with this drug. Isosorbide does not usually cause sleepiness or lethargy.

4 Answer: 1 Rationale: Atenolol increases blood flow to the myocardium, thereby increasing oxygen supply by reducing the heart rate and decreasing the contractility. Options 2, 3, and 4 are incorrect. Atenolol is a beta-adrenergic blocker, which decreases heart rate. This drug does not affect the sodium channels. Although this drug reduces blood pressure, the mechanism of action is not by blocking $alpha_2$ receptors.

5 Answer: 1, 3 Rationale: Verapamil decreases blood pressure and heart rate. The administration of this drug may cause significant hypotension and bradycardia in some patients. Options 2, 4, and 5 are incorrect. Verapamil may be used to treat fast heart rates and HTN in addition to angina. Tinnitus and hearing loss are not adverse effects associated with verapamil.

6 Answer: 1, 2, 3, 4 Rationale: Fibrinolytics are most effective when administered as soon as possible after the onset of MI symptoms, ideally less than 30 minutes. They have little to no benefit when administered 24 hours after MI. Because they interfere with normal clotting mechanisms, the risk for extreme bleeding requires frequent monitoring. Assessment before beginning drug therapy includes history of bleeding disorders, stroke within the past 3 months, or severe liver disease. Anticoagulants or antiplatelet drugs are used post-fibrinolytic therapy to maintain artery patency. Option 5 is incorrect. Fibrinolytic therapy is used to dissolve clots in the coronary artery, opening the vessel to blood flow. Calcium channel blockers are used in vasospastic angina where clots may not be present, but blood flow is hindered by vessel spasm.

Chapter 36

Patient Safety: After watching the patient take his pulse using the stethoscope, the nurse notes that he is counting rhythmically, counting "lub" and "dub" as two separate beats. The patient has been obtaining heart rates over 60, but his real rate is half of the value he obtains. He is experiencing syncope because his heart rate cannot compensate for the increased physical activity that results from the action of the carvedilol. The nurse should review the technique for pulse-taking with the patient and demonstrate the sites where he may locate his pulse. Some patients find it difficult to locate and measure a peripheral pulse and if this patient prefers to use a stethoscope, he should be taught that the two separate heart sounds comprise only one heartbeat. Having the patient teach back the technique will allow the nurse to assess that he has understood the teaching.

Making the Patient Connection

1 Dobutamine is a positive inotropic drug and will increase myocardial contractility and CO. It is used for the short-term treatment of patients with acute decompensated HF.

2 Sacubitril with valsartan combines an ARB (valsartan) with an angiotensin receptor neprilysin inhibitor. By blocking neprilysin, cardiac efficiency improves. Combined with an ARB, the drugs have been shown to reduce mortality and the number of hospitalizations in patients with HF.

3 Because Thelma has been taking furosemide at home, and has received another dose in the ED, the nurse will assess Thelma's fluid status for signs and symptoms of hypovolemia such as hypotension. Her blood pressure, urine output, lung sounds, and the severity of her peripheral edema will be assessed and continuously monitored. Renal function laboratory studies may be ordered to assess for renal impairment. The low potassium level of 3.1 mEq/L must be corrected but thereafter should be monitored closely as the valsartan may cause potassium retention. In addition, valsartan may cause angioedema and she should be assessed for increasing edema of the face, mouth, and throat.

Additional Case Study

1 The combination of carvedilol, furosemide, and potassium supplementation is common. The purpose of the carvedilol is to slow the heart rate and reduce blood pressure, thus decreasing cardiac workload and improving CO. The diuretic (furosemide) eliminates excessive body fluid and also reduces the workload of the failing heart. The potassium supplement is prescribed to replace the loss of potassium caused by the diuretic.

2 There is an increased risk of hypotension due to the decreased blood pressure from the carvedilol and the lessened fluid volume from the furosemide. Cardiac dysrhythmias may occur if hypokalemia occurs from the furosemide and the potassium supplementation is insufficient to maintain normal levels.

3 Heart failure patients with normal renal function should be encouraged to consume foods rich in potassium, such as bananas, tomatoes, citrus fruits and juices, prunes, potatoes, and broccoli.

Chapter Review

1 Answer: 2 Rationale: ACE inhibitors such as enalapril lower peripheral resistance through the inhibition of angiotensin II formation and reduce blood volume through inhibition of aldosterone secretion. This reduces arterial blood pressure, decreasing afterload and increasing CO. Options 1, 3, and 4 are incorrect. Enalapril is not a positive inotropic agent and does not strengthen the force of myocardial contraction. It does not slow heart rate

(negative chronotropic and dromotropic effects) and it does not have diuretic effects.

2 Answer: 2 Rationale: The patient will be taught to take the pulse daily and to contact the prescriber if the pulse rate is less than 60 or greater than 100 beats per minute. Options 1, 3, and 4 are incorrect. The medication should be taken at the same time each day, preferably after the patient has been active for a period of time. Typically, the pulse rate will be lower in the morning before the patient rises. Digoxin should be withheld if the pulse rate is below 60 beats per minute. A high-fiber diet may decrease the absorption of digoxin, and the drug should not be taken along with meals high in fiber. Furthermore, foods high in calcium may create hypercalcemia, which will potentiate the possibility of digoxin toxicity.

3 Answer: 4 Rationale: Concurrent use of ARNIs with ACE inhibitors is contraindicated due to an increased risk for angioedema. ARNIs are also contraindicated in patients with a history of angioedema. Options 1, 2, and 3 are incorrect. The drug combination would have an additive effect due to the additional antihypertensive effects and hypotension may result. The ACE inhibitors and ARBs may cause hyperkalemia. Rebound hypertension may occur when certain antihypertensive drugs are stopped abruptly. This patient remains on both medications.

4 Answer: 4 Rationale: Hydralazine with isosorbide may cause hypotension with reflex tachycardia, resulting in dizziness and rapid heart rate. Options 1, 2, and 3 are incorrect. Hydralazine with isosorbide does not cause confusion, agitation, bleeding, or tingling of the extremities. If these occur, other causes should be investigated.

5 Answer: 1 Rationale: Beta-adrenergic blockers such as carvedilol must be started at 1/10 to 1/20 of a usual dose and gradually increased to a target dosage. Options 2, 3, and 4 are incorrect. Because lower dosages are required, a higher loading dose will not be given, and beta-adrenergic blockers are often combined with ACE inhibitors, although dosage will not be directly related to the ACE inhibitor. While caution is required if beta-adrenergic blockers are used to treat HF, they are an important drug group for managing heart failure.

6 Answer: 1, 2, 4 Rationale: Beta-adrenergic blockers require gradual increases in dosage amount approximately every 2 weeks to a target dosage. Significant improvement may not be noticed in early therapy and the patient may feel worse during initiation of therapy. Overall, however, the therapy has been proven to reduce the number of HF-related hospitalizations and mortalities. Options 3 and 5 are incorrect. Beta-adrenergic blocker therapy may require alterations in dosage for other cardiac drugs but not all drugs will be affected. Lifestyle changes may be advisable in HF but are not necessarily directly related to beta-adrenergic blocker use.

Chapter 37

Making the Patient Connection

1 Normally the electrical impulse is initiated in a bundle of cells located in the right atrium, called the sinoatrial (SA) node. The electrical impulse moves from cell to cell until it reaches the atrioventricular (AV) node. This area is located in the middle of the heart, between the atrium and ventricles. After the AV node, the impulses travel to the atrioventricular bundle (Bundle of His), that separates the two ventricles. Once the impulse reaches the base of the ventricle (apex), it travels upward and spreads across both ventricles through the Purkinje fibers. Jada's diagnosis tells what part of the conduction is affected. Atrial fibrillation is a condition that occurs in the upper chambers of the heart. Fibrillation is a rapid, uncoordinated twitching movement of the atrium, which impairs cardiac function. This abnormality may be manifested by the lack of clear P waves on the ECG.

2 Amiodarone is given IV usually over 2 to 3 days to achieve a rapid therapeutic blood level. Afterward, patients are often placed on the oral preparation of this drug. As you explain the mechanism of action to Jada, begin by saying that this drug helps to regulate the electrical conduction system of the heart. It slows the rate at which the heart's electrical system recharges and prolongs the electrical phase during which the heart is electrically stimulated. This, in turn, helps to restore the normal heartbeat.

3 For prevention of stroke, most patients with atrial fibrillation are placed on anticoagulation therapy with warfarin, Factor Xa inhibitors, or direct thrombin inhibitors.

4 It is important to take amiodarone exactly as directed by the prescriber. If a dose is missed, the patient should take the missed dose as soon as it is remembered; however, never double the doses. Amiodarone may cause dizziness, drowsiness, and blurred vision. Until the effects of the drug are fully known, the patient should avoid driving or operating machinery. Patients should check their pulse daily and report values less than 60 beats/min to the healthcare provider. Because some patients receiving amiodarone may suffer from photosensitivity, they should be advised to protect their skin from ultraviolet rays and to wear sunglasses.

Additional Case Study

1 Many drugs may be used to treat rapid heart rates and other types of dysrhythmias. The type of drug chosen will depend on the dysrhythmia and other conditions. In this case, the neighbor may have other conditions (e.g., HF) that make digoxin a better choice for their treatment.

2 CCBs work at the cellular level and prevent electrical impulses from traveling too quickly along the myocardium. CCBs do not affect the bones.

3 Nicotine and OTC medications such as cold remedies including phenylephrine can cause serious dysrhythmias. A list of all medications, both OTC and prescription, and any herbal products being taken by the patient should be given to the healthcare provider.

Review Questions

1 Answer: 4 Rationale: Procainamide should be avoided in patients suffering from severe HF since this drug can worsen the condition. Options 1, 2, and 3 are incorrect. Ventricular tachycardia, paroxysmal atrial tachycardia, and atrial fibrillation are indications for the use of procainamide.

2 Answer: 3 Rationale: Early signs of lidocaine toxicity include CNS effects such as paresthesias, drowsiness, confusion, anxiety, or tremors. Options 1, 2, and 4 are incorrect. Decreased platelet levels are not related to the administration of lidocaine. Unless the patient experiences hypotension, there is no need to keep the patient supine. Although coughing and deep breathing are effective nursing strategies to maintain pulmonary function, they are not pertinent for the administration of IV lidocaine.

3 Answer: 3 Rationale: The therapeutic goal of verapamil is to stabilize the dysrhythmia by slowing the electrical conduction. While the atrial dysrhythmia may continue, the rate should return to a normal range (e.g., 60 to 100 in an adult). Options 1, 2, and 4 are incorrect. Verapamil may cause hypotension, but as an adverse rather than a therapeutic effect. It should not cause increases in potassium levels or reduction in urine output.

4 Answer: 4 Rationale: Adenosine has an extremely short half-life and must be administered by rapid IV push over 1 to 2 seconds. Options 1, 2, and 3 are incorrect. Adenosine is not given by IV infusion or slowly. While potassium is an important

electrolyte to monitor in patients with dysrhythmias, adenosine does not cause hypo- or hyperkalemia.

5 Answer: 3 Rationale: Beta blockers such as propranolol are negative inotropic drugs and reduce myocardial contractility. In patients with existing HF, this has the potential to decrease cardiac output and worsen symptoms. Options 1, 2, and 4 are incorrect. Propranolol does not cause sodium retention and its adverse effects include hypotension rather than HTN. It may cause bronchoconstriction because it is a nonselective beta-adrenergic antagonist (blocker), but this effect does not worsen HF. It warrants caution or is contraindicated in patients with COPD and other respiratory conditions.

6 Answer: 3 Rationale: An adverse effect associated with amiodarone is photosensitivity. The patient should be instructed to avoid direct sunlight, wear protective clothing, and use adequate sunscreen lotions of SPF 15 or higher. Options 1, 2, and 4 are incorrect. Amiodarone is not known to cause immunosuppression or to interact with oral contraceptives. Increased bleeding tendencies are not an adverse effect of amiodarone.

Chapter 38

Making the Patient Connection

1 It is common for patients to think that anticoagulants dissolve blood clots. However, these drugs only prevent the thrombus from enlarging or additional thrombi from forming. The body has a natural mechanism called fibrinolysis that occurs on a continual basis. This mechanism slowly and naturally dissolves blood clots. However, in the meantime, the heparin will prevent the existing clot from increasing in size.

2 The major emphasis for patients receiving anticoagulation therapy is to prevent injury that may result in internal or external bleeding. These drugs decrease the patient's ability to form a blood clot, and injury prevention is essential to prevent hemorrhage. Here are a few patient education tips that you will want to share with Jihyo: Avoid activities that may cause traumatic injury; use soft cloths and mild soap when bathing; avoid wearing clothing that is tight or rubs; avoid blowing or picking the nose; avoid rectal suppositories; tampons; or enemas; watch for bleeding and examine all body fluids for the presence of blood; avoid drugs that contain aspirin; NSAIDs; or other anticoagulants.

3 An activated partial thromboplastin time (aPTT) is a laboratory test that reports the time required for clot formation in blood plasma after contact activation and the addition of platelet substitutes. This test measures factors in the intrinsic and common pathways of coagulation. Heparin is titrated according to the aPTT value, which should be between 1.5 and 2 times the patient's baseline when therapeutic anticoagulation is achieved.

4 Long airplane flights can be problematic, especially in patients who have varicose veins (varicosities), irregularly swollen or enlarged veins commonly found in the lower extremities. People who travel on flights that last 8 hours or more are four times more likely to develop DVT. Air travel may increase the risk of DVT through one or more of the following mechanisms: Prolonged sitting and pressure on the calves by the passenger's seat, which can lead to stagnant blood flow in the veins, dehydration as a result of low humidity in the cabin or the consumption of alcohol and caffeine, decreased air pressure and the release of nitric oxide in the plane's cabin.

5 Aspirin and NSAIDs such as ibuprofen and naproxen, are common OTC medications. Because both have an anticoagulation effect and can cause bleeding, they should be avoided when the patient is receiving anticoagulation therapy.

Additional Case Study

1 Atrial fibrillation is the rapid, uncoordinated firing of electrical impulses from multiple sites in the upper chambers of the heart. This condition causes ineffective cardiac contractions and the atria of the heart quiver instead of beating normally. When blood pools in parts of the atrium, subsequent to the poor pumping action, the risk of blood clots increases. Even small blood clots can cause stroke and heart attack if released into the general circulation. Warfarin reduces the risk that the clotting process will begin in the atria.

2 While taking this medication, Lewis should contact the healthcare provider immediately if any bleeding or bruising occurs. He should also be told not to take any prescriptions or OTC medications, such as aspirin, vitamins, or herbal preparations (especially those containing vitamin E or vitamin K), unless ordered by the healthcare provider because many of these medications may interact with warfarin. If Lewis forgets to take his medication, warn him not to try to catch up or double up on the dosage and to contact his healthcare provider for instructions. Before starting any new medication or having a medical or surgical procedure, Lewis should talk with the healthcare provider.

3 Foods high in vitamin K such as liver, broccoli, cabbage, cauliflower, spinach, lentils, chickpeas (garbanzo beans), turnip greens, soybean oil, seaweed, green tea, and herbal teas can interact with warfarin. Lewis should minimize his intake of these foods.

4 The effects of warfarin are evaluated using blood tests such as prothrombin time or international normalized ratio (INR). The INR is the ratio of a patient's prothrombin time to a normal (control) sample. Both blood tests measure how long it takes for blood to clot. The warfarin will be adjusted based on the time it takes for blood to clot.

Review Questions

1 Answer: 1 Rationale: An aPPT is the appropriate laboratory value that should be monitored with heparin infusions. When the patient is receiving this drug, the results should be 1.5 to 2 times the patient's baseline, or 60 to 80 seconds. Options 2, 3, and 4 are incorrect. A prothrombin time or INR is used to monitor the effectiveness of warfarin. Platelets are not affected by anticoagulants and are therefore not used in the monitoring of these drugs.

2 Answer: 1, 2, 3 Rationale: The patient should be taught proper injection technique, including the need to inject the heparin into the deep subcutaneous fat layer. A soft-bristle toothbrush should be used for oral hygiene. Puncture wounds or cuts will require longer than normal pressure held at the site to stop bleeding—15 minutes or longer. Options 4 and 5 are incorrect. Dental flossing can cause gum irritation and excessive bleeding and should be avoided while receiving anticoagulants. Aspirin has antiplatelet effects and concurrent use may increase the risk of hemorrhage.

3 Answer: 3 Rationale: Many drugs such as aspirin and ibuprofen have strong anticoagulant effects. When the patient on warfarin takes these drugs, the risk of bleeding can be increased. Options 1, 2, and 4 are incorrect. Drugs such as aspirin and ibuprofen do not neutralize the effect of an anticoagulant. Anticoagulants do not influence the half-life of any drugs. The pain associated with arthritis is not worsened by the combination of these drugs.

4 Answer: 2 Rationale: Because of the risk of hemorrhage, dysrhythmias, and hypotension, the patient should remain supine during and for up to 8 hours post–drug infusion. Options 1, 3, and 4 are incorrect. The patient will remain in the hospital for a minimum of 24 hours or longer post-procedure for monitoring per agency protocol. The risk of bleeding remains elevated for 2 to

4 days post-infusion. Oral anticoagulants such as warfarin or antiplatelet drugs will be ordered after the infusion; increasing vitamin K in the diet or by supplement may increase the risk of clotting.

5 Answer: 1 Rationale: Clopidogrel is an antiplatelet drug used to prevent blood clots from forming inside arteries by inhibiting platelet aggregation. Options 2, 3, and 4 are incorrect. Heparin is an anticoagulant that blocks the formation of blood clots by activating antithrombin III. Warfarin is a vitamin K antagonist used to prevent the blood from clotting. The drug alteplase is a tissue plasminogen activator that dissolves fibrin clots.

6 Answer: 1, 3, 4, 5 Rationale: Ginger, garlic, and green tea may all increase the risk of bleeding. Dabigatran may be used for DVT and is monitored by aPTT, similar to heparin. The drug is contraindicated in patients with gastritis because of the increased risk of bleeding. Option 2 is incorrect. Vitamin B_{12} does not enhance the response of dabigatran.

Chapter 39

Patient Safety: Unintentional iron poisoning is a leading cause of death by poisoning in children under 6 years of age. The FDA requires labelling of all iron-containing drugs to include a warning for young children, but many OTC vitamin products are still shaped and taste like candy. Iron is directly caustic to the liver and GI tract, causing nausea and vomiting, abdominal pain, and bleeding. Vitamins, should be kept in a secure storage location, out of reach of young children. The mother's statement would be concerning to the nurse. Parents should be encouraged to treat vitamins like any other medication and to refrain from referring to them as "candy" or "treats" to avoid unintentional poisoning. Encouraging a diet sufficient in iron with lean red meats, eggs, enriched cereals and pasta, beans, eggs, and leafy green and yellow vegetables will help provide adequate amounts of dietary iron.

Making the Patient Connection

1 This drug is given when certain WBCs, called neutrophils, are below the normal level. Neutrophils are the most plentiful type of WBC and are the primary infection-fighters. These cells are normally produced in the bone marrow. Filgrastim stimulates the bone marrow to produce these cells, which will reduce the risk of infections.

2 Patients with neutropenia must take multiple precautions to prevent contact with pathogens. These include avoiding crowds, people with known infections, or young children who have a higher risk of having an infection. Uncooked fruits and vegetables or undercooked meats are also possible sources of infection, and other caregivers should prepare these items and perform the cleanup afterward. Careful and frequent hand hygiene is essential for patients with neutropenia as well as for those caring for them. Patients who experience fever, sore throat, or flulike symptoms should report them immediately. The need for complete isolation from others is usually not needed unless the cell counts are extremely low, in which case hospitalization for a short time may be necessary.

3 Some common adverse effects of filgrastim include bone pain, nausea, and swelling or redness at the injection site.

Additional Case Study

1 Common adverse effects of oral iron preparations include constipation, darkened or green stools, diarrhea, nausea, and stomach upset. If the GI adverse effects become excessive, the patient should contact the prescriber. Although taking iron with food may reduce gastric distress, it will also decrease iron absorption.

2 If tolerated, oral iron preparations should be taken on an empty stomach, usually 1 h before a meal or 2 h after a meal to allow for optimal absorption of the iron. Instruct patients not to take iron within 1 h of bedtime. Iron preparations can cause esophageal irritation, which may be avoided by remaining upright for at least 1 h after taking iron. Lastly, iron supplements should be scheduled 1 to 2 h before or after other medications.

Chapter Review

1 Answer: 2 Rationale: The patient who receives epoetin alfa has anemia. This reduction in RBCs produces cellular oxygen deficiency, which causes severe fatigue and weakness. Patients receiving this drug should be taught to take scheduled rest periods to avoid overexertion. Options 1, 3, and 4 are incorrect. Avoiding fresh fruits and vegetables or uncooked meat would be instructions more appropriate for an individual with neutropenia. Epoetin alfa is not associated with photosensitivity. Patients with anemia are not necessarily thrombocytopenic and do not routinely need to avoid activities that may cause injury.

2 Answer: 2 Rationale: Darbepoetin should not be given to patients with uncontrolled HTN because hematopoietic growth factors can increase blood pressure. Options 1, 3, and 4 are incorrect. HIV patients may receive hematopoietic growth factors such as epoetin alfa to correct anemia caused by their HIV drug therapy. Patients with chronic kidney disease often suffer from anemia because they are unable to secrete sufficient erythropoietin. Hematopoietic growth factors are often prescribed for these patients. Chemotherapy also causes anemia and patients may require hematopoietic growth factors if the anemia is severe.

3 Answer: 3 Rationale: Neupogen increases WBC counts. The nurse would monitor for effectiveness by examining this laboratory value. Options 1, 2, and 4 are incorrect. Epoetin alfa increases RBC count. Corticosteroids such as prednisone may be given to increase platelet levels. Reticulocytes are immature RBCs and mean cell volume is a measure of the volume of RBCs.

4 Answer: 4 Rationale: Fostamatinib has been noted to cause fetal harm and the route of administration does not alter this drug's effect on fetal development. Options 1, 2, and 3 are incorrect. Fostamatinib reduces the destruction of platelets in ITP and may be used to increase platelet levels. Fostamatinib may cause HTN and respiratory infections, and blood pressure or signs of infection should be monitored.

5 Answer: 1 Rationale: Patients who regularly consume large amounts of alcohol often suffer from a nutritional deficit of vitamin B_{12}, which can manifest as abnormal neurologic symptoms. Options 2, 3, and 4 are incorrect. Alcohol interferes with folate metabolism in the liver, but lack of folate does not cause destruction of vitamin B_{12}. Pernicious anemia is caused by a lack of intrinsic factor, a substance needed to absorb vitamin B_{12} from the GI tract, which may lead to the anemia, not neutropenia. Vitamin B_{12} is a water-soluble vitamin and is not stored in the body.

6 Answer: 1, 4, 5 Rationale: Parenteral iron can be given to patients with malabsorption conditions or those who cannot tolerate oral iron preparations because they bypass the GI route. They may raise iron levels more quickly than oral formulations, and they may cause anaphylaxis or severe allergic reactions. Options 2 and 3 are incorrect. Common adverse effects are similar to those with oral formulations, and they do not raise Hgb or RBC levels more quickly than orals because the body is limited as to how quickly it can produce new cells.

Chapter 41

Making the Patient Connection

1 Acute inflammation begins as a response to the invasion of particulate matter, bacteria, or cell damage. Fever results from inflammatory chemical mediators or bacterial toxins.

2 Aspirin reduces fever by suppression of prostaglandins in the hypothalamus to lower the body temperature and indirectly by causing peripheral vasodilation and sweating, helping to dissipate heat.

3 Joycee should *not* take the aspirin. The use of aspirin for fever in patients under the age of 19 has been associated with an increased risk of Reye's syndrome, a potentially fatal condition causing increased pressure in the brain, liver and other organ damage. While it can occur at any age, it tends to occur most often in pediatric patients who have been administered aspirin in the presence of viral infections such as the flu or varicella.

4 Joycee should be told that aspirin is not an appropriate drug for her to take because the symptoms suggest she may have the flu as well. If she cannot reach her parents about an acceptable alternative such as obtaining more ibuprofen, she should rest, drink additional fluids throughout the day, and wear lightweight clothing but not so that she feels chilled. To limit the spread of the flu she should stay home from school to avoid exposing others. If her fever continues, increases, or she has additional symptoms, Joycee should call her parents or contact a healthcare provider to assess her need for more definitive treatment.

Additional Case Study

1 Acetaminophen reduces fever by direct action on the heat-regulating center of the hypothalamus. It promotes peripheral vasodilation, sweating, and heat dissipation.

2 The patient should not be administered any pain medications that contain acetaminophen such as "Tylenol #3" (codeine 30 mg with acetaminophen 300 mg). The potential for overdosage of acetaminophen is increased when administering pain medication that contains acetaminophen along with acetaminophen for fever reduction.

3 Instruct the patient to increase fluid intake, rest, practice proper hand hygiene, and for Tameeka, practice perineal care, especially after bowel movements. The temperature should be taken before and after the administration of acetaminophen.

Review Questions

1 Answer: 2 Rationale: Acetaminophen overdose is treated with PO or IV acetylcysteine. For maximum effectiveness, the antidote should be administered within 8 hours of acetaminophen ingestion. Options 1, 3, and 4 are incorrect. The administration of 1,000 mL per hour of normal saline IV would place the patient at risk for fluid volume overload. The patient will not require cardioversion to treat acetaminophen poisoning. The patient's hepatic enzymes will be assessed; however, these enzymes only provide information as to the extent of liver damage. They do not treat acute acetaminophen overdose; they merely monitor for the effectiveness of the treatment and any effects of the overdose itself.

2 Answer: 3 Rationale: Acetaminophen is the drug of choice for reduction of fever in the event the patient has a hypersensitivity to aspirin. Options 1, 2, and 4 are incorrect. A patient who has hypersensitivity to aspirin should not be administered ibuprofen or celecoxib due to the risk of hypersensitivity with the NSAIDs. Ketorolac is not administered for reduction of fever; it is administered for pain control.

3 Answer: 1 Rationale: Ketorolac is administered parenterally for pain. Options 2, 3, and 4 are incorrect. Ketoprofen, ibuprofen, and celecoxib are all administered PO.

4 Answer: 4 Rationale: Ibuprofen should be discontinued 7 to 14 days before surgery to reduce the risk of bleeding. Options 1, 2, and 3 are incorrect. Ibuprofen should not be continued until surgery and the patient should continue her anti-inflammatory agent until 7 to 14 days before surgery to maintain its antiarthritis effects.

5 Answer: 1 Rationale: Acetaminophen is metabolized in the liver. The patient with cirrhosis of the liver has impaired liver function and should not receive acetaminophen for pain or fever reduction. Options 2, 3, and 4 are incorrect. A patient who has COPD or breast cancer or who is taking warfarin can be administered acetaminophen for fever and analgesia.

6 Answer: 1, 2, 3, 4 Rationale: A patient who is experiencing toxic effects from aspirin may experience tinnitus, hyperventilation, GI bleeding, or decreased urine output related to renal impairment. Option 5 is incorrect. A patient with salicylate toxicity does not tend to experience peripheral neuropathy.

Chapter 42

Making the Patient Connection

1 Normally, interferon is produced by lymphocytes and macrophages to fight infection and tumors. Although unable to protect the infected cell, interferon warns nearby cells of an impending infection. Interferons slow the spread of viral infections, enhance the activity of existing leukocytes, and increase phagocytosis and cytotoxic T-cell activity.

2 Common adverse effects of Intron A include flulike symptoms, increased body temperature, feeling ill, fatigue, headache, muscle pain, convulsion, dizziness, hair thinning, and depression. Analgesics and antipyretics may help her feel better but will need to be carefully chosen by the provider to avoid potential hepatotoxicity. Allowing her to express feelings of anxiety or depression may also be therapeutic, and a referral to a mental health provider may be appropriate. Carole should be informed that the adverse effects are short term and usually diminish as therapy progresses.

3 Many patients are fearful of self-administering injectable medication. The nurse will be instrumental in providing Carole with information on injection techniques, followed by having Carole teach-back and demonstrate the technique. Additionally, she should be instructed to pace her daily activities to avoid overtiring. The nurse should assist Carole in identifying designated rest periods while performing activities of daily living. She should also be encouraged to notify the healthcare provider promptly if symptoms of infection develop, such as sore throat, fever, vomiting, and diarrhea.

Additional Case Study

1 Cyclosporine works by targeting the T lymphocytes and inhibiting calcineurin, which is a chemical mediator involved in the immune response. Cyclosporine suppresses the immune system and prevents actions of certain immune cells. It is used to prevent organ rejection following transplant.

2 Gordon should be instructed to take this medication with meals to reduce nausea or gastric irritation. Furthermore, he should take medication at the same time each day to maintain therapeutic blood levels. He should avoid sources of infection due to his induced immunosuppression and keep all scheduled follow-up appointments.

3 Because cyclosporine causes immunosuppression, Gordon's food should be well cooked and raw meats and cleanup tasks should be handled by other family members or caregivers. He should be instructed to avoid drinking grapefruit juice since this significantly increases the serum level of the drug. Gordon may be told to limit the amount of foods with potassium in his diet (bananas, prunes, raisins, and orange juice) because this drug may cause hyperkalemia.

Review Questions

1 Answer: 1 Rationale: Interferon alpha-2b causes flulike symptoms in up to 50% of patients receiving the drug. Options 2, 3, and 4 are incorrect. While depression with suicidal thoughts has been reported, it is not a common adverse effect. Hypotension or hypertension, edema, fluid volume overload, tachycardia, and renal insufficiency are not adverse effects commonly associated with this drug.

2 Answer: 2 Rationale: The patient's high fever and chills are indicative of an infectious process. The use of two immunosuppressant drugs (i.e., basiliximab and cyclosporine) increases the risk of infection related to the additional immunosuppressant effects. Options 1, 3, and 4 are incorrect. Basiliximab has fewer significant adverse effects than other monoclonal antibodies; however, GI effects (nausea and vomiting, abdominal pain) are common and anaphylaxis has been reported. Capillary leak syndrome, a condition in which fluid and protein leak out of tiny blood vessels and flow into surrounding tissue, is not associated with basiliximab administration. Graft-versus-host rejection is a type of transplant rejection, and androgen insensitivity is a genetically linked syndrome. Both are unrelated to the drug.

3 Answer: 2 Rationale: Cyclosporine is toxic to bone marrow, although less so than some other immunosuppressants. A decrease in WBCs to below 4,000/mm^3 should be reported to the provider. Options 1, 3, and 4 are incorrect. Cyclosporine does not cause an elevation in red blood cells. The provider should be notified if platelet counts drop below 75,000/mm^3, but a count of 100,000/mm^3 is within acceptable limits. A creatinine level of less than 1 mg/100 mL is within normal limits.

4 Answer: 3 Rationale: Azathioprine should be used with caution in patients with a previous history of varicella zoster (chickenpox, shingles) because the immunosuppression may reactivate the virus and cause a serious infection. Options 1, 2, and 4 are incorrect. Benign prostatic hyperplasia and cataracts are not contraindications for the drug. Azathioprine may be used as a treatment for severe RA.

5 Answer: 4 Rationale: Tacrolimus is a potent immunosuppressant and patients should decrease their risk for infection by taking precautions such as avoiding raw fruits and vegetables that may harbor pathogens on the skin or inside, and by eating only fully cooked meats after the heat of cooking has destroyed pathogens. Options 1, 2, and 3 are incorrect. Aspirin may increase GI irritation, placing the patient at risk for infections gaining entry through the inflamed mucosa. Physical activity is important to overall health, but this drug has no direct connection with weight gain. Tacrolimus is not known to have significant cardiac effects, although HTN is a possible adverse effect and the blood pressure should be monitored.

6 Answer: 3 Rationale: Aldesleukin causes capillary leak syndrome, which causes fluid to exit the capillary beds and vasculature, decreasing the circulating blood volume. As many as 70% of patients will develop hypotension. With the drop in blood pressure, organs may not perfuse adequately, and urine output will assess the adequacy of renal blood flow. Options 1, 2, and 4 are incorrect. Altered skin condition, rashes, increased pancreatic enzymes such as amylase and lipase, and alterations in vision and hearing are not symptoms of capillary leak syndrome.

Chapter 43

Patient Safety: MMR is a live virus vaccination against measles, mumps, and rubella. Because live virus vaccinations may be contraindicated or deferred in some patient populations, the patient's full medical history should be assessed before giving the vaccine. Causes for deferral or contraindication include pregnancy, immunosuppression from drugs or disease, or when others are living in the home environment with these conditions.

Making the Patient Connection

1 It would be important to ask the parents the nature of Samantha's reaction to her first immunization. This should be compared to her office visit record, her immunization schedule, dosage, and the manufacturer's information to determine the cause of the reaction.

2 Minor adverse effects are frequently seen with the administration of vaccines and are effectively managed with good education. Clarification of questions will also decrease the fear of the effects of the vaccine and increase adherence. Parental adherence to the recommended pediatric immunization schedule is very important for the health of the child.

3 It would be important to discuss the cause of the symptom(s) and the rationale for the administration of vaccines with the Abbotts. It would also be important to provide them with education regarding the management of symptoms and potential adverse effects in both verbal and written forms.

Additional Case Study

1 You received the HBV vaccine upon admission to nursing school 4 years prior to this exposure. The antibody testing is ordered to check for the presence of anti-HBV antibodies, which would have occurred following your initial vaccination. Because the patient has HBV and you have had a contaminated exposure, you will need antibody protection against HBV to prevent its development.

2 The patient is documented positive for HIV and you will need treatment to prevent your development of HIV. This serum analysis is ordered to indicate the presence of antibodies against HIV, which would indicate if you have had a prior exposure to HIV. There would be no need for antiviral prophylaxis if you are already have HIV; you would instead need ongoing HIV treatment.

3 Gamma globulins are a major class of immunoglobulins (proteins) found in the blood and include many of the most common antibodies. When gamma globulin is administered, passive immunity occurs. Antibodies are transferred or "donated" from one individual to another when gamma globulins are used. Because there is currently no immunization against HCV, you will need to receive a passive immunization against it to prevent its development. This is not a vaccination; instead, it is the use of another person's immunity and antibodies to prevent disease development.

4 Antiviral prophylaxis is necessary because you have had a potentially contaminated exposure to a viral infection. In addition to the administration of passive immunity with gamma globulin, antiviral prophylaxis is recommended and will follow individual institutional protocol for the prevention of viral replication.

Review Questions

1 Answer: 2 Rationale: A parent's preconceived ideas or reservations about accepting vaccinations will be most influential on whether the infant receives the scheduled injections. This also presents an excellent teaching opportunity for the nurse to answer questions, allay any fears the mother may have, and teach postvaccine care. Options 1, 3, and 4 are incorrect. An allergy history will be taken, but unless the infant has demonstrated an allergy to the components in the vaccine, allergies to other medications will not necessarily increase the risk of reaction, nor will the parents' allergies increase the risk. Nurses working with children should be knowledgeable about the recommended schedule and, when in doubt, verify the necessary immunizations needed.

2 Answer: 3 Rationale: The MMR vaccination is an attenuated (live) virus and there is a slight risk that the virus could be transmitted to the child's father because he is immunocompromised from the chemotherapy. The nurse would check with the provider about delaying the vaccine until the father is finished with the chemotherapy. Options 1, 2, and 4 are incorrect. The nurse would teach the mother the signs of reaction and when to report them, and the family can safely leave town if healthcare is available at their destination. Although additional teaching may be required to allay the mother's fears of reaction, the mother's reaction to MMR will not necessarily result in a reaction in the child. As long as the brother's immune system is healthy, he should not have any adverse effects from his sister's MMR because of his cold.

3 Answer: 3, 4 Rationale: This child would need to receive rabies immunoglobulin to provide passive immunity to the potential exposure. A series of five rabies vaccines will be started over a 28-day period unless it is confirmed that the dog did not have rabies. If the dog is shown not to have rabies, the series can be stopped. Options 1, 2, and 5 are incorrect. Tetanus and DTaP would not be required as long as the child is current on her vaccination schedule. Rabies is a viral disease and the use of rabies toxoid would be ineffective.

4 Answer: 4 Rationale: Acetaminophen or ibuprofen are appropriate analgesics to treat the soreness from post–tetanus toxoid vaccination. Options 1, 2, and 3 are incorrect. There is no requirement to keep the arm still; in fact, motion may help disperse the medication and help it to absorb. There is no need to restrict fluids or to avoid crowds with a toxoid vaccination.

5 Answer: 3 Rationale: Known hypersensitivity to yeast is an absolute contraindication for the HBV vaccine. Options 1, 2, and 4 are incorrect. Smoking and hypertension are not contraindications for the vaccine and present an opportunity for health teaching. The HBV vaccine is only available by injection and the nurse would explore methods to help the patient be less fearful of the injection prior to administration.

6 Answer: 1 Rationale: Hypersensitivity reactions are most likely to occur within the first 20 minutes of administration. The nurse should closely monitor the patient's vital signs during this period. Options 2, 3, and 4 are incorrect. RhoGAM does not cause thrombocytopenia or anemia or increase liver enzymes. There is no need for a low-saturated-fat, low-cholesterol diet after receiving Rho immune globulin, and RhoGAM does not cause a cough.

Chapter 44

Patient Safety: Because the inhaler was recently ordered and the patient reports using it only during the past 2 days, he may not be using it properly to obtain the bronchodilation benefit. Correct use of the inhaler is necessary for adequate therapeutic outcomes. Proper inhaler use can be a challenge for all patients; however, the older adult is more likely than a younger patient to have one or more factors that impede appropriate use. These factors include patient issues (e.g., cognitive ability, dexterity, presence of tremors, visual or hearing impairments), disease-based issues (e.g., ability to inhale adequately, decreased inspiratory volume), device issues (e.g., devices with differing instructions, use of multiple devices), and cost. For this patient the nurse should review the proper use of the inhaler, verify that is able to use it appropriately, and explore potential additional reasons for his increasing distress, such as continued infection.

Making the Patient Connection

1 Nathan's acute asthma attack began after competing in a swim meet. Potential triggers for the attack include exercise, inhaled chlorine or other substances from the pool, and the possibility of molds or other allergens in the air. Nathan admits to missing his budesonide dose and is not sure about the montelukast. The absence of these preventive medications may have factored into his acute attack.

2 Nathan will be given oxygen therapy, and a nebulizer treatment with albuterol or another quick-acting beta agonist may also be used. If these fail to abort the attack, Nathan may require more aggressive therapy with epinephrine or isoproterenol, adrenergic drugs used to achieve rapid bronchodilation.

3 Because Nathan had forgotten to use his preventive medications, the nurse should explore the need for methods to remind Nathan to take his medications. Involving Nathan and his family in determining strategies will help to ensure adherence. A long-acting beta-agonist inhaler such as salmeterol may be added to the routine to provide longer-term bronchodilation. Because allergens may have triggered the asthma attack, the provider may want to test Nathan for allergies. If allergy testing is ordered, the nurse will need to teach the rationale and methods used for the testing and check with the provider regarding any changes to Nathan's current drug regimen before testing is started. Short-term administration of oral corticosteroids may also be needed. If changes to his other medications do not achieve the desired results, omalizumab may be added to Nathan's routine. Since omalizumab is given subcutaneously, it may be less desirable than inhalers or oral drugs and may be considered only if the other options have not proven effective.

Additional Case Study

1 Theophylline therapy needs careful monitoring and early signs of toxicity include decreased appetite, nausea and vomiting, dizziness, and restlessness. Serum drug levels are monitored to ensure that the therapeutic level is maintained.

2 The list of things to avoid may include several items. First, many medications interact with methylxanthines. Additionally, patients receiving theophylline should limit their intake of foods, beverages, and OTC medications for pain relief that contain caffeine. Lastly, smoking increases the rate of drug clearance from the body, which may result in an inadequate therapeutic level of the drug.

3 The spacer serves two primary purposes. First, it holds drops that fall out of the aerosol so that less medication is deposited on the oropharynx and in the mouth. Second, because the spacer holds the medication, the patient does not have to precisely coordinate inhalation with activation, so that more drug reaches the site of action.

Chapter Review Answers

1 Answer: 1 Rationale: A quick-acting inhaled beta agonist such as albuterol is used to abort bronchospasm. Options 2, 3, and 4 are incorrect. Beclomethasone, ipratropium, and montelukast are drugs used to prevent long-term attacks and will not cause bronchodilation quickly enough to abort an acute attack.

2 Answer: 3 Rationale: Corticosteroids can decrease the beneficial oral flora and may allow for overgrowth of fungal infections such as *Candida*. Rinsing the mouth removes any corticosteroid drug deposited and prevents it from being swallowed, decreasing the likelihood of systemic absorption. Options 1, 2, and 4 are incorrect. Inhaled corticosteroids such as beclomethasone do not cause tachycardia, nervousness, or tremors, and caffeine does not need to be avoided while the drug is used.

3 Answer: 1 Rationale: Bronchodilators such as albuterol may have an adverse effect on heart rate elevation and palpitations related to dosage. Options 2, 3, and 4 are incorrect. Bronchodilators do not decrease the immune response or increase alertness. While some bronchodilators have been

known to cause unexpected problems and paradoxical bronchospasm, this is uncommon.

4 Answer: 2, 4, 5 Rationale: Adverse effects related to vilanterol, a LABA, include tremor and nervousness and dry mouth and hoarseness. These adverse effects are also associated with fluticasone, a corticosteroid, as well as oropharyngeal candidiasis and an increased risk of infections. Options 1 and 3 are incorrect. Corticosteroids and LABAs are not associated with hypotension, sedation and drowsiness. Because vilanterol is a LABA, insomnia may occur.

5 Answer: 3 Rationale: Leukotriene modifiers such as montelukast take up to 1 week or longer for full effects. The patient should continue to use her bronchodilator as needed while the drug reaches full therapeutic effects. If no change in effects is noted after 7 to 10 days, the therapy should be reevaluated. Options 1, 2, and 4 are incorrect. Because the drug is taken PO, the patient should be self-administering the montelukast correctly. More time is needed before determining whether the drug will have full effects, and it is often used as an adjunct to bronchodilation therapy.

6 Answer: 1 Rationale: Ipratropium is contraindicated in patients with hypersensitivity to soya lecithin or related food products such as soybean and peanut. Options 2, 3, and 4 are incorrect. A history of intolerance to albuterol or bronchospasms is an indication for ipratropium. A history of allergy to chocolate is not a contraindication for this drug.

Chapter 45

Making the Patient Connection

1 Additional assessment data to gather would include lung sounds; history of allergies, heart disease, or HTN; other medicines Nancy is taking for her cold; and whether the cough is productive.

2 Nancy has been taking Neo-Synephrine, an intranasal sympathomimetic. The intranasal sympathomimetic does not usually cause the elevated vital signs as an oral drug would, so she may have anxiety. Taking her vitals again in 5 to 10 minutes may result in a normal set of readings. If the vital signs remain elevated, the nurse practitioner should assess how frequently the Neo-Synephrine is used. If it is used frequently, a significant amount may have been swallowed, resulting in the elevated pulse and blood pressure.

3 Nancy may have an allergy to the dog. Because getting rid of the pet may not be an option, suggest that she keep the dog away from her bedroom or outside. Frequent cleaning of the home and bathing of the dog to remove dander may be helpful.

4 Flonase is effective in 90% of patients when usesd to prevent major symptoms of allergic rhinitis. It may take 1 to 3 weeks to see the full effects, but an initial effect can be seen within hours. Nancy's current worsening nasal stuffiness is probably due to the abrupt withdrawal of the Neo-Synephrine. The drug causes rebound congestion if used for longer than 3 to 5 days. Two cough preparations will be taken to help prevent the dry cough. One preparation with dextromethorphan can be used for daytime relief because it does not sedate. The one with diphenhydramine does have sedating effects and can be used at night to allow the patient to get a better night's sleep.

Additional Case Study

1 The patient is having an anaphylactic reaction to strawberries. While this is an allergic reaction, the major cause of the response is not from histamines but from the release of other chemical mediators from mast cells. As an adrenergic agonist, the epinephrine will cause an immediate bronchodilation.

2 Once the initial treatment of anaphylaxis with epinephrine is started, an antihistamine is given as an adjunct to treatment. It will help decrease bronchoconstriction and laryngeal edema that may be caused by small amounts of histamine.

Review Questions

1 Answer: 2, 4 Rationale: Before using intranasal preparations, the nose should be cleared by blowing to ensure the drug reaches the mucosa. Oxymetazoline should not be used for more than 3 to 5 days to prevent rebound congestion. Options 1, 3, and 5 are incorrect. The medication is inhaled so a full glass of water after the drug is not needed, although any liquid that drips into the oral pharynx should be spit out. Inhaled sympathomimetic drugs such as oxymetazoline work quickly, but inhaled corticosteroids may take up to 3 weeks to become fully effective. As a sympathomimetic, drowsiness is not an expected side effect.

2 Answer: 4 Rationale: Pseudoephedrine is a sympathomimetic and is used only for nasal decongestion. Options 1, 2, and 3 are incorrect. Both dextromethorphan and diphenhydramine are effective for some coughs associated with allergic rhinitis and the common cold. Mucolytics are used to loosen thick bronchial secretions in patients with cystic fibrosis and chronic bronchitis.

3 Answer: Because diphenhydramine may cause dizziness and drowsiness, an increased risk of falls is possible, particularly in the older adult.

4 Answer: 4 Rationale: Second-generation (nonsedating) antihistamines such as fexofenadine have been associated with dysrhythmias in the sensitive individual. Options 1, 2, and 3 are incorrect. A history of osteoporosis, peptic ulcer disease, or psoriasis is not a contraindication for the drug.

5 Answer: 3 Rationale: The phenylephrine should be used first to decrease intranasal swelling. After waiting 5 minutes to allow the phenylephrine to work, the fluticasone will reach deeper into the nasal passages for better effects. Options 1, 2, and 4 are incorrect. Fluticasone is used to prevent nasal congestion due to allergic rhinitis and should be used consistently. Instilling fluticasone first may not reach deeper nasal passages if congestion is present.

6 Answer: 4 Rationale: The syrup base of an antitussive cough syrup such as dextromethorphan will help to soothe throat irritation, and the patient should avoid drinking fluids immediately following drug administration. Increasing overall fluid intake throughout the day will help moisten irritated mucous membranes as well as loosen secretions for better effects from the expectorant, guaifenesin. Options 1, 2, and 3 are incorrect. The patient does not have to remain supine after administration and taking the drug with food will not enhance the effects. Avoiding fluid intake will not prevent cough and may cause additional respiratory tract dryness.

Chapter 47

Making the Patient Connection

1 Several factors may have contributed to the patient's wound infection. First, wet dressings are breeding sites for microorganisms because pathogens thrive in warm, moist, dark environments. Patients should be taught to change a wet dressing or return to the healthcare facility for routine dressing changes. Second, older adult patients have an increased risk for infection due to age-related declines in immune function. Furthermore, proper wound healing is dependent on adequate nutrition. Many older adults fail to consume adequate amounts of nutrients, particularly proteins, needed for wound healing.

2 Laboratory studies for this patient might include hematocrit, hemoglobin, and WBC counts. Additionally, serum albumin

levels may be evaluated. These laboratory values not only indicate the presence or degree of infection, but they may also indicate the degree of nutritional impairment that contributes to poor wound healing. Most likely a specimen of the wound drainage will be sent to the laboratory for C&S testing to determine the infecting organism, as well as the specific antibiotic therapy that is indicated.

3 Katie should be instructed about her prescribed medication including potential adverse effects, when and how to take it in relation to meals and food, when to stop taking it, and indicators that would warrant seeking additional healthcare.

4 Cefazolin inhibits bacterial wall synthesis. It is bactericidal and exhibits a broad spectrum of bacterial coverage.

Additional Case Study

1 Open communication may be facilitated by maintaining a calm, matter-of-fact approach to the situation. The nurse should engage the patient in a dialogue that would clarify the reason for the behavior. The problem of saving outdated antibiotics may be related to a lack of understanding or to the patient's concerns about the cost of the drugs.

2 The nurse should provide the patient with information about the danger of saving medication. Additionally, the nurse and patient should explore alternatives that would ensure the patient will have access to medication when needed.

Chapter Review

1 Answer: 3 Rationale: Ampicillin may decrease the effectiveness of oral contraceptives, and the patient should be instructed to use a barrier method to avoid unwanted pregnancies while on the antibiotic and until the next cycle of oral contraceptives is started. Options 1, 2, and 4 are incorrect. The combination of ampicillin and oral contraceptives will not increase the risk of adverse effects related to the antibiotic. Oral contraceptive effectiveness may be reduced during ampicillin therapy, and ampicillin will not create serious toxicity related to the use of oral contraceptives.

2 Answer: 3 Rationale: Ototoxicity is associated with high serum concentrations of vancomycin and manifests with tinnitus, dizziness, or balance and coordination effects. Options 1, 2, and 4 are incorrect. Redness of the ears, itching of the ears, and ocular pain are not symptoms related to ototoxicity caused by vancomycin.

3 Answer: 2 Rationale: A vaginal yeast infection with discharge may be a symptom of a superinfection. Superinfection is a possible adverse effect associated with all antibiotics and particularly with fungal and viral infections. Options 1, 3, and 4 are incorrect. Hypersensitivity reactions and antibiotic toxicity are not usually manifested by vaginal discharge. The symptoms associated with PMC are significant GI effects.

4 Answer: 4 Rationale: Watery diarrhea containing mucus, blood, or pus is symptomatic of CDAD and must be monitored closely for progressing to PMC; both are adverse effects related to antibiotic use. Options 1, 2, and 3 are incorrect. These symptoms are not related to peptic ulcers, malabsorption, or hypersensitivity reactions.

5 Answer: 1 Rationale: Shortness of breath, mouth and tongue swelling, and generalized itching are signs of hypersensitivity reaction. Options 2, 3, and 4 are incorrect. Blood dyscrasias include such problems as thrombocytopenia and neutropenia, and the drug does not cause these symptoms. Beta-lactamase is a substance secreted by some bacteria that renders the antibiotic ineffective. Drug toxicity may result from an excessive level of the medication or adverse effects on body organ systems related to age or other changes. Hypersensitivity is associated with antigen and antibody reactions.

6 Answer: 1 Rationale: Ampicillin should be taken on an empty stomach to ensure adequate absorption. Options 2, 3, and 4 are incorrect. A black and furry tongue is the symptom of an oral superinfection and should be reported. The patient should be taught to take the full prescription even if the symptoms subside. Patients should never take two doses because this will place them at risk for toxicity.

Chapter 48

Patient Safety: Nurses should educate patients about methods to protect the skin from damage and severe reactions to the sun, especially when taking drugs known to cause photosensitivity. Teaching about the proper use of protective clothing and sunscreens, and restrictions on the amount of time spent in direct sunlight, is needed to avoid these problems.

Making the Patient Connection

1 There are multiple reasons that an antibiotic may be ineffective, including bacterial resistance, inadequate dosage, the pathogen(s) is not sensitive to the antibiotic, or patient factors. The nurse should investigate possible patient factors and assess that John Travis has been taking his antibiotic as prescribed. Unpleasant adverse effects, the cost of the drug, or misunderstanding about how frequently to take the medication and any special instructions such as taking with regard to meals may be reasons for less-than-ideal adherence to the medication regimen.

2 Because his current antibiotic has been ineffective, it is necessary to obtain a sputum sample to culture for the pathogen responsible for his symptoms. A C&S test will determine the pathogen responsible for his infection and will determine what antibiotic may best treat his infection.

3 A peak and trough blood specimen measures drug concentration in John's system. Ideally the drug concentration is maintained at a therapeutic level but not at such a high level as to be toxic and cause adverse effects. Blood specimens for drug monitoring are taken at two different times: during the time estimated for the drug's highest therapeutic concentration (peak level) and at its lowest (trough level). Peak levels are usually obtained 1 to 2 hours after oral intake, approximately 1 hour after IM administration, and approximately 30 minutes after IV administration. Trough levels are usually obtained within 15 to 30 minutes prior to the next scheduled dose.

4 Specific symptoms that may indicate a worsening of John's condition include continuous or increasing fever, chest pain, increasing shortness of breath, abdominal pain, increase in sputum production, a change in the color and consistency of the sputum, cyanosis of the lips or nail beds, restlessness, confusion, anxiety, hypotension, or tachycardia. Because of the possibility that John's condition is SARS-CoV2 (COVID 19) infection, testing to detect the virus should also be conducted if it was not done on the first office visit.

Additional Case Study

1 Due to Mr. Klein's past history of alcohol abuse and possible decreased hepatic function, he is at greater risk for the development of cholestatic hepatitis.

2 The most common adverse effects possible for this patient receiving erythromycin may include nausea and vomiting, abdominal cramping, diarrhea, dark urine, pale-colored stools, jaundice, or drug-related hepatitis.

3 Monitoring the patient's liver function laboratory values will be particularly important. These laboratory values include a series of tests known as a liver panel, liver function tests, or LFT. These tests help to detect liver damage or disease.

Chapter Review

1 Answer: 4 Rationale: Tetracycline may cause photosensitivity. Options 1, 2, and 3 are incorrect. Calcium products should not be taken at the same time as tetracycline but taken 1 hour before or 2 hours after the dose. Brushing will not remove teeth staining caused by the drug. The staining of teeth due to medication can only be removed by a dental specialist. Ototoxicity is not associated with tetracycline use, and any tinnitus or dizziness may be related to other causes.

2 Answer: 1 Rationale: Longer duration of action is one of the benefits of azithromycin therapy. Options 2, 3, and 4 are incorrect. There is no evidence that azithromycin causes any more nausea than other antibiotics. Azithromycin is not affected by gastric contents and can be taken any time. Azithromycin is not affected by calcium-based foods.

3 Answer: 1 Rationale: Weight gain may be an early sign of kidney damage secondary to amikacin toxicity. Options 2, 3, and 4 are incorrect. Adverse effects of amikacin do not include visual disturbances, mental depression, or urinary frequency.

4 Answer: 1 Rationale: Drug-induced nephrotoxicity would cause an elevated serum creatinine level and should be reported to the provider. Options 2, 3, and 4 are incorrect. BUN level is more commonly associated with hepatotoxicity but would be elevated and not decreased if nephrotoxicity is present. Nephrotoxicity is not typically indicated via the WBC levels or changes in serum iron levels.

5 Answer: Rationale: Tetracycline antibiotics should not be taken concurrently with dairy products, iron-containing preparations such as multivitamins, or with antacids. If these products are to be consumed, they should be taken 1 hour before or 2 hours after the tetracycline.

6 Answer: 1, 2, 4, 5 Rationale: Aminoglycosides are renal, oto-, and neurotoxic. They may also cause neuromuscular blockade. Increases in serum creatinine may indicate nephrotoxicity. Urine output should also be monitored. Dizziness, vertigo, or tinnitus may be signs of ototoxicity. Muscle weakness may indicate neuromuscular blockade and may last for several days. Option 3 is incorrect. Gentamicin is not metabolized, and changes in liver function tests would not be drug related.

Chapter 49

Patient Safety: Before giving the next dose, the nurse should reassess the patient for drug allergies. Even though patients may initially report drug allergies, they sometimes forget to mention them during the admission process. Before the patient receives another dose of levofloxacin, the provider should be notified of the reaction, when it occurred in relation to the drug's administration, and the extent of the reaction. Hypersensitivity reactions can worsen with each exposure to an antigen (in this case the antibiotic). In the future, if a patient reports allergy-related symptoms such as itching, swelling, or urticaria during IV drug administration, the drug should be stopped, the IV line maintained with normal saline or D_5W as ordered, and the reaction reported to the provider.

Making the Patient Connection

1 The patient teaching handout for Mike should include the following information: Ciprofloxacin can be taken with food or on an empty stomach but should not be taken with dairy products or calcium-fortified juices. It should be taken at about the same time, morning and evening. Take ciprofloxacin for the entire time as prescribed by the healthcare provider, even after the patient starts to feel better, to be sure the infection is eliminated. If a dose is missed, do not take another or double dose of the medication, but take it at the time the next dosage is due. The most common adverse effects of ciprofloxacin are mild and include nausea and vomiting, diarrhea, and abdominal discomfort. Diarrhea that persists with a fever or that contains blood or excessive mucus should be immediately reported to the provider.

2 Inform the patient that this medication is known to cause tendon damage, although it is a rare occurrence. Mike should seek immediate medical attention if he develops joint, muscle, or tendon pain or has difficulty walking. Also, he should be advised that some OTC medications, multivitamins, and other dietary supplements may contain magnesium, calcium, aluminum, iron, or zinc, which can interfere with the absorption of ciprofloxacin.

3 Remembering to take medication can be problematic, especially when the patient begins to feel better. Daily reminders are helpful for scheduling medication doses. One approach is to take medicine around routine activities such as brushing teeth, setting an alarm clock, eating meals, or going to work. Other examples include: Set a timer, smartphone, or watch alarm to go off when it is time to take the medicine; place a sticky note in a highly visible place such as on the refrigerator, by the phone, on the medicine cabinet, or on the bathroom mirror (change the message frequently, move it to a new spot, or use different colors to get needed attention for adherence); ask a family member or a friend to call, email, or text message with a reminder to take the medication; set up a personal computer to send daily email reminders to take the medication; use a medication box that holds the entire day's supply of medicine and load the entire day at one time to decrease the opportunity of a missed or forgotten dose.

Additional Case Study

1 Find the expiration date on the bottle. If it is nearing, on, or after the date, it should be discarded and a new prescription obtained from the provider the next time it is needed. Although antibiotic ophthalmic drops do not usually grow bacteria, if it has been a while since the bottle was last used, it may be best to discard it.

2 When ophthalmic antibiotics are used, care should be taken to avoid contaminating the bottle by opening with a fingertip or by touching the drop dispenser to the eye or surrounding tissues. Increasing redness, swelling, or drainage in the treatment area should be reported to the provider because it may indicate increasing infection or antibiotic resistance.

Chapter Review

1 Answer: 2 Rationale: Because pathogens grow rapidly and are constantly proliferating, all antibiotic therapies should be taken around the clock. Taking the drug as evenly spaced apart during the day as possible will help ensure a steady serum drug level. Options 1, 3, and 4 are incorrect. Ciprofloxacin is not known to cause problems with patients' sleep patterns. Superinfections are a problem associated with antibiotic therapy in general but it is not caused by not adhering to the prescribed schedule. Allergic reactions are common with antibiotic therapy, but they do not result from failing to adhere to the medication schedule.

2 Answer: 3, 4, 5 Rationale: Itching, even without the presence of a rash, may indicate histamine release from a drug allergy. Swelling of the face, lips, or tongue (angioedema), is also a symptom of allergy. Nervousness or anxiety may indicate an adrenergic response secondary to an allergic reaction and, while they may have other causes, should be investigated further to rule out a developing allergic reaction. Options 1 and 2 are incorrect. Common adverse effects of ofloxacin are headache and nausea and vomiting.

3 Answer: 1, 2 Rationale: Ciprofloxacin is excreted by the kidneys and increasing fluid intake will help to prevent drug

accumulation in this organ. Dairy products and antacids taken concurrently may inhibit absorption of ciprofloxacin. Options 3, 4, and 5 are incorrect. Vitamin C does not need to be avoided while on ciprofloxacin; however, products containing iron or zinc should be avoided. An antihistamine does not need to be taken concurrently and may mask the symptoms of adverse effects such as allergy. Excessive caffeine intake may increase the chance of nervousness or anxiety and should be avoided.

4 Answer: 1 Rationale: Fluoroquinolones such as levofloxacin have been associated with tendinopathy , especially in patients over age 65. Any unusual joint or tendon pain or difficulty walking should be reported to the provider. Options 2, 3, and 4 are incorrect. Many multivitamins may contain iron and zinc, and concurrent administration with levofloxacin will impair the antibiotic's absorption. Fluoroquinolones do not impair vitamin D absorption and may cause dermatologic toxicities such as photosensitivity and photoallergy. Sunscreens and protective clothing should be used if sun exposure is anticipated. Fluoroquinolones may be nephrotoxic and increased fluid intake is advised.

5 Answer: 4 Rationale: Fluoroquinolones such as ciprofloxacin may cause profound muscle weakness in patients with myasthenia gravis. Options 1, 2, and 3 are incorrect. Anxiety and nervousness do not require cautious use and are not contraindications to ciprofloxacin. While the incidence of tendinopathy is higher in patients over age 65, the drug is not contraindicated in this population. However, more frequent monitoring may be needed. Cross-allergy between fluoroquinolones and penicillins is not likely and a history of penicillin is not a contraindication.

6 Answer: 1 Rationale: Polymyxin B is a topical antibiotic used to promote wound healing. Options 2, 3, and 4 are incorrect. Skin and mucous membranes cannot be made sterile. Polymyxin B will cause cell death of the invading pathogenic bacteria but will not completely sterilize the skin. Polymyxin B does not prevent allergic reaction nor does it provide pain relief to wounds.

Chapter 50

Patient Safety: Based on the patient's history of allergies to thiazide diuretics, the nurse should withhold the dose of medication and notify the healthcare provider. TMP-SMZ is contraindicated in patients with hypersensitivity to sulfonamides or chemically related agents such as thiazide diuretics.

Making the Patient Connection

1 Urinary tract infections are common in women due to the shorter length of the female urethra. Most infections arise from *E. coli*, which normally exists in the colon. Nearly 20% of women will have another UTI after their first occurrence. Women can reduce the risk of an infection by drinking 1 or 2 liters of water daily, urinating when the need is first present, taking showers instead of tub baths, cleansing the genital area before sexual intercourse, and wiping the perineal area from front to back after toileting to prevent bacteria around the anus from entering the vagina or urethra. Feminine hygiene sprays and routine douching should be avoided because they may irritate the urethra and reduce the beneficial flora that help reduce the risk of UTIs.

2 Health teaching for the patient receiving TMP-SMZ includes reporting skin rashes, nausea and vomiting, diarrhea, sore throat, or muscle aches. Teach the patient to avoid direct sunlight due to photosensitivity from the drug. The patient should be taught to drink 2.5 to 3 L of water daily to maintain dilute urine and reduce the chance of adverse drug effects. Teach the patient to take the entire prescription of antibiotic and to return to a provider for follow-up.

3 The patient should be taught to use the entire prescription and not save antibiotics for another time for several reasons. Inappropriate use of antibiotics may cause the development of antibiotic-resistant strains of common bacterial species. Misuse of antibiotics may result in serious adverse reactions such as diarrhea and abdominal symptoms, rash and allergic reactions, and potentially dangerous interference with other medications. Drugs may lose potency after expiration dates or become toxic and should be discarded when no longer used.

Additional Case Study

1 The nurse should explain that catheter-related bacteriuria in the older adult represents the most common source of infection. Dorothy is alert and oriented and other measures may help her to avoid accidents. Urinary catheters are only used as a last resort such as when skin breakdown has occurred and should be used for a short amount of time.

2 The nurse should first assure the patient and family members that several nursing interventions will be implemented to assist with elimination. Relieving anxiety related to urinary incontinence is an essential part of the nurse's response to the fears of the patient. The following interventions may be helpful to address this problem: Establish a time that nursing staff will check with the patient about toileting needs, such as every 1 to 2 hours; keep the "nurse call" button with the patient for immediate access and provide the patient with a bedside commode so that she can quickly reach it when help arrives; provide the patient with incontinence pads placed in undergarments to provide an extra measure of security; limit the intake of fluids 2 to 3 hours before sleep time and limit the ingestion of bladder irritants such as colas, coffee, and tea.

Chapter Review

1 Answer: 3 Rationale: Crystalluria is the excretion of crystals in the urine. To prevent this adverse effect, patients are instructed to consume approximately 2 to 3 L of fluid per day. This action will flush the crystals from the urinary system. Options 1, 2, and 4 are incorrect. Limiting foods high in calcium will not prevent crystalluria. Positional changes are not related to the adverse effects of crystalluria. Alcohol should be avoided when taking most medications. However, the effects attributed to alcohol consumption do not include crystalluria.

2 Answer: 1 Rationale: Nitrofurantoin is prescribed most commonly for the prophylaxis of recurrent UTIs. Options 2, 3, and 4 are incorrect. Furadantin has no analgesic effect. The excretion of urine is not affected by this drug, and the drug is not used for pyelonephritis.

3 Answer: 2, 4, 5 Rationale: Trimethoprim-sulfamethoxazole is a sulfonamide and would be contraindicated in a patient with a previous history of allergy. The drug may cause fetal harm and result in kernicterus in the newborn. For people with diabetes who are taking oral sulfonylureas, an increased risk of hypoglycemia is possible when TMP-SMZ is used; hence, blood sugars must be monitored closely. Options 1 and 3 are incorrect. The occurrence of migraine headaches is not affected by TMP-SMZ. Urinating before or after sexual intercourse will not affect the use of TMP-SMZ.

4 Answer: 3 Rationale: Nausea and vomiting are the most common adverse effects of oral sulfonamide therapy but should not occur with topical use. If they occur, the patient should be evaluated for possible systemic effects and for the proper self-administration of the topical drug. This statement indicates that the patient has understood the teaching and when to report potential adverse effects. Options 1, 2, and 4 are incorrect. The drug should be applied topically only to affected areas. Stinging and burning are common effects of the topical application. Excess potassium consumption should be avoided with the oral forms of sulfonamides but is not necessary with the topical drug.

5 Answer: 1 Rationale: Nitrofurantoin is associated with pulmonary toxicities such as interstitial pneumonitis and pulmonary fibrosis. The drug should be used with extreme caution or not at all in the patient with preexisting pulmonary disease. Options 2, 3, and 4 are incorrect. Diabetes, rheumatoid arthritis, or angina and HTN are not contraindications for the drug.

6 Answer: 3 Rationale: TMP-SMZ causes dermatologic toxicities including SJS. Unusual, blistering-type rashes with purplish-red discoloration should be immediately reported to the provider. Options 1, 2, and 4 are incorrect. Fungal superinfections may be wet or dry and are reddened, possibly denuded areas. Viral eruptions are most often vesicular rashes. Nonadherence with drug therapy would not result in a rash.

Chapter 51

Making the Patient Connection

1 Tuberculosis is a communicable disease caused by *M. tuberculosis*. The microorganism is acquired by inhalation of infectious particles. Coughing, talking, laughing, and sneezing transmit infected droplets. Although brief exposure to TB does not usually cause infection, frequent and repeated contact with an infected individual increases the risk. High-risk populations include low-income individuals, foreign-born populations, and residents of long-term care facilities or correctional institutions.

2 Sam possibly acquired TB while staying at the homeless shelter. In fact, Sam may have been infected many months before the disease actually developed because the microorganism remains dormant and may not produce symptoms. However, some special circumstances seem to play a role in the progression from dormant TB infection to active disease. These factors include HIV infections, low body weight, advanced age, corticosteroid therapy, and the presence of chronic illness such as diabetes or kidney disease.

3 Sam's TB is compounded by his chronic use of alcohol. Many TB drugs are metabolized in the liver and hepatic impairment due to alcohol consumption may affect the drug's metabolism.

Answers to Additional Case Study

1 It is important to reassure Georgia that multiple drugs are given for active TB infections. The nurse should clarify that combining drug therapies is essential because the bacteria grow slowly and commonly develop resistance to the medications.

2 Peripheral neuropathy is a common adverse effect associated with isoniazid therapy. Isoniazid frequently affects the nervous system and produces tingling and numbness of the hands and feet. Pyridoxine (vitamin B_6) is routinely prescribed to prevent the development of these symptoms.

3 People who have an active TB infection must take their medications consistently to adequately treat the infection and prevent its spread to others. Directly observing patients take their medications greatly improves adherence and limits the appearance of resistant TB bacteria. Georgia will be required to take her pills while a healthcare provider is present, and the nurse will work with her to find the most convenient time and place for that to occur.

Chapter Review

1 Answer: 2 Rationale: Peripheral neuropathy can be problematic during isoniazid therapy. This is due to a decrease in the activity of pyridoxine on the nervous tissue. Often supplemental vitamin B_6 is prescribed to prevent this adverse effect. Options 1, 3, and 4 are incorrect. Isoniazid does not cause an increase in the nerve ending sensitivity or accelerate the excretion of neurotransmitters. Isoniazid does not affect ascorbic acid.

2 Answer: 2, 3, 4, 5 Rationale: Once the diagnosis of pulmonary TB is verified, sputum specimens are routinely collected to determine the effectiveness of the drug therapy. Ethambutol may cause hepatotoxicity and decreases renal excretion of uric acid. Hepatic function tests and uric acid levels will be monitored before beginning the drug and routinely thereafter. It may also cause optic neuritis and vision acuity, and color vision sense will be tested during therapy. Option 1 is incorrect. Coagulation studies are not affected by ethambutol.

3 Answer: To ensure that the patient is not experiencing adverse effects related to the acetylation process, both hepatic function and serum drug level will be monitored frequently.

4 Answer: 4 Rationale: Treatment of MAC infections in patients who are HIV positive is prolonged and relapse rates are high. Options 1, 2, and 3 are incorrect. MAC is not considered a contagious infection. Treatment is prolonged and is indicated when CD4 counts drop below 50 cells/mL.

5 Answer: 1 Rationale: The nurse should observe for any reddish-brown discoloration of skin, cornea, conjunctiva, and body fluids. This adverse effect occurs in 75 to 90% of patients within a few weeks of treatment. Even after discontinuation of therapy, skin discoloration may take months or years to fade. Options 2, 3, and 4 are incorrect. The drug does not cause constipation, chills, dehydration, hypoglycemia, impaired memory, impotence, memory loss, nervousness, or pruritus.

6 Answer: 3 Rationale: Isoniazid may increase glucose levels and more frequent monitoring is required in patients with diabetes. Options 1, 2, and 4 are incorrect. Isoniazid does not cause a decrease or rapid rises and falls of glucose level.

Chapter 52

Making the Patient Connection

1 *Candida albicans* can reproduce in large numbers in the mouth. Signs and symptoms include slightly raised, red or white patches on mucous membranes, tongue, mouth, and throat. Underneath the patches, the area is raw, may bleed, and can be painful. The throat may be sore and swallowing may be difficult. Taste may diminish.

2 Pathogenic fungi attack hosts with compromised immune systems. Conditions that can weaken the immune system include chemotherapy and corticosteroid use, which both apply to Sarah.

3 Sarah will most likely be given a topical suspension with an antifungal drug. She should be taught to remove her dentures before using the medication and to swish the solution around her mouth and then swallow. She should not drink water or rinse her mouth immediately after using the medication and should leave her dentures out overnight.

Additional Case Study

1 Sean was started on both antibiotics and antifungal drugs IV because he is neutropenic and at greater risk for developing sepsis related to the lack of normal defense mechanisms to fight off opportunistic bacterial or fungal pathogens.

2 Fluconazole often causes nausea, vomiting and diarrhea, placing Sean at risk for dehydration or electrolyte imbalances. His creatinine level, skin turgor, urine output, and oral intake levels should be monitored. Fluconazole can be nephrotoxic and fluid intake should be increased. IV fluids should be given if Sean is unable to take fluids PO due to nausea or vomiting. Although rare, fluconazole may be hepatotoxic and liver function studies should be monitored. A thorough medication history should be obtained on admission because fluconazole is metabolized through the hepatic CYP450 pathways and affects the metabolism of many medications.

Chapter Review

1 Answer: 2, 3, 4 Rationale: When administered too rapidly, amphotericin B may cause hypotension, hypokalemia, and shock. Options 1 and 5 are incorrect. Amphotericin is not known to cause laryngeal spasms or hypoglycemia.

2 Answer: 1 Rationale: Patients who take fluconazole may experience nausea, vomiting and diarrhea. Nutritional intake is especially important to maintain optimal health in a patient with AIDS. Keeping a food diary will assist the provider in determining overall calorie and fluid intake. Antinausea medication may be helpful to reduce nausea or vomiting. Options 2, 3, and 4 are incorrect. Loss of muscle mass is not related to fluconazole therapy. The decision to wear a high-filtration mask is not related to fluconazole, and patients on this drug do not need to avoid fat-based soaps. Allowing adequate air circulation to body areas will help prevent surface fungal infections but is not required as part of fluconazole therapy.

3 Answer: 1, 2 Rationale: Unless otherwise directed by the provider, small amounts of water after a feeding will rinse the mouth of milk proteins and sugars that can provide an ideal medium for *Candida* to grow. The suspension should be applied to all surfaces of the mouth and tongue, by syringe or applicator, and the infant should swallow the remainder to treat possible GI *Candida*. Options 3, 4, and 5 are incorrect. Nystatin suspension does not require chilling before administration. The suspension should not be added to formula or given before feedings and should be administered after feedings so that it can be retained in the mouth to treat the area of infection.

4 Answer: 4 Rationale: Nails grow very slowly and lengthy treatment may be required to adequately treat the infection. Options 1, 2, and 3 are incorrect. The infection will be evaluated during the treatment period, but it will take many months to adequately treat the infection. Purchasing more pills at one time does not necessarily reduce the cost of the prescription. Toxic doses are never administered, even to shorten treatment cycles.

5 Answer: 3 Rationale: Amphotericin B can cause serious adverse effects including fever, chills, and headache. Pretreatment with corticosteroids, antihistamines, and antipyretics may reduce the severity of these adverse effects. Options 1, 2, and 4 are incorrect. Pretreatment does not enhance the effectiveness of this antifungal agent. The by-products of amphotericin are not affected by the pretreatment of the patient, and pretreatment does not affect the half-life of the drug.

6 Answer: 3 Rationale: Depending on which antidiabetes medication is used (e.g., glyburide), fluconazole may decrease blood sugar levels, and an adjustment in antidiabetes treatments may be required. Options 1, 2, and 4 are incorrect. Fluconazole has an effect when given concurrently with some antidiabetes drugs (e.g., glyburide) and may cause hypoglycemia. It does not antagonize the effect of antidiabetes medications and does not cause an increase in blood sugar level.

Chapter 53

Making the Patient Connection

1 For many diseases, prevention is often easier than treatment or a cure. Chloroquine is given for prophylaxis therapy to prevent malaria contracted from the *Anopheles* mosquito carrying *Plasmodium*. It kills by causing a concentration of toxic products inside the parasite.

2 Patients with a congenital G6PD deficiency may be at higher risk for hemolysis from chloroquine. Because chloroquine concentrates in the tissues, the drug may cause irreversible retinal damage, and a baseline retinal evaluation should be conducted before starting therapy. Eye examinations will also be required periodically during the posttreatment period.

3 The incubation period for malaria is from 1 to 6 weeks. To reduce the possibility of infection, the drug is taken 1 to 2 weeks ahead of a possible exposure to build up adequate levels in the body. It is continued at least 4 weeks after the exposure risk to prevent any remaining sporozoites from infecting the host's liver. Because not all *Plasmodia* species are sensitive to chloroquine, Trevor should continue to watch for signs and symptoms of malaria. Symptoms include a "cold stage" with intense chills and shivering; a "hot stage" with fever, headache, and vomiting; and a "sweating stage" with profuse diaphoresis followed by return to normal body temperature; and fatigue. Each stage lasts approximately 6 to 10 hours and repeats on a 48-hour cycle.

4 Adverse effects of chloroquine include nausea, vomiting, stomach upset, cramps, loss of appetite, diarrhea, tiredness, weakness, and headache. Visual changes such as blurring, difficulty focusing, or photophobia may occur. If they are severe, continue, or worsen, Trevor should immediately contact his provider for more extensive visual screening.

Additional Case Study

1 Trichomoniasis, a common STI, affects both women and men. The infection is much more common in women because the vagina is a more favorable environment for the pathogen compared to the male reproductive tract.

2 The nurse is in an ideal position to discuss sexual health with patients. The patient should be taught the importance of adherence to the drug therapy and follow-up care. A discussion related to sexual practices should follow. Sexual abstinence is the surest method to avoid any STI. The next level of protection includes a long-term, mutually monogamous relationship with a partner who is uninfected. The use of latex male condoms, when used correctly and consistently, can reduce the transmission of STIs. An individual diagnosed with an STI should be encouraged to notify all recent sex partners so they can see a provider and be treated. This reduces the risk of sex partners developing complications and reduces the risk of reinfection or of spreading the infection.

3 Common adverse effects of metronidazole include anorexia, nausea, vomiting, diarrhea, abdominal pain, dizziness, headache, dryness of mouth, and metallic taste. When alcohol is consumed while the patient is on metronidazole, a disulfiram-like reaction may occur with severe nausea, vomiting, potential hypotension and electrolyte imbalances.

Chapter Review

1 Answer: 1 Rationale: Atovaquone-proguanil therapy begins 1 or 2 days before entering a malaria-endemic area and continues during the stay and for 7 days after return. Options 2, 3, and 4 are incorrect. Three days is not a sufficient to ensure adequate protection against malaria. If the patient develops symptoms of malaria, prophylaxis is no longer indicated, but the drug may be continued as part of the treatment regimen.

2 Answer: 1, 4 Rationale: Hydroxychloroquine has anti-inflammatory effects and is used in the treatment of systemic lupus erythematosus, rheumatoid arthritis, and other inflammatory diseases. Options 2, 3, and 5 are incorrect. Hydroxychloroquine is not used to treat roundworm, leishmaniasis, or urinary tract infections.

3 Answer: 3 Rationale: Many patients complain of an unpleasant metallic taste caused by metronidazole. Options 1, 2, and 4 are incorrect. Flatus and intestinal bloating are not characteristic adverse effects of metronidazole. The drug does not cause bad halitosis and if it occurs, other causes should be considered. Alopecia is not associated with metronidazole.

4 Answer: 2 Rationale: The use of pyrimethamine is associated with megaloblastic anemia, leukopenia, thrombocytopenia,

and pancytopenia as possible adverse effects. Unusual bleeding or fatigue, sores that do not heal, or low-grade fevers may indicate that blood cell counts are low. Options 1, 3, and 4 are incorrect. Pyrimethamine is associated with nausea, vomiting and abdominal cramping and increasing fiber-rich foods will not affect these. Increasing fluid intake is important with most anti-infective drugs but 3 L per day is not required for this drug. Adverse eye effects are not associated with pyrimethamine and sulfadiazine.

5 Answer: 4 Rationale: To reduce the risk of reinfection, bed linens and undergarments should be washed thoroughly after treatment. Options 1, 2, and 3 are incorrect. Mebendazole is usually given as a single dose but may be repeated for up to 3 days. Family members are also at risk and should be evaluated or treated empirically. Although consuming citrus products may increase the risk of GI adverse effects, citrus and dairy do not need to be eliminated from the diet.

6 Answer: 1 Rationale: An acute onset of any CNS abnormality may indicate metronidazole toxicity. If ataxia and confusion suddenly develop after the initiation of this drug, the nurse should discontinue the medication and contact the provider. Options 2, 3, and 4 are incorrect. Adverse effects to metronidazole are rare; however, nausea and diarrhea can occur. Anorexia and dryness of the mouth are common adverse effects. However, these effects usually disappear as therapy continues. Weight gain and irritability are not typical adverse effects associated with metronidazole.

Chapter 54

Patient Safety Question: The shingles vaccination is a live-attenuated vaccine recommended for patients 60 years of age and older to prevent reactivation of varicella-zoster virus. Patients who are immunosuppressed may experience an increased risk of adverse effects from the vaccination, including activation of herpes zoster. Before giving any immunization, the provider should assess the immune status of the patient, including the use of immunosuppressant drugs or corticosteroids, especially when live-attenuated vaccines are used.

Making the Patient Connection

1 Herpesviruses are usually acquired through direct physical contact with an infected individual. HSV may remain in a latent, asymptomatic, nonreplicating state in nerve root ganglia for many years. Infection is lifelong. Immunosuppression, physical challenge, or emotional stress can promote active replication of the virus and reappearance of the characteristic lesions.

2 Antiviral agents are not routinely prescribed for prophylaxis due to the cost and potential adverse effects. Patients who experience particularly severe or recurrent episodes may receive low-dose antiviral agents.

3 Richard should apply the acyclovir as soon as symptoms appear. The medication should be applied to all sores every 3 hours (up to six times a day) for 7 days, or as directed. Sometimes, this medication may cause burning, stinging, and redness. Cold sores are contagious at all stages and can spread to others through kissing or sharing items that touch the lips, such as towels or utensils. Given the nature of his part-time job at a restaurant, Richard should use disposable gloves when applying the medication to avoid spreading the infection. Lastly, a healthy lifestyle may reduce the recurrence of cold sores. This would include a balanced diet, exercise, sufficient sleep, and managing emotional stress. The college where Richard is a student may have stress management and other support services available that may be helpful.

Additional Case Study

1 The timing and onset of symptoms are critical factors when considering drugs such as oseltamivir. If the drug is given within 48 hours of the onset of symptoms, it may shorten the normal 7-day duration of influenza to 5 days. Since Jeanie's symptoms developed 24 hours ago, the provider may consider this drug an option.

2 For most patients, flu is short lived. Prescription antiviral medications such as oseltamivir can shorten the duration of the flu. Jeanie should not return to work until her fever is gone and the main symptoms have disappeared to avoid transmitting the infection to others.

Chapter Review

1 Answer: 1 Rationale: Acyclovir is associated with nephrotoxicity, especially when given IV. The drug should be administered IV slowly, over a minimum of 1 hour, and increased fluid intake encouraged throughout the day to prevent adverse renal effects. Options 2, 3, and 4 are incorrect. Acyclovir is not associated with an increased risk of fungal infections or eye discomfort. Itching and skin irritation may occur with topical use but if it occurs with IV drug administration, drug allergy should be questioned and the administration stopped until evaluated.

2 Answer: 3 Rationale: Zepatier may be used in combination with ribavirin. Options 1, 2, and 4 are incorrect. Zepatier is a fixed-dose PO combination of elbasvir and is not a topical or IV drug. Zepatier is used for a 12- to 16-week course of therapy, not 12 to 16 months. The he most common adverse effects being fatigue, headache, and nausea.

3 Answer: 2, 3, 5 Rationale: Amantadine is associated with nephrotoxicity, possible severe CNS effects including seizures, psychosis and suicidal ideation, and peripheral edema and heart failure. Options 1 and 4 are incorrect. Amantadine is not known to affect the white blood cell or platelet count. Potassium and sodium levels are not affected by amantadine.

4 Answer: 4 Rationale: Zanamivir must be started within 48 hours after the onset of symptoms to be effective. Options 1, 2, and 3 are incorrect. Waiting to take the drug longer than 48 hours will not shorten the infection period. It should not be saved because any future infection should be evaluated at that time to ascertain it is the flu and that it will respond to zanamivir.

5 Answer: 2 Rationale: Tenofovir is known to cause lactic acidosis. Symptoms such as anxiety, fatigue, nausea and vomiting, palpitations, lethargy, rapid breathing and heart rate, weakness, chest pain, hypotension, or shortness of breath should be immediately reported. Options 1, 3, and 4 are incorrect. Tenofovir is not associated with systemic yeast infections, heart failure, or ventricular dysrhythmias.

6 Answer: 4 Rationale: Ribavirin is associated with an increased risk of hemolytic anemia. Increased fatigue, dizziness, headache, abdominal pain, pallor, and chest pain are associated with this anemia. Options 1, 2, and 3 are incorrect. Respiratory, dermatologic, or neurologic adverse effects may occur but are not as severe as the hemolytic anemia associated with this drug.

Chapter 55

Making the Patient Connection

1 The primary concern with this hospitalization is the treatment of the secondary infection. Ryan will most likely be placed on antibiotics and antifungal medication first. Rarely is antiretroviral medication initiated until the presenting infection is treated and under control. The optimal time to start antiretroviral therapy depends on many factors including the presentation of HIV symptoms, HIV RNA and CD4 cell counts, and the patient's ability to accept the HIV diagnosis and willingness to adhere to the therapy.

2 After HIV enters the body, it uses the host's own immune cells to replicate. His HIV RNA is high, indicating that he has an active HIV infection, but his CD4 count, the type of cell that the virus uses to replicate, is still within an acceptable level. HIV is the infection with the human immunodeficiency virus, and AIDS is the very last stage of HIV infection that occurs as the host's immune system can no longer function. As diagnosed by his provider, Ryan has an HIV infection but does not currently have AIDS.

3 The antiretroviral drugs used to treat HIV infections will be required long term and require the patient to be consistent with the treatment regimen to keep the infection from worsening or from being transmitted to others. These drugs have many adverse effects. The nurse and provider will provide specific instructions, ideally verbally as well as in written form, about administration needs, adverse effects, and when to notify the provider. The nurse should keep in mind that a new diagnosis of HIV may be difficult or devastating to the patient. Ryan has already expressed his fears about knowing other people who have died of AIDS and his fears that it will happen to him. At this point in time, teaching may need to be brief and repeated several times, with written materials and follow-up teaching provided on subsequent office visits to ensure that the information is processed by Ryan.

Additional Case Study

1 HIV is a virus that attacks cells of the immune system. HIV progressively destroys the body's ability to fight infections and certain cancers. People diagnosed with HIV may develop life-threatening opportunistic infections, which are caused by pathogens such as viruses, bacteria, protozoans, or fungi that usually do not make healthy people sick. Having HIV does not mean an individual has AIDS. AIDS occurs when the body can no longer resist infections because it has lost the cells needed to fight off disease. ART is used in the treatment of HIV infection and uses a combination of several drugs known as antiretrovirals. The drugs slow down the ability of HIV to multiply in the body and delay or prevent the development of AIDS.

2 The goal of drug therapy is to reduce the amount of virus in the body so that transmission to another person is unlikely. The goal is to reduce the amount or HIV RNA to undetectable levels or less than 200 copies/mL. Maintaining the viral load at or below this level prevents the sexual transmission of the virus to their partners. This is known as "treatment as prevention." Once this level is reached, the viral load will be assessed every 3 to 6 months. Treatment as prevention only applies to sexual transmission of HIV. It does not prevent the transmission of the virus from blood exposure such as sharing needles and it also does not apply to transmission during pregnancy to the baby or during breastfeeding.

3 Current guidelines recommend beginning ART by the 28th week of pregnancy or sooner. ART is the most effective way to lower viral load, reduce the incidence of viral resistance, and protect the health of the mother. A major advantage in treating pregnant patients with antiretrovirals is that when HIV viral load is reduced to less than 1000 copies/mL, risk of transmission of the virus to the baby is very low. ART therapy for pregnant women is the same as for nonpregnant women. If a pregnancy test confirms that Alexa is pregnant, starting ART will help ensure that she stays healthy and that her baby has a greatly reduced risk of being infected with HIV.

Chapter Review

1 Answer: 4 Rationale: The integrase inhibitor dolutegravir has become an important first-line drug in the treatment of HIV and is less likely to cause drug resistance than older drugs. It does not cure the infection and sexual abstinence or barrier methods must be used until the HIV RNA is maintained at below 200 copies/mL. Options 1, 2, and 3 are incorrect. Dolutegravir may cause hepatotoxicity and hepatic function will be assessed throughout drug treatment. It should not be stopped and should continue when HIV RNA reaches 200 copies/mL or below, and the drug should be taken without schedule adjustment so that it continues to maintain a low viral load and resistance does not develop.

2 Answer: 2, 3, 5 Rationale: Hyperglycemia, pancreatitis, and hepatic failure are adverse effects associated with lopinavir with ritonavir. Options 1 and 4 are incorrect. Renal failure and bone marrow suppression are not adverse effects associated with lopinavir with ritonavir.

3 Answer: 4 Rationale: Lactic acidosis is known to occur with all NRTIs, although the risk with emtricitabine is less than that of some drugs. It is one of the preferred drugs for initial HIV therapy. Options 1, 2, and 3 are incorrect. Ventricular dysrhythmias, pulmonary fibrosis, and necrotic bowel syndrome are not associated with emtricitabine.

4 Answer: 3 Rationale: Nausea and vomiting, diarrhea, abdominal pain, and headache are common with protease inhibitor regimens; fatigue, generalized weakness, and myalgia are common adverse effects for NRTIs and NtRTIs; headache, diarrhea, nausea, fatigue, and insomnia are common with integrase inhibitors; and respiratory tract infections, cough, pyrexia, rash, and dizziness are common with miscellaneous antiretrovirals.

5 Answer: 1, 2, 3 Rationale: Patients receiving ART are immunocompromised and should avoid crowds and individuals who have infections. The patient should be instructed to notify the provider at the first sign of a rash. Several antiretroviral medications may cause SJS, a dermatologic adverse effect that can be fatal. Current research has shown that ART, especially when started early in HIV infection, significantly reduces viral load, reducing the chance of transmission. Transmission is still possible and infection control measures should still be practiced. Options 4 and 5 are incorrect. Total discontinuation of medication is not recommended because viral load will increase when ART is discontinued. Some herbal supplements, such as St. John's wort, interfere with antiretroviral therapy.

6 Answer: 2, 3 Rationale: Drug therapy for HIV-infected women is begun as soon as possible once pregnancy is confirmed to decrease viral load and the potential to transmit the infection to the infant. Drug therapy is also started as soon as possible in infants born to HIV-infected mothers. Options 1, 4, and 5 are incorrect. Waiting to confirm the viral load in an infant born to an HIV-infected mother delays treatment and may allow the viral load to increase. Treatment of the infant whose mother was not taking antiretroviral drugs during pregnancy should be given over 6 weeks. The CDC does not recommend breastfeeding because the virus is present in breast milk and many antiretroviral drugs are also found in breast milk.

Chapter 56

Making the Patient Connection

1 Even though the surgeon has removed a large part of the tumor, any remaining cancer cells may repopulate. The goal of chemotherapy is to obtain a total cell kill of any remaining cancer cells after surgery before they have a chance to repopulate.

2 Staging and grading are used to establish treatment and prognosis for the patient with cancer. T1, N0, M0 tells us that the tumor is relatively small in size and not significantly invading surrounding tissues, no cancerous cells were found in the lymph nodes, and no metastases were found. G_2 tells us that the cells are moderately differentiated and look somewhat like the parent cells.

The staging and grading for Cheryl's cancer suggest she may have a good prognosis.

3 Hematologic changes that Cheryl may experience are thrombocytopenia, neutropenia, and anemia. Thrombocytopenia, a platelet count of less than 100,000 per mL of blood, can cause abnormal bleeding. If the platelet count drops to less than 20,000 per mL, the patient may begin to bruise easily and exhibit petechiae or purpura. If the platelet count continues to decrease, the patient may hemorrhage.

Neutropenia is a neutrophil count is less than 1500 cells. The chemotherapy may cause a decrease in all WBCs (leukopenia); however, the neutrophils are usually affected the most. Cheryl's nadir must be calculated prior to administering subseqyent chemotherapy.

Anemia is when the RBC count is less than 4.2 million/mm^3 for men or 3.6/mm^3 for women, or a hemoglobin less than 14 g/dL for men and 12 g/dL for women. Because hemoglobin carries oxygen to all tissues, anemia may affect every body system.

Additional Case Study

1 Jonah's children may be allowed to visit if they are free from illness and if Jonah does not become neutropenic. Hospitals vary on their policies for children visiting oncology units. Because the chemotherapy will suppress his immune system, the risk for Jonah acquiring a bacterial or viral infection is high.

2 The use of multiple drugs affects different stages of the cancer cells' lifecycle and attacks the various clones within the tumor via several mechanisms of action, thus increasing the percentage of cell kill. Combination chemotherapy also allows lower dosages of each agent, thus reducing toxicity and slowing the development of resistance.

3 Leukemia is a disseminated cancer, not a solid tumor. Only solid tumors may be staged. Leukemias may be graded.

Chapter Review

1 Answer: 3 Rationale: Stage 1 suggests that the tumor is relatively small in size, has not invaded the surrounding tissue, and has not been detected in surrounding lymph nodes; thus, it has been detected at an early stage. Options 1, 2, and 4 are incorrect. Stage 1 is the earliest staging and has the best prognosis. Cell differentiation refers to grading of cancer cells, not staging. Stage 1 suggests that the tumor is small and has not begun to invade surrounding tissue.

2 Answer: 4, 5 Rationale: Patients and family members should avoid receiving live virus vaccination or exposure to chickenpox. Varicella (chickenpox) vaccination is usually given to children between ages 12 and 18 months and the patient should not care for her granddaughter if immunization with live virus vaccines is planned. The patient should also avoid crowds, especially in enclosed areas, to minimize the risk of infection. Options 1, 2, and 3 are incorrect. Attending a support group, maintaining normal activities when possible, and eating small, frequent meals with sufficient protein are routine care measures during chemotherapy.

3 Answer: 1 Rationale: The use of multiple drugs affects different stages of the cancer cells' life cycle by several mechanisms of action, thus increasing the percentage of cell kill. Combination chemotherapy also allows lower dosages of each individual agent, thus reducing toxicity and slowing the development of resistance. Options 2, 3, and 4 are incorrect. Staging describes the process of determining the extent of cancer in the body and where the cancer is located. Antineoplastic drugs may kill only a small portion of the tumor, leaving some clones unaffected and able to repopulate the tumor with resistant cells. Combination chemotherapy allows lower dosages of each agent, thus reducing toxicity.

4 Answer: 3 Rationale: Mucositis is the painful inflammation and ulceration of the mucous membranes lining the digestive tract, an adverse effect of chemotherapy and radiation treatment. Patients experiencing this adverse effect should be instructed to eat a bland diet with low roughage and to use a soft-bristle toothbrush or plain water rinses for oral care if the mucositis is severe. Options 1, 2, and 4 are incorrect. Most OTC mouthwashes contain a significant amount of alcohol, which will further inflame the oral tissue. Citrus foods and beverages should be avoided because their acidic nature would cause pain. Mucositis can last the duration of the chemotherapy treatment and should be treated because it may prevent intake of adequate nutrition.

5 Answer: 1 Rationale: Myelosuppression is the most common dose-limiting adverse effect of chemotherapy and the one that most often causes discontinuation or delays of chemotherapy. Options 2, 3, and 4 are incorrect. Although alopecia may be distressing for the patient, its presence does not determine when the next round of chemotherapy can be administered. Mucositis is not a reason that subsequent rounds of chemotherapy should be delayed. Cachexia is the physical wasting with loss of weight and muscle mass caused by disease. It is not the most common reason for delaying chemotherapy.

6 Answer: 4 Rationale: Many antineoplastics are classified as vesicants that can cause serious tissue injury if they leak into the surrounding tissue during an infusion or injection. The nurse should closely monitor the infusion site for swelling and pain. Options 1, 2, and 3 are incorrect. Vesicants do not always cause nausea. The intake of calcium-rich foods this is not related to receiving a chemotherapy classified as a vesicant. Respiratory status is not related to the administration of a vesicant-type agent.

Chapter 57

Making the Patient Connection

1 The different drugs affect the various stages of the cancer's lifecycle, allowing for lower doses of each individual drug and possibly slowing the development of resistance. Cyclophosphamide is an alkylating agent of the nitrogen mustard class. Carboplatin is also an alkylating agent, a platinum compound. Vincristine is a natural product, a vinca alkaloid. Etoposide is also a natural product of the topoisomerase inhibitor class.

2 Overlapping toxicities often arise when multiple chemotherapy drugs are used that have similar adverse effects, especially bone marrow suppression. The chance for overlapping toxicities for Zack is also high for the neurologic system (e.g., decreased DTRs, peripheral neuropathies, weakness, cranial nerve effects). All four drugs are likely to cause these adverse effects, and given Zack's diminished DTRs at this clinic visit, he should be monitored closely for increasing motor effects such as clumsiness or difficulty holding heavy objects. Other overlapping toxicities include effects on the cardiovascular or respiratory systems.

3 Zack is at great risk for infection. Any ANC count of less than 500 is a concern, and scrupulous infection control measures should be taken. While neutropenic precautions may not be required at this time, extra care should be taken to avoid exposing Zack to any extra risk of infection. He should not have visitors with known infections and should avoid crowded indoor places. Previous teaching should be reviewed with Zack and his family: He should continue with mouth rinses and bathe daily with a mild soap, covering the PICC line insertion site. Excellent hand hygiene should be performed by Zack and his family, especially prior to his filgrastim injections. His PICC line care should be performed using aseptic technique. Any fever over 38.3°C (101°F) or three sequential temperatures taken 4 hours apart over 38.1°C (100.5°F) should be reported. Considering his age, this time may be very frustrating for Zack. The nurse could explore options to help Zack maintain contact with his friends, perhaps by

synchronous online games, video conferencing, or text messaging, until his WBC count increases. He is also at increased risk for bleeding with a platelet count of 55,000. While his fatigue prevent him from participating in activities that may cause direct injury (e.g., sports), he should be monitored for increased bruising, petechiae, or nosebleeds. Zack and his family should be reminded that if bleeding occurs, prolonged pressure will be required to stop it and the provider should be notified.

Additional Case Study

1 The nurse should how Ansen is taking the granisetron. If he consistently experiences nausea, taking the drug regularly rather than prn may provide better results. Additional antiemetic therapy, perhaps supplementing or switching to another drug group, may be needed. Small sips of ginger ale, without carbonation, may help relieve nausea. Supplementing his diet with high-protein drinks such as Boost or Ensure and eating smaller, more frequent meals may increase oral and caloric intake. Ansen may benefit from a dietary consult. Improved fluid and caloric intake will keep him in optimal health during the time of his chemotherapy and may help reduce some of the drug-related fatigue.

2 If Ansen's job allows him to work at home, this might be a viable option during periods of extreme fatigue. Frequent rest breaks while at work, especially if a room is available in which to lie down, may allow Ansen to continue to work during this time. His employer may be able to offer a shortened workweek, and he could explore medical leave options. If there are financial concerns, a social services referral may be advisable.

Chapter Review

1 Answer: 2 Rationale: The nadir indicates that myelosuppression has occurred and is indicated by decreased blood cell counts. WBC and ANC are sensitive indicators of the nadir. Options 1, 3, and 4 are incorrect. Blood urea nitrogen, creatinine, ionized calcium, and serum albumin are not indicators of the nadir and myelosuppression.

2 Answer: 1, 3, 4 Rationale: The main dose-limiting toxicity to occur with vincristine is neurotoxicity. Numbness of the hands and feet, constipation related to decreased peristalsis, and diminished reflexes are all signs of neurotoxicity. Options 2 and 5 are incorrect. Cardiac and pulmonary toxicities are not associated with vincristine.

3 Answer: 4 Rationale: Tamoxifen is associated with an increased risk of endometrial cancer and monitoring will be necessary to detect early endometrial changes. Options 1, 2, and 3 are incorrect. Paralytic ileus and pulmonary fibrosis are not associated with tamoxifen. Alopecia is a common adverse effect of many chemotherapy drugs but will not require long-term monitoring.

4 Answer: 3 Rationale: As with many chemotherapy drugs, doxorubicin is associated with mucositis. Daily mouth rinses will be prescribed to decrease the risk of opportunistic infections from yeast and mouth bacteria. Options 1, 2, and 4 are incorrect. Performing active or assisted ROM is an important intervention associated with drugs that cause neurotoxicity. Controlling pain is associated with chemotherapy that may cause pain as an adverse effect. Maintaining bedrest is not related to the use of chemotherapy but may be required for other reasons.

5 Answer: 1 Rationale: NSAIDs may cause severe and fatal myelosuppression when taken concurrently with methotrexate. Options 2, 3, and 4 are incorrect. Antihistamines, laxatives, and cough suppressants may be used with methotrexate. However, the provider should be consulted if they are needed because symptoms associated with these drugs may indicate a more serious condition that requires additional treatment.

6 Answer: 3 Rationale: Filgrastim increases neutrophil production and decreases the duration of neutropenia with associated infection risk. Options 1, 2, and 4 are incorrect. Filgrastim does not boost the action of carboplatin, prevent the formation of additional cancers, or prevent bone loss.

Chapter 59

Making the Patient Connection

1 Risk factors for the development of PUD include infection with *H. pylori*, use of NSAIDS, tobacco smoking, alcohol use, serious illness, and genetic factors.

2 Antibiotics are used to eradicate *H. pylori*. Although Hugh is allergic to penicillin, there are other combinations of drugs available to eradicate *H. pylori*, which may include combinations of the following: clarithromycin, tetracycline, metronidazole, and bismuth compounds. A PPI may be prescribed to further decrease bacterial load and suppress acid.

Patient adherence is necessary to eradicate the organism. Patients must complete the entire antibiotic regimen to fully treat the peptic ulcer and combat antibiotic resistance. They should be advised of adverse effects including nausea, diarrhea, and headache.

3 Use of NSAIDs has been shown to worsen HTN in some patients. The chief mechanism by which NSAIDs contribute to HTN and decrease the effectiveness of antihypertensive drugs appears to be the inhibition of prostaglandin synthesis. This inhibition results in an increase in sodium reabsorption and water retention.

Additional Case Study

1 OTC medications for GERD are available, and effective for patients with mild and intermittent symptoms. However, self-medicating may cause a delay in seeking treatment for more serious disease. Warning signs and symptoms of GERD that suggest a more complicated disease include unexplained weight loss, early satiety, anemia, vomiting, initial onset of symptoms after age 50, and prolonged anorexia.

2 The cause of GERD is usually transient relaxation of the lower esophageal sphincter, allowing reflux of gastric juice back into the esophagus when the stomach contracts. Since the gastric contents are acidic, they cause injury to the esophagus. Risk factors mentioned in this case study include being overweight, eating spicy foods and drinking red wine, and the use of the calcium channel blocker amlodipine. All are known to promote reflux. Other risk factors include tobacco use, pregnancy, and use of other medications including bisphosphonates and nitrates.

3 The PPIs are the most effective medications available for GERD and are safe drugs with few adverse effects. The prototype PPI is omeprazole, which is available by prescription and OTC. H_2 antagonists are also used to treat PUD.

Chapter Review

1 Answer: 2 Rationale: Magnesium compounds, especially in higher doses, often cause diarrhea. Options 1, 3, and 4 are incorrect. Aluminum compounds and calcium compounds may cause constipation. Sodium compounds may cause flatulence.

2 Answer: 1, 2, 4, 5 Rationale: Symptoms of GERD include dysphagia, dyspepsia, nausea, belching, heartburn, and chest pain. Option 3 is incorrect. The nurse would not expect a decrease in the patient's appetite due to this medication.

3 Answer: 3 Rationale: The proton pump is activated by food intake. Administering the PPI 20 to 30 minutes before the first

meal of the day allows peak drug serum levels to coincide with when the maximum levels of pumps are activated, allowing maximum efficiency of the PPI. Options 1, 2, and 4 are incorrect. The proton pumps are less active at night, in the fasting state, or between meals.

4 Answer: 2 Rationale: Blood dyscrasias have been reported, especially neutropenia and thrombocytopenia, with long-term use. Periodic blood counts should be performed. Options 1, 3, and 4 are incorrect. Famotidine does not cause photophobia and skin irritations. Dyspnea and productive cough are not expected adverse effects for this medication.

5 Answer: 1, 2, 4 Rationale: First-line therapy for *H. pylori* includes a combination of a PPI such as omeprazole; antibiotics such a metronidazole, clarithromycin, or amoxicillin; and bismuth subsalicylate. Options 3 and 5 are incorrect. Sucralfate stimulates mucus, bicarbonate, and prostaglandin secretion and acts locally to produce a thick protective barrier that coats and binds to the ulcer, protecting it against further erosion from acid and pepsin. It is not used as a first-line drug in *H. pylori* infections. Fluconazole is an antifungal drug and will not be effective against a bacterial infection such as *H. pylori*.

6 Answer: 3 Rationale: Antibiotics have no role in the treatment of GERD, although certain antibiotics are used in treating PUD to eradicate the *H. pylori* organism. Options 1, 2, and 4 are incorrect. H_2-receptor antagonists and PPIs are used routinely to relieve symptoms of GERD. OTC antacids provide intermittent relief for mild cases.

Chapter 60

Answers to Critical Thinking Questions in Making the Patient Connections

1 Dicyclomine is an antispasmodic that will relax smooth muscle spasms. Loperamide is an antidiarrheal similar to diphenoxylate with atropine that slows peristalsis but without analgesia or dependence effects. Both will slow peristalsis, reducing the abdominal cramping and diarrhea associated with IBS.

2 Dicyclomine and loperamide may cause drowsiness, dry mouth, and blurred vision. Kerry should take the drug before bed to prevent adverse effects that might interfere with her classroom study or attendance. If dry mouth is a problem, Kerry could take water to sip during class, chew gum, or suck on hard candy. If her vision is affected, she may need to sit in the front of the classroom or discuss other options with the nurse practitioner.

3 Some patients find relief of IBS symptoms from the ingestion of fiber via the diet or bulk-forming laxatives such as psyllium. For others, these remedies worsen the symptoms. During a weekend or break week, Kerry could try to introduce extra fiber into her diet and note the effects. Kerry should be taught to keep a diary to detect possible food triggers such as caffeine, wheat, or lactose. If stress seems to be a trigger, complementary and alternative therapies such as relaxation and biofeedback may be helpful.

Additional Case Study

1 Sulfasalazine is the combination of two substances: sulfapyridine and an aspirin-like compound. It works to reduce the inflammation in the colon caused by ulcerative colitis. The drug tends to be effective in preventing recurrences, however, it is not as effective for relieving severe flare-ups of the disease.

2 The most common adverse effects are nausea and abdominal discomfort, which tend to occur early in the course of treatment. In some cases, sulfasalazine may reduce the number of white blood cells in the body. Other common adverse effects include a skin rash or headache. Sulfasalazine can increase sensitivity to sunlight. Some people taking sulfasalazine develop an orange discoloration of their urine and, occasionally, of their skin. This is usually harmless because the discoloration is temporary and goes away after stopping the medication.

3 This drug is contraindicated in the presence of the following conditions: allergies to sulfonamide or aspirin; hematologic disorders such as anemia; hepatic impairment; and urinary obstruction.

Chapter Review

1 Answer: 3 Rationale: Diphenoxylate with atropine is given for diarrhea. The patient should report a decrease in the number of loose, watery stools after administration. Options 1, 2, and 4 are incorrect. Although diphenoxylate with atropine may decrease abdominal cramping and gas as a result of slowed peristalsis, it is not the main therapeutic effect desired from this drug. Slowing peristalsis may cause a decrease in bowel sounds rather than an increase.

2 Answer: 2 Rationale: One adverse effect of sulfasalazine is blood dyscrasias, which may include anemia, leukopenia, and thrombocytopenia. Fever, an increase in bruising, and sore throat are all possible symptoms of these decreased cell counts. Options 1, 3, and 4 are incorrect. SJS results in inflammation of the skin and mucous membranes and includes a sunburn-like appearance, blisters, and possible exfoliation of the dermis. Idiosyncratic reactions are aberrant reactions that cannot be explained by the known pharmacologic action of the drug and occur only in a small percentage of the population. This patient's symptoms are well documented as adverse effects. Hypersensitivity responses are due to stimulation of the immune system and are invoked by an antigen or antibody response. The symptoms presented do not reflect hypersensitivity to the drug.

3 Answer: 4 Rationale: Ondansetron is known to prolong the QT interval and may cause or worsen existing dysrhythmias. Options 1, 2, and 3 are incorrect. An allergy to soy or soy products, chronic constipation, or glaucoma does not present contraindications to the drug.

4 Answer: 1 Rationale: The enzymes in pancrelipase come from pork. If the patient is allergic to or has religious restrictions on pork, the drug is contraindicated. Options 2, 3, and 4 are incorrect. Pancrelipase is not contraindicated for individuals with HTN or coronary artery disease. Pancrelipase is not an iodine-based agent. There is no expected cross sensitivity.

5 Answer: 4 Rationale: Because magnesium hydroxide will stimulate peristalsis, it is important that the nurse assess for bowel sounds before giving the drug. If blockage or an ileus is suspected, the drug should be held and the provider notified. Options 1, 2, and 3 are incorrect. Blood pressure is an important vital sign to monitor postoperatively, but the magnesium hydroxide should not have direct effects. The dosage of the opioid drug and the patient's ability to ambulate to the bathroom will not impact the drug's use or action.

6 Answer: 1, 3 Rationale: The nurse should explore possible causes for the diarrhea with the mother before making a recommendation. If diarrhea is caused by infections, slowing motility may allow the infection to worsen. Salicylates, including bismuth subsalicylate, are contraindicated under the age of 19 because of an increased risk for Reye's syndrome. Options 2, 4, and 5 are incorrect. Activity level and weight are important growth and development parameters to assess but are unrelated to the drug's use. The school schedule would not have a direct impact on which drug is recommended.

Chapter 61

Making the Patient Connection

1 Additional assessment data that would assist in determining Charlene's need for vitamin therapy includes her current diet,

alcohol use, medication history, menstrual history including heavy periods, recent weight-loss plans or dieting, and the possibility of pregnancy.

2 Charlene should not take the prenatal vitamins without checking with her provider. Some vitamins degrade and become less effective if stored near heat or humidity. Prenatal vitamins also contain higher amounts of some vitamins and minerals that Charlene may not need. Depending on the possibility of pregnancy, a new prescription for prenatal vitamins may be required.

3 Charlene should be encouraged to seek dietary sources of vitamins and minerals whenever possible. A nutritional consult may be advisable. If she enjoys alcohol, she should be encouraged to limit her intake to a maximum of one glass per day. If symptoms continue, she should check with her provider about a more complete physical examination to detect other possible causes.

Additional Case Study

1 Blood calcium and phosphate levels are dependent on adequate intake of vitamin D, which enhances their intestinal absorption by promoting mobilization of calcium from bone and renal reabsorption of phosphate. Additionally, consider Jerrod's lack of outdoor activities (sunlight) and poor nutritional habits, which increase the potential for vitamin D deficiency.

2 When patients are prescribed vitamin D, the nurse should monitor for ataxia, muscle and joint pain, pruritus, headache, and GI upset.

3 Vitamin D is produced photochemically in the epidermis. Exposing Jerrod to short periods of sunlight daily would help to increase his level of vitamin D.

Chapter Review

1 Answer: 2 Rationale: Oral contraceptives may increase the levels of vitamin A. Options 1, 3, and 4 are incorrect. Vitamins D and E are also fat-soluble vitamins and may be taken along with vitamin A. Mineral oil may decrease the fat-soluble vitamins, including vitamin A. Antibiotics are not known to have an effect on the serum levels of vitamin A.

2 Answer: Vitamin C may cause a false-negative result in occult blood if taken within 48 to 72 hours of the stool collection.

3 Answer: 4 Rationale: Pyridoxine (vitamin B_6) may antagonize the effects of antiparkinson drugs. Options 1, 2, and 3 are incorrect. INH, oral contraceptives, and hydralazine may increase the need for pyridoxine.

4 Answer: 1 Rationale: Zinc is found in protein foods such as beans, lentils, nuts, meats, and dairy. Options 2, 3, and 4 are incorrect. Vegetables such as leafy greens, carrots, squash, and crucifers and citrus fruits are not high in zinc.

5 Answer: 1, 3 Rationale: Vitamin K is routinely given to newborn infants to prevent bleeding postdelivery. It decreases the anticoagulant effects of the drug warfarin. Options 2, 4, and 5 are incorrect. Vitamin K is not indicated for visual disturbances or in the treatment of hypothyroidism or chronic acne.

6 Answer: 3 Rationale: Muscle cramping and spasms may be early signs of hypocalcemia. Options 1, 2, and 4 are incorrect. Night blindness is a sign of possible vitamin A deficiency. Anemia may indicate an iron deficiency. Bleeding abnormalities may signal a deficiency in vitamin K.

Chapter 62

Making the Patient Connection

1 It may be possible for Christopher to continue to eat small amounts of food or drink, but he should check with his provider first. If the gastroparesis has resulted in complete stasis of foods and fluid in the stomach, he may need to wait until the results of the metoclopramide and erythromycin treatment have been determined. Christopher may also be able to sip small amounts of water, which may absorb more quickly. Eating or drinking when gastric emptying is not occurring increases the risk of regurgitation and aspiration.

2 Christopher should inspect the area around the tube insertion site daily for redness, streaking, swelling, drainage, or tenderness. If the tube is sutured in place, he should also inspect the suture sites as well. Depending on the provider, Christopher may be taught to care for the tube by gently wiping around the area with a nonirritating soap and plain water. Aseptic technique and dressing changes may be required in the immediate postoperative period.

3 The list should include aspiration, gastroesophageal reflux, diarrhea, metabolic and electrolyte disturbances, tube clogging, tube migration and dislodgment, localized infections, sepsis, nasal or esophageal irritation, fever, redness or tenderness at the insertion site, drainage from the site, constipation, and fluctuations in blood glucose. Christopher should be provided with a written list of instructions on what to assess for and when to call his provider.

Additional Case Study

1 Because this patient's GI tract is unusable, parenteral nutrition therapy is indicated. Her nutritional needs are too great for PPN; thus, a course of TPN is indicated.

2 Because of this patient's poor nutritional status, she is at risk for developing refeeding syndrome once the nutritional therapy is initiated.

3 The deficits in the patient's baseline electrolyte values should be corrected before initiating TPN. The therapy should be started slowly and progress slowly.

Chapter Review

1 Answer: 3 Rationale: A patient receiving enteral feedings is at risk for dehydration caused by an inadequate intake of free water. It is important to irrigate the tube with water as ordered, or per protocol (before and after an intermittent feeding or medication, or every 4 to 6 hours for continuous feedings), and to include additional free water throughout the day unless contraindicated. Options 1, 2, and 4 are incorrect. Daily weights are important to track fluid balance, but they do not maintain fluid balance. The NG tube should be irrigated more than just once a day. While assessment of the skin around a PEG tube site is important, it will not indicate the patient's fluid balance. This patient is receiving the feeding via an NG tube, which is passed through the nose.

2 Answer: 1, 3, 5 Rationale: In addition to the base solution, TPN contains electrolytes, trace minerals, and multivitamins. Options 2 and 4 are incorrect. If diuretics are needed because of an underlying medical condition, they should be administered separately and not added to the TPN solution. Regular insulin may be added to the bag, but not NPH insulin.

3 Answer: 4 Rationale: 10% dextrose in water contains the highest concentration of glucose and should be hung until the new TPN bag is available. The solution selected should minimize the risk of hypoglycemia. Options 1, 2, and 3 are incorrect. They will not be effective in preventing hypoglycemia.

4 Answer: 2 Rationale: The patient's temperature should be monitored for signs of infection and subsequent sepsis, which are complications of TPN therapy. The weight is monitored to assess

the nutritional effectiveness of the TPN and to detect signs of fluid overload. Options 1, 3, and 4 are incorrect. Blood pressure and pulse are important assessments but do not relate specifically to the effects of TPN.

5 Answer: 4 Rationale: The nurse should not hang the lipids if separation of the emulsion or fat globules is visible in the solution. The solution should be returned to the pharmacy. Options 1, 2, and 3 are incorrect. Rolling or shaking the container or running the container under warm water will not correct the separation and may increase the risk of harm if the solution is used after separation has occurred.

6 Answer: 1, 2 Rationale: Refrigerating unused enteral feeding solutions and limiting the length of time the solution is not refrigerated will prevent the growth of pathogens. Options 3, 4, and 5 are incorrect. Feeding bags and tubes are used for a limited length of time, most for 24 hours, and washing out the bag and tubing will not prevent or reduce the growth of harmful pathogens. Using plain water to irrigate the feeding tube is an accepted technique but won't necessarily reduce the risk. Sterile technique is not needed when working with enteral feedings because the solution enters the GI tract. Clean technique is adequate except in severely immunocompromised patients.

Chapter 63

Making the Patient Connection

1 Diet drugs, both prescription and OTC, have had a rocky history. Early drugs were amphetamines or amphetamine-like substances with cardiovascular complications and addiction potential. Later drugs such as fenfluramine and phentermine (Fen-Phen)and sibutramine weree also removed from the market because of cardiovascular adverse effects. Only a few drugs remain available to assist in weight loss.

2 Orlistat is available in both prescription and nonprescription strength (the one Rosemary has seen in stores). Since Rosemary's weight is in the "overweight" category but not yet classified as "obese," the OTC dose may be appropriate. Before starting on orlistat, she should be screened for a past history of gallbladder disease because the drug slows gallbladder contractions and can worsen cholestasis. Other medical causes for weight gain, such as hypothyroidism, should be ruled out. Orlistat is taken up to three times per day with or within 1 hour of a meal containing fat. The drug may be skipped if the meal does not contain fat. Common adverse effects include gas, oily and loose stools, urge to defecate and difficulty controlling bowel movements, stomach or rectal area pain, and headache. Rosemary may want to begin the drug on a Friday to determine what adverse effects she experiences over the weekend before returning to work.

3 Factors that may have contributed to Rosemary's weight gain include a sedentary lifestyle, a diet with high-calorie, low nutrient-dense foods, alcohol use, postmenopausal hormonal changes, and stress. She should be encouraged to make small changes in her daily eating and activity rather than large and sudden changes that may be more difficult to sustain. She may find that keeping a refillable water bottle at her desk to increase her consumption of water throughout the day may be helpful, and the extra activity of refilling the bottle and restroom trips will increase her activity level. At her desk, Rosemary can take hourly breaks to stretch and move about, perhaps going up and down one flight of stairs each hour. Packing healthy snacks such as carrots, peppers, celery, unbuttered popcorn, or rice cakes to eat at work may help her avoid the high-calorie take-out lunches. Having packets of instant plain oatmeal or other cereals to microwave before work may cut down on trips to the fast-food store. Using smaller plates and visualizing the plate with one-quarter protein source, one-quarter carbohydrates, and one-half vegetables and fruits may help limit caloric intake at dinner.

Additional Case Study

1 Orlistat does not have addiction or cardiovascular risks that older diet drugs carried. It blocks the absorption of lipids, lowering calorie intake.

2 Prescription-strength orlistat is double the dose of OTC orlistat. GI adverse effects are common, and hepatic adverse effects may occur. Kathryn should immediately report any change in the color of her stools, increasing weakness, yellowing of the eyes or skin, and right upper quadrant pain.

3 Orlistat inhibits absorption of the fat-soluble vitamins, A, D, E, and K. If a multivitamin supplement is prescribed, Kathryn should take the vitamin at least 2 h before or after taking the orlistat. She should also be taught to report any increase in bleeding or bruising, signs of a potential vitamin K deficiency.

Chapter Review

1 Answer: 1, 3, 4, 5 Rationale: It is recommended that if a 5% weight loss is not achieved after 12 weeks of therapy with any weight loss drug, the drug should be discontinued and other options considered. Bupropion with naltrexone increases BP, and may precipitate severe HTN in patients with existing HTN. Naltrexone is an opioid antagonist and may initiate a withdrawal syndrome in patients currently taking opioids. Bupropion has a black box warning because of an increased risk of suicidal behavior. Option 2 is incorrect. It is not known whether there are long-term adverse effects that arise after the time bupropion with naltrexone is taken or whether the risk continues after the drug is discontinued.

2 Answer: 4 Rationale: Phentermine may cause fetal harm and should not be used if the patient is pregnant or there is a possibility of pregnancy. Options 1, 2, and 3 are incorrect. Phentermine is used for short-term treatment of obesity and the presence of extreme obesity may be an indication for the drug. The drug is used cautiously in patients with diabetes and HTN, but neither is an absolute contraindication for the drug. Careful monitoring will be required if either of these conditions exist.

3 Answer: 4 Rationale: Typically, orlistat is taken just prior to meals containing fats so that the drug can inhibit lipase and thus the absorption of lipids in the meal. Options 1, 2, and 3 are incorrect. Orlistat is taken throughout the day with each meal. It does not decrease appetite; it interferes with the absorption of fat in the diet. Although exercise is a part of the treatment plan for obesity, orlistat does not have to be administered before exercise.

4 Answer: 4 Rationale: Liraglutide was originally approved as a treatment for type 2 diabetes. Options 1, 2, and 3 are incorrect. Liraglutide has the potential to produce serious adverse effects such as pancreatitis, hypoglycemia, and gallbladder disease and carries a black box warning that it may cause thyroid tumors. It has known teratogenic effects and should not be taken during pregnancy, if pregnancy is suspected, or during breastfeeding.

5 Answer: 1 Rationale: Flatus and oily stools are adverse effects that are often troubling to the patient. The nurse should inform the patient that these often occur when taking orlistat. Options 2, 3, and 4 are incorrect. Heartburn and dyspepsia, constipation, and nausea and vomiting are not common adverse effects associated with orlistat.

6 Answer: 1, 2, 3 Rationale: Body weight, BMI, and waist circumference are all indicators used to assess levels of obesity. Options 4 and 5 are incorrect. A treadmill test assesses physical fitness, not obesity. Buoyancy analysis is not a test used to determine the degree of obesity.

Chapter 65

Making the Patient Connection

1 Raj and his parents will need instruction on when, where, and how to give the injections, how to store the medication, and any signs or symptoms of adverse effects that should be reported. The medication will be given subcutaneously in the abdomen, anterior thigh, or buttocks and the injection sites should be rotated with each injection. Giving the injection in the evenings will help to mimic the body's own hormone rhythms. Raj may prefer to learn to give his own injections and he should be included while teaching his parents. Teach the parents about the need for follow-up assessments of height, weight, bone age, and laboratory testing. Provide information on potential adverse effects, especially those that must be reported to the provider immediately, such as sudden weight gain, swelling, flank pain, or severe bone and joint pain.

2 It is important and appropriate to discuss with the parents the ability to afford this medication. Therapy is expensive and is not covered by all insurance plans. Therapy is also long term, usually continuing several years until closure of the epiphyseal plates and attainment of final adult height. You might consider referring the family to a medical social worker who might be able to find sources of funding, if necessary. It is also important to discuss the realistic effects of therapy: The increases in height are often modest but are still important to the overall well-being of the patient.

3 The adverse effects to discuss are hyperglycemia and insulin resistance, with the possibility of developing diabetes mellitus, hypothyroidism, and calcium-based kidney stones. Routine testing will monitor for these conditions. Other possible adverse effects are edema, headache, and HTN. These usually resolve with continued treatment and dose adjustments. Other adverse effects are joint and bone pain, local pain at the injection site, and the rare possibility of developing antibodies to growth hormone.

Additional Case Study

1 You would anticipate treatment with desmopressin PO, once a day, at bedtime.

2 Edward and his parents will need information about drug administration, possible adverse effects, and nondrug treatment. The drug should be taken at bedtime with a few sips of water. Keeping a diary of nighttime trips to the bathroom and episodes of bedwetting may help with dosage adjustments. Although they occur infrequently, adverse effects include transient headaches, rhinitis, nausea, abdominal pain, and cramping. The drug may cause fluid retention, with water intoxication a serious adverse effect. Early symptoms are drowsiness, listlessness, and headache. These early symptoms should be reported immediately to the provider. The risk for water intoxication may be reduced by limiting evening fluid intake to no more than one 240-mL (8-oz.) cup at dinner and no more than one additional 240-mL cup between dinner and bedtime.

Chapter Review

1 Answer: 2 Rationale: GH cannot be given PO; it can only be administered subcutaneously. Options 1, 3, and 4 are incorrect. A lack of GH is not associated with intellectual disability. Children whose epiphyseal plates have closed are not candidates for GH therapy; therefore, most adolescents would see minimal gain in height. Periodic testing for blood hormone levels is required during therapy.

2 Answer: 1, 2, 3 Rationale: GH increases the length and width of long bones; promotes organ, muscle, and connective tissue growth; and increases the synthesis of proteins. Options 4 and 5 are incorrect. GH may cause an increase in serum glucose levels, not a decrease. It may decrease fat deposits around the abdomen and improve lipid levels.

3 Answer: 3 Rationale: Patients on desmopressin need to record a daily weight and should monitor for the presence of peripheral edema. Options 1, 2, and 4 are incorrect. Desmopressin must be given in regular doses for continued therapeutic effects. Increasing the dosage may cause an increased risk of vasoconstriction and other adverse effects. Leg cramping when walking may indicate adverse peripheral vascular effects and should be assessed by the provider. Taking NSAIDs concurrently may increase the antidiuretic effect, leading to adverse effects.

4 Answer: 1 Rationale: Octreotide prolongs intestinal transit time and stimulates reabsorption of fluids and electrolytes from the GI tract. These effects would have the therapeutic action of decreasing diarrhea. Options 2, 3, and 4 are incorrect. Octreotide will not slow cancer growth or metastasis or improve lean body mass or fat deposits. Hypo- and hyperglycemia are possible adverse effects of octreotide, not therapeutic effects.

5 Answer: 4 Rationale: Concurrent administration of octreotide with PO antidiabetic drugs or insulin can produce hypoglycemia. Glucose levels would have to be monitored closely and insulin dose adjustments made. Options 1, 2, and 3 are incorrect. Glaucoma, COPD, or alcoholism would not be contraindications for this drug.

6 Answer: 1 Rationale: A patient with diabetes insipidus (DI) who is responding to therapy with desmopressin would have decreasing signs of dehydration. Options 2, 3, and 4 are incorrect. DI is characterized by large volumes of urine output with a very low urine specific gravity accompanied by signs of dehydration, including complaints of thirst and an increased pulse rate. The patient would see a lowered pulse rate related to an increase in circulating volume secondary to the decrease in urine output. Desmopressin therapy would cause the urine specific gravity to increase, not decrease. Blood glucose levels are not affected by desmopressin.

Chapter 66

Patient Safety: Humulin R (regular) insulin and Humalog (insulin lispro) have similar names and require special caution to avoid exchanging the vials and administering the incorrect insulin. Most healthcare facilities require insulin dosages to be checked by two nurses or licensed personnel before administration to the patient, with both members verifying the accuracy of the type and dose of insulin. Depending on agency policy, individual vials of insulin may be kept in the patient's room in a secured storage area to help prevent error. Direct observation of the insulin preparation by the patient, family, or caregiver may reduce the chance for errors and provides the nurse an opportunity for patient teaching.

Making the Patient Connection

1 Oral antidiabetic drugs are often used in combination to better treat type 2 diabetes. Glyburide stimulates the release of insulin and increases the sensitivity to insulin in peripheral tissues. Metformin reduces blood glucose by reducing glucogenolysis and decreasing the intestinal reabsorption of glucose. Together they work by different mechanisms to lower blood glucose levels.

2 Eileen should take the drugs before her morning meal. If the metformin prescription is not an extended-release formulation, additional doses throughout the day around mealtime may be required. Hypoglycemia is a possible adverse effect, particularly from the glyburide, and Eileen should be taught how to monitor her blood glucose levels. Appropriate care when ill or if Eileen changes her exercise routine should also be discussed.

3 Patients with type 2 diabetes produce their own insulin but it is either insufficient to meet their body's needs or their cells have developed a resistance to it. Providing oral drug therapy that assists her own insulin to work more efficiently is a goal of therapy for type 2 diabetes. While insulin may not be needed at this time, it may be needed in the future, particularly if illness or stress cause blood glucose levels to increase.

4 Occasional small amounts of alcohol may be allowed but Eileen should discuss this with her provider. Alcohol consumption increases the risk of hyper- and hypoglycemia and it is known to produce disulfiram-type reactions in patients taking glyburide. She should be taught to consume any alcohol with meals so that the food balances the alcohol consumption. She should also be taught the symptoms of a disulfiram-type reaction and to notify the provider if they occur.

Additional Case Study

1 Only regular insulin can be used for IV administration.

2 Nicholas is currently NPO and receiving an IV of 0.45 normal saline along with the IV insulin. Although this will replace the fluids he has lost due to the polyuria and vomiting, it supplies no carbohydrates. Because Nicholas's blood glucose may continue to fall as the insulin exerts therapeutic effects, the insulin will be stopped before his blood glucose levels have returned to the normal range to prevent hypoglycemia.

3 Essential teaching includes information on type 1 diabetes, including the symptoms Nicholas was having and how they relate to the diagnosis. They will need instruction on Nicholas's diet and a dietary consult should be arranged. As the nurse, when you give Nicholas his subcutaneous insulin doses, you can use the opportunity to discuss the need for insulin, why it is required, and how to give the injections. As Nicholas becomes more comfortable with the injections, he can begin practicing insulin administration along with his parents. Because this is a new diagnosis, short, frequent teaching sessions will help to cover the large amount of information they will need before going home. Planning for outpatient instruction through an agency-based diabetes education program or sessions with a Certified Diabetes Educator will also help ensure that Nicholas is able to return to his active lifestyle and manage his diabetes.

Chapter Review

1 Answer: 2 Rationale: Insulin peaks are the times of maximum insulin utilization with the greatest risk of hypoglycemia. Options 1, 3, and 4 are incorrect. Because the risk for hypoglycemia is highest at peak serum insulin levels, exercise or additional insulin may increase the risk further. Insulin schedules for the patient are developed by the provider and the patient should not self-select a schedule for insulin use.

2 Answer: 2, 3, 5 Rationale: The blood glucose level should be checked prior to administering any type of insulin. Because lispro is a rapid-acting insulin, the nurse should ensure that a meal is available and that the patient will be able to eat shortly after receiving a dose. If signs of hypoglycemia are present, the insulin dose should be held and the patient treated for hypoglycemia. Options 1 and 4 are incorrect. Urine testing for glucose and ketones gives non-specific data, and patients vary on the degree to which glucose and ketones will enter the urine. While a check of the pulse or blood pressure may be included in routine vital signs or to further assess symptoms of hypoglycemia, they do not provide information directly pertinent to the administration of insulin.

3 Answer: 3 Rationale: A serious adverse effect of metformin is the risk for developing lactic acidosis. Renal insufficiency and failure, excess alcohol use, and IV contrast agents increase the risk for lactic acidosis and are contraindications to the use of metformin. Options 1, 2, and 4 are incorrect. Hypoglycemia, GI distress, and weight loss are common adverse effects to most oral antidiabetic drugs and are not specific to metformin.

4 Answer: 2 Rationale: It can take several weeks for rosiglitazone to provide full therapeutic effects, so the appropriate response would be to give it more time to reach effectiveness. Options 1, 3, and 4 are incorrect. It is not within a nurse's scope of practice to prescribe additional drugs or change the dosage. The provider should be consulted about any change to the patient's drug regimen.

5 Answer: 4 Rationale: Glucagon injections can be repeated if one dose is not effective. Hypoglycemia is a medical emergency, and because this woman has not fully recovered, medical attention is needed. Options 1, 2, and 3 are incorrect. The patient is still experiencing symptoms of hypoglycemia, and continued treatment is indicated. Because she is still groggy and disoriented, it would not be safe to give anything by mouth.

6 Answer: 4 Rationale: Insulin glargine has no definite peak, so there is a minimal risk for hypoglycemic reaction. Options 1, 2, and 3 are incorrect. Insulin glargine must be given by subcutaneous injection, it cannot be given by IM injection, and blood glucose monitoring is required for all patients taking any insulin.

Chapter 67

Making the Patient Connection

1 It is anticipated that Helen's laboratory reports may reveal abnormal values consistent with hypothyroidism. Other possible testing the provider may order include an ultrasound of her thyroid gland, a radioactive iodine uptake test, or a test for antithyroid antibodies.

2 Helen should take the levothyroxine in the morning on awakening and as close as possible to the same time each morning to mimic the body's own natural thyroid hormone rhythm. If she forgets to take a dose, it should be taken as soon as remembered. If she is unable to take the drug for more than one day because of illness, she should contact the provider for further instructions.

3 Because the symptoms of hypothyroidism occur after the thyroid is no longer producing enough thyroid hormone, replacement therapy will be required lifelong.

4 Because replacing a hormone does not precisely mimic the body's own hormone levels, there may be times when Helen experiences symptoms of hyperthyroidism or return of symptoms similar to the ones she experienced from hypothyroidism. Symptoms of hypothyroidism do not need to be immediately reported to the provider unless they are significantly worse than previously experienced. If they continue for longer than a few days, Helen should inform the provider because a dosage adjustment may be required. Symptoms she should immediately report to her provider are similar to hyperthyroidism: rapid heart rate, palpitations, headache, shortness of breath, anxiety, and intolerance to heat.

Additional Case Study

1 The nurse would expect to see orders for the following diagnostic tests: serum T_4, T_3, and TSH levels. Radiologic exams such as magnetic resonance imaging or computed tomography may also be ordered.

2 Drug therapy for this patient would likely include propylthiouracil to decrease thyroid hormone production and secretion, a beta-adrenergic blocker for blood pressure control and to decrease sympathetic stimulation, and acetaminophen for fever control. Note that aspirin is not given to patients with hyperthyroid because it would displace T_3 and T_4 from their protein binding

sites. This would increase the amount of free, active thyroid hormone, worsening the patient's condition.

3 Long-term therapy for this patient would include antithyroid drugs, suppressive therapy with radioactive iodine, or surgical removal of all or part of the thyroid gland. These therapies may induce hypothyroidism, which is then treated with replacement therapy.

Chapter Review

1 Answer: 4 Rationale: The administration of too much levothyroxine may cause cause hyperthyroidism with nervousness, palpitations, weight loss, diarrhea, and muscle tremors. Before altering the dosage, thyroid function studies will be performed to verify this condition. Options 1, 2, and 3 are incorrect. Nervousness, palpitations, and tremors are not symptoms of hypothyroidism or normal thyroid states. While these symptoms may occur with diabetes and hyperglycemia, other symptoms would dominate and would be noted before these symptoms occurred.

2 Answer: 3, 4, 5 Rationale: A euthyroid (normal) state is indicated by a return to normal performance of ADLs without fatigue, normalizing cholesterol levels, and vital signs within normal limits with a pulse rate between 60 and 100 beats/minute. Options 1 and 2 are incorrect. Constipation and weight gain are symptoms of hypothyroidism. Decreased blinking and exophthalmos are symptoms of hyperthyroidism.

3 Answer: 1 Rationale: Low-grade fever, sore throat, and chills are symptoms of a possible infection. Because propylthiouracil may cause agranulocytosis, these symptoms should be reported to the provider. Options 2, 3, and 4 are incorrect. Increased appetite and caloric intake signal a return to a more euthyroid state. Tinnitus, altered taste, thickened saliva, insomnia, nightmares, and night sweats are not effects usually associated with propylthiouracil and if they occur, other causes should be investigated.

4 Answer: 3 Rationale: A heart rate of 110 beats/minute would cause the nurse to hold the scheduled dose of levothyroxine because it could indicate an excessive level of thyroid hormone. Options 1, 2, and 4 are incorrect. A low level of thyroid hormone could cause weight gain or decreased blood pressure. These are symptoms of hypothyroidism and would not cause the nurse to hold the medication. An elevated temperature without other signs of hyperthyroidism would not warrant withholding the medication.

5 Answer: 2 Rationale: The high levels of iodine found in potassium iodide solution will inhibit the synthesis and release of thyroid hormone. The effectiveness decreases over time so it is only used short term before more definitive treatment can be accomplished. Options 1, 3, and 4 are incorrect. Iodine deficiency is rare and does not cause symptoms of hyperthyroidism, the indication for the patient's potassium iodide solution. High-dose iodine is not always used prior to thyroid surgery and the thyroidectomy is not related to a loss of iodine. High doses of iodine will not prevent diabetes.

6 Answer: 3 Rationale: To closely approximate the body's own hormone levels, levothyroxine should be taken in the morning, at the same time each day. Options 1, 2, and 4 are incorrect. Taking levothyroxine along with food or meals containing high fiber may affect the absorption of the drug. Foods such as strawberries, spinach, and kale may inhibit thyroid secretion, reducing the effectiveness of the drug. If diarrhea occurs, the provider should be notified to determine the need to alter the dose.

Chapter 68

Making the Patient Connection

1 Some people believe that they have been exposed to poison ivy many times and have never gotten a rash, but that does not mean they are not allergic. Poison ivy reactions are triggered by an allergic response to urushiol, the oil found in the sap of poison ivy, oak, and sumac. Sometimes the allergy does not emerge until someone receives multiple exposures. Sensitivity to urushiol changes over time, and children who were not sensitive to poison ivy, oak, or sumac become allergic as adults. Allergic inflammation, or hypersensitivity, is caused by the immune system attacking the skin containing the plant oil, producing symptoms such as rashes, oozing blisters, and itching. This allergic response can occur 12 to 48 hours after exposure to the oil.

2 A Medrol Dosepak is too low of a starting dose and the duration of therapy is too short for poison ivy allergic dermatitis. The prednisone taper the nurse practitioner prescribed will help prevent a rebound reaction.

3 It is important to teach Charlie that abrupt discontinuation of the prednisone may cause an exacerbation of symptoms and, depending on the frequency and length of time on the corticosteroids, may also cause his adrenal glands to slow or stop producing normal amounts of cortisol.

4 Even though poison ivy, oak, and sumac rashes are not contagious and you cannot get them from another individual or the blister fluid, the urushiol oil from the plant can remain on objects for long periods of time. Since urushiol can stay active for years, it is important to wash any item that has come in contact with the poisonous plant. This includes garden tools, lawnmowers, shoes, camping equipment, and even pet fur.

Additional Case Study

Because Monica has been taking prednisone for a significant length of time, she has probably experienced atrophy of the adrenal glands. To avoid adrenal insufficiency or adrenal crisis, the drug must be tapered off gradually to allow normal adrenal function to return.

Chapter Review

1 Answer: 1, 3, 5 Rationale: Edema, eye pain or vision changes, and abdominal pain are symptoms of possible adverse effects from the methylprednisolone. Options 2 and 4 are incorrect. Tinnitus is not an adverse effect commonly associated with methylprednisolone and if it occurs, other causes should be investigated. Dizziness upon standing indicates possible *hypo*tension. *Hyper*tension is a possible adverse effect from methylprednisolone.

2 Answer: 1 Rationale: An irregular heart rate and rhythm is a symptom of hypokalemia. Hydrocortisone given concurrently with diuretics such as thiazides, which cause loss of potassium, increases the risk of hypokalemia. Options 2, 3, and 4 are incorrect. While these are common adverse effects of hydrocortisone, they do not require immediate attention.

3 Answer: 1, 2 Rationale: Weight-bearing exercise three to four times weekly and increased dietary intake of calcium and vitamin D may help prevent bone loss and osteoporosis. Options 3, 4, and 5 are incorrect. Remaining sedentary is not advisable and may increase the risk of osteoporosis and other adverse effects such as thrombophlebitis. Increased fluid intake and avoidance of alcohol are advised, but carbonated sodas should also be avoided because they have been linked to an increased risk of osteoporosis. While a bisphosphonate may be needed if bone density studies indicate the development of osteoporosis, it is not necessarily required at this time.

4 Answer: 4 Rationale: The patient should obtain a daily weight, at the same time each day to assess for excessive fluid retention. Fludrocortisone is a mineralocorticoid and may cause fluid retention, edema, and HTN. Options 1, 2, and 3 are incorrect. Abdominal pain and changes to the stool color may indicate GI

bleeding, which is an adverse effect associated with glucocorticoids. Increased lipid levels and mood changes are also associated with glucocorticoids.

5 Answer: 3 Rationale: The patient is experiencing symptoms of acute adrenal insufficiency related to the inability to take the prescribed drug for several days and will require immediate IV administration of hydrocortisone. Options 1, 2, and 4 are incorrect. Fludrocortisone is a mineralocorticoid and is not indicated in this emergency situation. Ketoconazole and pasireotide have antiadrenal effects and would worsen the situation.

6 Answer: 4 Rationale: Patients receiving replacement therapy for chronic adrenal insufficiency should carry PO and parenteral forms of the prescribed drugs in case of emergencies where the drugs may not be readily available. Options 1, 2, and 3 are incorrect. Checking BP, avoiding crowds and infections, and monitoring for visual changes are appropriate interventions when hyperphysiologic doses are given to treat disease and other conditions. Patients on replacement therapy for adrenal insufficiency receive lower, physiologic doses and should not experience adverse effects.

Chapter 69

Patient Safety: Although this order is within the normal dose range for oxytocin, there is no notation as to a maximum dose to be given or corresponding patient-specific parameters to be assessed, such as duration of contractions or fetal heart rate. Oxytocin is a "high-alert medication" recognized by The Joint Commission and the Institute for Safe Medication Practices as requiring special care for administration.

Making the Patient Connection

1 Maureen is over age 35 and smokes cigarettes, both of which place her at greater risk for thromboembolic events related to HT. The provider and Maureen will decide on HT after discussing the therapy and considering other factors such as a previous history of thrombus or embolism, a personal and family history of cardiovascular disease, and her blood pressure and heart rate.

2 Maureen may be a candidate for HT. Estrogen, progesterone, and testosterone decrease as a woman approaches menopause. She may also choose to take natural therapies such as black cohosh. Should Maureen choose to begin HT, the goal would be to normalize the ratio between estrogen and progesterone. Testosterone is useful in elevating a woman's mood, sex drive, and energy. The overall goal is to restore balance between the hormones and to diminish the unpleasant symptoms of menopause. Likely drugs are Premarin and Prempro.

3 Should Maureen choose to begin HT she will need to adjust her lifestyle. She should discontinue smoking because it greatly increases the risk for thromboembolic events. She should monitor for unusual symptoms in the first year of HT such as headache, pain or warmth in her calf, or sudden chest pain. She should reduce or discontinue caffeine intake because estrogen and caffeine may lead to increased CNS stimulation, further accentuating her nervousness, anxiety, and insomnia. Additionally she should begin a regular exercise program including walking, which retards the chances for osteoporosis.

Additional Case Study

1 Female infertility is multifactorial and accounts for 50 to 60% of infertility problems in couples. Some of the most common reasons include irregular or absent ovulation, pelvic inflammatory disease, and obstruction of the uterine tubes. Testing for endocrine causes should be carried out. Endocrine causes can be due to conditions in the hypothalamus, pituitary, or ovary. A sperm count and complete health exam should also be conducted on Prithi's husband. Having a child previously does not necessarily rule out male infertility as a current cause.

2 Before administration of clomiphene the nurse would complete a medical history and physical examination. Therapy is started with a low dose of 50 mg/day for 5 days. If ovulation does not occur, the dose is increased to 100 mg, and possibly to the maximum of 150 mg/day. If this regimen fails, HCG may be initiated. Inform Prithi that the pregnancy rate of persons taking this drug is about 90% and twins occur in about 5% of treated patients. Prithi should take the medication at the same time each day, and if a dose is missed it should be taken as soon as remembered. If not remembered until the next day, then take two doses. She should immediately report any abnormal bleeding or signs of jaundice and discontinue therapy immediately if pregnancy is suspected.

Chapter Review

1 Answer: 2, 3, 4 Rationale: A history of thromboembolic conditions, breast cancer, or hyperlipidemia may be contraindications for the use of HT and will require further assessment by the provider before prescribing conjugated estrogen. Options 1 and 5 are incorrect. Because conjugated estrogen is metabolized through CYP450 pathways and the drug may have hepatic effects, women with diabetes may need to more closely monitor blood glucose to ensure that their diabetes medications are effective, but this is not considered a contraindication to the drug. A past history of caesarean birth is also not a contraindication.

2 Answer: 3 Rationale: Regular contractions increasing in occurrence indicate that the oxytocin is exerting a therapeutic effect. Options 1, 2, and 4 are incorrect. Control of postpartum hemorrhage is a therapeutic effect of oxytocin but would not be considered a therapeutic effect during labor. Sustained contractions are an adverse effect of oxytocin and immediate intervention is needed to prevent serious injury to the mother or baby should they occur. Oxytocin stimulates the milk letdown reflex in nursing, but this would not be considered a therapeutic effect during labor.

3 Answer: 4 Rationale: Clomiphene is given over six ovulatory-menstrual cycles in increasing doses with HCG added as needed. If no pregnancy has occurred after six cycles, other treatment options will be considered. Options 1, 2, and 3 are incorrect. The drug will not be continued for 1 year if pregnancy has not occurred, and the dosage may be increased after each cycle. Clomiphene can cause fetal harm and should be discontinued if pregnancy occurs.

4 Answer: 3 Rationale: Medroxyprogesterone can decrease bone density over time. The patient should be taught to report any bone, joint, or musculoskeletal pain and to report any difficulty or pain with movement or ambulation. Options 1, 2, and 4 are incorrect. Insomnia or sleep difficulty and mouth, eye, or vaginal dryness are not related adverse effects. The drug may cause breakthrough spotting between menstrual cycles but this is a common effect and does not require evaluation unless the bleeding is heavy or continuous.

5 Answer: 2 Rationale: The standard treatment with clomiphene is to begin with a low dose for 5 days beginning on the fifth day of the menstrual cycle. Options 1, 3, and 4 are incorrect. Starting therapy on the first day of the menstrual cycle would not be as effective in stimulating ovulation because this occurs closer to midcycle. Because women experience menstrual periods of varying length, starting the drug on the "last day" would vary, and the drug might be started sooner or later than the recommended fifth day of the menstrual cycle. Many women do not know when ovulation occurs to be able to take it based on an ovulatory cycle and there is a possibility this patient is not experiencing ovulation.

6 Answer: 4 Rationale: Sedation, intense thirst, flushing of the skin, confusion, and muscle weakness are early symptoms of magnesium toxicity and should be immediately reported. Options 1, 2, and 3 are incorrect. The drug decreases deep tendon reflexes and CNS stimulation, and hyperactivity or seizure activity would not be expected. Chest congestion and cough are not associated with the drug and other causes should be explored.

Chapter 70

Making the Patient Connection

1 Lila is within the 72-hour timeframe for emergency contraceptive use with Plan B. If ulipristal is prescribed, it is effective for up to 5 days after intercourse.

2 Levonorgestrel (Plan B) works to prevent pregnancy by preventing ovulation. Another option Lila could have prescribed is ulipristal, which also prevents ovulation. Plan B is available OTC to women over the age of 18, although they must ask for it from the pharmacist so that age can be verified. Ulipristal is available only by prescription.

3 You will give Lila instructions for taking Plan B. If Lila prefers the Plan B One Step form, she will take one single pill; two pills 12 hours apart if regular Plan B is taken. Nausea is the most common adverse effect, although vomiting, abdominal pain, fatigue, headache, irregular menstrual bleeding, and dizziness may occur. Serious adverse effects are not common and if any symptoms other than the previous ones are noted, Lila should contact her healthcare provider. If Lila experiences vomiting within 2 hours of taking Plan B, she should contact the pharmacist or healthcare provider for advice on taking another dose. If she experiences severe abdominal pain, she should immediately contact her provider to rule out an ectopic pregnancy. Plan B does not protect against STIs and Lila should discuss STI screening with the provider if she has concerns. Plan B is not 100% effective, but the chance of pregnancy is reduced to approximately 1 to 2%. If she does not experience her menstrual period at the expected time and is more than 1 week late, she may be pregnant and should be assessed at that time.

Additional Case Study

1 Broad-spectrum antibiotics such as tetracyclines and penicillin can alter the effectiveness of OCs, resulting in an increased risk of pregnancy.

2 You would advise Gina that in addition to her OC dose, she should use additional precautions during antibiotic therapy. Condoms and spermicidal agents are possible choices until she starts another monthly cycle of her OC.

Chapter Review

1 Answer: 3, 4 Rationale: Smokers have a significantly increased risk of serious thromboembolic events when taking OCs. Mood disorders, including depression, may worsen in patients taking OCs, and additional monitoring may be advised. Options 1, 2, and 5 are incorrect. Obesity is a risk factor for both treatment failure and thromboembolic events; however, this patient is considered overweight and is not in the high-risk category. Patients with asthma are not high risk, and a healthy 42-year-old woman with no significant health history is not considered high risk.

2 Answer: 1 Rationale: If 2 consecutive days are missed, the patient should take two pills on the day it is discovered, two pills the following day, then resume the normal one pill per day routine. A second method of contraception should be used for 7 days after resuming the pills. Options 2, 3, and 4 are incorrect. Taking only one pill, skipping additional doses, or stopping the drug will not allow continued contraception. If the patient is concerned about pregnancy due to the missed pills, a pregnancy test may be conducted.

3 Answer: 4 Rationale: Levonorgestrel/estradiol is taken for 84 days followed by a lower dose of estrogen included in the pill package for 7 days. Options 1, 2, and 3 are incorrect. Taking levonorgestrel/estradiol for 3 weeks, year-round, or for 2 months would be incorrect administration cycles.

4 Answer: 3 Rationale: The patient takes mifepristone, followed by an assessment by the healthcare provider 2 days later. If abortion has not occurred, the misoprostol is taken. The patient returns to the healthcare provider in 14 days to confirm that abortion is complete. Options 1, 2, and 4 are incorrect. Two doses of mifepristone are not taken and the patient must be assessed by the provider before taking the misoprostol dose. Bleeding is a common effect of both drugs and is not an indication of when or whether to take the misoprostol.

5 Answer: 2 Rationale: Patients should be informed that spermicidal agents have relatively low levels of efficacy when used alone and should therefore be used only in conjunction with barrier methods such as condoms and diaphragms. Options 1, 3, and 4 are incorrect. Spermicides such as nonoxynol-9 are not highly effective in preventing pregnancy, do not cause or protect against HIV or PID, and do not prevent ectopic pregnancies.

6 Answer: 5, 1, 4, 3, 2 The correct ranking from most effective to least effective with typical use of the method is 1) Transdermal OCs 2) Depo-Provera 3) Oral contraceptives 4) Calendar rhythm 5) Spermicides.

Chapter 71

Patient Safety: The patient's normal diet includes a significant amount of grapefruit juice, which is known to increase the plasma level of sildenafil. The nurse should explore dietary options as replacements for grapefruit juice to avoid potential adverse reactions related to enhanced drug plasma levels in the future.

Making the Patient Connection

1 Common contributing factors to the diagnosis of ED include recent divorce, a diagnosis of depression, job-related stress, use of antidepressants, and a history of HTN.

2 The nurse needs to discuss the effects of tadalafil with Mike. The combination of this drug along with antidepressants and his antihypertensive, nifedipine, must be evaluated so as to avoid severe adverse effects. Instruct Mike on the correct administration of the drug and that its effects last up to 36 hours. Encourage continued visits with the psychiatrist.

3 Teach Mike about the differences between these drugs. Sildenafil has an onset that is relatively rapid, less than 1 hour, and its effects last up to 4 hours. Tadalafil acts within 30 to 60 minutes and has a longer duration of action than sildenafil: up to 36 hours. The longer duration of tadalafil allows for more spontaneity of sexual activity. Contraindications include patients who take nitrates, and dosing can be prescribed every 72 hours. Tadalafil produces less blood pressure change than other drugs in this class, making it safer for patients like Mike with HTN who are already taking other medications for this condition. Sildenafil is contraindicated in patients who are also taking nitrates, although Mike is not currently on a nitrate drug.

Additional Case Study

1 Finasteride acts in the prostrate to shrink the prostatic tissue, which decreases any mechanical obstruction in the urethra.

This drug is usually well tolerated but does decrease ejaculate volume and libido in some patients.

2 Avoid caffeine and alcohol intake, eliminate drugs that worsen BPH such as testosterone and other anabolic steroids, and restrict fluids close to bedtime. Morrie should know that the drug may take up to 6 months to reach full effect, but he should continue taking it consistently during that time. He will need to have more frequent laboratory tests for PSA levels because the drug is known to cause changes that make the detection of prostate cancer more difficult.

3 Other assessment findings for Mr. Jones may include complaints of increased urgency to urinate, postvoid leakage, decreased force of the urine stream, and a sensation that the bladder is not completely empty. A review of Mr. Jones's history and current medications should include the use of OTC and herbal preparations; a health history, especially for HTN; and an assessment of his laboratory studies to help prevent adverse effects.

Chapter Review

1 Answer: 2 Rationale: Primary hypogonadism results in patients with normal pituitary function and testes that are either diseased or unresponsive to FSH and LH. A primary goal of therapy would be an increased sperm count with an increase in male masculinization. Options 1, 3, and 4 are incorrect. Testosterone should not affect RBC count. Administering testosterone to the patient will not increase FSH or LH levels.

2 Answer: 1 Rationale: The use of nitrates is contraindicated with sildenafil because dangerous hypotension may result. Options 2, 3, and 4 are incorrect. A history of diabetes would not be of concern and may be an indication for treatment if ED occurs. An allergy to penicillin products is not a contraindication for use of sildenafil. There are no expected adverse reactions with sildenafil and the use of antiulcer medication.

3 Answer: 2, 3, 5 Rationale: Women and children should avoid skin contact with areas where testosterone gels or creams have been applied to avoid drug absorption. Testosterones may trigger sodium and water retention and a weight gain of 2 kg (5 lb) or more per week should be reported. They may also increase blood lipid levels. Therefore, the patient should follow a low-fat diet and have periodic blood lipid level assessments. Options 1 and 4 are incorrect. Testosterone gel should be applied to the upper arms, shoulders, or abdomen and never to the scrotum, perineal area, or on broken or irritated skin. Showering or swimming should be avoided for several hours after application to allow drug absorption, but a wait of 12 to 14 hours is excessive.

4 Answer: 2 Rationale: For sildenafil to be effective, the ED must be physiologic in nature. It is not effective if the dysfunction has solely psychologic origins and therefore does not always cause an erection. Options 1, 3, and 4 are incorrect. Sildenafil simply enhances, rather than causes, an erection. Prolonged use does not result in less intense feelings over time. Use of sildenafil by men will not have effects on female sexual function.

5 Answer: 3, 4, 5 Rationale: Silodosin relaxes smooth muscle in the prostate gland, bladder neck, and urethra, thus easing the urinary obstruction to restore urinary function. The drug should not be stopped abruptly because rebound HTN may occur. Dizziness and hypotension may occur, as well as a first-dose effect of hypotension and reflex tachycardia. The patient should sit or lie down until the sensation passes. Options 1 and 2 are incorrect. The drug does not cause shrinkage of the prostate gland and has no adverse effects if handled by women.

6 Answer: 4 Rationale: Full effects of finasteride are realized within 6 to 12 months of therapy. Because the symptoms of dysuria have suddenly increased, the patient should be assessed for possible prostate cancer. Options 1, 2, and 3 are incorrect. Continuing to take the drug after full therapeutic results should have been realized is not appropriate, given the sudden increase in symptoms. Decreasing fluid irritants such as caffeine and alcohol may help overall but will not cause the sudden symptoms. A low-dose diuretic may not be appropriate in this situation and may worsen the dysuria.

Chapter 72

Making the Patient Connection

1 Charlene's recent loss in height may explain why her pants seem longer and you should explain the details of this condition to the patient. Include these points in your discussion: 1) Risk factors: menopause, age over 60, family history of osteoporosis, high alcohol intake, estrogen deficiency, smoking history, androgen deficiency, anorexia nervosa, low calcium or vitamin D intake, physical inactivity, and thin, lean body build. 2) Signs and symptoms: fractures seen in the hips, wrists, forearms, or spine and height loss. 3) Diagnosis: height loss, bone fractures, and BMD values. 4) Treatments: Many drugs may be helpful. These include calcium and vitamin D, estrogen receptor modulators, statins, slow-release sodium fluoride, bisphosphonates, and calcitonin.

2 The nurse should encourage the patient to participate in preventive measures, which include adequate intake of calcium and vitamin D, physical exercise, routine healthcare follow-up especially in evaluating estrogen needs, use of OTC calcium supplements as recommended by a provider, and avoiding alcohol.

Additional Case Study

1 Etanercept is given by subcutaneous injection twice per week.

2 If the daughter has never given an injection before, she should be instructed on appropriate technique, followed by teach-back until she feels comfortable giving the injection. There may be discomfort, pain, swelling, or bruising at the site of injection, all of which tend to diminish over the length of therapy. Ice or hydrocortisone cream applied to the site may decrease these effects. The daughter should be advised that these are common reactions not related to her technique of giving the injection. Injection sites should be rotated with each injection.

3 In addition to localized pain, swelling, and bruising at the injection site, additional adverse effects include serious infections, reactivation of latent TB infection, HF, and blood dyscrasias.

4 Methotrexate is a potent immunosuppressant. Potential adverse effects related to methotrexate include increased susceptibility to infections, gastric irritation and stomatitis, pneumonitis, nephrotoxicity and hepatotoxicity, and bone marrow suppression.

Chapter Review

1 Answer: 3 Rationale: Alendronate may cause severe GI adverse effects. To decrease the risk, for esophageal irritation, and to promote the absorption of the medication, alendronate should be taken with a full glass of water after rising in the morning. The patient should not eat or drink anything or remain upright for 30 minutes after administration. Options 1, 2, and 4 are incorrect. The medication should be taken before breakfast, not before lunch or at bedtime. The patient should not lie down for at least 30 minutes after taking alendronate.

2 Answer: 1 Rationale: Headache, dizziness, and blurred vision are all early symptoms of toxicity to methotrexate. Options 2, 3, and 4 are incorrect. Hematuria, jaundice, and ascites are not associated with the use of methotrexate. While stomatitis may occur, constipation would be unrelated to methotrexate.

3 Answer: 2 Rationale: Colchicine prevents the migration of neutrophils into the area of inflammation caused by uric acid crystals, reducing further inflammation and relieving the symptoms of gout and gouty arthritis. Options 1, 3, and 4 are incorrect. Colchicine does not increase uric acid deposits in the synovial spaces of the joints, prevent accumulation of uric acid crystals in the joints, or increase renal excretion of uric acid crystals. Patients feel better from decreased inflammation secondary to fewer uric acid crystal deposits. Renal excretion of uric acid is not a mechanism of action of colchicine.

4 Answer: 1 Rationale: The patient with osteomalacia has low serum calcium and phosphate levels. An indicator that replacement therapy is achieving therapeutic benefits would be increasing serum calcium and phosphate levels. Options 2, 3, and 4 are incorrect. Increasing or decreasing actions of the serum calcium and phosphate levels are incorrectly stated.

5 Answer: 1 Rationale: Vitamin D toxicity may occur in the patient receiving calcitriol. Symptoms to assess include muscle weakness, fatigue, nausea and vomiting, and changes in the color or amount of urine. Options 2, 3, and 4 are incorrect. Diarrhea, abdominal pain, stomatitis, joint stiffness, photosensitivity, and tinnitus are not symptoms that would be associated with the effects of vitamin D therapy. Bone pain and fever are symptoms of vitamin D deficiency.

6 Answer: 1, 3, 4 Rationale: DMARDs modify immune and inflammatory responses but may increase the risk of infections and malignancies and reactivate latent TB. Injection-site reactions such as pain, swelling, and bruising are common adverse effects. Options 2 and 5 are incorrect. Adalimumab has not been associated with an increased risk of osteoporosis and is given subcutaneously every other week.

Chapter 73

Making the Patient Connection

1 Acne vulgaris is a common skin condition in the teenage years. It is thought to occur as hair follicles become blocked and trapped sebum interacts with the bacterium *P. acnes* in the hair follicle, causing inflammation and the classic papular acne lesion. Topical keratolytic drugs such as benzoyl peroxide help dry the skin and act as an antibacterial against *P. acnes*. Topical antibiotics may also be used. In severe cases, tretinoin may be required to adequately treat the condition.

2 Danny's increased acne at this time may be linked to rising androgen levels as he progresses through puberty. Because he is active in outdoor sports, sweat, dust and dirt from athletic fields, and the use of sunscreen may also be aggravating the condition.

3 Danny should wash his face gently with mild soap and water, especially after participating in sports practices or games. He should apply a thin layer of the tretinoin to the acne. He should discontinue benzoyl peroxide or other topical drugs while he is using the tretinoin to avoid excessive dryness. Tretinoin often causes redness, peeling, or a temporary hyperpigmentation. Danny should limit sun exposure to the treated areas and should consult with his provider about the use of sunscreens.

Additional Case Study

1 Psoriasis is a skin condition that results in a rapid turnover of skin cells and red, raised patches of skin covered with flaky, thick, silvery scales known as plaques. The scales will shed on their own but if scraped, may result in bleeding. Psoriasis is a genetic autoimmune disorder. It is not contagious, although because of the genetic link, other members of the family may also have the condition.

2 Stephanie should apply the betamethasone cream in thin layers to the affected areas. Warm, moist dressings may also be applied over the cream and wrapped with plastic wrap to increase the absorption. The wrap should not remain in place for more than 8 hours and the site should be inspected at each dressing change for skin breakdown, hyperpigmentation, or other signs of irritation.

3 Calcipotriene is a derivative of vitamin D that is applied topically to the skin to decrease cell turnover. It is applied in thin layers and is not recommended for use over large surface areas because hypocalcemia may result. Excessive sun exposure to the areas should be avoided, and it may take 2 to 3 weeks to see improvement. Because Stephanie is within childbearing age, she should be taught to consult with the provider if she plans to be or is pregnant.

Chapter Review

1 Answer: 4 Rationale: Lice and nits can live in areas of the body other than scalp hair. Options 1, 2, and 3 are incorrect. Permethrin should not be applied after body lotions and should not be used on eyelashes or eyebrows. Lice can survive for up to 24 to 48 hours on inanimate objects.

2 Answer: 1 Rationale: Patients taking topical corticosteroids for the treatment of atopic dermatitis may experience burning and stinging in the affected area. Options 2, 3, and 4 are incorrect. Localized pruritus and hives, a loss of hair in the application area, or a worsening of acne vulgaris are not symptoms related specifically to the effects of therapy.

3 Answer: 1, 2, 3 Rationale: Benzoyl peroxide suppresses sebum production and has antimicrobial action against the bacteria that cause acne. It also has a keratolytic effect, drying and encouraging more rapid cell turnover in the outer layer of the epidermis. Options 4 and 5 are incorrect. Microdermal abrasion is not a primary mechanism of action of the drug and benzoyl peroxide does not have sunscreen activity.

4 Answer: 3 Rationale: Tretinoin may cause dryness, irritation, and erythema. Mild soaps, gentle cleansing, warm but not hot water, and gentle drying should be used during tretinoin therapy. Options 1, 2, and 4 are incorrect. Antiacne soaps often contain compounds that dry the skin and may cause further irritation. Sunscreens with an SPF of 15 and coverings should be used while on tretinoin to avoid sunburn. Alternating tretinoin with benzoyl peroxide can cause excessive dryness and irritation and increase the risk of adverse effects.

5 Answer: 3 Rationale: A small test area should be used if benzocaine has not been used before to assess for allergy. If no symptoms are noted within 30 to 60 minutes, it may be applied to a wider area. Options 1, 2, and 4 are incorrect. Benzocaine should not be used on partial-thickness burns because of the risk of open blistered areas. The solution should not be warmed to avoid further heat and damage to the area of the burn. The burn should not be covered with plastic wrap to avoid heat trapping, potentially increasing the damage.

6 Answer: A patient who has been prescribed isotretinoin must comply with the iPledge Program because of the risk of teratogenic effects.

Chapter 74

Making the Patient Connection

1 Predisposing factors include that she is an African American and an older adult with a history of diabetes. Other general predisposing factors that may not apply to Mrs. Duclos include HTN, migraines, refractive disorders with a high degree of

nearsightedness or farsightedness, and the normal aging process . Long-term use of topical corticosteroids, some antihypertensives, antihistamines, and antidepressants may also contribute to the development or progression of glaucoma.

2 Wash hands prior to administering eyedrops and avoid touching the eye or eyelashes with any part of the eyedropper to avoid cross-contamination. Administer the eyedrop solution into the conjunctival sac. Apply gentle pressure over the lacrimal duct for 1 minute. Apply to only the affected eye(s). Ensure that only one drop is instilled unless ordered otherwise. Wait at least 5 minutes before instilling other eyedrops.

3 If eyedrops for glaucoma are given frequently or if the tear duct is not held after administering the drop and the solution is swallowed, systemic effects may occur. Adverse effects from beta-adrenergic blocker drops include angina, anxiety, bronchoconstriction, hypotension, and dysrhythmias. Systemic adverse effects from prostaglandin drops include respiratory infection, angina, and muscle or joint pain. Cholinergic agonist drops may cause systemic adverse effects such as salivation, tachycardia, hypotension, bronchospasm, nausea and vomiting.

Additional Case Study

A patient information sheet could include the following information: Wash hands prior to administering the medication; Pull the pinna of the ear gently up and back to straighten the ear canal for a child of this age (4 years old); Instill the desired number of drops into the ear. Do not instill the drops directly into the canal but allow them to flow down the side to prevent dizziness and nausea from the drop falling on the tympanic membrane; Gently massage the area just anterior to the ear) to facilitate movement of the medication into the ear canal. A cotton ball may be loosely placed in the ear to promote retention of the medication; Keep the child supine for 4 to 5 minutes to prevent leakage of the medication; Report any increase in pain, drainage, fever, dizziness, or difficulty hearing to the provider.

Chapter Review

1 Answer: 4 Rationale: Timolol is a beta-adrenergic blocker. To prevent swallowing and systemic absorption, pressure is to be applied to the inner canthus of the eye after instilling the drop. Options 1, 2, and 3 are incorrect. No other eyedrops or ointments should be used when taking timolol or other drops for glaucoma without the approval of the provider. Eye solutions for allergies may contain adrenergic drugs that may worsen glaucoma. Timolol is not contraindicated during seasonal allergies. It is not known to worsen seasonal allergies, although it may cause bronchoconstriction in the sensitive individual or if swallowed and systemic effects occur.

2 Answer: 1, 2, 4 Rationale: Latanoprost (Xalatan) may cause thickening and darkening of the eyelashes and upper eyelid and may cause darkening of the iris, especially noticeable in patients with light eye colors. Options 3 and 5 are incorrect. Latanoprost will not cause lightening of the iris or darkening of the sclera or a permanent bluish tint to the conjunctiva.

3 Answer: Pilocarpine causes miosis, which stretches the trabecular meshwork, allowing greater outflow of aqueous humor and decreasing the IOP.

4 Answer: 2, 3, 1, 4 Rationale: The ear should be pulled gently upward and back and the drop instilled, allowing it to flow down the side of the canal. Dropping the solution directly on the tympanic membrane may cause dizziness or nausea. The area in front of the ear should be gently massaged. The patient should remain in a side-lying position for 5 minutes to allow complete absorption of the solution. A dry cotton ball may be placed in the outer ear area to prevent leakage of solution.

5 Answer: 4 Rationale: Increasing pain, particularly around the ear area, may indicate worsening infection or mastoiditis and should be immediately reported. Options 1, 2, and 3 are incorrect. Mild itching and irritation may occur, but severe itching or swelling should be reported. Gradually decreasing pain is a therapeutic effect as the infection clears. Dizziness may occur if the eardrop is instilled directly onto the tympanic membrane.

6 Answer: Phenylephrine causes mydriasis, allowing better visualization of the area of the lens during cataract surgery.

Chapter 75

Making the Patient Connection

1 Because smallpox is caused by the variola virus, there is no specific treatment for it and vaccination is the only prevention. The virus can be spread from one individual to another by direct and prolonged face-to-face contact. Smallpox also can be spread through direct contact with infected body fluids or contaminated objects such as bedding or clothing. Exposure to smallpox is followed by an incubation period of 7 to 17 days. Initially, symptoms of smallpox include high fever, malaise, head and body aches, and sometimes vomiting. Often the development of a rash begins in the mouth. However, it quickly spreads to the face and moves to the arms and legs.

2 The method of transmission affects the symptoms of anthrax contamination. The most common (cutaneous anthrax) and the most serious (inhalation anthrax) forms of anthrax are transmitted through open skin and inhalation, respectively. The nurse should examine the patient's skin for open wounds that may be contaminated. Respiratory assessment and support are imperative for the patient who may have contracted anthrax via respiratory exposure. The CDC recommends standard contact precautions be maintained for patients suspected of exposure to anthrax.

3 *Yersinia pestis* is an anaerobic bacterium that causes a life-threatening condition known as pneumonic plague. The isolation of this disease is extremely difficult because it can be spread by aerosol. Individuals with this disease would be infectious to everyone with whom they have come in contact within 1 to 6 days after exposure. If untreated, pneumonic plague will result in respiratory failure with subsequent shock and death. Bubonic plague, a more common form, results in enlarged, painful lymph nodes.

Additional Case Study

1 Poison-proofing a home is the key to preventing childhood poisonings. Always close medication, cleaning product, and other hazardous material containers immediately after using them. Properly secure child-resistant packaging, and immediately store containers in a place where children cannot reach them. Keep iron-containing tablets and all medications out of reach and out of sight of children. Never keep medicines on a countertop or bedside table. Buy the least hazardous products for cleaning purposes and look for products that are safe for children. Never transfer cleaning solutions to other containers. The kitchen and bathroom are the most likely unsafe areas. Keep any cabinet containing a potentially poisonous item locked. Remember that child-resistant caps are child resistant, not childproof. Garages and utility rooms should also be checked for potential poison hazards. To be on the safe side, keep houseplants out of the reach of young children. Include your provider's phone number and the numbers of your regional poison control center in the phone.

2 Never administer ipecac syrup without first consulting a provider or poison control center. It is no longer recommended and may actually delay more appropriate treatment.

Chapter Review

1 Answer: 1 Rationale: No antidote or specific treatment exists for radiation poisoning. Supportive therapy for the associated symptoms is the only treatment available. Options 2, 3, and 4 are incorrect. Ultraviolet light does not affect individuals who experience radiation poisoning. An individual with radiation toxicity is incapable of contaminating other individuals. No antiradiation medications exist.

2 Answer: 1 Rationale: The preferred drug for *Y. pestis* exposure is doxycycline. Options 2, 3, and 4 are incorrect. Trivalent and heptavalent botulinum antitoxin are the two available treatments for botulism. Ribavirin is an antiviral agent that may be used to treat serious virus infections. Atropine sulfate is used as an antidote for organophosphate poisoning.

3 Answer: 3 Rationale: Time is a critical factor in acute poisonings. The emergency should be called into 911 and the rescue squad should transport the child to the nearest healthcare facility immediately. Options 1, 2, and 4 are incorrect. Instructions for poisoning may have changed since the packaging was printed. Based on the information provided in the question, the nurse does not know what chemicals the child has ingested. Forced vomiting is contraindicated for most poisonings. Waiting for the child to develop seizures or shortness of breath is too late since the development of these symptoms most likely represents a toxic level of the poison.

4 Answer: 3 Rationale: Patients with decreased sensorium are at high risk for pulmonary aspiration. Activated charcoal should only be given to these patients if the airway is maintained with an endotracheal tube. Options 1, 2, and 4 are incorrect. Activated charcoal is not absorbed in the GI tract and therefore would not be contraindicated in patients with liver pathology. Activated charcoal is eliminated in the feces and therefore would not be contraindicated in patients with renal impairment. Anxiety and nervousness are not reasons to withhold the administration of activated charcoal.

5 Answer: 1 Rationale: Chelating agents capture the toxic metal through a bonding process. The kidneys remove both the chelator and the metal bound to it from the body. Options 2, 3, and 4 are incorrect. A chelator binds heavy metals but does not deactivate any chemical reactions. Chelation therapy is not involved in metabolism. Glomerular filtration is not affected by chelation therapy.

6 Answer: 2 Rationale: EDTA may produce renal damage that may be reduced by ensuring adequate diuresis before therapy begins. Options 1, 3, and 4 are incorrect. Bowel function is not a critical parameter to consider prior to giving this drug. EDTA administration is not based on visual acuity. Skin integrity is not a critical parameter to consider prior to giving EDTA.

Glossary

A

Abortifacients drugs used to induce abortion

Absorption the process by which drug molecules move from their site of administration to the blood; movement of nutrients and other substances from the alimentary canal to the circulation

Abuse-deterrent formulations forms of opioid tablets or capsules that are resistant to crushing in order to discourage drug misuse

Accessory organs of digestion include the salivary glands, liver, gallbladder, and pancreas

Acetylation a biochemical process that adds a two-carbon chain to a drug molecule, which usually renders the drug less effective

Acetylcholine (ACh) primary neurotransmitter of the autonomic nervous system

Acetylcholinesterase (AChE) enzyme that resides in the synaptic cleft and catalyzes the destruction of ACh

Acetylcholinesterase (AChE) inhibitors indirect-acting cholinergic agonists that are nonselective and affect all ACh synapses

Acidosis condition of having too much acid in the blood; plasma pH below 7.35

Acne vulgaris disorder of the hair follicles and sebaceous glands characterized by small inflamed bumps that appear on the surface of the skin

Acquired immunodeficiency syndrome (AIDS) infection caused by the human immunodeficiency virus (HIV)

Acquired resistance ability of an organism to become unresponsive over time to the effects of an anti-infective

Acromegaly excessive growth hormone disorder in which bones become deformed

Activated partial thromboplastin time (aPTT) laboratory test used to measure blood coagulation

Active immunity resistance resulting from a previous exposure to an antigen

Acute dystonia occurs during pharmacotherapy with antipsychotics and involves severe muscle spasms, particularly of the back, neck, tongue, and face

Acute gouty arthritis condition in which uric acid crystals accumulate in the joints of the big toes, ankles, wrists, fingers, knees, or elbows, resulting in extremely painful, inflamed tissue

Acute retroviral syndrome symptoms during the initial phase of HIV infection

Adaptive defenses immune responses that are specific to certain threats

Addiction the continued use of a substance despite serious health and social consequences

Addison's disease hyposecretion of glucocorticoids and mineralocorticoids by the adrenal cortex

Additive effect type of drug interaction in which two drugs combine to produce a summation response

Adherence taking medications in the manner prescribed by the healthcare provider, or in the case of OTC drugs, following the instructions on the label

Adhesins chemicals produced by *H. pylori* that allow the organism to penetrate the GI mucosa and cause inflammation

Adipocytes fat cells that are the primary storage sites for lipids

Adverse Event Reporting System (FAERS) a voluntary program that encourages healthcare providers and consumers to report suspected adverse effects directly to the FDA or the product manufacturer

Adjuvant analgesics drugs that have indications other than pain but are used to enhance analgesia

Adjuvant chemotherapy administration of antineoplastic drugs after surgery or radiation therapy

Adrenal atrophy condition in which the adrenal cortex shrinks and stops secreting endogenous corticosteroids due to lack of stimulation by adrenocorticotropic hormone (ACTH)

Adrenal crisis condition that occurs when corticosteroid medication is abruptly withdrawn

Adrenergic receptors at the ends of postganglionic sympathetic neurons

Adrenergic agonists drugs that activate adrenergic receptors in the sympathetic nervous system; also known as sympathomimetics

Adrenergic antagonists drugs that block norepinephrine from reaching its receptors

Adrenocortical insufficiency lack of adequate corticosteroid secretion by the adrenal cortex

Adrenocorticotropic hormone (ACTH) hormone secreted by the anterior pituitary that stimulates the release of glucocorticoids by the adrenal cortex

Adverse drug effect an undesirable and potentially harmful action caused by the administration of medication

Aerobic pertaining to an oxygen environment

Aerosol suspension of minute liquid droplets or fine solid particles in a gas

Affinity the ability of some tissues to attract, accumulate, and store drugs in high concentrations relative to other tissues

Afterload pressure in the aorta that must be overcome for blood to be ejected from the left ventricle

Agonist drug that activates a receptor and produces the same type of response as the endogenous substance

Agoraphobia an extreme avoidance of closed places where a panic attack might occur such as airplanes, public meetings, or elevators

Akathisia inability to rest or relax; constantly moving

Alcohol use disorder dependence on alcohol (ethanol)

Alimentary canal a long, continuous, hollow tube of the GI tract that extends from the mouth to the anu

Alkalosis plasma pH above 7.45

Alkylating agents drugs that kill cancer cells by altering the shape of the DNA double helix and preventing the DNA from duplicating during cell division

Allergic rhinitis inflammation of the nasal mucosa due to exposure to allergens

Alopecia hair loss

Alpha-adrenergic antagonists drugs that block alpha-adrenergic receptors in the sympathetic nervous system

Alzheimer's disease (AD) neurodegenerative disease that involves a chronic progressive loss of cognitive function

Amide anesthetic local anesthetic that has the same mechanism of action as esters but has less effect on myocardial contraction and fewer allergic reactions

Amygdala located in the temporal lobe, it is essential for the ability to feel certain emotions and to perceive them in other people

Anabolic effects ability of a drug such as testosterone to accelerate the growth of red blood cells, muscle, bone, and neural tissues

Anabolic steroids testosterone-like substances with hormonal activity that are commonly abused by athletes

Anaerobic pertaining to an environment without oxygen

Analgesics drugs used to relieve pain

Anaphylaxis life-threatening allergic response that may cause cardiovascular shock and death

Androgens steroid sex hormones that promote the appearance of masculine characteristics

Anemia decreased oxygen-carrying capacity of the blood

Angina pectoris acute chest pain caused by myocardial ischemia

Angioedema rapid swelling of the throat, face, larynx, and tongue that can lead to airway obstruction and death

Angiogenesis the formation of new blood vessels

Angiotensin I a precursor to the formation of angiotensin II that is produced when angiotensinogen is split by the enzyme renin

Angiotensin II vasopressor substance released in response to falling blood pressure that causes vasoconstriction and release of aldosterone

Angiotensin-converting enzyme (ACE) inhibitor drug that blocks the formation of angiotensin II, decreasing blood pressure

Angiotensinogen protein synthesized by the liver that is continuously circulating in the bloodstream

Anorexiants drugs used to suppress appetite

Anovulatory cycles menstrual cycles lacking ovulation

Antacids inorganic compounds containing aluminum, magnesium, sodium, or calcium that neutralize gastric acid and inactivate pepsin

Antagonist drug that blocks or inhibits the response of another drug

Antagonistic effect type of drug interaction in which adding a second drug results in a diminished pharmacologic response

Anterior pituitary gland (adenohypophysis) consists of glandular tissue that manufactures and secretes hormones that control major body functions and systems

Anterograde amnesia type of short-term memory loss where the user cannot remember events that occurred while under the influence of a drug

Anthrax an acute infectious disease that results from exposure to the spore-forming bacterium *Bacillus anthracis*

Antibiotic natural substance produced by a microorganism that can kill other microorganisms

Antibodies proteins produced by the body in response to an antigen; used interchangeably with the term immunoglobulin

Anticholinergic syndrome symptoms such as dry mouth, blurred vision, photophobia, visual changes, difficulty swallowing, agitation, and hallucinations, caused by an overdose of anticholinergic substances

Anticoagulants natural substances or drugs that inhibit the formation of blood clots

Antidepressants drugs used to enhance, elevate, or stabilize mood

Antidiuretic hormone (ADH) hormone released by the posterior pituitary gland when blood pressure falls or when the osmotic pressure of the blood increases; most important means by which the body maintains fluid homeostasis

Antigens microbes and foreign substances that elicit an immune response

Anti-infective general term for any medication that is effective against pathogens

Antipyretics medications used to reduce body temperature

Antiretroviral therapy (ART) therapy designed to reduce the replication of HIV as much as possible, as measured by a reduction in plasma HIV RNA to its lowest possible (or undetectable) level; formerly called highly active antiretroviral therapy (HAART)

Antiretrovirals drugs that are effective against retroviruses

Antithrombin III (AT-III) protein that prevents abnormal clotting by inhibiting thrombin and other clotting factors

Antitussives medications that control cough

Anxiety state of apprehension, tension, or uneasiness that stems from the anticipation of danger, the source of which is largely unknown or unrecognized

Anxiolytic drugs that relieve anxiety

Apoprotein protein component of a lipoprotein

Appetite a psychologic response that drives food intake based on associations and memory

Aqueous humor fluid that fills the anterior and posterior chambers of the eye

Arteriosclerotic cardiovascular disease (ASCVD) event disease such as stroke, angina pectoris or myocardial infarction caused by plaque in arteries

Asthma chronic inflammatory disease of the lungs characterized by airway obstruction

Atherosclerosis condition characterized by the presence of plaque within the walls of arteries

Atonic seizures very short-lasting seizures during which the patient may stumble and fall for no apparent reason

Atrial natriuretic peptide (ANP) hormone secreted by specialized cells in the right atrium when large increases in blood volume produce excessive stretch on the atrial wall

Atrial reflex causes the heart rate and CO to increase until the backlog of venous blood (or IV fluid) is distributed throughout the body

Attention-deficit/hyperactivity disorder (ADHD) disorder typically diagnosed in childhood characterized by hyperactivity as well as attention, organization, and behavior control issues

Attenuated viruses that have been rendered unable to cause disease through the application of heat or chemicals from which effective vaccines can be developed

Atypical antidepressants diverse class of drugs that act by mechanisms other than those of the selective serotonin reuptake inhibitors, tricyclic antidepressants, and monoamine oxidase inhibitors

Atypical mycobacterial infections (AMIs) nontuberculosis opportunistic diseases caused by mycobacteria

Auras sensory warnings such as flashing lights, visual blind spots, and arm or leg tingling that precede a migraine

Automaticity ability of certain myocardial cells to spontaneously generate an action potential without an outside signal from the nervous system

Automatisms repetitive arm movements, leg movements, head rolling, chewing, lip smacking, or swallowing that occur in complex partial seizures

Autonomic nervous system (ANS) portion of the peripheral nervous system that provides for the involuntary control of vital functions of the cardiovascular, digestive, respiratory, and genitourinary systems

Autonomic tone the background level of autonomic activity that occurs in the absence of stimuli

Azole term for the major class of drugs used to treat mycoses

Azoospermia complete absence of sperm in an ejaculate

B

β-glucan an essential component that shapes and strengthens the cell walls of fungi

B cell lymphocyte responsible for humoral immunity

Bactericidal drug that kills bacteria

Bacteriostatic drug that inhibits the growth of bacteria

Bacteriuria bacteria found in the urine

Balanced anesthesia use of multiple medications to produce general anesthesia, provide sedation, rapid induction of unconsciousness, muscle relaxation, and analgesia

Baroreceptors receptors in the aorta and carotid artery that sense changes in blood pressure

Barrett's esophagus precancerous condition of the esophagus

Basal nuclei area of the brain responsible for starting and stopping synchronized motor activity such as leg and arm motions during walking; also called basal ganglia

Beers criteria list of drugs compiled by the American Geriatrics Society that may produce a high incidence of adverse effects in older adults

Belladonna natural source of alkaloids with anticholinergic activity acquired from the deadly nightshade plant, *Atropa belladonna*.

Benign prostatic hyperplasia (BPH) nonmalignant abnormal enlargement of the prostate gland

Best Pharmaceuticals for Children Act authorizes the FDA to contract for the testing of already approved pediatric drugs.

Beta-adrenergic antagonists drugs that block beta-adrenergic receptors; may be nonselective or selective; also called beta blockers

Beta-lactam ring portion of the chemical structure of penicillin and some other antibiotics that is responsible for their antibacterial activity

Beta-lactamase enzymes produced by bacteria that renders certain antibiotics ineffective

Bioavailability the rate and extent to which the active ingredient is absorbed from a drug product and becomes available at the site of drug action to produce its effect

Biologic response modifiers natural cytokines that boost specific functions of the immune system

Biosimilar drug drug that has comparable effectiveness and safety to an FDA-approved biologic product

Bioterrorism intentional release of an infectious agent for the purpose of causing harm to a large number of people

Bipolar disorder syndrome characterized by extreme and opposite moods, such as euphoria and depression

Bisphosphonates class of drugs for treating osteoporosis that inhibit bone resorption by suppressing osteoclast activity

Black box warning in some drug inserts, a statement by the FDA that warns prescribers that the drug carries a risk for serious or fatal adverse effects

Blood–brain barrier network of capillaries in the CNS that inhibits many chemicals and drugs from gaining access to the brain

Body mass index (BMI) measurement of obesity determined by dividing body weight (in kilograms) by the square of height (in meters)

Body surface area (BSA) method method of calculating pediatric dosages using an estimate of the child's BSA

Body weight method method of calculating pediatric dosages that requires a calculation of the number of milligrams of drug, based on the child's weight in kilograms (mg/kg)

Bone deposition opposite of bone resorption; bone building

Bone resorption process of bone demineralization or the breaking down of bone into mineral components

Boosters follow-up doses of vaccines that provide prolonged protection

Botanical plant extract used to treat or prevent illness

Botulism condition caused by *Clostridium botulinum*, an organism that secretes a potent toxin that paralyzes the muscles after an individual is poisoned

Bradydysrhythmias disorders characterized by a heart rate less than 60 beats/min

Bradykinesia difficulty initiating movement and controlling fine muscle movements

Bradykinin chemical released by cells during inflammation that produces pain and side effects similar to those of histamine

Bright-light therapy exposure to bright light for treating patients with seasonal affective disorder

Broad-spectrum antibiotic an anti-infective that is effective against a wide variety of different microbial species

Bronchospasm sudden contraction of the smooth muscle of the airways that causes acute dyspnea

Buffers chemicals that help maintain normal body pH by neutralizing strong acids or bases

C

Cachexia general wasting of muscle and other tissue

Calcineurin intracellular messenger enzyme that is activated when a T cell encounters an antigen

Calcitonin hormone secreted by the thyroid gland that decreases plasma levels of calcium by inhibiting resorption of calcium from bone and increasing excretion of calcium by the kidneys

Calcitonin gene–related peptide (CGRP) inhibitors medications used to treat migraines that act by blocking the CGRP protein in sensory nerves

Calcitriol the active form of vitamin D

Calcium channel type of voltage-gated channel in cardiac muscle and smooth muscles

Cannabis use disorder dependence on marijuana or hashish

Cancer malignant disease characterized by abnormal, uncontrolled cell division

Capillary leak syndrome a serious condition in which plasma proteins and other substances leave the blood and enter the interstitial spaces because of porous capillaries

Capsid protein coat that surrounds a virus

Carbonic anhydrase enzyme that forms carbonic acid by combining carbon dioxide and water

Carcinogens agents that cause cancer

Cardiac output (CO) amount of blood pumped by a ventricle per minute

Cardiac remodeling change in the size, shape, and structure of the myocardial cells (myocytes) that occurs over time in heart failure

Cardiotonic drugs drugs that increase the force of cardiac contraction; also called inotropic drugs

Cardioversion electrical shock of the heart that under ideal conditions will allow the return to a normal heart rhythm; also called defibrillation

Cataplexy sudden loss of muscle strength manifested as slurred speech, sagging of the jaw, head nodding, or complete collapse of the body

Catecholamines class of endogenous hormones involved in neurotransmission that include epinephrine, norepinephrine, and dopamine

Catechol-O-methyltransferase (COMT) enzyme that destroys catecholamines such as norepinephrine in brain, kidney and liver cells

Cathartic substance that causes accelerated, stronger, and more complete bowel emptying

CD4 receptor protein that accepts HIV and allows entry of the virus into the T_4 lymphocyte

Cell-kill hypothesis theoretical model that predicts the ability of antineoplastic drugs to eliminate cancer cells

Central nervous system (CNS) stimulants drugs that raise the general alertness level of the brain

Cerumenolytics agents used to loosen and remove impacted cerumen from the ear canal

Chelation therapy use of drugs to detoxify poisonous metals such as mercury, arsenic, and lead by converting them to a chemically inert form that can be easily excreted

Chemical names standard nomenclature for drugs assigned by the International Union of Pure and Applied Chemistry (IUPAC)

Chemoreceptor trigger zone (CTZ) location in the cerebral cortex that sends sensory signals to the vomiting center

Chemoreceptors sensory receptors in the aorta and carotid artery that recognize levels of oxygen, pH, or carbon dioxide in the blood

Chemotherapy pharmacotherapy of cancer

Chief cells cells located in the mucosa of the stomach that secrete pepsinogen, an inactive form of the enzyme pepsin that chemically breaks down proteins

Chloasma darkened pigmentation found on the forehead, temples, cheeks, and upper lips

Cholecalciferol inactive form of vitamin D

Cholestatic hepatitis type of liver inflammation caused by obstruction of the bile ducts

Cholinergic relating to neurons that release acetylcholine (ACh)

Cholinergic agonists drugs and chemicals that increase the action of acetylcholine (ACh) at a cholinergic receptor; also called parasympathomimetics

Cholinergic crisis caused by an overdosage with acetylcholinesterase (AChE) inhibitors or poisoning with organophosphate insecticides or toxic nerve gases; characterized by intense signs of parasympathetic stimulation such as miosis, nausea, vomiting, urinary incontinence, increased exocrine secretions, abdominal cramping, and diarrhea

Cholinesterase inhibitors drugs that block transmission at neurons that release acetylcholine

Chronic bronchitis recurrent disease of the lungs characterized by excess mucus production, inflammation, and coughing

Chronic kidney disease condition characterized by a gradual loss of kidney function, usually over a period of months or years; also called renal failure

Chronic obstructive pulmonary disease (COPD) progressive pulmonary disorder characterized by chronic obstructive airflow

Chyme partly digested food that is passed from the stomach to the small intestine

Cinchonism syndrome with symptoms such as tinnitus, headache, diarrhea, blurred vision, hearing loss, and dysrhythmias, caused by high doses of quinidine

Circadian rhythm cyclic basis by which body temperature, blood pressure, hormone levels, and respiration all fluctuate throughout the 24-hour day

Clinical phase trials the second stage of new drug testing in a clinical investigation

Closed-angle glaucoma acute intraocular pressure that is caused by obstruction of drainage of aqueous humor through the canal of Schlemm

Club drug a diverse group of abused substances taken by people at dance clubs, all-night parties, and raves

Colloids proteins, starches, or other large molecules that remain in the blood for a long time because they are too large to cross capillary membranes

Colony-stimulating factors (CSFs) hormones that activate white blood cells to fight an infection and stimulate the growth and differentiation of one or more types of leukocytes

Combination products drugs that contain more than one active generic ingredient

Comedolytics drugs that prevent and break up the formation of clogged pores

Comedones types of acne lesions that develop just beneath the surface of the skin (whitehead) or as a result of a plugged oil gland (blackhead)

Complement system part of the innate immune system that consists of a cluster of 20 plasma proteins that combine in a specific sequence and order when an infection occurs

Complementary and alternative medicine (CAM) diverse set of therapies and healing systems that are considered to be outside of mainstream healthcare

Complex partial (focal impaired awareness) seizures seizures that originate from a single focus and involve sensory, motor, or autonomic symptoms with some degree of altered or impaired consciousness

COMT inhibitors drugs that prevent the destruction of catechol-O-methyltransferase (COMT) in peripheral tissues, thus increasing the amount of levodopa available to enter the brain

Conjugation the direct transfer of small pieces of DNA from one bacterium to another

Constipation infrequent passage of abnormally hard and dry stools

Contraception the use of devices, drugs, or surgery to prevent pregnancy

Contractility the strength with which the myocardial fibers contract

Controlled substances drugs whose use is restricted by the Comprehensive Drug Abuse Prevention and Control Act

Convulsions involuntary violent spasms of the face, neck, arms, and legs

Coronary artery disease (CAD) a narrowing or occlusion of one or more coronary arteries

Corpora cavernosa tissue in the penis that fills with blood during an erection

Corpus luteum endocrine tissue formed from a ruptured follicle that remains in the ovary after ovulation and secretes progesterone

Cretinism condition marked by profound mental retardation and impaired growth that results from untreated congenital hypothyroidism

Cross-tolerance situation in which tolerance to one drug makes the patient tolerant to another closely-related drug

Crystalloids IV solutions that contain electrolytes and other agents in concentrations that mimic the body's extracellular fluid

Crystalluria crystals that form in the urine and potentially obstruct the kidneys or ureters

Culture set of beliefs, values, religious rituals, language, customs, and behavioral expectations that provide meaning for an individual or group

Culture and sensitivity (C&S) testing a laboratory test used to identify bacteria and the most effective antibiotic

Curare the first neuromuscular blocker, which was initially extracted from several different plant species native to the rain forests of South America

Cushing's syndrome condition caused by high levels of corticosteroids in the body over a prolonged period of time

Cyclooxygenase (COX) key enzyme in the synthesis of prostaglandin that is blocked by aspirin and other NSAIDs

Cycloplegics drugs that relax or temporarily paralyze ciliary muscles and cause blurred vision

Cystitis bladder infection

Cysts protective capsules formed by some protozoa that allow the organisms to survive in harsh environments in a dormant state for prolonged time periods

Cytokine release syndrome an acute inflammatory response that occurs 30 to 60 minutes following the IV administration of a drug due to massive cytokine release

Cytokines proteins produced by T cells, such as interleukins, leukotrienes, interferon, and tumor necrosis factor, that guide the immune response

D

Deep vein thrombosis (DVT) blood clot that occurs in the legs

Defecation elimination of indigestible substances from the body

Defibrillation electrical shock of the heart that allows the return to a normal heart rhythm; also called cardioversion

Delirium tremens a syndrome of intense agitation, confusion, terrifying hallucinations, uncontrollable tremors, panic attacks, and paranoia caused by alcohol withdrawal

Delusions false ideas and beliefs not founded in reality

Dementia degenerative disorder characterized by progressive memory loss, confusion, and the inability to think or communicate effectively

Dependence a powerful physiologic or psychologic need for a substance

Depolarization loss of membrane potential in a cell

Depression characterized by a sad or despondent mood that becomes out of proportion to actual life events

Dermatitis superficial inflammatory disorders of the skin characterized by redness, pain, and pruritus

Dermatophytosis fungal infection of the skin and hair

Diabetes insipidus (DI) disorder marked by production of large volumes of urine, usually accompanied by increased thirst

Diabetes mellitus metabolic disorder characterized by an imbalance between insulin availability and insulin need

Diabetic ketoacidosis (DKA) acute condition that occurs primarily in patients with type 1 diabetes characterized by hyperglycemia, metabolic acidosis, and osmotic diuresis

Diarrhea increase in the frequency and fluidity of bowel movements

Dietary Supplement and Nonprescription Drug Consumer Protection Act law that requires companies that market herbal and dietary supplements to include their address and phone number on the product labels so consumers can report adverse events

Dietary Supplement Health and Education Act of 1994 (DSHEA) primary law in the United States regulating herbal and dietary supplements

Dietary supplements products available over the counter that are intended to add to or supplement the nutritional value of the diet

Diffusion the movement of a chemical from an area of higher concentration to an area of lower concentration

Digestion the mechanical and chemical breakdown of food into a form that may be absorbed into the systemic circulation

Digitalization procedure in which the dose of digoxin is gradually increased until tissues become saturated with the drug, and the symptoms of heart failure diminish

Dihydropyridines the largest class of calcium channel blockers that bind reversibly to closed-type (inactivated) calcium channels to make them unresponsive to depolarization

Directly observed therapy (DOT) requires that a healthcare provider directly observe the patient swallowing the pills, whether it is in the hospital, office, or home care setting

Disease-modifying antirheumatic drugs (DMARDs) drugs that slow or modify the progression of rheumatoid arthritis

Dissociative anesthesia a trance-like feeling of being separated from the environment produced by an anesthetic

Distribution the transport of drugs throughout the body after they are absorbed

Diuretic substance that increases the rate of urine flow

DNA gyrase (topoisomerase II) in bacterial DNA replication, the enzyme that relaxes the supercoil

DNA helicase in bacterial DNA replication, the enzyme that unwinds the two DNA strands after the supercoil is relaxed

DNA polymerase in bacterial DNA replication, the enzyme that adds the precursor bases to replicate the original DNA and form new DNA strands

Dopamine chemical precursor in the synthesis of norepinephrine; classified as a catecholamine

Dopamine system stabilizers (DSSs) partial agonists that reduce the hyperactivity of dopamine in certain regions of the brain (to produce therapeutic effects), while at the same time restoring normal dopamine activity in other regions (to lower the incidence of adverse effects)

Dopamine type 2 (D_2) receptors receptors for dopamine in the basal nuclei of the brain that are associated with schizophrenia and antipsychotic drugs

Dose–response relationship the way a patient responds to varying doses of a drug

Down-regulation the process by which cells make fewer receptors on their surface

Drug any substance that is taken to prevent, cure, or reduce symptoms of a medical condition

Drug allergies a hyperresponse of body defenses to a drug that may result in a diverse range of patient symptoms

Drug interaction occurs when a medication interacts with another substance such as another drug, a dietary supplement, an herbal product, or food that is taken concurrently with the medication, and the drug's actions are affected

Drug misuse improper use of drugs, including overuse, underuse, or, in some cases, erratic use

Drug–protein complex formed when a drug that binds reversibly to a plasma protein, particularly albumin, makes the drug unavailable for distribution to its site of action

Drug monograph detailed description of a drug's active ingredient, acceptable forms, dosages or concentrations, and required labeling

Dry powder inhaler (DPI) device used to convert a solid drug to a fine powder for the purpose of inhalation

Dwarfism a growth hormone deficiency disorder in children associated with normal birth length followed by a slowing of the growth rate

Dysfunctional uterine bleeding hemorrhage that occurs on a noncyclic basis or in abnormal amounts

Dyslipidemia a general term that refers to abnormal amounts of lipids in the body

Dysrhythmias disorders of cardiac rhythm characterized by an abnormal heart rate or irregular contractions

Dystonia chronic neurologic disorder that is characterized by involuntary muscle contraction that forces body parts into abnormal painful movements or postures

E

Eclampsia pregnancy-induced hypertensive disorder

Ectopic foci regions of the myocardium outside the normal cardiac conduction pathway that may send impulses across the myocardium

Eczema chronic, inflammatory skin disorder

Efficacy the ability of a drug to produce a desired or intended response

Electrocardiogram (ECG) graphic recording of the wave of electrical conduction across the myocardium

Electroconvulsive therapy (ECT) treatment used for serious and life-threatening mood disorders in patients who are unresponsive to pharmacotherapy and psychotherapy

Electrolyte charged substance in the blood such as sodium, potassium, calcium, chloride, and phosphate

Elemental (monomeric) formulas enteral products that are usually lactose free and contain only a small percentage of calories from fat

Emergency contraception (EC) the prevention of implantation following unprotected intercourse or contraceptive failure

Emergency preparedness the ability to respond quickly and effectively to an unexpected event that may impact human health

Emetogenic potential usually applied to antineoplastic drugs; degree to which an agent is likely to trigger the vomiting center in the medulla, resulting in nausea and vomiting

Emphysema lung disease characterized by loss of bronchiolar elasticity and destruction of alveolar walls

Endocrine system body system that consists of various glands that secrete hormones

Endometriosis presence of endometrial tissue in nonuterine locations such as the pelvis and ovaries; a common cause of infertility

Endorphins a group of neurotransmitters that function as endogenous opioids or natural pain modifiers in the CNS

Endotoxins harmful nonproteins that are part of the normal cell wall of gram-negative bacteria

Enteral nutrition (EN) nutritional support used for patients with functioning GI tracts but who are unable to orally ingest adequate amounts of nutrients to meet their metabolic needs

Enteral route administration of drugs orally or through nasogastric or gastrostomy tubes

Enteric-coated tablets that have a hard, waxy coating designed to dissolve in the alkaline environment of the small intestine

Enteric nervous system (ENS) network of neurons in the submucosa of the alimentary canal that has sensory and motor functions that regulate the GI tract

Enteroendocrine cells specialized cells in the GI tract that secrete hormones that modify digestive processes

Enterohepatic recirculation occurs when a substance is recycled after biliary excretion back to the liver. Extends the half-life of drugs

Enzyme induction process by which a drug increases the activity of the hepatic microsomal enzymes

Epilepsy disruption of the activity of clusters of neurons in the brain that is characterized by two or more seizures

Erectile dysfunction (ED) consistent inability to either attain an erection or to sustain an erection long enough to achieve satisfactory sexual intercourse

Ergosterol lipid substance in fungal cell membranes

Erythema redness associated with skin irritation or allergy

Erythrocytic stage phase in malaria during which infected red blood cells rupture, releasing more merozoites and causing acute symptoms

Erythropoietin hormone secreted by the kidney that stimulates the body's production of erythrocytes (red blood cells)

Ester anesthetics local anesthetics that act by decreasing the amount of sodium that enters the neuron

Estrogen general term that refers to three different steroid hormones secreted by the ovary: estradiol, estrone, and estriol

Ethnicity social and historical experiences that apply to a community of people of common heritage and ancestry

Euphoria an intense sense of happiness and well-being

Exclusivity a period of time when competing companies are not allowed to market generic versions of a drug

Excoriation scratches that break the skin surface and fill with blood or serous fluid to form crusty scales

Excretion the process of removing substances from the body

Exophthalmos an outward bulging of the eyes

Exotoxins proteins released by bacteria into surrounding tissues that have the ability to inactivate or kill host cells

Expectorants drugs used to increase bronchial secretions

Extended release tablets or capsules designed to dissolve very slowly, resulting in a longer duration of action for the medication; also called long-acting or sustained release

Extracellular fluid (ECF) compartment of body fluid lying outside cells, which includes plasma and interstitial fluid

Extrapyramidal symptoms (EPS) symptoms of acute dystonia, akathisia, parkinsonism, and tardive dyskinesia often caused by antipsychotic drugs

Extrapyramidal system part of the CNS that controls locomotion, complex muscular movements, and posture

Extrinsic pathway activated in response to injury when blood leaks out of a vessel and enters tissue spaces; the pathway takes several seconds to complete

F

Fasting plasma glucose (FPG) test a primary blood test for diagnosing diabetes

Fat-soluble vitamins group of vitamins stored in the liver and fatty tissue that includes A, D, E, and K

FDA Adverse Event Reporting System (FAERS) a voluntary program that encourages healthcare providers and consumers to report suspected adverse effects directly to the FDA or the product manufacturer

Febrile seizures tonic–clonic motor activity lasting 1 to 2 minutes with rapid return of consciousness that occurs in conjunction with fever

Ferritin one of two protein complexes that maintain iron stores inside cells (hemosiderin is the other)

Fetal–placental barrier special anatomic barrier that inhibits many chemicals and drugs from entering the fetus

Fibrin an insoluble protein formed from fibrinogen by the action of thrombin in the blood clotting process

Fibrinogen blood protein that is converted to fibrin by the action of thrombin in the blood coagulation process

Fibrinolysis physiologic process that limits clot formation and removes existing clots

Fight-or-flight response characteristic set of actions produced when the sympathetic nervous system is activated that prepares the body for heightened activity and for an immediate response to a threat

Filtrate fluid in the nephron that is filtered into the Bowman's capsule

First-dose phenomenon orthostatic hypotension that occurs with the initial doses of $alpha_1$-adrenergic blockers

First-pass effect mechanism whereby drugs are absorbed, enter into the hepatic portal circulation, and are inactivated by the liver before they reach the general circulation

Folate see Folic acid

Folic acid B vitamin that is essential for normal DNA and RNA synthesis; also called folate

Food and Drug Administration (FDA) Modernization Act act that gave financial incentives to pharmaceutical companies to conduct pediatric research in pharmacology; in exchange for providing pediatric labeling, the legislation gives drug companies the ability to exclusively market the drug for an additional 6 months

Formulary list of drug and drug recipes commonly used by pharmacists

Frequency distribution curve a graphic representation of the actual number of patients responding to a particular drug action at different doses

Fungi kingdom of organisms that includes mushrooms, yeasts, and molds

G

Gamma aminobutyric acid (GABA) neurotransmitter in the CNS

Ganglia collection of neuron cell bodies located outside the CNS

Ganglionic blockers drugs that inhibit transmission at the ganglia in the sympathetic and parasympathetic nervous systems

Gastroesophageal reflux disease (GERD) regurgitation of acidic stomach contents into the esophagus

Gate control theory mechanism for explaining the transmission of pain in the spinal cord

Generalized absence seizures seizures with a reduction of normal activity, including staring and transient loss of responsiveness

General anesthesia medical procedure that produces unconsciousness and complete loss of sensation

Generalized anxiety disorder (GAD) difficult-to-control, excessive anxiety that lasts for 6 months or longer

Generalized seizures seizures that travel throughout the entire brain

Generalized tonic–clonic seizures seizures characterized by intense muscle contractions and loss of consciousness

Generic name name assigned to a drug by the U.S. Adopted Name Council

Genetic polymorphism changes in enzyme structure and function due to mutation of the encoding gene

Gestational diabetes condition resulting from glucose intolerance with an onset during pregnancy

Gigantism unusual tallness due to excessive growth hormone

Glaucoma condition that is characterized by optic neuropathy with gradual loss of peripheral vision caused by increased intraocular pressure

Glomerular filtration rate (GFR) the volume of water filtered through the Bowman's capsules per minute

Glomerulus a specialized capillary in the Bowman's capsule of the kidney that filters the blood during urine formation

Glucocorticoids class of hormones secreted by the adrenal cortex that prepare the body for long-term stress; also called corticosteroids

Gluconeogenesis the production of new glucose from noncarbohydrate molecules

Glutamate amino acid that is the most common neurotransmitter in the CNS

Glycoprotein IIb/IIIa receptor found on the surface of platelets

Goiter refers to an increase in the size of the thyroid gland

Gonadocorticoids sex hormones secreted by the adrenal cortex

Gout accumulation of uric acid (urate) crystals in the joints and other body tissues

Grading process that examines potential cancer cells under a microscope and compares their appearance to normal parent cells

Gram-negative bacteria that do not retain a violet stain because they have thin cell walls

Gram-positive bacteria that contain a thick cell wall composed of peptidoglycan and retain the violet color after staining

Graves' disease syndrome caused by hypersecretion of thyroid hormone

Gray baby syndrome condition seen most often in premature or newborn infants that occurs when the baby's liver is unable to metabolize or excrete chloramphenicol

Growth fraction the ratio of the number of replicating cells to resting cells in a tumor

Growth hormone (GH) hormone that is produced and secreted by the anterior pituitary gland; also called somatotropin or somatropin

H

H^+, K^+-ATPase enzyme secreting hydrochloride acid in the stomach

H_1 receptors histamine receptors that, when activated, produce allergy symptoms

H_2-receptor antagonists drugs that suppress gastric acid by blocking histamine receptors in the stomach

Hallucinations seeing, hearing, or feeling things that are not there

Hallucinogens chemicals that have the ability to produce an altered, dreamlike state of consciousness

Hashimoto's thyroiditis an autoimmune disorder that is the most common cause of hypothyroidism

Healthcare-associated infections (HAIs) infections acquired in a healthcare setting that are often resistant to common antibiotics

Healthcare failure mode and effect analysis (HFMEA) a tool that helps healthcare agencies identify processes where medication errors may occur related to prescription, dispensing, and administration

Heart failure (HF) inability of the heart to pump enough blood to meet the body's metabolic needs

Helminths various species of parasitic worms

Hemagglutinin an enzyme that facilitates the attachment of the virus to host cells

Hematopoiesis production and maturation of blood cells that occurs in red bone marrow; also called hemopoiesis

Hematopoietic growth factors drugs that promote the formation of specific blood cells and enhance the ability of the immune system to reduce some of the myelosuppression caused by antineoplastic medications

Hemoglobin A1C test (A1C) a laboratory test used in diabetic management; also called glycosylated hemoglobin

Hemophilia series of coagulation disorders caused by genetic mutations

Hemopoiesis production and maturation of blood cells that occurs in red bone marrow; also called hematopoiesis

Hemosiderin one of two protein complexes that maintain iron stores inside cells (ferritin is the other)

Hemostasis the slowing or stopping of blood flow

Hepatic microsomal enzyme system liver enzymes that metabolize drugs as well as nutrients and other endogenous substances; sometimes called the CYP450 system

Hepatic portal system a network of venous vessels that collects blood draining from the stomach, small intestine, and most of the large intestine

Hepatitis inflammation of the liver

Herb plant with a soft stem that is used for healing or as a seasoning

High-alert medications drugs that have a high risk of causing significant harm to the patient when used in error

High-density lipoprotein cholesterol (HDL-C) lipid-carrying particle in the blood that transports excess cholesterol away from body tissues or back to the liver for metabolism

Histamine chemical released by mast cells in response to foreign agents or injury that initiates the inflammatory response within seconds

HMG-CoA reductase primary regulatory enzyme for the biosynthesis of cholesterol

Hormones chemicals secreted by endocrine glands that act as chemical messengers to maintain homeostasis

Host flora microorganisms that normally inhabit the human body

Human immunodeficiency virus (HIV) the causative agent for AIDS

Hyperaldosteronism excessive secretion of aldosterone

Hypercholesterolemia high levels of cholesterol in the blood

Hyperemesis gravidarum condition of continual vomiting during pregnancy

Hyperkalemia elevated serum potassium level above 5 mEq/L

Hyperlipidemia elevated level of lipids in the blood

Hypernatremia elevated serum sodium level

Hyperosmolar hyperglycemic syndrome (HHS) acute complication of type 2 diabetes that is characterized by extreme hyperglycemia, hyperosmolarity with dehydration, the absence of ketoacidosis, and CNS dysfunction

Hypertension (HTN) consistent elevation of systemic arterial blood pressure

Hypertensive emergency (HTN-E) a diastolic pressure of greater than 120 mmHg, with evidence of target-organ system damage; also called hypertensive crisis

Hypertensive urgency severe hypertension, but with no evidence of target-organ damage

Hypertrichosis the elongation, thickening, and increased pigmentation of body hair

Hypertriglyceridemia elevated serum triglyceride level

Hyperuricemia elevated serum uric acid level 7 mg/dL or higher

Hypervitaminosis intake of toxic levels of vitamins

Hypnagogic hallucinations vivid, fearful illusions that may be experienced at the onset of sleep or on awakening

Hypnozoite dormant stage of *Plasmodium* in the liver

Hypoaldosteronism lack of adequate aldosterone secretion

Hypogonadism lack of sufficient testosterone by the testes

Hypokalemia serum potassium level below 3.5 mEq/L

Hypomania characterized by the same symptoms as bipolar disorder, but they are less severe and do not cause impaired functioning

Hyponatremia low sodium level in the blood

I

Idiosyncratic response unpredictable and unexplained drug reaction

Immunity ability to resist injury and infections

Immunization process of disease prevention in which the body produces antibodies in response to initial exposure to antigens

Immunomodulator general term referring to any drug or therapy that affects body defenses

Immunostimulants drugs that increase the ability of the immune system to fight infection and disease

Immunosuppressants drugs that diminish the ability of the immune system to fight infection and disease

Impotence inability to obtain or sustain an erection; also called erectile dysfunction

Incretins hormones released by the mucosa of the small intestine after a meal that stimulate the secretion of insulin

Incubation period following the first exposure to an antigen, the time needed for the body to process the antigen and mount an effective response

Indications the medical conditions for which a drug is approved

Infantile (epileptic) spasm usually occurs in the first year of life and is characterized by a sudden bending forward, body stiffening, or arching of the torso; also called West syndrome

Infertility inability to become pregnant after at least 1 year of frequent, unprotected intercourse

Inflammation nonspecific body defense that occurs in response to an injury or antigen

Inflammatory bowel disease (IBD) characterized by the presence of ulcers in the distal portion of the small intestine (Crohn's disease) or mucosal erosions in the large intestine (ulcerative colitis)

Influenza a viral infection characterized by acute symptoms that include sore throat, sneezing, coughing, fever, and chills; also called flu

Ingestion the process of taking food into the body by mouth

Innate body defenses nonspecific internal defenses which provide the first line of protection from pathogens

Inoculation the placement of a foreign substance on or in an individual for the purpose of disease prevention using "live" virus particles obtained from an infected patient

Inotropic drugs drugs that increase the force of contraction of the heart; also called cardiotonic drugs

Insomnia inability to fall asleep or stay asleep

Insulin pancreatic hormone that acts to decrease blood glucose levels

Insulin resistance occurs in type 2 diabetes mellitus; cells become unresponsive to insulin due to a defect in insulin receptor function

Insulin-like growth factor (IGF) a family of peptides that promote cartilage and bone growth

Integrase an enzyme unique to HIV that incorporates the viral DNA into the host's chromosomes

Interchangeable product a biosimilar drug that has undergone additional testing to show it produces the same clinical result when switched back and forth with its reference product

Interferons (IFNs) type of cytokine secreted by T cells in response to antigens to protect uninfected cells

Interleukins (ILs) class of cytokines synthesized by lymphocytes, monocytes, macrophages, and certain other cells in response to antigen exposure

Intermittent claudication (IC) pain or cramping in the lower legs that worsens with walking or exercise

Intracellular fluid (ICF) compartment contains water that is inside cells

Intracellular parasites infectious microbes that live inside host cells

Intrinsic activity the ability of a drug to bind to a receptor and produce a strong action

Intrinsic factor chemical substance secreted by stomach cells that is essential for the absorption of vitamin B_{12}

Intrinsic pathway coagulation pathway activated in response to injury; it takes several minutes to complete

Intrinsic sympathomimetic activity (ISA) low level of beta-agonist activity possessed by certain beta-adrenergic blockers

Invasiveness the ability of a pathogen to grow extremely rapidly and cause direct damage to surrounding tissues by virtue of sheer numbers

Investigational New Drug (IND) application to the FDA that contains all the animal and cell testing data

Iodism toxicity to Lugol's iodine solution therapy

Ion trapping phenomenon in which alkalinizing drugs are used to aid in the renal excretion of toxic substances

Irritable bowel syndrome (IBS) disease of the lower GI tract, characterized by abdominal pain, bloating, gas, cramping, and alternating diarrhea and constipation

Irritative voiding symptoms cluster of complaints that accompanies cystitis

Isozymes multiple, similar forms of an enzyme that perform slightly different metabolic functions

J

Juxtaglomerular (JG) cells specialized smooth muscle cells found in the afferent arteriole that sense blood pressure and release renin

K

Kappa receptors a type of opioid receptor in the CNS through which opioids produce their actions

Keratolytic action that promotes shedding of the outer layer of the epidermis

L

Laxatives drugs that promote defecation

Lennox-Gastaut syndrome mixed seizure that has characteristics of tonic–clonic, atonic, and atypical absence seizures

Leprosy a chronic infection caused by *Mycobacterium leprae*

Leptin hormone that regulates hunger and weight balance

Leucovorin rescue therapy drug therapy administered following chemotherapy with toxic folic acid analogs such as methotrexate to rescue normal cells

Leukotrienes chemical mediators of inflammation stored and released by mast cells

Leydig cells the primary cells in the testes that are responsible for androgen secretion

Libido interest in sexual activity

Limbic system area in the brain responsible for emotional expression, learning, and memory

Lipodystrophy a disorder in which fat is redistributed in specific areas in the body

Lipoproteins substances that carry lipids in the bloodstream that are composed of fat bound to carrier proteins

Loading dose relatively large dose of a drug given at the beginning of treatment to rapidly obtain a therapeutic response

Local anesthesia loss of sensation to a limited part of the body without loss of consciousness

Locus coeruleus located within the brainstem, monitors internal and external signals and is the principal site for norepinephrine synthesis in the brain

Long-acting reversible contraceptives (LARCs) devices that provide contraceptive protection for periods lasting from weeks to years

Low-density lipoprotein cholesterol (LDL-C) lipoprotein that carries the highest amount of cholesterol

Lymph nodes the principal lymphoid organs in the body that contain B cells and T cells

Lymphatic system consists of a network of cells, vessels, and tissues that provide immune surveillance

M

Macrominerals inorganic compounds needed by the body in amounts of 100 mg or more daily

Macula densa specialized cells in the distal convoluted tubule of the nephron that sense the flow rate and osmolality in the filtrate and send a message to the juxtaglomerular cells to release more renin

Maintenance dose amount of drug that keeps the plasma drug concentration in the therapeutic range

Major depressive disorder a depressed mood lasting for a minimum of 2 weeks that is present for most of the day, every day, or almost every day

Malaria disease characterized by severe fever and chills caused by the protozoan *Plasmodium*

Malignant hyperthermia rare but potentially fatal condition that is an adverse effect of some general anesthetics; characterized by a rapid onset of extremely high fever with muscle rigidity

Mania condition characterized by an inflated self-esteem, decreased need for sleep or food, distractibility, increased activity, excessive pursuit of pleasurable activities, increased talkativeness, delusions, paranoia, hallucinations, and bizarre behavior

Margin of safety (MOS) the amount of drug that is lethal to 1% of animals (LD_1) divided by the amount of drug that produces a therapeutic effect in 99% of the animals (ED_{99})

Mast cell stabilizers drugs that inhibit the release of inflammatory mediators from mast cells

Mastoiditis inflammation of the mastoid sinus

Median effective dose (ED_{50}) the dose of a drug required to produce a specific therapeutic response in 50% of a group of patients

Median lethal dose (LD_{50}) the dose of a drug that will kill 50% of a group of animals

Median toxicity dose (TD_{50}) the dose of a drug that will produce a given toxicity in 50% of a group of patients

Medication administration record (MAR) legal documentation of all pharmacotherapies received by a patient

Medication error any preventable event that may cause or lead to inappropriate medication use or patient harm while the medication is in the control of the healthcare provider, patient, or consumer

Medication error index categorization of medication errors according to the degree of harm an error can cause

Medication reconciliation the process of comparing a patient's medications with newly ordered medications to address duplications, omissions, and interactions, and the need to continue current medications

Menopause progressive decrease in estrogen secretion by the ovaries resulting in the permanent cessation of menses

Merozoites transformation of sporozoites carried by the blood to the liver inside the human host where they multiply into millions of progeny

Metabolic bone disease (MBD) refers to a cluster of disorders that have in common defects in the structure of bone

Metabolic syndrome a group of abnormalities that tend to occur together that places the patient at increased risk for developing diabetes and vascular complications

Metabolism the process used by the body to chemically change a drug molecule; also called biotransformation

Metastasis travel of cancer cells from their original site to a distant site

Metered-dose inhaler (MDI) device used to deliver a precise amount of medicine to the respiratory system

Methylxanthines chemical class for theophylline and caffeine and theobromine

Microbial antagonism condition of various host flora in competition with each other for physical space and nutrients that helps protect the host from being overrun by pathogenic organisms

Microminerals inorganic compounds needed by the body in amounts of 20 mg or less daily

Migraine severe headache preceded by auras and that may include nausea and vomiting

Milk-alkali syndrome syndrome caused by the administration of calcium carbonate antacids with milk or food containing vitamin D; symptoms include headache, urinary frequency, anorexia, nausea, and fatigue

Mineralocorticoids hormones secreted by the adrenal glands that affect the secretion of sodium and water

Minerals essential substances that constitute about 4% of an individual's body weight and serve many diverse functions

Minimum alveolar concentration describes the potency of inhalation anesthetics

Minimum effective concentration amount of drug required to produce a therapeutic effect

Miosis constriction of the pupil

Mitochondrial toxicity specific type of adverse effects resulting from a drug's toxic actions on mitochondria

Modular formulas enteral feedings that contain nutrients that are designed to meet a specific nutrient deficiency or disease state

Monitored anesthesia care (MAC) use of sedatives, analgesics, and other low-dose drugs that allow patients to remain responsive and breathe without assistance

Monoamine oxidase (MAO) enzyme that destroys catecholamines such as norepinephrine in the nerve terminal

Monoamine oxidase inhibitor (MAOI) drug inhibiting monoamine oxidase, an enzyme that slows the destruction of norepinephrine, dopamine, and serotonin

Monoclonal antibody (MAB) antibody made by cloning a single B cell that targets a specific cell or receptor

Mood disorder change in emotion that impairs the patient's ability to effectively deal with normal activities of daily living

Mood stabilizers drugs for bipolar disorder that can moderate extreme shifts in emotions and relieve symptoms of mania and depression during acute episodes

Motor end plate cholinergic synapse on skeletal muscle that allows for communication between the nervous system and skeletal muscle

Mu receptors a type of opioid receptor in the CNS through which opioids produce their actions

Mucolytics drugs used to remove mucus by loosening thick bronchial secretions

Mucositis inflammation of the epithelial lining of the digestive tract

Muscarinic type of cholinergic receptor found at postganglionic nerve endings in the parasympathetic nervous system that, when activated, results in stimulation

Muscarinic agonist drug that is selective for muscarinic receptors

Muscarinic antagonist drug that blocks receptors at cholinergic synapses in the parasympathetic nervous system and at a few target organs in the sympathetic nervous system

Muscle rigidity stiffness occurring in Parkinson's disease that causes difficulty bending over and moving limbs, changes in facial expression, or a lack of facial expression

Muscle spasms involuntary contractions that cause sudden, intense muscle pain, which slowly diminishes after a few minutes

Muscle spasticity condition caused by damage to the CNS in which certain muscle groups remain in a continuous state of contraction

Mutations errors made by bacteria while duplicating their genetic code

Myasthenia gravis (MG) muscular disorder caused by a destruction of nicotinic synapses on skeletal muscles and characterized by extreme fatigue, double vision, speech impairment, and difficulty chewing or swallowing

Myasthenic crisis extreme muscular weakness with symptoms similar to those of cholinergic crisis; caused by abrupt discontinuation of medication for myasthenia gravis

***Mycobacterium avium* complex (MAC)** infection that usually arises as a secondary infection due to the immunosuppression caused by HIV or AIDS

Mycolic acid a complex lipid that covers the cell surfaces of the genus *Mycobacterium* to protect them and make them resistant to many disinfectants

Mycoses diseases caused by fungi

Mydriasis pupil dilation

Mydriatics drugs that cause pupil dilation

Myocardial infarctions (MIs) blood clots blocking a portion of a coronary artery that cause necrosis of cardiac muscle

Myocardial ischemia condition in which the heart is receiving an insufficient amount of oxygen to meet its metabolic needs

Myoclonic seizures seizures characterized by brief, sudden contractions of major muscle groups

Myxedema swelling of the skin and other symptoms associated with hypothyroidism

Myxedema coma a life-threatening end-stage condition of hypothyroidism

N

Nadir lowest values of erythrocyte, leukocyte, and platelet counts resulting from chemotherapy

Narcolepsy sleep disorder that is characterized by severe daytime sleepiness and inability to stay awake

Narcotic natural or synthetic drug related to morphine; may be used as a broader legal term referring to hallucinogens, CNS stimulants, marijuana, and other illegal drugs

Narrow-spectrum antibiotic an anti-infective that is effective against only one or a small number of organisms

Natriuresis sodium excretion in the urine

Natriuretic peptides substances secreted in response to increased pressure in the heart

Nausea unpleasant feeling of the need to vomit accompanied by weakness, diaphoresis, dizziness, and hyperproduction of saliva

Nebulizer machine that delivers medication as a fine mist for the purpose of inhalation; also called small-volume nebulizer

Negative chronotropic effect the property of slowing the speed of electrical conduction across the myocardium

Negative feedback controls secretion and release of hormones by signaling the endocrine system once homeostasis is restored

Negative inotropic effect a reduction in the force of myocardial contraction

Negative symptoms in schizophrenia, symptoms associated with a loss of normal functioning, including a lack of interest, motivation, responsiveness, or pleasure in daily activities

Neoadjuvant chemotherapy the administration of antineoplastic drugs before surgery or radiation therapy with the goal of shrinking a large tumor to a manageable size

Neoplasm swelling, abnormal enlargement or mass; same as tumor

Nephrons structural and functional units of the kidney

Neuraminidase an enzyme that assists the virus in exiting the host cell

Neurodegenerative diseases degenerative diseases of the CNS that include a diverse set of disorders differing in their causes and outcomes

Neuroeffector junction synapse where the postganglionic neuron terminates on smooth muscle, cardiac muscle, or a gland

Neurofibrillary tangles bundles of nerve fibers found in the brain of patients with Alzheimer's disease on autopsy

Neurolept analgesia type of general anesthesia that combines fentanyl with droperidol to produce a state in which patients are conscious though insensitive to pain and unconnected with surroundings

Neuroleptic malignant syndrome (NMS) potentially fatal condition caused by certain antipsychotic medications characterized by high fever, sweating, fluctuating blood pressure, tachycardia, and muscle rigidity

Neuromuscular blockers drugs that inhibit transmission at the neuromuscular junctions on skeletal muscles in the somatic nervous system

Neuron the primary functional cell in all portions of the nervous system; its purpose is to communicate messages through conduction of an action potential

Neuropathic pain pain caused by injury or irritation to nerve tissue described as burning, shooting, or numbing pain

Neurotransmitters chemicals utilized in the communication of a message from one cell to another, or synaptic transmission

New Drug Application (NDA) application submitted to the FDA that signals that a pharmaceutical company is ready to market a new drug

New molecular entities medications that are truly unique and structurally different from existing drugs

Nicotinic agonist drug that selectively activates nicotinic receptors

Nicotinic antagonist drug that blocks receptors at cholinergic synapses in the ganglia or in the somatic nervous system at the neuromuscular junction

Nicotinic receptor receptor for acetylcholine in the ganglia of both the sympathetic and parasympathetic nervous systems

Nitric oxide in vascular smooth muscle, a cell-signaling molecule and potent vasodilator that causes relaxation of both arterial and venous smooth muscle

Nits eggs of the louse parasite

Nociceptor pain pain produced by injury to body tissue

Nociceptors sensory nerve receptors located throughout the body that initiate pain transmission when stimulated

Nondepolarizing neuromuscular blockers (NDNBs) class of nicotinic antagonists that bind to ACh receptors at motor end plates in skeletal muscle and prevent ACh from reaching its receptors

Nondihydropyridines largest class of calcium channel blockers that block closed-type calcium channels

Nonopioid analgesics analgesics that have a peripheral site of action, have no dependence potential; include NSAIDs, acetaminophen, and a few centrally acting medications

Non–rapid eye movement (NREM) sleep phase of sleep during which respirations slow, heart rate and blood pressure decrease, oxygen consumption by muscles decreases, and urine formation decreases

Norepinephrine (NE) primary neurotransmitter in the sympathetic and autonomic nervous systems

O

Obsessive-compulsive disorder (OCD) recurrent, intrusive thoughts or repetitive behaviors that interfere with normal activities or relationships

Oligospermia presence of less than 20 million sperm per milliliter of ejaculate

On–off syndrome occurs when a patient with Parkinson's disease alternates between symptom-free periods (on) and times when the drugs stop working and symptoms abruptly reappear (off)

Onychomycosis the invasion of the nail plate by a fungus; also called tinea unguium

Open-angle glaucoma form of glaucoma caused by the partial obstruction of the outflow of aqueous humor through the canal of Schlemm

Opiates natural substances obtained from opium, such as morphine and codeine

Opioid class of drugs that includes natural substances obtained from the seeds of the poppy plant such as opium, morphine, and codeine, and synthetic drugs such as meperidine, oxycodone, fentanyl, methadone, and heroin

Opioid use disorder dependence on opioids

Opium a milky substance extracted from the unripe seeds of the poppy plant that contains over 20 different chemicals having pharmacologic activity

Oral glucose tolerance test (OGTT) a primary blood test for diagnosing diabetes

Orexin neurons neurons that help regulate the balance between sleep and wakefulness

Orphan product a drug or biologic for treating rare diseases that affect fewer than 200,000 people in the United States

Orthostatic hypotension fall in blood pressure that occurs when changing position from recumbent to upright

Osmolality number of dissolved particles, or solutes, in 1 kg (1 L) of water

Osmosis process by which water moves from areas of low solute concentration (low osmolality) to areas of high solute concentration (high osmolality)

Osmotic pressure creates a force that moves substances between body compartments or across a membrane

Osteoarthritis (OA) progressive, degenerative joint disease caused by the breakdown of articular cartilage

Osteomalacia rickets in children; caused by vitamin D deficiency and characterized by softening of the bones without alteration of basic bone structure

Osteoporosis metabolic bone disease characterized by bone demineralization, decreased bone density, and subsequent fractures

Otitis externa an inflammation of the outer ear; commonly called swimmer's ear

Otitis interna infection of the inner ear; also called labyrinthitis

Otitis media inflammation of the middle ear

Ototoxicity drug-induced hearing impairment

Ovarian hyperstimulation syndrome (OHS) serious complication of certain fertility drugs characterized by rapid, massive enlargement of the ovaries accompanied by physical symptoms

Ovulation release of an oocyte (egg) by the ovary

Ovulatory dysfunction the presence of abnormal, irregular, or absent ovulation

Oxytocics drugs that stimulate uterine contractions and promote the induction of labor

P

Paget's disease chronic progressive condition characterized by accelerated remodeling of the bone, producing enlarged and softened bones; also called osteitis deformans

Palliation form of cancer chemotherapy intended to alleviate symptoms rather than cure the disease

Pancreatitis inflammation of the pancreas

Panic disorder anxiety disorder characterized by intense feelings of immediate apprehension, fearfulness, terror, or impending doom, accompanied by increased autonomic nervous system activity

Para-aminobenzoic acid (PABA) precursor molecule used by bacteria to make their own folic acid

Parasympathetic nervous system portion of the autonomic nervous system that is activated during nonstressful conditions and produces a set of symptoms known as the rest-and-digest response

Parenteral nutrition the administration of high-calorie nutrients via a central vein, such as the subclavian vein

Parenteral route method of administration that requires needles for drug delivery

Parietal cells cells in the stomach mucosa that secrete hydrochloric acid

Parkinsonism condition characterized by tremor, loss of fine motor skills, muscle rigidity, stooped posture, and a shuffling gait

Parkinson's disease (PD) degenerative disorder of the nervous system characterized by tremor, muscle rigidity, hypokinesia, masklike face, and a slow, shuffling gait

Paroxysmal supraventricular tachycardia (PSVT) occurs when episodes of atrial tachycardia alternate with periods of normal rhythm; also called paroxysmal atrial tachycardia (PAT)

Partial agonist medication that produces a weaker, or less efficacious, response than an agonist

Partial fatty-acid oxidation inhibitors a class of drugs used in the treatment of coronary artery disease

Partial (focal) seizures seizures that start on one side of the brain and travel a short distance before stopping

Partial parenteral nutrition a parenteral solution that lacks an essential element, usually fats or lipids

Passive immunity immune defense that lasts 2 to 3 weeks; obtained by administering antibodies

Patent medicines in early America before drug regulation, products that contained an easily identified trade name that falsely claimed to cure almost any symptom or disease

Pathogenicity ability of an organism to cause disease in humans

Pathogens microbes that are capable of causing disease

Patient safety event an event, incident, or condition that could have resulted or did result in harm to a patient

Pediatric Research Equity Act of 2003 (PREA) act that authorizes the FDA to require research of pediatric uses for new drugs

Pediculicides drugs that kill lice

Pegylation process that attaches polyethylene glycol to a drug molecule to extend its duration of activity

Penicillinase enzyme present in certain bacteria that is able to make penicillin ineffective

Penicillin-binding proteins (PBPs) enzymes used by bacteria to build bacterial cell walls that are targets for penicillins and related antibiotics

Pepsin digestive enzyme that breaks down proteins from food

Peptic ulcer erosion of the mucosa in the stomach or small intestine

Peptidoglycan substance containing sugars bound to peptides that is only found in bacteria

Peripartum depression depressed mood that occurs during pregnancy or within 4 weeks after delivery

Peripheral parenteral nutrition (PPN) delivery system used when a central venous line cannot be accessed or when it is not appropriate for the patient

Peripheral resistance amount of friction encountered by blood in the arteries

Peripherally inserted central catheter (PICC) line a central catheter that is threaded into the vena cava for administration of chemotherapy

Peristalsis rhythmic contractions of layers of smooth muscle

Pernicious anemia type of anemia usually caused by a deficiency of vitamin B_{12}

Phagocytes cells that engulf and destroy pathogens and other foreign substances

Pharmacodynamics study of the mechanisms of drug action and how the body responds to drugs

Pharmacogenetics the study of genetic variations that alter patients' responses to medications; branch of pharmacology that examines the role of genetics in drug response

Pharmacokinetic enhancers drugs such as ritonavir and cobicistat, that are given concurrently with antiretrovirals primarily for the purpose of inhibiting liver enzymes that would inactivate the antiretroviral; also called boosters

Pharmacokinetics study of drug movement throughout the body

Pharmacologic classification method of organizing drugs on the basis of their mechanisms of action

Pharmacology the study of medicines, ranging from how drugs are administered, to where they travel in the body, to the actual responses they produce

Pharmacopoeia a medical reference summarizing standards of drug purity, strength, and directions for synthesis

Pharmacotherapy the application of drugs for the purpose of disease prevention and treatment of suffering; also called pharmacotherapeutics

Pharmacy-level substitution when pharmacists may routinely substitute a generic drug when the prescription calls for a trade name

Pheochromocytoma a tumor arising from the adrenal medulla that is characterized by excessive secretion of catecholamines

Phobia fearful feeling attached to situations or objects such as snakes, spiders, crowds, or heights

Phosphodiesterase III enzyme in cardiac and smooth muscle; inhibition increases cardiac output due to an increase in myocardial contractility and a decrease in left ventricular afterload

Phospholipids type of lipid that contains two fatty acids, a phosphate group, and a chemical backbone of glycerol

Phototherapy therapy used for the treatment of seasonal affective disorder that consists of artificial lighting approximately 5 to 20 times brighter than normal indoor lighting

Physical dependence condition of experiencing unpleasant withdrawal symptoms when a substance is discontinued after repeated use

Pill rolling common behavior in Parkinson's disease, in which patients rub the thumb and forefinger together in a circular motion, resembling the motion of rolling a tablet between two fingers

Placebo in drug testing, an inert substance that serves as a control "nontreatment" group used to compare the effectiveness of the new drug

Placenta organ that allows for nutrition and gas exchange between a mother and her fetus

Plaque fibrous, fatty material that builds up in the walls of arteries

Plaques psoriatic lesions characterized by red, raised patches of skin covered with flaky, thick, silver scales

Plasma cells cells derived from B lymphocytes that secrete antibodies

Plasma half-life ($t_{1/2}$) the length of time required for the plasma concentration of a drug to decrease by one half after administration

Plasminogen inactive protein that is present in fibrin clot formation; precursor of plasmin

Pluripotent stem cells (hemocytoblasts) cells that are capable of maturing (differentiating) into any blood cell type

Pneumonic plague life-threatening infectious lung disease that occurs after breathing *Yersinia pestis*, a bacterium found on rodents and their fleas that is responsible for the bubonic plague

Polarized describes a cell that has negative membrane potential

Polyclonal antibodies contain a wide mixture of different antibodies that attack the T cells or T-cell receptors

Polycystic ovary syndrome a condition in which the ovaries are filled with follicular cysts and the patient has elevated levels of androgens and estrogen

Polydipsia excessive thirst

Polyherbacy use of multiple herbal and other supplements

Polymeric formulas solutions that contain various mixtures of proteins, lipids, and carbohydrates in high-molecular-weight form and are considered the most common enteral preparation

Polyphagia excessive appetite

Polypharmacy taking multiple drugs concurrently

Polyuria excessive urine production

Positive symptoms in schizophrenia, symptoms associated with an excess of distortion of normal function, including hallucinations, delusions, disorganized thought or speech patterns, and movement disorders

Postantibiotic effect antimicrobial activity that continues for a time after discontinuation of a drug

Posterior pituitary gland (neurohypophysis) consists of nervous tissue and is an extension of the hypothalamus that secretes antidiuretic hormone and oxytocin

Postherpetic neuralgia a serious form of shingles caused by herpes zoster in which the nerve pain lasts for years

Postictal state period immediately following a seizure

Postmarketing surveillance stage 4 of the drug approval process during which testing is done to survey for harmful drug effects in a large population

Postpartum depression major depression experienced by new mothers following delivery that is related to hormonal shifts and situational stresses that occur during that period

Post-traumatic stress disorder (PTSD) type of anxiety that develops in response to reexperiencing a previous life event that was psychologically traumatic

Potency the strength of a drug at a specified concentration or dose

Preclinical research first stage of drug development that involves extensive laboratory testing by the pharmaceutical company on human and microbial cells

Prediabetes condition in which serum glucose levels are elevated but are not high enough to be diagnosed as diabetes

Preeclampsia occurs during pregnancy when blood pressure increases to 140/90 mmHg or higher on two separate occasions, and 300 mg of protein is found in the urine over a 24-hour period

Pregnancy and Lactation Labeling Rule (PLLR) replaced the pregnancy risk letter system with narrative sections and subsections

Pregnancy categories five classifications developed by the FDA that rate medication risks during pregnancy; has been replaced by the Pregnancy and Lactation Labeling Rule.

Preload degree of stretch of the cardiac muscle fibers just before they contract

Preterm labor the initiation of labor prior to week 37 of gestation

Primary hypertension hypertension having no identifiable cause

Procoagulants natural substances that promote the formation of blood clots

Prodrugs drugs that become more active after they are metabolized

Prodysrhythmics conditions that promote the formation of cardiac rhythm abnormalities

Progesterone a natural progestin secreted by the corpus luteum

Prostaglandin E_2 hormone that stimulates the secretion of mucus and bicarbonate, promotes repair of damaged gastric mucosal cells, and increases blood flow to the mucosa to help maintain optimal mucosal conditions

Prostaglandins local hormones that have diverse functions depending on the location

Prostatitis bacterial infection of the prostate gland

Protease viral enzyme that is responsible for the final assembly of the HIV virions

Prothrombin blood clotting factor that is converted to the enzyme thrombin

Prothrombin time (PT) laboratory test used to measure blood coagulation

Proton pump inhibitors (PPIs) drugs that inhibit the enzyme H^+, K^+-ATPase

Prototype drug well-understood model drug to which other drugs in a pharmacologic class are compared

Protozoan single-celled organism that inhabits water, soil, and animal hosts

Provirus stage of a virus in which the viral DNA integrates into the host chromosome

Pruritus itching associated with dry, scaly skin or a parasite infection

Pseudocholinesterase enzyme produced by the liver that destroys acetylcholine and certain drugs such as succinylcholine and mivacurium

Pseudomembranous colitis (PMC) caused by *Clostridoides difficile*, a potentially severe disorder resulting from therapy with tetracyclines and other classes of antibiotics

Psoralens drugs used along with phototherapy for the treatment of severe psoriasis

Psychologic dependence desire to continue using a drug despite obvious negative economic, physical, or social consequences

Psychosis general term used in medicine to describe a loss of contact with reality

Psychosocial describes an individual's psychologic development in the context of one's social environment

Pulmonary embolism a venous clot dislodges, migrates to the pulmonary vessels, and blocks arterial circulation to the lungs

Pulmonary perfusion blood flow through the lung

Purified protein derivative (PPD) tuberculin skin test

Pyelonephritis an inflammation of the kidney due to a urinary tract infection

R

Radiation sickness occurs after exposure to ionizing radiation; symptoms include nausea, vomiting, diarrhea, weight loss, anorexia, fatigue, and suppression of the bone marrow

Radical cure complete removal of all forms of *Plasmodium* from a malaria patient

Rapid eye movement (REM) sleep stage of sleep characterized by diminished muscle tone, movements of the eyes, and irregular heart rate and breathing

Raynaud's disease vasospasms of vessels serving the fingers and toes that can lead to intermittent pain and cyanosis of the digits

Reabsorption movement of filtered substances from the kidney tubule back into the blood

Rebound congestion prolonged use of intranasal decongestants that causes hypersecretion of mucus and worsening nasal congestion once the drug effects wear off

Rebound effects symptoms of lethargy and fatigue caused by withdrawal of methamphetamine and other stimulants

Rebound insomnia increased sleeplessness that occurs when long-term sedative medication is discontinued abruptly

Receptor cellular molecule to which a drug binds to produce its effects

Recommended dietary allowances (RDAs) minimum amount of vitamins and minerals needed each day to prevent disease

Refeeding syndrome metabolic complications that can occur when nutritional support, including enteral nutrition therapy, is introduced to severely malnourished patients

Reference product an original biological product approved by the FDA based on a thorough evaluation of its safety and effectiveness

Reflex tachycardia temporary increase in heart rate that occurs when blood pressure falls

Refractory period time during which the myocardial cells rest and are not able to contract

Regional anesthesia similar to local anesthesia except that it encompasses a larger body area, such as an entire limb

Renin an enzyme that is synthesized, stored, and secreted by juxtaglomerular cells in the kidney

Renin-angiotensin-aldosterone system (RAAS) series of enzymatic steps by which the body raises blood pressure

Repetitive transcranial magnetic stimulation (rTMS) therapy for major depression that passes an electromagnetic pulse through a coil placed on the scalp

Replacement therapy hormones administered to patients who are unable to secrete sufficient quantities of their own endogenous hormones

Repolarization return of a negative resting membrane potential to the cell

Rest-and-digest response signs and symptoms produced when the parasympathetic nervous system is activated; they promote relaxation and maintenance activities

Reticular activating system (RAS) responsible for sleeping and wakefulness and performs an alerting function for the cerebral cortex

Retinoids drug class related to vitamin A used in the treatment of inflammatory skin conditions, dermatologic malignancies, and acne

Reverse cholesterol transport the process by which cholesterol is transported away from body tissues to the liver

Reverse remodeling occurs after several months of therapy with beta-adrenergic antagonists, when heart size, shape, and function return to normal

Reverse transcriptase viral enzyme that converts RNA to DNA

Rhabdomyolysis breakdown of muscle fibers usually due to muscle trauma or ischemia

Rheumatoid arthritis (RA) chronic, progressive, autoimmune disease that causes inflammation of the joints

Rhinophyma reddened, bulbous, irregular swelling of the nose

Rifamycin derivatives include rifampin, rifabutin, and rifapentine; used in combination with other antituberculosis medications

Risk management system of reducing medication errors by modifying policies and procedures within the institution

Risk–benefit ratio determination of whether the risks from a drug outweigh the potential benefits received by taking the medication

Root-cause analysis (RCA) focuses attention on the causes of a medication error, rather than on the individual responsible for the error

Rosacea inflammatory skin disorder affecting mainly the face, characterized by small papules that swell, thicken, and become painful

S

Salicylates the chemical family to which aspirin belongs

Salicylism acute or chronic overdose of aspirin

Sarcolemma the membrane surrounding muscles

Sarcoplasmic reticula structures within cells that store calcium ions that are released by depolarization

Satiety the psychologic feeling of fullness or satisfaction following a meal

Satiety center region of the hypothalamus that recognizes satiety

Scabicides drugs that kill scabies mites

Scheduled drugs drugs that are frequently abused or have a high potential for dependence are classified and regulated according to their potential for abuse

Schizoaffective disorder psychosis with symptoms of both schizophrenia and mood disorders

Schizophrenia psychosis characterized by abnormal thoughts and thought processes, withdrawal from people and the outside environment, an inability to independently perform ADLs, and a high risk of suicide

Sclerosing abnormal tissue hardening of the veins

Seasonal affective disorder a type of depression experienced during the dark winter months

Seborrhea skin condition characterized by overproduction of sebum by the oil glands

Second messenger cascade of biochemical events that initiates a drug's action by either stimulating or inhibiting a normal activity of the cell

Secondary hypertension hypertension having a specific identifiable cause

Secretion in the kidney, movement of substances from the blood into the tubule after filtration has occurred

Sedative–hypnotic drug with the ability to produce a calming effect at low doses and sleep at high doses

Sedatives substances that depress the CNS and cause drowsiness or sleep

Seizure symptom of epilepsy characterized by abnormal neuronal discharges within the brain

Seizure clusters three or more seizures in a 24-hour period

Selective estrogen receptor modulators (SERMs) drugs that produce an action similar to estrogen in body tissues; used for the treatment of osteoporosis in postmenopausal women

Semielemental (oligomeric) formulas enteral solutions that contain larger molecules than elemental products and a higher percentage of fat

Sentinel event a risk caused by a medication error that may result in death, permanent harm, or severe temporary harm to the patient

Separation anxiety disorder excessive, inappropriate fear when separated from home or an attachment figure

Serotonin a neurotransmitter that is found in high concentrations in the hypothalamus, limbic system, medulla, and spinal cord

Serotonin syndrome (SES) set of symptoms associated with overmedication with antidepressants that includes altered mental status, fever, hypertension, tremors, sweating, and lack of muscular coordination

Shingles painful herpes zoster infection caused by reactivation of the varicella-zoster virus or chickenpox

Short stature height below the fifth percentile for age and gender, or more than two standard deviations below the mean (average) for age and gender

Side effects types of drug effects that are less serious than adverse effects, are predictable, and may occur even at therapeutic doses

Silent ischemia myocardial ischemia that occurs in the absence of pain

Simple partial (focal aware) seizures seizures with an onset that begins as a small, regional focus, and subsequently progress to a generalized seizure

Sinus rhythm number of beats per minute normally generated by the SA node

Situational anxiety anxiety experienced by people faced with a temporarily stressful environment

Sjögren's syndrome chronic autoimmune disorder characterized by excessive dryness of mucous membranes

Sleep attacks sudden bouts of sleep that last 10 to 30 minutes and may occur during the daytime without warning

Sleep paralysis the temporary inability to move after waking from sleep

Small-molecule therapies types of targeted therapies used to treat cancer

Small volume nebulizer machine that delivers medication as a fine mist for the purpose of inhalation; also called nebulizer

Smallpox serious, contagious potentially fatal disease that is caused by the variola virus

Social anxiety disorder unreasonable and persistent fear of crowds or of being judged, ridiculed, or embarrassed by others; also called social phobia

Somatic nervous system nerves that provide for voluntary control of the skeletal muscles

Somatostatin hormone released by the hypothalamus, stomach, intestine, and pancreas that inhibits the effects of growth hormone and lowers acid secretion; also known as growth hormone-inhibiting hormone

Specialty supplements dietary products used to enhance or complement a specific function in the body, such as supporting joint health or immune function.

Specific (Simple) phobia an irrational and intense fear attached to certain situations or objects

Spermicides drugs that kill sperm

Sporozoite mature and infective form of *Plasmodium* that resides in the gut of the female *Anopheles* mosquito

Stable angina type of angina that occurs in a predictable pattern of frequency, intensity, and duration, usually relieved by rest

Staging the process of determining where a cancer is located and the extent of its invasion

Status asthmaticus emergency situation in which acute asthma attacks are unresponsive to drug treatment; may lead to respiratory failure

Status epilepticus medical emergency that occurs when a seizure continues for more than 30 minutes or when two successive seizures occur without full recovery of consciousness between seizures

Steatorrhea the passing of bulky, foul-smelling fatty stools

Steroids types of lipids having a characteristic ring structure

Strategic National Stockpile (SNS) national repository of antibiotics, chemical antidotes, antitoxins, antiviral drugs and other essential medical supplies for use in a major health emergency

Striatum location in the brain where dopamine encounters its receptors and produces multiple actions

Stroke volume amount of blood pumped by a ventricle in a single contraction

Substance abuse self-administration of a drug that does not conform to the medical or social norms within the patient's given culture or society

Substantia nigra location in the brain where dopamine is produced that is responsible for regulation of unconscious muscle movement

Substrate drug that is metabolized by a CYP450 enzyme

Suicide the intentional act of ending one's life

Supercoil the highly twisted arrangement of the DNA helix in bacteria

Superinfections new infections caused when an antibiotic kills the host's normal flora, making additional space and nutrients available for pathogenic organisms to grow unchecked

Supplements additional vitamins or minerals that some people take to complement their diets by providing missing nutrients

Surgical anesthesia stage 3 of anesthesia, in which most major surgery is conducted

Svedberg unit a unit of measurement represented by the letter "S" that indicates the size or sedimentation rate of the bacterial 70S ribosome

Sympathetic nervous system portion of the autonomic nervous system that is activated under emergency conditions or stress and produces a set of actions called the fight-or-flight response

Sympathomimetics drugs that activate adrenergic receptors in the sympathetic nervous system

Symporter a membrane protein that transports two molecules at the same time

Synapse a junction between two neurons or a neuron and a muscle

Synaptic cleft space where neurotransmitters enter that must be crossed for the impulse to reach the postganglionic neuron or organ

Syndrome of inappropriate antidiuretic hormone (SIADH) condition characterized by marked fluid retention, elevated urine osmolality, low serum osmolality, and sodium loss in the urine

Synergistic effect type of drug interaction in which two drugs produce an effect that is much greater than would be expected from simply adding the two individual drugs' responses

T

T cells lymphocytes that secrete cytokines essential to the cell-mediated immune response

Tachydysrhythmias disorders exhibiting a heart rate greater than 100 beats/min

Tachyphylaxis the rapid development of tolerance to any action of a drug, either adverse or therapeutic effects

Tardive dyskinesia (TD) unusual tongue and face movements such as lip smacking, rapid eye blinking, and wormlike motions of the tongue that occur during pharmacotherapy with certain antipsychotics

Target cells cells affected by hormones

Targeted therapies drugs that block specific gene products involved in the growth, progression, and survival of cancer cells

Telomerase an enzyme contained in certain human stem cells that can lengthen the DNA chains and allow continued replication

Telomeres regions in chromosomes that prevent the vital sequences of DNA from being destroyed each time a cell divides

Tension headache common type of head pain caused by stress and relieved by over-the-counter analgesics

Teratogen agent that causes birth defects

Tetrahydrocannabinol (THC) the active chemical in marijuana

Therapeutic classification method of organizing drugs on the basis of what condition is being treated by the drug

Therapeutic drug monitoring practice of monitoring plasma levels of drugs that have low safety profiles and using the data to predict drug action or toxicity

Therapeutic index (TI) the ratio of a drug's LD_{50} to its ED_{50}

Therapeutic range dosage that produces the desired effects of a drug

Threshold potential an action potential triggered by the membrane potential during myocardial electrical conduction

Thrombin enzyme that causes clotting by catalyzing the conversion of fibrinogen to fibrin

Thrombocytopenia coagulation disorder in which there is a deficiency of platelets

Thromboembolic disorder condition in which the body forms undesirable clots

Thrombopoietin hormone that promotes the formation of platelets in the blood

Thyroid crisis a rare, life-threatening form of thyrotoxicosis; also called thyroid storm

Thyroid storm see Thyroid crisis

Thyroid-stimulating hormone (TSH) hormone secreted by the anterior pituitary when stimulated by thyrotropin-releasing hormone

Thyroid-stimulating immunoglobulins (TSIs) stimulate the thyroid gland in Graves' disease

Thyrotoxicosis an acute condition caused by very high levels of circulating thyroid hormone

Thyrotropin-releasing hormone (TRH) hormone secreted by the hypothalamus when blood levels of thyroid hormone are low

Thyroxine (T_4) thyroid hormone that is synthesized from the amino acid tyrosine and 4 atoms of iodine

Thyroxine-binding globulin (TBG) a plasma protein produced in the liver that carries thyroid hormone through the bloodstream

Tocolytics drugs used to delay preterm labor

Tolerance process of adapting to a drug over a period of time and subsequently requiring higher doses to achieve the same effect

Tonicity the ability of a solution to cause a change in water movement across a membrane owing to osmotic forces

Tonometry technique that tests for glaucoma by measuring intraocular pressure

Topical route medications applied to the skin or the membranous linings of the eye, ear, nose, respiratory tract, urinary tract, vagina, and rectum

Topoisomerase IV in DNA replication, the enzyme that frees the newly formed interlocked strands, allowing them to migrate into the two daughter cells

Torsades de pointe type of ventricular tachycardia that is characterized by rates between 200 and 250 beats/min and "twisting of the points" of the QRS complex on the ECG

Total parenteral nutrition (TPN) nutrition provided through a peripheral or central vein

Toxic concentration level of drug that results in serious adverse effects

Toxoids type of vaccine that uses bacterial toxins that have been chemically modified to be incapable of causing disease

Trade name name assigned by the pharmaceutical company marketing a drug; sometimes called the proprietary, product, or brand name

Transdermal patches topical delivery method that uses patches that contain a specified amount of medication that is released over a specified time period

Transferrin protein complex that transports iron to sites in the body where it is needed

Translation basic steps in protein synthesis

Transplant rejection recognition by the immune system of a transplanted tissue as foreign and subsequent attack on the tissue

Treatment as prevention reducing HIV-RNA to less than 200 copies/mL or undetectable levels to prevent sexual transmission of HIV

Tricyclic antidepressants (TCAs) class of drugs used in the pharmacotherapy of depression

Triglycerides types of lipids that contain three fatty acids attached to a chemical backbone of glycerol

Tri-iodothyronine (T_3) thyroid hormone that is synthesized from the amino acid tyrosine and 3 atoms of iodine

Trophozoite the active, growing stage during which a protozoan organism feeds, often at the expense of its host

Tropic hormones ability of the anterior pituitary gland hormones to regulate the secretory actions of other endocrine glands

Tubercles cavity-like lesions in the lung characteristic of infection by *Mycobacterium tuberculosis*

Tuberculosis (TB) a highly contagious infection caused by the organism *Mycobacterium tuberculosis*

Tularemia serious infectious disease found in rodents, rabbits, and hares that is caused by the organism *Francisella tularensis*

Tumor abnormal swelling, enlargement, or mass; also called neoplasm

Tumor agnostic therapies drugs that treat certain genomic mutations or molecular features regardless of where the cancer is located

Type 1 diabetes metabolic disorder characterized by hyperglycemia caused by a lack of secretion of insulin by the pancreas in which glucose cannot enter cells and fatty acids are used as the primary energy source

Type 2 diabetes chronic metabolic disease characterized by hyperglycemia and insulin resistance

Tyramine form of the amino acid tyrosine that is found in foods such as cheese, beer, wine, and yeast products

U

Unstable angina angina that occurs suddenly, has added intensity, and occurs during periods of rest

Up-regulation process by which cells create more receptors on their surface to capture hormone molecules

Urethritis infection of the urethra

Uricosurics drugs that increase the rate of excretion of uric acid by blocking its reabsorption in the kidney

Uropathogens harmful microorganisms that invade the urinary system

Urticaria hypersensitivity response that is characterized by hives and is often accompanied by pruritus (itching)

U.S. Food and Drug Administration (FDA) U.S. regulatory agency responsible for ensuring that drugs and medical devices are safe and effective

USP verification program mark on the label of a dietary supplement that indicates to consumers that the product has been manufactured under acceptable standards of purity, has been tested for active ingredients stated on the label, and is free of harmful contaminants

V

Vaccination process of introducing foreign proteins or inactive cells (vaccines) into the body to trigger immune activation before the patient is exposed to the real pathogen

Vagus nerve stimulation (VNS) Type of therapy for major depression that involves surgical implantation of battery-powered device into the patient's chest with an electrode that stimulates the vagus nerve

Variant (Prinzmetal's) angina type of angina in which the decreased myocardial blood flow is caused by spasms of the coronary arteries; also called vasospastic angina

Vasomotor center cluster of neurons in the medulla that controls baseline blood pressure

Vectors organism or vehicle that transmits pathogens by carrying them from one host to another

Venous return the volume of blood returning to the heart from the veins

Venous thromboembolism (VTE) blood clots that occur when blood flow through a vein is very slow (stasis)

Ventilation process of moving air into and out of the lungs

Very low-density lipoprotein cholesterol (VLDL-C) primary carrier of triglycerides in the blood that is converted to LDL in the liver

Vesicants agents that can cause serious tissue injury if they escape from an artery or vein during an infusion or injection; many antineoplastics are vesicants

Viral load a measurement of HIV RNA levels in the blood that provides an estimate of how rapidly the virus is replicating

Virilization appearance of the male sex characteristics

Virion mature infective virus particle

Virologic failure a plasma HIV RNA level that rises above 200 copies/mL during HIV treatment

Virulence quantitative measure of an organism's pathogenicity

Viruses nonliving agents that contain DNA or RNA and are capable of causing disease

Vitamins organic nutrient substances required for the health of the human body

Vomiting emesis in which the stomach contents are forced upward into the esophagus and out of the mouth

Vomiting center area in the medulla that controls the vomiting reflex

von Willebrand's disease (vWD) bleeding disorder resulting from a decrease in quantity or quality of von Willebrand factor

W

Water-soluble vitamins group of vitamins stored briefly in the body and then excreted in the urine, including the C and B-complex vitamins

Wearing-off effect appears gradually near the end of a dosing interval; symptoms become worse because the concentration of the drug has fallen below the therapeutic level

Withdrawal syndrome symptoms that result when a patient discontinues taking a substance on which he or she was dependent

X

Xanthine oxidase enzyme responsible for the formation of uric acid

Xerostomia dry mouth

Z

Zollinger-Ellison syndrome (ZES) disorder of excess acid secretion in the stomach resulting in peptic ulcer disease

Credits

Unit Opener Sources

1 Diego Cervo/Shutterstock; Pearson Education, Inc; Pearson Education, Inc; Thinkstock Images/Getty Images
2 Pathdoc/Shutterstock; ucchie79/Shutterstock; Lisa F. Young/Shutterstock; Katrina Brown/Shutterstock
3 StudioSmart/Shutterstock; Fotorobs/Shutterstock; Image Point Fr/Shutterstock; Tani_Bel/Shutterstock
4 Koraysa/Shutterstock; AJR_photo/Shutterstock; Imagesbybarbara/Getty Images; Fotoluminate LLC/Shutterstock
5 Jeff Cleveland/Shutterstock; AshTproductions/Shutterstock; Petersemler-Photography/Shutterstock; T-Design/Shutterstock
6 SomkiatFakmee/Getty images; Iakov Filimonov/Shutterstock; Image Point Fr/Shutterstock; Christo/Shutterstock
7 Carol Urban; leungchopan/Shutterstock
8 Andrey_Popov/Shutterstock; wavebreakmedia/Shutterstock; Kim Reinick/Shutterstock; Carol Urban
9 Alexander Raths/Shutterstock; Michael Jung/Shutterstock; Carol Urban; LStockStudio/Shutterstock
10 Rocketclips, Inc./Shutterstock; Chaphot/Shutterstock; fizkes/Shutterstock; Yuri Arcurs/Shutterstock
11 PT Images/Shutterstock; travelview/Shutterstock; Jeffrey B. Banke/Shutterstock; RichVintage/Getty Images

Chapter Opener Sources

1 Diego Cervo/Shutterstock
2 Ruslan Huzau/Shutterstock
3 Tyler Olson/Shutterstock
4 Iakov Filimonov/Shutterstock
5 Pearson Education, Inc
6 Thinkstock Images/Getty Images
7 Alexander Raths/Shutterstock
8 Pathdoc/Shutterstock
9 ucchie79/Shutterstock
10 Lisa F. Young/Shutterstock
11 Katrina Brown/Shutterstock
12 StudioSmart/Shutterstock
13 Nika Art/Shutterstock
14 fotorobs/Shutterstock
15 Image Point Fr/Shutterstock
16 WAYHOME studio/Shutterstock
17 Digital Storm/Shuttestock
18 Koraysa/Shutterstock
19 michaelheim/Shutterstock
20 kevinruss/Getty Images
21 Denise Andersen/Shutterstock
22 AJR_photo/Shutterstock
23 Valua Vitaly/Shutterstock
24 Imagesbybarbara/Getty Images
25 Fotoluminate LLC/Shutterstock
26 Rocketclips, Inc/Shutterstock
27 John Sommer/Getty Images
28 Sebastian Kaulitzki/Shutterstock
29 Jeff Cleveland/Shutterstock
30 AshTproductions/Shutterstock
31 Real Deal Photo/Shutterstock
32 Ocskay Mark/Shutterstock
33 Michael Jung/Shutterstock
34 Nadino/Shutterstock
35 Wavebreak Media Ltd/123RF
36 Photographee.eu/Shutterstock
37 Jeep5d/Shutterstock
38 Kimberrywood/Shutterstock
39 T-Design/Shutterstock
40 SomkiatFakmee/Getty images
41 Iakov Filimonov/Shutterstock
42 Image Point Fr/Shutterstock
43 Christo/Shutterstock
44 Carol Urban
45 leungchopan/Shutterstock
46 Lotus_studio/Shutterstock
47 Ragne Kabanova/Shutterstock
48 Andrey_Popov/Shutterstock
49 andersonrise/123RF
50 wavebreakmedia/Shutterstock
51 Kim Reinick/Shutterstock
52 Image Point Fr/Shutterstock
53 oliveromg/Shutterstock
54 Portra/Getty Images
55 rui vale sousa/Shutterstock
56 sdominick/Getty Images
57 Carol Urban
58 decade3d - anatomy online/Shutterstock
59 wavebreakmedia/Shutterstock
60 Alexander Raths/Shutterstock
61 Michael Jung/Shutterstock
62 Carol Urban
63 L stock Studio/Shutterstock
64 Shyamalamuralinath/Shutterstock
65 Shyamalamuralinath/Shutterstock
66 Rocketclips, Inc./Shutterstock
67 Marcos Mesa Sam Wordley/Shutterstock
68 chaphot/Shutterstock
69 wavebreakmedia/Shutterstock
70 fizkes/Shutterstock
71 Dmitri Ma/Shutterstock
72 PT Images/Shutterstock
73 Travelview/Shutterstock
74 Jeffrey B. Banke/Shutterstock
75 CarlosDavid/Shutterstock

Index

Page numbers followed by an *f* indicate figures, and those followed by a *t* indicate tables.

B

C

F

G

M

N

P

Q

R

S

T

U

W

X

Y

Z

Special Features

Connections: Advanced Practice Application

Connections: Applied Clinical Judgment

Connections: Community-Oriented Practice

Connections: Complementary and Alternative Therapies

Connections: Lifespan Considerations

Connections: Patient Safety

Connections: Treating the Diverse Patient